Olay Pro X
Anthelios

CASTLE CONNOLLY
TOP DOCTORS
New York Metro Area

14th Edition

Doctors Make A Difference

America's Trusted Source For Identifying Top Doctors

For more information, please contact:

Castle Connolly Medical Ltd., 42 West 24th St, New York, New York 10010
212-367-8400x10
E-mail: info@castleconnolly.com
Web site: http://www.castleconnolly.com.

Library of Congress Control Number: 2010940283

| ISBN | 0-9845670-4-6; | 978-0-9845670-4-1 | (paperback) |
| ISBN | 0-9845670-5-4; | 978-0-9845670-5-8 | (hardcover) |

Printed in the United States of America

Table of Contents

Table of Contents

Table of Contents

Table of Contents

Table of Contents

Table of Contents

Hippocratic Oath

I swear by Apollo the physician, and Asklepios, and health, and All-Heal and all the gods and goddesses, that, according to my ability and judgement, I will keep this Oath and this stipulation — to reckon him who taught me this Art equally dear to me as my parents, to share my substance with him, and relieve his necessities if required; to look upon his offspring in the same footing as my own brothers, and to teach them this Art, if they should wish to learn it, without fee or stipulation; and that by precept, lecture and every other mode of instruction, I will impart a knowledge of the Art to my own sons, and those of my teachers, and to disciples bound by a stipulation and oath according to the law of medicine, but to none others.

I will follow that system of regimen which, according to my ability and judgement, I consider for the benefit of my patients, and abstain from whatever is deleterious and mischievous. I will give no deadly medicine to anyone if asked nor suggest any such counsel; and in like manner I will not give to a woman a pessary to produce abortion. With purity and wholeness I will pass my life and practice my Art.

I will not cut persons labouring under the stone, but will leave this to be done by men who are practitioners of this work. Into whatever houses I enter, I will go into them for the benefit of the sick, and will abstain from every voluntary act of mischief and corruption; and, further, from the seduction of females or males, of freemen and slaves. Whatever, in connection with my professional practice, or not in connection with it, I see or hear, in the life of men, which ought not to be spoken of abroad, I will not divulge, as reckoning that all such should be kept secret. While I continue to keep this Oath unviolated, may it be granted to me to enjoy life and the practice of the art, respected by all men, in all times! But should I trespass and violate this Oath, may the reverse be my lot!

From Dorland's Illustrated Medical Dictionary. 27th ed. (Philadelphia) W.B. Saunders Co., 1988. Hippocratic Oath. [Hippocrates. Greek physician, 460-377 B.C.]

About the Publishers

John K. Castle, the Chairman of Castle Connolly Medical Ltd., has spent much of the last three decades involved with healthcare institutions and issues. Mr. Castle served as Chairman of the Board of New York Medical College for eleven years, an institution where he served on the Board of Trustees for twenty-two years.

Mr. Castle has been extensively involved in other healthcare and voluntary activities as well. He served for five years as a commissioner and officer of the Joint Commission formerly known as (JCAHO), the body which accredits most public and private hospitals throughout the United States. Mr. Castle has also served as a trustee of five different hospitals in the metropolitan New York region, including NewYork Presbyterian Hospital, where he continues to serve.

Mr. Castle has also served as the Chairman of the Columbia Presbyterian Science Advisory Council and as a Director of the Whitehead Institute for Biomedical Research. He is a Fellow of New York Academy of Medicine and has served as a Trustee of the Academy. He was Chairman of the United Hospital Fund of New York's Capital Campaign and continues as Director Emeritus of the United Hospital Fund. He is a Life Member of the MIT Corporation, the governing body of the Massachusetts Institute of Technology.

Mr. Castle's goal, as is the goal of Dr. John Connolly and all the Castle Connolly team, is to publish *America's Top Doctors®, America's Top Doctors® for Cancer, Top Doctors: New York Metro Area*, and other materials as well as build websites to help the public identify the very best in healthcare resources.

Mr. Castle received his bachelor's degree from the Massachusetts Institute of Technology, his MBA as a Baker Scholar with High Distinction from Harvard, and two Honorary Doctorate degrees.

John J. Connolly, Ed.D. is the President & CEO of Castle Connolly Medical Ltd., and is the nation's foremost authority on identifying top physicians. Dr. Connolly's experience in healthcare is extensive.

For more than a decade he served as President of New York Medical College, the nation's second largest private medical college. He is a Fellow of the New York Academy of Medicine, a Fellow of the New York Academy of Sciences, a Director of the Northeast Business Group on Health, a member of the President's Council of the United Hospital Fund, and a member of the Board of Advisors of Funding First, a Lasker Foundation initiative. Dr. Connolly has served as a trustee of two hospitals and as Chairman of the Board of one. He is extensively involved in healthcare and community activities and has served on a number of voluntary and corporate boards including the Board of the American Lyme Disease Foundation, of which he is a founder and past chairman, and the Board of Advisors of the Whitehead Institute for Biomedical Research. He is also a Director and Chairman of the Professional Examination Service. He holds a Bachelor of Science degree from Worcester State College, a Master's degree from the University of Connecticut, and a Doctor of Education degree in College and University Administration from Teacher's College, Columbia University.

Dr. Connolly has appeared on or been interviewed by over 100 television and radio stations nationwide including *The Today Show* (NBC-TV), *Good Morning America* (ABC-TV), *20/20* (ABC-TV), *48 Hours* (CBS-TV), *Fox Cable News* (national), *Morning News* (CNN) and *Weekend Today in New York* (WNBC-TV). *The New York Times*, the *Chicago Tribune*, the *Daily News* (New York), the *Boston Herald* and other newspapers, as well as many national and regional magazines, have featured Castle Connolly Guides and/or Dr. Connolly in stories. He is the author and/or editor of eight books, all written to help families and individuals find the best healthcare.

Medical Advisory Board

Castle Connolly Medical Ltd. is pleased to be associated with a distinguished group of medical leaders who offer invaluable advice and wisdom in its efforts to assist consumers in making good healthcare choices. We thank each member of the Medical Advisory Board for their valuable contributions.

Jeremiah A. Barondess, M.D.
President Emeritus
New York Academy of Medicine,
Professor of Clinical Medicine
Emeritus,
Weill-Cornell Medical College

Roger Bulger, M.D.
National Institutes of Health (ret.)

Menard M. Gertler, M.D., D. Sc.
Clinical Professor of Medicine
Cornell University
Medical School

Leo Henikoff, M.D.
President and CEO (Ret.)
Rush Presbyterian-St. Luke's
Medical Center

Yutaka Kikkawa, M.D.
Professor and Chairman (Emeritus)
Department of Pathology
University of California, Irvine
College of Medicine

David Paige, M.D.
Professor
Bloomberg School of
Public Health
Johns Hopkins University

Ronald Pion, M.D.
Chairman and CEO
Medical Telecommunications
Associates

Richard L. Reece, M.D.
Editor
Physician Practice Options

Leon G. Smith, M.D.
Chairman of Medicine
St. Michael's Medical Center, NJ

Helen Smits, M.D.
Former Deputy Director
HealthCare Financing
Administration (HCFA)

Ralph Snyderman, M.D.
Former President and CEO
Duke University Health System

Foreword

Dear Reader:

Choosing a doctor is one of the most important choices in your life. However, most of us put little effort into this selection. We simply pick a name from a list or get a recommendation from a friend.

Most of us have very little information about our doctors, and/or don't know where to get it. With the publication of this Castle Connolly Guide—Top Doctors: New York Metro Area, you can learn about doctors' medical school education, residency, training, fellowships, board certifications, hospital appointments and much more. The Guide also describes in simple terms what information you should ascertain about each doctor and how to evaluate it. This information gathering is essential for anyone who wants to find a good doctor to truly meet his or her healthcare needs.

As an administrator and nurse who deals with the problems of health on a daily basis, I know well the importance of getting the best healthcare. Our center assists medical malpractice victims. The human tragedy we often encounter is heartbreaking.

In many cases, had the patient taken a few minutes to make a modest effort to learn more about his or her doctor's background, a serious incident may have been avoided.

That is why *Top Doctors: New York Metro Area* is so important to consumers. In this new and rapidly changing healthcare environment, patients must be well informed. Many do not trust the healthcare system. They are not confident that their HMO, their hospital, or even their doctor, is motivated to protect them and to ensure that they get excellent care.

The Castle Connolly Guide is a comprehensive guide chock full of valuable information. It is completely consumer-friendly, giving readers all that they need to know to make intelligent, informed choices.

Use it well and in good health!

Sincerely,

Sandra Gainer, R.N.
Associate Director
National Center for Patient Rights

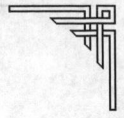

The Best in American Medicine
www.CastleConnolly.com

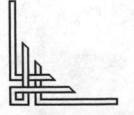
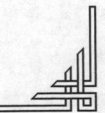

Introduction

A savvy consumer, searching for a car, restaurant, house or even a spouse, can easily find a guidebook to help. Yet, when it comes to choosing healthcare providers, the bookshelves are nearly bare.

Top Doctors: New York Metro Area has been written to fill that void. It will guide you in making critical —even lifesaving—choices.

This Guide Has Two Goals:

- To provide you with a base of information and a framework of understanding so that you can participate in the important healthcare choices that will maximize your own health, your family's health and the quality of your life.

- To provide detailed information on more than 6,000 well-trained, highly competent physicians from which you may confidently choose your personal best doctors for your own healthcare needs and those of your family.

Medicine is often described as a combination of art and science. This description holds true for the process of selecting the best medical care. This book describes the "science" of making that selection. It is not magical or even difficult. It is simply a matter of knowing what information you should have and where to find it.

The "art" is what you will bring to the selection process. It is based upon your feelings, your needs and the chemistry that develops between you and those who provide your healthcare. Castle Connolly's *Top Doctors: New York Metro Area* will help you prepare for that interaction and will guide you in getting the most from it.

Most importantly, Castle Connolly's *Top Doctors: New York Metro Area* will tell you how to combine the art and science so that you can make the best choices.

How to Use This Guide

This book has been written as a basic, "how to" guide for selecting the best healthcare. Section One provides important information on how to choose the best doctors. Doctors are the most important providers of healthcare and whether you are part of an HMO or covered by traditional medical insurance, you want the very best doctors to attend to your healthcare needs. Section Three contains listings of doctors as well as information on hospitals invited to participate in the Guide's Partnership for Excellence program. Section Four includes information on "Centers of Excellence"—special programs and services—offered by a number of the hospitals participating in the Partnership for Excellence program. Section Five contains seven appendices with important and interesting information.

Introduction

There Are Two Effective Ways to Use This Guide:

- Start at the beginning. This method will give you a broad understanding of the healthcare field and a clearer perspective of where you, the patient, fit in it. This method will arm you with necessary information for making informed choices and will help you find the best doctors.

- Study the doctor listings. While at least a brief reading of some or all of the introductory chapters is recommended so that, in the end, you will make well-informed choices, it is understandable that you may wish to go straight to the physician listings. The organization of these listings is outlined on pages 71 to 79. You will find guidelines for effectively using the listings on these pages.

Each chapter begins with explanations of terms that may be new to you. Reviewing these terms will help you read the section more easily.

In preparing this book, we've left little to chance or question. We hope to inspire you to assume a curious and insistent attitude as you make the healthcare choices that will take you and your family through life.

The Doctor of Choice

Primary Care Physicians

Quick Tips

The time to establish a relationship with a doctor is while you are healthy. The top doctor to establish your relationship with is the one who is most likely to keep you healthy: A primary care doctor.

Primary means first, so a primary care doctor is the first one you see for most health problems.

It is difficult for any doctor, however skilled, to make judgements based on only one visit or a single test.

Your primary care doctor can educate you about the "hows" and "whys" of health maintenance and disease prevention and follow up to help you stay faithful to the course the two of you have agreed upon.

Any doctor with a license can practice in any specialty he/she chooses. Board certification is your assurance that the doctor has appropriate training in the specialty.

When considering recommendations, use the old navigational technique of triangulation: focus on doctors whose names are mentioned by three or more people.

Hospital telephone referral lines are not designed to distinguish among hundreds of doctors who may be more or less well regarded by other doctors, or who may be better suited to a particular caller when factors other than location, insurance coverage and office hours are taken into consideration.

Many local medical societies publish directories, some of which are intended primarily for doctor-to-doctor referrals, while others are distributed to the public. They provide information but do not address quality.

The internet provides many websites that provide lists of doctors: some are of questionable quality. Be careful that the information is from a trusted source.

Quick Take

... Primary care physician. That's a hot term in healthcare today. Who is this physician? How do you find one?...

Key Terms

Lupus Erythematosus - An autoimmune disorder, also referred to as SLE, or simply "lupus". It can cause inflammation and possible damage to a number of vital organs and is commonly marked by joint pain, facial and other rashes, abnormally high antibody levels, and diminished red blood cell levels.

Lyme Disease - An infectious disease, transmitted through the bite of a deer tick, which may or may not produce a distinctive bull's-eye rash at the site of the tick bite. First identified in Lyme, Connecticut, the infection may also produce other symptoms, including flu-like aches, arthritic joint pain, and, in complicated cases, cardiac abnormalities.

Managed Care - The process of integrating the finance and delivery of healthcare to control costs and improve quality. A managed care plan typically involves a group of practitioners who "manage" care for a specified population.

Osteopath - A healthcare professional who has earned a degree in osteopathic medicine, a D.O. Osteopathic medicine emphasizes massage and bone manipulation while traditional western allopathic medicine emphasizes treatment with drugs and surgery.

Preventive Medicine/Care - Health services that are aimed at maintaining good health and preventing illness. These services include routine physical examinations, immunizations, certain screening tests such as mammograms or Pap tests, as well as the practice of good health habits.

Primary Care Physician - The first doctor consulted for any health problem, a Primary Care Physician is a specialist who offers basic, including preventive, medical care. It is important to maintain an ongoing relationship with your primary care physician.

Specialist - A physician who practices in one or more of the 25 specialties defined by the American Board of Medical Specialties (ABMS). The term is also used to denote a physician's area of practice, such as pediatrics, geriatrics, surgery, etc.

Subspecialist - A specialist who obtains further training and certification in one or more of the 70 subspecialties approved by the American Board of Medical Specialties. The physician must first be certified in a specialty. For example, a board certified internist may become certified in cardiology or gastroenterology.

Primary Care Physicians

When it comes to choosing a doctor, too many people let the decision slide until they are sick or hurt and need immediate medical attention. That's unfortunate if an illness that could have been managed successfully develops to a stage where it becomes difficult to control or cure. It's even more unfortunate if the illness could have been prevented in the first place.

The time to establish a relationship with a doctor is while you are healthy, and the best one to establish your relationship with is the one who is most likely to keep you healthy: a primary care doctor.

Primary means first, so a primary care doctor is the first one you see for any health problem. Primary also means basic, so a primary care doctor offers the kind of fundamental care that can keep you healthy.

Yes, You Do Need a Doctor When You're Healthy.

Here are four good reasons why you should start your search for a primary care doctor now:

Reason One

A primary care doctor can put your current medical condition into a context that consists of your medical history, current condition as compared with past medical status, and changes in your body and environment over time. It is difficult for any doctor, however skilled, to make informed medical judgments based on only one visit or a single test. Conditions well out of normal range are easy to pick up, but extreme variations do not always occur and a serious illness may develop slowly with only a gradual increase in symptoms. The operative word is continuity: ideally, your medical care should not be interrupted by changes in providers.

Reason Two

A primary care doctor is better able to treat you as a whole person. Medicine has become very specialized and procedure-oriented, but the human body is not a loose collection of unrelated parts. It is a "whole" with strong interrelationships among all biological systems. Some of the poorest medical care results from people jumping from subspecialist to subspecialist. Despite talent, skill and training, no specialist knows the patient well enough, or for long enough, to be able to take the whole person into consideration and track the normal patterns of evolution and change. We end up with a specialist for every organ and system instead of a doctor who will care for the whole person.

Reason Three

A primary care doctor can establish preventive programs. Our healthcare system does not place enough emphasis on preventing illness; most healthcare dollars are spent on curative, rather than preventive, medicine. However, the status quo is slowly changing, and it is within primary care that the change is most evident. Your primary care doctor can educate you about the hows and whys of health maintenance and disease prevention and can follow up to help you stay faithful to the course the two of you have agreed upon. Only an ongoing relationship makes this possible.

Reason Four

A primary care doctor can save you money. Managed care advocates, among others, have long deplored the waste inherent in a system in which patients can simply call any specialist any time they have an ache or pain or are not feeling well. Primary care doctors can monitor referrals to specialists, following the patient closely to put together a variety of observations, opinions, and test results in order to treat each person on an individual basis. This improves the quality of care and also controls costs.

Patients who visit specialists without some guidance from a primary care doctor may choose the wrong specialist based on a general observation and self-diagnosis about the problem or illness they're experiencing. While in some cases the problem may be obvious (for example, an eye injury), in others it may be more subtle. Diseases such as lupus erythematosus and Lyme disease, for example, often have a myriad of symptoms that are easily misinterpreted by laypersons; in fact, they are often difficult even for doctors to diagnose accurately. While certain problems may require the collaboration of several specialists, it is important to have a primary care doctor navigating the course.

Finally, it is estimated that almost half of all emergency room visits in some areas are for non-emergencies; it's the most expensive place to receive primary care. When people have primary care doctors, they tend to turn to them rather than to hospital emergency departments.

If you are enrolled in any kind of managed care program, health maintenance organization (HMO) or other program, you will almost always be required to select a primary care doctor from its roster. Managed care executives recognize the necessity of a primary care doctor, not only for delivering quality healthcare, but also for controlling costs.

How to Find a Doctor

Unless you already have a primary care doctor you are satisfied with, you will have to find one. How? Here are five possible avenues to begin the process of finding the doctor that best suits your needs; each has limits, however.

Doctor Referrals

If you are moving and are leaving a trusted doctor behind, get a recommendation or two before you go. Furthermore, ask in what context and how well your doctor knows the new doctor—they may not have met since medical school.

Friends and Relatives

Always keep in mind that such recommendations are based largely on what may be "simpatico," or a personal affinity. Ask why your friend likes the doctor. It might be because the fees are low or the doctor makes house calls or is warm and sociable—all valid considerations, but certainly not principal determinants. So be wary of the generalized recommendation that "Dr. Jones is just wonderful." When considering recommendations, use the old navigational technique of triangulation: focus on doctors whose names are mentioned by three or more people.

Hospital Referral Services

Hospital telephone referral lines are not designed to distinguish among hundreds of doctors who may be more or less well regarded by other doctors, or who may be better suited to a particular caller when factors other than location, insurance coverage and office hours are taken into consideration. It would be impolitic for hospital referral services to rate their doctors. Their recommendations are based on specialty and geographic proximity, usually by way of a computer that rotates through the lists to "recommend" the next three names in line, and all members of the medical staff are eligible to participate.

Medical Society Directories

Many local medical societies publish directories, some of which are intended primarily for doctor-to-doctor referrals, while others are distributed to the public. These directories usually provide names, addresses, phone numbers and specialties and can be useful sources. However, they do not distinguish among doctors in any way. All members of the medical society, usually a countywide organization, are eligible for inclusion. This also applies to the referral lines offered by many medical societies.

Advertising

Responding to advertising is the least effective way to find a doctor. While more and more health professionals now advertise, a practice which is no longer considered unethical, some stigma still remains. Advertising could lead you to a doctor who receives few or no referrals from colleagues and whose orientation to the profession is more entrepreneurial than medical. Most referral lines not sponsored by hospitals charge a fee to doctors who want to be listed. This is simply another form of advertising.

The Internet

There are many websites that provide information on doctors. Some are directories or internet phone books. These can be helpful. Some claim to be based on quality measures. Many of these require physicians to pay, others are of questionable quality. Be sure the site sponsor or source is a trusted one.

Many Ways to Say Doctor

In this guide, the term "doctor" is used to describe only medical doctors who have received a Doctor of Medicine degree (MD) and osteopaths who have received a Doctor of Osteopathic Medicine degree (DO). Doctors who have been trained in the British system may hold a degree of Bachelor of Medicine (MB), Bachelor of Surgery (BS), or Bachelor of Chirurgia (BCh), which is based on the ancient Greek term that refers to surgery.

The more formal term for any of these practitioners is "physician." However, most people use the more popular term "doctor," which is the one generally used in this book. Our discussions do not include other kinds of doctors such as dentists, podiatrists, psychologists or chiropractors, who also deliver healthcare.

Primary Care: The Fundamental Four

There is not complete agreement in medicine on which specialties are practiced by the group of doctors known as primary care specialists. For the purposes of this book, we have included the following specialties: Internal Medicine, Pediatrics, Family Practice and Obstetrics and Gynecology. Most adults choose general internists as their primary care doctors and select pediatricians for their children. There is also another type of specialist, the family practitioner, who cares for both children and adults. In addition to such generalists, many women also select an obstetrician/gynecologist as their primary care providers.

- A **general internist**, specializing in internal medicine, is trained to treat all internal organs and systems of the body. Many internists also are board certified in a subspecialty such as cardiology, gastroenterology or geriatric medicine. Therefore, if you have a history of heart disease, you may wish to select an internist who has additional training in cardiology, but who primarily practices general internal medicine. On the other hand, your primary care doctor may refer you to a cardiologist when necessary, and both may treat you over a period of years. In fact, it is not unusual for a patient with a serious or complex illness to be followed by two or three doctors, with the primary care doctor "quarterbacking" the team.

- A **family practitioner** is very broadly trained. Such doctors come closest to the general practitioner of the past. They are qualified to treat all family members, including children.

- A **pediatrician** is the doctor you would choose for the care of your children. As with doctors in internal medicine, pediatricians often have a subspecialty such as cardiology, rheumatology or endocrinology.

- **Obstetricians and Gynecologists** are the subject of significant debate in terms of their appropriateness as primary care doctors. The American Board of Obstetrics and Gynecology states that these doctors are specialists and are not generally trained for primary care. However, the reality is that many, particularly those who solely practice gynecology, often serve as a woman's primary care doctor. Gynecologists are divided on the issue. One recent study showed that 95 percent of visits to ob-gyns are self-referred and that about 60 percent of visits to these specialists are for diagnostic services and preventive services. Another study, by the American College of Obstetricians and Gynecologists, showed that 54 percent of women who see a gynecologist use these doctors for primary care. Reflecting the reality of current medical practice, we have included these specialists in the primary care category.

A businessman in his late fifties, a long-time competitive runner, had surgery in one of New York's top hospitals to repair a badly torn Achilles tendon. At his first follow-up visit to the orthopaedic surgeon, he was assured that "everything was healing perfectly," that he had nothing to be concerned about, and that he would soon be up and running again. Shortly thereafter, just before a summer camping trip, he decided to have his yearly physical examination. The primary care doctor examined the site of the surgery, probing up and down the whole length of the leg. Explaining that he was concerned about certain swelling and discoloration, the doctor arranged for a further examination with ultrasound imaging. This sophisticated test showed that a blood clot had formed in the upper part of the leg, which could have caused severe disability and even death had it gotten into the bloodstream and traveled to the heart or brain. It was the primary care doctor, who knew the patient well, who discovered the potentially fatal condition while carefully conducting a full physical exam.

What Makes A "Top" Doctor

Quick Tips

If in doubt about a doctor's training, ask the doctor if the residency completed was in the specialty of his/her practice. If not, ask why not.

Board certification and recertification are the best ways to measure competence and training.

The easiest way you can assess the quality of a doctor's residency program is to see if it took place in a large medical center with a name you recognize.

If a doctor does not have admitting privileges or is not on the attending staff of a hospital, you might consider choosing another doctor.

There are many excellent, well-trained doctors at community hospitals and they should be as carefully evaluated and considered in your search as a doctor at a teaching hospital.

Doctors who are full-time academicians may be in the forefront of new techniques and research, but they are not necessarily better doctors.

The best care is provided by a combination of primary care doctors and other specialists and subspecialists.

Do not hesitate to ask how frequently your doctor has performed a procedure and with what degree of success. Practice may not lead to perfection, but it improves skills and enhances the probability of success.

Check the date of graduation from medical school or completion of residency if you want to know precisely how long a doctor has been in practice.

Quick Take

... If a doctor does not have admitting privileges or is not on the attending staff of a hospital, you might consider choosing another doctor. ...

Key Terms

Academic Medical Center - A large medical complex that centers around a teaching hospital in which residency and fellowship programs are offered, where the medical school faculty practices full time and where major clinical research activities occur.

Board Certified - Term signifying that a doctor is qualified for specialization by one of the American Board of Medical Specialties (ABMS) boards. Qualification includes completing an approved residency and passing a rigid exam.

Board Eligible - Term signifying that a doctor has completed an approved residency but has not yet taken the exam given by one of the ABMS recognized boards. The term conveys no official status in the eyes of the ABMS.

Clinical - Medical care that involves direct contact with patients.

Credentialing - A process of screening conducted by hospitals wherein they review the training and licenses of doctors applying to practice on their medical staffs.

Indemnity - A form of health insurance coverage that pays for healthcare but permits the patients to select their provider. Until 1990, indemnity insurance covered most insured people in the United States.

Licensure - Official credentials by individual states that permit a doctor to practice medicine in that state. In some states, doctors may be licensed with no more than one year of post-graduate training.

Residency - A training period spent in a hospital by a graduate of a medical school before going into practice. Residents have earned a medical degree and, therefore, are doctors, but must complete an approved residency and pass an exam to become board certified.

Tertiary Care - Medical services provided by a hospital or medical center that include complex treatments and procedures such as open heart surgery, organ transplants and burn care.

What Makes A "Top" Doctor

Castle Connolly's Top Doctors™ selection process begins with surveys of physicians and healthcare professionals. Each year, Castle Connolly surveys thousands of physicians and other healthcare professionals and asks them to identify excellent doctors in every specialty in their region and throughout the nation. When we began the research for the first edition of America's Top Doctors®, we surveyed over 230,000 of the nation's leading medical specialists, department chairs, residency program directors, vice presidents of medical affairs and presidents of the nation's leading medical centers and specialty hospitals.

In addition to mail and online surveys, the Castle Connolly physician-led research team makes thousands of phone calls each year, talking with leading specialists, chairs of clinical departments and vice presidents of medical affairs, seeking to identify top specialists for most diseases and procedures.

The Castle Connolly physician-led research team carefully reviews the credentials of every physician being considered for inclusion in Castle Connolly Guides, magazine articles and website. The review includes, among other factors, scrutiny of medical education, training, hospital appointments, administrative posts, professional achievements, and malpractice and disciplinary history.

Information on outcomes, procedure volume and malpractice is becoming increasingly available, but the public disclosure varies from state to state. Castle Connolly uses its best efforts to gather the information that is available and use it effectively. Ultimately, however, it is the professional judgment of the Castle Connolly editors, the Chief Medical and Research Officer and the research staff, which determines Castle Connolly Top Doctor™ selection.

Physicians may also be removed from the Castle Connolly lists if, in the judgment of the selection team, that is warranted. Some of the reasons physicians are removed include retirement, change in practice (taking a full time administrative post, for example), unavailability to patients, malpractice or disciplinary issues, negative physician or patient feedback, professional demeanor or a change in the "mix" of specialists Castle Connolly will present for a given community. Being removed from a Castle Connolly list does not necessarily indicate something negative about the physician. At the same time, Castle Connolly does not claim to identify every excellent physician in the nation or a region. The physicians identified through the Castle Connolly research process are clearly among the very best, but there are always other very good physicians not identified by Castle Connolly and that is why our guides, websites and other distribution channels for this critical information describe a process whereby consumers can identify excellent physicians using their own efforts.

There are four basic criteria for selecting your own best doctor: professional preparation, professional reputation, office and practice arrangements and personal or bedside manner. The first three of these assessments can be made prior to your first visit, which is when you can make your fourth evaluation.

Professional Preparation

Education

Your review of your prospective doctor's education and training should begin with medical school. While you may feel that the institution where someone earned a bachelor's degree could be an indication of the quality of the doctor, most people in the medical field do not believe it plays a major role. A degree from a highly selective undergraduate college or university will help an aspiring doctor gain admission to a medical school, but once there, all students are peers. However, the information on undergraduate colleges, if important to you, is available in the American Board of Medical Specialties (ABMS) Compendium of Certified Medical Specialists and other medical directories.

American medical schools are highly standardized, at least in terms of minimum quality. All U.S. medical schools that grant medical degrees (MDs) and osteopathic degrees (DOs) are accredited by a group known as the LCME (Liaison Committee for Medical Education). Most are also accredited by the appropriate state agency, if one exists, and by regional accrediting agencies that accredit colleges and universities of all kinds.

Furthermore, U.S. medical schools have universally high standards for admission, including success on the undergraduate level and on the Medical College Admissions Tests (MCATs). Although frequently criticized for being slow to change and for training too many specialists, the system of medical education in the United States has insured high quality in medical practice. One recent positive change is a strong effort in most medical schools to diversify the composition of the student body. While these schools have been less successful in enrolling racial minorities, the number of women in U.S. medical schools has increased to the point where they now make up about 50 percent of most classes. In certain specialties preferred by female medical graduates (pediatrics, for example), it is possible that, in coming years, the majority of specialists will be female.

Most doctors practicing in the United States are graduates of U.S. medical schools. There are two other groups of doctors in practice who make up a relatively small proportion of the total doctor population. They are: (1) foreign nationals who graduated from foreign schools; and (2) U.S. nationals who graduated from foreign schools (Canadian medical schools are not considered foreign).

Foreign Medical Graduates

Foreign medical schools vary greatly in quality. Even some of the oldest and finest European schools have become virtually "open door institutions," with huge numbers of unscreened students who make teaching and learning difficult. Others are excellent and provided the model for our own system of medical education.

The fact that someone graduated from a foreign school does not mean that he or she is a poor doctor. Foreign schools, like U.S. schools, produce good doctors and poor doctors. Foreign medical graduates must pass the same exam taken by U.S. graduates for licensure, but the failure rate for foreign graduates is significantly higher. In the first year of using the new United States Medical Licensing Exam (USMLE), 93 percent of U.S. medical school graduates passed Step II, the clinical exam, as compared with 39 percent of foreign graduates. It is clear that the quality of foreign schools, if not individual doctors, is not the same as U.S. medical schools, at least as measured by our standards. Nonetheless, many communities and patients have been well served by foreign medical graduates practicing in this country—often in areas where it has been difficult to attract graduates of American schools.

Residency

Most doctors practicing today have at least three years of postgraduate training (following the MD or DO) in an approved residency program. This is not only an important step in the process of becoming a competent doctor, but it is also a requirement for board (specialty) certification. Most people assume that a prospective doctor needs to complete a three-year residency program to obtain a medical license. This is not true in some states. New York State, for example, requires only one postgraduate year. However, since all approved residencies last at least three years, and some, such as neurosurgery, general surgery, orthopaedic surgery and urology, may extend for five or more years, it is important to know the details of a doctor's training. Licensure alone is not enough of a basis on which to make a good choice.

Without undertaking extensive and detailed research on every residency program, the best assessment you can make of a doctor's residency program is to see if it took place in a large medical center whose name you recognize. The more prestigious institutions tend to attract the best medical students, sometimes regardless of the quality of the individual residency program. If in doubt about a doctor's training, ask the doctor if the residency completed was in the specialty of his/her practice. If not, ask why.

It is also important to be certain that a doctor completed a residency that has been approved by the appropriate governing board of the specialty such as the American Board of Surgery, the American Board of Radiology or the American Osteopathic Board of Pediatrics. These board groups are listed in Appendix A. If you are really concerned about a doctor's training, you should first call the hospital that offered the residency and ask if the residency was approved by the appropriate specialty group. If still in doubt, review the publication Directory of Graduate Medical Education Programs, often called the "green book," found in medical school or hospital libraries, which lists all approved residencies.

Board Certification

With an MD or DO degree and a license, an individual may practice any kind of medicine—with or without additional special training. For example, doctors with a license but no special training may call themselves cardiologists or pediatricians. This is why board certification is such an important factor. Twenty-five specialties are recognized by the American Board of Medical Specialties (ABMS). (Visit www.abms.org or call 866-275-2267 for more information.) Eighteen boards certify in 106 specialties under the aegis of the American Osteopathic Association (AOA). (Visit www.osteopathic.org or call 800-621-1773 for more information.) Doctors who have qualified for such specialization are called board certified; they have completed an approved residency and passed the board's exam. (See Appendix A for an approved ABMS and AOA list; see pages 81-87 for a description of each specialty and subspecialty.) While many doctors who are not board certified do call themselves specialists, board certification is the best standard by which to measure competence and training.

You can be confident that doctors who are board certified have at a minimum the proper training in their specialty and have demonstrated their proficiency through supervision and testing. While there are many non-board certified doctors who are highly competent, it is more difficult to assess the level of their training. Board certification alone does not guarantee competence, but it is a standard that reflects successful completion of an appropriate training program.

Recertification

A relatively new focus of the specialty boards is the area of recertification. Until recently, board certification lasted for an unlimited time period. Now, almost all of the boards have put time limits on the certification period. For example, in internal medicine, it is ten years; in family practice seven years. In osteopathic medicine, some of the boards need to set a recertification period within 10 years. Many have done so already. These more stringent standards reflect an increasing emphasis, by both the medical boards and state agencies responsible for licensing doctors, on recertification.

Since the policies of the boards vary widely, it is good procedure to ask a doctor if certification was awarded and when. If the date was seven to ten years ago, ask if he/she has been recertified. Note: The most recent date of board certification or recertification is indicated in each physician's listing in this guide.

Unfortunately, many boards permit "grandfathering," whereby already certified doctors do not have to be recertified, and recertification demands apply only to newly certified doctors. Appendix A contains a list of the names and addresses of the boards and the certification period for each board specialty. Even if recertification is not required, it is good professional practice for doctors to undertake the process. It assures you, the patient, that they are attempting to stay current.

Many states have a continuing medical education (CME) requirement for doctors. These states typically require a minimum number of CME credits for a doctor to maintain a medical license. Seven states require 150 CME credits over a three-year period. Osteopathic doctors are required to take 120 hours of CME credits within three years to maintain certification.

Board Eligibility

Many doctors who have been recently trained are waiting to take the boards. They are sometimes described as "board eligible," a common term that the ABMS advocates abandoning because of its ambiguity. Board eligible means that the doctor has completed an approved residency and is qualified to sit for the related board's exam.

Each member board of the ABMS has its own policy regarding the use and recognition of the board eligible term. Therefore, the description "board eligible" should not be viewed as a genuine qualification, especially if a doctor has been out of medical school long enough to have taken the certification exam. To the boards, a doctor is either board certified or not. Furthermore, most of the specialty boards permit unlimited attempts to pass the exam and, in some cases, doctors who have failed the exam twice or even ten times continue to call themselves board eligible. In osteopathic medicine, the board eligible status is recognized only for the first six years after completion of a residency.

Self-Designated Medical Specialties

In addition to the ABMS and AOA-approved list of specialties and subspecialties, there is a wide variety of other doctors, and groups of doctors, who may call themselves "specialists". There are, at present, at least 100 such groups called self-designated medical specialties. They range from doctors who are working to create a recognized body of knowledge and subspecialty training to less formal groups interested in a particular approach to the practice of medicine. These groups may or may not have standards for membership. There is no way of determining the true extent of their members' training, and they are not recognized by the ABMS* or the AOA. While you should be cautious of doctors who claim they are specialists in these areas, many do have advanced training and the groups at least offer a listing of people interested in a particular approach to medical care. Rely on board certification to assure yourself of basic competence and use membership in one of these groups to indicate strong interest and possible additional training in a particular aspect of medicine. A list of these self-designated medical specialties may be found in Appendix B.

Fellowships

The purpose of a fellowship is to provide advanced training in the clinical techniques and research of a particular subspecialty. In the U.S. there are a variety of fellowship programs available to doctors, and they fall into two broad categories: approved and unapproved. Approved fellowships are those approved by the appropriate medical specialty board (e.g., the American Board of Radiology) and that lead to a subspecialty certificate. Fellowship programs that are not approved are often in the same areas of training as those that are, but they do not lead to a subspecialty

---

* One subspecialty, not yet recognized by the ABMS - Pediatric Neurosurgery - has been included because the retaining and certification process is rigorous and meaningful.

certificate. Unfortunately, all too often, unapproved fellowships exist only to provide relatively inexpensive labor for the research and/or patient care activities of a clinical department in a medical school or hospital. In such cases, the learning that takes place is secondary and may be a good deal less than in an approved fellowship. On the other hand, any fellowship is better than none at all and some unapproved fellowships have that status for a valid reason, which should not reflect negatively on the program. For example, the fellowship may have been recently created with approval being sought. To check that a fellowship is an approved one, call the hospital where the training took place or the medical board for that specialty.

Professional Reputation

There are doctors who meet every professional standard on paper, but who are simply not good doctors. In all probability, the medical community has ascertained that while the individual may still practice medicine, his or her reputation will reflect that collective assessment. There are also doctors who are outstanding leaders in their fields because of research or professional activities, but who are not particularly strong or perhaps even active in patient care. It is important to distinguish that kind of professional reputation from a reputation as a competent, caring doctor in delivering patient care. In a consumer survey conducted by the management consulting firm Towers Perrin, the chief criterion by which the respondents selected doctors was reputation. This was the most important factor for those enrolled in either managed care or indemnity plans.

Hospital Appointment

Most doctors are on the medical staff of one or more hospitals and are known as attendings. If a doctor does not have admitting privileges or is not on the attending staff of a hospital, you may wish to consider choosing another doctor. It can be very difficult to ascertain whether the lack of hospital appointment is for a good reason or not. For example, it is understandable that some doctors who are raising families or heading toward retirement choose not to meet the demands (meetings, committees, etc.) of being an attending. However, if you need care in a hospital, the lack of such an appointment means that another doctor will have to oversee that care. In some specialties such as dermatology and psychiatry, doctors may conduct their entire practices in the office, and a hospital appointment is not as essential, or as good a criterion for assessment, as in other specialties.

While mistakes are made, most hospitals are quite careful about admissions to their medical staffs. The best hospitals are highly selective, so a degree of screening (or "credentialing") has been done for you. In other words, the best doctors practice at the best hospitals. Since caring for a patient in the hospital is often a team effort involving a number of specialists, the reputation of the hospital where the doctor admits patients carries special weight. Hospital medical staffs also review their colleagues credentials before authorizing them to perform specific procedures. In addition, they typically reappoint their medical staffs—and review them—every two or three years. In effect, this is an additional screening to protect patients. It is especially true of hospitals that have what are known as closed staffs, where it is impossible to obtain admitting privileges unless there is a vacancy that the administration and medical staff deem necessary to fill. If you are having some type of surgical procedure and are concerned about the doctor's skill or experience with it, it may be worthwhile to call the Medical Affairs office at the doctor's hospital to see if he or she is authorized to perform that procedure in the hospital.

The reasons for a hospital's selectivity are easy to understand: every hospital wants to have the best reputation possible in order to attract patients, and no hospital, excellent or not, wishes to expose itself to liability. Obviously, the quality of the medical staff is immensely important in creating that reputation. Unfortunately, some hospitals are less diligent when a major group practice of doctors, all of whom have previously been affiliated with the institution, adds new members. In such cases, the hospital may almost automatically grant privileges without conducting the same intensive review given to individual doctors who are not members of a group practice. Also, some hospitals are less selective in granting privileges when beds are empty than when beds are full, since additional attendings provide additional patients.

A last and very important reason why a hospital appointment is an essential requirement in your choice of a doctor is that many states permit doctors to practice without malpractice insurance. If you are injured as a result of the doctor's poor care, you could be without recourse. However, few hospitals permit doctors to practice in them unless they carry malpractice insurance. This not only protects the hospital, but the patient as well.

Many people believe that they should choose a doctor with an appointment at a major medical center as opposed to a community hospital. This assumption is incorrect on two counts. For one thing, there are many excellent, well-trained doctors at community hospitals and they should be as carefully evaluated and considered in your search as a doctor at a large institution. What's more, the term "medical center" has less significance today than it did years ago when the term was used to describe only the major university hospitals of medical schools. A true medical center is a teaching hospital that offers multiple residency programs and at which the medical school faculty practices full-time, with fellowship programs and major clinical research activities an integral part of the teaching of medical students. These large centers also are involved in tertiary care, offering services such as organ transplants, burn care and cardiovascular surgery.

Today many community hospitals have added the term medical center to their name. They do this for two purposes: to indicate that they, too, offer advanced and sophisticated medical programs, and to compete for patients with the academic medical centers. With academic medical centers turning out many well-trained specialists and subspecialists who establish practices in nearby communities and then want to continue the highly specialized techniques they have learned, many community hospitals have initiated tertiary care programs of their own, further blurring the distinction between medical centers and hospitals.

In any case, most of our healthcare today is delivered outside of the hospital in ambulatory outpatient settings. Those who are hospitalized for acute illness (e.g., surgery, serious infection) will find that community hospitals and their staffs are well-suited to the task.

When extremely difficult and complex problems develop, or when tertiary care is needed, many communities have excellent academic medical centers. Of course, they offer primary care as well, especially to those who live nearby. This illustrates the point, once again, that medical care is a local issue.

Medical School Faculty Appointment

Many doctors have appointments on the faculties of medical schools. There is a range of categories from "straight" appointments—meaning full-time appointment as professor, associate professor, assistant professor or instructor—to clinical ranks that may reflect lesser degrees of involvement in teaching or research. If someone carries what is known as a straight academic rank (i.e., professor of surgery, without "clinical" in the title), this usually means that the individual is engaged full-time in medical school research and/or teaching activities. The title "professor of clinical surgery" usually describes a doctor who has a full-time appointment in a medical school, but who puts a greater emphasis on clinical practice (patient care) than on research or teaching. The title "clinical professor of surgery" usually specifies a part-time or adjunct appointment and less direct involvement in medical school activities.

Doctors who are full-time academicians may be in the forefront of new techniques and research, but they are not necessarily better doctors. Nonetheless, you can be assured that they have the support of other faculty, residents and medical students.

When you are seeking a subspecialist, a doctor's relationship to a medical school becomes more meaningful since medical school faculties tend to be made up of subspecialists. You are less likely to find large numbers of general or primary care practitioners engaged full-time on a medical school faculty. The newest approaches and techniques in medicine, for the most part, are explored and developed by medical school faculties in their laboratories and clinical practice settings. This is where they practice their subspecialties, as well as teach and perform research. Such leading specialists are not necessarily better doctors than community doctors—they are trained to provide a different kind of medical care. The best care is provided by a combination of primary care doctors and other specialists and subspecialists.

Medical Society Membership

Most medical society memberships sound very prestigious and some are; however, there are many societies that are not selective and which virtually any doctor can join. In addition, membership in many of the more prestigious societies is based on research and publication, or on leadership in the field, and may have little to do with direct patient care. While it is clearly an honor to be invited to join these groups, membership may be less than helpful in discerning whether a doctor can meet your needs.

Board certified doctors are referred to as Diplomates of the Board. Some of the colleges of medical specialties (e.g., the American College of Radiology and the American College of Surgeons) have multiple levels of recognition. The first is basic membership and the second, more prestigious and difficult to obtain, is status as a Fellow. Fellowship status in the colleges is meaningful and is based on experience, professional achievement and recognition by one's peers, including extensive experience in patient care. It should be viewed as a significant professional qualification.

Experience

Experience is difficult to assess. Obviously, in most cases, an older doctor has more experience; on the other hand, a younger doctor has been more recently immersed in residency, the challenge of medical school, or even a fellowship, and may be the most up-to-date. If a doctor is board certified, you may assume that assures at least a minimal amount of experience, but it could be as little as a year. In this guide the board certification date may reflect a doctor's most recent recertification, so check the date of graduation from medical school or completion of residency if you want to know precisely how long a doctor has been in practice.

There is a good deal of evidence that there is a positive relationship between quantity of experience and quality of care. That is, the more often a doctor performs a procedure, the better he/she becomes at it. That is why it is important to ask a doctor about his or her experience with the procedure that you need. Does the doctor see and treat similar cases every day, every week or only rarely? Of course, with some rare conditions, rarely is the only possible answer, but it is relative frequency that is critical. Major metropolitan areas, especially New York and San Francisco, became leaders in the treatment of AIDS because of the large number of patients seen in those metropolitan areas. Doctors in the suburbs of New York City (especially in New York's Westchester, Nassau and Suffolk counties) and in Fairfield County, Connecticut became leaders in the research and treatment of Lyme disease because that region is the epicenter of the disease.

In some states, data is available on volume or numbers of certain procedures performed at hospitals. For this information in New York you can call the Center for Medical Consumers, a non-profit advocacy organization, or visit its website at www.medicalconsumers.org. For volume and outcome information in other states, visit the Website of Health Care Choices at www.healthcarechoices.com. There is a good deal of controversy, however, on the validity and usefulness of such data. Opponents cite the fact that some of the data is produced from Medicare patient records only and, thus, is based solely on an elderly population that does not represent the total activity of a hospital or doctor. Proponents of the use of such volume data agree that it is not perfect, but suggest that it can be one useful criterion in selecting the best places to receive care for these specific problems. Recognizing the limitations of such data, the healthcare consumer may, nonetheless, find it of interest and use.

Office and Practice Arrangements

Although clearly not as important as training or reputation, office and practice arrangements are usually of great significance to patients. Practice arrangements include office hours, office location, billing procedures and office testing among the many factors that result in how well the office is run.

Many years ago most doctors practiced independently in private offices. They were called solo practitioners and usually had agreements with other doctors to respond to their patients' calls when they were unavailable. In recent decades, most doctors have entered group practices; indeed, this is becoming the most common way for young doctors to begin to practice. Two or more doctors in the same specialty, or in different specialties (a multi-specialty group), share offices and staff to lower their costs of operations. They also cover for each other on rotation for weekends, evenings and vacations. As a patient you may prefer one of the following: a solo practitioner who is covered occasionally; a group where you usually, but not always, see the same doctor; or a multi-specialty group where, if a consultation or referral is necessary, the specialist is at the same location. The choice is really one of personal preference.

There are other factors relating to practice arrangements that may or may not be important to an individual when choosing a doctor. One is the location of the office. A consumer poll conducted for the Robert Wood Johnson Foundation identified office location as one of the two most important factors in the selection of a doctor (the other was a recommendation by a relative or friend). Actually, the site of the office can be very important in choosing a doctor you may visit on a regular basis. If the location is inconvenient, you may be discouraged from making needed visits.

Another important factor concerns the use of nurse practitioners and physician's assistants in the office. Licensed nurse practitioners are advanced practice nurses in primary care. They have additional training beyond the basic requirements for nursing licensure, usually a master's degree or special certificate. They perform a broad range of nursing functions as well as functions that, historically, have been performed by doctors, including assessing and diagnosing, conducting physical examinations, ordering diagnostic tests, implementing treatment plans and monitoring patient status. Physician's assistants are licensed to provide medical care in many states. However, unlike nurses, they may practice only under a doctor's direction and supervision. According to an article in the professional journal Family Practice Management, these "midlevel providers," as they are called, "can handle 80 to 90 percent of the problems that occasion office visits." These providers have become more of a presence in healthcare in recent years, especially in medical groups and HMOs. If you don't think you will be satisfied having your office visit and examination conducted by anyone but the doctor, you should determine up front how many midlevel providers are on staff and how extensive their responsibilities are.

Narrowing the Choice

Here are 10 additional questions that will guide you in assessing if the practice patterns or arrangements of a doctor meet your needs. If there are other items not listed that are important to you, add them to the list before you make your initial appointment. You should try to obtain as much of the information as possible from the staff.

- Are you currently accepting new patients and, if so, is a referral required?
- On average, how long does a patient have to wait for an appointment?
- Are you open on weekends? In the evening?
- If lab work and X-rays are performed in the office what are the qualifications of the people doing the tests?
- Are full payment, deductibles or co-payments required at the time of the appointment?
- Do you accept my insurance plan? Medicare? Medicaid? Workers' compensation? No-fault insurance?
- Do you accept credit cards and, if so, which do you accept?
- Do you accept patient phone calls?
- Will you care for patients in their homes?
- Is your office handicapped-accessible?

If you have a chronic illness or disease, there may be certain additional aspects of a doctor's practice that could be particularly important to you. You should discuss any chronic problems when first establishing a relationship with a doctor. In fact, you may want to find a doctor with special interest or training in that problem.

House calls also continue to be important to some people. Yes, some doctors still do make house calls! In fact, a recent American Medical News article suggested that 43 percent of internal medicine specialists and 65 percent of family practice specialists made one or more house calls a year. However, it is important to point out that the number of doctors making house calls has declined because of technology, liability risks and time pressures. Important diagnostic equipment often cannot be carried around in a doctor's little black bag and is only available in the office or hospital. Also, the time required to visit one patient at home markedly reduces the time available to see other patients.

Personal or Bedside Manner

To many patients, once they have determined that a doctor is competent, the doctor's professional manner—also known as bedside manner—is the most important part of their choice. The Towers Perrin report cited earlier indicated that after reputation, skill in communicating was the most important factor sought in doctors. Patients prefer sensitive and caring doctors who listen carefully and demonstrate their concern. Studies show that such doctors are sued less often than others!

What characteristics make up a doctor's personal manner? The four described below may, when considered together, give you a clear idea of whether a particular doctor will be your personal "top" doctor.

- **Listening**. Professional manner includes the doctor's willingness to listen to patients, be supportive and understanding, explain procedures and exhibit concern and respect. These skills are expressed at the bedside, in the office, or in any setting where there is doctor/patient contact. Listening is also a valuable diagnostic tool. Unfortunately, these skills often have not been taught well in medical schools and the lack of them forms the primary basis for complaints from patients. However, there is growing emphasis on these vital interpersonal and communications skills in medical schools today and with good reason. They are critically important to most patients.

- **Cultural Sensitivity.** Some patients may prefer doctors who speak their language or are familiar with their cultural background. The term "culturally competent physician" is a relatively new one describing doctors who have the needed skills and attitudes to effectively treat patients from minority cultures.

- **Ethical, Religious and Philosophical Views.** Religion, or at least views on issues such as abortion, utilization of life-sustaining measures, natural childbirth, breast-feeding and other such matters can also be important. It is perfectly appropriate to ask doctors their views on sensitive issues.

- **Decision-making Procedures.** Years ago patients took the words of the doctor as law, not to be questioned or perhaps even discussed. That is not the case today. Consumers are better informed about health issues and may want to be actively involved in the decision making that affects their health. Some patients do not feel this way and are comfortable accepting a doctor's diagnosis or course of treatment without question. Some doctors—in diminishing numbers, thankfully—feel uncomfortable with patients who want everything explained to them or want to be involved in decision-making. Consider how you feel about this issue and discuss it with your doctor to be certain you are on compatible wavelengths.

Of course, what ultimately makes a "top" doctor are the results, the "outcomes," of care. Unfortunately, there is relatively little information available to consumers on the outcomes of physicians and hospitals. Some states, New York for example, have produced studies on outcomes for cardiac surgery. Also, some HMOs are talking about producing report cards for doctors. Generally, however, consumers will have difficulty finding outcome studies for individual doctors.

On the other hand, there is a growing movement to track and publish outcomes data on hospitals. The federal government has taken the lead by releasing outcomes data by hospitals for selected procedures. Visit www.hospitalcompare.hhs.gov.

*O*ne woman—a long-time City resident who moved to the suburbs to be near her children—found out the hard way about advice when she selected a doctor on the basis of her neighbor's glowing praise. During the initial visit, the patient's numerous questions about her chronic arthritis condition went unanswered while the doctor merely patted her on the shoulder and assured her that he would "take care of everything." While the paternalistic attitude might have suited the neighbor's needs, it fell far short for this senior patient, who was used to a good give-and-take with her former internist. She resumed her search for a doctor—this time with the assistance of the Castle Connolly guide, a more reliable source than a friend's recommendation.

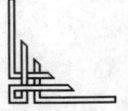

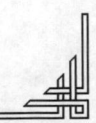

The Best in American Medicine
www.CastleConnolly.com

You And Your Doctor: A Team

Quick Tips

- Always obtain copies of all medical records and tests for your files.

- When selecting a doctor, especially a primary care doctor, it is appropriate to request an interview to get acquainted.

- Good doctors listen, good patients talk.

- Always bring a pad and pencil with you to medical appointments. When the doctor gives you instructions, take notes.

- The Physician's Desk Reference, commonly known as the PDR, is available in most libraries and is an excellent resource for learning more about medications. (The PDR web page is at http://www.pdr.net)

- Do not hesitate to ask your pharmacist about side effects, generic substitutions and other questions related to your medications.

Quick Take

... The best doctor-patient relationship is based on a two-way dialogue. Be open and honest and seek a doctor who is the same. ...

Key Terms

American Medical Association - A membership organization of physicians and their professional associations dedicated to promoting the art and science of medicine and the betterment of public health through establishing and promoting ethical, educational, and clinical standards for the medical profession. It represents the interests of physicians on the national level.

Baseline Tests - A series of basic, routine medical tests—such as electrocardiogram, complete blood count, blood pressure measurement, weight measurement, and chest X-ray—that are usually completed by a physician upon a patient's initial visit in order to provide a standard for comparison during subsequent health examinations.

Generic Drugs - Prescription medications that have been marketed by one company under a proprietary or brand name and which may be sold, after the original exclusive patent expires, under a generic name or the name assigned to it during an early stage of development. Most generic drugs are less expensive than proprietary versions and are just as effective except in cases when, because of different manufacturing processes, they are not bioequivalent or handled by the body in an identical manner.

Third Party Payer - An organization such as indemnity insurance company or managed care organization that provides individual and group health insurance, or a governmental department which assumes responsibility for the payment of an individual's healthcare, either directly to the healthcare provider or by means of reimbursement to the individual (Medicare and Medicaid are such government programs).

You And Your Doctor: A Team

Trust and respect between doctors and patients have reached a low point in modern American society. A recent poll of consumers sponsored by the American Medical Association (AMA) concluded that approximately 70 percent of those who responded agreed with the statement that "people are beginning to lose faith in their doctors." (Despite concerns about doctors in general, much research has shown that patients tend to rate their own doctors well.)

Trust between doctors and patients has declined for many reasons, including unrealistic expectations on the part of some patients and the patronizing attitudes of some doctors, which clash with the higher education level and medical sophistication of many patients. This has been further complicated by changing financial arrangements, particularly those involving the government and third-party payers, and the perception that some doctors seem to be motivated not by the values of the Hippocratic Oath (See page xiii), but by those of the marketplace. The AMA poll cited earlier found that 69 percent of respondents agreed that doctors "are too interested in making money." Perhaps a significant factor in creating this atmosphere is that in many cases the relationship between doctor and patient now has another dimension, the managed care organization. Another significant contributor is the huge amount of paperwork required from doctors. Generated by quality-assurance efforts, regulation, complex billing and managed care procedures, this burden reduces the time doctors are able to spend with patients.

Given the formidable obstacles, it might seem impossible to find a primary care doctor who is well suited to your needs. If you have carefully read the preceding chapters, your work is half done. What remains is to find that special individual who fits the criteria.

The Initial Interview

When selecting a doctor, especially a primary care doctor, it is appropriate to request an exploratory interview. Frequently, doctors will engage in such brief interviews at no charge, at a reduced fee or by telephone. It is preferable to find out about a doctor's credentials, office hours and billing procedures from the staff beforehand so you don't waste time asking about basic facts. This leaves time to ask the doctor questions that will allow you to determine what kind of relationship could develop. It is interesting that many parents will insist on interviewing a pediatrician for their child but wouldn't think of interviewing a physician for themselves.

Ask the Right Questions

The most important aspect of this session is to see if you can develop a positive doctor/patient relationship. Are you comfortable with the doctor's manner, style and general personality? Do you feel a strong sense of trust in the doctor? Here are five questions to ask the doctor plus two questions to ask yourself that may lead you closer to a selection.

- What is your experience in treating _____ (if you are seeking care for a particular illness or condition)?

- Are you open to treatments and therapies that do not rely heavily on medication?

- What preventive programs do you suggest for someone of my age, sex and health status?

- How do you feel about involving patients in decision-making?

- What are your views on_____(ethical and moral issues of importance to you as a patient)?

Even when the doctor is responding to your questions, you should ask yourself:

- Is the doctor paying attention to me and really considering my questions or do the impersonal "stock" answers indicate that the doctor's thoughts are elsewhere?

- Does this doctor speak about good health and prevention with the personal knowledge of someone who seems to practice it?

If your prospective doctor seems to measure up to your standards, get the relationship off to a good start by making an appointment for a complete check-up. During this appointment, you will have an opportunity to share your medical and family history and baseline tests will be performed to serve as a standard in the years ahead.

Talking with Your Doctor

After you have selected your doctor, your first appointment should include an extensive review of your medical history. Your doctor should spend time with you, ask questions and listen to your responses carefully.

Medical students are often told, "Listen to your patients. They'll tell you what's wrong with them." This conveys an important lesson not only for doctors, but for patients: Good doctors listen; good patients talk.

Analysis of doctor/patient conversations has revealed that many patients wait until the end of a conversation, even until they are saying goodbye, to tell their doctors what is really bothering them. This is just a small example of the dynamics of doctor/patient relationships. It is also a good example of a waste of valuable time— the doctor's and the patient's. One reason doctors need to be trained to be good listeners is that they frequently must ascertain what is troubling the patient not by what is said directly, but by what is said indirectly, not at all or through body language and other signs. However, it is always easier, less time-consuming and certainly more effective if a patient can describe problems completely and accurately.

Before you even see a doctor, you should prepare thoroughly. You should have a complete record of your medical history, including a record of X-rays and any other diagnostic tests, as well as blood workups. You need information about childhood diseases, chronic conditions, hospitalizations, past and present medications, doses and drug reactions, if any, and, if possible, something about the health history of your parents and even their siblings. Except for the last item, these are available to patients from their previous doctors or hospitals. That is why it is useful to obtain copies of all medical records and tests for your own files. Not only will this save you time and effort, but may avoid additional testing and expense. Your doctor will also ask many seemingly personal questions about your work, education, sex life and even drug and alcohol use. These are all part of a complete medical history and will help your doctor better understand you and your state of health.

If you have a particular problem or concern, describe all your symptoms. Try not to minimize or exaggerate and, most of all, don't deny.

If you have questions to ask your doctor, make a list. Always bring a pad and pencil with you to medical appointments. When the doctor gives you instructions, take notes or ask the doctor to write them down for you. If a prescription is written, ask about doses, side effects, efficacy and alternative medications as well as generic substitutes. The Physician's Desk Reference, commonly known as the PDR, is available in most libraries and is an excellent resource for learning more about medications. There is also a PDR web page on the Internet at http://www.pdr.net. You can also get a great deal of information on medications from another health professional, your pharmacist. Do not hesitate to ask your pharmacist about side effects, generic substitutions and other questions related to your medications. However, if the information you receive conflicts with that given by your doctor, consult with the doctor and follow his or her directions.

A Matter of Time

Patients want and expect doctors who listen, express concern, explain conditions and procedures in a clear and understandable manner, discuss medications and their effects and side effects thoroughly, return calls, are available when needed and, perhaps most importantly, spend sufficient time with them. With increasing demands on their time, many doctors are left with an uneasy feeling of "running to stay in place." The end result may be a tendency, unintended for the most part, to rush through a patient visit. This situation contributes to the erosion of the doctor/patient relationship.

Also contributing to this problem is pervasive lateness on the part of doctors. Patients frequently complain that they spend hours in a doctor's waiting room, long past the appointed hour (research has shown the average wait is 20 minutes).

Unfortunately, the duration of a patient visit is not always predictable and unexpected delays may occur if the diagnosis is complicated or if a patient needs to discuss what is on his or her mind. The doctor who spends extra time with another patient is probably the doctor you want for yourself. If the lateness is excessive, persistent and without apparent good reason, discuss it with your doctor and, if it is interfering with your relationship, consider changing doctors.

After a delay of two hours in his doctor's office, one patient, a self-employed marketing consultant, made sure that it would never happen again. Did he have a showdown with the doctor? Did he decide never to return? Not at all. He simply made it a point to call the doctor's office two hours before his scheduled appointment to see how the schedule was running. He then adjusted his own schedule to coincide with the doctor's.

Strengthening
Your Team

Quick Tips

The more complex and difficult the problem, the more important reputation is. In fact, you might well narrow your focus to doctors on the staffs of certain medical centers noted for excellence with specific problems.

Doctors typically refer patients to doctors on the staffs of the same hospitals where they practice.

If the lateness of your doctor is excessive, persistent and without apparent good reason, discuss it with him or her.

If you are not comfortable with your primary care doctor's referral, ask for a number of options. If necessary, you may consider going "out of network" even if you have to pay some or all of the fee.

In many cases, insurance companies will pay for second opinions, but check ahead of time to make sure your insurance plan does cover them.

One way HMOs control costs is by limiting second opinions.

Doctors may have different solutions to the same problem — and any one or more could work.

Quick Take

... The old adage, two heads are better than one, often applies in healthcare, too. Expanded options include referrals, second opinions, alternative therapies and clinical trials. ...

Key Terms

Alternative Therapy - Non-traditional forms of healthcare — including acupuncture, homeopathy, naturopathy, massage, reflexology, biofeedback, hypnotherapy, herbology, therapeutic touc, and prayer — that are often based on ancient healing methods and have not been tested in a conventional scientific manner.

Clinical Trial - An experimental trial of a new drug or therapy in a selected group of human volunteers who suffer from the condition for which the experimental drug or treatment is to be used.

Double Blind Study - One form of a clinical trial in which two groups of volunteers — one group receiving the real drug or treatment and the other receiving a placebo or dummy — are followed for a specific period of time by researchers who do not know themselves who is receiving which therapy.

Protocol - A rigid set of rules set up for a clinical trial by the Food and Drug Administration (FDA) which must be followed strictly by all researchers and volunteers participating in the trial.

Strengthening Your Team

When You Need a Specialist

For the most part, selecting a specialist is similar to choosing a primary care doctor. There is one major difference, however; typically you will be referred to a specialist by your primary care doctor. Suggesting a consultation does not show a weakness on the part of the doctor. On the contrary, the real weakness lies in a doctor's reluctance to suggest consultations when advisable. Your primary care doctor will receive a written report from any consultation or referral. You should request a copy as well.

Ask your doctor why this particular specialist is being recommended. Find out about the specialist's training and experience. If your doctor has sent many patients to the same doctor for the same treatment, you should find out how successful the treatment was and if the patients were satisfied. You might also ask if the specialist would be the one selected for your doctor's own personal care. You should feel comfortable about seeing the specialist and, if you are not, ask for another recommendation or find a different one on your own.

Frequently, patients do seek out specialists on their own. If you are attempting to find a specialist or subspecialist without the guidance of your primary care doctor, use the various selection procedures described in Chapters One, Two and Three. When selecting a physician on your own, even greater emphasis should be placed on board certification in the relevant specialty. If you are trying to find someone to treat a very specific problem, make certain that the individual is well trained in that area. You may check to see if a doctor is board certified by calling the American Board of Medical Specialties at (866) 275-2267 or visiting their web site at www.abms.org.

You will also want to know if the specialist you select is well respected. The more complex and difficult the problem, the more important reputation is. In fact, you might narrow your focus to doctors on the staffs of certain medical centers noted for excellence in treating your specific problem. There are a number of books and magazine articles such as the annual U.S. News & World Report issue on America's best hospitals that offer views on the best medical centers for specific problems.

Finally, make certain your doctor and the specialist communicate easily about your case. If you should have a problem with a specialist, or if you are not pleased with the care given, let your primary care doctor know about it right away.

Doctors typically refer patients to doctors on the staffs of the same hospitals at which they practice. There are good and poor reasons for this, as explained below.

Why Doctors Usually Refer to Doctors in the Same Hospitals

Good Reasons:

- They know the doctors better.

- They continue to be involved in the case.

- Coordination of multiple specialists may be easier.

Poor Reasons:

- It is easier.

- They will get referrals back.

- It reduces the chance of losing the patient to another doctor.

- It may help build social or professional relationships.

- The hospital may pressure doctors to refer within the institution.

In today's managed care environment doctor referrals usually are restricted to other doctors in the managed care organization's network. Sometimes the referring doctor may not even be familiar with the other doctor's qualifications. If you are not comfortable with your primary care doctor's referral, ask for a number of options. If necessary, you may consider going "out of network" even if you have to pay some or all of the fee.

Second Opinions

Second opinions are a valuable medical tool, infrequently used in many instances, overused in others. Clearly, you do not want to get another doctor's opinion on every ailment or problem, but there are definitely times you should seek out a second opinion:

- Before major surgery.

- When the diagnosis is serious or life-threatening.

- If a rare disease is diagnosed.

- If the diagnosis is uncertain.

- If you think the number of tests or procedures recommended is excessive.

- If a test result has serious implications—a positive Pap smear for example—have the test re-done immediately before taking further action.

- If the treatment suggested is risky or expensive.

- If you are uncomfortable with the diagnosis and treatment recommended.
- If a course of treatment is not working.
- If you question your doctor's competence.
- If your insurance company requires it.

Most doctors will be supportive if you request a second opinion and many will even recommend it. In many cases, insurance companies will pay for second opinions, but check ahead of time to make sure your insurance plan does indeed cover them. In an HMO, you may have to be more assertive because one way that HMOs control costs is by limiting second opinions. This is especially true if you want an opinion outside the plan's network.

Often, the opinion of a second doctor will affirm the opinion of the first, but the reassurance may be worth the time and extra cost. On the other hand, if the second opinion differs from the first, you have two remaining alternatives: seek the opinion of a third doctor, or educate yourself as much as possible by talking with both doctors and reading up on the problem (trusting your instincts about which diagnosis is correct). If the diagnosis is the same but the recommended treatments differ, remember that doctors may have different solutions to the same problem—and any one or more could be efficient. For example, an orthopaedic surgeon may recommend surgery to correct a knee injury while a physiatrist (a doctor certified in physical medicine and rehabilitation) may recommend rehabilitation. One might work better than the other or they could both work equally well. The choice may be based on your preference. Remember, however, that surgical solutions can rarely be reversed. It usually is best to try a non-surgical solution first, if possible.

Complementary Medicine: Exploring Your Options

A recent study conducted by the University of Florida estimated that 86 percent of households in the U.S. use some type of complementary therapies (a term that implies that these therapies are used along with conventional medical treatment rather than in place of them). Total out-of-pocket expenditures for complementary/alternative medicine approach $30 billion annually, estimates David Eisenberg, MD and colleagues at the Harvard/Beth Israel Center for the Study of Alternative Medicine Research. They further point out that total visits to complementary/alternative providers numbered 629 million in 1997 as compared to 386 million visits to primary care physicians.

One of the reasons conventional medical therapies are conventional is that most have been proven to be effective in a rigorous scientific manner, while many complementary/alternative therapies have not been tested under accepted scientific conditions. You should always consider the possibility that some alternative therapies, since they are unproven, may do more harm than good. The alternative approaches in use today range from legitimate searches for new therapies to outright quackery and fraud. Without the guidance of the scientific and medical community, it is sometimes impossible for doctors, let alone consumers, to tell the difference.

Nonetheless, doctors are becoming more open to the use of complementary/alternative approaches. One study reported that about 30 percent of doctors questioned in the Los Angeles area said that they were open to complementary/alternative practices in one form or another and that acceptance is growing. Medical scientists are also indicating a new interest in studying approaches to health that may complement the strengths of Western medicine. Some of the therapies being explored include mind-body medicine, hypnotherapy, biofeedback, chiropractic, vital energy, metabolic therapy, naturopathy, homeopathy, therapeutic touch, acupuncture, prayer and the use of herbs.

Alternative healthcare often complements rather than replaces Western medicine. As such, the terms complementary or integrative, which accurately describe the relationship between Western and alternative healthcare, are used with increased frequency as this type of approach towards medicine becomes more commonplace.

In a New England Journal of Medicine study, 72 percent of the respondents who used unconventional therapies did not inform their medical doctor that they had done so. That is unfortunate, because such treatments could be greatly enhanced with the support and advice of a primary care doctor. More worrisome is the great danger that some people may use alternative treatments in lieu of, rather than as a supplement to, more conventional and proven medical therapies. A classic and tragic example of this was the surge of patients who traveled to Mexico to seek a "magic bullet" cure for cancer promised by the drug Laetrile (made from apricot pits). There was no magic; indeed, patients lost money, hope and, in some cases, the opportunity for timely use of proven treatment. If you do explore alternative therapies, be certain to let your doctor know about it. Some may be harmful, especially if you are undergoing another treatment under your doctor's direction.

To learn more about complementary/alternative medicine, contact the National Center for Complementary and Alternative Medicine Clearinghouse to locate a source of reliable information on the practice you are considering (see Appendix E).

How to Use Complementary/Alternative Medicine Wisely and Well

- Try to learn everything you can about the particular therapy that interests you. Your local library and the Internet both have substantial materials on complementary/alternative medicine.

- Discuss your plans with your doctor. You might gain some insight into the therapy in terms of its possible risks. Furthermore, if you are currently under medical treatment, you should make certain that the two approaches will not conflict in some way.

- If you start an alternative therapy and it does not appear to be providing relief, or seems to be worsening the condition, contact your doctor immediately.

Clinical Trials: Should You Participate?

Each year, more than half a million Americans, some of them sick, but even more of them healthy, volunteer to take part in experimental trials of new drugs and therapies. Before drugs, vaccines, biological agents and medical devices are made available for general use by doctors and their patients, they must go through extensive testing on animals and humans called "clinical trials." There is probably at least one clinical trial in process at some medical center for almost every serious disease.

On the plus side, a clinical trial offers the opportunity for prompt use of a drug or other treatment that seems promising, and comes with the bonus of regular and thorough medical examinations at no cost to you (some trials even make allowances for participants' travel and other expenses). Moreover, patients are encouraged to discuss all of their experiences regarding the trial. You will probably learn more about your condition and feel more in control, which can have a very positive effect. On the downside, you may be giving up standard treatment for something that may or may not be better. There is even the possibility that you will not get a drug at all, because most trials are conducted by the double-blind method, in which half of the participants get the drug and half get a placebo, or "dummy" medicine. Even the doctors conducting the trials do not know who is getting which drug.

What to Know Before You Get Involved

If you are considering participating in a clinical trial, you will want to know:

- Who is the sponsor? Look for a federal government, major health organization, drug company or university-sponsored trial.

- Do any impartial authorities monitor the trial? Every hospital conducting research has an institutional review board (IRB) consisting of medical professionals and community leaders who approve that hospital's participation. There are also data and safety monitoring boards that oversee trials.

- What is the financial relationship, if any, between the doctor, hospital and the company or agency sponsoring the trial?

- Will there be pain or discomfort? Will diagnostic tests be involved? Get detailed answers to these concerns before you sign any form.

- How often will I be examined? This depends on the guidelines of the trial (called the protocol). You should make every effort to keep your appointments.

- Does my own doctor get a record of my participation in the trial? Routine health information is sent to your doctor, but details relevant to a "blinded" trial are not disclosed until the trial is over.

- Is the drug in this trial approved for treatment of any other disorder? If the answer is yes, you then know that the drug has a prior safety record.

- After the study has ended, if I have responded well to the drug, will I be able to continue using it, even before it is approved?

- Can I drop out?

If you are interested in participating in a clinical trial, make your desire known to your doctor, who can track down openings in trials being conducted by medical centers, private foundations, drug companies, physician groups and the federal government. You can also access information on clinical trials by visiting the CenterWatch Clinical Trials Listing Service at www.centerwatch.com or the web site of the National Cancer Institute at www.cancer.gov/clinicaltrials.

Easy Access to specialists and subspecialists, especially in large metropolitan areas, presents certain problems in coordination of care that a patient should be aware of. This difficulty is probably epitomized by one woman who was treated by a dermatologist, an ophthalmologist, a rheumatologist, a psychiatrist and an allergist, all of whom had office space in her very large apartment complex on Manhattan's upper west side-thus eliminating her need to even put on her coat. Fortunately, all were quite competent and had all the necessary qualifications. Unfortunately, each was affiliated with a different medical center, which made coordinating her care with her primary care doctor very complex.

Changing Your Doctor

Quick Tips

Surgical solutions can rarely be reversed. It usually is best to try a non-surgical solution first, if possible.

You should always consider the possibility that alternative therapies - simply because they are unproven - may do more harm than good.

If you do explore alternative therapies, be certain to let your doctor know about it. Some may be harmful, especially if you are undergoing another treatment under your doctor's direction.

Before you decide to part company with your doctor, ask yourself if you've been a responsible patient.

A doctor-patient relationship is like a marriage — both sides have to work to make it successful.

Expressing your dissatisfaction may open the communication lines between you and your doctor; you might even end up in a better relationship with your present doctor

Unless the situation is intolerable or the doctor is impaired, stay with your current doctor until you have found another one that you like

When changing doctors, you may have to sign a release with your new doctor approving the transfer of all your medical records to the new office. These records cannot be withheld for any reason, even if you have not yet paid your last bill.

Quick Take

... There's a big difference between doctor-hopping and changing doctors for a good reason. Most failed doctor-patient relationships can be attributed to some common complaints but sometimes are a matter of self-defense...

Key Terms

National Practitioner Data Bank - A computerized listing, created by an Act of Congress, to track health professionals who are disciplined for unprofessional behavior and to deter them from simply moving their practicies from one state to another.

Public Citizen Health Research Group - A Washington, D.C. based consumer advocacy group that has been publicly critical of many medical practices that the group considers detrimental to public healthcare.

Changing Your Doctor

Obviously, at times there are good reasons for changing doctors. Some are very simple and straightforward, such as a doctor's retirement, illness or death, your own relocation or a change in your health plan. About 40 percent of people enrolling in managed care plans have to change their doctor to one who is affiliated with their plan.

The onset of a chronic condition may also prompt a change to a different medical specialist, such as a rheumatologist or cardiologist, if a condition needs to be managed by a specialist other than a primary care doctor.

If you have continuing symptoms that your doctor has been unable to diagnose or if, after a diagnosis, your problems continue to linger without improvement, you should at least consider getting a second opinion and, depending on that opinion, possibly change doctors. Doctors often have different approaches to the same problem. A different doctor may offer a different perspective and, perhaps, a solution.

You might also change doctors in order to find one who includes complementary/alternative medicine in the treatment or to find one who can help you enroll in a clinical trial.

People who have hostile feelings toward organized medicine tend to change doctors frequently; their complaints then become a self-fulfilling prophecy. They don't get continuous, quality care because it's impossible for anyone to deliver it. On the other hand, negative feelings may be prompted by unfortunate encounters with incompetent doctors or by the patronizing or otherwise inappropriate attitudes expressed by some doctors toward patients. Patients on the receiving end of such a relationship should continue their search for a doctor who better meets their needs.

Eight Reasons to Say Goodbye

Here are the eight most common complaints about "doctors I don't go to anymore."

Poor Bedside Manner

Good medical care is more than diagnosis and treatment; it's also an attitude on the part of the doctor that sparks a sense of trust in the patient. Being under the care of a doctor who is impersonal, abrupt, bored, arrogant, condescending or sarcastic may, in the end, be counterproductive.

The doctor's aloofness could have a more serious explanation: substance abuse or psychological impairment, which, according to a recent American Medical Association report, affect 30,000 to 40,000 physicians. Mood swings and detachment are signs to watch for.

Too Vague and Evasive

A doctor who dismisses problems with "it's nothing to worry about" or "let me take care of it" or who uses medical jargon isn't interested in having you as a partner in your healthcare. The effect of this evasiveness can be anger, fear and confusion, leading to failure to follow directions and failure of treatment.

Never on Schedule

Medical emergencies can make appointment scheduling an inexact science, but when snafus become chronic, it's a sign of trouble. An explanation can ease the frustration, but make-up time should not be at your expense.

Couldn't Diagnose the Problem

Some conditions can't be diagnosed on-the-spot. Others aren't attributable to one specific cause. That doesn't excuse an incomplete workup, however, which may leave you with a condition that could have been treated earlier.

Ordered too Many Tests

Sophisticated technology is available and doctors tend to use it, although some testing may not be necessary. The number of tests performed for diagnosis seems to be reduced in patient-doctor relationships where communication is strong.

Discouraged Second Opinions

A doctor who dissuades you from talking to another doctor may perceive it as questioning his or her professional abilities.

Didn't Protect My Medical Privacy

No patient should have to discuss the reason for a visit, payment or payment problems within earshot of other patients or staff.

Under certain conditions, medical records can be requested by and turned over to insurance companies, lawyers, employers and certain others without your consent, but you can certainly see them, too, to make sure they contain the proper information. In all 50 states and the District of Columbia, federal law grants patients access to their medical records.

Unpleasant Office Staff

Repeated incidents such as rudeness over the telephone, a brusque physician's assistant or being kept waiting in an examining room for a long time before the doctor shows up are all annoying indications that a staff could do better.

The staff takes its cues from the chief. A doctor who doesn't demand the highest level of performance from a staff may be sending a message about his or her own laxity in diagnosis and treatment.

Should You Switch?

If these conditions exist in your doctor-patient relationship, it may be time to consider finding a new doctor. But before you decide to part company with your doctor, ask yourself if you've been a responsible patient. Often problems arise when patients don't reveal their full medical history or if they forget to alert their doctor about other drugs they are taking. A doctor-patient relationship is like a marriage—both sides have to work to make it successful.

If you're sure the problem isn't on your side, however, confront your doctor with your grievances. Or, if it's easier for you, you may want to write them in a letter. Expressing your dissatisfaction may open the communication lines between you and your doctor. You might even end up in a better relationship with your present doctor. Sometimes doctors aren't aware that they are in the midst of a deteriorating relationship until a patient wants to leave.

But if you are still unhappy with your doctor and you've decided a change is necessary, you can make a clean break by simply going to another doctor. Keep in mind, however, that your most important concern should be continuity of care. So, unless the situation is intolerable or the doctor is impaired, stay with your current doctor until you have found another one that you like.

Generally, medical records are kept by your doctor until you have found a new one. You will then have to sign a release with your new doctor approving the transfer of all your medical records to the new office. These records cannot be withheld for any reason, even if you have not yet paid your last bill.

Finally, don't feel embarrassed or guilty if you decide to change doctors. Remember, good quality medical care is your right!

Self Defense: Avoiding Questionable Doctors

In addition to finding good doctors, you also want to be able to identify and avoid doctors who have a history of professional problems. One way to do this is to make certain a doctor has not been disciplined by your state or, in fact, any state. You can call the appropriate state agency (listed in Appendix E) or check the web sites of those state agencies that make this information available. These sites list the names of doctors who have been disciplined by their state or by the federal government. The disciplinary actions were taken for a variety of reasons, including overprescribing or misprescribing medications, criminal convictions, alcohol or drug abuse and patient sexual abuse.

You also may visit the 'Vital Healthcare Info' section of the Castle Connolly Medical Ltd. web site (www.CastleConnolly.com) for links to those states with discipline information on their sites. You may also visit the American Medical Association (AMA) at www.ama-assn.org and American Board of Medical Specialities (ABMS) at www.abms.org. For the websites for biographical information about doctors, including board certification see Appendix D.

The Public Citizen Health Research Group, which publishes a report on the number of physicians disciplined in each state, believes that many states are not aggressive enough in monitoring doctors. They have been leading the call for public access to the National Practitioner Data Bank. The Data Bank was created in 1986 by an Act of Congress to track professionals who are disciplined for unprofessional behavior and to deter them from simply moving their practices from one state to another. The Data Bank became operational in 1990 and contains a record of adverse actions such as license removal, loss of clinical privileges and professional society membership actions taken against doctors and other licensed health professionals such as dentists. It contains the names of more than 170,000 health practitioners who have either a licensing action or malpractice judgment or settlement against them. There is strong pressure from some medical groups either to do away with the Data Bank or to place even stricter controls on access to it. They support their position with examples of errors in the handling of sensitive information. It is unlikely that Congress would permit the elimination of the Data Bank, however. In fact, it is possible that at some time in the future, access may be made more available to the public. However, at the present time there is no public access to this information.

A data service used by lawyers to check on a doctor's or hospital's malpractice history is LEXIS/NEXIS, the computerized legal information service. Some libraries will do a LEXIS/NEXIS search for a fee, usually more than $75.00. Public access to the listing of malpractice payments is one issue on which doctors are very sensitive, and rightfully so. Many malpractice payments are made by insurance companies over the objections of doctors because the insurers feel it's cheaper to settle than to fight. Yet, doctors who feel they are blameless contend that these settlements reflect negatively on them. Also, since so many specialists, such as those in obstetrics and gynecology, are subject to more frequent lawsuits because of the nature of their practices, doctors are concerned about how patients will interpret a malpractice settlement. A few states, for example Massachussetts, make this information available on the State Health Department website. Check to see if it is available in your state. (See Vital Healthcare Information on the Castle Connolly Medical Ltd website (www.CastleConnolly.com.)

People who believe they have a problem with a doctor, whether in regard to fees, treatment or ethics, may contact the appropriate local medical society in the county in which the doctor practices or the state medical society. State health departments are also places consumers may turn to for assistance or information on disciplinary actions taken against doctors. The health department, typically, will only divulge that an action has been taken but will not give you any specific information about it (See Appendix E for phone numbers and addresses).

Changing your doctor should not be considered a setback in your search for the best doctor to meet your needs. As you may have come to understand throughout preceding chapters in this book, the personal and treatment styles doctors bring to their practices vary greatly. What is important for you, as a patient, to realize is that these subtle and immeasurable characteristics can be as important as clinical skills.

There is, in fact, substantial empirical and anecdotal evidence demonstrating that confidence in the healer and the healing process plays a major role in many cures. Your main objective is to find the therapy—in combination with the professional who is providing the therapy—that works best for you.

*I*n one case involving a woman in her mid-thirties, the doctor-patient relationship was severed over what was basically a conflict in personalities: the woman wished to have more control over her healthcare, and the doctor was reluctant to give it. The impasse was reached before the two could attempt any kind of a compromise, and the woman went off in search of a doctor who would better suit her personal needs. A year later, after a fruitless search for a doctor whose medical expertise she respected, she returned to her original doctor.

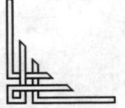

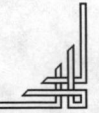

The Best in American Medicine
www.CastleConnolly.com

Choosing a Doctor
in an HMO

Quick Tips

A data service used by lawyers to check on a doctor's or hospital's malpractice history is Lexis/Nexis, the computerized legal information service. Lexis will do a search and issue a report on any malpractice awards or settlements ordered by a court.

State health departments are also places consumers may turn to for assistance or information on disciplinary actions taken against doctors.

There is substantial empirical and anecdotal evidence demonstrating that confidence in the healer and the healing process plays a major role in many cures.

People who belive they have a problem with a doctor in regard to fees, treatment, or ethics, may contact the appropriate local medical society in the county in which the doctor practices, or the state medical society.

When choosing a doctor in an HMO, use the same criteria you would apply to selecting a doctor in a fee-for-service practice.

Typically, you will be sent a list with little information other than the doctor's name, specialty and address. Find out more about those doctors you may be considering.

In some cases, an HMO will agree to pay at least a consultation fee if you feel strongly that you need to discuss your problem with another doctor outside of the HMO network

If method of HMO payment to physicians is an issue of concern to you, it may be wise to ask your doctor about the method of compensation in the HMO in which you are enrolled.

Quick Take

... The rules are different but they are not difficult to play by. The first step is to sort out the alphabet soup of models. The model of HMO usually determines how your care will be delivered and often your satisfaction with it ...

Key Terms

Capitation - A method of payment to physicians and other healthcare providers whereby a fixed amount of money is allotted for each patient served.

EPO - An Exclusive Provider Organization is similar to a PPO except the patients must use only providers in the EPO.

Group Model HMO - A model of an HMO in which the HMO contracts with large multi-specialty groups of doctors to provide care, usually from a number of central locations.

Health Maintenance Organization (HMO) - One type of managed care organization that provides for a wide range of comprehensive healthcare services for its members in return for a fixed, predetermined fee. The care is provided by a network or group of physicians affiliated with the organization and possibly other healthcare professionals.

IPA - An Independent Practice Association is one model of health maintenance organization (HMO) in which the organization contracts with individual doctors, or groups of doctors, to provide care for the enrolled patients in the doctors' own offices.

PHO - A Physician Hospital Organization is an organization of a hospital and its physicians that may contract with managed care organizations (MCO) or may become licensed as an MCO itself.

PPO - A Preferred Provider Organization is a managed care model that offers healthcare provided by a group of doctors and/or hospitals that have negotiated discounted rates, either capitated or fee-for-service, for enrollees while continuing to provide care for other patients. Patients typically pay less if they use the PPO provider.

PSO - A Provider Service Organization, sometimes called a provider service network (PSN), is a group of doctors that are organized to provide care to a large number of patients, typically under contract to managed care organizations.

Staff Model HMO - A managed care model where the HMO employs the doctors, usally on salary. Care is provided out of a number of centralized locations.

Choosing a Doctor in an HMO

At one time only doctors looking for new patients joined HMOs. Today, there is a new reality. Almost all doctors—more than 80 percent—participate in some kind of managed care arrangement. So it is likely that you will find the best for your own care if you know how to work the system.

When managed care achieves a significant market penetration and begins to control the flow of large numbers of patients, more doctors sign on. Also, many hospitals encourage their doctors to sign on with as many different plans as possible in order to ensure that the hospital does not lose any potential patients. Managed care now enrolls more than one out of every three people in the country, and more than 80 percent of workers who get health insurance through their employer are in some form of managed care. Today, more people are enrolled in PPOs (Preferred Provider Organization), which tend to be more flexible in choices of physicians, than are enrolled in HMOs. However, we will use HMO as "shorthand" for both.

The main factors to focus on in assessing an HMO or a PPO are its resources, primarily doctors and hospitals. First, is there an ample selection of primary care doctors near where you live and work? Second, are the doctors well qualified? This can be answered by following the approach outlined in this book for finding the best doctors. When choosing doctors, it is usually a good idea to call their offices to confirm they are still affiliated with the particular plan. Doctors frequently change affiliations with managed care plans. Also, it is a good idea to check on the procedure for using the doctor listed.

HMOs may list hundreds of doctors but not all of them are necessarily accessible to all members. A large HMO, for example, may restrict the number of specialists that primary care doctors can refer to for various reasons, including location, hospital capacity and general resource allocation. So although you may see the name of an ophthalmologist, gynecologist or other specialist you want to use, and indeed that doctor may be affiliated with the HMO, it does not necessarily follow that your primary care doctor is free to refer you to them. Those specialists may see HMO patients only on a certain basis—for specific procedures, for example, or in a certain geographic region—and then possibly only after a rigorous screening process. These possibilities illustrate the varying styles of operation you will find in managed care plans.

Doctors in HMOs are bound by the same professional ethics that guide all doctors. However, there is a major difference; in an HMO, the plan is responsible for providing you with care as well as with a doctor. If your doctor leaves the plan, you don't follow him or her. The plan provides a new doctor for you.

Selecting Doctors in an HMO

Selecting a doctor in an HMO can be a greater challenge than selecting one when you have indemnity insurance that leaves you free to select a doctor without the restrictions of the plan. Obviously, in an HMO arrangement you need to select a doctor who belongs to that plan. Studies have shown that about 40 percent of enrollees in managed care plans have to choose a new doctor when they join. However, even in a plan of small size, you will usually have the option of choosing among a number of primary care doctors as well as other specialists and subspecialists. In doing so, utilize the same criteria you would apply to selecting a doctor in a fee-for-service practice.

The first doctor you select in an HMO plan is your primary care doctor. Typically, you will be sent a list with little information other than the doctor's name, specialty and address. Find out more about those doctors you may be considering. Use the process described earlier in this book. If you make a selection and are not satisfied, request a change. Ask about the procedure for changing doctors before you join the plan.

When you need a specialist, it is your primary care doctor who will refer you, as in traditional indemnity plans. But, unlike indemnity plans in which you can find a specialist on your own if you choose, in managed care plans you must be referred to see a specialist. Again, your choices will be limited in selecting specialists, but be assertive. Ask for a choice of doctors and ask why your primary care doctor recommends a particular specialist. One disadvantage to the IPA model and the network referral process is that primary care doctors can end up making referrals to specialists and/or subspecialists that they do not know. This may result in poor communication between the primary care doctor and the specialist, which is not in the patient's best interest. If you are not satisfied with the choices offered, ask to go outside the plan. Choice of providers outside a plan is built into certain managed care plans (PPOs or POS, Point of Service) and is permitted in many others under certain conditions.

However, if you do not have a choice, or if the choices are not ones with which you agree, consider going outside the HMO. Although you are likely to have to pay more, it may be worth it if you get a correct diagnosis and appropriate treatment for your problem. In some cases, the HMO will agree to pay at least a consultation fee if you feel strongly that you need to discuss your problem with another doctor outside the HMO network. After the consultation, if you still feel the need for a different doctor, at least your choice will be based on more complete information.

One of the most popular plans offered by HMOs permits going outside of the network of doctors and hospitals—but at an added cost. The point of service, or POS plan, one of the fastest growing offerings of many HMOs, permits the HMO member to use doctors, hospitals, and other services that are not part of the HMO network. Typically, the member will pay an additional fee for this choice—for example, 20 percent or 30 percent of the cost—whereas if the member stays "in-network" the HMO will pay all or close to all of the cost.

When leaving the network of a POS, however, patients should find out exactly how much it will cost to do so. Some HMOs will pay a percentage of "usual and customary fees" while others will pay a percentage of their own fee schedule, which is usually lower.

HMO Models

Although a large alphabet soup of HMO models has appeared since the big move toward managed care began in the late 1980s, and we now have PPOs, PSOs, and EPOs, two models are most important to the healthcare consumer. One is the staff or group model where patients visit their doctors in a single, or perhaps in a few, locations and where all the doctors and most, if not all, diagnostic and treatment facilities are located. The second is the independent practice association or IPA model where doctors see patients in their private offices. Organizations such as PPOs, EPOs and PSOs tend to be organized on the IPA model.

Whether a group/staff model or an IPA, all HMOs require a primary care physician and all have certain protocols, usually involving referral by the primary care physician, to access a specialist.

Doctor Compensation

There is virtually no difference in the types of doctors who practice in the two HMO models and each should be evaluated in terms of benefits to the individual patient. There is, however, a separate matter of how doctors in HMOs are compensated, and this issue has become a major concern to both patients and doctors.

HMOs compensate doctors in a number of ways. Doctors who are employed by staff model HMOs are usually on salary, perhaps with a quality bonus based on patient satisfaction. In group model HMOs, the physician group has a contract with the HMO and the doctors are employed by the group, usually on salary and, again, often with a quality bonus.

In the IPA model HMOs, or in PPOs, EPOs, PSOs and other types of managed care organizations the doctors are usually paid in one of two ways. In the past, the predominant payment method was a negotiated fee schedule, typically designed at some discount to the doctor's normal fee. Doctors simply traded the promise of higher volume for a reduced fee. Today, a major method of payment in an IPA is capitation. While this is fast becoming the most common method of payment in IPAs it is also the one generating the most controversy.

Under a capitated or capitation system doctors are paid a set amount per month or per year to provide care to a patient during that time period. So, for example, a primary care physician may be paid $25 per member per month.

HMOs have moved toward capitation as a method of payment because they found that discounted fee-for-service payment methods did not reduce costs as much as had been hoped, if at all. To make up for discounted fees of 20 percent, for instance, some doctors simply scheduled 20 percent more patient visits so that their incomes would not decrease. Doctors openly comment that discounted fees translate to discounted time with patients!

Capitation has helped to control costs. However, it also has introduced a number of important ethical issues for doctors, other healthcare providers, and for patients. Many are troubled by the notion that a doctor could be placed in a situation that appears to promise rewards for not providing care. It is generally recognized that under a fee-for-service system doctors have an incentive to provide more care, even if it is not necessary, because they are paid by the amount of care they deliver. But the reverse is not accepted in such a benign fashion: the concept of a doctor being rewarded to provide less care is of major concern to many people, including many doctors.

Another technique involved in payment systems utilized by managed care companies is called "withholds" or "set-asides." This method is also used to motivate doctors to control costs and, as in capitation, raises similar ethical concerns. Under this method, for example, a group of pediatricians is contracted to care for 1,000 children. That contract is based on a budget of $15,000 a month. A certain amount of that budget, say 20 percent, is reserved for referrals to subspecialists and another 20 percent is set aside or withheld. If the group of doctors uses fewer subspecialist referrals than budgeted they receive the 20 percent that was set aside. If they use more subspecialist referrals than were budgeted the extra amount comes out of the set-aside. The more set-aside that is used for referrals, the less doctors will be able to receive from it.

A great deal of controversy has ensued over these payment mechanisms. Some states, in fact, are legislating to prohibit or restrict these practices. Individual "horror stories" of patients who have been denied appropriate care, such as not being referred to a subspecialist in a timely manner, have been used to demonstrate the issue in human terms.

Some studies demonstrate that when physician-run health plans are paid by capitation and are in control they reduce costs more substantially than other plans. Some doctors strongly support capitation. They believe it makes them, rather than managers, responsible for allocating resources and making medical decisions.

And, despite the outcry, most of the studies of HMO patients versus non-HMO patients demonstrate no differences in their health status.

In fact, there is a substantial body of research suggesting that HMO members receive more in the way of preventive services than do non-HMO populations.

If method of payment is an issue of concern to you, it may be wise to ask your doctor about the method of compensation in the HMO in which you are enrolled. If you believe the method would work against you as a patient you should discuss it with your doctor and ask if and how it influences the manner of care for patients. If you are not satisfied by the answer you may want to change doctors or, better yet, change HMOs, if possible.

While the wisest course of action is to ask about this issue before joining an HMO, rather than after you have become a member, most HMO members have not done this. If you believe you are not receiving appropriate care because of an HMO policy, you can contact your state health insurance department (see Appendix E).

In response to patient and physician concerns about payment policies, groups of doctors in various parts of the country have formed organizations to receive and investigate complaints against HMOs. You can contact them with any grievances you have about your HMO (see Physicians Who Care, Appendix D).

How Doctors and Patients Feel about Managed Care

People enrolled in HMOs tend to like them. However, most doctors do not like managed care—and understandably so! Managed care organizations negotiate deep discounts in fees for doctors. There is no reason doctors should prefer this process, but when managed care controls so many patients there is little choice but to join managed care and negotiate.

Managed care organizations also require doctors to do a substantial amount of paperwork and to follow policies and procedures that control costs and monitor quality. All of this creates a level of business management most doctors resent.

At least a portion of these negative attitudes toward managed care can be ascribed to differences in the organization of medical practices in different parts of the country.

The northeast, south, and southwest regions have been the slowest to accept managed care because doctors generally resisted it more strongly than those in other parts of the country. Doctors in large group practices, which are more common in the far west and midwest than in the east, adapted to managed care more readily. In the northeast, where doctors practice solo or in small groups, the change has been greater and the adjustment more difficult.

Most doctors have adapted and learned to practice successfully in this new medical environment. According to a survey conducted by the American Medical Association, just over a third (210,811) of physicians in this country are now members of group practices. In 1995 group practices numbered 19,788, an increase of 361 percent since 1965. From 1991 to 1995, the number of groups increased by 16.4 percent and the number of group physicians by 14.3 percent.

The survey shows that, in an environment that is organizationally complex, medical groups have changed how they are organized legally, with partnerships declining to 13.8 percent and professional corporations increasing to 77.9 percent. In the latter group, control of decision making remains largely in the physician's hands. This ability to retain decision making power has dramatically altered physicians' attitudes towards managed care.

The view of patients and the public, however, is decidedly more positive about managed care.

A study sponsored by the Medstat Group, J.D. Power and Associates and the New England Medical Center reported that in 20 markets across the United States, HMOs received more top scores than PPOs and fee-for-service plans.

The study asked plan members to assess their health plans on choice of providers, physician care, premiums and deductibles and access to care. HMOs topped fee-for-service and point-of-service plans in more than half of the markets.

One of the findings uncovered in a Louis Harris Associates poll of consumers was that of the majority surveyed, 59 percent, believed the trend toward managed care was a good thing as compared to 28 percent who viewed it as a bad thing. Also, 48 percent as compared to 39 percent believed managed care would improve quality, and 59 percent versus 30 percent believed it would help contain the costs of care. Of note was that the response of those people in communities with a high penetration by managed care tended to be the most positive!

There are many studies that have examined the quality of care and the satisfaction of patients in managed care settings. Most show that members of HMOs and other managed care organizations are at least as satisfied or more satisfied with their care than people covered by indemnity insurance. Some studies have shown indemnity-covered people are more satisfied, particularly when it relates to choice of doctors. In fact, the issue of greatest concern to HMO enrollees is usually access, particularly to specialists. Advocates of either view can point to studies to support managed care or to criticize it. The key may lay in the studies that have demonstrated that when individuals have a choice, and select a managed care plan, they tend to be more satisfied than those who have no choice.

In terms of quality, the conclusion is similar. While critics may contend that the care delivered by managed care organizations is not adequate, and a study of Medicaid patients is frequently cited to support this view, the overwhelming majority of studies demonstrate no difference in the health status and quality of care of those people covered by managed care plans or by indemnity insurance.

The variability in the results of all of the studies on quality and satisfaction in managed care reinforces the important premise that, as there are good doctors and poor doctors, there are good HMOs and poor HMOs. It is important for consumers to know how to discern the difference and to put some effort, however modest, into finding the best.

Points to Remember

- To summarize, there is basically no difference in quality between doctors in HMOs and those in private practice. You can find excellent doctors if you're a member of an HMO and you can find poor ones, just as you can find excellent and poor doctors if you carry indemnity insurance. The key is making sure that you find the best available for your own needs and the needs of your family.

Some simple guidelines to remember:

- Review the credentials and training of any doctor who cares for you.

- Make certain that a doctor you select is taking new patients and the waiting period for an appointment is not unreasonable.

- Be sure the HMO has a sufficient number of specialists and subspecialists you may need to see and that they are of high quality. For example, if you have diabetes, you will want to make sure that the HMO has endocrinologists on staff or as part of its network. If you have coronary heart disease, you will want to make sure that the HMO has first rate cardiologists and an arrangement with an outstanding center where the doctors perform invasive and non-invasive diagnostic techniques and which has a good record for open heart surgery.

- Determine beforehand the HMO's policy for patient referral to subspecialists, especially whether or not you will have a choice and how it may be exercised.

- Inquire about the rules for changing doctors in the HMO if you are not satisfied with your initial choice. You will want to know not only the procedure but how often such change is allowed.

- Ask about your options to go out of network and what your additional percentage of payment will be if you exercise this option. In determining what percentage the HMO pays, try to find out whether their payment is based on the HMO fee scale or "usual and customary" fees.

- Ask your doctor about the HMO's compensation system. You want to be sure that the system for paying your doctor will not have a negative influence on your care.

The Best in American Medicine
www.CastleConnolly.com

Directory of Doctors

Includes
Partnership for Excellence
Program

The Best in American Medicine
www.CastleConnolly.com

How to use the Directory of Doctors

Castle Connolly Medical Ltd. provides healthcare consumers with an invaluable source of information to identify leading physicians in their own community. This thirteenth edition of the Castle Connolly Guide, *Top Doctors: New York Metro Area*, contains vital information on more than 6,000 of the finest doctors in the region. Our guides are the result of a methodical process requiring a complete credential, licensing and disciplinary review of all doctors nominated for inclusion in the guide.

Why This Book Is Your Best Guide

Top Doctors: New York Metro Area is unique in a number of ways. The first edition of the Guide, published in 1994, was the first selective directory of doctors who practice in the New York metropolitan region. Castle Connolly recognizes that most healthcare is provided locally and people generally obtain their healthcare where they live or work. Therefore, by identifying excellent, caring physicians in every community and in every hospital, we apprise consumers of the best healthcare available to them within their own communities. Healthcare consumers in the New York metropolitan region are very fortunate with the abundance of doctors—approximately 55,000—who practice in the area. On the other hand, making a selection of one out of such a multitude can be a daunting task; it's hard even to know where to start. With *Top Doctors: New York Metro Area* in hand, you are already well on your way to finding the very best doctor for your individual needs and the needs of your family members.

With the profusion of outstanding academic medical centers, tertiary care teaching hospitals and fine regional hospitals in the New York metropolitan area, virtually any medical procedure or treatment can be found close to home. By virtue of this fact, it would be a simple matter to compile a book identifying the outstanding leaders in medical research and academic medicine in the region. Although many of these doctors are included in the listings, their names are to be found among the many excellent and caring doctors who deliver outstanding patient care in every community in the area. The goal—first and foremost—is to help you find the best doctors to meet your healthcare needs where you live and work. Again, a good reason why the Castle Connolly Guide is exceptional.

Further, the Castle Connolly Guide is different from most other listings of doctors in its selection process. Our selection is predicated on an extensive nomination procedure and a set of exacting standards which each nominated doctor was required to meet. To you, this means that the basis for inclusion of every one of the doctors in the listings was twofold: respect of their peers and medical excellence. Doctors do not pay to be listed. Our goal is to serve consumers, not doctors, hospitals or health plans.

How Castle Connolly Selects the Top Doctors

The basis of the Castle Connolly selection process is peer nomination. In some ways, this resembles an enhancement of the process in which a personal physician provides a patient with a referral to another physician for a particular problem. However, if the recommendation of one doctor is good, the recommendation of many doctors is even better. So, we ask thousands of randomly-selected physicians in the New York metropolitan area for their nominations.

How do we accomplish this enormous task? Over the years, the Castle Connolly physician-directed research team developed its extensive database of physicians through periodic mail, telephone and email surveys in the following counties:

New York State: New York, Bronx, Kings, Queens, Richmond, Nassau, Suffolk, Rockland, Westchester

New Jersey: Bergen, Essex, Hudson, Mercer, Middlesex, Monmouth, Morris, Passaic, Somerset, Union

Connecticut: Fairfield, New Haven

This cumulative database is systematically maintained and continuously updated. Surveyed physicians nominate top doctors in both their own and related specialties—especially those to whom they would refer their patients and their own family members. The database is also updated through further mail and telephone surveys. Each year we build on our prior research and supplement our database by inviting leading physicians at major medical centers in the metropolitan area, the thousands of top doctors included in earlier editions of our guide, and local leaders in the various medical specialties to offer their nominations for *Top Doctors: New York Metro Area.*

In addition to nominations obtained directly from practicing physicians, Castle Connolly solicits nominations from each area hospital's:

- President or Chief Executive Officer
- Vice President of Medical Affairs or the equivalent position
- Chief of Service in:
  - Anesthesiology
  - Medicine
  - Neurology
  - Obstetrics/Gynecology
  - Pathology
  - Pediatrics
  - Radiology
  - Surgery

Considerations for Inclusion Among the Top Doctors

Castle Connolly considers the following among the varied criteria used to determine physician eligibility for inclusion in our guides.

Professional Qualifications

- Education
- Residency
- Board certification
- Fellowships
- Professional Reputation
- Hospital appointment
- Medical school faculty appointment
- Experience
- Disciplinary history

Personal Characteristics/Qualities

Not only do we seek nominations of physicians who excel in academic medicine and research, but most importantly, those who exhibit excellence in patient care. We ask physicians in our survey to consider not only the training and clinical skills of the physicians they nominate, but also interpersonal skills such as the following:

- Listening and communicating effectively
- Demonstrating empathy
- Educating and informing
- Instilling trust and confidence

Verification/Credential Review

The Castle Connolly research staff reviews and refines the pool of nominated physicians in a region, validates nominations and verifies credentials. This results in the development of a preliminary list of physicians. Each provisionally selected physician is then required to complete a comprehensive professional biographical form including their special practice interests (see the "SPECIAL EXPERTISE INDEX"). The information contained in the biographical form becomes an integral part of each selected physician's listing in the guide.

The last phase of the process refines the list of provisionally selected doctors by cross-referencing their names against a variety of databases providing confirmation of:

- Board certification and recertification

- Licensing

- Disciplinary history

In some regions, a small number of peer-nominated physicians who are not board-certified may be included in a guide. These are doctors recognized by their colleagues as having exceptional demonstrated clinical practice experience.

Physicians ultimately selected for inclusion in *Top Doctors: New York Metro Area* receive formal notification of their nomination for listing upon completion of the final confirmation of their professional credentials.

How You Can Select the Top Doctors

How can you begin to make a choice from such a compilation of names? There is, in fact, a basic step-by-step process which varies somewhat depending on your individual needs as you approach the list. Here are the possibilities:

ONE: **If You are Looking for a Doctor in a Particular County**

The key: Physicians listed in the following pages are organized under the county in which their office is located so that you can go directly to the section listing doctors in your county of residence.

Key fact: Like most healthcare consumers, you probably receive your healthcare locally. If you think about it, you usually have been treated by doctors close to where you live and in community hospitals. If necessary, you may be referred to regional specialists and nearby medical centers.

TWO: **If You are Looking for a Primary Care Physician — a Generalist**

The key: The doctors who practice predominantly primary care, in the specialties of internal medicine, family practice, pediatrics, and obstetrics/gynecology, are designated by the notation a in the listing.

Key fact: Every board certified physician is a specialist. The term "having boards" signifies that a physician has completed an approved residency in a given specialty and has passed a rigorous examination given by that particular board. Therefore, doctors who practice primary care—internists, family practitioners, pediatricians, and Ob/Gyns—are specialists in their respective fields, as are urologists, otolaryngologists and radiologists. These specialists are considered primary care physicians.

THREE: **If You are Looking for a Physician in a Particular Specialty**

The key: Each entry contains the specialty practiced by the doctor and, in most cases, the most recent year of board certification.

Key fact: Many physicians specialize in fields of medicine that are not primary care. These specialists have completed an approved residency in a given specialty and have passed a rigorous exam given by that specialty board. For example, some physicians are board certified in psychiatry, surgery, allergy and immunology or dermatology.

Many doctors choose to specialize further. They choose an additional training program called a fellowship and upon completion of the program, they are required to take another exam in order to be certified as a subspecialist. An example of such subspecialization is an internist (initially board certified in internal medicine) who subspecialize in nephrology or cardiology. This doctor would be termed "double boarded" and would very likely practice nephrology or cardiology rather than internal medicine as a primary care physician.

FOUR: **If You are Looking for a Doctor with Expertise in a Particular Disease or Technique**

The key: Particular skills and interests of the doctors are found under the heading "SPECIAL EXPERTISE INDEX."

Key fact: A physician may have a special expertise interest in a particular field of medicine without actually being board certified in that area. Special expertise interests should not be confused with a board certified medical specialty. For example, cosmetic surgery is not an American Board of Medical Specialties recognized specialty, but it may constitute a major practice activity for many plastic surgeons. Certain doctors may develop a reputation as "specialists" in AIDS, diabetes or arthroscopic surgery. None of these are recognized medical specialties, yet they are indications of a doctor's expertise in a disease or medical or surgical procedure which may be helpful if you have the disease or need the procedure.

Many doctors who have a strong interest in, or consider themselves "specializing in," a particular health problem or medical technique form special interest groups referred to as "self-designated medical specialties." These groups are often confused with recognized medical specialties, which they are not. Some of the groups would like to be recognized by the ABMS and may even work toward that goal. For example, adolescent medicine was a special interest and self-designated specialty that is now an ABMS recognized subspecialty.

Choosing a doctor with a special practice interest is an additional step to be considered after you have already narrowed your choices to particular specialists and/or subspecialists. The "SPECIAL EXPERTISE INDEX" lists the doctors' special area or areas of expertise and can be particularly useful in identifying physicians who embrace alternative or complementary practices. Self-designated medical specialties are listed in Appendix B.

FIVE: **If You are Looking for a Doctor by Name**

The key: The "ALPHABETICAL LISTING OF DOCTORS" indicates the page on which information on the doctor's credentials can be found. The listing is arranged in last name, first name order.

Key fact: Most people start their search for a doctor through recommendation by family and friends. As a savvy healthcare consumer you realize that such recommendations are often based on personal "chemistry" and may be made by someone who actually knows very little about doctors or healthcare. Therefore, you will want to check the credentials of any recommended doctor and follow the additional recommendations that we have outlined in Sections one and two.

SIX: **If You want Detailed Information on a Particular Doctor**

The key: Each doctor's listing includes a substantial amount of information about the doctor.

Key fact: Wise choices in healthcare are made by consumers who have gathered as much information as possible about a particular doctor. If a professional information form was not returned by a doctor in time for inclusion in the book, our research staff verified certain major points of information (name, address, telephone, hospital affiliation, and specialty) from public sources and we have included this limited information. Even if a doctor's full credentials are included in this book, it is possible that, since the time of publication, the doctor has moved his or her office(s), changed telephone number(s), joined new medical groups, resigned from or joined hospital staffs, and, especially, changed relationships with HMOs and PPOs. Nonetheless, you can, in most cases, track down the doctor by using the following sources:

- Doctor's office—call the office number listed in the directory and ask for a new number.

- Hospitals—call the hospital listed in the directory and ask for help in locating a particular doctor.

- State Health Department—all state health department numbers are listed in Appendix E.

- American Board of Medical Specialties—a complete listing of ABMS Specialty Boards is found in Appendix A.

- American Osteopathic Association—a complete listing of AOA Specialty Boards is found in Appendix A.

Conclusion

You are now ready to work with our directory of more than 5,000 of the finest doctors in the New York metropolitan area. Although you may be well-informed as a result of reading Sections one and two of this book, it is possible that choosing the doctor will seem to be a complex endeavor. The tendency might be to try to get the job done as quickly as possible by choosing a doctor based solely on the convenience of the office's location. To do so would be a big mistake. You want the best healthcare. You deserve it. A little effort will help you to get the best.

There are many excellent doctors in the region not listed in this book. You can identify them by using the process we have described in Sections one and two or, if a doctor in this book is unable to meet your needs, ask about other physicians highly regarded by that doctor.

We believe that this book will educate and enlighten you throughout its pages and that it will prove its value in the end—when you decide on the doctor with whom you plan to have a lasting relationship.

Obtaining Additional Doctor Information

You may wish to call a doctor's office to make an appointment or to help determine if the doctor is the one you want to care for you. Here are some questions you may want to ask:

1. Is a referral required?

2. Are you accepting new patients?

3. Which health plans/insurance do you accept?

4. Do you accept Medicare? Medicaid? Workers' compensation? No-fault insurance?

5. Are payments of deductible and co-payments required at the time of appointment?

6. Do you accept credit cards?

7. Do you see patients in the evening? On weekends?

8. Is the office handicapped-accessible?

9. Do you accept phone calls from patients?

10 Do you communicate with patients via the internet?

11. If you are not comfortable addressing the doctor in English, ask if your native language is spoken by the doctor or by someone else in the office.

Sample Listing

Smith, John MD [IM] *PCP - Spec Exp: Ulcers; Crohn's Disease;*
<u>   </u>   <u>   </u>
     Name [specialty] &   Special Expertise(s)
  Primary Care Physician indication

Hospital: NYU Med Ctr (page 130); Address: 100 Tenth St, FL 5 - Ste 3A, MC-1234, New York, NY 10010;
    admitting hospital(s) &   Office address   Mail code   City, state zip
  Hospital Information page(s)

Phone: (904) 296-0000; Board Cert: IM 70, GE 74; Med School: U Fla Coll Med 66;
    Office phone   *Board certification(s) & date(s)   Medical school & year of degree

Resid: IM, NYU Med Ctr, 69; Fellow: GE, Lenox Hill Hosp, 72;
  Residency(ies) & location(s)   Fellowship(s) & location(s)

Fac Appt: Assoc Clin Prof Med, NYU Sch Med
    Faculty appointment & location

* Indicates the most recent date of board certification or recertification.

In our listings of the professional information on doctors, we have abbreviated hospitals and medical schools. The abbreviations are designed to be self-explanatory, but if you need assistance, refer to Appendix D: Hospitals Listings.

Note on Special Expertise(s):

These are not medical specialties as described on pages 81-87, but the areas of expertise or practice interests indicated by the doctor.

The information reported in each doctor's listing is, for the most part, provided by the doctor or his/her office staff. Castle Connolly attempts to verify the data through other sources but cannot guarantee that in all cases all data have been so verified or are accurate. All such information is subject to change from time to time due to changes in physician practices. Many doctors participate in several health plans and/or switch plans frequently. Therefore, you should verify with the doctor's office whether your health plan is currently accepted.

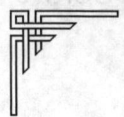

The Best in American Medicine
www.CastleConnolly.com

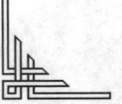
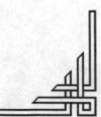

Medical Specialties and Subspecialties

In the pages that follow, each list of doctors in a medical specialty or subspecialty is preceded by a brief description of that specialty (or subspecialty) and the training required for board certification.

Critical Care Medicine has been excluded because in emergency situations there is neither time nor opportunity for choice. A number of other specialities not relevant to most patients (e.g., Forensic Psychiatry) have not been included as well.

The following descriptions of medical specialties and subspecialties were provided by the American Board of Medical Specialties (ABMS), an organization comprised of the 24 medical specialty boards that provide certification in 25 medical specialties. A complete listing of all specialists certified by the ABMS can be found in The Official ABMS Directory of Board Certified Medical Specialists, is published by Marquis Who's Who. It is available (either in a multi-volume directory or on CD-ROM) in most public libraries, hospital libraries, university libraries and medical libraries. The ABMS also operates a toll-free phone line at 1-866-275-2267 and a website at www.abms.org to verify the certification status of individual doctors.

The following important policy statement, approved by the ABMS Assembly on March 19, 1987, remains valid.

The Purpose Of Certification

The intent of the certification process, as defined by the member boards of the American Board of Medical Specialties, is to provide assurance to the public that a certified medical specialist has successfully completed an approved educational program and an evaluation, including an examination process designed to assess the knowledge, experience and skills requisite to the provision of high quality patient care in that specialty.

Medical Specialties and Subspecialties

Medical Specialty and Subspecialty Descriptions and Abbreviations

The following medical specialties and subspecialties are indicated in the doctors' listings by their abbreviations. Specialties are indicated in bold, subspecialties in italics, and the four primary care specialties in bold capitals. To review the official American Board of Medical Specialties (ABMS) organization of specialties, refer to Appendix A.

Addiction Psychiatry   AdP
Deals with habitual psychological and physiological dependence on a substance or practice which is beyond voluntary control.

Adolescent Medicine   AM
Involves the primary care treatment of adolescents and young adults.

Allergy & Immunology   **A&I**
Diagnosis and treatment of allergies, asthma and skin problems such as hives and contact dermatitis.

Anesthesiology   **Anes**
Provides pain relief in maintenance or restoration of a stable condition during and following an operation. Anesthesiologists also diagnose and treat acute and long standing pain problems.

Cardiac Electrophysiology (Clinical)   CE
Involves complicated technical procedures to evaluate heart rhythms and determine appropriate treatment for them.

Cardiovascular Disease   Cv
Involves the diagnosis and treatment of disorders of the heart, lungs and blood vessels.

Child & Adolescent Psychiatry   ChAP
Deals with the diagnosis and treatment of mental diseases in children and adolescents.

Child Neurology   ChiN
Diagnosis and medical treatment of disorders of the brain, spinal cord and nervous system in children.

Clinical Genetics   **CG**
Deals with identifying the genetic causes of inherited diseases and ailments and preventing, when possible, their occurrence.

Colon and Rectal Surgery   **CRS**
Surgical treatment of diseases of the intestinal tract, colon and rectum, anal canal and perianal area.

Critical Care Medicine   CCM
Involves diagnosing and taking immediate action to prevent death or further injury of a patient. Examples of critical injuries include shock, heart attack, drug overdose and massive bleeding.

Dermatology   D

Diagnosis and treatment of benign and malignant disorders of the skin, mouth, external genitalia, hair and nails, as well as a number of sexually transmitted diseases.

Diagnostic Radiology   DR

Involves the study of all modalities of radiant energy in medical diagnoses and therapeutic procedures utilizing radiologic guidance.

Endocrinology, Diabetes & Metabolism   EDM

Involves the study and treatment of patients suffering from hormonal and chemical disorders.

FAMILY MEDICINE   FP

Deals with and oversees the total healthcare of individual patients and their family members. Family practitioners are more common in rural areas and may perform procedures more commonly performed by specialists (e.g., minor surgery).

Forensic Psychiatry   FPsy

Concerns the evaluation of certain diagnostic groups of patients that include those with sexual disorders, antisocial personality disorders, paranoid disorders and addictive disorders.

Gastroenterology   Ge

The study, diagnosis and treatment of diseases of the digestive organs including the stomach, bowels, liver and gallbladder.

Geriatric Medicine   Ger

Deals with diseases of the elderly and the problems associated with aging.

Geriatric Psychiatry   GerPsy

Involves the diagnosis, prevention and treatment of mental illness in the elderly.

Gynecologic Oncology   GO

Deals with cancers of the female genital tract and reproductive systems.

Hand Surgery   HS

Involves the treatment of injury to the hand through surgical techniques.

Hematology   Hem

Involves the diagnosis and treatment of diseases and disorders of the blood, bone marrow, spleen and lymph glands.

Infectious Disease   Inf

The study and treatment of diseases caused by a bacterium, virus, fungus or animal parasite.

INTERNAL MEDICINE   IM

Diagnosis and nonsurgical treatment of diseases, especially those of adults. Internists may act as primary care specialists, highly trained family doctors or they may subspecialize in specialties such as cardiology or nephrology.

Maternal & Fetal Medicine   MF

Involves the care of women with high-risk pregnancies and their unborn fetuses.

Medical Specialties and Subspecialties

Medical Oncology   Onc
Refers to the study and treatment of tumors and other cancers.

Neonatal-Perinatal Medicine   NP
Involves the diagnosis and treatments of infants prior to, during and one month
beyond birth.

Nephrology   Nep
Concerned with disorders of the kidneys, high blood pressure, fluid and mineral
balance, dialysis of body wastes when the kidneys do not function and consultation
with surgeons about kidney transplantation.

Neurological Surgery   **NS**
Involves surgery of the brain, spinal cord and nervous system.

Neurology   **N**
Diagnosis and medical treatment of disorders of the brain, spinal cord and nervous
system.

Neuroradiology   NRad
Involves the utilization of imaging procedures during diagnosis as they relate to the
brain, spine and spinal cord, head, neck and organs of special sense in adults and
children.

Nuclear Medicine   **NuM**
Evaluation of the functions of all the organs in the body and treatment of thyroid
disease, benign and malignant tumors and radiation exposure through the use of
radioactive substances.

Nuclear Radiology   NR
Involves the use of radioactive substances to diagnose and treat certain functions and
diseases of the body.

OBSTETRICS & GYNECOLOGY   **ObG**
Deals with the medical aspects of and intervention in pregnancy and labor and the
overall health of the female reproductive system.

Occupational Medicine   OM
Concentrates on the effect of the work environment on the health of employees.

Ophthalmology   **Oph**
Diagnosis and treatment of diseases of and injuries to the eye.

Orthopaedic Surgery   **OrS**
Involves operations to correct injuries which interfere with the form and function of
the extremities, spine and associated structures.

Otolaryngology   **Oto**
Explores and treats diseases in the interrelated areas of the ears, nose and throat.

Otology/Neurotology   ON
Concentrates on the management, prevention, cure and care of patients with diseases
of the ear and temporal bone, including disorders of hearing and balance.

Pain Medicine
PM

Involves providing a high level of care for patients experiencing problems with acute or chronic pain in both hospital and ambulatory settings.

Pediatric Cardiology
PCd

Involves the diagnosis and treatment of heart disease in children.

Pediatric Critical Care Medicine
PCCM

Involves the care of children who are victims of life threatening disorders such as severe accidents, shock and diabetes acidosis.

Pediatric Dermatology
PD

Diagnosis and treatment of benign and malignant disorders of the skin, mouth, external genitalia, hair and nails in children.

Pediatric Endocrinology
PEn

Involves the study and treatment of children with hormonal and chemical disorders.

Pediatric Gastroenterology
PGe

The study, diagnosis and treatment of diseases of the digestive tract in children.

Pediatric Hematology-Oncology
PHO

The study and treatment of cancers of the blood and blood-forming parts of the body in children.

Pediatric Infectious Disease
PInf

The study and treatment of diseases caused by a virus, bacterium, fungus or animal parasite in children.

Pediatric Nephrology
PNep

Deals with the diagnosis and treatment of disorders of the kidneys in children.

Pediatric Otolaryngology
POto

Involves the diagnosis and treatment of disorders of the ear, nose and throat which affect children.

Pediatric Pulmonology
PPul

Involves the diagnosis and treatment of diseases of the chest, lungs, and chest tissue in children.

Pediatric Radiology
PR

Involves diagnostic imaging as it pertains to the newborn, infant, child and adolescent.

Pediatric Rheumatology
PRhu

Involves the treatment of diseases of the joints and connective tissues in children.

Pediatric Surgery
PS

Treatment of disease, injury or deformity in children through surgical techniques.

PEDIATRICS
Ped

Diagnosis and treatment of diseases of childhood and monitoring of the growth, development and well-being of preadolescent.

Medical Specialties and Subspecialties

Physical Medicine & Rehabilitation   **PMR**

The use of physical therapy and physical agents such as water, heat, light electricity and mechanical manipulations in the diagnosis, treatment and prevention of disease and body disorders.

Plastic Surgery   **PlS**

Involves reconstructive and cosmetic surgery of the face and other body parts.

Preventive Medicine   **PrM**

A specialty focusing on the prevention of illness and on the health of groups rather than individuals.

Psychiatry   **Psyc**

Examination, treatment and prevention of mental illness through the use of psychoanalysis and/or drugs.

Public Health & General Preventive Medicine   PHGPM

Involves the investigation of the causes of epidemic disease and the prevention of a wide variety of acute and chronic illness.

Pulmonary Disease   Pul

Involves the diagnosis and treatment of diseases of the chest, lungs and airways.

Radiation Oncology   RadRo

Involves the use of radiant energy and isotopes in the study and treatment of disease, especially malignant cancer.

Reproductive Endocrinology   RE

Deals with the endocrine system (including the pituitary, thyroid, parathyroid, adrenal glands, placenta, ovaries and testes) and how its failure relates to infertility.

Rheumatology   Rhu

Involves the treatment of diseases of the joints, muscles, bones and associated structures.

Sleep Medicine   Sleep Med

Involves the investigation and of patients with sleep disorders.

Spinal Cord Injury Medicine   SpCdInj

Involves the prevention, diagnosis, treatment and management of traumatic spinal cord injuries.

Sports Medicine   SM

Refers to the practice of an orthopedist or other physician who specializes in injuries to the bone or other soft tissues (muscles, tendons, ligaments) caused by participation in athletic active.

Surgery   **S**

Treatment of disease, injury and deformity by surgical procedures.

Surgery of the Hand   SHd

Involves providing appropriate care for all structures in the upper extremity directly affecting the hand and wrist function.

Surgical Critical Care   SCC

Involves specialized care in the management of the critically ill patient, particularly the trauma victim and postoperative patient in the emergency department, intensive care unit, trauma unit, burn unit and other similar settings.

Thoracic Surgery (includes open heart surgery)   **TS**

Involves surgery on the heart, lungs and chest area.

Urology   **U**

Diagnosis and treatment of diseases of the genitals in men and disorders of the urinary tract and bladder in both men and women.

Vascular & Interventional Radiology   VIR

Involves diagnosing and treating diseases by percutaneous methods guided by various radiologic imaging modalities.

Vascular Surgery   VascS

Involves the operative treatment of disorders of the blood vessels excluding those to the heart, lungs or brain.

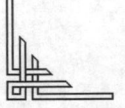

The Best in American Medicine
www.CastleConnolly.com

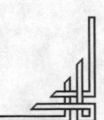

Partnership for Excellence
The Hospital Information Program

There are more than 200 acute care and specialty hospitals in the New York metropolitan area, many of which have extraordinary capabilities for superior patient care. Castle Connolly Medical Ltd. has received many requests from book buyers to provide information about hospitals. In response, we have invited a select group of outstanding hospitals to profile their services in this guide through the medium of paid advertorials. This program, called the Hospital Information Program is totally separate from the physician selection process, which is based upon a completely independent review system. Hospitals that sponsored pages in the Hospital Information Program are organized into three groups: Major Medical Centers, Specialty Hospitals and Regional Medical Centers.

Major Medical Centers begin on the next page and are followed by the Specialty Hospital pages. This section is followed by the listings of doctors. Regional Medical Centers and Hospitals are found at the beginning of each county section - within the doctor listings. The information gives you an overview of programs and services offered by these hospitals, as well as vital information related to their accreditation and sponsorship. Each hospital profile also contains a physician referral number, should you wish to ask the hospitals for recommendations of physicians not listed in the Castle Connolly Guide.

The "Centers of Excellence" section was also developed in response to requests from our readers who want to know which hospitals have special programs or services focusing on a particular illness or health need. The "Centers of Excellence" described here are also offered by hospitals participating in the Partnership for Excellence section of this guide. They reflect the depth of commitment of these hospitals, which provides the staff, resources and financial support necessary to develop these special programs. We believe you will find this information helpful in your search for the best healthcare — from both physicians and hospitals— for you and your family.

We are pleased to have these distinguished institutions as partners in our effort to help you meet your healthcare needs.

The following pages contain vital information on eight of the region's Major Medical Centers. A Major Medical Center is an acute care hospital with tertiary care services, residency programs, a major affiliation with a medical school and clinical research programs. A major medical center draws its patients from a broad geographic region, even nationally and internationally and, in many instances, is the center of a network or consortium of hospitals.

The New York metropolitan region is nationally and internationally known for its major medical centers and their excellent programs and services. Some of the nation's leading academic centers are in this region and, in addition to superior patient care and cutting edge patient research, they produce thousands of talented, well trained physicians and other health professionals each year. Castle Connolly Medical Ltd. has invited a number of major medical centers in the region to sponsor the profiles and information that follows.

Major Medical Centers

Atlantic Health System

Continuum Health Partners

Hackensack University Medical Center

Maimonides Medical Center

Montefiore Medical Center

Mount Sinai Medical Center

NewYork-Presbyterian Hospital

NYU Langone Medical Center

The Best in American Medicine
www.CastleConnolly.com

ATLANTIC HEALTH

Morristown Memorial Hospital • Overlook Hospital

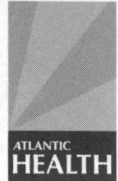

Goryeb Children's Hospital • Atlantic Neuroscience Institute
Carol G. Simon Cancer Center • Gagnon Cardiovascular Institute
Atlantic Rehabilitation Institute

P.O. Box 1905, Morristown, NJ 07962 • www.atlantichealth.org

To find a doctor, call 800-247-9580 or visit us online

Sponsorship:	Voluntary Not–for–Profit
Beds:	1,197
Accreditation:	Joint Commission

Atlantic Health is at the forefront of medicine, setting standards for quality health care in New Jersey and beyond. Our nationally recognized physicians, experienced nurses and skilled staff provide outstanding and compassionate care.

Renowned for its breadth of cardiac services, Morristown Memorial Hospital has the largest cardiac surgery program in the state of New Jersey. Overlook Hospital, the regional leader in comprehensive stroke care and neurosciences, was the first hospital in the Northeast to use revolutionary CyberKnife® technology and the first hospital to be designated a Comprehensive Stroke Center by the New Jersey Department of Health and Senior Services. Atlantic Health's stroke centers are recipients of the prestigious Gold Seal of Approval from the Joint Commission for Primary Stroke Centers.

In all our specialties such as pediatrics, orthopedics, cancer care, rehabilitation medicine, women's health, cardiovascular care and neuroscience, Atlantic Health physicians are leaders in their fields, always searching for the most effective diagnosis and treatment options for each patient. Our world-class facilities feature state-of-the-art equipment in a comfortable, family-friendly environment that puts patients first.

◢ MORRISTOWN MEMORIAL HOSPITAL – 100 Madison Avenue, Morristown, NJ 07962

Morristown Memorial Hospital has been serving the Morris County community for more than 100 years, providing high level patient care in first-rate facilities with a full range of medical specialties and services. Named a Level I Regional Trauma Center by the American College of Surgeons and a Level II Trauma Center by the state of NJ, Morristown Memorial offers superlative care with our highly trained trauma teams. Our cardiac surgery program is the largest in the state. Our Level III Regional Perinatal Center provides specialized care to sick or premature infants, and Goryeb Children's Hospital has helped over 50,000 children get well last year alone. Our mission at Carol G. Simon Cancer Center, where we treat all types of cancer with the most advanced methods, is to provide comprehensive, compassionate and individualized service. Our quality of care has earned us national recognition. Recently, Morristown Memorial was re-designated a Magnet Hospital for Excellence in Nursing Service, the highest level of recognition by American Nurses Credentialing Center for facilities that provide acute care services. Less than five percent of US hospitals receive the prestigious Magnet designation. Morristown Memorial is accredited by the Joint Commission. We are a clinical and academic affiliate of The Mount Sinai Hospital and Mount Sinai School of Medicine and a Major Clinical Research Affiliate of the Cancer Institute of New Jersey.

◢ OVERLOOK HOSPITAL - 99 Beauvoir Avenue, Summit, NJ 07902

Overlook Hospital is a pioneer in medical technology. We have the state's first combined PET/CT scanner and stereotactic radiosurgery cancer treatment program; our Neuroscience Institute offers a Brain Tumor Center, Comprehensive Stroke Center and a comprehensive Level IV Epilepsy Center, as well as comprehensive programs in Movement and Memory Disorders. In addition to the largest neurointerventional radiology service in New Jersey, we were the first center in the NYC area to offer the revolutionary CyberKnife. Nationally recognized for our Emergency Department, we are one of five New Jersey hospitals approved to provide emergency angioplasty in a community hospital setting. Overlook is a Circle of Excellence award winner for community service from the American Association of Critical Care Nurses, and the Atlantic Health Weight & Wellness Center at Overlook was named a Center of Excellence in Bariatric Surgery by the American Society of Metabolic and Bariatric Surgery.

Overlook is a clinical and academic affiliate of The Mount Sinai Hospital and Mount Sinai School of Medicine. We are also a Major Clinical Research Affiliate of The Cancer Institute of New Jersey. Overlook is accredited by The Joint Commission.

◢ GORYEB CHILDREN'S HOSPITAL

At Goryeb Children's Hospital, we know there is nothing more important than a child's health. That's why we are committed to delivering the finest personalized pediatric specialty care in a patient- and family-centered environment to more than 50,000 children, from infants to young adults, each year. Your child will benefit from the expertise of nationally recognized, board-certified pediatric specialists who are actively involved in clinical research, enabling them to offer your child the newest medications, treatments and technologies. We have over 100 specialty physicians in 20 concentrated areas of pediatric medical and surgical care.

◢ ATLANTIC NEUROSCIENCE INSTITUTE

Atlantic Neuroscience Institute integrates the broad range of neuroscience services of Atlantic Health. Based at Overlook Hospital, the Institute uses the expertise of adult and pediatric neurologists and neurosurgeons, neuroradiologists and specialists in related fields at Morristown Memorial and Overlook. We provide exceptional, comprehensive, compassionate care for individuals with neurologic disease and participate in related research, which elevates neuroscience knowledge and enables the Institute to offer the most advanced technology available for endovascular treatment of stroke, aneurysms and brain vascular malformations. We were the first center in the NYC region to offer the CyberKnife for the treatment of tumors and lesions in the brain, spine, lung, liver, pancreas and prostate.

◢ CAROL G. SIMON CANCER CENTER

The Carol G. Simon Cancer Center at Morristown Memorial and Overlook hospitals offers the most advanced methods to diagnose, treat and manage all types of cancers. Our highly trained physicians and oncology professionals work together in a collaborative setting that promotes a coordinated, multidisciplinary approach to care. We provide state-of-the-art medical and radiation oncology, including CyberKnife, the latest in intensity-modulated and external beam therapies and brachytherapy. We also offer the most sophisticated imaging technologies including digital mammography and PET/CT. Our cancer program at both hospitals was awarded the American College of Surgeon's Outstanding Achievement Awards for Cancer Care, given to fewer than 15 percent of centers nationwide, and our cancer program houses two state-of-the-art facilities lauded for innovation and achievement.

◢ GAGNON CARDIOVASCULAR INSTITUTE

We are a national leader in the research and treatment of cardiac disease. Expert care and comprehensive cardiovascular services are available at Gagnon Cardiovascular Institute, which encompasses all cardiovascular services at Overlook Hospital and at Morristown Memorial Hospital. Our cardiac surgery program – the state's largest – is based at Morristown Memorial. The Institute's new flagship facility in Morristown, which opened in January 2009, features 106 private patient rooms, new operating and procedure rooms, the most advanced diagnostic tools and convenient access to all facets of cardiac care.

Our Cardiac Care Units provide a full range of diagnostic testing procedures, including the 320-slice Cardiac CT Angiography - the latest technology in non-invasive cardiac imaging - and our cardiac specialists develop comprehensive treatment and recovery plans for each patient. During the recovery process, you have the benefit of cardiac rehabilitation experts who help you to gain physical and emotional strength, and to plan heart-healthy routines when you return home.

Sponsorship: Voluntary Not-for-profit **Beds:** 2,255 certified beds
Accreditation: Joint Commission of Accreditation of Healthcare Organizations (JCAHO), Accreditation Council for Graduate Medical Education, Medical Society of New York, in conjunction with the Accreditation Council for Continuing Medical Education

A STRONG PARTNERSHIP WITH A PROUD HERITAGE

Continuum Health Partners is a partnership of five venerable health care providers: Beth Israel Medical Center-Milton and Carroll Petrie Division, Beth Israel Medical Center-Kings Highway Division, St. Luke's Hospital, Roosevelt Hospital, and The New York Eye and Ear Infirmary. Each of the five partner institutions was established more than a century ago by individuals committed to improving health and health care in their communities. Today, the system represents over 4,000 physicians and dentists and is superbly equipped to respond to the health care needs of the populations we serve. Continuum providers also see patients in group and private practice settings and in ambulatory centers in New York City and Westchester County.

LOCATIONS

Continuum Health Partners has campuses in Manhattan and Brooklyn. Beth Israel Medical Center has two divisions: the Milton and Caroll Petrie Division on the East Side, and the Kings Highway Division in Brooklyn. The Phillips Ambulatory Care Center, a state-of-the-art outpatient center, is located at Union Square. St. Luke's Hospital is in Morningside Heights and Roosevelt Hospital is in the Columbus Circle and Lincoln Center neighborhoods on the West Side. The New York Eye and Ear Infirmary is located on Second Avenue and 14th Street.

ACADEMIC AFFILIATIONS

Beth Israel Medical Center is the University Hospital and Manhattan Campus for the Albert Einstein College of Medicine. St. Luke's-Roosevelt Hospital Center is an Academic Affiliate of Columbia University College of Physicians and Surgeons. The New York Eye and Ear Infirmary is the primary teaching center of the New York Medical College and affiliated teaching hospitals in the areas of ophthalmology and otolaryngology.

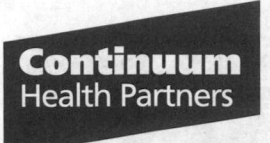

Continuum
Health Partners

For a referral to a great doctor in your neighborhood, call (800) 420-4004. Our Physician Referral Service can help you find a primary care physician or specialist affiliated with Beth Israel, St. Luke's, Roosevelt, or The New York Eye and Ear Infirmary. Visit our Website at www.chpnyc.org

Centers of Excellence at Continuum Health Partners

Cancer

The Continuum Cancer Centers of New York offer early detection, diagnosis, and treatment of a wide range of cancers. Our nationally recognized physicians offer innovative and highly successful programs coupled with superb support services. Our cancer services are state of the art, supported by sophisticated programs in medical oncology, surgical oncology, and radiation oncology.

Cardiac Services

The cardiology, cardiac surgery, and cardiac rehabilitation experts at Continuum offer a full range of diagnostic and treatment services. Some highlights of our cardiac programs are minimally invasive robotic cardiac surgery, arrhythmia services, 24-hour cardiac catheterization labs, and expertise in congestive heart failure.

Neurological Services

Continuum is home to many world leaders in neurology, neurosurgery and interventional neuroradiology. Our physicians are recognized authorities who establish innovative care protocols, chart new venues in therapy and develop the technologies that set the standards in the neuroscience fields.

Orthopedic Services

Continuum's orthopedic physicians are leading providers of general orthopedic, sports medicine, spine and rheumatologic care. Our specialists offer state-of-the-art care to patients throughout the New York metropolitan region. Many of our orthopedic surgeons are leaders in their field and are fellowship trained in their areas of sub-specialty.

Ear, Nose and Throat

Continuum offers eye, ear, nose and throat services throughout our system. The New York Eye and Ear Infirmary and Beth Israel are both ranked by US News & World Report among the Best Hospitals in the nation for the specialty of ear, nose and throat. New York Eye and Ear is also ranked 13th in the nation for excellence in ophthalmology.

HIV/AIDS

We are one of the largest providers of HIV/AIDS care in New York City, with comprehensive-care clinics and facilities in multiple locations. Our facilities offer a complete range of health care services for individuals with HIV: diagnostic procedures, the latest treatments, and support services.

Pain Management

Our Department of Pain Medicine and Palliative Care offers a broad array of therapies for chronic pain of all types. The highly trained medical team includes pain specialists with backgrounds in neurology, rehabilitation medicine, anesthesiology and psychology.

Substance Abuse

Continuum offers extensive chemical dependency treatment services through The Addiction Institute of New York, the Stuyvesant Square Chemical Dependency Treatment Program, and the Department of Psychiatry and Behavioral Health. Our services include inpatient detoxification and outpatient programs, services for the mentally ill, family services, and after-care programs.

HACKENSACK UNIVERSITY MEDICAL CENTER

30 Prospect Avenue
Hackensack, New Jersey 07601
phone 201-996-3760
fax 201-996-3452

www.humc.com

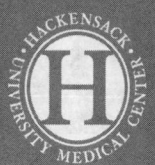

Sponsorship	**A not-for-profit, teaching and research hospital affiliated with the University of Medicine and Dentistry of New Jersey – New Jersey Medical School.**
Beds	**A 775-bed, Level II Trauma Center, providing tertiary and regional services for the New York/New Jersey metropolitan area.**
Accreditation	**Joint Commission on the Accreditation of Healthcare Organizations (JCAHO).**

Hackensack University Medical Center (HUMC) is also the recipient of 15 Gold Seals of Approval™ for healthcare quality from JCAHO, the only medical facility in the United States to achieve this record number of JCAHO Disease-Specific Care Certifications.

The medical center holds JCAHO Disease-Specific Care Certifications in: Acute Myocardial Infarction, Asthma, Bone Marrow Transplantation, Chronic Obstructive Pulmonary Disease, Coronary Artery Disease, Depression Program, End Stage Renal Disease, Heart Failure, Hip Replacement, Inpatient Diabetes Program, Knee Replacement, Pediatric Asthma, Pneumonia Disease, Primary Stroke Center, and Trauma.

HUMC is a nationally recognized healthcare organization offering patients the most comprehensive services, state-of-the-art technologies, and facilities. A leader in providing the highest quality patient-centered care, the medical center has been recognized for performance excellence encompassing the entire spectrum of hospital quality and service issues. These honors include being named one of America's 50 Best Hospitals by HealthGrades® for four years in a row. HUMC is the only hospital in New Jersey, New York, and New England to receive this honor. NJBIZ, New Jersey's premiere business news publication, honored HUMC as the "2010 Hospital of the Year," recognized for its excellence, innovation, and efforts which are making a significant impact on the quality of healthcare in New Jersey. *Hospital Newspaper* has also named HUMC "Hospital of the Year" in its December 2010 edition. *Hospital Newspaper* is the leading provider of local hospitals and healthcare community news and information for hospital executives, doctors, nurses, and other healthcare professionals. Additionally, HUMC was named to The Leapfrog Group's annual class of top hospitals and health systems and is one of only two hospitals in New Jersey to receive this national designation. HUMC is the hometown hospital of the New York Giants (NFL) and New Jersey Nets (NBA).

MEDICAL AND DENTAL STAFF

Since HUMC is one of the region's most comprehensive and progressive medical centers, it easily attracts many of the area's leading physicians. These doctors, many of whom are on the cutting edge in their fields and have received their training at our nation's most prominent institutions, have selected HUMC as their place to practice their best medicine.

NURSING EXCELLENCE

Our medical staff is joined by a team of extraordinary nurses. As a Magnet® Hospital, HUMC attracts and retains nurses who are tops in their fields.

Making history in 1995 as the first official Magnet Hospital in New Jersey. HUMC is the only hospital in New Jersey with four designations from the American Nurses Credentialing Center and named one of the Top 100 Hospitals to Work For by *Nursing Professionals* magazine.

NATIONAL RECOGNITIONS HIGHLIGHT SUPERIOR PATIENT CARE

Throughout its history, HUMC has been recognized by many of the nation's most prestigious organizations for its high level of clinical and organizational excellence. Not only do these recognitions set us apart from our competitors, more importantly they provide consumers with valuable objective data on which to make informed decisions about their healthcare. More than a plaque on the wall, our vast recognitions, rankings, and ratings highlight medical excellence at HUMC – the hallmark of our success.

One of America's 50 Best Hospitals for four years in a row – HUMC has been recognized as one of America's 50 Best Hospitals by HealthGrades, one of the nation's leading independent healthcare ratings company. These hospitals have achieved better survival rates and lower complication rates across dozens of medical procedures and diagnoses, from cardiac care to orthopedic surgery, consistently ranking among the top five percent in the nation for overall clinical outcomes. HUMC is the only hospital in New Jersey, New York, and New England to be named one of America's 50 Best Hospitals.

WORLD-CLASS CARDIAC CARE

HUMC is one of America's most comprehensive cardiac and vascular hospitals. Heart and Vascular Hospital provides a full-range of state-of-the-art invasive and non-invasive diagnostic and treatment services including electrophysiology studies, a state-designated cardiac catheterization center, and one of the largest cardiac surgery programs in the state.

HUMC opened a new state-of-the-art Heart and Vascular Hospital. This "hospital within a hospital" consolidates the medical center's full range of award-winning heart, vascular, and neurovascular services.

The Heart and Vascular Hospital integrates preventive, diagnostic, and treatment services, with a special focus on cardiovascular disease management and breakthrough research. Inpatients and outpatients are treated for all types of cardiac and vascular diseases, including heart problems, such as blocked arteries and irregular heartbeats; peripheral vascular disease; and neurovascular diseases, such as stroke and aneurysm. Housing all these services within one specialized location allows for more efficient, effective patient care.

ONE OF THE NATION'S LARGEST AND MOST COMPREHENSIVE CANCER CENTERS

The John Theurer Cancer Center at HUMC is one of the nation's largest and most comprehensive and is among the nation's top 10 in patient volume. The Cancer Center is composed of 14 specialized teams on-site fully engaged in the medical and emotional care of their patients and loved ones. Each of the 14 divisions features teams of physicians, nurses, technologists, and support staff with clinical and research expertise in a specific type of cancer such as leukemia or breast cancer. This approach – which brings together a close-knit team of medical, research, nursing, and support staff with specialized expertise – translates into more advanced, focused care for patients.

The new John Theurer Cancer Center opened to patients on December 27, 2010. This 155,000-square-foot facility houses outpatient cancer services and incorporates diagnostic facilities, chemotherapy preparation and infusion areas, pharmacy and laboratory resources, as well as a full spectrum of radiation oncology services. In keeping with its commitment to green and sustainable buildings, the new facility, complete with a rooftop garden, follows guidelines outlined by the Leadership in Energy and Environmental Design and developed by the U. S. Green Building Council.

ONE OF THE NATION'S RENOWNED PEDIATRIC PROGRAMS

HUMC is a state-designated New Jersey Children's Hospital. It is also a full-voting member in the National Association of Children's Hospitals and Related Institutions, the non-profit association that speaks on behalf of children's health needs and their caregivers.

The Joseph M. Sanzari Children's Hospital is located in the Sarkis and Siran Gabrellian Women's and Children's Pavilion, a 300,000-square-foot pavilion that also houses the Donna A. Sanzari Women's Hospital and the Mark Messier Skyway for Tomorrows Children. This facility is one of the country's first environmentally responsible and sustainable healthcare facilities and is ranked as one of the Top 10 Green Hospitals by *The Green Guide*.

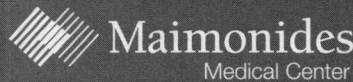

Cardiac Institute

Renowned for its Catheterization Lab and pioneering new surgical procedures, the Institute includes an electrophysiology (EP) lab, two ICUs, Chest Pain Observation Unit, Advanced Cardiac Care Unit, Congestive Heart Failure program and Atrial Fibrillation Center. The first successful heart transplant in America was performed at Maimonides in 1967. Today, its Cardiology division continues to innovate. Maimonides has been ranked by the Centers for Medicare & Medicaid Services among those hospitals achieving excellent ratings in both heart attack and heart failure patient outcomes.

Stroke Center

The Stroke Center at Maimonides is ranked among the best in the nation. It is currently the site of clinical trials for new stroke medications, medical devices, and stroke protocols. The Center is one of the few that provides interventional neuroradiology techniques to remove stroke-causing blood clots from the brain – without surgery – significantly reducing the debilitating effects of stroke.

Infants & Children's Hospital

The Maimonides Infants & Children's Hospital, one of only five accredited children's hospitals in NYC, includes comprehensive inpatient services and over 30 pediatric subspecialties. With a Child Life program fully integrated with family-centered care, the Maimonides Infants & Children's Hospital also provides a Pediatric ICU, Neonatal ICU, Outpatient Services and Pediatric ER.

Vascular Institute

The Vascular Institute at Maimonides provides comprehensive diagnostic, clinical, and vascular surgical services for patients with circulatory complications related to hypertension, diabetes, arteriosclerosis, and other diseases. One of only five centers in New York certified to train vascular surgeons, the Institute includes a Diagnostic Lab, Vein Center, Vascular Surgery Center and Wound Center.

Stella & Joseph Payson Birthing Center

More babies are delivered at Maimonides than at any other single-campus hospital in New York State. The Payson Birthing Center offers a home-like setting with physicians, nurses, midwives, and doulas, combined with advanced technology that includes a perinatal testing center with 3-D ultrasound and 24/7 neonatology.

Geriatrics Program

Maimonides serves one of the oldest inpatient populations in New York City, with one quarter of inpatients over the age of 75. The Geriatrics Program is fully equipped to meet the special needs of these seniors, including the assessment of memory loss and expertise in geriatric syndromes such as incontinence, falls, and frailty. The Program encompasses inpatient and outpatient services, features the Acute Care for Elderly (ACE) Unit, the Safe at Home program and home-visiting service.

Montefiore

Inspired Medicine

111 East 210th Street
Bronx, New York 10467
1-800-MD-MONTE
www.montefiore.org

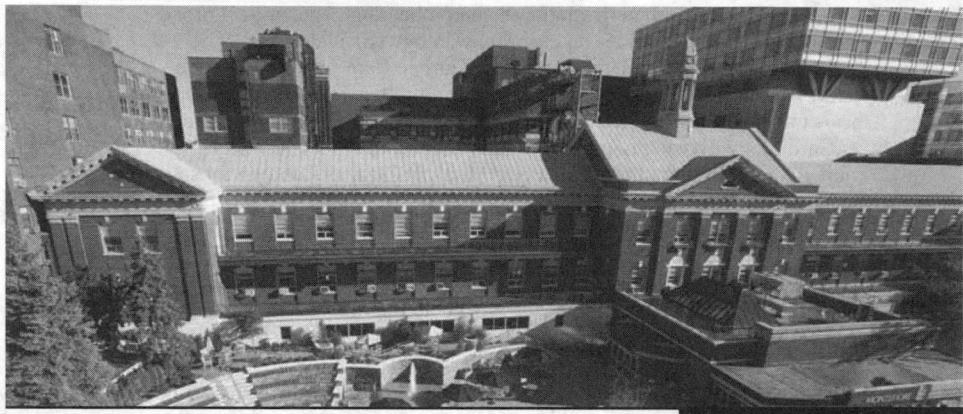

Montefiore, the University Hospital and academic medical center for Albert Einstein College of Medicine, is recognized by *U.S.News & World Report* as a leader in specialty and chronic care as well as in children's health. Montefiore was named among the top 50 hospitals in the country in Geriatrics, Diabetes and Endocrinology, and Neurology and Neurosurgery in "America's Best Hospitals." The Children's Hospital at Montefiore—recently listed among the top 10 in the nation in Kidney Disorders and among the top 25 in the nation in Neurology and Neurosurgery—has been consistently ranked in "America's Best Children's Hospitals."

Montefiore combines state-of-the-art technology with exceptional medical and nursing care in a teaching and research environment to provide patients with access to world-class medical experts, the most innovative treatments and the best patient experience available. This 1,491-bed medical center includes four hospitals; a large home healthcare agency; the largest school health program in the U.S.; a 23-site medical group practice integrated throughout the Bronx and Westchester; and a care management organization providing services to 179,000 health plan members.

Montefiore is a national leader in the research and treatment of acute and chronic diseases and is renowned for its model of care emphasizing accountability and interdisciplinary programs. With distinguished Centers of Excellence in heart and vascular care, cancer care, transplantation, children's health, surgery and neurosciences, Montefiore provides family-centered healthcare in a nurturing environment that extends well beyond its walls.

Montefiore's advanced programs include:

Adult and Pediatric Cardiology

Cardiac and Vascular Surgery

Cancer Care

Diabetes Management

Tissue and Organ Transplantation

Children's Health

Perinatal Care

Reproductive Medicine

Surgery and Surgical Subspecialties

Rehabilitation and Home Care

Neurology and Neurosurgery

Centers of Excellence

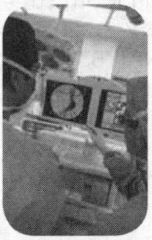

Montefiore Einstein Center for Heart and Vascular Care
The renowned expertise of the Center's clinicians, researchers and educators provide comprehensive, quality care to all patients. As a leader in cardiovascular care, our team continues to be a pioneer in the development of treatments for complex arrhythmias, hybrid approaches to coronary revascularization, minimally invasive techniques for heart valve repair and replacement, and mechanical assist devices for end-stage heart failure. Directed by world-renowned visionaries recruited from the nation's elite cardiac programs, Montefiore Einstein Center for Heart and Vascular Care provides innovative treatment options for all stages of cardiovascular care.

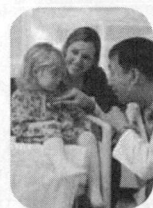

The Children's Hospital at Montefiore
One of the most advanced hospitals for children in the nation, The Children's Hospital at Montefiore (CHAM) is consistently ranked among the nation's leading institutions by *U.S.News & World Report*. Led by an internationally-recognized staff of physician and scientists, CHAM combines supreme clinical expertise, innovative research and leading-edge technology with an integrated, family-centric approach. As part of a premier academic medical center, CHAM trains the next generation of pediatric healthcare professionals and is transforming the future of children's health.

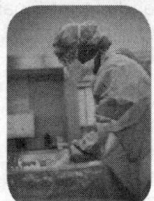

Montefiore Einstein Center for Transplantation
Through a novel approach, The Center for Transplantation unites Montefiore's clinical and surgical practices with the world-renowned expertise of Albert Einstein College of Medicine. Montefiore and Einstein have committed substantial resources to developing a center that includes transplantation for heart, liver, kidney and pancreas. We are a Center of Excellence with more than 40 years of experience. Our goals extend well beyond the integration of clinical practice and science, and include a holistic understanding of the on-going, medical and social needs of transplant patients.

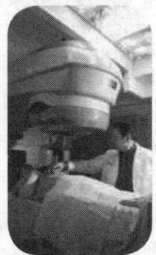

Montefiore Einstein Center for Cancer Care
Bringing together internationally-renowned experts with the latest technologies and cutting-edge research, the Montefiore Einstein Center for Cancer Care is known for its achievements in the prevention, diagnosis and treatment of rare and common cancers. Our multidisciplinary teams include medical, surgical and radiation oncologists, along with pathologists, radiologists and support specialists. They work together to provide each patient with the most effective, individualized treatment plan possible. The Montefiore Einstein Center for Cancer Care and its research partner, the National Cancer Institute-designated Albert Einstein Cancer Center, together develop groundbreaking approaches that are helping to revolutionize the stndard of cancer care.

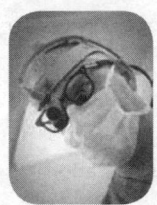

Surgery at Montefiore
Montefiore is a recognized world leader in the development of innovative new surgical procedures. With a proven reputation for performing even the most complex surgeries, our renowned surgeons provide both adults and children with extensive expertise in every surgical discipline. Employing state-of-the-art diagnostic, minimally invasive and robotic technologies, Montefiore continues to enhance surgical precision, reduce patient discomfort and speed recovery. Through leading-edge research, our surgeons offer the most advanced surgical procedures available anywhere today.

Montefiore Hospitals

Henry and Lucy Moses Division	Jack D. Weiler Division	North Division	The Children's Hospital at Montefiore
111 East 210th Street	1825 Eastchester Road	600 East 233rd Street	3415 Bainbridge Avenue
Bronx, New York 10467	Bronx, New York 10461	Bronx, New York 10466	Bronx, New York 10467

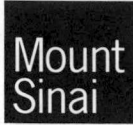
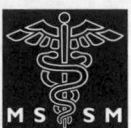

THE MOUNT SINAI MEDICAL CENTER
One Gustave L. Levy Place
Fifth Avenue and 100th Street
New York, NY 10029-6574
Physician Referral: 1-800-MD-SINAI (637-4624)
www.mountsinai.org

MOUNT SINAI SCHOOL OF MEDICINE

Sponsorship: Voluntary Not-for-Profit
Beds: 1,171
Accreditation: The Joint Commission;
Commission for Accreditation of Rehabilitation Facilities;
Magnet Award for Nursing Excellence

Since its founding over 150 years ago, The Mount Sinai Medical Center has been a leader in patient care and translational research. Generations of our patients have benefited as teams of physicians and scientists have always worked together to rapidly translate laboratory research into new treatments.

Located between the Upper East Side, and East and Central Harlem—New York City's most and least affluent communities—Mount Sinai provides a broad range of services that meet the needs of every patient we treat. The Medical Center consists of The Mount Sinai Hospital and Mount Sinai School of Medicine, both of which continue to be ranked by *U.S. News & World Report* as premier institutions in the nation.

In 2010, Mount Sinai was named among America's Best Hospitals, as determined by *U.S. News & World Report*. Mount Sinai was also ranked in 13 specialties: geriatric care; digestive disorders; neurology and neurosurgery; ear, nose and throat; heart and heart surgery; kidney disorders; gynecology; cancer; diabetes/endocrinology; psychiatry; rehabilitation; pulmonology; and urology. In addition, the School of Medicine was ranked 18th by the *Best Graduate Schools* edition.

Mount Sinai Heart, under the direction of Valentin Fuster, MD, PhD, combines Mount Sinai's world-class resources with innovative thinking, comprehensive and interdisciplinary programs, and an unwavering commitment to the prevention and treatment of cardiovascular disease. Mount Sinai became the first hospital in the country to successfully perform two unique procedures to treat atrial fibrillation: a non-surgical procedure to tie off the left atrial appendage, and a visually guided laser balloon catheter to ablate the condition. In a statewide study, our Cardiac Catheterization Laboratory was determined to be the busiest in New York State, and the safest, with the lowest 30-day risk-adjusted mortality rate. Building on the talent and expertise of internationally renowned Mount Sinai physicians David H. Adams, MD; Michael L. Marin, MD; Samin K. Sharma, MD; Eric A. Rose, MD; Vivek Y. Reddy, MD; and a host of other highly regarded cardiac surgeons, interventionalists, and cardiologists, Mount Sinai Heart provides patients with the most advanced approach to their care.

The Tisch Cancer Institute coordinates a full-service diagnostic and treatment program for cancer patients. Current clinical programs include those in cancer of the liver, breast, prostate, head and neck, as well as hematological malignancies, such as myeloproliferative disorders. In 2011, Mount Sinai will open the Dubin Breast Center to provide state-of-the-art detection and treatment, and address every aspect of breast health, in one centralized location.

Recognized as a national leader in organ transplantation, **The Recanati/Miller Transplantation Institute** is one of the few places in the country that provides multi-organ transplantation. Mount Sinai surgeons were the first in New York State to perform many combined transplant procedures, including liver and kidney transplantation, pediatric liver transplantation, and living adult- and pediatric-donor liver transplantation.

Geriatrics and Palliative Medicine specialists at Mount Sinai promote healthy aging and provide a balanced and integrated approach to improving the quality of life for New York's elderly. Ranked first in the country for geriatrics by *U.S. News & World Report*, Mount Sinai remains a national pioneer in geriatric medicine.

Mount Sinai's Neurology and Neurosurgery specialists are experts in skull base surgery and neuroendoscopy for adults and children with primary brain tumors and cerebrovascular, pituitary, and acoustic conditions, as well as epilepsy, disorders in neuromuscular transmission, peripheral nerve problems, and spinal reconstruction. Computerized stereotactic techniques allow three-dimensional localization of specific sites within the nervous system. Functional neurosurgery precisely targets abnormalities in the brain and spinal cord in combination with minimally invasive surgical approaches. Outpatient radiosurgery uses computer-assisted radiation to treat lesions without opening the skull.

Mount Sinai's **Gastrointestinal and Surgical Specialties** have developed and advanced numerous techniques to help patients with Crohn's disease and other digestive disorders lead healthier lives.

Rehabilitation Medicine at Mount Sinai offers comprehensive care for spinal cord injuries, brain injuries, and a variety of neuromuscular, musculoskeletal, and chronic conditions. Mount Sinai's Department of Rehabilitation Medicine is accredited by the Commission on Accreditation of Rehabilitation Facilities for the treatment of inpatient spinal cord and brain injury, and is home to a comprehensive physical and occupational therapy outpatient facility.

Mount Sinai's **Department of Orthopaedics** is dedicated to the preservation and restoration of the musculoskeletal system. Experts in surgery of the foot and ankle, knee, hip, hand, elbow, shoulder, and spine; total joint replacement; and microvascular, cancer, and minimally invasive surgeries provide personalized treatments using the latest technological innovations. In 2010, Mount Sinai opened a 5,000-square-foot Joint Replacement Center that offers easy access to care at all levels: pre-operative assessment, recovery, and therapy.

Minimally Invasive Surgery specializes in advanced procedures using state-of-the-art instruments. Mount Sinai surgeons are also adept at traditional surgical options.

A leader in the field of diabetes treatment, management, and research, Mount Sinai's **Division of Endocrinology, Diabetes, and Bone Disease** provides a full range of services to treat this growing public health epidemic. Children and adults with type 1 or type 2 diabetes are cared for by accomplished endocrinologists, nurse practitioners, and registered dietitians who provide specialized, state-of-the-art treatment to help patients safely manage their condition.

Mount Sinai's HIV/AIDS specialists offer cutting-edge treatments for the disease and common co-morbid conditions, such as Hepatitis-C, HIV-associated renal and neurologic disease, and cardiovascular disease — as well as care for the whole person, including primary and mental health care and prevention. In 2010, Mount Sinai merged with the former St. Vincent's Hospital HIV Center, which continues to operate at the same downtown location under the **Mount Sinai HIV Program,** making it one of the country's largest HIV programs with an anticipated 36,000 patient visits annually. The program is expanding access to research programs for new treatment regimens, and improving screening and treatment for emerging conditions.

The Kravis Children's Hospital was named among the best children's hospitals in the country by *U.S. News & World Report*, and ranked in the Top 25 in two specialties, gastroenterology and kidney diseases. Mount Sinai's health professionals offer advanced multidisciplinary treatment, supported by innovative research, effective community outreach, and advocacy programs. Mount Sinai offers pediatric treatment for heart, brain, and spine disorders; epilepsy, cancers and blood diseases; diabetes; gastrointestinal tract conditions; the full spectrum of renal disease and hypertension; asthma and other respiratory system illnesses; sleep problems; allergies; fetal and newborn conditions, and performs life-saving organ transplantations.

Under the direction of Angela Diaz, MD, MPH, **The Mount Sinai Adolescent Health Center** is the largest adolescent health facility of its kind in the United States, and is a national model and training site for health care professionals from around the world. Each year, it provides free and confidential services to more than 10,000 adolescents and young adults, from ages 10 to 24. The multidisciplinary team provides routine care, treatment of acute problems, mental health services, sexual health and reproductive health care, substance abuse prevention and treatment, HIV prevention and treatment, and medical-legal services. A multimillion dollar renovation in 2010 will allow the center to offer free dental and optical services, and treat an additional 5,000 patients a year.

⌐ NewYork-Presbyterian
⌐ The University Hospital of Columbia and Cornell

Affiliated with Columbia University College of Physicians and Surgeons and Weill Cornell Medical College

NewYork-Presbyterian Hospital
Weill Cornell Medical Center
525 East 68th Street
New York, NY 10065

NewYork-Presbyterian Hospital
Columbia University Medical Center
622 West 168th Street
New York, NY 10032

Sponsorship:	Voluntary Not-for-Profit
Beds:	2,369
Accreditation:	Joint Commission on Accreditation of Healthcare Organizations (JCAHO), Commission on Accreditation of Rehabilitation Facilities (CARF) and College of American Pathologists (CAP)

The *U.S. News & World Report* has ranked NewYork-Presbyterian Hospital higher in more specialties than any other hospital in the New York area. NewYork-Presbyterian Hospital was named to the *Honor Roll of America's Best Hospitals*.

OVERVIEW:

NewYork-Presbyterian Hospital is the largest hospital in New York and one of the most comprehensive healthcare institutions in the nation with 5,500 physicians, approximately 120,000 discharges and nearly 1.5 million outpatient visits annually, and with its affiliated medical schools, more than $600 million in research support. NewYork-Presbyterian is dedicated to providing top-quality care with sensitivity, warmth and compassion. The Hospital's world-class medical staff provides state-of-the-art diagnosis and treatment in all areas of medicine — including preventive and primary care—and in all specialties and subspecialties. The Hospital also offers inpatient and outpatient services at The Allen Pavilion in northern Manhattan, and at the Westchester Division, one of the nation's top ranked and the region's largest psychiatric facility.

AMONG ITS RENOWNED CENTERS OF EXCELLENCE ARE:

Morgan Stanley Children's Hospital and the Komansky Center for Children's Health— One of the largest, most comprehensive children's hospitals in the world providing highly sophisticated pediatric medical, surgical and intensive care, including a pediatric cardiovascular center, in a compassionate environment.

NewYork-Presbyterian Cancer Centers — Coordinated, multidisciplinary care and the latest therapeutic options and clinical trials. The Herbert Irving Comprehensive Cancer Center, located at Columbia Presbyterian, is one of only two cancer centers in the metropolitan area to have received the designation "comprehensive" from the National Cancer Institute.

NewYork-Presbyterian Heart — Expert diagnostic capabilities and medical and surgical innovations for simple to complex heart conditions. The Hospital's cardiac surgical mortality rates are among the lowest in the nation.

NewYork-Presbyterian Neuroscience Centers — Latest research, diagnosis and treatment capabilities in Alzheimer's disease, Multiple Sclerosis, Parkinson's disease, aneurysms, epilepsy, brain tumors, stokes and other neurological disorders.

NewYork-Presbyterian Psychiatry — World-renowned center of excellence in psychiatric treatment, research and education.

NewYork-Presbyterian Transplant Institute — Adult and pediatric heart, liver and kidney, and adult lung and pancreas transplantation and cutting-edge research.

NewYork-Presbyterian Vascular Care Center — Comprehensive and integrated preventive, diagnostic and treatment program for diverse problems related to arteries and veins throughout the body.

NewYork-Presbyterian Digestive Disease Services — Expert capabilities in the broad range of conditions that affect the organs as well as other components of the digestive system.

William Randolph Hearst Burn Center — Largest and busiest burn center in the nation which also conducts research to improve survival and enhance quality of life for burn victims.

In addition, the Hospital offers extraordinary expertise, comprehensive programs and specialized resources in the fields of:

AIDS — The Center for Special Studies at NewYork Weill Cornell and the AIDS Care Program at Columbia Presbyterian provide continuous, comprehensive care for men, women and children with HIV/AIDS. Both sites are designated AIDS centers by New York State and by the National Institutes of Health.

Gene Therapy — Research by Hospital physicians and scientists have made possible advances in the treatment of cardiac ischemia, atherosclerosis, breast cancer and cystic fibrosis.

Reproductive Medicine and Infertility — National leader in the field, the Hospital's prestigious IVF programs enjoy outstanding success rates.

Trauma Center — Level 1 designations as an Adult Trauma Unit and a Pediatric Trauma Unit ensure the Hospital upholds the highest standards of 24-hour preparedness and treatment.

Women's Health Care — One of the first hospitals dedicated to women's health, NewYork-Presbyterian has established comprehensive programs which provide healthcare to women through all stages of their lives.

ACADEMIC AFFILIATIONS:
NewYork-Presbyterian is the only hospital in the world affiliated with two Ivy League medical schools; The Joan and Sanford I Weill Medical College of Cornell University and the Columbia University College of Physicians and Surgeons.

NEWYORK-PRESBYTERIAN HEALTHCARE SYSTEM:
NewYork-Presbyterian Hospital is at the center of a premier healthcare system, which provides a comprehensive network of healthcare providers throughout the New York metropolitan area, including northern New Jersey, Westchester, the Hudson Valley and Fairfield, Connecticut. The full-service system includes 23 acute-care and community hospitals, 2 specialty institutions, 4 long-term facilities, and over 100 ambulatory-care centers.

Physician Referral: To find a NewYork-Presbyterian Hospital affiliated physician to meet your needs, call toll free **1-877-NYP-WELL** (1-877-697-9355) or visit our website at **www.nyp.org.**

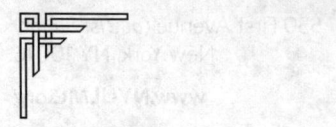

The Best in American Medicine
www.CastleConnolly.com

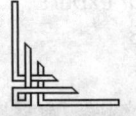
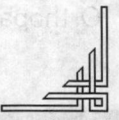

The New York metropolitan region is unique in its concentration of excellent Specialty Hospitals. Specialty Hospitals include those with a specific patient and disease focus such as cardiac care, psychiatric care and care of diseases and problems of eyes and ears. Many of these hospitals are nationally and internationally known for their outstanding care in these specialty areas and draw patients from the region and beyond who seek their excellent specialized care.

Castle Connolly Medical Ltd. has invited the following outstanding Specialty Hospitals to present important facts and information on their hospitals by sponsoring the profiles that follow.

Specialty Hospitals

Calvary Hospital

Hospital for Special Surgery

Memorial Sloan-Kettering Cancer Center

New York Eye & Ear Infirmary

Rusk Institute of Rehabilitation Medicine

St Francis Hospital - The Heart Center

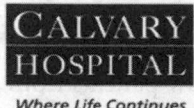

CALVARY HOSPITAL
Where Life Continues

1740 Eastchester Road
Bronx, NY 10461
Tel: (718) 518-2000
Fax: (718) 518-2674

150 55th Street
Brooklyn, NY 11220
Tel: (718) 518-2000
Fax: (718) 518-2670

www.calvaryhospital.org

Beds:	225 (200 in Bronx, 25 at Brooklyn Satellite located at Lutheran Medical Center)
Accreditation:	The Joint Commission, College of American Pathologists (CAP)

SETTING THE STANDARD FOR PALLIATIVE CARE

Founded in 1899, Calvary Hospital is the nation's only fully accredited acute care specialty hospital dedicated to providing palliative care to adult advanced cancer patients. We care for patients at a 200-bed Bronx facility and a 25-bed satellite at Lutheran Medical Center in Brooklyn. Calvary's family-centric approach helps more than 5,500 patients and families each year with inpatient care, outpatient care, Calvary@Home (Home Care and Hospice), and the Center for Curative and Palliative Wound Care. The Joint Commission gave Calvary Hospital and our Home Care/Hospice program the Gold Seal of Approval™ in 2009. Press Ganey consistently ranks Calvary in the top one percent of its peers in patient satisfaction. To learn more or sign up for the e-newsletter, *Calvary Life*, please go to www.calvaryhospital.org.

Palliative Care Institute
Calvary's research and education arm, offers a curriculum for medical students, residents, and postdoctoral fellows, and health lectures for the community.

Acute Inpatient Care
One-page form expedites admissions process. Adults with advanced cancer are assigned a primary physician and a care team: nurse, social worker, dietitian, and case manager. Goal is to maximize physical, spiritual, and emotional comfort. Pastoral care and bereavement support are integral to care.

Outpatient and Wound Care
Outpatient clinic for cancer patients undergoing active treatment or who do not require acute inpatient care. The Center for Curative and Palliative Wound Care treats complex wounds related to cancer, diabetes, vascular disease, and other illnesses.

Calvary@Home: Home Care, Hospice, Nursing Home Hospice

Certified Home Health Agency
We provides a full range of home care services, not limited to patients with advanced cancer, in Bronx, Queens, northern Manhattan, and southern Westchester. Our home care patients approaching the end of life have access to palliative care services such as pain and symptom management, assistance with advance care planning, and psychosocial support. Care is coordinated by patient's community physician or Calvary doctor. Nurse is available 24/7 for telephone consults.

Hospice & Nursing Home Hospice (NHH)
For people with all terminal diagnoses who are primarily cared for at home. Emphasis on quality of life, control of pain and symptoms, and support for family. Serves patients in Bronx, Brooklyn, Manhattan, Queens, Westchester, Nassau, and Rockland. Care may be coordinated by community physician or Calvary doctor. Nurse is available 24/7 by telephone. Bereavement support. Short-term hospitalization is available for acute symptom management.

NHH is for nursing home residents suffering from all end-stage illnesses. Goal is to promote quality of life.

Satellite Program
Calvary plans to develop new satellites in metropolitan New York to serve increasing numbers of people in our area.

Family Care
Focuses on the impact of cancer on the family. Extensive bereavement support for adults, teens, and children, including bereavement camp for children and teens who participate in our support groups.

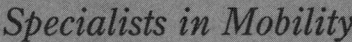

Memorial Sloan-Kettering Cancer Center

The Best Cancer Care. Anywhere.

1275 York Avenue
New York, NY 10065
Phone: (212) 639-2000
Make an Appointment: (800) 525-2225
www.mskcc.org

Beds: 434
Sponsorship/Network Affiliation: Private, Non-Profit
Make an Appointment: (800) 525-2225

THE MEMORIAL SLOAN-KETTERING ADVANTAGE: CANCER IS OUR ONLY FOCUS

At Memorial Sloan-Kettering Cancer Center (MSKCC), our only focus is cancer. Internationally recognized as one of the world's premier facilities for cancer care, we are consistently ranked as one of the nation's top cancer centers by *U.S. News & World Report*. We are proud to be a National Cancer Institute (NCI) Comprehensive Cancer Center and a member of the National Comprehensive Cancer Network.

A TEAM APPROACH TO CANCER CARE

Patients at MSKCC benefit from individualized treatment plans developed by a team of specialists with an unsurpassed depth and breadth of experience. The teams include surgeons, medical and radiation oncologists, radiologists, pathologists, nurses, and others who are specialists in treating patients with a specific type of cancer. They develop treatment plans that reflect their combined expertise, so that patients who need several different types of therapy will receive the best combination for them.

GREATER PRECISION IN DIAGNOSIS

Getting the correct diagnosis right from the start is crucial. At MSKCC, we use the most advanced imaging technologies, such as combined PET/CT and nuclear medicine scans, to accurately detect and precisely locate cancer. Our highly specialized pathologists analyze some 40,000 tumor samples annually to determine an exact diagnosis and the extent of disease. Increasingly, they use new technology to identify the molecular differences among tumors, allowing even greater precision in diagnosis.

UNPARALLELED SURGICAL EXPERTISE

Recent studies have shown that, for many cancers, patients have fewer complications and better outcomes if they have surgery at a hospital where high volumes of these operations are performed by surgeons with much experience in the procedure. MSKCC surgeons are among the most experienced cancer surgeons in the world. They use the latest surgical technology, including robotic and minimally invasive techniques, as well as interventional radiology for embolization, thermal ablation, and chemical ablation of tumors. In their quest to spare or reconstruct organs and preserve function, they are renowned for not only saving lives, but preserving the quality of life.

ADVANCES IN CHEMOTHERAPY

Our medical oncologists are leaders in developing new chemotherapy drugs that are safer and more effective than standard therapies. They also help manage any side effects of chemotherapy, such as nausea and fatigue, so patients can continue their usual activities wherever possible. Increasingly, our medical oncologists use advanced technologies, such as immunotherapies or vaccines, often in combination with chemotherapy.

LEADERS IN RADIATION THERAPY

MSKCC's radiation oncologists are highly skilled in complex treatment planning and sophisticated delivery techniques. For example, they have furthered intensity-modulated radiation therapy with image guidance (IGRT). IGRT enables them to image a tumor just before or even during a radiation treatment so they can adjust the radiation beams to pinpoint tumors with extreme accuracy. In some cases, our doctors may use radiation therapy combined with chemotherapy to make tumors more sensitive to the radiation, thus enhancing the chances of success.

RESEARCH EXPANDS TREATMENT OPTIONS

Through close collaboration between clinicians and research scientists, new therapies developed in the laboratory can be quickly translated into improved treatment options for patients.

INSURANCE

Memorial Sloan-Kettering Cancer Center is in-network with most New York–area insurance plans.

Make an Appointment: (800) 525-2225

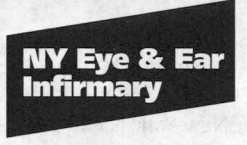

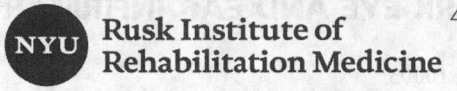

NYU Rusk Institute of Rehabilitation Medicine
NYU LANGONE MEDICAL CENTER

400 East 34th Street *(between 1st Avenue and FDR Drive)*
New York, NY 10016
HJD: 301 East 17th Street (at 2nd Avenue):
New York, NY 10003
www.RUSKINSTITUTE.org • (212) 598-6252

The rehabilitation care at the Rusk Institute of Rehabilitation Medicine at NYU Langone Medical Center is the best in New York and among the best in the world. Voted the best rehabilitation hospital in New York and among the top ten in the country for more than 20 years by U.S. News & World Report, it was founded in 1948 and is the largest center of its kind for the treatment of adults and children with disabilities in New York City. *We specialize in the following areas:*

Inpatient Programs:
The Brain Injury Program provides a structured therapeutic program tailored to meet the medical and rehabilitative needs of patients who have sustained a brain injury or neurological illness.
Specialized limb deficiency programs are available to patients who have undergone amputations.
The Medically Complex Conditions Unit offers individualized treatment programs for patients with a variety of medically complex conditions such as spinal cord injuries, multiple sclerosis, Parkinson's disease, amputations and pain syndrome.
Specialized pediatric therapy programs are available to newborns, children and young adults, including communication programs, educational services, occupational therapy, physical therapy, psychology and speech-language pathology services.
The Joan and Joel Smilow Cardiac Rehabilitation & Prevention Center provides personalized cardiac rehabilitation.
The William Randolph Hearst Foundation Stroke Rehabilitation Unit treats all aspects of stroke rehabilitation.

Outpatient Programs and Specialty Services:
The Adult Physical Therapy Outpatient Program offers evaluation and treatment for musculoskeletal and neurological disorders through individual and group programs.
The Chest Physical Therapy Program provides programs to individuals with lung congestion, secretion retention or areas of lung collapse. Occupational therapists work with individuals to devise a comprehensive treatment program to help them regain their independence in daily tasks.
The Outpatient Rehabilitation Psychology Service is the largest of its kind in the region, providing care to patients with neurological and medical conditions on an outpatient basis.
The Physical Therapy Department provides an array of outpatient programs designed to address concerns associated with pregnancy, osteoporosis, pelvic floor dysfunction and some cancers.
The Speech-Language Pathology Department offers rehabilitation services to patients with communication disorders due to neurological problems.
The Swallowing Disorders Center is dedicated to the diagnosis and therapeutic management of swallowing and feeding disorders.
The Vestibular Rehabilitation Program is the first program of its kind in the tri-state area, providing diagnosis and treatment for patients suffering from dizziness and imbalance.
The Vocational Services Department provides individuals with disabilities with the competencies needed to return to school, work and to lead a productive lifestyle.

Specialty Clinics:
The Adult Spasticity Clinic provides examination and treatment to patients with spasticity, resulting from cerebral palsy, traumatic brain injury, spinal cord injury, multiple sclerosis and stroke. Patients with neuromuscular disease receivephysical and occupational therapies, vocational counseling, equipment and seating and mobility services.

St. Francis Hospital The Heart Center®
100 Port Washington Blvd.
Roslyn, New York 11576
www.stfrancisheartcenter.com
(516) 562-6000   1-888-HEARTNY

St. Francis Hospital, The Heart Center® is New York State's only specialty designated cardiac center, offering one of the leading cardiac care programs in the nation. Founded in 1922 by the Franciscan Missionaries of Mary, the Hospital is recognized as an innovator in the delivery of specialized cardiovascular services in an environment where excellence and compassion are emphasized. St. Francis also offers a superb program in non-cardiac surgery, including some of the most advanced technology and minimally invasive techniques available for vascular, prostate, ear-nose-throat (ENT), abdominal, oncologic, and orthopedic surgery.

Cardiac Diagnostics and Treatment
St. Francis Hospital performs one of the highest volumes of cardiac surgical, interventional and arrhythmia procedures in the nation and has been consistently recognized for its outstanding quality of care. In 2010, St. Francis Hospital was ranked as one of America's best hospitals by *U.S. News & World Report*.

Cardiac surgery: In 2009, 1,597 open-heart surgeries were performed at St. Francis Hospital. The Hospital's seven cardiothoracic surgeons have the combined experience of over 20,000 open-heart procedures in the last 10 years alone and are experts in all types of heart surgery, from conventional, open-heart bypass to off-pump coronary artery bypass (OPCAB) to the newest, minimally invasive valve procedures, including surgical techniques designed to treat certain cardiac arrhythmias or irregular heart rhythms.

Cardiac catheterization: In 2009, St. Francis interventional cardiologists performed 8,739 cardiac catheterizations and 3,591 percutaneous coronary interventions (angioplasty and insertion of stents). The Hospital is also recognized as one of the East Coast's highest volume centers for catheter-based techniques to close atrial septal defects (ASDs) and patent foramen ovale (PFO).

Arrhythmia and Pacemaker Center: St. Francis has a leading national program for pacemaker implantation and the diagnosis and treatment of cardiac rhythm abnormalities. The Center has unparalleled expertise in radiofrequency cardiac ablation, including treatment of atrial fibrillation.

Research and Technology: At the St. Francis Cardiac Research Institute, a team of world-renowned researchers is working with the latest non-invasive imaging technology, including advanced techniques and world-class expertise in cardiac CT angiography, cardiac magnetic resonance imaging, cardiac PET/CT and three-dimensional echocardiography. This multimodality approach to investigating the heart's function and disease processes is aimed at improving methods of diagnosing heart disease.

Prevention and Education
St. Francis Hospital's satellite campus, The DeMatteis Center for Cardiac Research and Education, in Greenvale, New York, is one of the few freestanding campuses in the U.S. dedicated to the prevention of heart disease. It is the site of community health lectures, as well as the largest medically staffed cardiac fitness and rehabilitation program on Long Island.

Physician referral: **1-888-HEARTNY**
Sponsorship: Voluntary not-for-profit
Beds: 316
Accreditation: Awarded accreditation from the Joint Commission.

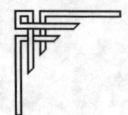

The Best in American Medicine
www.CastleConnolly.com

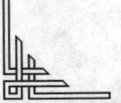
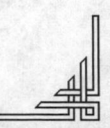

New York State Metropolitan Regional Medical Centers and Hospitals

The New York metropolitan region is fortunate to have a large number of truly excellent Regional Medical Centers and Hospitals. Many of these institutions offer sophisticated services that in years past were offered only at academic medical centers. However, with advancements in medical technology, Regional Medical Centers and Hospitals have access to the equipment, and by virtue of the medical schools and teaching hospitals in the region, the well-trained physicians and staff, to offer these programs.

Regional Medical Centers and Hospitals range in size from the small (100 beds) to the very large (800 beds) but they share a common theme: a primary focus on patient care.

We have invited a select number of excellent Regional Medical Centers and Hospitals to provide readers of the Castle Connolly Guide with information on their institutions and services by sponsoring profiles, which are included at the end of individual county sections in the physician listings that follow.

Regional Medical Centers and Hospitals

Englewood Hospital & Medical Center

Greenwich Hospital

Holy Name Hospital

New York Methodist Hospital

Phelps Memorial Hospital Center

Stamford Hospital

SUNY Downstate Medical Center

Trinitas Regional Medical Center

The Valley Hospital

SECTION THREE

Physician Listings

The State of New York

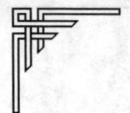

The Best in American Medicine
www.CastleConnolly.com

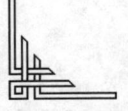
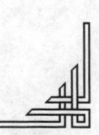

New York (Manhattan)

Addiction Psychiatry

Frances, Richard J MD (AdP) - **Spec Exp:** Addiction/Substance Abuse; Anxiety & Mood Disorders; Forensic Psychiatry; **Hospital:** Silver Hill Hosp, NYU Langone Med Ctr (page 106); **Address:** 510 E 86th St, Ste 1D, New York, NY 10028; **Phone:** 212-861-0570; **Board Cert:** Psychiatry 1976; Addiction Psychiatry 2002; **Med School:** NYU Sch Med 1971; **Resid:** Psychiatry, Bronx Meml Hosp 1974; **Fellow:** Psychoanalysis, NY Psychoanalitic Inst 1984; **Fac Appt:** Clin Prof Psyc, NYU Sch Med

Galanter, Marc MD (AdP) - **Spec Exp:** Alcohol Abuse; Drug Abuse; **Hospital:** NYU Langone Med Ctr (page 106), Bellevue Hosp Ctr; **Address:** 285 Central Park West, New York, NY 10024-3006; **Phone:** 212-877-4093; **Board Cert:** Psychiatry 1974; Addiction Psychiatry 2002; **Med School:** Albert Einstein Coll Med 1967; **Resid:** Psychiatry, Bronx Muni Hosp-Einstein 1971; **Fac Appt:** Prof Psyc, NYU Sch Med

Kleber, Herbert MD (AdP) - **Spec Exp:** Opiate Addiction; Cocaine Addiction; Marijuana Abuse; Drug Abuse; **Hospital:** NY-Presby Hosp/Columbia (page 104), NY State Psychiatric Inst; **Address:** NY State Psychiatric Inst, 1051 Riverside Drive, Room 3713, Unit 66, New York, NY 10032-1007; **Phone:** 212-543-5570; **Med School:** Jefferson Med Coll 1960; **Resid:** Psychiatry, Yale-New Haven Hosp 1964; **Fac Appt:** Prof Psyc, Columbia P&S

Levin, Frances R MD (AdP) - **Spec Exp:** Addiction/Substance Abuse; Dual Diagnosis; Substance Abuse in ADHD Patients; **Hospital:** NY State Psychiatric Inst, NY-Presby Hosp/Columbia (page 104); **Address:** NYSPI, Dept Psychiatry-RFMH, 1051 Riverside Drive, Box 66, New York, NY 10032; **Phone:** 212-923-3031; **Board Cert:** Psychiatry 1990; Addiction Psychiatry 2002; **Med School:** Cornell Univ-Weill Med Coll 1985; **Resid:** Psychiatry, Payne Whitney Clin 1989; **Fellow:** Substance Abuse, Univ Maryland/NIDA 1990; **Fac Appt:** Assoc Prof Psyc, Columbia P&S

Paul, Edward MD (AdP) - **Spec Exp:** Opiate Addiction; Alcohol Abuse; Smoking Cessation; **Hospital:** NYU Langone Med Ctr (page 106); **Address:** 155 E 31st St, Ste 25J, New York, NY 10016; **Phone:** 212-447-5712; **Board Cert:** Psychiatry 1987; Addiction Psychiatry 2003; **Med School:** Columbia P&S 1982; **Resid:** Psychiatry, Payne Whitney Clinic 1987; Psychoanalysis, NYU Med Ctr 1993; **Fellow:** Substance Abuse, New York Hosp 1987; **Fac Appt:** Asst Clin Prof Psyc, NYU Sch Med

Rosenberg, Kenneth P MD (AdP) - **Spec Exp:** Addiction/Substance Abuse; Sexual Dysfunction; Physicians' Health-Psychiatric; **Hospital:** NY-Presby Hosp/Weill Cornell (page 104); **Address:** 49 E 78th St, Ste 2A, New York, NY 10075; **Phone:** 212-861-8807; **Board Cert:** Psychiatry 1992; Addiction Psychiatry 2009; **Med School:** Albert Einstein Coll Med 1983; **Resid:** Psychiatry, NY Hosp-Cornell Med Ctr 1988; **Fellow:** Substance Abuse, NY Hosp-Cornell Med Ctr 1991; Public Health, NY Hosp-Cornell Med Ctr 1992; **Fac Appt:** Assoc Clin Prof Psyc, Cornell Univ-Weill Med Coll

Weiss, Carol J MD (AdP) - **Spec Exp:** Drug Abuse; Alcohol Abuse; **Hospital:** NY-Presby Hosp/Weill Cornell (page 104); **Address:** 1044 Madison Ave, Ste PH1, New York, NY 10075; **Phone:** 212-988-1209; **Board Cert:** Psychiatry 1989; Addiction Psychiatry 2003; Addiction Medicine 2009; **Med School:** Johns Hopkins Univ 1983; **Resid:** Psychiatry, New York Hosp 1987; **Fellow:** Addiction Psychiatry, New York Hosp 1989; **Fac Appt:** Asst Clin Prof Psyc, Cornell Univ-Weill Med Coll

Adolescent Medicine

Diaz, Angela MD (AM) - **Spec Exp:** Adolescent Gynecology; Abuse/Neglect; **Hospital:** Mount Sinai Med Ctr (page 102); **Address:** 320 E 94th St Fl 2, New York, NY 10128-5604; **Phone:** 212-423-2900; **Board Cert:** Pediatrics 1987; Adolescent Medicine 2004; **Med School:** Columbia P&S 1981; **Resid:** Pediatrics, Mt Sinai Med Ctr 1984; **Fellow:** Adolescent Medicine, Mt Sinai Med Ctr 1985; **Fac Appt:** Prof Ped, Mount Sinai Sch Med

Lopez, Ralph I MD (AM) - **Spec Exp:** Growth/Development Disorders; Eating Disorders; Learning Disorders; Parenting Issues; **Hospital:** NY-Presby Hosp/Weill Cornell (page 104), Lenox Hill Hosp; **Address:** 418 E 71st St, New York, NY 10021-4894; **Phone:** 212-772-8989; **Board Cert:** Pediatrics 1972; **Med School:** NYU Sch Med 1967; **Resid:** Pediatrics, Bellevue Hosp 1969; Pediatrics, Chldns Hosp 1970; **Fellow:** Adolescent Medicine, Chldns Hosp 1971; **Fac Appt:** Clin Prof Ped, Cornell Univ-Weill Med Coll

Marks, Andrea M MD (AM) - **Spec Exp:** Eating Disorders; Adolescent Gynecology; Psychosomatic Disorders; Parenting Issues; **Hospital:** Mount Sinai Med Ctr (page 102); **Address:** 14 E 90th St, Ste 1-B, New York, NY 10128-0671; **Phone:** 212-987-1414; **Board Cert:** Pediatrics 1977; **Med School:** Univ Pennsylvania 1972; **Resid:** Pediatrics, Chldns Hosp 1974; **Fellow:** Adolescent Medicine, Chldns Hosp 1975; **Fac Appt:** Assoc Clin Prof Ped, Mount Sinai Sch Med

Nucci, Anne T MD (AM) - **Spec Exp:** Adolescent Gynecology; Vaccines; **Hospital:** Mount Sinai Med Ctr (page 102); **Address:** 312 E 94th St, New York, NY 10128; **Phone:** 212-423-3000; **Board Cert:** Pediatrics 1986; Adolescent Medicine 2009; **Med School:** NY Med Coll 1981; **Resid:** Pediatrics, Bronx Municipal Hosp 1984; **Fellow:** Adolescent Medicine, Montefiore Hosp 1990; **Fac Appt:** Asst Prof Ped, Mount Sinai Sch Med

Pegler, Cynthia R MD (AM) - **Spec Exp:** Adolescent Gynecology; Eating Disorders; **Hospital:** Lenox Hill Hosp, NY-Presby Hosp/Weill Cornell (page 104); **Address:** 992 5th Ave, New York, NY 10028; **Phone:** 212-517-5313; **Board Cert:** Pediatrics 2005; Adolescent Medicine 2008; **Med School:** Albany Med Coll 1984; **Resid:** Pediatrics, N Shore Univ Hosp 1987; **Fellow:** Adolescent Medicine, N Shore Univ Hosp 1990

Allergy & Immunology

Bassett, Clifford MD (A&I) - **Spec Exp:** Asthma & Sinusitis; Food Allergy; Pet Allergy; **Hospital:** NYU Langone Med Ctr (page 106), Long Island Coll Hosp (page 94); **Address:** 381 Park Ave S, New York, NY 10010; **Phone:** 212-260-6078; **Board Cert:** Allergy & Immunology 2006; **Med School:** Mexico 1984; **Resid:** Internal Medicine, Hackensack Med Ctr 1989; **Fellow:** Allergy & Immunology, LI College Hosp 1993; **Fac Appt:** Asst Clin Prof Med, SUNY Hlth Sci Ctr

Buchbinder, Ellen MD (A&I) - **Spec Exp:** Asthma & Allergy; Rhinitis; Hives; Food & Drug Allergy; **Hospital:** Mount Sinai Med Ctr (page 102); **Address:** 111B E 88th St, New York, NY 10128; **Phone:** 212-410-3246; **Board Cert:** Internal Medicine 1981; Allergy & Immunology 1983; **Med School:** Tulane Univ 1978; **Resid:** Internal Medicine, New England Deaconess Hosp 1981; **Fellow:** Allergy & Immunology, Mass Genl Hosp 1983; **Fac Appt:** Asst Clin Prof Med, Mount Sinai Sch Med

Burton, Daniel A MD (A&I) - **Spec Exp:** Rhinitis; Asthma; Food & Drug Allergy; Urticaria; **Hospital:** NY-Presby Hosp/Weill Cornell (page 104), Hosp For Special Surgery (page 111); **Address:** 235 E 67th St, Ste 203, New York, NY 10065; **Phone:** 212-288-9300; **Board Cert:** Internal Medicine 1989; Allergy & Immunology 2003; **Med School:** Wright State Univ 1984; **Resid:** Internal Medicine, St Lukes-Roosevelt Hosp Ctr 1987; **Fellow:** Allergy & Immunology, NY Hosp 1989; **Fac Appt:** Asst Prof Med, Cornell Univ-Weill Med Coll

Chandler, Michael MD (A&I) - **Spec Exp:** Asthma; Sinus Disorders; Airway Disorders; **Hospital:** Mount Sinai Med Ctr (page 102); **Address:** 115 E 61st St Fl 12, New York, NY 10021-8183; **Phone:** 212-486-6715; **Board Cert:** Internal Medicine 1984; Allergy & Immunology 1987; **Med School:** Wayne State Univ 1981; **Resid:** Internal Medicine, Northwestern Meml Hosp 1984; **Fellow:** Allergy & Immunology, Northwestern Meml Hosp 1986; **Fac Appt:** Asst Clin Prof Med, Mount Sinai Sch Med

Corn, Beth E MD (A&I) - **Spec Exp:** Asthma; **Hospital:** Mount Sinai Med Ctr (page 102); **Address:** 5 E 98th St, Box 1089, New York, NY 10029; **Phone:** 212-241-0764; **Board Cert:** Allergy & Immunology 2005; **Med School:** Albert Einstein Coll Med 1989; **Resid:** Internal Medicine, St Lukes-Roosevelt Hosp 1992; **Fellow:** Clinical Immunology, Mt Sinai Med Ctr 1994; **Fac Appt:** Asst Prof Med, Mount Sinai Sch Med

Cunningham-Rundles, Charlotte MD/PhD (A&I) - **Spec Exp:** Immunotherapy; Immunodeficiency Disorders; **Hospital:** Mount Sinai Med Ctr (page 102); **Address:** 5 E 98th St, New York, NY 10029; **Phone:** 212-659-9268; **Board Cert:** Internal Medicine 1972; **Med School:** Columbia P&S 1969; **Resid:** Internal Medicine, Bellevue Hosp Ctr 1972; **Fellow:** Allergy & Immunology, NYU Med Ctr 1974; **Fac Appt:** Prof Med, Mount Sinai Sch Med

Feldman, B Robert MD (A&I) - **Spec Exp:** Asthma; Allergic Rhinitis; Food Allergy; Eczema; **Hospital:** NYPresby-Morgan Stanley Children's Hosp (page 104); **Address:** Morgan Stanley Chlds Hosp NY-Presby, 3959 Broadway, New York, NY 10032; **Phone:** 212-305-2300; **Board Cert:** Pediatrics 1965; Allergy & Immunology 1972; **Med School:** Ros Franklin Univ/Chicago Med Sch 1959; **Resid:** Pediatrics, Michael Reese Hosp 1962; Allergy & Immunology, Michael Reese Hosp 1963; **Fellow:** Allergy & Immunology, Columbia-Presby Med Ctr 1964; **Fac Appt:** Clin Prof Ped, Columbia P&S

Frenkel, Renata MD (A&I) - **Spec Exp:** Asthma; Allergy; Sinus Disorders; Urticaria; **Hospital:** St Luke's - Roosevelt Hosp Ctr - Roosevelt Div (page 94), Lenox Hill Hosp; **Address:** 30 W 60th St, Ste 1U, New York, NY 10023-7906; **Phone:** 212-265-1990; **Board Cert:** Allergy & Immunology 1979; **Med School:** Austria 1968; **Resid:** Allergy & Immunology, Roosevelt Hosp 1975; **Fac Appt:** Assoc Clin Prof Ped, Columbia P&S

Grubman, Samuel MD (A&I) - **Spec Exp:** Asthma & Allergy; Food Allergy; Immunodeficiency Disorders; Pediatric Allergy & Immunology; **Hospital:** NYU Langone Med Ctr (page 106); **Address:** 154 W 14th St Fl 4, New York, NY 10011; **Phone:** 212-616-4122; **Board Cert:** Pediatrics 1987; Allergy & Immunology 2009; **Med School:** Mount Sinai Sch Med 1983; **Resid:** Pediatrics, NYU Med Ctr 1986; **Fellow:** Allergy & Immunology, Montefiore Med Ctr 1988; **Fac Appt:** Asst Prof Ped, NYU Sch Med

Lubitz, Arthur M MD (A&I) - **Spec Exp:** Allergy; Asthma; Immunotherapy; **Hospital:** Lenox Hill Hosp, NY Downtown Hosp; **Address:** 250 W 57th St, Ste 1231, New York, NY 10107; **Phone:** 212-247-7447; **Board Cert:** Internal Medicine 1984; Allergy & Immunology 2001; **Med School:** SUNY Downstate 1980; **Resid:** Internal Medicine, Coney Island Hosp 1983; **Fellow:** Allergy & Immunology, Long Island Coll Hosp 1985; **Fac Appt:** Asst Clin Prof

Mazza, David S MD (A&I) - **Spec Exp:** Asthma; Sinus Disorders; Eczema; **Hospital:** St Luke's - Roosevelt Hosp Ctr - Roosevelt Div (page 94); **Address:** 7 Lexington Ave, Ste 3, New York, NY 10010-5517; **Phone:** 212-677-7170; **Board Cert:** Pediatrics 1983; Allergy & Immunology 2008; **Med School:** Univ VT Coll Med 1977; **Resid:** Pediatrics, NYU-Bellevue Hosp 1980; **Fellow:** Pediatric Allergy & Immunology, Bellevue Hosp 1982; **Fac Appt:** Assoc Prof Ped, Columbia P&S

Resnick, David J MD (A&I) - **Spec Exp:** Asthma; Eczema; Nasal Allergies; Food Allergy; **Hospital:** NY-Presby Hosp/Columbia (page 104); **Address:** 3959 Broadway, rm 107N, New York, NY 10032; **Phone:** 718-796-9393; **Board Cert:** Allergy & Immunology 2001; Pediatrics 2005; **Med School:** SUNY Hlth Sci Ctr 1986; **Resid:** Pediatrics, Brookdale Hosp 1989; **Fellow:** Allergy & Immunology, Columbia-Presby Med Ctr 1991; **Fac Appt:** Assoc Clin Prof Ped, Columbia P&S

Rubin, James MD (A&I) - **Spec Exp:** Asthma; Rhinitis; Sinus Disorders; **Hospital:** Beth Israel Med Ctr - Petrie Division (page 94); **Address:** 35 E 35th St, Ste 202, New York, NY 10016-3823; **Phone:** 212-685-4225; **Board Cert:** Internal Medicine 1968; Allergy & Immunology 1972; **Med School:** NY Med Coll 1960; **Resid:** Internal Medicine, Beth Israel Hosp 1964; **Fellow:** Allergy & Immunology, Jewish Hosp 1965; **Fac Appt:** Assoc Clin Prof Med, Albert Einstein Coll Med

Shepherd, Gillian M MD (A&I) - **Spec Exp:** Food & Drug Allergy; Rhinosinusitis & Asthma; Urticaria; Insect Allergies; **Hospital:** NY-Presby Hosp/Weill Cornell (page 104); **Address:** 235 E 67th St, Ste 203, New York, NY 10021-6040; **Phone:** 212-288-9300; **Board Cert:** Internal Medicine 1979; Allergy & Immunology 1981; **Med School:** NY Med Coll 1976; **Resid:** Internal Medicine, Lenox Hill Hosp 1979; **Fellow:** Allergy & Immunology, New York Hosp-Cornell 1981; **Fac Appt:** Assoc Clin Prof Med, Cornell Univ-Weill Med Coll

Siegal, Frederick P MD (A&I) - **Spec Exp:** AIDS/HIV; Immune Deficiency; **Hospital:** Mount Sinai Med Ctr (page 102); **Address:** 36 Seventh Ave, Ste 572, New York, NY 10011; **Phone:** 877-344-4908; **Board Cert:** Internal Medicine 1971; Allergy & Immunology 1979; **Med School:** Columbia P&S 1965; **Resid:** Internal Medicine, Mt Sinai Hosp 1970; **Fellow:** Immunology, Rockefeller Univ 1973

Slankard, Marjorie MD (A&I) - **Spec Exp:** Sinus Disorders; Asthma; Food Allergy; Hereditary Angioedema; **Hospital:** NY-Presby Hosp/Columbia (page 104), Valley Hosp (page 658); **Address:** 16 E 60th St, Ste 321, New York, NY 10022-1002; **Phone:** 212-326-8410; **Board Cert:** Internal Medicine 1974; Allergy & Immunology 1977; **Med School:** Univ MO-Columbia Sch Med 1971; **Resid:** Internal Medicine, New York Hosp 1974; Internal Medicine, Rockefeller Univ Hosp 1974; **Fellow:** Immunology, New York Hosp-Cornell 1976; Immunology, Mount Sinai Med Ctr 1980; **Fac Appt:** Clin Prof Med, Columbia P&S

Tolston, Evelyn MD (A&I) - **Spec Exp:** Rhinitis; Asthma; Allergy; Sinusitis; **Hospital:** NYU Langone Med Ctr (page 106), Beth Israel Med Ctr - Petrie Division (page 94); **Address:** 161 Madison Ave, Ste 3A, New York, NY 10016; **Phone:** 646-424-0400; **Board Cert:** Allergy & Immunology 2005; **Med School:** Ukraine 1982; **Resid:** Internal Medicine, Cabrini Med Ctr 1993; Allergy & Immunology, Albert Einstein Coll Med 1995

Young, Stuart H MD (A&I) - **Spec Exp:** Asthma; Nasal & Sinus Disorders; Urticaria; Eczema; **Hospital:** Mount Sinai Med Ctr (page 102); **Address:** 121 E 60th St, Ste 1D, New York, NY 10022-1102; **Phone:** 212-826-0815; **Board Cert:** Pediatrics 1968; Allergy & Immunology 1972; **Med School:** SUNY Downstate 1963; **Resid:** Pediatrics, Kings Co Hosp 1966; **Fellow:** Allergy & Immunology, Natl Jewish Hosp 1970; **Fac Appt:** Assoc Clin Prof Med, Mount Sinai Sch Med

Cardiac Electrophysiology

Chinitz, Larry MD (CE) - **Spec Exp:** Arrhythmias; Pacemakers; Defibrillators; Atrial Fibrillation; **Hospital:** NYU Langone Med Ctr (page 106); **Address:** 403 E 34th St, Heart Rhythm Center, 4th Fl, New York, NY 10016-6402; **Phone:** 212-263-7149; **Board Cert:** Internal Medicine 1982; Cardiovascular Disease 1985; **Med School:** NYU Sch Med 1979; **Resid:** Internal Medicine, Bellevue Hosp Ctr 1983; **Fellow:** Cardiovascular Disease, Bellevue Hosp Ctr 1986; Cardiac Electrophysiology, Montefiore Hosp 1985; **Fac Appt:** Assoc Prof Med, NYU Sch Med

Garan, Hasan MD (CE) - **Spec Exp:** Arrhythmias; Cardiac Catheterization; Pacemakers/Defibrillators; **Hospital:** NY-Presby Hosp/Columbia (page 104); **Address:** 173 Fort Washington Ave Fl 4 - rm 640, New York, NY 10032; **Phone:** 212-305-8559; **Board Cert:** Internal Medicine 1977; Cardiovascular Disease 1979; **Med School:** Harvard Med Sch 1974; **Resid:** Internal Medicine, Hosp Univ Penn 1976; **Fellow:** Cardiovascular Disease, Mass Genl Hosp 1978; Cardiac Electrophysiology, Mass Genl Hosp 1979; **Fac Appt:** Prof Med, Columbia P&S

Gomes, J Anthony MD (CE) - **Spec Exp:** Arrhythmias; Heart Attack; Atrial Fibrillation; Pacemakers; **Hospital:** Mount Sinai Med Ctr (page 102); **Address:** Mount Sinai Medical Ctr, One Gustave L Levy Pl, Box 1054, New York, NY 10029-6500; **Phone:** 212-241-7272; **Board Cert:** Internal Medicine 1974; Cardiovascular Disease 1975; **Med School:** India 1970; **Resid:** Internal Medicine, Mt Sinai Med Ctr 1973; **Fellow:** Cardiovascular Disease, Mt Sinai Med Ctr 1975; Cardiac Electrophysiology, USPHS Cardio-Pulmonary Lab 1976; **Fac Appt:** Prof Med, Mount Sinai Sch Med

Lerman, Bruce MD (CE) - **Spec Exp:** Catheter Ablation; Defibrillators; Arrhythmias; **Hospital:** NY-Presby Hosp/Weill Cornell (page 104); **Address:** NY Weill Cornell Med Ctr, 520 E 70th St, Starr 4, New York, NY 10021-9800; **Phone:** 212-746-2169; **Board Cert:** Internal Medicine 1980; Cardiovascular Disease 1985; Cardiac Electrophysiology 2002; **Med School:** Loyola Univ-Stritch Sch Med 1977; **Resid:** Internal Medicine, Northwestern Univ Hosp 1980; Internal Medicine, Univ Michigan Med Ctr 1981; **Fellow:** Cardiovascular Disease, Hosp Univ Penn 1982; Cardiovascular Disease, Johns Hopkins Hosp 1983; **Fac Appt:** Prof Med, Cornell Univ-Weill Med Coll

Markowitz, Steven M MD (CE) - **Spec Exp:** Arrhythmias; **Hospital:** NY-Presby Hosp/Weill Cornell (page 104); **Address:** Cardiac Electrophysiology, 520 E 70th St, Starr Fl 4, New York, NY 10021; **Phone:** 212-746-2655; **Board Cert:** Internal Medicine 2001; Cardiovascular Disease 2005; Cardiac Electrophysiology 2006; **Med School:** Harvard Med Sch 1988; **Resid:** Internal Medicine, New York Hosp 1991; **Fellow:** Cardiovascular Disease, New York Hosp-Cornell 1995; Cardiac Electrophysiology, New York Hosp-Cornell 1996; **Fac Appt:** Assoc Prof Med, Cornell Univ-Weill Med Coll

Matos, Jeffrey A MD (CE) - **Spec Exp:** Arrhythmias; Pacemakers; Defibrillators; **Hospital:** Lenox Hill Hosp; **Address:** Arrhythmia Associates, 1421 Third Ave Fl 5, New York, NY 10028; **Phone:** 212-772-6384; **Board Cert:** Internal Medicine 1980; Cardiovascular Disease 1983; **Med School:** Harvard Med Sch 1975; **Resid:** Internal Medicine, Beth Israel Hosp 1978; **Fellow:** Cardiovascular Disease, Peter Bent Brigham Hosp 1980; **Fac Appt:** Assoc Clin Prof Med, NYU Sch Med

Mehta, Davendra MD/PhD (CE) - **Spec Exp:** Arrhythmias; Congenital Heart Disease-Adult; Atrial Fibrillation; Heart Failure; **Hospital:** Mount Sinai Med Ctr (page 102), VA Med Ctr - Bronx; **Address:** One Gustave L Levy Pl Fl 3, New York, NY 10029-6501; **Phone:** 212-241-7272; **Board Cert:** Cardiovascular Disease 2009; Cardiac Electrophysiology 2010; **Med School:** India 1979; **Resid:** Internal Medicine, Leicester Royal Infirmary 1983; **Fellow:** Cardiovascular Disease, Groby Road Hosp 1986; Electrocardiography, St George's Hosp 1989; **Fac Appt:** Prof Med, Mount Sinai Sch Med

Steinberg, Jonathan S MD (CE) - **Spec Exp:** Atrial Fibrillation; Catheter Ablation; Defibrillators; Arrhythmias; **Hospital:** St Luke's - Roosevelt Hosp Ctr - Roosevelt Div (page 94), Valley Hosp (page 658); **Address:** St Luke's-Roosevelt Hospital S&R Bldg, 1111 W 114th St Fl 3 - rm 8-325, New York, NY 10025; **Phone:** 212-523-4007; **Board Cert:** Internal Medicine 1983; Cardiovascular Disease 1987; Cardiac Electrophysiology 2002; **Med School:** Mount Sinai Sch Med 1980; **Resid:** Internal Medicine, NYU Med Ctr/Manhattan VA Hosp 1984; **Fellow:** Cardiovascular Disease, Geo Wash Univ Med Ctr 1986; Cardiac Electrophysiology, Columbia Presby Med Ctr 1988; **Fac Appt:** Prof Med, Columbia P&S

Suri, Ranjit MD (CE) - **Spec Exp:** Arrhythmias; Atrial Fibrillation; Pacemakers; Heart Failure; **Hospital:** Lenox Hill Hosp, NY Hosp Queens; **Address:** Cardiac Arrythmia Ctr, Lenox Hill Hosp, 100 E 77th St, Bayside, NY 10075; **Phone:** 212-434-6500; **Board Cert:** Internal Medicine 2007; Cardiovascular Disease 2006; Cardiac Electrophysiology 2001; **Med School:** India 1982; **Resid:** Internal Medicine, Univ Conn Sch Med 1994; **Fellow:** Cardiovascular Disease, Univ Conn Sch Med 1993; Cardiac Electrophysiology, Mass Genl Hosp 2000; **Fac Appt:** Asst Clin Prof Med, Cornell Univ-Weill Med Coll

Cardiovascular Disease

Andersen, Holly S MD (Cv) - **Spec Exp:** Preventive Cardiology; Women's Health; Mitral Valve Prolapse; **Hospital:** NY-Presby Hosp/Weill Cornell (page 104); **Address:** 125 E 72nd St, New York, NY 10021; **Phone:** 212-628-6100; **Board Cert:** Internal Medicine 2002; Cardiovascular Disease 2005; **Med School:** Univ Rochester 1989; **Resid:** Internal Medicine, Ny Presby-Cornell Med Ctr 1992; **Fellow:** Cardiovascular Disease, NY Presby-Cornell Med Ctr 1995; **Fac Appt:** Assoc Clin Prof Med, Cornell Univ-Weill Med Coll

Askanas, Alexander MD (Cv) - **Spec Exp:** Arrhythmias; Angina; Congestive Heart Failure; **Hospital:** Beth Israel Med Ctr - Petrie Division (page 94), NYU Langone Med Ctr (page 106); **Address:** 242 E 19th St, Office #1, New York, NY 10003; **Phone:** 212-369-3080; **Board Cert:** Internal Medicine 1972; Cardiovascular Disease 1974; **Med School:** Poland 1960; **Resid:** Internal Medicine, VA Med Ctr 1971; **Fellow:** Cardiovascular Disease, VA Med Ctr 1972; **Fac Appt:** Asst Prof Med, Mount Sinai Sch Med

Berdoff, Russell L MD (Cv) - **Spec Exp:** Coronary Artery Disease; Heart Valve Disease; Preventive Cardiology; **Hospital:** Beth Israel Med Ctr - Petrie Division (page 94); **Address:** 67 Irving Pl, Fl 7, New York, NY 10003-2202; **Phone:** 212-979-9224; **Board Cert:** Internal Medicine 1978; Cardiovascular Disease 1981; **Med School:** NY Med Coll 1975; **Resid:** Internal Medicine, DC Genl Hosp 1978; **Fellow:** Cardiovascular Disease, Johns Hopkins Hosp 1980; **Fac Appt:** Assoc Clin Prof Med, Albert Einstein Coll Med

Berger, Marvin MD (Cv) - **Spec Exp:** Echocardiography; **Hospital:** Beth Israel Med Ctr - Petrie Division (page 94); **Address:** 1 St Ave & 16th St, New York, NY 10003; **Phone:** 212-420-2068; **Board Cert:** Internal Medicine 1969; Cardiovascular Disease 1977; **Med School:** Ros Franklin Univ/Chicago Med Sch 1961; **Resid:** Internal Medicine, Beth Israel Hosp 1964; **Fellow:** Cardiovascular Disease, Mount Sinai Hosp 1965; **Fac Appt:** Clin Prof Med, Albert Einstein Coll Med

Bergmann, Steven R MD (Cv) - **Spec Exp:** Nuclear Cardiology; Cardiac Imaging; **Hospital:** Beth Israel Med Ctr - Petrie Division (page 94); **Address:** Beth Israel Med Ctr, Heart Institute, 1st Ave at 16th St, Baird Hall, 5th fl, New York, NY 10003; **Phone:** 212-420-4681; **Board Cert:** Internal Medicine 1998; Nuclear Cardiology 1999; **Med School:** Washington Univ, St Louis 1985; **Resid:** Internal Medicine, Barnes-Jewish Hosp 1988; **Fellow:** Cardiovascular Disease, Barnes-Jewish Hosp 1990; **Fac Appt:** Prof Med, Albert Einstein Coll Med

Blake, James A MD (Cv) - **Spec Exp:** Congestive Heart Failure; Nuclear Cardiology; Echocardiography; Hypertension; **Hospital:** NY-Presby Hosp/Weill Cornell (page 104), Hosp For Special Surgery (page 111); **Address:** 328 E 61st St, New York, NY 10021; **Phone:** 212-755-8700; **Board Cert:** Internal Medicine 1984; Cardiovascular Disease 1987; Echocardiography 2009; Nuclear Cardiology 2009; **Med School:** Albert Einstein Coll Med 1981; **Resid:** Internal Medicine, NY Hosp 1984; **Fellow:** Cardiovascular Disease, NY Hosp 1987; **Fac Appt:** Assoc Clin Prof Med, Cornell Univ-Weill Med Coll

Blumenthal, David S MD (Cv) - **Spec Exp:** Heart Valve Disease; Preventive Cardiology; Coronary Artery Disease; **Hospital:** NY-Presby Hosp/Weill Cornell (page 104); **Address:** 407 E 70th St, Fl 1, New York, NY 10021-5302; **Phone:** 212-861-3222; **Board Cert:** Internal Medicine 1978; Cardiovascular Disease 1981; **Med School:** Cornell Univ-Weill Med Coll 1975; **Resid:** Internal Medicine, NY Hosp 1978; Internal Medicine, NY Hosp 1981; **Fellow:** Cardiovascular Disease, Johns Hopkins Hosp 1980; **Fac Appt:** Clin Prof Med, Cornell Univ-Weill Med Coll

Braff, Robert MD (Cv) - **Spec Exp:** Angiography-Coronary; Echocardiography; **Address:** 275 7th Ave Fl 3, New York, NY 10001; **Phone:** 646-660-9999; **Board Cert:** Internal Medicine 1976; Cardiovascular Disease 1981; **Med School:** SUNY Hlth Sci Ctr 1973; **Resid:** Internal Medicine, St Vincents Hosp 1976; **Fellow:** Cardiovascular Disease, Georgetown Univ Hosp 1978; **Fac Appt:** Asst Clin Prof Med, NY Med Coll

Cemaletin, Nevber S MD (Cv) - **Hospital:** Lenox Hill Hosp, Lenox Hill Hosp (Manh Eye, Ear & Throat Hosp); **Address:** 110 E 59th St, Ste 9B, New York, NY 10022; **Phone:** 212-583-2899; **Board Cert:** Internal Medicine 1988; Cardiovascular Disease 1989; **Med School:** NY Med Coll 1984; **Resid:** Internal Medicine, Lenox Hill Hosp 1987; **Fellow:** Cardiovascular Disease, Lenox Hill Hosp 1989

Cohen, Howard A MD (Cv) - **Spec Exp:** Interventional Cardiology; Carotid Artery Stent Placement; **Hospital:** Lenox Hill Hosp; **Address:** Lenox Hill Hospital, Interventional Cardiology, 130 E 77th St Fl 9, New York, NY 10021; **Phone:** 212-434-6973; **Board Cert:** Internal Medicine 1976; Cardiovascular Disease 1977; **Med School:** NYU Sch Med 1970; **Resid:** Internal Medicine, Bellevue Hosp Ctr 1974; **Fellow:** Cardiovascular Disease, Johns Hopkins Hosp 1976

Cohen, Michael H MD (Cv) - **Spec Exp:** Congestive Heart Failure; Coronary Artery Disease; Hypertension; Cholesterol/Lipid Disorders; **Hospital:** NY-Presby Hosp/Columbia (page 104); **Address:** 161 Fort Washington Ave, rm 328, New York, NY 10032-3713; **Phone:** 212-305-5440; **Board Cert:** Internal Medicine 1971; **Med School:** Johns Hopkins Univ 1965; **Resid:** Internal Medicine, NY-Presby Hosp/Columbia Univ 1971; **Fellow:** Cardiovascular Disease, NY-Presby Hosp/Columbia Univ 1970; **Fac Appt:** Clin Prof Med, Johns Hopkins Univ

Cole, William J MD (Cv) - **Spec Exp:** Coronary Artery Disease; Hypertension; Cholesterol/Lipid Disorders; **Hospital:** NYU Langone Med Ctr (page 106); **Address:** 530 First Ave, Ste 3-D, New York, NY 10016; **Phone:** 212-263-7071; **Board Cert:** Internal Medicine 1983; Cardiovascular Disease 1987; **Med School:** NYU Sch Med 1980; **Resid:** Cardiovascular Disease, NYU Med Ctr 1984; **Fac Appt:** Asst Clin Prof Med, NYU Sch Med

Coppola, John T MD (Cv) - **Spec Exp:** Cardiac Catheterization; Angioplasty; **Hospital:** NYU Langone Med Ctr (page 106), Bellevue Hosp Ctr; **Address:** 275 7th Ave Fl 3, New York, NY 10001; **Phone:** 646-660-9999; **Board Cert:** Internal Medicine 1981; Cardiovascular Disease 1983; Interventional Cardiology 2009; **Med School:** NY Med Coll 1978; **Resid:** Internal Medicine, St Vincent Catholic Med Ctr 1981; **Fellow:** Cardiovascular Disease, St Vincent Catholic Med Ctr 1983

Deutsch, Adam MD (Cv) - **Spec Exp:** Hypertension; Cholesterol/Lipid Disorders; Echocardiography; Congestive Heart Failure; **Hospital:** NY-Presby Hosp/Weill Cornell (page 104), Lenox Hill Hosp; **Address:** Park Avenue Cardiology, 1036 Park Ave at 86th St, New York, NY 10028; **Phone:** 212-879-9000; **Board Cert:** Internal Medicine 2006; Cardiovascular Disease 2009; **Med School:** Albert Einstein Coll Med 1992; **Resid:** Internal Medicine, Columbia Presby Med Ctr 1995; **Fellow:** Cardiovascular Disease, Columbia Presby Med Ctr 1998

Devereux, Richard B MD (Cv) - **Spec Exp:** Marfan's Syndrome; **Hospital:** NY-Presby Hosp/Weill Cornell (page 104); **Address:** 525 E 68th St, rm K-415, New York, NY 10065; **Phone:** 212-746-4655; **Board Cert:** Internal Medicine 1974; Cardiovascular Disease 1977; **Med School:** Univ Pennsylvania 1971; **Resid:** Internal Medicine, New York Hosp 1974; **Fellow:** Cardiovascular Disease, Hosp Univ Penn 1976; **Fac Appt:** Prof Med, Cornell Univ-Weill Med Coll

Drusin, Ronald MD (Cv) - **Spec Exp:** Heart Failure; Coronary Artery Disease; Heart Valve Disease; Transplant Medicine-Heart; **Hospital:** NY-Presby Hosp/Columbia (page 104); **Address:** 161 Fort Washington Ave, Ste 527, New York, NY 10032; **Phone:** 212-305-5371; **Board Cert:** Internal Medicine 1973; Cardiovascular Disease 1975; **Med School:** Columbia P&S 1966; **Resid:** Internal Medicine, Presby Hosp 1969; **Fellow:** Cardiovascular Disease, Columbia-Presby Hosp 1973; **Fac Appt:** Clin Prof Med, Columbia P&S

ElMasri, Bassem M MD (Cv) - **Spec Exp:** Cholesterol/Lipid Disorders; Coronary Artery Disease; Preventive Cardiology; Hypertension; **Hospital:** NY-Presby Hosp/Weill Cornell (page 104); **Address:** New York Presbyterian-Cornell Med Ctr, 1305 York Ave Fl 8, Cardiac Disease Prevention Ctr, New York, NY 10021; **Phone:** 646-962-6004; **Med School:** Lebanon 1988; **Resid:** Internal Medicine, American Univ of Beirut 1991; **Fellow:** Cardiovascular Disease, Baylor Coll Medicine; **Fac Appt:** Assoc Prof Med, Cornell Univ-Weill Med Coll

Epstein, Stanley MD (Cv) - **Spec Exp:** Non-Invasive Cardiology; Preventive Cardiology; Hypertension; Cholesterol/Lipid Disorders; **Hospital:** NY-Presby Hosp/Columbia (page 104), Montefiore Med Ctr - Div. Moses (page 100); **Address:** 15 W 72 St, Ste 22B, New York, NY 10023; **Phone:** 212-362-2079; **Board Cert:** Internal Medicine 1967; Cardiovascular Disease 1975; **Med School:** Ros Franklin Univ/Chicago Med Sch 1958; **Resid:** Internal Medicine, Jewish Hosp 1960; Internal Medicine, San Francisco Genl Hosp 1961; **Fellow:** Cardiovascular Disease, Montefiore Hosp Med Ctr 1967; **Fac Appt:** Clin Prof Med, Columbia P&S

Friedman, Howard S MD (Cv) - **Spec Exp:** Atrial Fibrillation; Coronary Artery Disease; Hypertension; **Hospital:** NYU Langone Med Ctr (page 106); **Address:** 650 First Ave, Fl 3, New York, NY 10016-3240; **Phone:** 212-889-9393; **Board Cert:** Internal Medicine 1971; Cardiovascular Disease 1974; Critical Care Medicine 2001; Geriatric Medicine 2004; **Med School:** SUNY Buffalo 1966; **Resid:** Internal Medicine, Mt Sinai Med Ctr 1969; Cardiovascular Disease, Mt Sinai Med Ctr 1973; **Fac Appt:** Clin Prof Med, NYU Sch Med

Friedman, Sanford MD (Cv) - **Spec Exp:** Preventive Cardiology; **Hospital:** Mount Sinai Med Ctr (page 102); **Address:** 103 E 81st St, New York, NY 10028; **Phone:** 212-988-3772; **Board Cert:** Internal Medicine 1980; Cardiovascular Disease 1977; **Med School:** Tufts Univ 1971; **Resid:** Internal Medicine, Mt Sinai Med Ctr 1974; **Fellow:** Cardiovascular Disease, Mt Sinai Med Ctr 1976; **Fac Appt:** Assoc Clin Prof Med, Mount Sinai Sch Med

Fuchs, Richard MD (Cv) - **Spec Exp:** Coronary Artery Disease; Heart Valve Disease; Preventive Cardiology; **Hospital:** NY-Presby Hosp/Weill Cornell (page 104); **Address:** 310 E 72nd St, New York, NY 10021; **Phone:** 212-717-2254; **Board Cert:** Internal Medicine 1979; Cardiovascular Disease 1981; **Med School:** Harvard Med Sch 1976; **Resid:** Internal Medicine, New York Hosp 1979; **Fellow:** Cardiovascular Disease, Johns Hopkins Hosp 1982; **Fac Appt:** Clin Prof Med, Cornell Univ-Weill Med Coll

Fuster, Valentin MD/PhD (Cv) - **Spec Exp:** Coronary Artery Disease; Heart Valve Disease; Congenital Heart Disease; Preventive Cardiology; **Hospital:** Mount Sinai Med Ctr (page 102); **Address:** One Gustave L Levy Pl, Box 1030, New York, NY 10029-6500; **Phone:** 212-241-7911; **Board Cert:** Internal Medicine 1976; Cardiovascular Disease 1977; **Med School:** Spain 1967; **Resid:** Internal Medicine, Mayo Clin 1972; Cardiovascular Disease, Mayo Cli 1974; **Fellow:** Cardiovascular Disease, Univ Edinburgh 1971; **Fac Appt:** Prof Med, Mount Sinai Sch Med

Giardina, Elsa-Grace MD (Cv) - **Spec Exp:** Heart Disease in Women; Arrhythmias; Preventive Cardiology; **Hospital:** NY-Presby Hosp/Columbia (page 104); **Address:** Herbert Irving Pavillion, 161 Fort Washington Ave, New York, NY 10032; **Phone:** 212-305-7934; **Board Cert:** Internal Medicine 1971; Cardiovascular Disease 1983; **Med School:** NY Med Coll 1965; **Resid:** Internal Medicine, St Luke's-Roosevelt Hosp 1969; **Fellow:** Cardiovascular Disease, Columbia-Presby Hosp 1971; **Fac Appt:** Prof Med, Columbia P&S

Gliklich, Jerry MD (Cv) - **Spec Exp:** Heart Valve Disease; Arrhythmias; **Hospital:** NY-Presby Hosp/Columbia (page 104); **Address:** 161 Fort Washington Ave, Ste 535, New York, NY 10032-3713; **Phone:** 212-305-5588; **Board Cert:** Internal Medicine 1978; Cardiovascular Disease 1981; **Med School:** Columbia P&S 1975; **Resid:** Internal Medicine, NY Hosp 1978; **Fellow:** Cardiovascular Disease, Columbia-Presby Med Ctr 1981; **Fac Appt:** Clin Prof Med, Columbia P&S

Goldberg, Harvey MD (Cv) - **Hospital:** NY-Presby Hosp/Weill Cornell (page 104), Lenox Hill Hosp; **Address:** 425 E 61st St Fl 6, New York, NY 10021-8795; **Phone:** 212-752-2000; **Board Cert:** Internal Medicine 1979; Cardiovascular Disease 1981; **Med School:** Cornell Univ-Weill Med Coll 1976; **Resid:** Internal Medicine, NY Hosp 1979; **Fellow:** Cardiovascular Disease, NY Hosp 1981; **Fac Appt:** Assoc Clin Prof Med, Cornell Univ-Weill Med Coll

Goldberg, Nieca MD (Cv) - **Spec Exp:** Heart Disease in Women; Preventive Cardiology; Echocardiography; **Hospital:** NYU Langone Med Ctr (page 106), Lenox Hill Hosp; **Address:** 177 E 87th St, New York, NY 10128; **Phone:** 212-289-2045; **Board Cert:** Internal Medicine 1987; Cardiovascular Disease 2005; **Med School:** SUNY Downstate 1984; **Resid:** Internal Medicine, St Lukes Roosevelt Hosp Ctr 1987; **Fellow:** Cardiovascular Disease, SUNY Hlth Sci Ctr 1990; **Fac Appt:** Assoc Clin Prof Med, NYU Sch Med

Goldman, Martin E MD (Cv) - **Spec Exp:** Heart Valve Disease; Echocardiography; Diagnostic Problems; **Hospital:** Mount Sinai Med Ctr (page 102); **Address:** 1 Gustave Levy Pl, Box 1030, New York, NY 10029-6504; **Phone:** 212-241-3078; **Board Cert:** Internal Medicine 1979; Cardiovascular Disease 1981; **Med School:** Albert Einstein Coll Med 1976; **Resid:** Internal Medicine, Peter Bent Brigham Hosp 1978; **Fellow:** Cardiovascular Disease, Mount Sinai Hosp 1980; **Fac Appt:** Prof Med, NYU Sch Med

Gotto Jr, Antonio M MD (Cv) - **Spec Exp:** Cholesterol/Lipid Disorders; **Hospital:** NY-Presby Hosp/Weill Cornell (page 104); **Address:** New York Presbyterian-Cornell Med Ctr, 1305 York Ave Fl 8, Cardiac Disease Prevention Ctr, New York, NY 10021; **Phone:** 646-962-6004; **Board Cert:** Internal Medicine 1980; **Med School:** Vanderbilt Univ 1965; **Resid:** Internal Medicine, Mass Genl Hosp 1967; **Fac Appt:** Prof Med, Cornell Univ-Weill Med Coll

Guyer, David E MD (Cv) - **Spec Exp:** Heart Valve Disease; Coronary Artery Disease; Hypertension; **Hospital:** NY-Presby Hosp/Weill Cornell (page 104); **Address:** NY Presby-Cornell Medical Ctr, 520 E 70th St, Starr 443, New York, NY 10021; **Phone:** 212-746-2240; **Board Cert:** Internal Medicine 1979; Cardiovascular Disease 1981; **Med School:** Case West Res Univ 1976; **Resid:** Internal Medicine, Peter Bent Brigham Hosp 1979; **Fellow:** Cardiovascular Disease, Mass Genl Hosp 1981

Halperin, Jonathan L MD (Cv) - **Spec Exp:** Peripheral Vascular Disease; Atrial Fibrillation; **Hospital:** Mount Sinai Med Ctr (page 102); **Address:** 1190 5th Ave, New York, NY 10029; **Phone:** 212-241-7243; **Board Cert:** Internal Medicine 1980; Cardiovascular Disease 1981; **Med School:** Boston Univ 1975; **Resid:** Internal Medicine, Mass Genl Hosp 1977; **Fellow:** Vascular Medicine, Boston Univ Med Ctr 1978; Cardiovascular Disease, Boston Univ Med Ctr 1980; **Fac Appt:** Prof Med, Mount Sinai Sch Med

Hecht, Alan MD (Cv) - **Spec Exp:** Heart Valve Disease; Coronary Artery Disease; Arrhythmias; **Hospital:** Mount Sinai Med Ctr (page 102); **Address:** 1075 Park Ave, New York, NY 10128; **Phone:** 212-876-0845; **Board Cert:** Internal Medicine 1984; Cardiovascular Disease 1987; **Med School:** Northwestern Univ 1981; **Resid:** Internal Medicine, Mt Sinai Hosp 1984; **Fellow:** Cardiovascular Disease, Mt Sinai Hosp 1986; **Fac Appt:** Assoc Clin Prof Med, Mount Sinai Sch Med

Horn, Evelyn M MD (Cv) - **Spec Exp:** Pulmonary Hypertension; Heart Failure; Ventricular Assist Device (LVAD); Heart Disease-Complex; **Hospital:** NY-Presby Hosp/Weill Cornell (page 104); **Address:** Perkins Heart Failure Ctr-Weill Cornell, 1305 York Ave Fl 8, New York, NY 10021; **Phone:** 212-746-2381; **Board Cert:** Internal Medicine 1983; Cardiovascular Disease 1985; **Med School:** Mount Sinai Sch Med 1980; **Resid:** Internal Medicine, Mt Sinai Hosp 1983; **Fellow:** Cardiovascular Disease, Cedars-Sinai Med Ctr 1985; **Fac Appt:** Clin Prof Med, Cornell Univ-Weill Med Coll

Infantino, Michael MD (Cv) - **Spec Exp:** Cholesterol/Lipid Disorders; Acute Coronary Syndromes; Echocardiography; **Hospital:** NYU Langone Med Ctr (page 106); **Address:** New York Cardiovascular Associate, PHC, 275 Seventh Ave Fl 3, New York, NY 10001; **Phone:** 646-660-9999; **Board Cert:** Cardiovascular Disease 1987; Internal Medicine 1984; **Med School:** SUNY Hlth Sci Ctr 1981; **Resid:** Internal Medicine, Staten Island Hosp 1984; **Fellow:** Cardiovascular Disease, St Vincent's Hosp & Med Ctr 1986

Inra, Lawrence A MD (Cv) - **Spec Exp:** Coronary Artery Disease; Heart Valve Disease; Cholesterol/Lipid Disorders; Hypertension; **Hospital:** NY-Presby Hosp/Weill Cornell (page 104), Hosp For Special Surgery (page 111); **Address:** 407 E 70th St, New York, NY 10021; **Phone:** 212-249-1011; **Board Cert:** Internal Medicine 1979; Cardiovascular Disease 1981; **Med School:** Johns Hopkins Univ 1976; **Resid:** Internal Medicine, NY Hosp 1979; **Fellow:** Cardiovascular Disease, Mt Sinai Hosp 1981; **Fac Appt:** Assoc Clin Prof Med, Cornell Univ-Weill Med Coll

Kalman, Jill MD (Cv) - **Spec Exp:** Heart Failure; Transplant Medicine-Heart; Heart Disease in Women; **Hospital:** Mount Sinai Med Ctr (page 102); **Address:** 5 E 98th St Fl 3, New York, NY 10029-6501; **Phone:** 212-241-0511; **Board Cert:** Internal Medicine 2000; Cardiovascular Disease 2005; **Med School:** Mount Sinai Sch Med 1987; **Resid:** Internal Medicine, Mt Sinai Med Ctr 1991; **Fellow:** Cardiovascular Disease, Mt Sinai Med Ctr 1995

Kamen, Mazen MD (Cv) - **Spec Exp:** Heart Valve Disease; Cholesterol/Lipid Disorders; Hypertension; Congenital Heart Disease; **Hospital:** NY-Presby Hosp/Weill Cornell (page 104); **Address:** 1021 Park Ave, Ste 101, New York, NY 10028; **Phone:** 212-427-5800; **Board Cert:** Cardiovascular Disease 2006; **Med School:** NYU Sch Med 1983; **Resid:** Internal Medicine, NYU Med Ctr 1986; **Fellow:** Cardiovascular Disease, NY Cornell Med Ctr 1990; **Fac Appt:** Asst Prof Med, Cornell Univ-Weill Med Coll

Katz, Edward MD (Cv) - **Spec Exp:** Echocardiography; Cholesterol/Lipid Disorders; Coronary Artery Disease; **Hospital:** NYU Langone Med Ctr (page 106), NYU Hosp For Joint Diseases (page 106); **Address:** Skirball Inst, 530 1st Ave, New York, NY 10016; **Phone:** 212-263-7751; **Board Cert:** Cardiovascular Disease 2009; Internal Medicine 1988; Echocardiography 2005; **Med School:** NYU Sch Med 1985; **Resid:** Internal Medicine, NYU Med Ctr 1988; **Fellow:** Cardiovascular Disease, NYU Med Ctr 1991; **Fac Appt:** Assoc Prof Med, NYU Sch Med

Katz, Stuart D MD (Cv) - **Spec Exp:** Heart Failure; Transplant Medicine-Heart; **Hospital:** NYU Langone Med Ctr (page 106); **Address:** NYU Cardiology Assocs, 530 First Ave, Skirball 9R, New York, NY 10016; **Phone:** 212-263-7751; **Board Cert:** Internal Medicine 1986; Cardiovascular Disease 1989; **Med School:** SUNY Downstate 1983; **Resid:** Internal Medicine, Francis Scott Key Med Ctr 1986; **Fellow:** Cardiovascular Disease, Montefiore Med Ctr 1989; **Fac Appt:** Prof Med, NYU Sch Med

Kligfield, Paul MD (Cv) - **Hospital:** NY-Presby Hosp/Weill Cornell (page 104); **Address:** Dept Cardiology, 525 E 68th St, rm L195, New York, NY 10021; **Phone:** 212-746-4686; **Board Cert:** Internal Medicine 1973; Cardiovascular Disease 1975; **Med School:** Harvard Med Sch 1970; **Resid:** Internal Medicine, Beth Israel Hosp 1972; Cardiovascular Disease, St George's Hosp 1973; **Fellow:** Cardiovascular Disease, New York Hosp 1975; **Fac Appt:** Prof Med, Cornell Univ-Weill Med Coll

Kronzon, Itzhak MD (Cv) - **Spec Exp:** Heart Valve Disease; Echocardiography; Cardiac Imaging; Pericardial Diseases; **Hospital:** Lenox Hill Hosp; **Address:** 100 E 77th St Fl 2 - Ste 2E, New York, NY 10075; **Phone:** 212-434-6119; **Board Cert:** Internal Medicine 1979; Cardiovascular Disease 1981; Echocardiography 2002; **Med School:** Israel 1964; **Resid:** Internal Medicine, Hadassah Hosp 1969; **Fellow:** Cardiovascular Disease, Montefiore Med Ctr 1973; Cardiovascular Disease, NYU Med Ctr 1974; **Fac Appt:** Prof Med, NYU Sch Med

Kutnick, Richard T MD (Cv) - **Spec Exp:** Echocardiography; **Hospital:** Lenox Hill Hosp; **Address:** 898 Park Ave, New York, NY 10021-2897; **Phone:** 212-879-2628; **Board Cert:** Internal Medicine 1979; Cardiovascular Disease 1981; **Med School:** Tufts Univ 1976; **Resid:** Internal Medicine, Lenox Hill Hosp 1979; **Fellow:** Cardiovascular Disease, Lenox Hill Hosp 1981; **Fac Appt:** Asst Prof Med, NYU Sch Med

Lazar, Eliot J MD (Cv) - **Spec Exp:** Hypertension; Coronary Artery Disease; **Hospital:** NY-Presby Hosp/Weill Cornell (page 104); **Address:** 525 E 68th St, Box 569 NYPH, New York, NY 10021; **Phone:** 212-746-0386; **Board Cert:** Internal Medicine 1984; Cardiovascular Disease 1987; Critical Care Medicine 2000; Geriatric Medicine 2006; **Med School:** SUNY Upstate Med Univ 1981; **Resid:** Internal Medicine, Bronx Muni Hosp 1984; **Fellow:** Cardiovascular Disease, Mount Sinai Hosp 1987; **Fac Appt:** Assoc Clin Prof Med, Cornell Univ-Weill Med Coll

Lewis, Benjamin H MD (Cv) - **Spec Exp:** Cardiac Stress Testing; Heart Disease & Gender; Echocardiography; Preventive Cardiology; **Hospital:** NY-Presby Hosp/Columbia (page 104), Lenox Hill Hosp; **Address:** 16 E 60th St Fl 3, New York, NY 10022-1002; **Phone:** 212-326-8425; **Board Cert:** Internal Medicine 1980; Cardiovascular Disease 1983; **Med School:** UCSF 1977; **Resid:** Internal Medicine, Columbia-Presby Hosp 1980; **Fellow:** Cardiovascular Disease, Brigham Womens Hosp 1982; **Fac Appt:** Assoc Prof Med, Columbia P&S

Mancini, Donna M MD (Cv) - **Spec Exp:** Congestive Heart Failure; Transplant Medicine-Heart; **Hospital:** NY-Presby Hosp/Columbia (page 104); **Address:** 622 W 168 St Fl 12 West - rm 134, New York, NY 10032; **Phone:** 212-305-4600; **Board Cert:** Internal Medicine 1983; Cardiovascular Disease 1987; **Med School:** Albert Einstein Coll Med 1980; **Resid:** Internal Medicine, Bronx Municipal Hosp 1983; **Fellow:** Cardiovascular Disease, Montefiore Med Ctr 1986; **Fac Appt:** Prof Med, Columbia P&S

Matta, Raymond J MD (Cv) - **Hospital:** Mount Sinai Med Ctr (page 102); **Address:** 1120 Park Ave, Ste 1C, New York, NY 10128-1242; **Phone:** 212-410-4800; **Board Cert:** Internal Medicine 1973; Cardiovascular Disease 1975; **Med School:** Univ Pittsburgh 1969; **Resid:** Internal Medicine, Mass Genl Hosp 1971; **Fellow:** Cardiovascular Disease, Peter Bent Brigham Hosp 1975; **Fac Appt:** Assoc Clin Prof Med, Mount Sinai Sch Med

Mattes, Leonard MD (Cv) - **Hospital:** Mount Sinai Med Ctr (page 102); **Address:** 1199 Park Ave, Ste 1F, New York, NY 10128-1713; **Phone:** 212-876-7045; **Board Cert:** Internal Medicine 1972; Cardiovascular Disease 1975; **Med School:** Tulane Univ 1962; **Resid:** Internal Medicine, Mt Sinai Hosp 1967; Cardiovascular Disease, Mt Sinai Hosp 1969; **Fellow:** Cardiovascular Disease, Mt Sinai Hosp 1968; **Fac Appt:** Asst Clin Prof Med, Mount Sinai Sch Med

Meller, Jose MD (Cv) - **Spec Exp:** Cardiac Catheterization; Hypertension; Angioplasty; **Hospital:** Mount Sinai Med Ctr (page 102); **Address:** 941 Park Ave, New York, NY 10028; **Phone:** 212-988-3772; **Board Cert:** Internal Medicine 1973; Cardiovascular Disease 1975; **Med School:** Chile 1969; **Resid:** Internal Medicine, Elmhurst Hosp 1971; Internal Medicine, Mt Sinai Med Ctr 1972; **Fellow:** Cardiovascular Disease, Mt Sinai Med Ctr 1974; **Fac Appt:** Prof Med, Mount Sinai Sch Med

Miller, David H MD (Cv) - **Spec Exp:** Hypertension; **Hospital:** NY-Presby Hosp/Weill Cornell (page 104); **Address:** 520 E 70th St, Starr 443, New York, NY 10021; **Phone:** 212-746-2144; **Board Cert:** Internal Medicine 1980; Cardiovascular Disease 1981; **Med School:** Univ VA Sch Med 1976; **Resid:** Internal Medicine, NY Hosp-Cornell Med Ctr 1979; **Fellow:** Cardiovascular Disease, NY Hosp-Cornell Med Ctr 1981; **Fac Appt:** Assoc Prof Med, Cornell Univ-Weill Med Coll

Mueller, Richard L MD (Cv) - **Spec Exp:** Vein Disorders; Stress Echocardiography; Hypertension; Echocardiography; **Hospital:** NY-Presby Hosp/Weill Cornell (page 104), St Luke's - Roosevelt Hosp Ctr - St Luke's Hosp (page 94); **Address:** Cardiovascular Diagnostics, PC, Cosmetic Vein Solutions, 401 E 55th St, New York, NY 10022-1236; **Phone:** 212-593-9800; **Board Cert:** Internal Medicine 2000; Cardiovascular Disease 2000; Echocardiography 1999; Vascular Medicine 2006; **Med School:** UCSF 1987; **Resid:** Internal Medicine, North Shore Univ Hosp 1991; Internal Medicine, Meml Sloan Kettering Cancer Ctr 1990; **Fellow:** Cardiovascular Disease, New York Hosp 1994; **Fac Appt:** Asst Clin Prof Med, Cornell Univ-Weill Med Coll

Nash, Ira MD (Cv) - **Spec Exp:** Preventive Cardiology; Coronary Artery Disease; **Hospital:** Mount Sinai Med Ctr (page 102); **Address:** Mt Sinai Medical Ctr, One Gustave Levy Pl, Box 1238, New York, NY 10029; **Phone:** 212-241-3282; **Board Cert:** Internal Medicine 1987; Cardiovascular Disease 1989; **Med School:** Harvard Med Sch 1984; **Resid:** Internal Medicine, Beth Israel Hosp 1987; **Fellow:** Cardiovascular Disease, Beth Israel Hosp 1990; **Fac Appt:** Assoc Prof Med, Mount Sinai Sch Med

O'Brien, Francis J MD (Cv) - **Spec Exp:** Preventive Cardiology; **Hospital:** NYU Langone Med Ctr (page 106), Bellevue Hosp Ctr; **Address:** 347 E 37th St Fl 2, New York, NY 10016; **Phone:** 212-726-7457; **Board Cert:** Internal Medicine 1985; Cardiovascular Disease 1989; **Med School:** Harvard Med Sch 1982; **Resid:** Internal Medicine, NYU Med Ctr 1983; **Fellow:** Cardiovascular Disease, Bellevue-NYU Hosp 1988; **Fac Appt:** Assoc Clin Prof Med, NYU Sch Med

Pinney, Sean MD (Cv) - **Spec Exp:** Transplant Medicine-Heart; Heart Failure; Pulmonary Hypertension; Congenital Heart Disease; **Hospital:** Mount Sinai Med Ctr (page 102); **Address:** Mount Sinai Cardiovascular Inst, One Gustave L Levy Pl, Box 1030, New York, NY 10029; **Phone:** 212-241-7300; **Board Cert:** Cardiovascular Disease 2001; **Med School:** Georgetown Univ 1994; **Resid:** Internal Medicine, Bet Israel Deaconess Med Ctr 1999; **Fellow:** Cardiovascular Disease, Columbia Presby Hosp 2001; Transplant Medicine, Columbia Presby Hosp 2002; **Fac Appt:** Asst Prof Med, Mount Sinai Sch Med

Porder, Joseph B MD (Cv) - **Spec Exp:** Preventive Cardiology; Nutrition; Echocardiography; Preventive Medicine; **Hospital:** Mount Sinai Med Ctr (page 102); **Address:** 1160 5th Ave, Ste 102, New York, NY 10029; **Phone:** 212-860-5500; **Board Cert:** Internal Medicine 1985; Cardiovascular Disease 1987; **Med School:** Columbia P&S 1982; **Resid:** Internal Medicine, Mt Sinai Hosp 1985; **Fellow:** Cardiovascular Disease, Mt Sinai Hosp 1987

Post, Martin R MD (Cv) - **Spec Exp:** Coronary Artery Disease; Cholesterol/Lipid Disorders; **Hospital:** NY-Presby Hosp/Weill Cornell (page 104); **Address:** 425 E 61st St, New York, NY 10021-8722; **Phone:** 212-752-2000; **Board Cert:** Internal Medicine 1974; Cardiovascular Disease 1974; **Med School:** SUNY Upstate Med Univ 1967; **Resid:** Internal Medicine, Ohio State Univ Hosp 1970; **Fellow:** Cardiovascular Disease, New York Hosp 1972; **Fac Appt:** Asst Prof Med, Cornell Univ-Weill Med Coll

Radwaner, Bradley A MD (Cv) - **Spec Exp:** Preventive Cardiology; Cholesterol/Lipid Disorders; Interventional Cardiology; **Hospital:** Lenox Hill Hosp; **Address:** 885 Park Ave, New York, NY 10075; **Phone:** 212-717-0666; **Board Cert:** Internal Medicine 1983; Cardiovascular Disease 1985; **Med School:** Cornell Univ-Weill Med Coll 1980; **Resid:** Internal Medicine, Lenox Hill Hosp 1983; **Fellow:** Cardiovascular Disease, St Lukes Hosp 1985; Interventional Cardiology, NYU Med Ctr 1986; **Fac Appt:** Asst Clin Prof Med, Cornell Univ-Weill Med Coll

Reichstein, Robert P MD (Cv) - **Spec Exp:** Preventive Cardiology; Cholesterol/Lipid Disorders; Aneurysm-Aortic; **Hospital:** Mount Sinai Med Ctr (page 102); **Address:** 1185 Park Ave, Ste 1L, New York, NY 10128; **Phone:** 212-996-2900; **Board Cert:** Internal Medicine 1980; Cardiovascular Disease 1983; **Med School:** Ros Franklin Univ/Chicago Med Sch 1977; **Resid:** Internal Medicine, Mt Sinai Hosp 1981; **Fellow:** Cardiovascular Disease, Mt Sinai Hosp 1984; **Fac Appt:** Asst Clin Prof Med, Mount Sinai Sch Med

Reiffel, James MD (Cv) - **Spec Exp:** Arrhythmias; **Hospital:** NY-Presby Hosp/Columbia (page 104); **Address:** 161 Fort Washington Ave, New York, NY 10032-3713; **Phone:** 212-305-5206; **Board Cert:** Internal Medicine 1972; Cardiovascular Disease 1975; **Med School:** Columbia P&S 1969; **Resid:** Internal Medicine, Columbia-Presby Med Ctr 1972; **Fellow:** Cardiovascular Disease, Columbia-Presby Med Ctr 1974; **Fac Appt:** Prof Med, Columbia P&S

Rentrop, K Peter MD (Cv) - **Hospital:** Lenox Hill Hosp, NYU Langone Med Ctr (page 106); **Address:** 920 Broadway, Ste 600, New York, NY 10010; **Phone:** 212-475-8066; **Board Cert:** Internal Medicine 1973; Nuclear Medicine 2002; **Med School:** Germany 1966; **Resid:** Internal Medicine, Detroit Med Ctr 1970; Internal Medicine, Cleveland Clinic 1971; **Fellow:** Cardiovascular Disease, Cleveland Clinic 1973; **Fac Appt:** Prof Med, NY Med Coll

Romanello, Paul P MD (Cv) - **Spec Exp:** Cholesterol/Lipid Disorders; Coronary Artery Disease; Hypertension; Nuclear Cardiology; **Hospital:** Lenox Hill Hosp; **Address:** 158 E 84th St, New York, NY 10028; **Phone:** 212-535-6340; **Board Cert:** Internal Medicine 1987; Cardiovascular Disease 1989; Nuclear Cardiology 2008; **Med School:** SUNY Upstate Med Univ 1983; **Resid:** Internal Medicine, Lenox Hill Hosp 1987; **Fellow:** Cardiovascular Disease, Lenox Hill Hosp 1989

Rosenbaum, Marlon S MD (Cv) - **Spec Exp:** Congenital Heart Disease-Adult; Heart Valve Disease; **Hospital:** NY-Presby Hosp/Columbia (page 104); **Address:** 161 Fort Washington Ave, rm 557, New York, NY 10032-3729; **Phone:** 212-305-6936; **Board Cert:** Internal Medicine 1983; Cardiovascular Disease 1985; **Med School:** NYU Sch Med 1980; **Resid:** Internal Medicine, Columbia-Presby Med Ctr 1983; **Fellow:** Cardiovascular Disease, Westchester Med Ctr 1985; Cardiovascular Disease, Mass Genl Hosp 1986; **Fac Appt:** Assoc Clin Prof Med, Columbia P&S

Schiffer, Mark B MD (Cv) - **Spec Exp:** Preventive Cardiology; Coronary Artery Disease; Cholesterol/Lipid Disorders; **Hospital:** Lenox Hill Hosp; **Address:** 158 E 84th St, New York, NY 10028-1802; **Phone:** 212-535-6340; **Board Cert:** Internal Medicine 1980; Cardiovascular Disease 1983; **Med School:** Northwestern Univ 1977; **Resid:** Internal Medicine, Lenox Hill Hosp 1981; **Fellow:** Cardiovascular Disease, Lenox Hill Hosp 1983

Schulman, Ira MD (Cv) - **Spec Exp:** Angina; Heart Failure; Cholesterol/Lipid Disorders; **Hospital:** NYU Langone Med Ctr (page 106), NY Downtown Hosp; **Address:** 111 Broadway Fl 2, New York, NY 10006; **Phone:** 212-263-9700; **Board Cert:** Internal Medicine 1977; Cardiovascular Disease 1979; **Med School:** NYU Sch Med 1974; **Resid:** Internal Medicine, Bellevue Hosp 1977; **Fellow:** Cardiovascular Disease, Montefiore Med Ctr 1979; **Fac Appt:** Assoc Prof Med, NYU Sch Med

Schulze, Paul Christian MD/PhD (Cv) - **Spec Exp:** Heart Failure; Vascular Medicine; Vasculitis; **Hospital:** NY-Presby Hosp/Columbia (page 104); **Address:** Columbia Presbyterian Hosp, 622 W 168th St, rm PH-1267, New York, NY 10032; **Phone:** 212-305-7912; **Board Cert:** Internal Medicine 2008; Cardiovascular Disease 2009; Echocardiography 2009; Nuclear Cardiology 2009; **Med School:** Germany 1998; **Resid:** Internal Medicine, Boston Univ Med Ctr 2007; **Fellow:** Cardiovascular Disease, NY Presby-Columbia Med Ctr 2009; **Fac Appt:** Asst Prof Med, Columbia P&S

Schwartz, Allan MD (Cv) - **Hospital:** NY-Presby Hosp/Columbia (page 104); **Address:** 161 Ft Washington Ave, Ste 551, New York, NY 10032-3713; **Phone:** 212-305-5367; **Board Cert:** Internal Medicine 1977; Cardiovascular Disease 1979; **Med School:** Columbia P&S 1974; **Resid:** Internal Medicine, Columbia-Presby Med Ctr 1976; **Fellow:** Cardiovascular Disease, Mass Genl Hosp 1978; **Fac Appt:** Clin Prof Med, Columbia P&S

Schwartz, William J MD (Cv) - **Spec Exp:** Coronary Artery Disease; Cardiac Catheterization; Congestive Heart Failure; **Hospital:** Mount Sinai Med Ctr (page 102), Lenox Hill Hosp; **Address:** Mt Sinai Multispecialty Physicians, 150 E 77th St, Ste 1E, New York, NY 10075; **Phone:** 212-439-6000; **Board Cert:** Internal Medicine 1978; Cardiovascular Disease 1981; **Med School:** Albert Einstein Coll Med 1975; **Resid:** Internal Medicine, Bronx Municipal Hosp 1978; **Fellow:** Cardiovascular Disease, Bronx Municipal Hosp 1979

Seinfeld, David MD (Cv) - **Spec Exp:** Preventive Cardiology; **Hospital:** Lenox Hill Hosp, Montefiore Med Ctr - Div. Moses (page 100); **Address:** 20 E 68th St, Ste 214, New York, NY 10065-5841; **Phone:** 212-288-1538; **Board Cert:** Internal Medicine 1976; Cardiovascular Disease 1979; **Med School:** Albert Einstein Coll Med 1973; **Resid:** Internal Medicine, Montefiore Med Ctr 1976; **Fellow:** Cardiovascular Disease, Montefiore Med Ctr 1978; **Fac Appt:** Assoc Clin Prof Med, Albert Einstein Coll Med

Sherman, Warren MD (Cv) - **Spec Exp:** Angioplasty; Interventional Cardiology; **Hospital:** NY-Presby Hosp/Columbia (page 104); **Address:** 161 Fort Washington Ave Fl 4, New York, NY 10032; **Phone:** 212-305-7060; **Board Cert:** Internal Medicine 1980; Cardiovascular Disease 1983; Interventional Cardiology 2000; **Med School:** SUNY Upstate Med Univ 1977; **Resid:** Internal Medicine, Rochester Genl Hosp 1980; **Fellow:** Cardiovascular Disease, Oregon Hlth Sci Univ 1982; **Fac Appt:** Assoc Clin Prof Med, Columbia P&S

Shimony, Rony MD (Cv) - **Spec Exp:** Coronary Artery Disease; Arrhythmias; Heart Failure; Non-Invasive Cardiology; **Hospital:** Lenox Hill Hosp, NY-Presby Hosp/Weill Cornell (page 104); **Address:** Lenox Hill Heart & Vascular Disease Ctr, 110 E 59th St Fl 8, New York, NY 10022; **Phone:** 212-434-6160; **Board Cert:** Internal Medicine 1987; Cardiovascular Disease 1989; **Med School:** SUNY Buffalo 1984; **Resid:** Internal Medicine, Lenox Hill Hosp 1987; **Fellow:** Cardiovascular Disease, Lenox Hill Hosp 1989; Cardiac Electrophysiology, Lenox Hill Hosp 1992

Siegal, Michael S MD (Cv) - **Spec Exp:** Coronary Artery Disease; **Hospital:** St Luke's - Roosevelt Hosp Ctr - Roosevelt Div (page 94); **Address:** 37 Central Park S, Ste 13A, New York, NY 10022; **Phone:** 212-319-1700; **Board Cert:** Internal Medicine 1980; Cardiovascular Disease 1983; **Med School:** Columbia P&S 1977; **Resid:** Internal Medicine, Bellevue/NYU Med Ctr 1980; **Fellow:** Cardiovascular Disease, Mt Sinai Hosp 1982

Siegel, Stephen MD (Cv) - **Spec Exp:** Sports Medicine-Cardiology; Preventive Cardiology; Cholesterol/Lipid Disorders; Hypertension; **Hospital:** NYU Langone Med Ctr (page 106); **Address:** 245 E 35th St, New York, NY 10016; **Phone:** 212-684-1108; **Board Cert:** Internal Medicine 1981; Cardiovascular Disease 1983; **Med School:** Med Coll VA 1978; **Resid:** Internal Medicine, NYU Med Ctr/Bellevue Hosp Ctr 1981; **Fellow:** Cardiovascular Disease, NYU Med Ctr/Bellevue Hosp Ctr 1983; **Fac Appt:** Asst Clin Prof Med, NYU Sch Med

Sklaroff, Herschel J MD (Cv) - **Spec Exp:** Angina; Syncope; Hypertension; Diagnostic Problems; **Hospital:** Mount Sinai Med Ctr (page 102); **Address:** 1175 Park Ave, New York, NY 10128-1211; **Phone:** 212-289-6500 x2; **Board Cert:** Internal Medicine 1969; Cardiovascular Disease 1977; **Med School:** Univ Pennsylvania 1961; **Resid:** Internal Medicine, Mt Sinai Hosp 1965; Cardiovascular Disease, Mt Sinai Hosp 1966; **Fac Appt:** Clin Prof Med, Mount Sinai Sch Med

Slater, William R MD (Cv) - **Spec Exp:** Arrhythmias; Heart Valve Disease; Electrophysiologic Testing; **Hospital:** NYU Langone Med Ctr (page 106); **Address:** NYU Medical Ctr, Div Cardiology, 530 First Ave, Ste 9U, New York, NY 10016; **Phone:** 212-263-7463; **Board Cert:** Internal Medicine 1981; Cardiovascular Disease 1985; Cardiac Electrophysiology 2002; **Med School:** Harvard Med Sch 1978; **Resid:** Internal Medicine, NYU-Bellevue Med Ctr 1981; **Fellow:** Cardiovascular Disease, Mt Sinai Hosp 1984; Cardiovascular Disease, Mass Genl Hosp/Brigham-Womens Hops 1986; **Fac Appt:** Assoc Prof Med, NYU Sch Med

Stein, Richard A MD (Cv) - **Spec Exp:** Preventive Cardiology; Coronary Artery Disease; Cardiac Rehabilitation; **Hospital:** NYU Langone Med Ctr (page 106); **Address:** NYU Cardiology Assocs, 530 First Ave, Skirball 9R, New York, NY 10016; **Phone:** 212-263-7751; **Board Cert:** Internal Medicine 1973; Cardiovascular Disease 1975; Sports Medicine 2007; **Med School:** NYU Sch Med 1967; **Resid:** Internal Medicine, Univ Hosp 1969; **Fellow:** Cardiovascular Disease, Univ Hosp 1974; **Fac Appt:** Prof Med, NYU Sch Med

Steingart, Richard MD (Cv) - **Spec Exp:** Heart Failure; Nuclear Cardiology; Heart Disease in Cancer Patients; Cardiac Effects of Cancer/Cancer Therapy; **Hospital:** Meml Sloan-Kettering Cancer Ctr (page 112); **Address:** 1275 York Avenue, New York, NY 10065; **Phone:** 800-525-2225; **Board Cert:** Internal Medicine 1977; Cardiovascular Disease 1979; **Med School:** Mount Sinai Sch Med 1974; **Resid:** Internal Medicine, Yale-New Haven Hosp 1977; **Fellow:** Cardiovascular Disease, Mt Sinai Med Ctr 1979; **Fac Appt:** Prof Med, Cornell Univ-Weill Med Coll

Tenenbaum, Joseph MD (Cv) - **Spec Exp:** Heart Valve Disease; Coronary Artery Disease; Atrial Fibrillation; **Hospital:** NY-Presby Hosp/Columbia (page 104); **Address:** 161 Ft Washington Ave, Ste 535, Irving Pavilion, New York, NY 10032-3713; **Phone:** 212-305-5288; **Board Cert:** Internal Medicine 1977; Cardiovascular Disease 1979; **Med School:** Harvard Med Sch 1974; **Resid:** Internal Medicine, Columbia-Presby Med Ctr 1977; **Fellow:** Cardiovascular Disease, Mt Sinai Hosp 1979; **Fac Appt:** Prof Med, Columbia P&S

Tyberg, Theodore MD (Cv) - **Spec Exp:** Coronary Artery Disease; Cholesterol/Lipid Disorders; **Hospital:** NY-Presby Hosp/Weill Cornell (page 104); **Address:** 425 E 61st St, Fl 6, New York, NY 10065; **Phone:** 212-752-2000; **Board Cert:** Internal Medicine 1978; Cardiovascular Disease 1981; **Med School:** Rush Med Coll 1975; **Resid:** Internal Medicine, New York Hosp 1978; **Fellow:** Cardiovascular Disease, Yale-New Haven Hosp 1980; **Fac Appt:** Assoc Clin Prof Med, Cornell Univ-Weill Med Coll

Unger, Allen MD (Cv) - **Spec Exp:** Cholesterol/Lipid Disorders; Hypertension; Preventive Cardiology; Coronary Artery Disease; **Hospital:** Mount Sinai Med Ctr (page 102); **Address:** 12 E 86th St, New York, NY 10028-0506; **Phone:** 212-734-6000; **Board Cert:** Internal Medicine 1968; Cardiovascular Disease 1977; **Med School:** SUNY Upstate Med Univ 1960; **Resid:** Internal Medicine, Mount Sinai Hosp 1967; **Fellow:** Cardiovascular Disease, Mount Sinai Hosp 1966; **Fac Appt:** Asst Clin Prof Med, Mount Sinai Sch Med

Varriale, Philip MD (Cv) - **Spec Exp:** Coronary Artery Disease; Arrhythmias; Congestive Heart Failure; Pacemakers; **Hospital:** Beth Israel Med Ctr - Petrie Division (page 94); **Address:** 222 E 19th St, Ste 2D, New York, NY 10003-2666; **Phone:** 212-777-3219; **Board Cert:** Internal Medicine 1966; Cardiovascular Disease 1970; **Med School:** SUNY Hlth Sci Ctr 1959; **Resid:** Internal Medicine, St Vincent's Hosp 1963; Cardiovascular Disease, St Vincent's Hosp 1964; **Fac Appt:** Assoc Clin Prof Med, Mount Sinai Sch Med

Weintraub, Howard S MD (Cv) - **Spec Exp:** Hypertension; Echocardiography; Preventive Cardiology; Cholesterol/Lipid Disorders; **Hospital:** NYU Langone Med Ctr (page 106); **Address:** 345 E 37th St, Ste 308, New York, NY 10016-3217; **Phone:** 212-599-5030; **Board Cert:** Internal Medicine 1979; Cardiovascular Disease 1985; **Med School:** NYU Sch Med 1976; **Resid:** Internal Medicine, NYU Med Ctr 1979; **Fellow:** Pulmonary Disease, NYU Med Ctr 1980; Cardiovascular Disease, NYU Med Ctr 1982; **Fac Appt:** Assoc Clin Prof Med, NYU Sch Med

Weisenseel, Arthur C MD (Cv) - **Spec Exp:** Coronary Artery Disease; Cholesterol/Lipid Disorders; Congestive Heart Failure; Preventive Cardiology; **Hospital:** Mount Sinai Med Ctr (page 102); **Address:** 12 E 86th St, New York, NY 10028-0506; **Phone:** 212-734-6000; **Board Cert:** Internal Medicine 1969; Cardiovascular Disease 1973; **Med School:** Georgetown Univ 1963; **Resid:** Internal Medicine, Mount Sinai Hosp 1966; **Fellow:** Cardiovascular Disease, Mount Sinai 1967; **Fac Appt:** Assoc Clin Prof Med, Mount Sinai Sch Med

Wolk, Michael MD (Cv) - **Spec Exp:** Coronary Artery Disease; Heart Failure; Hypertension; **Hospital:** NY-Presby Hosp/Weill Cornell (page 104); **Address:** 425 E 61st St Fl 6, New York, NY 10021; **Phone:** 212-752-2000; **Board Cert:** Internal Medicine 1971; Cardiovascular Disease 1973; **Med School:** Columbia P&S 1964; **Resid:** Internal Medicine, Univ Hosp 1967; **Fellow:** Cardiovascular Disease, New England Med Ctr 1969; Cardiovascular Disease, New York Hosp-Cornell 1970; **Fac Appt:** Clin Prof Med, Cornell Univ-Weill Med Coll

Zaremski, Benjamin MD (Cv) *PCP* - **Hospital:** Beth Israel Med Ctr - Petrie Division (page 94), Lenox Hill Hosp; **Address:** 510 E 80th St, New York, NY 10075; **Phone:** 212-517-0022; **Board Cert:** Internal Medicine 1986; **Med School:** Dominican Republic 1981; **Resid:** Internal Medicine, Metropolitan Hosp 1984; **Fellow:** Cardiovascular Disease, St Francis Hosp/Metropolitan Hosp 1986

Child & Adolescent Psychiatry

Abright, Arthur R MD (ChAP) - **Spec Exp:** Bipolar/Mood Disorders; ADD/ADHD; Anxiety Disorders; **Address:** 144 W 12th St, New York, NY 10011-8202; **Phone:** 212-604-8213; **Board Cert:** Psychiatry 1978; Child & Adolescent Psychiatry 1981; **Med School:** Univ Tex SW, Dallas 1973; **Resid:** Psychiatry, St Vincent's Hosp 1974; Psychiatry, NY Hosp-Cornell Med Ctr 1977; **Fellow:** Child & Adolescent Psychiatry, NY Hosp-Cornell Med Ctr 1979; **Fac Appt:** Clin Prof Psyc, NY Med Coll

Bird, Hector MD (ChAP) - **Spec Exp:** ADD/ADHD; Anxiety & Depression; Personality Disorders; **Hospital:** NY-Presby Hosp/Columbia (page 104); **Address:** 300 W 72nd St, Ste 1F, New York, NY 10023-2004; **Phone:** 212-874-5311; **Board Cert:** Psychiatry 1975; Child & Adolescent Psychiatry 1977; **Med School:** Yale Univ 1965; **Resid:** Psychiatry, NY State Psych Inst 1971 NY State Psych Inst 1972; **Fellow:** Psychoanalysis, WA White Institute 1977; **Fac Appt:** Prof Emeritus Psyc, Columbia P&S

Burkes, Lynn MD (ChAP) - **Spec Exp:** Diagnostic Problems; ADD/ADHD; Divorce/Family Issues; Developmental Disorders; **Hospital:** NYU Langone Med Ctr (page 106); **Address:** 185 West End Ave, New York, NY 10023-5539; **Phone:** 212-362-5920; **Board Cert:** Psychiatry 1977; Child & Adolescent Psychiatry 1978; **Med School:** Drexel Univ Coll Med 1970; **Resid:** Psychiatry, Albert Einstein 1973; **Fellow:** Psychiatry, Bellevue Hosp 1975; **Fac Appt:** Assoc Clin Prof Psyc, NYU Sch Med

Coffey, Barbara J MD (ChAP) - **Spec Exp:** Tourette's Syndrome; ADD/ADHD; Obsessive-Compulsive Disorder; Psychopharmacology; **Hospital:** NYU Langone Med Ctr (page 106); **Address:** NYU Child Study Ctr, 577 1st Ave, New York, NY 10016; **Phone:** 212-263-3926; **Board Cert:** Psychiatry 1981; Child & Adolescent Psychiatry 1986; **Med School:** Tufts Univ 1975; **Resid:** Psychiatry, Boston Univ Med Ctr 1978; **Fellow:** Child & Adolescent Psychiatry, Tufts Univ 1980; **Fac Appt:** Assoc Prof Psyc, NYU Sch Med

Gabbay, Vilma MD (ChAP) - **Spec Exp:** Depression; **Hospital:** NYU Langone Med Ctr (page 106), Bellevue Hosp Ctr; **Address:** NYU Child Study Ctr, 577 First Ave, New York, NY 10016; **Phone:** 212-263-3654; **Board Cert:** Psychiatry 2005; Child & Adolescent Psychiatry 2007; **Med School:** Israel 1994; **Resid:** Psychiatry, Montefiore Med Ctr 2001; **Fellow:** Child & Adolescent Psychiatry, NYU Med Ctr 2003; **Fac Appt:** Asst Prof ChAP, NYU Sch Med

Havens, Jennifer MD (ChAP) - **Spec Exp:** Anxiety Disorders; Bereavement/Traumatic Grief; **Hospital:** NYU Langone Med Ctr (page 106), Bellevue Hosp Ctr; **Address:** NYU Child Study Ctr, 577 First Ave, New York, NY 10016; **Phone:** 212-562-2156; **Board Cert:** Psychiatry 1991; Child & Adolescent Psychiatry 1993; **Med School:** Tufts Univ 1986; **Resid:** Psychiatry, Payne Witney Clinic/Cornell Med Ctr 1988; **Fellow:** Child & Adolescent Psychiatry, Columbia Presby Med Ctr 1991

Hertzig, Margaret MD (ChAP) - **Spec Exp:** Developmental Disorders; ADD/ADHD; **Hospital:** NY-Presby Hosp/Weill Cornell (page 104); **Address:** 525 E 68th St, Box 140, New York, NY 10021-4870; **Phone:** 212-746-5712; **Board Cert:** Psychiatry 1968; Child & Adolescent Psychiatry 1975; **Med School:** NYU Sch Med 1960; **Resid:** Pediatrics, Jewish Hosp 1962; Psychiatry, Bellevue Psych Hosp 1964; **Fellow:** Psychiatric Research, NYU Sch Med 1966; **Fac Appt:** Prof Psyc, Cornell Univ-Weill Med Coll

Hirsch, Glenn S MD (ChAP) - **Spec Exp:** Anxiety & Mood Disorders; Tourette's Syndrome; Bipolar/Mood Disorders; ADD/ADHD; **Hospital:** NYU Langone Med Ctr (page 106), Bellevue Hosp Ctr; **Address:** NYU Child Study Center, 577 First Ave, New York, NY 10016; **Phone:** 212-263-8704; **Board Cert:** Psychiatry 1984; Child & Adolescent Psychiatry 1985; **Med School:** Albert Einstein Coll Med 1979; **Resid:** Psychiatry, New York Hosp-Cornell 1982; **Fellow:** Child & Adolescent Psychiatry, Columbia-Presby Med Ctr 1984; **Fac Appt:** Asst Prof ChAP, NYU Sch Med

Kron, Leo L MD (ChAP) - **Spec Exp:** Psychopharmacology; Psychotherapy; **Hospital:** St Luke's - Roosevelt Hosp Ctr - Roosevelt Div (page 94); **Address:** 30 E 76th St, Ste 3A, New York, NY 10021; **Phone:** 212-861-7001; **Board Cert:** Psychiatry 1977; Child & Adolescent Psychiatry 1986; **Med School:** Univ British Columbia Fac Med 1971; **Resid:** Psychiatry, Albert Einstein Affil Hosp 1976; **Fellow:** Child & Adolescent Psychiatry, St Lukes Hosp 1978; **Fac Appt:** Asst Clin Prof Psyc, Columbia P&S

Leventhal, Bennett MD (ChAP) - **Spec Exp:** Autism; ADD/ADHD; Psychopharmacology; **Hospital:** NYU Langone Med Ctr (page 106); **Address:** 577 First Ave, New York, NY 10016; **Phone:** 212-263-8696; **Board Cert:** Psychiatry 1979; Child & Adolescent Psychiatry 1980; **Med School:** Louisiana State U, New Orleans 1974; **Resid:** Psychiatry, Duke Univ Med Ctr 1978; **Fellow:** Child & Adolescent Psychiatry, Duke Univ Med Ctr 1977; **Fac Appt:** Prof Psyc, NYU Sch Med

Lewis, Owen MD (ChAP) - **Spec Exp:** Psychotherapy; Psychopharmacology; **Hospital:** NY-Presby Hosp/Columbia (page 104); **Address:** 11 E 87th St, New York, NY 10128-0527; **Phone:** 212-996-8196; **Board Cert:** Psychiatry 1982; Child & Adolescent Psychiatry 1986; **Med School:** Mount Sinai Sch Med 1976; **Resid:** Psychiatry, NY Hosp 1980; **Fellow:** Child & Adolescent Psychiatry, NY Hosp 1982; **Fac Appt:** Clin Prof Psyc, Columbia P&S

Moreau, Donna L MD (ChAP) - **Spec Exp:** Psychotherapy & Psychopharmacology; Anxiety & Mood Disorders; **Hospital:** NYPresby-Morgan Stanley Children's Hosp (page 104); **Address:** 110 East End Ave, New York, NY 10028-7412; **Phone:** 212-772-9205; **Board Cert:** Psychiatry 1985; Child & Adolescent Psychiatry 1991; **Med School:** SUNY Hlth Sci Ctr 1980; **Resid:** Psychiatry, NY Hosp 1984; **Fellow:** Child & Adolescent Psychiatry, NY Hosp 1986; **Fac Appt:** Assoc Clin Prof Psyc, Columbia P&S

Newcorn, Jeffrey H MD (ChAP) - **Spec Exp:** Psychopharmacology; ADD/ADHD; Developmental Disorders; Behavioral Disorders; **Hospital:** Mount Sinai Med Ctr (page 102); **Address:** Mount Sinai Hosp, Dept Psychiatry, One Gustave Levy Pl, Box 1230, New York, NY 10029; **Phone:** 212-659-8705; **Board Cert:** Psychiatry 1982; Child & Adolescent Psychiatry 1984; **Med School:** Univ Rochester 1977; **Resid:** Psychiatry, Tufts-New England Med Ctr 1980; **Fellow:** Child & Adolescent Psychiatry, Tufts-New England Med Ctr 1982; **Fac Appt:** Assoc Prof Psyc, Mount Sinai Sch Med

Perry, Richard MD (ChAP) - **Spec Exp:** Pervasive Development Disorders; Behavioral Disorders; Psychopharmacology; **Hospital:** Bellevue Hosp Ctr; **Address:** 55 W 74th St, New York, NY 10023-2429; **Phone:** 212-595-0116; **Board Cert:** Psychiatry 1976; Child & Adolescent Psychiatry 1985; **Med School:** Belgium 1970; **Resid:** Psychiatry, Bellevue Hosp 1972; **Fellow:** Child & Adolescent Psychiatry, Bellevue Hosp 1974; **Fac Appt:** Clin Prof Psyc, NYU Sch Med

Shatkin, Jess P MD (ChAP) - **Spec Exp:** Autism; Anxiety & Mood Disorders; ADD/ADHD; **Hospital:** NYU Langone Med Ctr (page 106), Bellevue Hosp Ctr; **Address:** 577 First Ave, New York, NY 10016; **Phone:** 212-263-4769; **Board Cert:** Psychiatry 2001; Child & Adolescent Psychiatry 2003; **Med School:** SUNY Hlth Sci Ctr 1996; **Resid:** Psychiatry, UCLA NPI 1999; **Fellow:** Child & Adolescent Psychiatry, UCLA NPI 2001; **Fac Appt:** Asst Prof Psyc, NYU Sch Med

Spencer, Elizabeth Kay MD (ChAP) - **Hospital:** NYU Langone Med Ctr (page 106); **Address:** 121 E 31st St, Ste 1B, New York, NY 10016-6835; **Phone:** 212-684-3810; **Board Cert:** Psychiatry 1990; Child & Adolescent Psychiatry 1992; **Med School:** Geo Wash Univ 1979; **Resid:** Pediatrics, Univ Maryland Hosp 1982; Psychiatry, NYU Med Ctr 1986; **Fellow:** Behavioral Pediatrics, Univ Maryland Hosp 1984; Child & Adolescent Psychiatry, NYU Med Ctr 1988; **Fac Appt:** Asst Clin Prof Psyc, NYU Sch Med

Turecki, Stanley K MD (ChAP) - **Spec Exp:** Temperamentally Difficult Child; ADD/ADHD; Parenting Issues; **Hospital:** Lenox Hill Hosp, Beth Israel Med Ctr - Petrie Division (page 94); **Address:** 136 E 64th St, Ste 1B, New York, NY 10021-2137; **Phone:** 212-355-2535; **Board Cert:** Psychiatry 1978; Child & Adolescent Psychiatry 1981; **Med School:** South Africa 1961; **Resid:** Psychiatry, Tara Hospital 1969; Psychiatry, Mt Sinai Hosp 1971

Child Neurology

Allen, Jeffrey MD (ChiN) - **Spec Exp:** Neuro-Oncology; Brain Tumors; **Hospital:** NYU Langone Med Ctr (page 106); **Address:** Hassenfeld Childrens Ctr, 160 E 32nd St Fl 2nd - Ste L3, New York, NY 10016; **Phone:** 212-263-9907; **Board Cert:** Child Neurology 1977; **Med School:** Harvard Med Sch 1969; **Resid:** Pediatrics, Montreal Chldns Hosp 1973; Pediatric Neurology, Montreal Neur Inst/McGill 1976; **Fac Appt:** Prof Ped, NYU Sch Med

De Vivo, Darryl C MD (ChiN) - **Spec Exp:** Metabolic Disorders; Neuromuscular Disorders; Spinal Muscular Atrophy (SMA); **Hospital:** NY-Presby Hosp/Columbia (page 104); **Address:** Neurological Institute, 710 W 168th St, rm 201, New York, NY 10032; **Phone:** 212-305-5244; **Board Cert:** Child Neurology 1972; **Med School:** Univ VA Sch Med 1964; **Resid:** Pediatrics, Mass Genl Hosp 1966; Neurology, Mass Genl Hosp 1967; **Fellow:** Neurology, Natl Inst Hlth 1969; Child Neurology, Children's Hosp 1970; **Fac Appt:** Prof N, Columbia P&S

Kaufman, David M MD (ChiN) - **Spec Exp:** Epilepsy/Seizure Disorders; Headache; Learning Disorders; Autism; **Hospital:** Mount Sinai Med Ctr (page 102), Lenox Hill Hosp; **Address:** 3 E 83rd St, New York, NY 10028-0459; **Phone:** 212-737-4911; **Board Cert:** Pediatrics 1980; **Med School:** Boston Univ 1975; **Resid:** Pediatrics, New York Hosp 1977; Neurology, Mount Sinai Hosp 1978; **Fellow:** Child Neurology, Mount Sinai Hosp 1980; **Fac Appt:** Assoc Clin Prof N, Mount Sinai Sch Med

Kosofsky, Barry MD/PhD (ChiN) - **Spec Exp:** Developmental Disorders; Autism; Stroke; **Hospital:** NY-Presby Hosp/Weill Cornell (page 104); **Address:** NY-Cornell Med Ctr, Dept Pediatrics, 525 E 68th St, Box 91, New York, NY 10065; **Phone:** 212-746-3278; **Board Cert:** Child Neurology 1993; **Med School:** Johns Hopkins Univ 1985; **Resid:** Pediatrics, Chldns Hosp 1987; Child Neurology, Mass Genl Hosp 1990; **Fellow:** Neurological Biology, Mass Genl Hosp 1992; **Fac Appt:** Prof Ped, Cornell Univ-Weill Med Coll

Miles, Daniel K MD (ChiN) - **Spec Exp:** Pediatric Neurology; Tuberous Sclerosis; Epilepsy; **Hospital:** NYU Langone Med Ctr (page 106); **Address:** NYU Comprehensive Epilepsy Ctr, 403 E 34th St Fl 4, New York, NY 10016; **Phone:** 212-263-8318; **Board Cert:** Child Neurology 1994; **Med School:** UMDNJ-NJ Med Sch, Newark 1983; **Resid:** Pediatrics, St Christopher's Hosp 1986; Pediatric Neurology, Chlds Meml Hosp 1989; **Fellow:** Epilepsy, Boston Chlds Hosp 1990

Molofsky, Walter MD (ChiN) - **Spec Exp:** Seizure Disorders; Headache; ADD/ADHD; Stroke; **Hospital:** Beth Israel Med Ctr - Petrie Division (page 94), St Luke's - Roosevelt Hosp Ctr - Roosevelt Div (page 94); **Address:** Phillips Ambulatory Care Center, 10 Union Square E, Ste 5J, New York, NY 10003; **Phone:** 212-844-6910; **Board Cert:** Pediatrics 1982; Child Neurology 1986; **Med School:** NYU Sch Med 1976; **Resid:** Pediatrics, Columbia-Presby Med Ctr 1978; **Fellow:** Child Neurology, Columbia-Presby Med Ctr 1981; **Fac Appt:** Assoc Prof N, Albert Einstein Coll Med

Nass, Ruth MD (ChiN) - **Spec Exp:** Autism; ADD/ADHD; Learning Disorders; Migraine; **Hospital:** NYU Langone Med Ctr (page 106); **Address:** 400 E 34th St, rm 311, New York, NY 10016-4901; **Phone:** 212-263-7753; **Board Cert:** Pediatrics 1980; Child Neurology 1981; **Med School:** Albert Einstein Coll Med 1975; **Resid:** Pediatrics, NY Hosp 1977; Child Neurology, Columbia-Presby 1980; **Fellow:** Neurology, NY Hosp 1982; **Fac Appt:** Prof N, NYU Sch Med

Wolf, Steven M MD (ChiN) - **Spec Exp:** Epilepsy; Headache; Migraine; **Hospital:** Beth Israel Med Ctr - Petrie Division (page 94), St Luke's - Roosevelt Hosp Ctr - Roosevelt Div (page 94); **Address:** Beth Israel Med Ctr, Dept Ped Neurology, 10 Union Square East, Ste 5J, New York, NY 10003; **Phone:** 212-844-6944; **Board Cert:** Child Neurology 2006; Pediatrics 2004; Clinical Neurophysiology 2008; **Med School:** Albany Med Coll 1989; **Resid:** Pediatrics, Montefiore Med Ctr 1991; Child Neurology, Montefiore Med Ctr 1994; **Fellow:** Epilepsy, Montefiore Med Ctr 1995; **Fac Appt:** Asst Prof N, Albert Einstein Coll Med

Clinical Genetics

Anyane-Yeboa, Kwame MD (CG) - **Spec Exp:** Dysmorphology; Prenatal Diagnosis; **Hospital:** NYPresby-Morgan Stanley Children's Hosp (page 104), St Luke's - Roosevelt Hosp Ctr - Roosevelt Div (page 94); **Address:** Morgan Stanley Children's Hospital of NY, 3959 Broadway Fl 6N - rm 601A, New York, NY 10032; **Phone:** 212-305-6731; **Board Cert:** Pediatrics 1979; Clinical Genetics 1982; **Med School:** Ghana 1972; **Resid:** Pediatrics, Harlem Hosp 1977; **Fellow:** Clinical Genetics, Babies Hosp-Columbia Presby 1980; **Fac Appt:** Assoc Prof Ped, Columbia P&S

Davis, Jessica G MD (CG) - **Spec Exp:** Marfan's Syndrome; Mental Retardation; Neurofibromatosis; Ehlers-Danlos Syndrome; **Hospital:** NY-Presby Hosp/Weill Cornell (page 104), Hosp For Special Surgery (page 111); **Address:** 505 E 70th St, Box 128, New York, NY 10065; **Phone:** 646-962-2205; **Board Cert:** Clinical Genetics 1984; **Med School:** Columbia P&S 1959; **Resid:** Pediatrics, St Luke's Hosp 1962; Clinical Genetics, Albert Einstein Coll Med 1965; **Fellow:** Cytogenetics, Albert Einstein Coll Med 1966; Pediatrics, Albert Einstein Col Med 1968; **Fac Appt:** Assoc Clin Prof Ped, Cornell Univ-Weill Med Coll

Desnick, Robert J MD/PhD (CG) - **Spec Exp:** Inherited Metabolic Disorders; Fabry's Disease; Gaucher Disease; Porphyria; **Hospital:** Mount Sinai Med Ctr (page 102), Beth Israel Med Ctr - Petrie Division (page 94); **Address:** Mt Sinai Sch Med, Box 1498, Fifth Ave @ 100th St, New York, NY 10029; **Phone:** 212-241-6947; **Board Cert:** Clinical Genetics 1982; Clinical Molecular Genetics 2009; Clinical Biochemical Genetics 1982; **Med School:** Univ Minn 1971; **Resid:** Pediatrics, Univ Minn Hosps 1973; **Fac Appt:** Prof CG, Mount Sinai Sch Med

Gilbert, Fred MD (CG) - **Spec Exp:** Cancer Genetics; Prenatal Diagnosis; **Hospital:** NY-Presby Hosp/Weill Cornell (page 104), Brooklyn Hosp Ctr-Downtown; **Address:** 1300 York Ave, Box 128, New York, NY 10065; **Phone:** 646-962-2205; **Board Cert:** Clinical Genetics 1982; Clinical Cytogenetics 1982; Clinical Molecular Genetics 2006; **Med School:** Albert Einstein Coll Med 1966; **Resid:** Internal Medicine, Barnes Hosp 1968; Internal Medicine, Natl Inst Hlth 1971; **Fellow:** Clinical Genetics, Yale-New Haven Hosp 1974; **Fac Appt:** Assoc Prof Ped, Cornell Univ-Weill Med Coll

Ostrer, Harry MD (CG) - **Spec Exp:** Genetic Disorders; Hereditary Cancer; **Hospital:** NYU Langone Med Ctr (page 106); **Address:** NYU Medical Ctr, 550 1st Ave, rm MSB136, New York, NY 10016; **Phone:** 212-263-5746; **Board Cert:** Clinical Genetics 1984; Pediatrics 1985; Clinical Cytogenetics 1990; Clinical Molecular Genetics 2010; **Med School:** Columbia P&S 1976; **Resid:** Pediatrics, Johns Hopkins Hosp 1978; Clinical Genetics, Natl Inst Health 1981; **Fellow:** Molecular Genetics, Johns Hopkins Hosp 1983; **Fac Appt:** Prof Ped, NYU Sch Med

Colon & Rectal Surgery

Arnell, Tracey D MD (CRS) - **Spec Exp:** Laparoscopic Surgery; Diverticulitis; Inflammatory Bowel Disease; Anorectal Disorders; **Hospital:** NY-Presby Hosp/Columbia (page 104); **Address:** 161 Fort Washington Ave Fl 8, New York, NY 10032; **Phone:** 212-342-1734; **Board Cert:** Surgery 2009; Colon & Rectal Surgery 2000; **Med School:** Univ Wash 1992; **Resid:** Surgery, Harbor-UCLA Med Ctr 1998; **Fellow:** Colon & Rectal Surgery, Lahey Clinic 1999; **Fac Appt:** Asst Prof S, Columbia P&S

Brandeis, Steven MD (CRS) - **Spec Exp:** Hemorrhoids; Anal Disorders & Reconstruction; Colon & Rectal Cancer; Anorectal Disorders; **Hospital:** NY Downtown Hosp, NYU Langone Med Ctr (page 106); **Address:** 251 E 33rd St Fl 2 - Ste 2N, New York, NY 10016; **Phone:** 212-696-5411; **Board Cert:** Surgery 1981; Colon & Rectal Surgery 2001; **Med School:** NYU Sch Med 1975; **Resid:** Surgery, NYU Med Ctr-Bellevue Hosp 1980; **Fellow:** Colon & Rectal Surgery, RWJ Univ Hosp 1981; **Fac Appt:** Asst Prof S, NYU Sch Med

Gorfine, Stephen R MD (CRS) - **Spec Exp:** Anal Disorders & Reconstruction; Hemorrhoids; Rectal Cancer; Anal Cancer; **Hospital:** Mount Sinai Med Ctr (page 102), Lenox Hill Hosp; **Address:** 25 E 69th St, New York, NY 10021-4925; **Phone:** 212-517-8600; **Board Cert:** Internal Medicine 1981; Surgery 2007; Colon & Rectal Surgery 1988; **Med School:** Univ Mass Sch Med 1978; **Resid:** Internal Medicine, Mt Sinai Hosp 1981; Surgery, Mt Sinai Hosp 1985; **Fellow:** Colon & Rectal Surgery, Ferguson Hosp 1987; **Fac Appt:** Clin Prof S, Mount Sinai Sch Med

Gottesman, Lester MD (CRS) - **Spec Exp:** Anorectal Disorders; Incontinence-Fecal; Colonoscopy; **Hospital:** St Luke's - Roosevelt Hosp Ctr - Roosevelt Div (page 94); **Address:** 425 W 59th St, Ste 9A, New York, NY 10019-1104; **Phone:** 212-523-8417; **Board Cert:** Colon & Rectal Surgery 2009; **Med School:** Univ Pittsburgh 1978; **Resid:** Surgery, St Luke's-Roosevelt Hosp Ctr 1983; **Fellow:** Surgery, Meml Sloan Kettering Cancer Ctr 1985; Colon & Rectal Surgery, Ferguson Clinic 1987; **Fac Appt:** Assoc Prof S, Columbia P&S

Guillem, Jose MD (CRS) - **Spec Exp:** Colon & Rectal Cancer; Rectal Cancer/Sphincter Preservation; Colon & Rectal Cancer-Hereditary; Peritoneal Mucinous Carcinomatosis; **Hospital:** Meml Sloan-Kettering Cancer Ctr (page 112); **Address:** 1275 York Avenue, New York, NY 10065; **Phone:** 212-639-8278; **Board Cert:** Colon & Rectal Surgery 2005; Surgery 2004; **Med School:** Yale Univ 1983; **Resid:** Surgery, Columbia-Presby Med Ctr 1990; **Fellow:** Colon & Rectal Surgery, Lahey Clinic 1991; **Fac Appt:** Prof CRS, Cornell Univ-Weill Med Coll

Milsom, Jeffrey W MD (CRS) - **Spec Exp:** Inflammatory Bowel Disease; Laparoscopic Surgery; Colon & Rectal Cancer; Crohn's Disease; **Hospital:** NY-Presby Hosp/Weill Cornell (page 104); **Address:** NY Cornell Med Ctr, Div Colorectal Surgery, 1315 York Ave Fl 2, New York, NY 10065-5304; **Phone:** 212-746-6030; **Board Cert:** Colon & Rectal Surgery 1986; **Med School:** Univ Pittsburgh 1979; **Resid:** Surgery, Roosevelt Hosp 1981; Surgery, Univ Virginia Med Ctr 1984; **Fellow:** Colon & Rectal Surgery, Ferguson Hosp 1985; **Fac Appt:** Prof S, Cornell Univ-Weill Med Coll

Penzer, Jason MD (CRS) - **Spec Exp:** Hemorrhoids; Colon & Rectal Cancer; Diverticulitis; Inflammatory Bowel Disease; **Hospital:** Lenox Hill Hosp, Beth Israel Med Ctr - Petrie Division (page 94); **Address:** 36 7th Ave, Ste 522, New York, NY 10011; **Phone:** 212-675-2997; **Board Cert:** Surgery 2002; Colon & Rectal Surgery 2003; **Med School:** Yale Univ 1996; **Resid:** Surgery, St Vincent's Hosp 2001; **Fellow:** Colon & Rectal Surgery, UMDNJ Med Ctr 2002; **Fac Appt:** Asst Clin Prof S, NY Med Coll

Sonoda, Toyooki MD (CRS) - **Spec Exp:** Inflammatory Bowel Disease; Laparoscopic Surgery; Colon & Rectal Cancer & Surgery; Crohn's Disease; **Hospital:** NY-Presby Hosp/Weill Cornell (page 104); **Address:** NY Presbyterian-Cornell Medical Ctr, 1315 York Ave, Box 172, New York, NY 10021; **Phone:** 212-746-6030; **Board Cert:** Surgery 1999; Colon & Rectal Surgery 2001; **Med School:** Yale Univ 1993; **Resid:** Surgery, UCSF Med Ctr 1995; Surgery, Cleveland Clinic 1998; **Fellow:** Laparoscopic Surgery, Mt Sinai Med Ctr 1999; Colon & Rectal Surgery, Cleveland Clinic 2000; **Fac Appt:** Asst Prof S, Cornell Univ-Weill Med Coll

Steinhagen, Randolph MD (CRS) - **Spec Exp:** Colostomy Avoidance; Colon & Rectal Cancer; Inflammatory Bowel Disease/Crohn's; Ulcerative Colitis; **Hospital:** Mount Sinai Med Ctr (page 102), St John's Riverside Hosp; **Address:** Div Colon & Rectal Surgery, 5 E 98th St Fl 14, Box 1259, New York, NY 10029-6501; **Phone:** 212-241-3547; **Board Cert:** Surgery 2002; Colon & Rectal Surgery 1985; **Med School:** Wayne State Univ 1977; **Resid:** Surgery, Mount Sinai Hosp 1982; **Fellow:** Colon & Rectal Surgery, Cleveland Clinic 1983; **Fac Appt:** Prof S, Mount Sinai Sch Med

Temple, Larissa MD (CRS) - **Spec Exp:** Colon & Rectal Cancer; Anal Cancer; Laparoscopic Surgery; **Hospital:** Meml Sloan-Kettering Cancer Ctr (page 112); **Address:** 1275 York Ave, New York, NY 10065; **Phone:** 212-639-6081; **Board Cert:** Surgery 2001; Colon & Rectal Surgery 2005; **Med School:** Univ Calgary 1994; **Resid:** Surgery, Univ Toronto 2000; **Fellow:** Surgical Oncology, Meml Sloan Kettering Cancer Ctr 2002

Weiser, Martin R MD (CRS) - **Spec Exp:** Colon & Rectal Cancer; Minimally Invasive Surgery; Cancer Surgery; **Hospital:** Meml Sloan-Kettering Cancer Ctr (page 112); **Address:** Meml Sloan Kettering Cancer Ctr, 1275 York Ave, New York, NY 10021; **Phone:** 800-525-2225; **Board Cert:** Surgery 2009; Colon & Rectal Surgery 2002; **Med School:** Univ Chicago-Pritzker Sch Med 1991; **Resid:** Surgery, Brigham & Women's Hosp 1998; Colon & Rectal Surgery, Mount Sinai Med Ctr 2002; **Fellow:** Research, Harvard Med Sch 1995; Surgical Oncology, Meml Sloan Kettering Cancer Ctr 2000; **Fac Appt:** Assoc Prof S, Cornell Univ-Weill Med Coll

Whelan, Richard L MD (CRS) - **Spec Exp:** Laparoscopic Surgery; Colon & Rectal Cancer; **Hospital:** St Luke's - Roosevelt Hosp Ctr - Roosevelt Div (page 94); **Address:** 425 W 59th St, Ste 7B, New York, NY 10019; **Phone:** 212-523-8172; **Board Cert:** Surgery 1997; Colon & Rectal Surgery 1989; **Med School:** Columbia P&S 1982; **Resid:** Surgery, Columbia Presby Hosp 1987; **Fellow:** Colon & Rectal Surgery, Univ Minn Med Ctr 1988; **Fac Appt:** Assoc Clin Prof S, Columbia P&S

Critical Care Medicine

Bahr, Gerald S MD (CCM) - **Spec Exp:** Ethics; Critical Care-Complex; **Hospital:** Lenox Hill Hosp; **Address:** Lenox Hill Hosp - Medicine, 110 E 59th St, Ste 9A, New York, NY 10022-1304; **Phone:** 212-583-2878; **Board Cert:** Internal Medicine 1976; Critical Care Medicine 2009; **Med School:** NY Med Coll 1972; **Resid:** Internal Medicine, Lenox Hill Hosp 1976; **Fellow:** Internal Medicine, Lenox Hill Hosp 1976; **Fac Appt:** Assoc Clin Prof Med, NYU Sch Med

Benjamin, Ernest MD (CCM) - **Spec Exp:** Respiratory Distress Syndrome; Sepsis; **Hospital:** Mount Sinai Med Ctr (page 102); **Address:** Mount Sinai Hosp, SICU, 1 Gustave Levy Pl, Box 1264, New York, NY 10029; **Phone:** 212-241-8867; **Board Cert:** Anesthesiology 1988; Critical Care Medicine 1989; **Med School:** France 1971; **Resid:** Critical Care Medicine, Univ Lyon Affil Hosps 1978; Internal Medicine, North Genl Hosp 1982; **Fellow:** Anesthesiology, Mount Sinai Hosp 1983; **Fac Appt:** Prof S, Mount Sinai Sch Med

Halpern, Neil MD (CCM) - **Hospital:** Meml Sloan-Kettering Cancer Ctr (page 112), Mount Sinai Med Ctr (page 102); **Address:** 1275 York Avenue, New York, NY 10065; **Phone:** 212-639-6731; **Board Cert:** Internal Medicine 1984; Critical Care Medicine 1998; **Med School:** Mount Sinai Sch Med 1981; **Resid:** Internal Medicine, Mount Sinai Hosp 1984; **Fellow:** Critical Care Medicine, Univ Pittsburgh 1985; **Fac Appt:** Prof Med, Cornell Univ-Weill Med Coll

Dermatology

Albom, Michael J MD (D) - **Spec Exp:** Mohs' Surgery; Cosmetic Dermatology; Botox Therapy; Reconstructive Surgery; **Hospital:** NYU Langone Med Ctr (page 106), Lenox Hill Hosp (Manh Eye, Ear & Throat Hosp); **Address:** 33 E 70th St, New York, NY 10021; **Phone:** 212-517-2121; **Board Cert:** Dermatology 1976; **Med School:** Boston Univ 1970; **Resid:** Dermatology, Boston Univ Med Ctr 1974; **Fellow:** Mohs Surgery, NYU Med Ctr 1975; **Fac Appt:** Clin Prof D, NYU Sch Med

Aranoff, Shera M MD (D) - **Spec Exp:** Skin Cancer; Cosmetic Dermatology; Acne; Dermatologic Surgery; **Hospital:** Lenox Hill Hosp; **Address:** 975 Park Ave, Ste 1-A, New York, NY 10028; **Phone:** 212-772-9305; **Board Cert:** Dermatology 1980; **Med School:** NY Med Coll 1973; **Resid:** Dermatology, Westchester Co Med Ctr 1980

Avram, Marc R MD (D) - **Spec Exp:** Hair Restoration/Transplant; Skin Laser Surgery; Cosmetic Dermatology; Botox Therapy; **Hospital:** NY-Presby Hosp/Weill Cornell (page 104), Long Island Coll Hosp (page 94); **Address:** 905 5th Ave, New York, NY 10021-2650; **Phone:** 212-734-4007; **Board Cert:** Dermatology 2005; Hair Restoration Surgery 1997; **Med School:** SUNY Downstate 1989; **Resid:** Dermatology, Mass Genl Hosp 1994; **Fac Appt:** Assoc Prof D, Cornell Univ-Weill Med Coll

Bernstein, Robert M MD (D) - **Spec Exp:** Hair Restoration/Transplant; Hair Loss in Women; **Hospital:** NY-Presby Hosp/Columbia (page 104); **Address:** 110 E 55th St Fl 11, New York, NY 10022; **Phone:** 212-826-2400; **Board Cert:** Dermatology 1982; Hair Restoration Surgery 1998; **Med School:** UMDNJ-NJ Med Sch, Newark 1978; **Resid:** Dermatology, Albert Einstein Hosp 1982; **Fac Appt:** Clin Prof D, Columbia P&S

Berson, Diane S MD (D) - **Spec Exp:** Aging Skin; Acne; Skin Cancer; **Hospital:** NY-Presby Hosp/Weill Cornell (page 104); **Address:** 211 E 53rd St, Ste 3, New York, NY 10022-4803; **Phone:** 212-355-3511; **Board Cert:** Dermatology 1988; **Med School:** NYU Sch Med 1984; **Resid:** Dermatology, SUNY Hlth Sci Ctr 1988; **Fac Appt:** Assoc Prof D, Cornell Univ-Weill Med Coll

Bickers, David MD (D) - **Spec Exp:** Skin Cancer; Photodynamic Therapy; Psoriasis; Phototherapy; **Hospital:** NY-Presby Hosp/Columbia (page 104); **Address:** 16 E 60th St, Ste 300, New York, NY 10022-1002; **Phone:** 212-326-8465; **Board Cert:** Dermatology 1974; **Med School:** Univ VA Sch Med 1967; **Resid:** Dermatology, NYU Med Ctr 1973; **Fellow:** Pharmacology, Rockefeller Univ Hosp 1974; **Fac Appt:** Prof D, Columbia P&S

Brademas, Mary Ellen MD (D) - **Spec Exp:** Skin Diseases; Cosmetic Dermatology; Nail Diseases; **Hospital:** NYU Langone Med Ctr (page 106), Bellevue Hosp Ctr; **Address:** 11 5th Ave, Ste F, New York, NY 10003; **Phone:** 212-477-1515; **Board Cert:** Dermatology 1983; **Med School:** Georgetown Univ 1979; **Resid:** Dermatology, Johns Hopkins Hosp 1981; Dermatology, NYU Med Ctr 1983; **Fac Appt:** Assoc Clin Prof D, NYU Sch Med

Brandt, Fredric S MD (D) - **Spec Exp:** Botox Therapy; Cosmetic Dermatology; **Address:** Laser & Skin Surgery Ctr, 323 E 34th St Fl 6, New York, NY 10016; **Phone:** 212-889-7096; **Board Cert:** Internal Medicine 1978; Dermatology 1981; **Med School:** Hahnemann Univ 1975; **Resid:** Internal Medicine, VA Hosp 1981; Dermatology, Univ Miami Hosps 1983

Buchness, Mary Ruth MD (D) - **Spec Exp:** Skin Infections; Skin Cancer; Cosmetic Dermatology; Psoriasis; **Hospital:** NY-Presby Hosp (page 104); **Address:** 560 Broadway, Ste 406, New York, NY 10012; **Phone:** 212-822-3515; **Board Cert:** Dermatology 1986; **Med School:** Columbia P&S 1982; **Resid:** Dermatology, Columbia Univ Med Ctr 1986; **Fac Appt:** Assoc Prof Med, NY Med Coll

Burke, Karen E MD/PhD (D) - **Spec Exp:** Skin Cancer; Cosmetic Dermatology; Aging Skin; **Hospital:** Mount Sinai Med Ctr (page 102); **Address:** 429 E 52nd St, New York, NY 10022-6430; **Phone:** 212-754-1100; **Board Cert:** Dermatology 1985; **Med School:** NYU Sch Med 1978; **Resid:** Dermatology, NYU Med Ctr 1983; **Fac Appt:** Asst Clin Prof D, Mount Sinai Sch Med

Bystryn, Jean-Claude MD (D) - **Spec Exp:** Melanoma; Blistering Diseases; Skin Cancer; Hair Loss; **Hospital:** NYU Langone Med Ctr (page 106); **Address:** 530 1st Ave, Ste 7F, New York, NY 10016; **Phone:** 212-889-3846; **Board Cert:** Dermatology 1970; Clinical & Laboratory Dermatologic Immunology 1985; **Med School:** NYU Sch Med 1962; **Resid:** Internal Medicine, Montefiore Med Ctr 1964; Dermatology, NYU Med Ctr 1969; **Fellow:** Immunology, NYU Med Ctr 1972; **Fac Appt:** Prof D, NYU Sch Med

Carucci, John A MD/PhD (D) - **Spec Exp:** Mohs' Surgery; **Hospital:** NY-Presby Hosp/Weill Cornell (page 104); **Address:** 1305 York Ave Fl 9, New York, NY 10021; **Phone:** 646-962-3376; **Board Cert:** Dermatology 2007; **Med School:** SUNY Downstate 1994; **Resid:** Dermatology, NYU Med Ctr 1998; **Fellow:** Mohs Surgery, Yale-New Haven Hosp 2000; **Fac Appt:** Asst Prof D, Cornell Univ-Weill Med Coll

Clark, Sheryl MD (D) - **Spec Exp:** Melanoma; Skin Cancer; Skin Laser Surgery; Cosmetic Dermatology; **Hospital:** NY-Presby Hosp/Weill Cornell (page 104); **Address:** 109 E 61st St, New York, NY 10065; **Phone:** 212-750-2905; **Board Cert:** Dermatology 1988; **Med School:** Case West Res Univ 1982; **Resid:** Internal Medicine, Mount Sinai-Univ Hosp 1983; Dermatology, Barnes Hosp-Wash Univ 1988; **Fellow:** Dermatology, Barnes Hosp-Wash Univ 1988; **Fac Appt:** Asst Clin Prof D, Cornell Univ-Weill Med Coll

Cohen, David E MD (D) - **Spec Exp:** Occupational Dermatology; Contact Dermatitis; **Hospital:** NYU Langone Med Ctr (page 106); **Address:** NYU Dermatologic Assocs, 530 1st Ave, Ste 7R, New York, NY 10016; **Phone:** 212-263-5889; **Board Cert:** Dermatology 2003; Occupational Medicine 1996; **Med School:** SUNY Stony Brook 1989; **Resid:** Dermatology, NYU Med Ctr 1993; **Fellow:** Occupational Medicine, Columbia Univ Sch of Public Hlth 1994; **Fac Appt:** Assoc Prof D, NYU Sch Med

Davis, Joyce MD (D) - **Spec Exp:** Acne; Hair loss; Cosmetic Dermatology; **Hospital:** Beth Israel Med Ctr - Petrie Division (page 94), Mount Sinai Med Ctr (page 102); **Address:** 69 Fifth Avenue at 15th St, New York, NY 10003; **Phone:** 212-242-3066; **Board Cert:** Dermatology 1983; **Med School:** Albert Einstein Coll Med 1979; **Resid:** Dermatology, Mount Sinai Med Ctr 1983

DeLeo, Vincent A MD (D) - **Spec Exp:** Photosensitive Skin Diseases; Contact Dermatitis; Facial Rejuvenation; Eczema; **Hospital:** St Luke's - Roosevelt Hosp Ctr - Roosevelt Div (page 94), Beth Israel Med Ctr - Petrie Division (page 94); **Address:** 1090 Amsterdam Ave Fl 11, New York, NY 10025; **Phone:** 212-523-5898; **Board Cert:** Dermatology 1976; **Med School:** Louisiana State U, New Orleans 1969; **Resid:** Dermatology, Columbia-Presby Med Ctr 1976; **Fac Appt:** Clin Prof D, Columbia P&S

Demar, Leon K MD (D) - **Spec Exp:** Skin Cancer; Acne; Cosmetic Dermatology; Pediatric Dermatology; **Hospital:** Lenox Hill Hosp, NY-Presby Hosp/Columbia (page 104); **Address:** 985 5th Ave, New York, NY 10075; **Phone:** 212-988-9010; **Board Cert:** Dermatology 1977; **Med School:** NYU Sch Med 1973; **Resid:** Dermatology, Stanford Med Ctr 1975; Dermatology, Columbia-Presby Med Ctr 1977; **Fac Appt:** Assoc Clin Prof D, Columbia P&S

Felderman, Lenora MD (D) - **Spec Exp:** Cosmetic Dermatology; Facian Rejuvenation; Acne & Rosacea; Skin Cancer; **Hospital:** NY-Presby Hosp/Weill Cornell (page 104); **Address:** 1317 3rd Ave Fl 8, New York, NY 10021-2995; **Phone:** 212-734-0091; **Board Cert:** Dermatology 2009; **Med School:** NY Med Coll 1981; **Resid:** Internal Medicine, Montefiore Med Ctr 1982; Dermatology, Montefiore Med Ctr 1985; **Fac Appt:** Asst Clin Prof D, Cornell Univ-Weill Med Coll

Franks Jr, Andrew G MD (D) - **Spec Exp:** Lupus/SLE; Raynaud's Disease; Scleroderma; Dermatomyositis; **Hospital:** NYU Langone Med Ctr (page 106); **Address:** NYU Dermatologic Assocs, Faculty Practice Tower, 530 First Ave Fl 7 - Ste 7R, New York, NY 10016; **Phone:** 212-263-5889; **Board Cert:** Internal Medicine 1975; Dermatology 1977; Rheumatology 1978; **Med School:** NY Med Coll 1971; **Resid:** Internal Medicine, Beth Israel Med Ctr 1974; Dermatology, Columbia-Presby Med Ctr 1975; **Fellow:** Rheumatology, Columbia-Presby Med Ctr 1977; **Fac Appt:** Prof D, NYU Sch Med

Friedman-Kien, Alvin MD (D) - **Spec Exp:** AIDS/HIV; Herpes Simplex; Warts; **Hospital:** NYU Langone Med Ctr (page 106); **Address:** 530 1st Ave, Ste 7C, New York, NY 10016-6402; **Phone:** 212-263-7380; **Board Cert:** Dermatology 1965; **Med School:** Yale Univ 1960; **Resid:** Dermatology, Mass Genl Hosp 1962; Dermatology, Natl Inst Health 1964; **Fellow:** Dermatology, NYU Med Ctr 1967; **Fac Appt:** Prof D, NY Med Coll

Garzon, Maria C MD (D) - **Spec Exp:** Pediatric Dermatology; Vascular Anomalies; Mycosis Fungoides; **Hospital:** NY-Presby Hosp/Columbia (page 104); **Address:** Columbia Univ, Dept Dermatology, 161 Ft Washington Ave Fl 12, New York, NY 10032; **Phone:** 212-305-5293; **Board Cert:** Dermatology 2004; Pediatric Dermatology 2004; **Med School:** Columbia P&S 1988; **Resid:** Pediatrics, Columbia Presby-Babies Hosp 1991; **Fellow:** Dermatology, Columbia Presby Med Ctr 1995; **Fac Appt:** Assoc Clin Prof D, Columbia P&S

Gendler, Ellen C MD (D) - **Spec Exp:** Cosmetic Dermatology; Contact Dermatitis; Botox Therapy; Facial Rejuvenation; **Hospital:** NYU Langone Med Ctr (page 106); **Address:** 1035 Fifth Ave, New York, NY 10028; **Phone:** 212-288-8222; **Board Cert:** Dermatology 1985; **Med School:** Columbia P&S 1981; **Resid:** Dermatology, NYU Med Ctr 1985; **Fac Appt:** Assoc Clin Prof D, NYU Sch Med

Geronemus, Roy MD (D) - **Spec Exp:** Skin Laser Surgery; Cosmetic Dermatology; Mohs' Surgery; Skin Cancer; **Hospital:** NYU Langone Med Ctr (page 106), New York Eye & Ear Infirm (page 113); **Address:** 317 E 34 St, Ste 11N, New York, NY 10016-4974; **Phone:** 212-686-7306; **Board Cert:** Dermatology 1983; **Med School:** Univ Miami Sch Med 1979; **Resid:** Dermatology, NYU-Skin Cancer Unit 1983; **Fellow:** Mohs Surgery, NYU-Skin Cancer Unit 1984; **Fac Appt:** Clin Prof D, NYU Sch Med

Goldberg, David J MD (D) - **Spec Exp:** Mohs' Surgery; Skin Cancer; Cosmetic Dermatology; Laser Surgery; **Hospital:** Mount Sinai Med Ctr (page 102), Hackensack Univ Med Ctr (page 96); **Address:** 115 E 57th St, Ste 710, New York, NY 10022; **Phone:** 212-750-8900; **Board Cert:** Dermatology 1984; Clinical & Laboratory Dematologic Immunology 1987; **Med School:** Yale Univ 1980; **Resid:** Dermatology, NYU Med Ctr 1984; **Fellow:** Mohs Surgery, NYU Med Ctr 1985; **Fac Appt:** Clin Prof D, Mount Sinai Sch Med

Gordon, Marsha MD (D) - **Spec Exp:** Cosmetic Dermatology; Botox Therapy; Facial Rejuvenation; **Hospital:** Mount Sinai Med Ctr (page 102); **Address:** 5 E 98th St Fl 5, New York, NY 10029-6501; **Phone:** 212-241-9728; **Board Cert:** Dermatology 1988; **Med School:** Univ Pennsylvania 1984; **Resid:** Dermatology, Mt Sinai Hosp 1988; **Fac Appt:** Clin Prof D, Mount Sinai Sch Med

Granstein, Richard D MD (D) - **Spec Exp:** Autoimmune Disease; Skin Cancer; Psoriasis; **Hospital:** NY-Presby Hosp/Weill Cornell (page 104); **Address:** 1305 York Ave Fl 9, New York, NY 10021; **Phone:** 646-962-7546; **Board Cert:** Dermatology 2009; Clinical & Laboratory Dematologic Immunology 1985; **Med School:** UCLA 1978; **Resid:** Dermatology, Mass Genl Hosp 1981; **Fellow:** Research, Natl Cancer Inst 1982; Dermatology, Mass Genl Hosp 1983; **Fac Appt:** Prof D, Cornell Univ-Weill Med Coll

Greenberg, Robert MD (D) - **Spec Exp:** Skin Laser Surgery; Cosmetic Dermatology; Botox Therapy; **Hospital:** NYU Langone Med Ctr (page 106); **Address:** 117 E 72nd St, New York, NY 10021-4249; **Phone:** 212-861-2580; **Board Cert:** Dermatology 1977; **Med School:** Univ Mich Med Sch 1970; **Resid:** Dermatology, Univ of Miami Hosps 1975; Dermatology, New York Univ 1977; **Fellow:** Dermatology, Univ Miami Hosp 1974; **Fac Appt:** Asst Clin Prof D, NYU Sch Med

Greenspan, Alan H MD (D) - **Spec Exp:** Skin Cancer; Dermatologic Surgery; Phototherapy; **Hospital:** NYU Langone Med Ctr (page 106), NY Downtown Hosp; **Address:** 39 Broadway, Ste 3005, New York, NY 10006; **Phone:** 212-509-5200; **Board Cert:** Dermatology 2009; **Med School:** Northwestern Univ 1979; **Resid:** Internal Medicine, Northwestern Univ 1981; Dermatology, NYU Med Ctr 1984; **Fac Appt:** Asst Clin Prof D, NYU Sch Med

Gross, Dennis F MD (D) - **Hospital:** NYU Langone Med Ctr (page 106); **Address:** 105 E 37th St, Ground Fl, New York, NY 10016; **Phone:** 212-725-4555; **Board Cert:** Dermatology 1990; **Med School:** SUNY Stony Brook 1986; **Resid:** Dermatology, NYU Med Ctr 1990; **Fac Appt:** Asst Clin Prof D, NYU Sch Med

Grossman, Melanie MD (D) - **Spec Exp:** Skin Laser Surgery; Tattoo Removal; Skin Laser Surgery; Facial Rejuvenation; **Hospital:** NY-Presby Hosp/Columbia (page 104); **Address:** 161 Madison Ave, Ste 4NW, New York, NY 10016-5405; **Phone:** 212-725-8600; **Board Cert:** Dermatology 1999; **Med School:** NYU Sch Med 1988; **Resid:** Internal Medicine, Yale-New Haven Hosp 1989; Dermatology, Columbia-Presby Med Ctr 1992; **Fellow:** Laser Surgery, Mass Genl Hosp 1995; **Fac Appt:** Asst Clin Prof D, Columbia P&S

Halpern, Allan C MD (D) - **Spec Exp:** Skin Cancer; Melanoma; Melanoma Early Detection/Prevention; **Hospital:** Meml Sloan-Kettering Cancer Ctr (page 112); **Address:** 160 E 53rd St Fl 2, Dermatology, New York, NY 10022; **Phone:** 212-610-0766; **Board Cert:** Internal Medicine 1984; Dermatology 1988; **Med School:** Albert Einstein Coll Med 1981; **Resid:** Internal Medicine, Montefiore Hosp 1985; Dermatology, Hosp Univ Penn 1989; **Fellow:** Epidemiology, Hosp Univ Penn 1989; **Fac Appt:** Assoc Prof Med, Cornell Univ-Weill Med Coll

Hatcher, Virgil MD (D) - **Spec Exp:** Cosmetic Dermatology; Psoriasis; Viral Infections; **Hospital:** NYU Langone Med Ctr (page 106); **Address:** 420 W 23rd St, Ste A-GF, New York, NY 10011-2172; **Phone:** 212-675-4244; **Board Cert:** Dermatology 1982; **Med School:** UCSF 1978; **Resid:** Dermatology, NYU Med Ctr 1982; **Fellow:** Virology, NYU Med Ctr 1983; **Fac Appt:** Asst Clin Prof D, NYU Sch Med

Hochman, Herbert MD (D) - **Spec Exp:** Cosmetic Dermatology; Skin Laser Surgery; Skin Cancer; **Hospital:** Lenox Hill Hosp; **Address:** 1020 Park Ave, New York, NY 10028-0913; **Phone:** 212-861-1656; **Board Cert:** Dermatology 1977; **Med School:** Tulane Univ 1970; **Resid:** Dermatology, Montefiore Med Ctr 1976

Jacobs, Michael Ira MD (D) - **Spec Exp:** Skin Cancer; Melanoma; Cosmetic Dermatology; **Hospital:** NY-Presby Hosp/Weill Cornell (page 104), Hosp For Special Surgery (page 111); **Address:** 407 E 70th St Fl 2, New York, NY 10021-5302; **Phone:** 212-772-7190; **Board Cert:** Dermatology 1981; **Med School:** Cornell Univ-Weill Med Coll 1977; **Resid:** Dermatology, New York Hosp-Cornell 1981; **Fac Appt:** Assoc Clin Prof D, Cornell Univ-Weill Med Coll

Katz, Bruce MD (D) - **Spec Exp:** Skin Laser Surgery; Cosmetic Dermatology; Laser Surgery; **Hospital:** Mount Sinai Med Ctr (page 102); **Address:** 60 E 56th St Fl 2, New York, NY 10022-3350; **Phone:** 212-688-5882; **Board Cert:** Dermatology 1983; **Med School:** McGill Univ 1977; **Resid:** Internal Medicine, Columbia Presby Med Ctr 1979; Dermatology, Columbia Presby Med Ctr 1982; **Fac Appt:** Clin Prof D, Mount Sinai Sch Med

Kauvar, Arielle MD (D) - **Spec Exp:** Laser Surgery; Cosmetic Dermatology; Mohs' Surgery; Botox Therapy; **Hospital:** NYU Langone Med Ctr (page 106), New York Eye & Ear Infirm (page 113); **Address:** 1044 Fifth Ave, New York, NY 10028; **Phone:** 212-249-9440; **Board Cert:** Dermatology 2001; **Med School:** Harvard Med Sch 1989; **Resid:** Dermatology, NYU Med Ctr 1993; **Fellow:** Mohs Surgery, Laser & Skin Surgery Ctr 1994; **Fac Appt:** Assoc Clin Prof D, NYU Sch Med

Kenet, Barney J MD (D) - **Spec Exp:** Dermatologic Surgery; Cosmetic Dermatology; Liposuction; **Hospital:** NY-Presby Hosp/Weill Cornell (page 104); **Address:** 25 E 86th St, New York, NY 10028; **Phone:** 212-535-9753; **Board Cert:** Dermatology 2001; **Med School:** Brown Univ 1988; **Resid:** Dermatology, New York Hosp 1992

Kline, Mitchell A MD (D) - **Spec Exp:** Melanoma; Skin Cancer; Mohs' Surgery; Cosmetic Dermatology; **Hospital:** NY-Presby Hosp/Weill Cornell (page 104); **Address:** 700 Park Ave, New York, NY 10021; **Phone:** 212-517-6555; **Board Cert:** Dermatology 2009; **Med School:** Univ Pennsylvania 1985; **Resid:** Internal Medicine, Graduate Hosp 1987; Dermatology, New York Hosp 1990

Kriegel, David MD (D) - **Spec Exp:** Mohs' Surgery; Botox Therapy; Skin Laser Surgery; Cosmetic Dermatology; **Hospital:** Mount Sinai Med Ctr (page 102); **Address:** 250 W 57th St, Ste 825, New York, NY 10107-0809; **Phone:** 212-489-6669; **Board Cert:** Dermatology 2003; **Med School:** Boston Univ 1987; **Resid:** Dermatology, New England Med Ctr 1991; **Fellow:** Mohs Surgery, Stony Brook Univ Hosp 1993; **Fac Appt:** Assoc Prof D, Mount Sinai Sch Med

Lebwohl, Mark MD (D) - **Spec Exp:** Skin Cancer; Psoriasis; Cutaneous Lymphoma; Pseudoxanthoma Elasticum; **Hospital:** Mount Sinai Med Ctr (page 102); **Address:** 5 E 98th St Fl 5, New York, NY 10029-6501; **Phone:** 212-241-9728; **Board Cert:** Internal Medicine 1981; Dermatology 1983; **Med School:** Harvard Med Sch 1978; **Resid:** Internal Medicine, Mt Sinai Hosp 1981; **Fellow:** Dermatology, Mt Sinai Hosp 1983; **Fac Appt:** Prof D, Mount Sinai Sch Med

Lombardo, Peter C MD (D) - **Spec Exp:** Skin Laser Surgery; Skin Cancer; Cosmetic Dermatology; **Hospital:** St Luke's - Roosevelt Hosp Ctr - Roosevelt Div (page 94), NY-Presby Hosp/Columbia (page 104); **Address:** Sutton Place Dermatology, 445 E 58th St, New York, NY 10022-2302; **Phone:** 212-838-0270; **Board Cert:** Dermatology 2009; **Med School:** Albany Med Coll 1959; **Resid:** Dermatology, Columbia-Presby 1965; Internal Medicine, St Luke's-Roosevelt Hosp Ctr 1966; **Fac Appt:** Assoc Clin Prof D, Columbia P&S

Marmur, Ellen S MD (D) - **Spec Exp:** Cosmetic Dermatology; Mohs' Surgery; Laser Surgery; **Hospital:** Mount Sinai Med Ctr (page 102); **Address:** 5 E 98th St Fl 5, Box 1048, New York, NY 10029; **Phone:** 212-241-6189; **Board Cert:** Dermatology 2003; **Med School:** Albert Einstein Coll Med 1999; **Resid:** Dermatology, NY Hosp-Cornell Univ 2003; **Fellow:** Cosmetic Plastic Surgery, Hackensack Hosp 2004; **Fac Appt:** Assoc Prof D, Mount Sinai Sch Med

Myskowski, Patricia L MD (D) - **Spec Exp:** AIDS-Kaposi's Sarcoma; Cutaneous Lymphoma; Skin Cancer; **Hospital:** Meml Sloan-Kettering Cancer Ctr (page 112); **Address:** 1275 York Avenue, New York, NY 10065; **Phone:** 212-610-0768; **Board Cert:** Dermatology 1980; Clinical & Laboratory Dermatologic Immunology 1985; **Med School:** Brown Univ 1975; **Resid:** Internal Medicine, Bronx VA Hosp; Dermatology, NY Hosp-Cornell Med Ctr 1980; **Fellow:** Dermatology, Meml Sloan Kettering Cancer Ctr 1981; **Fac Appt:** Assoc Prof D, Cornell Univ-Weill Med Coll

Orbuch, Philip MD (D) - **Spec Exp:** Pediatric Dermatology; Skin Cancer; **Hospital:** NYU Langone Med Ctr (page 106), Bellevue Hosp Ctr; **Address:** 345 E 37th St, Ste 307, New York, NY 10016; **Phone:** 212-532-5355; **Board Cert:** Dermatology 1986; **Med School:** Israel 1981; **Resid:** Dermatology, NYU Med Ctr 1985; **Fellow:** Dermatology, NYU Med Ctr 1986; **Fac Appt:** Assoc Clin Prof D, NYU Sch Med

Orentreich, David S MD (D) - **Spec Exp:** Dermatologic Surgery; Liposuction; Hair Restoration/Transplant; Laser Surgery; **Hospital:** Mount Sinai Med Ctr (page 102); **Address:** 909 5th Ave, New York, NY 10021; **Phone:** 212-794-0800; **Board Cert:** Dermatology 1984; **Med School:** Columbia P&S 1980; **Resid:** Dermatology, Mt Sinai Med Ctr 1984; **Fac Appt:** Asst Clin Prof D, Mount Sinai Sch Med

Orlow, Seth J MD/PhD (D) - **Spec Exp:** Pediatric Dermatology; Birthmarks/Hemangiomas; Psoriasis/Eczema; **Hospital:** NYU Langone Med Ctr (page 106); **Address:** 530 1st Ave, Ste 7R, New York, NY 10016-6402; **Phone:** 212-263-5889; **Board Cert:** Dermatology 2009; Pediatric Dermatology 2004; **Med School:** Albert Einstein Coll Med 1986; **Resid:** Pediatrics, Mt Sinai Hosp 1987; Dermatology, Yale-New Haven Hosp 1989; **Fellow:** Pediatric Dermatology, Yale-New Haven Hosp 1990; **Fac Appt:** Prof D, NYU Sch Med

Ostad, Ariel MD (D) - **Spec Exp:** Skin Cancer; Mohs' Surgery; Skin Laser Surgery; Cosmetic Dermatology; **Hospital:** NYU Langone Med Ctr (page 106), Lenox Hill Hosp; **Address:** 897 Lexington Ave, New York, NY 10021; **Phone:** 212-517-7900; **Board Cert:** Dermatology 2004; **Med School:** NYU Sch Med 1991; **Resid:** Dermatology, NYU Med Ctr 1995; **Fellow:** Dermatologic Surgery, UCLA Med Ctr 1996; **Fac Appt:** Asst Prof D, NYU Sch Med

Podwal, Mark H MD (D) - **Spec Exp:** Skin Cancer; **Hospital:** NYU Langone Med Ctr (page 106); **Address:** 55 E 73rd St, New York, NY 10021; **Phone:** 212-288-7488; **Board Cert:** Dermatology 1975; **Med School:** NYU Sch Med 1970; **Resid:** Dermatology, Kings Co Hosp Ctr 1972; Dermatology, Bellevue Hosp 1974; **Fac Appt:** Assoc Clin Prof D, NYU Sch Med

Polis, Laurie MD (D) - **Spec Exp:** Cosmetic Dermatology; Skin Laser Surgery; Facial Rejuvenation; **Hospital:** Mount Sinai Med Ctr (page 102); **Address:** 62 Crosby St, New York, NY 10012; **Phone:** 212-431-1600 x227; **Board Cert:** Dermatology 1989; **Med School:** Mount Sinai Sch Med 1983; **Resid:** Dermatology, Montefiore Med Ctr 1989; **Fac Appt:** Asst Prof D, Mount Sinai Sch Med

Prioleau, Philip G MD (D) - **Spec Exp:** Melanoma; Skin Cancer; Mohs' Surgery; **Hospital:** NY-Presby Hosp/Weill Cornell (page 104); **Address:** 1035 Fifth Ave, Ste C, New York, NY 10028; **Phone:** 212-794-3548; **Board Cert:** Surgery 1973; Anatomic Pathology 1979; Dermatopathology 1980; Dermatology 1983; **Med School:** Med Univ SC 1967; **Resid:** Surgery, Univ Va Hosp 1972; Plastic Surgery, Duke Univ Hosp 1975; **Fellow:** Pathology, Barnes Jewish Hosp 1980; Dermatopathology, NYU Med Ctr 1981; **Fac Appt:** Assoc Prof D, Cornell Univ-Weill Med Coll

Prystowsky, Janet MD (D) - **Spec Exp:** Mohs' Surgery; Cosmetic Dermatology; Skin Cancer; Laser Surgery; **Hospital:** St Luke's - Roosevelt Hosp Ctr - Roosevelt Div (page 94); **Address:** 110 E 55th St Fl 7, New York, NY 10022; **Phone:** 212-230-1212; **Board Cert:** Dermatology 1987; **Med School:** Univ Chicago-Pritzker Sch Med 1983; **Resid:** Internal Medicine, Univ Chicago 1984; Dermatology, Hosp Univ Penn 1987; **Fellow:** Mohs Surgery, SUNY Stony Brook

Ramsay, David L MD (D) - **Spec Exp:** Cutaneous Lymphoma; Skin Cancer; **Hospital:** NYU Langone Med Ctr (page 106); **Address:** 530 1st Ave, Ste 7G, New York, NY 10016-6402; **Phone:** 212-683-6283; **Board Cert:** Dermatology 1974; **Med School:** Indiana Univ 1969; **Resid:** Dermatology, NYU Med Ctr 1973; **Fellow:** Dermatology, Univ Ill Hosp 1973; **Fac Appt:** Clin Prof D, NYU Sch Med

Ratner, Desiree MD (D) - **Spec Exp:** Mohs' Surgery; Skin Cancer; Dermatologic Surgery; **Hospital:** NY-Presby Hosp/Columbia (page 104); **Address:** Columbia Presbyterian Med Ctr, 161 Fort Washington Ave Fl 12, New York, NY 10032; **Phone:** 212-305-3625; **Board Cert:** Dermatology 2003; **Med School:** Johns Hopkins Univ 1989; **Resid:** Dermatology, Univ Michigan Med Ctr 1993; **Fellow:** Mohs Surgery, New England Med Ctr 1994; Mohs Surgery, Lahey Clinic 1995; **Fac Appt:** Prof D, Columbia P&S

Rigel, Darrell S MD (D) - **Spec Exp:** Melanoma; Skin Cancer; Cosmetic Dermatology; **Hospital:** NYU Langone Med Ctr (page 106), Mount Sinai Med Ctr (page 102); **Address:** 35 E 35th Street, Ste 208, New York, NY 10016-3823; **Phone:** 212-684-5964; **Board Cert:** Dermatology 1983; **Med School:** Geo Wash Univ 1978; **Resid:** Dermatology, NYU Med Ctr 1982; **Fellow:** Dermatologic Surgery, NYU Med Ctr 1983; **Fac Appt:** Clin Prof D, NYU Sch Med

Robins, Perry MD (D) - **Spec Exp:** Mohs' Surgery; Skin Cancer; Melanoma; **Hospital:** NYU Langone Med Ctr (page 106), Bellevue Hosp Ctr; **Address:** 345 E 37 St, Ste 209, New York, NY 10016; **Phone:** 212-263-7222; **Med School:** Germany 1961; **Resid:** Dermatology, VA Med Ctr 1964; **Fellow:** Dermatology, NYU Med Ctr 1967; **Fac Appt:** Prof Emeritus D, NYU Sch Med

Romano, John MD (D) - **Spec Exp:** Cosmetic Dermatology; Botox Therapy; **Hospital:** NY-Presby Hosp/Weill Cornell (page 104); **Address:** 36 7th Ave, Ste 423, New York, NY 10011-6688; **Phone:** 212-242-5815; **Board Cert:** Dermatology 1980; **Med School:** Cornell Univ-Weill Med Coll 1973; **Resid:** Internal Medicine, St. Vincents Hosp 1976; Dermatology, New York Hosp 1978; **Fac Appt:** Asst Clin Prof D, Cornell Univ-Weill Med Coll

Safai, Bijan MD (D) - **Spec Exp:** Dermatologic Surgery; Skin Cancer; Skin Laser Surgery; Cosmetic Surgery; **Hospital:** Metropolitan Hosp Ctr - NY, Montefiore Med Ctr - Div. North (page 100); **Address:** 625 Park Ave, New York, NY 10021-6545; **Phone:** 212-988-8918; **Board Cert:** Dermatology 1974; **Med School:** Iran 1965; **Resid:** Internal Medicine, VA Med Ctr 1970; Dermatology, NYU Med Ctr 1973; **Fellow:** Immunology, Meml Sloan-Kettering Cancer Ctr 1974; **Fac Appt:** Prof D, NY Med Coll

Schultz, Neal MD (D) - **Spec Exp:** Cosmetic Dermatology; Melanoma Early Detection/Prevention; Skin Laser Surgery; Tattoo Removal; **Hospital:** Mount Sinai Med Ctr (page 102), Lenox Hill Hosp; **Address:** 1130 Park Ave, New York, NY 10128; **Phone:** 212-369-9600; **Board Cert:** Dermatology 1978; **Med School:** Columbia P&S 1973; **Resid:** Internal Medicine, Mt Sinai Hosp 1975; Dermatology, Mt Sinai Hosp 1978; **Fac Appt:** Asst Clin Prof D, Mount Sinai Sch Med

Seidenberg, Roy Stern MD (D) - **Spec Exp:** Cosmetic Dermatology; Acne; **Hospital:** VA Med Ctr - Manhattan; **Address:** 800A 5th Ave, Ste 403, New York, NY 10065; **Phone:** 212-421-7546; **Board Cert:** Dermatology 2008; **Med School:** NY Med Coll 1991; **Resid:** Internal Medicine, Montefiore Med Ctr 1994; Dermatology, Cooper Hosp 1998; **Fellow:** Dermatologic Surgery, Boston Univ Med Ctr 1995; **Fac Appt:** Asst Clin Prof D, NYU Sch Med

Shelton, Ronald M MD (D) - **Spec Exp:** Cosmetic Dermatology; Mohs' Surgery; Skin Laser Surgery; **Hospital:** Mount Sinai Med Ctr (page 102); **Address:** 260 E 66 St, New York, NY 10065; **Phone:** 212-593-1818; **Board Cert:** Dermatology 1990; **Med School:** SUNY Upstate Med Univ 1984; **Resid:** Dermatology, Brooke Army Med Ctr 1990; **Fellow:** Mohs Surgery, UCSF Med Ctr 1993; **Fac Appt:** Assoc Clin Prof D, Mount Sinai Sch Med

Shim-Chang, Helen MD (D) - **Spec Exp:** Dermatopathology; **Hospital:** Mount Sinai Med Ctr (page 102); **Address:** Dermatology Assocs, 5 E 98th St Fl 5, New York, NY 10029; **Phone:** 212-241-9728; **Board Cert:** Anatomic Pathology 1997; Dermatopathology 1998; Dermatology 2008; **Med School:** Hahnemann Univ 1991; **Resid:** Internal Medicine, Mt Sinai Sch Med 1993; Dermatology, Mt Sinai Sch Med 1997; **Fellow:** Dermatopathology, Mt Sinai Hosp 1998

Shupack, Jerome L MD (D) - **Spec Exp:** Rare Skin Disorders; Psoriasis; Eczema; Blistering Diseases; **Hospital:** NYU Langone Med Ctr (page 106); **Address:** 530 1st Ave, HCC 7F, New York, NY 10016-6402; **Phone:** 212-263-7344; **Board Cert:** Dermatology 1970; **Med School:** Columbia P&S 1963; **Resid:** Internal Medicine, Mt Sinai Hosp 1965; Dermatology, NYU Med Ctr 1970; **Fac Appt:** Prof D, NYU Sch Med

Sibulkin, David MD (D) - **Hospital:** St Luke's - Roosevelt Hosp Ctr - Roosevelt Div (page 94), NY-Presby Hosp/Columbia (page 104); **Address:** 240 Central Park S, New York, NY 10019; **Phone:** 212-753-1470; **Board Cert:** Dermatology 1973; **Med School:** NYU Sch Med 1966; **Resid:** Dermatology, Bellevue Hosp 1972; **Fac Appt:** Assoc Clin Prof D, Columbia P&S

Silverberg, Nanette B MD (D) - **Spec Exp:** Pediatric Dermatology; Eczema; Vitiligo; Alopecia Areata; **Hospital:** St Luke's - Roosevelt Hosp Ctr - Roosevelt Div (page 94), Beth Israel Med Ctr - Petrie Division (page 94); **Address:** 425 W 59th St, Ste 5C, New York, NY 10019; **Phone:** 212-523-5898; **Board Cert:** Dermatology 2006; Pediatric Dermatology 2004; **Med School:** SUNY Downstate 1994; **Resid:** Dermatology, SUNY Downstate 1998; **Fellow:** Pediatric Dermatology, Chldn's Meml Hosp 1999; **Fac Appt:** Clin Prof D, Columbia P&S

Silvers, David MD (D) - **Spec Exp:** Dermatopathology; **Hospital:** NY-Presby Hosp/Columbia (page 104); **Address:** Vanderbilt Clinic 15, 630 W 168th St, rm 207, New York, NY 10032-3725; **Phone:** 212-305-2155; **Board Cert:** Dermatology 1973; Dermatopathology 1974; **Med School:** Duke Univ 1968; **Resid:** Dermatology, NYU Med Ctr 1971; **Fellow:** Dermatopathology, Armed Forces Inst Path 1973; **Fac Appt:** Clin Prof D, Columbia P&S

Sobel, Howard MD (D) - **Spec Exp:** Cosmetic Dermatology; Botox Therapy; Liposuction; Laser Surgery; **Hospital:** Lenox Hill Hosp, Beth Israel Med Ctr - Petrie Division (page 94); **Address:** 960A Park Ave, New York, NY 10028-0325; **Phone:** 212-288-0060; **Med School:** Albert Einstein Coll Med 1975; **Resid:** Dermatology, Emory Univ Hosp 1979

Soter, Nicholas A MD (D) - **Spec Exp:** Urticaria; Psoriasis; Vasculitis; **Hospital:** NYU Langone Med Ctr (page 106); **Address:** 530 1st Ave, Ste 7R, Dermatology Assocs-Langone, New York, NY 10016-6402; **Phone:** 212-263-5889; **Board Cert:** Dermatology 1970; Diagnostic Lab Immunology 1985; **Med School:** Univ Tex SW, Dallas 1965; **Resid:** Dermatology, Baylor Med Ctr 1968; Dermatology, Mass Genl Hosp 1969; **Fac Appt:** Prof D, NYU Sch Med

Tanenbaum, Diane MD (D) - **Spec Exp:** Skin Cancer; **Hospital:** Lenox Hill Hosp, NYU Langone Med Ctr (page 106); **Address:** 16 E 79th St, Ste 22, New York, NY 10021-0150; **Phone:** 212-249-6122; **Board Cert:** Dermatology 1971; **Med School:** SUNY Downstate 1964; **Resid:** Dermatology, NYU Med Ctr 1970; **Fac Appt:** Assoc Clin Prof D, NYU Sch Med

Tesser, Mark F MD (D) - **Spec Exp:** Cosmetic Dermatology; Skin Cancer; **Hospital:** Mount Sinai Med Ctr (page 102), Beth Israel Med Ctr - Petrie Division (page 94); **Address:** 1107 Park Ave, New York, NY 10128; **Phone:** 212-996-9600; **Board Cert:** Internal Medicine 1977; Dermatology 1980; **Med School:** Albert Einstein Coll Med 1974; **Resid:** Internal Medicine, Mount Sinai Hosp 1977; Dermatology, Mount Sinai Hosp 1979; **Fac Appt:** Asst Clin Prof D, Mount Sinai Sch Med

Unger, Walter P MD (D) - **Spec Exp:** Hair Restoration/Transplant; **Hospital:** Mount Sinai Med Ctr (page 102); **Address:** 710 Park Ave, New York, NY 10021-6591; **Phone:** 212-249-9393; **Board Cert:** Dermatology 1968; Hair Restoration Surgery 2008; **Med School:** Univ Toronto 1963; **Resid:** Dermatology, Philadelphia Skin-Cancer Hosp 1967; Internal Medicine, Sunny Brook Hosp 1968; **Fac Appt:** Clin Prof D, Mount Sinai Sch Med

Vogel, Louis MD (D) - **Spec Exp:** Cosmetic Dermatology; Botox Therapy; Hair Removal-Laser; **Hospital:** NYU Langone Med Ctr (page 106); **Address:** 16 Park Ave, Ste 1D, New York, NY 10016-4329; **Phone:** 212-447-5443; **Board Cert:** Internal Medicine 1980; Dermatology 1983; **Med School:** Boston Univ 1977; **Resid:** Internal Medicine, NYU Med Ctr 1980; Dermatology, NYU Med Ctr 1983; **Fac Appt:** Asst Clin Prof D, NYU Sch Med

Walther, Robert MD (D) - **Spec Exp:** Acne; Skin Cancer; Psoriasis; **Hospital:** NY-Presby Hosp/Columbia (page 104); **Address:** 16 E 60th St, Ste 300, New York, NY 10022; **Phone:** 212-326-8465; **Board Cert:** Dermatology 2009; Internal Medicine 1977; **Med School:** Univ NC Sch Med 1973; **Resid:** Internal Medicine, Univ Miami Hosps 1975; Dermatology, Columbia-Presby Hosp 1978; **Fellow:** Dermatology, Rockefeller Univ Hosp 1980; **Fac Appt:** Clin Prof D, Columbia P&S

Warner, Robert MD (D) - **Spec Exp:** Laser Surgery; Hair Removal-Laser; Cosmetic Dermatology; Botox Therapy; **Hospital:** Mount Sinai Med Ctr (page 102); **Address:** 580 Park Ave, New York, NY 10021-7313; **Phone:** 212-752-3692; **Board Cert:** Dermatology 1981; **Med School:** SUNY Hlth Sci Ctr 1977; **Resid:** Dermatology, Mount Sinai Hosp 1981; **Fac Appt:** Asst Clin Prof D, Mount Sinai Sch Med

Wattenberg, Debra J MD (D) - **Spec Exp:** Cosmetic Dermatology; Botox Therapy; Skin Laser Surgery; Acne; **Hospital:** Mount Sinai Med Ctr (page 102); **Address:** 875 Fifth Ave, New York, NY 10065; **Phone:** 212-288-3200; **Board Cert:** Dermatology 2001; **Med School:** Mount Sinai Sch Med 1988; **Resid:** Internal Medicine, Beth Israel Med Ctr 1989; Dermatology, Mount Sinai Hosp 1992; **Fac Appt:** Assoc Clin Prof D, Mount Sinai Sch Med

Wexler, Patricia MD (D) - **Spec Exp:** Facial Rejuvenation; Liposuction; Botox Therapy; Acne; **Hospital:** Mount Sinai Med Ctr (page 102); **Address:** 145 E 32nd St Fl 7, New York, NY 10016; **Phone:** 212-684-2626; **Board Cert:** Internal Medicine 1983; Dermatology 1986; **Med School:** Belgium 1979; **Resid:** Internal Medicine, Beth Israel Med Ctr 1982; Dermatology, Mt Sinai Hosp 1986; **Fellow:** Infectious Disease, Beth Israel Med Ctr 1983; **Fac Appt:** Assoc Clin Prof D, Mount Sinai Sch Med

Diagnostic Radiology

Abramson, Sara MD (DR) - **Spec Exp:** Pediatric Radiology; **Hospital:** Meml Sloan-Kettering Cancer Ctr (page 112); **Address:** 1275 York Avenue, New York, NY 10065; **Phone:** 800-525-2225; **Board Cert:** Diagnostic Radiology 1976; **Med School:** Mount Sinai Sch Med 1971; **Resid:** Pediatrics, Mt Sinai Hosp 1973; Diagnostic Radiology, Chldns Mercy Hosp 1976; **Fellow:** Pediatric Radiology, Chldns Hosp 1981; **Fac Appt:** Prof Rad, Cornell Univ-Weill Med Coll

Adler, Ronald S MD/PhD (DR) - **Spec Exp:** Musculoskeletal Imaging; Ultrasound; Power Doppler Imaging; **Hospital:** Hosp For Special Surgery (page 111), NY-Presby Hosp/Weill Cornell (page 104); **Address:** Hosp for Special Surgery, 535 E 70th St, New York, NY 10021; **Phone:** 212-606-1635; **Board Cert:** Diagnostic Radiology 1988; **Med School:** Wayne State Univ 1984; **Resid:** Diagnostic Radiology, Univ Mich Med Ctr 1988; **Fellow:** Ultrasound/CT/MRI, Univ Mich Med Ctr 1989; **Fac Appt:** Prof Rad, Cornell Univ-Weill Med Coll

Austin, John H M MD (DR) - **Spec Exp:** Lung Cancer; Thoracic Radiology; **Hospital:** NY-Presby Hosp/Columbia (page 104); **Address:** Columbia Presby Hosp, Dept Radiology, 622 W 168th St, HP 3-305, New York, NY 10032-3784; **Phone:** 212-305-2986; **Board Cert:** Diagnostic Radiology 1970; **Med School:** Yale Univ 1965; **Resid:** Diagnostic Radiology, UCSF Med Ctr 1968; **Fellow:** Diagnostic Radiology, UCSF Med Ctr 1970; **Fac Appt:** Prof Rad, Columbia P&S

Baer, Jeanne W MD (DR) - **Spec Exp:** Abdominal Imaging; **Hospital:** St Luke's - Roosevelt Hosp Ctr - St Luke's Hosp (page 94); **Address:** St Luke's Hosp, Dept Radiology, 440 W 114th St Fl 3, New York, NY 10025; **Phone:** 212-523-4272; **Board Cert:** Diagnostic Radiology 1971; **Med School:** Columbia P&S 1964; **Resid:** Internal Medicine, Geo Wash Univ Med Ctr 1967; **Fellow:** Diagnostic Radiology, St Luke's-Roosevelt Hosp Ctr 1970; **Fac Appt:** Assoc Clin Prof Rad, Columbia P&S

Barone, Clement MD (DR) - **Spec Exp:** Women's Imaging; Mammography; Bone Densitometry; **Address:** 1440 York Ave, Ste P-1, New York, NY 10075; **Phone:** 212-988-1303; **Board Cert:** Diagnostic Radiology 1974; **Med School:** NY Med Coll 1968; **Resid:** Diagnostic Radiology, Mt Sinai Hosp 1970; Diagnostic Radiology, Mt Sinai Hosp 1974; **Fac Appt:** Asst Clin Prof, Mount Sinai Sch Med

Berson, Barry MD (DR) - **Spec Exp:** Mammography; Breast Imaging; Bone Densitometry; **Hospital:** Mount Sinai Med Ctr (page 102); **Address:** 165 E 84th St, New York, NY 10028-0302; **Phone:** 212-535-9770; **Board Cert:** Diagnostic Radiology 1990; **Med School:** Mount Sinai Sch Med 1984; **Resid:** Diagnostic Radiology, Mount Sinai Hosp 1990; **Fellow:** Neuroradiology, NYU Med Ctr 1992

Brill, Paula MD (DR) - **Spec Exp:** Pediatric Radiology; Bone Imaging; **Hospital:** NY-Presby Hosp/Weill Cornell (page 104); **Address:** 525 E 68th St, New York, NY 10021-4873; **Phone:** 212-746-2554; **Board Cert:** Pediatrics 1970; Diagnostic Radiology 1971; Pediatric Radiology 2005; **Med School:** Cornell Univ-Weill Med Coll 1962; **Resid:** Pediatrics, New York Hosp 1968; Diagnostic Radiology, New York Hosp 1971; **Fellow:** Diagnostic Radiology, Cornell Univ 1971; **Fac Appt:** Prof, Cornell Univ-Weill Med Coll

Cohen, Burton A MD (DR) - **Spec Exp:** CT Scan; MRI; PET Imaging; **Hospital:** Mount Sinai Med Ctr (page 102); **Address:** 165 E 84th St, New York, NY 10028; **Phone:** 212-535-9770; **Board Cert:** Diagnostic Radiology 1979; **Med School:** NY Med Coll 1975; **Resid:** Diagnostic Radiology, Mt Sinai Hosp 1979; **Fac Appt:** Assoc Clin Prof Rad, Mount Sinai Sch Med

Dershaw, D David MD (DR) - **Spec Exp:** Breast Imaging; Breast Cancer; Mammography; **Hospital:** Meml Sloan-Kettering Cancer Ctr (page 112); **Address:** 300 E 66th St, New York, NY 10065; **Phone:** 800-525-2225; **Board Cert:** Diagnostic Radiology 1978; **Med School:** Jefferson Med Coll 1974; **Resid:** Diagnostic Radiology, New York Hosp 1978; **Fellow:** Ultrasound, Thos Jefferson Univ Hosp 1979; **Fac Appt:** Prof Rad, Cornell Univ-Weill Med Coll

Edelstein, Barbara A MD (DR) - **Spec Exp:** Breast Cancer; Women's Imaging; **Address:** 1045 Park Ave, New York, NY 10028; **Phone:** 212-860-7700; **Board Cert:** Diagnostic Radiology 1983; **Med School:** NY Med Coll 1977; **Resid:** Diagnostic Radiology, Montefiore Hosp 1982

Fefferman, Nancy R MD (DR) - **Spec Exp:** Pediatric Radiology; **Hospital:** NYU Rusk Inst (page 114); **Address:** Rusk Institute, 560 First Ave Fl 22 - Ste 234, New York, NY 10016; **Phone:** 212-263-5362; **Board Cert:** Radiology 1996; Pediatric Radiology 2008; **Med School:** NYU Sch Med 1991; **Resid:** Radiology, NYU Langone Med Ctr 1996; **Fellow:** Pediatric Radiology, NYU Langone Med Ctr 1997; **Fac Appt:** Asst Prof Rad, NYU Sch Med

Fried, Karen O MD (DR) - **Spec Exp:** Ultrasound; Thyroid Ultrasound; Vascular Ultrasound; **Address:** Lenox Hill Radiology, 61 E 77th St, New York, NY 10075; **Phone:** 212-772-3111; **Board Cert:** Diagnostic Radiology 1990; **Med School:** Albany Med Coll 1985; **Resid:** Diagnostic Radiology, LIJ Med Ctr 1990; **Fellow:** Cross Sectional Imaging, LIJ Med Ctr 1991

Genieser, Nancy B MD (DR) - **Spec Exp:** Neonatal Radiology; Pediatric Radiology; Child Abuse Imaging; **Hospital:** NYU Langone Med Ctr (page 106), Bellevue Hosp Ctr; **Address:** 462 1st Ave, NBV 3W33, New York, NY 10016-9196; **Phone:** 212-263-6373; **Board Cert:** Pediatric Radiology 2005; Diagnostic Radiology 1967; **Med School:** Med Coll PA Hahnemann 1962; **Resid:** Diagnostic Radiology, NYU Med Ctr 1966; **Fac Appt:** Prof Rad, NYU Sch Med

Ginsberg, Michelle MD (DR) - **Spec Exp:** Lung Cancer; Thoracic Radiology; Pulmonary Embolism; Gastrointestinal Imaging; **Hospital:** Meml Sloan-Kettering Cancer Ctr (page 112); **Address:** Meml Sloan Kettering Cancer Ctr, 1275 Dept Rad- York Ave, New York, NY 10021; **Phone:** 800-525-2225; **Board Cert:** Diagnostic Radiology 1995; **Med School:** Brown Univ 1990; **Resid:** Radiology, Montefiore Med Ctr- Weiler Div 1995; **Fellow:** Diagnostic Radiology, Meml Sloan Kettering Cancer Ctr 1996; **Fac Appt:** Assoc Prof Rad, Cornell Univ-Weill Med Coll

Hann, Lucy MD (DR) - **Spec Exp:** Liver & Biliary Cancer Ultrasound; Ovarian Cancer Ultrasound Diagnosis; Thyroid Ultrasound; **Hospital:** Meml Sloan-Kettering Cancer Ctr (page 112); **Address:** 1275 York Avenue, New York, NY 10065; **Phone:** 800-525-2225; **Board Cert:** Diagnostic Radiology 1977; **Med School:** Harvard Med Sch 1971; **Resid:** Diagnostic Radiology, Hosp Univ Penn 1974; Diagnostic Radiology, Mass Genl Hosp 1977; **Fellow:** Body Imaging, Mass Genl Hosp 1978; **Fac Appt:** Prof Rad, Cornell Univ-Weill Med Coll

Henschke, Claudia L MD/PhD (DR) - **Spec Exp:** Lung Cancer; Lung Disease; Thoracic Radiology; **Hospital:** Mount Sinai Med Ctr (page 102); **Address:** Mt Sinai Med Ctr, Radiology Dept, 1 Gustave Levy Pl, Box 1234, New York, NY 10029; **Phone:** 212-241-2420; **Board Cert:** Diagnostic Radiology 1981; **Med School:** Howard Univ 1977; **Resid:** Diagnostic Radiology, Brigham & Womens Hosp 1983; **Fac Appt:** Prof Rad, Cornell Univ-Weill Med Coll

Herman, Zeva W MD (DR) - **Spec Exp:** Mammography; Breast Imaging; **Hospital:** Mount Sinai Med Ctr (page 102); **Address:** Park Avenue Radiologists, 525 Park Ave, New York, NY 10065; **Phone:** 212-888-1000; **Board Cert:** Diagnostic Radiology 1993; **Med School:** Mount Sinai Sch Med 1989; **Resid:** Diagnostic Radiology, Lenox Hill Hosp 1992; **Fellow:** Breast Imaging, Meml Sloan Kettering Cancer Ctr 1993

Holliday, Roy MD (DR) - **Spec Exp:** Head & Neck Imaging; **Hospital:** New York Eye & Ear Infirm (page 113), Beth Israel Med Ctr - Petrie Division (page 94); **Address:** 310 E 14th St, New York, NY 10003; **Phone:** 212-979-4397; **Board Cert:** Diagnostic Radiology 1986; **Med School:** NYU Sch Med 1982; **Resid:** Diagnostic Radiology, NYU Med Ctr 1986; **Fellow:** Neurological Radiology, NYU Med Ctr 1987; **Fac Appt:** Clin Prof Rad, NYU Sch Med

Hricak, Hedvig MD/PhD (DR) - **Spec Exp:** Prostate Cancer-MR Spectroscopy (MRSI); Breast Imaging; Breast Cancer; **Hospital:** Meml Sloan-Kettering Cancer Ctr (page 112); **Address:** 1275 York Ave, Ste C278, New York, NY 10065; **Phone:** 800-525-2225; **Board Cert:** Diagnostic Radiology 1978; **Med School:** Yugoslavia 1970; **Resid:** Diagnostic Radiology, St Joseph Mercy Hosp 1977; **Fellow:** Ultrasound/CT, Henry Ford Hosp 1978; **Fac Appt:** Prof Rad, Cornell Univ-Weill Med Coll

Jacobs, Morton MD (DR) - **Spec Exp:** Neuroradiology; Head & Neck Imaging; Musculoskeletal Imaging; **Address:** Manhattan Diagnostic Radiology, 400 E 66th St, New York, NY 10065; **Phone:** 212-838-4243; **Board Cert:** Diagnostic Radiology 1976; Neuroradiology 1996; **Med School:** Univ Chicago-Pritzker Sch Med 1972; **Resid:** Diagnostic Radiology, New York Hosp 1976; **Fellow:** Neuroradiology, New York Hosp 1979

Kazam, Elias MD (DR) - **Spec Exp:** CT Scan; Ultrasound; MRI; **Hospital:** NY-Presby Hosp/Weill Cornell (page 104); **Address:** 400 E 66th St, New York, NY 10065; **Phone:** 212-838-4243; **Board Cert:** Diagnostic Radiology 1974; Nuclear Medicine 1976; **Med School:** Albert Einstein Coll Med 1966; **Resid:** Diagnostic Radiology, Peter Bent Brigham Hosp 1972; Diagnostic Radiology, New York Hosp 1973; **Fellow:** Biostatistics, Natl Cancer Inst-NIH 1969; **Fac Appt:** Prof Emeritus Rad, Cornell Univ-Weill Med Coll

Knopp, Edmond A MD (DR) - **Spec Exp:** MRI; Neuroradiology; Endocrine Radiology; CT Scan; **Hospital:** NYU Langone Med Ctr (page 106); **Address:** NYU Med Ctr, Neuro MRI Dept, 560 First Ave Fl 2, New York, NY 10016; **Phone:** 212-263-8723; **Board Cert:** Diagnostic Radiology 1992; Neuroradiology 2005; **Med School:** SUNY Downstate 1986; **Resid:** Surgery, Maimonides Med Ctr 1988; Diagnostic Radiology, St Lukes\Roosevelt Hosp 1992; **Fellow:** Neuroradiology, NYU Med Ctr 1994; **Fac Appt:** Assoc Prof Rad, NYU Sch Med

Levy, Miriam MD (DR) - **Spec Exp:** Breast Imaging; Mammography; Women's Imaging; **Hospital:** Mount Sinai Med Ctr (page 102); **Address:** 635 Madison Ave Fl 16, New York, NY 10022; **Phone:** 212-794-2500; **Board Cert:** Diagnostic Radiology 1983; **Med School:** Albert Einstein Coll Med 1979; **Resid:** Diagnostic Radiology, Geo Wash Univ Hosp 1982; Diagnostic Radiology, St Vincents Hosp 1983; **Fellow:** Ultrasound/CT/MRI, New York Hosp 1984; **Fac Appt:** Asst Clin Prof Path, Mount Sinai Sch Med

Liberman, Laura MD (DR) - **Spec Exp:** Breast Imaging; Breast Cancer; **Hospital:** Meml Sloan-Kettering Cancer Ctr (page 112); **Address:** 300 E 66th St Fl 7, New York, NY 10065; **Phone:** 646-888-4504; **Board Cert:** Diagnostic Radiology 1990; **Med School:** Columbia P&S 1984; **Resid:** Diagnostic Radiology, NY Hosp-Cornell Med Ctr 1990; **Fac Appt:** Assoc Prof Rad, Cornell Univ-Weill Med Coll

Megibow, Alec J MD (DR) - **Spec Exp:** Abdominal Imaging; Gastrointestinal Imaging; CT Body Scan; **Hospital:** NYU Langone Med Ctr (page 106), Bellevue Hosp Ctr; **Address:** 550 1st Ave, HHC 232, New York, NY 10016; **Phone:** 212-263-5222; **Board Cert:** Diagnostic Radiology 1978; **Med School:** SUNY Upstate Med Univ 1974; **Resid:** Diagnostic Radiology, Bellevue/NYU Med Ctr 1978; **Fellow:** Abdominal Imaging, NYU Med Ctr 1978; **Fac Appt:** Prof Rad, NYU Sch Med

Miller, Theodore MD (DR) - **Spec Exp:** Musculoskeletal Imaging; Ultrasound; **Hospital:** Hosp For Special Surgery (page 111); **Address:** Dept Radiology, 535 E 70th St, New York, NY 10021; **Phone:** 212-606-1127; **Board Cert:** Diagnostic Radiology 1993; **Med School:** Vanderbilt Univ 1987; **Resid:** Radiology, Mt Sinai Hosp 1992; **Fellow:** Radiology, Hosp for Spec Surg 1993; **Fac Appt:** Assoc Prof Rad, Cornell Univ-Weill Med Coll

Mitnick, Julie MD (DR) - **Spec Exp:** Mammography; Breast Cancer; **Address:** 650 1st Ave, New York, NY 10016; **Phone:** 212-686-4440; **Board Cert:** Diagnostic Radiology 1977; **Med School:** NYU Sch Med 1973; **Resid:** Diagnostic Radiology, NYU Med Ctr 1977; **Fellow:** Pediatric Radiology, NYU Med Ctr 1978; **Fac Appt:** Assoc Clin Prof Rad, NYU Sch Med

Morris, Elizabeth A MD (DR) - **Spec Exp:** Breast Imaging; Breast MRI; Breast Cancer; **Hospital:** Meml Sloan-Kettering Cancer Ctr (page 112); **Address:** 1275 York Avenue, New York, NY 10065; **Phone:** 800-525-2225; **Board Cert:** Diagnostic Radiology 1994; **Med School:** UCSF 1989; **Resid:** Diagnostic Radiology, NY-Cornell Med Ctr 1993; **Fellow:** Breast Imaging, Meml Sloan-Kettering Cancer Ctr 1994; **Fac Appt:** Assoc Prof Rad, Cornell Univ-Weill Med Coll

Naidich, David P MD (DR) - **Spec Exp:** Chest Radiology; Chronic Lung Disease; Lung Cancer; Pulmonary Embolism; **Hospital:** NYU Langone Med Ctr (page 106), Bellevue Hosp Ctr; **Address:** NYU Medical Center, Dept Radiology, 560 1st Ave, rm 236, New York, NY 10016; **Phone:** 212-263-5229; **Board Cert:** Diagnostic Radiology 1980; **Med School:** NYU Sch Med 1975; **Resid:** Diagnostic Radiology, Johns Hopkins Hosp 1979; **Fellow:** Cross Sectional Imaging, Johns Hopkins Hosp 1980; **Fac Appt:** Prof Rad, NYU Sch Med

Neistadt, L Daniel MD (DR) - **Spec Exp:** CT Body Scan; Gastroentestinal Imaging; Ultrasound; PET Imaging; **Address:** Manhattan Diagnostic Radiology, 400 E 66th St, New York, NY 10065; **Phone:** 212-838-4243; **Board Cert:** Internal Medicine 1975; Nuclear Medicine 1977; Diagnostic Radiology 1980; **Med School:** Stanford Univ 1972; **Resid:** Nuclear Medicine, New York Hosp 1977; Diagnostic Radiology, New York Hosp 1980; **Fellow:** Ultrasound/CT, New York Hosp 1981

Newhouse, Jeffrey MD (DR) - **Spec Exp:** Abdominal Imaging; Pelvic Imaging; **Hospital:** NY-Presby Hosp/Columbia (page 104); **Address:** 177 Fort Washington Ave, Millstein Bldg, 3rd Fl-Radiology, New York, NY 10032; **Phone:** 212-305-7898; **Board Cert:** Diagnostic Radiology 1972; **Med School:** Harvard Med Sch 1967; **Resid:** Diagnostic Radiology, Mass Genl Hosp 1972; **Fac Appt:** Prof, Columbia P&S

Panicek, David M MD (DR) - **Spec Exp:** Bone Cancer; Soft Tissue Tumors; Musculoskeletal Tumor Imaging; **Hospital:** Meml Sloan-Kettering Cancer Ctr (page 112); **Address:** 1275 York Avenue, New York, NY 10065; **Phone:** 800-525-2225; **Board Cert:** Diagnostic Radiology 1984; **Med School:** Cornell Univ-Weill Med Coll 1980; **Resid:** Diagnostic Radiology, NY Hosp-Cornell Med Ctr 1984; **Fac Appt:** Prof Rad, Cornell Univ-Weill Med Coll

Pavlov, Helene MD (DR) - **Spec Exp:** Sports Medicine Radiology; Musculoskeletal Imaging; Orthopaedic Imaging; **Hospital:** Hosp For Special Surgery (page 111), NY-Presby Hosp/Weill Cornell (page 104); **Address:** Hosp for Special Surgery, 535 E 70th St, New York, NY 10021-4892; **Phone:** 212-606-1132; **Board Cert:** Diagnostic Radiology 1976; **Med School:** Temple Univ 1972; **Resid:** Diagnostic Radiology, Germantown Hosp 1976; **Fellow:** Musculoskeletal Imaging, Hosp For Special Surg 1977; **Fac Appt:** Prof Rad, Cornell Univ-Weill Med Coll

Potter, Hollis G MD (DR) - **Spec Exp:** Musculoskeletal Imaging; Cartilage Damage; Arthroplasty Imaging; **Hospital:** Hosp For Special Surgery (page 111); **Address:** Hosp for Special Surgery, MRI-basement, 535 E 70th St, New York, NY 10021-4892; **Phone:** 212-606-1882; **Board Cert:** Diagnostic Radiology 1990; **Med School:** NY Med Coll 1985; **Resid:** Diagnostic Radiology, North Shore Univ Hosp 1990; **Fellow:** Diagnostic Radiology, Hosp Special Surgery 1991; **Fac Appt:** Prof Rad, Cornell Univ-Weill Med Coll

Prince, Martin R MD/PhD (DR) - **Spec Exp:** MRI Angiography; Vascular Ultrasound; **Hospital:** NY-Presby Hosp/Weill Cornell (page 104), NY-Presby Hosp/Columbia (page 104); **Address:** 416 E 55th St, New York, NY 10022; **Phone:** 212-746-6000; **Board Cert:** Diagnostic Radiology 1993; **Med School:** Harvard Med Sch 1985; **Resid:** Radiology, Mass Genl Hosp 1993; **Fellow:** Magnetic Resonance Imaging, Mass Genl Hosp 1993; **Fac Appt:** Prof Rad, Cornell Univ-Weill Med Coll

Recht, Michael MD (DR) - **Spec Exp:** Musculoskeletal Imaging; **Hospital:** NYU Langone Med Ctr (page 106); **Address:** NYU Sch Med, Dept Radiology, rm IRM 229, New York, NY 10016; **Phone:** 212-263-9530; **Board Cert:** Diagnostic Radiology 1987; **Med School:** Univ Pennsylvania 1983; **Resid:** Radiology, Hosp Univ Penn 1987; **Fellow:** Interventional Radiology, Hosp Univ Penn 1987; Musculoskeletal Imaging, UCSD Med Ctr 1992

Rosenberg, Zehava MD (DR) - **Spec Exp:** Musculoskeletal Imaging; **Hospital:** NYU Langone Med Ctr (page 106), NYU Hosp For Joint Diseases (page 106); **Address:** 301 E 17th St Bldg 600, NYU Hosp for Joint Diseases,, New York, NY 10003-3804; **Phone:** 212-598-6112; **Board Cert:** Diagnostic Radiology 1985; **Med School:** Univ Conn 1980; **Resid:** Diagnostic Radiology, Einstein Affil Hosp 1984; **Fellow:** Musculoskeletal Imaging, NY Columbia-Presby Hosp 1986; **Fac Appt:** Prof Rad, NYU Sch Med

Rosenblatt, Ruth MD (DR) - **Spec Exp:** Breast Cancer; **Hospital:** NY-Presby Hosp/Weill Cornell (page 104); **Address:** 425 E 61st St Fl 9, New York, NY 10021; **Phone:** 212-821-0600; **Board Cert:** Diagnostic Radiology 1969; **Med School:** Med Coll PA Hahnemann 1964; **Resid:** Diagnostic Radiology, Montefiore Med Ctr 1968; **Fac Appt:** Clin Prof, Cornell Univ-Weill Med Coll

Rosenfeld, Stanley MD (DR) - **Spec Exp:** Mammography; Ultrasound; Breast MRI; **Hospital:** Mount Sinai Med Ctr (page 102); **Address:** 1421 3rd Ave, New York, NY 10028; **Phone:** 212-744-5538; **Board Cert:** Diagnostic Radiology 1978; **Med School:** Albert Einstein Coll Med 1974; **Resid:** Diagnostic Radiology, Montefiore Hosp Med Ctr 1978

Ruzal-Shapiro, Carrie MD (DR) - **Spec Exp:** Pediatric Radiology; **Hospital:** NY-Presby Hosp/Columbia (page 104); **Address:** 3959 Broadway, New York, NY 10032; **Phone:** 212-305-9665; **Board Cert:** Diagnostic Radiology 1988; Pediatric Radiology 2004; **Med School:** Columbia P&S 1982; **Resid:** Radiology, Columbia-Presby Med Ctr 1988; **Fellow:** Pediatric Radiology, Columbia-Presby Med Ctr 1989; **Fac Appt:** Clin Prof Rad, Columbia P&S

Schwartz, Lawrence H MD (DR) - **Spec Exp:** Prostate Cancer; MRI; **Hospital:** NY-Presby Hosp/Columbia (page 104); **Address:** 630 W 168th St, MC 28, New York, NY 10032; **Phone:** 212-639-5511; **Board Cert:** Diagnostic Radiology 1991; **Med School:** Boston Univ 1986; **Resid:** Diagnostic Radiology, NY Hosp-Cornell Med Ctr 1991; **Fellow:** Ultrasound/CT/MRI, Brigham & Women's Hosp 1991; **Fac Appt:** Prof Rad, Cornell Univ-Weill Med Coll

Som, Peter MD (DR) - **Spec Exp:** Head & Neck Imaging; **Hospital:** Mount Sinai Med Ctr (page 102); **Address:** Mount Sinai Med Ctr, Dept Radiology, 1 Gustave Levy Pl, New York, NY 10029-6504; **Phone:** 212-241-7420; **Board Cert:** Diagnostic Radiology 1972; **Med School:** NYU Sch Med 1967; **Resid:** Diagnostic Radiology, Mt Sinai Hosp 1971; **Fac Appt:** Prof, Mount Sinai Sch Med

Sonnenblick, Emily B MD (DR) - **Spec Exp:** Women's Imaging; Breast MRI; **Hospital:** Mount Sinai Med Ctr (page 102); **Address:** 1421 3rd Ave, New York, NY 10028; **Phone:** 212-744-5538; **Board Cert:** Diagnostic Radiology 1987; **Med School:** Cornell Univ-Weill Med Coll 1982; **Resid:** Diagnostic Radiology, Hosp Univ Penn 1984; Diagnostic Radiology, Columbia-Presby Hosp 1986; **Fellow:** Ultrasound, Mt Sinai Hosp 1987

Wolff, Steven D MD/PhD (DR) - **Spec Exp:** Cardiovascular Imaging; Cardiac MRI; **Hospital:** Lenox Hill Hosp; **Address:** 62 E 88th St, Lower Level, New York, NY 10128; **Phone:** 212-369-9200; **Board Cert:** Diagnostic Radiology 1994; **Med School:** Duke Univ 1989; **Resid:** Diagnostic Radiology, Johns Hopkins Hosp 1994

Yankelevitz, David MD (DR) - **Spec Exp:** Lung Cancer; Thoracic Radiology; **Hospital:** NY-Presby Hosp/Weill Cornell (page 104); **Address:** Mt Sinai Med Ctr, Radiology Dept, 1 Gustave Levy Pl, Box 1234, New York, NY 10029; **Phone:** 212-241-2420; **Board Cert:** Diagnostic Radiology 1987; Nuclear Medicine 1987; **Med School:** SUNY Hlth Sci Ctr 1981; **Resid:** Diagnostic Radiology, Long Island Coll Hosp 1984; Nuclear Medicine, NY-Cornell Med Ctr 1987; **Fellow:** Diagnostic Radiology, NY-Cornell Med Ctr 1987; **Fac Appt:** Prof Rad, Cornell Univ-Weill Med Coll

Endocrinology, Diabetes & Metabolism

Bergman, Donald MD (EDM) - **Spec Exp:** Osteoporosis; Thyroid Disorders; Calcium Disorders; Paget's Disease of Bone; **Hospital:** Mount Sinai Med Ctr (page 102); **Address:** 1199 Park Ave, Ste 1F, New York, NY 10128; **Phone:** 212-876-7333; **Board Cert:** Internal Medicine 1975; Endocrinology, Diabetes & Metabolism 1977; **Med School:** Jefferson Med Coll 1971; **Resid:** Obstetrics & Gynecology, Mt Sinai Hosp 1972; Internal Medicine, Mt Sinai Hosp 1975; **Fellow:** Endocrinology, Diabetes & Metabolism, Mt Sinai Hosp 1977; **Fac Appt:** Clin Prof Med, Mount Sinai Sch Med

Bilezikian, John P MD (EDM) - **Spec Exp:** Osteoporosis; Bone Disorders-Metabolic; Parathyroid Disorders; **Hospital:** NY-Presby Hosp/Columbia (page 104); **Address:** Columbia Metabolic Bone Disease Program, Harkness Pavilion, 180 Ft Washington Ave Fl 9 - Ste 904, New York, NY 10032; **Phone:** 212-305-2663; **Board Cert:** Internal Medicine 1975; Endocrinology, Diabetes & Metabolism 1977; **Med School:** Columbia P&S 1969; **Resid:** Internal Medicine, Columbia-Presby Hosp 1975; **Fellow:** Endocrinology, Diabetes & Metabolism, Natl Inst Health 1977; **Fac Appt:** Prof Med, Columbia P&S

Bloomgarden, Zachary MD (EDM) - **Spec Exp:** Diabetes; Diabetic Kidney Disease; Cholesterol/Lipid Disorders; **Hospital:** Mount Sinai Med Ctr (page 102); **Address:** 35 E 85th St, New York, NY 10028-0954; **Phone:** 212-879-5933; **Board Cert:** Internal Medicine 1977; Endocrinology, Diabetes & Metabolism 1979; **Med School:** Albert Einstein Coll Med 1974; **Resid:** Internal Medicine, Montefiore Med Ctr 1977; **Fellow:** Endocrinology, Diabetes & Metabolism, Vanderbilt Univ Med Ctr 1979; **Fac Appt:** Assoc Clin Prof Med, Mount Sinai Sch Med

Blum, Conrad B MD (EDM) - **Spec Exp:** Cholesterol/Lipid Disorders; Thyroid Disorders; Diabetes; **Hospital:** NY-Presby Hosp/Columbia (page 104); **Address:** 16 E 60th St, Ste 320, New York, NY 10022-1002; **Phone:** 212-326-8421; **Board Cert:** Internal Medicine 1976; Endocrinology, Diabetes & Metabolism 1977; **Med School:** Northwestern Univ 1971; **Resid:** Internal Medicine, Brigham Women & Chldn's Hosp 1976; **Fellow:** Endocrinology, Diabetes & Metabolism, Northwestern Univ Med Sch 1977; **Fac Appt:** Clin Prof Med, Columbia P&S

Bockman, Richard MD/PhD (EDM) - **Spec Exp:** Bone Disorders-Metabolic; Osteoporosis; Parathyroid Disorders; Paget's Disease of Bone; **Hospital:** Hosp For Special Surgery (page 111), NY-Presby Hosp/Weill Cornell (page 104); **Address:** 519 E 72nd St, Ste 206, New York, NY 10021; **Phone:** 212-606-1458; **Board Cert:** Internal Medicine 1975; **Med School:** Yale Univ 1968; **Resid:** Internal Medicine, NYU Med Ctr 1975; **Fellow:** Internal Medicine, NY-Cornell Med Ctr 1973; **Fac Appt:** Prof Med, Cornell Univ-Weill Med Coll

Brillon, David MD (EDM) - **Spec Exp:** Diabetes; Thyroid Disorders; **Hospital:** NY-Presby Hosp/Weill Cornell (page 104); **Address:** NY Presby-Cornell, Div Endocrinology, 525 E 68th St, Box 136, Box 136, New York, NY 10065; **Phone:** 212-746-6290; **Board Cert:** Internal Medicine 1983; Endocrinology, Diabetes & Metabolism 1987; **Med School:** Brown Univ 1980; **Resid:** Internal Medicine, Rochester Genl Hosp 1983; **Fellow:** Endocrinology, Rochester Genl Hosp 1986; Endocrinology, Diabetes & Metabolism, UCSD Med Ctr 1988; **Fac Appt:** Assoc Clin Prof Med, Cornell Univ-Weill Med Coll

Bukberg, Phillip MD (EDM) - **Spec Exp:** Diabetes; Cholesterol/Lipid Disorders; **Address:** 36 7th Ave, Ste 517, New York, NY 10011-6688; **Phone:** 212-420-2777; **Board Cert:** Internal Medicine 1977; Endocrinology, Diabetes & Metabolism 1979; **Med School:** SUNY Downstate 1973; **Resid:** Internal Medicine, St Vincent's Hosp & Med Ctr 1977; **Fellow:** Endocrinology, Meml Sloan Kettering Cancer Ctr 1979; Endocrinology, Mt Sinai Hosp 1982

Davies, Terry MD (EDM) - **Spec Exp:** Thyroid Disorders in Pregnancy; Graves' Disease; Hashimoto's Disease; Thyroid Cancer; **Hospital:** Mount Sinai Med Ctr (page 102), VA Med Ctr - Manhattan; **Address:** 5 E 98th St, Box 1055, New York, NY 10029-6500; **Phone:** 212-241-7975; **Med School:** England, UK 1971; **Resid:** Internal Medicine, Univ Newcastle 1975; **Fellow:** Endocrinology, Diabetes & Metabolism, Univ Newcastle 1977; Endocrinology, Diabetes & Metabolism, Natl Inst Hlth 1979; **Fac Appt:** Prof Med, Mount Sinai Sch Med

Felig, Philip MD (EDM) - **Spec Exp:** Diabetes; Thyroid Disorders; Osteoporosis; **Hospital:** Lenox Hill Hosp, Beth Israel Med Ctr - Petrie Division (page 94); **Address:** 1056 5th Ave, New York, NY 10028-0112; **Phone:** 212-534-5900; **Board Cert:** Internal Medicine 1968; **Med School:** Yale Univ 1961; **Resid:** Internal Medicine, Yale-New Haven Hosp 1967; **Fellow:** Endocrinology, Diabetes & Metabolism, Peter Bent Brigham Hosp 1969

Goland, Robin MD (EDM) - **Spec Exp:** Diabetes; **Hospital:** NY-Presby Hosp/Columbia (page 104); **Address:** 1150 St Nicholas Ave Fl 2, Naomi Bone Diabetic Ctr, New York, NY 10032; **Phone:** 212-851-5494; **Board Cert:** Internal Medicine 1983; Endocrinology 1989; **Med School:** Columbia P&S 1980; **Resid:** Internal Medicine, Columbia-Presby Med Ctr 1984; **Fellow:** Endocrinology, Diabetes & Metabolism, Columbia-Presby Med Ctr 1987; **Fac Appt:** Assoc Prof Med, Columbia P&S

Greene, Loren Wissner MD (EDM) - **Spec Exp:** Thyroid Disorders; Osteoporosis; Pituitary Disorders; Diabetes; **Hospital:** NYU Langone Med Ctr (page 106), NY Downtown Hosp; **Address:** 530 1st Ave, Ste 4B, New York, NY 10016-6402; **Phone:** 212-263-7449; **Board Cert:** Internal Medicine 1978; Endocrinology, Diabetes & Metabolism 1981; **Med School:** NYU Sch Med 1975; **Resid:** Internal Medicine, Bellevue Hosp Ctr-NYU 1978; **Fellow:** Endocrinology, Bellevue Hosp Ctr-NYU 1980; **Fac Appt:** Assoc Clin Prof Med, NYU Sch Med

Hembree III, Wylie C MD (EDM) - **Spec Exp:** Reproductive Endocrinology-Male; Andrology; **Hospital:** NY-Presby Hosp/Columbia (page 104); **Address:** 101 Central Park West, Ste 1-B, New York, NY 10023; **Phone:** 212-721-3622; **Board Cert:** Internal Medicine 1972; Endocrinology 1973; **Med School:** Washington Univ, St Louis 1964; **Resid:** Internal Medicine, Boston City Hosp 1966; Internal Medicine, Columbia-Presby Hosp 1971; **Fellow:** Endocrinology, NIH Endo Br/Natl Cancer Inst 1968; **Fac Appt:** Assoc Clin Prof Med, Columbia P&S

Jacobs, Thomas MD (EDM) - **Spec Exp:** Adrenal Disorders; Pituitary Disorders; Calcium Disorders; Thyroid Disorders; **Hospital:** NY-Presby Hosp/Columbia (page 104); **Address:** 161 Fort Washington Ave, rm 210, New York, NY 10032-3713; **Phone:** 212-305-5578; **Board Cert:** Internal Medicine 1973; Endocrinology, Diabetes & Metabolism 1975; **Med School:** Johns Hopkins Univ 1968; **Resid:** Internal Medicine, Columbia Presby Hosp 1973; **Fellow:** Endocrinology, Diabetes & Metabolism, Univ Wash Med Ctr 1975; **Fac Appt:** Clin Prof Med, Columbia P&S

Kleinberg, David L MD (EDM) - **Spec Exp:** Neuroendocrinology; Pituitary Disorders; **Hospital:** NYU Langone Med Ctr (page 106); **Address:** 530 1st Ave, Ste 4C, New York, NY 10016; **Phone:** 212-263-6772; **Board Cert:** Internal Medicine 1972; Endocrinology 1975; **Med School:** Univ Miami Sch Med 1966; **Resid:** Internal Medicine, Maimonides Med Ctr 1968; Internal Medicine, Columbia-Presby Med Ctr 1971; **Fellow:** Endocrinology, Diabetes & Metabolism, Columbia-Presby Med Ctr 1970; **Fac Appt:** Prof Med, NYU Sch Med

Klyde, Barry J MD (EDM) - **Spec Exp:** Thyroid Disorders; Adrenal Disorders; Reproductive Endocrinology; Bone Disorders-Metabolic; **Hospital:** NY-Presby Hosp/Weill Cornell (page 104); **Address:** 520 E 72nd St, Ste L0, New York, NY 10021-4840; **Phone:** 212-772-3333; **Board Cert:** Internal Medicine 1977; Endocrinology, Diabetes & Metabolism 1981; **Med School:** Stanford Univ 1974; **Resid:** Internal Medicine, New York Hosp 1977; **Fellow:** Endocrinology, Diabetes & Metabolism, New York Hosp & Rockefeller Univ 1979; **Fac Appt:** Asst Clin Prof Med, Cornell Univ-Weill Med Coll

Mahler, Richard J MD (EDM) - **Spec Exp:** Diabetes; Thyroid Disorders; **Hospital:** NY-Presby Hosp/Weill Cornell (page 104); **Address:** 220 E 69th St, New York, NY 10021-5737; **Phone:** 212-879-4073; **Board Cert:** Internal Medicine 1987; **Med School:** NY Med Coll 1959; **Resid:** Internal Medicine, NY Med-Metro Med 1962; Endocrinology, Diabetes & Metabolism, NY Med Coll 1963; **Fellow:** Endocrinology, Diabetes & Metabolism, Univ Durham/Univ New Castle 1964; **Fac Appt:** Assoc Clin Prof Med, Cornell Univ-Weill Med Coll

McConnell, Robert John MD (EDM) - **Spec Exp:** Thyroid Disorders; Thyroid Ultrasound; **Hospital:** NY-Presby Hosp/Columbia (page 104); **Address:** 161 Fort Washington Ave, Ste 210, New York, NY 10032-3713; **Phone:** 212-305-5579; **Board Cert:** Internal Medicine 1978; Endocrinology, Diabetes & Metabolism 1981; **Med School:** Columbia P&S 1973; **Resid:** Internal Medicine, Barnes Hosp 1975; **Fellow:** Endocrinology, Diabetes & Metabolism, Columbia-Presby Hosp 1978; **Fac Appt:** Prof Med, Columbia P&S

Mechanick, Jeffrey I MD (EDM) - **Spec Exp:** Nutrition; Thyroid Disorders; Thyroid Cancer; Bone Disorders-Metabolic; **Hospital:** Mount Sinai Med Ctr (page 102); **Address:** 1192 Park Ave, New York, NY 10128; **Phone:** 212-831-2100; **Board Cert:** Internal Medicine 1988; Endocrinology, Diabetes & Metabolism 2003; Clinical Nutrition 2001; **Med School:** Mount Sinai Sch Med 1985; **Resid:** Internal Medicine, Baylor Affil Hosp 1988; **Fellow:** Endocrinology, Diabetes & Metabolism, Mt Sinai Hosp 1990; **Fac Appt:** Clin Prof Med, Mount Sinai Sch Med

Park, Constance MD/PhD (EDM) - **Spec Exp:** Thyroid Disorders; Osteoporosis; Menopause Problems; Complementary Medicine; **Hospital:** NY-Presby Hosp/Columbia (page 104), Harlem Hosp Ctr; **Address:** 903 Park Ave, New York, NY 10021; **Phone:** 212-639-9850; **Board Cert:** Internal Medicine 1980; Endocrinology, Diabetes & Metabolism 2007; **Med School:** Albert Einstein Coll Med 1974; **Resid:** Internal Medicine, Bellevue Hosp 1976; **Fellow:** Endocrinology, Diabetes & Metabolism, Albert Einstein 1978; **Fac Appt:** Assoc Clin Prof Med, Columbia P&S

Peck, Valerie H MD (EDM) - **Spec Exp:** Osteoporosis; Thyroid Disorders; Obesity; Weight Management; **Hospital:** NYU Langone Med Ctr (page 106); **Address:** 135 E 37th St, New York, NY 10016; **Phone:** 212-213-3233; **Board Cert:** Internal Medicine 1977; Endocrinology, Diabetes & Metabolism 1979; **Med School:** NYU Sch Med 1974; **Resid:** Internal Medicine, Bellevue Hosp Ctr 1977; **Fellow:** Endocrinology, Bellevue Hosp Ctr 1978; **Fac Appt:** Assoc Clin Prof Med, NYU Sch Med

Poretsky, Leonid MD (EDM) - **Spec Exp:** Diabetes; Thyroid Disorders; **Hospital:** Beth Israel Med Ctr - Petrie Division (page 94); **Address:** 317 E 17th St Fl 7, New York, NY 10003; **Phone:** 212-420-2226; **Board Cert:** Internal Medicine 1983; Endocrinology, Diabetes & Metabolism 1985; **Med School:** Russia 1977; **Resid:** Internal Medicine, Coney Island Hosp 1983; **Fellow:** Endocrinology, Beth Israel Hosp 1985; **Fac Appt:** Prof Med, Albert Einstein Coll Med

Seltzer, Terry MD (EDM) - **Spec Exp:** Diabetes; Thyroid Disorders; Calcium Disorders; Pheochromocytoma; **Hospital:** NYU Langone Med Ctr (page 106); **Address:** 530 1st Ave, Ste 4D, New York, NY 10016-6402; **Phone:** 212-263-8717; **Board Cert:** Internal Medicine 1980; Endocrinology 1983; **Med School:** Harvard Med Sch 1977; **Resid:** Internal Medicine, NYU-Bellevue Hosp 1980; **Fellow:** Endocrinology, Diabetes & Metabolism, NYU-Bellevue Hosp 1982; **Fac Appt:** Asst Prof Med, NYU Sch Med

Seplowitz, Alan H MD (EDM) - **Spec Exp:** Thyroid Disorders; Cholesterol/Lipid Disorders; Diabetes; **Hospital:** NY-Presby Hosp/Columbia (page 104); **Address:** 161 Fort Washington Ave, New York, NY 10032-3729; **Phone:** 212-305-5503; **Board Cert:** Internal Medicine 1975; Endocrinology 1977; **Med School:** Columbia P&S 1972; **Resid:** Internal Medicine, Columbia-Presby Med Ctr 1974; **Fellow:** Endocrinology, Diabetes & Metabolism, Columbia-Presby Med Ctr 1978; **Fac Appt:** Assoc Clin Prof Med, Columbia P&S

Shane, Elizabeth MD (EDM) - **Spec Exp:** Bone Disorders-Metabolic; Osteoporosis; Parathyroid Disorders; **Hospital:** NY-Presby Hosp/Columbia (page 104); **Address:** 180 Ft Washington Ave Fl 9 - rm 910, New York, NY 10032; **Phone:** 212-305-2663; **Board Cert:** Internal Medicine 1978; Endocrinology 1981; **Med School:** Univ Toronto 1975; **Resid:** Internal Medicine, Columbia-Presby Hosp 1978; **Fellow:** Endocrinology, Columbia-Presby Hosp 1981; **Fac Appt:** Clin Prof Med, Columbia P&S

Silverberg, Shonni J MD (EDM) - **Spec Exp:** Osteoporosis; Parathyroid Disorders; Calcium Disorders; **Hospital:** NY-Presby Hosp/Columbia (page 104); **Address:** 180 Fort Washington Ave, Ste 9-904, New York, NY 10032; **Phone:** 212-305-2663; **Board Cert:** Internal Medicine 1983; Endocrinology, Diabetes & Metabolism 1985; **Med School:** Cornell Univ-Weill Med Coll 1980; **Resid:** Internal Medicine, NY Hosp 1983; **Fellow:** Endocrinology, Diabetes & Metabolism, Columbia-Presby Med Ctr 1986; **Fac Appt:** Prof Med, Columbia P&S

Siris, Ethel MD (EDM) - **Spec Exp:** Osteoporosis; Paget's Disease of Bone; Bone Disorders-Metabolic; **Hospital:** NY-Presby Hosp/Columbia (page 104); **Address:** 180 Ft Washington Ave, Harkness Bldg - Ste 904, New York, NY 10032-3710; **Phone:** 212-305-9531; **Board Cert:** Internal Medicine 1974; Endocrinology, Diabetes & Metabolism 1977; **Med School:** Columbia P&S 1971; **Resid:** Internal Medicine, Columbia-Presby Med Ctr 1974; **Fellow:** Research, Natl Inst Hlth 1976; Endocrinology, Diabetes & Metabolism, Columbia-Presby Med Ctr 1977; **Fac Appt:** Prof Med, Columbia P&S

Szabo, Andrew John MD (EDM) - **Spec Exp:** Diabetes; Thyroid Disorders; **Hospital:** Lenox Hill Hosp, NY-Presby Hosp/Weill Cornell (page 104); **Address:** 860 Fifth Ave, New York, NY 10022-1304; **Phone:** 212-583-2816; **Board Cert:** Internal Medicine 1987; Endocrinology, Diabetes & Metabolism 1989; **Med School:** McGill Univ 1959; **Resid:** Internal Medicine, Montreal General Hosp 1962; Internal Medicine, Queen Mary Veteran's Hosp 1962; **Fellow:** Endocrinology, Diabetes & Metabolism, Montreal General Hosp 1964; Endocrinology, Diabetes & Metabolism, New England Med Ctr-Deaconess Hosp 1965; **Fac Appt:** Assoc Clin Prof Med, Cornell Univ-Weill Med Coll

Tuttle, R Michael MD (EDM) - **Spec Exp:** Thyroid Cancer; **Hospital:** Meml Sloan-Kettering Cancer Ctr (page 112); **Address:** 1275 York Avenue, New York, NY 10065; **Phone:** 800-525-2225; **Board Cert:** Endocrinology, Diabetes & Metabolism 2004; **Med School:** Univ Louisville Sch Med 1987; **Resid:** Internal Medicine, DD Eisenhower Army Med Ctr 1990; **Fellow:** Endocrinology, Diabetes & Metabolism, Madigan Army Med Ctr 1993; **Fac Appt:** Assoc Prof Med, Cornell Univ-Weill Med Coll

Wardlaw, Sharon MD (EDM) - **Spec Exp:** Pituitary Disorders; Neuroendocrinology; **Hospital:** NY-Presby Hosp/Columbia (page 104); **Address:** 180 Fort Washington Ave, rm 970, New York, NY 10032; **Phone:** 212-305-2254; **Board Cert:** Internal Medicine 1978; Endocrinology, Diabetes & Metabolism 1979; **Med School:** Cornell Univ-Weill Med Coll 1975; **Resid:** Internal Medicine, Case Western Univ Hosp 1977; **Fellow:** Endocrinology, Diabetes & Metabolism, Columbia-Presby 1980; **Fac Appt:** Prof Med, Columbia P&S

Young, Iven MD (EDM) - **Spec Exp:** Thyroid Disorders; Osteoporosis; Pituitary Disorders; **Hospital:** NYU Langone Med Ctr (page 106); **Address:** 36th 7th Ave, rm 507, New York, NY 10011-8253; **Phone:** 212-675-9332; **Board Cert:** Internal Medicine 1966; Endocrinology, Diabetes & Metabolism 1973; **Med School:** NYU Sch Med 1959; **Resid:** Internal Medicine, VA Med Ctr 1963; **Fellow:** Endocrinology, NYU Med Ctr 1966; **Fac Appt:** Assoc Clin Prof Med, NYU Sch Med

Family Medicine

Calman, Neil S MD (FMed) *PCP* - **Hospital:** Beth Israel Med Ctr - Petrie Division (page 94), Montefiore Med Ctr - Div. Moses (page 100); **Address:** Sidney Hillman Family Practice, 16 E 16th St Fl 3, New York, NY 10003-3105; **Phone:** 212-924-7744; **Board Cert:** Family Medicine 2003; **Med School:** Rush Med Coll 1975; **Resid:** Family Medicine, Montefiore Hosp Med Ctr 1978; **Fac Appt:** Prof FMed, Albert Einstein Coll Med

Kligler, Benjamin E MD (FMed) *PCP* - **Spec Exp:** Complementary Medicine; Acupuncture; **Hospital:** Beth Israel Med Ctr - Petrie Division (page 94); **Address:** Continuum Ctr for Health & Healing, 245 Fifth Ave Fl 2, New York, NY 10016; **Phone:** 646-935-2257; **Board Cert:** Family Medicine 2008; **Med School:** Boston Univ 1990; **Resid:** Family Medicine, Albert Einstein Affil Hosps 1994; **Fac Appt:** Asst Prof FMed, Albert Einstein Coll Med

Leeds, Gary E MD (FMed) *PCP* - **Spec Exp:** Asthma & Allergy; Hypertension; Cholesterol/Lipid Disorders; **Hospital:** Beth Israel Med Ctr - Petrie Division (page 94); **Address:** 22 W 15th St, New York, NY 10011-6842; **Phone:** 212-206-7717; **Board Cert:** Family Medicine 2002; **Med School:** Brown Univ 1978; **Resid:** Family Medicine, Georgetown Univ Hosp 1981

Levy, Albert MD (FMed) *PCP* - **Spec Exp:** Hypertension; Diabetes; Sexual Dysfunction; **Hospital:** Mount Sinai Med Ctr (page 102), Lenox Hill Hosp; **Address:** 911 Park Ave, New York, NY 10021-0337; **Phone:** 212-288-7193; **Board Cert:** Family Medicine 2006; **Med School:** Brazil 1973; **Resid:** Surgery, Maimonides Hosp 1978; Family Medicine, Kings County Hosp 1980; **Fac Appt:** Asst Clin Prof Med, Mount Sinai Sch Med

Lyon, Valerie K MD (FMed) *PCP* - **Spec Exp:** Preventive Medicine; **Hospital:** Lenox Hill Hosp; **Address:** 59 E 54th St Fl 2, New York, NY 10022; **Phone:** 212-750-8330; **Board Cert:** Family Medicine 2006; **Med School:** Temple Univ 1986; **Resid:** Family Medicine, South Nassau Comm Hosp 1989

Schiller, Robert MD (FMed) *PCP* - **Spec Exp:** Complementary Medicine; Pediatrics; **Hospital:** Beth Israel Med Ctr - Petrie Division (page 94), Long Island Coll Hosp (page 94); **Address:** Sidney Hillman Family Practice, 16 E 16th St Fl 3, New York, NY 10003-3105; **Phone:** 212-924-7744; **Board Cert:** Family Medicine 2006; **Med School:** NYU Sch Med 1982; **Resid:** Family Medicine, Montefiore Med Ctr 1985; **Fac Appt:** Asst Prof FMed, Albert Einstein Coll Med

Gastroenterology

Ackert, John MD (Ge) - **Spec Exp:** Endoscopy; Colonoscopy; Gastroesophageal Reflux Disease (GERD); **Hospital:** NYU Langone Med Ctr (page 106); **Address:** 232 E 30th St, Ground Level, New York, NY 10016; **Phone:** 212-889-5544; **Board Cert:** Internal Medicine 1975; Gastroenterology 1977; **Med School:** NYU Sch Med 1972; **Resid:** Internal Medicine, NYU Med Ctr 1975; **Fellow:** Gastroenterology, NYU Med Ctr 1977; **Fac Appt:** Asst Prof Med, NYU Sch Med

Adler, Howard MD (Ge) - **Spec Exp:** Colon Cancer; Colonoscopy; Endoscopy; **Hospital:** Lenox Hill Hosp, Beth Israel Med Ctr - Petrie Division (page 94); **Address:** 35 Sutton Pl, New York, NY 10022-2464; **Phone:** 212-421-3696; **Board Cert:** Internal Medicine 1967; Gastroenterology 1977; **Med School:** Albert Einstein Coll Med 1960; **Resid:** Internal Medicine, Herbert C Moffitt Hosp 1962; Internal Medicine, Bronx Municipal Hosp 1965; **Fellow:** Gastroenterology, Cornell U-Bellevue Hosp 1967; **Fac Appt:** Assoc Clin Prof Med, Albert Einstein Coll Med

Aisenberg, James MD (Ge) - **Spec Exp:** Colon Cancer Screening; Inflammatory Bowel Disease; Gastroesophageal Reflux Disease (GERD); Crohn's Disease; **Hospital:** Mount Sinai Med Ctr (page 102); **Address:** 311 E 79th St, Ste 2-A, New York, NY 10075; **Phone:** 212-996-6633; **Board Cert:** Internal Medicine 2000; Gastroenterology 2000; **Med School:** Harvard Med Sch 1987; **Resid:** Internal Medicine, Columbia-Presby Med Ctr 1990; **Fellow:** Gastroenterology, Mt Sinai Hosp 1993; **Fac Appt:** Assoc Prof Med, Mount Sinai Sch Med

Baiocco, Peter J MD (Ge) - **Spec Exp:** Inflammatory Bowel Disease; Colon Cancer Screening; Gastroesophageal Reflux Disease (GERD); Endoscopy; **Hospital:** Lenox Hill Hosp; **Address:** 1317 3rd Ave Fl 5, New York, NY 10021-2995; **Phone:** 212-734-8811; **Board Cert:** Internal Medicine 1981; Gastroenterology 1983; **Med School:** Mount Sinai Sch Med 1978; **Resid:** Internal Medicine, Lenox Hill Hosp 1981; **Fellow:** Gastroenterology, Lenox Hill Hosp 1983; **Fac Appt:** Asst Clin Prof Med, NYU Sch Med

Basuk, Paul M MD (Ge) - **Spec Exp:** Gallbladder Disease; Pancreatic Disease; Esophageal Disorders; **Hospital:** NY-Presby Hosp/Weill Cornell (page 104); **Address:** 210 E 86th St, Ste 201, New York, NY 10028; **Phone:** 212-861-9715; **Board Cert:** Internal Medicine 1983; Gastroenterology 1987; **Med School:** Northwestern Univ 1980; **Resid:** Internal Medicine, UCSF Med Ctr 1983; **Fellow:** Gastroenterology, UCSF Med Ctr 1987; **Fac Appt:** Asst Prof Med, Cornell Univ-Weill Med Coll

Bednarek, Karl MD (Ge) - **Spec Exp:** Liver Disease; **Hospital:** Beth Israel Med Ctr - Petrie Division (page 94); **Address:** 10 Union Square E, Ste 2G, New York, NY 10003; **Phone:** 212-844-6335; **Board Cert:** Internal Medicine 1985; **Med School:** Mount Sinai Sch Med 1982; **Resid:** Internal Medicine, Beth Israel Med Ctr 1986; **Fellow:** Gastroenterology, Beth Israel Med Ctr 1988

Ben-Zvi, Jeffrey MD (Ge) - **Spec Exp:** Inflammatory Bowel Disease/Crohn's; Gastroe-sophageal Reflux Disease (GERD); Pancreatic/Biliary Endoscopy (ERCP); **Hospital:** Lenox Hill Hosp, NY-Presby Hosp/Columbia (page 104); **Address:** 212 E 70th St, New York, NY 10075; **Phone:** 212-772-8730; **Board Cert:** Internal Medicine 2004; Gastroenterology 2004; Geriatric Medicine 2004; **Med School:** Columbia P&S 1983; **Resid:** Internal Medicine, St Lukes-Roosevelt Hosp 1986; **Fellow:** Gastroenterology, St Lukes-Roosevelt Hosp 1988; **Fac Appt:** Asst Clin Prof Med, Columbia P&S

Bernstein, Brett B MD (Ge) - **Spec Exp:** Gastroesophageal Reflux Disease (GERD); Capsule Endoscopy; Colon Cancer Screening; **Hospital:** Beth Israel Med Ctr - Petrie Division (page 94); **Address:** 10 Union Square East, Ste 2G, New York, NY 10003; **Phone:** 212-844-6330; **Board Cert:** Internal Medicine 2001; Gastroenterology 2005; **Med School:** Mount Sinai Sch Med 1988; **Resid:** Internal Medicine, Beth Israel Med Ctr 1991; **Fellow:** Gastroenterology, Beth Israel Med Ctr 1994; **Fac Appt:** Asst Prof Med, Albert Einstein Coll Med

Bodenheimer Jr, Henry C MD (Ge) - **Spec Exp:** Liver & Biliary Disease; Transplant Medi-cine-Liver; Hepatitis; Toxicology; **Hospital:** Beth Israel Med Ctr - Petrie Division (page 94); **Address:** Beth Israel Med Ctr Dept of Med, 1st Ave @ 16th St, New York, NY 10003; **Phone:** 212-420-4077; **Board Cert:** Internal Medicine 1978; Gastroenterology 1981; Transplant Hepatology 2006; **Med School:** Tufts Univ 1975; **Resid:** Internal Medicine, Mount Sinai Hosp 1978; **Fellow:** Gastroenterol-ogy, Mount Sinai Hosp 1979; Gastroenterology, Rhode Island Hosp 1981; **Fac Appt:** Prof Med, Al-bert Einstein Coll Med

Borcich, Anthony S MD (Ge) - **Spec Exp:** Liver Disease; Hepatitis C; HIV & Hepatitis co-infec-tion; **Hospital:** Mount Sinai Med Ctr (page 102), Lenox Hill Hosp; **Address:** 1049 Park Ave, Ste 1-C, New York, NY 10028; **Phone:** 212-722-8400; **Board Cert:** Internal Medicine 1987; Gastroenterology 1989; **Med School:** Northwestern Univ-Feinberg Sch Med 1984; **Resid:** Internal Medicine, St Lukes-Roosevelt Hosp 1987; **Fellow:** Gastroenterology, St Lukes-Roosevelt Hosp 1989; **Fac Appt:** Asst Clin Prof Med, Mount Sinai Sch Med

Brown Jr, Robert S MD (Ge) - **Spec Exp:** Hepatitis; Liver Disease; Transplant Medicine-Liver; **Hospital:** NY-Presby Hosp/Columbia (page 104); **Address:** Ctr for Liver Disease & Transplantation, 622 W 168th St Fl 14 - rm 105, New York, NY 10032; **Phone:** 212-305-1305; **Board Cert:** Inter-nal Medicine 2002; Gastroenterology 2005; **Med School:** NYU Sch Med 1989; **Resid:** Internal Medicine, Beth Israel Deaconess Med Ctr 1992; **Fellow:** Gastroenterology, UCSF Med Ctr 1994; He-patology, UCSF Med Ctr 1995; **Fac Appt:** Prof Med, Columbia P&S

Cantor, Michael C MD (Ge) - **Spec Exp:** Colon Cancer; Hepatitis; Liver Disease; **Hospital:** NY-Presby Hosp/Weill Cornell (page 104); **Address:** 310 E 72nd St Fl Level C, New York, NY 10021-4703; **Phone:** 212-472-3333; **Board Cert:** Internal Medicine 1985; Gastroenterology 1989; **Med School:** Columbia P&S 1982; **Resid:** Internal Medicine, New York Hosp 1985; **Fellow:** Gastroenterology, New York Hosp 1988; **Fac Appt:** Asst Clin Prof Med, Cornell Univ-Weill Med Coll

Carr-Locke, David L MD (Ge) - **Spec Exp:** Pancreatic/Biliary Endoscopy (ERCP); Pancreatic & Biliary Disease; Endoscopy; **Hospital:** Beth Israel Med Ctr - Petrie Division (page 94); **Address:** 1st & 16th St, New York, NY 10003; **Phone:** 212-420-4015; **Board Cert:** Internal Medicine 1974; **Med School:** England, UK 1972; **Resid:** Obstetrics & Gynecology, Orsett Hosp 1974; Internal Medi-cine, Leicester Hosp 1976; **Fellow:** Gastroenterology, Leicester Hosp 1978; Research, New Eng Bap-tist Hosp 1979; **Fac Appt:** Assoc Prof Med, Harvard Med Sch

Chapman, Mark L MD (Ge) - **Spec Exp:** Inflammatory Bowel Disease/Crohn's; Peptic Ulcer Disease; Gastrointestinal Motility Disorders; **Hospital:** Mount Sinai Med Ctr (page 102); **Address:** 12 E 86th St, New York, NY 10028-0506; **Phone:** 212-861-2000; **Board Cert:** Internal Medicine 1968; Gastroenterology 1970; **Med School:** SUNY Downstate 1961; **Resid:** Internal Medicine, Montefiore Med Ctr 1963; Internal Medicine, Mt Sinai Hosp 1964; **Fellow:** Gastroenterology, Mt Sinai Hosp 1966; **Fac Appt:** Assoc Clin Prof Med, Mount Sinai Sch Med

Clain, David J MD (Ge) - **Spec Exp:** Liver Disease; Hepatitis; Pancreatic/Biliary Endoscopy (ERCP); Colonoscopy; **Hospital:** Beth Israel Med Ctr - Petrie Division (page 94); **Address:** Beth Israel Med Ctr-Digestive Diseases, 1st Ave at 16th St E, New York, NY 10003; **Phone:** 212-420-4521; **Board Cert:** Internal Medicine 1980; Gastroenterology 1981; **Med School:** South Africa 1959; **Resid:** Internal Medicine, Birmingham General 1964; Internal Medicine, Charing Cross 1965; **Fellow:** Gastroenterology, Royal Free Hosp 1966; **Fac Appt:** Prof Med, Albert Einstein Coll Med

Cohen, Jonathan MD (Ge) - **Spec Exp:** Pancreatic/Biliary Endoscopy (ERCP); Pancreatic Disease; Barrett's Esophagus; Colonoscopy; **Hospital:** NYU Langone Med Ctr (page 106); **Address:** 232 E 30th St, New York, NY 10016-8202; **Phone:** 212-889-5544; **Board Cert:** Gastroenterology 2005; **Med School:** Harvard Med Sch 1990; **Resid:** Internal Medicine, Beth Israel Hosp 1993; **Fellow:** Gastroenterology, UCLA Med Ctr 1995; Endoscopy, Wellesley Hosp 1995; **Fac Appt:** Clin Prof Med, NYU Sch Med

Cohen, Lawrence B MD (Ge) - **Spec Exp:** Gastroesophageal Reflux Disease (GERD); Esophageal Disorders; Colon & Rectal Cancer; Endoscopy; **Hospital:** Mount Sinai Med Ctr (page 102); **Address:** 311 E 79th St, Ste 2A, New York, NY 10021-0903; **Phone:** 212-996-6633; **Board Cert:** Internal Medicine 1981; Gastroenterology 1983; **Med School:** Hahnemann Univ 1978; **Resid:** Internal Medicine, Mt Sinai Hosp 1981; **Fellow:** Gastroenterology, Mt Sinai Hosp 1983; **Fac Appt:** Assoc Clin Prof Med, Mount Sinai Sch Med

Cohen, Seth A MD (Ge) - **Spec Exp:** Pancreatic/Biliary Endoscopy (ERCP); Colonoscopy; Endoscopy; **Hospital:** Beth Israel Med Ctr - Petrie Division (page 94), Mount Sinai Med Ctr (page 102); **Address:** 60 East End Ave, New York, NY 10028-0305; **Phone:** 212-734-8874; **Board Cert:** Internal Medicine 1989; Gastroenterology 2004; **Med School:** Columbia P&S 1986; **Resid:** Internal Medicine, Mount Sinai Med Ctr 1989; Gastroenterology, St Luke's-Roosevelt Hosp Ctr 1991; **Fellow:** Gastroenterology, Beth Israel Hosp 1992

Connor, Bradley A MD (Ge) - **Spec Exp:** Travel Medicine; Parasitic Infections; Diarrheal Diseases; **Hospital:** NY-Presby Hosp/Weill Cornell (page 104); **Address:** 50 E 69th St, New York, NY 10021; **Phone:** 212-988-2800; **Board Cert:** Internal Medicine 1982; Gastroenterology 1985; **Med School:** Univ Tex SW, Dallas 1978; **Resid:** Internal Medicine, Univ Tex Hlth Sci Ctr-San Antonio Co/A Murphy VA Hosps 1981; **Fellow:** Gastroenterology, NY Hosp 1984; **Fac Appt:** Assoc Clin Prof Med, Cornell Univ-Weill Med Coll

Cooper, Robert B MD (Ge) - **Spec Exp:** Colon Cancer Screening; Gastroesophageal Reflux Disease (GERD); Celiac Disease; Gallbladder Disease; **Hospital:** NY-Presby Hosp/Weill Cornell (page 104); **Address:** 635 Madison Ave Fl 17, New York, NY 10022; **Phone:** 212-717-4967; **Board Cert:** Internal Medicine 1984; Gastroenterology 1989; **Med School:** Cornell Univ-Weill Med Coll 1981; **Resid:** Internal Medicine, NY Hosp 1984; **Fellow:** Gastroenterology, NY Hosp 1987; **Fac Appt:** Asst Prof Med, Cornell Univ-Weill Med Coll

Dieterich, Douglas T MD (Ge) - **Spec Exp:** Hepatitis; AIDS/HIV-Gastrointestinal Complications; Liver Disease; Endoscopy; **Hospital:** Mount Sinai Med Ctr (page 102); **Address:** 5 E 98th St Fl 8, New York, NY 10029; **Phone:** 212-241-7270; **Board Cert:** Internal Medicine 1981; Gastroenterology 1987; **Med School:** NYU Sch Med 1978; **Resid:** Internal Medicine, Bellevue Hosp Ctr-NYU 1981; **Fellow:** Gastroenterology, Bellevue Hosp Ctr-NYU 1983; **Fac Appt:** Prof Med, Mount Sinai Sch Med

Faust, Michael J MD (Ge) - **Spec Exp:** Gastrointestinal Disorders; **Hospital:** NYU Langone Med Ctr (page 106); **Address:** 345 E 37th St, Ste 207, New York, NY 10016-3256; **Phone:** 212-986-3330; **Board Cert:** Internal Medicine 1981; Gastroenterology 1983; **Med School:** NYU Sch Med 1978; **Resid:** Internal Medicine, Bellevue Hosp/NYU Med Ctr 1981; **Fellow:** Gastroenterology, Bellevue Hosp/NYU Med Ctr 1983; **Fac Appt:** Asst Prof Med, NYU Sch Med

Ferran, Elena Nascimbeni MD (Ge) - **Spec Exp:** Gastroesophageal Reflux Disease (GERD); Peptic Ulcer Disease; Liver Disease; **Hospital:** Lenox Hill Hosp; **Address:** 121 E 69th St, New York, NY 10021; **Phone:** 212-861-9268; **Board Cert:** Gastroenterology 2008; **Med School:** Italy 1989; **Resid:** Internal Medicine, St Vincent's Hosp 1994; **Fellow:** Gastroenterology, St Vincent's Hosp 1997Mt. Sinai Hosp 1998

Field, Steven P MD (Ge) - **Spec Exp:** Irritable Bowel Syndrome; **Hospital:** NYU Langone Med Ctr (page 106); **Address:** 245 E 35th St, New York, NY 10016; **Phone:** 212-686-9477; **Board Cert:** Internal Medicine 1980; Gastroenterology 1983; **Med School:** NYU Sch Med 1977; **Resid:** Internal Medicine, Bellevue Hosp 1981; **Fellow:** Gastroenterology, Mt Sinai Hosp 1983; **Fac Appt:** Asst Clin Prof Med, NYU Sch Med

Fochios, Steven E MD (Ge) - **Spec Exp:** Endoscopy; **Hospital:** Lenox Hill Hosp; **Address:** 117 E 65th St, New York, NY 10065; **Phone:** 212-861-4278; **Board Cert:** Internal Medicine 1980; Gastroenterology 1985; **Med School:** Geo Wash Univ 1976; **Resid:** Internal Medicine, Lenox Hill Hosp 1979; **Fellow:** Gastroenterology, Lenox Hill Hosp 1981

Foong, Anthony MD (Ge) - **Spec Exp:** Endoscopy; Colonoscopy; Gastrointestinal Disorders; Hemorrhoids; **Hospital:** Beth Israel Med Ctr - Petrie Division (page 94); **Address:** 210 Canal St, Ste 601, New York, NY 10013; **Phone:** 212-693-2100; **Board Cert:** Internal Medicine 1984; Gastroenterology 1987; **Med School:** Tufts Univ 1981; **Resid:** Internal Medicine, Univ Md Hosp 1984; **Fellow:** Gastroenterology, St Luke's-Roosevelt Hosp Ctr 1986

Frank, Michael MD (Ge) - **Spec Exp:** Inflammatory Bowel Disease/Crohn's; Colonoscopy; Endoscopy; **Hospital:** Lenox Hill Hosp; **Address:** 9 E 63rd St, New York, NY 10021-7236; **Phone:** 212-593-7170; **Board Cert:** Internal Medicine 1977; Gastroenterology 1979; **Med School:** Albert Einstein Coll Med 1974; **Resid:** Internal Medicine, Bronx Municipal Hosp Ctr 1977; **Fellow:** Gastroenterology, Montefiore Hosp Med Ctr 1979; **Fac Appt:** Assoc Clin Prof Med, Albert Einstein Coll Med

Freiman, Hal MD (Ge) - **Spec Exp:** Gastroesophageal Reflux Disease (GERD); Biliary Disease; Pancreatic/Biliary Endoscopy (ERCP); Hepatitis; **Hospital:** Beth Israel Med Ctr - Petrie Division (page 94), NYU Langone Med Ctr (page 106); **Address:** 59 W 12th St, Ste 1D, New York, NY 10011-8520; **Phone:** 212-206-0074; **Board Cert:** Internal Medicine 1981; Gastroenterology 1983; **Med School:** Albany Med Coll 1978; **Resid:** Internal Medicine, St Vincent's Hosp 1981; **Fellow:** Gastroenterology, Westchester Co Med Ctr 1983; **Fac Appt:** Asst Clin Prof Med, NY Med Coll

Friedlander, Charles N MD (Ge) - **Spec Exp:** Colonoscopy; Irritable Bowel Syndrome; **Hospital:** NYU Langone Med Ctr (page 106); **Address:** 232 E 30th St, New York, NY 10016-8202; **Phone:** 212-889-5544; **Board Cert:** Internal Medicine 1974; Gastroenterology 1977; **Med School:** SUNY Downstate 1968; **Resid:** Internal Medicine, Bellevue Hosp 1971; Internal Medicine, Bellevue Hosp 1974; **Fellow:** Gastroenterology, NYU Med Ctr 1976; **Fac Appt:** Assoc Prof Med, NYU Sch Med

Friedman, Scott L MD (Ge) - **Spec Exp:** Liver Disease; Hepatitis; **Hospital:** Mount Sinai Med Ctr (page 102); **Address:** Mt Sinai Med Ctr, Div Liver Diseases, 1475 Madison Ave, rm 1170, Box 1123, New York, NY 10029; **Phone:** 212-659-9501; **Board Cert:** Internal Medicine 1982; Gastroenterology 1985; **Med School:** Mount Sinai Sch Med 1979; **Resid:** Internal Medicine, Beth Israel Hosp 1982; **Fellow:** Gastroenterology, UCSF Med Ctr 1985; **Fac Appt:** Prof Med, Mount Sinai Sch Med

Gerdes, Hans MD (Ge) - **Spec Exp:** Endoscopy; Endoscopic Ultrasound; Barrett's Esophagus; Gastrointestinal Cancer; **Hospital:** Meml Sloan-Kettering Cancer Ctr (page 112); **Address:** 1275 York Avenue, New York, NY 10065; **Phone:** 800-525-2225; **Board Cert:** Internal Medicine 1987; Gastroenterology 1989; **Med School:** Cornell Univ-Weill Med Coll 1983; **Resid:** Internal Medicine, New York Hosp 1986; **Fellow:** Gastroenterology, Meml Sloan Kettering Cancer Ctr 1989

Gerson, Charles MD (Ge) - **Spec Exp:** Irritable Bowel Syndrome; Diarrheal Diseases; **Hospital:** Mount Sinai Med Ctr (page 102); **Address:** 80 Central Park West, Ste B, New York, NY 10023-5204; **Phone:** 212-496-6161; **Board Cert:** Internal Medicine 1970; Gastroenterology 1972; **Med School:** SUNY Downstate 1962; **Resid:** Internal Medicine, Bellevue Hosp 1964; Internal Medicine, Mount Sinai Hosp 1965; **Fellow:** Gastroenterology, Bellevue Hosp 1968; Gastroenterology, Mount Sinai Hosp 1969; **Fac Appt:** Clin Prof Med, Mount Sinai Sch Med

Goldberg, Myron D MD (Ge) - **Spec Exp:** Colon Cancer Screening; Colonoscopy; Endoscopy; Hepatitis B & C; **Hospital:** Lenox Hill Hosp; **Address:** 110 E 59th St, Ste 10D, New York, NY 10022-1304; **Phone:** 212-583-2900; **Board Cert:** Internal Medicine 1977; Gastroenterology 1979; **Med School:** Albert Einstein Coll Med 1971; **Resid:** Internal Medicine, Montefiore Med Ctr 1973; Internal Medicine, Lenox Hill Hosp 1974; **Fellow:** Gastroenterology, Columbia-Presby Hosp 1977; Gastroenterology, Lenox Hill Hosp 1978; **Fac Appt:** Asst Clin Prof Med, NYU Sch Med

Goldin, Howard MD (Ge) - **Spec Exp:** Inflammatory Bowel Disease/Crohn's; Endoscopy; Liver Disease; **Hospital:** NY-Presby Hosp/Weill Cornell (page 104), Rockefeller Univ; **Address:** 646 Park Ave, New York, NY 10065; **Phone:** 212-249-0404; **Board Cert:** Internal Medicine 1968; Gastroenterology 1973; **Med School:** Cornell Univ-Weill Med Coll 1961; **Resid:** Internal Medicine, New York Hosp 1964; **Fellow:** Gastroenterology, New York Hosp 1966; **Fac Appt:** Clin Prof Med, Cornell Univ-Weill Med Coll

Green, Peter H-R MD (Ge) - **Spec Exp:** Celiac Disease; Endoscopy; Colonoscopy; Malabsorption; **Hospital:** NY-Presby Hosp/Columbia (page 104); **Address:** Celiac Disease Ctr, Harkness Bldg, 180 Fort Washington Ave, rm 956, New York, NY 10032-3713; **Phone:** 212-305-5590; **Med School:** Australia 1970; **Resid:** Internal Medicine, North Shore Med Ctr 1974; **Fellow:** Gastroenterology, North Shore Med Ctr 1976; Gastroenterology, Beth Israel Hosp 1977; **Fac Appt:** Clin Prof Med, Columbia P&S

Haber, Gregory B MD (Ge) - **Spec Exp:** Endoscopy; Pancreatic/Biliary Endoscopy (ERCP); Endoscopic Ultrasound; Barrett's Esophagus; **Hospital:** Lenox Hill Hosp; **Address:** 100 E 77th St, New York, NY 10075; **Phone:** 212-434-6279; **Med School:** Univ Toronto 1970; **Resid:** Internal Medicine, Univ Toronto Med Ctr 1975; **Fellow:** Gastroenterology, Univ Toronto Med Ctr 1978

Hammerman, Hillel S MD (Ge) - **Spec Exp:** Swallowing Disorders; Liver Disease; Colonoscopy; **Hospital:** Lenox Hill Hosp; **Address:** 210 E 73rd St, Ste 1C, New York, NY 10021; **Phone:** 212-288-1030; **Board Cert:** Internal Medicine 1981; Gastroenterology 1983; **Med School:** Cornell Univ-Weill Med Coll 1978; **Resid:** Internal Medicine, Baltimore City Hosps 1981; **Fellow:** Gastroenterology, Lahey Clin 1983

Harary, Albert M MD (Ge) - **Spec Exp:** Endoscopy & Colonoscopy; Gastroesophageal Reflux Disease (GERD); Swallowing Disorders; **Hospital:** Lenox Hill Hosp, NYU Langone Med Ctr (page 106); **Address:** 654 Madison Ave, Fl 6, New York, NY 10065; **Phone:** 212-702-0123; **Board Cert:** Internal Medicine 1982; Gastroenterology 1985; **Med School:** Columbia P&S 1979; **Resid:** Internal Medicine, Univ Miami Affil Hosp 1982; **Fellow:** Gastroenterology, Univ Miami Affil Hosp 1984; **Fac Appt:** Asst Clin Prof Med, NYU Sch Med

Itzkowitz, Steven H MD (Ge) - **Spec Exp:** Colon & Rectal Cancer; Colon & Rectal Cancer Detection; Inflammatory Bowel Disease; **Hospital:** Mount Sinai Med Ctr (page 102); **Address:** 5 E 98th St, Box 1625, New York, NY 10029-6501; **Phone:** 212-241-4299; **Board Cert:** Internal Medicine 1982; Gastroenterology 1985; **Med School:** Mount Sinai Sch Med 1979; **Resid:** Internal Medicine, Bellevue Hosp/NYU Med Ctr 1982; **Fellow:** Gastroenterology, UCSF Med Ctr 1984; **Fac Appt:** Prof Med, Mount Sinai Sch Med

Jacobson, Ira MD (Ge) - **Spec Exp:** Liver & Biliary Disease; Pancreatic Disease; Colonoscopy; Hepatitis; **Hospital:** NY-Presby Hosp/Weill Cornell (page 104); **Address:** 1305 York Ave Fl 4, New York, NY 10021-5016; **Phone:** 646-962-4040; **Board Cert:** Internal Medicine 1982; Gastroenterology 1985; Transplant Hepatology 2006; **Med School:** Columbia P&S 1979; **Resid:** Internal Medicine, UCSF Med Ctr 1982; **Fellow:** Gastroenterology, Mass Genl Hosp 1984; **Fac Appt:** Prof Med, Cornell Univ-Weill Med Coll

Jaffin, Barry W MD (Ge) - **Spec Exp:** Gastrointestinal Motility Disorders; Inflammatory Bowel Disease; **Hospital:** Mount Sinai Med Ctr (page 102); **Address:** 620 Columbus Ave, New York, NY 10024; **Phone:** 212-721-2600; **Board Cert:** Internal Medicine 1984; Gastroenterology 1987; **Med School:** Mount Sinai Sch Med 1981; **Resid:** Internal Medicine, Med Ctr Hosp 1984; **Fellow:** Gastroenterology, Boston Univ Med Ctr 1986; **Fac Appt:** Asst Clin Prof Med, Mount Sinai Sch Med

Kairam, Indira MD (Ge) - **Spec Exp:** Colon Cancer; Peptic Ulcer Disease; Hepatitis C; **Hospital:** St Luke's - Roosevelt Hosp Ctr - St Luke's Hosp (page 94), St Luke's - Roosevelt Hosp Ctr - Roosevelt Div (page 94); **Address:** 945 West End Ave, Ste 1D, New York, NY 10025-3573; **Phone:** 212-865-7355; **Board Cert:** Internal Medicine 1978; **Med School:** India 1973; **Resid:** Internal Medicine, St Clare's Hosp 1978; **Fellow:** Gastroenterology, Lahey Clinic 1980; **Fac Appt:** Asst Prof Med, NY Med Coll

Kimball, Annetta MD (Ge) - **Spec Exp:** Hepatitis; Inflammatory Bowel Disease/Crohn's; Irritable Bowel Syndrome; **Hospital:** St Luke's - Roosevelt Hosp Ctr - Roosevelt Div (page 94); **Address:** 315 W 57th St, Ste 301, New York, NY 10019; **Phone:** 212-371-8900; **Board Cert:** Internal Medicine 1972; Gastroenterology 1973; **Med School:** Boston Univ 1968; **Resid:** Internal Medicine, Roosevelt Hosp 1970; Internal Medicine, Mount Sinai Hosp 1971; **Fellow:** Gastroenterology, Mount Sinai Hosp 1973; **Fac Appt:** Assoc Clin Prof Med, Columbia P&S

Knapp, Albert B MD (Ge) - **Spec Exp:** Colonoscopy/Polypectomy; Endoscopy; Liver Disease; Transplant Medicine-Liver; **Hospital:** NYU Langone Med Ctr (page 106), Lenox Hill Hosp; **Address:** 760 Park Ave, New York, NY 10021-4152; **Phone:** 212-737-3446; **Board Cert:** Internal Medicine 1982; Gastroenterology 1987; **Med School:** Columbia P&S 1979; **Resid:** Internal Medicine, Albert Einstein Med Ctr 1982; **Fellow:** Gastroenterology, Brigham & Women's Hosp 1985; Virology, Pasteur Inst 1975; **Fac Appt:** Clin Prof Med, NYU Sch Med

Kotler, Donald P MD (Ge) - **Spec Exp:** Esophageal Disorders; Nutrition & AIDS; Hepatitis; **Hospital:** St Luke's - Roosevelt Hosp Ctr - St Luke's Hosp (page 94); **Address:** 1111 Amsterdam Ave, SR 12, New York, NY 10025; **Phone:** 212-523-3670; **Board Cert:** Internal Medicine 1976; Gastroenterology 1979; **Med School:** Albert Einstein Coll Med 1973; **Resid:** Internal Medicine, Jacobi Med Ctr 1976; **Fellow:** Gastroenterology, Hosp Univ Penn 1978; **Fac Appt:** Prof Med, Columbia P&S

Krumholz, Michael MD (Ge) - **Spec Exp:** Colonoscopy; Colon Cancer Screening; **Hospital:** Lenox Hill Hosp; **Address:** 111 E 80th St, Ste 1C, New York, NY 10021-0350; **Phone:** 212-734-5533; **Board Cert:** Internal Medicine 1983; Gastroenterology 1987; **Med School:** Mount Sinai Sch Med 1980; **Resid:** Internal Medicine, Beth Israel Hosp 1984; **Fellow:** Gastroenterology, Lenox Hill Hosp 1986; **Fac Appt:** Med, NYU Sch Med

Kummer, Bart A MD (Ge) - **Spec Exp:** Colonoscopy; Endoscopy; **Hospital:** NYU Langone Med Ctr (page 106), NY Downtown Hosp; **Address:** Trinity Center at Broadway, 111 Broadway Fl 2, New York, NY 10006; **Phone:** 212-263-9700; **Board Cert:** Internal Medicine 1982; Gastroenterology 1985; **Med School:** Cornell Univ-Weill Med Coll 1979; **Resid:** Internal Medicine, Harlem Hosp 1982; **Fellow:** Gastroenterology, St Luke's-Roosevelt Hosp Ctr 1985; **Fac Appt:** Asst Prof Med, NYU Sch Med

Kurtz, Robert C MD (Ge) - **Spec Exp:** Pancreatic Cancer(Familial); Gastrointestinal Cancer; Endoscopy; Nutrition & Cancer Prevention/Control; **Hospital:** Meml Sloan-Kettering Cancer Ctr (page 112); **Address:** 1275 York Avenue, New York, NY 10065; **Phone:** 212-639-8286; **Board Cert:** Internal Medicine 1971; Gastroenterology 1977; **Med School:** Jefferson Med Coll 1968; **Resid:** Internal Medicine, NY Hosp/Meml Sloan Kettering Cancer Ctr 1971; **Fellow:** Gastroenterology, Meml Sloan Kettering Cancer Ctr 1973; **Fac Appt:** Prof Med, Cornell Univ-Weill Med Coll

Lambroza, Arnon MD (Ge) - **Spec Exp:** Swallowing Disorders; Gastroesophageal Reflux Disease (GERD); Barrett's Esophagus; Achalasia; **Hospital:** NY-Presby Hosp/Weill Cornell (page 104), Lenox Hill Hosp; **Address:** 950 Park Ave, New York, NY 10028-0320; **Phone:** 212-517-7570; **Board Cert:** Internal Medicine 1987; Gastroenterology 2001; **Med School:** Albert Einstein Coll Med 1984; **Resid:** Internal Medicine, Hosp Univ Penn 1987; **Fellow:** Gastroenterology, New York Hosp 1990; **Fac Appt:** Assoc Clin Prof Med, Cornell Univ-Weill Med Coll

Lax, James D MD (Ge) - **Spec Exp:** Liver Disease; Gastroesophageal Reflux Disease (GERD); Barrett's Esophagus; Eosinophilic Esophogitis; **Hospital:** St Luke's - Roosevelt Hosp Ctr - Roosevelt Div (page 94), Lenox Hill Hosp; **Address:** 160 E 72nd St, New York, NY 10021-4364; **Phone:** 212-988-5740; **Board Cert:** Internal Medicine 1984; Gastroenterology 1987; **Med School:** NYU Sch Med 1981; **Resid:** Internal Medicine, St Luke's-Roosevelt Hosp Ctr 1984; **Fellow:** Gastroenterology, St Luke's-Roosevelt Hosp Ctr 1986; **Fac Appt:** Asst Clin Prof Med, Columbia P&S

Lebwohl, Oscar MD (Ge) - **Spec Exp:** Endoscopy; Inflammatory Bowel Disease/Crohn's; Ulcerative Colitis; Gastrointestinal Cancer; **Hospital:** NY-Presby Hosp/Columbia (page 104); **Address:** 161 Fort Washington Ave, rm 420, New York, NY 10032-3713; **Phone:** 212-305-5363; **Board Cert:** Internal Medicine 1975; Gastroenterology 1977; **Med School:** Harvard Med Sch 1972; **Resid:** Internal Medicine, Mt Sinai Med Ctr 1975; **Fellow:** Gastroenterology, Columbia-Presby Med Ctr 1976; Hepatology, Mt Sinai Med Ctr 1977; **Fac Appt:** Clin Prof Med, Columbia P&S

Lewis, Blair MD (Ge) - **Spec Exp:** Endoscopy; Capsule Endoscopy; **Hospital:** Mount Sinai Med Ctr (page 102); **Address:** 1067 5th Ave, New York, NY 10128-0101; **Phone:** 212-369-6600; **Board Cert:** Internal Medicine 1985; Gastroenterology 1987; **Med School:** Albert Einstein Coll Med 1982; **Resid:** Internal Medicine, Montefiore Med Ctr 1985; **Fellow:** Gastroenterology, Mt Sinai Med Ctr 1987; **Fac Appt:** Clin Prof Med, Mount Sinai Sch Med

Lightdale, Charles J MD (Ge) - **Spec Exp:** Barrett's Esophagus; Gastrointestinal Cancer; Endoscopic Ultrasound; **Hospital:** NY-Presby Hosp/Columbia (page 104); **Address:** Columbia-Presby Med Ctr, Irving Pavilion, 161 Fort Washington Ave, rm 812, New York, NY 10032-3713; **Phone:** 212-305-3423; **Board Cert:** Internal Medicine 1972; Gastroenterology 1973; **Med School:** Columbia P&S 1966; **Resid:** Internal Medicine, Yale-New Haven Hosp 1968; Internal Medicine, NY Hosp-Cornell 1969; **Fellow:** Gastroenterology, NY Hosp-Cornell 1973; **Fac Appt:** Clin Prof Med, Columbia P&S

Lucak, Susan L MD (Ge) - **Spec Exp:** Irritable Bowel Syndrome; Liver Disease; **Hospital:** Lenox Hill Hosp, St Luke's - Roosevelt Hosp Ctr - Roosevelt Div (page 94); **Address:** 121 E 69th St, New York, NY 10021; **Phone:** 212-861-0481; **Board Cert:** Internal Medicine 1984; Gastroenterology 2001; **Med School:** Albert Einstein Coll Med 1981; **Resid:** Internal Medicine, Montefiore Med Ctr 1985; **Fellow:** Gastroenterology, Montefiore Med Ctr 1987; Research, Columbia Presby Med Ctr 1991; **Fac Appt:** Asst Clin Prof Med, Columbia P&S

Lustbader, Ian J MD (Ge) - **Spec Exp:** Hepatitis C; Colonoscopy; Ulcerative Colitis/Crohn's; **Hospital:** NYU Langone Med Ctr (page 106); **Address:** 245 E 35th St, New York, NY 10016-4283; **Phone:** 212-685-5252; **Board Cert:** Internal Medicine 1985; Gastroenterology 1987; **Med School:** Columbia P&S 1982; **Resid:** Internal Medicine, St Luke's-Roosevelt Hosp Ctr 1985; **Fellow:** Gastroenterology, Bellevue Hosp 1987; **Fac Appt:** Asst Clin Prof Med, NYU Sch Med

Magun, Arthur M MD (Ge) - **Spec Exp:** Hepatitis; Ulcerative Colitis; Endoscopy; Crohn's Disease; **Hospital:** NY-Presby Hosp/Columbia (page 104); **Address:** 161 Fort Washington Ave, rm 338, New York, NY 10032-3713; **Phone:** 212-305-5287; **Board Cert:** Internal Medicine 1980; Gastroenterology 1983; **Med School:** Mount Sinai Sch Med 1977; **Resid:** Internal Medicine, Columbia-Presby Med Ctr 1980; **Fellow:** Gastroenterology, Columbia-Presby Med Ctr 1983; **Fac Appt:** Clin Prof Med, Columbia P&S

Marion, James MD (Ge) - **Spec Exp:** Colonoscopy; Colitis; Crohn's Disease; **Hospital:** Mount Sinai Med Ctr (page 102); **Address:** 12 E 86th St, New York, NY 10028; **Phone:** 212-861-2000; **Board Cert:** Internal Medicine 2003; Gastroenterology 2005; **Med School:** Columbia P&S 1989; **Resid:** Internal Medicine, Columbia Presby Hosp 1992; **Fellow:** Gastroenterology, Mt Sinai Hosp 1995; **Fac Appt:** Assoc Clin Prof Med, Mount Sinai Sch Med

Markowitz, Arnold J MD (Ge) - **Spec Exp:** Endoscopy; Gastrointestinal Cancer; **Hospital:** Meml Sloan-Kettering Cancer Ctr (page 112); **Address:** 1275 York Avenue, New York, NY 10065; **Phone:** 800-525-2225; **Board Cert:** Gastroenterology 2003; **Med School:** NYU Sch Med 1987; **Resid:** Internal Medicine, NYU Med Ctr 1990; **Fellow:** Gastroenterology, Univ Mich Med Ctr 1992; Gastroenterology, Univ Penn Med Ctr 1994; **Fac Appt:** Asst Prof Med, Cornell Univ-Weill Med Coll

Markowitz, David D MD (Ge) - **Spec Exp:** Gastroesophageal Reflux Disease (GERD); Esophageal Disorders; Endoscopy; **Hospital:** NY-Presby Hosp/Columbia (page 104); **Address:** 161 Ft Washington Ave, Ste 853, New York, NY 10032; **Phone:** 212-305-1024; **Board Cert:** Internal Medicine 1988; Gastroenterology 2001; **Med School:** Columbia P&S 1985; **Resid:** Internal Medicine, Columbia-Presby Hosp 1988; **Fellow:** Gastroenterology, Columbia-Presby Hosp 1991; **Fac Appt:** Assoc Prof Med, Columbia P&S

Marsh Jr, Franklin MD (Ge) - **Spec Exp:** Colon Cancer; Liver Disease; Gastrointestinal Motility Disorders; **Hospital:** NY-Presby Hosp/Weill Cornell (page 104), N Genl Hosp; **Address:** 342 E 67th St, Ste 1D, New York, NY 10065-6238; **Phone:** 212-288-8820; **Board Cert:** Internal Medicine 1981; Gastroenterology 1985; Geriatric Medicine 2000; **Med School:** SUNY Buffalo 1978; **Resid:** Internal Medicine, Harlem Hosp 1982; **Fellow:** Gastroenterology, New York Hosp 1984; **Fac Appt:** Asst Clin Prof Med, Cornell Univ-Weill Med Coll

Mayer, Lloyd MD (Ge) - **Spec Exp:** Inflammatory Bowel Disease/Crohn's; Ulcerative Colitis; **Hospital:** Mount Sinai Med Ctr (page 102); **Address:** 1425 Madison Ave, rm 11-20, Box 1089, New York, NY 10029; **Phone:** 212-659-9266; **Board Cert:** Internal Medicine 1979; Gastroenterology 1981; **Med School:** Mount Sinai Sch Med 1976; **Resid:** Internal Medicine, Bellevue Hosp 1979; **Fellow:** Gastroenterology, Mt Sinai Hosp 1981; **Fac Appt:** Prof Med, Mount Sinai Sch Med

Milano, Andrew MD (Ge) - **Spec Exp:** Endoscopy; Inflammatory Bowel Disease/Crohn's; Esophageal Disorders; **Hospital:** NYU Langone Med Ctr (page 106); **Address:** 530 1st Ave, Ste 4K, New York, NY 10016-6402; **Phone:** 212-263-7483; **Board Cert:** Internal Medicine 1977; Gastroenterology 1972; **Med School:** NYU Sch Med 1964; **Resid:** Internal Medicine, NYU-Bellevue Hosp 1967; **Fellow:** Gastroenterology, NYU-Bellevue Hosp 1968; **Fac Appt:** Clin Prof Med, NYU Sch Med

Min, Albert D MD (Ge) - **Spec Exp:** Hepatitis B & C; Liver Disease; **Hospital:** Beth Israel Med Ctr - Petrie Division (page 94); **Address:** Beth Israel Medical Ctr, 1st Ave at 16th St, New York, NY 10003; **Phone:** 212-420-4751; **Board Cert:** Internal Medicine 1988; Gastroenterology 2002; **Med School:** Univ Rochester 1985; **Resid:** Gastroenterology, SUNY Stony Brook 1988; **Fellow:** Hepatology, Montefiore Med Ctr 1991; **Fac Appt:** Assoc Clin Prof Med, Albert Einstein Coll Med

Miskovitz, Paul MD (Ge) - **Spec Exp:** Endoscopy; Liver Disease; Biliary Disease; **Hospital:** NY-Presby Hosp/Weill Cornell (page 104); **Address:** 635 Madison Ave Fl 17, New York, NY 10022; **Phone:** 212-717-4966; **Board Cert:** Internal Medicine 1978; Gastroenterology 1981; **Med School:** Cornell Univ-Weill Med Coll 1975; **Resid:** Internal Medicine, NY Hosp 1978; **Fellow:** Gastroenterology, NY Hosp 1980; **Fac Appt:** Clin Prof Med, Cornell Univ-Weill Med Coll

Nagler, Jerry MD (Ge) - **Spec Exp:** Inflammatory Bowel Disease; Irritable Bowel Syndrome; **Hospital:** NY-Presby Hosp/Weill Cornell (page 104); **Address:** 407 E 70th St, FL 5, New York, NY 10021-5302; **Phone:** 212-628-7777; **Board Cert:** Internal Medicine 1976; Gastroenterology 1983; **Med School:** Yale Univ 1973; **Resid:** Internal Medicine, Columbia-Presby Hosp 1976; **Fellow:** Gastroenterology, NY Hosp/Cornell Med Ctr 1978; **Fac Appt:** Asst Clin Prof Med, Cornell Univ-Weill Med Coll

Ottaviano, Lawrence MD (Ge) - **Spec Exp:** Peptic Ulcer Disease; Colitis; **Address:** 60 Gramercy Park N, Ste 1B, New York, NY 10010; **Phone:** 212-254-1220; **Board Cert:** Internal Medicine 1988; Gastroenterology 2006; **Med School:** West Indies 1984; **Resid:** Internal Medicine, Cabrini Med Ctr 1987; **Fellow:** Gastroenterology, Cabrini Med Ctr 1989; **Fac Appt:** Asst Clin Prof Med, NY Med Coll

Pochapin, Mark B MD (Ge) - **Spec Exp:** Pancreatic Cancer; Endoscopic Ultrasound; Colon & Rectal Cancer Detection; Diarrheal Diseases; **Hospital:** NY-Presby Hosp/Weill Cornell (page 104); **Address:** The Jay Monahan Ctr for GI Hlth, 1315 York Ave Fl Ground, New York, NY 10021; **Phone:** 212-746-4014; **Board Cert:** Gastroenterology 2004; **Med School:** Cornell Univ-Weill Med Coll 1988; **Resid:** Internal Medicine, NY Hosp-Cornell Med Ctr 1991; **Fellow:** Gastroenterology, Montefiore Med Ctr 1993; **Fac Appt:** Assoc Clin Prof Med, Cornell Univ-Weill Med Coll

Robilotti, James G MD (Ge) - **Spec Exp:** Irritable Bowel Syndrome; Peptic Ulcer Disease; Gastroesophageal Reflux Disease (GERD); Colon Cancer Screening; **Address:** 29 Washington Sq West, New York, NY 10011-9180; **Phone:** 212-475-4030; **Board Cert:** Internal Medicine 1972; Gastroenterology 1981; **Med School:** UMDNJ-NJ Med Sch, Newark 1965; **Resid:** Internal Medicine, St Vincent's Hosp 1968; **Fellow:** Gastroenterology, St Vincent's Hosp 1970; **Fac Appt:** Assoc Clin Prof Med, NY Med Coll

Romeu, Jose MD (Ge) - **Spec Exp:** Colonoscopy/Polypectomy; Gastroscopy; Gastrointestinal Cancer; Gastroesophageal Reflux Disease (GERD); **Hospital:** Mount Sinai Med Ctr (page 102), Lenox Hill Hosp; **Address:** 1107 5th Ave, New York, NY 10128-0145; **Phone:** 212-534-6747; **Board Cert:** Internal Medicine 1973; Gastroenterology 1975; **Med School:** NYU Sch Med 1970; **Resid:** Internal Medicine, Mt Sinai Hosp 1973; **Fellow:** Gastroenterology, Mt Sinai Hosp 1976; **Fac Appt:** Asst Prof Med, Mount Sinai Sch Med

Rubin, Moshe MD (Ge) - **Spec Exp:** Capsule Endoscopy; Colonoscopy; Celiac Disease; Inflammatory Bowel Disease; **Hospital:** NY Hosp Queens, Lenox Hill Hosp; **Address:** 1020 Park Ave Fl 1, New York, NY 10028; **Phone:** 212-772-1012; **Board Cert:** Internal Medicine 1986; Gastroenterology 1989; **Med School:** Yale Univ 1983; **Resid:** Internal Medicine, NY Hosp 1986; **Fellow:** Gastroenterology, Columbia-Presby Hosp 1988; **Fac Appt:** Assoc Clin Prof Med, Cornell Univ-Weill Med Coll

Ruoff, Michael MD (Ge) - **Spec Exp:** Esophageal Disorders; Malabsorption; **Hospital:** NYU Langone Med Ctr (page 106); **Address:** 232 E 30 St, New York, NY 10016-8202; **Phone:** 212-889-5544; **Board Cert:** Internal Medicine 1980; Gastroenterology 1972; **Med School:** NYU Sch Med 1963; **Resid:** Internal Medicine, Bellevue Hosp 1966; **Fellow:** Gastroenterology, NYU Med Ctr 1967; **Fac Appt:** Clin Prof Med, NYU Sch Med

Sachar, David MD (Ge) - **Spec Exp:** Inflammatory Bowel Disease-Consult; Crohn's Disease; Ulcerative Colitis; **Hospital:** Mount Sinai Med Ctr (page 102); **Address:** 5 E 98th St Fl 11, New York, NY 10029; **Phone:** 212-241-4299; **Board Cert:** Internal Medicine 1969; Gastroenterology 1972; **Med School:** Harvard Med Sch 1963; **Resid:** Internal Medicine, Beth Israel Hosp 1965; Internal Medicine, Beth Israel Hosp 1968; **Fellow:** Gastroenterology, Mount Sinai Hosp 1970; **Fac Appt:** Clin Prof Med, Mount Sinai Sch Med

Salik, James MD (Ge) - **Spec Exp:** Colonoscopy; Liver Disease; Inflammatory Bowel Disease; **Hospital:** NYU Langone Med Ctr (page 106); **Address:** 232 E 30th St, New York, NY 10016-8202; **Phone:** 212-889-5544; **Board Cert:** Internal Medicine 1983; Gastroenterology 1985; **Med School:** NYU Sch Med 1980; **Resid:** Internal Medicine, Bellevue Hosp 1983; **Fellow:** Gastroenterology, Bellevue Hosp 1985; **Fac Appt:** Asst Prof Med, NYU Sch Med

Scherl, Ellen MD (Ge) - **Spec Exp:** Inflammatory Bowel Disease; Crohn's Disease; Colitis; **Hospital:** NY-Presby Hosp/Weill Cornell (page 104), Beth Israel Med Ctr - Petrie Division (page 94); **Address:** 1315 York Ave, Mezzanine Level, New York, NY 10021; **Phone:** 212-746-5077; **Board Cert:** Internal Medicine 1983; **Med School:** NY Med Coll 1977; **Resid:** Internal Medicine, Beth Israel Med Ctr 1981; **Fellow:** Gastroenterology, Mt Sinai Med Ctr 1983; **Fac Appt:** Asst Prof Med, Cornell Univ-Weill Med Coll

Schiano, Thomas D MD (Ge) - **Spec Exp:** Liver Disease; Transplant Medicine-Liver; Transplant Medicine-Bowel; Hepatitis; **Hospital:** Mount Sinai Med Ctr (page 102); **Address:** Mount Sinai Medical Ctr, One Gustave L Levy Pl, Box 1104, New York, NY 10029; **Phone:** 212-241-8035; **Board Cert:** Internal Medicine 2000; Gastroenterology 2005; Transplant Hepatology 2006; **Med School:** Mexico 1987; **Resid:** Internal Medicine, Maimonides Med Ctr 1992; Gastroenterology, Temple Univ 1995; **Fellow:** Nutrition, Meml Sloan-Kettering Cancer Ctr 1993; Hepatology, Mt Sinai Med Ctr 1996; **Fac Appt:** Prof Med, Mount Sinai Sch Med

Schmerin, Michael J MD (Ge) - **Spec Exp:** Colonoscopy; Gastroscopy; Gastroesophageal Reflux Disease (GERD); **Hospital:** NY-Presby Hosp/Weill Cornell (page 104), Lenox Hill Hosp; **Address:** 1060 Park Ave, Ste 1G, New York, NY 10128-1095; **Phone:** 212-348-3166; **Board Cert:** Internal Medicine 1976; Gastroenterology 1977; **Med School:** Jefferson Med Coll 1973; **Resid:** Internal Medicine, New York Hosp 1976; **Fellow:** Gastroenterology, New York Hosp-Cornell 1977; **Fac Appt:** Asst Prof Med, Cornell Univ-Weill Med Coll

Schneebaum, Cary MD (Ge) - **Spec Exp:** Colon Cancer Screening; **Hospital:** Beth Israel Med Ctr - Petrie Division (page 94); **Address:** 22 W 15th St, New York, NY 10011; **Phone:** 212-741-6100; **Board Cert:** Internal Medicine 1984; **Med School:** SUNY Hlth Sci Ctr 1981; **Resid:** Internal Medicine, Beth Israel Med Ctr 1984; **Fellow:** Gastroenterology, Beth Israel Med Ctr 1986

Schneider, Lewis MD (Ge) - **Spec Exp:** Colon Cancer; Gastrointestinal Cancer; Esophageal Cancer; **Hospital:** NY-Presby Hosp/Columbia (page 104); **Address:** 16 E 60th St, rm 322, New York, NY 10022; **Phone:** 212-326-8426; **Board Cert:** Internal Medicine 1981; **Med School:** SUNY Downstate 1978; **Resid:** Internal Medicine, Columbia-Presby Hosp 1981; **Fellow:** Gastroenterology, Columbia-Presby Hosp 1983

Shike, Moshe MD (Ge) - **Spec Exp:** Gastrointestinal Cancer; Nutrition & Cancer Prevention; Endoscopy; **Hospital:** Meml Sloan-Kettering Cancer Ctr (page 112); **Address:** 1275 York Ave, rm 224, New York, NY 10065; **Phone:** 800-525-2225; **Board Cert:** Internal Medicine 1977; Gastroenterology 1981; **Med School:** Israel 1975; **Resid:** Internal Medicine, Mt Auburn Hosp 1977; **Fellow:** Gastroenterology, Toronto Genl Hosp 1981; **Fac Appt:** Prof Med, Cornell Univ-Weill Med Coll

Starpoli, Anthony MD (Ge) - **Spec Exp:** Gastroesophageal Reflux Disease (GERD); **Hospital:** Lenox Hill Hosp, NYU Langone Med Ctr (page 106); **Address:** 29 Washington Square W, New York, NY 10011; **Phone:** 212-673-2721; **Board Cert:** Internal Medicine 1989; Gastroenterology 2003; **Med School:** Univ IL Coll Med 1986; **Resid:** Internal Medicine, Sound Shore Med Ctr 1989; **Fellow:** Gastroenterology, St Vincents Hosp 1991; **Fac Appt:** Asst Clin Prof Med, NY Med Coll

Stein, Jeffrey A MD (Ge) - **Spec Exp:** Gallbladder Disease; Pancreatic Disease; **Hospital:** NY-Presby Hosp/Columbia (page 104); **Address:** 161 Ft Washington Ave, rm 328, New York, NY 10032; **Phone:** 212-305-5444; **Board Cert:** Internal Medicine 1971; Gastroenterology 1973; **Med School:** Harvard Med Sch 1965; **Resid:** Internal Medicine, Presbyterian Hosp 1970; **Fellow:** Gastroenterology, Presbyterian Hosp 1971; **Fac Appt:** Clin Prof Med, Columbia P&S

Stevens, Peter D MD (Ge) - **Spec Exp:** Endoscopy; Pancreatic Disease; Pancreatic/Biliary Endoscopy (ERCP); **Hospital:** NY-Presby Hosp/Columbia (page 104); **Address:** NY Presby-Columbia Presbyterian Med Ctr, 161 Fort Washington Ave, Ste 864, New York, NY 10032; **Phone:** 212-305-1909; **Board Cert:** Gastroenterology 2003; **Med School:** Columbia P&S 1987; **Resid:** Internal Medicine, Columbia Presby Med Ctr 1991; **Fellow:** Gastroenterology, Columbia Presby Med Ctr 1993; Endoscopy, Columbia Presby Med Ctr 1994; **Fac Appt:** Asst Clin Prof Med, Columbia P&S

Tobias, Hillel MD (Ge) - **Spec Exp:** Liver Disease; Hepatitis B & C; Liver & Biliary Disease; **Hospital:** NYU Langone Med Ctr (page 106); **Address:** 232 E 30th St, New York, NY 10016-8202; **Phone:** 212-889-5544; **Board Cert:** Internal Medicine 1967; Gastroenterology 1979; **Med School:** Washington Univ, St Louis 1960; **Resid:** Internal Medicine, Bellevue Hosp 1963; **Fellow:** Hepatology, Royal Free Hosp 1965; Hepatology, Mount Sinai Hosp 1967; **Fac Appt:** Prof Med, NYU Sch Med

Traube, Morris MD (Ge) - **Spec Exp:** Esophageal Disorders; Swallowing Disorders; Gastroesophageal Reflux Disease (GERD); **Hospital:** NYU Langone Med Ctr (page 106); **Address:** NYU Gastroenterology Associates, 530 First Ave Skirball Bldg - Ste 9N, New York, NY 10016; **Phone:** 212-263-3095; **Board Cert:** Internal Medicine 1981; Gastroenterology 1983; **Med School:** SUNY Downstate 1978; **Resid:** Internal Medicine, Maimonides Med Ctr 1981; **Fellow:** Gastroenterology, Yale-New Haven Hosp 1984; **Fac Appt:** Prof Med, NYU Sch Med

Ullman, Thomas A MD (Ge) - **Spec Exp:** Irritable Bowel Syndrome; Ulcerative Colitis; Inflammatory Bowel Disease/Crohn's; Colon & Rectal Cancer; **Hospital:** Mount Sinai Med Ctr (page 102); **Address:** 5 E 98th St Fl 11, New York, NY 10029; **Phone:** 212-241-4299; **Board Cert:** Gastroenterology 2009; **Med School:** Cornell Univ-Weill Med Coll 1992; **Resid:** Internal Medicine, New York Hosp 1995; **Fellow:** Gastroenterology, Yale-New Haven Hosp 1999; **Fac Appt:** Assoc Prof Med, Mount Sinai Sch Med

Wang, Timothy C MD (Ge) - **Hospital:** NY-Presby Hosp/Columbia (page 104); **Address:** 161 Fort Washington Ave, New York, NY 10032; **Phone:** 212-305-1021; **Board Cert:** Internal Medicine 1986; Gastroenterology 1989; **Med School:** Columbia P&S 1983; **Resid:** Internal Medicine, Barnes Jewish Hosp 1986; **Fellow:** Gastroenterology, Mass General Hosp 1989; **Fac Appt:** Prof Med, Columbia P&S

Waye, Jerome MD (Ge) - **Spec Exp:** Endoscopy; Colon Cancer; Colonoscopy; **Hospital:** Mount Sinai Med Ctr (page 102), Lenox Hill Hosp; **Address:** 650 Park Ave, New York, NY 10065; **Phone:** 212-439-7779; **Board Cert:** Internal Medicine 1965; Gastroenterology 1970; **Med School:** Boston Univ 1958; **Resid:** Internal Medicine, Mt Sinai Hosp 1961; **Fellow:** Gastroenterology, Mt Sinai Hosp 1962; **Fac Appt:** Clin Prof Med, Mount Sinai Sch Med

Weiss, Robert A MD (Ge) - **Spec Exp:** Colon Cancer; Gastroesophageal Reflux Disease (GERD); Endoscopy; **Hospital:** Beth Israel Med Ctr - Petrie Division (page 94); **Address:** 380 2nd Ave, Ste 1004, New York, NY 10010; **Phone:** 212-473-4100; **Board Cert:** Internal Medicine 1987; Gastroenterology 1989; **Med School:** Mount Sinai Sch Med 1983; **Resid:** Internal Medicine, Beth Israel Med Ctr 1986; **Fellow:** Gastroenterology, Elmhurst Hosp Ctr-Mt Sinai 1988; **Fac Appt:** Asst Clin Prof Med, Albert Einstein Coll Med

Geriatric Medicine

Adelman, Ronald MD (Ger) - **Hospital:** NY-Presby Hosp/Weill Cornell (page 104); **Address:** 1484 1st Ave, New York, NY 10021; **Phone:** 212-746-7000; **Board Cert:** Internal Medicine 1982; Geriatric Medicine 2009; **Med School:** Albert Einstein Coll Med 1978; **Resid:** Internal Medicine, Montefiore Med Ctr 1981

Bloom, Patricia A MD (Ger) - **Spec Exp:** Complementary Medicine; Dementia; **Hospital:** Mount Sinai Med Ctr (page 102); **Address:** 1440 Madison Ave, New York, NY 10029-6542; **Phone:** 212-659-8552; **Board Cert:** Internal Medicine 1978; Geriatric Medicine 1998; **Med School:** Univ Minn 1975; **Resid:** Internal Medicine, Montefiore Med Ctr 1978; **Fac Appt:** Assoc Prof Med, Mount Sinai Sch Med

Callahan, Eileen MD (Ger) - **Spec Exp:** Frail Elderly; Preventive Medicine; Dementia; **Hospital:** Mount Sinai Med Ctr (page 102); **Address:** 1 Gustave L Levy Pl, Box 1470, New York, NY 10029; **Phone:** 212-659-8552; **Board Cert:** Internal Medicine 2004; Geriatric Medicine 2008; Hospice & Palliative Medicine 2005; **Med School:** UMDNJ-NJ Med Sch, Newark 1991; **Resid:** Internal Medicine, St Vincents Hosp Med Ctr 1994; **Fellow:** Geriatric Medicine, Mount Sinai Hosp 1996; **Fac Appt:** Assoc Prof Med, Mount Sinai Sch Med

Chai, Emily MD (Ger) - **Spec Exp:** Palliative Care; **Hospital:** Mount Sinai Med Ctr (page 102); **Address:** Mount Sinai Med Ctr, One Gustave L Levy Pl, Box 1070, New York, NY 10029; **Phone:** 212-241-1446; **Board Cert:** Internal Medicine 2001; Geriatric Medicine 2002; Hospice & Palliative Medicine 2008; **Med School:** NYU Sch Med 1998; **Resid:** Internal Medicine, Mt Sinai Hosp 2001; **Fellow:** Geriatric Medicine, Mt Sinai Hosp 2003; **Fac Appt:** Asst Prof Med, Mount Sinai Sch Med

Chang, Christine MD (Ger) - **Spec Exp:** Alzheimer's Disease; Dementia; **Hospital:** Mount Sinai Med Ctr (page 102); **Address:** 1440 Madison Ave, New York, NY 10029; **Phone:** 212-659-8552; **Board Cert:** Internal Medicine 2008; Geriatric Medicine 2000; **Med School:** Duke Univ 1995; **Resid:** Internal Medicine, Univ Pitt Hlth Sys 1998; **Fellow:** Geriatric Medicine, Johns Hopkins Hosp 2000; **Fac Appt:** Asst Prof Med, Mount Sinai Sch Med

Chun, Audrey K MD (Ger) - **Spec Exp:** Dementia; Depression; **Hospital:** Mount Sinai Med Ctr (page 102); **Address:** One Gustave Levy Pl, Box 1070, New York, NY 10029; **Phone:** 212-659-8552; **Board Cert:** Internal Medicine 2001; Geriatric Medicine 2002; **Med School:** Baylor Coll Med 1998; **Resid:** Internal Medicine, Baylor Affil Hosp 2001; **Fellow:** Geriatric Medicine, Mt Sinai Hosp 2003; **Fac Appt:** Asst Prof Med, Mount Sinai Sch Med

Finkelstein, Martin S MD (Ger) - **Hospital:** NYU Langone Med Ctr (page 106); **Address:** 314 E 30th St, New York, NY 10016-6402; **Phone:** 646-370-2000; **Board Cert:** Internal Medicine 1970; **Med School:** NYU Sch Med 1964; **Resid:** Internal Medicine, Bellevue Hosp 1966; Internal Medicine, Stanford Univ Med Ctr 1967; **Fellow:** Infectious Disease, Stanford Univ Med Ctr 1968; **Fac Appt:** Assoc Clin Prof Med, NYU Sch Med

Fogel, Joyce MD (Ger) *PCP* - **Spec Exp:** Memory Disorders; Geriatric Functional Assessment; Preventive Medicine; **Hospital:** Beth Israel Med Ctr- Kings Hwy Div (page 94); **Address:** 275 8th Ave, New York, NY 10011-8305; **Phone:** 212-463-0101; **Board Cert:** Internal Medicine 1986; Geriatric Medicine 2000; **Med School:** SUNY Downstate 1982; **Resid:** Internal Medicine, Kings Co Hosp 1986; **Fellow:** Geriatric Medicine, Bellevue/NYU Med Ctr 1989; **Fac Appt:** Assoc Clin Prof Med, NY Med Coll

Karp, Adam H MD (Ger) *PCP* - **Hospital:** NYU Hosp For Joint Diseases (page 106), NYU Langone Med Ctr (page 106); **Address:** 301 E 17th St, rm 208, New York, NY 10003; **Phone:** 212-598-6738; **Board Cert:** Internal Medicine 1999; Geriatric Medicine 2002; **Med School:** Albert Einstein Coll Med 1987; **Resid:** Internal Medicine, Maimonides Med Ctr 1990; **Fellow:** Geriatric Medicine, Bellevue Hosp/NYU Med Ctr 1992; **Fac Appt:** Asst Prof Med, NYU Sch Med

Kellogg, F Russell MD (Ger) *PCP* - **Spec Exp:** Hypertension; Dementia; **Address:** 36 7th Ave, Ste C512, New York, NY 10011; **Phone:** 212-604-6513; **Board Cert:** Internal Medicine 1998; **Med School:** NY Med Coll 1974; **Resid:** Internal Medicine, St Vincent's Hosp 1977; **Fac Appt:** Asst Prof Med, NY Med Coll

Korc, Beatriz MD/PhD (Ger) - **Spec Exp:** Alzheimer's Disease; Diabetes; Preventive Medicine; **Hospital:** Mount Sinai Med Ctr (page 102); **Address:** One Gustave Levy Pl, Box 1070, New York, NY 10029; **Phone:** 212-659-8552; **Board Cert:** Internal Medicine 2007; Geriatric Medicine 2002; **Med School:** Uruguay 1983; **Resid:** Internal Medicine, Univ Rochester Med Ctr 1997; **Fellow:** Geriatric Medicine, Univ Rochester 2002; **Fac Appt:** Asst Prof Med, Mount Sinai Sch Med

Lachs, Mark S MD (Ger) - **Spec Exp:** Abuse/Neglect; **Hospital:** NY-Presby Hosp/Weill Cornell (page 104); **Address:** Irving Sherwood Wright Center on Aging, 1484 First Ave, New York, NY 10075; **Phone:** 212-746-7000; **Board Cert:** Internal Medicine 1988; Geriatric Medicine 2002; **Med School:** NYU Sch Med 1985; **Resid:** Internal Medicine, Hosp Univ Penn 1988; **Fellow:** Geriatric Medicine, Yale-New Haven Hosp 1990; **Fac Appt:** Prof Med, Cornell Univ-Weill Med Coll

Leipzig, Rosanne M MD (Ger) *PCP* - **Spec Exp:** Medications in the Elderly; **Hospital:** Mount Sinai Med Ctr (page 102); **Address:** 1468 Madison Ave, Box 1070, New York, NY 10029; **Phone:** 212-689-8552; **Board Cert:** Internal Medicine 1982; Geriatric Medicine 2008; **Med School:** Univ Mich Med Sch 1978; **Resid:** Internal Medicine, Strong Meml Hosp 1982; **Fellow:** Clinical Pharmacology, New York Hosp 1985; **Fac Appt:** Prof Med, Mount Sinai Sch Med

Meier, Diane E MD (Ger) - **Spec Exp:** Palliative Care; **Hospital:** Mount Sinai Med Ctr (page 102); **Address:** Mt Sinai School Medicine, Box 1070, New York, NY 10029-6501; **Phone:** 212-241-1446; **Board Cert:** Internal Medicine 1981; Geriatric Medicine 1999; Hospice & Palliative Medicine 2008; **Med School:** Northwestern Univ 1977; **Resid:** Internal Medicine, Oregon Hlth Sci Univ 1981; **Fellow:** Geriatric Medicine, VA Med Ctr 1983; **Fac Appt:** Prof Med, Mount Sinai Sch Med

Morrison, R Sean MD (Ger) - **Spec Exp:** Palliative Care; **Hospital:** Mount Sinai Med Ctr (page 102); **Address:** 1470 Madison Ave, New York, NY 10029; **Phone:** 212-659-8552; **Board Cert:** Internal Medicine 2003; Geriatric Medicine 2006; Hospice & Palliative Medicine 2008; **Med School:** Univ Chicago-Pritzker Sch Med 1990; **Resid:** Internal Medicine, NY Hosp/Cornell Med Ctr 1993; **Fellow:** Geriatric Medicine, Mt Sinai Med Ctr; **Fac Appt:** Prof Med, Mount Sinai Sch Med

Nichols, Jeffrey MD (Ger) - **Spec Exp:** Dementia; Long Term Care; Home Care; **Hospital:** Beth Israel Med Ctr - Petrie Division (page 94); **Address:** 220 E 19th St, New York, NY 10003-2601; **Phone:** 212-358-6255; **Board Cert:** Internal Medicine 1979; Geriatric Medicine 1998; **Med School:** Cornell Univ-Weill Med Coll 1976; **Resid:** Internal Medicine, St Vincent's Hosp & Med Ctr 1979; **Fac Appt:** Assoc Clin Prof Med, Mount Sinai Sch Med

Raman, Bharathi MD (Ger) - **Hospital:** NY-Presby Hosp/Weill Cornell (page 104); **Address:** 1484 1st Ave, New York, NY 10021; **Phone:** 212-746-7000; **Board Cert:** Internal Medicine 1988; Geriatric Medicine 2001; **Med School:** India 1973; **Resid:** Internal Medicine, Woodhill Med Ctr 1988; **Fellow:** Geriatric Medicine, Mt Sinai Med Ctr 1990; **Fac Appt:** Asst Prof Med, Cornell Univ-Weill Med Coll

Sherman, Fredrick T MD (Ger) *PCP* - **Spec Exp:** Frail Elderly; Falls in the Elderly; Polypharmacology (Excess Medications); Memory Disorders; **Hospital:** Mount Sinai Med Ctr (page 102); **Address:** Archcare Senior Life, 1432 5th Ave, New York, NY 10026; **Phone:** 646-289-7700; **Board Cert:** Internal Medicine 1975; Geriatric Medicine 1998; **Med School:** Temple Univ 1972; **Resid:** Internal Medicine, Med Coll Penn Hosp 1975; **Fac Appt:** Clin Prof Med, Mount Sinai Sch Med

Siegler, Eugenia L MD (Ger) *PCP* - **Spec Exp:** Dementia; **Hospital:** NY-Presby Hosp/Weill Cornell (page 104); **Address:** Irving Sherwood Wright Ctr on Aging, 1484 First Ave, New York, NY 10021; **Phone:** 212-746-7000; **Board Cert:** Internal Medicine 1986; Geriatric Medicine 1998; **Med School:** Johns Hopkins Univ 1983; **Resid:** Internal Medicine, Bellevue Hosp 1987; **Fellow:** Geriatric Medicine, Hosp Univ Penn 1989; **Fac Appt:** Assoc Prof Med, Cornell Univ-Weill Med Coll

Geriatric Psychiatry

Reisberg, Barry MD (GerPsy) - **Spec Exp:** Alzheimer's Disease; Dementia; Cognitive Loss in Aging; Depression; **Hospital:** NYU Langone Med Ctr (page 106); **Address:** Aging & Dementia Rsch Ctr - NYU, 145 E 32nd St, rm 508, New York, NY 10016-6055; **Phone:** 212-263-8550; **Board Cert:** Psychiatry 1976; Geriatric Psychiatry 2000; **Med School:** NY Med Coll 1972; **Resid:** Psychiatry, Metropolitan Hosp 1975; **Fellow:** Psychiatric Research, Univ London 1975; **Fac Appt:** Prof Psyc, NYU Sch Med

Serby, Michael J MD (GerPsy) - **Spec Exp:** Alzheimer's Disease; Depression; Parkinson's Disease; **Hospital:** Beth Israel Med Ctr - Petrie Division (page 94); **Address:** 317 E 17th St Fl 9, New York, NY 10003; **Phone:** 212-420-2421; **Board Cert:** Psychiatry 1979; Geriatric Psychiatry 2000; **Med School:** Emory Univ 1969; **Resid:** Psychiatry, Bellevue Hosp-NYU 1976; **Fac Appt:** Clin Prof Psyc, Albert Einstein Coll Med

Gynecologic Oncology

Abu-Rustum, Nadeem R MD (GO) - **Spec Exp:** Ovarian Cancer; Uterine Cancer; Cervical Cancer; Vulvar Disease/Cancer; **Hospital:** Meml Sloan-Kettering Cancer Ctr (page 112); **Address:** 1275 York Avenue, New York, NY 10065; **Phone:** 212-639-7051; **Board Cert:** Obstetrics & Gynecology 2008; Gynecologic Oncology 2008; **Med School:** Lebanon 1990; **Resid:** Obstetrics & Gynecology, Greater Baltimore Med Ctr 1994; **Fellow:** Gynecologic Oncology, Meml Sloan-Kettering Cancer Ctr 1997; **Fac Appt:** Assoc Prof ObG, Cornell Univ-Weill Med Coll

Barakat, Richard R MD (GO) - **Spec Exp:** Laparoscopic Surgery; Ovarian Cancer; Uterine Cancer; **Hospital:** Meml Sloan-Kettering Cancer Ctr (page 112); **Address:** 1275 York Ave, rm H1305, New York, NY 10065; **Phone:** 800-525-2225; **Board Cert:** Obstetrics & Gynecology 2006; Gynecologic Oncology 2006; **Med School:** SUNY Hlth Sci Ctr 1985; **Resid:** Obstetrics & Gynecology, Bellevue Hosp 1989; **Fellow:** Gynecologic Oncology, Meml Sloan Kettering Cancer Ctr 1991; **Fac Appt:** Assoc Prof ObG, Cornell Univ-Weill Med Coll

Brown, Carol MD (GO) - **Spec Exp:** Ovarian Cancer; Cervical Cancer; Uterine Cancer; Laparoscopic Surgery; **Hospital:** Meml Sloan-Kettering Cancer Ctr (page 112); **Address:** 1275 York Avenue, New York, NY 10065; **Phone:** 646-497-9055; **Board Cert:** Obstetrics & Gynecology 2009; Gynecologic Oncology 2009; **Med School:** Columbia P&S 1986; **Resid:** Obstetrics & Gynecology, Hosp Univ Penn 1990; **Fellow:** Gynecologic Oncology, Meml Sloan Kettering Cancer Ctr 1992; Research, Meml Sloan Kettering Cancer Ctr 1994; **Fac Appt:** Asst Prof ObG, Cornell Univ-Weill Med Coll

Caputo, Thomas A MD (GO) - **Spec Exp:** Cervical Cancer; Ovarian Cancer; Uterine Cancer; Vulvar Disease/Cancer; **Hospital:** NY-Presby Hosp/Weill Cornell (page 104); **Address:** NY Presby Hosp-Weill Cornell, 525 E 68th St, Ste J130, New York, NY 10021; **Phone:** 212-746-3179; **Board Cert:** Obstetrics & Gynecology 1993; Gynecologic Oncology 1977; **Med School:** UMDNJ-NJ Med Sch, Newark 1965; **Resid:** Obstetrics & Gynecology, Martland Hosp 1969; **Fellow:** Gynecologic Oncology, Emory Univ Hosp 1974; **Fac Appt:** Clin Prof ObG, Cornell Univ-Weill Med Coll

Curtin, John P MD (GO) - **Spec Exp:** Uterine Cancer; Ovarian Cancer; Laparoscopic Surgery; Gestational Trophoblastic Disease; **Hospital:** NYU Langone Med Ctr (page 106), Bellevue Hosp Ctr; **Address:** NYU Clin Cancer Ctr, 160 E 34th St Fl 4, New York, NY 10016-6402; **Phone:** 212-731-5345; **Board Cert:** Obstetrics & Gynecology 2008; Gynecologic Oncology 2009; **Med School:** Creighton Univ 1979; **Resid:** Obstetrics & Gynecology, Univ Minn Med Ctr 1984; **Fellow:** Gynecologic Oncology, Meml Sloan-Kettering Cancer Ctr 1988; **Fac Appt:** Prof ObG, NYU Sch Med

Dottino, Peter R MD (GO) - **Spec Exp:** Laparoscopic Surgery; Gynecologic Cancer; **Hospital:** Mount Sinai Med Ctr (page 102), Hackensack Univ Med Ctr (page 96); **Address:** 800-A 5th Ave, Ste 405, New York, NY 10065; **Phone:** 212-888-8439; **Board Cert:** Obstetrics & Gynecology 2007; Gynecologic Oncology 2007; **Med School:** Georgetown Univ 1979; **Resid:** Obstetrics & Gynecology, SUNY Downstate Med Ctr 1983; **Fellow:** Gynecologic Oncology, Mt Sinai Hosp 1985

Fishman, David A MD (GO) - **Spec Exp:** Ovarian Cancer; Ovarian Cancer-Early Detection; Gynecologic Cancer; **Hospital:** Mount Sinai Med Ctr (page 102); **Address:** 1190 Fifth Ave, New York, NY 10029; **Phone:** 212-427-9898; **Board Cert:** Obstetrics & Gynecology 2008; Gynecologic Oncology 2008; **Med School:** Texas Tech Univ 1988; **Resid:** Obstetrics & Gynecology, Yale-New Haven Hosp 1992; **Fellow:** Gynecologic Oncology, Yale-New Haven Hosp 1994; **Fac Appt:** Prof ObG, Mount Sinai Sch Med

Herzog, Thomas J MD (GO) - **Spec Exp:** Cervical Cancer; Gynecologic Cancer; Laparoscopic Surgery; Ovarian Cancer; **Hospital:** NY-Presby Hosp/Columbia (page 104); **Address:** Herbert Irving Pavilion, 161 Fort Washington Ave, 8-837, New York, NY 10032; **Phone:** 212-305-3410; **Board Cert:** Obstetrics & Gynecology 2008; Gynecologic Oncology 2008; **Med School:** Univ Cincinnati 1986; **Resid:** Obstetrics & Gynecology, Good Samaritan Hosp 1990; **Fellow:** Gynecologic Oncology, Barnes Jewish Hosp 1993; **Fac Appt:** Prof ObG, Columbia P&S

Holcomb, Kevin M MD (GO) - **Spec Exp:** Cervical Cancer; Laparoscopic Surgery; Robotic Surgery; **Hospital:** NY-Presby Hosp/Weill Cornell (page 104); **Address:** Weill Cornell Physicians - Ob/Gyn, 525 E 68th St, Ste J-130, New York, NY 10021; **Phone:** 212-746-7553; **Board Cert:** Obstetrics & Gynecology 2000; Gynecologic Oncology 2002; **Med School:** NY Med Coll 1992; **Resid:** Obstetrics & Gynecology, NY Hosp-Cornell Med Ctr 1996; **Fellow:** Gynecologic Oncology, Downstate Med Ctr 1999; **Fac Appt:** Assoc Clin Prof ObG, Cornell Univ-Weill Med Coll

Koulos, John MD (GO) - **Spec Exp:** Uterine Cancer; Ovarian Cancer; Cervical Cancer; **Hospital:** Beth Israel Med Ctr - Petrie Division (page 94); **Address:** Beth Israel Hosp Cancer Ctr, 10 Union Square E, Ste 4C, New York, NY 10003; **Phone:** 212-844-5729; **Board Cert:** Obstetrics & Gynecology 2006; Gynecologic Oncology 2006; **Med School:** Northwestern Univ 1978; **Resid:** Obstetrics & Gynecology, Northwestern Univ Med Sch 1982; **Fellow:** Gynecologic Oncology, Meml Sloan Kettering Cancer Ctr 1984; **Fac Appt:** Assoc Prof ObG, NY Med Coll

Poynor, Elizabeth A MD/PhD (GO) - **Spec Exp:** Gynecologic Cancer; Gynecologic Surgery-Complex; Laparoscopic Surgery; Breast Cancer; **Hospital:** Lenox Hill Hosp; **Address:** 1050 5th Ave, New York, NY 10028; **Phone:** 212-426-2700; **Board Cert:** Obstetrics & Gynecology 2009; Gynecologic Oncology 2009; **Med School:** Columbia P&S 1988; **Resid:** Obstetrics & Gynecology, Hosp Univ Penn 1992; **Fellow:** Gynecologic Oncology, Meml Sloan-Kettering Cancer Ctr 1995

Rahaman, Jamal MD (GO) - **Spec Exp:** Minimally Invasive Surgery; Gynecologic Cancer; Robotic Surgery; Laparoscopic Surgery; **Hospital:** Mount Sinai Med Ctr (page 102); **Address:** 11360 Fifth Ave, New York, NY 10029; **Phone:** 212-427-1415; **Board Cert:** Obstetrics & Gynecology 2009; Gynecologic Oncology 2009; **Med School:** Jamaica 1984; **Resid:** Obstetrics & Gynecology, Lincoln Med Ctr 1991; Obstetrics & Gynecology, Mt Sinai Med Ctr 1993; **Fellow:** Cardiovascular Surgery, Texas Heart Inst 1990; Gynecologic Oncology, Mt Sinai Med Ctr 1995; **Fac Appt:** Assoc Prof ObG, Mount Sinai Sch Med

Wallach, Robert C MD (GO) - **Spec Exp:** Vulvar & Vaginal Cancer; Ovarian Cancer; Cervical Cancer; Peritoneal Carcinomatosis; **Hospital:** NYU Langone Med Ctr (page 106), Bellevue Hosp Ctr; **Address:** NYU Clinical Cancer Ctr, 160 E 34th St, New York, NY 10016; **Phone:** 212-731-5345; **Board Cert:** Obstetrics & Gynecology 1967; Gynecologic Oncology 1974; **Med School:** Yale Univ 1960; **Resid:** Obstetrics & Gynecology, Beth Israel Med Ctr 1965; **Fellow:** Gynecologic Oncology, SUNY Downstate Med Ctr 1966; **Fac Appt:** Prof ObG, NYU Sch Med

Hand Surgery

Athanasian, Edward MD (HS) - **Spec Exp:** Bone & Soft Tissue Tumors; Hand & Upper Extremity Tumors; Hand & Upper Extremity Surgery; **Hospital:** Hosp For Special Surgery (page 111), Meml Sloan-Kettering Cancer Ctr (page 112); **Address:** Hospital for Special Surgery, 535 E 70th St, New York, NY 10021; **Phone:** 212-606-1962; **Board Cert:** Orthopaedic Surgery 2008; Hand Surgery 2008; **Med School:** Columbia P&S 1988; **Resid:** Surgery, Beth Israel Hosp 1989; Orthopaedic Surgery, Hosp Special Surgery 1993; **Fellow:** Hand Surgery, Mayo Clinic 1994; Orthopaedic Oncology, Meml Sloan Kettering Cancer Ctr 1995; **Fac Appt:** Asst Prof OrS, Cornell Univ-Weill Med Coll

Barron, O Alton MD (HS) - **Spec Exp:** Shoulder Arthroscopic Surgery; Elbow Surgery; Nerve & Tendon Reconstruction; Shoulder Reconstruction; **Hospital:** St Luke's - Roosevelt Hosp Ctr - Roosevelt Div (page 94); **Address:** CV Starr Hand Surgery Ctr, 1000 10th Ave, New York, NY 10019; **Phone:** 212-523-7590; **Board Cert:** Orthopaedic Surgery 2009; Hand Surgery 2009; **Med School:** Tulane Univ 1989; **Resid:** Surgery, Tulane Univ Affil Hosps 1994; **Fellow:** Shoulder Surgery, Columbia Presby Hosp 1995; Hand Surgery, St Lukes Roosevelt Hosp 1996; **Fac Appt:** Asst Clin Prof S, Columbia P&S

Beldner, Steven MD (HS) - **Spec Exp:** Elbow Surgery; **Hospital:** Beth Israel Med Ctr - Petrie Division (page 94), St Luke's - Roosevelt Hosp Ctr - St Luke's Hosp (page 94); **Address:** 321 E 34th St, New York, NY 10016; **Phone:** 212-340-0000; **Board Cert:** Orthopaedic Surgery 1999; Hand Surgery 2001; **Med School:** UMDNJ-NJ Med Sch, Newark 1991; **Resid:** Orthopaedic Surgery, Bellevue Hosp 1996; **Fellow:** Hand Surgery, NYU Med Ctr 1997; **Fac Appt:** Asst Prof OrS, Albert Einstein Coll Med

Botwinick, Nelson MD (HS) - **Spec Exp:** Trauma; Carpal Tunnel Syndrome; Arthritis Hand Surgery; **Hospital:** NY Downtown Hosp, NYU Hosp For Joint Diseases (page 106); **Address:** 19 Beekman St, New York, NY 10038-1522; **Phone:** 212-513-7711; **Board Cert:** Orthopaedic Surgery 2009; Hand Surgery 2009; **Med School:** NYU Sch Med 1980; **Resid:** Orthopaedic Surgery, NYU Med Ctr 1985; **Fellow:** Orthopaedic Surgery, NYU Med Ctr 1986; **Fac Appt:** Assoc Clin Prof OrS, NYU Sch Med

Carlson, Michelle Gerwin MD (HS) - **Spec Exp:** Sports Injuries; Hand & Upper Extremity Surgery; Pediatric Hand/Arm Surgery; Cerebral Palsy; **Hospital:** Hosp For Special Surgery (page 111), NY-Presby Hosp/Weill Cornell (page 104); **Address:** 523 E 72nd St Fl 4 - rm 439, New York, NY 10021; **Phone:** 212-606-1546; **Board Cert:** Orthopaedic Surgery 2007; Hand Surgery 2007; **Med School:** Cornell Univ-Weill Med Coll 1989; **Resid:** Surgery, Hosp Special Surg 1992; **Fellow:** Hand Surgery, Hosp Special Surg 1993; **Fac Appt:** Assoc Prof OrS, Cornell Univ-Weill Med Coll

Glickel, Steven Z MD (HS) - **Spec Exp:** Hand & Wrist Surgery; Elbow Surgery; Peripheral Nerve Surgery; **Hospital:** St Luke's - Roosevelt Hosp Ctr - Roosevelt Div (page 94); **Address:** 1000 10th Ave Fl 3, New York, NY 10019-1147; **Phone:** 212-523-7590; **Board Cert:** Orthopaedic Surgery 1985; Hand Surgery 2010; **Med School:** Harvard Med Sch 1976; **Resid:** Surgery, Columbia Presby Hosp 1978; Orthopaedic Surgery, Harvard Comb Ortho 1981; **Fellow:** Hand Surgery, St Luke's-Roosevelt Hosp Ctr 1983; Research, Columbia Presby Hosp 1982; **Fac Appt:** Assoc Clin Prof OrS, Columbia P&S

King, William MD (HS) - **Spec Exp:** Carpal Tunnel Syndrome; Hand Reconstruction; Microvascular Surgery; Fractures; **Hospital:** NYU Hosp For Joint Diseases (page 106), Lenox Hill Hosp; **Address:** 424 Madison Ave Fl 9, New York, NY 10017; **Phone:** 212-813-2104; **Board Cert:** Orthopaedic Surgery 2009; **Med School:** Columbia P&S 1974; **Resid:** Surgery, St Lukes-Roosevelt Hosp Ctr 1976; Orthopaedic Surgery, Columbia-Presby Med Ctr 1979; **Fellow:** Hand & Microvascular Surgery, Univ Colorado Hosp 1980; **Fac Appt:** Asst Prof OrS, NYU Sch Med

Lee, Steve K MD (HS) - **Spec Exp:** Carpal Tunnel Syndrome; Sports Injuries; Microsurgery; Tendon Surgery; **Hospital:** NYU Hosp For Joint Diseases (page 106), NYU Langone Med Ctr (page 106); **Address:** NYU Hosp for Joint Diseases, Fl 4 - Ste 400, 301 E 17th St, New York, NY 10003; **Phone:** 212-598-6697; **Board Cert:** Orthopaedic Surgery 2010; Hand Surgery 2010; **Med School:** Duke Univ 1993; **Resid:** Orthopaedic Surgery, Yale-New Haven Hosp 1998; **Fellow:** Hand Surgery, NYU Hosp for Joint Diseases 2003; **Fac Appt:** Asst Prof OrS, NYU Sch Med

Lenzo, Salvatore MD (HS) - **Spec Exp:** Carpal Tunnel Syndrome; Arthritis Hand Surgery; Hand & Wrist Injuries; Congenital Hand Deformities; **Hospital:** NYU Hosp For Joint Diseases (page 106), NYU Langone Med Ctr (page 106); **Address:** 955 5th Ave, New York, NY 10021; **Phone:** 212-734-9949; **Board Cert:** Orthopaedic Surgery 2009; Hand Surgery 2009; **Med School:** NYU Sch Med 1981; **Resid:** Orthopaedic Surgery, Bellevue Hosp 1986; **Fellow:** Hand Surgery, Bellevue Hosp 1987; **Fac Appt:** Assoc Prof OrS, NYU Sch Med

Melone Jr, Charles P MD (HS) - **Spec Exp:** Arthritis; Wrist Surgery; Fractures; **Hospital:** Beth Israel Med Ctr - Petrie Division (page 94); **Address:** 321 E 34th St, New York, NY 10016; **Phone:** 212-340-0000; **Board Cert:** Orthopaedic Surgery 1976; Hand Surgery 2004; **Med School:** Georgetown Univ 1969; **Resid:** Surgery, Nassau Co Med Ctr 1971; Orthopaedic Surgery, Nassau Co Med Ctr 1974; **Fellow:** Hand Surgery, NYU Langone Med Ctr 1975; **Fac Appt:** Clin Prof OrS, Albert Einstein Coll Med

Pruzansky, Mark E MD (HS) - **Spec Exp:** Arthritis Hand Surgery; Carpal Tunnel Syndrome; Sports Injuries; Wrist Surgery; **Hospital:** Mount Sinai Med Ctr (page 102), Lenox Hill Hosp; **Address:** 975 Park Ave, New York, NY 10028; **Phone:** 212-249-8700; **Board Cert:** Orthopaedic Surgery 1980; Hand Surgery 2003; Orthopaedic Sports Medicine 2007; **Med School:** Mount Sinai Sch Med 1974; **Resid:** Orthopaedic Surgery, Mount Sinai Med Ctr 1978; **Fellow:** Hand Surgery, South Baptist Hosp 1978; Hand Surgery, Pacific Presby Hosp 1979; **Fac Appt:** Asst Prof OrS, Mount Sinai Sch Med

Raskin, Keith B MD (HS) - **Spec Exp:** Wrist/Hand Injuries; Arthritis; Carpal Tunnel Syndrome; Elbow Surgery; **Hospital:** NYU Langone Med Ctr (page 106), NYU Hosp For Joint Diseases (page 106); **Address:** 317 E 34th St, Fl 3, New York, NY 10016; **Phone:** 212-263-4263; **Board Cert:** Orthopaedic Surgery 2002; Hand Surgery 2002; **Med School:** Geo Wash Univ 1983; **Resid:** Orthopaedic Surgery, NYU Med Ctr 1988; **Fellow:** Hand Surgery, Union Mem Hosp 1989; **Fac Appt:** Assoc Clin Prof OrS, NYU Sch Med

Rettig, Michael MD (HS) - **Spec Exp:** Fractures; Arthritis; Nerve Disorders/Surgery; **Hospital:** NYU Langone Med Ctr (page 106), NYU Hosp For Joint Diseases (page 106); **Address:** 317 E 34th St Fl 3, New York, NY 10016-4974; **Phone:** 212-263-4263; **Board Cert:** Orthopaedic Surgery 2005; Hand Surgery 2005; **Med School:** SUNY Upstate Med Univ 1986; **Resid:** Orthopaedic Surgery, NYU Med Ctr 1991; **Fellow:** Hand Surgery, Mayo Clinic 1992; **Fac Appt:** Asst Prof OrS, NYU Sch Med

Rosenwasser, Melvin P MD (HS) - **Spec Exp:** Carpal Tunnel Syndrome; Sports Injuries; Elbow Surgery; Trauma; **Hospital:** NY-Presby Hosp/Columbia (page 104); **Address:** 622 W 168th St, PH 11, New York, NY 10032; **Phone:** 212-305-8036; **Board Cert:** Orthopaedic Surgery 1999; Hand Surgery 1999; **Med School:** Columbia P&S 1976; **Resid:** Surgery, Roosevelt Hosp 1979; Orthopaedic Surgery, Columbia Presby Hosp 1982; **Fellow:** Hand Surgery, Columbia Presby Hosp 1983; **Fac Appt:** Prof OrS, Columbia P&S

Strauch, Robert MD (HS) - **Spec Exp:** Hand Reconstruction; Hand & Elbow Nerve Disorders; Hand & Wrist Surgery; Elbow Surgery; **Hospital:** NY-Presby Hosp/Columbia (page 104); **Address:** 622 W 168th St, rm PH-11, New York, NY 10032; **Phone:** 212-305-4272; **Board Cert:** Orthopaedic Surgery 2005; Hand Surgery 2005; **Med School:** Columbia P&S 1986; **Resid:** Orthopaedic Surgery, Columbia-Presby Hosp 1991; **Fellow:** Hand Surgery, Indiana Hand Center 1992; **Fac Appt:** Prof OrS, Columbia P&S

Weiland, Andrew J MD (HS) - **Spec Exp:** Wrist/Hand Injuries; Hand Reconstruction; **Hospital:** Hosp For Special Surgery (page 111), NY-Presby Hosp/Weill Cornell (page 104); **Address:** Hospital for Special Surgery, 535 E 70th St, New York, NY 10021-4872; **Phone:** 212-606-1575; **Board Cert:** Orthopaedic Surgery 1992; **Med School:** Wake Forest Univ 1968; **Resid:** Surgery, Univ Michigan Med Ctr 1970; Orthopaedic Surgery, Johns Hopkins Hosp 1975; **Fellow:** Hand Surgery, Kleinert Hosp 1975; **Fac Appt:** Prof OrS, Cornell Univ-Weill Med Coll

Wolfe, Scott W MD (HS) - **Spec Exp:** Wrist Surgery; Nerve Disorders/Surgery; Fractures; **Hospital:** Hosp For Special Surgery (page 111); **Address:** Hospital for Special Surgery, 523 E 72 St Fl 4, New York, NY 10021; **Phone:** 212-606-1529; **Board Cert:** Orthopaedic Surgery 2003; Hand Surgery 2003; **Med School:** Cornell Univ-Weill Med Coll 1984; **Resid:** Orthopaedic Surgery, Hosp Special Surg 1989; **Fellow:** Hand & Microvascular Surgery, Columbia Presby Med Ctr 1990; **Fac Appt:** Prof OrS, Cornell Univ-Weill Med Coll

Yang, S Steven MD (HS) - **Spec Exp:** Hand Surgery; Shoulder Surgery; Congenital Hand Deformities; **Hospital:** Lenox Hill Hosp, NYU Hosp For Joint Diseases (page 106); **Address:** 130 E 77th St Fl 7, New York, NY 10021; **Phone:** 212-744-8114; **Board Cert:** Orthopaedic Surgery 2009; Hand Surgery 2003; **Med School:** Duke Univ 1988; **Resid:** Orthopaedic Surgery, Lenox Hill Hosp 1994; **Fellow:** Hand Surgery, Hosp for Special Surgery 1995; **Fac Appt:** Asst Clin Prof OrS, NYU Sch Med

Hematology

Aledort, Louis M MD (Hem) - **Spec Exp:** Bleeding/Coagulation Disorders; Platelet Disorders; **Hospital:** Mount Sinai Med Ctr (page 102); **Address:** Mount Sinai Med Ctr, 1190 Fifth Ave, Box 1006, New York, NY 10029; **Phone:** 212-860-0205; **Board Cert:** Internal Medicine 1966; Hematology 1972; **Med School:** Albert Einstein Coll Med 1959; **Resid:** Internal Medicine, Univ Va Hlth Sci Ctr 1961; Hematology, Nat Inst Health 1963; **Fellow:** Internal Medicine, Strong Meml Hosp 1964; Hematology, Strong Meml Hosp 1966; **Fac Appt:** Prof Med, Mount Sinai Sch Med

Amorosi, Edward L MD (Hem) - **Hospital:** NYU Langone Med Ctr (page 106); **Address:** NYU Clinical Cancer Ctr, 160 E 34th St, New York, NY 10016; **Phone:** 212-731-5187; **Board Cert:** Internal Medicine 1966; Hematology 1972; Medical Oncology 1977; **Med School:** NYU Sch Med 1959; **Resid:** Internal Medicine, Bellevue Hosp Ctr- NYU 1962; Internal Medicine, Francis Delafield Hosp 1963; **Fellow:** Hematology, NYU Med Ctr 1965; **Fac Appt:** Prof Med, NYU Sch Med

Ansell, Jack Edward MD (Hem) - **Spec Exp:** Thrombotic Disorders; **Hospital:** Lenox Hill Hosp; **Address:** 100 E 77th St, New York, NY 10075; **Phone:** 212-434-2140; **Board Cert:** Internal Medicine 1975; Hematology 1976; **Med School:** Univ VA Sch Med 1972; **Resid:** Internal Medicine, Tufts- New England Med Ctr 1974; **Fellow:** Hematology, Boston Univ/Boston City Hosp 1975; Hematology, Boston VA Hosp 1977

Brower, Mark MD (Hem) - **Spec Exp:** Breast Cancer; Bleeding/Coagulation Disorders; Hematologic Malignancies; **Hospital:** NY-Presby Hosp/Weill Cornell (page 104); **Address:** 310 E 72nd St, New York, NY 10021-4703; **Phone:** 212-717-2995; **Board Cert:** Internal Medicine 1977; Hematology 1982; Medical Oncology 1979; **Med School:** Johns Hopkins Univ 1974; **Resid:** Internal Medicine, NY Hosp/Cornell Med Ctr 1977; **Fellow:** Hematology & Oncology, NY Hosp/Cornell Med Ctr 1980; **Fac Appt:** Clin Prof Med, Cornell Univ-Weill Med Coll

Castro-Malaspina, Hugo MD (Hem) - **Spec Exp:** Myelodysplastic Syndromes; Bone Marrow Failure Disorders; Bone Marrow Transplant; Anemia-Aplastic; **Hospital:** Meml Sloan-Kettering Cancer Ctr (page 112); **Address:** 1275 York Avenue, New York, NY 10065; **Phone:** 800-525-2225; **Med School:** Peru 1971; **Resid:** Internal Medicine, St Louis Hosp; **Fellow:** Hematology & Oncology, Andean Biology Inst; Pediatric Hematology-Oncology, St Louis Hosp

Coller, Barry MD (Hem) - **Spec Exp:** Glanzmann's Thrombasthenia; Bleeding/Coagulation Disorders; **Hospital:** Rockefeller Univ, Mount Sinai Med Ctr (page 102); **Address:** Rockefeller Univ, 1230 York Ave, New York, NY 10065; **Phone:** 212-327-7490; **Board Cert:** Internal Medicine 1973; Hematology 1975; **Med School:** NYU Sch Med 1970; **Resid:** Internal Medicine, Bellevue Hosp 1972; **Fellow:** Hematology, Natl Inst Hlth Clin Ctr 1974; **Fac Appt:** Clin Prof Med, Mount Sinai Sch Med

Cook, Perry MD (Hem) - **Spec Exp:** Bone Marrow Transplant; Leukemia; Lymphoma; **Hospital:** NYU Langone Med Ctr (page 106); **Address:** 160 E 34th St Fl 7, New York, NY 10016; **Phone:** 212-731-5184; **Board Cert:** Internal Medicine 1980; Hematology 1982; Medical Oncology 1983; **Med School:** Univ Iowa Coll Med 1977; **Resid:** Internal Medicine, St Luke's-Roosevelt Hosp Ctr 1979; Internal Medicine, Columbia-Presby Med Ctr 1980; **Fellow:** Hematology & Oncology, Columbia-Presby Med Ctr 1983; **Fac Appt:** Assoc Clin Prof Med, NYU Sch Med

Diaz, Michael MD (Hem) - **Spec Exp:** Anemia; Bleeding/Coagulation Disorders; Lymphoma; **Hospital:** Mount Sinai Med Ctr (page 102); **Address:** 1112 Park Ave, New York, NY 10128; **Phone:** 212-876-4500; **Board Cert:** Internal Medicine 1979; Hematology 1986; **Med School:** St Louis Univ 1971; **Resid:** Internal Medicine, Lenox Hill Hosp 1974; **Fellow:** Hematology, Elmhurst Hosp 1976; **Fac Appt:** Asst Clin Prof Med, Mount Sinai Sch Med

Diuguid, David L MD (Hem) - **Spec Exp:** Bleeding/Coagulation Disorders; **Hospital:** NY-Presby Hosp/Columbia (page 104); **Address:** 161 Ft Washington Ave, Irving 10, New York, NY 10032; **Phone:** 212-305-0527; **Board Cert:** Internal Medicine 1982; Hematology 1986; Medical Oncology 1985; **Med School:** Cornell Univ-Weill Med Coll 1979; **Resid:** Internal Medicine, Boston Univ Med Ctr 1983; **Fellow:** Hematology & Oncology, New England Med Ctr 1986; **Fac Appt:** Assoc Prof Med, Columbia P&S

Fruchtman, Steven M MD (Hem) - **Spec Exp:** Myeloproliferative Disorders; Polycythemia Rubra Vera; **Address:** 1111 Park Ave, New York, NY 10128; **Phone:** 212-427-7700; **Board Cert:** Internal Medicine 1980; Hematology 1984; **Med School:** NY Med Coll 1977; **Resid:** Internal Medicine, Univ Hosp 1981; **Fellow:** Hematology, Mount Sinai Med Ctr 1984; Hematology, Meml Sloan Kettering Cancer Ctr 1985; **Fac Appt:** Assoc Prof Med, NY Med Coll

Goldenberg, Alec MD (Hem) - **Spec Exp:** Breast Cancer; Lymphoma; Bleeding/Coagulation Disorders; **Hospital:** NYU Langone Med Ctr (page 106); **Address:** 157 E 32nd St Fl 2, New York, NY 10016; **Phone:** 212-689-6791; **Board Cert:** Internal Medicine 1986; Medical Oncology 1987; **Med School:** Johns Hopkins Univ 1980; **Resid:** Internal Medicine, Bellevue Hosp-NYU 1984; **Fellow:** Hematology & Oncology, Meml Sloan Kettering Canc Ctr 1988; **Fac Appt:** Assoc Clin Prof Med, NYU Sch Med

Gruenstein, Steven MD (Hem) - **Spec Exp:** Hematologic Malignancies; Breast Cancer; Gastrointestinal Cancer; Lung Cancer; **Hospital:** Mount Sinai Med Ctr (page 102), Lenox Hill Hosp; **Address:** 12 E 86th St, New York, NY 10028-0506; **Phone:** 212-861-6660; **Board Cert:** Internal Medicine 1988; Medical Oncology 2001; **Med School:** Italy 1984; **Resid:** Internal Medicine, Metropolitan Hosp Ctr 1987; **Fellow:** Hematology & Oncology, Beth Israel Med Ctr 1990; **Fac Appt:** Assoc Clin Prof Med, Mount Sinai Sch Med

Halperin, Ira MD (Hem) - **Spec Exp:** Leukemia; Myeloproliferative Disorders; **Hospital:** Beth Israel Med Ctr - Petrie Division (page 94); **Address:** 2 Fifth Ave, Ste 9, New York, NY 10011-8855; **Phone:** 212-254-5940; **Board Cert:** Internal Medicine 1970; Hematology 1976; Medical Oncology 1979; **Med School:** NYU Sch Med 1962; **Resid:** Internal Medicine, St Vincents Hosp 1966; **Fellow:** Hematology, Mt Sinai Hosp 1969

Hymes, Kenneth MD (Hem) - **Spec Exp:** Bleeding/Coagulation Disorders; Leukemia & Lymphoma; Cutaneous Lymphoma, T-cell; Mycosis Fungoides; **Hospital:** NYU Langone Med Ctr (page 106); **Address:** NYU Clinical Cancer Center, 160 E 34th St Fl 7, New York, NY 10016-6402; **Phone:** 212-731-5189; **Board Cert:** Internal Medicine 1978; Hematology 1980; Medical Oncology 1981; **Med School:** SUNY Upstate Med Univ 1975; **Resid:** Internal Medicine, Barnes Hosp 1978; **Fellow:** Hematology, NYU Med Ctr 1980; Medical Oncology, NYU Med Ctr 1981; **Fac Appt:** Assoc Prof Med, NYU Sch Med

Isola, Luis M MD (Hem) - **Spec Exp:** Bone Marrow Transplant; Stem Cell Transplant; Myelodysplastic Syndromes; Anemia; **Hospital:** Mount Sinai Med Ctr (page 102); **Address:** Mount Sinai Med Ctr, 19 E 98th St, Ste 3D, New York, NY 10029; **Phone:** 212-241-6021; **Board Cert:** Internal Medicine 1986; Hematology 1988; **Med School:** Argentina 1979; **Resid:** Internal Medicine, Ctr for Med Education 1983; **Fellow:** Hematology, Mt Sinai Med Ctr 1985; **Fac Appt:** Assoc Prof Med, Mount Sinai Sch Med

Kempin, Sanford J MD (Hem) - **Spec Exp:** Bleeding/Coagulation Disorders; Leukemia; Lymphoma; Thrombotic Disorders; **Hospital:** Beth Israel Med Ctr - Petrie Division (page 94), St Luke's - Roosevelt Hosp Ctr - Roosevelt Div (page 94); **Address:** St Vincents Cancer Ctr, 325 W 15th St, New York, NY 10011; **Phone:** 212-604-6010; **Board Cert:** Internal Medicine 1976; Medical Oncology 1977; Hematology 1978; **Med School:** Belgium 1971; **Resid:** Internal Medicine, Lemuel Shattuck Hosp 1972; **Fellow:** Hematology, St Jude Chldns Hosp 1975; Medical Oncology, Meml Sloan Kettering Cancer Ctr 1976; **Fac Appt:** Asst Prof Med, NY Med Coll

Leonard, John P MD (Hem) - **Spec Exp:** Lymphoma; Multiple Myeloma; Hematologic Malignancies; Leukemia; **Hospital:** NY-Presby Hosp/Weill Cornell (page 104); **Address:** NY Presby Hosp-NY Weill Cornell Med Ctr, 525 E 68th St, Payson 3, New York, NY 10065; **Phone:** 646-962-2068; **Board Cert:** Hematology 2006; Medical Oncology 2007; **Med School:** Univ VA Sch Med 1990; **Resid:** Internal Medicine, NY Hosp-Cornell Med Ctr 1993; **Fellow:** Hematology & Oncology, NY Hosp-Cornell Med Ctr 1996; **Fac Appt:** Prof Med, Cornell Univ-Weill Med Coll

Levine, Randy MD (Hem) - **Spec Exp:** Hematologic Malignancies; Bleeding/Coagulation Disorders; **Hospital:** Lenox Hill Hosp, St Luke's - Roosevelt Hosp Ctr - Roosevelt Div (page 94); **Address:** 4 E 76th St, New York, NY 10021-2611; **Phone:** 212-717-1020; **Board Cert:** Internal Medicine 1982; Hematology 1984; Blood Banking 1985; **Med School:** SUNY Buffalo 1979; **Resid:** Internal Medicine, Montefiore Hosp Med Ctr 1982; **Fellow:** Hematology, Montefiore Hosp Med Ctr 1983; Blood Banking, Mt Sinai Hosp 1984; **Fac Appt:** Assoc Clin Prof Med, NYU Sch Med

Mears, John Gregory MD (Hem) - **Spec Exp:** Lymphoma; Leukemia; Multiple Myeloma; Breast Cancer; **Hospital:** NY-Presby Hosp/Columbia (page 104); **Address:** 161 Ft Washington Ave, Ste 923, New York, NY 10032; **Phone:** 212-305-3506; **Board Cert:** Internal Medicine 1976; Hematology 1978; **Med School:** Columbia P&S 1973; **Resid:** Internal Medicine, Boston Univ Med Ctr 1975; **Fellow:** Hematology & Oncology, Columbia-Presby Med Ctr 1978; **Fac Appt:** Clin Prof Med, Columbia P&S

Meyer, Richard MD (Hem) - **Spec Exp:** Lymphoma; Leukemia; Multiple Myeloma; Head & Neck Cancer; **Hospital:** Mount Sinai Med Ctr (page 102); **Address:** 1111 Park Ave, New York, NY 10128-1234; **Phone:** 212-427-7700; **Board Cert:** Internal Medicine 1975; Hematology 1978; Medical Oncology 1979; **Med School:** Mount Sinai Sch Med 1972; **Resid:** Internal Medicine, Mt Sinai Hosp 1975; Hematology, Mt Sinai Hosp 1977; **Fellow:** Medical Oncology, Mt Sinai Hosp 1977; **Fac Appt:** Assoc Clin Prof Med, Mount Sinai Sch Med

Moskovits, Tibor MD (Hem) - **Spec Exp:** Lymphoma; Breast Cancer; Lung Cancer; **Hospital:** NYU Langone Med Ctr (page 106), NY Downtown Hosp; **Address:** NYU Clinical Cancer Center, 160 E 34th St Fl 7, New York, NY 10016; **Phone:** 212-731-5191; **Board Cert:** Internal Medicine 1988; Hematology 2003; Medical Oncology 2004; **Med School:** SUNY Downstate 1985; **Resid:** Internal Medicine, Beth Israel Med Ctr 1989; **Fellow:** Hematology & Oncology, NYU Med Ctr 1992; **Fac Appt:** Asst Clin Prof Med, NYU Sch Med

Nimer, Stephen D MD (Hem) - **Spec Exp:** Bone Marrow Transplant; Myelodysplastic Syndromes; Leukemia; Stem Cell Transplant; **Hospital:** Meml Sloan-Kettering Cancer Ctr (page 112); **Address:** 1275 York Avenue, New York, NY 10065; **Phone:** 800-525-2225; **Board Cert:** Internal Medicine 1982; Hematology 1986; Medical Oncology 1985; **Med School:** Univ Chicago-Pritzker Sch Med 1979; **Resid:** Internal Medicine, UCLA Med Ctr 1982; **Fellow:** Hematology & Oncology, UCLA Med Ctr 1986; **Fac Appt:** Prof Med, Cornell Univ-Weill Med Coll

Ossias, A Lawrence MD (Hem) - **Spec Exp:** Lymphoma; Leukemia; Coagulation/Bleeding Disorders; **Hospital:** Mount Sinai Med Ctr (page 102); **Address:** 1112 Park Ave, New York, NY 10128; **Phone:** 212-427-9333; **Board Cert:** Internal Medicine 1972; Hematology 1977; Medical Oncology 1979; **Med School:** Yale Univ 1965; **Resid:** Internal Medicine, Montefiore Med Ctr 1970; **Fellow:** Hematology & Oncology, Mt Sinai Med Ctr 1972; **Fac Appt:** Asst Clin Prof Med, Mount Sinai Sch Med

Raphael, Bruce MD (Hem) - **Spec Exp:** Lymphoma; Leukemia; Multiple Myeloma; **Hospital:** NYU Langone Med Ctr (page 106), NY Downtown Hosp; **Address:** 160 E 34th Street Ave Fl 7, NYU Clinical Cancer Ctr, New York, NY 10016-6402; **Phone:** 212-731-5185; **Board Cert:** Internal Medicine 1978; Hematology 1980; Medical Oncology 1981; **Med School:** McGill Univ 1975; **Resid:** Internal Medicine, Jewish Genl Hosp 1977; **Fellow:** Medical Oncology, Meml Sloan Kettering Cancer Ctr 1978; Hematology, NYU Med Ctr 1980; **Fac Appt:** Assoc Prof Med, NYU Sch Med

Savage, David G MD (Hem) - **Spec Exp:** Stem Cell Transplant; Multiple Myeloma; Lymphoma; **Hospital:** NY-Presby Hosp/Columbia (page 104); **Address:** 177 Fort Washington Ave, Millstein Bldg Fl 6 - rm 435, New York, NY 10032; **Phone:** 212-305-9783; **Board Cert:** Internal Medicine 1977; Hematology 1982; Medical Oncology 1985; **Med School:** Columbia P&S 1974; **Resid:** Internal Medicine, Harlem Hosp/Columbia Presby Med Ctr 1977; **Fellow:** Hematology & Oncology, Harlem Hosp/Columbia Presby Med Ctr 1979; **Fac Appt:** Assoc Prof Med, Columbia P&S

Scigliano, Eileen MD (Hem) - **Spec Exp:** Bone Marrow Transplant; **Hospital:** Mount Sinai Med Ctr (page 102); **Address:** 19 E 98th St, Box 1410, New York, NY 10029; **Phone:** 212-241-6021; **Board Cert:** Internal Medicine 1984; Hematology 1988; **Med School:** Israel 1981; **Resid:** Internal Medicine, Kings County Hosp 1984; **Fellow:** Medical Oncology, VA Med Ctr 1985; Hematology, Mount Sinai Hosp 1988; **Fac Appt:** Asst Clin Prof Med, Mount Sinai Sch Med

Tallman, Martin S MD (Hem) - **Spec Exp:** Bone Marrow Transplant; Leukemia; Hairy Cell Leukemia; **Hospital:** Meml Sloan-Kettering Cancer Ctr (page 112); **Address:** 1275 York Ave, Box 380, Ste 21-100, New York, NY 10065; **Phone:** 212-639-3842; **Board Cert:** Internal Medicine 1983; Medical Oncology 1987; Hematology 1988; **Med School:** Ros Franklin Univ/Chicago Med Sch 1980; **Resid:** Internal Medicine, Evanston Hosp 1983; **Fellow:** Medical Oncology, Fred Hutchinson Cancer Ctr 1987; **Fac Appt:** Prof Med, Cornell Univ-Weill Med Coll

Troy, Kevin M MD (Hem) - **Spec Exp:** Leukemia; Lymphoma; Multiple Myeloma; **Hospital:** Mount Sinai Med Ctr (page 102); **Address:** 1735 York Ave, Ste P2, New York, NY 10128; **Phone:** 212-860-9055; **Board Cert:** Internal Medicine 1982; Hematology 1984; **Med School:** Univ Conn 1979; **Resid:** Internal Medicine, Lenox Hill Hosp 1982; **Fellow:** Hematology, Mount Sinai Hosp 1984; **Fac Appt:** Assoc Clin Prof Med, Mount Sinai Sch Med

Vogel, James M MD (Hem) - **Spec Exp:** Breast Cancer; Colon Cancer; Leukemia & Lymphoma; Platelet Disorders; **Hospital:** Mount Sinai Med Ctr (page 102), Mount Sinai Hosp of Queens (page 102); **Address:** 1125 Park Ave, New York, NY 10128-1243; **Phone:** 212-369-4250; **Board Cert:** Internal Medicine 1969; Hematology 1972; Medical Oncology 1973; **Med School:** Columbia P&S 1962; **Resid:** Internal Medicine, Mount Sinai Hosp 1964; Internal Medicine, Mount Sinai Hosp 1967; **Fellow:** Medical Oncology, Natl Cancer Inst 1966; Hematology, Mount Sinai Hosp 1968; **Fac Appt:** Assoc Prof Med, Mount Sinai Sch Med

Wisch, Nathaniel MD (Hem) - **Spec Exp:** Lymphoma; Breast Cancer; Leukemia; Anemia-Cancer Related; **Hospital:** Lenox Hill Hosp, Mount Sinai Med Ctr (page 102); **Address:** 12 E 86th St, New York, NY 10028-0506; **Phone:** 212-861-6660; **Board Cert:** Internal Medicine 1965; Hematology 1972; Medical Oncology 1977; **Med School:** Northwestern Univ 1958; **Resid:** Internal Medicine, VA Hosp 1960; Internal Medicine, Montefiore Hosp 1961; **Fellow:** Hematology, Mount Sinai Hosp 1962; **Fac Appt:** Clin Prof Med, Mount Sinai Sch Med

Wolf, David J MD (Hem) - **Spec Exp:** Hematologic Malignancies; Hematology-Benign; Solid Tumors; **Hospital:** NY-Presby Hosp/Weill Cornell (page 104); **Address:** 115 E 61st St Fl 11, New York, NY 10021; **Phone:** 212-688-7100; **Board Cert:** Internal Medicine 1976; Hematology 1978; Medical Oncology 1979; **Med School:** SUNY Hlth Sci Ctr 1973; **Resid:** Internal Medicine, NY Hosp/Meml Hosp 1976; **Fellow:** Hematology, NY Hosp 1976; **Fac Appt:** Asst Clin Prof Med, Cornell Univ-Weill Med Coll

Infectious Disease

Aberg, Judith MD (Inf) - **Spec Exp:** AIDS/HIV; **Hospital:** Bellevue Hosp Ctr; **Address:** Bellevue C&D Bldg, 5, rm 558, 550 First Ave, New York, NY 10016; **Phone:** 212-263-6565; **Board Cert:** Infectious Disease 2006; **Med School:** Penn State Univ-Hershey Med Ctr 1990; **Resid:** Internal Medicine, Cleveland Clinic Fdn 1994; **Fellow:** Infectious Disease, Washington Univ Sch Med 1996; **Fac Appt:** Assoc Prof Med, NYU Sch Med

Badshah, Cyrus S MD/PhD (Inf) - **Spec Exp:** Tuberculosis; AIDS/HIV; **Hospital:** Harlem Hosp Ctr, Montefiore Med Ctr - Div. Moses (page 100); **Address:** Harlem Hospital, MLK Bldg, 506 Lenox Ave, rm 3101A, New York, NY 10037; **Phone:** 212-939-2310; **Board Cert:** Internal Medicine 2009; Infectious Disease 2001; **Med School:** India 1986; **Resid:** Internal Medicine, Montefiore-Weiler Einstein Med Ctr 1999; **Fellow:** Infectious Disease, Cornell Univ/Meml Sloan-Kettering Cancer Ctr 2001

Brause, Barry MD (Inf) - **Spec Exp:** Bone/Joint Infections; Skin/Soft Tissue Infections; Infections in Prosthetic Devices; **Hospital:** Hosp For Special Surgery (page 111), NY-Presby Hosp/Weill Cornell (page 104); **Address:** 535 E 70th St, New York, NY 10021-5718; **Phone:** 212-774-7411; **Board Cert:** Internal Medicine 1973; Infectious Disease 1976; **Med School:** Univ Pittsburgh 1970; **Resid:** Internal Medicine, NY Hosp 1973; **Fellow:** Infectious Disease, NY Hosp 1975; **Fac Appt:** Clin Prof Med, Cornell Univ-Weill Med Coll

Brown, Arthur E MD (Inf) - **Spec Exp:** Infections in Cancer Patients; Fungal Infections; Infections in Immunocompromised Patients; **Hospital:** Meml Sloan-Kettering Cancer Ctr (page 112); **Address:** 1275 York Avenue, New York, NY 10065; **Phone:** 212-639-8475; **Med School:** Jefferson Med Coll 1971; **Resid:** Internal Medicine, Roosevelt Hosp 1972; Internal Medicine, USPHS Hosp-Staten Island NY & USPHS Hosp 1974; **Fellow:** Internal Medicine, Roosevelt Hosp 1976; Infectious Disease, Mem Sloan Kettering Cancer Ctr 1978; **Fac Appt:** Clin Prof Med, Cornell Univ-Weill Med Coll

Busillo, Christopher MD (Inf) - **Spec Exp:** AIDS/HIV; Travel Medicine; Lyme Disease; **Hospital:** NY Downtown Hosp; **Address:** 19 Beekman St Fl 6th, New York, NY 10038-2668; **Phone:** 212-374-2145; **Board Cert:** Internal Medicine 2000; Infectious Disease 2000; **Med School:** Italy 1986; **Resid:** Internal Medicine, Cabrini Med Ctr 1989; **Fellow:** Infectious Disease, Cabrini Med Ctr 1991

El-Sadr, Wafaa M MD (Inf) - **Spec Exp:** AIDS/HIV; Tuberculosis; **Hospital:** Harlem Hosp Ctr; **Address:** Harlem Hospital, 506 Lenox Ave MLK Bldg - rm 310A, New York, NY 10037; **Phone:** 212-939-2936; **Board Cert:** Internal Medicine 1979; Infectious Disease 1982; **Med School:** Egypt 1974; **Resid:** Internal Medicine, Columbia-Presby Med Ctr 1982; **Fellow:** Infectious Disease, VA Medical Ctr 1983

Flood, Mary T MD/PhD (Inf) - **Spec Exp:** Infectious Disease; HIV; Hepatitis; Herpes Simplex; **Hospital:** NY-Presby Hosp/Columbia (page 104); **Address:** 161 Fort Washington Ave, rm 215, New York, NY 10032-3702; **Phone:** 212-305-8039; **Board Cert:** Internal Medicine 2002; Infectious Disease 2004; **Med School:** Columbia P&S 1987; **Resid:** Internal Medicine, NY-Presby Hosp 1991; **Fellow:** Infectious Disease, NY-Presby Hosp 1993; **Fac Appt:** Assoc Clin Prof Med, Columbia P&S

Greene, Jeffrey MD (Inf) - **Spec Exp:** AIDS/HIV; **Hospital:** NYU Langone Med Ctr (page 106); **Address:** 104 E 40th St, Ste 603, New York, NY 10016; **Phone:** 212-375-2940; **Board Cert:** Internal Medicine 1979; Infectious Disease 1982; **Med School:** NYU Sch Med 1976; **Resid:** Internal Medicine, Bellevue Hosp 1980; **Fellow:** Infectious Disease, Bellevue Hosp 1982; **Fac Appt:** Assoc Clin Prof Med, NYU Sch Med

Gumprecht, Jeffrey P MD (Inf) - **Spec Exp:** AIDS/HIV; Travel Medicine; Infections-Surgical; **Hospital:** Mount Sinai Med Ctr (page 102); **Address:** 1100 Park Ave, New York, NY 10128; **Phone:** 212-427-9550; **Board Cert:** Internal Medicine 1987; Infectious Disease 2003; **Med School:** Albany Med Coll 1983; **Resid:** Internal Medicine, Mt Sinai Hosp 1987; **Fellow:** Infectious Disease, Montefiore Med Ctr 1990; **Fac Appt:** Asst Clin Prof Med, Mount Sinai Sch Med

Hammer, Glenn MD (Inf) - **Spec Exp:** AIDS/HIV; Hospital Acquired Infections; Infections-Surgical; **Hospital:** Mount Sinai Med Ctr (page 102); **Address:** 1100 Park Ave, New York, NY 10128-1202; **Phone:** 212-427-9550; **Board Cert:** Infectious Disease 1974; Internal Medicine 1973; **Med School:** NYU Sch Med 1969; **Resid:** Internal Medicine, Mount Sinai Hosp 1972; **Fellow:** Infectious Disease, Mount Sinai Hosp 1974; **Fac Appt:** Asst Clin Prof Med, Mount Sinai Sch Med

Hammer, Scott M MD (Inf) - **Spec Exp:** AIDS/HIV; **Hospital:** NY-Presby Hosp/Columbia (page 104); **Address:** 630 W 168th St, P&S Box 82, New York, NY 10032; **Phone:** 212-305-8039; **Board Cert:** Internal Medicine 1975; Infectious Disease 1980; **Med School:** Columbia P&S 1972; **Resid:** Internal Medicine, Columbia-Presby Hosp 1975; Internal Medicine, Stanford Univ Hosp 1975; **Fellow:** Infectious Disease, Mass Genl Hosp 1981; **Fac Appt:** Prof Med, Columbia P&S

Hartman, Barry Jay MD (Inf) - **Spec Exp:** Endocarditis; Infections-Surgical; Parasitic Infections; **Hospital:** NY-Presby Hosp/Weill Cornell (page 104); **Address:** 407 E 70th St, Fl 4, New York, NY 10021-5302; **Phone:** 212-744-4882; **Board Cert:** Internal Medicine 1976; Infectious Disease 1980; **Med School:** Penn State Univ-Hershey Med Ctr 1973; **Resid:** Internal Medicine, NY Hosp/Cornell Med Ctr 1976; **Fellow:** Infectious Disease, NY Hosp/Cornell Med Ctr 1981; **Fac Appt:** Clin Prof Med, Cornell Univ-Weill Med Coll

Helfgott, David MD (Inf) - **Spec Exp:** Infections in Immunocompromised Patients; Travel Medicine; Skin/Soft Tissue Infections; **Hospital:** NY-Presby Hosp/Weill Cornell (page 104); **Address:** 212 E 68th St, New York, NY 10065; **Phone:** 212-879-6004; **Board Cert:** Internal Medicine 1986; Infectious Disease 1988; **Med School:** Yale Univ 1983; **Resid:** Internal Medicine, NY Hosp/Cornell Med Ctr 1986; Internal Medicine, NY Hosp 1990; **Fellow:** Infectious Disease, NY Hosp/Cornell Med Ctr 1989; **Fac Appt:** Asst Clin Prof Med, Cornell Univ-Weill Med Coll

Horowitz, Harold MD (Inf) - **Spec Exp:** AIDS/HIV; Tick-borne Diseases; Travel Medicine; **Hospital:** NYU Langone Med Ctr (page 106); **Address:** NYU School Medicine, 550 First Ave, NBV 16 S 5, New York, NY 10016; **Phone:** 212-263-2115; **Board Cert:** Internal Medicine 1983; Infectious Disease 1988; **Med School:** NYU Sch Med 1979; **Resid:** Internal Medicine, Univ Wisconsin Hosp 1983; **Fellow:** Infectious Disease, New England Med Ctr 1986; **Fac Appt:** Prof Med, NYU Sch Med

Huprikar, Shirish S MD (Inf) - **Spec Exp:** Infections in Transplant Patients; Infections in Immunocompromised Patients; Infections in Transplant Patients w/HIV; **Hospital:** Mount Sinai Med Ctr (page 102); **Address:** Mt Sinai Med Ctr, One Gustave L Levy Pl, Box 1090, New York, NY 10029; **Phone:** 212-241-7968; **Board Cert:** Internal Medicine 2010; Infectious Disease 2001; **Med School:** Northwestern Univ 1996; **Resid:** Internal Medicine, Mt Sinai Med Ctr 1999; **Fellow:** Infectious Disease, Mt Sinai Med Ctr 2001; **Fac Appt:** Assoc Prof Med, Mount Sinai Sch Med

Jacobs, Jonathan MD (Inf) - **Spec Exp:** AIDS/HIV; **Hospital:** NY-Presby Hosp/Weill Cornell (page 104); **Address:** 449 E 68th St, Ground Fl, New York, NY 10065; **Phone:** 212-734-1365; **Board Cert:** Internal Medicine 1983; Infectious Disease 1986; **Med School:** Yale Univ 1980; **Resid:** Internal Medicine, NY Hosp/Cornell Med Ctr 1983; **Fellow:** Infectious Disease, NY Hosp/Cornell Med Ctr 1986; **Fac Appt:** Clin Prof Med, Cornell Univ-Weill Med Coll

Lerner, Chester MD (Inf) - **Spec Exp:** AIDS/HIV; Travel Medicine; Sexually Transmitted Diseases; **Hospital:** NY Downtown Hosp; **Address:** 170 William St Fl 7, New York, NY 10038-2612; **Phone:** 212-238-0106; **Board Cert:** Internal Medicine 1981; Infectious Disease 1984; **Med School:** Univ Pittsburgh 1978; **Resid:** Internal Medicine, Lenox Hill Hosp 1981; **Fellow:** Infectious Disease, Lenox Hill Hosp 1983; **Fac Appt:** Asst Clin Prof Med, NYU Sch Med

Louie, Eddie MD (Inf) - **Spec Exp:** Lyme Disease; AIDS/HIV; Hospital Acquired Infections; **Hospital:** NYU Langone Med Ctr (page 106); **Address:** 345 E 37th St, Ste 207, New York, NY 10016-3256; **Phone:** 212-682-9202; **Board Cert:** Internal Medicine 1982; Infectious Disease 1986; **Med School:** NYU Sch Med 1979; **Resid:** Internal Medicine, Kings County Hosp 1983; **Fellow:** Infectious Disease, NYU Med Ctr 1985; **Fac Appt:** Assoc Clin Prof Med, NYU Sch Med

McMeeking, Alexander MD (Inf) - **Spec Exp:** AIDS/HIV; Hepatitis B & C; Herpes Simplex; Antibiotic Resistance; **Hospital:** NYU Langone Med Ctr (page 106); **Address:** 104 E 40th St, Ste 507, New York, NY 10016; **Phone:** 212-375-2560; **Board Cert:** Internal Medicine 1985; Infectious Disease 1988; **Med School:** UMDNJ-NJ Med Sch, Newark 1982; **Resid:** Internal Medicine, St Luke's-Roosevelt Hosp 1985; **Fellow:** Infectious Disease, Bellvue/NYU Med Ctr 1986

Mildvan, Donna MD (Inf) - **Spec Exp:** AIDS/HIV; Clinical Trials; Infectious Disease; **Hospital:** Beth Israel Med Ctr - Petrie Division (page 94); **Address:** Beth Israel Med Ctr, Div Infectious Dis, 1st Ave at 16th St, 19BH17, New York, NY 10003; **Phone:** 212-420-4005; **Board Cert:** Internal Medicine 1972; Infectious Disease 1972; **Med School:** Johns Hopkins Univ 1967; **Resid:** Internal Medicine, Mt Sinai Hosp 1970; **Fellow:** Infectious Disease, Mt Sinai Hosp 1972; **Fac Appt:** Prof Med, Albert Einstein Coll Med

Miller, Dennis K MD (Inf) - **Spec Exp:** Lyme Disease; AIDS/HIV; Travel Medicine; **Hospital:** Lenox Hill Hosp; **Address:** 4 E 76th St, New York, NY 10021-1811; **Phone:** 212-472-1237; **Board Cert:** Internal Medicine 1985; Infectious Disease 1988; **Med School:** Rush Med Coll 1982; **Resid:** Internal Medicine, Lenox Hill Hosp 1985; **Fellow:** Infectious Disease, Lenox Hill Hosp 1987

Mullen, Michael P MD (Inf) - **Spec Exp:** Osteomyelitis; AIDS/HIV; **Hospital:** Mount Sinai Med Ctr (page 102); **Address:** Mount Sinai Faculty Practice Assocs, 5 E 98th St Fl 8, New York, NY 10029; **Phone:** 212-241-3150; **Board Cert:** Internal Medicine 1985; Infectious Disease 1986; **Med School:** Spain 1981; **Resid:** Internal Medicine, Jewish Hosp Med Ctr 1984; **Fellow:** Infectious Disease, Cabrini Med Ctr 1986; **Fac Appt:** Assoc Clin Prof Med, Mount Sinai Sch Med

Murray, Henry W MD (Inf) - **Spec Exp:** Parasitic Infections; Travel Medicine; **Hospital:** NY-Presby Hosp/Weill Cornell (page 104); **Address:** NY Presby-Cornell Med Ctr, 525 E 68th St, Box 136, New York, NY 10065; **Phone:** 212-746-6330; **Board Cert:** Internal Medicine 1975; Infectious Disease 1978; **Med School:** Cornell Univ-Weill Med Coll 1972; **Resid:** Internal Medicine, New York Hosp 1974; Internal Medicine, Johns Hopkins Hosp 1975; **Fellow:** Infectious Disease, New York Hosp 1977; **Fac Appt:** Prof Med, Cornell Univ-Weill Med Coll

Neibart, Eric MD (Inf) - **Spec Exp:** Travel Medicine; AIDS/HIV; Fungal Infections; **Hospital:** Mount Sinai Med Ctr (page 102); **Address:** 1100 Park Ave, New York, NY 10128-1202; **Phone:** 212-427-9550; **Board Cert:** Internal Medicine 1983; Infectious Disease 1986; **Med School:** UMDNJ-NJ Med Sch, Newark 1980; **Resid:** Internal Medicine, Mt Sinai Med Ctr 1983; **Fellow:** Infectious Disease, Mt Sinai Med Ctr 1986; **Fac Appt:** Asst Prof Med, Mount Sinai Sch Med

Perlman, David MD (Inf) - **Spec Exp:** AIDS/HIV; Lyme Disease; Travel Medicine; Infectious Disease; **Hospital:** Beth Israel Med Ctr - Petrie Division (page 94), Lenox Hill Hosp; **Address:** Beth Israel Med Ctr, 1st Ave at 16th St, New York, NY 10003; **Phone:** 212-844-8549; **Board Cert:** Internal Medicine 1986; Infectious Disease 1988; **Med School:** Albert Einstein Coll Med 1983; **Resid:** Internal Medicine, New York Hosp/Meml Sloan Kettering 1986; **Fellow:** Infectious Disease, Montefiore Hosp 1988; **Fac Appt:** Prof Med, Albert Einstein Coll Med

Pollock, Alan MD (Inf) - **Hospital:** Lenox Hill Hosp; **Address:** 184 E 70th St, Level B1, New York, NY 10021-5110; **Phone:** 212-988-2702; **Board Cert:** Internal Medicine 1975; Infectious Disease 1978; **Med School:** NY Med Coll 1972; **Resid:** Internal Medicine, Lenox Hill Hosp 1975; **Fellow:** Infectious Disease, Manhattan VA Hosp 1977; **Fac Appt:** Asst Clin Prof Med, NYU Sch Med

Polsky, Bruce W MD (Inf) - **Spec Exp:** AIDS/HIV; Viral Infections; Infections in Cancer Patients; AIDS Related Cancers; **Hospital:** St Luke's - Roosevelt Hosp Ctr - Roosevelt Div (page 94); **Address:** 1111 Amsterdam Ave, New York, NY 10025; **Phone:** 212-523-2525; **Board Cert:** Internal Medicine 1983; Infectious Disease 1986; **Med School:** Wayne State Univ 1980; **Resid:** Internal Medicine, Montefiore Hosp 1983; **Fellow:** Infectious Disease, Meml Sloan Kettering Cancer Ctr 1986; **Fac Appt:** Prof Med, Columbia P&S

Press, Robert A MD (Inf) - **Spec Exp:** Infections-Surgical; Hospital Acquired Infections; **Hospital:** NYU Langone Med Ctr (page 106); **Address:** 530 1st Ave, Ste 4G, New York, NY 10016-6402; **Phone:** 212-263-7229; **Board Cert:** Internal Medicine 1976; Infectious Disease 1999; **Med School:** NYU Sch Med 1973; **Resid:** Internal Medicine, Beth Israel Hosp 1975; Internal Medicine, Bellevue Hosp 1976; **Fellow:** Infectious Disease, Montefiore Hosp Med Ctr 1978; **Fac Appt:** Assoc Clin Prof Med, NYU Sch Med

Romagnoli, Mario MD (Inf) - **Spec Exp:** AIDS/HIV; Bone/Joint Infections; **Hospital:** Lenox Hill Hosp; **Address:** 903 Park Ave, New York, NY 10021; **Phone:** 212-396-3390; **Board Cert:** Internal Medicine 1979; Infectious Disease 1982; **Med School:** Columbia P&S 1976; **Resid:** Internal Medicine, Columbia-Presby Med Ctr 1979; **Fellow:** Infectious Disease, Beth Israel Med Ctr 1981; **Fac Appt:** Assoc Prof Med, Columbia P&S

Scully, Brian MD (Inf) - **Spec Exp:** Lyme Disease; **Hospital:** NY-Presby Hosp/Columbia (page 104); **Address:** 161 Fort Washington Ave, rm 215, New York, NY 10032; **Phone:** 212-305-8039; **Board Cert:** Internal Medicine 1975; Infectious Disease 1982; **Med School:** Ireland 1971; **Resid:** Internal Medicine, St Luke's-Roosevelt Hosp Ctr 1975; **Fellow:** Infectious Disease, Columbia Presby Med Ctr 1982

Sepkowitz, Kent MD (Inf) - **Spec Exp:** Tuberculosis; Infections in Cancer Patients; Fungal Infections; **Hospital:** Meml Sloan-Kettering Cancer Ctr (page 112); **Address:** 1275 York Avenue, New York, NY 10065; **Phone:** 800-525-2225; **Board Cert:** Internal Medicine 1983; Infectious Disease 2000; **Med School:** Univ Okla Coll Med 1980; **Resid:** Internal Medicine, Roosevelt Hosp 1984; **Fellow:** Infectious Disease, Meml Sloan Kettering Cancer Ctr 1991; **Fac Appt:** Prof Med, Cornell Univ-Weill Med Coll

Simberkoff, Michael S MD (Inf) - **Spec Exp:** AIDS/HIV; Pneumonia; **Hospital:** VA Med Ctr - Manhattan, NYU Langone Med Ctr (page 106); **Address:** 423 E 23rd St, 3 West Executive Office, New York, NY 10010; **Phone:** 212-951-3417; **Board Cert:** Internal Medicine 1980; Infectious Disease 1972; **Med School:** NYU Sch Med 1962; **Resid:** Internal Medicine, Bellevue Hosp 1967; **Fellow:** Infectious Disease, NYU Med Ctr 1969; **Fac Appt:** Assoc Prof Med, NYU Sch Med

Smith, Paul T MD (Inf) - **Spec Exp:** AIDS/HIV; Skin/Soft Tissue Infections; **Hospital:** NY-Presby Hosp/Weill Cornell (page 104), Hosp For Special Surgery (page 111); **Address:** 943 Lexington Ave, New York, NY 10021; **Phone:** 212-396-4077; **Board Cert:** Internal Medicine 2005; Infectious Disease 2007; **Med School:** Hahnemann Univ 1992; **Resid:** Internal Medicine, NY Hosp-Cornell Med Ctr 1995; **Fellow:** Infectious Disease, Yale-New Haven Hosp 1997; **Fac Appt:** Asst Clin Prof Med, Cornell Univ-Weill Med Coll

Wallach, Frances MD (Inf) - **Spec Exp:** AIDS/HIV; Infection Control; HIV & Blood Transfusions; **Hospital:** Mount Sinai Med Ctr (page 102); **Address:** Mount Sinai Medical Ctr, One Gustave L Levy Pl, Box 1090, New York, NY 10029; **Phone:** 212-241-7968; **Board Cert:** Internal Medicine 1989; Infectious Disease 2002; **Med School:** Albany Med Coll 1985; **Resid:** Internal Medicine, Montefiore Med Ctr 1989; **Fellow:** Nuclear Medicine, Montefiore Med Ctr 1990; Infectious Disease, NY Hosp-Cornell Med Ctr 1992; **Fac Appt:** Asst Prof Med, Mount Sinai Sch Med

Wetherbee, Roger MD (Inf) - **Spec Exp:** Infections-Transplant; AIDS/HIV; Staphylococcal Infections; Travel Medicine; **Hospital:** NYU Langone Med Ctr (page 106); **Address:** 530 1st Ave, Ste 4C, New York, NY 10016; **Phone:** 212-263-7243; **Board Cert:** Internal Medicine 1974; **Med School:** NYU Sch Med 1969; **Resid:** Internal Medicine, Bellevue Hosp 1974; Internal Medicine, VA Hosp 1974; **Fellow:** Infectious Disease, Natl Inst Hlth 1972; Infectious Disease, VA Hosp 1975; **Fac Appt:** Assoc Clin Prof Med, NYU Sch Med

Yancovitz, Stanley MD (Inf) - **Spec Exp:** Lyme Disease; AIDS/HIV; **Hospital:** Beth Israel Med Ctr - Petrie Division (page 94); **Address:** 1st Ave at 16th St, Ste 17 BH10, New York, NY 10003; **Phone:** 212-420-2600; **Board Cert:** Internal Medicine 1973; Infectious Disease 1976; **Med School:** SUNY Downstate 1967; **Resid:** Internal Medicine, Metropolitan Hosp 1969; Internal Medicine, Beth Israel Med Ctr 1972; **Fellow:** Infectious Disease, Mt Sinai Hosp 1975; **Fac Appt:** Clin Prof Med, Albert Einstein Coll Med

Internal Medicine

Adler, Mitchell MD (IM) *PCP* - **Spec Exp:** Sports Medicine; Geriatric Rehabilitation; **Hospital:** NYU Langone Med Ctr (page 106); **Address:** 317 E 34th St Fl 10, New York, NY 10016; **Phone:** 212-726-7499; **Board Cert:** Internal Medicine 1983; **Med School:** NYU Sch Med 1980; **Resid:** Internal Medicine, Bellevue Hosp 1984; **Fac Appt:** Asst Clin Prof Med, NYU Sch Med

Aronne, Louis J MD (IM) - **Spec Exp:** Obesity; Diabetes; Weight Management; **Hospital:** NY-Presby Hosp/Weill Cornell (page 104); **Address:** 1165 York Ave, New York, NY 10065; **Phone:** 212-583-1000; **Board Cert:** Internal Medicine 1984; **Med School:** Johns Hopkins Univ 1981; **Resid:** Internal Medicine, Bronx Muni Hosp 1984; **Fellow:** Internal Medicine, New York Hosp 1986; **Fac Appt:** Assoc Clin Prof Med, Cornell Univ-Weill Med Coll

Ascheim, Robert S MD (IM) - **Spec Exp:** Coronary Artery Disease; Congestive Heart Failure; **Hospital:** NY-Presby Hosp/Weill Cornell (page 104); **Address:** 10 Rockefeller Plaza Fl 4, New York, NY 10020; **Phone:** 212-332-3774; **Board Cert:** Internal Medicine 1969; **Med School:** Tufts Univ 1962; **Resid:** Internal Medicine, Bellevue Hosp 1968; Cardiovascular Disease, Mem Sloan-Kettering Med Ctr 1967; **Fellow:** Cardiovascular Disease, New York Hosp 1970; **Fac Appt:** Assoc Prof Med, Cornell Univ-Weill Med Coll

Babitz, Lisa E MD (IM) *PCP* - **Spec Exp:** Geriatric Medicine; **Hospital:** St Luke's - Roosevelt Hosp Ctr - Roosevelt Div (page 94); **Address:** 457 W 57th St, New York, NY 10019; **Phone:** 212-265-1471; **Board Cert:** Internal Medicine 1984; Geriatric Medicine 1998; **Med School:** Yale Univ 1981; **Resid:** Internal Medicine, Yale-New Haven Hosp 1984; **Fellow:** Geriatric Medicine, NYU Med Ctr 1986; **Fac Appt:** Assoc Clin Prof Med, Columbia P&S

Barley, Christopher L MD (IM) - **Hospital:** NY-Presby Hosp/Weill Cornell (page 104); **Address:** 30 Central Park S, New York, NY 10019; **Phone:** 212-758-3590; **Board Cert:** Internal Medicine 2006; **Med School:** Geo Wash Univ 1993; **Resid:** Internal Medicine, NY Hosp Cornell Med Ctr 1996; **Fac Appt:** Asst Clin Prof Med, Cornell Univ-Weill Med Coll

Baskin, David H MD (IM) *PCP* - **Spec Exp:** Preventive Medicine; Cholesterol/Lipid Disorders; **Hospital:** St Luke's - Roosevelt Hosp Ctr - Roosevelt Div (page 94); **Address:** 185 W End Ave, Ste 1M, New York, NY 10023-5540; **Phone:** 212-595-7701; **Board Cert:** Internal Medicine 1985; **Med School:** Boston Univ 1982; **Resid:** Internal Medicine, St Lukes Roosevelt Hosp 1985; **Fac Appt:** Asst Clin Prof Med, Columbia P&S

Bregman, Zachary MD (IM) *PCP* - **Spec Exp:** Pulmonary Disease; AIDS/HIV; **Hospital:** Beth Israel Med Ctr - Petrie Division (page 94); **Address:** 247 3rd Ave, Ste 304, New York, NY 10010; **Phone:** 212-505-6663; **Board Cert:** Internal Medicine 1986; **Med School:** Univ Pennsylvania 1981; **Resid:** Internal Medicine, Beth Israel Med Ctr 1984; **Fellow:** Pulmonary Disease, Beth Israel Med Ctr 1986; **Fac Appt:** Asst Clin Prof Med, Albert Einstein Coll Med

Bush, Michael N MD (IM) *PCP* - **Spec Exp:** Preventive Medicine; **Hospital:** Lenox Hill Hosp, NYU Langone Med Ctr (page 106); **Address:** 115 E 57th St, Ste 630, New York, NY 10022; **Phone:** 212-583-2990; **Board Cert:** Internal Medicine 1981; **Med School:** SUNY Downstate 1978; **Resid:** Internal Medicine, Lenox Hill Hosp 1982; **Fac Appt:** Asst Clin Prof Med, NYU Sch Med

Carmichael, L David MD (IM) *PCP* - **Spec Exp:** Preventive Medicine; Travel Medicine; Hemochromatosis; **Hospital:** NY-Presby Hosp/Columbia (page 104); **Address:** 903 Park Ave, New York, NY 10021; **Phone:** 212-639-9850; **Board Cert:** Internal Medicine 1979; **Med School:** Albert Einstein Coll Med 1976; **Resid:** Internal Medicine, Bronx Lebanon Hosp 1979; Epidemiology, Columbia Sch Pub Health 1983; **Fellow:** Internal Medicine, Columbia Presby Med Ctr 1980; **Fac Appt:** Assoc Clin Prof Med, Columbia P&S

Case, David B MD (IM) *PCP* - **Spec Exp:** Hypertension; Preventive Cardiology; **Hospital:** NY-Presby Hosp/Columbia (page 104); **Address:** 635 Madison Ave Fl 7, New York, NY 10022-1009; **Phone:** 212-857-4660; **Board Cert:** Internal Medicine 1974; **Med School:** Columbia P&S 1968; **Resid:** Internal Medicine, Johns Hopkins Hosp 1970; **Fellow:** Cardiovascular Disease, Columbia-Presby Med Ctr 1972; **Fac Appt:** Assoc Clin Prof Med, Cornell Univ-Weill Med Coll

Charap, Mitchell MD (IM) *PCP* - **Hospital:** NYU Langone Med Ctr (page 106); **Address:** 530 1st Ave, Ste 7B, New York, NY 10016; **Phone:** 212-263-7442; **Board Cert:** Internal Medicine 2002; **Med School:** NYU Sch Med 1977; **Resid:** Internal Medicine, NYU Med Ctr 1981; **Fac Appt:** Assoc Clin Prof Med, NYU Sch Med

Charap, Peter MD (IM) *PCP* - **Spec Exp:** Preventive Medicine; **Hospital:** Mount Sinai Med Ctr (page 102); **Address:** 234 Central Park West, New York, NY 10024; **Phone:** 212-579-2200; **Board Cert:** Internal Medicine 1987; **Med School:** Mount Sinai Sch Med 1984; **Resid:** Internal Medicine, Mount Sinai Hosp 1987; **Fellow:** Public Health & Genl Preventive Med, Mount Sinai Hosp 1988; **Fac Appt:** Asst Clin Prof Med, Mount Sinai Sch Med

Cohen, Richard P MD (IM) *PCP* - **Spec Exp:** Complex Diagnosis; Preventive Medicine; **Hospital:** NY-Presby Hosp/Weill Cornell (page 104), Hosp For Special Surgery (page 111); **Address:** 235 E 67th St, New York, NY 10021-6040; **Phone:** 212-734-6464; **Board Cert:** Internal Medicine 1978; **Med School:** Cornell Univ-Weill Med Coll 1975; **Resid:** Internal Medicine, NY Hosp 1978; **Fellow:** Infectious Disease, NY Hosp 1979; **Fac Appt:** Prof Med, Cornell Univ-Weill Med Coll

Cohen, Robert L MD (IM) - ; **Address:** 314 W 14th St, FL 5, New York, NY 10014-5002; **Phone:** 212-620-0144; **Board Cert:** Internal Medicine 1978; **Med School:** Rush Med Coll 1975; **Resid:** Internal Medicine, Cook County Hosp 1979; **Fac Appt:** Asst Prof Med, Albert Einstein Coll Med

Cohn, Symra A MD (IM) *PCP* - **Spec Exp:** Women's Health; **Hospital:** NY-Presby Hosp/Weill Cornell (page 104); **Address:** 3 E 71st St Fl 1, New York, NY 10021; **Phone:** 212-288-1302; **Board Cert:** Internal Medicine 2005; **Med School:** NY Med Coll 1991; **Resid:** Internal Medicine, NY Hosp-Cornell Med Ctr 1994; **Fac Appt:** Asst Clin Prof Med, Cornell Univ-Weill Med Coll

Constantiner, Arturo MD (IM) *PCP* - **Spec Exp:** Hypertension; Kidney Disease; Kidney Stones; Dialysis Care; **Hospital:** NY Downtown Hosp; **Address:** 19 Beekman St, Fl 6, New York, NY 10038-1522; **Phone:** 212-349-8455; **Board Cert:** Internal Medicine 1979; Nephrology 2006; **Med School:** Mexico 1975; **Resid:** Internal Medicine, Elmhurst Hosp 1979; **Fellow:** Nephrology, Mount Sinai Hosp 1981; **Fac Appt:** Asst Clin Prof Med, NYU Sch Med

Cunningham-Rundles, Ward MD (IM) *PCP* - **Spec Exp:** Allergy & Immunology; **Hospital:** NY-Presby Hosp/Weill Cornell (page 104), Mount Sinai Med Ctr (page 102); **Address:** 240 E 68th St, New York, NY 10065-6001; **Phone:** 212-737-8973; **Board Cert:** Internal Medicine 1976; **Med School:** NYU Sch Med 1971; **Resid:** Internal Medicine, Bellevue Hosp 1973; **Fellow:** Immunology, Meml Sloan Kettering Cancer Ctr 1975; Medical Oncology, Meml Sloan Kettering Cancer Ctr 1976; **Fac Appt:** Asst Clin Prof Med, Mount Sinai Sch Med

Dhalla, Satish MD (IM) *PCP* - **Spec Exp:** Hypertension; Cholesterol/Lipid Disorders; Diabetes; Travel Medicine; **Hospital:** NYU Langone Med Ctr (page 106), NY Downtown Hosp; **Address:** 111 Broadway Fl 2, NYU-Trinity Ctr, New York, NY 10006; **Phone:** 212-263-9700; **Board Cert:** Internal Medicine 1976; **Med School:** India 1972; **Resid:** Internal Medicine, Beekman Downtown Hosp 1976; **Fac Appt:** Assoc Clin Prof Med, NYU Sch Med

Dolinsky, Jason H MD (IM) *PCP* - **Hospital:** Beth Israel Med Ctr - Petrie Division (page 94), Mount Sinai Med Ctr (page 102); **Address:** 899 Lexington Ave, New York, NY 10065; **Phone:** 212-737-1102; **Board Cert:** Internal Medicine 2007; **Med School:** NYU Sch Med 1994; **Resid:** Internal Medicine, Hosp Univ Penn 1997

Ehrlich, Martin Harvey MD (IM) *PCP* - **Spec Exp:** Complementary Medicine; Preventive Medicine; Acupuncture; **Hospital:** Beth Israel Med Ctr - Petrie Division (page 94); **Address:** Center for Health & Healing, 245 Fifth Ave Fl 2, New York, NY 10016; **Phone:** 646-935-2265; **Board Cert:** Internal Medicine 1988; **Med School:** Columbia P&S 1985; **Resid:** Internal Medicine, Harlem Hosp 1989; **Fac Appt:** Asst Prof Med, Albert Einstein Coll Med

Etingin, Orli MD (IM) *PCP* - **Spec Exp:** Preventive Medicine; Bleeding/Coagulation Disorders; Women's Health; **Hospital:** NY-Presby Hosp/Weill Cornell (page 104); **Address:** 425 E 61st St Fl 11, New York, NY 10065; **Phone:** 212-821-0926; **Board Cert:** Internal Medicine 1984; Hematology 1988; **Med School:** Albert Einstein Coll Med 1980; **Resid:** Internal Medicine, NY Hosp 1983; **Fellow:** Hematology & Oncology, NY Hosp 1986; **Fac Appt:** Clin Prof Med, Cornell Univ-Weill Med Coll

Feltheimer, Seth MD (IM) *PCP* - **Spec Exp:** Preventive Medicine; Perioperative Medical Care; **Hospital:** NY-Presby Hosp/Columbia (page 104); **Address:** 161 Ft Washington Ave, Ste 336, New York, NY 10032; **Phone:** 212-305-8669; **Board Cert:** Internal Medicine 1984; **Med School:** Spain 1981; **Resid:** Internal Medicine, Interfaith Med Ctr 1984; **Fellow:** Internal Medicine, Columbia-Presby Med Ctr 1985; **Fac Appt:** Assoc Clin Prof Med, Columbia P&S

Fiedler, Robert P MD (IM) *PCP* - **Spec Exp:** Thyroid Disorders; Diabetes; **Hospital:** Mount Sinai Med Ctr (page 102); **Address:** 1175 Park Ave, New York, NY 10128-1211; **Phone:** 212-289-6500; **Board Cert:** Internal Medicine 1970; Endocrinology, Diabetes & Metabolism 1972; **Med School:** Albert Einstein Coll Med 1964; **Resid:** Internal Medicine, DC Gen Hosp 1966; Internal Medicine, VA Med Ctr 1967; **Fellow:** Endocrinology, Mount Sinai Med Ctr 1969; **Fac Appt:** Assoc Clin Prof Med, Mount Sinai Sch Med

Fisher, Laura MD (IM) *PCP* - **Spec Exp:** Preventive Medicine; Lyme Disease; Women's Health; **Hospital:** NY-Presby Hosp/Weill Cornell (page 104); **Address:** 1385 York Ave, New York, NY 10021; **Phone:** 212-717-5920; **Board Cert:** Internal Medicine 1987; **Med School:** Brown Univ 1984; **Resid:** Internal Medicine, NY Hosp-Cornell Med Ctr 1987; **Fellow:** Infectious Disease, Mass Genl Hosp 1989; **Fac Appt:** Asst Clin Prof Med, Cornell Univ-Weill Med Coll

Fried, Richard P MD (IM) *PCP* - **Spec Exp:** Lyme Disease; Fevers of Unknown Origin; Infectious Disease; **Hospital:** St Luke's - Roosevelt Hosp Ctr - Roosevelt Div (page 94); **Address:** 15 W 72nd St, Ste 1N, New York, NY 10023; **Phone:** 212-580-4840; **Board Cert:** Internal Medicine 1972; Infectious Disease 1974; **Med School:** Columbia P&S 1968; **Resid:** Internal Medicine, St Lukes Hosp 1972; **Fellow:** Infectious Disease, Stanford Med Ctr 1974; **Fac Appt:** Assoc Clin Prof Med, Columbia P&S

Friedman, Jeffrey Paul MD (IM) *PCP* - **Spec Exp:** Preventive Medicine; Travel Medicine; **Hospital:** NYU Langone Med Ctr (page 106); **Address:** 317 E 34th St Fl 10, New York, NY 10016; **Phone:** 212-726-7440; **Board Cert:** Internal Medicine 1986; **Med School:** NYU Sch Med 1983; **Resid:** Internal Medicine, Bellevue Hosp 1987; **Fac Appt:** Prof Med, NYU Sch Med

Galland, Leo MD (IM) - **Spec Exp:** Nutrition; Chronic Illness; Complementary Medicine; **Address:** 156 5th Ave, Ste 820, New York, NY 10010; **Phone:** 212-989-6733; **Board Cert:** Internal Medicine 1972; **Med School:** NYU Sch Med 1968; **Resid:** Internal Medicine, Bellevue Hosp 1972; **Fellow:** Behavioral Medicine, Univ Conn Hlth Ctr 1981

Golden, Flavia A MD (IM) *PCP* - **Spec Exp:** Women's Health; **Hospital:** NY-Presby Hosp/Weill Cornell (page 104); **Address:** 310 E 72nd St, New York, NY 10021; **Phone:** 212-396-3016; **Board Cert:** Internal Medicine 2003; **Med School:** NYU Sch Med 1990; **Resid:** Internal Medicine, New York Hosp 1993; **Fac Appt:** Asst Prof Med, Cornell Univ-Weill Med Coll

Goldstein, Paul H MD (IM) *PCP* - **Spec Exp:** Preventive Medicine; **Hospital:** NYU Langone Med Ctr (page 106); **Address:** 80 5th Ave, Ste 1601, New York, NY 10011; **Phone:** 212-645-8500; **Board Cert:** Internal Medicine 1985; **Med School:** NY Med Coll 1982; **Resid:** Internal Medicine, St Vincent's Hosp & Med Ctr 1985; **Fac Appt:** Assoc Prof Med, NY Med Coll

Greaney, Edward J MD (IM) *PCP* - **Spec Exp:** Preventive Medicine; Nutrition; **Hospital:** NYU Langone Med Ctr (page 106); **Address:** 317 E 34th St, Fl 4th, New York, NY 10016; **Phone:** 212-726-7488; **Board Cert:** Internal Medicine 1998; **Med School:** NYU Sch Med 1995; **Resid:** Internal Medicine, NYU Med Ctr-Bellevue Hosp 1999; **Fac Appt:** Asst Clin Prof Med, NYU Sch Med

Haber, Stuart MD (IM) *PCP* - **Spec Exp:** AIDS/HIV; Travel Medicine; Infectious Disease; **Address:** 12-A Sheridan Square, New York, NY 10014; **Phone:** 212-929-2370; **Board Cert:** Internal Medicine 1986; Infectious Disease 2000; **Med School:** NYU Sch Med 1983; **Resid:** Internal Medicine, Emory Univ Hosp 1986; **Fellow:** Infectious Disease, Emory Univ Hosp 1989

Hart, Catherine MD (IM) *PCP* - **Spec Exp:** Infectious Disease; **Hospital:** NY-Presby Hosp/Weill Cornell (page 104); **Address:** 310 E 72nd St, Fl 2, New York, NY 10021; **Phone:** 212-396-3272; **Board Cert:** Internal Medicine 1984; Infectious Disease 1986; **Med School:** Univ Pennsylvania 1980; **Resid:** Internal Medicine, NY Hosp 1983; **Fellow:** Infectious Disease, NY Hosp 1985; **Fac Appt:** Asst Clin Prof Med, Cornell Univ-Weill Med Coll

Hauptman, Allen S MD (IM) *PCP* - **Spec Exp:** Preventive Medicine; **Hospital:** NYU Langone Med Ctr (page 106); **Address:** 317 E 34th St, New York, NY 10016-4974; **Phone:** 212-726-7494; **Board Cert:** Internal Medicine 1981; **Med School:** NYU Sch Med 1978; **Resid:** Internal Medicine, Bellevue Hosp 1982; **Fac Appt:** Asst Clin Prof Med, NYU Sch Med

Hoffman, Eileen M MD (IM) - **Spec Exp:** Women's Health; **Hospital:** NYU Langone Med Ctr (page 106); **Address:** 35 E 35 St, Ste 1J, New York, NY 10016; **Phone:** 646-424-1530; **Board Cert:** Internal Medicine 1982; **Med School:** SUNY Stony Brook 1979; **Resid:** Internal Medicine, Bellevue Hosp Ctr 1982; **Fellow:** Immunology, Rockefeller Univ 1983; **Fac Appt:** Asst Clin Prof Med, NYU Sch Med

Horbar, Gary M MD (IM) *PCP* - **Hospital:** Lenox Hill Hosp; **Address:** 6 E 85th St, New York, NY 10028; **Phone:** 212-570-9119; **Board Cert:** Internal Medicine 1979; **Med School:** NY Med Coll 1976; **Resid:** Internal Medicine, Lenox Hill Hosp 1980; **Fac Appt:** Asst Clin Prof Med, NYU Sch Med

Horovitz, Len H MD (IM) *PCP* - **Spec Exp:** Bronchoscopy; Asthma; Emphysema; Asthma; **Hospital:** Lenox Hill Hosp, Lenox Hill Hosp (Manh Eye, Ear & Throat Hosp); **Address:** 47 E 77th St, Ste 201, New York, NY 10021; **Phone:** 212-744-3001; **Board Cert:** Internal Medicine 1980; Pulmonary Disease 1984; **Med School:** NYU Sch Med 1976; **Resid:** Internal Medicine, Lenox Hill Hosp 1980; **Fellow:** Pulmonary Disease, Lenox Hill Hosp 1982

Kaminsky, Donald L MD (IM) - **Spec Exp:** AIDS/HIV; Tropical Diseases; Travel Medicine; **Hospital:** Beth Israel Med Ctr - Petrie Division (page 94); **Address:** 10 Union Square East, Ste 5M-1, New York, NY 10003-3314; **Phone:** 212-253-6800; **Board Cert:** Internal Medicine 1982; **Med School:** Geo Wash Univ 1979; **Resid:** Internal Medicine, Beth Israel Hosp 1982; **Fellow:** Infectious Disease, Beth Israel Hosp 1984; **Fac Appt:** Asst Clin Prof Med, Albert Einstein Coll Med

Kaufman, David L MD (IM) *PCP* - **Spec Exp:** AIDS/HIV; Hepatitis C; Lyme Disease; **Hospital:** NYU Langone Med Ctr (page 106), Mount Sinai Med Ctr (page 102); **Address:** 37 Washington Square W, New York, NY 10011; **Phone:** 212-982-4070; **Board Cert:** Internal Medicine 1980; **Med School:** NY Med Coll 1977; **Resid:** Internal Medicine, St Vincents Med Ctr 1980; **Fac Appt:** Asst Clin Prof Med, NY Med Coll

Kennedy, James T MD (IM) *PCP* - **Spec Exp:** Thyroid Disorders; Diabetes; **Hospital:** NYU Langone Med Ctr (page 106); **Address:** 650 1st Ave, Fl 4th, New York, NY 10016; **Phone:** 212-689-7768; **Board Cert:** Internal Medicine 1978; **Med School:** NYU Sch Med 1972; **Resid:** Internal Medicine, Bellevue Hosp 1977; **Fac Appt:** Clin Prof Med, NYU Sch Med

Kennish, Arthur J MD (IM) *PCP* - **Spec Exp:** Mitral Valve Disease; Coronary Artery Disease; **Hospital:** Mount Sinai Med Ctr (page 102); **Address:** 108 E 96th St, New York, NY 10128-6217; **Phone:** 212-410-6610; **Board Cert:** Internal Medicine 1980; Cardiovascular Disease 1983; **Med School:** Albert Einstein Coll Med 1977; **Resid:** Internal Medicine, Mt Sinai Hosp 1980; **Fellow:** Cardiovascular Disease, Mt Sinai Hosp 1982; **Fac Appt:** Asst Clin Prof Med, Mount Sinai Sch Med

Korenstein, Deborah R MD (IM) - **Spec Exp:** Women's Health; Eating Disorders; **Hospital:** Mount Sinai Med Ctr (page 102); **Address:** One Gustave Levy Pl, Box 1087, New York, NY 10029; **Phone:** 212-659-8551; **Board Cert:** Internal Medicine 2006; **Med School:** Columbia P&S 1993; **Resid:** Internal Medicine, Beth Israel Hosp 1996; **Fac Appt:** Assoc Prof Med, Mount Sinai Sch Med

Lamm, Steven MD (IM) *PCP* - **Spec Exp:** Obesity; Sexual Dysfunction; Preventive Medicine; **Hospital:** NYU Langone Med Ctr (page 106), Lenox Hill Hosp; **Address:** 12 E 86th St, New York, NY 10028-0506; **Phone:** 212-988-1146; **Board Cert:** Internal Medicine 1977; **Med School:** NYU Sch Med 1974; **Resid:** Internal Medicine, NYU Med Ctr 1979; **Fellow:** Rheumatology, NYU Med Ctr 1978; **Fac Appt:** Asst Clin Prof Med, NYU Sch Med

Lee, Roberta A MD (IM) - **Spec Exp:** Complementary Medicine; **Hospital:** Beth Israel Med Ctr - Petrie Division (page 94); **Address:** Center for Health & Healing, 245 Fifth Ave Fl 2, New York, NY 10016; **Phone:** 646-935-2265; **Board Cert:** Internal Medicine 1996; **Med School:** Geo Wash Univ 1985; **Resid:** Internal Medicine, Washington Hosp Ctr 1988; **Fellow:** Complementary Medicine, Univ Arizona Med Ctr 1999

Legato, Marianne J MD (IM) - **Spec Exp:** Cardiovascular Disease; Women's Health; Gender Specific Medicine; **Hospital:** NY-Presby Hosp/Columbia (page 104), St Luke's - Roosevelt Hosp Ctr - Roosevelt Div (page 94); **Address:** 903 Park Ave, Ste 2A, New York, NY 10075; **Phone:** 212-737-5663; **Board Cert:** Internal Medicine 2003; **Med School:** NYU Sch Med 1962; **Resid:** Internal Medicine, Columbia-Presby Med Ctr 1965; **Fellow:** Cardiovascular Disease, Columbia-Presby Med Ctr 1968; **Fac Appt:** Prof Emeritus Med, Columbia P&S

Lewin, Margaret MD (IM) *PCP* - **Spec Exp:** Preventive Medicine; Women's Health; Travel Medicine; **Hospital:** NY-Presby Hosp/Weill Cornell (page 104), Hosp For Special Surgery (page 111); **Address:** 635 Madison Ave Fl 8, New York, NY 10022; **Phone:** 212-857-4505; **Board Cert:** Internal Medicine 1980; Hematology 1982; Medical Oncology 1983; **Med School:** Case West Res Univ 1977; **Resid:** Internal Medicine, NY Hosp/Cornell Med Ctr 1980; **Fellow:** Hematology & Oncology, NY Hosp/Cornell Med Ctr 1983; **Fac Appt:** Assoc Clin Prof Med, Cornell Univ-Weill Med Coll

Lewin, Neal A MD (IM) *PCP* - **Spec Exp:** Preventive Medicine; Headache; Complex Diagnosis; **Hospital:** NYU Langone Med Ctr (page 106); **Address:** 120 E 36th St, Ste 1B, New York, NY 10016-3426; **Phone:** 212-889-2813; **Board Cert:** Internal Medicine 1977; Emergency Medicine 2002; Medical Toxicology 1983; **Med School:** SUNY Downstate 1974; **Resid:** Internal Medicine, NYU-Bellevue Hosp 1977; **Fac Appt:** Prof Med, NYU Sch Med

Lewin, Sharon MD (IM) *PCP* - **Spec Exp:** AIDS/HIV; Travel Medicine; Women's Health; Fevers of Unknown Origin; **Hospital:** St Luke's - Roosevelt Hosp Ctr - Roosevelt Div (page 94), NY-Presby Hosp/Weill Cornell (page 104); **Address:** 139 W 82nd St, New York, NY 10024-5544; **Phone:** 212-496-7200; **Board Cert:** Internal Medicine 1978; Infectious Disease 1980; **Med School:** Univ Toronto 1975; **Resid:** Internal Medicine, Wadsworth VA Hosp 1978; **Fellow:** Infectious Disease, Bellevue Hosp/NYU Med Ctr 1980; **Fac Appt:** Asst Clin Prof Med, Columbia P&S

Liguori, Michael MD (IM) *PCP* - **Spec Exp:** Geriatric Rehabilitation; AIDS/HIV; **Hospital:** NYU Langone Med Ctr (page 106); **Address:** 80 5th Ave, Ste 1601, New York, NY 10011-8002; **Phone:** 212-645-8500; **Board Cert:** Internal Medicine 1985; **Med School:** Mount Sinai Sch Med 1981; **Resid:** Internal Medicine, St Vincents Hosp 1984; **Fac Appt:** Asst Clin Prof Med, NY Med Coll

Lipton, Mark S MD (IM) *PCP* - **Spec Exp:** Preventive Cardiology; Coronary Artery Disease; Non-Invasive Cardiology; **Hospital:** NYU Langone Med Ctr (page 106); **Address:** 635 Madison Ave Fl 3, New York, NY 10022-1009; **Phone:** 212-570-2077; **Board Cert:** Internal Medicine 1981; Cardiovascular Disease 1985; **Med School:** NYU Sch Med 1978; **Resid:** Internal Medicine, Bellevue Hosp 1981; **Fellow:** Cardiovascular Disease, NYU Med Ctr 1985; **Fac Appt:** Assoc Clin Prof Med, NYU Sch Med

Liu, George C K MD (IM) *PCP* - **Spec Exp:** Endocrinology; Chinese Community Health; Diabetes; **Hospital:** NY Downtown Hosp, NYU Langone Med Ctr (page 106); **Address:** 185 Canal St Fl 6, New York, NY 10013-4513; **Phone:** 212-343-7323; **Board Cert:** Internal Medicine 1983; **Med School:** Cornell Univ-Weill Med Coll 1978; **Resid:** Internal Medicine, NYU Med Ctr-Manhattan VA Hosp 1981; **Fellow:** Endocrinology, Stanford Univ Med Ctr 1983; **Fac Appt:** Asst Clin Prof Med, NYU Sch Med

Lodge Jr, Henry S MD (IM) *PCP* - **Spec Exp:** Preventive Medicine; **Hospital:** NY-Presby Hosp/Columbia (page 104); **Address:** New York Physicians, 635 Madison Ave Fl 8, New York, NY 10022-1009; **Phone:** 212-857-4555; **Board Cert:** Internal Medicine 1988; **Med School:** Columbia P&S 1985; **Resid:** Internal Medicine, Columbia-Presby Hosp 1988; **Fac Appt:** Assoc Clin Prof Med, Columbia P&S

Logan, Bruce D MD (IM) *PCP* - **Spec Exp:** Preventive Medicine; Hypertension; Diabetes; Cholesterol/Lipid Disorders; **Hospital:** NY Downtown Hosp, NY-Presby Hosp/Weill Cornell (page 104); **Address:** 19 Beekman St, Fl 6, New York, NY 10038; **Phone:** 212-608-6634; **Board Cert:** Internal Medicine 1978; **Med School:** Columbia P&S 1972; **Resid:** Internal Medicine, Harlem Hosp Ctr 1978; **Fac Appt:** Assoc Clin Prof Med, Cornell Univ-Weill Med Coll

Mackenzie, C Ronald MD (IM) *PCP* - **Spec Exp:** Complementary Medicine; **Hospital:** Hosp For Special Surgery (page 111), NY-Presby Hosp/Weill Cornell (page 104); **Address:** 535 E 70th St, New York, NY 10021; **Phone:** 212-606-1669; **Board Cert:** Internal Medicine 1981; Rheumatology 2002; **Med School:** Univ Calgary 1977; **Resid:** Family Medicine, Calgary Gen Hosp 1978; Internal Medicine, Univ Manitoba Hosp 1981; **Fellow:** Internal Medicine, New York Hosp/Cornell 1983; Rheumatology, Hosp For Spec Surg 1992; **Fac Appt:** Assoc Clin Prof Med, Cornell Univ-Weill Med Coll

Mann, Samuel J MD (IM) - **Spec Exp:** Hypertension; **Hospital:** NY-Presby Hosp/Weill Cornell (page 104); **Address:** Weill-Cornell Hypertension Clinic, 450 E 69th St, New York, NY 10021; **Phone:** 212-746-2200; **Board Cert:** Internal Medicine 1975; **Med School:** SUNY Downstate 1972; **Resid:** Internal Medicine, St Lukes Roosevelt Hosp 1975; **Fellow:** Hypertension, Mt Sinai Hosp 1983; **Fac Appt:** Clin Prof Med, Cornell Univ-Weill Med Coll

Minkowitz, Susan MD (IM) *PCP* - **Spec Exp:** Asthma; Emphysema; Hypertension; Chronic Obstructive Lung Disease (COPD); **Hospital:** NYU Langone Med Ctr (page 106); **Address:** 355 W 52nd St Fl 7th, New York, NY 10019; **Phone:** 212-604-1866; **Board Cert:** Internal Medicine 1988; **Med School:** NY Med Coll 1984; **Resid:** Internal Medicine, Metropolitan Hosp Ctr 1987; **Fellow:** Pulmonary Disease, Montefiore Med Ctr 1989; **Fac Appt:** Asst Prof Med, NY Med Coll

Nelson, Deena J MD (IM) *PCP* - **Spec Exp:** Cancer Survivors-Late Effects of Therapy; Cancer Prevention; **Hospital:** NY-Presby Hosp/Weill Cornell (page 104); **Address:** 635 Madison Ave Fl 8, New York, NY 10022-1009; **Phone:** 212-857-4670; **Board Cert:** Internal Medicine 1980; **Med School:** Albert Einstein Coll Med 1977; **Resid:** Internal Medicine, New York Hosp 1979; Internal Medicine, Barnes Hosp 1980; **Fac Appt:** Asst Clin Prof Med, Cornell Univ-Weill Med Coll

Olichney, John J MD (IM) - **Hospital:** St Luke's - Roosevelt Hosp Ctr - Roosevelt Div (page 94); **Address:** 350 W 58th St Fl Ground, New York, NY 10019-1804; **Phone:** 212-246-9101; **Board Cert:** Internal Medicine 1974; **Med School:** Albany Med Coll 1969; **Resid:** Internal Medicine, Roosevelt Hosp 1972; **Fellow:** Hematology, St Luke's-Roosevelt Hosp Ctr 1973; **Fac Appt:** Clin Prof Med, Columbia P&S

Orsher, Stuart MD (IM) *PCP* - **Hospital:** Lenox Hill Hosp; **Address:** 9 E 79th St, New York, NY 10075; **Phone:** 212-535-7763; **Board Cert:** Internal Medicine 1983; **Med School:** Hahnemann Univ 1975; **Resid:** Internal Medicine, Lenox Hill Hosp 1978

Pardi, Desiree A MD (IM) - **Spec Exp:** Palliative Care; **Hospital:** NY-Presby Hosp/Weill Cornell (page 104); **Address:** 1484 1st Ave, New York, NY 10075; **Phone:** 212-746-7000; **Board Cert:** Internal Medicine 2005; Hospice & Palliative Medicine 2006; **Med School:** Mount Sinai Sch Med 2002; **Resid:** Internal Medicine, NY Presby-Cornell Med Ctr 2005; **Fellow:** Hospice & Palliative Medicine, NY Presby-Cornell Med Ctr 2006; **Fac Appt:** Asst Prof Med, Cornell Univ-Weill Med Coll

Pecker, Mark S MD (IM) - **Spec Exp:** Hypertension; **Hospital:** NY-Presby Hosp/Weill Cornell (page 104); **Address:** NY-Cornell Medical Ctr, Hypertension Ctr, 450 E 69th St, New York, NY 10021; **Phone:** 212-746-2210; **Board Cert:** Internal Medicine 1980; **Med School:** NYU Sch Med 1977; **Resid:** Internal Medicine, Univ Texas SW Affil Hosps 1980; **Fac Appt:** Clin Prof Med, Cornell Univ-Weill Med Coll

Postley, John E MD (IM) *PCP* - **Spec Exp:** Preventive Medicine; **Hospital:** NY-Presby Hosp/Columbia (page 104); **Address:** 635 Madison Ave Fl 7, New York, NY 10022; **Phone:** 212-317-4646; **Board Cert:** Internal Medicine 1973; **Med School:** Columbia P&S 1968; **Resid:** Internal Medicine, Columbia-Presby Med Ctr 1973; **Fac Appt:** Asst Clin Prof Med, Columbia P&S

Rivlin, Richard S MD (IM) - **Spec Exp:** Nutrition & Cancer Prevention/Control; Breast Cancer; Prostate Cancer; Colon Cancer; **Hospital:** NY-Presby Hosp/Weill Cornell (page 104); **Address:** 1167 York Ave, New York, NY 10065; **Phone:** 646-898-2749; **Board Cert:** Internal Medicine 1969; **Med School:** Harvard Med Sch 1959; **Resid:** Internal Medicine, Johns Hopkins Hosp 1961; Internal Medicine, Johns Hopkins Hosp 1964; **Fellow:** Endocrinology, Diabetes & Metabolism, Natl Inst Hlth 1963; Biochemistry, Johns Hopkins Hosp 1966; **Fac Appt:** Prof Med, Cornell Univ-Weill Med Coll

Rosen, Nedra J MD (IM) *PCP* - **Hospital:** Lenox Hill Hosp, NYU Langone Med Ctr (page 106); **Address:** 115 E 57th St, Ste 630, New York, NY 10022; **Phone:** 212-583-2990; **Board Cert:** Internal Medicine 1983; **Med School:** NY Med Coll 1980; **Resid:** Internal Medicine, Lenox Hill Hosp 1984

Salsitz, Edwin A MD (IM) - **Spec Exp:** Addiction/Substance Abuse; Opiate Addiction; **Hospital:** Beth Israel Med Ctr - Petrie Division (page 94); **Address:** Beth Israel Med Ctr, 1st Ave at 16th St, 10 Bernstein Pavilion, Dept Medicine, New York, NY 10003; **Phone:** 212-420-4400; **Board Cert:** Internal Medicine 1977; Pulmonary Disease 1980; **Med School:** SUNY Buffalo 1972; **Resid:** Obstetrics & Gynecology, Beth Israel Med Ctr 1974; Internal Medicine, Beth Israel Med Ctr 1977; **Fellow:** Pulmonary Disease, Beth Israel Med Ctr 1979; **Fac Appt:** Asst Clin Prof Med, Albert Einstein Coll Med

Schneider, Steven J MD (IM) *PCP* - **Spec Exp:** Travel Medicine; Occupational Medicine; Lyme Disease; **Hospital:** Lenox Hill Hosp, Mount Sinai Med Ctr (page 102); **Address:** 115 E 57th St, Ste 630, New York, NY 10022; **Phone:** 212-583-2880; **Board Cert:** Internal Medicine 1979; **Med School:** Johns Hopkins Univ 1976; **Resid:** Internal Medicine, Presby Med Ctr 1979

Silverman, David MD (IM) *PCP* - **Spec Exp:** Infectious Disease; Preventive Medicine; **Hospital:** NYU Langone Med Ctr (page 106), Mount Sinai Med Ctr (page 102); **Address:** 239 Central Park West, Ste 1A-N, New York, NY 10024; **Phone:** 212-496-1929; **Board Cert:** Internal Medicine 1979; **Med School:** Columbia P&S 1976; **Resid:** Internal Medicine, NYU/Bellevue Hosp 1980; **Fellow:** Infectious Disease, NYU/Bellevue Hosp 1981; **Fac Appt:** Assoc Clin Prof Med, NYU Sch Med

Smith, Sharon E MD (IM) *PCP* - **Hospital:** St Luke's - Roosevelt Hosp Ctr - Roosevelt Div (page 94); **Address:** Manhattan Phys Grp, 1865 Amsterdam Ave, New York, NY 10031; **Phone:** 212-491-2400; **Board Cert:** Internal Medicine 1999; **Med School:** Howard Univ 1996; **Resid:** Internal Medicine, St. Vincent's Hosp 1999

Solomon, Gregory W MD (IM) *PCP* - **Spec Exp:** Preventive Medicine; Hypertension; Cholesterol/Lipid Disorders; **Hospital:** Mount Sinai Med Ctr (page 102); **Address:** 899 Lexington Ave, New York, NY 10021-6103; **Phone:** 212-717-9205; **Board Cert:** Internal Medicine 2005; **Med School:** NYU Sch Med 1991; **Resid:** Internal Medicine, Montefiore Med Ctr 1995; **Fac Appt:** Assoc Clin Prof Med, Mount Sinai Sch Med

Spero, Marc MD (IM) *PCP* - **Spec Exp:** Pulmonary Disease; Diving Medicine; Asthma; **Hospital:** NYU Langone Med Ctr (page 106), Lenox Hill Hosp; **Address:** 654 Madison Ave, FL 6, New York, NY 10021-8404; **Phone:** 212-355-8315; **Board Cert:** Internal Medicine 1977; Pulmonary Disease 1980; **Med School:** Albert Einstein Coll Med 1973; **Resid:** Internal Medicine, St Lukes Hosp 1977; **Fellow:** Pulmonary Disease, St Lukes Hosp 1979

Strauss, Michael L MD (IM) *PCP* - **Spec Exp:** Acupuncture; **Hospital:** Beth Israel Med Ctr - Petrie Division (page 94), New York Eye & Ear Infirm (page 113); **Address:** 310 E 14th St, Fl 3 North, New York, NY 10003; **Phone:** 212-979-4204; **Board Cert:** Internal Medicine 1983; **Med School:** Belgium 1980; **Resid:** Internal Medicine, Cabrini Med Ctr 1983

Tay, Steven I MD (IM) *PCP* - **Spec Exp:** Geriatric Care; **Hospital:** Beth Israel Med Ctr - Petrie Division (page 94); **Address:** 10 Union Square E, Ste 5M2, New York, NY 10003; **Phone:** 212-253-9322; **Board Cert:** Internal Medicine 1977; Geriatric Medicine 2004; **Med School:** SUNY Downstate 1974; **Resid:** Internal Medicine, Kings Co Hosp 1977

Underberg, James MD (IM) - **Spec Exp:** Cholesterol/Lipid Disorders; Hypertension; Preventive Cardiology; **Hospital:** NYU Langone Med Ctr (page 106); **Address:** Murray Hill Medical Group, 317 E 34th St Fl 7, New York, NY 10016-4974; **Phone:** 212-726-7430; **Board Cert:** Internal Medicine 1989; **Med School:** Univ Pennsylvania 1986; **Resid:** Internal Medicine, NYU Med Ctr/Bellevue Hosp Ctr 1993; **Fac Appt:** Asst Clin Prof Med, NYU Sch Med

Walfish, Jacob S MD (IM) *PCP* - **Spec Exp:** Gastrointestinal Disorders; Irritable Bowel Syndrome; Diagnostic Problems; **Hospital:** NYU Langone Med Ctr (page 106); **Address:** NYU-Williamsburg, 101 Broadway, Ste 301, Brooklyn, NY 11211; **Phone:** 718-384-5179; **Board Cert:** Internal Medicine 1977; Gastroenterology 1979; **Med School:** Harvard Med Sch 1974; **Resid:** Internal Medicine, Mount Sinai Hosp 1977; **Fellow:** Gastroenterology, Mount Sinai Hosp 1979; **Fac Appt:** Asst Clin Prof Med, NYU Sch Med

Weinstein, Jay MD (IM) *PCP* - **Hospital:** Beth Israel Med Ctr - Petrie Division (page 94); **Address:** Beth Israel Medical Group, 222 W 14th St Fl Ground, New York, NY 10011; **Phone:** 212-604-1800 x8; **Board Cert:** Internal Medicine 2000; **Med School:** Hahnemann Univ 1987; **Resid:** Internal Medicine, St Vincents Hosp Med Ctr 1990

Wiseman, Paul E MD (IM) *PCP* - **Spec Exp:** Preventive Medicine; **Hospital:** St Luke's - Roosevelt Hosp Ctr - Roosevelt Div (page 94); **Address:** 101 Central Park West, New York, NY 10023-4204; **Phone:** 212-496-5800; **Board Cert:** Internal Medicine 1987; **Med School:** Albert Einstein Coll Med 1981; **Resid:** Internal Medicine, Montefiore Med Ctr 1984

Witt III, Marvin MD (IM) *PCP* - **Spec Exp:** Diabetes; Hypertension; **Hospital:** Lenox Hill Hosp; **Address:** Manhattan's Physician Grp, 590 5th Ave, New York, NY 10036; **Phone:** 212-582-7117; **Board Cert:** Internal Medicine 1986; **Med School:** Germany 1983; **Resid:** Internal Medicine, Bridgeport Hosp 1986

Yaffe, Bruce MD (IM) - **Spec Exp:** Gastroscopy; Colonoscopy; **Hospital:** Lenox Hill Hosp; **Address:** 201 E 65th St, New York, NY 10021-6701; **Phone:** 212-879-4700; **Board Cert:** Internal Medicine 1979; Gastroenterology 1981; **Med School:** Geo Wash Univ 1976; **Resid:** Internal Medicine, Mount Sinai Hosp 1979; Hepatology, Mount Sinai Hosp 1980; **Fellow:** Gastroenterology, Lenox Hill Hosp 1982

Zackson, David A MD (IM) - **Spec Exp:** Osteoporosis; Parathyroid Disorders; Bone Disorders-Metabolic; Kidney Stones; **Hospital:** NY-Presby Hosp/Weill Cornell (page 104); **Address:** NY Presbyterian Hospital, 525 E 68th St, New York, NY 10021; **Phone:** 212-746-6292; **Board Cert:** Internal Medicine 1964; **Med School:** NYU Sch Med 1957; **Resid:** Internal Medicine, Kingsbridge VA Med Ctr 1960; **Fellow:** Nephrology, Montefiore Med Ctr 1961

Zeale, Peter J MD (IM) *PCP* - **Spec Exp:** Hypertension; Cholesterol/Lipid Disorders; **Hospital:** NYU Langone Med Ctr (page 106); **Address:** 275 W 7th Ave Fl 3, New York, NY 10011; **Phone:** 646-660-9998; **Board Cert:** Internal Medicine 1982; **Med School:** Georgetown Univ 1979; **Resid:** Internal Medicine, St Vincent's Hosp 1983

Interventional Cardiology

Fox, John T MD (IC) - **Hospital:** Beth Israel Med Ctr - Petrie Division (page 94), Long Island Coll Hosp (page 94); **Address:** Betrh Israel Heart Inst, First Ave at 16th St, 11 Dazian, New York, NY 10003; **Phone:** 212-420-2416; **Board Cert:** Cardiovascular Disease 2007; Interventional Cardiology 2001; **Med School:** NY Med Coll 1989; **Resid:** Internal Medicine, Beth Israel Med Ctr 1993; **Fellow:** Cardiovascular Disease, Beth Israel Med Ctr 1996; Interventional Cardiology, Beth Israel Med Ctr 1997; **Fac Appt:** Asst Prof Med, Albert Einstein Coll Med

Gray, William A MD (IC) - **Spec Exp:** Percutaneous Valve Repair; Peripheral Vascular Disease; Patent Foramen Ovale; **Hospital:** NY-Presby Hosp/Columbia (page 104); **Address:** Ctr for Interventional Vascular Therapy, 161 Fort Washington Ave Fl 5, New York, NY 10032; **Phone:** 212-305-7060; **Board Cert:** Internal Medicine 1987; Cardiovascular Disease 2002; Interventional Cardiology 1999; **Med School:** Temple Univ 1984; **Resid:** Internal Medicine, Rhode Island Hosp 1988; **Fellow:** Cardiovascular Disease, Brown Univ 1992; **Fac Appt:** Assoc Clin Prof Med, Columbia P&S

Leon, Martin MD (IC) - **Hospital:** NY-Presby Hosp/Columbia (page 104); **Address:** 161 Ft Washington Ave Fl 5, New York, NY 10032; **Phone:** 212-305-7060; **Board Cert:** Internal Medicine 1979; Cardiovascular Disease 1983; Interventional Cardiology 1999; **Med School:** Yale Univ 1975; **Resid:** Internal Medicine, Yale-New Haven Hosp 1978; **Fellow:** Cardiovascular Disease, Yale-New Haven Hosp 1980

Moses, Jeffrey W MD (IC) - **Spec Exp:** Angiography-Coronary; Angioplasty & Stent Placement; Heart Valve Disease; **Hospital:** NY-Presby Hosp/Columbia (page 104); **Address:** 161 Fort Washington Fl 5, New York, NY 10032; **Phone:** 212-305-7060; **Board Cert:** Internal Medicine 1977; Cardiovascular Disease 1981; Interventional Cardiology 1999; **Med School:** Univ Pennsylvania 1974; **Resid:** Internal Medicine, Penn Presby Med Ctr 1977; **Fellow:** Cardiovascular Disease, Penn Presby Med Ctr 1980

Parikh, Manish A MD (IC) - **Spec Exp:** Coronary Angioplasty/Stents; **Hospital:** Lenox Hill Hosp; **Address:** 16 E 60th St, Ste 322, New York, NY 10022; **Phone:** 212-326-8532; **Board Cert:** Cardiovascular Disease 2010; Interventional Cardiology 2010; **Med School:** UMDNJ-NJ Med Sch, Newark 1990; **Resid:** Internal Medicine, New York Hosp 1993; **Fellow:** Cardiovascular Disease, New York Hosp 1997; **Fac Appt:** Asst Prof Med, Cornell Univ-Weill Med Coll

Roubin, Gary MD/PhD (IC) - **Spec Exp:** Coronary Angioplasty/Stents; Carotid Artery Stent Placement; Peripheral Vascular Disease; **Hospital:** Lenox Hill Hosp; **Address:** 130 E 77th St Fl 9th, New York, NY 10021; **Phone:** 212-434-2606; **Med School:** Australia 1975; **Resid:** Internal Medicine, Royal Prince Albert Hosp 1979; Cardiovascular Disease, Hallstrom Inst of Cardiology 1981; **Fellow:** Cardiology Research, Natl Heart Fdn 1983; Interventional Cardiology, Emory Univ 1985; **Fac Appt:** Clin Prof Med, NYU Sch Med

Sharma, Samin K MD (IC) - **Spec Exp:** Angioplasty & Stent Placement; Heart Valve Disease; **Hospital:** Mount Sinai Med Ctr (page 102); **Address:** One Gustave L Levy Pl, Box 1030, New York, NY 10029; **Phone:** 212-241-4021; **Board Cert:** Internal Medicine 1986; Cardiovascular Disease 1989; Interventional Cardiology 1999; **Med School:** India 1978; **Resid:** Internal Medicine, SMS Hosp 1982; Internal Medicine, NYU Downtown Hosp 1986; **Fellow:** Cardiovascular Disease, City Hosp Ctr at Elmhurst 1988; Interventional Cardiology, Mt Sinai Hosp 2000; **Fac Appt:** Prof Med, Mount Sinai Sch Med

Slater, James N MD (IC) - **Spec Exp:** Coronary Angioplasty/Stents; Heart Valve Disease; **Hospital:** NYU Langone Med Ctr (page 106), St Luke's - Roosevelt Hosp Ctr - St Luke's Hosp (page 94); **Address:** 426 W 58th St Fl Ground, New York, NY 10019; **Phone:** 212-247-0790; **Board Cert:** Internal Medicine 1980; Cardiovascular Disease 1985; Interventional Cardiology 1999; **Med School:** Univ Rochester 1977; **Resid:** Internal Medicine, Bellevue Hosp Ctr-NYU 1981; **Fellow:** Cardiovascular Disease, Bellevue Hosp Ctr-NYU 1983; **Fac Appt:** Assoc Prof Med, NYU Sch Med

Stone, Gregg W MD (IC) - **Spec Exp:** Angioplasty & Stent Placement; Coronary Artery Disease; **Hospital:** NY-Presby Hosp/Columbia (page 104); **Address:** 173 Ft. Washington Ave, The Heart Ctr-2nd Flr, New York, NY 10032; **Phone:** 646-434-4134; **Board Cert:** Internal Medicine 1985; Cardiovascular Disease 1987; Interventional Cardiology 1999; **Med School:** Johns Hopkins Univ 1982; **Resid:** Internal Medicine, NY Hosp-Cornell Medical Ctr 1985; **Fellow:** Cardiovascular Disease, Cedars-Sinai Medical Ctr 1988; Coronary Angioplasty, Mid-America Heart Inst 1989

Weinberger, Judah Z MD/PhD (IC) - **Spec Exp:** Cardiac Catheterization; Peripheral Vascular Disease; Coronary Artery Disease; Heart Valve Disease; **Hospital:** NY-Presby Hosp/Columbia (page 104); **Address:** NY Presbyterian-Columbia Med Ctr, 173 Fort Washington Ave, Ste 4-602, Milstein Hospital Bldg, New York, NY 10032; **Phone:** 212-305-1581; **Board Cert:** Internal Medicine 1984; Cardiovascular Disease 1985; Interventional Cardiology 2009; **Med School:** Harvard Med Sch 1980; **Resid:** Internal Medicine, Brigham & Womens Hosp 1982; **Fellow:** Cardiovascular Disease, Brigham & Womens Hosp 1985; Interventional Cardiology, MIT 1987; **Fac Appt:** Assoc Prof Med, Columbia P&S

Maternal & Fetal Medicine

Berkowitz, Richard MD (MF) - **Spec Exp:** Fetal Therapy; Multiple Gestation; Pregnancy & Hematologic Abnormalities; **Hospital:** NY-Presby Hosp/Columbia (page 104); **Address:** 16 E 60th St Fl 4, New York, NY 10022; **Phone:** 212-326-8951; **Board Cert:** Obstetrics & Gynecology 2005; Maternal & Fetal Medicine 2005; **Med School:** NYU Sch Med 1965; **Resid:** Obstetrics & Gynecology, NY Hosp-Cornell Med Ctr 1972; **Fac Appt:** Prof ObG, Columbia P&S

Chervenak, Francis A MD (MF) - **Spec Exp:** Ultrasound; Pregnancy-High Risk; Ethics; **Hospital:** NY-Presby Hosp/Weill Cornell (page 104); **Address:** 525 E 68th St, Ste J-130, New York, NY 10021-4870; **Phone:** 212-746-3184; **Board Cert:** Obstetrics & Gynecology 1984; Maternal & Fetal Medicine 1985; **Med School:** Jefferson Med Coll 1976; **Resid:** Obstetrics & Gynecology, NY Med Coll-Flower Fifth Ave Hosp 1979; Obstetrics & Gynecology, St Lukes Hosp 1981; **Fellow:** Maternal & Fetal Medicine, Yale-New Haven Hosp 1983; **Fac Appt:** Prof ObG, Cornell Univ-Weill Med Coll

D'Alton, Mary E MD (MF) - **Spec Exp:** Pregnancy-High Risk; Multiple Gestation; Prenatal Diagnosis; **Hospital:** NY-Presby Hosp/Columbia (page 104); **Address:** 16 E 60th St, Ste 480, New York, NY 10022; **Phone:** 212-326-8951; **Board Cert:** Obstetrics & Gynecology 2001; Maternal & Fetal Medicine 2001; **Med School:** Ireland 1976; **Resid:** Obstetrics & Gynecology, Ottowa Genl Hosp 1982; **Fellow:** Maternal & Fetal Medicine, Tufts-New Eng Med Ctr 1984; **Fac Appt:** Clin Prof ObG, Columbia P&S

Eddleman, Keith A MD (MF) - **Spec Exp:** Obstetric Ultrasound; Pregnancy-High Risk; Fetal Therapy; Reproductive Genetics; **Hospital:** Mount Sinai Med Ctr (page 102); **Address:** Mount Sinai Medical Ctr, 5 E 98th St, Box 1170, New York, NY 10029; **Phone:** 212-241-5681; **Board Cert:** Obstetrics & Gynecology 2009; Maternal & Fetal Medicine 2009; Clinical Genetics 2009; **Med School:** Wake Forest Univ 1985; **Resid:** Obstetrics & Gynecology, George Washington Univ Med Ctr 1989; **Fellow:** Maternal & Fetal Medicine, Mt Sinai Med Ctr 1991; Genetics, NY-Cornell Med Ctr 1996; **Fac Appt:** Prof ObG, Mount Sinai Sch Med

Grunebaum, Amos MD (MF) - **Spec Exp:** Pregnancy-High Risk; Amniocentesis; **Hospital:** NY-Presby Hosp/Weill Cornell (page 104); **Address:** Dept Obstetrics & Gynecology, 525 E 68th St, Ste J-130, New York, NY 10065; **Phone:** 212-746-0714; **Board Cert:** Obstetrics & Gynecology 2008; Maternal & Fetal Medicine 2008; **Med School:** Germany 1974; **Resid:** Anesthesiology, Maimonides Med Ctr 1978; Obstetrics & Gynecology, Downstate Med Ctr 1982; **Fellow:** Maternal & Fetal Medicine, Downstate Med Ctr 1984; **Fac Appt:** Assoc Prof ObG, Columbia P&S

Hutson, J Milton MD (MF) - **Spec Exp:** Multiple Gestation; Pregnancy After Age 35; Amniocentesis; **Hospital:** NY-Presby Hosp/Weill Cornell (page 104); **Address:** 523 E 72nd St, FL 9, New York, NY 10021-4099; **Phone:** 212-472-5340; **Board Cert:** Obstetrics & Gynecology 1997; Maternal & Fetal Medicine 1997; **Med School:** Univ Alabama 1975; **Resid:** Obstetrics & Gynecology, Univ Hosp 1979; **Fellow:** Maternal & Fetal Medicine, Columbia-Presby Med Ctr 1982; **Fac Appt:** Asst Clin Prof ObG, Cornell Univ-Weill Med Coll

Lysikiewicz, Andrzej J MD (MF) - **Spec Exp:** Prenatal Ultrasound; Prenatal Diagnosis; Pregnancy-High Risk; **Hospital:** St Luke's - Roosevelt Hosp Ctr - Roosevelt Div (page 94); **Address:** 1000 Tenth Ave, Ste 11A61, New York, NY 10019; **Phone:** 212-523-7579; **Board Cert:** Obstetrics & Gynecology 2008; Maternal & Fetal Medicine 2008; **Med School:** Poland 1968; **Resid:** Obstetrics & Gynecology, Toronto Genl Hosp 1985; **Fellow:** Maternal & Fetal Medicine, Case Western Res Univ 1987; **Fac Appt:** Prof ObG, Columbia P&S

Patrick, Sharon MD (MF) - **Spec Exp:** Pregnancy-High Risk; Premature Labor; **Hospital:** St Luke's - Roosevelt Hosp Ctr - Roosevelt Div (page 94); **Address:** 800-A Fifth Ave, Ste 503, New York, NY 10021; **Phone:** 212-230-1785; **Board Cert:** Obstetrics & Gynecology 2009; Maternal & Fetal Medicine 2009; **Med School:** Case West Res Univ 1986; **Resid:** Obstetrics & Gynecology, Columbia Presby Hosp 1990; **Fellow:** Maternal & Fetal Medicine, Columbia Presby Hosp 1992; **Fac Appt:** Asst Clin Prof ObG, Columbia P&S

Rebarber, Andrei MD (MF) - **Spec Exp:** Pregnancy-High Risk; Ultrasound; Clotting Disorders in Pregnancy; **Hospital:** Mount Sinai Med Ctr (page 102), Valley Hosp (page 658); **Address:** 70 E 90th St, New York, NY 10128; **Phone:** 212-722-7409; **Board Cert:** Obstetrics & Gynecology 2009; Maternal & Fetal Medicine 2009; **Med School:** SUNY Hlth Sci Ctr 1991; **Resid:** Obstetrics & Gynecology, Beth Israel Med Ctr 1995; **Fellow:** Maternal & Fetal Medicine, Yale-New Haven Hosp 1997; **Fac Appt:** Assoc Prof ObG, Mount Sinai Sch Med

Roshan, Daniel MD (MF) - **Spec Exp:** Pregnancy-High Risk; Pregnancy Loss; Thrombotic Disorders; Multiple Gestation; **Hospital:** NYU Langone Med Ctr (page 106), N Shore Univ Hosp; **Address:** 213 Madison Ave, Ste 1-A, New York, NY 10016; **Phone:** 212-725-0123; **Board Cert:** Obstetrics & Gynecology 1999; Maternal & Fetal Medicine 2001; **Med School:** Israel 1992; **Resid:** Obstetrics & Gynecology, Maimonides Med Ctr 1996; **Fellow:** Maternal & Fetal Medicine, Johns Hopkins Hosp 1998; **Fac Appt:** Asst Prof ObG, NYU Sch Med

Saltzman, Daniel MD (MF) - **Spec Exp:** Pregnancy-High Risk; Prenatal Diagnosis; Ultrasound; **Hospital:** Mount Sinai Med Ctr (page 102); **Address:** 70 E 90th St, New York, NY 10128; **Phone:** 212-722-7409; **Board Cert:** Obstetrics & Gynecology 2009; Maternal & Fetal Medicine 2009; **Med School:** SUNY Buffalo 1979; **Resid:** Obstetrics & Gynecology, Geo Wash Med Ctr 1983; **Fellow:** Maternal & Fetal Medicine, Brigham & Women's Hosp 1985; **Fac Appt:** Clin Prof ObG, Mount Sinai Sch Med

Stone, Joanne L MD (MF) - **Spec Exp:** Prenatal Ultrasound; Twin to Twin Transfusion Syndrome (TTTS); **Hospital:** Mount Sinai Med Ctr (page 102); **Address:** Mount Sinai Medical Ctr, 5 E 98th St, Box 1170, New York, NY 10029; **Phone:** 212-241-5681; **Board Cert:** Obstetrics & Gynecology 2009; Maternal & Fetal Medicine 2009; **Med School:** Columbia P&S 1987; **Resid:** Obstetrics & Gynecology, Mt Sinai Med Ctr 1991; **Fellow:** Maternal & Fetal Medicine, Mt Sinai Med Ctr 1993; **Fac Appt:** Assoc Prof ObG, Mount Sinai Sch Med

Wapner, Ronald J MD (MF) - **Spec Exp:** Perinatal Medicine; Genetic Disorders; Multiple Gestation; Vomiting-Cyclic; **Hospital:** NY-Presby Hosp/Columbia (page 104); **Address:** Div Maternal/Fetal Medicine, 16 E 60th St, rm 480, New York, NY 10022; **Phone:** 212-326-8951; **Board Cert:** Obstetrics & Gynecology 2000; Maternal & Fetal Medicine 2000; Clinical Genetics 2006; **Med School:** Jefferson Med Coll 1972; **Resid:** Obstetrics & Gynecology, Jefferson Univ Hosp 1976; **Fellow:** Maternal & Fetal Medicine, Jefferson Med Coll 1978; **Fac Appt:** Prof ObG, Columbia P&S

Medical Oncology

Aghajanian, Carol A MD (Onc) - **Spec Exp:** Ovarian Cancer; Gynecologic Cancer; Trophoblastic Disease; **Hospital:** Meml Sloan-Kettering Cancer Ctr (page 112); **Address:** 1275 York Ave, Ste H905, New York, NY 10065; **Phone:** 212-639-2252; **Board Cert:** Internal Medicine 2002; Medical Oncology 2005; **Med School:** SUNY Downstate 1989; **Resid:** Internal Medicine, Mt Sinai Med Ctr 1993; **Fellow:** Medical Oncology, Meml Sloan Kettering Cancer Ctr 1995; **Fac Appt:** Assoc Prof Med, Cornell Univ-Weill Med Coll

Bajorin, Dean F MD (Onc) - **Spec Exp:** Genitourinary Cancer; Bladder Cancer; Testicular Cancer; **Hospital:** Meml Sloan-Kettering Cancer Ctr (page 112); **Address:** 1275 York Avenue, New York, NY 10065; **Phone:** 646-422-4333; **Board Cert:** Internal Medicine 1981; Medical Oncology 1985; **Med School:** NY Med Coll 1978; **Resid:** Internal Medicine, Hartford Hosp 1981; **Fellow:** Medical Oncology, Meml Sloan Kettering Ctr 1986; **Fac Appt:** Prof Med, Cornell Univ-Weill Med Coll

Barbasch, Avi MD (Onc) - **Spec Exp:** Breast Cancer; Colon & Rectal Cancer; Lung Cancer; Gastrointestinal Cancer; **Hospital:** Mount Sinai Med Ctr (page 102), Lenox Hill Hosp; **Address:** 1050 Park Ave, New York, NY 10028-1031; **Phone:** 212-860-3292; **Board Cert:** Medical Oncology 2010; **Med School:** Mexico 1975; **Resid:** Internal Medicine, Elmhurst Hosp Ctr 1980; **Fellow:** Medical Oncology, Roswell Park Cancer Inst 1982; **Fac Appt:** Assoc Clin Prof Med, Mount Sinai Sch Med

Berman, Ellin MD (Onc) - **Spec Exp:** Leukemia; Lymphoma; **Hospital:** Meml Sloan-Kettering Cancer Ctr (page 112); **Address:** 1275 York Avenue, New York, NY 10065; **Phone:** 212-639-7762; **Board Cert:** Internal Medicine 1980; Medical Oncology 1985; Hematology 1984; **Med School:** Harvard Med Sch 1977; **Resid:** Internal Medicine, Boston Univ Med Ctr 1980; **Fellow:** Medical Oncology, Meml Sloan Kettering Cancer Ctr 1983; **Fac Appt:** Prof Med, Cornell Univ-Weill Med Coll

Blum, Ronald MD (Onc) - **Spec Exp:** Melanoma; Sarcoma; Lung Cancer; Breast Cancer; **Hospital:** Beth Israel Med Ctr - Petrie Division (page 94); **Address:** 10 Union Square East, Ste 4C, New York, NY 10003-3314; **Phone:** 212-844-8282; **Board Cert:** Internal Medicine 1975; Medical Oncology 1975; **Med School:** SUNY Buffalo 1970; **Resid:** Internal Medicine, Boston City Hosp 1974; **Fellow:** Medical Oncology, Dana Farber Cancer Ctr 1975; **Fac Appt:** Prof Med, Albert Einstein Coll Med

Bosl, George MD (Onc) - **Spec Exp:** Testicular Cancer; **Hospital:** Meml Sloan-Kettering Cancer Ctr (page 112); **Address:** 1275 York Avenue, New York, NY 10065; **Phone:** 212-639-8473; **Board Cert:** Internal Medicine 1976; Medical Oncology 1979; **Med School:** Creighton Univ 1973; **Resid:** Internal Medicine, NY Hosp 1975; Internal Medicine, Meml Sloan-Kettering Cancer Ctr 1977; **Fellow:** Medical Oncology, Univ Minn Hosps 1979; **Fac Appt:** Prof Med, Cornell Univ-Weill Med Coll

Bruckner, Howard W MD (Onc) - **Spec Exp:** Pancreatic Cancer; **Hospital:** NY Downtown Hosp; **Address:** 170 William St, Ste 4B, New York, NY 10038; **Phone:** 212-228-4800; **Board Cert:** Internal Medicine 1972; Medical Oncology 1973; **Med School:** Albert Einstein Coll Med 1966; **Resid:** Internal Medicine, Montefiore/Weiler-Einstein Div 1970; **Fellow:** Medical Oncology, Yale-New Haven Hosp 1971

Brunckhorst, Keith R MD (Onc) - **Hospital:** Lenox Hill Hosp; **Address:** 110 E 59th St, Ste 9B, New York, NY 10022-1304; **Phone:** 212-583-2858; **Board Cert:** Internal Medicine 1979; Hematology 1982; Medical Oncology 1983; **Med School:** NY Med Coll 1976; **Resid:** Internal Medicine, Stamford Hosp 1979; **Fellow:** Hematology & Oncology, Lenox Hill Hosp 1983

Chachoua, Abraham MD (Onc) - **Spec Exp:** Lung Cancer; **Hospital:** NYU Langone Med Ctr (page 106); **Address:** NYU Clinical Cancer Ctr, 160 E 34th St Fl 8, New York, NY 10016; **Phone:** 212-731-5388; **Med School:** Australia 1978; **Resid:** Internal Medicine, Alfred Hosp 1982; **Fellow:** Hematology & Oncology, Alfred Hosp 1985; Hematology & Oncology, NYU Med Ctr 1988; **Fac Appt:** Asst Prof Med, NYU Sch Med

Chapman, Paul B MD (Onc) - **Spec Exp:** Melanoma; Immunotherapy; Clinical Trials; **Hospital:** Meml Sloan-Kettering Cancer Ctr (page 112); **Address:** 1275 York Avenue, New York, NY 10065; **Phone:** 646-888-2378; **Board Cert:** Internal Medicine 1984; Medical Oncology 1987; **Med School:** Cornell Univ-Weill Med Coll 1981; **Resid:** Internal Medicine, Univ Chicago Hosps 1984; **Fellow:** Medical Oncology, Meml Sloan-Kettering Cancer Ctr 1987; **Fac Appt:** Prof Med, Cornell Univ-Weill Med Coll

Cohen, Seymour M MD (Onc) - **Spec Exp:** Breast Cancer; Melanoma; Lung Cancer; Lymphoma; **Hospital:** Mount Sinai Med Ctr (page 102); **Address:** 1150 5th Ave, New York, NY 10128; **Phone:** 212-249-9141; **Board Cert:** Internal Medicine 1971; Medical Oncology 1973; **Med School:** Univ Pittsburgh 1962; **Resid:** Internal Medicine, Montefiore Med Ctr 1964; Internal Medicine, Mount Sinai Med Ctr 1965; **Fellow:** Hematology, Mount Sinai Med Ctr 1966; Hematology & Oncology, LI Jewish Hosp 1969; **Fac Appt:** Assoc Clin Prof Med, Mount Sinai Sch Med

Coleman, Morton MD (Onc) - **Spec Exp:** Leukemia & Lymphoma; Hodgkin's Disease; Multiple Myeloma; Waldenstrom's Macroglobulinemia; **Hospital:** NY-Presby Hosp/Weill Cornell (page 104); **Address:** 407 E 70th St, FL 3, New York, NY 10021-5302; **Phone:** 212-517-5900; **Board Cert:** Internal Medicine 1971; Hematology 1972; Medical Oncology 1973; **Med School:** Med Coll VA 1963; **Resid:** Internal Medicine, Grady Meml Hosp-Emory 1965; Internal Medicine, NY Hosp-Cornell 1968; **Fellow:** Hematology & Oncology, NY Hosp-Cornell 1970; **Fac Appt:** Clin Prof Med, Cornell Univ-Weill Med Coll

Decter, Julian A MD (Onc) - **Spec Exp:** Leukemia & Lymphoma; Multiple Myeloma; Myelodysplastic Syndromes; Colon Cancer; **Hospital:** NY-Presby Hosp/Weill Cornell (page 104); **Address:** NY Presby Hosp, Div Hem/Onc, 407 E 70th St, New York, NY 10021; **Phone:** 212-517-5900; **Board Cert:** Internal Medicine 1972; Hematology 1974; Medical Oncology 1975; **Med School:** NYU Sch Med 1966; **Resid:** Internal Medicine, Ohio State Hosps 1968; **Fellow:** Hematology, NYU Med Ctr 1970; Medical Oncology, Nat Cancer Inst 1974; **Fac Appt:** Assoc Clin Prof Med, Cornell Univ-Weill Med Coll

Dickler, Maura MD (Onc) - **Spec Exp:** Breast Cancer; **Hospital:** Meml Sloan-Kettering Cancer Ctr (page 112); **Address:** 300 E 66th St, New York, NY 10065; **Phone:** 646-497-9064; **Board Cert:** Medical Oncology 2008; **Med School:** Univ Chicago-Pritzker Sch Med 1991; **Resid:** Internal Medicine, Univ Chicago Hosps 1994; **Fellow:** Medical Oncology, Meml Sloan Kettering Cancer Ctr 1998; **Fac Appt:** Asst Prof Med, Cornell Univ-Weill Med Coll

Fanucchi, Michael P MD (Onc) - **Spec Exp:** Sarcoma; Aerodigestive Tract Cancer; Lung Cancer; **Address:** 325 W 15th St, New York, NY 10011; **Phone:** 212-604-6011; **Board Cert:** Internal Medicine 1980; Medical Oncology 1985; **Med School:** Columbia P&S 1977; **Resid:** Internal Medicine, Bronx Muni Hosp Ctr 1981; **Fellow:** Medical Oncology, Meml Sloan-Kettering Cancer Ctr 1984; **Fac Appt:** Assoc Prof Med, Emory Univ

Feldman, Eric MD (Onc) - **Spec Exp:** Leukemia; Stem Cell Transplant; **Hospital:** NY-Presby Hosp/Weill Cornell (page 104); **Address:** 520 E 70th St, New York, NY 10021; **Phone:** 212-746-6736; **Board Cert:** Internal Medicine 1984; Medical Oncology 1987; **Med School:** NY Med Coll 1981; **Resid:** Internal Medicine, Westchester Co Med Ctr 1984; **Fellow:** Medical Oncology, Westchester Co Med Ctr 1986 Fred Hutchinson Cancer Rsch Ctr 1987; **Fac Appt:** Prof Med, Cornell Univ-Weill Med Coll

Fine, Robert MD (Onc) - **Spec Exp:** Pancreatic Cancer; Drug Development; Brain Tumors; Clinical Trials; **Hospital:** NY-Presby Hosp/Columbia (page 104); **Address:** Columbia Univ Comprehensive Cancer Ctr, 650 W 168th St, rm BB 20-05, New York, NY 10032; **Phone:** 212-305-1168; **Board Cert:** Internal Medicine 1983; Medical Oncology 1985; **Med School:** Univ Chicago-Pritzker Sch Med 1979; **Resid:** Internal Medicine, Stanford Univ Med Ctr 1982; **Fellow:** Medical Oncology, National Cancer Inst 1988; **Fac Appt:** Assoc Prof Med, Columbia P&S

Gabrilove, Janice MD (Onc) - **Spec Exp:** Myelodysplastic Syndromes; Leukemia; Hematologic Malignancies; Myeloproliferative Disorders; **Hospital:** Mount Sinai Med Ctr (page 102); **Address:** Mount Sinai Med Ctr, One Gustave L Levy Pl, Box 1079, Dept Hem Onc, New York, NY 10029-6574; **Phone:** 212-241-9650; **Board Cert:** Internal Medicine 1980; Medical Oncology 1983; **Med School:** Mount Sinai Sch Med 1977; **Resid:** Internal Medicine, Columbia-Presby Med Ctr 1980; **Fellow:** Hematology & Oncology, Meml Sloan-Kettering Cancer Ctr 1983; **Fac Appt:** Prof Med, Mount Sinai Sch Med

Gaynor, Mitchell MD (Onc) - **Spec Exp:** Breast Cancer; Lung Cancer; Nutrition & Cancer; Complementary Medicine; **Hospital:** NY-Presby Hosp/Weill Cornell (page 104); **Address:** 215 E 72nd St, New York, NY 10021; **Phone:** 212-472-2828; **Board Cert:** Internal Medicine 1985; Medical Oncology 1987; Hematology 1988; **Med School:** Univ Tex SW, Dallas 1982; **Resid:** Internal Medicine, New York Hosp 1985; **Fellow:** Hematology & Oncology, New York Hosp 1988; **Fac Appt:** Asst Clin Prof Med, Cornell Univ-Weill Med Coll

Gelmann, Edward P MD (Onc) - **Spec Exp:** Prostate Cancer; Testicular Cancer; Bladder Cancer; Kidney Cancer; **Hospital:** NY-Presby Hosp/Columbia (page 104); **Address:** Columbia Univ Med Ctr, Milstein Hosp Bldg 6-435, 177 Fort Washington Ave, New York, NY 10032; **Phone:** 212-305-8602; **Board Cert:** Internal Medicine 1979; Medical Oncology 1981; **Med School:** Stanford Univ 1976; **Resid:** Internal Medicine, Univ Chicago Hosps 1978; **Fellow:** Medical Oncology, National Cancer Inst 1981; **Fac Appt:** Prof Med, Columbia P&S

Goldberg, Arthur I MD (Onc) - **Spec Exp:** Breast Cancer; Prostate Cancer; Colon & Rectal Cancer; Anal Cancer; **Hospital:** Lenox Hill Hosp, Mount Sinai Med Ctr (page 102); **Address:** 121 E 79th St, New York, NY 10075; **Phone:** 212-249-0030; **Board Cert:** Internal Medicine 1974; Medical Oncology 1975; **Med School:** SUNY Hlth Sci Ctr 1969; **Resid:** Internal Medicine, Bellevue/NYU Med Ctr 1973; **Fellow:** Cancer Immunology, Natl Cancer Inst 1972; Medical Oncology, Meml Sloan Kettering Cancer Ctr 1975

Grace, William MD (Onc) - **Spec Exp:** Breast Cancer; Liver Cancer; Pancreatic Cancer; Lung Cancer; **Address:** 36 7th Ave, Ste 511, New York, NY 10011; **Phone:** 212-675-6826; **Board Cert:** Medical Oncology 1977; Internal Medicine 1976; **Med School:** Boston Univ 1969; **Resid:** Internal Medicine, St Vincent's Hosp & Med Ctr 1971; **Fellow:** Hematology & Oncology, Dartmouth-Hitchcock Med Ctr 1976; **Fac Appt:** Assoc Clin Prof Med, NY Med Coll

Grossbard, Lionel MD (Onc) - **Spec Exp:** Lymphoma; Anemia; Breast Cancer; **Hospital:** NY-Presby Hosp/Columbia (page 104); **Address:** 161 Fort Washington Ave, New York, NY 10032-3713; **Phone:** 212-305-8399; **Board Cert:** Internal Medicine 1973; Hematology 1974; Medical Oncology 1975; **Med School:** Columbia P&S 1961; **Resid:** Internal Medicine, Columbia-Presby Med Ctr 1964; **Fellow:** Hematology, Columbia-Presby Med Ctr 1968; **Fac Appt:** Clin Prof Med, Columbia P&S

Grossbard, Michael L MD (Onc) - **Spec Exp:** Lymphoma; Breast Cancer; Gastrointestinal Cancer; **Hospital:** St Luke's - Roosevelt Hosp Ctr - Roosevelt Div (page 94), Beth Israel Med Ctr - Petrie Division (page 94); **Address:** 1000 10th Ave Fl 11 - Ste C02, New York, NY 10019; **Phone:** 212-523-5419; **Board Cert:** Internal Medicine 1989; Medical Oncology 2001; **Med School:** Yale Univ 1986; **Resid:** Internal Medicine, Mass Genl Hosp 1989; **Fellow:** Medical Oncology, Dana Farber Cancer Inst 1991; **Fac Appt:** Clin Prof Med, Columbia P&S

Gulati, Subhash C MD/PhD (Onc) - **Spec Exp:** Breast Cancer; Lymphoma; Lung Cancer; **Hospital:** NY-Presby Hosp/Weill Cornell (page 104), Wyckoff Heights Med Ctr; **Address:** 331 E 65th St, New York, NY 10065; **Phone:** 212-535-1514; **Board Cert:** Internal Medicine 1980; Hematology 1986; Medical Oncology 1983; **Med School:** Univ Miami Sch Med 1976; **Resid:** Internal Medicine, Buffalo Genl Hosp 1978; **Fellow:** Hematology & Oncology, Meml Sloan Kettering Cancer Ctr 1980; **Fac Appt:** Clin Prof Med, Cornell Univ-Weill Med Coll

Hassoun, Hani MD (Onc) - **Spec Exp:** Hematologic Malignancies; Multiple Myeloma; Lymphoma; Stem Cell Transplant; **Hospital:** Meml Sloan-Kettering Cancer Ctr (page 112); **Address:** 1275 York Avenue, New York, NY 10065; **Phone:** 800-525-2225; **Board Cert:** Internal Medicine 1986; Medical Oncology 1989; **Med School:** France 1983; **Resid:** Internal Medicine, Brigham & Womens Hosp 1986; **Fellow:** Hematology & Oncology, Tufts-St Elizabeth Hosp 1991; **Fac Appt:** Assoc Prof Med, Cornell Univ-Weill Med Coll

Hershman, Dawn L MD (Onc) - **Spec Exp:** Breast Cancer; Cancer Survivors-Late Effects of Therapy; Clinical Trials; **Hospital:** NY-Presby Hosp/Columbia (page 104); **Address:** Columbia Univ Med Ctr, Hematology/Oncology, 161 Fort Washington Ave, HIP 10 1068, New York, NY 10032; **Phone:** 212-305-5098; **Board Cert:** Internal Medicine 2007; Medical Oncology 2001; **Med School:** Albert Einstein Coll Med 1994; **Resid:** Internal Medicine, Columbia Univ Med Ctr 1998; **Fellow:** Medical Oncology, Columbia Univ Med Ctr 2001; **Fac Appt:** Asst Prof Med, Columbia P&S

Hirschman, Richard J MD (Onc) - **Spec Exp:** Breast Cancer; Colon Cancer; Lung Cancer; **Hospital:** Beth Israel Med Ctr - Petrie Division (page 94); **Address:** 247 3rd Ave, Ste 401, New York, NY 10010-7455; **Phone:** 212-228-0471; **Board Cert:** Internal Medicine 1971; Hematology 1972; Medical Oncology 1973; **Med School:** Johns Hopkins Univ 1965; **Resid:** Internal Medicine, Bellevue Hosp Ctr 1967; Internal Medicine, Columbia-Presby Hosp 1970; **Fellow:** Hematology & Oncology, Columbia-Presby Hosp 1971; **Fac Appt:** Assoc Clin Prof Med, Mount Sinai Sch Med

Hirshaut, Yashar MD (Onc) - **Spec Exp:** Breast Cancer; Lung Cancer; Colon Cancer; **Hospital:** Lenox Hill Hosp, NY-Presby Hosp/Weill Cornell (page 104); **Address:** 860 5th Ave, New York, NY 10021-5856; **Phone:** 212-861-1799; **Board Cert:** Internal Medicine 1972; Medical Oncology 1975; **Med School:** Albert Einstein Coll Med 1963; **Resid:** Internal Medicine, Montefiore Hosp Med Ctr 1965; **Fellow:** Medical Oncology, Natl Cancer Inst 1968; Medical Oncology, Meml Sloan Kettering Cancer Ctr 1970; **Fac Appt:** Assoc Clin Prof Med, Cornell Univ-Weill Med Coll

Holland, James F MD (Onc) - **Spec Exp:** Breast Cancer; Colon Cancer; Lung Cancer; Pancreatic Cancer; **Hospital:** Mount Sinai Med Ctr (page 102); **Address:** Ruttenberg Cancer Ctr, 1190 5th Ave, Box 1129, New York, NY 10029; **Phone:** 212-241-6756; **Board Cert:** Internal Medicine 1955; **Med School:** Columbia P&S 1947; **Resid:** Internal Medicine, Columbia-Presby Hosp 1949; **Fellow:** Medical Oncology, Francis Delafield Hosp 1953; **Fac Appt:** Prof Med, Mount Sinai Sch Med

Horwitz, Steven MD (Onc) - **Spec Exp:** Lymphoma, Cutaneous T Cell (CTCL); **Hospital:** Meml Sloan-Kettering Cancer Ctr (page 112); **Address:** Meml Sloan-Kettering Cancer Ctr, 1275 York Ave, New York, NY 10065; **Phone:** 212-639-3045; **Board Cert:** Medical Oncology 2001; **Med School:** Case West Res Univ 1993; **Resid:** Internal Medicine, Strong Memorial Hosp 1996; **Fellow:** Medical Oncology, Stanford Univ Med Ctr 1999

Hudis, Clifford A MD (Onc) - **Spec Exp:** Breast Cancer; **Hospital:** Meml Sloan-Kettering Cancer Ctr (page 112); **Address:** 1275 York Avenue, New York, NY 10065; **Phone:** 800-525-2225; **Board Cert:** Internal Medicine 1986; Medical Oncology 2001; **Med School:** Med Coll PA Hahnemann 1983; **Resid:** Internal Medicine, Hosp Med Coll Penn 1987; **Fellow:** Medical Oncology, Meml Sloan Kettering Cancer Ctr 1991; **Fac Appt:** Prof Med, Cornell Univ-Weill Med Coll

Ilson, David H MD (Onc) - **Spec Exp:** Esophageal Cancer; Colon & Rectal Cancer; Mesothelioma; Unknown Primary Cancer; **Hospital:** Meml Sloan-Kettering Cancer Ctr (page 112); **Address:** 1275 York Avenue, New York, NY 10065; **Phone:** 212-639-8306; **Board Cert:** Internal Medicine 1989; Medical Oncology 2002; **Med School:** NYU Sch Med 1986; **Resid:** Internal Medicine, Bellevue-NYU Sch Med 1989; **Fellow:** Medical Oncology, Meml Sloan Kettering Hosp 1992; **Fac Appt:** Assoc Prof Med, Cornell Univ-Weill Med Coll

Jagannath, Sundar MD (Onc) - **Spec Exp:** Multiple Myeloma; **Address:** 325 W 15th St, New York, NY 10011; **Phone:** 212-604-6068; **Board Cert:** Internal Medicine 1980; Medical Oncology 1985; **Med School:** India 1976; **Resid:** Internal Medicine, Bronx Lebanon Hosp 1979; Internal Medicine, Harper-Grace Hosp 1980; **Fellow:** Medical Oncology, MD Anderson Cancer Ctr 1982; **Fac Appt:** Prof Med, NY Med Coll

Jakubowski, Ann MD (Onc) - **Spec Exp:** Leukemia; Bone Marrow Transplant; **Hospital:** Meml Sloan-Kettering Cancer Ctr (page 112); **Address:** 1275 York Ave, New York, NY 10065; **Phone:** 212-639-5013; **Board Cert:** Internal Medicine 1984; Medical Oncology 1987; Hematology 1986; **Med School:** Univ Conn 1981; **Resid:** Internal Medicine, Mt Sinai Hosp 1984; **Fellow:** Hematology, Montefiore Hosp 1985; Medical Oncology, Meml Sloan-Kettering Cancer Ctr 1988

Jarowski, Charles MD (Onc) - **Spec Exp:** Breast Cancer; Lung Cancer; Colon Cancer; **Hospital:** NY-Presby Hosp/Weill Cornell (page 104), Hosp For Special Surgery (page 111); **Address:** 400 E 77th St, Ste 1A, New York, NY 10075; **Phone:** 212-794-9500; **Board Cert:** Internal Medicine 1975; Medical Oncology 1977; Hematology 1978; **Med School:** Cornell Univ-Weill Med Coll 1972; **Resid:** Internal Medicine, New York Hosp 1975; **Fellow:** Hematology & Oncology, New York Hosp 1978; **Fac Appt:** Asst Prof Med, Cornell Univ-Weill Med Coll

Jurcic, Joseph G MD (Onc) - **Spec Exp:** Leukemia; Myelodysplastic Syndromes; Clinical Trials; **Hospital:** Meml Sloan-Kettering Cancer Ctr (page 112); **Address:** 1275 York Avenue, New York, NY 10065; **Phone:** 800-525-2225; **Board Cert:** Internal Medicine 2001; Medical Oncology 2005; Hematology 2008; **Med School:** Univ Pennsylvania 1988; **Resid:** Internal Medicine, Barnes Hosp 1991; **Fellow:** Hematology & Oncology, Meml Sloan Kettering Cancer Ctr 1994; **Fac Appt:** Assoc Prof Med, Cornell Univ-Weill Med Coll

Kelsen, David MD (Onc) - **Spec Exp:** Gastrointestinal Cancer; Neuroendocrine Tumors; Unknown Primary Cancer; Merkel Cell Carcinoma; **Hospital:** Meml Sloan-Kettering Cancer Ctr (page 112); **Address:** 1275 York Avenue, New York, NY 10065; **Phone:** 212-639-8470; **Board Cert:** Internal Medicine 1976; Medical Oncology 1979; **Med School:** Hahnemann Univ 1972; **Resid:** Internal Medicine, Temple Univ Hosp 1976; **Fellow:** Medical Oncology, Meml Sloan Kettering Cancer Ctr 1978; **Fac Appt:** Prof Med, Cornell Univ-Weill Med Coll

Kemeny, Nancy MD (Onc) - **Spec Exp:** Colon Cancer; Rectal Cancer; Liver Cancer; **Hospital:** Meml Sloan-Kettering Cancer Ctr (page 112); **Address:** 1275 York Avenue, New York, NY 10065; **Phone:** 800-525-2225; **Board Cert:** Internal Medicine 1974; Medical Oncology 1981; **Med School:** UMDNJ-NJ Med Sch, Newark 1971; **Resid:** Internal Medicine, St Luke's Hosp 1974; **Fellow:** Medical Oncology, Mem Sloan Kettering Cancer Ctr 1976; **Fac Appt:** Prof Med, Cornell Univ-Weill Med Coll

Kozuch, Peter S MD (Onc) - **Spec Exp:** Gastrointestinal Cancer; **Hospital:** Beth Israel Med Ctr - Petrie Division (page 94); **Address:** 10 Union Square, Fl 4 - Ste 4C, New York, NY 10003; **Phone:** 212-844-8070; **Board Cert:** Medical Oncology 2000; Hematology 2004; **Med School:** Hahnemann Univ 1994; **Resid:** Internal Medicine, Boston Univ Sch Med 1997; **Fellow:** Medical Oncology, UT MD Anderson Cancer Ctr 2000; **Fac Appt:** Assoc Clin Prof Med, Albert Einstein Coll Med

Kris, Mark G MD (Onc) - **Spec Exp:** Lung Cancer; Mediastinal Tumors; Thymoma; Thoracic Cancers; **Hospital:** Meml Sloan-Kettering Cancer Ctr (page 112); **Address:** 1275 York Avenue, New York, NY 10065; **Phone:** 212-639-7590; **Board Cert:** Internal Medicine 1980; Medical Oncology 1983; **Med School:** Cornell Univ-Weill Med Coll 1977; **Resid:** Internal Medicine, New York Hosp 1980; **Fellow:** Medical Oncology, Meml Sloan Kettering Cancer Ctr 1983; **Fac Appt:** Prof Med, Cornell Univ-Weill Med Coll

Krown, Susan MD (Onc) - **Spec Exp:** AIDS/HIV; AIDS-Kaposi's Sarcoma; **Hospital:** Meml Sloan-Kettering Cancer Ctr (page 112); **Address:** 1275 York Avenue, New York, NY 10065; **Phone:** 800-525-2225; **Board Cert:** Internal Medicine 1974; Medical Oncology 1977; **Med School:** SUNY Hlth Sci Ctr 1971; **Resid:** Internal Medicine, Mount Sinai Hosp 1974; **Fellow:** Medical Oncology, Meml Sloan Kettering Cancer Ctr 1977; Clinical Immunology, Meml Sloan Kettering Cancer Ctr 1975; **Fac Appt:** Prof Med, Cornell Univ-Weill Med Coll

Krug, Lee M MD (Onc) - **Spec Exp:** Small Cell Lung Cancer; Mesothelioma; Clinical Trials; **Hospital:** Meml Sloan-Kettering Cancer Ctr (page 112); **Address:** Meml Sloan-Kettering Cancer Center, Dept Thoracic Oncology, 1275 York Ave, New York, NY 10065; **Phone:** 212-639-8420; **Board Cert:** Internal Medicine 2007; Medical Oncology 2009; **Med School:** Washington Univ, St Louis 1994; **Resid:** Internal Medicine, Johns Hopkins Hosp 1997; **Fellow:** Medical Oncology, Meml Sloan Kettering Canc Ctr 1997

Kruger, Bernard M MD (Onc) - **Spec Exp:** Breast Cancer; **Hospital:** Lenox Hill Hosp; **Address:** 170 E 78th St, New York, NY 10075; **Phone:** 212-772-9222; **Board Cert:** Internal Medicine 1974; Medical Oncology 1979; **Med School:** Univ Colorado 1968; **Resid:** Internal Medicine, Boston City Hosp 1972; Internal Medicine, Georgetown Hosp 1974; **Fellow:** Medical Oncology, Mt Sinai Hosp 1976

Livingston, Philip O MD (Onc) - **Spec Exp:** Melanoma; Vaccine Therapy; Immunotherapy; **Hospital:** Meml Sloan-Kettering Cancer Ctr (page 112); **Address:** 1275 York Avenue, New York, NY 10065; **Phone:** 800-525-2225; **Board Cert:** Internal Medicine 1980; Allergy & Immunology 1974; Rheumatology 1974; Medical Oncology 1981; **Med School:** Harvard Med Sch 1969; **Resid:** Internal Medicine, North Shore Hosp-Cornell 1971; **Fellow:** Immunology, NYU Med Ctr 1973; Medical Oncology, Meml Sloan Kettering Cancer Inst 1977; **Fac Appt:** Prof Med, Cornell Univ-Weill Med Coll

Malamud, Stephen C MD (Onc) - **Spec Exp:** Lung Cancer; Gastrointestinal Cancer; **Hospital:** Beth Israel Med Ctr - Petrie Division (page 94), NYU Hosp For Joint Diseases (page 106); **Address:** 10 Union Square E, Ste 4A, New York, NY 10003; **Phone:** 212-844-8280; **Board Cert:** Internal Medicine 1981; Medical Oncology 1983; **Med School:** Albert Einstein Coll Med 1978; **Resid:** Internal Medicine, Beth Israel Med Ctr 1981; **Fellow:** Medical Oncology, Mt Sinai Hosp 1983; **Fac Appt:** Assoc Clin Prof Med, Albert Einstein Coll Med

Maslak, Peter G MD (Onc) - **Spec Exp:** Leukemia; Stem Cell Transplant; Myelodysplastic Syndromes; Clinical Trials; **Hospital:** Meml Sloan-Kettering Cancer Ctr (page 112); **Address:** 1275 York Avenue, New York, NY 10065; **Phone:** 800-525-2225; **Board Cert:** Internal Medicine 1987; Hematology 2000; Medical Oncology 1989; **Med School:** Mount Sinai Sch Med 1984; **Resid:** Internal Medicine, Univ Michigan Med Ctr 1987; **Fellow:** Hematology & Oncology, Meml Sloan Kettering Cancer Ctr 1990

Miller, Vincent A MD (Onc) - **Spec Exp:** Lung Cancer; Drug Development; **Hospital:** Meml Sloan-Kettering Cancer Ctr (page 112); **Address:** Memorial Sloan-Kettering Cancer Ctr, 1275 York Ave, New York, NY 10065; **Phone:** 800-525-2225; **Board Cert:** Internal Medicine 2002; Medical Oncology 2005; **Med School:** UMDNJ-NJ Med Sch, Newark 1987; **Resid:** Internal Medicine, Thos Jefferson Univ Hosp 1991; **Fellow:** Medical Oncology, Meml Sloan Kettering Cancer Ctr 1994; **Fac Appt:** Assoc Prof Med, Cornell Univ-Weill Med Coll

Milowsky, Matthew I MD (Onc) - **Spec Exp:** Genitourinary Cancer; Bladder Cancer; Prostate Cancer; Kidney Cancer; **Hospital:** Meml Sloan-Kettering Cancer Ctr (page 112); **Address:** 1275 York Avenue, New York, NY 10065; **Phone:** 646-422-4461; **Board Cert:** Internal Medicine 2009; Medical Oncology 2002; Hematology 2002; **Med School:** SUNY Downstate 1996; **Resid:** Internal Medicine, New Eng Med Ctr 1999; **Fellow:** Hematology & Oncology, NY Presby Hosp-Cornell Univ 2002; **Fac Appt:** Asst Prof Med, Cornell Univ-Weill Med Coll

Moore, Anne MD (Onc) - **Spec Exp:** Breast Cancer; **Hospital:** NY-Presby Hosp/Weill Cornell (page 104); **Address:** Weill Cornell Breast Ctr, 425 E 61st St Fl 8, New York, NY 10065; **Phone:** 212-821-0550; **Board Cert:** Internal Medicine 1973; Hematology 1976; Medical Oncology 2008; **Med School:** Columbia P&S 1969; **Resid:** Internal Medicine, Cornell Univ Med Ctr 1973; **Fellow:** Medical Oncology, Rockefeller Univ 1973; **Fac Appt:** Prof Med, Cornell Univ-Weill Med Coll

Motzer, Robert J MD (Onc) - **Spec Exp:** Kidney Cancer; Testicular Cancer; Prostate Cancer; **Hospital:** Meml Sloan-Kettering Cancer Ctr (page 112); **Address:** 1275 York Avenue, New York, NY 10065; **Phone:** 800-525-2225; **Board Cert:** Internal Medicine 1984; Medical Oncology 1987; **Med School:** Univ Mich Med Sch 1981; **Resid:** Internal Medicine, Meml Sloan Kettering Cancer Ctr 1984; **Fellow:** Medical Oncology, Meml Sloan Kettering Cancer Ctr 1987; **Fac Appt:** Assoc Prof Med, Cornell Univ-Weill Med Coll

Muggia, Franco MD (Onc) - **Spec Exp:** Gynecologic Cancer; **Hospital:** NYU Langone Med Ctr (page 106); **Address:** NYU Clinical Cancer Ctr, 160 E 34th St Fl 4, New York, NY 10016; **Phone:** 212-731-5433; **Board Cert:** Internal Medicine 1968; Medical Oncology 1973; Hematology 1974; **Med School:** Cornell Univ-Weill Med Coll 1961; **Resid:** Internal Medicine, Hartford Hosp 1964; Internal Medicine, Francis A Delafield Hosp 1966; **Fac Appt:** Prof Med, NYU Sch Med

Nanus, David M MD (Onc) - **Spec Exp:** Prostate Cancer; Bladder Cancer; Testicular Cancer; Genitourinary Cancer; **Hospital:** NY-Presby Hosp/Weill Cornell (page 104); **Address:** NY Hosp-Cornell Med Ctr, Payson Pavilion, 525 E 68th St Fl 3 - Ste 341, New York, NY 10021; **Phone:** 646-962-2072; **Board Cert:** Internal Medicine 1985; Medical Oncology 1987; **Med School:** Univ Hlth Scis, Chicago Med Sch 1982; **Resid:** Internal Medicine, Bronx Muni Hosp 1985; **Fellow:** Medical Oncology, Meml Sloan Kettering Canc Ctr 1989; **Fac Appt:** Prof Med, Cornell Univ-Weill Med Coll

Norton, Larry MD (Onc) - **Spec Exp:** Breast Cancer; **Hospital:** Meml Sloan-Kettering Cancer Ctr (page 112); **Address:** 300 E 66th St, New York, NY 10065; **Phone:** 800-525-2225; **Board Cert:** Internal Medicine 1975; Medical Oncology 1977; **Med School:** Columbia P&S 1972; **Resid:** Internal Medicine, Bronx Muni Hosp 1974; **Fellow:** Medical Oncology, Natl Cancer Inst 1977; **Fac Appt:** Prof Med, Cornell Univ-Weill Med Coll

O'Reilly, Eileen M MD (Onc) - **Spec Exp:** Pancreatic Cancer; Liver Cancer; Biliary Cancer; Neuroendocrine Tumors; **Hospital:** Meml Sloan-Kettering Cancer Ctr (page 112); **Address:** 1275 York Avenue, Meml Sloan-Kettering Cancer Ctr, New York, NY 10065; **Phone:** 212-639-6672; **Med School:** Ireland 1990; **Resid:** Internal Medicine, St Vincent's Hosp 1994; **Fellow:** Hematology, St Vincent's Hosp 1995; Medical Oncology, Memorial-Sloan Kettering Cancer Ctr 1997; **Fac Appt:** Assoc Prof Med, Cornell Univ-Weill Med Coll

Offit, Kenneth MD (Onc) - **Spec Exp:** Cancer Genetics; Breast Cancer; Lymphoma; **Hospital:** Meml Sloan-Kettering Cancer Ctr (page 112); **Address:** 1275 York Avenue, New York, NY 10065; **Phone:** 646-888-4050; **Board Cert:** Internal Medicine 1985; Medical Oncology 1987; **Med School:** Harvard Med Sch 1982; **Resid:** Internal Medicine, Lenox Hill Hosp 1985; **Fellow:** Hematology & Oncology, Meml Sloan Kettering Cancer Ctr 1988; **Fac Appt:** Prof Med, Cornell Univ-Weill Med Coll

Oh, William K MD (Onc) - **Spec Exp:** Genitourinary Cancer; Prostate Cancer; Testicular Cancer; Adrenal Cancer; **Hospital:** Mount Sinai Med Ctr (page 102); **Address:** Mount Sinai Medical Ctr, Gustave Levy Pl, Box 1079, New York, NY 10029; **Phone:** 212-241-5293; **Board Cert:** Medical Oncology 1998; **Med School:** NYU Sch Med 1992; **Resid:** Internal Medicine, Brigham & Womens Hosp 1995; **Fellow:** Medical Oncology, Dana-Farber Cancer Inst 1997; **Fac Appt:** Prof Med, Mount Sinai Sch Med

Oratz, Ruth MD (Onc) - **Spec Exp:** Breast Cancer; Ovarian Cancer; **Hospital:** NYU Langone Med Ctr (page 106); **Address:** 345 E 37th St, Ste 202, New York, NY 10016; **Phone:** 212-400-4904; **Board Cert:** Internal Medicine 1985; Medical Oncology 1989; **Med School:** Albert Einstein Coll Med 1982; **Resid:** Internal Medicine, NYU Med Ctr 1982; **Fellow:** Medical Oncology, NYU Med Ctr 1985; **Fac Appt:** Assoc Clin Prof Med, NYU Sch Med

Oster, Martin W MD (Onc) - **Spec Exp:** Breast Cancer; Gastrointestinal Cancer; Head & Neck Cancer; **Hospital:** NY-Presby Hosp/Columbia (page 104); **Address:** NY Presby Hosp-Columbia Presby Med Ctr, 161 Fort Washington Ave, New York, NY 10032-3713; **Phone:** 212-305-8231; **Board Cert:** Internal Medicine 1974; Medical Oncology 1975; **Med School:** Columbia P&S 1971; **Resid:** Internal Medicine, Mass Genl Hosp 1973; **Fellow:** Medical Oncology, Natl Cancer Inst/NIH 1976; **Fac Appt:** Assoc Clin Prof Med, Columbia P&S

Ott, Patrick MD (Onc) - **Spec Exp:** Melanoma; **Hospital:** NYU Langone Med Ctr (page 106); **Address:** NYU Cancer Ctr, 160 E 34th St Fl 9, New York, NY 10016; **Phone:** 212-731-6564; **Board Cert:** Internal Medicine 2005; Hematology 2008; Medical Oncology 2008; **Med School:** Germany 1996; **Resid:** Internal Medicine, Case Western Reserve Med Ctr 2005; **Fellow:** Hematology & Oncology, NYU Med Ctr 2007

Pasmantier, Mark W MD (Onc) - **Spec Exp:** Lung Cancer; Ovarian Cancer; Breast Cancer; Lymphoma; **Hospital:** NY-Presby Hosp/Weill Cornell (page 104); **Address:** 407 E 70th St Fl 3, New York, NY 10021-5302; **Phone:** 212-517-5900; **Board Cert:** Internal Medicine 1972; Hematology 1974; Medical Oncology 1975; **Med School:** NYU Sch Med 1966; **Resid:** Internal Medicine, Harlem Hosp 1970; **Fellow:** Hematology, Montefiore Med Ctr 1971; Medical Oncology, NY Hosp 1972; **Fac Appt:** Clin Prof Med, Cornell Univ-Weill Med Coll

Pavlick, Anna C DO (Onc) - **Spec Exp:** Melanoma; Skin Cancer; **Hospital:** NYU Langone Med Ctr (page 106); **Address:** NYU Cancer Ctr, 160 E 34th St Fl 9, New York, NY 10016; **Phone:** 212-731-5431; **Board Cert:** Medical Oncology 2008; **Med School:** UMDNJ Sch Osteo Med 1990; **Resid:** Internal Medicine, Hackensack Med Ctr 1993; **Fellow:** Hematology & Oncology, Meml Sloan Kettering Cancer Ctr 1996; **Fac Appt:** Assoc Prof Med, NYU Sch Med

Petrylak, Daniel P MD (Onc) - **Spec Exp:** Genitourinary Cancer; Prostate Cancer; Bladder Cancer; Kidney Cancer; **Hospital:** NY-Presby Hosp/Columbia (page 104); **Address:** 161 Fort Washington Ave Fl 9, New York, NY 10032-3729; **Phone:** 212-305-1731; **Board Cert:** Internal Medicine 2001; Medical Oncology 2003; **Med School:** Case West Res Univ 1985; **Resid:** Internal Medicine, Jacobi Med Ctr 1988; **Fellow:** Oncology, Meml-Sloan Kettering Cancer Ctr 1991; **Fac Appt:** Assoc Prof Med, Columbia P&S

Pfister, David G MD (Onc) - **Spec Exp:** Head & Neck Cancer; Laryngeal Cancer; Thyroid Cancer; Skin Cancer; **Hospital:** Meml Sloan-Kettering Cancer Ctr (page 112); **Address:** 1275 York Avenue, New York, NY 10065; **Phone:** 800-525-2225; **Board Cert:** Internal Medicine 1985; Medical Oncology 1989; **Med School:** Univ Pennsylvania 1982; **Resid:** Internal Medicine, Hosp Univ Penn 1985; **Fellow:** Epidemiology, Yale-New Haven Hosp 1987; Hematology & Oncology, Meml Sloan Kettering Cancer Ctr 1989; **Fac Appt:** Prof Med, Cornell Univ-Weill Med Coll

Portlock, Carol S MD (Onc) - **Spec Exp:** Lymphoma; Hodgkin's Disease; **Hospital:** Meml Sloan-Kettering Cancer Ctr (page 112); **Address:** 1275 York Avenue, New York, NY 10065; **Phone:** 800-525-2225; **Board Cert:** Internal Medicine 1976; Medical Oncology 1978; **Med School:** Stanford Univ 1971; **Resid:** Internal Medicine, Stanford U Med Ctr 1974; **Fellow:** Medical Oncology, Stanford U Med Ctr 1976; **Fac Appt:** Clin Prof Med, Cornell Univ-Weill Med Coll

Posner, Marshall R MD (Onc) - **Spec Exp:** Head & Neck Cancer; Skin Cancer-Head & Neck; **Hospital:** Mount Sinai Med Ctr (page 102); **Address:** Mount Sinai Med Ctr, 1 Gustave L Levy Pl, Box 1128, New York, NY 10029; **Phone:** 212-241-6756; **Board Cert:** Internal Medicine 1978; Medical Oncology 1981; **Med School:** Tufts Univ 1975; **Resid:** Internal Medicine, Boston City Hosp 1978; **Fellow:** Oncology, Dana-Farber Cancer Inst 1981; **Fac Appt:** Assoc Prof Med, Mount Sinai Sch Med

Raptis, George MD (Onc) - **Spec Exp:** Breast Cancer; **Hospital:** Mount Sinai Med Ctr (page 102); **Address:** Ruttenberg Treatment Ctr, 1190 5th Ave, Box 1129, New York, NY 10029; **Phone:** 212-241-6756; **Board Cert:** Medical Oncology 2003; **Med School:** Mount Sinai Sch Med 1987; **Resid:** Internal Medicine, Mt Sinai Med Ctr 1990; **Fellow:** Hematology & Oncology, Meml Sloan-Kettering Canc Ctr 1993; **Fac Appt:** Assoc Prof Med, Mount Sinai Sch Med

Ratner, Lynn H MD (Onc) - **Spec Exp:** Breast Cancer; Carcinoid Tumors; Neuroendocrine Tumors; Gliomas; **Hospital:** Mount Sinai Med Ctr (page 102), Lenox Hill Hosp; **Address:** 112 E 83rd St, New York, NY 10028-0506; **Phone:** 212-396-0400; **Board Cert:** Internal Medicine 1971; Medical Oncology 1973; **Med School:** Albert Einstein Coll Med 1964; **Resid:** Internal Medicine, Bellevue Hosp 1966; Internal Medicine, Bellevue Hosp 1970; **Fellow:** Medical Oncology, Meml Sloan Kettering Cancer Ctr 1970

Raza, Azra MD (Onc) - **Spec Exp:** Myelodysplastic Syndromes; Leukemia; **Address:** 325 W 15th St, New York, NY 10011; **Phone:** 212-604-6004; **Board Cert:** Internal Medicine 1980; Medical Oncology 1985; **Med School:** Pakistan 1976; **Resid:** Internal Medicine, Franklin Sq Hosp 1979; Internal Medicine, Georgetown Univ/VA Med Ctr 1980; **Fellow:** Medical Oncology, Roswell Park Cancer Inst 1982

Rizvi, Naiyer A MD (Onc) - **Spec Exp:** Thoracic Cancers; Thymoma; Lung Cancer; Clinical Trials; **Hospital:** Meml Sloan-Kettering Cancer Ctr (page 112); **Address:** 1275 York Avenue, New York, NY 10065; **Phone:** 800-525-2225; **Board Cert:** Internal Medicine 2002; Medical Oncology 2003; **Med School:** Canada 1987; **Resid:** Internal Medicine, University of Manitoba Med Ctr 1992; **Fellow:** Medical Oncology, Beth Israel Med Ctr 1994

Robson, Mark Emerson MD (Onc) - **Spec Exp:** Breast Cancer; Cancer Genetics; **Hospital:** Meml Sloan-Kettering Cancer Ctr (page 112); **Address:** 1275 York Avenue, New York, NY 10065; **Phone:** 646-888-4058; **Board Cert:** Internal Medicine 1989; Medical Oncology 2001; Hematology 2002; **Med School:** Univ VA Sch Med 1986; **Resid:** Internal Medicine, Walter Reed AMC 1989; **Fellow:** Hematology & Oncology, Walter Reed AMC 1991

Ruggiero, Joseph T MD (Onc) - **Spec Exp:** Gastrointestinal Cancer; **Hospital:** NY-Presby Hosp/Weill Cornell (page 104); **Address:** 428 E 72nd St, Ste 300, New York, NY 10021-4635; **Phone:** 212-746-2083; **Board Cert:** Internal Medicine 1980; Hematology 1982; Medical Oncology 1983; **Med School:** NYU Sch Med 1977; **Resid:** Internal Medicine, New York Hosp 1980; **Fellow:** Hematology & Oncology, New York Hosp/Cornell 1983; **Fac Appt:** Assoc Clin Prof Med, Cornell Univ-Weill Med Coll

Sabbatini, Paul J MD (Onc) - **Spec Exp:** Gynecologic Cancer; Uterine Cancer; Ovarian Cancer; **Hospital:** Meml Sloan-Kettering Cancer Ctr (page 112); **Address:** Meml Sloan Kettering Cancer Ctr, 1275 York Ave, Ste H906, New York, NY 10021; **Phone:** 212-639-6423; **Board Cert:** Internal Medicine 1992; Medical Oncology 1997; **Med School:** Univ Miss 1989; **Resid:** Internal Medicine, Vanderbilt Univ Med Ctr; **Fellow:** Medical Oncology, Meml Sloan-Kettering Cancer Ctr; **Fac Appt:** Asst Prof Med, Cornell Univ-Weill Med Coll

Saltz, Leonard B MD (Onc) - **Spec Exp:** Colon & Rectal Cancer; Gastrointestinal Cancer & Rare Tumors; Liver Cancer; Neuroendocrine Tumors; **Hospital:** Meml Sloan-Kettering Cancer Ctr (page 112); **Address:** 1275 York Avenue, New York, NY 10065; **Phone:** 646-497-9053; **Board Cert:** Internal Medicine 1986; Hematology 1988; Medical Oncology 1989; **Med School:** Yale Univ 1983; **Resid:** Internal Medicine, New Yor Hosp 1986; **Fellow:** Hematology & Oncology, New York Hosp-Cornell/Rockefeller Univ 1987; **Fac Appt:** Prof Med, Cornell Univ-Weill Med Coll

Sara, Gabriel MD (Onc) - **Spec Exp:** Breast Cancer; Lung Cancer; Lymphoma; Gastrointestinal Cancer; **Hospital:** St Luke's - Roosevelt Hosp Ctr - Roosevelt Div (page 94); **Address:** 1000 10th Ave Fl 11, New York, NY 10023; **Phone:** 212-523-7580; **Board Cert:** Internal Medicine 1984; Hematology 1986; Medical Oncology 1987; **Med School:** Lebanon 1980; **Resid:** Internal Medicine, SUNY Downstate Med Ctr 1984; **Fellow:** Hematology & Oncology, St Luke's-Roosevelt Med Ctr 1986; Hematology & Oncology, Columbia-Presby Med Ctr 1987; **Fac Appt:** Asst Clin Prof Med, Columbia P&S

Scheinberg, David MD/PhD (Onc) - **Spec Exp:** Leukemia; Immunotherapy; Vaccine Therapy; **Hospital:** Meml Sloan-Kettering Cancer Ctr (page 112); **Address:** 1275 York Avenue, New York, NY 10065; **Phone:** 646-888-2190; **Board Cert:** Internal Medicine 1986; Medical Oncology 2005; **Med School:** Johns Hopkins Univ 1983; **Resid:** Internal Medicine, NY Hosp-Cornell Med Ctr 1985; **Fellow:** Medical Oncology, Meml Sloan Kettering Cancer Ctr 1987; **Fac Appt:** Prof Med, Cornell Univ-Weill Med Coll

Scher, Howard MD (Onc) - **Spec Exp:** Genitourinary Cancer; Prostate Cancer; Bladder Cancer; **Hospital:** Meml Sloan-Kettering Cancer Ctr (page 112); **Address:** 1275 York Avenue, New York, NY 10065; **Phone:** 800-525-2225; **Board Cert:** Internal Medicine 1979; Medical Oncology 1985; **Med School:** NYU Sch Med 1976; **Resid:** Internal Medicine, Bellevue Hosp 1980; **Fellow:** Medical Oncology, Meml Sloan Kettering Cancer Ctr 1983; **Fac Appt:** Prof Med, Cornell Univ-Weill Med Coll

Sherman, William H MD (Onc) - **Spec Exp:** Pancreatic Cancer; Multiple Myeloma; Melanoma; **Hospital:** NY-Presby Hosp/Columbia (page 104); **Address:** 161 Fort Washington Ave, Ste 922, New York, NY 10032-3729; **Phone:** 212-305-3856; **Board Cert:** Internal Medicine 1975; Medical Oncology 1979; **Med School:** Jefferson Med Coll 1969; **Resid:** Internal Medicine, Univ Illinois Hosp 1971; **Fellow:** Medical Oncology, Columbia-Presby Hosp 1977; **Fac Appt:** Assoc Clin Prof Med, Columbia P&S

Silverman, Lewis R MD (Onc) - **Spec Exp:** Myelodysplastic Syndromes; Leukemia & Lymphoma; Multiple Myeloma; **Hospital:** Mount Sinai Med Ctr (page 102); **Address:** Ruttenberg Treatment Ctr, 1190 5th Ave, Box 1129, New York, NY 10029; **Phone:** 212-241-6756; **Board Cert:** Internal Medicine 1981; Medical Oncology 1987; **Med School:** Belgium 1978; **Resid:** Internal Medicine, Metro Hospital 1980; Internal Medicine, Montefiore Med Ctr 1981; **Fellow:** Hematology, Montefiore Med Ctr 1982; Neoplastic Diseases, Mt Sinai Med Ctr 1984; **Fac Appt:** Assoc Prof Med, Mount Sinai Sch Med

Sklarin, Nancy MD (Onc) - **Spec Exp:** Breast Cancer; **Hospital:** Meml Sloan-Kettering Cancer Ctr (page 112); **Address:** 1275 York Avenue, New York, NY 10065; **Phone:** 800-525-2225; **Board Cert:** Internal Medicine 1984; Medical Oncology 1987; **Med School:** Albert Einstein Coll Med 1981; **Resid:** Internal Medicine, LI Jewish Hospital 1984; **Fellow:** Hematology & Oncology, Mount Sinai Hospital 1987; **Fac Appt:** Asst Prof Med, Cornell Univ-Weill Med Coll

Slovin, Susan F MD/PhD (Onc) - **Spec Exp:** Prostate Cancer; Genitourinary Cancer; Immunotherapy; **Hospital:** Meml Sloan-Kettering Cancer Ctr (page 112), NY-Presby Hosp/Weill Cornell (page 104); **Address:** 1275 York Avenue, New York, NY 10065; **Phone:** 646-422-4470; **Board Cert:** Internal Medicine 2005; Medical Oncology 1999; **Med School:** Jefferson Med Coll 1990; **Resid:** Internal Medicine, Mt Sinai Hosp 1993; **Fellow:** Medical Oncology, Meml Sloan Kettering Cancer Ctr 1996; **Fac Appt:** Assoc Prof Med, Cornell Univ-Weill Med Coll

Smith, Julia A MD/PhD (Onc) - **Spec Exp:** Breast Cancer; Breast Cancer-High Risk Women; **Hospital:** NYU Langone Med Ctr (page 106), Bellevue Hosp Ctr; **Address:** 530 First Ave, Ste 4-G, NYU Medical Ctr, New York, NY 10016; **Phone:** 212-263-7269; **Board Cert:** Internal Medicine 1985; Medical Oncology 1989; **Med School:** NYU Sch Med 1980; **Resid:** Internal Medicine, Brigham & Womens Hosp 1983; **Fellow:** Hematology & Oncology, Meml Sloan Kettering Cancer Ctr 1986; **Fac Appt:** Asst Clin Prof Med, NYU Sch Med

Speyer, James MD (Onc) - **Spec Exp:** Ovarian Cancer; Breast Cancer; Cardiac Toxicity in Cancer Therapy; **Hospital:** NYU Langone Med Ctr (page 106); **Address:** NYU Clinical Cancer Center, 160 E 34th St Fl 8, New York, NY 10016-4750; **Phone:** 212-731-5432; **Board Cert:** Internal Medicine 1977; Hematology 1978; Medical Oncology 1979; **Med School:** Johns Hopkins Univ 1974; **Resid:** Internal Medicine, Columbia-Presby Med Ctr 1976; Hematology, Columbia-Presby Med Ctr 1977; **Fellow:** Medical Oncology, Natl Cancer Inst 1979; **Fac Appt:** Prof Med, NYU Sch Med

Spriggs, David R MD (Onc) - **Spec Exp:** Ovarian Cancer; Drug Development; Uterine Cancer; Gynecologic Cancer; **Hospital:** Meml Sloan-Kettering Cancer Ctr (page 112); **Address:** 1275 York Avenue, New York, NY 10065; **Phone:** 800-525-2225; **Board Cert:** Internal Medicine 1981; Medical Oncology 2006; **Med School:** Univ Wisc 1977; **Resid:** Internal Medicine, Columbia-Presby Hosp 1981; **Fellow:** Medical Oncology, Dana-Farber Cancer Inst 1985; **Fac Appt:** Prof Med, Cornell Univ-Weill Med Coll

Stoopler, Mark MD (Onc) - **Spec Exp:** Lung Cancer; Esophageal Cancer; Unknown Primary Cancer; **Hospital:** NY-Presby Hosp/Columbia (page 104); **Address:** 161 Fort Washington Ave, Ste 936, New York, NY 10032-3713; **Phone:** 212-305-8230; **Board Cert:** Internal Medicine 1978; Medical Oncology 1981; **Med School:** Cornell Univ-Weill Med Coll 1975; **Resid:** Internal Medicine, North Shore Univ Hosp 1978; Internal Medicine, NY Meml Hosp 1978; **Fellow:** Medical Oncology, Meml-Sloan Kettering Cancer Ctr 1980; **Fac Appt:** Assoc Clin Prof Med, Columbia P&S

Straus, David J MD (Onc) - **Spec Exp:** Lymphoma; Multiple Myeloma; **Hospital:** Meml Sloan-Kettering Cancer Ctr (page 112); **Address:** 1275 York Avenue, New York, NY 10065; **Phone:** 212-639-8365; **Board Cert:** Internal Medicine 1972; Hematology 1976; Medical Oncology 1977; **Med School:** Marquette Sch Med 1969; **Resid:** Internal Medicine, Montefiore Med Ctr 1972; Medical Oncology, Meml Sloan Kettering Cancer Ctr 1977; **Fellow:** Hematology, Beth Israel Hosp 1973; **Fac Appt:** Prof Med, Cornell Univ-Weill Med Coll

Tagawa, Scott T MD (Onc) - **Spec Exp:** Prostate Cancer; Bladder Cancer; Kidney Cancer; Urologic Cancer; **Hospital:** NY-Presby Hosp/Weill Cornell (page 104); **Address:** NY Presby-Cornell Medical Ctr, 525 E 68th St, Starr Bldg - Ste 341, New York, NY 10065; **Phone:** 212-746-5360; **Board Cert:** Internal Medicine 2001; Medical Oncology 2005; Hematology 2006; **Med School:** USC-Keck School of Medicine 1998; **Resid:** Internal Medicine, USC Med Ctr 2001; **Fellow:** Medical Oncology, USC Med Ctr 2003; Hematology, USC Med Ctr 2004; **Fac Appt:** Asst Prof Med, Cornell Univ-Weill Med Coll

Vahdat, Linda MD (Onc) - **Spec Exp:** Breast Cancer; **Hospital:** NY-Presby Hosp/Weill Cornell (page 104); **Address:** 425 E 61st St Fl 8, New York, NY 10021; **Phone:** 212-821-0644; **Board Cert:** Medical Oncology 2005; **Med School:** Mount Sinai Sch Med 1987; **Resid:** Internal Medicine, Mt Sinai Hosp 1990; **Fellow:** Hematology & Oncology, Meml Sloan Kettering Cancer Ctr 1994; **Fac Appt:** Assoc Prof Med, Cornell Univ-Weill Med Coll

Zelenetz, Andrew D MD/PhD (Onc) - **Spec Exp:** Lymphoma; **Hospital:** Meml Sloan-Kettering Cancer Ctr (page 112); **Address:** 1275 York Avenue, New York, NY 10065; **Phone:** 800-525-2225; **Board Cert:** Medical Oncology 2009; **Med School:** Harvard Med Sch 1984; **Resid:** Internal Medicine, Stanford Univ Med Ctr 1986; **Fellow:** Medical Oncology, Stanford Univ Med Ctr 1991; **Fac Appt:** Asst Prof Med, Cornell Univ-Weill Med Coll

Neonatal-Perinatal Medicine

Bateman, David MD (NP) - **Spec Exp:** Critical Care; **Hospital:** NY-Presby Hosp/Columbia (page 104); **Address:** 3959 Broadway, CHN1-115, New York, NY 10037; **Phone:** 212-305-5827; **Board Cert:** Pediatrics 1979; Neonatal-Perinatal Medicine 1981; **Med School:** Tufts Univ 1973; **Resid:** Pediatrics, Lincoln Hosp 1975; Pediatrics, Boston Fltg Hosp 1977; **Fellow:** Neonatal-Perinatal Medicine, Colum-Presby Med Ctr 1982; **Fac Appt:** Assoc Prof Ped, Columbia P&S

Hendricks-Munoz, Karen MD (NP) - **Spec Exp:** Breathing Disorders; Neonatal Neurology; Retinopathy of Prematurity; **Hospital:** NYU Langone Med Ctr (page 106), Bellevue Hosp Ctr; **Address:** NYU Med Ctr, Dept Neonatology, 530 1st Ave, Ste HCC-7A, New York, NY 10016-6402; **Phone:** 212-263-7477; **Board Cert:** Pediatrics 1985; Neonatal-Perinatal Medicine 2009; **Med School:** Yale Univ 1978; **Resid:** Pediatrics, Yale-New Haven Hosp 1981; **Fellow:** Neonatology, Strong Meml Hosp 1984; **Fac Appt:** Assoc Prof Ped, NYU Sch Med

Marron-Corwin, Mary MD (NP) - **Spec Exp:** Neonatal Respiratory Care; Critical Care; Neonatal Liver Disease; **Hospital:** Harlem Hosp Ctr; **Address:** 506 Lenox Ave, MLK Pavilion, Ste 4419, New York, NY 10037; **Phone:** 212-939-8457; **Board Cert:** Pediatrics 2001; Neonatal-Perinatal Medicine 2008; **Med School:** Philippines 1985; **Resid:** Pediatrics, St Vincents Hosp Med Ctr 1988; **Fellow:** Neonatal-Perinatal Medicine, Babies Hosp/Colum-Presby Med Ctr 1990; **Fac Appt:** Assoc Prof Ped, Columbia P&S

Perlman, Jeffrey M MD (NP) - **Spec Exp:** Neonatal Critical Care; Prematurity/Low Birth Weight Infants; Neonatal Neurology; Lung Disease in Newborns; **Hospital:** NY-Presby Hosp/Weill Cornell (page 104); **Address:** 525 E 68th St, Ste N 506, New York, NY 10065; **Phone:** 212-746-3530; **Board Cert:** Pediatrics 1983; Neonatal-Perinatal Medicine 1983; **Med School:** South Africa 1974; **Resid:** Pediatrics, Johannesburg Chldns Hosp 1979; Pediatrics, St Louis Chldns Hosp 1981; **Fellow:** Neonatology, St Louis Chldns Hosp 1983; **Fac Appt:** Prof Ped, Cornell Univ-Weill Med Coll

Polin, Richard A MD (NP) - **Spec Exp:** Neonatal Infections; **Hospital:** NYPresby-Morgan Stanley Children's Hosp (page 104); **Address:** Morgan Stanley Chlds Hosp, 3959 Broadway, CHC 115, New York, NY 10032; **Phone:** 212-305-5827; **Board Cert:** Pediatrics 1975; Neonatal-Perinatal Medicine 1977; **Med School:** Temple Univ 1970; **Resid:** Pediatrics, Chldns Meml Hosp 1972; Pediatrics, Babies Hosp 1975; **Fellow:** Neonatal-Perinatal Medicine, Babies Hosp-Columbia 1974; **Fac Appt:** Prof Ped, Columbia P&S

Rosen, Tove S MD (NP) - **Spec Exp:** Neonatology; Substance Abuse Effects in Newborn; Ethics; **Hospital:** NYPresby-Morgan Stanley Children's Hosp (page 104); **Address:** Morgan Stanley Chldns Hosp of NY-Presby, 3959 Broadway, CHN 1201, New York, NY 10032-1559; **Phone:** 212-305-8500; **Board Cert:** Pediatrics 1971; Neonatal-Perinatal Medicine 1975; **Med School:** SUNY Hlth Sci Ctr 1965; **Resid:** Pediatrics, St Luke's Hosp 1970; **Fellow:** Neonatal-Perinatal Medicine, Columbia-Presby Med Ctr 1974; **Fac Appt:** Clin Prof Ped, Columbia P&S

Shahrivar, Farrokh MD (NP) - **Spec Exp:** Neonatology; Prematurity/Low Birth Weight Infants; **Hospital:** St Luke's - Roosevelt Hosp Ctr - Roosevelt Div (page 94), Beth Israel Med Ctr - Petrie Division (page 94); **Address:** 1000 10th Ave NICU Fl 12, New York, NY 10019-1192; **Phone:** 212-523-3760; **Board Cert:** Pediatrics 1974; Neonatal-Perinatal Medicine 1975; **Med School:** Iran 1966; **Resid:** Pediatrics, St Luke's-Roosevelt Hosp Ctr 1971; Pediatrics, St Luke's-Roosevelt Hosp Ctr 1972; **Fellow:** Neonatal-Perinatal Medicine, St Christopher's Hosp 1973; Neonatal-Perinatal Medicine, Montefiore Med Ctr 1973; **Fac Appt:** Assoc Clin Prof Ped, Columbia P&S

Nephrology

Ames, Richard MD (Nep) - **Spec Exp:** Hypertension; Kidney Disease; Dialysis Care; **Hospital:** St Luke's - Roosevelt Hosp Ctr - Roosevelt Div (page 94); **Address:** 1886 Broadway, New York, NY 10023-7033; **Phone:** 917-224-4270; **Board Cert:** Internal Medicine 1974; Nephrology 1972; Medical Oncology 1973; Hematology 1974; **Med School:** Columbia P&S 1958; **Resid:** Internal Medicine, Boston Med Ctr 1961; **Fellow:** Nephrology, Columbia-Presby Hosp 1963; **Fac Appt:** Clin Prof Med, Columbia P&S

Appel, Gerald MD (Nep) - **Spec Exp:** Glomerulonephritis; Lupus Nephritis; Nephrotic Syndrome; **Hospital:** NY-Presby Hosp/Columbia (page 104); **Address:** 622 W 168th St, Ste PH4-124, New York, NY 10032-3720; **Phone:** 212-305-0320; **Board Cert:** Internal Medicine 1975; Nephrology 1978; **Med School:** Albert Einstein Coll Med 1972; **Resid:** Internal Medicine, Columbia Presby Hosp 1975; **Fellow:** Nephrology, Columbia Presby Hosp 1976; Nephrology, Yale-New Haven Hosp 1978; **Fac Appt:** Clin Prof Med, Columbia P&S

August, Phyllis MD (Nep) - **Spec Exp:** Hypertension; Hypertension in Pregnancy; **Hospital:** NY-Presby Hosp/Weill Cornell (page 104); **Address:** 450 E 69th St, Hypertension Center, New York, NY 10021-4870; **Phone:** 212-746-2210; **Board Cert:** Internal Medicine 1980; Nephrology 1982; **Med School:** Yale Univ 1977; **Resid:** Internal Medicine, NY Hosp-Cornell Med Ctr 1980; **Fellow:** Nephrology, NY Hosp-Cornell Med Ctr 1983; **Fac Appt:** Prof Med, Cornell Univ-Weill Med Coll

Blumenfeld, Jon D MD (Nep) - **Spec Exp:** Hypertension; Polycystic Kidney Disease; Adrenal Disorders; **Hospital:** NY-Presby Hosp/Weill Cornell (page 104), Rockefeller Univ; **Address:** The Rogosin Institute, 505 E 70th St Fl 2, New York, NY 10021; **Phone:** 212-746-1495; **Board Cert:** Internal Medicine 1984; Nephrology 1986; **Med School:** Yale Univ 1981; **Resid:** Internal Medicine, New York Hosp 1984; **Fellow:** Nephrology, Brigham & Womens Hosp 1988; **Fac Appt:** Prof Med, Cornell Univ-Weill Med Coll

Cohen, David J MD (Nep) - **Spec Exp:** Transplant Medicine-Kidney; Glomerulonephritis; **Hospital:** NY-Presby Hosp/Columbia (page 104); **Address:** Columbia Univ Med Ctr, 622 W 168th St, rm PH 4-124, New York, NY 10032-3720; **Phone:** 212-305-0320; **Board Cert:** Internal Medicine 1980; Nephrology 1984; **Med School:** Albert Einstein Coll Med 1977; **Resid:** Internal Medicine, Mount Sinai Hosp 1980; **Fellow:** Nephrology, Columbia-Presby Hosp 1981; Transplant Immunobiology, Brigham & Womens Hosp 1983; **Fac Appt:** Clin Prof Med, Columbia P&S

De Fabritus, Albert MD (Nep) - **Spec Exp:** Kidney Disease-Chronic; Hypertension; Anemia in Chronic Kidney Disease; **Address:** 36 7th Ave, rm 418, New York, NY 10011; **Phone:** 212-807-8817; **Board Cert:** Internal Medicine 1976; Nephrology 1978; **Med School:** NY Med Coll 1973; **Resid:** Internal Medicine, St Vincent's Hosp & Med Ctr 1976; **Fellow:** Nephrology, New York Hosp 1978; **Fac Appt:** Asst Clin Prof Med, NY Med Coll

Devita, Maria V MD (Nep) - **Spec Exp:** Glomerulonephritis; Dialysis Care; Hypertension; Kidney Disease-Chronic; **Hospital:** Lenox Hill Hosp; **Address:** 130 E 77th St, New York, NY 10075; **Phone:** 212-439-9251; **Board Cert:** Internal Medicine 1988; Nephrology 2002; **Med School:** Georgetown Univ 1984; **Resid:** Internal Medicine, Lenox Hill Hosp 1987; **Fellow:** Nephrology, Lenox Hill Hosp 1989; **Fac Appt:** Assoc Clin Prof Med, NYU Sch Med

Gardenswartz, Mark MD (Nep) - **Spec Exp:** Hypertension; Hypertension in Pregnancy; Polycystic Kidney Disease; **Hospital:** Lenox Hill Hosp, Mount Sinai Med Ctr (page 102); **Address:** 110 E 59th St, Ste 10B, New York, NY 10022; **Phone:** 212-583-2930; **Board Cert:** Internal Medicine 1978; Nephrology 1980; Critical Care Medicine 2002; **Med School:** Univ Colorado 1975; **Resid:** Internal Medicine, Columbia Presby Med Ctr 1978; **Fellow:** Nephrology, Univ Colorado Hosp 1978; **Fac Appt:** Asst Clin Prof Med, NY Med Coll

Garvey, Michael MD (Nep) - **Spec Exp:** Dialysis Care; **Hospital:** Beth Israel Med Ctr - Petrie Division (page 94); **Address:** 510-526 6th Ave, Ste 5C, New York, NY 10011; **Phone:** 212-807-7920; **Board Cert:** Internal Medicine 1979; Nephrology 1982; **Med School:** NY Med Coll 1975; **Resid:** Internal Medicine, St Vincent's Hosp & Med Ctr 1979; **Fellow:** Nephrology, NYU Med Ctr 1981

Liu, David T MD (Nep) - **Spec Exp:** Glomerulonephritis; Nephrotic Syndrome; Kidney Failure; Hypertension; **Hospital:** NYU Langone Med Ctr (page 106); **Address:** 530 1st Ave, Ste 4B, New York, NY 10016-6402; **Phone:** 212-263-0705; **Board Cert:** Internal Medicine 1980; Nephrology 1984; **Med School:** SUNY Buffalo 1977; **Resid:** Internal Medicine, Univ Miami Hosps 1980; **Fellow:** Nephrology, NYU Med Ctr 1984; **Fac Appt:** Asst Clin Prof Med, NYU Sch Med

Matalon, Robert MD (Nep) - **Spec Exp:** Dialysis Care; Kidney Failure; **Hospital:** NYU Langone Med Ctr (page 106), NY Downtown Hosp; **Address:** 530 1st Ave, Ste 4A, New York, NY 10016-6402; **Phone:** 212-263-7239; **Board Cert:** Internal Medicine 1970; Nephrology 1974; **Med School:** NYU Sch Med 1964; **Resid:** Internal Medicine, Bellevue Hosp 1967; **Fellow:** Nephrology, NYU Med Ctr 1969; **Fac Appt:** Assoc Prof Med, NYU Sch Med

Michelis, Michael F MD (Nep) - **Spec Exp:** Kidney Disease; Hypertension; Dialysis Care; **Hospital:** Lenox Hill Hosp; **Address:** 130 E 77th St, FL 5, New York, NY 10075-1851; **Phone:** 212-988-3506; **Board Cert:** Internal Medicine 1969; **Med School:** Geo Wash Univ 1963; **Resid:** Internal Medicine, Lenox Hill Hosp 1965; Internal Medicine, Hosp Med Coll Penn 1967; **Fellow:** Renal Disease, Univ Pittsburgh 1970; **Fac Appt:** Clin Prof Med, NYU Sch Med

Murphy, Barbara MD (Nep) - **Spec Exp:** Transplant Medicine-Kidney; **Hospital:** Mount Sinai Med Ctr (page 102); **Address:** 5 E 98th St Fl 12, New York, NY 10029; **Phone:** 212-659-8086; **Med School:** Ireland 1989; **Resid:** Internal Medicine, Beaumont Hosp 1992; **Fellow:** Nephrology, Beaumont Hosp 1993; Nephrology, Brigham & Women's Hosp 1997; **Fac Appt:** Prof Med, Mount Sinai Sch Med

Saal, Stuart MD (Nep) - **Spec Exp:** Transplant Medicine-Kidney; **Hospital:** NY-Presby Hosp/Weill Cornell (page 104); **Address:** 505 E 70th St, Ste 230, New York, NY 10021-4872; **Phone:** 212-746-1553; **Board Cert:** Internal Medicine 1974; Nephrology 1978; **Med School:** NY Med Coll 1971; **Resid:** Internal Medicine, St Luke's-Roosevelt Hosp Ctr 1974; **Fellow:** Nephrology, NY Hosp 1976; **Fac Appt:** Assoc Clin Prof Med, Cornell Univ-Weill Med Coll

Sherman, Raymond MD (Nep) - **Spec Exp:** Glomerulonephritis; Hypertension; Kidney Failure-Chronic; **Hospital:** NY-Presby Hosp/Weill Cornell (page 104); **Address:** 407 E 70th St Fl 4, New York, NY 10021-5302; **Phone:** 212-879-8245; **Board Cert:** Internal Medicine 1969; Nephrology 1974; **Med School:** SUNY Hlth Sci Ctr 1961; **Resid:** Internal Medicine, St Luke's-Roosevelt Hosp Ctr 1965; Nephrology, Strong Meml Hosp 1965; **Fellow:** Nephrology, NY Hosp/Cornell Med Ctr 1969; **Fac Appt:** Clin Prof Med, Cornell Univ-Weill Med Coll

Stern, Leonard MD (Nep) - **Spec Exp:** Kidney Failure-Chronic; Transplant Medicine-Kidney; Bone Disorders-Metabolic; Dialysis Care; **Hospital:** NY-Presby Hosp/Columbia (page 104); **Address:** 622 W 168th St, rm PH4-124, New York, NY 10032-3702; **Phone:** 212-305-0559; **Board Cert:** Internal Medicine 1978; Nephrology 1980; **Med School:** NY Med Coll 1975; **Resid:** Internal Medicine, Jacobi Med Ctr 1978; **Fellow:** Nephrology, Montefiore Med Ctr 1979; Nephrology, Yale-New Haven Hosp 1981; **Fac Appt:** Assoc Clin Prof Med, Columbia P&S

Wang, John C MD (Nep) - **Spec Exp:** Hypertension; **Hospital:** NY-Presby Hosp/Weill Cornell (page 104); **Address:** 505 E 70th St, rm 213, New York, NY 10021; **Phone:** 212-746-3097; **Board Cert:** Internal Medicine 1985; Nephrology 1986; **Med School:** Cornell Univ-Weill Med Coll 1979; **Resid:** Internal Medicine, Laguardia Hosp 1982; **Fellow:** Nephrology, NY Hosp 1984

Weisstuch, Joseph M MD (Nep) - **Hospital:** NYU Langone Med Ctr (page 106), NYU Hosp For Joint Diseases (page 106); **Address:** 530 1st Ave, Ste 4B, New York, NY 10016-6402; **Phone:** 212-263-0705; **Board Cert:** Internal Medicine 1988; Nephrology 2002; **Med School:** NYU Sch Med 1985; **Resid:** Internal Medicine, NYU Med Ctr 1989; **Fellow:** Nephrology, Bellevue Hosp 1991; **Fac Appt:** Asst Clin Prof Med, NYU Sch Med

Winchester, James F MD (Nep) - **Spec Exp:** Dialysis Care; **Hospital:** Beth Israel Med Ctr - Petrie Division (page 94); **Address:** 10 Union Square E, Ste 2F, New York, NY 10003; **Phone:** 212-420-4070; **Board Cert:** Internal Medicine 2007; **Med School:** Scotland, UK 1969; **Resid:** Internal Medicine, Royal Infirmiry 1972; **Fellow:** Nephrology, Royal Infirmiry 1974

Winston, Jonathan MD (Nep) - **Spec Exp:** Kidney Disease-Chronic; Kidney Failure; HIV Related Kidney Disease; Glomerulonephritis; **Hospital:** Mount Sinai Med Ctr (page 102); **Address:** 5 E 98th St Fl 11, New York, NY 10029-6501; **Phone:** 212-241-4060; **Board Cert:** Internal Medicine 1980; Nephrology 1984; **Med School:** Geo Wash Univ 1977; **Resid:** Internal Medicine, LI Jewish Med Ctr 1980; **Fellow:** Nephrology, Mt Sinai Hosp 1982; **Fac Appt:** Assoc Prof Med, Mount Sinai Sch Med

Neurological Surgery

Bederson, Joshua B MD (NS) - **Spec Exp:** Brain & Spinal Cord Tumors; Aneurysm-Cerebral; Meningioma; Pituitary Tumors; **Hospital:** Mount Sinai Med Ctr (page 102); **Address:** Mount Sinai Med Ctr, 1 Gustave Levy Pl, Box 1136, New York, NY 10029; **Phone:** 212-241-2377; **Board Cert:** Neurological Surgery 1993; **Med School:** UCSF 1984; **Resid:** Neurological Surgery, UCSF Med Ctr 1990; **Fellow:** Neurological Vascular Surgery, Barrow Neur Inst 1990; Neurological Vascular Surgery, Univ Hosp Zurich 1990; **Fac Appt:** Prof NS, Mount Sinai Sch Med

Bilsky, Mark H MD (NS) - **Spec Exp:** Spinal Tumors; Skull Base Tumors; Brain Tumors; Spinal Reconstructive Surgery; **Hospital:** Meml Sloan-Kettering Cancer Ctr (page 112), NY-Presby Hosp/Weill Cornell (page 104); **Address:** 1275 York Avenue, New York, NY 10065; **Phone:** 212-639-8526; **Board Cert:** Neurological Surgery 1999; **Med School:** Emory Univ 1988; **Resid:** Neurological Surgery, NY Hosp-Cornell Med Ctr 1994; **Fellow:** Neuro-Oncology, Louisville Univ Med Ctr 1995; **Fac Appt:** Assoc Prof NS, Cornell Univ-Weill Med Coll

Boockvar, John MD (NS) - **Spec Exp:** Brain Tumors; Gliomas; Pituitary Tumors; Minimally Invasive Surgery; **Hospital:** NY-Presby Hosp/Weill Cornell (page 104); **Address:** 525 68 St, Box 99, New York, NY 10065; **Phone:** 212-746-1996; **Board Cert:** Neurological Surgery 2007; **Med School:** SUNY Downstate 1997; **Resid:** Neurological Surgery, Hosp Univ Penn 2003; **Fellow:** Neuro-Oncology, Univ Penn Cancer Ctr 2004; **Fac Appt:** Asst Prof NS, Cornell Univ-Weill Med Coll

Bruce, Jeffrey MD (NS) - **Spec Exp:** Brain Tumors; Pituitary Tumors; Skull Base Surgery; Meningioma; **Hospital:** NY-Presby Hosp/Columbia (page 104); **Address:** NY Presby Hosp, Dept Neurosurgery, 710 W 168th St N1 Bldg Fl 4 - rm 434, New York, NY 10032; **Phone:** 212-305-7346; **Board Cert:** Neurological Surgery 1993; **Med School:** UMDNJ-RW Johnson Med Sch 1983; **Resid:** Neurological Surgery, Columbia-Presby Med Ctr 1990; **Fellow:** Neurological Surgery, Nat Inst Hlth 1985; **Fac Appt:** Prof NS, Columbia P&S

Chen, Chun Siang MD (NS) - **Spec Exp:** Skull Base Tumors; Skull Base Surgery; Microsurgery; Brain & Spinal Surgery; **Hospital:** Mount Sinai Med Ctr (page 102); **Address:** Mount Sinai Med Ctr, Annenberg Bldg, One Gustave L Levy Pl Fl 8 - rm 10, New York, NY 10029; **Phone:** 212-241-8480; **Med School:** Brazil 1978; **Resid:** Neurological Surgery, Santa Casa de Misericordia of Sao Paulo Med Sch 1983; Neurological Surgery, Mt Sinai Med Ctr 2005; **Fellow:** Skull Base Surgery, St Lukes Roosevelt Hosp 2006; **Fac Appt:** Asst Prof NS, Mount Sinai Sch Med

Di Giacinto, George V MD (NS) - **Spec Exp:** Spinal Surgery; Pain Management; **Hospital:** St Luke's - Roosevelt Hosp Ctr - Roosevelt Div (page 94); **Address:** 425 W 59th St, Ste 4E, New York, NY 10019; **Phone:** 212-523-8500; **Board Cert:** Neurological Surgery 1981; **Med School:** Harvard Med Sch 1970; **Resid:** Neurological Surgery, Columbia-Presby Hosp 1978

Feldstein, Neil A MD (NS) - **Spec Exp:** Pediatric Neurosurgery; Chiari's Deformity; Brain Tumors-Pediatric; Spinal Cord Surgery-Pediatric; **Hospital:** NY-Presby Hosp/Columbia (page 104); **Address:** Neurological Inst, 710 W 168th St Fl 2 - rm 213, New York, NY 10032; **Phone:** 212-305-1396; **Board Cert:** Neurological Surgery 1995; Pediatric Neurological Surgery 2007; **Med School:** NYU Sch Med 1984; **Resid:** Neurological Surgery, Baylor Coll Med 1989; **Fellow:** Pediatric Neurological Surgery, NYU Med Ctr 1991; **Fac Appt:** Assoc Prof NS, Columbia P&S

Frempong-Boadu, Anthony K MD (NS) - **Spec Exp:** Spinal Cord Injury-Complex; Minimally Invasive Spinal Surgery; Spinal Cord Tumors; Spinal Reconstructive Surgery; **Hospital:** NYU Langone Med Ctr (page 106); **Address:** NYU Med Ctr, Dept Neurosurgery, 550 1st Ave, New York, NY 10016; **Phone:** 212-263-6514; **Board Cert:** Neurological Surgery 2004; **Med School:** Temple Univ 1992; **Resid:** Neurological Surgery, NYU Med Ctr 1998; **Fellow:** Spinal Surgery, NYU Med Ctr 1999; Minimally Invasive Surgery, Univ Florida/Shands Hosp 2000; **Fac Appt:** Asst Prof NS, NYU Sch Med

Gamache Jr, Francis W MD (NS) - **Spec Exp:** Brain & Spinal Cord Tumors; Spinal Surgery-Neck; **Hospital:** NY-Presby Hosp/Weill Cornell (page 104), Hosp For Special Surgery (page 111); **Address:** 523 E 72nd St Fl 8, New York, NY 10021-4099; **Phone:** 212-988-5200; **Board Cert:** Neurological Surgery 1982; **Med School:** Cornell Univ-Weill Med Coll 1971; **Resid:** Surgery, NY Hosp-Cornell Med Ctr 1975; Neurological Surgery, NY Hosp-Cornell Med Ctr 1979; **Fellow:** Trauma, MD Inst Emerg Med Serv 1979; Neurological Vascular Surgery, Univ West Ontario 1980; **Fac Appt:** Clin Prof NS, Cornell Univ-Weill Med Coll

Golfinos, John G MD (NS) - **Spec Exp:** Brain Tumors; Acoustic Neuroma; Stereotactic Radiosurgery; Skull Base Surgery; **Hospital:** NYU Langone Med Ctr (page 106), Lenox Hill Hosp; **Address:** NYU Med Ctr, Dept Neurosurgery, 530 1st Ave, Ste 8R, New York, NY 10016-6402; **Phone:** 212-263-2950; **Board Cert:** Neurological Surgery 1998; **Med School:** Columbia P&S 1988; **Resid:** Neurological Surgery, Barrow Neuro Inst 1995

Goodman, Robert R MD/PhD (NS) - **Spec Exp:** Parkinson's Disease/Movement Disorders; Epilepsy; Trigeminal Neuralgia; Hydrocephalus-Adult; **Hospital:** NY-Presby Hosp/Columbia (page 104), Valley Hosp (page 658); **Address:** 710 W 168th St, rm 426, New York, NY 10032-2603; **Phone:** 212-305-3774; **Board Cert:** Neurological Surgery 1993; **Med School:** Johns Hopkins Univ 1982; **Resid:** Neurological Surgery, Columbia-Presby Med Ctr 1989; **Fac Appt:** Assoc Prof NS, Columbia P&S

Gutin, Philip MD (NS) - **Spec Exp:** Brain Tumors; Meningioma; Acoustic Neuroma; **Hospital:** Meml Sloan-Kettering Cancer Ctr (page 112), NY-Presby Hosp/Weill Cornell (page 104); **Address:** 1275 York Avenue, New York, NY 10065; **Phone:** 212-639-8556; **Board Cert:** Neurological Surgery 1981; **Med School:** Univ Pennsylvania 1971; **Resid:** Neurological Surgery, UCSF Med Ctr 1979; **Fellow:** Neurological Surgery, Natl Cancer Inst 1976; **Fac Appt:** Prof NS, Cornell Univ-Weill Med Coll

Hartl, Roger MD (NS) - **Spec Exp:** Spinal Surgery-Complex; Minimally Invasive Spinal Surgery; Spinal Disc Replacement; **Hospital:** NY-Presby Hosp/Weill Cornell (page 104); **Address:** Cornell Neurosurgery, 525 E 68th St, Starr 651, New York, NY 10065; **Phone:** 212-746-2152; **Board Cert:** Neurological Surgery 2008; **Med School:** Germany 1993; **Resid:** Neurological Surgery, NY Presby-Cornell Med Ctr 2003; **Fellow:** Spinal Surgery, Barrow Neurological Inst

Hirschfeld, Alan D MD (NS) - **Spec Exp:** Brain Tumors; **Hospital:** Lutheran Med Ctr - Brooklyn; **Address:** Dept Neurosurgery, 170 W 12th St NR Bldg - rm 809, New York, NY 10011; **Phone:** 212-604-7767; **Board Cert:** Neurological Surgery 1986; **Med School:** NYU Sch Med 1977; **Resid:** Surgery, NYU-Bellevue Hosp 1978; Neurological Surgery, NYU-Bellevue Hosp 1982; **Fac Appt:** Assoc Prof S, NY Med Coll

Holtzman, Robert N N MD (NS) - **Spec Exp:** Brain & Spinal Cord Tumors; Spinal Surgery; Aneurysm-Cerebral; Chiari's Deformity; **Hospital:** Lenox Hill Hosp, NY-Presby Hosp/Columbia (page 104); **Address:** 247 3rd Ave, Ste 403, New York, NY 10010-7455; **Phone:** 212-529-3580; **Board Cert:** Neurology 1978; Neurological Surgery 1980; **Med School:** Columbia P&S 1969; **Resid:** Surgery, Harbor Genl Hosp 1973; Neurological Surgery, New York Neurological Inst 1977; **Fac Appt:** Assoc Clin Prof NS, Columbia P&S

Huang, Paul MD (NS) - **Spec Exp:** Brain Tumors; Spinal Disorders-Degenerative; Vascular Neurosurgery; Pituitary Tumors; **Hospital:** NY Downtown Hosp, NYU Langone Med Ctr (page 106); **Address:** 170 Williams St, New York, NY 10038; **Phone:** 212-312-5321; **Board Cert:** Neurological Surgery 1998; **Med School:** Columbia P&S 1989; **Resid:** Neurological Surgery, NYU Med Ctr 1996

Jafar, Jafar J MD (NS) - **Spec Exp:** Aneurysm-Cerebral; Brain Tumors; Skull Base Tumors; Acoustic Neuroma; **Hospital:** NYU Langone Med Ctr (page 106), Lenox Hill Hosp; **Address:** 530 1st Ave, Ste 8R, New York, NY 10016-6402; **Phone:** 212-263-6312; **Board Cert:** Neurological Surgery 1984; **Med School:** Iran 1976; **Resid:** Neurological Surgery, Univ Chicago Hosps 1982; Neurological Surgery, Natl Hosp for Nervous Disease; **Fac Appt:** Prof NS, NYU Sch Med

Kaiser, Michael G MD (NS) - **Spec Exp:** Spinal Surgery-Complex; Minimally Invasive Spinal Surgery; Spinal Disc Replacement; **Hospital:** NY-Presby Hosp/Columbia (page 104); **Address:** Neurological Institute, Dept Neurological Surgery, 710 W 168th St, New York, NY 10032; **Phone:** 212-305-0378; **Board Cert:** Neurological Surgery 2004; **Med School:** Yale Univ 1994; **Resid:** Neurological Surgery, Columbia Neuro Inst 2000; **Fellow:** Spinal Surgery, Emory Univ 2001; **Fac Appt:** Asst Prof NS, Columbia P&S

Kaplitt, Michael G MD/PhD (NS) - **Spec Exp:** Parkinson's Disease/Movement Disorders; Deep Brain Stimulation; Trigeminal Neuralgia; Hydrocephalus; **Hospital:** NY-Presby Hosp/Weill Cornell (page 104); **Address:** 525 E 68th St, Box 99, New York, NY 10065; **Phone:** 212-746-4966; **Board Cert:** Neurological Surgery 2005; **Med School:** Cornell Univ-Weill Med Coll 1995; **Resid:** Neurological Surgery, New York Hosp 2000; **Fellow:** Stereo Neurological Surgery, Toronto Western Hosp 2001; **Fac Appt:** Assoc Prof NS, Cornell Univ-Weill Med Coll

Lavyne, Michael H MD (NS) - **Spec Exp:** Spinal Surgery; Spinal Tumors; Spinal Disorders; **Hospital:** NY-Presby Hosp/Weill Cornell (page 104), Hosp For Special Surgery (page 111); **Address:** 110 E 55th St Fl 9, New York, NY 10022; **Phone:** 212-486-9100; **Board Cert:** Neurological Surgery 1982; **Med School:** Cornell Univ-Weill Med Coll 1972; **Resid:** Neurological Surgery, Mass Genl Hosp 1979; **Fellow:** Neurology, Beth Israel Hosp 1974; **Fac Appt:** Clin Prof NS, Cornell Univ-Weill Med Coll

McCormick, Paul C MD (NS) - **Spec Exp:** Spinal Surgery; Spinal Tumors; **Hospital:** NY-Presby Hosp/Columbia (page 104), Valley Hosp (page 658); **Address:** 710 W 168th St, Ste 506, New York, NY 10032-2603; **Phone:** 212-305-7976; **Board Cert:** Neurological Surgery 1993; **Med School:** Columbia P&S 1982; **Resid:** Neurological Surgery, Columbia Presby Med Ctr 1989; **Fellow:** Neurological Surgery, Natl Inst Hlth 1984; Spinal Surgery, Med Coll Wisconsin 1990; **Fac Appt:** Prof NS, Columbia P&S

Moore, Frank M MD (NS) - **Spec Exp:** Aneurysm-Cerebral; Brain Tumors; Spinal Cord Tumors; Spinal Surgery; **Hospital:** Mount Sinai Med Ctr (page 102), Englewood Hosp & Med Ctr (page 656); **Address:** 1158 5th Ave, New York, NY 10029-6917; **Phone:** 212-410-6990; **Board Cert:** Neurological Surgery 1992; **Med School:** France 1983; **Resid:** Neurological Surgery, Mt Sinai Hosp 1988; **Fac Appt:** Assoc Prof NS, Mount Sinai Sch Med

Patel, Aman B MD (NS) - **Spec Exp:** Interventional Neuroradiology; Endovascular Neurosurgery; Aneurysm-Cerebral; Arteriovenous Malformations; **Hospital:** Mount Sinai Med Ctr (page 102); **Address:** One Gustave L Levy Place, Box 1136, New York, NY 10029; **Phone:** 212-241-3457; **Board Cert:** Neurological Surgery 2004; **Med School:** UCLA 1993; **Resid:** Neurological Surgery, UCLA Med Ctr 1999; **Fellow:** Interventional Neuroradiology, UCLA Med Ctr 2001; **Fac Appt:** Assoc Prof NS, Mount Sinai Sch Med

Perin, Noel I MD (NS) - **Spec Exp:** Spinal Surgery-Minimally Invasive; Spinal Tumors; **Hospital:** St Luke's - Roosevelt Hosp Ctr - Roosevelt Div (page 94); **Address:** Dept Neurosurgery, 1000 10th Ave, Ste 5G80, New York, NY 10019; **Phone:** 212-523-6720; **Board Cert:** Neurological Surgery 1995; **Med School:** Sri Lanka 1973; **Resid:** Neurological Surgery, NYU Med Ctr 1990; **Fellow:** Spinal Surgery, NYU Med Ctr 1991; **Fac Appt:** Asst Prof NS, Mount Sinai Sch Med

Quest, Donald O MD (NS) - **Spec Exp:** Spinal Surgery; Neurovascular Surgery; Carotid Artery Surgery; **Hospital:** NY-Presby Hosp/Columbia (page 104), Valley Hosp (page 658); **Address:** 710 W 168th St, Ste 440, New York, NY 10032; **Phone:** 212-305-5582; **Board Cert:** Neurological Surgery 1978; **Med School:** Columbia P&S 1970; **Resid:** Surgery, Mass Genl Hosp 1972; Neurological Surgery, Columbia-Presby Hosp 1976; **Fac Appt:** Clin Prof NS, Columbia P&S

Riina, Howard A MD (NS) - **Spec Exp:** Neuroradiology; Aneurysm-Cerebral; Cerebrovascular Malformations; Stroke; **Hospital:** NY-Presby Hosp/Weill Cornell (page 104); **Address:** 525 E 68th St, Starr 651, Nwe York, NY 10021; **Phone:** 212-746-5149; **Board Cert:** Neurological Surgery 2004; **Med School:** Temple Univ 1993; **Resid:** Neurological Surgery, Hosp Univ Penn 2000; **Fellow:** Interventional Neuroradiology, Beth Israel Med Ctr 1997; Skull Base Surgery, Barrow Neuro Inst 2001; **Fac Appt:** Assoc Prof NS, Cornell Univ-Weill Med Coll

Schwartz, Theodore H MD (NS) - **Spec Exp:** Brain Tumors; Pituitary Tumors; Epilepsy; Endoscopic Surgery; **Hospital:** NY-Presby Hosp/Weill Cornell (page 104); **Address:** Cornell Neurosurgery, 525 E 68th St, Starr Pavilion, rm 651, New York, NY 10021; **Phone:** 212-746-5620; **Board Cert:** Neurological Surgery 2002; **Med School:** Harvard Med Sch 1993; **Resid:** Neurological Surgery, Columbia-Presby Med Ctr 1999; **Fellow:** Neurological Surgery, Yale-New Haven Med Ctr 2000; **Fac Appt:** Assoc Prof NS, Cornell Univ-Weill Med Coll

Sen, Chandranath MD (NS) - **Spec Exp:** Brain Tumors; Skull Base Tumors; Skull Base Surgery; **Hospital:** St Luke's - Roosevelt Hosp Ctr - Roosevelt Div (page 94); **Address:** St Lukes Roosevelt Hosp Ctr, Dept Neurosurgery, 1000 10th Ave, Ste 5G-80, New York, NY 10019; **Phone:** 212-523-6720; **Board Cert:** Neurological Surgery 1989; **Med School:** India 1976; **Resid:** Surgery, Univ Wisconsin Hosps 1980; Neurological Surgery, Univ Wisconsin Hosps 1985; **Fellow:** Microsurgery, Univ Pittsburgh Med Ctr 1986

Sisti, Michael B MD (NS) - **Spec Exp:** Acoustic Neuroma; Brain Tumors; Stereotactic Radiosurgery; Meningioma; **Hospital:** NY-Presby Hosp/Columbia (page 104); **Address:** 710 W 168th St, New York, NY 10032-2603; **Phone:** 212-305-1728; **Board Cert:** Neurological Surgery 1991; **Med School:** Columbia P&S 1981; **Resid:** Neurological Surgery, Neuro Inst-Columbia-Presby Med Ctr 1988; **Fellow:** Neurological Surgery, Natl Inst Hlth 1983; **Fac Appt:** Assoc Prof NS, Columbia P&S

Snow, Robert MD (NS) - **Spec Exp:** Spinal Surgery; Spinal Cord Tumors; Minimally Invasive Surgery; **Hospital:** NY-Presby Hosp/Weill Cornell (page 104); **Address:** 55 E 72nd St, New York, NY 10021-4099; **Phone:** 212-717-0256; **Board Cert:** Neurological Surgery 1989; **Med School:** Stanford Univ 1981; **Resid:** Neurological Surgery, New York Hosp 1986; **Fac Appt:** Prof NS, Cornell Univ-Weill Med Coll

Solomon, Robert A MD (NS) - **Spec Exp:** Aneurysm-Cerebral; Arteriovenous Malformations; **Hospital:** NY-Presby Hosp/Columbia (page 104); **Address:** 710 W 168th St, Ste 439, New York, NY 10032; **Phone:** 212-305-4118; **Board Cert:** Neurological Surgery 1988; **Med School:** Johns Hopkins Univ 1980; **Resid:** Neurological Surgery, Neuro Inst-Columbia 1986; **Fac Appt:** Prof NS, Columbia P&S

Souweidane, Mark M MD (NS) - **Spec Exp:** Pediatric Neurosurgery; Minimally Invasive Neurosurgery; Endoscopic Surgery; Brain Tumors-Pediatric; **Hospital:** NY-Presby Hosp/Weill Cornell (page 104), Meml Sloan-Kettering Cancer Ctr (page 112); **Address:** 525 E 68th St, Box 99, New York, NY 10065-4870; **Phone:** 212-746-2363; **Board Cert:** Neurological Surgery 1999; Pediatric Neurological Surgery 2000; **Med School:** Wayne State Univ 1988; **Resid:** Neurological Surgery, NYU Med Ctr 1994; **Fellow:** Pediatric Neurological Surgery, Hosp Sick Chldn 1995; **Fac Appt:** Prof NS, Cornell Univ-Weill Med Coll

Steinberger, Alfred A MD (NS) - **Spec Exp:** Spinal Cord Tumors; Aneurysm; Brain Tumors; Spinal Surgery; **Hospital:** Mount Sinai Med Ctr (page 102), Englewood Hosp & Med Ctr (page 656); **Address:** 1158 5th Ave, New York, NY 10029-6917; **Phone:** 212-410-6990; **Board Cert:** Neurological Surgery 1985; **Med School:** Columbia P&S 1976; **Resid:** Neurological Surgery, Neuro Inst-Columbia-Presby 1982; **Fac Appt:** Asst Clin Prof NS, Mount Sinai Sch Med

Stieg, Philip E MD/PhD (NS) - **Spec Exp:** Cerebrovascular Surgery; Acoustic Neuroma; Skull Base Surgery; Brain Tumors; **Hospital:** NY-Presby Hosp/Weill Cornell (page 104), Hosp For Special Surgery (page 111); **Address:** 525 E 68th St, STARR 651, New York, NY 10021-9800; **Phone:** 212-746-4684; **Board Cert:** Neurological Surgery 1992; **Med School:** Med Coll Wisc 1983; **Resid:** Neurological Surgery, Dallas Chldns Hosp/Parkland Meml Hosp 1988; **Fellow:** Neurological Biology, Karolinska Inst 1988; **Fac Appt:** Prof NS, Cornell Univ-Weill Med Coll

Tabar, Viviane MD (NS) - **Spec Exp:** Brain Tumors; **Hospital:** Meml Sloan-Kettering Cancer Ctr (page 112); **Address:** 1275 York Ave, New York, NY 10065; **Phone:** 212-639-3006; **Board Cert:** Neurological Surgery 2006; **Med School:** Amer Univ Beirut 1989; **Resid:** Neurological Surgery, Univ Mass Med Ctr 1998; **Fellow:** NIH/Natl Inst Neuro Dis & StrokeMeml Sloan Kettering Cancer Ctr

Weiner, Howard L MD (NS) - **Spec Exp:** Pediatric Neurosurgery; Epilepsy; Brain Tumors; Tuberous Sclerosis; **Hospital:** NYU Langone Med Ctr (page 106); **Address:** NYU Med Ctr, Div Pediatric Neurosurgery, 317 E 34th St, Ste 1002, New York, NY 10016; **Phone:** 212-263-6419; **Board Cert:** Neurological Surgery 2001; **Med School:** Cornell Univ 1989; **Resid:** Neurological Surgery, NYU Med Ctr 1996; **Fellow:** Pediatric Neurological Surgery, NYU Med Ctr 1997; **Fac Appt:** Prof NS, NYU Sch Med

Wisoff, Jeffrey H MD (NS) - **Spec Exp:** Pediatric Neurosurgery; Brain Tumors-Pediatric; Hydrocephalus; Chiari's Deformity; **Hospital:** NYU Langone Med Ctr (page 106), Maimonides Med Ctr (page 98); **Address:** 317 E 34th St, Ste 1002, New York, NY 10016-4974; **Phone:** 212-263-6419; **Board Cert:** Neurological Surgery 1990; Pediatric Neurological Surgery 2008; **Med School:** Geo Wash Univ 1978; **Resid:** Neurological Surgery, NYU/Bellevue Hosp 1984; **Fellow:** Pediatric Neurological Surgery, NYU Med Ctr 1985; **Fac Appt:** Assoc Prof NS, NYU Sch Med

Neurology

Apatoff, Brian R MD/PhD (N) - **Spec Exp:** Multiple Sclerosis; Neuro-Immunology; **Hospital:** NY-Presby Hosp/Weill Cornell (page 104); **Address:** Multiple Sclerosis Inst, Ctr for Neurologic Disease, 401 E 55th St, New York, NY 10022; **Phone:** 212-593-6262; **Board Cert:** Neurology 1991; **Med School:** Univ Chicago-Pritzker Sch Med 1984; **Resid:** Neurology, Columbia Presby Med Ctr 1990; **Fellow:** Multiple Sclerosis, Neuro Inst-Columbia Univ 1992; **Fac Appt:** Assoc Prof N, Cornell Univ-Weill Med Coll

Belok, Lennart C MD (N) - **Spec Exp:** Carpal Tunnel Syndrome; **Hospital:** Beth Israel Med Ctr - Petrie Division (page 94); **Address:** 410 E 20th St, New York, NY 10009-8113; **Phone:** 212-254-9716; **Board Cert:** Neurology 1983; Internal Medicine 1977; **Med School:** NY Med Coll 1973; **Resid:** Internal Medicine, Beth Israel Med Ctr 1976; Nephrology, New York Univ Med Ctr 1979

Brannagan III, Thomas H MD (N) - **Spec Exp:** Peripheral Neuropathy; Diabetic Neuropathy; **Hospital:** NY-Presby Hosp/Columbia (page 104); **Address:** Ciolumbia Univ Dept Neurology, 710 W 168th St, New York, NY 10032; **Phone:** 212-305-0405; **Board Cert:** Neurology 2005; Clinical Neurophysiology 2009; Electrodiagnostic Medicine ; **Med School:** Univ VA Sch Med 1990; **Resid:** Neurology, Columbia-Presby Med Ctr 1994; **Fellow:** Neuromuscular Disease, Columbia; Neurological Immunology, Columbia; **Fac Appt:** Assoc Clin Prof N, Columbia P&S

Bressman, Susan MD (N) - **Spec Exp:** Parkinson's Disease; Movement Disorders; Dystonia; **Hospital:** Beth Israel Med Ctr - Petrie Division (page 94); **Address:** 10 Union Square East, Ste 5J, New York, NY 10003-3314; **Phone:** 212-844-8379; **Board Cert:** Neurology 1983; **Med School:** Columbia P&S 1977; **Resid:** Neurology, Columbia-Presby Med Ctr 1981; **Fellow:** Movement Disorders, Columbia-Presby Med Ctr 1983; **Fac Appt:** Prof N, Albert Einstein Coll Med

Britton, Carolyn B MD (N) - **Spec Exp:** Neurologic Complications-HIV/Infections; Lyme Disease; Multiple Sclerosis; **Hospital:** NY-Presby Hosp/Columbia (page 104); **Address:** 710 W 168th St, Ste 232, New York, NY 10032-2603; **Phone:** 212-305-5220; **Board Cert:** Internal Medicine 1979; Neurology 1982; **Med School:** NYU Sch Med 1975; **Resid:** Internal Medicine, Harlem Hosp 1977; Neurology, Columbia-Presby Hosp 1980; **Fellow:** Neurology, Columbia-Presby Hosp 1983; **Fac Appt:** Assoc Prof N, Columbia P&S

Bronster, David J MD (N) - **Spec Exp:** Headache; Dizziness; Seizure Disorders; **Hospital:** Mount Sinai Med Ctr (page 102); **Address:** 3 E 83rd St, New York, NY 10028-0459; **Phone:** 212-772-0008; **Board Cert:** Neurology 1984; **Med School:** Mount Sinai Sch Med 1979; **Resid:** Neurology, Mount Sinai Hosp 1983; **Fac Appt:** Assoc Clin Prof N, Mount Sinai Sch Med

Brust, John C M MD (N) - **Spec Exp:** Stroke; Substance Abuse; Behavioral Neurology; **Hospital:** Harlem Hosp Ctr, NY-Presby Hosp/Columbia (page 104); **Address:** 506 Lenox Ave, rm 16-101, New York, NY 10037-1802; **Phone:** 212-939-4244; **Board Cert:** Neurology 2004; **Med School:** Columbia P&S 1962; **Resid:** Internal Medicine, Columbia Presby 1966; Neurology, Columbia Presby 1969; **Fac Appt:** Clin Prof N, Columbia P&S

Cafferty, Maureen S MD (N) - **Hospital:** St Luke's - Roosevelt Hosp Ctr - Roosevelt Div (page 94); **Address:** 1090 Amsterdam Ave, Ste 8B, New York, NY 10025-1737; **Phone:** 212-523-6770; **Board Cert:** Internal Medicine 1982; Neurology 1987; **Med School:** Columbia P&S 1979; **Resid:** Internal Medicine, St Luke's-Roosevelt Hosp Ctr 1982; Neurology, Columbia-Presby Hosp 1985; **Fac Appt:** Asst Prof N, Columbia P&S

Charney, Jonathan Z MD (N) - **Spec Exp:** Headache; Stroke; **Hospital:** Mount Sinai Med Ctr (page 102); **Address:** 1111 Park Ave, Ste 1H, New York, NY 10128-1234; **Phone:** 212-831-2886; **Board Cert:** Neurology 1977; **Med School:** NY Med Coll 1969; **Resid:** Neurology, Methodist Hosp-Baylor 1971; Neurology, Columbia-Presby Med Ctr 1973; **Fac Appt:** Asst Prof N, Mount Sinai Sch Med

Coll, Raymond MD (N) - **Spec Exp:** Multiple Sclerosis; Headache; Stroke; **Hospital:** NY-Presby Hosp/Weill Cornell (page 104); **Address:** 1365 York Ave, New York, NY 10021-4035; **Phone:** 212-249-0840; **Board Cert:** Neurology 1974; **Med School:** South Africa 1961; **Resid:** Neurology, NY Hosp 1971; **Fac Appt:** Assoc Clin Prof N, Cornell Univ-Weill Med Coll

Daras, Michael MD (N) - **Spec Exp:** Neuromuscular Disorders; **Hospital:** NY-Presby Hosp/Columbia (page 104); **Address:** 710 W 168 St, rm 246, New York, NY 10032; **Phone:** 212-305-6876; **Board Cert:** Neurology 1980; **Med School:** Greece 1969; **Resid:** Psychiatry, Elmhurst City Hosp 1976; Neurology, Metropolitan Hosp 1979; **Fellow:** Clinical Neurophysiology, Albert Einstein 1980; **Fac Appt:** Prof N, Columbia P&S

De Angelis, Lisa M MD (N) - **Spec Exp:** Neuro-Oncology; **Hospital:** Meml Sloan-Kettering Cancer Ctr (page 112); **Address:** 1275 York Avenue, New York, NY 10065; **Phone:** 212-639-7123; **Board Cert:** Neurology 1986; **Med School:** Columbia P&S 1980; **Resid:** Neurology, Neuro Inst-Presby Hosp 1984; **Fellow:** Neuro-Oncology, Neuro Inst-Presby Hosp 1985; Neuro-Oncology, Meml Sloan-Kettering Cancer Ctr 1986; **Fac Appt:** Prof N, Cornell Univ-Weill Med Coll

Devinsky, Orrin MD (N) - **Spec Exp:** Epilepsy; Tuberous Sclerosis; Behavioral Neurology; **Hospital:** NYU Langone Med Ctr (page 106), Saint Barnabas Med Ctr; **Address:** 223 E 34th St Fl Ground, New York, NY 10016-4972; **Phone:** 646-558-0803; **Board Cert:** Neurology 1987; Clinical Neurophysiology 1990; **Med School:** Harvard Med Sch 1982; **Resid:** Neurology, NY Hosp-Cornell Med Ctr 1986; **Fellow:** Epilepsy, Natl Inst Health 1988; **Fac Appt:** Prof N, NYU Sch Med

Engel, Murray MD (N) - **Hospital:** NY-Presby Hosp/Weill Cornell (page 104), Stamford Hosp (page 863); **Address:** 525 E 68th St, Box 91, New York, NY 10021; **Phone:** 212-746-3278; **Board Cert:** Pediatrics 1979; Neurology 1980; Neurodevelopmental Disabilities 2001; Clinical Neurophysiology 2005; **Med School:** Univ Chicago-Pritzker Sch Med 1972; **Resid:** Neurology, Yale-New Haven Hosp 1976; Neurology, Columbia Presby Med Ctr 1977; **Fac Appt:** Clin Prof Ped, Cornell Univ-Weill Med Coll

Fahn, Stanley MD (N) - **Spec Exp:** Movement Disorders; Parkinson's Disease; **Hospital:** NY-Presby Hosp/Columbia (page 104); **Address:** Neurological Institute, 710 W 168th St Fl 3 - rm 350, New York, NY 10032; **Phone:** 212-305-5277; **Board Cert:** Neurology 1968; **Med School:** UCSF 1958; **Resid:** Neurology, Neuro Inst-Columbia 1962; **Fellow:** Neurological Chemistry, Natl Inst Hlth 1968; **Fac Appt:** Prof N, Columbia P&S

Feinberg, Todd E MD (N) - **Spec Exp:** Alzheimer's Disease; Dementia; **Hospital:** Beth Israel Med Ctr - Petrie Division (page 94); **Address:** Beth Israel Med Ctr, Yarmon Neurobehavioral Ctr, First Ave at 16th St, New York, NY 10003; **Phone:** 212-420-4111; **Board Cert:** Psychiatry 1984; Neurology 1987; **Med School:** Mount Sinai Sch Med 1978; **Resid:** Psychiatry, Mt Sinai Med Ctr 1982; Neurology, Mt Sinai Med Ctr 1984; **Fellow:** Behavioral Neurology, Univ Florida 1986; **Fac Appt:** Clin Prof N, Albert Einstein Coll Med

Fink, Matthew E MD (N) - **Spec Exp:** Cerebrovascular Disease; Stroke; **Hospital:** NY-Presby Hosp/Weill Cornell (page 104); **Address:** NY Cornell Med Ctr Dept Neurology, 525 E 68th St, New York, NY 10065; **Phone:** 212-746-4564; **Board Cert:** Internal Medicine 1980; Neurology 1983; Vascular Neurology 2005; **Med School:** Univ Pittsburgh 1976; **Resid:** Internal Medicine, Boston Med Ctr 1980; Neurology, Columbia-Presby Hosp 1982; **Fac Appt:** Prof N, Cornell Univ

Foo, Sun-Hoo MD (N) - **Spec Exp:** Stroke; Headache; Parkinson's Disease; Dementia; **Hospital:** NYU Langone Med Ctr (page 106), NY Downtown Hosp; **Address:** 650 1st Ave, FL 4, New York, NY 10016-3240; **Phone:** 212-213-0270; **Board Cert:** Internal Medicine 1976; Neurology 1980; **Med School:** Taiwan 1972; **Resid:** Internal Medicine, St Vincent's Hosp 1976; Neurology, NYU Med Ctr 1979; **Fac Appt:** Prof N, NYU Sch Med

Forster, George MD (N) - **Spec Exp:** Multiple Sclerosis; Parkinson's Disease; Brain Tumors; Pain-Back; **Hospital:** Mount Sinai Med Ctr (page 102); **Address:** 5 E 98 St, Fl 7, Box 1139, New York, NY 10029; **Phone:** 212-241-7076; **Board Cert:** Neurology 1980; **Med School:** Italy 1971; **Resid:** Internal Medicine, Maimonides Med Ctr 1974; Neurology, Mt Sinai Hosp 1977; **Fac Appt:** Asst Prof N, Mount Sinai Sch Med

French, Jacqueline MD (N) - **Spec Exp:** Epilepsy/Seizure Disorders; **Hospital:** NYU Langone Med Ctr (page 106); **Address:** 223 E 34th St, New York, NY 10016; **Phone:** 646-558-0805; **Board Cert:** Neurology 1987; **Med School:** Brown Univ 1982; **Resid:** Neurology, Mount Sinai Hosp 1986; **Fellow:** Epilepsy, Mount Sinai Hosp 1988; Epilepsy, Yale-New Haven Hosp 1989; **Fac Appt:** Prof N, NYU Sch Med

Gendelman, Seymour MD (N) - **Spec Exp:** Parkinson's Disease; Dementia; Headache; **Hospital:** Mount Sinai Med Ctr (page 102); **Address:** 5 E 98th St Fl 7, Box 1139, New York, NY 10029-6501; **Phone:** 212-241-8172; **Board Cert:** Neurology 1971; **Med School:** Geo Wash Univ 1964; **Resid:** Neurology, Mt Sinai Hosp 1968; **Fac Appt:** Clin Prof N, Mount Sinai Sch Med

Goodgold, Albert MD (N) - **Spec Exp:** Parkinson's Disease; Spinal Cord Disorders; Multiple Sclerosis; Movement Disorders; **Hospital:** NYU Langone Med Ctr (page 106); **Address:** 530 First Ave Fl 5 - Ste 5A, New York, NY 10016; **Phone:** 212-263-7205; **Med School:** Switzerland 1955; **Resid:** Neurology, Bellevue Hosp 1960; **Fac Appt:** Prof N, NYU Sch Med

Green, Mark W MD (N) - **Spec Exp:** Headache; Pain-Facial; **Hospital:** Mount Sinai Med Ctr (page 102); **Address:** Mount Sinai Sch Med, 5 S 98th St Fl 7, New York, NY 10029; **Phone:** 212-241-7076; **Board Cert:** Neurology 1979; Headache Medicine 1976; **Med School:** Albert Einstein Coll Med 1974; **Resid:** Neurology, Albert Einstein Affil Hosp 1978; **Fac Appt:** Prof N, Mount Sinai Sch Med

Gruber, Michael L MD (N) - **Spec Exp:** Neuro-Oncology; Headache; Pain-Back; **Hospital:** NYU Langone Med Ctr (page 106), Overlook Hosp (page 92); **Address:** NYU Clinical Cancer Ctr, 160 E 34th St Fl 7, New York, NY 10016; **Phone:** 212-731-5577; **Board Cert:** Neurology 1975; **Med School:** Temple Univ 1966; **Resid:** Pediatrics, Columbia-Presby Med Ctr 1968; Neurology, Columbia-Presby Med Ctr 1973; **Fellow:** Neuro-Oncology, Mass Genl Hosp 1990; **Fac Appt:** Prof N, NYU Sch Med

Herbert, Joseph MD (N) - **Spec Exp:** Multiple Sclerosis; Neuromuscular Disorders; Neuro-Rehabilitation; **Hospital:** NYU Hosp For Joint Diseases (page 106); **Address:** 301 E 17th St, Ste 544, New York, NY 10003; **Phone:** 212-598-6305; **Board Cert:** Neurology 1987; **Med School:** Israel 1974; **Resid:** Neurology, Longwood/Harvard U Sch Med 1983; Neuropathology, Children's Hosp 1984; **Fellow:** Clinical Genetics, Columbia Presby Med Ctr 1986; **Fac Appt:** Assoc Prof N, NYU Sch Med

Herbstein, Diego MD (N) - **Spec Exp:** Parkinson's Disease; Cerebrovascular Disease; **Hospital:** Lenox Hill Hosp, NY Hosp Queens; **Address:** 162 E 78th St, New York, NY 10075; **Phone:** 212-794-2281; **Board Cert:** Neurology 1976; **Med School:** Argentina 1968; **Resid:** Internal Medicine, Fernandez 1970; Neurology, Albert Einstein 1973; **Fellow:** Neurology, Jacobi Med Ctr 1974; **Fac Appt:** Asst Clin Prof N, Cornell Univ-Weill Med Coll

Heublum, Michael MD (N) - **Spec Exp:** Neuromuscular Disorders; Electrodiagnosis; **Hospital:** Mount Sinai Med Ctr (page 102), Beth Israel Med Ctr - Petrie Division (page 94); **Address:** 247 3rd Ave, Ste 203, New York, NY 10010; **Phone:** 212-505-9800; **Board Cert:** Internal Medicine 1989; Neurology 1993; **Med School:** SUNY Downstate 1986; **Resid:** Internal Medicine, Staten Island Univ Hosp 1989; Neurology, Mt Sinai Med Ctr 1992; **Fellow:** Neuromuscular Disease, Univ Michigan Med Ctr 1993

Hiesiger, Emile MD (N) - **Spec Exp:** Pain Management; Neuro-Oncology; **Hospital:** NYU Langone Med Ctr (page 106), VA Med Ctr - Manhattan; **Address:** 530 1st Ave, Ste 5A, New York, NY 10016-6402; **Phone:** 212-263-6123; **Board Cert:** Neurology 1983; **Med School:** NY Med Coll 1978; **Resid:** Neurology, NYU Med Ctr 1982; **Fellow:** Neurology, Meml Sloan-Kettering Cancer Ctr 1984; **Fac Appt:** Assoc Clin Prof N, NYU Sch Med

Horvath, Susanna E MD (N) - **Spec Exp:** Stroke; **Hospital:** NY-Presby Hosp/Columbia (page 104), NY-Presby Hosp/The Allen Hosp (page 104); **Address:** Columbia Univ Med Ctr, Neurological Inst Stroke Div, 710 W 168th St Fl 6th, New York, NY 10032; **Phone:** 212-932-4254; **Board Cert:** Neurology 2003; Vascular Neurology 2005; **Med School:** Hungary 1990; **Resid:** Internal Medicine, Kaleida/Millard Fillmore Hosp 1995; Neurology, SUNY-Buffalo Med Ctr 2000; **Fac Appt:** Asst Clin Prof N, Columbia P&S

Kolodny, Edwin H MD (N) - **Spec Exp:** Pediatric Neurology; Inherited Disorders of Nervous System; Gaucher Disease; Fabry's Disease; **Hospital:** NYU Langone Med Ctr (page 106), Bellevue Hosp Ctr; **Address:** 403 E 34 St Fl 2, New York, NY 10016-6402; **Phone:** 212-263-8344; **Board Cert:** Neurology 1971; Clinical Genetics 1984; Clinical Biochemical Genetics 1987; **Med School:** NYU Sch Med 1962; **Resid:** Internal Medicine, Bellevue Hosp 1964; Neurology, Mass Genl Hosp 1967; **Fellow:** Neurological Pathology, Mass Genl Hosp 1966; Neurology, Nat Inst Neurol Dis & Stroke 1970; **Fac Appt:** Prof N, NYU Sch Med

Koppel, Barbara MD (N) - **Spec Exp:** Epilepsy; Headache; Stroke; AIDS/HIV; **Hospital:** Metropolitan Hosp Ctr - NY; **Address:** Metropolitan Hospital, 1901 First Ave, rm 7C5, New York, NY 10029; **Phone:** 212-423-6676; **Board Cert:** Neurology 1983; **Med School:** Columbia P&S 1978; **Resid:** Internal Medicine, Montefiore Med Ctr 1979; Neurology, Columbia-Presby Hosp 1982; **Fac Appt:** Prof N, NY Med Coll

Kuzniecky, Ruben MD (N) - **Spec Exp:** Epilepsy/Seizure Disorders; MRI; Developmental Disorders; **Hospital:** NYU Langone Med Ctr (page 106); **Address:** 223 E 34th St Fl Ground, New York, NY 10016; **Phone:** 646-558-0802; **Board Cert:** Neurology 1990; **Med School:** Argentina 1980; **Resid:** Neurology, McGill Univ 1986; **Fellow:** Epilepsy, McGill Univ 1988; **Fac Appt:** Prof N, NYU Sch Med

Labar, Douglas R MD/PhD (N) - **Spec Exp:** Epilepsy/Seizure Disorders; **Hospital:** NY-Presby Hosp/Weill Cornell (page 104); **Address:** NY Weill Cornell Med Ctr, 525 E 68th St, Ste K619, New York, NY 10021; **Phone:** 212-746-2359; **Board Cert:** Neurology 1987; **Med School:** Med Coll PA 1982; **Resid:** Neurology, Columbia Presby Med Ctr 1986; **Fellow:** Epilepsy, Columbia Presby Med Ctr 1988; **Fac Appt:** Prof N, Cornell Univ-Weill Med Coll

Lange, Dale J MD (N) - **Spec Exp:** Neuromuscular Disorders; Amyotrophic Lateral Sclerosis (ALS); Electromyography; **Hospital:** NY-Presby Hosp/Weill Cornell (page 104); **Address:** Hosp For Special Surgery, 535 E 70th St, New York, NY 10021; **Phone:** 646-797-8917; **Board Cert:** Neurology 1985; Neuromuscular Medicine 2008; **Med School:** NY Med Coll 1978; **Resid:** Neurology, New England Med Ctr 1982; **Fellow:** Neuromuscular Medicine, Columbia-Presby Med Ctr 1983; **Fac Appt:** Prof N, Cornell Univ-Weill Med Coll

Latov, Norman MD/PhD (N) - **Spec Exp:** Peripheral Neuropathy; Neuro-Immunology; **Hospital:** NY-Presby Hosp/Weill Cornell (page 104); **Address:** 1305 York Ave Fl 2, New York, NY 10021; **Phone:** 646-962-3202; **Board Cert:** Neurology 1989; **Med School:** Univ Pennsylvania 1975; **Resid:** Internal Medicine, Boston City Hosp 1976; Neurology, Columbia-Presby Med Ctr 1979; **Fellow:** Immunology, Columbia-Presby Med Ctr 1981; **Fac Appt:** Prof N, Cornell Univ-Weill Med Coll

Levine, David N MD (N) - **Spec Exp:** Dementia; Stroke; Spinal Cord Disorders; **Hospital:** NYU Langone Med Ctr (page 106); **Address:** 400 E 34th St, Ste RIRM-311, New York, NY 10016-4901; **Phone:** 212-263-7744; **Board Cert:** Neurology 1976; **Med School:** Harvard Med Sch 1968; **Resid:** Neurology, Mass Genl Hosp 1974; **Fellow:** Neurology, Mass Genl Hosp 1976; **Fac Appt:** Prof N, NYU Sch Med

Levine, Steven R MD (N) - **Spec Exp:** Stroke; Cerebrovascular Disease; **Hospital:** Mount Sinai Med Ctr (page 102); **Address:** SUNY Downstate Univ Hosp of Brooklyn, 5 E 98th St, 7th Flr, Box 1139, Brooklyn, NY 10029-6500; **Phone:** 212-241-1970; **Board Cert:** Neurology 1986; Vascular Neurology 2005; **Med School:** Med Coll Wisc 1981; **Resid:** Neurology, Univ Mich Hosps 1985; **Fellow:** Cerebrovascular Disease, Henry Ford Hosp 1987; **Fac Appt:** Prof N, Mount Sinai Sch Med

Lin, Michael Tai-Ju MD (N) - **Spec Exp:** Memory Disorders; Neurodegenerative Disorders; **Hospital:** NY-Presby Hosp/Weill Cornell (page 104); **Address:** 428 E 72nd St, Ste 500, New York, NY 10021; **Phone:** 212-746-2441; **Board Cert:** Neurology 2007; **Med School:** UCSF 1992; **Resid:** Neurology, Mass General Hosp 1996; **Fellow:** Memory Disorders, Mass General Hosp 1997; **Fac Appt:** Asst Prof N, Cornell Univ-Weill Med Coll

Lublin, Fred D MD (N) - **Spec Exp:** Multiple Sclerosis; **Hospital:** Mount Sinai Med Ctr (page 102); **Address:** Dickinson Ctr for Multiple Sclerosis, 5 E 98th St, Box 1138, New York, NY 10029-6574; **Phone:** 212-241-6854; **Board Cert:** Neurology 1977; **Med School:** Jefferson Med Coll 1972; **Resid:** Neurology, New York Hosp/Cornell 1976; **Fac Appt:** Prof N, Mount Sinai Sch Med

Luciano, Daniel J MD (N) - **Spec Exp:** Epilepsy/Seizure Disorders; **Hospital:** NYU Langone Med Ctr (page 106); **Address:** 223 E 34th St, New York, NY 10016; **Phone:** 646-558-0805; **Board Cert:** Neurology 1992; Clinical Neurophysiology 2004; **Med School:** UMDNJ-NJ Med Sch, Newark 1984; **Resid:** Neurology, Mt Sinai Med Ctr 1988; **Fellow:** Epilepsy, Mt Sinai Med Ctr 1990; **Fac Appt:** Asst Prof N, NYU Sch Med

Marder, Karen S MD (N) - **Spec Exp:** Huntington's Disease; Alzheimer's Disease; Dementia; **Hospital:** NY-Presby Hosp/Columbia (page 104); **Address:** Neurological Institute, 710 W 168th St, Ste 104, New York, NY 10032-2603; **Phone:** 212-305-6939; **Board Cert:** Neurology 1989; **Med School:** Cornell Univ-Weill Med Coll 1983; **Resid:** Neurology, Columbia Presby Med Ctr 1987; **Fellow:** Behavioral Neurology, Columbia Presby Med Ctr 1989; **Fac Appt:** Assoc Prof N, Columbia P&S

Mauskop, Alexander MD (N) - **Spec Exp:** Headache; Migraine; Botox Therapy; **Hospital:** Beth Israel Med Ctr - Petrie Division (page 94); **Address:** New York Headache Ctr, 30 E 76th St, New York, NY 10021; **Phone:** 212-794-3550; **Board Cert:** Neurology 1987; Headache Medicine 2006; **Med School:** Ukraine 1979; **Resid:** Internal Medicine, Brookdale Hosp 1981; Neurology, Univ Hosp 1984; **Fellow:** Pain Management, Meml Sloan Kettering Cancer Ctr 1986; **Fac Appt:** Assoc Clin Prof N, SUNY Downstate

Mayer, Stephan A MD (N) - **Spec Exp:** Neurologic Critical Care; Stroke; Coma; **Hospital:** NY-Presby Hosp/Columbia (page 104); **Address:** 177 Fort Washington Ave Fl 8, Milstene Hosp Bldg, rm 300 Center, New York, NY 10032-2603; **Phone:** 212-305-7236; **Board Cert:** Neurology 1993; **Med School:** Cornell Univ-Weill Med Coll 1988; **Resid:** Neurology, Columbia-Presby Med Ctr 1992; **Fellow:** Critical Care Neurology, Columbia-Presby Med Ctr 1993; **Fac Appt:** Assoc Prof N, Columbia P&S

Miller, Aaron MD (N) - **Spec Exp:** Multiple Sclerosis; Alzheimer's Disease; Autoimmune Disease; **Hospital:** Mount Sinai Med Ctr (page 102), Maimonides Med Ctr (page 98); **Address:** Corinne Goldsmith Dickinson Ctr for MS, 5 E 98th St, Box 1138, New York, NY 10029; **Phone:** 212-241-6854; **Board Cert:** Internal Medicine 1972; Neurology 1977; **Med School:** NYU Sch Med 1968; **Resid:** Internal Medicine, Jacobi Med Ctr 1970; Neurology, Montefiore Med Ctr 1975; **Fellow:** Neurovirology, Johns Hopkins Hosp 1977; **Fac Appt:** Prof N, Mount Sinai Sch Med

Mitsumoto, Hiroshi MD (N) - **Spec Exp:** Amyotrophic Lateral Sclerosis (ALS); Neuromuscular Disorders; Clinical Trials; **Hospital:** NY-Presby Hosp/Columbia (page 104); **Address:** Neurological Inst, 710 W 168th St Fl 9 - rm 9001, New York, NY 10032; **Phone:** 212-305-1319; **Board Cert:** Neurology 1978; **Med School:** Japan 1968; **Resid:** Internal Medicine, Toho Univ Hosps 1972; Neurology, Univ Hosps 1976; **Fellow:** Neurological Pathology, Cleveland Clinic 1978; Neuromuscular Medicine, New England Med Ctr 1981; **Fac Appt:** Prof N, Columbia P&S

Mohr, JP MD (N) - **Spec Exp:** Aphasia; Stroke; Arteriovenous Malformations; Moya Moya; **Hospital:** NY-Presby Hosp/Columbia (page 104); **Address:** Neurological Inst-Dept Neurology, 710 W 168 St, Ste 615, New York, NY 10032-2603; **Phone:** 212-305-8033; **Board Cert:** Neurology 1971; Vascular Neurology 2005; **Med School:** Univ VA Sch Med 1963; **Resid:** Neurology, Columbia Presby Med Ctr 1966; Neurology, Mass Genl Hosp 1968; **Fellow:** Neurology, Mass Genl Hosp 1969; **Fac Appt:** Clin Prof N, Columbia P&S

Motiwala, Rajeev S MD (N) - **Hospital:** NY-Presby Hosp/Columbia (page 104); **Address:** 710 W 168 St, rm 246, New York, NY 10032; **Phone:** 212-305-6876; **Board Cert:** Neurology 1990; **Med School:** India 1979; **Resid:** Neurology, UMDMNJ Med Ctr 1988

Nealon, Nancy MD (N) - **Spec Exp:** Multiple Sclerosis; Migraine; **Hospital:** NY-Presby Hosp/Weill Cornell (page 104); **Address:** 1305 York Ave, rm Y217, New York, NY 10021; **Phone:** 646-962-9800; **Board Cert:** Internal Medicine 1978; Neurology 1984; **Med School:** Penn State Univ-Hershey Med Ctr 1975; **Resid:** Neurology, NY Hosp 1981; **Fellow:** Neuromuscular Disease, Columbia-Presby Med Ctr 1982; Neuromuscular Medicine, Meml Sloan Kettering Cancer Ctr 1983; **Fac Appt:** Asst Prof N, Cornell Univ-Weill Med Coll

Neophytides, Andreas MD (N) - **Spec Exp:** Spinal Disorders; Stroke; **Hospital:** NYU Langone Med Ctr (page 106); **Address:** 650 1st Ave, New York, NY 10016; **Phone:** 212-213-9581; **Board Cert:** Neurology 1978; **Med School:** Greece 1970; **Resid:** Surgery, LIJ Med Ctr 1973; Neurology, NYU Med Ctr 1976; **Fellow:** Neurological Pharmacology, Natl Inst Hlth 1978; **Fac Appt:** Clin Prof N, NYU Sch Med

Newman, Lawrence C MD (N) - **Spec Exp:** Headache; Pain-Facial; **Hospital:** St Luke's - Roosevelt Hosp Ctr - Roosevelt Div (page 94); **Address:** St Luke's-Roosevelt Hosp-Headache Inst, 425 W 59th St, Ste 4A, New York, NY 10019; **Phone:** 212-523-5869; **Board Cert:** Neurology 2005; Headache Medicine 2006; **Med School:** Mexico 1983; **Resid:** Internal Medicine, Elmhurst Hosp 1986; Neurology, Montefiore Med Ctr 1989; **Fellow:** Headache, Montefiore Med Ctr 1990; **Fac Appt:** Prof N, Albert Einstein Coll Med

Olanow, C Warren MD (N) - **Spec Exp:** Parkinson's Disease; Movement Disorders; **Hospital:** Mount Sinai Med Ctr (page 102); **Address:** 5 E 98th St, New York, NY 10029; **Phone:** 212-241-8435; **Med School:** Univ Toronto 1965; **Resid:** Neurology, Toronto Genl Hosp 1968; Neurology, Columbia Presby Hosp 1970; **Fellow:** Neurological Anatomy, Columbia Presby Hosp 1971; **Fac Appt:** Prof N, Mount Sinai Sch Med

Olarte, Marcelo R MD (N) - **Spec Exp:** Myasthenia Gravis; Electrodiagnosis; Headache; Neuromuscular Disorders; **Hospital:** NY-Presby Hosp/Columbia (page 104); **Address:** 710 W 168th St Fl 2 - rm 246, New York, NY 10032; **Phone:** 212-305-1832; **Board Cert:** Neurology 1976; **Med School:** Argentina 1970; **Resid:** Neurology, St Vincent's Hosp 1974; **Fellow:** Neuromuscular Medicine, Columbia-Presby Hosp 1975; **Fac Appt:** Clin Prof N, Columbia P&S

Oribe, Emilio M MD (N) - **Spec Exp:** Movement Disorders; Stroke; **Hospital:** NY Hosp Queens, NY-Presby Hosp/Weill Cornell (page 104); **Address:** 162 E 78th St, New York, NY 10075; **Phone:** 718-606-9193; **Board Cert:** Internal Medicine 1986; Neurology 1991; **Med School:** Uruguay 1981; **Resid:** Internal Medicine, NYU Downtown Hosp 1986; Neurology, Mt Sinai Med Ctr 1989; **Fellow:** Movement Disorders, Mt Sinai Med Ctr 1991

Pacia, Steven MD (N) - **Spec Exp:** Epilepsy/Seizure Disorders; **Hospital:** NYU Langone Med Ctr (page 106), Lenox Hill Hosp; **Address:** 223 E 34th St Fl 1, New York, NY 10016; **Phone:** 646-558-0867; **Board Cert:** Neurology 1992; Clinical Neurophysiology 2007; **Med School:** Yale Univ 1989; **Resid:** Neurology, Yale-New Haven Hosp 1992; **Fellow:** Epilepsy, Yale-New Haven Hosp 1992; **Fac Appt:** Assoc Prof N, NYU Sch Med

Pedley, Timothy A MD (N) - **Spec Exp:** Epilepsy/Seizure Disorders; **Hospital:** NY-Presby Hosp/Columbia (page 104); **Address:** The Neurological Inst, 710 W 168th St, rm 1406, New York, NY 10032; **Phone:** 212-305-6489; **Board Cert:** Neurology 1975; **Med School:** Yale Univ 1969; **Resid:** Neurology, Stanford Univ Hosp 1973; **Fellow:** Clinical Neurophysiology, Stanford Univ Hosp 1975; **Fac Appt:** Prof N, Columbia P&S

Petito, Frank A MD (N) - **Spec Exp:** Multiple Sclerosis; Headache; Lyme Disease; **Hospital:** NY-Presby Hosp/Weill Cornell (page 104); **Address:** 525 E 68th St, Ste 615, New York, NY 10065; **Phone:** 212-746-2309; **Board Cert:** Neurology 1974; **Med School:** Columbia P&S 1967; **Resid:** Neurology, New York Hosp 1971; **Fac Appt:** Prof N, Cornell Univ-Weill Med Coll

Posner, Jerome MD (N) - **Spec Exp:** Neuro-Oncology; Brain Tumors; **Hospital:** Meml Sloan-Kettering Cancer Ctr (page 112); **Address:** 1275 York Ave, rm C731, New York, NY 10065; **Phone:** 212-639-7047; **Board Cert:** Neurology 1962; **Med School:** Univ Wash 1955; **Resid:** Neurology, Univ WA Affil Hosp 1959; **Fellow:** Biochemistry, Univ WA Affil Hosp 1963; **Fac Appt:** Prof N, Cornell Univ-Weill Med Coll

Rapoport, Samuel MD/PhD (N) - **Spec Exp:** Peripheral Neuropathy; Pain-Back & Neck; Electromyography; **Hospital:** NY-Presby Hosp/Weill Cornell (page 104), Lenox Hill Hosp; **Address:** 354 E 76th St, New York, NY 10021-2505; **Phone:** 212-570-0642; **Board Cert:** Neurology 1986; **Med School:** Cornell Univ-Weill Med Coll 1976; **Resid:** Neurology, New York Hosp-Cornell 1982; **Fac Appt:** Assoc Prof N, Cornell Univ-Weill Med Coll

Relkin, Norman R MD/PhD (N) - **Spec Exp:** Alzheimer's Disease; Dementia; Memory Disorders; **Hospital:** NY-Presby Hosp/Weill Cornell (page 104); **Address:** Weill Cornell Memory Disorders Program, 428 E 72nd St, Ste 500, New York, NY 10021; **Phone:** 212-746-2441; **Board Cert:** Neurology 1992; **Med School:** Albert Einstein Coll Med 1987; **Resid:** Neurology, New York Hosp 1991; **Fellow:** Behavioral Neurology, New York Hosp-Cornell 1992; **Fac Appt:** Asst Prof N, Cornell Univ-Weill Med Coll

Rosenfeld, Steven S MD (N) - **Spec Exp:** Brain Tumors; Gliomas; Neuro-Oncology; **Hospital:** NY-Presby Hosp/Columbia (page 104); **Address:** Neurological Inst of NY-Brain Tumor Ctr, 710 W 168th St, rm 204, New York, NY 10032; **Phone:** 212-305-1718; **Board Cert:** Neurology 1994; **Med School:** Northwestern Univ 1985; **Resid:** Neurology, Duke Univ Med Ctr 1989; **Fellow:** Neuro-Oncology, Duke Univ Med Ctr 1990; **Fac Appt:** Prof N, Columbia P&S

Sadiq, Saud MD (N) - **Spec Exp:** Multiple Sclerosis; **Hospital:** St Luke's - Roosevelt Hosp Ctr - Roosevelt Div (page 94); **Address:** International MS Management Practice, 521 W 57th St Fl 4, New York, NY 10019; **Phone:** 212-265-8070; **Board Cert:** Neurology 2009; **Med School:** Africa 1979; **Resid:** Neurology, Univ TX Med Branch 1988; **Fellow:** Neurological Immunology, Ny Presby-Columbia Med Ctr 1991; **Fac Appt:** , Albert Einstein Coll Med

Sander, Howard W MD (N) - **Spec Exp:** Electromyography; Peripheral Neuropathy; Neuromuscular Disorders; **Hospital:** NYU Langone Med Ctr (page 106); **Address:** New York Univ Med Ctr, 1st E 34th St, Dept of Neurology,RR-311, New York, NY 10011; **Phone:** 212-263-3895; **Board Cert:** Neurology 1993; Pain Medicine 2000; Clinical Neurophysiology 2005; Vascular Neurology 2008; **Med School:** SUNY Downstate 1988; **Resid:** Neurology, Albert Einstein Coll of Med 1992; **Fellow:** Electromyography, Mass Genl Hosp 1993; **Fac Appt:** Assoc Prof N, Cornell Univ-Weill Med Coll

Schaefer, John A MD (N) - **Spec Exp:** Spinal Disorders; Multiple Sclerosis; Stroke; Cerebrovascular Disease; **Hospital:** NY-Presby Hosp/Weill Cornell (page 104), Hosp For Special Surgery (page 111); **Address:** 523 E 72nd St Fl 8, New York, NY 10021-4099; **Phone:** 212-717-0231; **Board Cert:** Neurology 1979; **Med School:** Australia 1968; **Resid:** Neurology, St Vincents Hosp 1973; **Fellow:** Neurology, New York Hosp 1978; **Fac Appt:** Assoc Clin Prof N, Cornell Univ-Weill Med Coll

Sheinart, Kara F MD (N) - **Spec Exp:** Cerebrovascular Disease; Stroke; **Hospital:** Mount Sinai Med Ctr (page 102); **Address:** 5 E 98th St Fl 7th, New York, NY 10029; **Phone:** 212-241-7076; **Board Cert:** Neurology 2005; **Med School:** SUNY Downstate 1989; **Resid:** Internal Medicine, Mt Sinai Med Ctr 1990; Neurology, Mt Sinai Med Ctr 1993; **Fellow:** Cerebrovascular Disease, Mt Sinai Med Ctr 1995; **Fac Appt:** Asst Clin Prof N, Mount Sinai Sch Med

Shulman, Melanie MD (N) - **Spec Exp:** Memory Disorders; Epilepsy; **Hospital:** NYU Langone Med Ctr (page 106); **Address:** Barlow Center, 145 E 32 St, New York, NY 10016; **Phone:** 212-263-3210; **Board Cert:** Neurology 2007; **Med School:** Univ Pennsylvania 1991; **Resid:** Neurology, Brigham & Women's Hosp 1995; **Fac Appt:** Asst Clin Prof N, NYU Sch Med

Simpson, David M MD (N) - **Spec Exp:** Infections-CNS; AIDS-Neurologic Complications; Peripheral Neuropathy; Neuromuscular Disorders; **Hospital:** Mount Sinai Med Ctr (page 102); **Address:** Mt Sinai Med Ctr, Dept Neurology, 1 Gustave L Levy Pl, Box 1052, Annenberg, 2nd Flr, New York, NY 10029; **Phone:** 212-241-8748; **Board Cert:** Neurology 1984; Clinical Neurophysiology 2005; Neuromuscular Medicine 2008; **Med School:** SUNY Buffalo 1979; **Resid:** Neurology, New York Hosp-Cornell Med Ctr 1983; **Fellow:** Clinical Neurophysiology, Mass Genl Hosp 1984; **Fac Appt:** Prof N, Mount Sinai Sch Med

Sivak, Mark A MD (N) - **Spec Exp:** Myasthenia Gravis; Amyotrophic Lateral Sclerosis (ALS); Neuromuscular Disorders; **Hospital:** Mount Sinai Med Ctr (page 102); **Address:** 5 E 98th St Fl 7, Box 1139, New York, NY 10029-6501; **Phone:** 212-241-8747; **Board Cert:** Neurology 1978; Clinical Neurophysiology 1999; Neuromuscular Medicine 2008; **Med School:** Univ Louisville Sch Med 1971; **Resid:** Neurology, Mt Sinai Med Ctr 1975; **Fellow:** Electromyography, Mt Sinai Med Ctr 1976; Clinical Neurophysiology, Uppsala Univ 1986; **Fac Appt:** Asst Prof N, Mount Sinai Sch Med

Smallberg, Gerald MD (N) - **Spec Exp:** Spinal Disorders; **Hospital:** Lenox Hill Hosp, Hosp For Special Surgery (page 111); **Address:** 1010 5th Ave, New York, NY 10028-0130; **Phone:** 212-535-5348; **Board Cert:** Neurology 1977; **Med School:** Yale Univ 1969; **Resid:** Internal Medicine, Univ Mich Med Ctr 1971; Neurology, Hosp Univ Penn 1975; **Fellow:** Neurology, Columbia-Presby Med Ctr 1976

Snyder, David H MD (N) - **Spec Exp:** Multiple Sclerosis; **Hospital:** NY Hosp Queens, Lenox Hill Hosp; **Address:** 162 E 78th St, New York, NY 10075; **Phone:** 212-794-2281; **Board Cert:** Neurology 1975; **Med School:** Univ MD Sch Med 1969; **Resid:** Neurology, Univ Maryland Hosp 1973; **Fellow:** Neuropathology, Albert Einstein Med Ctr 1975; **Fac Appt:** Asst Clin Prof N, Cornell Univ-Weill Med Coll

Stubgen, Joerg-Patrick MD (N) - **Spec Exp:** Amyotrophic Lateral Sclerosis (ALS); Peripheral Neuropathy; Neuromuscular Disorders; **Hospital:** NY-Presby Hosp/Weill Cornell (page 104), Hosp For Special Surgery (page 111); **Address:** Dept Neur Starr 607, 520 E 70th St, New York, NY 10021; **Phone:** 212-746-2334; **Board Cert:** Neurology 2006; Clinical Neurophysiology 1999; **Med School:** South Africa 1983; **Resid:** Neurology, Univ Pretoria Med Ctr 1989; Neurology, New York Hosp 1995; **Fellow:** Clinical Neurophysiology, Menl Sloan Kettering Cancer Ctr 1995; **Fac Appt:** Clin Prof N, Cornell Univ-Weill Med Coll

Tuchman, Alan MD (N) - **Spec Exp:** Epilepsy; Multiple Sclerosis; **Hospital:** Montefiore Med Ctr - Div. North (page 100); **Address:** 975 Park Ave, New York, NY 10028; **Phone:** 212-772-9305; **Board Cert:** Neurology 1979; **Med School:** Univ Cincinnati 1972; **Resid:** Neurology, Mt Sinai Med Ctr 1976; **Fellow:** Multiple Sclerosis, Albert Einstein Med Ctr 1979; **Fac Appt:** Clin Prof N, NY Med Coll

Tuhrim, Stanley MD (N) - **Spec Exp:** Stroke; Cerebrovascular Disease; Fibromuscular Dysplasia; **Hospital:** Mount Sinai Med Ctr (page 102); **Address:** 5 E 98th St, Box 1139, New York, NY 10029-6501; **Phone:** 212-241-7076; **Board Cert:** Neurology 1984; Vascular Neurology 2005; **Med School:** Mount Sinai Sch Med 1979; **Resid:** Neurology, Mt Sinai Med Ctr 1983; **Fellow:** Cerebrovascular Disease, Univ MD Sch Med 1984; **Fac Appt:** Prof N, Mount Sinai Sch Med

Waters, Cheryl H MD (N) - **Spec Exp:** Parkinson's Disease; Movement Disorders; **Hospital:** NY-Presby Hosp/Columbia (page 104); **Address:** 710 W 168th St Fl 3, New York, NY 10032; **Phone:** 212-305-3665; **Board Cert:** Neurology 1986; **Med School:** Univ Toronto 1980; **Resid:** Internal Medicine, Univ Toronto Med Ctr 1982; Neurology, Univ Toronto Med Ctr 1985; **Fellow:** Neurological Pharmacology, Univ Toronto Med Ctr 1987; **Fac Appt:** Prof N, Columbia P&S

Weinberg, Harold J MD (N) - **Spec Exp:** Stroke; Spinal Disorders; Neuromuscular Disorders; Memory Disorders; **Hospital:** NYU Langone Med Ctr (page 106); **Address:** 650 1st Ave Fl 4, New York, NY 10016-3240; **Phone:** 212-213-9339; **Board Cert:** Neurology 1983; Electrodiagnostic Medicine 1989; **Med School:** Albert Einstein Coll Med 1978; **Resid:** Neurology, Columbia-Presby Med Ctr 1982; **Fellow:** Neuromuscular Medicine, Columbia-Presby Med Ctr 1982; **Fac Appt:** Clin Prof N, NYU Sch Med

Weinberger, Jesse MD (N) - **Spec Exp:** Stroke; **Hospital:** Mount Sinai Med Ctr (page 102), N Genl Hosp; **Address:** 5 E 98th St Fl 7, New York, NY 10029-6501; **Phone:** 212-241-4529; **Board Cert:** Neurology 1976; Vascular Neurology 2005; **Med School:** Johns Hopkins Univ 1971; **Resid:** Neurology, Mt Sinai Med Ctr 1975; **Fellow:** Cerebrovascular Disease, Univ Penn 1978; **Fac Appt:** Prof N, Mount Sinai Sch Med

Neuroradiology

Berenstein, Alejandro MD (NRad) - **Spec Exp:** Interventional Neuroradiology; Aneurysm-Cerebral; Endovascular Surgery; Vascular Malformations; **Hospital:** St Luke's - Roosevelt Hosp Ctr - Roosevelt Div (page 94); **Address:** Center for Endovascular Surgery, 1000 10th Ave, 10th Fl, Ste 10G - INN, New York, NY 10019; **Phone:** 212-636-3400; **Board Cert:** Diagnostic Radiology 1976; **Med School:** Mexico 1970; **Resid:** Diagnostic Radiology, Mt Sinai Med Ctr 1976; **Fellow:** Neuroradiology, NYU Med Ctr 1978; **Fac Appt:** Prof Rad, Albert Einstein Coll Med

Drayer, Burton P MD (NRad) - **Spec Exp:** Stroke; Parkinson's Disease/Aging Brain; MRI & CT of Brain & Spine; **Hospital:** Mount Sinai Med Ctr (page 102); **Address:** 1 Gustave Levy Pl, Box 1234, New York, NY 10029; **Phone:** 212-241-6403; **Board Cert:** Neurology 1976; Diagnostic Radiology 1978; Neuroradiology 2006; **Med School:** Ros Franklin Univ/Chicago Med Sch 1971; **Resid:** Neurology, Univ Vt Med Ctr 1975; Diagnostic Radiology, Univ Pitt Hlth Ctr 1978; **Fellow:** Neuroradiology, Univ Pitt Hlth Ctr 1978; **Fac Appt:** Prof Rad, Mount Sinai Sch Med

Jahre, Caren MD (NRad) - **Spec Exp:** Cardiac CT Angiography; **Address:** Lenox Hill Radiology & Med Assocs, 61 E 77th St, New York, NY 10075; **Phone:** 212-772-3111; **Board Cert:** Diagnostic Radiology 1988; Neuroradiology 2005; **Med School:** Cornell Univ-Weill Med Coll 1982; **Resid:** Pathology, New York Hosp 1984; Diagnostic Radiology, New York Hosp 1988; **Fellow:** Neuroradiology, New York Hosp 1990; **Fac Appt:** Asst Prof Rad, NYU Sch Med

Kelly, Anna B MD (NRad) - **Hospital:** NY-Presby Hosp/Columbia (page 104); **Address:** Columbia Presbyterian Eastside Radiology, 16 E 60th St, New York, NY 10022; **Phone:** 212-326-8518; **Board Cert:** Diagnostic Radiology 1986; Neuroradiology 2005; **Med School:** Univ Cincinnati 1982; **Resid:** Diagnostic Radiology, NY Hosp-Cornell Med Ctr 1986; **Fellow:** Neurological Radiology, NY Hosp-Cornell Med Ctr 1989

Khandji, Alexander G MD (NRad) - **Spec Exp:** Pituitary Disorders; Spine Imaging & Intervention; MRI; Brain Tumors; **Hospital:** NY-Presby Hosp/Columbia (page 104); **Address:** 177 Ft Washington Ave, Ste 4-156, New York, NY 10032-3173; **Phone:** 212-305-7669; **Board Cert:** Diagnostic Radiology 1985; Neuroradiology 2006; **Med School:** SUNY Downstate 1980; **Resid:** Surgery, MS Hershey Med Ctr 1982; Diagnostic Radiology, Columbia-Presby Med Ctr 1985; **Fellow:** Neuroradiology, Columbia-Presby Med Ctr 1987; **Fac Appt:** Clin Prof Rad, Columbia P&S

Meyers, Philip M MD (NRad) - **Spec Exp:** Interventional Neuroradiology; Endovascular Surgery; Aneurysm-Cerebral; Arteriovenous Malformations; **Hospital:** NY-Presby Hosp/Columbia (page 104); **Address:** Neurological Institute, 710 168th St, rm 428, New York, NY 10032; **Phone:** 212-305-6384; **Board Cert:** Diagnostic Radiology 1997; Neuroradiology 2002; **Med School:** Case West Res Univ 1989; **Resid:** Neurological Surgery, Univ Cincinnati Med Ctr 1990; Diagnostic Radiology, Univ Cincinnati Med Ctr 1997; **Fellow:** Neurological Radiology, Univ Cincinnati Med Ctr 1998; Vascular Neurology, UCSF Med Ctr 1999; **Fac Appt:** Assoc Prof Rad, Columbia P&S

Nuclear Medicine

Carrasquillo, Jorge A MD (NuM) - **Spec Exp:** Radioimmunotherapy of Cancer; PET Imaging; **Hospital:** Meml Sloan-Kettering Cancer Ctr (page 112); **Address:** 1275 York Avenue, Nuclear Medicine Svc, Box 77, New York, NY 10065; **Phone:** 212-639-2459; **Board Cert:** Internal Medicine 1977; Nuclear Medicine 1982; **Med School:** Univ Puerto Rico 1974; **Resid:** Internal Medicine, Univ Dist Hosp 1977; Nuclear Medicine, Univ Wash Hosp 1982

Fawwaz, Rashid MD/PhD (NuM) - **Spec Exp:** PET Imaging; Brain Imaging; Radioimmunotherapy of Cancer; **Hospital:** NY-Presby Hosp/Columbia (page 104); **Address:** Columbia Presby Med Ctr, Dept Rad, 177 Ft Washington Ave, MHB 3-202A, New York, NY 10032-3713; **Phone:** 212-305-7138; **Board Cert:** Nuclear Medicine 1975; **Med School:** Amer Univ Beirut 1961; **Resid:** Diagnostic Radiology, American Univ Hosp 1963; **Fellow:** Nuclear Medicine, Donner Lab-UC 1966; **Fac Appt:** Clin Prof, Columbia P&S

Goldfarb, C Richard MD (NuM) - **Spec Exp:** Thyroid Disorders; **Hospital:** Beth Israel Med Ctr - Petrie Division (page 94); **Address:** Beth Israel Med Ctr, Dept Radiology, 1st Ave at 16th St, New York, NY 10003; **Phone:** 212-252-6070; **Board Cert:** Nuclear Medicine 1974; Diagnostic Radiology 1975; **Med School:** NY Med Coll 1970; **Resid:** Diagnostic Radiology, St Lukes Hosp 1974; **Fellow:** Nuclear Medicine, St Lukes Hosp 1975; **Fac Appt:** Assoc Prof NuM, Albert Einstein Coll Med

Goldsmith, Stanley J MD (NuM) - **Spec Exp:** Thyroid Cancer; Neuroendocrine Tumors; PET Imaging; Lymphoma, Non-Hodgkin's; **Hospital:** NY-Presby Hosp/Weill Cornell (page 104); **Address:** 525 E 68th St Starr Bldg - rm 2-21, New York, NY 10021-9800; **Phone:** 212-746-4588; **Board Cert:** Internal Medicine 1969; Nuclear Medicine 1972; Endocrinology 1972; **Med School:** SUNY Downstate 1962; **Resid:** Internal Medicine, Kings Co Hosp 1967; **Fellow:** Endocrinology, Diabetes & Metabolism, Mt Sinai Hosp 1968; Nuclear Medicine, Bronx VA Hosp 1969; **Fac Appt:** Prof Rad, Cornell Univ-Weill Med Coll

Larson, Steven M MD (NuM) - **Spec Exp:** Thyroid Cancer; PET Imaging; **Hospital:** Meml Sloan-Kettering Cancer Ctr (page 112); **Address:** 1275 York Avenue, New York, NY 10065; **Phone:** 800-525-2225; **Board Cert:** Nuclear Medicine 1972; Internal Medicine 1973; **Med School:** Univ Wash 1965; **Resid:** Internal Medicine, Virginia Mason Hosp 1970; Nuclear Medicine, Natl Inst Hlth 1972; **Fac Appt:** Prof NuM, Cornell Univ-Weill Med Coll

Sanger, Joseph J MD (NuM) - **Spec Exp:** Nuclear Cardiology; Nuclear Oncology; **Hospital:** NYU Langone Med Ctr (page 106), Bellevue Hosp Ctr; **Address:** Old Bellevue C & D Bldg, 1st Floor, rm 7, 462 First Ave, New York, NY 10016-6402; **Phone:** 212-731-5001; **Board Cert:** Nuclear Medicine 1981; **Med School:** NYU Sch Med 1977; **Resid:** Diagnostic Radiology, NYU Med Ctr 1979; **Fellow:** Nuclear Medicine, NYU Med Ctr 1981; **Fac Appt:** Assoc Prof Rad, NYU Sch Med

Scharf, Stephen MD (NuM) - **Spec Exp:** Thyroid & Parathyroid Imaging; Kidney Imaging; Bone Imaging; CT Scan; **Hospital:** Lenox Hill Hosp; **Address:** Lenox Hill Hospital, Dept Nuclear Medicine, 100 E 77th St Fl 3, New York, NY 10075; **Phone:** 212-434-2630; **Board Cert:** Internal Medicine 1977; Nuclear Medicine 1979; **Med School:** Albert Einstein Coll Med 1974; **Resid:** Internal Medicine, Bronx Municipal Hosp 1976; Nuclear Medicine, Montefiore Med Ctr 1978; **Fellow:** Nephrology, Montefiore Med Ctr 1979; **Fac Appt:** Asst Clin Prof NuM, Albert Einstein Coll Med

Strauss, H William MD (NuM) - **Spec Exp:** Cardiac Imaging in Cancer Therapy; Thyroid Disorders; Cardiac Imaging; **Hospital:** Meml Sloan-Kettering Cancer Ctr (page 112); **Address:** 1275 York Avenue, New York, NY 10065; **Phone:** 212-639-7238; **Board Cert:** Nuclear Medicine 1988; **Med School:** SUNY Downstate 1965; **Resid:** Internal Medicine, Downstate Med Ctr 1967; Internal Medicine, Bellevue Hosp 1968; **Fellow:** Nuclear Medicine, Johns Hopkins Hosp 1970; **Fac Appt:** Prof NuM, Cornell Univ-Weill Med Coll

Vanheertum, Ronald L MD (NuM) - **Spec Exp:** PET Imaging; PET Imaging-Brain; Neurologic Imaging; **Hospital:** NY-Presby Hosp/Columbia (page 104); **Address:** NY Presby Hosp, Dept Radiology, 622 W 168th St, HP319, New York, NY 10032; **Phone:** 212-305-7132; **Board Cert:** Diagnostic Radiology 1971; Nuclear Medicine 1973; **Med School:** UMDNJ-NJ Med Sch, Newark 1966; **Resid:** Diagnostic Radiology, St Vincents Hosp 1970; **Fellow:** Diagnostic Radiology, St Vincents Hosp Med Ctr 1971; Nuclear Medicine, SUNY-Upstate Med Ctr 1975; **Fac Appt:** Prof Rad, Columbia P&S

Obstetrics & Gynecology

Ascher-Walsh, Charles J MD (ObG) - **Spec Exp:** Uro-Gynecology; Gynecologic Surgery; Pelvic Surgery; Robotic Surgery; **Hospital:** Mount Sinai Med Ctr (page 102); **Address:** 5 E 98th St Fl 2, New York, NY 10029; **Phone:** 212-241-7952; **Board Cert:** Obstetrics & Gynecology 2009; **Med School:** SUNY Hlth Sci Ctr 1995; **Resid:** Obstetrics & Gynecology, NY Presby Hosp-Columbia 1999; **Fellow:** Uro-Gynecology, NY Presby Hosp-Columbia 2000; **Fac Appt:** Asst Clin Prof ObG, Mount Sinai Sch Med

Bacall, Charles J MD (ObG) - **Hospital:** Mount Sinai Med Ctr (page 102); **Address:** 1150 5th Ave, Ste 1B, New York, NY 10128-2920; **Phone:** 212-996-9100; **Board Cert:** Obstetrics & Gynecology 1981; **Med School:** NY Med Coll 1975; **Resid:** Obstetrics & Gynecology, Mt Sinai Hosp 1979; **Fac Appt:** Asst Clin Prof ObG, Mount Sinai Sch Med

Berman, Alvin MD (ObG) - **Spec Exp:** Menopause Problems; Osteoporosis; Sexual Dysfunction; Women's Health over age 40; **Hospital:** Mount Sinai Med Ctr (page 102); **Address:** 111B E 88th St, New York, NY 10128; **Phone:** 212-722-5757; **Board Cert:** Obstetrics & Gynecology 1978; **Med School:** South Africa 1969; **Resid:** Obstetrics & Gynecology, Mount Sinai Hosp 1976; **Fellow:** Neonatal-Perinatal Medicine, Mount Sinai Hosp 1977; **Fac Appt:** Asst Clin Prof ObG, Mount Sinai Sch Med

Blanco, Jody MD (ObG) - **Spec Exp:** Uro-Gynecology; Uterine Fibroids; Colposcopy; **Hospital:** NY-Presby Hosp/Columbia (page 104); **Address:** 161 Fort Washington Ave, rm 447, Herbert Irving Pavilion, New York, NY 10032-3713; **Phone:** 212-305-1107; **Board Cert:** Obstetrics & Gynecology 2009; **Med School:** SUNY Hlth Sci Ctr 1981; **Resid:** Obstetrics & Gynecology, Columbia-Presby Med Ctr 1985; **Fellow:** Uro-Gynecology, UC Irvine 1986; **Fac Appt:** Asst Clin Prof ObG, Columbia P&S

Brightman, Rebecca MD (ObG) - **Spec Exp:** Preconception Planning; Menopause Problems; Pregnancy-High Risk; **Hospital:** Mount Sinai Med Ctr (page 102); **Address:** 134 E 93rd St, New York, NY 10128; **Phone:** 212-348-7800; **Board Cert:** Obstetrics & Gynecology 2009; **Med School:** Mount Sinai Sch Med 1986; **Resid:** Obstetrics & Gynecology, Mt Sinai Med Ctr 1990

Brodman, Michael L MD (ObG) - **Spec Exp:** Incontinence-Female; Laparoscopic Surgery; Pelvic Organ Prolapse Repair; Uro-Gynecology; **Hospital:** Mount Sinai Med Ctr (page 102); **Address:** Dept Gynecology/Urogynecology, 5 E 98th St Fl 2, New York, NY 10029; **Phone:** 212-241-7952; **Board Cert:** Obstetrics & Gynecology 2008; **Med School:** Mount Sinai Sch Med 1982; **Resid:** Obstetrics & Gynecology, Mt Sinai Hosp 1986; **Fellow:** Pelvic Surgery, Mt Sinai Hosp 1987; **Fac Appt:** Assoc Prof ObG, Mount Sinai Sch Med

Brustman, Lois MD (ObG) - **Spec Exp:** Prematurity/Low Birth Weight Infants; Diabetes in Pregnancy; Preconception Planning; Maternal & Fetal Medicine; **Hospital:** St Luke's - Roosevelt Hosp Ctr - Roosevelt Div (page 94); **Address:** 1000 Tenth Ave, Ste 11A-61, New York, NY 10019-1147; **Phone:** 212-523-7579; **Board Cert:** Obstetrics & Gynecology 2009; Maternal & Fetal Medicine 2009; **Med School:** NY Med Coll 1979; **Resid:** Obstetrics & Gynecology, Montefiore Med Ctr 1984; **Fellow:** Maternal & Fetal Medicine, Montefiore Med Ctr 1988; **Fac Appt:** Assoc Prof ObG, NY Med Coll

Buterman, Irving MD (ObG) - **Spec Exp:** Women's Health; Pregnancy-High Risk; **Hospital:** Lenox Hill Hosp, Beth Israel Med Ctr - Petrie Division (page 94); **Address:** 950 Park Ave, New York, NY 10028-0320; **Phone:** 212-472-8200; **Board Cert:** Obstetrics & Gynecology 1983; **Med School:** Netherlands 1971; **Resid:** Obstetrics & Gynecology, Lenox Hill Hosp 1976; **Fellow:** Gynecologic Oncology, Lenox Hill Hosp 1977; **Fac Appt:** Asst Clin Prof ObG, NY Med Coll

Cherry, Sheldon MD (ObG) - **Spec Exp:** Cancer Prevention; Infertility; Menopause Problems; **Hospital:** Mount Sinai Med Ctr (page 102); **Address:** 1160 Park Ave, New York, NY 10128-1212; **Phone:** 212-860-2600; **Board Cert:** Obstetrics & Gynecology 1981; **Med School:** Columbia P&S 1958; **Resid:** Obstetrics & Gynecology, Columbia-Presby Hosp 1962; **Fac Appt:** Clin Prof ObG, Mount Sinai Sch Med

Chin, Jean MD (ObG) *PCP* - **Spec Exp:** Menopause Problems; **Hospital:** Mount Sinai Med Ctr (page 102); **Address:** 785 Park Ave, New York, NY 10021; **Phone:** 212-249-7800; **Board Cert:** Obstetrics & Gynecology 1982; **Med School:** Columbia P&S 1976; **Resid:** Obstetrics & Gynecology, Mt Sinai Hosp 1980; **Fac Appt:** Asst Clin Prof ObG, Columbia P&S

Coady, Deborah MD (ObG) - **Spec Exp:** Gynecology Only; Vulvar Disease; Pain-Pelvic; Uterine Fibroids; **Hospital:** NYU Langone Med Ctr (page 106); **Address:** 430 West Broadway Fl 2, New York, NY 10012; **Phone:** 212-941-0011; **Board Cert:** Obstetrics & Gynecology 2006; **Med School:** Mount Sinai Sch Med 1980; **Resid:** Obstetrics & Gynecology, NYU-Bellevue Hosp 1984; **Fac Appt:** Asst Clin Prof ObG, NYU Sch Med

Cox, Kathryn A MD (ObG) - **Spec Exp:** Menopause Problems; Gynecologic Surgery; **Hospital:** NY-Presby Hosp/Weill Cornell (page 104); **Address:** 449 E 68th St, Ste 8, New York, NY 10021; **Phone:** 212-535-2600; **Board Cert:** Obstetrics & Gynecology 1981; **Med School:** Univ Mich Med Sch 1975; **Resid:** Obstetrics & Gynecology, New York Hosp/Cornell 1979

Diamond, Sharon MD (ObG) *PCP* - **Spec Exp:** Menopause Problems; Pap Smear Abnormalities; Gynecology Only; **Hospital:** Mount Sinai Med Ctr (page 102); **Address:** 61 E 86th St, Ste 1, New York, NY 10028-1003; **Phone:** 212-876-2200; **Board Cert:** Obstetrics & Gynecology 2009; **Med School:** Mount Sinai Sch Med 1979; **Resid:** Obstetrics & Gynecology, Mt Sinai Med Ctr 1983; **Fac Appt:** Asst Clin Prof ObG, Mount Sinai Sch Med

Evans, Mark I MD (ObG) - **Spec Exp:** Reproductive Genetics; Fetal Diagnosis & Therapy; Multiple Gestation; Ultrasound; **Hospital:** Mount Sinai Med Ctr (page 102); **Address:** Comprehensive Genetics, 131 E 65th St, New York, NY 10065; **Phone:** 212-288-1422; **Board Cert:** Obstetrics & Gynecology 2009; Clinical Genetics 1984; **Med School:** SUNY Downstate 1978; **Resid:** Obstetrics & Gynecology, Lying-In Hosp 1982; **Fellow:** Clinical Genetics, Natl Inst Hlth 1984; **Fac Appt:** Prof ObG, Mount Sinai Sch Med

Friedman, Lynn MD (ObG) *PCP* - **Spec Exp:** Miscarriage-Recurrent; Infertility; Pregnancy After Age 35; Pap Smear Abnormalities; **Hospital:** Mount Sinai Med Ctr (page 102); **Address:** 885 Park Ave, Ste 1-D, New York, NY 10021-0325; **Phone:** 212-737-3282; **Board Cert:** Obstetrics & Gynecology 2009; **Med School:** NYU Sch Med 1984; **Resid:** Obstetrics & Gynecology, Mt Sinai Med Ctr 1988; **Fac Appt:** Asst Clin Prof ObG, Mount Sinai Sch Med

Friedman, Ricky MD (ObG) *PCP* - **Spec Exp:** Women's Health; Pap Smear Abnormalities; **Hospital:** Mount Sinai Med Ctr (page 102); **Address:** 47 E 88th St. 1st Fl, New York, NY 10128-1152; **Phone:** 212-534-0200; **Board Cert:** Obstetrics & Gynecology 2000; **Med School:** SUNY Hlth Sci Ctr 1985; **Resid:** Obstetrics & Gynecology, Mount Sinai Hosp 1989; **Fac Appt:** Assoc Clin Prof ObG, Mount Sinai Sch Med

Goldman, Gary MD (ObG) - **Spec Exp:** Endometriosis; Laparoscopic Surgery-Complex; Hysterectomy Alternatives; **Hospital:** NY-Presby Hosp/Weill Cornell (page 104); **Address:** 715 Park Ave, New York, NY 10021; **Phone:** 212-535-6100; **Board Cert:** Obstetrics & Gynecology 2009; **Med School:** SUNY Stony Brook 1986; **Resid:** Obstetrics & Gynecology, New York Hosp 1990; **Fac Appt:** Asst Clin Prof ObG, Cornell Univ-Weill Med Coll

Goldstein, Martin S MD (ObG) - **Spec Exp:** Uterine Fibroids; Laparoscopic Surgery; Pelvic Organ Prolapse Repair; Endometriosis; **Hospital:** Mount Sinai Med Ctr (page 102); **Address:** 40 E 84th St, New York, NY 10028-1314; **Phone:** 212-472-6500; **Board Cert:** Obstetrics & Gynecology 1980; **Med School:** SUNY Hlth Sci Ctr 1966; **Resid:** Obstetrics & Gynecology, Mount Sinai Hosp 1971; **Fac Appt:** Assoc Clin Prof ObG, Mount Sinai Sch Med

Goldstein, Steven R MD (ObG) - **Spec Exp:** Gynecologic Ultrasound; Menopause Problems; Uterine Fibroids; **Hospital:** NYU Langone Med Ctr (page 106); **Address:** 530 1st Avenue Ste 10N, New York, NY 10016-6402; **Phone:** 212-263-7416; **Board Cert:** Obstetrics & Gynecology 2008; **Med School:** NYU Sch Med 1975; **Resid:** Obstetrics & Gynecology, NYU Affil Hosps 1980; **Fac Appt:** Prof ObG, NYU Sch Med

Gruss, Leslie MD (ObG) *PCP* - **Spec Exp:** HPV-Human Papillomavirus; Pap Smear Abnormalities; **Hospital:** NYU Langone Med Ctr (page 106); **Address:** 568 Broadway, Ste 304, New York, NY 10012; **Phone:** 212-966-7600; **Board Cert:** Obstetrics & Gynecology 2007; **Med School:** Med Coll PA Hahnemann 1983; **Resid:** Obstetrics & Gynecology, Montefiore Hosp Med Ctr 1987

Gubernick, Martin MD (ObG) - **Spec Exp:** Pregnancy-High Risk; **Hospital:** Mount Sinai Med Ctr (page 102); **Address:** 131 E 65th St, New York, NY 10021; **Phone:** 212-288-1422; **Board Cert:** Obstetrics & Gynecology 2008; **Med School:** Northwestern Univ 1982; **Resid:** Obstetrics & Gynecology, NY Presby-Cornell Med Ctr 1986

Harris, Dena E MD (ObG) *PCP* - **Spec Exp:** Gynecology Only; Menopause Problems; Vulvar Disease; **Hospital:** NYU Langone Med Ctr (page 106); **Address:** 430 W Broadway Fl 2, New York, NY 10012; **Phone:** 212-941-0011; **Board Cert:** Obstetrics & Gynecology 2009; **Med School:** Hahnemann Univ 1976; **Resid:** Obstetrics & Gynecology, NYU Med Ctr 1980; **Fac Appt:** Asst Clin Prof ObG, NYU Sch Med

Hirsch, Lissa B MD (ObG) - **Spec Exp:** Menopause Problems; **Hospital:** Lenox Hill Hosp; **Address:** 755 Park Ave, New York, NY 10021-4255; **Phone:** 212-570-2222; **Board Cert:** Obstetrics & Gynecology 1985; **Med School:** UMDNJ-NJ Med Sch, Newark 1979; **Resid:** Obstetrics & Gynecology, NYU Med Ctr 1983

Hockstein, Steven MD (ObG) - **Spec Exp:** Uterine Fibroids; **Hospital:** NY-Presby Hosp/Weill Cornell (page 104); **Address:** 425 E 61st St Fl 11, New York, NY 10065; **Phone:** 212-821-0810; **Board Cert:** Obstetrics & Gynecology 2009; **Med School:** Univ MD Sch Med 1993; **Resid:** Obstetrics & Gynecology, McGaw Med Ctr 1997; **Fac Appt:** Asst Clin Prof ObG, Cornell Univ-Weill Med Coll

Holland, Claudia MD (ObG) *PCP* - **Hospital:** St Luke's - Roosevelt Hosp Ctr - Roosevelt Div (page 94); **Address:** 800A 5th Ave, Ste 503, New York, NY 10021; **Phone:** 212-230-1760; **Board Cert:** Obstetrics & Gynecology 2009; **Med School:** Mount Sinai Sch Med 1981; **Resid:** Obstetrics & Gynecology, NYU Med Ctr 1985

Karamitsos, Harry MD (ObG) - **Hospital:** Lenox Hill Hosp; **Address:** Manhattan's Physician Group, 215 E 95th St, New York, NY 10128; **Phone:** 212-996-8000; **Board Cert:** Obstetrics & Gynecology 1999; **Med School:** NY Med Coll 1993; **Resid:** Obstetrics & Gynecology, Montefiore Med Ctr 1997

Kent, Joan L MD (ObG) - **Hospital:** NY-Presby Hosp/Weill Cornell (page 104); **Address:** 235 E 67th St, Ste 204, New York, NY 10021; **Phone:** 212-772-2900; **Board Cert:** Obstetrics & Gynecology 2009; **Med School:** Cornell Univ-Weill Med Coll 1984; **Resid:** Obstetrics & Gynecology, New York Hosp 1988; **Fac Appt:** Assoc Prof ObG, Cornell Univ-Weill Med Coll

Kessler, Alan A MD (ObG) - **Spec Exp:** Multiple Gestation; Pregnancy-High Risk; **Hospital:** NY-Presby Hosp/Weill Cornell (page 104); **Address:** 523 East 72nd St Fl 9, New York, NY 10021-4099; **Phone:** 212-472-5340; **Board Cert:** Obstetrics & Gynecology 2008; **Med School:** Mexico 1978; **Resid:** Obstetrics & Gynecology, New York Hosp 1983; **Fac Appt:** Assoc Prof ObG, Cornell Univ-Weill Med Coll

Kim, Joyce M MD (ObG) *PCP* - **Spec Exp:** Pregnancy-High Risk; **Hospital:** Mount Sinai Med Ctr (page 102); **Address:** 885 Park Ave St, Ste 1D, New York, NY 10021; **Phone:** 212-737-3282; **Board Cert:** Obstetrics & Gynecology 2008; **Med School:** Mount Sinai Sch Med 1986; **Resid:** Obstetrics & Gynecology, Mount Sinai Hosp 1990

Krause, Cynthia MD (ObG) *PCP* - **Spec Exp:** Menopause Problems; Pap Smear Abnormalities; Ovarian Cancer Genetics; Breast Cancer Genetics; **Hospital:** Mount Sinai Med Ctr (page 102); **Address:** 1185 Park Ave, Ste 1L, New York, NY 10128; **Phone:** 212-369-0602; **Board Cert:** Obstetrics & Gynecology 2008; **Med School:** Duke Univ 1980; **Resid:** Internal Medicine, Baltimore City Hosp 1982; Obstetrics & Gynecology, Mount Sinai Med Ctr 1986; **Fac Appt:** Asst Clin Prof ObG, Mount Sinai Sch Med

Leiter, Gila MD (ObG) - **Spec Exp:** Osteoporosis; Multiple Gestation; Menopause Problems; Uterine Fibroids; **Hospital:** Mount Sinai Med Ctr (page 102), Beth Israel Med Ctr - Petrie Division (page 94); **Address:** 1160 Park Ave, New York, NY 10028; **Phone:** 212-860-2600; **Board Cert:** Obstetrics & Gynecology 2010; **Med School:** Albert Einstein Coll Med 1983; **Resid:** Obstetrics & Gynecology, Mt Sinai Hosp 1987; **Fac Appt:** Asst Clin Prof ObG, Mount Sinai Sch Med

Levine, Richard U MD (ObG) - **Spec Exp:** Uterine Fibroids; Gynecologic Surgery; HPV-Human Papillomavirus; **Hospital:** NY-Presby Hosp/Columbia (page 104); **Address:** 16 E 60th St Fl 4 - rm 480, New York, NY 10022; **Phone:** 212-326-8491; **Board Cert:** Obstetrics & Gynecology 1994; **Med School:** Cornell Univ-Weill Med Coll 1966; **Resid:** Obstetrics & Gynecology, Columbia-Presby Med Ctr 1975; **Fellow:** Obstetrics & Gynecology, Karolinska Inst 1970; **Fac Appt:** Prof ObG, Columbia P&S

Lind, Lawrence R MD (ObG) - **Spec Exp:** Uro-Gynecology; Pelvic Reconstruction; **Hospital:** N Shore Univ Hosp; **Address:** 865 Northern Blvd, Ste 202, Great Neck, NY 10021; **Phone:** 516-622-5114; **Board Cert:** Obstetrics & Gynecology 2009; **Med School:** Cornell Univ-Weill Med Coll 1990; **Resid:** Obstetrics & Gynecology, N Shore Univ Hosp 1994; **Fellow:** Gynecologic Urology, UCLA Med Ctr 1996

Lustig, Ilana MD (ObG) - **Spec Exp:** Gynecology Only; **Hospital:** NYU Langone Med Ctr (page 106); **Address:** 233 E 31st St, New York, NY 10016-6302; **Phone:** 212-696-9536; **Board Cert:** Obstetrics & Gynecology 1984; **Med School:** Geo Wash Univ 1977; **Resid:** Obstetrics & Gynecology, Yale-New Haven 1981; **Fellow:** Maternal & Fetal Medicine, Bellevue Hosp 1983; **Fac Appt:** Assoc Prof ObG, NYU Sch Med

Maidman, Jack MD (ObG) *PCP* - **Spec Exp:** Maternal & Fetal Medicine; Genetic Disorders; Pregnancy-High Risk; **Hospital:** NY-Presby Hosp/Columbia (page 104); **Address:** 16 E 60th St, Ste 480, New York, NY 10022; **Phone:** 212-326-8951; **Board Cert:** Obstetrics & Gynecology 1970; Maternal & Fetal Medicine 1977; Clinical Genetics 1982; **Med School:** UCSF 1962; **Resid:** Obstetrics & Gynecology, Kings Co Hosp 1968; **Fellow:** Gynecologic Oncology, Kings Co Hosp 1969; Clinical Genetics, Hosp Univ Penn 1970; **Fac Appt:** Assoc Clin Prof ObG, Columbia P&S

Mazlin, Jeffrey A MD (ObG) - **Hospital:** Lenox Hill Hosp; **Address:** 53 E 67th St, New York, NY 10065; **Phone:** 212-517-9048; **Board Cert:** Obstetrics & Gynecology 2009; **Med School:** NY Med Coll 1983; **Resid:** Obstetrics & Gynecology, Lenox Hill Hosp 1987

Melnick, Hugh D MD (ObG) - **Spec Exp:** Infertility-IVF; Infertility-Male; Impotence; **Hospital:** Lenox Hill Hosp; **Address:** Advanced Fertility Services, 1625 Third Ave, Ground Fl, New York, NY 10128-3603; **Phone:** 212-369-8700; **Board Cert:** Obstetrics & Gynecology 1978; **Med School:** Temple Univ 1972; **Resid:** Obstetrics & Gynecology, Lenox Hill Hosp 1976; **Fellow:** Immunopathology, Univ Birmingham 1971

Michel, Ketly MD (ObG) - **Hospital:** Lenox Hill Hosp; **Address:** 261 E 78th St, New York, NY 10075; **Phone:** 212-249-4501; **Board Cert:** Obstetrics & Gynecology 2009; **Med School:** SUNY Upstate Med Univ 1984; **Resid:** Obstetrics & Gynecology, Metropolitan Hosp 1988

Ordorica, Steven A MD (ObG) - **Spec Exp:** Pregnancy-High Risk; Miscarriage-Recurrent; Maternal & Fetal Medicine; **Hospital:** NYU Langone Med Ctr (page 106); **Address:** NYU Med Ctr, 530 1st Ave, Ste 10Q, New York, NY 10016-6402; **Phone:** 212-263-5982; **Board Cert:** Obstetrics & Gynecology 2009; Maternal & Fetal Medicine 2009; **Med School:** SUNY Stony Brook 1983; **Resid:** Obstetrics & Gynecology, NYU Med Ctr 1987; **Fellow:** Maternal & Fetal Medicine, NYU Med Ctr 1989; **Fac Appt:** Assoc Prof ObG, NYU Sch Med

Phillips, Robin N MD (ObG) - **Spec Exp:** Gynecology Only; Menopause Problems; **Hospital:** Mount Sinai Med Ctr (page 102); **Address:** 1126 Park Ave, New York, NY 10128; **Phone:** 212-534-5300; **Board Cert:** Obstetrics & Gynecology 2000; **Med School:** Mount Sinai Sch Med 1977; **Resid:** Obstetrics & Gynecology, Mount Sinai Med Ctr 1982; **Fac Appt:** Asst Clin Prof ObG, Mount Sinai Sch Med

Rodke, Gae MD (ObG) *PCP* - **Spec Exp:** Vulvar Disease; Gynecologic Surgery; **Hospital:** St Luke's - Roosevelt Hosp Ctr - Roosevelt Div (page 94); **Address:** 185 West End Ave, Ste 1D, New York, NY 10023-2005; **Phone:** 212-496-9800; **Board Cert:** Obstetrics & Gynecology 2008; **Med School:** Albert Einstein Coll Med 1981; **Resid:** Family Medicine, Univ Hosp 1982; Obstetrics & Gynecology, Univ Hosp 1986; **Fac Appt:** Asst Clin Prof ObG, Columbia P&S

Sadarangani, Balvinder MD (ObG) - **Spec Exp:** Gynecology Only; Minimally Invasive Surgery; **Hospital:** Beth Israel Med Ctr - Petrie Division (page 94); **Address:** 247 3rd Ave, Ste 503, New York, NY 10010; **Phone:** 212-982-4100; **Board Cert:** Obstetrics & Gynecology 1980; **Med School:** India 1968; **Resid:** Obstetrics & Gynecology, St Vincent's Hosp & Med Ctr 1978

Sailon, Peter S MD (ObG) - **Spec Exp:** Gynecology Only; Hysteroscopic Surgery; Laparoscopic Surgery; **Hospital:** Lenox Hill Hosp; **Address:** 955 Park Ave, New York, NY 10028-0321; **Phone:** 212-879-9191; **Board Cert:** Obstetrics & Gynecology 1982; **Med School:** Italy 1976; **Resid:** Surgery, Univ Hosp Downstate 1977; Obstetrics & Gynecology, St Luke's-Roosevelt Hosp Ctr 1980; **Fellow:** Reproductive Endocrinology, St Luke's-Roosevelt Hosp Ctr 1981

Sassoon, Robert I MD (ObG) - **Spec Exp:** Laparoscopic Surgery; Pregnancy-High Risk; Gynecologic Surgery; **Hospital:** NY-Presby Hosp/Weill Cornell (page 104); **Address:** 449 E 68th St, New York, NY 10021; **Phone:** 212-628-1500; **Board Cert:** Obstetrics & Gynecology 2008; **Med School:** Cornell Univ-Weill Med Coll 1981; **Resid:** Obstetrics & Gynecology, New York Hosp 1985; **Fac Appt:** Clin Prof ObG, Cornell Univ-Weill Med Coll

Scher, Jonathan MD (ObG) - **Spec Exp:** Miscarriage-Recurrent; Pregnancy-High Risk; Infertility-IVF Failure; **Hospital:** Mount Sinai Med Ctr (page 102); **Address:** 1126 Park Ave, New York, NY 10128-1203; **Phone:** 212-427-7400; **Board Cert:** Obstetrics & Gynecology 1981; **Med School:** South Africa 1964; **Resid:** Obstetrics & Gynecology, Groote Schuur Hosp 1970; Obstetrics & Gynecology, Kings College Hosp 1972; **Fac Appt:** Asst Clin Prof ObG, Mount Sinai Sch Med

Schwartz, Judith W MD (ObG) - **Spec Exp:** Gynecologic Surgery; Menopause Problems; **Hospital:** Mount Sinai Med Ctr (page 102); **Address:** 45 E 82nd St Fl 1, New York, NY 10028; **Phone:** 212-879-5959; **Board Cert:** Obstetrics & Gynecology 2009; **Med School:** Mount Sinai Sch Med 1982; **Resid:** Obstetrics & Gynecology, Mount Sinai Hosp 1986; **Fac Appt:** Asst Clin Prof ObG, Mount Sinai Sch Med

Segarra, Pedro R MD (ObG) - **Spec Exp:** Pelvic Organ Prolapse Repair; Breast Disease; Gynecologic Surgery; Vaginal Reconstruction; **Hospital:** Lenox Hill Hosp; **Address:** 1430 2nd Ave, Ste 101, New York, NY 10021; **Phone:** 212-737-0641; **Board Cert:** Obstetrics & Gynecology 2009; **Med School:** NY Med Coll 1983; **Resid:** Obstetrics & Gynecology, Lenox Hill Hosp 1987

Smilen, Scott W MD (ObG) - **Spec Exp:** Uro-Gynecology; Pelvic Organ Prolapse Repair; Minimally Invasive Surgery; Incontinence; **Hospital:** NYU Langone Med Ctr (page 106), Valley Hosp (page 658); **Address:** NYU Med Ctr, Urogynecology, 530 1st Ave, Ste 5F, New York, NY 10016-6497; **Phone:** 212-263-0395; **Board Cert:** Obstetrics & Gynecology 2009; **Med School:** NYU Sch Med 1988; **Resid:** Obstetrics & Gynecology, NYU Med Ctr 1992; **Fellow:** Uro-Gynecology, NYU Med Ctr 1993; **Fac Appt:** Assoc Prof ObG, NYU Sch Med

Snyder, Jon R MD (ObG) - **Spec Exp:** Menopause Problems; Menstrual Disorders; Gynecology Only; **Hospital:** NYU Langone Med Ctr (page 106), Bellevue Hosp Ctr; **Address:** 530 1st Ave, Ste 10N, New York, NY 10016-6402; **Phone:** 212-263-6356; **Board Cert:** Obstetrics & Gynecology 2005; **Med School:** NYU Sch Med 1972; **Resid:** Obstetrics & Gynecology, Bellevue Hosp 1976; **Fac Appt:** Assoc Clin Prof ObG, NYU Sch Med

Sullum, Stanford MD (ObG) *PCP* - **Spec Exp:** Gynecology Only; **Hospital:** Mount Sinai Med Ctr (page 102); **Address:** 1136 5th Ave, New York, NY 10128-0122; **Phone:** 212-876-4630; **Board Cert:** Obstetrics & Gynecology 1979; **Med School:** Jefferson Med Coll 1973; **Resid:** Obstetrics & Gynecology, Mount Sinai Hosp 1977; **Fac Appt:** Asst Clin Prof ObG, Mount Sinai Sch Med

Yale, Suzanne I MD (ObG) - **Hospital:** Lenox Hill Hosp; **Address:** 16 E 82nd St, New York, NY 10028; **Phone:** 212-744-9300; **Board Cert:** Obstetrics & Gynecology 1984; **Med School:** UMDNJ-RW Johnson Med Sch 1977; **Resid:** Obstetrics & Gynecology, Lenox Hill Hosp 1981

Yarberry Allen, Patricia MD (ObG) - **Spec Exp:** Gynecology Only; Menopause Problems; Women's Health; Vulvar & Vaginal Disorders; **Hospital:** NY-Presby Hosp/Weill Cornell (page 104); **Address:** 16 E 90th St, New York, NY 10128-0676; **Phone:** 212-410-4280; **Board Cert:** Obstetrics & Gynecology 1985; **Med School:** Univ Louisville Sch Med 1976; **Resid:** Obstetrics & Gynecology, New York Hosp 1982; **Fellow:** Infectious Disease, New York Hosp 1980; Gynecology, NEw York Hosp 1980

Young, Bruce MD (ObG) - **Spec Exp:** Infertility; Minimally Invasive Surgery; Twin to Twin Transfusion Syndrome (TTTS); Miscarriage-Recurrent; **Hospital:** NYU Langone Med Ctr (page 106), Bellevue Hosp Ctr; **Address:** 530 1st Ave, HCC-5th Fl, Ste 5G, New York, NY 10016; **Phone:** 212-263-6359; **Board Cert:** Obstetrics & Gynecology 1970; Maternal & Fetal Medicine 1975; **Med School:** NYU Sch Med 1963; **Resid:** Obstetrics & Gynecology, NYU Med Ctr 1968; **Fellow:** Reproductive Endocrinology, NYU Med Ctr 1968; **Fac Appt:** Prof ObG, NYU Sch Med

Occupational Medicine

Landrigan, Philip MD (OM) - **Spec Exp:** Environmental Health in Children; **Hospital:** Mount Sinai Med Ctr (page 102); **Address:** Dept Preventive Med, One Gustave L Levy Pl, Box 1057, New York, NY 10029-6500; **Phone:** 212-824-7018; **Board Cert:** Pediatrics 1973; Public Health & Genl Preventive Med 1979; Occupational Medicine 1983; **Med School:** Harvard Med Sch 1967; **Resid:** Internal Medicine, Metro Genl Hosp 1968; Pediatrics, Chldns Hosp 1970; **Fellow:** Epidemiology, Ctrs for Disease Control 1973; Occupational Medicine, Univ London 1977; **Fac Appt:** Prof Ped, Mount Sinai Sch Med

Ophthalmology

Abramson, David H MD (Oph) - **Spec Exp:** Eye Tumors/Cancer; Orbital Tumors/Cancer; Retinoblastoma; Melanoma-Choroidal (eye); **Hospital:** Meml Sloan-Kettering Cancer Ctr (page 112), NY-Presby Hosp/Weill Cornell (page 104); **Address:** 70 E 66th St, New York, NY 10065; **Phone:** 212-744-1700; **Board Cert:** Ophthalmology 1975; **Med School:** Albert Einstein Coll Med 1969; **Resid:** Ophthalmology, Harkness Eye Inst 1974; **Fellow:** Ocular Oncology, Columbia-Presby Med Ctr 1975; **Fac Appt:** Prof Oph, Cornell Univ-Weill Med Coll

Accardi, Frank E MD (Oph) - **Spec Exp:** Cataract Surgery; Refractive Surgery; **Hospital:** New York Eye & Ear Infirm (page 113), Lenox Hill Hosp (Manh Eye, Ear & Throat Hosp); **Address:** 114 E 27th St, New York, NY 10016; **Phone:** 212-481-4000; **Board Cert:** Ophthalmology 1987; **Med School:** Italy 1979; **Resid:** Internal Medicine, Cabrini Med Ctr 1982; Ophthalmology, SUNY-Downstate Med Ctr 1985; **Fellow:** Cornea, SUNY-Downstate Med Ctr 1986; **Fac Appt:** Asst Clin Prof Oph, NY Med Coll

Angioletti, Louis V MD (Oph) - **Spec Exp:** Retinal Disorders; Diabetic Eye Disease/Retinopathy; Macular Degeneration; **Hospital:** New York Eye & Ear Infirm (page 113); **Address:** 7 Gramercy Park, New York, NY 10003-1759; **Phone:** 212-505-8510; **Board Cert:** Ophthalmology 1975; **Med School:** NY Med Coll 1966; **Resid:** Ophthalmology, NY Eye & Ear Infirm 1973; **Fellow:** Retina, NY Eye & Ear Infirm 1974; **Fac Appt:** Asst Clin Prof Oph, NY Med Coll

Asbell, Penny A MD (Oph) - **Spec Exp:** Corneal Disease & Transplant; LASIK-Refractive Surgery; Cataract Surgery; Keratoconus; **Hospital:** Mount Sinai Med Ctr (page 102); **Address:** Mt Sinai School of Medicine, 1190 Fifth Ave, Box 1183, Annenberg Bldg 22-86, New York, NY 10029-6574; **Phone:** 212-241-7977; **Board Cert:** Ophthalmology 1980; **Med School:** SUNY Buffalo 1975; **Resid:** Ophthalmology, NYU Med Ctr 1979; **Fellow:** Immunology, NYU Med Ctr 1980; Cornea & Ext Eye Disease, LSU Eye Ctr 1982; **Fac Appt:** Prof Oph, Mount Sinai Sch Med

Auran, James D MD (Oph) - **Spec Exp:** Corneal Disease; Cataract Surgery; Acanthamoeba Keratitis; Dry Eye Syndrome; **Hospital:** NY-Presby Hosp/Columbia (page 104); **Address:** 635 W 165th St, New York, NY 10032-3701; **Phone:** 212-342-0943; **Board Cert:** Ophthalmology 1989; **Med School:** Cornell Univ-Weill Med Coll 1983; **Resid:** Ophthalmology, Manhattan EET Hosp 1987; **Fellow:** Ophthalmology, Manhattan EET Hosp 1988; **Fac Appt:** Clin Prof Oph, Columbia P&S

Barile, Gaetano R MD (Oph) - **Spec Exp:** Macular Disease/Degeneration; Retinal Disorders; Diabetic Eye Disease/Retinopathy; Retina/Vitreous Consultation; **Hospital:** NY-Presby Hosp/Columbia (page 104); **Address:** Columbia Ophthalmic Consultants, 635 W 165th St, Flanzer Ste, New York, NY 10033; **Phone:** 212-305-9535; **Board Cert:** Ophthalmology 2008; **Med School:** Cornell Univ-Weill Med Coll 1991; **Resid:** Ophthalmology, Manhattan EET Hosp 1995; **Fellow:** Retina/Vitreous, Roosevelt Hosp/Harkness Eye Inst 1997; Retina, Moorfields Eye Hosp 1997; **Fac Appt:** Assoc Prof Oph, Columbia P&S

Barker, Barbara Ann MD (Oph) - **Spec Exp:** Glaucoma; Corneal Disease; **Hospital:** New York Eye & Ear Infirm (page 113), Beth Israel Med Ctr - Petrie Division (page 94); **Address:** 90 E 96th St, New York, NY 10028; **Phone:** 212-289-2244; **Board Cert:** Ophthalmology 1981; **Med School:** Mount Sinai Sch Med 1976; **Resid:** Ophthalmology, Mt Sinai Med Ctr 1980; **Fellow:** Glaucoma, Beth Israel 1981; Cornea, Beth Israel 1983; **Fac Appt:** Asst Clin Prof Oph, Mount Sinai Sch Med

Behrens, Myles MD (Oph) - **Spec Exp:** Neuro-Ophthalmology; **Hospital:** NY-Presby Hosp/Columbia (page 104); **Address:** 635 W 165th St, New York, NY 10032-3701; **Phone:** 212-305-5415; **Board Cert:** Ophthalmology 1971; **Med School:** Columbia P&S 1962; **Resid:** Internal Medicine, Columbia Presby Hosp 1964; Ophthalmology, Columbia Presby Hosp 1970; **Fellow:** Neuro-Ophthalmology, UCSF Med Ctr 1971; **Fac Appt:** Clin Prof Oph, Columbia P&S

Braunstein, Richard E MD (Oph) - **Spec Exp:** LASIK-Refractive Surgery; Corneal Disease & Transplant; Cataract Surgery; **Hospital:** NY-Presby Hosp/Columbia (page 104), Lenox Hill Hosp; **Address:** Harkness Eye Inst, 635 W 165th St, Box 39, New York, NY 10032; **Phone:** 212-305-3015; **Board Cert:** Ophthalmology 2006; **Med School:** Columbia P&S 1989; **Resid:** Ophthalmology, Harkness Eye Inst 1993; **Fellow:** Cornea & Ext Eye Disease, Wilmer Inst/Johns Hopkins Hosp 1994; **Fac Appt:** Assoc Prof Oph, Columbia P&S

Buxton, Douglas F MD (Oph) - **Spec Exp:** Corneal Disease & Transplant; LASIK-Refractive Surgery; Cataract Surgery-Lens Implant; Glaucoma-Pediatric; **Hospital:** New York Eye & Ear Infirm (page 113), Lenox Hill Hosp (Manh Eye, Ear & Throat Hosp); **Address:** 310 E 14th St, Ste 403, New York, NY 10003-4201; **Phone:** 212-979-4410; **Board Cert:** Ophthalmology 2008; Penetrating Keratoplasty 1998; Cataract/Implant Surgery 2002; Refractive Surgery(LASIK) 2002; **Med School:** Cornell Univ-Weill Med Coll 1982; **Resid:** Ophthalmology, New York Eye & Ear Infirm 1986; **Fellow:** Cornea & Ext Eye Disease, New York Eye & Ear Infirm 1988; **Fac Appt:** Assoc Clin Prof Oph, NY Med Coll

Campolattaro, Brian MD (Oph) - **Spec Exp:** Pediatric Ophthalmology; Strabismus; Tear Duct Problems; Eye Muscle Disorders; **Hospital:** New York Eye & Ear Infirm (page 113); **Address:** 30 E 40th St, Ste 405, New York, NY 10016-3507; **Phone:** 212-684-3980; **Board Cert:** Ophthalmology 2006; **Med School:** UMDNJ-NJ Med Sch, Newark 1990; **Resid:** Ophthalmology, New York Eye & Ear Infirm 1994; **Fellow:** Pediatrics, St Louis Chldns Hosp 1995; **Fac Appt:** Asst Prof Oph, NY Med Coll

Carr, Ronald MD (Oph) - **Spec Exp:** Macular Disease/Degeneration; Retinal Disorders; Electrophysiologic Testing; **Hospital:** NYU Langone Med Ctr (page 106), Bellevue Hosp Ctr; **Address:** 530 1st Ave, Ste 3B, New York, NY 10016-6402; **Phone:** 212-263-7360; **Board Cert:** Ophthalmology 1964; **Med School:** Johns Hopkins Univ 1958; **Resid:** Ophthalmology, Bellevue Hosp-NYU 1963; **Fellow:** Ophthalmology, Natl Inst Hlth 1965; **Fac Appt:** Prof Oph, NYU Sch Med

Casper, Daniel S MD/PhD (Oph) - **Spec Exp:** Diabetic Eye Disease; **Hospital:** NY-Presby Hosp/Columbia (page 104); **Address:** N Berrie Diabetes Ctr-Columbia-Presby, 1150 St Nicholas Ave Fl 2, New York, NY 10032-3822; **Phone:** 212-851-5494; **Board Cert:** Ophthalmology 1991; **Med School:** Albany Med Coll 1985; **Resid:** Ophthalmology, Harkness Eye Inst-Columbia 1989; **Fellow:** Oculoplastic Surgery, Harkness Eye Inst-Columbia 1990; **Fac Appt:** Assoc Clin Prof Oph, Columbia P&S

Chaiken, Barry MD (Oph) - **Spec Exp:** Cataract Surgery; LASIK-Refractive Surgery; **Hospital:** New York Eye & Ear Infirm (page 113), Lenox Hill Hosp (Manh Eye, Ear & Throat Hosp); **Address:** 625 Park Ave, New York, NY 10065; **Phone:** 212-249-1976; **Board Cert:** Ophthalmology 1981; **Med School:** Columbia P&S 1976; **Resid:** Ophthalmology, Mt Sinai Hosp 1980

Chang, Stanley MD (Oph) - **Spec Exp:** Diabetic Eye Disease/Retinopathy; Macular Disease/Degeneration; Retina/Vitreous Surgery; Retinal Disorders; **Hospital:** NY-Presby Hosp/Columbia (page 104); **Address:** 635 W 165th St, Box 20, New York, NY 10032; **Phone:** 212-305-9535; **Board Cert:** Ophthalmology 1979; **Med School:** Columbia P&S 1974; **Resid:** Ophthalmology, Mass Eye & Ear Infirm 1978; **Fellow:** Vitreoretinal Surgery, Bascom Palmer Eye Inst 1979; **Fac Appt:** Prof Oph, Columbia P&S

Charles, Norman MD (Oph) - **Spec Exp:** Glaucoma; Eyelid Tumors/Cancer; Contact Lenses; Cornea & External Eye Disease; **Hospital:** NYU Langone Med Ctr (page 106); **Address:** 620 Park Ave, New York, NY 10021-6591; **Phone:** 212-772-6920; **Board Cert:** Ophthalmology 1971; **Med School:** NYU Sch Med 1963; **Resid:** Ophthalmology, NYU Med Ctr 1970; **Fac Appt:** Clin Prof Oph, NYU Sch Med

Chern, Relly MD (Oph) - **Spec Exp:** Cataract Surgery; Ophthalmic Plastic Surgery; **Hospital:** Montefiore Med Ctr - Div. Moses (page 100), New York Eye & Ear Infirm (page 113); **Address:** 923 5th Ave, New York, NY 10021; **Phone:** 212-628-0160; **Board Cert:** Ophthalmology 1983; **Med School:** Albert Einstein Coll Med 1976; **Resid:** Ophthalmology, Montefiore Hosp Med Ctr 1980; **Fac Appt:** Asst Clin Prof Oph, Albert Einstein Coll Med

Chu, Wing MD (Oph) - **Spec Exp:** Corneal Disease & Transplant; Cataract Surgery; **Hospital:** Lenox Hill Hosp (Manh Eye, Ear & Throat Hosp), New York Eye & Ear Infirm (page 113); **Address:** 17 E 72nd St, New York, NY 10021-4145; **Phone:** 212-288-3301; **Board Cert:** Ophthalmology 1978; **Med School:** SUNY Hlth Sci Ctr 1972; **Resid:** Internal Medicine, N Shore Univ & Meml Hosp 1974; Ophthalmology, NY Eye & Ear Infirm 1977; **Fellow:** Cornea & Ext Eye Disease, Mass Eye & Ear Infirm 1979; **Fac Appt:** Assoc Clin Prof Oph, Columbia P&S

Cohen, Ben MD (Oph) - **Spec Exp:** Retina/Vitreous Surgery; Macular Degeneration; Diabetic Eye Disease/Retinopathy; **Hospital:** New York Eye & Ear Infirm (page 113); **Address:** 140 E 80th St, FL 1, New York, NY 10075; **Phone:** 212-772-0600; **Board Cert:** Ophthalmology 1981; **Med School:** NY Med Coll 1976; **Resid:** Ophthalmology, Univ Chicago Hosps 1980; **Fellow:** Retina, Manhattan Eye & Ear Infirmary 1981; Retina, Mass Eye & Ear Infirmary 1983

Cohen, Leeber MD (Oph) - **Spec Exp:** Cataract Surgery; AIDS Related Eye Diseases; Botox Therapy; **Hospital:** New York Eye & Ear Infirm (page 113); **Address:** 11 5th Ave, Ste B, New York, NY 10003-4342; **Phone:** 212-777-1644; **Board Cert:** Ophthalmology 1989; **Med School:** SUNY Hlth Sci Ctr 1983; **Resid:** Ophthalmology, Kings Co Hosp/SUNY Downstate 1987; **Fac Appt:** Asst Clin Prof Med, SUNY Downstate

Coleman, D Jackson MD (Oph) - **Spec Exp:** Retina/Vitreous Surgery; Ultrasound-Eye; Melanoma-Choroidal (eye); **Hospital:** NY-Presby Hosp/Weill Cornell (page 104); **Address:** 1305 York Ave, New York, NY 10021; **Phone:** 646-962-5588; **Board Cert:** Ophthalmology 1969; **Med School:** SUNY Buffalo 1960; **Resid:** Ophthalmology, Columbia-Presby Med Ctr 1967; **Fellow:** Retina, Columbia-Presby Med Ctr 1968; **Fac Appt:** Prof Oph, Cornell Univ-Weill Med Coll

Cykiert, Robert C MD (Oph) - **Spec Exp:** LASIK-Refractive Surgery; Cataract Surgery; Corneal Disease; **Hospital:** NYU Langone Med Ctr (page 106), New York Eye & Ear Infirm (page 113); **Address:** 345 E 37th St, Ste 210, New York, NY 10016-3217; **Phone:** 212-922-1430; **Board Cert:** Ophthalmology 1981; **Med School:** NY Med Coll 1976; **Resid:** Ophthalmology, Montefiore Med Ctr 1980; **Fellow:** Cornea, Wills Eye Hosp 1981; **Fac Appt:** Assoc Clin Prof Oph, NYU Sch Med

D'Amico, Donald J MD (Oph) - **Spec Exp:** Diabetic Eye Disease/Retinopathy; Retinal Detachment; Retinal Disorders; **Hospital:** NY-Presby Hosp/Weill Cornell (page 104); **Address:** Weill Cornell Medical College, Dept of Ophthalmology, 1305 York Ave Fl 11th, New York, NY 10021; **Phone:** 646-962-2020; **Board Cert:** Ophthalmology 1982; **Med School:** Univ IL Coll Med 1977; **Resid:** Ophthalmology, Mass Eye & Ear Infirm 1981; **Fellow:** Vitreoretinal Surgery, Bascom Palmer Eye Inst 1982; **Fac Appt:** Prof Oph, Cornell Univ-Weill Med Coll

Del Priore, Lucian MD/PhD (Oph) - **Spec Exp:** Diabetic Eye Disease/Retinopathy; Macular Degeneration; Retinal Detachment; Retina-Artificial; **Hospital:** NY-Presby Hosp/Columbia (page 104), Lenox Hill Hosp (Manh Eye, Ear & Throat Hosp); **Address:** Harkness Eye Inst, 635 W 165th St, New York, NY 10032; **Phone:** 212-305-9535; **Board Cert:** Ophthalmology 1989; **Med School:** Univ Rochester 1982; **Resid:** Ophthalmology, Wilmer Eye Inst/Johns HopkinsHosp 1987; **Fellow:** Glaucoma, Wilmer Eye Inst/Johns Hopkins Hosp 1988; Vitreoretinal Surgery, Wilmer Eye Inst/Johns Hopkins Hosp 1989; **Fac Appt:** Prof Oph, Columbia P&S

Delerme, Milton MD (Oph) - **Hospital:** Harlem Hosp Ctr; **Address:** 75 E 116th St, New York, NY 10029; **Phone:** 212-828-7700; **Board Cert:** Ophthalmology 1987; **Med School:** UMDNJ-NJ Med Sch, Newark 1978; **Resid:** Surgery, UMDNJ-Univ Hosp 1980; Ophthalmology, Harlem Hosp 1984; **Fellow:** Anterior Segment - External Disease, St Francis Hosp 1985

Della Rocca, Robert C MD (Oph) - **Spec Exp:** Orbital Tumors/Cancer; Eyelid Tumors/Cancer; Thyroid Eye Disease; Oculoplastic Surgery; **Hospital:** New York Eye & Ear Infirm (page 113), Sound Shore Med Ctr - Westchester; **Address:** 310 E 14th St, South Bldg, rm 319, New York, NY 10003; **Phone:** 212-979-4575; **Board Cert:** Ophthalmology 1975; **Med School:** Creighton Univ 1967; **Resid:** Ophthalmology, NY Eye & Ear Infirm 1973; **Fellow:** Oculoplastic Surgery, Albany Med Ctr

Dinnerstein, Stephen R MD (Oph) - **Spec Exp:** Cataract Surgery; Glaucoma; **Hospital:** New York Eye & Ear Infirm (page 113), Mount Sinai Med Ctr (page 102); **Address:** 36 E 36th St, Ste 1J, New York, NY 10016; **Phone:** 212-889-4944; **Board Cert:** Ophthalmology 1976; **Med School:** NY Med Coll 1970; **Resid:** Ophthalmology, Downstate-Kings Co Hosp Ctr 1974

Dodick, Jack M MD (Oph) - **Spec Exp:** Cataract Surgery-Lens Implant; Laser Vision Surgery; **Hospital:** Lenox Hill Hosp (Manh Eye, Ear & Throat Hosp), NYU Langone Med Ctr (page 106); **Address:** 535 Park Ave, New York, NY 10021-8167; **Phone:** 212-288-7638; **Board Cert:** Ophthalmology 1969; **Med School:** Univ Toronto 1963; **Resid:** Ophthalmology, Manhattan EE&T Hosp 1967; **Fellow:** Anterior Segment - External Disease, Westchester Co Med Ctr 1968; **Fac Appt:** Prof Oph, NYU Sch Med

Eggers, Howard M MD (Oph) - **Spec Exp:** Pediatric Ophthalmology; Strabismus-Adult & Pediatric; **Hospital:** NY-Presby Hosp/Columbia (page 104); **Address:** Harkness Eye Institute, 635 W 165th St, New York, NY 10032-3724; **Phone:** 212-305-5409; **Board Cert:** Ophthalmology 1978; **Med School:** Columbia P&S 1971; **Resid:** Ophthalmology, Harkness Inst-Presby Hosp 1975; **Fac Appt:** Prof Oph, Columbia P&S

Eichenbaum, Joseph MD (Oph) - **Spec Exp:** Uveitis; **Hospital:** Mount Sinai Med Ctr (page 102), Lenox Hill Hosp (Manh Eye, Ear & Throat Hosp); **Address:** 1050 Park Ave, New York, NY 10028; **Phone:** 212-289-7200; **Board Cert:** Ophthalmology 1980; **Med School:** Yale Univ 1973; **Resid:** Ophthalmology, NYU Med Ctr 1977; **Fac Appt:** Assoc Clin Prof Oph, Mount Sinai Sch Med

Elahi, Ebrahim MD (Oph) - **Spec Exp:** Oculoplastic Surgery; Orbital Surgery/Tumors; Facial Plastic Surgery; Thyroid Eye Disease; **Hospital:** Mount Sinai Med Ctr (page 102); **Address:** Fifth Avenue Eye Assocs, 1034 Fifth Ave, New York, NY 10028; **Phone:** 212-570-0707; **Board Cert:** Ophthalmology 2001; **Med School:** Mount Sinai Sch Med 1996; **Resid:** Ophthalmology, Mt Sinai Hosp 2000; **Fellow:** Ophthalmic Plastic & Reconstructive Surgery, Manhattan EE&T Infirmary 2001; **Fac Appt:** Assoc Clin Prof Oph, Mount Sinai Sch Med

Engel, Harry MD (Oph) - **Spec Exp:** Retinal Disorders; **Hospital:** Montefiore Med Ctr - Div. Moses (page 100), New York Eye & Ear Infirm (page 113); **Address:** 40 W 72nd St, New York, NY 10023; **Phone:** 212-724-2555; **Board Cert:** Ophthalmology 1981; **Med School:** NY Med Coll 1976; **Resid:** Ophthalmology, U Michigan Med Ctr 1980; **Fellow:** Eye Pathology, Wilmer Inst 1981; Retina/Vitreous, Barnes Jewish Hosp 1982; **Fac Appt:** Clin Prof Oph, Albert Einstein Coll Med

Esposito, Donna A MD (Oph) - **Spec Exp:** Glaucoma; **Hospital:** New York Eye & Ear Infirm (page 113); **Address:** 49 W 23rd St Fl 12th, New York, NY 10011; **Phone:** 212-255-4373; **Board Cert:** Ophthalmology 1991; **Med School:** NY Med Coll 1983; **Resid:** Surgery, St Vincent's Hosp 1985; Ophthalmology, St Vincent's Hosp 1989; **Fellow:** Glaucoma, NY Hosp 1990

Finger, Paul T MD (Oph) - **Spec Exp:** Eye Tumors/Cancer; Melanoma-Choroidal (eye); Retinoblastoma; Orbital Tumors/Cancer; **Hospital:** New York Eye & Ear Infirm (page 113), NYU Langone Med Ctr (page 106); **Address:** The New York Eye Cancer Ctr, 115 E 61st St, Ste 5D, New York, NY 10065; **Phone:** 212-832-8170; **Board Cert:** Ophthalmology 1990; **Med School:** Tulane Univ 1982; **Resid:** Ophthalmology, Manhattan EET Hosp 1986; **Fellow:** Ocular Oncology, N Shore Univ Hosp 1987; **Fac Appt:** Clin Prof Oph, NYU Sch Med

Fisher, Yale MD (Oph) - **Spec Exp:** Retina/Vitreous Consultation; Diabetic Eye Disease; Ocular Ultrasound; **Hospital:** Lenox Hill Hosp (Manh Eye, Ear & Throat Hosp), NY-Presby Hosp/Weill Cornell (page 104); **Address:** 460 Park Ave, New York, NY 10022; **Phone:** 212-861-9797; **Board Cert:** Ophthalmology 1973; **Med School:** Cornell Univ-Weill Med Coll 1967; **Resid:** Ophthalmology, Manhattan EET Hosp 1971; **Fac Appt:** Clin Prof Oph, Cornell Univ-Weill Med Coll

Florakis, George J MD (Oph) - **Spec Exp:** Cornea Transplant; Corneal Disease; Keratoconus; Anterior Segment Trauma/Reconstruction; **Hospital:** NY-Presby Hosp/Columbia (page 104), White Plains Hosp Ctr; **Address:** Harkness Eye Institute, 635 W 165th St, Ste 303, New York, NY 10032; **Phone:** 212-927-2394; **Board Cert:** Ophthalmology 1989; **Med School:** Columbia P&S 1983; **Resid:** Ophthalmology, Harkness Eye Inst 1987; **Fellow:** Cornea & Ext Eye Disease, Univ Iowa Hosps & Clins 1988; **Fac Appt:** Clin Prof Oph, Columbia P&S

Fong, Raymond MD (Oph) - **Spec Exp:** Cataract Surgery; LASIK-Refractive Surgery; Glaucoma; **Hospital:** Lenox Hill Hosp (Manh Eye, Ear & Throat Hosp), NY Downtown Hosp; **Address:** 109 Lafayette St Fl 4, New York, NY 10013-4154; **Phone:** 212-274-1900; **Board Cert:** Ophthalmology 1987; **Med School:** Cornell Univ 1981; **Resid:** Ophthalmology, Manhattan EET Hosp 1985

Fox, Martin L MD (Oph) - **Spec Exp:** LASIK-Refractive Surgery; Cornea Transplant; Corneal Ring Implants; **Hospital:** New York Eye & Ear Infirm (page 113); **Address:** 425 Madison Ave, Ste 1501, New York, NY 10017; **Phone:** 212-838-1053; **Board Cert:** Ophthalmology 1981; **Med School:** Hahnemann Univ 1976; **Resid:** Ophthalmology, Boston Univ Med Ctr 1980; **Fellow:** Cornea, NY Eye & Ear Infirmary 1981

Friedman, Alan H MD (Oph) - **Spec Exp:** Uveitis; Eye Tumors/Cancer; Retinal Disorders; Ophthalmic Pathology; **Hospital:** Mount Sinai Med Ctr (page 102), Lenox Hill Hosp; **Address:** 888 Park Ave, Ste 1A, New York, NY 10075; **Phone:** 212-794-2277; **Board Cert:** Ophthalmology 1971; **Med School:** NYU Sch Med 1963; **Resid:** Ophthalmology, NYU Med Ctr 1969; **Fellow:** Pathology, Hammersmith Hosp 1972; Ocular Pathology, NYU Med Ctr 1970; **Fac Appt:** Clin Prof Oph, Mount Sinai Sch Med

Friedman, Alan J MD (Oph) - **Spec Exp:** Glaucoma; Migraine; **Hospital:** New York Eye & Ear Infirm (page 113), NYU Langone Med Ctr (page 106); **Address:** 120 E 36th St, Ste 1C, New York, NY 10016-3423; **Phone:** 212-683-5180; **Board Cert:** Ophthalmology 1965; **Med School:** Harvard Med Sch 1959; **Resid:** Ophthalmology, NYU-Bellevue Hosp 1963; **Fellow:** Glaucoma, NYU-Bellevue Hosp 1964; **Fac Appt:** Assoc Clin Prof Oph, NYU Sch Med

Friedman, Robert MD (Oph) - **Spec Exp:** Laser Refractive Surgery; Cataract Surgery; Retina/Vitreous Surgery; Macular Disease/Degeneration; **Hospital:** Lenox Hill Hosp, Mount Sinai Med Ctr (page 102); **Address:** 1001 Park Ave, New York, NY 10028-0935; **Phone:** 212-772-6202; **Board Cert:** Ophthalmology 1989; **Med School:** Albert Einstein Coll Med 1983; **Resid:** Ophthalmology, Lenox Hill Hosp 1987; **Fellow:** Vitreoretinal Surgery, Manhattan EET Hosp 1988

Fromer, Mark D MD (Oph) - **Spec Exp:** Retinal Disorders; Laser Vision Surgery; Cataract Surgery; Diabetic Eye Disease/Retinopathy; **Hospital:** New York Eye & Ear Infirm (page 113), Lenox Hill Hosp (Manh Eye, Ear & Throat Hosp); **Address:** 550 Park Ave, New York, NY 10021-8183; **Phone:** 212-832-9228; **Board Cert:** Ophthalmology 1989; **Med School:** UMDNJ-Rutgers Med Sch 1984; **Resid:** Ophthalmology, St Vincents Hosp 1988; **Fellow:** Vitreoretinal Surgery, Manhattan EE&T Hosp 1989; **Fac Appt:** Clin Prof Oph, NY Med Coll

Fuchs, Wayne MD (Oph) - **Spec Exp:** Diabetic Eye Disease/Retinopathy; Macular Disease/Degeneration; Retinal Disorders; Pseudoxanthoma Elasticum; **Hospital:** Mount Sinai Med Ctr (page 102), Lenox Hill Hosp (Manh Eye, Ear & Throat Hosp); **Address:** 121 E 60th St, Ste 5B, New York, NY 10022-1186; **Phone:** 212-319-8205; **Board Cert:** Ophthalmology 1985; **Med School:** Mount Sinai Sch Med 1979; **Resid:** Ophthalmology, Mt Sinai Hosp 1983; **Fellow:** Vitreoretinal Surgery & Disease, NY Hosp-Cornell Med Ctr 1984; **Fac Appt:** Clin Prof Oph, Mount Sinai Sch Med

Gallin, Pamela F MD (Oph) - **Spec Exp:** Pediatric Ophthalmology; Amblyopia; Strabismus; Lacrimal Gland Disorders; **Hospital:** NY-Presby Hosp/Columbia (page 104), Lenox Hill Hosp (Manh Eye, Ear & Throat Hosp); **Address:** NY Presby/Columbia Univ, 635 W 165th St, Ste 224, New York, NY 10032-3701; **Phone:** 212-305-5407; **Board Cert:** Ophthalmology 1983; **Med School:** Washington Univ, St Louis 1978; **Resid:** Ophthalmology, Mount Sinai Med Ctr 1982; **Fellow:** Pediatric Ophthalmology, Chldns Natl Med Ctr 1983; Strabismus, Columbia-Presby Med Ctr 1983; **Fac Appt:** Clin Prof Oph, Columbia P&S

Gentile, Ronald MD (Oph) - **Spec Exp:** Retina/Vitreous Surgery; Diabetic Eye Disease/Retinopathy; Macular Degeneration; Retinal Disorders; **Hospital:** New York Eye & Ear Infirm (page 113); **Address:** 2nd Ave at 14th St, South Bldg - Ste 319, New York, NY 10003-4201; **Phone:** 212-979-4120; **Board Cert:** Ophthalmology 2008; **Med School:** SUNY Downstate 1991; **Resid:** Ophthalmology, NY Eye & Ear Infirm 1995; **Fellow:** Vitreoretinal Surgery & Disease, Kresge Eye Inst 1998; **Fac Appt:** Prof Oph, NY Med Coll

Gibralter, Richard P MD (Oph) - **Spec Exp:** Cataract Surgery; Laser Vision Surgery; Cornea Transplant; Corneal Disease & Surgery; **Hospital:** Lenox Hill Hosp (Manh Eye, Ear & Throat Hosp), New York Eye & Ear Infirm (page 113); **Address:** 154 E 71st St, New York, NY 10021-5123; **Phone:** 212-628-2202; **Board Cert:** Ophthalmology 1981; **Med School:** Mount Sinai Sch Med 1976; **Resid:** Ophthalmology, Manhattan EE&T Hosp 1980; **Fellow:** Cornea, Manhattan EE&T Hosp 1981; **Fac Appt:** Assoc Clin Prof Oph, NYU Sch Med

Grayson, Douglas K MD (Oph) - **Spec Exp:** Cataract Surgery; Glaucoma; **Hospital:** New York Eye & Ear Infirm (page 113); **Address:** 36 E 36th St, New York, NY 10016-3463; **Phone:** 212-353-0030; **Board Cert:** Ophthalmology 2006; **Med School:** Brown Univ 1989; **Resid:** Ophthalmology, NY Eye & Ear Infirm 1993; **Fellow:** Glaucoma, NY Eye & Ear Infirm 1994; **Fac Appt:** Asst Prof Oph, NY Med Coll

Guillory, Samuel L MD (Oph) - **Spec Exp:** LASIK-Refractive Surgery; PRK-Refractive Surgery; Pediatric Ophthalmology; **Hospital:** Mount Sinai Med Ctr (page 102); **Address:** 1103 Park Ave, New York, NY 10128-1236; **Phone:** 212-860-5400; **Board Cert:** Ophthalmology 1980; **Med School:** Mount Sinai Sch Med 1975; **Resid:** Ophthalmology, Mount Sinai Med Ctr 1979; **Fellow:** Ophthalmology, Cornell Med Ctr 1981; **Fac Appt:** Assoc Clin Prof Oph, Mount Sinai Sch Med

Haight, David MD (Oph) - **Spec Exp:** Laser Vision Surgery; Cornea Transplant; Cataract Surgery; **Hospital:** Lenox Hill Hosp, NY-Presby Hosp/Weill Cornell (page 104); **Address:** 155 E 72nd St, New York, NY 10021-4371; **Phone:** 212-772-9474; **Board Cert:** Ophthalmology 1985; **Med School:** Johns Hopkins Univ 1980; **Resid:** Ophthalmology, Manhattan EE&T Hosp 1984; **Fellow:** Cornea, Manhattan EE&T Hosp 1985; **Fac Appt:** Clin Prof Oph, NYU Sch Med

Hall, Lisabeth S MD (Oph) - **Spec Exp:** Pediatric Ophthalmology; Strabismus-Adult & Pediatric; Eye Muscle Disorders; Cataract-Pediatric; **Hospital:** New York Eye & Ear Infirm (page 113), NYU Langone Med Ctr (page 106); **Address:** 40 W 72nd St, New York, NY 10023; **Phone:** 212-979-4614; **Board Cert:** Ophthalmology 2009; **Med School:** SUNY Stony Brook 1992; **Resid:** Ophthalmology, Manhattan Eye & Ear Infirm 1996; **Fellow:** Pediatric Ophthalmology, Jules Stein Eye Inst 1997; **Fac Appt:** Assoc Prof Oph, NY Med Coll

Harmon, Gregory K MD (Oph) - **Spec Exp:** Cataract Surgery; Glaucoma; **Hospital:** NY-Presby Hosp/Weill Cornell (page 104); **Address:** 205 E 64 St, Ste 101, New York, NY 10065; **Phone:** 212-888-4100; **Board Cert:** Ophthalmology 1991; **Med School:** Mount Sinai Sch Med 1982; **Resid:** Ophthalmology, NY Hosp 1986; **Fellow:** Glaucoma, NY Hosp 1987

Heinemann, Murk Hein MD (Oph) - **Hospital:** Meml Sloan-Kettering Cancer Ctr (page 112), NY-Presby Hosp/Weill Cornell (page 104); **Address:** 1275 York Avenue, New York, NY 10065; **Phone:** 800-525-2225; **Board Cert:** Ophthalmology 1982; **Med School:** Cornell Univ-Weill Med Coll 1976; **Resid:** Ophthalmology, Yale-New Haven Hosp 1980; **Fellow:** Ophthalmology, New York Hosp 1982; **Fac Appt:** Assoc Prof Oph, Cornell Univ-Weill Med Coll

Jabs, Douglas MD (Oph) - **Spec Exp:** Uveitis; **Hospital:** Mount Sinai Med Ctr (page 102); **Address:** 17 E 102 St Fl 8, New York, NY 10029; **Phone:** 212-241-6752; **Board Cert:** Ophthalmology 1982; Internal Medicine 1983; **Med School:** Johns Hopkins Univ 1977; **Resid:** Ophthalmology, Wilmer Eye Inst 1981; Internal Medicine, Johns Hopkins Hosp 1983; **Fellow:** Rheumatology, Johns Hopkins Hosp 1984; **Fac Appt:** Prof Oph, Mount Sinai Sch Med

Kazim, Michael MD (Oph) - **Spec Exp:** Thyroid Eye Disease; Oculoplastic Surgery; Orbital Tumors/Cancer; Eyelid Tumors/Cancer; **Hospital:** NY-Presby Hosp/Columbia (page 104), New York Eye & Ear Infirm (page 113); **Address:** 635 W 165th St, New York, NY 10032-3701; **Phone:** 212-305-5477; **Board Cert:** Ophthalmology 1989; **Med School:** Columbia P&S 1984; **Resid:** Ophthalmology, Columbia-Presby Hosp 1988; **Fellow:** Oculoplastic Surgery, Univ Penn-Childrens Hosp 1989; Orbital Surgery, Allegheny Genl Hosp 1990; **Fac Appt:** Clin Prof Oph, Columbia P&S

Kelly, Stephen E MD (Oph) - **Spec Exp:** LASIK-Refractive Surgery; Cataract Surgery; Corneal Disease; **Hospital:** New York Eye & Ear Infirm (page 113), Lenox Hill Hosp (Manh Eye, Ear & Throat Hosp); **Address:** 154 E 71st St, New York, NY 10021-5125; **Phone:** 212-628-2202; **Board Cert:** Ophthalmology 1976; **Med School:** Washington Univ, St Louis 1970; **Resid:** Ophthalmology, NY Eye & Ear Infirmary 1975; **Fellow:** Cornea, Manhattan EET Hosp 1976

Klapper, Daniel MD (Oph) - **Spec Exp:** Laser-Refractive Surgery; Glaucoma; Cataract Surgery; **Hospital:** Lenox Hill Hosp (Manh Eye, Ear & Throat Hosp), Holy Name Med Ctr (page 657); **Address:** 7 W 81st St, Ste 1A, New York, NY 10024; **Phone:** 212-874-2726; **Board Cert:** Ophthalmology 1991; **Med School:** Albert Einstein Coll Med 1984; **Resid:** Ophthalmology, Brookdale Univ Hosp 1988

Klein, Noah MD (Oph) - **Spec Exp:** Glaucoma; Cataract Surgery; LASIK-Refractive Surgery; **Hospital:** New York Eye & Ear Infirm (page 113), Beth Israel Med Ctr - Petrie Division (page 94); **Address:** 51 E 25th St Fl 3, New York, NY 10010; **Phone:** 212-696-9013; **Board Cert:** Ophthalmology 1985; **Med School:** Albert Einstein Coll Med 1980; **Resid:** Ophthalmology, LI Jewish Med Ctr 1985

Koplin, Richard MD (Oph) - **Spec Exp:** Cataract Surgery; Laser Refractive Surgery; Eye Trauma; Eye Infections; **Hospital:** New York Eye & Ear Infirm (page 113); **Address:** 310 E 14th St South Bldg Fl 2, New York, NY 10003-4201; **Phone:** 212-979-4428; **Board Cert:** Ophthalmology 1975; **Med School:** NY Med Coll 1969; **Resid:** Ophthalmology, NY Eye & Ear Infirm 1973; **Fac Appt:** Clin Prof Oph, NY Med Coll

Kupersmith, Mark J MD (Oph) - **Spec Exp:** Neuro-Ophthalmology; **Hospital:** St Luke's - Roosevelt Hosp Ctr - Roosevelt Div (page 94); **Address:** Roosevelt Hosp, 1000 10th Ave, 10th Fl - INN, New York, NY 10019; **Phone:** 212-870-9418; **Board Cert:** Ophthalmology 1981; Neurology 1981; **Med School:** Northwestern Univ 1974; **Resid:** Neurology, NYU Med Ctr 1978; Ophthalmology, NYU Med Ctr 1980; **Fac Appt:** Prof Oph, Albert Einstein Coll Med

Lauer, Simeon A MD (Oph) - **Spec Exp:** Oculoplastic Surgery; Ophthalmic Plastic Surgery; Lacrimal Gland Disorders; Orbital Surgery; **Hospital:** Montefiore Med Ctr - Div. Moses (page 100), Hackensack Univ Med Ctr (page 96); **Address:** 130 E 67th St, New York, NY 10021; **Phone:** 212-879-6824; **Board Cert:** Ophthalmology 1991; **Med School:** SUNY Downstate 1984; **Resid:** Ophthalmology, Montefiore Med Ctr 1989; **Fellow:** Oculoplastic & Reconstructive Surgery, LSU Eye Ctr 1990; **Fac Appt:** Assoc Clin Prof Oph, Albert Einstein Coll Med

Lee, Carol M MD (Oph) - **Spec Exp:** Retina/Vitreous Surgery; Diabetic Eye Disease/Retinopathy; **Hospital:** NYU Langone Med Ctr (page 106); **Address:** 161 Madison Ave, Ste 5NE, New York, NY 10016-5405; **Phone:** 212-684-2424; **Board Cert:** Ophthalmology 1991; **Med School:** SUNY Downstate 1984; **Resid:** Research, Univ Illinois E&E Inst 1986; Ophthalmology, NYU Med Ctr 1989; **Fellow:** Vitreoretinal Surgery & Disease, Washington Univ Barnes Hosp 1991; **Fac Appt:** Clin Prof Oph, NYU Sch Med

Leib, Martin L MD (Oph) - **Spec Exp:** Cataract Surgery; Laser Refractive Surgery; Oculoplastic & Orbital Surgery; Laser Surgery; **Hospital:** NY-Presby Hosp/Columbia (page 104), St Luke's - Roosevelt Hosp Ctr - Roosevelt Div (page 94); **Address:** 635 W 165th St, Ste 230, New York, NY 10032; **Phone:** 212-305-2303; **Board Cert:** Ophthalmology 1982; **Med School:** NY Med Coll 1974; **Resid:** Surgery, Mount Sinai Med Ctr 1976; Ophthalmology, McGill Univ Teaching Hosps 1979; **Fellow:** Ophthalmic Plastic Surgery, Columbia-Presby Med Ctr 1980; Orbital Surgery, Columbia-Presby Med Ctr 1980; **Fac Appt:** Clin Prof Oph, Columbia P&S

Lewis, Hilel MD (Oph) - **Spec Exp:** Retinal Detachment; Diabetic Eye Disease/Retinopathy; Macular Disease/Degeneration; **Hospital:** NY-Presby Hosp/Columbia (page 104); **Address:** Edward Harkness Eye Inst, 635 W 165th St, rm 516, New York, NY 10032; **Phone:** 212-305-4606; **Board Cert:** Ophthalmology 1990; **Med School:** Mexico 1980; **Resid:** Ophthalmology, Jules Stein Eye Inst-UCLA 1986; **Fellow:** Ocular Pathology, Jules Stein Eye Inst-UCLA 1983; Vitreoretinal Surgery, Med Coll Wisconsin 1987; **Fac Appt:** Prof Oph, Columbia P&S

Liebmann, Jeffrey M MD (Oph) - **Spec Exp:** Glaucoma; Cataract Surgery; **Hospital:** New York Eye & Ear Infirm (page 113), Lenox Hill Hosp (Manh Eye, Ear & Throat Hosp); **Address:** 121 E 60th St Fl 8, New York, NY 10022; **Phone:** 212-477-7540; **Board Cert:** Ophthalmology 1989; **Med School:** Boston Univ 1983; **Resid:** Ophthalmology, SUNY Downstate Med Ctr 1987; **Fellow:** Glaucoma, New York EE Infirmary 1988; **Fac Appt:** Clin Prof Oph, NYU Sch Med

Lisman, Richard D MD (Oph) - **Spec Exp:** Oculoplastic Surgery; Eyelid/Tear Duct Reconstruction; Eyelid Cosmetic & Reconstructive Surgery; Orbital & Eyelid Tumors/Cancer; **Hospital:** NYU Langone Med Ctr (page 106), Lenox Hill Hosp (Manh Eye, Ear & Throat Hosp); **Address:** 635 Park Ave, New York, NY 10021-6546; **Phone:** 212-585-1405; **Board Cert:** Ophthalmology 1981; **Med School:** NYU Sch Med 1976; **Resid:** Ophthalmology, Manhattan EE Hosp 1980; **Fellow:** Ophthalmic Plastic Surgery, NY Eye & Ear Infirmary 1981; Plastic Surgery, Manhattan EE&T Hosp 1982; **Fac Appt:** Clin Prof Oph, NYU Sch Med

MacKay, Cynthia J MD (Oph) - **Spec Exp:** Diabetic Eye Disease/Retinopathy; Macular Degeneration; Laser Surgery; Retinitis Pigmentosa; **Hospital:** NY-Presby Hosp/Columbia (page 104), Lenox Hill Hosp (Manh Eye, Ear & Throat Hosp); **Address:** 315 W Central Park West, Ste 1B, New York, NY 10025; **Phone:** 212-772-6050; **Board Cert:** Ophthalmology 1982; **Med School:** SUNY Hlth Sci Ctr 1977; **Resid:** Ophthalmology, Columbia-Presby Med Ctr 1981; **Fellow:** Retina, NYU Med Ctr 1982; **Fac Appt:** Clin Prof Oph, Columbia P&S

Magramm, Irene MD (Oph) - **Spec Exp:** Pediatric Ophthalmology; Strabismus; Cataract Surgery; Diplopia; **Hospital:** Lenox Hill Hosp (Manh Eye, Ear & Throat Hosp), New York Eye & Ear Infirm (page 113); **Address:** 225 E 64th St, New York, NY 10021; **Phone:** 212-644-5100; **Board Cert:** Ophthalmology 1987; **Med School:** Cornell Univ-Weill Med Coll 1981; **Resid:** Ophthalmology, North Shore Univ Hosp 1985; **Fellow:** Pediatric Ophthalmology, Manhattan EE&T Hosp 1986; **Fac Appt:** Asst Clin Prof Oph, Cornell Univ-Weill Med Coll

Mandel, Eric R MD (Oph) - **Spec Exp:** LASIK-Refractive Surgery; Corneal Disease; PRK-Refractive Surgery; **Hospital:** Lenox Hill Hosp; **Address:** 211 E 70th St, New York, NY 10021-5106; **Phone:** 212-734-0111; **Board Cert:** Ophthalmology 1988; **Med School:** SUNY Stony Brook 1982; **Resid:** Ophthalmology, Lenox Hill Hosp 1986; **Fellow:** Cornea & Ext Eye Disease, Mass EE Infirm 1987

Mandelbaum, Sidney MD (Oph) - **Spec Exp:** Cataract Surgery; Cornea Transplant; **Hospital:** New York Eye & Ear Infirm (page 113), Long Island Jewish Med Ctr; **Address:** 178 E 71st St, New York, NY 10021; **Phone:** 212-650-0400; **Board Cert:** Ophthalmology 1982; **Med School:** Yale Univ 1976; **Resid:** Ophthalmology, Los Angeles Chldn's Hosp 1981; **Fellow:** Cornea, Bascom Palmer Eye Inst 1982; **Fac Appt:** Assoc Clin Prof Oph, Albert Einstein Coll Med

McDermott, John A MD (Oph) - **Spec Exp:** Glaucoma; Laser Vision Surgery; **Hospital:** New York Eye & Ear Infirm (page 113); **Address:** 310 E 14th St, New York, NY 10003; **Phone:** 212-979-4446; **Board Cert:** Ophthalmology 1982; **Med School:** NY Med Coll 1976; **Resid:** Ophthalmology, NY Eye & Ear Infirm 1981; Ophthalmology; **Fellow:** Glaucoma, Mass Eye & Ear Infirm 1983; **Fac Appt:** Asst Clin Prof Oph, NY Med Coll

McVeigh, Anne Marie MD (Oph) - ; **Address:** 36 7th Ave, Ste 519, New York, NY 10011; **Phone:** 212-929-3747; **Board Cert:** Ophthalmology 1989; **Med School:** NY Med Coll 1982; **Resid:** Ophthalmology, St Vincent's Hosp & Med Ctr 1986

Medow, Norman MD (Oph) - **Spec Exp:** Cataract-Pediatric; Glaucoma-Pediatric; Corneal Disease-Pediatric; **Hospital:** Lenox Hill Hosp (Manh Eye, Ear & Throat Hosp), NY-Presby Hosp/Weill Cornell (page 104); **Address:** 225 E 64th St, Ste 8, New York, NY 10021-6690; **Phone:** 212-644-5100; **Board Cert:** Ophthalmology 1975; **Med School:** SUNY Hlth Sci Ctr 1966; **Resid:** Ophthalmology, Manhattan EE&T Hosp 1972; **Fellow:** Cataract/Lens Implant Surgery, Charles Kelman, MD 1973; **Fac Appt:** Assoc Clin Prof Oph, Cornell Univ-Weill Med Coll

Melton, R Christine MD (Oph) - **Hospital:** NY-Presby Hosp/Weill Cornell (page 104); **Address:** 247 3rd Ave, Ste 202, New York, NY 10010-7454; **Phone:** 212-475-3791; **Board Cert:** Ophthalmology 1982; **Med School:** Canada 1977; **Resid:** Ophthalmology, St Vincent's Hosp & Med Ctr 1981; **Fac Appt:** Asst Clin Prof Oph, Cornell Univ-Weill Med Coll

Merhige, Kenneth E MD (Oph) - **Hospital:** St Luke's - Roosevelt Hosp Ctr - Roosevelt Div (page 94); **Address:** St. Luke's-Roosevelt Hosp Ctr, 1111 Amsterdam Ave, rm 4207, Stuyvesant 2, rm S-4207, New York, NY 10025; **Phone:** 212-523-2562; **Board Cert:** Ophthalmology 1985; **Med School:** Cornell Univ-Weill Med Coll 1980; **Resid:** Ophthalmology, St Luke's Hosp 1984; **Fellow:** Vitreoretinal Surgery, NY Hosp-Cornell 1985

Merriam, John C MD (Oph) - **Spec Exp:** Cataract Surgery; Reconstructive Surgery; **Hospital:** NY-Presby Hosp/Columbia (page 104), Lenox Hill Hosp (Manh Eye, Ear & Throat Hosp); **Address:** Edward S Harkness Eye Inst, 635 W 165th St, rm 305, New York, NY 10032-3724; **Phone:** 212-305-5402; **Board Cert:** Ophthalmology 1983; **Med School:** Harvard Med Sch 1977; **Resid:** Plastic Surgery, Brigham-Boston Chldns Hosp 1979; Ophthalmology, Mass Eye & Ear Infirm 1982; **Fellow:** Ophthalmology, UCSF Med Ctr 1983; Ophthalmology, Moorefields Eye Hosp; **Fac Appt:** Clin Prof Oph, Columbia P&S

Milite, James MD (Oph) - **Spec Exp:** Oculoplastic Surgery; Eyelid Cosmetic Surgery; Eyelid Tumors/Cancer; Thyroid Eye Disease; **Hospital:** New York Eye & Ear Infirm (page 113); **Address:** 36 E 36th St, New York, NY 10016; **Phone:** 212-353-0030; **Board Cert:** Ophthalmology 2006; **Med School:** NYU Sch Med 1990; **Resid:** Ophthalmology, NY Eye & Ear Infirm 1994; **Fellow:** Ocular Pathology, NY Eye & Ear Infirm 1995; Ophthalmic Plastic Surgery, NY Eye & Ear Infirm 1996; **Fac Appt:** Asst Prof Oph, NY Med Coll

Mindel, Joel MD/PhD (Oph) - **Spec Exp:** Neuro-Ophthalmology; **Hospital:** Mount Sinai Med Ctr (page 102), VA Med Ctr - Bronx; **Address:** One E Gustave Levy Pl, Box 1183, New York, NY 10029; **Phone:** 212-241-0939; **Board Cert:** Ophthalmology 1970; **Med School:** Univ MD Sch Med 1964; **Resid:** Ophthalmology, Univ Michigan Med Ctr 1969; **Fellow:** Neuro-Ophthalmology, Columbia-Presby Med Ctr 1966; Ocular Pharmacology, Mount Sinai Med Ctr 1973; **Fac Appt:** Prof Oph, Mount Sinai Sch Med

Mitchell, John P MD (Oph) - **Spec Exp:** Neuro-Ophthalmology; Cataract Surgery; Glaucoma; **Hospital:** NY-Presby Hosp/Columbia (page 104); **Address:** 226 W 135th St, New York, NY 10030; **Phone:** 212-281-8400; **Board Cert:** Ophthalmology 1978; **Med School:** Cornell Univ-Weill Med Coll 1973; **Resid:** Ophthalmology, Harlem Hosp 1977; **Fellow:** Neuro-Ophthalmology, Columbia-Presby Med Ctr 1978; **Fac Appt:** Asst Prof Oph, Columbia P&S

Moazed, Kambiz T MD (Oph) - **Spec Exp:** Cataract Surgery; Eyelid/Tear Duct Reconstruction; **Hospital:** St Luke's - Roosevelt Hosp Ctr - Roosevelt Div (page 94); **Address:** Manhattan's Physician Group, 2465 Broadway, New York, NY 10025; **Phone:** 212-712-1000; **Board Cert:** Ophthalmology 1983; **Med School:** Iran 1973; **Resid:** Ophthalmology, Mass EE Infirm 1982; **Fellow:** Eye Pathology, Stanford Univ Med Ctr 1977; Oculoplastic Surgery, Edward Harkness Eye Inst 1983; **Fac Appt:** Asst Clin Prof Oph, Columbia P&S

Moskowitz, Bruce K MD (Oph) - **Spec Exp:** Oculoplastic Surgery; Reconstructive Surgery; **Hospital:** New York Eye & Ear Infirm (page 113); **Address:** 310 E 14th St, Ste 401, New York, NY 10003; **Phone:** 212-979-4586; **Board Cert:** Ophthalmology 2003; **Med School:** SUNY Downstate 1987; **Resid:** Ophthalmology, SUNY Downstate 1991; **Fellow:** Ophthalmology, Kingsbrook Jewish Med Ctr 1992; **Fac Appt:** Asst Clin Prof Oph, NY Med Coll

Muchnick, Richard S MD (Oph) - **Spec Exp:** Pediatric Ophthalmology; Strabismus; **Hospital:** NY-Presby Hosp/Weill Cornell (page 104), Lenox Hill Hosp; **Address:** 69 E 71st St, New York, NY 10021-4213; **Phone:** 212-744-1726; **Board Cert:** Ophthalmology 1975; **Med School:** Cornell Univ-Weill Med Coll 1967; **Resid:** Ophthalmology, NY Hosp 1973; **Fellow:** Ophthalmic Plastic Surgery, UCSF Med Ctr 1974; Pediatric Ophthalmology, Manhattan EE&T Hosp 1975; **Fac Appt:** Clin Prof Oph, Cornell Univ-Weill Med Coll

Muldoon, Thomas O MD (Oph) - **Spec Exp:** Retina/Vitreous Surgery; Macular Disease/Degeneration; Diabetic Eye Disease/Retinopathy; **Hospital:** New York Eye & Ear Infirm (page 113); **Address:** 310 E 14th St, Ste 402, New York, NY 10003-4201; **Phone:** 212-979-4595; **Board Cert:** Ophthalmology 1971; **Med School:** Univ Rochester 1962; **Resid:** Surgery, St Lukes Hosp 1966; Ophthalmology, NY EE Infirm 1969; **Fellow:** Retinal Surgery, NY EE Infirm 1970; **Fac Appt:** Assoc Clin Prof Oph, NY Med Coll

Newton, Michael MD (Oph) - **Spec Exp:** Cornea & Cataract Surgery; Refractive Surgery; Eye Infections; **Hospital:** New York Eye & Ear Infirm (page 113), Mount Sinai Med Ctr (page 102); **Address:** 799 Park Ave, New York, NY 10021-3275; **Phone:** 212-861-0146; **Board Cert:** Ophthalmology 1978; **Med School:** Tufts Univ 1971; **Resid:** Ophthalmology, Mount Sinai Hosp 1977; **Fellow:** Cornea & Ext Eye Disease, AB Nesburn MD 1978; **Fac Appt:** Assoc Clin Prof Oph, Mount Sinai Sch Med

Nightingale, Jeffrey MD (Oph) - **Spec Exp:** LASIK-Refractive Surgery; Cataract Surgery; **Hospital:** New York Eye & Ear Infirm (page 113); **Address:** 211 Central Park West, New York, NY 10024-6020; **Phone:** 212-877-7188; **Board Cert:** Ophthalmology 1977; **Med School:** SUNY Hlth Sci Ctr 1972; **Resid:** Ophthalmology, Bronx Lebanon Hosp 1976; **Fellow:** Oculoplastic Surgery, NY Eye & Ear Infirmary 1977

Obstbaum, Stephen A MD (Oph) - **Spec Exp:** Cataract Surgery; Glaucoma; **Hospital:** Lenox Hill Hosp, Lenox Hill Hosp (Manh Eye, Ear & Throat Hosp); **Address:** 121 E 60th St Fl 2, New York, NY 10022; **Phone:** 212-477-7540; **Board Cert:** Ophthalmology 1974; **Med School:** NY Med Coll 1967; **Resid:** Ophthalmology, Flower Fifth Ave Hosp 1972; **Fellow:** Glaucoma, Washington Univ 1973; **Fac Appt:** Prof Oph, NYU Sch Med

Odel, Jeffrey G MD (Oph) - **Spec Exp:** Neuro-Ophthalmology; Retinal Disorders; Optic Nerve Disorders; **Hospital:** NY-Presby Hosp/Columbia (page 104); **Address:** Harkness Eye Institute, 635 W 165th St, rm 316, New York, NY 10032-3701; **Phone:** 212-305-5415; **Board Cert:** Ophthalmology 1981; **Med School:** Univ Rochester 1975; **Resid:** Ophthalmology, Mt Sinai Hosp 1981; **Fellow:** Ophthalmology, Bascom-Palmer Eye Inst 1977; Ophthalmology, Columbia Presby Med Ctr 1982; **Fac Appt:** Assoc Clin Prof Oph, Columbia P&S

Paccione, Jeffrey C MD (Oph) - **Spec Exp:** Retinal Disorders; Macular Degeneration; **Hospital:** Lenox Hill Hosp (Manh Eye, Ear & Throat Hosp), New York Eye & Ear Infirm (page 113); **Address:** Retina Associates of New York, 140 E 80th St, New York, NY 10075; **Phone:** 212-772-0600; **Board Cert:** Ophthalmology 2010; **Med School:** Columbia P&S 1989; **Resid:** Ophthalmology, Manhattan EE&T Hosp 1992; **Fellow:** Vitreoretinal Disease, Mt Sinai Med Ctr 1998; **Fac Appt:** Assoc Clin Prof Oph, Mount Sinai Sch Med

Prince, Andrew MD (Oph) - **Spec Exp:** Glaucoma; Cataract Surgery; **Hospital:** New York Eye & Ear Infirm (page 113), Lenox Hill Hosp (Manh Eye, Ear & Throat Hosp); **Address:** 178 E 71st St, New York, NY 10021-5119; **Phone:** 212-717-2200; **Board Cert:** Ophthalmology 1987; **Med School:** SUNY Downstate 1981; **Resid:** Ophthalmology, SUNY Downstate Med Ctr 1985; **Fellow:** Glaucoma, NY Eye & Ear Infirmary 1986; **Fac Appt:** Assoc Prof Oph, NYU Sch Med

Raab, Edward L MD (Oph) - **Spec Exp:** Pediatric Ophthalmology; Strabismus-Adult & Pediatric; Glaucoma-Pediatric; **Hospital:** Mount Sinai Med Ctr (page 102); **Address:** 17 E 102nd St Fl 8th, New York, NY 10029-6501; **Phone:** 212-369-0988; **Board Cert:** Ophthalmology 1966; **Med School:** NYU Sch Med 1958; **Resid:** Ophthalmology, Mount Sinai 1964; **Fellow:** Pediatric Ophthalmology, Chldns Natl Med Ctr 1967; **Fac Appt:** Prof Oph, Mount Sinai Sch Med

Relland, Maureen MD (Oph) - **Spec Exp:** Oculoplastic Surgery; Eyelid Cosmetic Surgery; Cataract Surgery; **Hospital:** New York Eye & Ear Infirm (page 113); **Address:** 36 7th Ave, Ste 506, New York, NY 10011; **Phone:** 212-645-7771; **Board Cert:** Ophthalmology 1971; **Med School:** NY Med Coll 1964; **Resid:** Ophthalmology, St Vincent's Hosp & Med Ctr 1968; **Fac Appt:** Asst Clin Prof Oph, NY Med Coll

Ritch, Robert MD (Oph) - **Spec Exp:** Glaucoma; **Hospital:** New York Eye & Ear Infirm (page 113); **Address:** 310 E 14th St, rm 304S, New York, NY 10003-4201; **Phone:** 212-477-7540; **Board Cert:** Ophthalmology 1977; **Med School:** Albert Einstein Coll Med 1972; **Resid:** Ophthalmology, Mt Sinai Hosp 1976; **Fellow:** Glaucoma, Mt Sinai Hosp 1978; **Fac Appt:** Clin Prof Oph, NY Med Coll

Ritterband, David MD (Oph) - **Spec Exp:** Eye Infections; Corneal Disease; Refractive Surgery; **Hospital:** New York Eye & Ear Infirm (page 113); **Address:** 310 E 14th St, South Bldg Fl 2, New York, NY 10003-4201; **Phone:** 212-979-4428; **Board Cert:** Ophthalmology 2006; **Med School:** NY Med Coll 1990; **Resid:** Ophthalmology, NY Med Coll 1994; **Fellow:** Cornea & Ext Eye Disease, Eye & Ear Inst 1995

Rodgers, I Rand MD (Oph) - **Spec Exp:** Oculoplastic Surgery; Eyelid Cosmetic & Reconstructive Surgery; Eyelid/Tear Duct Disorders; **Hospital:** Mount Sinai Med Ctr (page 102), N Shore Univ Hosp; **Address:** 229 E 79 St, New York, NY 10021; **Phone:** 212-249-7600; **Board Cert:** Ophthalmology 1989; **Med School:** Mount Sinai Sch Med 1983; **Resid:** Surgery, Mt Sinai Med Ctr 1984; Ophthalmology, Mt Sinai Med Ctr 1987; **Fellow:** Ocular Oncology, Manhattan Eye, Ear & Throat 1988; Ophthalmic Plastic Surgery, Mass E&E Infirm 1990; **Fac Appt:** Asst Clin Prof Oph, Mount Sinai Sch Med

Rodriguez-Sains, Rene S MD (Oph) - **Spec Exp:** Eyelid Cosmetic & Reconstructive Surgery; Eyelid Tumors/Cancer; Melanoma; Eye Tumors/Cancer; **Hospital:** New York Eye & Ear Infirm (page 113), NYU Langone Med Ctr (page 106); **Address:** 799 Park Ave, New York, NY 10021-3275; **Phone:** 212-535-0315; **Board Cert:** Ophthalmology 1982; **Med School:** NYU Sch Med 1977; **Resid:** Ophthalmology, Manhattan EET Hosp 1981; **Fellow:** Plastic Surgery, Manhattan EET Hosp 1982; Ophthalmic Oncololgy, Manhattan EET Hosp 1982; **Fac Appt:** Asst Clin Prof Oph, NYU Sch Med

Rosenthal, Jeanne L MD (Oph) - **Spec Exp:** Retina/Vitreous Surgery; Macular Degeneration; Diabetic Eye Disease/Retinopathy; **Hospital:** New York Eye & Ear Infirm (page 113); **Address:** 20 E 9th St, New York, NY 10003-5944; **Phone:** 212-674-2970; **Board Cert:** Ophthalmology 1985; **Med School:** SUNY Downstate 1979; **Resid:** Ophthalmology, NY Eye & Ear Infirm 1983; **Fellow:** Retina, NY Eye & Ear Infirm 1985; **Fac Appt:** Clin Prof Oph, NY Med Coll

Rudick Jr, A Joseph MD (Oph) - **Spec Exp:** LASIK-Refractive Surgery; Cataract Surgery; Glaucoma; Dry Eye Syndrome; **Hospital:** New York Eye & Ear Infirm (page 113), NY Downtown Hosp; **Address:** 150 Broadway, Ste 1800, New York, NY 10038; **Phone:** 212-233-2344; **Board Cert:** Ophthalmology 1989; **Med School:** Univ Pennsylvania 1983; **Resid:** Ophthalmology, Manhattan EE&T Hosp 1988

Samson, C Michael MD (Oph) - **Spec Exp:** Uveitis; Immunotherapy; Eye Infections; **Hospital:** New York Eye & Ear Infirm (page 113); **Address:** 310 E 14th St, Ste 319 S, New York, NY 10003; **Phone:** 212-979-4515; **Board Cert:** Ophthalmology 2000; **Med School:** SUNY Downstate 1994; **Resid:** Ophthalmology, NY Eye & Ear Infirm 1998; **Fellow:** Ophthalmology, Mass Eye & Ear Infirm 1999

Schiff, William M MD (Oph) - **Spec Exp:** Macular Disease/Degeneration; Diabetic Eye Disease/Retinopathy; Retinal Detachment; Macular Disease/Degeneration; **Hospital:** NY-Presby Hosp/Columbia (page 104), St Luke's - Roosevelt Hosp Ctr - Roosevelt Div (page 94); **Address:** Columbia Ophthalmic Consultants, 635 W 165th St, New York, NY 10032; **Phone:** 212-305-9535; **Board Cert:** Ophthalmology 2006; **Med School:** NYU Sch Med 1988; **Resid:** Ophthalmology, New York Eye & Ear Infirm 1994; **Fellow:** Retina/Vitreous, NY Hosp-Harkness Eye Inst 1996; **Fac Appt:** Prof Oph, Columbia P&S

Schubert, Hermann D MD (Oph) - **Spec Exp:** Diabetic Eye Disease/Retinopathy; Macular Degeneration; Retinal Disorders; Retinal Detachment; **Hospital:** NY-Presby Hosp/Columbia (page 104), Southampton Hosp; **Address:** 635 W 165th St, Rm 206, New York, NY 10032-3701; **Phone:** 212-305-6534; **Board Cert:** Ophthalmology 1987; Anatomic Pathology 1981; **Med School:** Germany 1974; **Resid:** Pathology, Columbia-Presby Hosp 1979; Ophthalmology, Columbia-Presby Hosp 1985; **Fellow:** Retina, Wills Eye Hosp 1987; **Fac Appt:** Prof Oph, Columbia P&S

Seedor, John A MD (Oph) - **Spec Exp:** Cornea & External Eye Disease; Laser Vision Surgery; **Hospital:** New York Eye & Ear Infirm (page 113); **Address:** 310 E 14th St South Bldg Fl 2, New York, NY 10003-4201; **Phone:** 212-979-4428; **Board Cert:** Ophthalmology 1987; **Med School:** Hahnemann Univ 1981; **Resid:** Ophthalmology, NY Eye & Ear Infirm 1985; **Fellow:** Cornea, Emory Univ Hosp 1987; **Fac Appt:** Assoc Clin Prof Oph, NY Med Coll

Serle, Janet B MD (Oph) - **Spec Exp:** Glaucoma; **Hospital:** Mount Sinai Med Ctr (page 102), Syosset Hosp; **Address:** 17 E 102 St, 8th Fl, Box 1183, New York, NY 10029; **Phone:** 212-241-0939; **Board Cert:** Ophthalmology 1987; **Med School:** Harvard Med Sch 1980; **Resid:** Ophthalmology, Mount Sinai Hosp 1985; **Fellow:** Glaucoma, Mount Sinai Hosp 1982; Glaucoma, Mount Sinai Hosp 1986; **Fac Appt:** Prof Oph, Mount Sinai Sch Med

Shabto, Uri MD (Oph) - **Spec Exp:** Retinopathy of Prematurity; Macular Disease/Degeneration; Diabetic Eye Disease/Retinopathy; **Hospital:** New York Eye & Ear Infirm (page 113); **Address:** 310 E 14th St South Bldg - Ste 419, New York, NY 10003-4201; **Phone:** 212-677-2000; **Board Cert:** Ophthalmology 1991; **Med School:** Harvard Med Sch 1986; **Resid:** Ophthalmology, NY Eye & Ear Infirm 1990; **Fellow:** Vitreoretinal Surgery, Montefiore Hosp 1991; **Fac Appt:** Asst Prof Oph, NYU Sch Med

Sherman, Spencer E MD (Oph) - **Spec Exp:** Cataract Surgery; Glaucoma; Contact Lenses; Refractive Surgery; **Hospital:** Lenox Hill Hosp (Manh Eye, Ear & Throat Hosp), Mount Sinai Med Ctr (page 102); **Address:** 166 E 63rd St, New York, NY 10021-7636; **Phone:** 212-753-8300; **Board Cert:** Ophthalmology 1970; **Med School:** Columbia P&S 1962; **Resid:** Ophthalmology, Mt Sinai Hosp 1968; **Fac Appt:** Asst Clin Prof Oph, Mount Sinai Sch Med

Shulman, Julius MD (Oph) - **Spec Exp:** Cataract Surgery; LASIK-Refractive Surgery; Contact Lenses; Glaucoma; **Hospital:** Mount Sinai Med Ctr (page 102); **Address:** 229 E 79th St, Apt 1L, New York, NY 10075; **Phone:** 212-861-6200; **Board Cert:** Ophthalmology 2006; **Med School:** SUNY Hlth Sci Ctr 1969; **Resid:** Ophthalmology, Mt Sinai Med Ctr 1975; **Fac Appt:** Asst Clin Prof Oph, Mount Sinai Sch Med

Sidoti, Paul MD (Oph) - **Spec Exp:** Glaucoma; **Hospital:** New York Eye & Ear Infirm (page 113), Beth Israel Med Ctr - Petrie Division (page 94); **Address:** New York Eye & Ear Infirmary, 310 E 14th St, Ste 319, New York, NY 10003-4201; **Phone:** 212-979-4590; **Board Cert:** Ophthalmology 2005; **Med School:** Albert Einstein Coll Med 1988; **Resid:** Ophthalmology, NY Eye & Ear Infirm 1992; **Fellow:** Glaucoma, Doheny Eye Inst-USC 1994; **Fac Appt:** Prof Oph, NY Med Coll

Slakter, Jason MD (Oph) - **Spec Exp:** Retinal Disorders; Macular Degeneration; **Hospital:** Lenox Hill Hosp (Manh Eye, Ear & Throat Hosp); **Address:** 460 Park Ave Fl 5, New York, NY 10022; **Phone:** 212-861-9797; **Board Cert:** Ophthalmology 1989; **Med School:** Albert Einstein Coll Med 1983; **Resid:** Ophthalmology, Manhattan Eye & Ear Infirm 1987; **Fellow:** Retina/Vitreous, Manhattan Eye & Ear Infirm 1988; **Fac Appt:** Clin Prof Oph, NYU Sch Med

Smith, R Theodore MD (Oph) - **Spec Exp:** Retinal Disorders; Macular Degeneration; **Hospital:** NY-Presby Hosp/Columbia (page 104); **Address:** Harkness Eye Institute, 635 W 165th St, Ste 314, New York, NY 10032; **Phone:** 212-342-1849; **Board Cert:** Ophthalmology 1986; **Med School:** Albert Einstein Coll Med 1981; **Resid:** Ophthalmology, Montefiore Hosp 1982; Ophthalmology, Columbia-Presby Hosp 1985; **Fellow:** Retina, Illinois Eye&Ear Infirm 1986; **Fac Appt:** Assoc Clin Prof Oph, Columbia P&S

Smith, Scott D MD (Oph) - **Spec Exp:** Glaucoma; **Hospital:** NY-Presby Hosp/Columbia (page 104); **Address:** Edward Harkness Eye Inst, 635 W 165th St, New York, NY 10030; **Phone:** 212-305-9535; **Board Cert:** Ophthalmology 2006; **Med School:** Yale Univ 1990; **Resid:** Ophthalmology, Mass Eye & Ear Infirm 1994; **Fellow:** Glaucoma, Wilmer Eye Inst 1996; **Fac Appt:** Assoc Prof Oph, Columbia P&S

Solomon, Joel M MD (Oph) - **Spec Exp:** Cornea & Cataract Surgery; Refractive Surgery; **Hospital:** NYU Langone Med Ctr (page 106), Bellevue Hosp Ctr; **Address:** 323 E 34th St Fl 4, New York, NY 10016; **Phone:** 212-689-5080; **Board Cert:** Ophthalmology 1987; **Med School:** Cornell Univ-Weill Med Coll 1981; **Resid:** Internal Medicine, Albany Med Ctr 1983; Ophthalmology, NYU Med Ctr 1986; **Fellow:** Cornea & Ext Eye Disease, Med Coll Wisc 1987; **Fac Appt:** Clin Prof Oph, NYU Sch Med

Soloway, Barrie D MD (Oph) - **Spec Exp:** LASIK-Refractive Surgery; Corneal Disease; Glaucoma; **Hospital:** New York Eye & Ear Infirm (page 113), Lenox Hill Hosp; **Address:** 160 E 56th St, Fl 9th, New York, NY 10022; **Phone:** 212-758-3838; **Board Cert:** Ophthalmology 1987; **Med School:** Penn State Univ-Hershey Med Ctr 1980; **Resid:** Ophthalmology, NY Eye & Ear Infirm 1985; **Fellow:** Cornea, NY Eye & Ear Infirm 1986; **Fac Appt:** Asst Prof Oph, Mount Sinai Sch Med

Spaide, Richard MD (Oph) - **Spec Exp:** Retinal Disorders; Macular Degeneration; Diabetic Eye Disease/Retinopathy; **Hospital:** Lenox Hill Hosp (Manh Eye, Ear & Throat Hosp); **Address:** 460 Park Ave Fl 5th, New York, NY 10022; **Phone:** 212-861-9797; **Board Cert:** Ophthalmology 1987; **Med School:** Jefferson Med Coll 1981; **Resid:** Ophthalmology, St Vincent's Hosp & Med Ctr 1985; **Fellow:** Vitreoretinal Surgery & Disease, Manhattan EET Hosp 1990; **Fac Appt:** Assoc Clin Prof Oph, NY Med Coll

Starr, Michael B MD (Oph) - **Spec Exp:** LASIK-Refractive Surgery; Cornea & Cataract Surgery; Eye Infections; **Hospital:** Lenox Hill Hosp, Lenox Hill Hosp (Manh Eye, Ear & Throat Hosp); **Address:** 67 E 78th St, New York, NY 10021; **Phone:** 212-717-0222; **Board Cert:** Ophthalmology 1978; **Med School:** Mount Sinai Sch Med 1972; **Resid:** Neurology, Mount Sinai 1974; Ophthalmology, Lenox Hill Hosp 1977; **Fellow:** Cornea, UCSF Med Ctr 1979; **Fac Appt:** Assoc Clin Prof Oph, Mount Sinai Sch Med

Steele, Mark MD (Oph) - **Spec Exp:** Pediatric Ophthalmology; Strabismus; Eye Muscle Disorders; **Hospital:** NYU Langone Med Ctr (page 106), New York Eye & Ear Infirm (page 113); **Address:** 40 W 72nd St, New York, NY 10023; **Phone:** 212-981-9800; **Board Cert:** Ophthalmology 1991; **Med School:** NYU Sch Med 1986; **Resid:** Ophthalmology, NYU Med Ctr 1990; **Fellow:** Pediatric Ophthalmology, Wills Eye Hosp 1991; **Fac Appt:** Assoc Clin Prof Oph, NYU Sch Med

Tello, Celso MD (Oph) - **Spec Exp:** Glaucoma; **Hospital:** New York Eye & Ear Infirm (page 113); **Address:** 310 E 14th St, Ste 304, New York, NY 10003; **Phone:** 212-477-7540; **Board Cert:** Ophthalmology 2000; **Med School:** Ecuador 1988; **Resid:** Ophthalmology, NY Eye & Ear Infirm 1993; **Fellow:** Glaucoma, NY Eye & Ear Infirm 1994; **Fac Appt:** Asst Prof Oph, NYU Sch Med

Walsh, Joseph B MD (Oph) - **Spec Exp:** Diabetic Eye Disease/Retinopathy; Macular Degeneration; Retinal Disorders; **Hospital:** New York Eye & Ear Infirm (page 113), Beth Israel Med Ctr - Petrie Division (page 94); **Address:** 310 E 14th St Bldg S Fl 3, New York, NY 10003-4201; **Phone:** 212-979-4500; **Board Cert:** Ophthalmology 2005; **Med School:** Georgetown Univ 1966; **Resid:** Internal Medicine, Univ Hosp 1968; Ophthalmology, NY Eye & Ear Infirm 1973; **Fellow:** Retina, Montefiore Med Ctr 1974; **Fac Appt:** Prof Oph, NY Med Coll

Wang, Frederick MD (Oph) - **Spec Exp:** Pediatric Ophthalmology; Strabismus; Eye Muscle Disorders; **Hospital:** New York Eye & Ear Infirm (page 113), Montefiore Med Ctr - Div. Moses (page 100); **Address:** 30 E 40th St, Ste 405, New York, NY 10016-1201; **Phone:** 212-684-3980; **Board Cert:** Pediatrics 1978; Ophthalmology 1980; **Med School:** Albert Einstein Coll Med 1972; **Resid:** Pediatrics, Jacobi Med Ctr 1974; Ophthalmology, Albert Einstein 1979; **Fellow:** Pediatric Ophthalmology, Children's Hosp Natl Med Ctr 1980; **Fac Appt:** Clin Prof Oph, Albert Einstein Coll Med

Warren, Floyd A MD (Oph) - **Spec Exp:** Neuro-Ophthalmology; Optic Nerve Disorders; Orbital Diseases; **Hospital:** NYU Langone Med Ctr (page 106), Lenox Hill Hosp (Manh Eye, Ear & Throat Hosp); **Address:** Schwartz Health Care Ctr, 530 First Ave, Ste 3B, New York, NY 10016; **Phone:** 212-263-7030; **Board Cert:** Ophthalmology 1985; **Med School:** NYU Sch Med 1979; **Resid:** Ophthalmology, St Vincents Hosp 1983; **Fellow:** Neuro-Ophthalmology, Bellevue Hosp 1984; Orbital Disease, Univ Pittsburgh 1985; **Fac Appt:** Clin Prof Oph, NYU Sch Med

Weiss, Michael J MD/PhD (Oph) - **Spec Exp:** Uveitis; Retinal Disorders; Cataract Surgery; **Hospital:** NY-Presby Hosp/Columbia (page 104); **Address:** 635 W 165th St, Ste 101, New York, NY 10032-3701; **Phone:** 212-305-9925; **Board Cert:** Ophthalmology 1987; **Med School:** Columbia P&S 1981; **Resid:** Ophthalmology, Columbia-Presby Med Ctr 1985; **Fac Appt:** Clin Prof Oph, Columbia P&S

Weseley, Peter E MD (Oph) - **Spec Exp:** Retina/Vitreous Surgery; **Hospital:** New York Eye & Ear Infirm (page 113); **Address:** 310 E 14th St, Ste 419, New York, NY 10003; **Phone:** 212-979-4286; **Board Cert:** Ophthalmology 2003; **Med School:** Tulane Univ 1987; **Resid:** Ophthalmology, NY E&E Infirm 1991; **Fellow:** Vitreoretinal Surgery, Devers Eye Inst 1993

Whitmore, Wayne G MD (Oph) - **Spec Exp:** Cataract Surgery; Glaucoma; Corneal Disease; **Hospital:** NY-Presby Hosp/Weill Cornell (page 104), Lenox Hill Hosp (Manh Eye, Ear & Throat Hosp); **Address:** 116 E 68th St, New York, NY 10065; **Phone:** 212-249-3030; **Board Cert:** Ophthalmology 1982; **Med School:** Dartmouth Med Sch 1977; **Resid:** Ophthalmology, NY Hosp 1981; **Fellow:** Ophthalmic Oncololgy, NY Hosp 1982; **Fac Appt:** Asst Clin Prof Oph, Cornell Univ-Weill Med Coll

Winterkorn, Jacqueline MD/PhD (Oph) - **Spec Exp:** Neuro-Ophthalmology; Brain Tumors; Eye Muscle Disorders; **Hospital:** NY-Presby Hosp/Weill Cornell (page 104); **Address:** 1305 York Ave Fl 11, New York, NY 10021; **Phone:** 212-746-3072; **Board Cert:** Ophthalmology 1989; **Med School:** Cornell Univ-Weill Med Coll 1983; **Resid:** Ophthalmology, Mount Sinai Med Ctr 1987; **Fellow:** Neuro-Ophthalmology, Columbia Presby Med Ctr 1988; **Fac Appt:** Clin Prof Oph, Cornell Univ-Weill Med Coll

Wisnicki, H Jay MD (Oph) - **Spec Exp:** Strabismus; Eye Muscle Disorders; Pediatric Ophthalmology; **Hospital:** Beth Israel Med Ctr - Petrie Division (page 94), New York Eye & Ear Infirm (page 113); **Address:** 235 Park Ave S Fl 2nd, Phillips Ambulatory Care Ctr, New York, NY 10003; **Phone:** 212-844-2020; **Board Cert:** Ophthalmology 1987; **Med School:** SUNY Hlth Sci Ctr 1981; **Resid:** Ophthalmology, Mount Sinai Med Ctr 1985; **Fellow:** Strabismus, Johns Hopkins Hosp 1986; **Fac Appt:** Assoc Prof Oph, Albert Einstein Coll Med

Wong, Raymond F MD (Oph) - **Spec Exp:** Diabetic Eye Disease/Retinopathy; Retinal Detachment; Macular Disease/Degeneration; **Hospital:** New York Eye & Ear Infirm (page 113); **Address:** 210 Canal St, rm 409, New York, NY 10013-4159; **Phone:** 212-227-5451; **Board Cert:** Ophthalmology 1990; **Med School:** SUNY Hlth Sci Ctr 1984; **Resid:** Ophthalmology, Yale-New Haven Hosp 1988; **Fellow:** Retina, USC-Doheny Eye Inst 1990; **Fac Appt:** Asst Clin Prof Oph, NY Med Coll

Yagoda, Arnold D MD (Oph) - **Spec Exp:** Macular Degeneration; Laser Vision Surgery; Diabetic Eye Disease/Retinopathy; **Hospital:** Lenox Hill Hosp, New York Eye & Ear Infirm (page 113); **Address:** 67 E 78th St, New York, NY 10075; **Phone:** 212-744-2513; **Board Cert:** Ophthalmology 1980; **Med School:** Cornell Univ-Weill Med Coll 1975; **Resid:** Ophthalmology, Lenox Hill Hosp 1979; **Fellow:** Vitreoretinal Disease, Montefiore Hosp Med Ctr 1980; **Fac Appt:** Asst Clin Prof Oph, Albert Einstein Coll Med

Yannuzzi, Lawrence MD (Oph) - **Spec Exp:** Retina/Vitreous Surgery; Macular Disease/Degeneration; Diabetic Eye Disease/Retinopathy; **Hospital:** NY-Presby Hosp/Columbia (page 104), Lenox Hill Hosp (Manh Eye, Ear & Throat Hosp); **Address:** 460 Park Ave Fl 5, New York, NY 10021-4028; **Phone:** 212-861-9797; **Board Cert:** Ophthalmology 1970; **Med School:** Boston Univ 1964; **Resid:** Ophthalmology, Manhattan EE&T Hosp 1968; **Fellow:** Ophthalmology, Manhattan EE&T Hosp 1971; **Fac Appt:** Clin Prof Oph, Columbia P&S

Young, Joshua A MD (Oph) - **Spec Exp:** Cataract Surgery; PRK-Refractive Surgery; Contact Lenses; **Hospital:** NYU Langone Med Ctr (page 106), Lenox Hill Hosp (Manh Eye, Ear & Throat Hosp); **Address:** 161 Madison Ave, Ste 5 SE, New York, NY 10016; **Phone:** 212-448-0101; **Board Cert:** Ophthalmology 2008; **Med School:** NYU Sch Med 1990; **Resid:** Ophthalmology, NYU Med Ctr 1994; **Fellow:** Ophthalmology, Mass Eye & Ear Infirm/Harvard 1996; **Fac Appt:** Assoc Prof Oph, NYU Sch Med

Zweifach, Philip H MD (Oph) - **Spec Exp:** Cataract Surgery; Neuro-Ophthalmology; Glaucoma; **Hospital:** NY-Presby Hosp/Weill Cornell (page 104); **Address:** 131 E 69th St, New York, NY 10021-5158; **Phone:** 212-535-1508; **Board Cert:** Ophthalmology 1968; **Med School:** Cornell Univ-Weill Med Coll 1961; **Resid:** Neurology, Boston City Hosp 1963; Ophthalmology, New York Hosp 1966; **Fellow:** Neuro-Ophthalmology, Mass Eye & Ear Infirmary 1967; **Fac Appt:** Clin Prof Oph, Cornell Univ-Weill Med Coll

Orthopaedic Surgery

Adler, Edward MD (OrS) - **Spec Exp:** Hip Replacement; Knee Replacement; Foot & Ankle Surgery; **Hospital:** NYU Hosp For Joint Diseases (page 106), NYU Langone Med Ctr (page 106); **Address:** 145 E 32nd St Fl 4, New York, NY 10016; **Phone:** 212-427-3986; **Board Cert:** Orthopaedic Surgery 2003; **Med School:** UMDNJ-NJ Med Sch, Newark 1984; **Resid:** Orthopaedic Surgery, UMDNJ-NJ Sch Med 1989; **Fellow:** Joint Replacement Surgery, Hosp for Joint Dis 1990; **Fac Appt:** Asst Clin Prof OrS, NYU Sch Med

Alexiades, Michael M MD (OrS) - **Spec Exp:** Hip Replacement; Knee Replacement; Arthroscopic Surgery; Minimally Invasive Surgery; **Hospital:** Lenox Hill Hosp, Hosp For Special Surgery (page 111); **Address:** 523 E 72nd St Fl 7, New York, NY 10021; **Phone:** 212-774-7557; **Board Cert:** Orthopaedic Surgery 2002; **Med School:** Cornell Univ-Weill Med Coll 1983; **Resid:** Orthopaedic Surgery, Lenox Hill Hosp 1988; Surgery, Children's Hosp 1986; **Fellow:** Arthritis Surgery, Hosp for Special Surgery 1989; **Fac Appt:** Asst Prof OrS, Cornell Univ-Weill Med Coll

Bauman, Phillip A MD (OrS) - **Spec Exp:** Foot & Ankle Surgery; Knee Surgery; Dance/Sports Medicine; Arthroscopic Surgery; **Hospital:** St Luke's - Roosevelt Hosp Ctr - Roosevelt Div (page 94), NY-Presby Hosp/Columbia (page 104); **Address:** Orthopaedic Assocs of NY, 343 W 58th St, rm 1, New York, NY 10019; **Phone:** 212-506-0228; **Board Cert:** Orthopaedic Surgery 2009; **Med School:** Columbia P&S 1981; **Resid:** Surgery, St Lukes-Roosevelt Hosp Ctr 1983; Orthopaedic Surgery, Columbia-Presby Med Ctr 1987; **Fac Appt:** Asst Prof OrS, Columbia P&S

Bendo, John A MD (OrS) - **Spec Exp:** Spinal Surgery-Minimally Invasive; Scoliosis; Spinal Disc Replacement; **Hospital:** NYU Hosp For Joint Diseases (page 106), NYU Langone Med Ctr (page 106); **Address:** Hosp for Joint Diseases-Spine Ctr, 301 E 17th St, Ste 400, New York, NY 10003; **Phone:** 212-598-6625; **Board Cert:** Orthopaedic Surgery 2007; **Med School:** Mount Sinai Sch Med 1989; **Resid:** Orthopaedic Surgery, Mt Sinai Hosp 1994; **Fellow:** Spinal Surgery, Hosp Joint Diseases 1996; **Fac Appt:** Asst Prof OrS, NYU Sch Med

Bigliani, Louis U MD (OrS) - **Spec Exp:** Shoulder Surgery; Sports Medicine; Arthroscopic Surgery; Rotator Cuff Surgery; **Hospital:** NY-Presby Hosp/Columbia (page 104); **Address:** 622 W 168th St, rm 1130, New York, NY 10032-3720; **Phone:** 212-305-0998; **Board Cert:** Orthopaedic Surgery 1979; **Med School:** Loyola Univ-Stritch Sch Med 1973; **Resid:** Surgery, Roosevelt Hosp 1974; Orthopaedic Surgery, Columbia Presby Med Ctr 1977; **Fac Appt:** Prof OrS, Columbia P&S

Bitan, Fabien D MD (OrS) - **Spec Exp:** Spinal Surgery-Pediatric & Adult; Spinal Disc Replacement; Spinal Deformity; Spinal Disorders-Degenerative; **Hospital:** Lenox Hill Hosp, Beth Israel Med Ctr - Petrie Division (page 94); **Address:** Manhattan Orthopaedics, 130 E 77th St Fl 7, New York, NY 10075; **Phone:** 212-744-8114; **Med School:** France 1981; **Resid:** Orthopaedic Surgery, Hospital Beaujon 1987; Pediatric Orthopaedic Surgery, Hosp des Enfants Malades 1990; **Fellow:** Pediatric Orthopaedic Surgery, Hosp Special Surgery 1997; Spinal Surgery, Beth Israel Med Ctr 1998

Boachie-Adjei, Oheneba MD (OrS) - **Spec Exp:** Spinal Surgery; Scoliosis; **Hospital:** Hosp For Special Surgery (page 111); **Address:** Hosp for Special Surgery, 535 E 70th St, New York, NY 10021; **Phone:** 212-606-1948; **Board Cert:** Orthopaedic Surgery 2000; **Med School:** Columbia P&S 1980; **Resid:** Surgery, St Vincents Hosp 1982; Orthopaedic Surgery, Hosp Spec Surg 1986; **Fellow:** Orthopaedic Pathology, Hosp Spec Surg 1983; Spinal Surgery, Twin Cities Scoliosis Ctr/Minn Spine Ctr 1987; **Fac Appt:** Assoc Clin Prof S, Cornell Univ-Weill Med Coll

Bosco, Joseph MD (OrS) - **Spec Exp:** Sports Medicine; Knee Surgery; Shoulder Surgery; **Hospital:** NYU Hosp For Joint Diseases (page 106), Jamaica Hosp Med Ctr; **Address:** 530 1st Ave, Ste 8U, New York, NY 10016; **Phone:** 212-263-2192; **Board Cert:** Orthopaedic Surgery 2006; **Med School:** Univ VT Coll Med 1986; **Resid:** Orthopaedic Surgery, Univ NC Med Ctr 1991; **Fellow:** Reconstructive Surgery, Univ Ariz Coll Med 1992; **Fac Appt:** Asst Prof OrS, NYU Sch Med

Bostrom, Mathias P MD (OrS) - **Spec Exp:** Knee Replacement; Hip Replacement; Hip & Knee Reconstruction; Joint Replacement; **Hospital:** Hosp For Special Surgery (page 111), NY-Presby Hosp/Weill Cornell (page 104); **Address:** 535 E 70th St, New York, NY 10021; **Phone:** 212-606-1674; **Board Cert:** Orthopaedic Surgery 2009; **Med School:** Johns Hopkins Univ 1989; **Resid:** Orthopaedic Surgery, Hosp for Spec Surg 1995; **Fellow:** Reconstructive Surgery, Hosp for Spec Surg 1996; **Fac Appt:** Prof OrS, Cornell Univ-Weill Med Coll

Brisson, Paul M MD (OrS) - **Spec Exp:** Spinal Surgery; **Hospital:** Brooklyn Hosp Ctr-Downtown, NY Downtown Hosp; **Address:** 160 E 56th St Fl 11, New York, NY 10022; **Phone:** 212-813-3632; **Board Cert:** Orthopaedic Surgery 2004; **Med School:** Univ Montreal 1979; **Resid:** Orthopaedic Surgery, McGill Med Ctr 1987; **Fellow:** Spinal Surgery, Hosp Joint Diseases 1988; Spinal Surgery, Buffalo Genl Hosp 1989

Bronson, Michael J MD (OrS) - **Spec Exp:** Joint Replacement; Knee Replacement; Hip Replacement; Arthritis; **Hospital:** Mount Sinai Med Ctr (page 102); **Address:** Mt Sinai Med Ctr, Dept Orthopedic Surgery, 5 E 98th St, Box 1188, New York, NY 10029; **Phone:** 212-241-1640; **Board Cert:** Orthopaedic Surgery 1984; **Med School:** NY Med Coll 1976; **Resid:** Orthopaedic Surgery, Lenox Hill Hosp 1980; **Fellow:** Hip & Knee Surgery, Columbia-Presby Med Ctr 1981; **Fac Appt:** Assoc Prof OrS, Mount Sinai Sch Med

Buly, Robert L MD (OrS) - **Spec Exp:** Hip Replacement; Minimally Invasive Surgery; Arthritis; Knee Replacement; **Hospital:** Hosp For Special Surgery (page 111), NY-Presby Hosp/Weill Cornell (page 104); **Address:** Hospital for Special Surgery, 535 E 70th St, New York, NY 10021; **Phone:** 212-606-1971; **Board Cert:** Orthopaedic Surgery 2004; **Med School:** Cornell Univ-Weill Med Coll 1985; **Resid:** Orthopaedic Surgery, Hosp for Special Surg 1990; **Fellow:** Hip Surgery, Mueller Fdn 1991; Joint Reconstruction, Case Western Res/ Univ Hosp 1992; **Fac Appt:** Assoc Prof OrS, Cornell Univ-Weill Med Coll

Cammisa Jr, Frank P MD (OrS) - **Spec Exp:** Spinal Surgery; Spinal Disc Replacement; Minimally Invasive Spinal Surgery; Scoliosis; **Hospital:** Hosp For Special Surgery (page 111), NY-Presby Hosp/Weill Cornell (page 104); **Address:** 523 E 72nd St, Fl 3, New York, NY 10021; **Phone:** 212-606-1946; **Board Cert:** Orthopaedic Surgery 2001; **Med School:** Columbia P&S 1982; **Resid:** Surgery, Columbia-Presby Hosp 1983; Orthopaedic Surgery, Hosp for Special Surgery 1987; **Fellow:** Spinal Surgery, Jackson Meml Hosp 1988; **Fac Appt:** Assoc Prof OrS, Cornell Univ-Weill Med Coll

Casden, Andrew M MD (OrS) - **Spec Exp:** Spinal Surgery; Spinal Disc Replacement; Minimally Invasive Spinal Surgery; Scoliosis; **Hospital:** Beth Israel Med Ctr - Petrie Division (page 94); **Address:** 10 Union Square East, Ste 5P, Spine Institute of New York, New York, NY 10003-3314; **Phone:** 212-844-8674; **Board Cert:** Orthopaedic Surgery 2002; **Med School:** Cornell Univ-Weill Med Coll 1983; **Resid:** Orthopaedic Surgery, Hosp Joint Diseases 1988; **Fellow:** Spinal Surgery, Rush-Presbyterian Med Ctr 1989; **Fac Appt:** Assoc Prof OrS, Albert Einstein Coll Med

Compito, Catherine MD (OrS) - **Spec Exp:** Shoulder Surgery; Elbow Surgery; Sports Medicine; Arthroscopic Surgery; **Hospital:** Beth Israel Med Ctr - Petrie Division (page 94); **Address:** 10 Union Square E Fl 3 - Ste 3K, New York, NY 10003; **Phone:** 212-844-8544; **Board Cert:** Orthopaedic Surgery 2009; **Med School:** Albert Einstein Coll Med 1986; **Resid:** Orthopaedic Surgery, Montefiore Med Ctr 1991; **Fellow:** Sports Medicine, Staten Island U Hosp 1992; Shoulder Surgery, NY Presby-Columbia Med Ctr 1993

Cordasco, Frank A MD (OrS) - **Spec Exp:** Sports Medicine; Arthroscopic Surgery-Knee; Arthroscopic Surgery-Shoulder; Rotator Cuff Surgery; **Hospital:** Hosp For Special Surgery (page 111); **Address:** Hospital for Special Surgery, 535 E 70th St, New York, NY 10021; **Phone:** 212-606-1636; **Board Cert:** Orthopaedic Surgery 2003; Sports Medicine 2009; **Med School:** UMDNJ-NJ Med Sch, Newark 1985; **Resid:** Orthopaedic Surgery, Columbia-Presby Hosp 1989; **Fellow:** Elbow & Shoulder Surgery, Columbia-Presby Hosp 1991; **Fac Appt:** Assoc Prof OrS, Cornell Univ-Weill Med Coll

Cornell, Charles MD (OrS) - **Spec Exp:** Trauma; Joint Replacement; Hip & Knee Replacement; **Hospital:** Hosp For Special Surgery (page 111); **Address:** 535 E 70th St, New York, NY 10021; **Phone:** 212-606-1414; **Board Cert:** Orthopaedic Surgery 2009; **Med School:** Cornell Univ-Weill Med Coll 1980; **Resid:** Surgery, Presby Hosp 1982; Orthopaedic Surgery, Hosp For Special Surg/New York Hosp 1985; **Fellow:** Orthopaedic Surgery, Univ Wash Med Ctr 1986; **Fac Appt:** Clin Prof OrS, Cornell Univ-Weill Med Coll

Craig, Edward V MD (OrS) - **Spec Exp:** Shoulder Arthroscopic Surgery; Shoulder Replacement; Sports Medicine; Elbow Surgery; **Hospital:** Hosp For Special Surgery (page 111), NY-Presby Hosp/Weill Cornell (page 104); **Address:** 535 E 70th St, New York, NY 10021-4892; **Phone:** 212-606-1966; **Board Cert:** Orthopaedic Surgery 1984; **Med School:** Columbia P&S 1973; **Resid:** Internal Medicine, Columbia-Presby Hosp 1976; Orthopaedic Surgery, Columbia-Presby Hosp 1980; **Fellow:** Shoulder Surgery, Columbia-Presby Hosp 1981; Hand Surgery, Columbia-Presby Hosp 1982; **Fac Appt:** Clin Prof OrS, Cornell Univ-Weill Med Coll

Cuomo, Frances MD (OrS) - **Spec Exp:** Shoulder Surgery; Elbow Surgery; Sports Medicine; **Hospital:** Beth Israel Med Ctr - Petrie Division (page 94); **Address:** Beth Israel Orthpaedics & Sports Med, 10 Union Square E, Ste 3M, New York, NY 10003; **Phone:** 212-844-6938; **Board Cert:** Orthopaedic Surgery 2002; **Med School:** NYU Sch Med 1983; **Resid:** Orthopaedic Surgery, Lenox Hill Hosp 1988; **Fellow:** Shoulder Surgery, Columbia-Presby Med Ctr 1989; **Fac Appt:** Asst Prof OrS, Albert Einstein Coll Med

Cushner, Fred D MD (OrS) - **Spec Exp:** Knee Reconstruction; Knee Injuries/Ligament Surgery; Cartilage Damage; Sports Medicine; **Hospital:** Lenox Hill Hosp, Southside Hosp; **Address:** 210 E 64th St Fl 4, New York, NY 10021; **Phone:** 212-434-4312; **Board Cert:** Orthopaedic Surgery 2007; **Med School:** Med Univ SC 1988; **Resid:** Orthopaedic Surgery, Univ SC Med Ctr 1993; **Fellow:** Knee Reconstruction, Beth Israel Med Ctr 1994

Deland, Jonathan T MD (OrS) - **Spec Exp:** Foot & Ankle Surgery; Sports Medicine; Arthritis; **Hospital:** Hosp For Special Surgery (page 111); **Address:** Hosp Spec Surg, Foot & Ankle Service, 535 E 70th St, New York, NY 10021-4099; **Phone:** 212-606-1665; **Board Cert:** Orthopaedic Surgery 2003; **Med School:** Columbia P&S 1980; **Resid:** Orthopaedic Surgery, St Luke's-Roosevelt Hosp Ctr 1982; Orthopaedic Surgery, Mass Genl Hosp 1987; **Fac Appt:** Asst Prof S, Cornell Univ-Weill Med Coll

Egol, Kenneth A MD (OrS) - **Spec Exp:** Trauma; Reconstructive Surgery; Limb Lengthening (Ilizarov Procedure); **Hospital:** NYU Hosp For Joint Diseases (page 106), Jamaica Hosp Med Ctr; **Address:** 301 E 17th St, New York, NY 10003; **Phone:** 212-598-3889; **Board Cert:** Orthopaedic Surgery 2001; **Med School:** SUNY Upstate Med Univ 1993; **Resid:** Orthopaedic Surgery, Hosp For Joint Diseases 1998; **Fellow:** Trauma, Carolinas Med Ctr 1999; **Fac Appt:** Assoc Prof OrS, NYU Sch Med

Elliott, Andrew J MD (OrS) - **Spec Exp:** Foot & Ankle Surgery; Arthroscopic Surgery; Sports Injuries; **Hospital:** Hosp For Special Surgery (page 111); **Address:** 420 E 72nd St Fl Ground - Ste 1B, New York, NY 10021; **Phone:** 212-203-0740; **Board Cert:** Orthopaedic Surgery 2009; **Med School:** Harvard Med Sch 1991; **Resid:** Surgery, Yale/New Haven Hosp 1996; **Fellow:** Orthopaedic Surgery, Hosp For Special Surgery 1997; **Fac Appt:** Asst Clin Prof OrS, Cornell Univ-Weill Med Coll

Errico, Thomas J MD (OrS) - **Spec Exp:** Spinal Surgery; Spinal Disc Replacement; Scoliosis; **Hospital:** NYU Langone Med Ctr (page 106), NYU Hosp For Joint Diseases (page 106); **Address:** 530 1st Ave, Ste 8U, New York, NY 10016-6402; **Phone:** 212-263-7182; **Board Cert:** Orthopaedic Surgery 1986; **Med School:** UMDNJ-NJ Med Sch, Newark 1978; **Resid:** Orthopaedic Surgery, NYU Med Ctr 1983; **Fellow:** Spinal Surgery, Toronto Genl Hosp 1984; **Fac Appt:** Assoc Prof OrS, NYU Sch Med

Fealy, Stephen MD (OrS) - **Spec Exp:** Sports Medicine; Shoulder Arthroscopic Surgery; Shoulder Replacement; Knee Replacement; **Hospital:** Hosp For Special Surgery (page 111); **Address:** Hospital for Special Surgery, 535 E 70th St, New York, NY 10021; **Phone:** 212-606-1894; **Board Cert:** Orthopaedic Surgery 2004; **Med School:** Columbia P&S 1995; **Resid:** Orthopaedic Surgery, Hosp for Special Surg 2000; **Fellow:** Sports Medicine, Hosp for Special Surg 2001; **Fac Appt:** Asst Prof OrS, Cornell Univ-Weill Med Coll

Feldman, David S MD (OrS) - **Spec Exp:** Limb Deformities; Spinal Surgery; Pediatric Orthopaedic Surgery; Scoliosis; **Hospital:** NYU Hosp For Joint Diseases (page 106), NYU Langone Med Ctr (page 106); **Address:** 67 Irving Pl Fl 8, New York, NY 10003; **Phone:** 212-533-5310; **Board Cert:** Orthopaedic Surgery 2007; **Med School:** Albert Einstein Coll Med 1988; **Resid:** Orthopaedic Surgery, Hosp for Joint Diseases 1993; **Fellow:** Pediatric Surgery, Hosp For Sick Chldn 1994; **Fac Appt:** Asst Prof OrS, NYU Sch Med

Ferriter, Pierce MD (OrS) - **Spec Exp:** Spinal Surgery; **Hospital:** Lenox Hill Hosp; **Address:** 1421 3rd Ave Fl 5, New York, NY 10028; **Phone:** 212-772-9711; **Board Cert:** Orthopaedic Surgery 2009; **Med School:** UMDNJ-RW Johnson Med Sch 1979; **Resid:** Orthopaedic Surgery, Lenox Hill Hosp 1985; **Fellow:** Spinal Surgery, Buffalo Genl Hosp 1986

Figgie, Mark P MD (OrS) - **Spec Exp:** Joint Replacement; Minimally Invasive Surgery; Hip Surgery; Knee Surgery; **Hospital:** Hosp For Special Surgery (page 111), NY-Presby Hosp/Weill Cornell (page 104); **Address:** 535 E 70th St, Ste 328, New York, NY 10021; **Phone:** 212-606-1932; **Board Cert:** Orthopaedic Surgery 2001; **Med School:** Case West Res Univ 1981; **Resid:** Orthopaedic Surgery, Univ Hosp-Case Western Reserve 1986; **Fellow:** Biomedical Engineering, Hosp For Special Surgery 1987; Joint Replacement Surgery, Hosp For Special Surgery 1988; **Fac Appt:** Assoc Clin Prof OrS, Cornell Univ-Weill Med Coll

Flatow, Evan MD (OrS) - **Spec Exp:** Rotator Cuff Surgery; Shoulder Injuries; Shoulder Replacement; Shoulder Arthroscopic Surgery; **Hospital:** Mount Sinai Med Ctr (page 102); **Address:** 5 E 98th St Fl 9, Box 1188, New York, NY 10029; **Phone:** 212-241-1663; **Board Cert:** Orthopaedic Surgery 2010; **Med School:** Columbia P&S 1981; **Resid:** Surgery, Roosevelt Hosp 1983; Orthopaedic Surgery, Columbia-Presby Med Ctr 1985; **Fellow:** Shoulder Surgery, Columbia-Presby Med Ctr 1987; **Fac Appt:** Prof OrS, Mount Sinai Sch Med

Gladstone, James N MD (OrS) - **Spec Exp:** Shoulder & Knee Surgery; Cartilage Damage; Knee-Patella Problems; Arthritis; **Hospital:** Mount Sinai Med Ctr (page 102); **Address:** Mt Sinai Med Ctr, 5 E 98th St Fl 9, Box 1188, New York, NY 10029; **Phone:** 212-241-1645; **Board Cert:** Orthopaedic Surgery 2009; Orthopaedic Sports Medicine 2007; **Med School:** Tufts Univ 1990; **Resid:** Orthopaedic Surgery, Columbia-Presby Med Ctr 1995; **Fellow:** Sports Medicine, American Sports Med Inst 1996; **Fac Appt:** Assoc Prof OrS, Mount Sinai Sch Med

Glashow, Jonathan L MD (OrS) - **Spec Exp:** Sports Medicine; Shoulder Surgery; Knee Surgery; Arthroscopic Surgery; **Hospital:** Mount Sinai Med Ctr (page 102), Lenox Hill Hosp; **Address:** 737 Park Ave, Ste 1C, New York, NY 10021; **Phone:** 212-794-5096; **Board Cert:** Orthopaedic Surgery 2004; **Med School:** Cornell Univ-Weill Med Coll 1984; **Resid:** Orthopaedic Surgery, Lenox Hill Hosp 1989; **Fellow:** Arthroscopic Surgery, S Calif Ortho Inst 1990; Shoulder Surgery, Univ Texas Med Ctr 1990; **Fac Appt:** Assoc Clin Prof OrS, Mount Sinai Sch Med

Goldstein, Jeffrey A MD (OrS) - **Spec Exp:** Spinal Surgery; Minimally Invasive Spinal Surgery; Spinal Disc Replacement; Scoliosis; **Hospital:** NYU Hosp For Joint Diseases (page 106), NYU Langone Med Ctr (page 106); **Address:** NYU Hosp for Joint Diseases, 19 Beekman St Fl 5, New York, NY 10038; **Phone:** 212-513-7711; **Board Cert:** Orthopaedic Surgery 2004; **Med School:** SUNY Downstate 1990; **Resid:** Orthopaedic Surgery, Case West Univ Med Ctr 1995; **Fellow:** Spinal Surgery, Maryland Spine Ctr 1996; **Fac Appt:** Assoc Clin Prof OrS, NYU Sch Med

Goodwin, Charles MD (OrS) - **Spec Exp:** Spinal Surgery; Sports Medicine; Minimally Invasive Spinal Surgery; **Hospital:** Hosp For Special Surgery (page 111), St Luke's - Roosevelt Hosp Ctr - Roosevelt Div (page 94); **Address:** 635 Madison Ave Fl 7, New York, NY 10022-1009; **Phone:** 212-317-4600; **Board Cert:** Orthopaedic Surgery 1985; **Med School:** Univ Cincinnati 1976; **Resid:** Surgery, St Luke's Roosevelt Hosp Ctr 1979; Orthopaedic Surgery, NY Presby Hosp/ Columbia 1982; **Fellow:** Spinal Surgery, Univ Toronto Affil Hosp 1983; **Fac Appt:** Asst Prof OrS, Cornell Univ-Weill Med Coll

Green, Steven M MD (OrS) - **Spec Exp:** Hand & Wrist Surgery; Carpal Tunnel Syndrome; Hand Surgery; **Hospital:** Mount Sinai Med Ctr (page 102), NYU Hosp For Joint Diseases (page 106); **Address:** 2 E 88th St, New York, NY 10128-0555; **Phone:** 212-348-6644; **Board Cert:** Orthopaedic Surgery 1977; Hand Surgery 2000; **Med School:** Albert Einstein Coll Med 1970; **Resid:** Surgery, Georgia Bapt Hosp 1972; Orthopaedic Surgery, Mt Sinai Hosp 1975; **Fellow:** Hand Surgery, Thomas Jefferson Univ Hosp 1978; **Fac Appt:** Assoc Clin Prof OrS, NYU Sch Med

Grelsamer, Ronald P MD (OrS) - **Spec Exp:** Knee-Patella Problems; Sports Medicine; Knee Reconstruction; Arthritis-Hip & Knee; **Hospital:** Mount Sinai Med Ctr (page 102); **Address:** Mount Sinai Medical Ctr, Dept Orthopaedics, 5 E 98th St, Box 1188, New York, NY 10029-6574; **Phone:** 212-241-2914; **Board Cert:** Orthopaedic Surgery 2008; **Med School:** Columbia P&S 1979; **Resid:** Orthopaedic Surgery, Columbia Presby Med Ctr 1984; **Fellow:** Hip & Knee Surgery, Columbia Presby Med Ctr 1985; **Fac Appt:** Assoc Prof OrS, Mount Sinai Sch Med

Haas, Steven B MD (OrS) - **Spec Exp:** Knee Surgery; Knee Replacement; Minimally Invasive Surgery; **Hospital:** Hosp For Special Surgery (page 111); **Address:** Hospital for Special Surgery, 535 E 70th St Fl 3, New York, NY 10021; **Phone:** 212-606-1852; **Board Cert:** Orthopaedic Surgery 2004; **Med School:** Univ Rochester 1985; **Resid:** Orthopaedic Surgery, Hosp Special Surgery 1990; **Fellow:** Knee Surgery, Hosp Special Surgery 1991; **Fac Appt:** Assoc Prof OrS, Cornell Univ-Weill Med Coll

Hamilton, William G MD (OrS) - **Spec Exp:** Dance Medicine; Foot & Ankle Surgery; Sports Medicine; **Hospital:** St Luke's - Roosevelt Hosp Ctr - Roosevelt Div (page 94), Hosp For Special Surgery (page 111); **Address:** 343 W 58th St, New York, NY 10019-1173; **Phone:** 212-765-2260; **Board Cert:** Orthopaedic Surgery 1971; **Med School:** Columbia P&S 1964; **Resid:** Surgery, St Luke's-Roosevelt Hosp Ctr 1966; Orthopaedic Surgery, Columbia-Presby Hosp 1969; **Fellow:** Pediatric Orthopaedic Surgery, Newington Chldrn's Hosp 1970; **Fac Appt:** Clin Prof OrS, Columbia P&S

Hannafin, Jo A MD/PhD (OrS) - **Spec Exp:** Sports Medicine-Women; Shoulder Arthroscopic Surgery; Knee Injuries/Ligament Surgery; Ligament Reconstruction; **Hospital:** Hosp For Special Surgery (page 111), NY-Presby Hosp/Weill Cornell (page 104); **Address:** 535 E 70th St, New York, NY 10021-4872; **Phone:** 212-606-1004; **Board Cert:** Orthopaedic Surgery 2005; Orthopaedic Sports Medicine 2010; **Med School:** Albert Einstein Coll Med 1985; **Resid:** Orthopaedic Surgery, Montefiore Med Ctr 1990; **Fellow:** Sports Medicine, Hosp Special Sur 1992; **Fac Appt:** Assoc Prof OrS, Cornell Univ-Weill Med Coll

Harwin, Steven F MD (OrS) - **Spec Exp:** Hip & Knee Replacement; Arthroscopic Surgery; Rotator Cuff Surgery; Knee Injuries/ACL; **Hospital:** Beth Israel Med Ctr - Petrie Division (page 94); **Address:** Center for Reconstructive Joint Surgery, 910 Park Ave, New York, NY 10075; **Phone:** 212-861-9800; **Board Cert:** Orthopaedic Surgery 1976; **Med School:** SUNY Hlth Sci Ctr 1971; **Resid:** Orthopaedic Surgery, Albert Einstein Coll Med 1975; **Fellow:** Joint Replacement Surgery, Traveling Fellowship 1978; **Fac Appt:** Assoc Prof OrS, Albert Einstein Coll Med

Hausman, Michael R MD (OrS) - **Spec Exp:** Hand Reconstruction; Elbow Reconstruction; Reconstructive Microvascular Surgery; Arthroscopic Surgery; **Hospital:** Mount Sinai Med Ctr (page 102); **Address:** 5 E 98th St, Box 1188, New York, NY 10029-6501; **Phone:** 212-241-1658; **Board Cert:** Orthopaedic Surgery 2000; Hand Surgery 2000; **Med School:** Yale Univ 1979; **Resid:** Surgery, Yale-New Haven Hosp 1981; Orthopaedic Surgery, Yale-New Haven Hosp 1985; **Fellow:** Hand Surgery, Roosevelt Hosp 1987; **Fac Appt:** Assoc Clin Prof OrS, Mount Sinai Sch Med

Healey, John H MD (OrS) - **Spec Exp:** Bone Tumors; Hip & Knee Replacement in Bone Tumors; Sarcoma; Sarcoma-Soft Tissue; **Hospital:** Meml Sloan-Kettering Cancer Ctr (page 112), Hosp For Special Surgery (page 111); **Address:** 1275 York Avenue, New York, NY 10065; **Phone:** 800-525-2225; **Board Cert:** Orthopaedic Surgery 2007; **Med School:** Univ VT Coll Med 1978; **Resid:** Orthopaedic Surgery, Hosp Special Surg 1983; **Fellow:** Orthopaedic Oncology, Meml Sloan Kettering Cancer Ctr 1984; Orthopaedic Surgery, Hosp Special Surgery 1984; **Fac Appt:** Prof OrS, Cornell Univ-Weill Med Coll

Hecht, Andrew MD (OrS) - **Spec Exp:** Spinal Surgery; Spinal Disc Replacement; Minimally Invasive Spinal Surgery; **Hospital:** Mount Sinai Med Ctr (page 102); **Address:** Mount Sinai Med Ctr, Dept Orthopaedic Surg, 5 E 98th St Fl 9, Box 1188, New York, NY 10029; **Phone:** 212-241-0735; **Board Cert:** Orthopaedic Surgery 2003; **Med School:** Harvard Med Sch 1994; **Resid:** Orthopaedic Surgery, Mass Genl Hosp 1999; **Fellow:** Spinal Surgery, Emory Univ Spine Ctr 2001; **Fac Appt:** Asst Prof OrS, Mount Sinai Sch Med

Helfet, David L MD (OrS) - **Spec Exp:** Fractures-Complex; Fractures-Complex & Non Union; Fractures-Stress; Deformity Reconstruction; **Hospital:** Hosp For Special Surgery (page 111), NY-Presby Hosp/Weill Cornell (page 104); **Address:** 535 E 70th St, New York, NY 10021; **Phone:** 212-606-1888; **Board Cert:** Orthopaedic Surgery 1984; **Med School:** South Africa 1975; **Resid:** Surgery, Edendale Hosp 1977; Orthopaedic Surgery, Johns Hopkins Hosp 1981; **Fellow:** Orthopaedic Surgery, Inselspita Hosp 1981; Orthopaedic Surgery, UCLA Med Ctr 1982; **Fac Appt:** Prof OrS, Cornell Univ-Weill Med Coll

Hotchkiss, Robert N MD (OrS) - **Spec Exp:** Hand Surgery; Wrist Surgery; Elbow Reconstruction; Dupuytren's Contracture; **Hospital:** Hosp For Special Surgery (page 111), NY-Presby Hosp/Weill Cornell (page 104); **Address:** 523 E 72nd St Fl 4, New York, NY 10021-4099; **Phone:** 212-606-1964; **Board Cert:** Orthopaedic Surgery 2010; Hand Surgery 2010; **Med School:** Johns Hopkins Univ 1980; **Resid:** Surgery, Johns Hopkins Hosp 1982; Orthopaedic Surgery, Johns Hopkins Hosp 1985; **Fellow:** Hand Surgery, Union Meml Hosp 1987; **Fac Appt:** Assoc Prof OrS, Cornell Univ-Weill Med Coll

Hubbard, Christopher E MD (OrS) - **Spec Exp:** Foot & Ankle Surgery; Sports Medicine; Arthroscopic Surgery; **Hospital:** Beth Israel Med Ctr - Petrie Division (page 94); **Address:** Beth Israel Orthopaedics & Sports Med, 10 Union Square East, Ste 3M, New York, NY 10003-3314; **Phone:** 212-844-6940; **Board Cert:** Orthopaedic Surgery 2002; **Med School:** UMDNJ-NJ Med Sch, Newark 1994; **Resid:** Orthopaedic Surgery, Columbia-Presby Med Ctr 1999; **Fellow:** Foot & Ankle Surgery, Hosp for Special Surgery 2000; **Fac Appt:** Asst Prof S, Albert Einstein Coll Med

Hyman, Joshua E MD (OrS) - **Spec Exp:** Pediatric Orthopaedic Surgery; Fractures-Pediatric; Scoliosis; Clubfoot/Foot Deformities in Children; **Hospital:** NY-Presby Hosp/Columbia (page 104); **Address:** Chldn's Hosp New York, 3959 Broadway, Ste 8 North, New York, NY 10032-3784; **Phone:** 212-305-5475; **Board Cert:** Orthopaedic Surgery 2002; **Med School:** Columbia P&S 1990; **Resid:** Surgery, Beth Israel Hosp 1993; Orthopaedic Surgery, Mass Genl Hosp/Beth Israel Hosp 1998; **Fellow:** Pediatric Orthopaedic Surgery, Hosp for Sick Children 1999; **Fac Appt:** Assoc Prof OrS, Columbia P&S

Jaffe, Fredrick F MD (OrS) - **Spec Exp:** Hip Replacement; Knee Replacement; Hip & Knee Reconstruction; **Hospital:** NYU Hosp For Joint Diseases (page 106); **Address:** 301 E 17th St, Ste 213, New York, NY 10003-3804; **Phone:** 212-598-7605; **Board Cert:** Orthopaedic Surgery 1974; **Med School:** Tufts Univ 1968; **Resid:** Surgery, New York Hosp 1970; Orthopaedic Surgery, Hosp for Joint Diseases 1973; **Fellow:** Reconstructive Surgery, Hosp for Joint Diseases 1974; **Fac Appt:** Clin Prof OrS, NYU Sch Med

Kiernan, Howard MD (OrS) - **Hospital:** NY-Presby Hosp/Columbia (page 104); **Address:** 161 Fort Washington Ave, rm 249, New York, NY 10032; **Phone:** 212-305-5241; **Board Cert:** Orthopaedic Surgery 1975; **Med School:** NYU Sch Med 1966; **Resid:** Surgery, Bellevue Hosp Ctr-NYU 1970; Orthopaedic Surgery, Columbia-Presby Med Ctr 1974

Lane, Joseph MD (OrS) - **Spec Exp:** Bone Disorders-Metabolic; Osteoporosis Spine-Kyphoplasty; Bone Cancer; **Hospital:** Hosp For Special Surgery (page 111), NY-Presby Hosp/Weill Cornell (page 104); **Address:** Hosp for Special Surgery, 535 E 70th St, New York, NY 10021; **Phone:** 212-606-1172; **Board Cert:** Orthopaedic Surgery 1974; **Med School:** Harvard Med Sch 1965; **Resid:** Surgery, Hosp Univ Penn 1967; Orthopaedic Surgery, Hosp Univ Penn 1973; **Fac Appt:** Prof OrS, Cornell Univ-Weill Med Coll

Lee, Francis Y MD/PhD (OrS) - **Spec Exp:** Bone Tumors; Pediatric Orthopaedic Cancers; Pediatric Orthopaedic Surgery; **Hospital:** NYPresby-Morgan Stanley Children's Hosp (page 104), NY-Presby Hosp/Columbia (page 104); **Address:** 3959 Broadway, Ste 800N, New York, NY 10032; **Phone:** 212-305-3293; **Board Cert:** Orthopaedic Surgery 2001; **Med School:** South Korea 1986; **Resid:** Orthopaedic Surgery, NJ Med Ctr 1997; **Fellow:** Orthopaedic Oncology, Harvard Med Sch 1998; Pediatric Orthopaedic Surgery, Hosp for Sick Chldn/Univ Toronto 1999; **Fac Appt:** Asst Prof OrS, Columbia P&S

Levine, David S MD (OrS) - **Spec Exp:** Foot & Ankle Surgery; Ankle Reconstruction; **Hospital:** Hosp For Special Surgery (page 111); **Address:** Hospital for Special Surgery, 535 East 70th St, New York, NY 10021; **Phone:** 212-606-1940; **Board Cert:** Orthopaedic Surgery 2000; **Med School:** Cornell Univ-Weill Med Coll 1992; **Resid:** Orthopaedic Surgery, Hosp for Special Surgery 1997; **Fellow:** Foot & Ankle Surgery, Harborview Med Ctr 1998

Levy, Howard J MD (OrS) - **Spec Exp:** Knee Surgery; Shoulder Surgery; Sports Medicine; Arthroscopic Surgery; **Hospital:** Lenox Hill Hosp, Beth Israel Med Ctr - Petrie Division (page 94); **Address:** 130 E 77th St Fl 7, New York, NY 10021; **Phone:** 212-744-8114; **Board Cert:** Orthopaedic Surgery 2004; **Med School:** SUNY Hlth Sci Ctr 1983; **Resid:** Orthopaedic Surgery, Jackson Meml Hosp 1989; **Fellow:** Sports Medicine, American Sports Med Inst 1989; Hand Surgery, Roosevelt Hosp 1990; **Fac Appt:** Asst Clin Prof OrS, Albert Einstein Coll Med

Lonner, Baron S MD (OrS) - **Spec Exp:** Scoliosis; Minimally Invasive Surgery; Spinal Deformity; Spinal Surgery; **Hospital:** NYU Hosp For Joint Diseases (page 106); **Address:** 820 2nd Ave, Ste 7A, New York, NY 10017; **Phone:** 212-986-0140; **Board Cert:** Orthopaedic Surgery 2008; **Med School:** Boston Univ 1989; **Resid:** Orthopaedic Surgery, Montefiore Med Ctr 1994; **Fellow:** Orthopaedic Surgery, Hosp Special Surgery 1995; **Fac Appt:** Asst Prof OrS, NYU Sch Med

Lorich, Dean G MD (OrS) - **Spec Exp:** Trauma; Fractures-Complex; **Hospital:** Hosp For Special Surgery (page 111); **Address:** Hospital for Special Surgery, 535 E 70th St, New York, NY 10021; **Phone:** 212-746-4509; **Board Cert:** Orthopaedic Surgery 2010; **Med School:** Univ Pennsylvania 1990; **Resid:** Orthopaedic Surgery, Hosp Univ Penn 1995; **Fellow:** Orthopaedic Surgery, Hosp Special Surg 1996; **Fac Appt:** Assoc Prof OrS, Cornell Univ-Weill Med Coll

Lubliner, Jerry A MD (OrS) - **Spec Exp:** Arthroscopic Surgery; Shoulder Surgery; Knee Surgery; Rotator Cuff Surgery; **Hospital:** Beth Israel Med Ctr - Petrie Division (page 94), NYU Hosp For Joint Diseases (page 106); **Address:** 215 E 73rd St, Ste 1C, New York, NY 10021-3653; **Phone:** 212-249-8200; **Board Cert:** Orthopaedic Surgery 2009; Orthopaedic Sports Medicine 2008; **Med School:** SUNY Hlth Sci Ctr 1980; **Resid:** Orthopaedic Surgery, Hosp Joint Diseases 1985; **Fellow:** Sports Medicine, U West Ont Affil Hosps 1985; **Fac Appt:** Assoc Clin Prof S, NYU Sch Med

Lyden, John MD (OrS) - **Spec Exp:** Joint Replacement; Trauma; Arthroscopic Surgery; **Hospital:** Hosp For Special Surgery (page 111), NY-Presby Hosp/Weill Cornell (page 104); **Address:** 535 E 70th St, rm 355, New York, NY 10021-4872; **Phone:** 212-606-1126; **Board Cert:** Orthopaedic Surgery 1973; **Med School:** Columbia P&S 1965; **Resid:** Surgery, Roosevelt Hosp 1967; Orthopaedic Surgery, Hosp Special Surg 1972; **Fellow:** Hand Surgery, Hosp Special Surg 1973; **Fac Appt:** Assoc Prof OrS, NY Med Coll

Macaulay, William B MD (OrS) - **Spec Exp:** Hip Replacement; Knee Replacement; Minimally Invasive Surgery; Reconstructive Surgery; **Hospital:** NY-Presby Hosp/Columbia (page 104); **Address:** Columbia Orthopaedics, 161 Fort Washington Ave, Irving Pavilion Fl 2, New York, NY 10032; **Phone:** 212-305-6959; **Board Cert:** Orthopaedic Surgery 2001; **Med School:** Columbia P&S 1992; **Resid:** Orthopaedic Surgery, Univ Pittsburgh Med Ctr 1997; **Fellow:** Adult Reconstructive Surgery, Hosp for Special Surgery 1999; **Fac Appt:** Prof OrS, Columbia P&S

Marx, Robert G MD (OrS) - **Spec Exp:** Shoulder Surgery; Knee Surgery; Arthroscopic Surgery; Joint Replacement; **Hospital:** Hosp For Special Surgery (page 111); **Address:** Hospital for Special Surgery, 535 E 70th St, New York, NY 10021; **Phone:** 212-606-1645; **Board Cert:** Orthopaedic Surgery 2003; **Med School:** McGill Univ 1991; **Resid:** Orthopaedic Surgery, Univ Toronto 1996; **Fellow:** Sports Medicine, Hosp Special Surgery 1998; **Fac Appt:** Assoc Prof OrS, Cornell Univ-Weill Med Coll

McCann, Peter D MD (OrS) - **Spec Exp:** Shoulder Surgery; Elbow Surgery; **Hospital:** Beth Israel Med Ctr - Petrie Division (page 94); **Address:** 10 Union Square E, Ste 3M, New York, NY 10003; **Phone:** 212-844-6735; **Board Cert:** Orthopaedic Surgery 2009; **Med School:** Columbia P&S 1980; **Resid:** Surgery, St Vincent's Hosp 1982; Orthopaedic Surgery, Columbia-Presby Med Ctr 1985; **Fellow:** Shoulder Surgery, Columbia-Presby Med Ctr 1986; **Fac Appt:** Assoc Prof OrS, Albert Einstein Coll Med

McClelland, Shearwood J MD (OrS) - **Spec Exp:** Musculoskeletal Injuries; Joint Replacement; **Hospital:** Harlem Hosp Ctr; **Address:** Harlem Hosp Ctr, Dept Ortho Surgery, 506 Lenox Ave MLK Bldg Fl 9 - rm 9122, New York, NY 10037-1889; **Phone:** 212-939-3510; **Board Cert:** Orthopaedic Surgery 2007; **Med School:** Columbia P&S 1974; **Resid:** Surgery, St. Lukes Hosp 1976; Orthopaedic Surgery, NY Ortho Hosp-Columbia 1979; **Fellow:** Joint Arthroplasty, Ohio State Univ Med Ctr 1982; **Fac Appt:** Assoc Prof OrS, Columbia P&S

Meere, Patrick MD (OrS) - **Spec Exp:** Hip Replacement & Revision; Knee Replacement & Revision; Knee Meniscal Repair; Joint Infection; **Hospital:** NYU Hosp For Joint Diseases (page 106), NYU Langone Med Ctr (page 106); **Address:** 530 1st Ave FPO Bldg - Ste 5J, New York, NY 10016; **Phone:** 212-263-2366; **Board Cert:** Orthopaedic Surgery 2008; **Med School:** McGill Univ 1988; **Resid:** Orthopaedic Surgery, McGill Univ Med Ctr 1993; **Fellow:** Reconstructive Surgery, Hosp for Joint Diseases 1995; **Fac Appt:** Assoc Prof OrS, NYU Sch Med

Mendoza, Francis X MD (OrS) - **Spec Exp:** Shoulder & Elbow Surgery; Sports Medicine; **Hospital:** Lenox Hill Hosp; **Address:** 333 E 56th St, New York, NY 10021; **Phone:** 212-628-9600; **Board Cert:** Orthopaedic Surgery 1984; **Med School:** Columbia P&S 1976; **Resid:** Surgery, Roosevelt Hosp 1978; Orthopaedic Surgery, Columbia-Presby Hosp 1981; **Fellow:** Shoulder Surgery, Columbia-Presby Hosp 1982

Moskovich, Ronald MD (OrS) - **Spec Exp:** Scoliosis; Spinal Surgery-Pediatric & Adult; Spondylitis; Spinal Disorders; **Hospital:** NYU Hosp For Joint Diseases (page 106), NYU Langone Med Ctr (page 106); **Address:** 301 E 17th St, Ste 400, New York, NY 10003; **Phone:** 212-598-6622; **Board Cert:** Orthopaedic Surgery 2002; **Med School:** South Africa 1978; **Resid:** Surgery, St George's Hosp 1984; Orthopaedic Surgery, Hosp for Joint Diseases 1988; **Fellow:** Spinal Surgery, UC Davis Med Ctr 1989; Neurological Surgery, Natl Hosp 1989; **Fac Appt:** Asst Prof OrS, NYU Sch Med

Neuwirth, Michael MD (OrS) - **Spec Exp:** Scoliosis; Spinal Surgery; **Hospital:** Beth Israel Med Ctr - Petrie Division (page 94); **Address:** Beth Israel Med Ctr - Spine Institute, 10 Union Square E, Ste 5P, New York, NY 10003-3314; **Phone:** 212-844-8692; **Board Cert:** Orthopaedic Surgery 1980; **Med School:** SUNY Hlth Sci Ctr 1974; **Resid:** Orthopaedic Surgery, Hosp for Joint Diseases 1978; **Fellow:** Spinal Surgery, Rush-Presby Med Ctr 1979; **Fac Appt:** Assoc Clin Prof OrS, NYU Sch Med

Nicholas, Stephen J MD (OrS) - **Spec Exp:** Sports Medicine; Shoulder & Knee Surgery; Arthroscopic Surgery; **Hospital:** Lenox Hill Hosp; **Address:** 130 E 77 St, New York, NY 10075; **Phone:** 212-737-3301; **Board Cert:** Orthopaedic Surgery 2005; **Med School:** NY Med Coll 1986; **Resid:** Orthopaedic Surgery, Hosp for Special Surgery 1991; **Fellow:** Sports Medicine, Lenox Hill Hosp 1992

O'Leary, Patrick MD (OrS) - **Spec Exp:** Spinal Surgery; **Hospital:** Hosp For Special Surgery (page 111); **Address:** 1015 Madison Ave Fl 4, New York, NY 10021; **Phone:** 212-249-8100; **Board Cert:** Orthopaedic Surgery 1983; **Med School:** Ireland 1968; **Resid:** Surgery, Roosevelt Hosp 1972; Orthopaedic Surgery, Hosp Spec Surg-Cornell 1975; **Fellow:** Spinal Surgery, Univ Toronto Genl Ortho Hosp 1976; **Fac Appt:** Assoc Clin Prof OrS, Cornell Univ-Weill Med Coll

O'Malley, Martin J MD (OrS) - **Spec Exp:** Foot & Ankle Surgery; Sports Medicine; Ankle Replacement & Revision; Arthroscopic Surgery; **Hospital:** Hosp For Special Surgery (page 111), NY-Presby Hosp/Weill Cornell (page 104); **Address:** 420 E 72nd St, Ste 1B, New York, NY 10021; **Phone:** 212-203-0740; **Board Cert:** Orthopaedic Surgery 2006; **Med School:** Case West Res Univ 1986; **Resid:** Orthopaedic Surgery, Tufts-New Eng Med Ctr 1992; **Fellow:** Foot & Ankle Surgery, Hosp for Special Surg 1993; **Fac Appt:** Assoc Prof OrS, Cornell Univ-Weill Med Coll

Padgett, Douglas E MD (OrS) - **Spec Exp:** Hip & Knee Replacement; Arthroscopic Surgery-Hip; Arthroscopic Surgery-Knee; Dance Medicine; **Hospital:** Hosp For Special Surgery (page 111); **Address:** Hosp for Special Surgery, 535 E 70 St, New York, NY 10021; **Phone:** 212-606-1642; **Board Cert:** Orthopaedic Surgery 2003; **Med School:** NY Med Coll 1982; **Resid:** Orthopaedic Surgery, Hosp Spec Surg 1989; **Fellow:** Orthopaedic Surgery, Rush Presby Med Ctr 1990; **Fac Appt:** Assoc Prof OrS, Cornell Univ-Weill Med Coll

Parks, Michael MD (OrS) - **Spec Exp:** Hip & Knee Replacement; Joint Replacement; Reconstructive Surgery; **Hospital:** Hosp For Special Surgery (page 111), NY-Presby Hosp/Weill Cornell (page 104); **Address:** 535 E 70th St Fl 6, New York, NY 10021; **Phone:** 646-797-8995; **Board Cert:** Orthopaedic Surgery 2010; **Med School:** Med Univ SC 1990; **Resid:** Orthopaedic Surgery, Duke Univ Med Ctr 1996; **Fellow:** Orthopaedic Surgery, Hosp for Spec Surgery 1997; **Fac Appt:** Asst Prof OrS, Cornell Univ-Weill Med Coll

Pellicci, Paul M MD (OrS) - **Spec Exp:** Hip Replacement-Young Adults; Hip Resurfacing; Knee Replacement; Joint Replacement; **Hospital:** Hosp For Special Surgery (page 111), NY-Presby Hosp/Weill Cornell (page 104); **Address:** 535 E 70th St, New York, NY 10021-4872; **Phone:** 212-606-1010; **Board Cert:** Orthopaedic Surgery 1982; **Med School:** Cornell Univ-Weill Med Coll 1975; **Resid:** Surgery, NY Hosp 1977; Orthopaedic Surgery, Hosp Spec Surg 1980; **Fellow:** Joint Replacement Surgery, Brigham & Womens Hosp 1981; **Fac Appt:** Prof OrS, Cornell Univ-Weill Med Coll

Pianka, George MD (OrS) - **Spec Exp:** Hand Surgery; Wrist Surgery; Upper Extremity Surgery; Arthroscopic Surgery; **Hospital:** Lenox Hill Hosp, Phelps Meml Hosp Ctr (page 592); **Address:** 73 E 71st St, New York, NY 10021; **Phone:** 212-472-5899; **Board Cert:** Orthopaedic Surgery 2003; Hand Surgery 2003; **Med School:** Univ Conn 1984; **Resid:** Orthopaedic Surgery, Lenox Hill Hosp 1989; **Fellow:** Hand Surgery, Hosp For Joint Diseases 1990

Price, Andrew E MD (OrS) - **Spec Exp:** Erbs Palsy/Brachial Plexus Injuries; Cerebral Palsy; Fractures-Pediatric; Trauma-Pediatric; **Hospital:** NYU Langone Med Ctr (page 106), St Luke's - Roosevelt Hosp Ctr - Roosevelt Div (page 94); **Address:** 129A W 20th St, New York, NY 10011; **Phone:** 212-974-7242; **Board Cert:** Orthopaedic Surgery 2001; **Med School:** NYU Sch Med 1980; **Resid:** Orthopaedic Surgery, NYU Med Ctr 1985; **Fellow:** Pediatric Orthopaedic Surgery, Newington Chldns Hosp 1986; **Fac Appt:** Assoc Prof OrS, NYU Sch Med

Ranawat, Chitranjan MD (OrS) - **Spec Exp:** Hip Replacement; Knee Replacement; **Hospital:** Hosp For Special Surgery (page 111); **Address:** Hosp for Special Surgery, 535 E 70th St Fl 6, New York, NY 10021; **Phone:** 646-797-8700; **Board Cert:** Orthopaedic Surgery 1969; **Med School:** India 1958; **Resid:** Surgery, MY Hosp 1963; Orthopaedic Surgery, Albany Med Ctr 1965; **Fellow:** Orthopaedic Surgery, Hosp Special Surg 1969; **Fac Appt:** Prof OrS, Cornell Univ-Weill Med Coll

Rawlins, Bernard A MD (OrS) - **Spec Exp:** Scoliosis; Spinal Surgery; Chiari's Deformity; **Hospital:** Hosp For Special Surgery (page 111); **Address:** 535 E 70 St, New York, NY 10021; **Phone:** 212-606-1632; **Board Cert:** Orthopaedic Surgery 2006; **Med School:** Cornell Univ 1987; **Resid:** Orthopaedic Surgery, Columbia-Presby Hosp 1992; **Fellow:** Spinal Surgery, Minnesota Spine Ctr 1993; **Fac Appt:** Assoc Prof OrS, Cornell Univ-Weill Med Coll

Roberts, Matthew M MD (OrS) - **Spec Exp:** Foot & Ankle Surgery; Arthritis; Foot Deformities; Sports Medicine; **Hospital:** Hosp For Special Surgery (page 111); **Address:** Hospital for Special Surgery, 535 E 70th St, New York, NY 10021; **Phone:** 212-606-1181; **Board Cert:** Orthopaedic Surgery 2005; **Med School:** Univ Tex, Houston 1997; **Resid:** Orthopaedic Surgery, Hosp for Special Surg 2003; **Fellow:** Foot & Ankle Surgery, Hosp for Special Surg 2004; **Fac Appt:** Asst Prof OrS, Cornell Univ-Weill Med Coll

Rose, Donald J MD (OrS) - **Spec Exp:** Dance/Ballet Injuries; Arthroscopic Surgery; Sports Injuries; Hip Surgery; **Hospital:** NYU Hosp For Joint Diseases (page 106), NYU Langone Med Ctr (page 106); **Address:** 1095 Park Ave, New York, NY 10128-1154; **Phone:** 212-427-7750; **Board Cert:** Orthopaedic Surgery 2009; **Med School:** UMDNJ-RW Johnson Med Sch 1980; **Resid:** Surgery, Beth Israel Med Ctr 1981; Orthopaedic Surgery, Hosp for Joint Diseases 1985; **Fellow:** Sports Medicine, Temple Univ Hosp 1986; **Fac Appt:** Assoc Clin Prof OrS, NYU Sch Med

Rose, Howard A MD (OrS) - **Spec Exp:** Sports Medicine; Joint Replacement; Arthroscopic Surgery; **Hospital:** Hosp For Special Surgery (page 111), NY-Presby Hosp/Weill Cornell (page 104); **Address:** 535 E 70th St, New York, NY 10021; **Phone:** 212-606-1278; **Board Cert:** Orthopaedic Surgery 1985; **Med School:** Geo Wash Univ 1977; **Resid:** Orthopaedic Surgery, Hosp Special Surg 1982; **Fellow:** Sports Medicine, Brigham & Womens Hosp 1983; Joint Replacement Surgery, Brigham & Womens Hosp 1983; **Fac Appt:** Asst Prof OrS, Cornell Univ-Weill Med Coll

Roye, David MD (OrS) - **Spec Exp:** Pediatric Orthopaedic Surgery; Scoliosis; Hip Disorders-Pediatric; **Hospital:** NY-Presby Hosp/Columbia (page 104), White Plains Hosp Ctr; **Address:** Morgan Stanley Chlds Hosp NewYork-Presby, 3959 Broadway, 8 North, New York, NY 10032-1559; **Phone:** 212-305-5475; **Board Cert:** Orthopaedic Surgery 1981; **Med School:** Columbia P&S 1975; **Resid:** Orthopaedic Surgery, Columbia-Presby Med Ctr 1979; **Fellow:** Orthopaedic Surgery, Hosp for Sick Chldn 1980; **Fac Appt:** Prof OrS, Columbia P&S

Rozbruch, Jacob D MD (OrS) - **Spec Exp:** Spinal Surgery; Shoulder Surgery; Knee Surgery; **Hospital:** Beth Israel Med Ctr - Petrie Division (page 94); **Address:** 420 E 72nd St, Ste 1J, New York, NY 10021; **Phone:** 212-744-9857; **Board Cert:** Pediatrics 1979; Orthopaedic Surgery 1980; **Med School:** SUNY Buffalo 1973; **Resid:** Surgery, NY Hosp 1976; Orthopaedic Surgery, Hosp for Special Surg 1979; **Fac Appt:** Asst Clin Prof OrS, Albert Einstein Coll Med

Rozbruch, S Robert MD (OrS) - **Spec Exp:** Limb Lengthening; Limb Deformities; Limb Surgery/Reconstruction; Fractures-Complex & Non Union; **Hospital:** Hosp For Special Surgery (page 111), NY-Presby Hosp/Weill Cornell (page 104); **Address:** 535 E 70th St, New York, NY 10021; **Phone:** 212-606-1415; **Board Cert:** Orthopaedic Surgery 2009; **Med School:** Cornell Univ-Weill Med Coll 1990; **Resid:** Orthopaedic Surgery, Hosp Special Surgery 1995; **Fellow:** Trauma, Univ Bern Hosp 1997; Limb Lengthening, Intl Ctr Limb Length/Univ MD 1999; **Fac Appt:** Assoc Clin Prof OrS, Cornell Univ-Weill Med Coll

Salvati, Eduardo A MD (OrS) - **Spec Exp:** Hip Surgery; Hip & Knee Replacement; **Hospital:** Hosp For Special Surgery (page 111); **Address:** Hosp for Spec Surg, 535 E 70th Street, New York, NY 10021; **Phone:** 212-606-1472; **Board Cert:** Orthopaedic Surgery 1972; **Med School:** Argentina 1963; **Resid:** Orthopaedic Surgery, Univ Florence Ortho Clinic 1965; Orthopaedic Surgery, Hosp Buenos Aires 1969; **Fellow:** Hip Surgery, Hosp For Spec Surg 1972; **Fac Appt:** Clin Prof OrS, Cornell Univ-Weill Med Coll

Sandhu, Harvinder S MD (OrS) - **Spec Exp:** Minimally Invasive Surgery; Spinal Disc Replacement; Spinal Surgery; **Hospital:** Hosp For Special Surgery (page 111), NY-Presby Hosp/Weill Cornell (page 104); **Address:** 535 E 70th St, New York, NY 10021; **Phone:** 212-606-1798; **Board Cert:** Orthopaedic Surgery 2007; **Med School:** Northwestern Univ 1987; **Resid:** Orthopaedic Surgery, Univ Hosp-SUNY Hlth Sci Ctr 1992; **Fellow:** Spinal Surgery, UCLA Med Ctr 1993; **Fac Appt:** Assoc Prof OrS, Cornell Univ-Weill Med Coll

Sands, Andrew K MD (OrS) - **Spec Exp:** Foot & Ankle Surgery; Ankle Replacement & Revision; Arthroscopic Surgery; Sports Medicine; **Hospital:** NY Downtown Hosp, Kingsbrook Jewish Med Ctr; **Address:** 170 William St Fl 4, New York, NY 10038; **Phone:** 212-312-5966; **Board Cert:** Orthopaedic Surgery 2003; **Med School:** NY Med Coll 1985; **Resid:** Orthopaedic Surgery, Lenox Hill Hosp 1990; **Fellow:** Foot & Ankle Surgery, Harborview Med Ctr 1994

Scher, David M MD (OrS) - **Spec Exp:** Pediatric Orthopaedic Surgery; Musculoskeletal Disorders; Trauma; Gait Disorders; **Hospital:** Hosp For Special Surgery (page 111); **Address:** Hosp for Special Surgery, 535 E 70th St, New York, NY 10021; **Phone:** 212-606-1253; **Board Cert:** Orthopaedic Surgery 2002; **Med School:** Duke Univ 1993; **Resid:** Orthopaedic Surgery, Hosp Joint Diseases 1999; **Fellow:** Pediatric Orthopaedic Surgery, Childrens Hosp 2000; **Fac Appt:** Assoc Prof OrS, Cornell Univ-Weill Med Coll

Schwab, Frank J MD (OrS) - **Spec Exp:** Spinal Surgery; Pain-Back; Spinal Deformity; Scoliosis; **Hospital:** NYU Hosp For Joint Diseases (page 106), New York Methodist Hosp (page 404); **Address:** 306 E 15th St, Ste 1F, New York, NY 10003; **Phone:** 646-794-8646; **Board Cert:** Orthopaedic Surgery 2010; **Med School:** Columbia P&S 1990; **Resid:** Surgery, NY Presby-Columbia Med Ctr 1992; Orthopaedic Surgery, NY Presby-Columbia Med Ctr 1996; **Fellow:** Hospital Lariboisiere 1991; Spinal Surgery, Maimonides Med Ctr 1997

Scott, W Norman MD (OrS) - **Spec Exp:** Knee Injuries; Knee Replacement; Sports Medicine; **Hospital:** Lenox Hill Hosp, Franklin Hosp; **Address:** 210 E 64th St Fl 4, New York, NY 10065; **Phone:** 212-434-4301; **Board Cert:** Orthopaedic Surgery 1978; **Med School:** Cornell Univ-Weill Med Coll 1972; **Resid:** Surgery, St Lukes-Roosevelt Hosp Ctr 1974; Orthopaedic Surgery, Hosp Special Surg 1977; **Fac Appt:** Clin Prof OrS, Cornell Univ-Weill Med Coll

Scuderi, Giles R MD (OrS) - **Spec Exp:** Knee Replacement; Knee Reconstruction; Knee Injuries/Ligament Surgery; Sports Medicine; **Hospital:** Lenox Hill Hosp, Franklin Hosp; **Address:** 210 E 64th St Fl 4, New York, NY 10021-7471; **Phone:** 212-434-4310; **Board Cert:** Orthopaedic Surgery 2009; **Med School:** SUNY Downstate 1982; **Resid:** Orthopaedic Surgery, Lenox Hill Hosp 1987; **Fellow:** Knee Surgery, Hosp Special Surgery 1988; **Fac Appt:** Asst Clin Prof OrS, Albert Einstein Coll Med

Sculco, Thomas P MD (OrS) - **Spec Exp:** Hip Replacement; Knee Replacement; Minimally Invasive Surgery; Joint Replacement; **Hospital:** Hosp For Special Surgery (page 111); **Address:** 535 E 70th St, Ste 238, New York, NY 10021-4872; **Phone:** 212-606-1475; **Board Cert:** Orthopaedic Surgery 1976; **Med School:** Columbia P&S 1969; **Resid:** Surgery, Roosevelt Hosp 1971; Orthopaedic Surgery, Hosp For Special Surgery 1974; **Fellow:** Orthopaedic Surgery, The London Hosp 1975; **Fac Appt:** Prof OrS, Cornell Univ-Weill Med Coll

Simon, Sheldon R MD (OrS) - **Spec Exp:** Foot & Ankle Surgery; Pediatric Orthopaedic Surgery; **Hospital:** Beth Israel Med Ctr - Petrie Division (page 94), Long Island Coll Hosp (page 94); **Address:** Phillips Ambulatory Care Ctr, 10 Union Square E, Ste 3K, New York, NY 10003; **Phone:** 212-844-6756; **Board Cert:** Orthopaedic Surgery 1976; **Med School:** NYU Sch Med 1966; **Resid:** Surgery, Bellevue Hosp/NYU Med Ctr 1968; Orthopaedic Surgery, Mass Genl Hosp 1973; **Fac Appt:** Clin Prof OrS, Albert Einstein Coll Med

Spivak, Jeffrey M MD (OrS) - **Spec Exp:** Spinal Surgery; Scoliosis; Sports Medicine Back Injuries; **Hospital:** NYU Hosp For Joint Diseases (page 106), NYU Langone Med Ctr (page 106); **Address:** Hosp for Joint Diseases, Spine Ctr, 301 E 17th St, Ste 400, New York, NY 10003-3804; **Phone:** 212-598-6696; **Board Cert:** Orthopaedic Surgery 2006; **Med School:** Cornell Univ-Weill Med Coll 1986; **Resid:** Orthopaedic Surgery, Hosp for Joint Diseases 1992; **Fellow:** Spinal Surgery, Thomas Jefferson Univ Hosp 1993; **Fac Appt:** Asst Prof OrS, NYU Sch Med

Strauss, Elton MD (OrS) - **Spec Exp:** Fractures; Hip & Knee Replacement; Osteomyelitis; Geriatric Orthopaedic Surgery; **Hospital:** Mount Sinai Med Ctr (page 102); **Address:** Mount Sinai Dept Orthopaedic Surgery, 5 E 98 St, Box 1188, New York, NY 10029-6501; **Phone:** 212-241-1648; **Board Cert:** Orthopaedic Surgery 1981; **Med School:** Mexico 1974; **Resid:** Orthopaedic Surgery, Bronx Lebanon Hosp 1979; **Fac Appt:** Assoc Prof OrS, Mount Sinai Sch Med

Stuchin, Steven MD (OrS) - **Spec Exp:** Hand Surgery; Arthritis; Hip & Knee Replacement; Hip Resurfacing; **Hospital:** NYU Hosp For Joint Diseases (page 106), Lenox Hill Hosp; **Address:** 301 E 17th St, Ste 1402, New York, NY 10003-3804; **Phone:** 212-598-6708; **Board Cert:** Orthopaedic Surgery 1984; **Med School:** Columbia P&S 1976; **Resid:** Surgery, Roosevelt Hosp 1978; Orthopaedic Surgery, Hosp For Special Surg 1981; **Fellow:** Hand Surgery, Thomas Jefferson Univ Hosp 1982; **Fac Appt:** Assoc Prof OrS, NYU Sch Med

Tindel, Nathaniel L MD (OrS) - **Spec Exp:** Spinal Surgery; Scoliosis; Minimally Invasive Surgery; Spinal Reconstructive Surgery; **Hospital:** Lenox Hill Hosp; **Address:** NY Ctr for Spinal Disorders, 425 E 79th St, Ste 1H, New York, NY 10075; **Phone:** 212-249-3840; **Board Cert:** Orthopaedic Surgery 2009; **Med School:** Univ Pennsylvania 1989; **Resid:** Orthopaedic Surgery, Lenox Hill Hosp 1994; **Fellow:** Spinal Surgery, Univ Miami-Jackson Meml Hosp 1995; **Fac Appt:** Asst Prof OrS, Albert Einstein Coll Med

Turtel, Andrew H MD (OrS) - **Spec Exp:** Knee Surgery; Shoulder Surgery; Sports Medicine; Arthroscopic Surgery; **Hospital:** Lenox Hill Hosp, Beth Israel Med Ctr - Petrie Division (page 94); **Address:** 333 E 56th St, New York, NY 10022-3758; **Phone:** 212-319-6500; **Board Cert:** Orthopaedic Surgery 2005; **Med School:** SUNY Upstate Med Univ 1985; **Resid:** Surgery, SUNY Upstate Med Ctr 1987; Orthopaedic Surgery, LI Jewish Med Ctr 1991; **Fellow:** Sports Medicine, NYU Med Ctr 1992; **Fac Appt:** Assoc Clin Prof OrS, Albert Einstein Coll Med

Unis, George L MD (OrS) - **Spec Exp:** Sports Medicine; Arthroscopic Surgery; **Hospital:** St Luke's - Roosevelt Hosp Ctr - Roosevelt Div (page 94), St Luke's - Roosevelt Hosp Ctr - St Luke's Hosp (page 94); **Address:** 115 E 61st St, FL 8, New York, NY 10065; **Phone:** 212-688-3710; **Board Cert:** Orthopaedic Surgery 1973; **Med School:** UMDNJ-NJ Med Sch, Newark 1965; **Resid:** Surgery, St Lukes Roosevelt Hosp 1967; Orthopaedic Surgery, St Lukes Roosevelt Hosp 1970; **Fac Appt:** Clin Prof OrS, Columbia P&S

Vitale, Michael MD (OrS) - **Spec Exp:** Spinal Surgery-Pediatric; Scoliosis; Limb Lengthening (Ilizarov Procedure); Clubfoot/Foot Deformities in Children; **Hospital:** NYPresby-Morgan Stanley Children's Hosp (page 104), NY-Presby Hosp/Columbia (page 104); **Address:** Morgan Stanley Chldn's Hosp, 3959 Broadway, Ste 800N, New York, NY 10032; **Phone:** 212-305-5475; **Board Cert:** Orthopaedic Surgery 2003; **Med School:** Columbia P&S 1995; **Resid:** Orthopaedic Surgery, Columbia Presby Med Ctr 2000; **Fellow:** Orthopaedic Surgery, Chldn's Hosp of Los Angeles 2001

Warren, Russell MD (OrS) - **Spec Exp:** Knee Injuries/Ligament Surgery; Shoulder Surgery; Shoulder Replacement; Rotator Cuff Surgery; **Hospital:** Hosp For Special Surgery (page 111), NY-Presby Hosp/Weill Cornell (page 104); **Address:** 535 E 70th St, New York, NY 10021-4892; **Phone:** 212-606-1178; **Board Cert:** Orthopaedic Surgery 1974; **Med School:** SUNY Upstate Med Univ 1966; **Resid:** Surgery, St Lukes Hosp 1968; Orthopaedic Surgery, Hosp For Special Surgery 1973; **Fellow:** Shoulder Surgery, Columbia-Presby Med Ctr 1977; **Fac Appt:** Prof OrS, Cornell Univ-Weill Med Coll

Weiner, Lon S MD (OrS) - **Spec Exp:** Trauma; Fractures; **Hospital:** Lenox Hill Hosp, Mount Sinai Med Ctr (page 102); **Address:** 130 E 77th St, Black Hall, Fl 12, New York, NY 10075; **Phone:** 212-434-4880; **Board Cert:** Orthopaedic Surgery 2001; **Med School:** Mount Sinai Sch Med 1982; **Resid:** Orthopaedic Surgery, Mount Sinai Hosp 1987; **Fellow:** Pediatric Orthopaedic Surgery, Hosp Special Surg 1988

Weinfeld, Steven B MD (OrS) - **Spec Exp:** Foot & Ankle Surgery; Diabetic Leg/Foot; **Hospital:** Mount Sinai Med Ctr (page 102), Hackensack Univ Med Ctr (page 96); **Address:** 5 E 98th St Fl 9, Box 1188, New York, NY 10029; **Phone:** 212-241-1634; **Board Cert:** Orthopaedic Surgery 2009; **Med School:** Albany Med Coll 1990; **Resid:** Orthopaedic Surgery, Albany Med Ctr 1995; **Fellow:** Ankle and Foot Surgery, Union Meml Hosp 1996; **Fac Appt:** Assoc Prof OrS, Mount Sinai Sch Med

Westrich, Geoffrey H MD (OrS) - **Spec Exp:** Hip Replacement & Revision; Knee Replacement & Revision; Arthroscopic Surgery-Hip; Arthroscopic Surgery-Knee; **Hospital:** Hosp For Special Surgery (page 111), NY-Presby Hosp/Weill Cornell (page 104); **Address:** Hospital for Special Surgery, 535 E 70th St, New York, NY 10021; **Phone:** 212-606-1510; **Board Cert:** Orthopaedic Surgery 2009; **Med School:** Tufts Univ 1990; **Resid:** Orthopaedic Surgery, Hosp for Special Surg 1995; **Fellow:** Trauma, Inselspital 1995; Adult Reconstructive Surgery, Hosp for Special Surg 1996; **Fac Appt:** Assoc Prof OrS, Cornell Univ-Weill Med Coll

Wickiewicz, Thomas L MD (OrS) - **Spec Exp:** Shoulder Surgery; Sports Medicine; Knee Injuries/ACL; Rotator Cuff Surgery; **Hospital:** Hosp For Special Surgery (page 111), NY-Presby Hosp/Weill Cornell (page 104); **Address:** 535 E 70th St, New York, NY 10021; **Phone:** 212-606-1450; **Board Cert:** Orthopaedic Surgery 1984; **Med School:** UMDNJ-NJ Med Sch, Newark 1976; **Resid:** Orthopaedic Surgery, Hosp for Special Surg 1981; **Fellow:** Sports Medicine, UCLA Med Ctr 1982; **Fac Appt:** Clin Prof OrS, Cornell Univ-Weill Med Coll

Widmann, Roger F MD (OrS) - **Spec Exp:** Pediatric Orthopaedic Surgery; Scoliosis; Limb Lengthening; Limb Deformities; **Hospital:** Hosp For Special Surgery (page 111); **Address:** 535 E 70th St, New York, NY 10021; **Phone:** 212-606-1325; **Board Cert:** Orthopaedic Surgery 2008; **Med School:** Yale Univ 1989; **Resid:** Orthopaedic Surgery, Mass General Hosp 1994; **Fellow:** Pediatric Orthopaedic Surgery, Children's Hosp 1995; **Fac Appt:** Asst Prof OrS, Cornell Univ-Weill Med Coll

Williams, Riley J MD (OrS) - **Spec Exp:** Cartilage Damage & Transplant; Shoulder Arthroscopic Surgery; Knee Injuries/ACL; Knee Surgery; **Hospital:** Hosp For Special Surgery (page 111), NY-Presby Hosp/Weill Cornell (page 104); **Address:** Hospital For Special Surgery, 535 E 70th St, New York, NY 10021; **Phone:** 212-606-1855; **Board Cert:** Orthopaedic Surgery 2000; **Med School:** Stanford Univ 1992; **Resid:** Orthopaedic Surgery, Hosp Special Surgery 1997; **Fellow:** Sports Medicine & Shoulder Surgery, Hosp Special Surgery 1998; **Fac Appt:** Assoc Prof OrS, Cornell Univ-Weill Med Coll

Windsor, Russell E MD (OrS) - **Spec Exp:** Knee Replacement; Hip Replacement; Knee Injuries/Ligament Surgery; **Hospital:** Hosp For Special Surgery (page 111), NY-Presby Hosp/Weill Cornell (page 104); **Address:** Hosp for Special Surgery, 535 E 70th St, New York, NY 10021; **Phone:** 212-606-1166; **Board Cert:** Orthopaedic Surgery 2007; **Med School:** Georgetown Univ 1978; **Resid:** Orthopaedic Surgery, Hosp Univ Penn 1983; **Fellow:** Knee Surgery, Hosp For Special Surg 1984; **Fac Appt:** Prof OrS, Cornell Univ-Weill Med Coll

Wittig, James C MD (OrS) - **Spec Exp:** Bone Tumors; Sarcoma-Soft Tissue; Hip & Knee Replacement; Shoulder Tumors; **Hospital:** Mount Sinai Med Ctr (page 102), Hackensack Univ Med Ctr (page 96); **Address:** 5 E 98th St Fl 9, New York, NY 10029; **Phone:** 212-241-1807 x4817; **Board Cert:** Orthopaedic Surgery 2003; **Med School:** NYU Sch Med 1994; **Resid:** Orthopaedic Surgery, Columbia Presby Med Ctr 1999; **Fellow:** Orthopaedic Oncology, Washington Cancer Inst 2001; Orthopaedic Oncology, NIH 2001; **Fac Appt:** Assoc Prof OrS, Mount Sinai Sch Med

Zambetti Jr, George J MD (OrS) - **Spec Exp:** Knee Reconstruction; Shoulder Surgery; Sports Medicine; Arthroscopic Surgery; **Hospital:** St Luke's - Roosevelt Hosp Ctr - Roosevelt Div (page 94); **Address:** 343 W 58th St, New York, NY 10019-1173; **Phone:** 212-506-0236; **Board Cert:** Orthopaedic Surgery 1983; **Med School:** Albany Med Coll 1976; **Resid:** Orthopaedic Surgery, Columbia-Presby Med Ctr 1981

Zuckerman, Joseph D MD (OrS) - **Spec Exp:** Shoulder Surgery; Hip Replacement; Knee Replacement; Rotator Cuff Surgery; **Hospital:** NYU Hosp For Joint Diseases (page 106), NYU Langone Med Ctr (page 106); **Address:** NYU Hosp for Joint Diseases, Dept Ortho Surg, 301 E 17th St Fl 14 - Ste 1402, New York, NY 10003; **Phone:** 212-598-6674; **Board Cert:** Orthopaedic Surgery 2007; **Med School:** Med Coll Wisc 1978; **Resid:** Orthopaedic Surgery, Univ WA Med Ctr 1983; **Fellow:** Arthritis Surgery, Brigham & Womans Hosp 1984; Shoulder Surgery, Mayo Clinic 1984; **Fac Appt:** Prof OrS, NYU Sch Med

Otolaryngology

Amin, Milan R MD (Oto) - **Spec Exp:** Voice Disorders; Vocal Cord Disorders; Swallowing Disorders; Airway Disorders; **Hospital:** NYU Langone Med Ctr (page 106); **Address:** NYU Medical Ctr, 530 1st Ave, HCC 3C, New York, NY 10016; **Phone:** 212-263-3705; **Board Cert:** Otolaryngology 2000; **Med School:** Northwestern Univ 1994; **Resid:** Otolaryngology, Temple Univ Med Ctr 1999; **Fellow:** Wake Forest Univ Med Ctr 2000; **Fac Appt:** Asst Prof Oto, NYU Sch Med

Aviv, Jonathan MD (Oto) - **Spec Exp:** Voice Disorders; Swallowing Disorders; Cough; Endoscopy; **Hospital:** Mount Sinai Med Ctr (page 102); **Address:** 210 E 86th St Fl 9, New York, NY 10028; **Phone:** 212-722-5570; **Board Cert:** Otolaryngology 1990; **Med School:** Columbia P&S 1985; **Resid:** Surgery, Mt Sinai Med Ctr 1987; Otolaryngology, Mt Sinai Med Ctr 1990; **Fellow:** Otolaryngology, Mt Sinai Med Ctr 1991; **Fac Appt:** Prof Oto, Mount Sinai Sch Med

Blitzer, Andrew MD/DDS (Oto) - **Spec Exp:** Voice Disorders; Swallowing Disorders; Nasal & Sinus Surgery; Botox Therapy; **Hospital:** St Luke's - Roosevelt Hosp Ctr - Roosevelt Div (page 94); **Address:** 425 W 59th St Fl 10, New York, NY 10019-1104; **Phone:** 212-262-9500; **Board Cert:** Otolaryngology 1977; **Med School:** Mount Sinai Sch Med 1973; **Resid:** Surgery, Beth Israel Med Ctr 1974; Otolaryngology, Mt Sinai Hosp 1977; **Fac Appt:** Clin Prof Oto, Columbia P&S

Branovan, Daniel Igor MD (Oto) - **Spec Exp:** Sinus Disorders/Surgery; Endoscopic Sinus Surgery; Thyroid Cancer; **Hospital:** New York Eye & Ear Infirm (page 113), Beth Israel Med Ctr - Petrie Division (page 94); **Address:** NY Eye & Ear Infirm, Dept Otolaryngology, 310 E 14th St 2nd Ave Fl 6, New York, NY 10003-4201; **Phone:** 212-979-4200; **Board Cert:** Otolaryngology 1999; **Med School:** Stanford Univ 1992; **Resid:** Otolaryngology, NY E&E Infirm 1996

Carew, John F MD (Oto) - **Spec Exp:** Head & Neck Surgery; Head & Neck Cancer; **Hospital:** Lenox Hill Hosp, Mount Sinai Med Ctr (page 102); **Address:** 969 Park Ave, Ste 1C, New York, NY 10028; **Phone:** 212-744-1941; **Board Cert:** Otolaryngology 1998; **Med School:** Cornell Univ-Weill Med Coll 1991; **Resid:** Otolaryngology, Manhattan EE&T 1997; **Fellow:** Head & Neck Oncology, Meml Sloan Kettering Cancer Ctr 1998

Caruana, Salvatore MD (Oto) - **Spec Exp:** Head & Neck Cancer; Thyroid & Parathyroid Surgery; Nasal & Sinus Disorders; Laser Surgery; **Hospital:** NY-Presby Hosp/Columbia (page 104); **Address:** 180 Fort Washington Ave Fl 7, New York, NY 10032; **Phone:** 212-305-5335; **Board Cert:** Otolaryngology 1996; **Med School:** Mount Sinai Sch Med 1989; **Resid:** Otolaryngology, NY EE Infirm 1995; **Fellow:** Head & Neck Surgical Oncology, Meml Sloan-Kettering Canc Ctr 1997; **Fac Appt:** Asst Prof Oto, Columbia P&S

Chandrasekhar, Sujana MD (Oto) - **Spec Exp:** Hearing & Balance Disorders; Cochlear Implants; Acoustic Neuroma; Meniere's Disease; **Hospital:** Mount Sinai Med Ctr (page 102), New York Eye & Ear Infirm (page 113); **Address:** 364 E 69th St, New York, NY 10021; **Phone:** 212-249-3232; **Board Cert:** Otolaryngology 1993; **Med School:** Mount Sinai Sch Med 1986; **Resid:** Surgery, NYU Med Ctr 1988; Otolaryngology, NYU Med Ctr 1992; **Fellow:** Neurotology, House Ear Clinic 1993; **Fac Appt:** Assoc Clin Prof Oto, Mount Sinai Sch Med

Close, Lanny G MD (Oto) - **Spec Exp:** Skull Base Surgery; Head & Neck Cancer; Sinus Disorders/Surgery; Endoscopic Sinus Surgery; **Hospital:** NY-Presby Hosp/Columbia (page 104); **Address:** 16 E 60th St, Ste 470, New York, NY 10022; **Phone:** 212-326-8475; **Board Cert:** Otolaryngology 1977; **Med School:** Baylor Coll Med 1972; **Resid:** Surgery, Johns Hopkins Hosp 1974; Otolaryngology, Baylor Affil Hosps 1977; **Fellow:** Head and Neck Surgery, MD Anderson Cancer Ctr 1979; **Fac Appt:** Prof Oto, Columbia P&S

Constantinides, Minas MD (Oto) - **Spec Exp:** Rhinoplasty; Rhinoplasty Revision; Nasal Surgery; Facial Rejuvenation; **Hospital:** NYU Langone Med Ctr (page 106), Lenox Hill Hosp; **Address:** NYU Med Ctr, Div Facial Plastic Surg, 530 First Ave, Ste 7U, New York, NY 10016-6402; **Phone:** 866-557-9042; **Board Cert:** Otolaryngology 1994; Facial Plastic & Reconstr Surgery 1997; **Med School:** Columbia P&S 1987; **Resid:** Surgery, Harvard Surg Svcs 1989; Otolaryngology, NYU Medical Center 1993; **Fellow:** Facial Plastic Surgery, Univ Toronto 1994; **Fac Appt:** Asst Prof Oto, NYU Sch Med

Costantino, Peter D MD (Oto) - **Spec Exp:** Skull Base Tumors; Head & Neck Cancer; Craniofacial Surgery/Reconstruction; **Hospital:** St Luke's - Roosevelt Hosp Ctr - Roosevelt Div (page 94), NY-Presby Hosp/Columbia (page 104); **Address:** 1000 W 10th Ave, Ste 5G-80, New York, NY 10019-1104; **Phone:** 212-523-6756; **Board Cert:** Otolaryngology 1990; Facial Plastic & Reconstr Surgery 2000; **Med School:** Northwestern Univ 1984; **Resid:** Surgery, Northwestern Meml Hosp 1986; Otolaryngology, Northwestern Meml Hosp 1989; **Fellow:** Head and Neck Surgery, Northwestern Meml Hosp 1990; Skull Base Surgery, Univ Pittsburgh 1991; **Fac Appt:** Prof Oto, Columbia P&S

DeLacure, Mark D MD (Oto) - **Spec Exp:** Head & Neck Cancer; Head & Neck Cancer Reconstruction; Reconstructive Microsurgery; **Hospital:** NYU Langone Med Ctr (page 106), VA Med Ctr - Manhattan; **Address:** 160 E 34th St Fl 9, New York, NY 10016; **Phone:** 212-731-5329; **Board Cert:** Otolaryngology 1992; **Med School:** Univ Fla Coll Med 1986; **Resid:** Otolaryngology, Yale Univ Sch Med 1991; Plastic/Reconstructive Surgery, UCLA Med Ctr 1993; **Fellow:** Head & Neck Oncology, Meml Sloan-Kettering Cancer Ctr 1992; **Fac Appt:** Assoc Clin Prof Oto, NYU Sch Med

Dropkin, Lloyd MD (Oto) - **Hospital:** NY-Presby Hosp/Weill Cornell (page 104); **Address:** 449 E 68th St, Ste 11, New York, NY 10065; **Phone:** 212-535-9191; **Board Cert:** Otolaryngology 1976; **Med School:** Cornell Univ-Weill Med Coll 1970; **Resid:** Otolaryngology, New York Hosp 1976; **Fac Appt:** Assoc Prof Oto, Cornell Univ-Weill Med Coll

Edelstein, David R MD (Oto) - **Spec Exp:** Endoscopic Sinus Surgery; Nasal Reconstruction; Rhinoplasty; Sleep Disorders/Apnea; **Hospital:** Lenox Hill Hosp (Manh Eye, Ear & Throat Hosp), Lenox Hill Hosp; **Address:** 1421 3rd Ave Fl 4, New York, NY 10028; **Phone:** 212-452-1500; **Board Cert:** Otolaryngology 1985; **Med School:** Boston Univ 1980; **Resid:** Otolaryngology, Mount Sinai Hosp 1984; **Fac Appt:** Clin Prof Oto, Cornell Univ-Weill Med Coll

Genden, Eric M MD (Oto) - **Spec Exp:** Head & Neck Cancer & Surgery; Head & Neck Cancer Reconstruction; Airway Reconstruction; Thyroid & Parathyroid Cancer & Surgery; **Hospital:** Mount Sinai Med Ctr (page 102); **Address:** Mt Sinai Dept Otolaryngology, 1 Gustave L Levy Pl, Box 1191, New York, NY 10029; **Phone:** 212-241-9410; **Board Cert:** Otolaryngology 1999; Facial Plastic & Reconstr Surgery 2000; **Med School:** Mount Sinai Sch Med 1992; **Resid:** Otolaryngology, Barnes Jewish Hosp 1998; **Fellow:** Head and Neck Surgery, Mt Sinai Med Ctr 1999; **Fac Appt:** Assoc Prof Oto, Mount Sinai Sch Med

Gold, Scott D MD (Oto) - **Spec Exp:** Endoscopic Sinus Surgery; Sinus Disorders/Surgery; **Hospital:** Beth Israel Med Ctr - Petrie Division (page 94), Mount Sinai Med Ctr (page 102); **Address:** 36A E 36th St, Ste 200, New York, NY 10016-3401; **Phone:** 212-889-8575; **Board Cert:** Otolaryngology 1983; **Med School:** Mount Sinai Sch Med 1979; **Resid:** Otolaryngology, Mt Sinai Med Ctr 1983; **Fac Appt:** Asst Clin Prof Oto, Mount Sinai Sch Med

Green, Robert P MD (Oto) - **Spec Exp:** Sinus Disorders; Hearing Loss/Tinnitus; Throat Disorders; **Hospital:** Mount Sinai Med Ctr (page 102); **Address:** ENT & Allergy, 210 E 86th St Fl 9, New York, NY 10028; **Phone:** 212-722-5570; **Board Cert:** Otolaryngology 1981; **Med School:** Harvard Med Sch 1977; **Resid:** Otolaryngology, Mount Sinai Hosp 1981; **Fac Appt:** Assoc Clin Prof Oto, Mount Sinai Sch Med

Guida, Robert MD (Oto) - **Spec Exp:** Rhinoplasty; Nasal Surgery; Cosmetic Surgery-Face; Skin Laser Surgery; **Hospital:** NY-Presby Hosp/Weill Cornell (page 104), Lenox Hill Hosp (Manh Eye, Ear & Throat Hosp); **Address:** 1175 5th Ave, Ste 1-B, New York, NY 10128; **Phone:** 212-871-0900; **Board Cert:** Otolaryngology 1989; Facial Plastic & Reconstr Surgery 1994; **Med School:** Hahnemann Univ 1983; **Resid:** Surgery, Graduate Hosp 1985; Otolaryngology, NY Eye & Ear Infirm 1989; **Fellow:** Facial Plastic Surgery, Oregon Hlth Sci Ctr 1990; **Fac Appt:** Assoc Prof Oto, Cornell Univ-Weill Med Coll

Hammerschlag, Paul E MD (Oto) - **Spec Exp:** Cochlear Implants; Hearing Loss; Meniere's Disease; Balance Disorders; **Hospital:** NYU Langone Med Ctr (page 106), New York Eye & Ear Infirm (page 113); **Address:** 650 First Ave, New York, NY 10016-3240; **Phone:** 212-889-2600; **Board Cert:** Otolaryngology 1978; **Med School:** Albert Einstein Coll Med 1972; **Resid:** Surgery, Virginia Mason Hosp 1974; Otolaryngology, Mass Eye & Ear Infirm 1978; **Fellow:** Otolaryngology, Mass Eye & Ear Infirm 1978; **Fac Appt:** Assoc Clin Prof Oto, NYU Sch Med

Har-El, Gady MD (Oto) - **Spec Exp:** Head & Neck Cancer; Thyroid & Parathyroid Surgery; Sinus Tumors; Skull Base Tumors; **Hospital:** Lenox Hill Hosp, Lenox Hill Hosp (Manh Eye, Ear & Throat Hosp); **Address:** 186 E 76th St Fl 2, New York, NY 10021; **Phone:** 212-434-2323; **Board Cert:** Otolaryngology 1992; **Med School:** Israel 1982; **Resid:** Otolaryngology, SUNY Downstate Med Ctr 1991; **Fac Appt:** Prof Oto, SUNY Hlth Sci Ctr

Hoffman, Ronald MD (Oto) - **Spec Exp:** Cochlear Implants; Balance Disorders; Ear Disorders/Surgery; **Hospital:** New York Eye & Ear Infirm (page 113); **Address:** 310 14th St Fl 6th, New York, NY 10003; **Phone:** 212-614-8388; **Board Cert:** Otolaryngology 1976; **Med School:** Jefferson Med Coll 1971; **Resid:** Otolaryngology, NYU Med Ctr 1976; **Fellow:** Otology & Neurotology, Lenox Hill Hosp 1977; **Fac Appt:** Prof Oto, Albert Einstein Coll Med

Jacobs, Joseph B MD (Oto) - **Spec Exp:** Endoscopic Sinus Surgery; Sinus Disorders/Surgery; Sinus Surgery-Revision; **Hospital:** NYU Langone Med Ctr (page 106); **Address:** NYU Med Ctr, 530 1st Ave, Ste 3C, New York, NY 10016-6402; **Phone:** 212-263-7398; **Board Cert:** Otolaryngology 1978; **Med School:** Albert Einstein Coll Med 1974; **Resid:** Otolaryngology, NYU Med Ctr 1978; **Fellow:** Plastic/Reconstructive Surgery, UCLA Med Ctr 1979; **Fac Appt:** Prof Oto, NYU Sch Med

Jahn, Anthony MD (Oto) - **Spec Exp:** Voice Disorders/Professional Voice Care; Hearing Loss; Otology & Neuro-Otology; **Hospital:** St Luke's - Roosevelt Hosp Ctr - Roosevelt Div (page 94); **Address:** 425 W 59th St, New York, NY 10019; **Phone:** 212-262-4400; **Board Cert:** Otolaryngology 1979; **Med School:** Canada 1974; **Resid:** Otolaryngology, Toronto Genl Hosp 1979; **Fac Appt:** Prof Oto, Columbia P&S

Josephson, Jordan S MD (Oto) - **Spec Exp:** Rhinoplasty Revision; Endoscopic Sinus Surgery; Nasal & Sinus Disorders; Sleep Apnea; **Hospital:** Lenox Hill Hosp (Manh Eye, Ear & Throat Hosp), Lenox Hill Hosp; **Address:** 205 E 76th St, Ste M1, New York, NY 10021; **Phone:** 212-717-1773; **Board Cert:** Otolaryngology 1988; **Med School:** SUNY Downstate 1983; **Resid:** Otolaryngology, LI Jewish Med Ctr 1988; **Fellow:** Sinus Surgery, Johns Hopkins Hosp 1989

Kacker, Ashutosh MD (Oto) - **Spec Exp:** Sinus Surgery; **Hospital:** NY-Presby Hosp/Weill Cornell (page 104); **Address:** 1305 York Ave Fl 5, New York, NY 10021; **Phone:** 646-962-5097; **Board Cert:** Otolaryngology 2002; **Med School:** India 1989; **Resid:** Surgery, Lenox Hill Hosp 1997; **Fellow:** Otolaryngology, Manhattan Eye, Ear & Throat 2001; **Fac Appt:** Assoc Prof Oto, Cornell Univ

Kohan, Darius MD (Oto) - **Spec Exp:** Cochlear Implants; Acoustic Neuroma; Hearing Disorders; Ear Tumors; **Hospital:** New York Eye & Ear Infirm (page 113), NYU Langone Med Ctr (page 106); **Address:** 863 Park Ave, Ste 1E, New York, NY 10021; **Phone:** 212-472-1300; **Board Cert:** Otolaryngology 1990; **Med School:** NYU Sch Med 1984; **Resid:** Surgery, Beth Israel Med Ctr 1986; Otolaryngology, NYU Med Ctr 1990; **Fellow:** Otology, NYU Med Ctr 1991; **Fac Appt:** Assoc Prof Oto, NYU Sch Med

Komisar, Arnold MD/DDS (Oto) - **Spec Exp:** Thyroid & Parathyroid Surgery; Salivary Gland Tumors; Nasal & Sinus Surgery; **Hospital:** Lenox Hill Hosp, Lenox Hill Hosp (Manh Eye, Ear & Throat Hosp); **Address:** 1421 3rd Ave Fl 4, New York, NY 10021-2995; **Phone:** 212-861-8888; **Board Cert:** Otolaryngology 1979; **Med School:** Hahnemann Univ 1975; **Resid:** Surgery, Beth Israel Hosp 1976; Otolaryngology, Mt Sinai Med Ctr 1979; **Fac Appt:** Clin Prof Oto, NYU Sch Med

Koufman, Jamie A MD (Oto) - **Spec Exp:** Voice Disorders; Laryngeal Disorders; **Hospital:** New York Eye & Ear Infirm (page 113); **Address:** 200 W 57th St, Ste 1203, New York, NY 10019; **Phone:** 212-463-8014; **Board Cert:** Otolaryngology 1978; **Med School:** Boston Univ 1973; **Resid:** Surgery, Hartford Hosp 1975; Otolaryngology, Boston Univ Med Ctr 1978

Kraus, Dennis H MD (Oto) - **Spec Exp:** Head & Neck Cancer; Skull Base Tumors; Thyroid & Parathyroid Surgery; **Hospital:** Meml Sloan-Kettering Cancer Ctr (page 112); **Address:** 1275 York Avenue, New York, NY 10065; **Phone:** 800-525-2225; **Board Cert:** Otolaryngology 1990; **Med School:** Univ Rochester 1985; **Resid:** Surgery, Cleveland Clinic 1987; Otolaryngology, Cleveland Clinic 1990; **Fellow:** Head and Neck Surgery, Meml Sloan Kettering Cancer Ctr 1991; **Fac Appt:** Prof Oto, Cornell Univ-Weill Med Coll

Krespi, Yosef P MD (Oto) - **Spec Exp:** Nasal & Sinus Cancer & Surgery; Sleep Disorders/Apnea; Head & Neck Cancer & Surgery; Snoring/Sleep Apnea; **Hospital:** St Luke's - Roosevelt Hosp Ctr - Roosevelt Div (page 94); **Address:** 425 W 59th St Fl 10, New York, NY 10019-1128; **Phone:** 212-262-2929; **Board Cert:** Otolaryngology 1981; **Med School:** Israel 1973; **Resid:** Surgery, Mt Sinai Hosp 1976; Otolaryngology, Mt Sinai Hosp 1980; **Fellow:** Surgery, Northwestern Meml Hosp 1981; **Fac Appt:** Clin Prof Oto, Columbia P&S

Krevitt, Lane MD (Oto) - **Spec Exp:** Head & Neck Surgery; Endoscopic Sinus Surgery; Voice Disorders/Professional Voice Care; Sleep Medicine; **Hospital:** Beth Israel Med Ctr - Petrie Division (page 94); **Address:** 36A E 36th St, New York, NY 10016-3453; **Phone:** 212-889-8575; **Board Cert:** Otolaryngology 1999; **Med School:** Hahnemann Univ 1993; **Resid:** Surgery, Albert Einstein Univ & Affiliated Hosps 1994; Otolaryngology, Albert Einstein Univ & Affiliated Hosps 1998; **Fellow:** Head & Neck Surgical Oncology, Montefiore Med Ctr 1999; **Fac Appt:** Asst Prof Oto, Albert Einstein Coll Med

Kuhel, William I MD (Oto) - **Spec Exp:** Head & Neck Surgery; Thyroid Surgery; Parathyroid Surgery; **Hospital:** NY-Presby Hosp/Weill Cornell (page 104), Hosp For Special Surgery (page 111); **Address:** 1305 York Ave Fl 5, New York, NY 10021; **Phone:** 646-962-6325; **Board Cert:** Otolaryngology 1988; **Med School:** Univ Mich Med Sch 1983; **Resid:** Surgery, St Vincent's Hosp 1985; Otolaryngology, Indiana Univ 1988; **Fellow:** Head and Neck Surgery, MD Anderson Hosp 1989; **Fac Appt:** Assoc Clin Prof Oto, Cornell Univ-Weill Med Coll

Kuriloff, Daniel MD (Oto) - **Spec Exp:** Thyroid Surgery; Parathyroid Surgery; Minimally Invasive Surgery; Head & Neck Surgery; **Hospital:** St Luke's - Roosevelt Hosp Ctr - Roosevelt Div (page 94), NY-Presby Hosp/Columbia (page 104); **Address:** 425 W 59th St, Fl 10, New York, NY 10019-1104; **Phone:** 212-262-5555; **Board Cert:** Otolaryngology 1988; **Med School:** Mount Sinai Sch Med 1982; **Resid:** Surgery, Beth Israel Hosp 1984; Otolaryngology, NY Eye & Ear Infirmary 1988; **Fellow:** Head & Neck Surgical Oncology, Univ Mich Med Ctr 1990; **Fac Appt:** Assoc Prof Oto, Columbia P&S

Lalwani, Anil K MD (Oto) - **Spec Exp:** Ear Disorders/Surgery; Facial Nerve Disorders; Pediatric Otolaryngology; Skull Base Surgery; **Hospital:** NYU Langone Med Ctr (page 106); **Address:** 540 1st Ave, Ste 8S, New York, NY 10016; **Phone:** 212-263-7167; **Board Cert:** Otolaryngology 1992; Neurotology 2010; **Med School:** Univ Mich Med Sch 1985; **Resid:** Surgery, Duke Univ Med Ctr 1987; Otolaryngology, UCSF Med Ctr 1991; **Fellow:** Skull Base Surgery, UCSF Med Ctr 1992; **Fac Appt:** Prof Oto, NYU Sch Med

Lawson, William MD (Oto) - **Spec Exp:** Nasal & Sinus Surgery; Head & Neck Cancer; Skull Base Surgery; Head & Neck Inflammatory Disorders; **Hospital:** Mount Sinai Med Ctr (page 102); **Address:** 5 E 98th St Fl 8, Box 1191, New York, NY 10029-6501; **Phone:** 212-241-9410; **Board Cert:** Otolaryngology 1974; **Med School:** NYU Sch Med 1965; **Resid:** Surgery, Bronx VA Hosp 1967; Otolaryngology, Mt Sinai Hosp 1973; **Fellow:** Otolaryngology, Mt Sinai Hosp 1970; **Fac Appt:** Prof Oto, Mount Sinai Sch Med

Lebovics, Robert S MD (Oto) - **Spec Exp:** Head & Neck Inflammatory Disorders; Head & Neck Autoimmune Disease; Head & Neck Infectious Disease; Relapsing Polychondritis; **Hospital:** St Luke's - Roosevelt Hosp Ctr - Roosevelt Div (page 94); **Address:** 425 W 59th St Fl 10, New York, NY 10019; **Phone:** 212-262-2002; **Board Cert:** Otolaryngology 1988; **Med School:** SUNY Downstate 1982; **Resid:** Surgery, Montefiore-Weiler Einstein Div 1983; Otolaryngology, Montefiore-Weiler Einstein Div 1987

Linstrom, Christopher MD (Oto) - **Spec Exp:** Cochlear Implants; Acoustic Neuroma; Encephalocele; Cholesteatoma; **Hospital:** New York Eye & Ear Infirm (page 113); **Address:** NY Eye & Ear Infirmary, Dept Otolaryngology, 310 E 14th St Fl 6, New York, NY 10003-4201; **Phone:** 212-979-4200; **Board Cert:** Otolaryngology 1987; **Med School:** McGill Univ 1982; **Resid:** Surgery, Geo Wash Med Ctr 1984; Otolaryngology, NY Hosp 1987; **Fellow:** Otology & Neurotology, Michigan Ear Inst 1989; **Fac Appt:** Assoc Prof Oto, NY Med Coll

Markowitz, Arlene MD (Oto) - **Hospital:** NY-Presby Hosp/Columbia (page 104), Lenox Hill Hosp; **Address:** 110 E 82nd St, New York, NY 10028; **Phone:** 212-794-3999; **Board Cert:** Otolaryngology 1990; **Med School:** Columbia P&S 1984; **Resid:** Surgery, Columbia-Presby Med Ctr 1986; Otolaryngology, Columbia-Presby Med Ctr 1990; **Fac Appt:** Asst Clin Prof Oto, Columbia P&S

Miller, Philip J MD (Oto) - **Spec Exp:** Rhinoplasty; Cosmetic Surgery-Face; Facial Nerve Disorders; Facial Rejuvenation; **Hospital:** Lenox Hill Hosp (Manh Eye, Ear & Throat Hosp), NYU Langone Med Ctr (page 106); **Address:** 60 E 56 St Fl 3, New York, NY 10022; **Phone:** 212-750-7100; **Board Cert:** Otolaryngology 1996; Facial Plastic & Reconstr Surgery 1998; **Med School:** Univ Mass Sch Med 1989; **Resid:** Otolaryngology, NYU Med Ctr 1995; **Fellow:** Facial Plastic Surgery, Oregon Health Sci Ctr 1996; **Fac Appt:** Asst Prof Oto, NYU Sch Med

Myssiorek, David MD (Oto) - **Spec Exp:** Thyroid & Parathyroid Surgery; Laryngeal Disorders; Salivary Gland Surgery; Paragangliomas; **Hospital:** NYU Langone Med Ctr (page 106), Bellevue Hosp Ctr; **Address:** 160 E 34th St, New York, NY 10016; **Phone:** 212-731-6085; **Board Cert:** Otolaryngology 1985; **Med School:** NYU Sch Med 1980; **Resid:** Otolaryngology, Bellevue/NYU/VA Med Ctr 1984; **Fellow:** Head & Neck Oncology, Montefiore Hosp Med Ctr 1985; **Fac Appt:** Prof Oto, NYU Sch Med

Nass, Richard L MD (Oto) - **Spec Exp:** Sinus Disorders/Surgery; Nasal Surgery; Allergy; **Hospital:** NYU Langone Med Ctr (page 106), Lenox Hill Hosp; **Address:** 1430 2nd Ave, Ste 108, New York, NY 10021; **Phone:** 212-734-4515; **Board Cert:** Otolaryngology 1979; **Med School:** NYU Sch Med 1975; **Resid:** Otolaryngology, NYU-Bellevue Hosp 1979; **Fac Appt:** Assoc Clin Prof Oto, NYU Sch Med

Parisier, Simon C MD (Oto) - **Spec Exp:** Cochlear Implants; Hearing Loss; Ear Disorders/Surgery; Cholesteatoma; **Hospital:** New York Eye & Ear Infirm (page 113); **Address:** NY Eye & Ear Infirmary - Otolaryngology, 310 E 14th St, 6th Fl - Window 5, New York, NY 10003-4297; **Phone:** 212-979-4542; **Board Cert:** Otolaryngology 1967; **Med School:** Boston Univ 1961; **Resid:** Otolaryngology, Mount Sinai Hosp 1966; **Fac Appt:** Prof Oto, NY Med Coll

Persky, Mark S MD (Oto) - **Spec Exp:** Head & Neck Cancer; Skull Base Tumors; Thyroid Cancer; Vascular Lesions-Head & Neck; **Hospital:** Beth Israel Med Ctr - Petrie Division (page 94), New York Eye & Ear Infirm (page 113); **Address:** 10 Union Square East, Ste 4J, New York, NY 10003; **Phone:** 212-844-8648; **Board Cert:** Otolaryngology 1976; **Med School:** SUNY Upstate Med Univ 1972; **Resid:** Otolaryngology, Bellevue Hosp 1976; **Fellow:** Head and Neck Surgery, Beth Israel Med Ctr 1977; **Fac Appt:** Clin Prof Oto, Albert Einstein Coll Med

Pincus, Robert L MD (Oto) - **Spec Exp:** Sinus Disorders; Voice Disorders; Endoscopic Sinus Surgery; **Hospital:** Beth Israel Med Ctr - Petrie Division (page 94), Lenox Hill Hosp; **Address:** 36A E 36th St, Ste 200, New York, NY 10016-3401; **Phone:** 212-889-8575; **Board Cert:** Otolaryngology 1983; **Med School:** Univ Mich Med Sch 1978; **Resid:** Surgery, Lenox Hill Hosp 1980; Otolaryngology, Mt Sinai Med Ctr 1983; **Fac Appt:** Assoc Prof Oto, NY Med Coll

Pollack, Geoffrey MD (Oto) - **Spec Exp:** Head & Neck Surgery; **Hospital:** St Luke's - Roosevelt Hosp Ctr - St Luke's Hosp (page 94); **Address:** 211 Central Park West, New York, NY 10024; **Phone:** 212-873-6175; **Board Cert:** Otolaryngology 1984; **Med School:** Columbia P&S 1979; **Resid:** Otolaryngology, Columbia-Presby Med Ctr 1984

Portnoy, William M MD (Oto) - **Spec Exp:** Head & Neck Cancer & Surgery; Head & Neck Cancer Reconstruction; Facial Plastic & Reconstructive Surgery; **Hospital:** Beth Israel Med Ctr - Petrie Division (page 94), New York Eye & Ear Infirm (page 113); **Address:** 160 W 18th St, Ground Fl, New York, NY 10011; **Phone:** 212-366-0848 x201; **Board Cert:** Otolaryngology 1993; Facial Plastic & Reconstr Surgery 1993; **Med School:** Geo Wash Univ 1987; **Resid:** Otolaryngology, NY E&E Infirm 1992; Head and Neck Surgery, NY E&E Infirm 1992; **Fellow:** Head and Neck Surgery, Mercy Hosp 1993; Microvascular Surgery, Mercy Hosp 1993

Rizk, Samieh S MD (Oto) - **Spec Exp:** Facial Plastic & Reconstructive Surgery; Rhinoplasty Revision; Nasal Surgery; **Hospital:** Lenox Hill Hosp, Lenox Hill Hosp (Manh Eye, Ear & Throat Hosp); **Address:** 1040 Park Ave, New York, NY 10028; **Phone:** 212-452-3362; **Board Cert:** Facial Plastic & Reconstr Surgery 2000; Otolaryngology 2000; **Med School:** Univ Mich Med Sch 1993; **Resid:** Otolaryngology, Manhattan EE&T Hosp 1999; **Fellow:** Facial Plastic Surgery, Facial Surgery Center 2000

Roland Sr, J Thomas MD (Oto) - **Spec Exp:** Acoustic Neuroma; Cochlear Implants; Neuro-Otology; Facial Nerve Disorders; **Hospital:** NYU Langone Med Ctr (page 106), Bellevue Hosp Ctr; **Address:** 550 First Avenue, Ste 7Q, New York, NY 10016; **Phone:** 212-263-5565; **Board Cert:** Otolaryngology 1993; Neurotology 2004; **Med School:** Temple Univ 1983; **Resid:** Otolaryngology, NYU Med Ctr 1992; **Fellow:** Neurotology, NYU Med Ctr 1993; **Fac Appt:** Assoc Prof Oto, NYU Sch Med

Romo III, Thomas MD (Oto) - **Spec Exp:** Facial Plastic & Reconstructive Surgery; Cosmetic Surgery-Face; Rhinoplasty Revision; Ear Reconstruction/Microtia; **Hospital:** Lenox Hill Hosp, Lenox Hill Hosp (Manh Eye, Ear & Throat Hosp); **Address:** 135 E 74th St, New York, NY 10021; **Phone:** 212-288-1500; **Board Cert:** Otolaryngology 1985; Facial Plastic & Reconstr Surgery 1992; **Med School:** Baylor Coll Med 1979; **Resid:** Otolaryngology, Baylor Hosps 1982; Otolaryngology, New York Eye & Ear Infirm 1984; **Fellow:** Facial Plastic Surgery, New York Eye & Ear Infirm 1985; Facial Plastic Surgery, Tampa General Hosp 1987; **Fac Appt:** Asst Clin Prof Oto, NY Med Coll

Rosenberg, David B MD (Oto) - **Spec Exp:** Rhinoplasty Revision; Cosmetic Surgery-Face; Reconstructive Surgery; **Hospital:** Lenox Hill Hosp (Manh Eye, Ear & Throat Hosp); **Address:** 115 E 61st St Fl 12, New York, NY 10021; **Phone:** 212-832-8595; **Board Cert:** Otolaryngology 2000; Facial Plastic & Reconstr Surgery 2002; **Med School:** Cornell Univ-Weill Med Coll 1993; **Resid:** Otolaryngology, Manhattan EE&T Hosp 1999; **Fellow:** Facial Plastic Surgery, RWJohnson Univ Hosp 2000

Rothstein, Stephen G MD (Oto) - **Spec Exp:** Voice Disorders; Swallowing Disorders; Laser Surgery; **Hospital:** NYU Langone Med Ctr (page 106); **Address:** 530 1st Ave, Ste 3C, New York, NY 10016-6402; **Phone:** 212-263-7505; **Board Cert:** Surgical Critical Care 1988; **Med School:** Ros Franklin Univ/Chicago Med Sch 1982; **Resid:** Surgery, NYU Med Ctr 1984; Otolaryngology, NYU Med Ctr 1987; **Fellow:** Head and Neck Surgery, NYU Med Ctr 1988; **Fac Appt:** Assoc Clin Prof Oto, NYU Sch Med

Sacks, Steven H MD (Oto) - **Spec Exp:** Sinus Disorders/Surgery; Thyroid & Parathyroid Surgery; Salivary Gland Tumors & Surgery; **Hospital:** Mount Sinai Med Ctr (page 102); **Address:** ENT & Allergy Assocs, 210 E 86th St Fl 9, New York, NY 10028; **Phone:** 212-722-5570; **Board Cert:** Otolaryngology 1981; **Med School:** Washington Univ, St Louis 1977; **Resid:** Otolaryngology, Mt Sinai Hosp 1981; **Fac Appt:** Asst Clin Prof Oto, Mount Sinai Sch Med

Schaefer, Steven D MD (Oto) - **Spec Exp:** Sinus Disorders/Surgery; Head & Neck Surgery; Endoscopic Sinus Surgery; **Hospital:** New York Eye & Ear Infirm (page 113), Beth Israel Med Ctr - Petrie Division (page 94); **Address:** NY Eye & Ear Infirm, Dept Otolaryngology, 310 E 14th St, New York, NY 10003-4201; **Phone:** 212-979-4070; **Board Cert:** Otolaryngology 1978; **Med School:** UC Irvine 1972; **Resid:** Surgery, UCLA Med Ctr 1974; Otolaryngology, Stanford Med Ctr 1977; **Fac Appt:** Prof Oto, NY Med Coll

Schantz, Stimson P MD (Oto) - **Spec Exp:** Head & Neck Surgery; Head & Neck Cancer; Thyroid Cancer; **Hospital:** New York Eye & Ear Infirm (page 113), Beth Israel Med Ctr - Petrie Division (page 94); **Address:** 310 E 14th St Fl 6N, New YorkNew York, NY 10003; **Phone:** 212-979-4535; **Board Cert:** Surgery 2005; **Med School:** Univ Cincinnati 1975; **Resid:** Surgery, Georgetown Univ Med CtrGeorgetown Univ Med Ctr 1982; Otolaryngology, Univ Illinois Eye & Ear Infirm 1980; **Fellow:** Surgical Oncology, MD Anderson Cancer Ctr 1984; **Fac Appt:** Prof Oto, NY Med Coll

Schley, W Shain MD (Oto) - **Spec Exp:** Nasal & Sinus Disorders; Throat Disorders; Voice Disorders; Sleep Disorders; **Hospital:** NY-Presby Hosp/Weill Cornell (page 104); **Address:** 449 E 68th St Fl 2 - Ste DS 10, New York, NY 10065; **Phone:** 212-746-2223; **Board Cert:** Otolaryngology 1973; **Med School:** Emory Univ 1966; **Resid:** Surgery, Roosevelt Hosp 1968; Otolaryngology, New York Hosp 1973; **Fac Appt:** Assoc Clin Prof Oto, Cornell Univ-Weill Med Coll

Schneider, Kenneth L MD (Oto) - **Spec Exp:** Snoring/Sleep Apnea; Nasal & Sinus Disorders; Sleep Disorders/Apnea; **Hospital:** NYU Langone Med Ctr (page 106); **Address:** 530 1st Ave, Ste 3C, New York, NY 10016-6402; **Phone:** 212-263-7165; **Board Cert:** Otolaryngology 1982; **Med School:** SUNY Hlth Sci Ctr 1978; **Resid:** Otolaryngology, NYU Med Ctr 1982; **Fellow:** Head and Neck Surgery, Montefiore Med Ctr 1983; **Fac Appt:** Assoc Clin Prof Oto, NYU Sch Med

Sclafani, Anthony P MD (Oto) - **Spec Exp:** Cosmetic Surgery-Face; Botox Therapy; Rhinoplasty; Reconstructive Surgery; **Hospital:** New York Eye & Ear Infirm (page 113), Northern Westchester Hosp; **Address:** 310 E 14th St Fl 6, New York, NY 10003; **Phone:** 212-979-4534; **Board Cert:** Otolaryngology 1996; Facial Plastic & Reconstr Surgery 1999; **Med School:** Univ Pennsylvania 1989; **Resid:** Surgery, Beth Israel Med Ctr 1991; Otolaryngology, NY Eye & Ear Infirm 1995; **Fellow:** Facial Plastic Surgery, St Louis Univ 1996; **Fac Appt:** Prof Oto, NY Med Coll

Selesnick, Samuel H MD (Oto) - **Spec Exp:** Acoustic Neuroma; Cholesteatoma; Otosclerosis; **Hospital:** NY-Presby Hosp/Weill Cornell (page 104), Meml Sloan-Kettering Cancer Ctr (page 112); **Address:** 1305 York Ave Fl 5, New York, NY 10021; **Phone:** 646-962-3277; **Board Cert:** Otolaryngology 1990; Neurotology 2008; **Med School:** NYU Sch Med 1985; **Resid:** Surgery, St Vincent's Med Ctr 1987; Otolaryngology, Manhattan EE&T Hosp 1990; **Fellow:** Skull Base Surgery, UCSF Med Ctr 1991; **Fac Appt:** Prof Oto, Cornell Univ-Weill Med Coll

Shemen, Larry J MD (Oto) - **Spec Exp:** Head & Neck Cancer; Thyroid Cancer; Parathyroid Cancer; Snoring/Sleep Apnea; **Hospital:** NY Hosp Queens, Lenox Hill Hosp; **Address:** 233 E 69th St, Ste 1D, New York, NY 10021; **Phone:** 212-472-8882; **Board Cert:** Otolaryngology 1983; **Med School:** Univ Toronto 1978; **Resid:** Surgery, Cedar-Sinai Med Ctr 1982; Otolaryngology, St Michael's Med Ctr 1983; **Fellow:** Head and Neck Surgery, Meml Sloan-Kettering Cancer Ctr 1984; **Fac Appt:** Assoc Clin Prof Oto, Cornell Univ-Weill Med Coll

Shugar, Joel MD (Oto) - **Spec Exp:** Hearing & Balance Disorders; Head & Neck Surgery; Nasal & Sinus Disorders; **Hospital:** Mount Sinai Med Ctr (page 102); **Address:** 55 E 87th St, Ste 1K, New York, NY 10128-1043; **Phone:** 212-289-1731; **Board Cert:** Otolaryngology 1978; **Med School:** McGill Univ 1972; **Resid:** Surgery, Jewish Genl Hosp 1974; Otolaryngology, Mount Sinai Med Ctr 1978; **Fellow:** Otolaryngology, Mount Sinai Med Ctr 1975; **Fac Appt:** Assoc Clin Prof Oto, Mount Sinai Sch Med

Singh, Bhuvanesh MD/PhD (Oto) - **Spec Exp:** Head & Neck Cancer & Surgery; Thyroid Cancer; **Hospital:** Meml Sloan-Kettering Cancer Ctr (page 112); **Address:** 1275 York Ave, MC C1073, New York, NY 10065; **Phone:** 800-525-2225; **Board Cert:** Otolaryngology 1998; **Med School:** SUNY Downstate 1991; **Resid:** Otolaryngology, SUNY Downstate Med Ctr 1997; **Fellow:** Head and Neck Surgery, Meml Sloan-Kettering Canc Ctr 1999; **Fac Appt:** Assoc Prof Oto, Cornell Univ-Weill Med Coll

Slavit, David H MD (Oto) - **Spec Exp:** Voice Disorders; Nasal & Sinus Disorders; Head & Neck Surgery; Thyroid Surgery; **Hospital:** Lenox Hill Hosp, Lenox Hill Hosp (Manh Eye, Ear & Throat Hosp); **Address:** 787 Park Ave, New York, NY 10021-3552; **Phone:** 212-517-9177; **Board Cert:** Otolaryngology 1992; **Med School:** Mount Sinai Sch Med 1986; **Resid:** Otolaryngology, Mayo Clinic 1991; **Fac Appt:** Asst Prof Oto, SUNY Hlth Sci Ctr

Stewart, Michael G MD (Oto) - **Spec Exp:** Nasal & Sinus Disorders; Sleep Disorders/Apnea; Head & Neck Surgery; **Hospital:** NY-Presby Hosp/Weill Cornell (page 104); **Address:** Weill Cornell Physicians, 1305 York Ave, Ste 5, New York, NY 10011; **Phone:** 646-962-6673; **Board Cert:** Otolaryngology 1995; **Med School:** Johns Hopkins Univ 1988; **Resid:** Otolaryngology, Baylor Coll Med 1994; **Fac Appt:** Prof Oto, Cornell Univ-Weill Med Coll

Storper, Ian MD (Oto) - **Spec Exp:** Skull Base Surgery; Cochlear Implants; Acoustic Neuroma; **Hospital:** NY-Presby Hosp/Columbia (page 104); **Address:** 180 Fort Washington Ave Fl 7, New York, NY 10032-3173; **Phone:** 212-305-5335; **Board Cert:** Otolaryngology 1995; **Med School:** Univ Pennsylvania 1988; **Resid:** Otolaryngology, UCLA Med Ctr 1994; **Fellow:** Otology & Neurotology, Ear Foundation 1995; **Fac Appt:** Asst Prof Oto, Columbia P&S

Strome, Marshall MD (Oto) - **Spec Exp:** Sleep Disorders/Apnea; Voice Disorders; Head & Neck Cancer; Swallowing Disorders; **Hospital:** St Luke's - Roosevelt Hosp Ctr - St Luke's Hosp (page 94), Mount Sinai Med Ctr (page 102); **Address:** 110 E 59th St, Ste 10A, New York, NY 10022; **Phone:** 212-223-1333; **Board Cert:** Otolaryngology 1970; **Med School:** Univ Mich Med Sch 1964; **Resid:** Surgery, Harper Hosp 1966; Otolaryngology, Univ Michigan Hosp 1970; **Fac Appt:** Prof Oto

Sulica, Radu Lucian MD (Oto) - **Spec Exp:** Laryngeal & Vocal Cord Surgery; Voice Disorders; Vocal Cord Disorders; Botox Therapy; **Hospital:** NY-Presby Hosp/Weill Cornell (page 104); **Address:** Weill Cornell Otorhinolaryngology, 1305 York Ave Fl 5, New York, NY 10021; **Phone:** 646-962-4734; **Board Cert:** Otolaryngology 2000; **Med School:** Georgetown Univ 1993; **Resid:** Surgery, Georgetown Univ Hosp 1995; Otolaryngology, Georgetown Univ Hosp 1999; **Fellow:** Laryngology, St Lukes Roosevelt Hosp 2000; **Fac Appt:** Assoc Prof Oto, Cornell Univ-Weill Med Coll

Urken, Mark MD (Oto) - **Spec Exp:** Head & Neck Cancer & Surgery; Head & Neck Cancer Reconstruction; Thyroid & Parathyroid Cancer & Surgery; Salivary Gland Tumors; **Hospital:** Beth Israel Med Ctr - Petrie Division (page 94); **Address:** Inst for Head, Neck & Thyroid Cancer, 10 Union Square E, Ste 5B, New York, NY 10003-3314; **Phone:** 212-844-8775; **Board Cert:** Otolaryngology 1986; **Med School:** Univ VA Sch Med 1981; **Resid:** Otolaryngology, Mt Sinai Hosp 1986; **Fellow:** Microvascular Surgery, Mercy Hosp 1987; **Fac Appt:** Prof Oto, Albert Einstein Coll Med

Volpi, David O MD (Oto) - **Spec Exp:** Sinus Disorders; Sleep Disorders; Snoring/Sleep Apnea; **Hospital:** Lenox Hill Hosp, New York Eye & Ear Infirm (page 113); **Address:** 262 Central Park West, Ste 1H, New York, NY 10024; **Phone:** 212-873-6036; **Board Cert:** Otolaryngology 1988; **Med School:** Hahnemann Univ 1982; **Resid:** Otolaryngology, NY Eye & Ear Infirm 1988

Waner, Milton MD (Oto) - **Spec Exp:** Pediatric Facial Plastic Surgery; Birthmarks/Hemangiomas; Vascular Malformations; **Hospital:** St Luke's - Roosevelt Hosp Ctr - St Luke's Hosp (page 94), Beth Israel Med Ctr - Petrie Division (page 94); **Address:** Vascular Birthmark Institute, 126 W 60th St, New York, NY 10023; **Phone:** 212-636-3970; **Med School:** South Africa 1977; **Resid:** Surgery, Univ of Witwatersrand 1980; Otolaryngology, Univ of Witwatersrand 1984; **Fellow:** Otolaryngology, Univ Cincinnatti Med Ctr 1985

Woo, Peak MD (Oto) - **Spec Exp:** Voice Disorders; Laryngeal Disorders; Laryngeal Cancer; **Hospital:** Mount Sinai Med Ctr (page 102); **Address:** 300 Central Park West, Ste 1-H, New York, NY 10024; **Phone:** 212-580-1004; **Board Cert:** Otolaryngology 1983; **Med School:** Boston Univ 1978; **Resid:** Otolaryngology, Boston Univ Med Ctr 1983; **Fac Appt:** Clin Prof Oto, Mount Sinai Sch Med

Pain Medicine

Diwan, Sudhir MD (PM) - **Spec Exp:** Pain-after Spinal Intervention; Pain-Musculoskeletal; Pain-Neuropathic; Pain-Cancer; **Hospital:** NY-Presby Hosp/Weill Cornell (page 104); **Address:** 1305 York Ave Fl 10, Box 120, New York, NY 10021; **Phone:** 646-962-7246; **Board Cert:** Anesthesiology 2001; Pain Medicine 2002; **Med School:** India 1983; **Resid:** Surgery, St Luke's-Roosevelt Hosp Ctr 1994; Anesthesiology, St Luke's-Roosevelt Hosp Ctr 1997; **Fellow:** Pain Medicine, NY Presby Hosp 1998; **Fac Appt:** Assoc Prof Anes, Cornell Univ-Weill Med Coll

Dubois, Michel Y MD (PM) - **Spec Exp:** Pain-Back & Neck; Pain-Neuropathic; Pain-Cancer; **Hospital:** NYU Langone Med Ctr (page 106), Bellevue Hosp Ctr; **Address:** 317 E 34th St, Ste 902, New York, NY 10016-4974; **Phone:** 212-201-1004; **Board Cert:** Anesthesiology 1985; Pain Medicine 2004; **Med School:** France 1974; **Resid:** Anesthesiology, Georgetown Univ Hosp 1980; **Fellow:** Pain Medicine, Georgetown Univ Hosp 1983; **Fac Appt:** Prof Anes, NYU Sch Med

Freedman, Gordon MD (PM) - **Spec Exp:** Pain-Back & Neck; Pain-Cancer; Reflex Sympathetic Dystrophy (RSD); Pain-Neuropathic; **Hospital:** Mount Sinai Med Ctr (page 102), Mount Sinai Hosp of Queens (page 102); **Address:** 1540 York Ave, New York, NY 10028; **Phone:** 212-288-2180; **Board Cert:** Anesthesiology 1992; Pain Medicine 2004; **Med School:** Israel 1985; **Resid:** Anesthesiology, Mt Sinai Hosp 1991; **Fellow:** Pain Medicine, Mt Sinai Hosp 1991; **Fac Appt:** Assoc Prof Anes, Mount Sinai Sch Med

Gharibo, Christopher G MD (PM) - **Spec Exp:** Pain-Back & Neck; Pain-Neuropathic; Pain-Chronic; Complex Regional Pain Syndrome; **Hospital:** NYU Langone Med Ctr (page 106), NYU Hosp For Joint Diseases (page 106); **Address:** 301 E 17th St, Ste 1001, New York, NY 10003; **Phone:** 212-598-6174; **Board Cert:** Anesthesiology 1997; Pain Medicine 2009; **Med School:** UMDNJ-NJ Med Sch, Newark 1992; **Resid:** Anesthesiology, NYU Med Ctr 1995; **Fellow:** Pain Medicine, Jefferson Univ Hosp 1997; **Fac Appt:** Asst Prof Anes, NYU Sch Med

Gusmorino, Paul MD (PM) - **Spec Exp:** Pain-Chronic; Pain Rehabilitation & Psychiatry; **Hospital:** NYU Hosp For Joint Diseases (page 106); **Address:** 301 E 17th St, Ste 1029, New York, NY 10003-3804; **Phone:** 212-598-6204; **Board Cert:** Psychiatry 1980; Child & Adolescent Psychiatry 1982; Pain Medicine 2006; **Med School:** Italy 1974; **Resid:** Psychiatry, Kings County Hosp 1978; **Fellow:** Child & Adolescent Psychiatry, NY Hosp 1980; **Fac Appt:** Asst Clin Prof Psyc, NYU Sch Med

Jain, Subhash MD (PM) - **Spec Exp:** Pain-Cancer; Pain-Pelvic; Reflex Sympathetic Dystrophy; Complex Regional Pain Syndrome-CRPS; **Hospital:** Beth Israel Med Ctr - Petrie Division (page 94); **Address:** 360 E 72nd St, Ste C, New York, NY 10021; **Phone:** 212-439-6100; **Board Cert:** Anesthesiology 1994; Pain Medicine 1998; **Med School:** India 1968; **Resid:** Surgery, St Vincent Med Ctr 1977; Anesthesiology, New York Hosp 1979; **Fellow:** Pain Medicine, New York Hosp/Meml Sloan Kettering Cancer Ctr 1980; **Fac Appt:** Assoc Prof Anes, Cornell Univ-Weill Med Coll

Kaplan, Ronald MD (PM) - **Spec Exp:** Pain-Chronic; **Hospital:** Beth Israel Med Ctr - Petrie Division (page 94); **Address:** Pain Medicine & Palliative Care, 10 Union Square E, Ste 4K, New York, NY 10003-3314; **Phone:** 212-844-8074; **Board Cert:** Anesthesiology 2009; Pain Medicine 2004; **Med School:** Univ MD Sch Med 1974; **Resid:** Anesthesiology, Univ Maryland Hosp 1978; **Fellow:** Pediatric Anesthesiology, Childrens Hosp 1979; **Fac Appt:** Clin Prof Anes, Albert Einstein Coll Med

Kreitzer, Joel MD (PM) - **Spec Exp:** Pain-Back; Pain-Cancer; Pain-Neuropathic; **Hospital:** Mount Sinai Med Ctr (page 102), Mount Sinai Hosp of Queens (page 102); **Address:** Upper East Side Pain Medicine, 1540 York Ave, New York, NY 10028; **Phone:** 212-288-2180; **Board Cert:** Anesthesiology 1990; Pain Medicine 2004; **Med School:** Albert Einstein Coll Med 1985; **Resid:** Anesthesiology, Mt Sinai Hosp 1989; **Fellow:** Pain Medicine, Mt Sinai Hosp 1989; **Fac Appt:** Assoc Clin Prof Anes, Mount Sinai Sch Med

Marcus, Norman J MD (PM) - **Spec Exp:** Pain-Back & Neck; Headache; Pain-Musculoskeletal; Reflex Sympathetic Dystrophy (RSD); **Hospital:** NYU Langone Med Ctr (page 106), Lenox Hill Hosp; **Address:** 30 E 40th St, Ste 1100, New York, NY 10016-1201; **Phone:** 212-532-7999; **Board Cert:** Psychiatry 1974; Pain Medicine 1993; **Med School:** SUNY Upstate Med Univ 1967; **Resid:** Psychiatry, Montefiore Med Ctr 1971; **Fellow:** Psychosomatic Medicine, Montefiore Med Ctr 1973; Pain Medicine, Lenox Hill Hosp 1995; **Fac Appt:** Assoc Clin Prof Anes, NYU Sch Med

Moqtaderi, Farideh MD (PM) - **Spec Exp:** Acupuncture; Pain-Musculoskeletal; Herpetic Neuralgia (Shingles); Fibromyalgia; **Hospital:** Mount Sinai Med Ctr (page 102); **Address:** 520 E 72nd St, Ste 1C, New York, NY 10021-4850; **Phone:** 212-426-9200; **Board Cert:** Anesthesiology 1973; **Med School:** Iran 1966; **Resid:** Anesthesiology, Mount Sinai Hosp 1969; Anesthesiology, Meml Sloan Kettering Hosp 1971; **Fellow:** Pain Medicine, Westchester Co Med Ctr 1973; **Fac Appt:** Asst Clin Prof Anes, Mount Sinai Sch Med

Ngeow, Jeffrey MD (PM) - **Spec Exp:** Pain-Musculoskeletal-Spine & Neck; Acupuncture; Reflex Sympathetic Dystrophy (RSD); Pain-Neuropathic; **Hospital:** Hosp For Special Surgery (page 111); **Address:** 535 E 70th St, New York, NY 10021-4872; **Phone:** 212-606-1059; **Board Cert:** Anesthesiology 1980; Pain Medicine 2005; **Med School:** England, UK 1971; **Resid:** Anesthesiology, Peter Bent Brigham Hosp 1977; **Fellow:** Pain Medicine, Tufts New England Med Ctr 1978; **Fac Appt:** Assoc Clin Prof Anes, Cornell Univ-Weill Med Coll

Portenoy, Russell MD (PM) - **Spec Exp:** Pain-Cancer; Palliative Care; **Hospital:** Beth Israel Med Ctr - Petrie Division (page 94); **Address:** Beth Israel Med Ctr, Dept Pain Medicine/Palliative Care, First Ave at 16th St, New York, NY 10003; **Phone:** 212-844-1403; **Board Cert:** Neurology 1985; Hospice & Palliative Medicine 2008; **Med School:** Univ MD Sch Med 1980; **Resid:** Neurology, Montefiore Med Ctr 1984; **Fellow:** Pain Medicine, Meml Sloan-Kettering Cancer Ctr 1985; **Fac Appt:** Prof N, Albert Einstein Coll Med

Richman, Daniel MD (PM) - **Spec Exp:** Pain-Back & Neck; Complex Regional Pain Syndrome; Reflex Sympathetic Dystrophy (RSD); **Hospital:** Hosp For Special Surgery (page 111); **Address:** 535 E 70th St, rm 375, New York, NY 10021-4872; **Phone:** 212-606-1768; **Board Cert:** Anesthesiology 1991; Pain Medicine 2005; **Med School:** UMDNJ-NJ Med Sch, Newark 1986; **Resid:** Anesthesiology, Hartford Hosp 1990; **Fellow:** Pain Medicine, Hosp Special Surgery 1991; **Fac Appt:** Assoc Clin Prof Anes, Cornell Univ-Weill Med Coll

Sarno, John E MD (PM) - **Spec Exp:** Pain-Mind/Body Disorder; **Hospital:** NYU Langone Med Ctr (page 106); **Address:** Rusk Institute, Ground Floor, 400 E 34th St, rm 30, New York, NY 10016-4901; **Phone:** 212-263-6035; **Board Cert:** Physical Medicine & Rehabilitation 1965; **Med School:** Columbia P&S 1950; **Resid:** Physical Medicine & Rehabilitation, NYU Med Ctr 1952; Pediatrics, Babies Hosp/Columbia-Presby Med Ctr 1961; **Fellow:** Physical Medicine & Rehabilitation, NYU Med Ctr 1963; **Fac Appt:** Clin Prof PMR, NYU Sch Med

Thomas, Gary P MD (PM) - **Spec Exp:** Pain-Neuropathic; Fibromyalgia; Headache; Pain-after Spinal Intervention; **Hospital:** Beth Israel Med Ctr - Petrie Division (page 94), New York Methodist Hosp (page 404); **Address:** Comprehensive Pain Management, 10 Union Square E, Ste 4K, New York, NY 10003; **Phone:** 212-995-6495; **Board Cert:** Pain Medicine 2007; Anesthesiology 1996; **Med School:** Mount Sinai Sch Med 1991; **Resid:** Anesthesiology, Mount Sinai Med Ctr 1995; **Fellow:** Pain Medicine, Mount Sinai Med Ctr 1996

Waldman, Seth MD (PM) - **Spec Exp:** Pain-Spine; Pain-Neuropathic; Sciatica; **Hospital:** Hosp For Special Surgery (page 111), Burke Rehab Hosp; **Address:** Hosp For Special Surgery, 535 E 70th St, rm 442, New York, NY 10021-4872; **Phone:** 212-606-1686; **Board Cert:** Anesthesiology 1994; Pain Medicine 2005; **Med School:** Albany Med Coll 1988; **Resid:** Internal Medicine, Beth Israel Med Ctr 1990; Anesthesiology, Beth Israel Hosp 1993; **Fellow:** Pain Medicine, Beth Israel Hosp/Mass Genl Hosp 1994; **Fac Appt:** Asst Clin Prof Anes, Cornell Univ-Weill Med Coll

Weinberger, Michael L MD (PM) - **Spec Exp:** Pain-Cancer; Pain-Back; Palliative Care; **Hospital:** NY-Presby Hosp/Columbia (page 104); **Address:** 630 W 168th St, PH5, rm 500, New York, NY 10032-3720; **Phone:** 212-305-7114; **Board Cert:** Internal Medicine 1986; Anesthesiology 1990; Pain Medicine 2004; Hospice & Palliative Medicine 2006; **Med School:** Columbia P&S 1983; **Resid:** Internal Medicine, St Vincent's Hosp 1986; Anesthesiology, Columbia-Presby Med Ctr 1989; **Fellow:** Pain Medicine, Meml Sloan Kettering Cancer Ctr 1990; **Fac Appt:** Assoc Prof Anes, Columbia P&S

Pathology

Bleiweiss, Ira J MD (Path) - **Spec Exp:** Breast Pathology; Breast Cancer; **Hospital:** Mount Sinai Med Ctr (page 102); **Address:** Mt Sinai Med Ctr, Dept Pathology, 1 Gustave Levy Pl, Box 1194, New York, NY 10029-6504; **Phone:** 212-241-9159; **Board Cert:** Anatomic & Clinical Pathology 1988; **Med School:** West Indies 1984; **Resid:** Pathology, Mt Sinai Med Ctr 1988; **Fellow:** Surgical Pathology, Mt Sinai Med Ctr 1989; Surgical Pathology, Meml-Sloan Kettering Cancer Ctr 1990; **Fac Appt:** Prof Path, Mount Sinai Sch Med

Gottlieb, Geoffrey J MD (Path) - **Spec Exp:** Dermatopathology; Melanoma; **Address:** Ackerman Academy Dermatopathology, 145 E 32nd St Fl 10, New York, NY 10016; **Phone:** 212-889-6225; **Board Cert:** Anatomic Pathology 1979; Dermatopathology 1982; **Med School:** Cornell Univ-Weill Med Coll 1976; **Resid:** Pathology, NY Hosp-Cornell Med Ctr 1979; **Fellow:** Dermatopathology, NYU Med Ctr 1982

Harpaz, Noam MD (Path) - **Spec Exp:** Gastrointestinal Pathology; **Hospital:** Mount Sinai Med Ctr (page 102); **Address:** Mount Sinai Medical Ctr, Pathology, One Gustave L Levy Pl, Box 1194, New York, NY 10029; **Phone:** 212-241-6692; **Board Cert:** Anatomic & Clinical Pathology 1986; **Med School:** Univ Miami Sch Med 1981; **Resid:** Anatomic & Clinical Pathology, Mt Sinai Med Ctr 1984; **Fac Appt:** Prof Path, Mount Sinai Sch Med

Hoda, Syed A MD (Path) - **Spec Exp:** Breast Cancer; Surgical Pathology; **Hospital:** NY-Presby Hosp/Weill Cornell (page 104); **Address:** 525 E 68th St, 1028 Starr, New York, NY 10021-4870; **Phone:** 212-746-2700; **Board Cert:** Anatomic & Clinical Pathology 1990; Cytopathology 1991; Pathology 2001; **Med School:** Pakistan 1984; **Resid:** Anatomic & Clinical Pathology, Tulane Univ Affil Hosps 1990; **Fellow:** Cytopathology, Meml Sloan Kettering Cancer Ctr 1991; Pathology, Meml Sloan Kettering Cancer Ctr 1992; **Fac Appt:** Clin Prof Path, Cornell Univ-Weill Med Coll

Knowles, Daniel M MD (Path) - **Spec Exp:** Lymph Node Pathology; Bone Marrow Pathology; Lymphoma; Leukemia; **Hospital:** NY-Presby Hosp/Weill Cornell (page 104); **Address:** Cornell-Weill Med Coll- Dept Pathology, 1300 York Ave, rm C302, New York, NY 10021; **Phone:** 212-746-6464; **Board Cert:** Anatomic Pathology 1978; Immunopathology 1984; **Med School:** Univ Chicago-Pritzker Sch Med 1973; **Resid:** Anatomic Pathology, Columbia-Presby Med Ctr 1975; Anatomic Pathology, Columbia-Presby Med Ctr 1978; **Fellow:** Immunopathology, Rockefeller Univ 1977; **Fac Appt:** Prof Path, Cornell Univ-Weill Med Coll

Magro, Cynthia MD (Path) - **Spec Exp:** Cutaneous Lymphoma; **Hospital:** NY-Presby Hosp/Weill Cornell (page 104); **Address:** 1300 York Ave, Ste F309, New York, NY 10065; **Phone:** 212-746-6434; **Board Cert:** Anatomic Pathology 1988; Dermatopathology 1990; Cytopathology 1991; **Med School:** Univ Manitoba 1984; **Resid:** Anatomic Pathology, Mass Genl Hosp 1988; **Fellow:** Cytopathology, Mass Genl Hosp 1989; Dermatology, Mass Genl Hosp 1991

McNutt, N Scott MD (Path) - **Spec Exp:** Dermatopathology; **Hospital:** Rockefeller Univ; **Address:** Rockefeller Univ, Krueger Laboratory, 1230 York Ave, Box 175, New York, NY 10065; **Phone:** 212-327-8039; **Board Cert:** Anatomic Pathology 1973; Dermatopathology 1979; **Med School:** Harvard Med Sch 1966; **Resid:** Pathology, Mass Genl Hosp 1970; **Fellow:** Pathology, Mass Genl Hosp 1972

Melamed, Jonathan MD (Path) - **Spec Exp:** Prostate Cancer; Tumor Banking-Prostate; **Hospital:** NYU Langone Med Ctr (page 106); **Address:** NYU Medical Ctr, Dept Pathology, TH-461, 560 First Ave, New York, NY 10016; **Phone:** 212-263-8927; **Board Cert:** Anatomic & Clinical Pathology 1992; **Med School:** South Africa 1985; **Resid:** Pathology, Lenox Hill Hosp 1991; **Fellow:** Pathology, Meml Sloan Kettering Cancer Ctr 1992; Urologic Pathology, Meml Sloan Kettering Cancer Ctr 1993; **Fac Appt:** Assoc Prof Path, NYU Sch Med

Orazi, Attilio MD (Path) - **Spec Exp:** Hematopathology; Bone Marrow Pathology; Lymph Node Pathology; Spleen Pathology; **Hospital:** NY-Presby Hosp/Weill Cornell (page 104); **Address:** NY Presby-Cornell Medical Ctr, 525 E 68th St, Starr Pavilion, rm 715, New York, NY 10021; **Phone:** 212-746-2050; **Board Cert:** Anatomic Pathology 1997; Hematology 1998; **Med School:** Italy 1979; **Resid:** Internal Medicine, Leicester Royal Infirmary 1982; Histopathology, Northampton Genl Hosp 1983; **Fellow:** Anatomic Pathology, Natl Cancer Inst 1985; **Fac Appt:** Prof Path, Cornell Univ-Weill Med Coll

Reuter, Victor E MD (Path) - **Spec Exp:** Prostate Cancer; Genitourinary Pathology; Bladder Cancer; Testicular Cancer; **Hospital:** Meml Sloan-Kettering Cancer Ctr (page 112); **Address:** Memorial Sloan Kettering Cancer Ctr, Dept Pathology, 1275 York Ave, New York, NY 10021; **Phone:** 212-639-8225; **Board Cert:** Anatomic & Clinical Pathology 1983; **Med School:** Dominican Republic 1978; **Resid:** Anatomic Pathology, Thos Jefferson Univ Hosp 1981; Clinical Pathology, Thos Jefferson Univ Hosp 1983; **Fellow:** Surgical Pathology, Meml Sloan Kettering Cancer Ctr 1985; **Fac Appt:** Prof Path, Cornell Univ-Weill Med Coll

Rosenblum, Marc K MD (Path) - **Spec Exp:** Neuropathology; Brain Tumors; **Hospital:** Meml Sloan-Kettering Cancer Ctr (page 112); **Address:** 1275 York Avenue, New York, NY 10065; **Phone:** 212-639-5905; **Board Cert:** Anatomic Pathology 1984; Neuropathology 1988; **Med School:** Univ Miami Sch Med 1979; **Resid:** Anatomic Pathology, Mt Sinai Med Ctr 1984; **Fellow:** Pathology, Meml Sloan-Kettering Cancer Ctr 1985; Neurological Pathology, Bellevue-NYU Med Ctr 1987; **Fac Appt:** Prof Path, Cornell Univ-Weill Med Coll

Schiller, Alan L MD (Path) - **Spec Exp:** Bone & Joint Pathology; Soft Tissue Pathology; Bone Tumors; **Hospital:** Mount Sinai Med Ctr (page 102); **Address:** Mt Sinai Sch Med, Dept Pathology, 1 Gustave Levy Pl, Box 1194, New York, NY 10029-6500; **Phone:** 212-241-8014; **Board Cert:** Anatomic Pathology 1973; **Med School:** Ros Franklin Univ/Chicago Med Sch 1967; **Resid:** Pathology, Mass Genl Hosp 1972; **Fac Appt:** Prof Path, Mount Sinai Sch Med

Soslow, Robert A MD (Path) - **Spec Exp:** Gynecologic Pathology; **Hospital:** Meml Sloan-Kettering Cancer Ctr (page 112); **Address:** 1275 York Avenue, Pathology Department, New York, NY 10065; **Phone:** 800-525-2225; **Board Cert:** Anatomic Pathology 1995; **Med School:** Univ Pennsylvania 1991; **Resid:** Anatomic Pathology, Stanford Univ Med Ctr 1994; **Fellow:** Immunopathology, Stanford Univ Med Ctr 1995; **Fac Appt:** Assoc Prof Path, Cornell Univ

Travis, William MD (Path) - **Spec Exp:** Pulmonary Pathology; Lung Cancer; Interstitial Lung Disease; **Hospital:** Meml Sloan-Kettering Cancer Ctr (page 112); **Address:** 1275 York Avenue, Pathology Dept, New York, NY 10065; **Phone:** 212-639-6364; **Board Cert:** Anatomic & Clinical Pathology 1985; **Med School:** Univ Fla Coll Med 1981; **Resid:** Anatomic Pathology, New England Deaconess Hosp 1983; Clinical Pathology, Mayo Clinic 1985; **Fellow:** Surgical Pathology, Mayo Clinic 1986

Wenig, Bruce M MD (Path) - **Spec Exp:** Head & Neck Pathology; Surgical Pathology; Endocrine Pathology; **Hospital:** Beth Israel Med Ctr - Petrie Division (page 94), St Luke's - Roosevelt Hosp Ctr - St Luke's Hosp (page 94); **Address:** Beth Israel Med Ctr, Dept Pathology, First Ave at 16th St, 11 Silver, Rm 10, New York, NY 10003; **Phone:** 212-420-4031; **Board Cert:** Anatomic & Clinical Pathology 2003; **Med School:** Israel 1981; **Resid:** Pathology, Mt Sinai Med Ctr 1985; Surgical Pathology, Cedars-Sinai Med Ctr 1986; **Fellow:** Head and Neck Pathology, AFIP 1987; **Fac Appt:** Prof Path, Albert Einstein Coll Med

Zagzag, David MD/PhD (Path) - **Spec Exp:** Neuropathology; Brain Tumors; Tumor Banking-Brain; **Hospital:** NYU Langone Med Ctr (page 106), Bellevue Hosp Ctr; **Address:** NYU Med Ctr, Dept Pathology, 550 First Ave, Div Neuropathology, NB-4N30, New York, NY 10016; **Phone:** 212-263-6449; **Board Cert:** Anatomic Pathology 1993; Neuropathology 1993; **Med School:** France 1984; **Resid:** Surgical Pathology, NYU Med Ctr 1990; **Fellow:** Neurological Pathology, NYU Med Ctr 1992; **Fac Appt:** Assoc Prof Path, NYU Sch Med

Pediatric Allergy & Immunology

Ehrlich, Paul M MD (PA&I) - **Spec Exp:** Asthma; Food Allergy; **Hospital:** New York Eye & Ear Infirm (page 113), NYU Langone Med Ctr (page 106); **Address:** 35 E 35th St, Ste 202, New York, NY 10016-3823; **Phone:** 212-685-4225; **Board Cert:** Pediatrics 1975; Allergy & Immunology 1977; **Med School:** NYU Sch Med 1970; **Resid:** Pediatrics, Bellevue Hosp Ctr 1973; **Fellow:** Allergy & Immunology, Walter Reed Army Med Ctr 1976; **Fac Appt:** Assoc Clin Prof Ped, NYU Sch Med

Rappaport, Irwin MD (PA&I) - **Spec Exp:** Asthma; Food Allergy; Allergic Rhinitis; **Hospital:** NY-Presby Hosp/Weill Cornell (page 104), Lenox Hill Hosp; **Address:** 9 E 68th St, Ste 1A, New York, NY 10021; **Phone:** 212-777-8407; **Board Cert:** Pediatrics 1967; Allergy & Immunology 1977; **Med School:** Med Coll VA 1962; **Resid:** Pediatrics, NY Hosp 1965; **Fellow:** Allergy & Immunology, St Vincent's Hosp & Med Ctr 1966; **Fac Appt:** Clin Prof Ped, Cornell Univ-Weill Med Coll

Sampson, Hugh MD (PA&I) - **Spec Exp:** Food Allergy; Eczema; Atopic Dermatitis; **Hospital:** Mount Sinai Med Ctr (page 102); **Address:** Mt Sinai Sch Med, Dept Peds, 1 Gustave Levy Pl, Box 1198, New York, NY 10029-6500; **Phone:** 212-241-5548; **Board Cert:** Pediatrics 1980; Allergy & Immunology 1981; **Med School:** SUNY Buffalo 1975; **Resid:** Pediatrics, Chldns Meml Hosp 1979; **Fellow:** Allergy & Immunology, Duke Univ Med Ctr 1980; **Fac Appt:** Prof Ped, Mount Sinai Sch Med

Sicherer, Scott H MD (PA&I) - **Spec Exp:** Food Allergy; Drug Sensitivity; Eczema; **Hospital:** Mount Sinai Med Ctr (page 102); **Address:** 1 Gustave Levy Pl, Box 1198, New York, NY 10029-6500; **Phone:** 212-241-5548; **Board Cert:** Pediatrics 2008; Allergy & Immunology 2007; **Med School:** Johns Hopkins Univ 1990; **Resid:** Pediatrics, Mt Sinai Hosp 1994; **Fellow:** Allergy & Immunology, Johns Hopkins Hosp 1997; **Fac Appt:** Prof Ped, Mount Sinai Sch Med

Pediatric Cardiology

Addonizio, Linda J MD (PCd) - **Spec Exp:** Transplant Medicine-Heart; Heart Failure; Hypertrophic Cardiomyopathy; **Hospital:** NYPresby-Morgan Stanley Children's Hosp (page 104); **Address:** 3959 Broadway, Ste 229 N, New York, NY 10032; **Phone:** 212-305-6575; **Board Cert:** Pediatrics 1983; Pediatric Cardiology 1985; **Med School:** Columbia P&S 1978; **Resid:** Pediatrics, Columbia Presby/Babies Hosp 1981; **Fellow:** Pediatric Cardiology, Columbia Presby/Babies Hosp 1984; **Fac Appt:** Prof Ped, Columbia P&S

Arnon, Rica G MD (PCd) - **Spec Exp:** Congenital Heart Disease; Exercise Physiology; **Hospital:** Mount Sinai Med Ctr (page 102), Elmhurst Hosp Ctr; **Address:** 1 Gustave Levy Pl, Box 1201, New York, NY 10029-6504; **Phone:** 212-241-7578; **Board Cert:** Pediatrics 1970; Pediatric Cardiology 1973; **Med School:** SUNY Hlth Sci Ctr 1967; **Resid:** Pediatrics, Kings County Hosp 1970; **Fellow:** Pediatric Cardiology, Kings County Hosp 1973; **Fac Appt:** Assoc Prof Ped, Mount Sinai Sch Med

Borg, Morton D MD (PCd) - **Spec Exp:** Fetal Echocardiography; **Hospital:** Beth Israel Med Ctr - Petrie Division (page 94), Mount Sinai Med Ctr (page 102); **Address:** Phillips Amb Care Ctr, Dept Peds, 10 Union Square E, Ste 2J, New York, NY 10003-3314; **Phone:** 212-844-8300; **Board Cert:** Pediatrics 1986; Pediatric Cardiology 2003; **Med School:** Albert Einstein Coll Med 1981; **Resid:** Pediatrics, Brookdale Hosp 1984; **Fellow:** Pediatric Cardiology, New York Hosp 1986; **Fac Appt:** Asst Prof Ped, Albert Einstein Coll Med

Brick, David H MD (PCd) - **Spec Exp:** Fetal Echocardiography; Congenital Heart Disease; **Hospital:** NYU Langone Med Ctr (page 106); **Address:** St Vincents Hosp & Med Ctr, 154 W 14th St Fl 4, New York, NY 10011; **Phone:** 212-604-7880; **Board Cert:** Pediatrics 2004; Pediatric Cardiology 2008; **Med School:** Ohio State Univ 1993; **Resid:** Pediatrics, Univ Hosp Cleveland 1996; **Fellow:** Pediatric Cardiology, NY-Presby Hosp 2000

Flynn, Patrick MD (PCd) - **Spec Exp:** Congenital Heart Disease; Echocardiography; Marfan's Syndrome; Cardiac Catheterization; **Hospital:** NY-Presby Hosp/Weill Cornell (page 104); **Address:** 525 E 68th St, Ste F695B, New York, NY 10065; **Phone:** 212-746-3561; **Board Cert:** Pediatric Cardiology 2006; **Med School:** Univ MD Sch Med 1986; **Resid:** Pediatrics, NY Presby Hosp/Cornell Med Ctr 1990; **Fellow:** Pediatric Cardiology, NY Presby Hosp/Cornell Med Ctr 1993; **Fac Appt:** Assoc Prof Ped, Cornell Univ-Weill Med Coll

Gelb, Bruce D MD (PCd) - **Spec Exp:** Transplant Medicine-Heart; Marfan's Syndrome; Noonan Syndrome; **Hospital:** Mount Sinai Med Ctr (page 102); **Address:** 1 Gustave Levy Pl, Box 1201, New York, NY 10029; **Phone:** 212-241-8592; **Board Cert:** Pediatric Cardiology 2006; **Med School:** Univ Rochester 1984; **Resid:** Pediatrics, NY Presby Hosp 1987; **Fellow:** Pediatric Cardiology, Baylor College Med 1991; **Fac Appt:** Prof Ped, Mount Sinai Sch Med

Hellenbrand, William E MD (PCd) - **Spec Exp:** Interventional Cardiology; **Hospital:** NYPresby-Morgan Stanley Children's Hosp (page 104), Robert Wood Johnson Univ Hosp - New Brunswick; **Address:** Morgan Stanley Chlds Hosp, 3959 Broadway Fl 2N - rm 255, New York, NY 10032; **Phone:** 212-342-0610; **Board Cert:** Pediatrics 1975; Pediatric Cardiology 1977; **Med School:** SUNY Downstate 1970; **Resid:** Pediatrics, Yale-New Haven Hosp 1972; **Fellow:** Pediatric Cardiology, Yale-New Haven Hosp 1976; **Fac Appt:** Prof Ped, Columbia P&S

Hordof, Allan J MD (PCd) - **Spec Exp:** Arrhythmias; **Hospital:** NYPresby-Morgan Stanley Children's Hosp (page 104); **Address:** Morgan Stanley Chlds Hosp of NY-Presby, 3959 Broadway, Ste 255 N, New York, NY 10032; **Phone:** 212-305-4432; **Board Cert:** Pediatrics 1971; Pediatric Cardiology 1973; **Med School:** NYU Sch Med 1966; **Resid:** Pediatrics, Chldns Hosp 1968; Pediatrics, Babies Hosp 1969; **Fellow:** Pediatric Cardiology, Babies Hosp 1973; **Fac Appt:** Prof Ped, Columbia P&S

Love, Barry A MD (PCd) - **Spec Exp:** Cardiac Catheterization; Interventional Cardiology; Atrial Septal Defect; Arrhythmias; **Hospital:** Mount Sinai Med Ctr (page 102); **Address:** Mt Sinai Med Ctr, Div Ped Cardiology, 1 Gustave Levy Pl, Box 1201, New York, NY 10029; **Phone:** 212-241-3616; **Board Cert:** Pediatrics 2004; Pediatric Cardiology 2008; **Med School:** Univ Western Ontario 1993; **Resid:** Pediatrics, Chldns Hosp Montreal 1996; **Fellow:** Pediatric Cardiology, Chldns Hosp 2000; **Fac Appt:** Asst Prof Ped, Mount Sinai Sch Med

Parness, Ira A MD (PCd) - **Spec Exp:** Echocardiography; Congenital Heart Disease; Fetal Echocardiography; **Hospital:** Mount Sinai Med Ctr (page 102), Englewood Hosp & Med Ctr (page 656); **Address:** 1 Gustave Levy Pl, Box 1201, New York, NY 10029-6500; **Phone:** 212-241-6640; **Board Cert:** Pediatrics 1984; Pediatric Cardiology 1985; **Med School:** SUNY Downstate 1979; **Resid:** Pediatrics, Brookdale Hosp 1982; **Fellow:** Pediatric Cardiology, Chldns Hosp 1985; **Fac Appt:** Prof Ped, Mount Sinai Sch Med

Sommer, Robert J MD (PCd) - **Spec Exp:** Congenital Heart Disease; Atrial Septal Defect; Cardiac Catheterization; **Hospital:** NYPresby-Morgan Stanley Children's Hosp (page 104), St Joseph's Regl Med Ctr - Paterson; **Address:** 173 Fort Washington Ave Fl 4, New York, NY 10032; **Phone:** 212-342-0886; **Board Cert:** Pediatric Cardiology 2006; **Med School:** NYU Sch Med 1985; **Resid:** Pediatrics, Mt Sinai Med Ctr 1988; **Fellow:** Pediatric Cardiology, Mt Sinai Med Ctr 1991; Interventional Cardiology, Childrens Hosp 1991; **Fac Appt:** Assoc Prof Ped, Columbia P&S

Starc, Thomas J MD (PCd) - **Spec Exp:** Cholesterol/Lipid Disorders; **Hospital:** NYPresby-Morgan Stanley Children's Hosp (page 104); **Address:** NY Presby-Morgan Stanley Children's Hosp, 3959 Broadway, Ste 255 N, New York, NY 10032-1537; **Phone:** 212-305-4432; **Board Cert:** Pediatrics 1981; Pediatric Cardiology 1983; **Med School:** Mount Sinai Sch Med 1976; **Resid:** Pediatrics, USC Med Ctr 1980; **Fellow:** Pediatric Cardiology, NY Presby-Columbia Med Ctr 1984; **Fac Appt:** Clin Prof Ped, Columbia P&S

Steinberg, L Gary MD (PCd) - **Spec Exp:** Echocardiography; Congenital Heart Disease; **Hospital:** NY-Presby Hosp/Weill Cornell (page 104); **Address:** Pediatric Cardiovascular Services, NY Presby Hosp/ Weill Cornell, 525 E 68 St, Ste F695B, New York, NY 10065; **Phone:** 212-746-3561; **Board Cert:** Pediatrics 2006; Pediatric Cardiology 2006; **Med School:** Philippines 1985; **Resid:** Pediatrics, Elmhurst Hosp 1989; **Fellow:** Pediatric Cardiology, Mount Sinai Hosp 1992; **Fac Appt:** Asst Prof Ped, Cornell Univ-Weill Med Coll

Steinherz, Laurel MD (PCd) - **Spec Exp:** Cardiac Effects of Cancer/Cancer Therapy; **Hospital:** Meml Sloan-Kettering Cancer Ctr (page 112), NY-Presby Hosp/Weill Cornell (page 104); **Address:** 1275 York Avenue, New York, NY 10065; **Phone:** 212-639-8103; **Board Cert:** Pediatrics 1976; Pediatric Cardiology 1978; **Med School:** Albert Einstein Coll Med 1970; **Resid:** Pediatrics, Chldns Hosp 1972; **Fellow:** Pediatric Cardiology, NY Hosp-Cornell Med Ctr 1975; **Fac Appt:** Prof Ped, Cornell Univ-Weill Med Coll

Pediatric Critical Care Medicine

Conway Jr, Edward E MD (PCCM) - **Spec Exp:** Neurologic Critical Care; Respiratory Failure; Head Injury; **Hospital:** Beth Israel Med Ctr - Petrie Division (page 94); **Address:** Beth Israel Med Ctr, Dept Peds, 16th St @ 1st Ave, New York, NY 10003; **Phone:** 212-844-1824; **Board Cert:** Pediatrics 2008; Pediatric Critical Care Medicine 2005; **Med School:** SUNY Hlth Sci Ctr 1984; **Resid:** Pediatrics, Montefiore Med Ctr 1988; **Fellow:** Pediatric Critical Care Medicine, Montefiore Med Ctr-Albert Einstein 1990; **Fac Appt:** Prof Ped, Albert Einstein Coll Med

Greenwald, Bruce M MD (PCCM) - **Spec Exp:** Respiratory Failure; Sepsis & Septic Shock; Asthma; Diabetes Ketoacidosis; **Hospital:** NY-Presby Hosp/Weill Cornell (page 104), Meml Sloan-Kettering Cancer Ctr (page 112); **Address:** New York Presbyterian Hosp, Div Pediatric Critical Care Med, 525 E 68th St, rm M-508, New York, NY 10065; **Phone:** 212-746-3056; **Board Cert:** Pediatrics 1987; Pediatric Critical Care Medicine 2005; **Med School:** NYU Sch Med 1982; **Resid:** Pediatrics, NYU-Bellevue Hosp Ctr 1986; **Fellow:** Pediatric Critical Care Medicine, NY Hosp-Cornell 1988; **Fac Appt:** Clin Prof Ped, Cornell Univ-Weill Med Coll

Pediatric Endocrinology

Fennoy, Ilene MD (PEn) - **Spec Exp:** Growth/Development Disorders; Diabetes; Klinefelter's Syndrome; Obesity; **Hospital:** NYPresby-Morgan Stanley Children's Hosp (page 104), Harlem Hosp Ctr; **Address:** 622 W 168 St PH East Bldg Fl 5E - rm 522, New York, NY 10032; **Phone:** 212-305-6559; **Board Cert:** Pediatrics 1979; Pediatric Endocrinology 1980; **Med School:** UCSF 1973; **Resid:** Pediatrics, Montefiore Med Ctr 1975; **Fellow:** Nutrition, Columbia-Presby Med Ctr 1977; Endocrinology, Nat Inst Hlth 1979; **Fac Appt:** Assoc Clin Prof Ped, Columbia P&S

Franklin, Bonita H MD (PEn) - **Spec Exp:** Diabetes; Growth Disorders; Thyroid Disorders; **Hospital:** NYU Langone Med Ctr (page 106), Mount Sinai Med Ctr (page 102); **Address:** 109 Reade St, New York, NY 10013-3863; **Phone:** 212-732-2401; **Board Cert:** Pediatrics 1982; Pediatric Endocrinology 2009; **Med School:** SUNY Hlth Sci Ctr 1976; **Resid:** Pediatrics, Bronx Muni Hosp 1978; Pediatrics, Mt Sinai Hosp 1979; **Fellow:** Pediatric Endocrinology, Mt Sinai Hosp 1981; **Fac Appt:** Assoc Clin Prof Ped, NYU Sch Med

Gallagher, Mary Pat MD (PEn) - **Spec Exp:** Diabetes; **Hospital:** NYPresby-Morgan Stanley Children's Hosp (page 104); **Address:** 1150 St Nicholas Ave, New York, NY 10032; **Phone:** 212-851-5494; **Board Cert:** Pediatrics 2006; Pediatric Endocrinology 2003; **Med School:** UMDNJ-NJ Med Sch, Newark 1995; **Resid:** Pediatrics, NY Presby-Columbia Med Ctr 1998; **Fellow:** Pediatric Endocrinology, NY Presby-Columbia Med Ctr 2002; **Fac Appt:** Asst Prof Ped, Columbia P&S

Kohn, Brenda MD (PEn) - **Spec Exp:** Growth Disorders; Pituitary Disorders; Thyroid Disorders; Adrenal Disorders; **Hospital:** NYU Langone Med Ctr (page 106), Lenox Hill Hosp; **Address:** 530 1st Ave, Ste 3A, New York, NY 10016-6402; **Phone:** 212-263-7455; **Board Cert:** Pediatrics 1981; Pediatric Endocrinology 1983; **Med School:** Albert Einstein Coll Med 1976; **Resid:** Pediatrics, NYU Med Ctr 1979; **Fellow:** Endocrinology, Diabetes & Metabolism, NY-Cornell Med Ctr 1983; **Fac Appt:** Assoc Prof Ped, NYU Sch Med

Maclaren, Noel K MD (PEn) - **Spec Exp:** Diabetes; Obesity; Metabolic Syndrome; **Hospital:** Lenox Hill Hosp; **Address:** Bioseek Endocrine Clinic, 200 W 57th St, Ste 610, New York, NY 10019; **Phone:** 212-371-0658; **Board Cert:** Pediatrics 1977; Pediatric Endocrinology 1978; **Med School:** New Zealand 1963; **Resid:** Pediatrics, Wellington Public Hosp 1967; **Fellow:** Pediatric Endocrinology, Johns Hopkins Hosp 1973; **Fac Appt:** Prof Ped, Cornell Univ-Weill Med Coll

New, Maria I MD (PEn) - **Spec Exp:** Adrenal Disorders; Growth/Development Disorders; **Hospital:** Mount Sinai Med Ctr (page 102); **Address:** Mount Sinai Medical Ctr, 1 Gustave L Levy Pl, Box 1198, New York, NY 10029; **Phone:** 212-241-8210; **Board Cert:** Pediatrics 1960; **Med School:** Univ Pennsylvania 1954; **Resid:** Pediatrics, New York Hosp 1957; **Fellow:** Pediatric Endocrinology, New York Hosp 1958; Endocrinology, Diabetes & Metabolism, New York Hosp 1964; **Fac Appt:** Prof Ped, Cornell Univ-Weill Med Coll

Oberfield, Sharon E MD (PEn) - **Spec Exp:** Adrenal Disorders; Neuroendocrine Growth Disorders; Growth Disorders; **Hospital:** NYPresby-Morgan Stanley Children's Hosp (page 104); **Address:** 630 W 168th St PH East Bldg - Ste 522, New York, NY 10032; **Phone:** 212-305-6559; **Board Cert:** Pediatrics 1979; Pediatric Endocrinology 2000; **Med School:** Cornell Univ-Weill Med Coll 1974; **Resid:** Pediatrics, NY Hosp-Cornell 1976; **Fellow:** Pediatric Endocrinology, NY Hosp-Cornell 1979; **Fac Appt:** Prof Ped, Columbia P&S

Rapaport, Robert MD (PEn) - **Spec Exp:** Diabetes; Thyroid Disorders; Growth Disorders; **Hospital:** Mount Sinai Med Ctr (page 102); **Address:** 1 Gustave L Levy Pl, Box 1616, New York, NY 10029-6508; **Phone:** 212-241-8487 x4847; **Board Cert:** Pediatrics 1980; Pediatric Endocrinology 1983; **Med School:** SUNY Downstate 1974; **Resid:** Pediatrics, LIJ-Hillside Med Ctr 1977; **Fellow:** Pediatric Endocrinology, St Christopher's Hosp 1978; Pediatric Endocrinology, New York Hosp 1980; **Fac Appt:** Prof Ped, Mount Sinai Sch Med

Sklar, Charles A MD (PEn) - **Spec Exp:** Cancer Survivors-Late Effects of Therapy; Growth Disorders in Childhood Cancer; Pituitary Disorders; **Hospital:** Meml Sloan-Kettering Cancer Ctr (page 112); **Address:** 1275 York Avenue, New York, NY 10065; **Phone:** 800-525-2225; **Board Cert:** Pediatrics 1979; Pediatric Endocrinology 1980; **Med School:** USC Sch Med 1974; **Resid:** Pediatrics, Childrens Hosp 1976; **Fellow:** Pediatric Endocrinology, UCSF Med Ctr 1979; **Fac Appt:** Assoc Prof Ped, Cornell Univ-Weill Med Coll

Slonim, Alfred E MD (PEn) - **Spec Exp:** Muscular Disorders-Metabolic; Inflammatory Bowel Disease/Crohn's; Glycogen Storage Diseases; Chronic Fatigue Syndrome; **Hospital:** NYPresby-Morgan Stanley Children's Hosp (page 104); **Address:** NY Presby-Morgan Stanley Children's Hosp, 622 W 168th St, rm 517, New York, NY 10032; **Phone:** 212-305-5717; **Board Cert:** Pediatrics 1978; Pediatric Endocrinology 1986; **Med School:** Australia 1958; **Resid:** Pediatrics, Royal Chldns Hosp 1963; **Fellow:** Pediatrics, Royal Chldns Hosp 1965; Endocrinology, Hadassah Hosp 1970; **Fac Appt:** Prof Ped, Columbia P&S

Vargas, Ileana MD (PEn) - **Spec Exp:** Diabetes; **Hospital:** NY-Presby Hosp/Columbia (page 104); **Address:** 1150 St Nicholas Ave Fl 2, New York, NY 10032; **Phone:** 212-851-5494; **Board Cert:** Pediatric Endocrinology 2003; **Med School:** Albert Einstein Coll Med 1986; **Resid:** Pediatrics, Babies Hosp 1989; **Fellow:** Pediatric Endocrinology, Mt Sinai Hosp 1990

Vogiatzi, Maria G MD (PEn) - **Spec Exp:** Growth Disorders; Osteoporosis; Pubertal Disorders; Adrenal Disorders; **Hospital:** NY-Presby Hosp/Weill Cornell (page 104); **Address:** 525 E 68th St, Box 103, New York, NY 10065; **Phone:** 212-746-3462; **Board Cert:** Pediatrics 2007; Pediatric Endocrinology 2005; **Med School:** Greece 1987; **Resid:** Pediatrics, Univ Hosp 1991; **Fellow:** Pediatric Endocrinology, New York Hosp 1993; Pediatric Endocrinology, Baylor Coll Med 1995; **Fac Appt:** Assoc Clin Prof Ped, Cornell Univ-Weill Med Coll

Pediatric Gastroenterology

Bangaru, Babu S MD (PGe) - **Spec Exp:** Ulcerative Colitis/Crohn's; Liver Disease; Nutrition; Endoscopy; **Hospital:** NYU Langone Med Ctr (page 106), Flushing Hosp Med Ctr; **Address:** NYU Medical Center, 530 First Ave, Ste 3A, New York, NY 10016; **Phone:** 212-263-7868; **Board Cert:** Pediatrics 1978; Pediatric Gastroenterology 2006; **Med School:** India 1970; **Resid:** Pediatrics, St Lukes Hosp 1976; **Fellow:** Hepatology, Albert Einstein Coll Med 1978; Gastroenterology & Nutrition, Emory Univ Sch Med 1979; **Fac Appt:** Assoc Clin Prof Ped, NYU Sch Med

Benkov, Keith J MD (PGe) - **Spec Exp:** Inflammatory Bowel Disease/Crohn's; Liver Disease; Celiac Disease; **Hospital:** Mount Sinai Med Ctr (page 102), Englewood Hosp & Med Ctr (page 656); **Address:** Mt Sinai Div Ped Gastroenterology, 5 E 98th St Fl 10, New York, NY 10029; **Phone:** 212-241-5415; **Board Cert:** Pediatrics 1984; Pediatric Gastroenterology 2005; **Med School:** Mount Sinai Sch Med 1979; **Resid:** Pediatrics, Mt Sinai Hosp 1982; **Fellow:** Pediatric Gastroenterology, Mt Sinai Hosp 1984; **Fac Appt:** Assoc Prof Ped, Mount Sinai Sch Med

Kazlow, Philip MD (PGe) - **Spec Exp:** Inflammatory Bowel Disease; Celiac Disease; Nutrition; **Hospital:** NYPresby-Morgan Stanley Children's Hosp (page 104), Valley Hosp (page 658); **Address:** Morgan Stanley Chldns Hosp of NY-Presby, 3959 Broadway, CHN 702, New York, NY 10032; **Phone:** 212-305-5903; **Board Cert:** Pediatrics 1985; Pediatric Gastroenterology 2005; **Med School:** Mount Sinai Sch Med 1980; **Resid:** Pediatrics, Mt Sinai Hosp 1984; **Fellow:** Pediatric Gastroenterology, Mt Sinai Hosp 1986; **Fac Appt:** Assoc Clin Prof Ped, Columbia P&S

Levy, Joseph MD (PGe) - **Spec Exp:** Celiac Disease; Irritable Bowel Syndrome; Gastroesophageal Reflux Disease (GERD); Nutrition in Autism; **Hospital:** NYU Langone Med Ctr (page 106); **Address:** 160 E 32nd St Fl 2, New York, NY 10016; **Phone:** 212-263-5407; **Board Cert:** Pediatrics 1981; Pediatric Gastroenterology 2005; **Med School:** Israel 1973; **Resid:** Pediatrics, Beth Israel Med Ctr 1977; **Fellow:** Research, Columbia-Presby Med Ctr 1975; Pediatric Gastroenterology, Columbia-Presby Med Ctr 1979; **Fac Appt:** Prof Ped, NYU Sch Med

Sockolow, Robbyn MD (PGe) - **Spec Exp:** Constipation; Gastroesophageal Reflux Disease (GERD); Inflammatory Bowel Disease/Crohn's; Capsule Endoscopy; **Hospital:** NY-Presby Hosp/Weill Cornell (page 104); **Address:** Weill Med Coll, Dept Peds, 525 E 68th St, New York, NY 10021; **Phone:** 646-962-3869; **Board Cert:** Pediatrics 2005; Pediatric Gastroenterology 2003; **Med School:** NY Med Coll 1986; **Resid:** Pediatrics, Montefiore Med Ctr 1989; **Fellow:** Pediatric Gastroenterology, Mt Sinai 1990; Pediatric Gastroenterology, Montefiore Med Ctr 1992; **Fac Appt:** Assoc Clin Prof Ped, Cornell Univ-Weill Med Coll

Spivak, William MD (PGe) - **Spec Exp:** Inflammatory Bowel Disease/Crohn's; Ulcerative Colitis; Gastroesophageal Reflux Disease (GERD); Feeding Disorders; **Hospital:** NY-Presby Hosp/Weill Cornell (page 104), Lenox Hill Hosp; **Address:** 177 E 87th St, Ste 305, New York, NY 10128; **Phone:** 212-369-7700; **Board Cert:** Pediatrics 1981; Pediatric Gastroenterology 2005; **Med School:** Albert Einstein Coll Med 1976; **Resid:** Pediatrics, Jacobi Med Ctr 1979; **Fellow:** Gastroenterology, Childrens Hosp 1982; Research, Brigham & Womens Hosp 1982; **Fac Appt:** Clin Prof Ped, Cornell Univ-Weill Med Coll

Suchy, Frederick J MD (PGe) - **Spec Exp:** Hepatitis; Liver Disease; Neonatal Cholestasis; **Hospital:** Mount Sinai Med Ctr (page 102); **Address:** Mount Sinai Medical Ctr, 1 Gustave Levy Pl, Box 1198, New York, NY 10029; **Phone:** 212-241-6933; **Board Cert:** Pediatrics 1982; Pediatric Gastroenterology 2005; Pediatric Transplant Hepatology 2006; **Med School:** Univ Cincinnati 1974; **Resid:** Pediatrics, Chldns Hosp Med Ctr 1978; **Fellow:** Pediatric Gastroenterology, Chldns Hosp Med Ctr 1981; **Fac Appt:** Prof Ped, Mount Sinai Sch Med

Pediatric Hematology-Oncology

Aledo, Alexander MD (PHO) - **Spec Exp:** Leukemia; Lymphoma; Bone Tumors; **Hospital:** NY-Presby Hosp/Weill Cornell (page 104), NY Hosp Queens; **Address:** 525 E 68th St, rm P695, New York, NY 10021-4870; **Phone:** 212-746-3447; **Board Cert:** Pediatric Hematology-Oncology 2004; **Med School:** NYU Sch Med 1984; **Resid:** Pediatrics, NY Hosp 1987; **Fellow:** Pediatric Hematology-Oncology, Meml Sloan Kettering Cancer Ctr 1990; **Fac Appt:** Assoc Clin Prof Ped, Cornell Univ-Weill Med Coll

Blei, Francine MD (PHO) - **Spec Exp:** Hemangiomas; Vascular Anomalies; Vascular Malformations; Lymphedema; **Hospital:** NYU Langone Med Ctr (page 106), Bellevue Hosp Ctr; **Address:** Vascular Birthmark Inst, 126 W 60th St, New York, NY 10023; **Phone:** 212-523-8931; **Board Cert:** Pediatrics 1987; Pediatric Hematology-Oncology 1987; **Med School:** Israel 1982; **Resid:** Pediatrics, NYU-Bellevue 1985; **Fellow:** Pediatric Hematology-Oncology, Babies Hosp-Columbia Presby 1987; **Fac Appt:** Assoc Prof Ped, NYU Sch Med

Bussel, James MD (PHO) - **Spec Exp:** Autoimmune Disease; Bleeding/Coagulation Disorders; **Hospital:** NY-Presby Hosp/Weill Cornell (page 104), Lenox Hill Hosp; **Address:** 525 E 68th St, rm P-695, New York, NY 10065; **Phone:** 212-746-3474; **Board Cert:** Pediatrics 1979; Pediatric Hematology-Oncology 1980; **Med School:** Columbia P&S 1975; **Resid:** Pediatrics, Chldns Hosp 1978; **Fellow:** Pediatric Hematology-Oncology, NY Presby Hosp/Cornell 1981; **Fac Appt:** Prof Ped, Cornell Univ-Weill Med Coll

Cairo, Mitchell S MD (PHO) - **Spec Exp:** Bone Marrow Transplant; Leukemia; Lymphoma; **Hospital:** NYPresby-Morgan Stanley Children's Hosp (page 104); **Address:** Columbia Univ Med Ctr, 3959 Broadway, CHN 10-03, New York, NY 10032; **Phone:** 212-305-8316; **Board Cert:** Pediatrics 1980; Pediatric Hematology-Oncology 1982; **Med School:** UCSF 1976; **Resid:** Pediatrics, UCLA Med Ctr 1979; **Fellow:** Pediatric Hematology-Oncology, Indiana Univ Med Ctr 1981; **Fac Appt:** Prof Ped, Columbia P&S

Carroll, William L MD (PHO) - **Spec Exp:** Leukemia; **Hospital:** NYU Langone Med Ctr (page 106); **Address:** NYU Med Ctr, Div Ped Hem/Onc, 160 E 32nd St Fl 2, New York, NY 10016; **Phone:** 212-263-9947; **Board Cert:** Pediatrics 1984; Pediatric Hematology-Oncology 1987; **Med School:** UC Irvine 1978; **Resid:** Pediatrics, Chldns Hosp Med Ctr 1981; **Fellow:** Pediatric Hematology-Oncology, Stanford Univ 1987; **Fac Appt:** Prof Ped, NYU Sch Med

DiMichele, Donna MD (PHO) - **Spec Exp:** Hemophilia; **Hospital:** NY-Presby Hosp/Weill Cornell (page 104); **Address:** 525 E 68th St, rm P695, New York, NY 10065; **Phone:** 212-746-3421; **Board Cert:** Pediatrics 1985; Pediatric Hematology-Oncology 1987; **Med School:** McGill Univ 1978; **Resid:** Pediatrics, Univ Colo Hlth Sci Ctr 1983; **Fellow:** Hematology & Oncology, Univ Colo Hlth Sci Ctr 1987; **Fac Appt:** Prof Ped, Cornell Univ-Weill Med Coll

Dunkel, Ira J MD (PHO) - **Spec Exp:** Retinoblastoma; Brain & Spinal Cord Tumors; Brain Tumors; Pediatric Cancers; **Hospital:** Meml Sloan-Kettering Cancer Ctr (page 112); **Address:** 1275 York Avenue, New York, NY 10065; **Phone:** 800-525-2225; **Board Cert:** Pediatric Hematology-Oncology 2007; **Med School:** Duke Univ 1985; **Resid:** Pediatrics, Duke Univ Med Ctr 1988; **Fellow:** Pediatric Hematology-Oncology, Memorial-Sloan Kettering 1992; **Fac Appt:** Asst Prof Ped, Cornell Univ-Weill Med Coll

Garvin, James H MD/PhD (PHO) - **Spec Exp:** Brain Tumors; Pediatric Cancers; Bone Marrow Transplant; **Hospital:** NYPresby-Morgan Stanley Children's Hosp (page 104); **Address:** 161 Fort Washington Ave Fl 7 - rm 708, New York, NY 10032-3729; **Phone:** 212-305-8685; **Board Cert:** Pediatrics 1982; Pediatric Hematology-Oncology 1984; **Med School:** Jefferson Med Coll 1976; **Resid:** Pediatrics, Chldns Hosp 1978; Pediatrics, Middlesex Hosp 1979; **Fellow:** Pediatric Hematology-Oncology, Dana Farber Cancer Inst/Childrens Hosp 1982; **Fac Appt:** Clin Prof Ped, Columbia P&S

Giardina, Patricia J V MD (PHO) - **Spec Exp:** Thalassemia; **Hospital:** NY-Presby Hosp/Weill Cornell (page 104); **Address:** 525 E 68th St, Payson Pavilion 695, New York, NY 10065; **Phone:** 212-746-3400; **Board Cert:** Pediatrics 1973; Pediatric Hematology-Oncology 1974; **Med School:** NY Med Coll 1968; **Resid:** Pediatrics, New York Hosp 1971; **Fellow:** Pediatric Hematology-Oncology, New York Hosp-Cornell 1974; **Fac Appt:** Clin Prof Ped, Cornell Univ-Weill Med Coll

Kernan, Nancy A MD (PHO) - **Spec Exp:** Leukemia; Immune Deficiency; Bone Marrow Transplant; Stem Cell Transplant; **Hospital:** Meml Sloan-Kettering Cancer Ctr (page 112), NY-Presby Hosp/Weill Cornell (page 104); **Address:** 1275 York Avenue, New York, NY 10065; **Phone:** 212-639-7250; **Board Cert:** Pediatrics 1983; Pediatric Hematology-Oncology 1984; **Med School:** Cornell Univ-Weill Med Coll 1978; **Resid:** Pediatrics, Chldns Hosp Natl Med Ctr 1981; **Fellow:** Pediatric Hematology-Oncology, Meml Sloan Kettering Cancer Ctr 1984; **Fac Appt:** Assoc Prof Ped, Cornell Univ-Weill Med Coll

Kushner, Brian H MD (PHO) - **Spec Exp:** Neuroblastoma; Bone Marrow Transplant; Immunotherapy; **Hospital:** Meml Sloan-Kettering Cancer Ctr (page 112); **Address:** 1275 York Avenue, New York, NY 10065; **Phone:** 800-525-2225; **Board Cert:** Pediatrics 1983; Pediatric Hematology-Oncology 1987; **Med School:** Johns Hopkins Univ 1976; **Resid:** Pediatrics, Columbia-Presby Med Ctr 1978; Pediatrics, NY Hosp 1979; **Fellow:** Pediatric Hematology-Oncology, Boston Chldns Hosp 1980; Pediatric Hematology-Oncology, Meml Sloan Kettering Cancer Ctr 1986; **Fac Appt:** Prof Ped, Cornell Univ-Weill Med Coll

Marcus, Judith R MD (PHO) - **Spec Exp:** Leukemia; Lymphoma; Bleeding/Coagulation Disorders; Solid Tumors-Pediatric; **Hospital:** NYPresby-Morgan Stanley Children's Hosp (page 104), White Plains Hosp Ctr; **Address:** 161 Ft Wasthington Ave, Ste 7I, New York, NY 10032; **Phone:** 914-684-0220; **Board Cert:** Pediatrics 1997; Pediatric Hematology-Oncology 1997; **Med School:** NYU Sch Med 1971; **Resid:** Pediatrics, Bronx Muni Hosp-Albert Einstein 1974; **Fellow:** Pediatric Hematology-Oncology, Meml Sloan Kettering Cancer Ctr 1979; **Fac Appt:** Clin Prof Ped, Columbia P&S

Meyers, Paul A MD (PHO) - **Spec Exp:** Pediatric Cancers; Bone Tumors; Sarcoma; **Hospital:** Meml Sloan-Kettering Cancer Ctr (page 112), NY-Presby Hosp/Weill Cornell (page 104); **Address:** 1275 York Avenue, New York, NY 10065; **Phone:** 800-525-2225; **Board Cert:** Pediatrics 1978; Pediatric Hematology-Oncology 1978; **Med School:** Mount Sinai Sch Med 1973; **Resid:** Pediatrics, Mt Sinai Hosp 1976; **Fellow:** Pediatric Hematology-Oncology, NY Hosp-Cornell Med Ctr 1979; **Fac Appt:** Prof Ped, Cornell Univ-Weill Med Coll

O'Reilly, Richard MD (PHO) - **Spec Exp:** Bone Marrow Transplant; **Hospital:** Meml Sloan-Kettering Cancer Ctr (page 112), NY-Presby Hosp/Weill Cornell (page 104); **Address:** 1275 York Avenue, New York, NY 10065; **Phone:** 800-525-2225; **Board Cert:** Pediatrics 1974; **Med School:** Univ Rochester 1968; **Resid:** Pediatrics, Chldrns Hosp 1972; **Fellow:** Infectious Disease, Chldrns Hosp 1973; **Fac Appt:** Prof Ped, Cornell Univ-Weill Med Coll

Rausen, Aaron R MD (PHO) - **Spec Exp:** Leukemia & Lymphoma; Bone Tumors; Retinoblastoma; **Hospital:** NYU Langone Med Ctr (page 106), Lenox Hill Hosp; **Address:** NYU Medical Ctr, 160 E 32nd St Fl 2, New York, NY 10016; **Phone:** 212-263-7144; **Board Cert:** Pediatrics 1960; Pediatric Hematology-Oncology 1974; **Med School:** SUNY Downstate 1954; **Resid:** Pediatrics, Bellevue Hosp 1956; Pediatrics, Mount Sinai 1959; **Fellow:** Hematology, Chldns Hosp 1961; **Fac Appt:** Prof Ped, NYU Sch Med

Steinherz, Peter G MD (PHO) - **Spec Exp:** Leukemia & Lymphoma; Pediatric Cancers; Wilms' Tumor; **Hospital:** Meml Sloan-Kettering Cancer Ctr (page 112), NY-Presby Hosp/Weill Cornell (page 104); **Address:** 1275 York Avenue, New York, NY 10065; **Phone:** 212-639-7951; **Board Cert:** Pediatrics 1973; Pediatric Hematology-Oncology 1978; **Med School:** Albert Einstein Coll Med 1968; **Resid:** Pediatrics, NY Hosp-Cornell 1971; **Fellow:** Pediatric Hematology-Oncology, NY Hosp-Cornell 1975; **Fac Appt:** Prof Ped, Cornell Univ-Weill Med Coll

Weiner, Michael MD (PHO) - **Spec Exp:** Hodgkin's Disease; Lymphoma; Leukemia; **Hospital:** NY-Presby Hosp/Columbia (page 104); **Address:** 161 Fort Washington Ave, Irving Pavilion-FL 7, New York, NY 10032-3710; **Phone:** 212-305-9770; **Board Cert:** Pediatrics 1980; Pediatric Hematology-Oncology 1980; **Med School:** SUNY Hlth Sci Ctr 1972; **Resid:** Pediatrics, Montefiore Med Ctr 1974; **Fellow:** Pediatric Hematology-Oncology, NYU Med Ctr 1976; Pediatric Hematology-Oncology, Johns Hopkins Hosp 1977; **Fac Appt:** Prof Ped, Columbia P&S

Wexler, Leonard MD (PHO) - **Spec Exp:** Rhabdomyosarcoma; Bone Cancer; Gastrointestinal Stromal Tumors; Sarcoma-Soft Tissue; **Hospital:** Meml Sloan-Kettering Cancer Ctr (page 112); **Address:** 1275 York Avenue, New York, NY 10065; **Phone:** 800-525-2225; **Board Cert:** Pediatrics 2007; Pediatric Hematology-Oncology 2007; **Med School:** Boston Univ 1985; **Resid:** Pediatrics, Montefiore Med Ctr 1988; **Fellow:** Pediatric Hematology-Oncology, National Cancer Inst 1991; **Fac Appt:** Assoc Prof Ped, Columbia P&S

Pediatric Infectious Disease

Borkowsky, William MD (PInf) - **Spec Exp:** AIDS/HIV; **Hospital:** NYU Langone Med Ctr (page 106), Bellevue Hosp Ctr; **Address:** 550 1st Ave, Dept Pediatrics, New York, NY 10016; **Phone:** 212-263-6513; **Board Cert:** Pediatrics 1979; Pediatric Infectious Disease 2009; **Med School:** NYU Sch Med 1972; **Resid:** Pediatrics, Bellevue Hosp Ctr 1975; **Fellow:** Infectious Disease, Bellevue Hosp Ctr-NYU 1978; **Fac Appt:** Prof Ped, NYU Sch Med

Krasinski, Keith M MD (PInf) - **Spec Exp:** AIDS/HIV; Infections-CNS; **Hospital:** Bellevue Hosp Ctr, NYU Langone Med Ctr (page 106); **Address:** NYU Med Ctr, Dept Peds, 550 1st Ave, New York, NY 10016-6497; **Phone:** 212-263-6427; **Board Cert:** Pediatrics 1980; Pediatric Infectious Disease 2009; **Med School:** Univ IL Coll Med 1976; **Resid:** Pediatrics, Children's Med Ctr, Parkland Hosp 1979; **Fellow:** Pediatric Infectious Disease, Univ Texas SW Med Ctr 1981; **Fac Appt:** Prof Ped, NYU Sch Med

Larsen, John MD (PInf) - **Hospital:** Mount Sinai Med Ctr (page 102); **Address:** 1245 Park Ave, New York, NY 10128-1211; **Phone:** 212-427-0540; **Board Cert:** Pediatrics 1979; Pediatric Infectious Disease 2005; **Med School:** SUNY Hlth Sci Ctr 1974; **Resid:** Pediatrics, Mount Sinai Med Ctr 1977; **Fellow:** Pediatric Infectious Disease, Mount Sinai Med Ctr 1978; **Fac Appt:** Assoc Clin Prof Ped, Mount Sinai Sch Med

Neu, Natalie M MD (PInf) - **Spec Exp:** AIDS/HIV; Sexually Transmitted Diseases; **Hospital:** NY-Presby Hosp/Columbia (page 104); **Address:** Columbia Presbyterian Ctr, PH4-468, 622 W 168th St, New Yoek, NY 10032; **Phone:** 212-305-9683; **Board Cert:** Pediatrics 2009; Pediatric Infectious Disease 2005; **Med School:** Columbia P&S 1991; **Resid:** Pediatrics, Michigan State Med Ctr 1994; **Fellow:** Pediatric Infectious Disease, Columbia Presby Med Ctr 1997; **Fac Appt:** Assoc Clin Prof Ped, Columbia P&S

Saiman, Lisa MD (PInf) - **Spec Exp:** Cystic Fibrosis Infection; Fungal Infections; Tick-borne Diseases; Tuberculosis; **Hospital:** NYPresby-Morgan Stanley Children's Hosp (page 104); **Address:** Columbia University, 622 W 168th St Fl 4 PH4 W - rm 470, New York, NY 10032; **Phone:** 212-305-0635; **Board Cert:** Pediatrics 1987; Pediatric Infectious Disease 2009; **Med School:** Albert Einstein Coll Med 1983; **Resid:** Pediatrics, Babies Hosp/NY Presby 1986; **Fellow:** Infectious Disease, Babies Hosp/NY Presby 1989; **Fac Appt:** Assoc Clin Prof Ped, Columbia P&S

Pediatric Nephrology

Johnson, Valerie MD/PhD (PNep) - **Spec Exp:** Nephrotic Syndrome; Glomerulonephritis; Hypertension; Transplant Medicine-Kidney; **Hospital:** NY-Presby Hosp/Weill Cornell (page 104), Valley Hosp (page 658); **Address:** 525 E 68th St, Box 176, New York, NY 10021; **Phone:** 646-962-4344; **Board Cert:** Pediatrics 1984; Pediatric Nephrology 1985; **Med School:** Cornell Univ-Weill Med Coll 1977; **Resid:** Pediatrics, Mt Sinai Hosp 1979; **Fellow:** Nephrology, Montefiore Med Ctr 1982; **Fac Appt:** Assoc Clin Prof Ped, Cornell Univ-Weill Med Coll

Nash, Martin MD (PNep) - **Spec Exp:** Nephrotic Syndrome; Kidney Failure; Urinary Abnormalities; Kidney Disease; **Hospital:** NYPresby-Morgan Stanley Children's Hosp (page 104); **Address:** Morgan Stanley Chlds Hosp of NY-Presby, 3959 Broadway, rm 701, New York, NY 10032-1559; **Phone:** 212-305-5825; **Board Cert:** Pediatrics 1969; Nephrology 1974; **Med School:** Duke Univ 1964; **Resid:** Internal Medicine, Georgetown Univ Hosp 1965; Pediatrics, Columbia-Presby Med Ctr 1967; **Fellow:** Pediatric Nephrology, Montefiore Med Ctr 1971; **Fac Appt:** Clin Prof Ped, Columbia P&S

Perelstein, Eduardo MD (PNep) - **Spec Exp:** Kidney Failure; Glomerulonephritis; Hypertension; **Hospital:** NY-Presby Hosp/Weill Cornell (page 104), NY Hosp Queens; **Address:** 505 E 70th St Fl 3, New York, NY 10021; **Phone:** 646-962-4324; **Board Cert:** Pediatrics 2004; Pediatric Nephrology 2005; **Med School:** Argentina 1974; **Resid:** Pediatrics, Chldn's Hosp 1978; **Fellow:** Pediatric Nephrology, St Christopher's Hosp for Chldn 1985; Pediatric Nephrology, NY Hosp-Cornell Med Ctr 1987; **Fac Appt:** Assoc Prof Ped, Cornell Univ-Weill Med Coll

Saland, Jeffrey M MD (PNep) - **Spec Exp:** Transplant Medicine-Kidney; Kidney Disease; Hypertension in Children; Hemolytic Uremic Syndrome; **Hospital:** Mount Sinai Med Ctr (page 102); **Address:** Mt Sinai Medical Ctr, 5 E 98th St Fl 10, New York, NY 10029; **Phone:** 212-241-6187; **Board Cert:** Pediatric Nephrology 2003; **Med School:** Univ New Mexico 1995; **Resid:** Pediatrics, Chldns Hosp Med Ctr 1998; **Fellow:** Pediatric Nephrology, Univ TX-SW Med Ctr 2000; Pediatric Nephrology, Mt Sinai Med Ctr 2002; **Fac Appt:** Asst Prof Ped, Mount Sinai Sch Med

Satlin, Lisa M MD (PNep) - **Spec Exp:** Kidney Disease-Hereditary; Hypertension; Polycystic Kidney Disease; Electrolyte Disorders; **Hospital:** Mount Sinai Med Ctr (page 102); **Address:** Mount Sinai Med Ctr, Dept Pediatrics, One Gustave L Levy Pl, Box 1198, New York, NY 10029; **Phone:** 212-241-6187; **Board Cert:** Pediatric Nephrology 1985; Pediatrics 1985; **Med School:** Columbia P&S 1979; **Resid:** Pediatrics, Columbia-Presby Med Ctr 1982; **Fellow:** Nephrology, Montefiore Med Ctr 1986; **Fac Appt:** Prof Ped, Mount Sinai Sch Med

Seigle, Robert MD (PNep) - **Spec Exp:** Glomerulonephritis; Kidney Failure; Kidney Disease; **Hospital:** NYPresby-Morgan Stanley Children's Hosp (page 104); **Address:** Morgan Stanley Chldns Hosp, 3959 Broadway, rm 701B, New York, NY 10032; **Phone:** 212-305-5825; **Board Cert:** Pediatrics 1980; Pediatric Nephrology 1982; **Med School:** Columbia P&S 1974; **Resid:** Pediatrics, Columbia-Presby Med Ctr 1978; **Fellow:** Pediatric Nephrology, Albert Einstein Med Coll 1981; **Fac Appt:** Asst Prof Ped, Columbia P&S

Pediatric Otolaryngology

April, Max M MD (PO) - **Spec Exp:** Sinus Disorders; Neck Masses; Laryngeal Disorders; Sleep Apnea; **Hospital:** NY-Presby Hosp/Weill Cornell (page 104), Long Island Jewish Med Ctr; **Address:** 428 E 72nd St, Ste 100, New York, NY 10021; **Phone:** 646-962-2225; **Board Cert:** Otolaryngology 1990; **Med School:** Boston Univ 1985; **Resid:** Otolaryngology, Boston Univ Med Ctr 1990; **Fellow:** Pediatric Otolaryngology, Johns Hopkins Hosp 1991; **Fac Appt:** Clin Prof Oto, Cornell Univ-Weill Med Coll

Dolitsky, Jay MD (PO) - **Spec Exp:** Ear Infections; Neck Masses; Tonsil/Adenoid Disorders; Sleep Disorders; **Hospital:** New York Eye & Ear Infirm (page 113); **Address:** 404 Park Ave S Fl 12, New York, NY 10016; **Phone:** 212-679-3499; **Board Cert:** Otolaryngology 1990; **Med School:** SUNY Downstate 1981; **Resid:** Otolaryngology, Manhattan EET Hosp 1990; **Fellow:** Pediatric Otolaryngology, Children's Hosp 1992; **Fac Appt:** Assoc Prof Oto, NY Med Coll

Haddad Jr, Joseph MD (PO) - **Spec Exp:** Ear Infections; Sinus Disorders; Cleft Palate/Lip; **Hospital:** NYPresby-Morgan Stanley Children's Hosp (page 104); **Address:** Morgan Stanley Chldns Hosp of NY-Presby, 3959 Broadway, Ste 501N, New York, NY 10032-1559; **Phone:** 212-305-8933; **Board Cert:** Otolaryngology 1988; **Med School:** NYU Sch Med 1983; **Resid:** Surgery, Columbia-Presby Hosp 1985; Otolaryngology, Columbia-Presby Hosp 1988; **Fellow:** Pediatric Otolaryngology, Chldns Hosp 1990; **Fac Appt:** Clin Prof Oto, Columbia P&S

Jones, Jacqueline MD (PO) - **Spec Exp:** Sinus Disorders/Surgery; Ear Infections; **Hospital:** NY-Presby Hosp/Weill Cornell (page 104), Lenox Hill Hosp; **Address:** 1175 Park Ave, Ste 1A, New York, NY 10128; **Phone:** 212-996-2559; **Board Cert:** Otolaryngology 1989; **Med School:** Cornell Univ-Weill Med Coll 1984; **Resid:** Otolaryngology, Hosp Univ Penn 1989; **Fellow:** Pediatric Otolaryngology, Chldns Hosp 1990; **Fac Appt:** Assoc Prof Oto, Cornell Univ-Weill Med Coll

Rothschild, Michael A MD (PO) - **Spec Exp:** Choanal Atresia; Neck Masses; Sinusitis; Ear Disorders; **Hospital:** Mount Sinai Med Ctr (page 102); **Address:** Park Ave ENT, 1175 Park Ave, Ste 1A, New York, NY 10128; **Phone:** 212-996-2995; **Board Cert:** Otolaryngology 1994; **Med School:** Yale Univ 1988; **Resid:** Surgery, Mt Sinai Med Ctr 1990; Otolaryngology, Mt Sinai Med Ctr 1993; **Fellow:** Pediatric Otolaryngology, Chldn's Hosp 1994; **Fac Appt:** Clin Prof Oto, Mount Sinai Sch Med

Ward, Robert MD (PO) - **Spec Exp:** Airway Disorders; Sinus Disorders/Surgery; Choanal Atresia; **Hospital:** NY-Presby Hosp/Weill Cornell (page 104), Lenox Hill Hosp (Manh Eye, Ear & Throat Hosp); **Address:** Weill Cornell Med Ctr, Otolaryngology, 1305 York Ave Fl 5, New York, NY 10021; **Phone:** 646-962-2224; **Board Cert:** Otolaryngology 1986; **Med School:** Cornell Univ-Weill Med Coll 1981; **Resid:** Surgery, NY Hosp 1983; Otolaryngology, NY Hosp 1986; **Fellow:** Pediatric Otolaryngology, Chldns Hosp 1986; **Fac Appt:** Assoc Clin Prof Oto, Cornell Univ-Weill Med Coll

Pediatric Pulmonology

Bye, Michael R MD (PPul) - **Spec Exp:** Asthma; Pneumonia; Breathing Disorders; **Hospital:** NY-Presby Hosp/Columbia (page 104), Englewood Hosp & Med Ctr (page 656); **Address:** Morgan Stanley Chlds Hosp of NY-Presby, 3959 Broadway Bldg CH Fl 7S, New York, NY 10032-1559; **Phone:** 212-305-5122; **Board Cert:** Pediatrics 1980; Pediatric Pulmonology 2003; **Med School:** SUNY Buffalo 1976; **Resid:** Pediatrics, Childrens Hosp 1979; **Fellow:** Pediatric Pulmonology, Children's Hosp 1982; **Fac Appt:** Prof Ped, Columbia P&S

Dimaio, Mary MD (PPul) - **Spec Exp:** Cystic Fibrosis; Asthma; Allergy; **Hospital:** NY-Presby Hosp/Weill Cornell (page 104); **Address:** 1440 York Ave, Ste P5, New York, NY 10075; **Phone:** 212-988-5008; **Board Cert:** Pediatrics 1987; Pediatric Pulmonology 2007; Allergy & Immunology 2009; **Med School:** SUNY Hlth Sci Ctr 1981; **Resid:** Pediatrics, Kings Co Hosp/Downstate 1983; Pediatrics, N Shore Univ Hosp 1985; **Fellow:** Pediatric Pulmonology, Mt Sinai Hosp 1988

Kattan, Meyer MD (PPul) - **Spec Exp:** Asthma; Cystic Fibrosis; Chronic Lung Disease; **Hospital:** NY-Presby Hosp/Columbia (page 104), Englewood Hosp & Med Ctr (page 656); **Address:** 3959 Broadway, CHC 7-701, New York, NY 10032; **Phone:** 212-305-5122; **Board Cert:** Pediatrics 1980; Pediatric Pulmonology 2003; **Med School:** McGill Univ 1973; **Resid:** Pediatrics, Chldns Hosp 1975; Pediatrics, Hosp for Sick Chldn 1976; **Fellow:** Pulmonary Disease, Hosp for Sick Chldn 1978; **Fac Appt:** Prof Ped, Columbia P&S

Lamm, Carin MD (PPul) - **Spec Exp:** Sleep Disorders; Asthma; **Hospital:** NYPresby-Morgan Stanley Children's Hosp (page 104); **Address:** Columbia Univ Medical Ctr, 3959 Broadway Fl 7 Central, New York, NY 10032; **Phone:** 212-305-5122; **Board Cert:** Pediatrics 1980; Pediatric Pulmonology 2003; **Med School:** NYU Sch Med 1975; **Resid:** Pediatrics, Mt Sinai Med Ctr 1979; **Fellow:** Pediatric Pulmonology, Mt Sinai Med Ctr 1981; **Fac Appt:** Assoc Prof Ped, Mount Sinai Sch Med

Loughlin, Gerald M MD (PPul) - **Spec Exp:** Sleep Disorders/Apnea; Swallowing Disorders; Asthma & Chronic Lung Disease; Breathing Disorders; **Hospital:** NY-Presby Hosp/Weill Cornell (page 104); **Address:** Cornell Med Coll, Dept Peds, 525 E 68th St, rm M-622, New York, NY 10021-4870; **Phone:** 212-746-4111; **Board Cert:** Pediatrics 1993; Pediatric Pulmonology 2003; **Med School:** Univ Rochester 1973; **Resid:** Pediatrics, Univ Ariz Med Ctr 1973; **Fellow:** Pediatric Pulmonology, Univ Ariz Med Ctr 1977; **Fac Appt:** Prof Ped, Cornell Univ-Weill Med Coll

Quittell, Lynne MD (PPul) - **Spec Exp:** Cystic Fibrosis; Asthma; **Hospital:** NYPresby-Morgan Stanley Children's Hosp (page 104); **Address:** Morgan Stanley Chlds Hosp of NY-Presby, 3959 Broadway CHS Fl 7, New York, NY 10032-1551; **Phone:** 212-305-5122; **Board Cert:** Pediatrics 1986; Pediatric Pulmonology 2004; **Med School:** Israel 1981; **Resid:** Pediatrics, Schneider Chldns Hosp 1984; **Fellow:** Pediatric Pulmonology, St Christopher's Hosp 1988; **Fac Appt:** Assoc Prof Ped, Columbia P&S

Ting, Andrew S MD (PPul) - **Spec Exp:** Asthma; Cystic Fibrosis; Bronchoscopy; Cough; **Hospital:** Mount Sinai Med Ctr (page 102); **Address:** 5 E 98th St Fl 8, New York, NY 10029; **Phone:** 212-241-7788; **Board Cert:** Pediatric Pulmonology 2009; **Med School:** NYU Sch Med 1987; **Resid:** Pediatrics, Mt Sinai Med Ctr 1991; **Fellow:** Pediatric Pulmonology, Mt Sinai Med Ctr 1994; **Fac Appt:** Asst Prof Ped, Mount Sinai Sch Med

Pediatric Rheumatology

Eichenfield, Andrew H MD (PRhu) - **Spec Exp:** Juvenile Arthritis; Lyme Disease; Lupus/SLE; **Hospital:** NYPresby-Morgan Stanley Children's Hosp (page 104), Nyack Hosp; **Address:** Morgan Stanley Chldns Hosp, 3959 Broadway, CHN-106, Ped Rheumatology, New York, NY 10032; **Phone:** 212-305-9304; **Board Cert:** Pediatrics 1983; Pediatric Rheumatology 2007; **Med School:** Ros Franklin Univ/Chicago Med Sch 1978; **Resid:** Pediatrics, Mt Sinai Hosp 1982; **Fellow:** Pediatric Rheumatology, Chldns Hosp 1984; **Fac Appt:** Asst Clin Prof Ped, Columbia P&S

Lazarus, Herbert MD (PRhu) - **Spec Exp:** Juvenile Arthritis; Lyme Disease; Pain-Musculoskeletal; **Hospital:** NYU Langone Med Ctr (page 106), Lenox Hill Hosp; **Address:** 390 West End Ave, rm 1E, New York, NY 10024; **Phone:** 212-787-1444; **Board Cert:** Pediatrics 1987; Pediatric Rheumatology 2007; **Med School:** UMDNJ-NJ Med Sch, Newark 1983; **Resid:** Pediatrics, NYU Med Ctr 1986; **Fellow:** Pediatric Rheumatology, Hosp for Joint Diseases 1987; **Fac Appt:** Asst Clin Prof Ped, NYU Sch Med

Lehman, Thomas MD (PRhu) - **Spec Exp:** Arthritis; Scleroderma; Lupus/SLE; Rheumatoid Arthritis; **Hospital:** Hosp For Special Surgery (page 111), NY-Presby Hosp/Weill Cornell (page 104); **Address:** 535 E 70th St, New York, NY 10021-4872; **Phone:** 212-606-1151; **Board Cert:** Pediatrics 1979; Pediatric Rheumatology 2007; **Med School:** Jefferson Med Coll 1974; **Resid:** Pediatrics, Chldns Hosp 1976; Pediatrics, UCSF Med Ctr 1977; **Fellow:** Pediatric Rheumatology, Chldns Hosp 1979; Rheumatology, Natl Inst Hlth 1983; **Fac Appt:** Prof Ped, Cornell Univ-Weill Med Coll

Pediatric Surgery

Bodenstein, Lawrence MD/PhD (PS) - **Hospital:** NYPresby-Morgan Stanley Children's Hosp (page 104); **Address:** 3959 Broadway, CHN-215 Fl 2 North, New York, NY 10032; **Phone:** 212-305-2648; **Board Cert:** Surgery 2003; Pediatric Surgery 2005; **Med School:** Harvard Med Sch 1986; **Resid:** Surgery, Beth Israel Hosp 1991; **Fellow:** Critical Care Medicine, Beth Israel Hosp 1992; Pediatric Surgery, Babies Hosp-Columbia Presb 1994; **Fac Appt:** Asst Prof S, Columbia P&S

Cooper, Arthur MD (PS) - **Spec Exp:** Endoscopy; Trauma; Disaster Preparedness; Child Abuse; **Hospital:** Harlem Hosp Ctr, Metropolitan Hosp Ctr - NY; **Address:** Harlem Hospital, Dept Surgery, 506 Lenox Ave, New York, NY 10037; **Phone:** 212-939-4003; **Board Cert:** Surgery 2002; Pediatric Surgery 2003; Surgical Critical Care 2004; **Med School:** Univ Pennsylvania 1975; **Resid:** Surgery, Hosp Univ Penn 1981; Pediatric Surgery, Childrens Hosp 1984; **Fellow:** Pediatric Nutrition, Columbia P&S-Inst Human Nutrition 1982; **Fac Appt:** Prof S, Columbia P&S

Ginsburg, Howard B MD (PS) - **Spec Exp:** Neonatal Surgery; Tumor Surgery; Pediatric Urology; Gastrointestinal Surgery; **Hospital:** NYU Langone Med Ctr (page 106), Bellevue Hosp Ctr; **Address:** NYU Medical Ctr, Div Pediatric Surgery, 530 1st Ave, Ste 10W, New York, NY 10016-6402; **Phone:** 212-263-7391; **Board Cert:** Pediatric Surgery 2001; **Med School:** Univ Cincinnati 1972; **Resid:** Surgery, NYU-Bellvue Hosp 1977; Pediatric Surgery, Columbia-Presby Med Ctr 1979; **Fellow:** Pediatric Surgery, Mass Genl Hosp 1980; **Fac Appt:** Assoc Prof S, NYU Sch Med

La Quaglia, Michael MD (PS) - **Spec Exp:** Cancer Surgery; Neuroblastoma; Liver Cancer; Colon & Rectal Cancer; **Hospital:** Meml Sloan-Kettering Cancer Ctr (page 112), NY-Presby Hosp/Weill Cornell (page 104); **Address:** 1275 York Ave, Ste H1315, New York, NY 10065; **Phone:** 212-639-7002; **Board Cert:** Surgery 2003; Pediatric Surgery 2007; **Med School:** UMDNJ-NJ Med Sch, Newark 1976; **Resid:** Surgery, Mass Genl Hosp 1983; **Fellow:** Cardiothoracic Surgery, Broadgreen Ctr 1984; Pediatric Surgery, Chldns Hosp 1985; **Fac Appt:** Prof S, Cornell Univ-Weill Med Coll

Middlesworth, William MD (PS) - **Spec Exp:** Cancer Surgery; **Hospital:** NYPresby-Morgan Stanley Children's Hosp (page 104); **Address:** Morgan Stanley Children's Hospital, Div Pediatric Surgery, 3959 Broadway, CHN 206, New York, NY 10032-1537; **Phone:** 212-342-8585; **Board Cert:** Surgery 2007; Pediatric Surgery 2007; **Med School:** UMDNJ-RW Johnson Med Sch 1989; **Resid:** Surgery, Univ Maryland Hosps 1995; **Fellow:** Pediatric Surgery, Columbia Presby Med Ctr 1997; **Fac Appt:** Asst Prof S, Columbia P&S

Quaegebeur, Jan M MD (PS) - **Spec Exp:** Arterial Switch; Heart Valve Surgery; Pediatric Cardiac Surgery; **Hospital:** NYPresby-Morgan Stanley Children's Hosp (page 104); **Address:** Morgan Stanley Chlds Hosp of NY-Presby, 3959 Broadway, Ste 276, New York, NY 10032; **Phone:** 212-305-5975; **Med School:** Belgium 1969; **Resid:** Surgery, St Michel Clinic 1973; **Fellow:** Thoracic Surgery, Baylor Coll Med 1974; Thoracic Surgery, Univ Hosp 1978; **Fac Appt:** Prof S, Columbia P&S

Stolar, Charles J H MD (PS) - **Spec Exp:** Neonatal Surgery; Hernia; Pediatric Cancers; **Hospital:** NYPresby-Morgan Stanley Children's Hosp (page 104); **Address:** Morgan Stanley Chldns Hosp NY-Presby, 3959 Broadway, Fl 2 - rm 215 North, New York, NY 10032; **Phone:** 212-342-8586; **Board Cert:** Surgery 2001; Pediatric Surgery 2007; **Med School:** Georgetown Univ 1974; **Resid:** Surgery, Univ Illinois Hosp 1980; **Fellow:** Pediatric Surgery, Chldns Hosp Natl Med Ctr 1982; **Fac Appt:** Prof S, Columbia P&S

Velcek, Francisca T MD (PS) - **Spec Exp:** Anorectal Malformations; Pediatric Gynecology; Neonatal Surgery; Hernia; **Hospital:** Lenox Hill Hosp, Long Island Coll Hosp (page 94); **Address:** 965 5th Ave, New York, NY 10021; **Phone:** 212-744-9396; **Board Cert:** Surgery 1974; Pediatric Surgery 2007; **Med School:** Philippines 1966; **Resid:** Surgery, St Clares Hosp 1971; Pediatric Surgery, SUNY Downstate Med Ctr 1975; **Fellow:** Pediatric Surgery, SUNY Downstate Med Ctr 1973; **Fac Appt:** Prof S, SUNY Hlth Sci Ctr

Pediatrics

Allendorf, Dennis MD (Ped) *PCP* - **Spec Exp:** Congenital Anomalies; **Hospital:** NYPresby-Morgan Stanley Children's Hosp (page 104), St Luke's - Roosevelt Hosp Ctr - Roosevelt Div (page 94); **Address:** 401 W 118th St, Ste 2, New York, NY 10027-7216; **Phone:** 212-666-4610; **Board Cert:** Pediatrics 1987; **Med School:** NY Med Coll 1970; **Resid:** Pediatrics, St Luke's-Roosevelt Hosp Ctr 1972; Pediatrics, Columbia-Presby Hosp 1973; **Fac Appt:** Asst Clin Prof Ped, Columbia P&S

Arpadi, Stephen MD (Ped) *PCP* - **Spec Exp:** AIDS/HIV; **Hospital:** St Luke's - Roosevelt Hosp Ctr - St Luke's Hosp (page 94), NY-Presby Hosp/Columbia (page 104); **Address:** 1111 Amsterdam Ave at 114th St, New York, NY 10025; **Phone:** 212-523-3847; **Board Cert:** Pediatrics 1987; **Med School:** Geo Wash Univ 1982; **Resid:** Pediatrics, Chldns Hosp Natl Med Ctr 1985; **Fac Appt:** Assoc Prof Ped, Columbia P&S

Axelrod, Felicia B MD (Ped) - **Spec Exp:** Dysautonomia; **Hospital:** NYU Langone Med Ctr (page 106); **Address:** New York Med Ctr, 530 1St Av, Ste 9Q, New York, NY 10016-6402; **Phone:** 212-263-7225; **Board Cert:** Pediatrics 1971; **Med School:** NYU Sch Med 1966; **Resid:** Pediatrics, Bellevue/NYU Med Ctr 1969; **Fellow:** Genetics, Mt Sinai Med Ctr 1976; **Fac Appt:** Prof Ped, NYU Sch Med

Brovender, Bruce J MD (Ped) *PCP* - **Hospital:** NY-Presby Hosp/Weill Cornell (page 104), Mount Sinai Med Ctr (page 102); **Address:** 1559 York Ave, New York, NY 10028; **Phone:** 212-585-3329; **Board Cert:** Pediatrics 2004; **Med School:** Italy 1984; **Resid:** Pediatrics, Lenox Hill Hosp 1987; **Fellow:** Pediatric Hematology-Oncology, NYU/Bellvue Hosp 1988; **Fac Appt:** Asst Clin Prof Ped, Cornell Univ-Weill Med Coll

Burstin, Harris E MD (Ped) *PCP* - **Spec Exp:** Asthma; Allergy; Critical Care; **Hospital:** NYU Langone Med Ctr (page 106); **Address:** 317 E 34th St Fl 3, New York, NY 10016-4974; **Phone:** 212-725-6300; **Board Cert:** Pediatrics 1983; **Med School:** Mexico 1977; **Resid:** Pediatrics, Bellevue Hosp Ctr 1982; **Fac Appt:** Assoc Prof Ped, NYU Sch Med

Cohen, Michel A MD (Ped) *PCP* - **Spec Exp:** Child Development; Sleep Disorders; **Hospital:** NYU Langone Med Ctr (page 106), NY-Presby Hosp/Weill Cornell (page 104); **Address:** Tribeca Pediatrics, 46 Warren St, New York, NY 10007; **Phone:** 212-226-7666; **Board Cert:** Pediatrics 2003; **Med School:** France 1989; **Resid:** Pediatrics, New York Univ Med Ctr 1991; Pediatrics, Long Island Hosp 1993

Cross, Jennifer MD (Ped) - **Spec Exp:** Learning Disorders; Child Development; Behavioral Disorders; **Hospital:** NY-Presby Hosp/Weill Cornell (page 104); **Address:** 525 E 68th St, New York, NY 10065; **Phone:** 646-962-4303; **Board Cert:** Pediatrics 2005; Developmental-Behavioral Pediatrics 2002; **Med School:** England, UK 1983; **Resid:** Pediatrics, Lenox Hill Hosp 1988; **Fellow:** Neonatal-Perinatal Medicine, NY Hosp 1991; Developmental-Behavioral Pediatrics, Westchester Co Med Ctr 1994; **Fac Appt:** Asst Prof Ped, Cornell Univ-Weill Med Coll

Edelstein, Gary S MD (Ped) *PCP* - **Hospital:** NYPresby-Morgan Stanley Children's Hosp (page 104), NY-Presby Hosp/Weill Cornell (page 104); **Address:** Manhattan Pediatrics, 16 E 60th St, Ste 410, New York, NY 10022; **Phone:** 212-326-3351; **Board Cert:** Pediatrics 2008; **Med School:** NYU Sch Med 1990; **Resid:** Pediatrics, Columbia Presby Babies Hosp 1993; **Fellow:** Ambulatory Pediatrics, Columbia Presby Babies Hosp 1995

Ferrier, Genevieve MD (Ped) *PCP* - **Spec Exp:** Developmental & Behavioral Disorders; **Hospital:** NY Downtown Hosp, NYU Langone Med Ctr (page 106); **Address:** 46 W 11th St, New York, NY 10011-8602; **Phone:** 212-529-4330; **Board Cert:** Pediatrics 2006; **Med School:** Mount Sinai Sch Med 1988; **Resid:** Pediatrics, Chldn's Hosp 1991; **Fac Appt:** Asst Prof Ped, NY Med Coll

Goldstein, Judith MD (Ped) *PCP* - **Spec Exp:** Newborn Care; Infectious Disease; **Hospital:** NY-Presby Hosp/Weill Cornell (page 104), Lenox Hill Hosp; **Address:** 1559 York Ave, New York, NY 10028; **Phone:** 212-585-3329; **Board Cert:** Pediatrics 1977; **Med School:** SUNY Downstate 1972; **Resid:** Pediatrics, Lenox Hill Hosp 1975; **Fac Appt:** Asst Clin Prof Ped, Cornell Univ-Weill Med Coll

Inamdar, Sarla MD (Ped) *PCP* - **Spec Exp:** Pediatric Rheumatology; **Hospital:** Metropolitan Hosp Ctr - NY; **Address:** 1901 1st Ave, rm 523, New York, NY 10029-7404; **Phone:** 212-423-6228; **Board Cert:** Pediatrics 1974; **Med School:** India 1969; **Resid:** Pediatrics, Metropolitan Hosp Ctr 1972; **Fac Appt:** Clin Prof Ped, NY Med Coll

Kahn, Max MD (Ped) *PCP* - **Hospital:** NYU Langone Med Ctr (page 106), Lenox Hill Hosp; **Address:** 390 West End Ave, Ste 1E, New York, NY 10024; **Phone:** 212-787-1444; **Board Cert:** Pediatrics 1980; **Med School:** Columbia P&S 1975; **Resid:** Pediatrics, Bronx Muni Hosp 1978; **Fac Appt:** Assoc Clin Prof Ped, NYU Sch Med

Keith, Marie B MD (Ped) *PCP* - **Hospital:** NYU Langone Med Ctr (page 106); **Address:** 552 Broadway Fl 5, New York, NY 10012; **Phone:** 212-334-3366; **Board Cert:** Pediatrics 1979; **Med School:** Mount Sinai Sch Med 1974; **Resid:** Pediatrics, NY Presby-Columbia Presby Medical Ctr 1978

Kotin, Neal M MD (Ped) *PCP* - **Spec Exp:** Asthma; Bronchitis; Sleep Disorders; Pulmonary Disease; **Hospital:** Mount Sinai Med Ctr (page 102), Lenox Hill Hosp; **Address:** Carnegie Hill Pediatrics, 1125 Park Ave, New York, NY 10128-1243; **Phone:** 212-289-1400; **Board Cert:** Pediatrics 2005; Pediatric Pulmonology 2004; **Med School:** Albany Med Coll 1982; **Resid:** Pediatrics, Johns Hopkins Hosp 1985; **Fellow:** Pediatric Pulmonology, Mt Sinai Med Ctr 1988; **Fac Appt:** Asst Clin Prof Ped, Mount Sinai Sch Med

Laraque, Danielle MD (Ped) *PCP* - **Spec Exp:** Child Abuse; Mental Health-Child; Adolescent Behavior-High Risk; **Hospital:** Maimonides Med Ctr (page 98); **Address:** Maimonides Med Ctr, Dept Pediatrics, 977 48th St, Brooklyn, NY 11219; **Phone:** 718-283-6150; **Board Cert:** Pediatrics 1986; Child Abuse Pediatrics 2009; **Med School:** UCLA 1981; **Resid:** Pediatrics, Childrens Hosp 1984; **Fellow:** Academic Pediatrics, Childrens Hosp 1986

Larson, Signe S MD (Ped) *PCP* - **Spec Exp:** Pediatric Endocrinology; **Hospital:** Mount Sinai Med Ctr (page 102); **Address:** Uptowm Padiatrics, 1245 Park Ave, New York, NY 10128; **Phone:** 212-427-0540; **Board Cert:** Pediatrics 1984; Pediatric Endocrinology 2004; **Med School:** SUNY Stony Brook 1978; **Resid:** Family Medicine, Vancouver Genl Hosp 1979; Pediatrics, St Luke's Med Ctr 1982; **Fellow:** Pediatric Endocrinology, Mt Sinai Hosp 1984

Lazarus, George M MD (Ped) *PCP* - **Hospital:** NYPresby-Morgan Stanley Children's Hosp (page 104), NY-Presby Hosp/Weill Cornell (page 104); **Address:** 106 E 78th Street, New York, NY 10021-0302; **Phone:** 212-744-0840; **Board Cert:** Pediatrics 1976; **Med School:** Columbia P&S 1971; **Resid:** Pediatrics, NY Presby-Columbia Med Ctr 1974; **Fac Appt:** Assoc Clin Prof Ped, Columbia P&S

Levitzky, Susan L MD (Ped) *PCP* - **Spec Exp:** Asthma; Child Development; Adoption & Foster Care; **Hospital:** NYU Langone Med Ctr (page 106), Beth Israel Med Ctr - Petrie Division (page 94); **Address:** 161 Madison Ave, Ste 6W, New York, NY 10016-5405; **Phone:** 212-213-1960; **Board Cert:** Pediatrics 1972; **Med School:** Univ IL Coll Med 1967; **Resid:** Pediatrics, Beth Israel Hosp 1970; **Fac Appt:** Asst Clin Prof Ped, NYU Sch Med

McCarton, Cecelia MD (Ped) - **Spec Exp:** Autism; Learning Disorders; ADD/ADHD; Developmental Disorders; **Hospital:** Montefiore Med Ctr - Div. Weiler (page 100); **Address:** McCarton Ctr for Developmental Pediatrics, 350 E 82nd St, New York, NY 10028; **Phone:** 212-996-9019; **Board Cert:** Pediatrics 1988; **Med School:** Albert Einstein Coll Med 1970; **Resid:** Pediatrics, Bronx Muni Hosp Ctr 1974; **Fellow:** Developmental-Behavioral Pediatrics, Montefiore Med Ctr- Weiler Einstein Div 1977; **Fac Appt:** Prof Ped, Albert Einstein Coll Med

McHugh, Margaret T MD (Ped) - **Spec Exp:** Child Abuse; Adolescent Medicine; **Hospital:** Bellevue Hosp Ctr, NYU Langone Med Ctr (page 106); **Address:** Bellevue Hosp Ctr-Pediatrics, 462 First Ave, rm GC65, New York, NY 10016; **Phone:** 212-562-6073; **Board Cert:** Pediatrics 1975; **Med School:** Georgetown Univ 1970; **Resid:** Pediatrics, Metropolitan Hosp 1973; **Fellow:** Ambulatory Pediatrics, Columbia-Presby Med Ctr 1975; **Fac Appt:** Assoc Prof Ped, NYU Sch Med

Monti, Louis G MD (Ped) *PCP* - **Spec Exp:** Infectious Disease; **Hospital:** Mount Sinai Med Ctr (page 102); **Address:** 55 E 87th St, Ste 1G, New York, NY 10128-1049; **Phone:** 212-722-0707; **Board Cert:** Pediatrics 2009; **Med School:** Mount Sinai Sch Med 1980; **Resid:** Pediatrics, Mount Sinai Hosp 1983; **Fellow:** Infectious Disease, Childrens Hosp 1984; **Fac Appt:** Asst Clin Prof Ped, Mount Sinai Sch Med

Murphy, Ramon J C MD (Ped) *PCP* - **Spec Exp:** Community Medicine; **Hospital:** Mount Sinai Med Ctr (page 102); **Address:** Uptown Pediatrics, 1245 Park Ave, New York, NY 10128; **Phone:** 212-427-0540; **Board Cert:** Pediatrics 2009; **Med School:** Northwestern Univ 1969; **Resid:** Internal Medicine, Cook Co Hosp 1970; Pediatrics, Chldns Meml Hosp 1971; **Fellow:** Pediatrics, Babies Hosp 1973; Community Medicine, Mt Sinai Med Ctr 1974; **Fac Appt:** Clin Prof Ped, Mount Sinai Sch Med

Newman-Cedar, Meryl MD (Ped) *PCP* - **Spec Exp:** Child Development; **Hospital:** NY-Presby Hosp/Weill Cornell (page 104), Lenox Hill Hosp; **Address:** 215 E 79th St, Ste 1C, New York, NY 10075; **Phone:** 212-737-7800; **Board Cert:** Pediatrics 1987; **Med School:** SUNY Downstate 1981; **Resid:** Pediatrics, New York Hosp 1984; **Fellow:** Developmental-Behavioral Pediatrics, New York Hosp 1987

Oeffinger, Kevin MD (Ped) - **Spec Exp:** Cancer Survivors-Late Effects of Therapy; **Hospital:** Meml Sloan-Kettering Cancer Ctr (page 112); **Address:** 300 E 66th St, New York, NY 10065; **Phone:** 800-525-2225; **Board Cert:** Family Medicine 2006; **Med School:** Univ Tex, San Antonio 1984; **Resid:** Family Medicine, Baylor Coll Med 1985; **Fellow:** Family Medicine, Fam Practice Faculty Dev Ctr 1999Natl Cancer Inst 2000

Poon, Eric Sin-Kam MD (Ped) *PCP* - **Spec Exp:** Asthma; Pediatric Cardiology; Developmental Disorders; **Hospital:** NY Downtown Hosp, NY-Presby Hosp/Weill Cornell (page 104); **Address:** 170 William St Fl 3, New York, NY 10038-2612; **Phone:** 212-312-5350; **Board Cert:** Pediatrics 1988; **Med School:** Mexico 1982; **Resid:** Pediatrics, LI Coll Hosp 1986; **Fellow:** Pediatric Cardiology, NY Hosp-Cornell Med Ctr 1988; **Fac Appt:** Asst Clin Prof Ped, Cornell Univ-Weill Med Coll

Popper, Laura MD (Ped) *PCP* - **Hospital:** Mount Sinai Med Ctr (page 102); **Address:** 116 E 66th St, Ste 1C, New York, NY 10021-6547; **Phone:** 212-794-2136; **Board Cert:** Pediatrics 1981; **Med School:** Columbia P&S 1974; **Resid:** Pediatrics, Babies Hosp 1976; **Fellow:** Pediatrics, Babies Hosp 1977; **Fac Appt:** Asst Clin Prof Ped, NY Coll Osteo Med

Prezioso, Paula J MD (Ped) *PCP* - **Spec Exp:** Behavioral Disorders; **Hospital:** NYU Langone Med Ctr (page 106); **Address:** 317 E 34th St, Fl 3, New York, NY 10016-4974; **Phone:** 212-725-6300; **Board Cert:** Pediatrics 2006; **Med School:** SUNY Downstate 1987; **Resid:** Pediatrics, NYU-Bellevue Hosp 1991; **Fac Appt:** Asst Clin Prof Ped, NYU Sch Med

Prince, Alice MD (Ped) - **Spec Exp:** Pediatric Infectious Disease; **Hospital:** NYPresby-Morgan Stanley Children's Hosp (page 104); **Address:** 650 W 168th St, New York, NY 10032-3702; **Phone:** 212-305-4193; **Board Cert:** Pediatrics 1979; Pediatric Infectious Disease 2009; **Med School:** Columbia P&S 1975; **Resid:** Pediatrics, Babies Hosp 1978; **Fellow:** Infectious Disease, Columbia Univ 1981; **Fac Appt:** Prof Ped, Columbia P&S

Raucher, Harold S MD (Ped) *PCP* - **Spec Exp:** Infectious Disease; Travel Medicine; **Hospital:** Mount Sinai Med Ctr (page 102), Lenox Hill Hosp; **Address:** Carnegie Hill Pediatrics, 1125 Park Ave, New York, NY 10128-1243; **Phone:** 212-289-1400; **Board Cert:** Pediatrics 2006; Pediatric Infectious Disease 2009; **Med School:** Mount Sinai Sch Med 1978; **Resid:** Pediatrics, Mt Sinai Med Ctr 1980; **Fellow:** Pediatric Infectious Disease, Mt Sinai Med Ctr 1982; **Fac Appt:** Assoc Clin Prof Ped, Mount Sinai Sch Med

Rosello, Lori J MD (Ped) *PCP* - **Hospital:** NYU Langone Med Ctr (page 106); **Address:** 46 W 11th St, New York, NY 10011-8602; **Phone:** 212-529-4330; **Board Cert:** Pediatrics 2005; **Med School:** Albert Einstein Coll Med 1987; **Resid:** Pediatrics, Babies Hosp/Columbia 1990; **Fac Appt:** Asst Clin Prof Ped, NYU Sch Med

Rosenbaum, Michael MD (Ped) *PCP* - **Spec Exp:** Nutrition; Growth Disorders; Obesity; **Hospital:** NYPresby-Morgan Stanley Children's Hosp (page 104); **Address:** 450 West End Ave, New York, NY 10024-5307; **Phone:** 212-769-3070; **Board Cert:** Pediatrics 1988; **Med School:** Cornell Univ-Weill Med Coll 1982; **Resid:** Pediatrics, Columbia-Presby Med Ctr 1985; **Fellow:** Pediatric Endocrinology, New York Hosp 1988; **Fac Appt:** Assoc Prof Ped, Columbia P&S

Rosenfeld, Suzanne MD (Ped) *PCP* - **Spec Exp:** Developmental Disorders; Asthma; **Hospital:** NY-Presby Hosp/Weill Cornell (page 104), Lenox Hill Hosp; **Address:** 450 West End Ave, New York, NY 10024-5393; **Phone:** 212-769-3070; **Board Cert:** Pediatrics 1986; **Med School:** Columbia P&S 1980; **Resid:** Pediatrics, Columbia-Presby Med Ctr 1983; **Fellow:** Pediatrics, NY Hosp-Cornell Med Ctr 1984

Sacker, Ira MD (Ped) - **Spec Exp:** Eating Disorders; Obesity; **Hospital:** NYU Langone Med Ctr (page 106); **Address:** 19 W 34th St, Penthouse Fl, New York, NY 10016; **Phone:** 212-268-4440; **Board Cert:** Pediatrics 1982; **Med School:** UCLA 1968; **Resid:** Pediatrics, Bellevue Hosp/NYU Med Ctr 1972; **Fellow:** Adolescent Medicine, Chldns Hosp 1972; **Fac Appt:** Asst Clin Prof Ped, NYU Sch Med

Sanford, Marie MD (Ped) *PCP* - **Hospital:** Mount Sinai Med Ctr (page 102); **Address:** Westside Pediatrics, 620 Columbus Ave, Ste 1, New York, NY 10011; **Phone:** 212-874-4500; **Board Cert:** Pediatrics 2009; **Med School:** Mount Sinai Sch Med 1991; **Resid:** Pediatrics, Mount Sinai Med Ctr 1995; **Fac Appt:** Asst Clin Prof Ped, Mount Sinai Sch Med

Softness, Barney MD (Ped) *PCP* - **Spec Exp:** Diabetes; **Hospital:** NYPresby-Morgan Stanley Children's Hosp (page 104), NYU Langone Med Ctr (page 106); **Address:** 450 West End Ave, New York, NY 10024-5307; **Phone:** 212-769-3070; **Board Cert:** Pediatrics 1986; Pediatric Endocrinology 1986; **Med School:** Columbia P&S 1980; **Resid:** Pediatrics, Columbia Presby Med Ctr 1983; **Fellow:** Pediatric Endocrinology, NY Cornell Med Ctr 1985; **Fac Appt:** Assoc Clin Prof Ped, Columbia P&S

Stein, Barry B MD (Ped) *PCP* - **Spec Exp:** Developmental & Behavioral Disorders; **Hospital:** Mount Sinai Med Ctr (page 102), Lenox Hill Hosp; **Address:** Carnegie Hill Pediatrics, 1125 Park Ave, New York, NY 10128-1243; **Phone:** 212-289-1400; **Board Cert:** Pediatrics 1987; **Med School:** South Africa 1980; **Resid:** Pediatrics, Mt Sinai Hosp 1986; **Fac Appt:** Asst Clin Prof Ped, Mount Sinai Sch Med

Traister, Michael R MD (Ped) *PCP* - **Spec Exp:** Adoption & Foster Care; **Hospital:** NYU Langone Med Ctr (page 106), Lenox Hill Hosp; **Address:** 390 West End Ave, Ste 1E, New York, NY 10024; **Phone:** 212-787-1444; **Board Cert:** Pediatrics 1980; **Med School:** NY Med Coll 1975; **Resid:** Pediatrics, Bronx Municipal Hosp 1978; **Fellow:** Ambulatory Pediatrics, Bellevue Hosp 1979; **Fac Appt:** Asst Clin Prof Ped, NYU Sch Med

Weinberger, Sylvain M MD (Ped) *PCP* - **Spec Exp:** Prematurity/Low Birth Weight Infants; **Hospital:** NYU Langone Med Ctr (page 106), Beth Israel Med Ctr - Petrie Division (page 94); **Address:** 51 E 25 St Fl 3, New York, NY 10010; **Phone:** 212-598-0331; **Board Cert:** Pediatrics 1982; Neonatal-Perinatal Medicine 1983; **Med School:** Belgium 1977; **Resid:** Pediatrics, LI Jewish Med Ctr 1979; **Fellow:** Neonatal-Perinatal Medicine, LI Jewish Med Ctr 1981; **Fac Appt:** Asst Clin Prof Ped, NYU Sch Med

Zimmerman, Sol MD (Ped) *PCP* - **Spec Exp:** Growth/Development Disorders; Behavioral Disorders; Cough-Tic Syndrome; **Hospital:** NYU Langone Med Ctr (page 106); **Address:** 317 E 34th St, New York, NY 10016-4974; **Phone:** 212-725-6300; **Board Cert:** Pediatrics 1977; **Med School:** NYU Sch Med 1972; **Resid:** Pediatrics, Bellevue Hosp Ctr 1975; Pediatrics, Bellevue Hosp/NYU 1978; **Fac Appt:** Assoc Prof Ped, NYU Sch Med

Physical Medicine & Rehabilitation

Ahn, Jung Hwan MD (PMR) - **Spec Exp:** Spinal Cord Injury; Stroke Rehabilitation; Neurologic Rehabilitation; **Hospital:** NYU Langone Med Ctr (page 106); **Address:** 400 E 34th St, rm 421, New York, NY 10016-4901; **Phone:** 212-263-6122; **Board Cert:** Physical Medicine & Rehabilitation 1980; Spinal Cord Injury Medicine 1998; **Med School:** South Korea 1970; **Resid:** Obstetrics & Gynecology, Elmhurst City Hosp - Mt Sinai 1976; Physical Medicine & Rehabilitation, NYU Med Ctr 1979; **Fellow:** Spinal Cord Injury Medicine, NYU Med Ctr 1980; **Fac Appt:** Clin Prof PMR, NYU Sch Med

Brown, Andrew MD (PMR) - **Spec Exp:** Electromyography; **Hospital:** NY Downtown Hosp; **Address:** 19 Beekman St, New York, NY 10038; **Phone:** 212-513-7711; **Board Cert:** Physical Medicine & Rehabilitation 1988; **Med School:** West Indies 1982; **Resid:** Pediatrics, Univ Md Hosp 1984; Physical Medicine & Rehabilitation, Mount Sinai Med Ctr 1987

Bryce, Thomas MD (PMR) - **Spec Exp:** Spinal Cord Injury; Pain-Neuropathic; **Hospital:** Mount Sinai Med Ctr (page 102); **Address:** Rehab Medicine Assocs, 5 E 98th St, Box 1240B, New York, NY 10029; **Phone:** 212-241-6321; **Board Cert:** Physical Medicine & Rehabilitation 2008; Spinal Cord Injury Medicine 2000; Pain Medicine 2002; **Med School:** Albany Med Coll 1993; **Resid:** Physical Medicine & Rehabilitation, Thomas Jefferson Univ Hosp 1997

Dillard, James N MD (PMR) - **Spec Exp:** Pain Management; Acupuncture; Complementary Medicine; Nutrition; **Hospital:** Southampton Hosp; **Address:** 110 E 59th St, Ste 10A, New York, NY 10022; **Phone:** 212-265-4038; **Board Cert:** Physical Medicine & Rehabilitation 2005; **Med School:** Rush Med Coll 1990; **Resid:** Physical Medicine & Rehabilitation, Columbia-Presby Med Ctr 1994; **Fac Appt:** Asst Clin Prof PMR, Columbia P&S

Feinberg, Joseph H MD (PMR) - **Spec Exp:** Peripheral Neuropathy; Spinal Rehabilitation; Electrodiagnosis; Sports Medicine; **Hospital:** Hosp For Special Surgery (page 111), Kessler Inst for Rehab - W Orange; **Address:** 535 E 70th St, New York, NY 10021-4872; **Phone:** 212-606-1568; **Board Cert:** Physical Medicine & Rehabilitation 1991; **Med School:** Albany Med Coll 1983; **Resid:** Surgery, Mt Sinai Hosp 1985; Physical Medicine & Rehabilitation, Rusk Inst Rehab 1990; **Fellow:** Orthopaedic Pathology, Hosp Spec Surg 1986; Orthopaedic Biomechanics, Univ Iowa Hosp & Clins 1987; **Fac Appt:** Assoc Prof PMR, Cornell Univ-Weill Med Coll

Flanagan, Steven R MD (PMR) - **Spec Exp:** Brain Injury Rehabilitation; Stroke Rehabilitation; **Hospital:** NYU Langone Med Ctr (page 106), NYU Hosp For Joint Diseases (page 106); **Address:** Rusk Institute, 400 E 34th St, New York, NY 10016; **Phone:** 212-263-6105; **Board Cert:** Physical Medicine & Rehabilitation 2003; **Med School:** UMDNJ-NJ Med Sch, Newark 1988; **Resid:** Physical Medicine & Rehabilitation, Mt Sinai Hosp 1992; **Fac Appt:** Prof PMR, NYU Sch Med

Gold, Joan T MD (PMR) - **Spec Exp:** Cerebral Palsy; Spina Bifida; Pediatric Rehabilitation; **Hospital:** NYU Langone Med Ctr (page 106), NYU Hosp For Joint Diseases (page 106); **Address:** 400 E 34th St, Ste 518, New York, NY 10016-4901; **Phone:** 212-263-6519; **Board Cert:** Pediatrics 1979; Physical Medicine & Rehabilitation 1981; Pediatric Rehabilitation Medicine 2008; **Med School:** SUNY Downstate 1974; **Resid:** Pediatrics, Beth Israel Med Ctr 1977; Physical Medicine & Rehabilitation, Inst Rehab Med-NYU 1979; **Fac Appt:** Clin Prof PMR, NYU Sch Med

Gotlin, Robert S DO (PMR) - **Spec Exp:** Sports Medicine; Running Injuries; Pain-Coccyx; Pain-Knee & Shoulder; **Hospital:** Beth Israel Med Ctr - Petrie Division (page 94); **Address:** 245 Fifth Ave Fl 2, New York, NY 10016; **Phone:** 646-935-2255; **Board Cert:** Physical Medicine & Rehabilitation 1992; **Med School:** Southeastern Univ Coll Osteo Med 1987; **Resid:** Physical Medicine & Rehabilitation, Mount Sinai Hosp 1991; **Fac Appt:** Assoc Prof PMR, Albert Einstein Coll Med

Greenwald, Brian MD (PMR) - **Spec Exp:** Stroke Rehabilitation; Brain Injury Rehabilitation; **Hospital:** Mount Sinai Med Ctr (page 102), Elmhurst Hosp Ctr; **Address:** 5 E 98th St Fl 6, Box 1240B, New York, NY 10029; **Phone:** 212-241-3981; **Board Cert:** Physical Medicine & Rehabilitation 2000; **Med School:** SUNY Stony Brook 1995; **Resid:** Physical Medicine & Rehabilitation, UMDNJ-NJ Med Sch 1999; **Fellow:** Physical Medicine & Rehabilitation, Med Coll Va 2000; **Fac Appt:** Asst Prof PMR, Mount Sinai Sch Med

Inwald, Gary DO (PMR) - **Spec Exp:** Musculoskeletal Disorders; Pain Management; **Hospital:** Beth Israel Med Ctr - Petrie Division (page 94); **Address:** 24 E 12th St, Ste 302, New York, NY 10003; **Phone:** 212-807-6599; **Board Cert:** Physical Medicine & Rehabilitation 1983; **Med School:** Mich State Univ Coll Osteo Med 1976; **Resid:** Physical Medicine & Rehabilitation, St Vincents Hosp 1982

Lachmann, Elisabeth A MD (PMR) - **Spec Exp:** Pain-Back; Sports Medicine; Cancer Rehabilitation; **Hospital:** NY-Presby Hosp/Weill Cornell (page 104); **Address:** 115 E 64th St Fl 1, New York, NY 10065; **Phone:** 212-535-3005; **Board Cert:** Physical Medicine & Rehabilitation 1992; **Med School:** Med Coll PA Hahnemann 1987; **Resid:** Physical Medicine & Rehabilitation, NY-Cornell Med Ctr 1991; **Fac Appt:** Assoc Prof PMR, Cornell Univ-Weill Med Coll

Lee, Alexander J MD (PMR) - **Spec Exp:** Pain Management; **Hospital:** Beth Israel Med Ctr - Petrie Division (page 94); **Address:** NY Spine Inst, Beth Israel Med Ctr, 10 Union St E, Ste 5 P, New York, NY 10003; **Phone:** 212-844-8756; **Board Cert:** Physical Medicine & Rehabilitation 2009; Pain Medicine 2003; **Med School:** Wayne State Univ 1994; **Resid:** Physical Medicine & Rehabilitation, UMDNJ Affil Hosp 1998; **Fellow:** Pain Medicine, Beth Israel Med Ctr 1999

Lutz, Gregory MD (PMR) - **Spec Exp:** Spinal Rehabilitation; Sports Medicine; Pain-Low Back; **Hospital:** Hosp For Special Surgery (page 111), Univ Med Ctr - Princeton; **Address:** 535 E 70th St, New York, NY 10021; **Phone:** 212-606-1648; **Board Cert:** Physical Medicine & Rehabilitation 2003; **Med School:** Georgetown Univ 1988; **Resid:** Physical Medicine & Rehabilitation, Mayo Clinic 1992; **Fellow:** Sports Medicine, Hosp For Spec Surg 1993; **Fac Appt:** Assoc Prof PMR, Cornell Univ-Weill Med Coll

Ma, Dong M MD (PMR) - **Spec Exp:** Electromyography; Musculoskeletal Disorders; **Hospital:** NYU Rusk Inst (page 114), NYU Langone Med Ctr (page 106); **Address:** Rusk Institute, 400 E 34th St, rm 211, New York, NY 10016; **Phone:** 212-263-6338; **Board Cert:** Physical Medicine & Rehabilitation 1979; **Med School:** South Korea 1968; **Resid:** Physical Medicine & Rehabilitation, NYU Med Ctr 1975; **Fellow:** Physical Medicine & Rehabilitation, NYU Med Ctr 1977; **Fac Appt:** Clin Prof PMR, NYU Sch Med

Moldover, Jonathan MD (PMR) - **Spec Exp:** Spinal Rehabilitation; Pain-Chronic; Post Polio Syndrome/Rehabilitation; **Hospital:** Beth Israel Med Ctr - Petrie Division (page 94); **Address:** 200 W 57th St, Ste 608, New York, NY 10019-3211; **Phone:** 212-581-4488; **Board Cert:** Physical Medicine & Rehabilitation 1979; Pain Medicine 2002; **Med School:** Columbia P&S 1974; **Resid:** Internal Medicine, Strong Meml Hosp 1976; Physical Medicine & Rehabilitation, Columbia-Presby Med Ctr 1978; **Fac Appt:** Assoc Clin Prof PMR, Albert Einstein Coll Med

Ragnarsson, Kristjan T MD (PMR) - **Spec Exp:** Spinal Cord Injury; Brain Injury Rehabilitation; Pain-Back & Neck; **Hospital:** Mount Sinai Med Ctr (page 102); **Address:** 5 E 98th St Fl 6, New York, NY 10029-6501; **Phone:** 212-659-9370; **Board Cert:** Physical Medicine & Rehabilitation 1976; **Med School:** Iceland 1969; **Resid:** Physical Medicine & Rehabilitation, NYU Med Ctr 1974; **Fellow:** Spinal Cord & Brain Injury Rehab, NYU Med Ctr 1975; **Fac Appt:** Prof PMR, Mount Sinai Sch Med

Rho, Dae Sik MD (PMR) - **Spec Exp:** Sports Medicine; Pain Management; **Hospital:** Lenox Hill Hosp; **Address:** 100 E 77th St, New York, NY 10021; **Phone:** 212-434-2465; **Board Cert:** Physical Medicine & Rehabilitation 1980; **Med School:** South Korea 1962; **Resid:** Physical Medicine & Rehabilitation, NYU Med Ctr 1975; **Fac Appt:** Asst Clin Prof PMR, Cornell Univ-Weill Med Coll

Sheth, Parag MD (PMR) - **Spec Exp:** Musculoskeletal Disorders; **Hospital:** Mount Sinai Med Ctr (page 102); **Address:** Mount Sinai Medical Ctr, 5 E 98th St, Box 1240B, New York, NY 10029; **Phone:** 212-241-6321; **Board Cert:** Physical Medicine & Rehabilitation 2004; Pain Medicine 2002; **Med School:** SUNY Stony Brook 1987; **Resid:** Physical Medicine & Rehabilitation, St Vincent's Med Ctr 1993; **Fac Appt:** Asst Prof PMR, Mount Sinai Sch Med

Stein, Joel MD (PMR) - **Spec Exp:** Stroke Rehabilitation; **Hospital:** NY-Presby Hosp/Columbia (page 104); **Address:** 180 Fort Washington Ave, Ste 199, Harkness Pavilion, New York, NY 10032; **Phone:** 212-305-3535; **Board Cert:** Internal Medicine 1989; Physical Medicine & Rehabilitation 2003; **Med School:** Albert Einstein Coll Med 1986; **Resid:** Internal Medicine, Montefiore Med Ctr 1989; Physical Medicine & Rehabilitation, Columbia-Presby Med Ctr 1992

Strauss, Nancy E MD (PMR) - **Spec Exp:** Neuromuscular Disorders; **Hospital:** NY-Presby Hosp/Columbia (page 104), NY-Presby Hosp/Weill Cornell (page 104); **Address:** NY Presbyterian-Columbia Med Ctr, 180 Fort Washington Ave, New York, NY 10032; **Phone:** 212-305-3535; **Board Cert:** Physical Medicine & Rehabilitation 2003; Electrodiagnostic Medicine 2004; **Med School:** SUNY Upstate Med Univ 1988; **Resid:** Physical Medicine & Rehabilitation, Nassau Univ Med Ctr 1992; **Fac Appt:** Assoc Prof PMR, Columbia P&S

Stubblefield, Michael MD (PMR) - **Spec Exp:** Cancer Rehabilitation; Pain-Cancer; Pain-Neuropathic; Pain-Musculoskeletal; **Hospital:** Meml Sloan-Kettering Cancer Ctr (page 112), NY-Presby Hosp (page 104); **Address:** Meml Sloan-Kettering Cancer Ctr, 1275 York Ave, Box 349, New York, NY 10065; **Phone:** 646-888-1936; **Board Cert:** Internal Medicine 2001; Physical Medicine & Rehabilitation 2002; Electrodiagnostic Medicine 2003; **Med School:** Columbia P&S 1996; **Resid:** Internal Medicine, Columbia Presby Med Ctr 2001; Physical Medicine & Rehabilitation, Columbia Presby Med Ctr 2001; **Fac Appt:** Asst Prof PMR, Cornell Univ-Weill Med Coll

Thomas, David C MD (PMR) - **Hospital:** Mount Sinai Med Ctr (page 102); **Address:** Mount Sinai Med Ctr, 17 E 102nd St, Box 1087, New York, NY 10029; **Phone:** 212-824-7210; **Board Cert:** Internal Medicine 2007; Physical Medicine & Rehabilitation 2008; **Med School:** Hahnemann Univ 1991; **Resid:** Internal Medicine, Westchester Co Med Ctr 1996; Physical Medicine & Rehabilitation, Mount Sinai Hosp 1998; **Fac Appt:** Assoc Prof Med, Mount Sinai Sch Med

Vad, Vijay B MD (PMR) - **Spec Exp:** Sports Medicine-Golf & Tennis Injuries; Joint Pain-Minimally Invasive Therapy; Pain-Back; Pain-Knee & Shoulder; **Hospital:** Hosp For Special Surgery (page 111); **Address:** 535 E 70 St, New York, NY 10021; **Phone:** 212-606-1306; **Board Cert:** Physical Medicine & Rehabilitation 2007; Sports Medicine 2007; **Med School:** Univ Okla Coll Med 1992; **Resid:** Physical Medicine & Rehabilitation, Cornell Affil Hosp 1996; **Fellow:** Sports Medicine, Hosp Special Surgery 1997; **Fac Appt:** Asst Prof PMR, Cornell Univ-Weill Med Coll

Weiner, Kevin H MD (PMR) - **Hospital:** Beth Israel Med Ctr - Petrie Division (page 94); **Address:** 55 E 34 St Fl 3, New York, NY 10016; **Phone:** 212-252-6182; **Board Cert:** Physical Medicine & Rehabilitation 2009; **Med School:** Ros Franklin Univ/Chicago Med Sch 1994; **Resid:** Physical Medicine & Rehabilitation, NYU Med Ctr 1998

Plastic Surgery

Ahn, Christina Y MD (PIS) - **Spec Exp:** Breast Reconstruction; Cosmetic Surgery-Face; Cosmetic Surgery-Body; **Hospital:** NYU Langone Med Ctr (page 106), Lenox Hill Hosp (Manh Eye, Ear & Throat Hosp); **Address:** 150 E 77th St, New York, NY 10075; **Phone:** 212-717-8860; **Board Cert:** Plastic Surgery 1994; **Med School:** NYU Sch Med 1983; **Resid:** Surgery, Mt Sinai Med Ctr 1988; Plastic Surgery, Univ Pittsburgh Med Ctr 1990; **Fellow:** Microvascular Surgery, UCLA Med Ctr 1991; **Fac Appt:** Assoc Prof S, NYU Sch Med

Almeyda, Elizabeth MD (PIS) - **Spec Exp:** Abdominoplasty; Cosmetic Surgery-Breast; Liposuction; **Hospital:** St Luke's - Roosevelt Hosp Ctr - Roosevelt Div (page 94); **Address:** 75 Central Park West, New York, NY 10023-6011; **Phone:** 212-501-0600; **Board Cert:** Plastic Surgery 1988; **Med School:** Univ Rochester 1978; **Resid:** Surgery, Roosevelt Hosp 1983; **Fellow:** Plastic Surgery, New York Hosp 1985

Ascherman, Jeffrey MD (PIS) - **Spec Exp:** Cosmetic Surgery; Craniofacial Surgery; Breast Cosmetic & Reconstructive Surgery; **Hospital:** NY-Presby Hosp/Columbia (page 104), New York Eye & Ear Infirm (page 113); **Address:** 161 Ft Washington Ave, Ste 607, New York, NY 10032-3713; **Phone:** 212-305-9612; **Board Cert:** Plastic Surgery 2007; **Med School:** Columbia P&S 1988; **Resid:** Surgery, Columbia-Presby Med Ctr 1991; Plastic Surgery, Columbia-Presby Med Ctr 1994; **Fellow:** Craniofacial Surgery, Hosp Necke-Enfants Malades 1995; **Fac Appt:** Assoc Prof S, Columbia P&S

Aston, Sherrell MD (PIS) - **Spec Exp:** Cosmetic Surgery-Face & Body; Rhinoplasty; Cosmetic Surgery-Breast; Liposuction & Body Contouring; **Hospital:** Lenox Hill Hosp, NYU Langone Med Ctr (page 106); **Address:** 728 Park Ave, New York, NY 10021; **Phone:** 212-249-6000; **Board Cert:** Surgery 1974; Plastic Surgery 1978; **Med School:** Univ VA Sch Med 1968; **Resid:** Surgery, UCLA Med Ctr 1973; Plastic Surgery, NY Univ 1975; **Fellow:** Surgery, Johns Hopkins Hosp 1970; **Fac Appt:** Prof PIS, NYU Sch Med

Baker, Daniel MD (PIS) - **Spec Exp:** Cosmetic Surgery-Face; Reconstructive Surgery-Face; Rhinoplasty; **Hospital:** Lenox Hill Hosp (Manh Eye, Ear & Throat Hosp); **Address:** 65 E 66th St, New York, NY 10021; **Phone:** 212-734-9695; **Board Cert:** Plastic Surgery 1978; **Med School:** Columbia P&S 1968; **Resid:** Surgery, UCSF Med Ctr 1975; Plastic Surgery, NYU Med Ctr 1977; **Fellow:** Head and Neck Surgery, NYU Med Ctr/St Vincents Hosp 1978; **Fac Appt:** Assoc Prof PIS, NYU Sch Med

Birnbaum, Jay MD (PIS) - **Spec Exp:** Cosmetic Surgery-Face & Breast; Breast Reconstruction; Liposuction; **Hospital:** Mount Sinai Med Ctr (page 102), Beth Israel Med Ctr - Petrie Division (page 94); **Address:** 74 E 79th St, Ste 1A, New York, NY 10021-0266; **Phone:** 212-472-3040; **Board Cert:** Plastic Surgery 1989; **Med School:** Med Univ SC 1980; **Resid:** Surgery, Mount Sinai Hosp 1983; Plastic Surgery, Mount Sinai Hosp 1986; **Fac Appt:** Assoc Prof S, Mount Sinai Sch Med

Bromley, Gary S MD (PIS) - **Spec Exp:** Cosmetic Surgery; **Hospital:** NY-Presby Hosp/Weill Cornell (page 104), Jamaica Hosp Med Ctr; **Address:** 5 E 84th St, New York, NY 10028-0407; **Phone:** 212-570-5443; **Board Cert:** Plastic Surgery 1986; **Med School:** Cornell Univ-Weill Med Coll 1978; **Resid:** Surgery, New York Hosp 1981; Plastic Surgery, New York Hosp 1983; **Fellow:** Hand Surgery, NYU Med Ctr 1984

Broumand, Stafford MD (PlS) - **Spec Exp:** Eyelid Surgery; Breast Surgery; Liposuction & Body Contouring; Craniofacial Surgery/Reconstruction; **Hospital:** Mount Sinai Med Ctr (page 102); **Address:** 740 Park Ave, New York, NY 10021-4251; **Phone:** 212-879-7900; **Board Cert:** Plastic Surgery 2006; **Med School:** Yale Univ 1985; **Resid:** Surgery, Mt Sinai Med Ctr 1990; **Fellow:** Plastic Surgery, Mass Genl Hosp 1992; Cosmetic Plastic Surgery, Cran Hosp Necker 1993; **Fac Appt:** Assoc Clin Prof PlS, Mount Sinai Sch Med

Chiu, David T W MD (PlS) - **Spec Exp:** Hand & Microvascular Surgery; Cosmetic Surgery-Face; Peripheral Nerve Surgery; **Hospital:** NYU Langone Med Ctr (page 106), Lenox Hill Hosp; **Address:** 900 Park Ave, New York, NY 10021-0231; **Phone:** 212-879-8880; **Board Cert:** Plastic Surgery 1982; Hand Surgery 2000; **Med School:** Columbia P&S 1973; **Resid:** Surgery, Barnes Jewish Hosp 1977; Plastic Surgery, Columbia-Presby Med Ctr 1979; **Fellow:** Hand Surgery, NYU Med Ctr 1980; **Fac Appt:** Prof S, NYU Sch Med

Choi, Mihye MD (PlS) - **Spec Exp:** Breast Surgery; Cosmetic Surgery; Hand Surgery; Breast Reconstruction; **Hospital:** NYU Langone Med Ctr (page 106); **Address:** 305 E 47th St, Ste 1A, New York, NY 10017; **Phone:** 212-355-5779; **Board Cert:** Plastic Surgery 2008; Hand Surgery 2000; **Med School:** Univ Rochester 1987; **Resid:** Surgery, Beth Israel Hosp 1990; Plastic Surgery, Mt Sinai Med Ctr 1995; **Fellow:** Hand Surgery, NYU Med Ctr 1996; Research, Mass Genl Hosp 1992; **Fac Appt:** Assoc Prof S, NYU Sch Med

Chun, Jin K MD (PlS) - **Spec Exp:** Cosmetic Surgery-Face; Breast Cosmetic & Reconstructive Surgery; Facial Deformities/Reconstruction; Pediatric Plastic Surgery; **Hospital:** Mount Sinai Med Ctr (page 102); **Address:** Mount Sinai School of Medicine, 5 E 98 St Fl 14, Box 1259, New York, NY 10029-6501; **Phone:** 212-241-9161; **Board Cert:** Plastic Surgery 1993; **Med School:** Univ VA Sch Med 1983; **Resid:** Surgery, Eastern VA Med Coll Affil Hosp 1986; Plastic Surgery, Albany Meml Hosp 1990; **Fellow:** Microsurgery, Micro Surgery Rsrch Ctr 1987; Burn Surgery, Westchester Med Ctr 1988; **Fac Appt:** Assoc Prof PlS, Mount Sinai Sch Med

Colen, Helen S MD (PlS) - **Spec Exp:** Cosmetic Surgery-Face & Breast; Liposuction & Body Contouring; Vaginal Reconstructive Surgery; Poland Syndrome; **Hospital:** NYU Langone Med Ctr (page 106), Lenox Hill Hosp (Manh Eye, Ear & Throat Hosp); **Address:** 742 Park Ave, New York, NY 10021-4251; **Phone:** 212-772-1300; **Board Cert:** Plastic Surgery 1983; **Med School:** NYU Sch Med 1972; **Resid:** Surgery, Univ Colorado Med Ctr 1979; Plastic Surgery, St Lukes Hosp 1981; **Fellow:** Microsurgery, NYU Med Ctr 1982; **Fac Appt:** Assoc Clin Prof PlS, NYU Sch Med

Cordeiro, Peter G MD (PlS) - **Spec Exp:** Reconstructive Surgery; Breast Reconstruction; Facial Plastic & Reconstructive Surgery; **Hospital:** Meml Sloan-Kettering Cancer Ctr (page 112), Lenox Hill Hosp (Manh Eye, Ear & Throat Hosp); **Address:** 1275 York Avenue, New York, NY 10065; **Phone:** 800-525-2225; **Board Cert:** Surgery 1998; Plastic Surgery 1994; **Med School:** Harvard Med Sch 1983; **Resid:** Surgery, New Eng Deaconess Hosp-Harvard 1989; Plastic Surgery, NYU Med Ctr 1991; **Fellow:** Microsurgery, Meml Sloan-Kettering Cancer Ctr. 1992; Craniofacial Surgery, Univ Miami 1992; **Fac Appt:** Prof S, Cornell Univ-Weill Med Coll

Cutting, Court MD (PlS) - **Spec Exp:** Cleft Palate/Lip; Reconstructive Plastic Surgery; Rhinoplasty; Craniofacial Surgery/Reconstruction; **Hospital:** NYU Langone Med Ctr (page 106); **Address:** 333 E 34th St, Ste 1K, New York, NY 10016-6481; **Phone:** 212-447-6229; **Board Cert:** Otolaryngology 1980; Plastic Surgery 1986; **Med School:** Univ Chicago-Pritzker Sch Med 1975; **Resid:** Otolaryngology, Univ Iowa Hosps 1980; Plastic Surgery, NYU Langone Med Ctr 1983; **Fellow:** Craniofacial Surgery, NYU Langone Med Ctr 1984; **Fac Appt:** Prof PlS, NYU Sch Med

Diktaban, Theodore MD (PlS) - **Spec Exp:** Liposuction & Body Contouring; Rhinoplasty; Breast Augmentation; Facial Rejuvenation; **Hospital:** Lenox Hill Hosp, Lenox Hill Hosp (Manh Eye, Ear & Throat Hosp); **Address:** 911 Park Ave, New York, NY 10021; **Phone:** 212-988-5656; **Board Cert:** Otolaryngology 1981; Plastic Surgery 1988; **Med School:** NY Med Coll 1976; **Resid:** Otolaryngology, Mount Sinai Hosp 1981; Plastic Surgery, Lenox Hill Hosp 1983; **Fellow:** Reconstructive Microsurgery, Univ Louisville 1984

Disa, Joseph MD (PlS) - **Spec Exp:** Breast Surgery; Breast Reconstruction; Head & Neck Reconstruction; Microsurgery; **Hospital:** Meml Sloan-Kettering Cancer Ctr (page 112); **Address:** 1275 York Ave, New York, NY 10065; **Phone:** 212-639-5022; **Board Cert:** Surgery 2005; Plastic Surgery 2009; **Med School:** Univ Mass Sch Med 1988; **Resid:** Surgery, Univ Md Med Ctr 1994; Plastic Surgery, Johns Hopkins Univ 1996; **Fellow:** Reconstructive Microsurgery, Meml Sloan-Kettering Cancer Ctr.; **Fac Appt:** Prof PlS, Cornell Univ-Weill Med Coll

Forley, Bryan G MD (PlS) - **Spec Exp:** Cosmetic Surgery; Reconstructive Surgery; **Hospital:** Beth Israel Med Ctr - Petrie Division (page 94), New York Eye & Ear Infirm (page 113); **Address:** 5 E 82nd St, New York, NY 10028-0342; **Phone:** 212-861-3757; **Board Cert:** Plastic Surgery 2008; **Med School:** Mount Sinai Sch Med 1984; **Resid:** Surgery, NYU Med Ctr & Mt Sinai Med Ctr 1989; Plastic Surgery, Saint Francis Meml Hosp 1992; **Fellow:** Craniofacial Surgery, Hosp for Sick Children, Great Ormond St 1993

Foster, Craig A MD (PlS) - **Spec Exp:** Cosmetic Surgery-Face & Nose; Cosmetic Surgery-Breast; Rhinoplasty Revision; **Hospital:** Lenox Hill Hosp (Manh Eye, Ear & Throat Hosp), Lenox Hill Hosp; **Address:** 850 Park Ave, Ste 1A, New York, NY 10075; **Phone:** 212-744-5746; **Board Cert:** Otolaryngology 1980; Plastic Surgery 1984; **Med School:** Univ Minn 1974; **Resid:** Otolaryngology, Univ Minn Hosps 1980; Plastic Surgery, NYU Med Ctr 1982

Freund, Robert M MD (PlS) - **Spec Exp:** Cosmetic Surgery-Face & Neck; Cosmetic Surgery-Breast; Rhinoplasty Revision; **Hospital:** Lenox Hill Hosp, Long Island Jewish Med Ctr; **Address:** 220 E 63rd St, Ste LJ, New York, NY 10021; **Phone:** 212-583-1200; **Board Cert:** Plastic Surgery 2008; **Med School:** Cornell Univ-Weill Med Coll 1987; **Resid:** Surgery, NYU Med Ctr 1993; Plastic Surgery, NYU Med Ctr 1995; **Fellow:** Microvascular Surgery, NYU Med Ctr 1991

Friedman, David J MD (PlS) - **Spec Exp:** Cosmetic Surgery-Face; Liposuction & Body Contouring; Abdominoplasty; Breast Reconstruction; **Hospital:** Beth Israel Med Ctr - Petrie Division (page 94), Lenox Hill Hosp; **Address:** 630 Park Ave, New York, NY 10065; **Phone:** 212-439-1600; **Board Cert:** Plastic Surgery 2008; **Med School:** Albany Med Coll 1988; **Resid:** Surgery, Beth Israel Med Ctr 1993; Plastic Surgery, Mt Sinai Med Ctr 1994

Gayle, Lloyd MD (PlS) - **Spec Exp:** Breast Reconstruction & Augmentation; Hand Surgery; Cosmetic Surgery-Body; **Hospital:** NY-Presby Hosp/Weill Cornell (page 104), NY Hosp Queens; **Address:** 50 E 69th St, New York, NY 10021; **Phone:** 212-452-5121; **Board Cert:** Plastic Surgery 1993; **Med School:** NYU Sch Med 1983; **Resid:** Surgery, NYU Med Ctr 1988; Plastic Surgery, NY Hosp-Cornell Univ 1990; **Fellow:** Hand & Microvascular Surgery, Davies Med Ctr 1991; **Fac Appt:** Assoc Prof S, Cornell Univ-Weill Med Coll

Ginsberg, Gerald D MD (PlS) - **Spec Exp:** Cosmetic Surgery; Reconstructive Plastic Surgery; **Hospital:** NY Downtown Hosp; **Address:** Dept of Surgery, 170 William St Fl 5, New York, NY 10038; **Phone:** 212-452-3421; **Board Cert:** Plastic Surgery 1984; **Med School:** Northwestern Univ 1974; **Resid:** Surgery, NYU Med Ctr 1980; Plastic Surgery, NYU Med Ctr 1982; **Fellow:** Hand Surgery, NYU Med Ctr 1983; **Fac Appt:** Assoc Clin Prof PlS, NYU Sch Med

Godfrey, Norman V MD (PlS) - **Spec Exp:** Rhinoplasty; Eyelid Surgery; **Hospital:** NY-Presby Hosp/Weill Cornell (page 104); **Address:** 9 E 93rd St, New York, NY 10128-0666; **Phone:** 212-628-6600; **Board Cert:** Plastic Surgery 1984; **Med School:** Harvard Med Sch 1973; **Resid:** Surgery, Bellevue Hosp 1978; Plastic Surgery, Bellevue Hosp 1981; **Fac Appt:** Asst Clin Prof S, Cornell Univ-Weill Med Coll

Godfrey, Philip M MD/DMD (PlS) - **Spec Exp:** Cosmetic Surgery-Breast; Liposuction & Body Contouring; Congenital Breast Anomalies; **Hospital:** NY-Presby Hosp/Weill Cornell (page 104); **Address:** 9 E 93rd St, New York, NY 10128; **Phone:** 212-628-6600; **Board Cert:** Plastic Surgery 1988; **Med School:** Med Coll PA 1981; **Resid:** Surgery, Hartford Hosp 1984; Plastic Surgery, New York Hosp 1986; **Fellow:** Plastic Surgery, Meml Sloan Kettering Cancer Ctr 1987; **Fac Appt:** Asst Clin Prof S, Cornell Univ-Weill Med Coll

Grant, Robert T MD (PlS) - **Spec Exp:** Breast Reconstruction; Cosmetic Surgery; Microsurgery; **Hospital:** NY-Presby Hosp/Columbia (page 104), NY-Presby Hosp/Weill Cornell (page 104); **Address:** 161 Fort Washington Ave, rm 601, New York, NY 10032; **Phone:** 212-305-3103; **Board Cert:** Surgery 2001; Plastic Surgery 2003; **Med School:** Albany Med Coll 1983; **Resid:** Surgery, NY Hosp 1988; Plastic Surgery, NY Hosp 1990; **Fellow:** Microvascular Surgery, NYU Med Ctr/Bellevue Hosp 1991; **Fac Appt:** Assoc Clin Prof PlS, Columbia P&S

Hidalgo, David MD (PlS) - **Spec Exp:** Cosmetic Surgery-Face; Cosmetic Surgery-Breast; Rhinoplasty; Reconstructive Surgery; **Hospital:** NY-Presby Hosp/Weill Cornell (page 104), Lenox Hill Hosp; **Address:** 655 Park Ave Fl 1, New York, NY 10065; **Phone:** 212-517-9777; **Board Cert:** Plastic Surgery 1987; **Med School:** Georgetown Univ 1978; **Resid:** Surgery, NYU Med Ctr 1983; Plastic Surgery, NYU Med Ctr 1985; **Fellow:** Microsurgery, NYU Med Ctr 1986; **Fac Appt:** Clin Prof S, Cornell Univ-Weill Med Coll

Hoffman, Lloyd A MD (PlS) - **Spec Exp:** Cosmetic Surgery-Face; Liposuction; Breast Reconstruction; **Hospital:** NY-Presby Hosp/Columbia (page 104), Lenox Hill Hosp; **Address:** 12A E 68th St, New York, NY 10021; **Phone:** 212-861-1640; **Board Cert:** Plastic Surgery 1989; **Med School:** Northwestern Univ 1978; **Resid:** Surgery, New York Hosp 1983; Plastic Surgery, NYU Med Ctr 1986; **Fellow:** Hand Surgery, NYU Med Ctr 1987; **Fac Appt:** Assoc Prof PlS, Cornell Univ-Weill Med Coll

Hunter, John G MD (PlS) - **Spec Exp:** Female Genital Cosmetic Surgery; Cosmetic Surgery-Breast; Cosmetic Surgery-Body; **Hospital:** NY-Presby Hosp/Weill Cornell (page 104), New York Methodist Hosp (page 404); **Address:** 47 E 63rd St, New York, NY 10021-7315; **Phone:** 212-751-4444; **Board Cert:** Plastic Surgery 1991; **Med School:** SUNY Downstate 1983; **Resid:** Surgery, Mount Sinai Hosp 1986; **Fellow:** Plastic Surgery, Univ Hosp-SUNY Downstate 1988; **Fac Appt:** Assoc Clin Prof S, Cornell Univ-Weill Med Coll

Imber, Gerald MD (PlS) - **Spec Exp:** Cosmetic Surgery-Face; Eyelid Surgery; **Hospital:** NY-Presby Hosp/Weill Cornell (page 104); **Address:** 1009 5th Ave, New York, NY 10028; **Phone:** 212-472-1800; **Board Cert:** Plastic Surgery 1976; **Med School:** SUNY Downstate 1966; **Resid:** Surgery, LI Jewish Med Ctr 1972; Plastic Surgery, NY Hosp 1974; **Fac Appt:** Asst Clin Prof S, Cornell Univ-Weill Med Coll

Jacobs, Elliot W MD (PlS) - **Spec Exp:** Cosmetic Surgery-Face & Breast; Gynecomastia; Body Contouring; Rhinoplasty; **Hospital:** New York Eye & Ear Infirm (page 113), Beth Israel Med Ctr - Petrie Division (page 94); **Address:** 815 Park Ave, New York, NY 10021-3276; **Phone:** 212-570-6080; **Board Cert:** Plastic Surgery 1982; **Med School:** Mount Sinai Sch Med 1970; **Resid:** Surgery, Mt Sinai Med Ctr 1974; Plastic Surgery, Mt Sinai Med Ctr 1977

Karp, Nolan MD (PlS) - **Spec Exp:** Breast Cosmetic & Reconstructive Surgery; Liposuction & Body Contouring; Cosmetic Surgery; **Hospital:** NYU Langone Med Ctr (page 106); **Address:** 305 E 47th St, Ste 1A, New York, NY 10017; **Phone:** 212-355-5779; **Board Cert:** Plastic Surgery 1994; **Med School:** Northwestern Univ 1983; **Resid:** Surgery, NYU Med Ctr 1988; **Fellow:** Plastic Surgery, NYU Med Ctr 1991; **Fac Appt:** Assoc Prof PlS, NYU Sch Med

Karpinski, Richard MD (PlS) - **Spec Exp:** Cosmetic Surgery-Face; Cosmetic Surgery-Liposuction; Rhinoplasty; Hyperhidrosis; **Hospital:** St Luke's - Roosevelt Hosp Ctr - Roosevelt Div (page 94); **Address:** 200 Central Park South, Ste 108, New York, NY 10019-1436; **Phone:** 212-977-9797; **Board Cert:** Plastic Surgery 1983; **Med School:** Harvard Med Sch 1971; **Resid:** Surgery, Boston City Hosp 1973; Surgery, New England Deaconess 1977; **Fellow:** Plastic Surgery, NYU Med Ctr 1981; **Fac Appt:** Asst Clin Prof PlS, Columbia P&S

Kolker, Adam R MD (PlS) - **Spec Exp:** Cosmetic Surgery-Breast; Breast Reconstruction; Body Contouring after Weight Loss; Pediatric Plastic Surgery; **Hospital:** Mount Sinai Med Ctr (page 102), Lenox Hill Hosp; **Address:** 710 Park Ave, New York, NY 10021; **Phone:** 212-744-6500; **Board Cert:** Plastic Surgery 2001; Surgery 2005; **Med School:** Albany Med Coll 1990; **Resid:** Surgery, St Vincent's Hosp 1995; Plastic/Reconstructive Surgery, Beth Israel Med Ctr 1998; **Fellow:** Microsurgery, NYU Med Ctr 1996; Craniofacial Surgery, Univ Melbourne Chldns Hosp 2000; **Fac Appt:** Assoc Clin Prof S, Mount Sinai Sch Med

Lesesne, Carroll B MD (PlS) - **Spec Exp:** Cosmetic Surgery-Face; Rhinoplasty; Skin Cancer Reconstruction; Abdominoplasty; **Hospital:** Lenox Hill Hosp (Manh Eye, Ear & Throat Hosp), Lenox Hill Hosp; **Address:** 620 Park Ave, New York, NY 10021-6591; **Phone:** 212-570-6318; **Board Cert:** Plastic Surgery 1987; **Med School:** Duke Univ 1980; **Resid:** Surgery, Stanford Univ Med Ctr 1983; Plastic Surgery, New York Hosp 1985; **Fellow:** Plastic Surgery, Meml Sloan Kettering Cancer Ctr 1985; **Fac Appt:** Asst Clin Prof PlS, NYU Sch Med

Matarasso, Alan MD (PlS) - **Spec Exp:** Cosmetic Surgery-Face & Eyes; Rhinoplasty; Liposuction; Abdominoplasty; **Hospital:** Lenox Hill Hosp (Manh Eye, Ear & Throat Hosp); **Address:** 1009 Park Ave, New York, NY 10028-0936; **Phone:** 212-249-7500; **Board Cert:** Plastic Surgery 1986; **Med School:** Univ Miami Sch Med 1979; **Resid:** Surgery, Montefiore Med Ctr 1983; Plastic Surgery, Montefiore Med Ctr 1985; **Fellow:** Plastic Surgery, Manhattan EET Hosp/NYU 1985; **Fac Appt:** Clin Prof PlS, Albert Einstein Coll Med

McCarthy, Joseph G MD (PlS) - **Spec Exp:** Craniofacial Surgery-Pediatric; Reconstructive Surgery-Face; Cosmetic Surgery-Face; **Hospital:** NYU Langone Med Ctr (page 106), Lenox Hill Hosp (Manh Eye, Ear & Throat Hosp); **Address:** 722 Park Ave, New York, NY 10021-4954; **Phone:** 212-628-4420; **Board Cert:** Surgery 1972; Plastic Surgery 1974; **Med School:** Columbia P&S 1964; **Resid:** Surgery, Columbia-Presby Med Ctr 1971; Plastic Surgery, NYU Med Ctr 1973; **Fac Appt:** Prof PlS, NYU Sch Med

Mehrara, Babak J MD (PlS) - **Spec Exp:** Breast Reconstruction; Cancer Reconstruction; Microsurgery; Reconstructive Surgery-Face; **Hospital:** Meml Sloan-Kettering Cancer Ctr (page 112); **Address:** 1275 York Ave, New York, NY 10065; **Phone:** 212-639-8639; **Board Cert:** Plastic Surgery 2003; **Med School:** Columbia P&S 1993; **Resid:** Surgery, NYU Med Ctr 1996; Plastic Surgery, NYU Med Ctr 2001; **Fellow:** Microsurgery, UCLA Med Ctr 2002; **Fac Appt:** Assoc Prof S, Cornell Univ-Weill Med Coll

Perrotti, John A MD (PlS) - **Spec Exp:** Liposuction & Body Contouring; Cosmetic Surgery-Face & Breast; Abdominoplasty; **Hospital:** Lenox Hill Hosp (Manh Eye, Ear & Throat Hosp), Lenox Hill Hosp; **Address:** 125 E 69th St, New York, NY 10121; **Phone:** 212-258-2200; **Board Cert:** Plastic Surgery 2000; **Med School:** NY Med Coll 1991; **Resid:** Surgery, Westchester Medical Ctr 1996; Plastic Surgery, Cleveland Clinic 1998; **Fac Appt:** Asst Clin Prof S, NY Med Coll

Pitman, Gerald H MD (PlS) - **Spec Exp:** Cosmetic Surgery-Face; Liposuction; Abdominoplasty; **Hospital:** Lenox Hill Hosp (Manh Eye, Ear & Throat Hosp), NYU Langone Med Ctr (page 106); **Address:** 170 E 73rd St, New York, NY 10021; **Phone:** 212-517-2600; **Board Cert:** Plastic Surgery 1978; **Med School:** Univ Pennsylvania 1968; **Resid:** Surgery, Columbia-Presby Hosp 1975; Plastic Surgery, NYU Med Ctr 1977; **Fellow:** Microsurgery, NYU Med Ctr 1981; **Fac Appt:** Clin Prof PlS, NYU Sch Med

Razaboni, Rosa MD (PlS) - **Spec Exp:** Cosmetic Surgery; Breast Reconstruction; Body Contouring after Weight Loss; **Hospital:** Lenox Hill Hosp, Mount Sinai Med Ctr (page 102); **Address:** 14-A E 68th St, New York, NY 10021-5847; **Phone:** 212-772-0200; **Board Cert:** Plastic Surgery 1993; **Med School:** Brazil 1975; **Resid:** Surgery, St Vincents Hosp 1985; Plastic Surgery, NYU Med Ctr 1988; **Fellow:** Surgery, Hospital Trousseau 1986; **Fac Appt:** Asst Prof PlS, Mount Sinai Sch Med

Romita, Mauro C MD (PlS) - **Spec Exp:** Cosmetic Surgery-Face; Liposuction & Body Contouring; Reconstructive Plastic Surgery; **Hospital:** Lenox Hill Hosp; **Address:** 853 5th Ave, New York, NY 10065; **Phone:** 212-772-3220; **Board Cert:** Plastic Surgery 1983; **Med School:** Univ Miami Sch Med 1973; **Resid:** Surgery, NYU Med Ctr 1978; Plastic Surgery, NYU Med Ctr 1980; **Fellow:** Craniofacial Surgery, NYU Med Ctr 1981; Microsurgery, NYU Med Ctr 1982; **Fac Appt:** Asst Prof S, NY Med Coll

Rosenblatt, William B MD (PlS) - **Spec Exp:** Nasal Surgery; Cosmetic Surgery-Face & Body; Cosmetic Surgery-Breast; Rhinoplasty; **Hospital:** Lenox Hill Hosp, Lenox Hill Hosp (Manh Eye, Ear & Throat Hosp); **Address:** 308 E 79th St, Ste 1D, New York, NY 10075; **Phone:** 212-570-6100; **Board Cert:** Otolaryngology 1977; Plastic Surgery 1980; **Med School:** NY Med Coll 1973; **Resid:** Otolaryngology, Metropolitan Hosp 1977; Plastic Surgery, Lenox Hill Hosp 1979

Sabry, M Zakir MD (PlS) - **Spec Exp:** Cosmetic Surgery; Breast Reconstruction; Craniofacial Surgery; Cleft Palate/Lip; **Hospital:** Lenox Hill Hosp; **Address:** 1049 5th Ave at 86th St, New York, NY 10028; **Phone:** 212-737-1308; **Board Cert:** Plastic Surgery 2004; **Med School:** NY Med Coll 1993; **Resid:** Surgery, St Vincents Hosp 1999; Plastic Surgery, Med Coll Virginia 2001; **Fellow:** Craniofacial Surgery, Barnes Jewish Hosp 2002; **Fac Appt:** Asst Clin Prof PlS, Med Coll VA

Schulman, Matthew R MD (PlS) - **Spec Exp:** Body Contouring after Weight Loss; Breast Augmentation; Facial Rejuvenation; Liposuction; **Hospital:** Mount Sinai Med Ctr (page 102); **Address:** Mt Sinai Med Ctr, 21 E 87th St, New York, NY 10128; **Phone:** 212-289-1851; **Board Cert:** Plastic Surgery 2007; **Med School:** Jefferson Med Coll 2000; **Resid:** Surgery, Mt Sinai Med Ctr 2003; **Fellow:** Plastic Surgery, Mt Sinai Med Ctr 2006

Schulman, Norman H MD (PlS) - **Spec Exp:** Cosmetic Surgery-Face & Body; Breast Cosmetic & Reconstructive Surgery; Nasal Surgery; Tuberous Breast; **Hospital:** Lenox Hill Hosp, Lenox Hill Hosp (Manh Eye, Ear & Throat Hosp); **Address:** 308 E 79th St, New York, NY 10075; **Phone:** 212-861-5004; **Board Cert:** Surgery 1973; Plastic Surgery 1976; **Med School:** Tufts Univ 1965; **Resid:** Surgery, Jacobi Med Ctr 1972; Plastic Surgery, Lenox Hill Hosp 1974; **Fellow:** Plastic Surgery, Roswell Park Cancer Inst 1975; **Fac Appt:** Clin Prof PlS, Cornell Univ-Weill Med Coll

Scott, Susan M MD (PlS) - **Spec Exp:** Cosmetic Surgery-Face; Eyelid Surgery; Hand Reconstruction; **Hospital:** NYU Hosp For Joint Diseases (page 106), Lenox Hill Hosp; **Address:** 150 E 77th St, New York, NY 10075; **Phone:** 212-288-9922; **Board Cert:** Plastic Surgery 1987; Hand Surgery 2005; **Med School:** Columbia P&S 1974; **Resid:** Surgery, St Luke's-Roosevelt Hosp Ctr 1979; Plastic Surgery, NYU Med Ctr 1981; **Fellow:** Hand Surgery, St Luke's-Roosevelt Hosp Ctr 1982

Sherman, John E MD (PlS) - **Spec Exp:** Cosmetic Surgery-Face; Cosmetic Surgery-Liposuction; Facial Plastic & Reconstructive Surgery; **Hospital:** NY-Presby Hosp/Weill Cornell (page 104), Lenox Hill Hosp; **Address:** 1016 Fifth Ave, New York, NY 10028-0132; **Phone:** 212-535-2300; **Board Cert:** Plastic Surgery 1984; **Med School:** NY Med Coll 1975; **Resid:** Surgery, Montefiore Med Ctr 1978; Plastic Surgery, NY Hosp/Meml Sloan Kettering Cancer Ctr 1980; **Fac Appt:** Asst Clin Prof S, Cornell Univ-Weill Med Coll

Siebert, John W MD (PlS) - **Spec Exp:** Facial Plastic & Reconstructive Surgery; Microsurgery; Cosmetic Surgery-Face; **Hospital:** Lenox Hill Hosp (Manh Eye, Ear & Throat Hosp), Univ WI Hosp & Clins; **Address:** 630 Park Ave, New York, NY 10065; **Phone:** 212-737-8300; **Board Cert:** Plastic Surgery 1991; **Med School:** Univ Wisc 1981; **Resid:** Surgery, Mass Genl Hosp 1986; Plastic Surgery, NYU Med Ctr 1988; **Fellow:** Microsurgery, NYU Med Ctr 1989; **Fac Appt:** Assoc Prof S, Univ Wisc

Silich, Robert C MD (PlS) - **Spec Exp:** Cosmetic Surgery-Face & Eyes; Blepharoplasty; Rhino-plasty; **Hospital:** NY-Presby Hosp/Weill Cornell (page 104), Lenox Hill Hosp; **Address:** 1009 5th Ave, New York, NY 10028; **Phone:** 212-472-0082; **Board Cert:** Plastic Surgery 2010; **Med School:** Georgetown Univ 1993; **Resid:** Surgery, Cornell Med Ctr 1997; Plastic Surgery, Cornell Med Ctr 1999; **Fac Appt:** Asst Clin Prof PlS, Cornell Univ-Weill Med Coll

Silver, Lester MD (PlS) - **Spec Exp:** Cleft Palate/Lip; Pediatric Plastic Surgery; Reconstructive Surgery; **Hospital:** Mount Sinai Med Ctr (page 102); **Address:** 5 E 98th St, Box 1259, New York, NY 10029-6574; **Phone:** 212-241-1968; **Board Cert:** Plastic Surgery 1978; **Med School:** Ros Franklin Univ/Chicago Med Sch 1960; **Resid:** Surgery, Montefiore Med Ctr 1966; Plastic Surgery, Mt Sinai Med Ctr 1969; **Fac Appt:** Prof PlS, Mount Sinai Sch Med

Skolnik, Richard A MD (PlS) - **Spec Exp:** Cosmetic Surgery-Face; Cosmetic Surgery-Breast; Li-posuction & Body Contouring; **Hospital:** Mount Sinai Med Ctr (page 102); **Address:** 21 E 87th St, New York, NY 10128-0506; **Phone:** 212-722-1977; **Board Cert:** Plastic Surgery 1983; **Med School:** Cornell Univ-Weill Med Coll 1976; **Resid:** Surgery, Mt Sinai Hosp 1979; Plastic Surgery, Mt Sinai Hosp 1982; **Fac Appt:** Assoc Clin Prof PlS, Mount Sinai Sch Med

Spector, Jason A MD (PlS) - **Spec Exp:** Cosmetic Surgery; **Hospital:** NY-Presby Hosp/Weill Cornell (page 104); **Address:** New York Presby-Weill Cornell, 525 E 68th St, Ste 115, New York, NY 10065-4870; **Phone:** 212-746-4532; **Board Cert:** Plastic Surgery 2007; **Med School:** NYU Sch Med 1996; **Resid:** Surgery, NYU Medical Center 2002; Plastic Surgery, NYU Medical Center 2005; **Fellow:** Plastic Surgery, NYU Medical Center 2006; Microsurgery, NYU Medical Center 2006; **Fac Appt:** Asst Prof S, Cornell Univ-Weill Med Coll

Spinelli, Henry M MD (PlS) - **Spec Exp:** Cosmetic Surgery-Face; Craniofacial Surgery/Recon-struction; Oculoplastic & Orbital Surgery; **Hospital:** NY-Presby Hosp/Weill Cornell (page 104), Lenox Hill Hosp (Manh Eye, Ear & Throat Hosp); **Address:** 875 Fifth Ave, New York, NY 10021-4952; **Phone:** 212-570-6235; **Board Cert:** Ophthalmology 1987; Plastic Surgery 1993; **Med School:** NYU Sch Med 1981; **Resid:** Ophthalmology, Manhattan EET Hosp 1985; Plastic/Reconstructive Sur-gery, NYU-Bellevue Hosp 1990; **Fellow:** Craniofacial Surgery, NYU Med Ctr 1991; **Fac Appt:** Clin Prof S, Cornell Univ-Weill Med Coll

Sultan, Mark MD (PlS) - **Spec Exp:** Breast Reconstruction; Cosmetic Surgery-Breast; Cosmetic Surgery-Face; **Hospital:** St Luke's - Roosevelt Hosp Ctr - Roosevelt Div (page 94); **Address:** 1100 Park Ave, New York, NY 10128; **Phone:** 212-360-0700; **Board Cert:** Plastic Surgery 1992; **Med School:** Columbia P&S 1982; **Resid:** Surgery, Columbia-Presby Hosp 1987; Plastic Surgery, Colum-bia-Presby Hosp 1990; **Fellow:** Head and Neck Surgery, Emory Univ Hosp 1989; **Fac Appt:** Assoc Prof S, Columbia P&S

Tabbal, Nicolas MD (PlS) - **Spec Exp:** Rhinoplasty; Cosmetic Surgery-Face; Eyelid Surgery; **Hospital:** Lenox Hill Hosp (Manh Eye, Ear & Throat Hosp), NYU Langone Med Ctr (page 106); **Address:** 521 Park Ave, rm 1, New York, NY 10021-8140; **Phone:** 212-644-5800; **Board Cert:** Plastic Surgery 1980; **Med School:** Lebanon 1972; **Resid:** Surgery, Am Univ Med Ctr 1976; Plastic Surgery, Akron City Hosp 1979; **Fellow:** Surgery, Upstate Med Ctr 1977; Reconstructive Microsurgery, NYU Med Ctr 1980

Taub, Peter J MD (PlS) - **Spec Exp:** Pediatric Plastic Surgery; Craniofacial Surgery; Cosmetic Surgery; Maxillofacial Surgery; **Hospital:** Mount Sinai Med Ctr (page 102), Westchester Med Ctr; **Address:** Mount Sinai Medical Ctr, 5 E 98th St Fl 15, Box 1259, New York, NY 10029-6574; **Phone:** 212-241-4178; **Board Cert:** Surgery 2000; Plastic Surgery 2003; **Med School:** Albert Einstein Coll Med 1993; **Resid:** Surgery, Mt Sinai Med Ctr 1999; Plastic Surgery, UCLA Med Ctr 2001; **Fellow:** Craniofacial Surgery, UCLA Med Ctr 2002; **Fac Appt:** Assoc Prof PlS, Mount Sinai Sch Med

Thorne, Charles MD (PlS) - **Spec Exp:** Cosmetic Surgery-Face & Breast; Ear Reconstruction/Microtia; Craniofacial Surgery; Pediatric Plastic Surgery; **Hospital:** NYU Langone Med Ctr (page 106), Lenox Hill Hosp (Manh Eye, Ear & Throat Hosp); **Address:** 812 Park Ave, New York, NY 10021-2759; **Phone:** 212-794-0044; **Board Cert:** Plastic Surgery 1991; **Med School:** UCLA 1981; **Resid:** Surgery, Mass Genl Hosp 1986; Plastic Surgery, NYU Med Ctr 1988; **Fellow:** Craniofacial Surgery, NYU Med Ctr 1989; **Fac Appt:** Assoc Prof PlS, NYU Sch Med

Ting, Jess MD (PlS) - **Spec Exp:** Reconstructive Microvascular Surgery; Hand Surgery; Nerve Surgery & Transplantation; Breast Reconstruction; **Hospital:** Mount Sinai Med Ctr (page 102); **Address:** Dept of Surgery Mount Sinai Sch Med, 5 E 98th St, Box 1259, New York, NY 10029; **Phone:** 212-241-4410; **Board Cert:** Plastic Surgery 2002; Hand Surgery 2003; **Med School:** Columbia P&S 1995; **Resid:** Surgery, Columbia Presby Med Ctr 1998; Plastic Surgery, Univ Pittsburgh Med Ctr 2000; **Fellow:** Hand Surgery, Hosp Special Surgery 2001; **Fac Appt:** Asst Prof S, Mount Sinai Sch Med

Verga, Michele MD (PlS) - **Spec Exp:** Cosmetic Surgery-Face; Liposuction; Body Contouring; Reconstructive Surgery; **Hospital:** Mount Sinai Med Ctr (page 102); **Address:** 1010 5th Ave, New York, NY 10028-0130; **Phone:** 212-535-0470; **Board Cert:** Plastic Surgery 1984; **Med School:** Italy 1974; **Resid:** Surgery, Mt Sinai Hosp 1978; Surgery, Lutheran Med Ctr 1980; **Fellow:** Plastic Surgery, Mt Sinai Hosp 1983; **Fac Appt:** Asst Clin Prof S, Mount Sinai Sch Med

Vickery, Carlin MD (PlS) - **Spec Exp:** Breast Cosmetic & Reconstructive Surgery; Cosmetic Surgery-Body; Cosmetic Surgery-Face; **Hospital:** Mount Sinai Med Ctr (page 102); **Address:** 1125 5th Ave, New York, NY 10128; **Phone:** 212-288-9800; **Board Cert:** Plastic Surgery 1987; **Med School:** NYU Sch Med 1977; **Resid:** Surgery, New York Univ Med Ctr 1982; **Fellow:** Microsurgery, New York Univ Med Ctr 1985; **Fac Appt:** Assoc Clin Prof S, Mount Sinai Sch Med

Weiss, Paul R MD (PlS) - **Spec Exp:** Breast Cosmetic & Reconstructive Surgery; Cosmetic Surgery-Face; Cosmetic Surgery-Body; **Hospital:** Montefiore Med Ctr - Div. Moses (page 100), Montefiore Med Ctr - Div. Weiler (page 100); **Address:** 1049 5th Ave, Ste 2D, New York, NY 10028-0115; **Phone:** 212-861-8000; **Board Cert:** Surgery 1975; Plastic Surgery 1977; **Med School:** Tulane Univ 1969; **Resid:** Surgery, Montefiore Med Ctr/Bronx Muni Hosp 1974; Plastic Surgery, Montefiore Med Ctr 1976; **Fac Appt:** Clin Prof S, Albert Einstein Coll Med

Wells, Scott B MD (PlS) - **Spec Exp:** Cosmetic Surgery-Face; Abdominoplasty; Breast Augmentation; **Hospital:** Winthrop - Univ Hosp; **Address:** 655 Park Ave, New York, NY 10065; **Phone:** 212-794-3900; **Board Cert:** Plastic Surgery 2005; **Med School:** NY Med Coll 1985; **Resid:** Surgery, Beth Israel Med Ctr 1990; Plastic/Reconstructive Surgery, SUNY Hlth Sci Ctr 1992

Zevon, Scott MD (PlS) - **Spec Exp:** Breast Augmentation; Breast Surgery; Body Contouring; Liposuction; **Hospital:** St Luke's - Roosevelt Hosp Ctr - Roosevelt Div (page 94), Long Island Coll Hosp (page 94); **Address:** 75 Central Park West, New York, NY 10023; **Phone:** 212-496-6600; **Board Cert:** Plastic Surgery 1989; **Med School:** Boston Univ 1979; **Resid:** Surgery, St Luke's-Roosevelt Hosp Ctr 1984; Plastic Surgery, Nassau Co Med Ctr 1986; **Fellow:** Craniofacial Surgery, Mayo Clinic 1987

Zide, Barry M MD/DMD (PlS) - **Spec Exp:** Facial Surgery-Chin & Lip; Birthmarks/Hemangiomas; Facial Plastic & Reconstructive Surgery; Melanoma; **Hospital:** NYU Langone Med Ctr (page 106), Lenox Hill Hosp; **Address:** 420 E 55th St, Ste 1D, New York, NY 10022-5140; **Phone:** 212-421-2424; **Board Cert:** Plastic Surgery 1981; **Med School:** Tufts Univ 1973; **Resid:** Surgery, Stanford Med Ctr 1976; Plastic Surgery, U NC Hosp 1978; **Fellow:** Head & Neck Oncology, Roswell Park Cancer Inst 1979; Craniofacial Surgery, NYU Med Ctr 1980; **Fac Appt:** Prof PlS, NYU Sch Med

Preventive Medicine

Cahill, John MD (PrM) - **Spec Exp:** Tropical Diseases; Travel Medicine; Parasitic Infections; International Health; **Hospital:** St Luke's - Roosevelt Hosp Ctr - Roosevelt Div (page 94); **Address:** 425 W 59th St, Ste 8A, New York, NY 10019; **Phone:** 212-492-5500; **Board Cert:** Emergency Medicine 2001; **Med School:** Mount Sinai Sch Med 1996; **Resid:** Emergency Medicine, Rhode Island Hosp 1997; Emergency Medicine, Rhode Island Hosp 2000; **Fellow:** Tropical Medicine, Royal Coll Surgeons 1998; **Fac Appt:** Asst Clin Prof Med, Columbia P&S

Cahill, Kevin M MD (PrM) - **Spec Exp:** Tropical Diseases; International Health; Parasitic Infections; Tropical Diseases; **Hospital:** Lenox Hill Hosp; **Address:** 850 5th Ave, New York, NY 10021; **Phone:** 212-434-2477; **Board Cert:** Public Health & Genl Preventive Med 1970; **Med School:** Cornell Univ-Weill Med Coll 1961; **Resid:** Internal Medicine, US Navy Med Res Unit 1965; Public Health & Genl Preventive Med, US Navy Med Res Unit 1965; **Fac Appt:** Clin Prof Med, NYU Sch Med

Hoffman, Robert S MD (PrM) - **Spec Exp:** Poison Control; Disaster Preparedness; **Hospital:** NYU Langone Med Ctr (page 106), Bellevue Hosp Ctr; **Address:** NY Poison Control Ctr, 455 1st Ave, rm 123, New York, NY 10016; **Phone:** 212-340-4494; **Board Cert:** Internal Medicine 1987; Emergency Medicine 2005; Medical Toxicology 2008; **Med School:** NYU Sch Med 1984; **Resid:** Internal Medicine, NYU Med Ctr 1987; **Fellow:** Medical Toxicology, NYU Med Ctr 1989; **Fac Appt:** Assoc Prof Med, NYU Sch Med

Psychiatry

Adler, Lenard A MD (Psyc) - **Spec Exp:** ADD/ADHD; Psychopharmacology; **Hospital:** NYU Langone Med Ctr (page 106); **Address:** 403 E 34th St Fl 4, New York, NY 10016; **Phone:** 212-263-3580; **Board Cert:** Psychiatry 1987; **Med School:** Emory Univ 1982; **Resid:** Psychiatry, NYU Med Ctr 1986; **Fac Appt:** Assoc Prof Psyc, NYU Sch Med

Almeleh, Jack MD (Psyc) - **Spec Exp:** Cognitive Psychotherapy; Anxiety & Depression; **Hospital:** Mount Sinai Med Ctr (page 102); **Address:** 340 E 52nd St, New York, NY 10022; **Phone:** 212-355-4250; **Board Cert:** Psychiatry 1977; **Med School:** SUNY Buffalo 1969; **Resid:** Psychiatry, Temple Univ Hosp 1073; **Fac Appt:** Asst Clin Prof Psyc, Mount Sinai Sch Med

Alper, Kenneth R MD (Psyc) - **Spec Exp:** Psychopharmacology; Neuro-Psychiatry; **Hospital:** NYU Langone Med Ctr (page 106); **Address:** 150 E 58th St Fl 25, New York, NY 10155; **Phone:** 212-966-3506; **Board Cert:** Psychiatry 1989; **Med School:** Univ Tex, San Antonio 1984; **Resid:** Psychiatry, NYU Med Ctr 1988; **Fellow:** Clinical Neurophysiology, NYU Med Ctr 1990; **Fac Appt:** Assoc Prof Psyc, NYU Sch Med

Appelbaum, Paul S MD (Psyc) - **Spec Exp:** Forensic Psychiatry; Depression; Anxiety & Mood Disorders; **Hospital:** NY-Presby Hosp/Columbia (page 104); **Address:** NY State Psychiatric Inst, 1051 Riverside Drive, rm 6714, Box 122, New York, NY 10032; **Phone:** 212-543-4184; **Board Cert:** Psychiatry 1981; Forensic Psychiatry 2004; **Med School:** Harvard Med Sch 1976; **Resid:** Psychiatry, Mass Mental Health Ctr 1980; **Fac Appt:** Prof Psyc, Columbia P&S

Arkow, Stan D MD (Psyc) - **Spec Exp:** Psychotherapy; Psychopharmacology; **Hospital:** NY-Presby Hosp/Columbia (page 104); **Address:** 740 West End Ave, Ste 5-A, New York, NY 10025; **Phone:** 212-663-5185; **Board Cert:** Psychiatry 1985; **Med School:** Columbia P&S 1977; **Resid:** Psychiatry, Columbia-Presby Med Ctr/Psych Inst 1981; **Fac Appt:** Assoc Clin Prof Psyc, Columbia P&S

Aronoff, Michael S MD (Psyc) - **Spec Exp:** Sleep Disorders; Stress Management; Anxiety & Depression; Family & Couples Therapy; **Hospital:** Lenox Hill Hosp, NYU Langone Med Ctr (page 106); **Address:** 60 Riverside Drive, Ste 16E, New York, NY 10024-6171; **Phone:** 212-799-8257; **Board Cert:** Psychiatry 1977; **Med School:** Univ Pennsylvania 1966; **Resid:** Psychiatry, NY State Psych Inst 1972; **Fellow:** Psychoanalysis, Columbia-Presby Hosp 1976; **Fac Appt:** Clin Prof Psyc, NYU Sch Med

Attia, Evelyn MD (Psyc) - **Spec Exp:** Eating Disorders; Mood Disorders; **Hospital:** NY State Psychiatric Inst, NY-Presby Hosp/Columbia (page 104); **Address:** NYS Psychiatric Inst, Box 98, 1051 Riverside Drive, New York, NY 10032; **Phone:** 212-543-5923; **Board Cert:** Psychiatry 1992; **Med School:** Columbia P&S 1986; **Resid:** Psychiatry, Hosp Univ Penn 1987; Psychiatry, NY State Psych Inst 1990; **Fac Appt:** Assoc Clin Prof Psyc, Columbia P&S

Barbuto, Joseph MD (Psyc) - **Spec Exp:** Psychiatry in Cancer; Anxiety & Mood Disorders; Personality Disorders; **Hospital:** NY-Presby Hosp/Weill Cornell (page 104), Meml Sloan-Kettering Cancer Ctr (page 112); **Address:** 945 Fifth Ave, New York, NY 10021; **Phone:** 212-724-7366; **Board Cert:** Psychiatry 1983; **Med School:** Albert Einstein Coll Med 1978; **Resid:** Psychiatry, NY Hosp 1982; **Fellow:** Psychiatric Oncology, Meml Sloan-Kettering Cancer Ctr 1986; **Fac Appt:** Assoc Clin Prof Psyc, Cornell Univ-Weill Med Coll

Basch, Samuel MD (Psyc) - **Spec Exp:** Psychopharmacology; Psychiatry in Physical Illness; Psychiatry in Cancer; Psychoanalysis; **Hospital:** Mount Sinai Med Ctr (page 102); **Address:** 10 E 85th St, Ste 1B, New York, NY 10028-0412; **Phone:** 212-427-0344; **Board Cert:** Psychiatry 1970; **Med School:** Hahnemann Univ 1961; **Resid:** Psychiatry, Mount Sinai Hosp 1965; **Fellow:** Psychoanalysis, Columbia Presby Hosp 1976; **Fac Appt:** Clin Prof Psyc, Mount Sinai Sch Med

Bone, Stanley MD (Psyc) - **Spec Exp:** Psychotherapy; Psychoanalysis; **Hospital:** NY-Presby Hosp/Columbia (page 104); **Address:** 1155 Park Ave, New York, NY 10128-1209; **Phone:** 212-831-0917; **Board Cert:** Psychiatry 1979; **Med School:** Mount Sinai Sch Med 1974; **Resid:** Psychiatry, Columbia Presby 1978; **Fellow:** Psychoanalysis, Columbia Univ 1983; **Fac Appt:** Clin Prof Psyc, Columbia P&S

Borbely, Antal MD (Psyc) - **Spec Exp:** Career Related Problems; Relationship Problems; Creativity Enhancement; **Hospital:** Mount Sinai Med Ctr (page 102); **Address:** 675 W End Ave, Ste 1A, New York, NY 10028; **Phone:** 212-222-1678; **Board Cert:** Psychiatry 1976; **Med School:** Switzerland 1968; **Resid:** Psychiatry, NY State Psyc Inst 1972; Psychiatry, Albert Einstein Affil Hosp 1973; **Fellow:** Community Psychiatry, Albert Einstein Affil Hosp 1975

Breitbart, William MD (Psyc) - **Spec Exp:** Psychiatry in Cancer; AIDS Related Cancers; Pain-Cancer; Palliative Care; **Hospital:** Meml Sloan-Kettering Cancer Ctr (page 112); **Address:** 1275 York Avenue, New York, NY 10065; **Phone:** 646-888-0100; **Board Cert:** Internal Medicine 1982; Psychiatry 1986; Psychosomatic Medicine 2005; **Med School:** Albert Einstein Coll Med 1978; **Resid:** Internal Medicine, Bronx Muni Hosp Ctr 1982; Psychiatry, Bronx Muni Hosp Ctr 1984; **Fellow:** Psychiatric Oncology, Meml Sloan Kettering Cancer Ctr 1986; **Fac Appt:** Prof Psyc, Cornell Univ-Weill Med Coll

Brodie, Jonathan D MD (Psyc) - **Spec Exp:** Psychopharmacology; Anxiety & Depression; Neuro-Psychiatry; **Hospital:** NYU Langone Med Ctr (page 106); **Address:** 155 E 38th St, Ste 3L, New York, NY 10016; **Phone:** 212-986-6693; **Board Cert:** Psychiatry 1979; **Med School:** NYU Sch Med 1975; **Resid:** Psychiatry, NYU Med Ctr/Bellevue Hosp 1978; **Fac Appt:** Prof Psyc, NYU Sch Med

Bronheim, Harold MD (Psyc) - **Spec Exp:** Psychiatry in Body Image Awareness; Relationship Problems; Psychiatry in Physical Illness; Anxiety & Depression; **Hospital:** Mount Sinai Med Ctr (page 102); **Address:** 1155 Park Ave, New York, NY 10128-1209; **Phone:** 212-996-5777; **Board Cert:** Psychiatry 1985; Internal Medicine 1986; Psychosomatic Medicine 2005; Geriatric Psychiatry 2001; **Med School:** SUNY Downstate 1980; **Resid:** Psychiatry, Mount Sinai Hosp 1984; **Fellow:** Internal Medicine, Beth Israel Hosp 1985; **Fac Appt:** Clin Prof Psyc, Mount Sinai Sch Med

Brown, Richard P MD (Psyc) - **Spec Exp:** Psychopharmacology; Complementary Medicine; **Hospital:** NY-Presby Hosp/Columbia (page 104); **Address:** 30 East End Ave, Ste 1B, New York, NY 10028-7053; **Phone:** 212-737-0821; **Board Cert:** Psychiatry 1983; **Med School:** Columbia P&S 1977; **Resid:** Psychiatry, New York Hosp 1982; **Fellow:** Psychopharmacology, New York Hosp 1984; **Fac Appt:** Assoc Prof Psyc, Columbia P&S

Buckley, Peter J MD (Psyc) - **Spec Exp:** Psychoanalysis; **Hospital:** Montefiore Med Ctr - Div. Moses (page 100); **Address:** 336 Central Park W, Ste 5A, New York, NY 10025; **Phone:** 718-920-7967; **Board Cert:** Psychiatry 1974; **Med School:** New Zealand 1966; **Resid:** Psychiatry, Bronx Muni Hosp Ctr 1970; **Fellow:** Child & Adolescent Psychiatry, Bronx Muni Hosp Ctr 1972; **Fac Appt:** Prof Psyc, Albert Einstein Coll Med

Bukberg, Judith MD (Psyc) - **Spec Exp:** Psychotherapy; Psychoanalysis; **Address:** 3 E 10th St, Ste 1A, New York, NY 10003; **Phone:** 212-614-0312; **Board Cert:** Psychiatry 1979; **Med School:** Mount Sinai Sch Med 1974; **Resid:** Psychiatry, Mount Sinai Hosp 1978; **Fellow:** Liaison Psychiatry, Meml Sloan Kettering Cancer Ctr 1980; Psychoanalysis, NY Psych Inst 1996; **Fac Appt:** Assoc Clin Prof Psyc, NY Med Coll

Chung, Henry MD (Psyc) - **Spec Exp:** Depression; Anxiety Disorders; **Hospital:** NYU Langone Med Ctr (page 106); **Address:** 85 Fifth Ave, Ste 907, New York, NY 10003; **Phone:** 917-533-6908; **Board Cert:** Psychiatry 2004; **Med School:** SUNY Buffalo 1989; **Resid:** Psychiatry, NY Hosp 1994; **Fellow:** Research, NY Hosp 1995; **Fac Appt:** Assoc Clin Prof Psyc, NYU Sch Med

Cohen, Arnold R MD (Psyc) - **Spec Exp:** Psychotherapy; ADD/ADHD; Autism; **Hospital:** Mount Sinai Med Ctr (page 102); **Address:** 64 E 94th St, Apt 1A, New York, NY 10128; **Phone:** 212-289-6800; **Board Cert:** Psychiatry 1969; **Med School:** SUNY Hlth Sci Ctr 1963; **Resid:** Psychiatry, Mount Sinai Hosp 1966; **Fellow:** Child & Adolescent Psychiatry, Mount Sinai Hosp 1970; **Fac Appt:** Asst Clin Prof Psyc, Mount Sinai Sch Med

Cournos, Francine MD (Psyc) - **Spec Exp:** Aggression Disorders; Relationship Problems; Psychotherapy; **Hospital:** NY-Presby Hosp/Columbia (page 104), NY State Psychiatric Inst; **Address:** Mailman Sch Public Hlth, 722 W 168th St, rm 1030C, New York, NY 10032; **Phone:** 212-543-5412; **Board Cert:** Psychiatry 1978; **Med School:** NYU Sch Med 1971; **Resid:** Internal Medicine, Montefiore Hosp Med Ctr 1973; Psychiatry, NY State Psyc Inst 1976; **Fac Appt:** Prof Psyc, Columbia P&S

Devlin, Michael MD (Psyc) - **Spec Exp:** Eating Disorders; Obesity; **Hospital:** NY-Presby Hosp/Columbia (page 104); **Address:** New York State Psyc Inst, 1051 Riverside Dr, New York, NY 10032; **Phone:** 212-543-5748; **Board Cert:** Psychiatry 1987; **Med School:** Columbia P&S 1982; **Resid:** Psychiatry, NY State Psych Inst-Columbia P&S 1986; **Fellow:** Biological Psychiatry, NY State Psych Inst-Columbia P&S 1989; **Fac Appt:** Clin Prof Psyc, Columbia P&S

Douglas, Carolyn MD (Psyc) - **Spec Exp:** Depression; Anxiety Disorders; Relationship Problems; **Hospital:** NY-Presby Hosp/Columbia (page 104), NY-Presby Hosp/Weill Cornell (page 104); **Address:** 345 E 84th St, New York, NY 10028-4434; **Phone:** 212-396-9808; **Board Cert:** Psychiatry 1985; **Med School:** Harvard Med Sch 1980; **Resid:** Psychiatry, NY Hosp-Payne Whitney Clinic 1984; **Fac Appt:** Assoc Clin Prof Psyc, Columbia P&S

Eth, Spencer MD (Psyc) - **Spec Exp:** Forensic Psychiatry; Post Traumatic Stress Disorder; **Address:** 144 W 12th St, rm 174, New York, NY 10011-8202; **Phone:** 212-604-8196; **Board Cert:** Child & Adolescent Psychiatry 1982; Geriatric Psychiatry 2000; Forensic Psychiatry 2005; **Med School:** UCLA 1976; **Resid:** Psychiatry, NY Cornell Med Ctr 1979; **Fellow:** Child & Adolescent Psychiatry, Cedars-Sinai Med Ctr 1981; **Fac Appt:** Prof Psyc, NY Med Coll

Fallon, Brian A MD (Psyc) - **Spec Exp:** Lyme Disease-Neuro Complications; Psychosomatic Disorders; Obsessive-Compulsive Disorder; Psychiatry in Physical Illness; **Hospital:** NY-Presby Hosp/Columbia (page 104); **Address:** NYS Psychiatric Institute, 1051 Riverside Drive, Room 3724, Unit/Box 69, New York, NY 10032; **Phone:** 212-543-5487; **Board Cert:** Psychiatry 1991; **Med School:** Columbia P&S 1985; **Resid:** Psychiatry, NYS Psychiatric Inst 1989; **Fellow:** Psychiatric Research, NYS Psychiatric Inst 1992; Psychodynamic Psychotherapy, Columbia Univ Psychoanalytic Inst 1990; **Fac Appt:** Asst Clin Prof Psyc, Columbia P&S

Ferran Jr, Ernesto MD (Psyc) - **Spec Exp:** Cultural Psychiatry; Child & Adolescent Psychiatry; Mood Disorders; Couples Therapy; **Hospital:** NYU Langone Med Ctr (page 106); **Address:** 15 Charles St, Ste 6H, New York, NY 10014-3024; **Phone:** 212-924-2673; **Board Cert:** Psychiatry 1983; Child & Adolescent Psychiatry 1986; **Med School:** Albert Einstein Coll Med 1976; **Resid:** Psychiatry, Bellevue Hosp/NYU Med Ctr 1979; **Fellow:** Child & Adolescent Psychiatry, Bellevue Hosp/NYU Med Ctr 1981; **Fac Appt:** Clin Prof Psyc, NYU Sch Med

Finkel, Jay MD (Psyc) - **Spec Exp:** Anxiety Disorders; Mood Disorders; **Hospital:** Mount Sinai Med Ctr (page 102); **Address:** 108 E 91st St, New York, NY 10128-1657; **Phone:** 212-289-2077; **Board Cert:** Psychiatry 1985; **Med School:** NY Med Coll 1980; **Resid:** Psychiatry, Mount Sinai Hosp 1984; **Fac Appt:** Asst Clin Prof Psyc, Mount Sinai Sch Med

First, Michael B MD (Psyc) - **Spec Exp:** Psychotherapy; Psychopharmacology; Forensic Psychiatry; Sexual Addiction; **Hospital:** NY-Presby Hosp/Columbia (page 104); **Address:** NY State Psychiatric Inst, Unit 60, 1051 Riverside Drive, New York, NY 10032; **Phone:** 212-543-5531; **Board Cert:** Psychiatry 1989; **Med School:** Univ Pittsburgh 1983; **Resid:** Psychiatry, NY State Psych Inst 1987; **Fellow:** Psychiatric Research, NY State Psych Inst 1988; **Fac Appt:** Clin Prof Psyc, Columbia P&S

Fox, Herbert A MD (Psyc) - **Spec Exp:** Electroconvulsive Therapy (ECT); Psychotherapy; Psychopharmacology; **Hospital:** Lenox Hill Hosp, Gracie Square Hosp; **Address:** 416 E 76th St, New York, NY 10021-4032; **Phone:** 212-674-8622; **Board Cert:** Psychiatry 1976; **Med School:** Albert Einstein Coll Med 1969; **Resid:** Psychiatry, Montefiore Med Ctr 1973; **Fac Appt:** Assoc Prof Psyc, Cornell Univ-Weill Med Coll

Friedman, Richard Alan MD (Psyc) - **Spec Exp:** Psychopharmacology; Anxiety & Mood Disorders; Depression; **Hospital:** NY-Presby Hosp/Weill Cornell (page 104); **Address:** 525 E 68th St, Box 140, New York, NY 10021-4870; **Phone:** 212-746-5775; **Board Cert:** Psychiatry 1989; **Med School:** UMDNJ-RW Johnson Med Sch 1982; **Resid:** Psychiatry, Mount Sinai 1987; **Fac Appt:** Prof Psyc, Cornell Univ-Weill Med Coll

Fyer, Abby J MD (Psyc) - **Spec Exp:** Anxiety Disorders; Panic Disorder; **Hospital:** NY State Psychiatric Inst; **Address:** 1051 Riverside Dr, Box 82, New York, NY 10032; **Phone:** 212-543-5372; **Board Cert:** Psychiatry 1980; **Med School:** NYU Sch Med 1973; **Resid:** Psychiatry, Montefiore Med Ctr 1978; **Fac Appt:** Prof Psyc, Columbia P&S

Fyer, Minna R MD (Psyc) - **Spec Exp:** Anxiety Disorders; Mood Disorders; Menopause Problems; **Hospital:** NY-Presby Hosp/Weill Cornell (page 104); **Address:** 242 E 72nd St, New York, NY 10021-4574; **Phone:** 212-861-2586; **Board Cert:** Psychiatry 1985; **Med School:** SUNY Hlth Sci Ctr 1980; **Resid:** Psychiatry, NY Hosp/Payne Whitney Cl 1984; **Fellow:** Psychopharmacology, NY State Psych Inst/Columbia 1986; **Fac Appt:** Asst Prof Psyc, Cornell Univ-Weill Med Coll

Gershell, William J MD (Psyc) - **Spec Exp:** Psychopharmacology; Anxiety & Mood Disorders; Neuro-Psychiatry; **Hospital:** Mount Sinai Med Ctr (page 102); **Address:** 1100 Madison Ave, Ste 2C, New York, NY 10028-0338; **Phone:** 212-737-9300; **Board Cert:** Psychiatry 1975; Geriatric Psychiatry 2001; **Med School:** Switzerland 1965; **Resid:** Psychiatry, Mt Sinai Hosp 1968; **Fellow:** Child & Adolescent Psychiatry, Mt Sinai Hosp 1970; Psychoanalysis, William Alanson White Inst of Psychoanalysis 1977; **Fac Appt:** Asst Clin Prof Psyc, Mount Sinai Sch Med

Glassman, Alexander MD (Psyc) - **Spec Exp:** Depression; Psychopharmacology; Smoking Cessation; **Hospital:** NY State Psychiatric Inst, NYPresby-Morgan Stanley Children's Hosp (page 104); **Address:** 161 Fort Washington Ave, New York, NY 10032-1007; **Phone:** 212-543-5750; **Board Cert:** Psychiatry 1975; **Med School:** Univ IL Coll Med 1958; **Resid:** Psychiatry, Jacobi Med Ctr 1962; **Fellow:** Psychiatry, US Public Hlth Service 1964

Goldenberg, David B MD (Psyc) - **Spec Exp:** HIV Psychiatry; Psychoanalysis; Gender Issues; Psychiatry in Cancer; **Hospital:** NY-Presby Hosp/Weill Cornell (page 104); **Address:** 35 E 85th St, New York, NY 10028; **Phone:** 212-717-4834; **Board Cert:** Psychiatry 2007; Psychosomatic Medicine 2005; **Med School:** Univ MD Sch Med 1991; **Resid:** Psychiatry, Yale-New Haven Hosp 1996; **Fellow:** Psychiatry, Meml Sloan Kettering Cancer Ctr 1997

Goldman, Neil S MD (Psyc) - **Spec Exp:** Mood Disorders; Anxiety Disorders; Addiction/Substance Abuse; **Hospital:** N Shore Univ Hosp; **Address:** 235 W 48th St, New York, NY 10036; **Phone:** 212-929-4395; **Board Cert:** Psychiatry 1981; **Med School:** Ros Franklin Univ/Chicago Med Sch 1970; **Resid:** Psychiatry, Brookdale Hosp 1974; **Fellow:** Addiction Psychiatry, St Vincent's Hosp & Med Ctr 1979; **Fac Appt:** Asst Prof Psyc, NY Med Coll

Goldstein, Susanna K MD (Psyc) - **Spec Exp:** Psychopharmacology; Anxiety Disorders; **Hospital:** Lenox Hill Hosp; **Address:** 65 Central Park West, Ste 1BR, New York, NY 10023; **Phone:** 212-362-6657; **Board Cert:** Psychiatry 1985; **Med School:** Israel 1975; **Resid:** Psychiatry, Rambam Med Ctr 1980; Neurology, Rambam Med Ctr 1981; **Fellow:** Biological Psychiatry, Montefiore Med Ctr 1983; **Fac Appt:** Asst Clin Prof Psyc

Goodman, Berney MD (Psyc) - **Spec Exp:** Psychotherapy & Psychopharmacology; Psychiatry in Physical Illness; Psychosomatic Disorders; **Hospital:** Mount Sinai Med Ctr (page 102), Lenox Hill Hosp; **Address:** 11 E 68th St, New York, NY 10021-4955; **Phone:** 212-535-0111; **Board Cert:** Psychiatry 1971; **Med School:** South Africa 1957; **Resid:** Internal Medicine, Mount Sinai Hosp 1964; Psychiatry, Bronx Municipal/Montefiore 1969; **Fellow:** Physiology, Mount Sinai 1962; **Fac Appt:** Asst Clin Prof Psyc, Mount Sinai Sch Med

Gorman, Lauren K MD (Psyc) - **Spec Exp:** Psychopharmacology; Anxiety & Mood Disorders; **Hospital:** Mount Sinai Med Ctr (page 102); **Address:** 685 West End Ave, Ste 1AF, New York, NY 10025; **Phone:** 212-580-7713; **Board Cert:** Psychiatry 1983; **Med School:** Columbia P&S 1977; **Resid:** Ophthalmology, Bellevue Hosp 1979; Psychiatry, Mt Sinai Hosp 1982; **Fellow:** Biological Psychiatry, Montefiore Hosp Med Ctr 1984; **Fac Appt:** Asst Clin Prof Psyc, Mount Sinai Sch Med

Heller, Stanley S MD (Psyc) - **Spec Exp:** Panic Disorder; Depression; **Address:** 1136 Fifth Ave, New York, NY 10128; **Phone:** 212-831-5919; **Board Cert:** Psychiatry 1975; **Med School:** Columbia P&S 1960; **Resid:** Psychiatry, NYS Psych Inst-Columbia 1966; **Fac Appt:** Assoc Clin Prof Psyc, Columbia P&S

Hoffman, Joel MD (Psyc) - **Spec Exp:** Psychopharmacology; Depression; Treatment Resistant Mental Illness; **Hospital:** Lenox Hill Hosp, NY-Presby Hosp/Weill Cornell (page 104); **Address:** 1236 Park Ave, New York, NY 10128-1717; **Phone:** 212-722-3004; **Board Cert:** Psychiatry 1977; **Med School:** Columbia P&S 1963; **Resid:** Internal Medicine, Univ Michigan Med Ctr 1967; Psychiatry, NYS Psychiatric Inst 1972; **Fac Appt:** Asst Clin Prof Psyc, Columbia P&S

Hollander, Eric MD (Psyc) - **Spec Exp:** Obsessive-Compulsive Disorder; Anxiety Disorders; Autism; Body Dysmorphic Disorder (BDD); **Hospital:** Montefiore Med Ctr - Div. Moses (page 100); **Address:** 300 Central Park West, Ste 1C, New York, NY 10024-1513; **Phone:** 914-698-4696; **Board Cert:** Psychiatry 1987; **Med School:** SUNY Hlth Sci Ctr 1982; **Resid:** Internal Medicine, Mount Sinai Hosp 1983; Psychiatry, Mount Sinai Hosp 1986; **Fellow:** Psychiatry, Columbia-Presby Med Ctr 1988; **Fac Appt:** Prof Psyc, Albert Einstein Coll Med

Isay, Richard A MD (Psyc) - **Spec Exp:** Gay & Lesbian Issues; **Address:** 55 E End Ave, Ste 1G, New York, NY 10028-7933; **Phone:** 212-535-1863; **Board Cert:** Psychiatry 1969; **Med School:** Univ Rochester 1961; **Resid:** Psychiatry, Yale-New Haven Hosp 1965; **Fac Appt:** Clin Prof Psyc, Cornell Univ-Weill Med Coll

Kahn, David A MD (Psyc) - **Spec Exp:** Anxiety & Mood Disorders; Psychopharmacology; Psychotherapy; Schizophrenia; **Hospital:** NY-Presby Hosp/Columbia (page 104); **Address:** 180 Fort Washington Ave, rm HP242, New York, NY 10032; **Phone:** 212-472-0100; **Board Cert:** Psychiatry 1984; **Med School:** Columbia P&S 1979; **Resid:** Psychiatry, NY State Psych Inst 1983; **Fellow:** Biological Psychiatry, NY State Psych Inst 1984; **Fac Appt:** Clin Prof Psyc, Columbia P&S

Kalinich, Lila J MD (Psyc) - **Spec Exp:** Psychoanalysis; Psychotherapy; Adolescent Psychiatry; **Hospital:** NY-Presby Hosp/Columbia (page 104), NY State Psychiatric Inst; **Address:** 333 Central Park West, Ste 12, New York, NY 10025-7104; **Phone:** 212-866-0200; **Board Cert:** Psychiatry 1975; **Med School:** Northwestern Univ 1969; **Resid:** Psychiatry, Columbia-Presby Hosp 1973; **Fac Appt:** Clin Prof Psyc, Columbia P&S

Karasu, Sylvia R MD (Psyc) - **Spec Exp:** Weight Management; Eating Disorders; **Hospital:** NY-Presby Hosp/Weill Cornell (page 104); **Address:** 2 E 88th St, New York, NY 10128; **Phone:** 212-534-7822; **Board Cert:** Psychiatry 1981; Child & Adolescent Psychiatry 1982; **Med School:** Albert Einstein Coll Med 1976; **Resid:** Psychiatry, Payne Whitney-Cornell Univ 1979; **Fellow:** Child Psychiatry, Payne Whitney-Cornell Univ 1981; **Fac Appt:** Assoc Clin Prof Psyc

Karasu, T Byram MD (Psyc) - **Spec Exp:** Depression; Personality Disorders; Psychotherapy; **Hospital:** Montefiore Med Ctr - Div. Moses (page 100); **Address:** 2 E 88th St, New York, NY 10128-0555; **Phone:** 212-426-5208; **Board Cert:** Psychiatry 1972; **Med School:** Turkey 1959; **Resid:** Psychiatry, Yale-New Haven Hosp 1968; **Fellow:** Psychiatry, Yale-New Haven Hosp 1969; **Fac Appt:** Prof Psyc, Albert Einstein Coll Med

Kaufmann, Charles A MD (Psyc) - **Spec Exp:** Schizophrenia; Bipolar/Mood Disorders; Genetic Counseling-Psychiatric; **Hospital:** NY-Presby Hosp/Columbia (page 104), NY State Psychiatric Inst; **Address:** 161 Fort Washington Ave, Ste 211, New York, NY 10032; **Phone:** 914-238-7909; **Board Cert:** Psychiatry 1982; **Med School:** Columbia P&S 1977; **Resid:** Psychiatry, NY Hosp 1981; **Fellow:** Research, Natl Inst Hlth 1985; Research, Ctr for Neurobio & Behavior 1988; **Fac Appt:** Assoc Prof Psyc, Columbia P&S

Kavey, Neil B MD (Psyc) - **Spec Exp:** Sleep Medicine; Narcolepsy; Sleep Disorders/Apnea; **Hospital:** NY-Presby Hosp/Columbia (page 104), Rockefeller Univ; **Address:** Columbia Presby Med Ctr, Sleep Disorders Ctr, 161 Ft Washington Ave Fl 3 - rm 342, New York, NY 10032; **Phone:** 212-305-1860; **Board Cert:** Psychiatry 1976; Sleep Medicine 2003; **Med School:** Columbia P&S 1969; **Resid:** Psychiatry, Columbia Presby Med Ctr 1973; **Fac Appt:** Clin Prof Psyc, Columbia P&S

Kocsis, James MD (Psyc) - **Spec Exp:** Psychopharmacology; Mood Disorders; Anxiety Disorders; **Hospital:** NY-Presby Hosp/Weill Cornell (page 104); **Address:** 525 E 68th St, Box 140, New York, NY 10021-4885; **Phone:** 212-746-5913; **Board Cert:** Psychiatry 1977; **Med School:** Cornell Univ-Weill Med Coll 1968; **Resid:** Psychiatry, New York Hosp 1975; **Fac Appt:** Prof Psyc, Cornell Univ-Weill Med Coll

Kowallis, George MD (Psyc) - **Spec Exp:** Depression; Anxiety Disorders; ADD/ADHD; **Address:** 162 W 56th St, Ste 407, New York, NY 10019-3831; **Phone:** 212-757-0324; **Board Cert:** Psychiatry 1977; Child & Adolescent Psychiatry 1978; **Med School:** Univ Pennsylvania 1969; **Resid:** Psychiatry, St Luke's-Roosevelt Hosp Ctr 1974; **Fac Appt:** Asst Clin Prof Psyc, NY Med Coll

Kremberg, M Roy MD (Psyc) - **Spec Exp:** Mood Disorders; Anxiety Disorders; ADD/ADHD; **Hospital:** St Luke's - Roosevelt Hosp Ctr - Roosevelt Div (page 94), NY-Presby Hosp/Columbia (page 104); **Address:** 2109 Broadway, Ste 8144, New York, NY 10023-2106; **Phone:** 212-875-8568; **Board Cert:** Psychiatry 1980; Child & Adolescent Psychiatry 1982; **Med School:** Columbia P&S 1976; **Resid:** Psychiatry, St Luke's-Roosevelt Hosp Ctr 1978; **Fellow:** Child & Adolescent Psychiatry, St Luke's-Roosevelt Hosp Ctr 1980

Krueger, Richard B MD (Psyc) - **Spec Exp:** Sexual Behavior-Compulsive; **Hospital:** NY-Presby Hosp/Columbia (page 104); **Address:** 210 E 68th St, Ste 1H, New York, NY 10021-6047; **Phone:** 212-517-6624; **Board Cert:** Psychiatry 1984; Internal Medicine 1980; Addiction Psychiatry 2007; Forensic Psychiatry 2006; **Med School:** Harvard Med Sch 1977; **Resid:** Internal Medicine, Boston VA Hosp 1980; **Fellow:** Psychiatry, Boston Univ Hosp 1983; **Fac Appt:** Assoc Prof Psyc, Columbia P&S

Levitan, Stephan MD (Psyc) - **Spec Exp:** Psychotherapy; Psychopharmacology; Couples Therapy; Psychoanalysis; **Hospital:** NY-Presby Hosp/Columbia (page 104); **Address:** 185 E 85th St, Ste 29J, New York, NY 10028-2143; **Phone:** 212-722-4311; **Board Cert:** Psychiatry 1974; **Med School:** SUNY Buffalo 1965; **Resid:** Psychiatry, Hillside Hosp 1969; **Fellow:** Psychoanalysis, Columbia Presby Med Ctr 1973; **Fac Appt:** Clin Prof Psyc, Columbia P&S

Lindenmayer, Jean-Pierre MD (Psyc) - **Spec Exp:** Psychopharmacology; Schizophrenia; Bipolar/Mood Disorders; **Address:** 18 E 77th St, Ste B, New York, NY 10021-1700; **Phone:** 212-249-2720; **Board Cert:** Psychiatry 1975; **Med School:** Switzerland 1967; **Resid:** Psychiatry, Univ Hosp-Geneva Med Sch 1969; Psychiatry, SUNY Downstate Med Ctr 1973; **Fellow:** Research, SUNY Downstate Med Ctr 1975; **Fac Appt:** Clin Prof Psyc, NYU Sch Med

Lipton, Brian P MD (Psyc) - **Spec Exp:** Psychotherapy; Psychopharmacology; Anxiety & Mood Disorders; Psychosomatic Disorders; **Hospital:** Lenox Hill Hosp; **Address:** 1111 Park Ave, Ste 1A, New York, NY 10128-1234; **Phone:** 212-427-4499; **Board Cert:** Psychiatry 1970; **Med School:** SUNY Hlth Sci Ctr 1964; **Resid:** Psychiatry, Hillside Hosp 1968; **Fac Appt:** Asst Clin Prof Psyc, NYU Sch Med

Mahon, Eugene MD (Psyc) - **Spec Exp:** Psychoanalysis; **Address:** 6 E 96th St, New York, NY 10128-0706; **Phone:** 212-831-1414; **Med School:** Ireland 1964; **Resid:** Internal Medicine, Brooklyn Hosp 1969; Psychiatry, St Lukes Roosevelt Hosp Ctr 1974; **Fellow:** Psychoanalysis, Columbia Univ Psychoanalytic Ctr 1980; Child Psychiatry, Columbia Univ Psychoanalytic Ctr 1980

Manevitz, Alan MD (Psyc) - **Spec Exp:** Marital/Family/Sex Therapy; Depression-TMS Therapy; ADD/PTSD; Frbromyalgia Syndrome (FMS); **Hospital:** NY-Presby Hosp/Weill Cornell (page 104), Lenox Hill Hosp; **Address:** 60 Sutton Place South, Ste 1CN, New York, NY 10022; **Phone:** 212-751-5072; **Board Cert:** Psychiatry 1987; **Med School:** Columbia P&S 1980; **Resid:** Psychiatry, NY Hosp 1984; **Fellow:** Psychopharmacology, NY Hosp 1985; **Fac Appt:** Assoc Clin Prof Psyc, Cornell Univ-Weill Med Coll

Mann, J John MD/PhD (Psyc) - **Spec Exp:** Mood Disorders; Clinical Trials; Suicide; **Hospital:** NY-Presby Hosp/Columbia (page 104); **Address:** NYS Psychiatric Institute, 1051 Riverside Drive, Box 42, New York, NY 10032; **Phone:** 212-543-5571; **Board Cert:** Psychiatry 1980; **Med School:** Australia 1978; **Resid:** Psychiatry, Royal Melbourne Hosp 1976; **Fac Appt:** Prof Psyc, Columbia P&S

Marin, Deborah B MD (Psyc) - **Spec Exp:** Memory Disorders; Depression; Depression in the Elderly; Geriatric Psychiatry; **Hospital:** Mount Sinai Med Ctr (page 102); **Address:** Mount Sinai Hospital, One Gustave L Levy Pl, Box 1068, New York, NY 10029; **Phone:** 212-241-7139; **Board Cert:** Psychiatry 1990; **Med School:** Mount Sinai Sch Med 1984; **Resid:** Psychiatry, Mount Sinai Hosp 1988; **Fellow:** Psychiatry, NY Hosp-Cornell Med Ctr 1991; **Fac Appt:** Prof Psyc, Mount Sinai Sch Med

Markowitz, John MD (Psyc) - **Spec Exp:** Depression; Post Traumatic Stress Disorder; Cognitive Psychotherapy; Psychopharmacology; **Hospital:** NY-Presby Hosp/Columbia (page 104), NY State Psychiatric Inst; **Address:** 40 E 83rd St, New York, NY 10028; **Phone:** 212-288-3070; **Board Cert:** Psychiatry 1987; **Med School:** Columbia P&S 1982; **Resid:** Psychiatry, Payne Whitney Clin/New York Hosp 1987; **Fac Appt:** Clin Prof Psyc, Columbia P&S

McGowan, James M MD (Psyc) - **Spec Exp:** Alcohol Abuse; Drug Abuse; **Hospital:** NY-Presby Hosp/Weill Cornell (page 104); **Address:** 49 E 78th St, Ste 1-A, New York, NY 10021-0211; **Phone:** 212-517-3888; **Board Cert:** Psychiatry 1974; **Med School:** Univ KY Coll Med 1964; **Resid:** Internal Medicine, Bellevue Hosp 1968; Psychiatry, Albert Einstein Coll Med 1971; **Fellow:** Community Psychiatry, Albert Einstein Coll Med 1972; **Fac Appt:** Asst Clin Prof Psyc, Cornell Univ-Weill Med Coll

McGrath, Patrick J MD (Psyc) - **Spec Exp:** Psychopharmacology; Depression; **Hospital:** NY-Presby Hosp/Columbia (page 104), NY State Psychiatric Inst; **Address:** 161 Fort Washington Ave, New York, NY 10032-3713; **Phone:** 212-543-5764; **Board Cert:** Psychiatry 1979; **Med School:** Columbia P&S 1974; **Resid:** Surgery, NY State Psy Inst 1978; **Fac Appt:** Assoc Clin Prof Psyc, Columbia P&S

McMullen, Robert MD (Psyc) - **Spec Exp:** Psychopharmacology; Anxiety Disorders; Bipolar/Mood Disorders; Pain-Facial (TMJ); **Hospital:** NY-Presby Hosp/Columbia (page 104); **Address:** 171 W 79th St, Ste 2, New York, NY 10024-6449; **Phone:** 212-362-9635; **Board Cert:** Psychiatry 1982; **Med School:** Georgetown Univ 1976; **Resid:** Psychiatry, Columbia-Presby Med Ctr 1980; **Fac Appt:** Asst Prof Psyc, Columbia P&S

Mellman, Lisa A MD (Psyc) - **Spec Exp:** Anxiety & Depression; Relationship Problems; Work Problems; **Hospital:** NY-Presby Hosp/Columbia (page 104), NY State Psychiatric Inst; **Address:** Columbia Univ Med Ctr, 161 Ft Washington Ave, New York, NY 10032; **Phone:** 917-620-6010; **Board Cert:** Psychiatry 1986; **Med School:** Case West Res Univ 1981; **Resid:** Psychiatry, Psych Inst/Columbia-Presby Med Ctr 1985; **Fellow:** Psychoanalysis, Columbia Univ 1991; **Fac Appt:** Clin Prof Psyc, Columbia P&S

Michels, Robert MD (Psyc) - **Spec Exp:** Psychoanalysis; **Hospital:** NY-Presby Hosp/Weill Cornell (page 104); **Address:** 418 E 71st St, New York, NY 10021-4894; **Phone:** 212-746-6001; **Board Cert:** Psychiatry 1964; **Med School:** Northwestern Univ 1958; **Resid:** Psychiatry, Columbia-Presby Hosp 1962; **Fac Appt:** Prof Psyc, Cornell Univ-Weill Med Coll

Moore, Joanne MD (Psyc) - **Spec Exp:** Depression; Anxiety Disorders; **Hospital:** NY-Presby Hosp/Columbia (page 104); **Address:** 635 W 165th St, Ste 303, New York, NY 10032; **Phone:** 212-305-9499; **Board Cert:** Psychiatry 1988; Addiction Psychiatry 2006; **Med School:** Harvard Med Sch 1982; **Resid:** Psychiatry, Columbia-Presby Med Ctr 1987; **Fellow:** Geriatric Psychiatry, Columbia-Presby Med Ctr 1984; **Fac Appt:** Assoc Prof Psyc, Columbia P&S

Muhlbauer, Helen G MD (Psyc) - **Spec Exp:** Women's Health-Mental Health; Addiction/Substance Abuse; Psychosomatic Disorders; **Hospital:** NY-Presby Hosp/Columbia (page 104); **Address:** NY Presby Hosp-Dept Psychiatry, Allen Pavillion, 3 River E, 5141 Broadway, New York, NY 10034; **Phone:** 212-932-4642; **Board Cert:** Psychiatry 1991; Addiction Psychiatry 2008; Psychosomatic Medicine 2006; **Med School:** Albert Einstein Coll Med 1977; **Resid:** Psychiatry, Albert Einstein Affil Hosp 1981; **Fac Appt:** Asst Prof Psyc, Columbia P&S

Muskin, Philip MD (Psyc) - **Spec Exp:** Psychopharmacology; Anxiety & Depression; Psychiatry in Physical Illness; **Hospital:** NY-Presby Hosp/Columbia (page 104); **Address:** 1700 York Ave, New York, NY 10128-7820; **Phone:** 212-722-8438; **Board Cert:** Psychiatry 1979; Geriatric Psychiatry 2001; Psychosomatic Medicine 2005; **Med School:** NY Med Coll 1974; **Resid:** Psychiatry, NYS Psych Inst 1978; **Fellow:** Psychosomatic Medicine, Columbia-Presby Hosp 1979; Psychopharmacology, NY State Psych Inst 1979; **Fac Appt:** Prof Psyc, Columbia P&S

Nininger, James MD (Psyc) - **Spec Exp:** Psychotherapy; Psychopharmacology; Geriatric Psychiatry; **Hospital:** NY-Presby Hosp/Weill Cornell (page 104); **Address:** 10 E 78th St, Ste 5A, New York, NY 10075; **Phone:** 212-879-8338; **Board Cert:** Psychiatry 1978; **Med School:** Univ Cincinnati 1974; **Resid:** Psychiatry, Mount Sinai 1977; **Fac Appt:** Assoc Clin Prof Psyc, Cornell Univ-Weill Med Coll

Nunes, Edward MD (Psyc) - **Spec Exp:** Depression; Substance Abuse; **Hospital:** NY State Psychiatric Inst, NY-Presby Hosp/Columbia (page 104); **Address:** 1051 Riverside Drive, Mail Unit 51, New York, NY 10032-1007; **Phone:** 212-579-0339; **Board Cert:** Psychiatry 1986; Addiction Psychiatry 2002; **Med School:** Univ Conn 1981; **Resid:** Psychiatry, Columbia-Presby/NYS Psyc Inst 1985; **Fellow:** Psychopharmacology, Columbia-Presby/NYS Psyc Inst 1988; **Fac Appt:** Prof Psyc, Columbia P&S

Oberfield, Richard MD (Psyc) - **Spec Exp:** Child & Adolescent Psychiatry; Divorce/Family Issues; ADD/ADHD; **Hospital:** NYU Langone Med Ctr (page 106); **Address:** 200 E 33rd St, Ste 2J, New York, NY 10016-4874; **Phone:** 212-684-0148; **Board Cert:** Psychiatry 1979; Child & Adolescent Psychiatry 1980; Forensic Psychiatry 1999; **Med School:** Mount Sinai Sch Med 1974; **Resid:** Psychiatry, Bellevue Hosp 1976; **Fellow:** Child & Adolescent Psychiatry, Bellevue Hosp 1978; **Fac Appt:** Clin Prof Psyc, NYU Sch Med

Olds, David MD (Psyc) - **Spec Exp:** Psychoanalysis; Psychotherapy; **Hospital:** NY-Presby Hosp/Columbia (page 104); **Address:** 108 E 96th St, Ste 6F, New York, NY 10128; **Phone:** 212-427-9688; **Board Cert:** Psychiatry 1975; **Med School:** Columbia P&S 1967; **Resid:** Psychiatry, NY State Psych Inst 1971; **Fellow:** Psychiatry, Columbia-Psych Ctr 1977; **Fac Appt:** Clin Prof Psyc, Columbia P&S

Papp, Laszlo A MD (Psyc) - **Spec Exp:** Anxiety & Mood Disorders; Depression; Panic Disorder; Psychopharmacology; **Hospital:** NY-Presby Hosp/Columbia (page 104); **Address:** 124 E 84th St, Ste 1B, New York, NY 10028; **Phone:** 212-360-5750; **Board Cert:** Psychiatry 1993; **Med School:** Hungary 1978; **Resid:** Internal Medicine, Natl Inst of Rheumatology 1981; Psychiatry, Beth Israel Med Ctr 1986; **Fellow:** Psychopharmacology, Columbia Univ 1989; **Fac Appt:** Assoc Prof Psyc, Columbia P&S

Pawel, Michael A MD (Psyc) - **Spec Exp:** Adolescent Psychiatry; **Hospital:** St Luke's - Roosevelt Hosp Ctr - St Luke's Hosp (page 94); **Address:** 15 W 72nd St, New York, NY 10023; **Phone:** 212-873-9170; **Board Cert:** Psychiatry 1977; **Med School:** Albert Einstein Coll Med 1971; **Resid:** Psychiatry, Montefiore Hosp Med Ctr 1974; **Fac Appt:** Asst Prof Psyc, Columbia P&S

Pfeffer, Cynthia MD (Psyc) - **Spec Exp:** Child & Adolescent Psychiatry; Bereavement/Traumatic Grief; Anxiety & Depression; ADD/ADHD; **Hospital:** NY-Presby Hosp/Weill Cornell (page 104), NYU Langone Med Ctr (page 106); **Address:** 1100 Madison Ave, New York, NY 10028; **Phone:** 212-717-2334; **Board Cert:** Psychiatry 1975; Child & Adolescent Psychiatry 1976; **Med School:** NYU Sch Med 1968; **Resid:** Psychiatry, Montefiore Med Ctr 1973; **Fellow:** Child & Adolescent Psychiatry, Montefiore Med Ctr 1973; **Fac Appt:** Prof Psyc, Cornell Univ-Weill Med Coll

Pines, Jeffrey MD (Psyc) - **Spec Exp:** Substance Abuse; **Hospital:** NY-Presby Hosp/Columbia (page 104); **Address:** NY Presbyterian Hosp, 161 Fort Washington Ave, New York, NY 10032; **Phone:** 212-579-1913; **Board Cert:** Psychiatry 1982; **Med School:** Columbia P&S 1973; **Resid:** Internal Medicine, Presby Hosp 1976; Psychiatry, NY State Psych Inst 1980; **Fellow:** Rheumatology, Hosp For Special Surg 1977; Liaison Psychiatry, Columbia-Presby Med Ctr 1981; **Fac Appt:** Assoc Clin Prof Psyc, Columbia P&S

Preven, David W MD (Psyc) - **Spec Exp:** Forensic Psychiatry; Psychopharmacology; Psychotherapy; **Hospital:** Montefiore Med Ctr - Div. Moses (page 100); **Address:** 52 Riverside Drive, New York, NY 10024-6501; **Phone:** 212-799-4907; **Board Cert:** Psychiatry 1969; Forensic Psychiatry 2005; **Med School:** Harvard Med Sch 1963; **Resid:** Psychiatry, Jacobi Hosp/ Albert Einstein 1967; **Fellow:** Psychiatry, NIMH-Albert Einstein Affil Hosp 1971; **Fac Appt:** Clin Prof Psyc, Albert Einstein Coll Med

Rees, Ellen MD (Psyc) - **Spec Exp:** Psychoanalysis; Psychotherapy; **Hospital:** NY-Presby Hosp/Weill Cornell (page 104); **Address:** 108 E 96th St Fl 7 - Ste F, New York, NY 10128-6217; **Phone:** 212-722-5988; **Board Cert:** Psychiatry 1979; **Med School:** Albert Einstein Coll Med 1974; **Resid:** Psychiatry, Mt Sinai Hosp 1977; **Fellow:** Psychiatry, New York Hosp-Cornell 1978; Psychoanalysis, Columbia Univ Ctr Psych Trng 1991; **Fac Appt:** Assoc Clin Prof Psyc, Cornell Univ-Weill Med Coll

Resnick, Richard MD (Psyc) - **Spec Exp:** Anxiety & Depression; Addiction/Substance Abuse; Marital/Family Therapy; **Hospital:** NYU Langone Med Ctr (page 106); **Address:** Ctr for Psychiatry & Family Therapy, 43 W 94th St, New York, NY 10025-7113; **Phone:** 212-678-6949; **Board Cert:** Psychiatry 1965; **Med School:** NY Med Coll 1958; **Resid:** Psychiatry, Hillside Hosp 1961; Psychiatry, Montefiore Hosp 1962; **Fac Appt:** Assoc Clin Prof Psyc, NYU Sch Med

Roose, Steven MD (Psyc) - **Spec Exp:** Depression in the Elderly; **Hospital:** NY-Presby Hosp/Columbia (page 104); **Address:** NY State Psychiatric Institute, 1051 Riverside Drive, New York, NY 10032; **Phone:** 212-831-8644; **Board Cert:** Psychiatry 1979; **Med School:** Mount Sinai Sch Med 1974; **Resid:** Psychiatry, NY Psychiatric Inst 1978; **Fellow:** Research, Columbia-Presby Med Ctr 1981; **Fac Appt:** Clin Prof Psyc, Columbia P&S

Rosen, Arnold M MD (Psyc) - **Spec Exp:** Depression; Psychopharmacology; **Address:** 200 E 78th St, New York, NY 10021; **Phone:** 212-288-6380; **Board Cert:** Psychiatry 1976; **Med School:** Univ Tex SW, Dallas 1968; **Resid:** Psychiatry, Metropolitan Hosp Ctr 1970; Psychiatry, Metropolitan Hosp Ctr 1974; **Fellow:** Psychiatry, Metropolitan Hosp Ctr 1975

Rosenbloom, Charles MD (Psyc) - **Spec Exp:** Psychotherapy; **Hospital:** VA Med Ctr - Bklyn; **Address:** 50 E 86th St, Ste 2A, New York, NY 10028-1067; **Phone:** 212-472-8673; **Board Cert:** Psychiatry 1977; **Med School:** Italy 1964; **Resid:** Psychiatry, St Vincent's Hosp 1967; Psychiatry, Hillside Hosp 1968; **Fellow:** Psychiatry, Creedmoor Psych Ctr 1969

Rosenthal, Jesse MD (Psyc) - **Spec Exp:** ADD/ADHD; Anxiety Disorders; Depression; **Hospital:** Beth Israel Med Ctr - Petrie Division (page 94); **Address:** 21 E 93rd St, New York, NY 10128-0609; **Phone:** 212-876-3080; **Board Cert:** Psychiatry 1978; **Med School:** Geo Wash Univ 1973; **Resid:** Psychiatry, Mount Sinai Hosp 1976; **Fac Appt:** Asst Clin Prof Psyc, Mount Sinai Sch Med

Rosenthal, Richard N MD (Psyc) - **Spec Exp:** Anxiety & Mood Disorders; Addiction/Substance Abuse; **Hospital:** St Luke's - Roosevelt Hosp Ctr - Roosevelt Div (page 94), Beth Israel Med Ctr - Petrie Division (page 94); **Address:** 1090 Amerstdam Ave Fl 16 - Ste G, New York, NY 10025; **Phone:** 212-523-5366; **Board Cert:** Psychiatry 1985; Addiction Psychiatry 2002; **Med School:** SUNY Hlth Sci Ctr 1980; **Resid:** Psychiatry, Mount Sinai Hosp 1984; **Fac Appt:** Prof Psyc, Columbia P&S

Rosner, Richard MD (Psyc) - **Spec Exp:** Adolescent Psychiatry; Forensic Psychiatry; Addiction/Substance Abuse; **Hospital:** NYU Langone Med Ctr (page 106), Bellevue Hosp Ctr; **Address:** 140 E 83rd St, Ste 6A, New York, NY 10028-1928; **Phone:** 212-988-6014; **Board Cert:** Psychiatry 1974; Forensic Psychiatry 2004; Addiction Psychiatry 2004; **Med School:** NYU Sch Med 1966; **Resid:** Psychiatry, Mount Sinai Hosp 1970; **Fac Appt:** Clin Prof Psyc, NYU Sch Med

Roth, Andrew J MD (Psyc) - **Spec Exp:** Psychiatry of Prostate Cancer; Geriatic Psychiatry; **Hospital:** Meml Sloan-Kettering Cancer Ctr (page 112), NY-Presby Hosp (page 104); **Address:** 641 Lexington Ave Fl 7, New York, NY 10022; **Phone:** 646-888-0024; **Board Cert:** Psychiatry 1993; Geriatric Psychiatry 2007; Psychosomatic Medicine 2005; **Med School:** NY Med Coll 1988; **Resid:** Psychiatry, Mt Sinai Med Ctr 1992; **Fellow:** Liaison Psychiatry, Meml Sloan-Kettering Canc Ctr 1994; **Fac Appt:** Clin Prof Psyc, Cornell Univ-Weill Med Coll

Rubinstein, Mort MD (Psyc) - **Spec Exp:** Psychopharmacology; **Hospital:** VA Med Ctr - Manhattan; **Address:** 423 E 23rd St, New York, NY 10010-5013; **Phone:** 212-686-7500 x7991; **Board Cert:** Psychiatry 1988; **Med School:** NY Med Coll 1976; **Resid:** Psychiatry, NYU-Bellevue Hosp 1979; **Fellow:** Psychiatry, Mount Sinai Med Ctr 1980; **Fac Appt:** Assoc Clin Prof Psyc, NYU Sch Med

Sacks, Michael MD (Psyc) - **Spec Exp:** Personality Disorders; Relationship Problems; Anxiety & Depression; **Hospital:** NY-Presby Hosp/Weill Cornell (page 104); **Address:** 525 E 68th St, New York, NY 10021-4870; **Phone:** 212-746-3710; **Board Cert:** Psychiatry 1973; **Med School:** NYU Sch Med 1967; **Resid:** Psychiatry, NY State Psych Inst 1971; **Fellow:** Psychiatry, Natl Inst Mental Health 1973; **Fac Appt:** Prof Psyc, Cornell Univ-Weill Med Coll

Sadock, Virginia MD (Psyc) - **Spec Exp:** Psychotherapy; Sexual Dysfunction; Anxiety & Depression; Marital/Family/Sex Therapy; **Hospital:** NYU Langone Med Ctr (page 106); **Address:** 4 E 89th St, Ste 1E, New York, NY 10128; **Phone:** 212-427-0885; **Board Cert:** Psychiatry 1975; **Med School:** NY Med Coll 1970; **Resid:** Psychiatry, Metropolitan Hosp 1973; **Fac Appt:** Clin Prof Psyc, NYU Sch Med

Samberg, Eslee MD (Psyc) - **Spec Exp:** Psychoanalysis; **Hospital:** NY-Presby Hosp/Weill Cornell (page 104); **Address:** 2211 Broadway, Ste 1H, New York, NY 10024-6263; **Phone:** 212-874-7725; **Board Cert:** Psychiatry 1983; **Med School:** Cornell Univ-Weill Med Coll 1978; **Resid:** Psychiatry, NY Hosp-Cornell Med Ctr 1982; **Fac Appt:** Assoc Clin Prof Psyc, Cornell Univ-Weill Med Coll

Sawyer, David MD (Psyc) - **Spec Exp:** Psychoanalysis; Child & Adolescent Psychiatry; **Hospital:** NY-Presby Hosp/Weill Cornell (page 104); **Address:** 1 W 64th St, Ste 1C, New York, NY 10023; **Phone:** 212-787-8260; **Board Cert:** Psychiatry 1982; Child & Adolescent Psychiatry 1984; **Med School:** NY Med Coll 1977; **Resid:** Psychiatry, NY Hosp-Cornell-Westchester 1980; **Fellow:** Child & Adolescent Psychiatry, NY Hosp-Cornell-Westchester 1982

Scharf, Robert D MD (Psyc) - **Spec Exp:** Psychotherapy; Psychopharmacology; Psychoanalysis; **Hospital:** St Luke's - Roosevelt Hosp Ctr - Roosevelt Div (page 94); **Address:** 207 E 74th St, Ste 1L, New York, NY 10021-3341; **Phone:** 212-988-4145; **Board Cert:** Psychiatry 1976; **Med School:** Albert Einstein Coll Med 1960; **Resid:** Internal Medicine, Barnes Hosp/Straight Ward Med 1961; Psychiatry, Kings Co Hosp 1964; **Fellow:** Psychoanalysis, NY Psychoanalytic Inst 1973; **Fac Appt:** Asst Clin Prof Psyc, Columbia P&S

Schein, Jonah MD (Psyc) - **Spec Exp:** Depression; Anxiety Disorders; **Hospital:** NY-Presby Hosp/Weill Cornell (page 104); **Address:** 1349 Lexington Ave, Ste 1E, New York, NY 10128-1514; **Phone:** 212-876-2324; **Board Cert:** Psychiatry 1975; **Med School:** NYU Sch Med 1969; **Resid:** Psychiatry, NY State Psych Inst 1973; **Fac Appt:** Assoc Clin Prof Psyc, Cornell Univ-Weill Med Coll

Schore, Arthur MD (Psyc) - **Spec Exp:** Depression; Sexual Dysfunction; Eating Disorders; **Hospital:** NY-Presby Hosp/Columbia (page 104); **Address:** 905 5th Ave, New York, NY 10021-4156; **Phone:** 212-535-6070; **Board Cert:** Psychiatry 1980; **Med School:** Ros Franklin Univ/Chicago Med Sch 1965; **Resid:** Columbia-Presby 1969; **Fellow:** NYS Psychiatric Inst 1975; **Fac Appt:** Psyc, Cornell Univ-Weill Med Coll

Seaman, Cheryl MD (Psyc) - **Spec Exp:** Anxiety Disorders; Depression; Psychopharmacology; Psychotherapy; **Address:** 30 E 60th St, Ste 1002, New York, NY 10022; **Phone:** 917-687-8901; **Board Cert:** Psychiatry 1986; Geriatric Psychiatry 2001; **Med School:** Columbia P&S 1979; **Resid:** Psychiatry, NY Hosp-Westchester Div 1983

Shapiro, Peter A MD (Psyc) - **Spec Exp:** Depression; Psychiatry in Physical Illness; Liaison Psychiatry; **Hospital:** NY-Presby Hosp/Columbia (page 104); **Address:** 239 Central Park West, New York, NY 10024-6038; **Phone:** 212-874-6030; **Board Cert:** Psychiatry 1985; Geriatric Psychiatry 2001; Psychosomatic Medicine 2005; **Med School:** Columbia P&S 1980; **Resid:** Psychiatry, NY State Psych Inst 1984; **Fellow:** Liaison Psychiatry, Columbia-Presby Med Ctr 1986; **Fac Appt:** Prof Psyc, Columbia P&S

Shaw, Ronda R MD (Psyc) - **Spec Exp:** Psychoanalysis; Psychotherapy; **Hospital:** Mount Sinai Med Ctr (page 102); **Address:** 35 E 85th St, Profl, Ste 2, New York, NY 10028-0954; **Phone:** 212-772-0321; **Board Cert:** Psychiatry 1977; **Med School:** Wayne State Univ 1966; **Resid:** Psychiatry, Einstein Hosp 1970; **Fac Appt:** Assoc Clin Prof Psyc, Mount Sinai Sch Med

Shinbach, Kent MD (Psyc) - **Spec Exp:** Depression; Psychopharmacology; Geriatric Psychiatry; **Hospital:** Gracie Square Hosp, Bridgeport Hosp; **Address:** 435 E 79th St, Ste 1C, New York, NY 10075; **Phone:** 212-744-7100; **Board Cert:** Psychiatry 1970; **Med School:** Jefferson Med Coll 1963; **Resid:** Psychiatry, NY Med Coll 1968; **Fac Appt:** Asst Clin Prof Psyc, Albert Einstein Coll Med

Siever, Larry J MD (Psyc) - **Spec Exp:** Psychopharmacology; Depression; Personality Disorders; **Hospital:** Mount Sinai Med Ctr (page 102), VA Med Ctr - Bronx; **Address:** 1 Gustave L Levy Pl, Box 1230, New York, NY 10029-6500; **Phone:** 212-774-1722; **Board Cert:** Psychiatry 1980; **Med School:** Stanford Univ 1975; **Resid:** Psychiatry, McLean Hosp 1978; **Fellow:** Biological Psychiatry, Natl Inst Mntl Hlth 1982; **Fac Appt:** Prof Psyc, Mount Sinai Sch Med

Silver, Jonathan M MD (Psyc) - **Spec Exp:** Neuro-Psychiatry; Psychopharmacology; Brain Injury; **Hospital:** Lenox Hill Hosp; **Address:** 40 E 83rd St, Ste 1E, New York, NY 10028; **Phone:** 212-874-6453; **Board Cert:** Psychiatry 1984; Behavioral Neurology & Neuropsychiatry 2006; **Med School:** Albert Einstein Coll Med 1979; **Resid:** Psychiatry, NY State Psych Inst 1983; **Fellow:** Research, NY State Psych Inst 1985; **Fac Appt:** Clin Prof Psyc, NYU Sch Med

Spitz, Henry MD (Psyc) - **Spec Exp:** Family & Couples Therapy; Addiction/Substance Abuse; Anxiety Disorders; **Hospital:** NY-Presby Hosp/Columbia (page 104); **Address:** 101 Central Park West, Ste 1C, New York, NY 10023-4204; **Phone:** 212-873-1415; **Board Cert:** Psychiatry 1973; **Med School:** NY Med Coll 1965; **Resid:** Psychiatry, NY Med Coll 1969; **Fellow:** Psychiatry, NY Med Coll 1971; **Fac Appt:** Clin Prof Psyc, Columbia P&S

Stein, Stefan MD (Psyc) - **Spec Exp:** Couples Therapy; Psychotherapy & Psychopharmacology; **Hospital:** NY-Presby Hosp/Weill Cornell (page 104); **Address:** 850 Park Ave, Ste 1E, New York, NY 10021; **Phone:** 212-249-0200; **Board Cert:** Psychiatry 1970; **Med School:** NYU Sch Med 1963; **Resid:** Internal Medicine, Boston City Hosp 1964; Psychiatry, Albert Einstein Coll Med 1968; **Fellow:** Psychiatry, Mass Genl Hosp 1965; Psychoanalysis, NY Psychoan Inst 1974; **Fac Appt:** Prof Psyc, Cornell Univ-Weill Med Coll

Stone, Michael H MD (Psyc) - **Spec Exp:** Personality Disorders; Psychoanalysis; Forensic Psychiatry; Addiction/Substance Abuse; **Hospital:** NY-Presby Hosp/Columbia (page 104); **Address:** 225 Central Park West, Ste 114, New York, NY 10024-6027; **Phone:** 212-758-2000; **Board Cert:** Psychiatry 1971; **Med School:** Cornell Univ-Weill Med Coll 1958; **Resid:** Internal Medicine, Bellevue Hosp 1961; Psychiatry, NYS Psych Inst 1966; **Fellow:** Hematology, Meml Sloan Kettering Cancer Ctr 1962; Medical Oncology, Meml Sloan Kettering Cancer Ctr 1963; **Fac Appt:** Clin Prof Psyc, Columbia P&S

Strain, James J MD (Psyc) - **Spec Exp:** Psychiatry in Physical Illness; Psychoanalysis; **Hospital:** Mount Sinai Med Ctr (page 102); **Address:** Dept of Psychiatry, 1425 Madison Ave, New York, NY 10029; **Phone:** 212-659-8728; **Board Cert:** Psychiatry 1969; **Med School:** Case West Res Univ 1962; **Resid:** Psychiatry, Univ Hosps 1966; **Fellow:** Psychiatric Research, Univ Hosps 1967; Psychoanalysis, New York Psychoanal Inst 1972; **Fac Appt:** Prof Psyc, Mount Sinai Sch Med

Sussman, Norman MD (Psyc) - **Spec Exp:** Psychopharmacology; Anxiety & Mood Disorders; Bipolar/Mood Disorders; **Hospital:** NYU Langone Med Ctr (page 106); **Address:** 150 E 58th St, Fl 27, New York, NY 10155; **Phone:** 212-588-9722; **Board Cert:** Psychiatry 1980; **Med School:** NY Med Coll 1975; **Resid:** Psychiatry, Metropolitan Hosp Ctr 1977; Psychiatry, Westchester Co Med Ctr 1978; **Fac Appt:** Prof Psyc, NYU Sch Med

Swiller, Hillel MD (Psyc) - **Spec Exp:** Psychotherapy; Couples Therapy; **Hospital:** Mount Sinai Med Ctr (page 102); **Address:** 108 E 96th St, Ste 9F, New York, NY 10128; **Phone:** 212-534-5588; **Board Cert:** Psychiatry 1972; **Med School:** Cornell Univ-Weill Med Coll 1965; **Resid:** Psychiatry, Albert Einstein Coll Med 1969; **Fac Appt:** Clin Prof Psyc, Mount Sinai Sch Med

Tancredi, Laurence R MD (Psyc) - **Spec Exp:** Forensic Psychiatry; Anxiety & Depression; **Hospital:** Lenox Hill Hosp; **Address:** 129B E 71st St, New York, NY 10021-4201; **Phone:** 212-288-5197; **Board Cert:** Psychiatry 1979; **Med School:** Univ Pennsylvania 1966; **Resid:** Psychiatry, NYS Psych Inst 1975; Psychiatry, Yale-New Haven Hosp 1977; **Fac Appt:** Clin Prof Psyc, NYU Sch Med

Tardiff, Kenneth J MD (Psyc) - **Spec Exp:** Psychopharmacology; Forensic Psychiatry; Psychotherapy; **Hospital:** NY-Presby Hosp/Weill Cornell (page 104); **Address:** Payne Whitney Clinic-NY Hosp, Dept Psyc, 525 E 68th St, Psy Box 140, New York, NY 10021-4870; **Phone:** 212-746-3871; **Board Cert:** Psychiatry 1976; **Med School:** Tulane Univ 1969; **Resid:** Psychiatry, Mass Genl Hosp 1973; **Fellow:** Public Health, Harvard Sch Public Hlth 1973; **Fac Appt:** Prof Psyc, Cornell Univ-Weill Med Coll

Taylor, Noel MD (Psyc) - **Spec Exp:** Anxiety Disorders; Mood Disorders; **Address:** 150 E 58 St, Fl 27, New York, NY 10155; **Phone:** 212-888-9038; **Board Cert:** Psychiatry 1985; **Med School:** Johns Hopkins Univ 1980; **Resid:** Psychiatry, Johns Hopkins Hosp 1984; **Fac Appt:** Asst Prof Psyc, Albert Einstein Coll Med

Teusink, J Paul MD (Psyc) - **Spec Exp:** Geriatric Psychiatry; Depression; Dementia; **Hospital:** Beth Israel Med Ctr - Petrie Division (page 94); **Address:** 88 University Pl, Ste 705, New York, NY 10003; **Phone:** 347-466-2521; **Board Cert:** Psychiatry 1976; Geriatric Psychiatry 2001; **Med School:** Univ Mich Med Sch 1969; **Resid:** Psychiatry, Topeka State Hosp 1971; Psychiatry, CF Menninger Meml Hosp 1973; **Fac Appt:** Assoc Prof Psyc, Albert Einstein Coll Med

Tolchin, Joan G MD (Psyc) - **Spec Exp:** Child & Adolescent Psychiatry; Psychotherapy; **Hospital:** NY-Presby Hosp/Weill Cornell (page 104); **Address:** 35 E 84th St, New York, NY 10028-0871; **Phone:** 212-744-1446; **Board Cert:** Psychiatry 1979; Child & Adolescent Psychiatry 1982; **Med School:** NYU Sch Med 1972; **Resid:** Psychiatry, Bronx Municipal Hosp 1975; **Fellow:** Child & Adolescent Psychiatry, NY Presby Hosp 1977; **Fac Appt:** Assoc Clin Prof Psyc, Cornell Univ-Weill Med Coll

Wachtel, Alan B MD (Psyc) - **Spec Exp:** ADD/ADHD; Mood Disorders; Learning Disorders; **Hospital:** NYU Langone Med Ctr (page 106); **Address:** 201 E 87th St, Ste 16J, New York, NY 10128; **Phone:** 212-348-0175; **Board Cert:** Therapeutic Radiology 1977; **Med School:** Mount Sinai Sch Med 1972; **Resid:** Psychiatry, Mt Sinai Hosp 1976; **Fellow:** Liaison Psychiatry, NY Hosp-Cornell Med Ctr 1977; **Fac Appt:** Assoc Clin Prof Psyc, NYU Sch Med

Wager, Steven G MD (Psyc) - **Spec Exp:** Psychopharmacology; Depression; Anxiety Disorders; **Address:** 145 W 86th St, Ste 1B, New York, NY 10024-3421; **Phone:** 212-769-9620; **Board Cert:** Psychiatry 1986; **Med School:** Case West Res Univ 1980; **Resid:** Psychiatry, Columbia-Presby Med Ctr 1984; **Fellow:** Psychopharmacology, Columbia-Presby Med Ctr 1986

Wallack, Joel J MD (Psyc) - **Spec Exp:** Psychopharmacology; Psychiatry in Physical Illness; Anxiety & Depression; **Hospital:** Beth Israel Med Ctr - Petrie Division (page 94), Mount Sinai Med Ctr (page 102); **Address:** Beth Israel Med Ctr, 10 Union Square E, New York, NY 10003; **Phone:** 212-420-2398; **Board Cert:** Psychiatry 1979; Psychosomatic Medicine 2005; **Med School:** UMDNJ-NJ Med Sch, Newark 1974; **Resid:** Psychiatry, St Lukes Hosp 1978; **Fellow:** Liaison Psychiatry, Montefiore Med Ctr 1979; Psychosomatic Medicine, Mt Sinai Hosp 1980; **Fac Appt:** Prof Psyc, Mount Sinai Sch Med

Walsh, B Timothy MD (Psyc) - **Spec Exp:** Eating Disorders; **Hospital:** NY State Psychiatric Inst, NY-Presby Hosp/Columbia (page 104); **Address:** NY State Psychiatric Inst-Unit 98, 1051 Riverside Dr, New York, NY 10032-2695; **Phone:** 212-543-5739; **Board Cert:** Psychiatry 1978; **Med School:** Harvard Med Sch 1972; **Resid:** Internal Medicine, Dartmouth Affil Hosps 1973; Psychiatry, Bronx Muni Hosp Ctr 1977; **Fac Appt:** Prof Psyc, Columbia P&S

Weill, Terry L MD (Psyc) - **Spec Exp:** Bipolar/Mood Disorders; Psychiatry in Physical Illness; **Hospital:** Mount Sinai Med Ctr (page 102), Beth Israel Med Ctr - Petrie Division (page 94); **Address:** 350 Central Park West, New York, NY 10023-6547; **Phone:** 212-316-5818; **Board Cert:** Psychiatry 1985; Geriatric Psychiatry 2000; **Med School:** Hahnemann Univ 1980; **Resid:** Psychiatry, Mount Sinai Med Ctr 1984; **Fellow:** Psychoanalysis, NYS Psyc Inst 1991; **Fac Appt:** Asst Prof Psyc, Mount Sinai Sch Med

Welsh, Howard K MD (Psyc) - **Spec Exp:** Psychotherapy; Psychoanalysis; **Hospital:** NYU Langone Med Ctr (page 106); **Address:** 27 W 86th St, Ste C, New York, NY 10024-3615; **Phone:** 212-362-5846; **Board Cert:** Psychiatry 1976; **Med School:** Albert Einstein Coll Med 1971; **Resid:** Psychiatry, Kings County Hosp 1974; **Fac Appt:** Clin Prof Psyc, NYU Sch Med

Wilner, Philip MD (Psyc) - **Hospital:** NY-Presby Hosp/Weill Cornell (page 104); **Address:** 525 E 68th St, Box 140, New York, NY 10065; **Phone:** 212-746-3705; **Board Cert:** Psychiatry 1989; **Med School:** Columbia P&S 1983; **Resid:** Psychiatry, NY Hosp 1987; **Fellow:** Psychopharmacology, NY Hosp 1991; **Fac Appt:** Assoc Prof Psyc, Cornell Univ-Weill Med Coll

Wineburg, Elliot N MD (Psyc) - **Spec Exp:** Hypnosis; Smoking Cessation; **Hospital:** Mount Sinai Med Ctr (page 102); **Address:** 145 W 58th St, Ste 3F, Neuro-Psychiatric Offices, New York, NY 10019; **Phone:** 212-582-0720; **Board Cert:** Psychiatry 1966; **Med School:** Switzerland 1956; **Resid:** Psychiatry, Manhattan State Hosp 1960; **Fac Appt:** Asst Clin Prof Psyc, Mount Sinai Sch Med

Winters, Richard A MD (Psyc) - **Spec Exp:** Psychopharmacology; Crisis Intervention; Psychodynamic Psychotherapy; **Address:** 35 E 85th St, New York, NY 10028-0954; **Phone:** 212-744-1346; **Board Cert:** Psychiatry 1977; **Med School:** NY Med Coll 1972; **Resid:** Psychiatry, Metropolitan Hosp Ctr 1975; **Fac Appt:** Asst Prof Psyc, NY Med Coll

Zimberg, Sheldon MD (Psyc) - **Spec Exp:** Geriatric Psychiatry; Hypnosis; Addiction Psychiatry; **Hospital:** St Luke's - Roosevelt Hosp Ctr - St Luke's Hosp (page 94), Beth Israel Med Ctr - Petrie Division (page 94); **Address:** 245-A E 61st St, New York, NY 10021-8203; **Phone:** 212-988-5139; **Board Cert:** Psychiatry 1969; Addiction Psychiatry 2004; **Med School:** SUNY Hlth Sci Ctr 1961; **Resid:** Psychiatry, NYS Psych Inst/Colum-Presby Med Ctr 1965; **Fellow:** Community Psychiatry, Columbia Univ Sch Pub Hlth 1966; **Fac Appt:** Clin Prof Psyc, Columbia P&S

Pulmonary Disease

Acquista, Angelo J MD (Pul) - **Spec Exp:** Asthma; Disaster Preparedness; **Hospital:** Lenox Hill Hosp; **Address:** Madison Medical, 110 E 59th St, Ste 9C, New York, NY 10022; **Phone:** 212-583-2850; **Board Cert:** Internal Medicine 1984; Pulmonary Disease 1986; **Med School:** NYU Sch Med 1981; **Resid:** Internal Medicine, Lenox Hill Hosp 1984; **Fellow:** Pulmonary Disease, Lenox Hill Hosp 1986

Adams, Francis V MD (Pul) - **Spec Exp:** Asthma; Chronic Obstructive Lung Disease (COPD); Pulmonary Fibrosis; Sarcoidosis; **Hospital:** NYU Langone Med Ctr (page 106); **Address:** 650 First Ave, Fl 7, New York, NY 10016-3240; **Phone:** 212-447-0088; **Board Cert:** Internal Medicine 1974; Pulmonary Disease 1976; **Med School:** Cornell Univ-Weill Med Coll 1971; **Resid:** Internal Medicine, Georgetown Univ Hosp 1973; **Fellow:** Pulmonary Disease, Bellevue Hosp 1975; **Fac Appt:** Asst Prof Med, NYU Sch Med

Addrizzo-Harris, Doreen MD (Pul) - **Spec Exp:** Bronchoscopy; Tuberculosis; Lung Cancer; Interstitial Lung Disease; **Hospital:** NYU Langone Med Ctr (page 106), Bellevue Hosp Ctr; **Address:** 462 First Ave, New Bellevue, rm 7N24, New York, NY 10016; **Phone:** 212-263-7951; **Board Cert:** Internal Medicine 2002; Pulmonary Disease 2006; Critical Care Medicine 2007; **Med School:** NYU Sch Med 1989; **Resid:** Internal Medicine, Bellevue Hosp/NYU Med Ctr 1992; **Fellow:** Pulmonary Critical Care Medicine, Bellevue Hosp/NYU Med Ctr 1996; **Fac Appt:** Assoc Prof Med, NYU Sch Med

Adler, Jack MD (Pul) - **Spec Exp:** Asthma; Chronic Obstructive Lung Disease (COPD); Tuberculosis; **Hospital:** Mount Sinai Med Ctr (page 102), Lenox Hill Hosp; **Address:** 210 E 86th St, New York, NY 10021-0117; **Phone:** 212-535-3622; **Board Cert:** Internal Medicine 1970; Pulmonary Disease 1971; **Med School:** Univ Chicago-Pritzker Sch Med 1962; **Resid:** Internal Medicine, Philadelphia Genl Hosp 1967; Internal Medicine, Michael Reese Hosp Med Ctr 1968; **Fellow:** Pulmonary Disease, Bronx Municipal Hosp Ctr 1971; **Fac Appt:** Assoc Prof Med, Mount Sinai Sch Med

Arcasoy, Selim M MD (Pul) - **Spec Exp:** Transplant Medicine-Lung; Chronic Obstructive Lung Disease (COPD); Interstitial Lung Disease; Pulmonary Embolism; **Hospital:** NY-Presby Hosp/Columbia (page 104); **Address:** Ctr for Advanced Lung Dis/Transp, 622 W 168th St PH Bldg Fl 14E - rm 104, New York, NY 10032-3720; **Phone:** 212-305-6589; **Board Cert:** Internal Medicine 2003; Pulmonary Disease 2006; Critical Care Medicine 2007; **Med School:** Turkey 1990; **Resid:** Internal Medicine, SUNY Downstate Med Ctr 1994; **Fellow:** Pulmonary Critical Care Medicine, Univ Pittsburgh Med Ctr 1998; **Fac Appt:** Prof Med, Columbia P&S

Baskin, Martin MD (Pul) - **Spec Exp:** Asthma; Pneumonia; Emphysema; **Hospital:** St Luke's - Roosevelt Hosp Ctr - Roosevelt Div (page 94); **Address:** 185 W End Ave, Ste 1M, New York, NY 10023-5567; **Phone:** 212-595-7701; **Board Cert:** Internal Medicine 1985; Pulmonary Disease 1988; **Med School:** Mount Sinai Sch Med 1981; **Resid:** Internal Medicine, Beth Israel Med Ctr 1984; **Fellow:** Pulmonary Disease, St Luke's Roosevelt Hosp Ctr 1988; Critical Care Medicine, St Luke's Roosevelt Hosp Ctr 1989; **Fac Appt:** Asst Clin Prof Med, Columbia P&S

Bevelaqua, Frederick MD (Pul) - **Spec Exp:** Asthma; Lung Cancer; Chronic Obstructive Lung Disease (COPD); Sarcoidosis; **Hospital:** NYU Langone Med Ctr (page 106); **Address:** 35 A E 35th St, Ste 204, New York, NY 10016; **Phone:** 212-213-6796; **Board Cert:** Internal Medicine 1978; Pulmonary Disease 1980; **Med School:** NYU Sch Med 1974; **Resid:** Internal Medicine, NYU Med Ctr 1978; **Fellow:** Pulmonary Disease, NYU Med Ctr 1980; **Fac Appt:** Asst Clin Prof Med, NYU Sch Med

Blair, Lester W MD (Pul) - **Spec Exp:** Asthma; Sarcoidosis; Bronchitis; Chronic Obstructive Lung Disease (COPD); **Hospital:** NY Downtown Hosp, Bellevue Hosp Ctr; **Address:** 170 William St, Fl 7, New York, NY 10038-2668; **Phone:** 212-238-0101; **Board Cert:** Internal Medicine 1987; Pulmonary Disease 1980; Critical Care Medicine 2009; **Med School:** Columbia P&S 1974; **Resid:** Internal Medicine, Columbia-Presby Med Ctr 1977; **Fellow:** Pulmonary Disease, Bellevue Hosp 1979; **Fac Appt:** Asst Clin Prof Med, NYU Sch Med

Burschtin, Omar E MD (Pul) - **Spec Exp:** Sleep Disorders/Apnea; Airway Disorders; Asthma; **Hospital:** NYU Langone Med Ctr (page 106); **Address:** 11 E 26th St, Fl 13th, New York, NY 10010; **Phone:** 212-481-1818; **Board Cert:** Pulmonary Disease 2008; Sleep Medicine 2009; **Med School:** Uruguay 1988; **Resid:** Internal Medicine, NYU Downtown Hosp 1994; Pulmonary Disease, NYU Downtown Hosp 1998; **Fac Appt:** Asst Clin Prof Med, NYU Sch Med

Cooke, Joseph T MD (Pul) - **Spec Exp:** Asthma; Lung Cancer; Critical Care; Emphysema; **Hospital:** NY-Presby Hosp/Weill Cornell (page 104); **Address:** Pulmonary and Critical Medicine, 520 E 70th St Starr Bldg - rm 505, New York, NY 10021-9800; **Phone:** 646-962-2333; **Board Cert:** Internal Medicine 1989; Pulmonary Disease 2002; Critical Care Medicine 2003; **Med School:** SUNY Downstate 1985; **Resid:** Internal Medicine, NY Hosp 1988; **Fellow:** Pulmonary Intensive Care, NY Hosp 1991; **Fac Appt:** Assoc Clin Prof Med, Cornell Univ-Weill Med Coll

DiFabrizio, Larry MD (Pul) - **Hospital:** Lenox Hill Hosp; **Address:** 111 E 80th St, New York, NY 10075; **Phone:** 212-517-8488; **Board Cert:** Internal Medicine 1987; Critical Care Medicine 2002; Pulmonary Disease 2000; Sleep Medicine 2009; **Med School:** Washington Univ, St Louis 1984; **Resid:** Internal Medicine, Brigham & Womens Hosp 1987; **Fellow:** Pulmonary Critical Care Medicine, Brigham & Womens Hosp 1988; Rheumatology, Columbia-Presby Med Ctr 1990

Eden, Edward MD (Pul) - **Spec Exp:** Emphysema; Asthma; Sarcoidosis; Emphysema/Alpha-1 Antitrypsin Deficiency; **Hospital:** St Luke's - Roosevelt Hosp Ctr - Roosevelt Div (page 94); **Address:** 425 W 59th St, Ste 8A, New York, NY 10019-1104; **Phone:** 212-492-5500; **Board Cert:** Internal Medicine 1980; Pulmonary Disease 1982; Critical Care Medicine 2007; **Med School:** England, UK 1975; **Resid:** Internal Medicine, Wayne State Univ Affil Hosp 1978; Internal Medicine, Univ Hosp 1980; **Fellow:** Pulmonary Disease, Mount Sinai Hosp 1982; Pulmonary Disease, Columbia-Presby Med Ctr 1985; **Fac Appt:** Assoc Prof Med, Columbia P&S

Fishman, Donald MD (Pul) - **Spec Exp:** Asthma; Chronic Obstructive Lung Disease (COPD); Bronchoscopy; Interstitial Lung Disease; **Hospital:** St Luke's - Roosevelt Hosp Ctr - Roosevelt Div (page 94), Lenox Hill Hosp; **Address:** 200 W 57th St, Ste 1201, New York, NY 10019; **Phone:** 212-765-5151; **Board Cert:** Internal Medicine 1976; Pulmonary Disease 1978; **Med School:** Univ Pennsylvania 1973; **Resid:** Internal Medicine, Univ Mich Med Ctr 1976; **Fellow:** Pulmonary Disease, NYU Med Ctr 1978; **Fac Appt:** Asst Clin Prof Med, Columbia P&S

Gagliardi, Anthony MD (Pul) - **Spec Exp:** Asthma; Lung Cancer; Tuberculosis; **Address:** 170 W 12th St, Smith 502, New York, NY 10011; **Phone:** 212-604-7900; **Board Cert:** Internal Medicine 1984; Pulmonary Disease 1986; **Med School:** UMDNJ-NJ Med Sch, Newark 1981; **Resid:** Internal Medicine, St Vincent's Hosp & Med Ctr 1984; **Fellow:** Pulmonary Disease, Meml Sloan Kettering Cancer Ctr 1986; **Fac Appt:** Asst Clin Prof Med, NY Med Coll

Garay, Stuart M MD (Pul) - **Spec Exp:** Asthma; Chronic Obstructive Lung Disease (COPD); Sleep Apnea; **Hospital:** NYU Langone Med Ctr (page 106); **Address:** 436 3rd Ave Fl 2, New York, NY 10016-6025; **Phone:** 212-685-6001; **Board Cert:** Internal Medicine 1977; Pulmonary Disease 1980; **Med School:** Harvard Med Sch 1974; **Resid:** Internal Medicine, Mt Sinai Hosp 1977; **Fellow:** Pulmonary Disease, Bellevue Hosp 1979; **Fac Appt:** Clin Prof Med, NYU Sch Med

Kamelhar, David L MD (Pul) - **Spec Exp:** Chronic Obstructive Lung Disease (COPD); Bronchiectasis; Mycobacterial Infections; **Hospital:** NYU Langone Med Ctr (page 106); **Address:** 404 Park Ave S, Ste 701, New York, NY 10016; **Phone:** 212-685-6611; **Board Cert:** Internal Medicine 1977; Pulmonary Disease 1980; **Med School:** NYU Sch Med 1974; **Resid:** Internal Medicine, VA Hosp 1978; **Fellow:** Pulmonary Disease, Bellevue/NYU Med Ctr 1980; **Fac Appt:** Assoc Prof Med, NYU Sch Med

Klapholz, Ari MD (Pul) - **Spec Exp:** Lung Cancer; Sleep Disorders/Apnea; Emphysema; Asthma; **Hospital:** Beth Israel Med Ctr - Petrie Division (page 94); **Address:** 275 7th Ave Fl 3, New York, NY 10001; **Phone:** 646-660-9999; **Board Cert:** Internal Medicine 1987; Pulmonary Disease 2000; Critical Care Medicine 2000; Sleep Medicine 2007; **Med School:** NY Med Coll 1984; **Resid:** Internal Medicine, Beth Israel Med Ctr 1987; **Fellow:** Pulmonary Disease, Beth Israel Med Ctr 1989; Critical Care Medicine, Mount Sinai Hosp 1990; **Fac Appt:** Asst Prof Med, Mount Sinai Sch Med

Kolodny, Erwin MD (Pul) - **Spec Exp:** Asthma; Emphysema; Bronchitis; **Hospital:** NYU Langone Med Ctr (page 106); **Address:** 650 1st Ave, New York, NY 10016-3240; **Phone:** 212-213-0090; **Board Cert:** Internal Medicine 1977; Pulmonary Disease 1978; **Med School:** NYU Sch Med 1973; **Resid:** Internal Medicine, Bellevue Hosp 1976; **Fellow:** Pulmonary Disease, NYU Med Ctr 1978; **Fac Appt:** Asst Clin Prof Med, NYU Sch Med

Lee, Marjorie MD (Pul) - **Spec Exp:** Asthma; Emphysema; Sarcoidosis; **Hospital:** Beth Israel Med Ctr - Petrie Division (page 94); **Address:** 305 2nd Ave, Ste 12, New York, NY 10003; **Phone:** 212-533-1185; **Board Cert:** Internal Medicine 1976; Pulmonary Disease 1978; **Med School:** SUNY Hlth Sci Ctr 1973; **Resid:** Internal Medicine, Kaiser Hosp 1976; Pulmonary Disease, Cabrini Hosp 1977; **Fellow:** Pulmonary Disease, Yale-New Haven Hosp 1979

Libby, Daniel M MD (Pul) - **Spec Exp:** Asthma; Lung Cancer; Interstitial Lung Disease; Chronic Obstructive Lung Disease (COPD); **Hospital:** NY-Presby Hosp/Weill Cornell (page 104); **Address:** 635 Madison Ave, Ste 1101, New York, NY 10022; **Phone:** 212-628-6611; **Board Cert:** Internal Medicine 1977; Pulmonary Disease 1980; **Med School:** Baylor Coll Med 1974; **Resid:** Internal Medicine, NY Hosp 1977; **Fellow:** Pulmonary Disease, NY Hosp 1979; **Fac Appt:** Clin Prof Med, Cornell Univ-Weill Med Coll

Lowy, Joseph MD (Pul) - **Spec Exp:** Lung Cancer; Asthma; Chronic Obstructive Lung Disease (COPD); **Hospital:** NYU Langone Med Ctr (page 106); **Address:** 530 First Ave, HCC-Suite 6B, New York, NY 10016; **Phone:** 212-263-6202; **Board Cert:** Internal Medicine 1983; Pulmonary Disease 1986; Hospice & Palliative Medicine 2008; **Med School:** Univ Rochester 1980; **Resid:** Internal Medicine, Bellevue Hosp 1983; **Fellow:** Pulmonary Disease, UCSD Med Ctr 1986; **Fac Appt:** Assoc Clin Prof Med, NYU Sch Med

Maxfield, Roger MD (Pul) - **Spec Exp:** Emphysema & Asthma; Occupational Lung Disease; Lung Cancer; Bronchoscopy; **Hospital:** NY-Presby Hosp/Columbia (page 104); **Address:** Columbia Presbyterian Eastside, 16 E 60th St, Ste 320, New York, NY 10022-1002; **Phone:** 212-326-8415; **Board Cert:** Internal Medicine 1980; Pulmonary Disease 1986; **Med School:** Brown Univ 1977; **Resid:** Internal Medicine, Georgetown Univ Hosp 1980; **Fellow:** Pulmonary Disease, Bellevue-NYU Med Ctr 1985; **Fac Appt:** Clin Prof Med, Columbia P&S

Nash, Thomas MD (Pul) - **Spec Exp:** Asthma; Cough; Pneumonia; **Hospital:** NY-Presby Hosp/Weill Cornell (page 104), Hosp For Special Surgery (page 111); **Address:** 310 E 72nd St, New York, NY 10021-4726; **Phone:** 212-734-6612; **Board Cert:** Internal Medicine 1981; Infectious Disease 1984; Pulmonary Disease 1988; **Med School:** NYU Sch Med 1978; **Resid:** Internal Medicine, New York Hosp-Cornell 1981; **Fellow:** Infectious Disease, New York Hosp-Cornell 1983; Pulmonary Disease, Meml Sloan Kettering Cancer Ctr 1985; **Fac Appt:** Assoc Clin Prof Med, NYU Sch Med

Nelson, Judith E MD (Pul) - **Spec Exp:** Palliative Care; Critical Care; **Hospital:** Mount Sinai Med Ctr (page 102); **Address:** Mt Sinai Medical Ctr, One Gustave Levy Pl, Box 1232, New York, NY 10029; **Phone:** 212-241-2587; **Board Cert:** Internal Medicine 1989; Pulmonary Disease 2002; Critical Care Medicine 2003; Hospice & Palliative Medicine 2005; **Med School:** NYU Sch Med 1986; **Resid:** Internal Medicine, Mt Sinai Med Ctr 1989; **Fellow:** Pulmonary Critical Care Medicine, Mt Sinai Med Ctr 1992; **Fac Appt:** Assoc Prof Med, Mount Sinai Sch Med

Padilla, Maria L MD (Pul) - **Spec Exp:** Pulmonary Fibrosis; Transplant Medicine-Lung; Sarcoidosis; Pulmonary Hypertension; **Hospital:** Mount Sinai Med Ctr (page 102); **Address:** Mt Sinai Med Ctr, Div Pulmonology, One Gustave L Levy Pl, Box 1232, New York, NY 10029-6574; **Phone:** 212-241-5656; **Board Cert:** Internal Medicine 1978; Pulmonary Disease 1980; **Med School:** Mount Sinai Sch Med 1975; **Resid:** Internal Medicine, Mt Sinai Hosp 1978; **Fellow:** Pulmonary Disease, Mt Sinai Hosp 1980; Critical Care Medicine, Mt Sinai Hosp 1991; **Fac Appt:** Prof Med, Mount Sinai Sch Med

Posner, David H MD (Pul) - **Spec Exp:** Asthma; Lung Cancer; Sarcoidosis; Pulmonary Fibrosis; **Hospital:** Lenox Hill Hosp, NY-Presby Hosp/Weill Cornell (page 104); **Address:** 178 E 85th St Fl 3, New York, NY 10028-2119; **Phone:** 212-861-8976; **Board Cert:** Internal Medicine 1984; Pulmonary Disease 1988; **Med School:** NY Med Coll 1981; **Resid:** Internal Medicine, Lenox Hill Hosp 1985; **Fellow:** Pulmonary Disease, LI Jewish Med Ctr 1987; **Fac Appt:** Assoc Clin Prof Med, NYU Sch Med

Prager, Kenneth MD (Pul) - **Spec Exp:** Lung Disease; Asthma; Ethics; **Hospital:** NY-Presby Hosp/Columbia (page 104); **Address:** 161 Fort Washington Ave, New York, NY 10032-3713; **Phone:** 212-305-5535; **Board Cert:** Internal Medicine 1973; **Med School:** Harvard Med Sch 1968; **Resid:** Internal Medicine, Columbia-Presby Med Ctr 1972; Internal Medicine, Billings Hosp 1973; **Fac Appt:** Clin Prof Med, Columbia P&S

Rapoport, David M MD (Pul) - **Spec Exp:** Sleep Disorders/Apnea; Sleep Medicine; Hepatopulmonary Syndrome; **Hospital:** Bellevue Hosp Ctr, NYU Langone Med Ctr (page 106); **Address:** 462 1st Ave, rm 7N2, New York, NY 10016-6402; **Phone:** 212-263-6407; **Board Cert:** Internal Medicine 1977; Pulmonary Disease 1980; Sleep Medicine 2007; **Med School:** Albert Einstein Coll Med 1974; **Resid:** Internal Medicine, Roosevelt Hosp 1977; **Fellow:** Pulmonary Disease, NYU/Bellevue Med Ctr 1979; **Fac Appt:** Assoc Prof Med, NYU Sch Med

Raskin, Jonathan MD (Pul) - **Spec Exp:** Asthma; Chronic Obstructive Lung Disease (COPD); Pulmonary Rehabilitation; **Hospital:** Beth Israel Med Ctr - Petrie Division (page 94), Lenox Hill Hosp; **Address:** 1000 Park Ave, New York, NY 10028-0934; **Phone:** 212-288-4600; **Board Cert:** Internal Medicine 1982; Pulmonary Disease 1984; **Med School:** Mexico 1978; **Resid:** Internal Medicine, Beth Israel Med Ctr 1982; **Fellow:** Pulmonary Disease, Mount Sinai Hosp 1985; **Fac Appt:** Asst Clin Prof Med, Albert Einstein Coll Med

Sanders, Abraham MD (Pul) - **Hospital:** NY-Presby Hosp/Weill Cornell (page 104), Hosp For Special Surgery (page 111); **Address:** 1305 York Ave Fl 4, New York, NY 10001; **Phone:** 646-962-0110; **Board Cert:** Internal Medicine 1979; Pulmonary Disease 1982; Critical Care Medicine 2008; **Med School:** SUNY Downstate 1976; **Resid:** Internal Medicine, Univ Hosp/Kings County Hosp 1980; **Fellow:** Pulmonary Disease, Kings County Hosp 1980; Pulmonary Disease, Royal Postgraduate Sch Med 1981; **Fac Appt:** Assoc Prof Med, Cornell Univ-Weill Med Coll

Schluger, Neil MD (Pul) - **Spec Exp:** Tuberculosis; **Hospital:** NY-Presby Hosp/Columbia (page 104); **Address:** Div Pulm, Allergy & Crit Care Med, 630 W 168th St, PH-8 East, Rm 101, New York, NY 10032; **Phone:** 212-305-1544; **Board Cert:** Internal Medicine 1988; Pulmonary Disease 2003; **Med School:** Univ Pennsylvania 1985; **Resid:** Internal Medicine, St Lukes Hosp 1989; **Fellow:** Pulmonary Critical Care Medicine, NY Hosp-Cornell 1992; **Fac Appt:** Prof Med, Columbia P&S

Steiger, David MD (Pul) - **Spec Exp:** Rheumatologic Diseases of the Lung; Thromboembolic Disorders; Pulmonary Hypertension; Critical Care; **Hospital:** NYU Hosp For Joint Diseases (page 106), NYU Langone Med Ctr (page 106); **Address:** 305 2nd Ave, Ste 16, New York, NY 10003; **Phone:** 212-598-6091; **Board Cert:** Internal Medicine 1987; Pulmonary Disease 2002; Critical Care Medicine 2005; **Med School:** England, UK 1981; **Resid:** Internal Medicine, St Thomas's Hosp 1984; Internal Medicine, St Lukes Hosp 1989; **Fellow:** Pulmonary Disease, UCSF Med Ctr 1994; **Fac Appt:** Asst Prof Med, NYU Sch Med

Stein, Sidney MD (Pul) - **Spec Exp:** Asthma; Bronchitis; Emphysema; Hiccups-Chronic; **Hospital:** Beth Israel Med Ctr - Petrie Division (page 94); **Address:** 55 E 34th St Fl 6, New York, NY 10016-4337; **Phone:** 212-879-7777; **Board Cert:** Internal Medicine 1982; Pulmonary Disease 1988; **Med School:** SUNY Hlth Sci Ctr 1979; **Resid:** Internal Medicine, Beth Israel Med Ctr 1982; **Fellow:** Pulmonary Disease, Beth Israel Med Ctr 1984; **Fac Appt:** Asst Clin Prof Med, Albert Einstein Coll Med

Stover-Pepe, Diane E MD (Pul) - **Spec Exp:** Interstitial Lung Disease; Pulmonary Infections; Pulmonary Disease/Immunocompromised; **Hospital:** Meml Sloan-Kettering Cancer Ctr (page 112); **Address:** 1275 York Avenue, New York, NY 10065; **Phone:** 800-525-2225; **Board Cert:** Internal Medicine 1975; Pulmonary Disease 1978; **Med School:** Albert Einstein Coll Med 1970; **Resid:** Internal Medicine, Harlem Hosp Ctr 1972; Internal Medicine, NY Hosp-Cornell Med Ctr 1975; **Fellow:** Pulmonary Disease, Montefiore Med Ctr 1977; **Fac Appt:** Prof Med, Cornell Univ-Weill Med Coll

Sukumaran, Muthiah MD (Pul) - **Spec Exp:** Asthma; Chronic Obstructive Lung Disease (COPD); Lung Cancer; Tuberculosis; **Hospital:** NY Downtown Hosp, NYU Langone Med Ctr (page 106); **Address:** Trinty Medical Centre, 111 Broadway, New York, NY 10016; **Phone:** 212-263-9700; **Board Cert:** Internal Medicine 1976; Pulmonary Disease 1980; **Med School:** India 1973; **Resid:** Internal Medicine, Elmhurst City Hosp 1976; **Fellow:** Pulmonary Disease, Elmhurst City Hosp 1977; **Fac Appt:** Assoc Clin Prof Med, NY Med Coll

Teirstein, Alvin S MD (Pul) - **Spec Exp:** Sarcoidosis; Interstitial Lung Disease; Occupational Lung Disease; Lung Cancer; **Hospital:** Mount Sinai Med Ctr (page 102), VA Med Ctr - Bronx; **Address:** Mount Sinai Med Ctr, 1 Gustave Levy Pl, Box 1232, New York, NY 10029; **Phone:** 212-241-5656; **Board Cert:** Internal Medicine 1961; Pulmonary Disease 1969; **Med School:** SUNY Downstate 1953; **Resid:** Internal Medicine, Mt Sinai Med Ctr 1957; **Fellow:** Pulmonary Disease, Mt Sinai Med Ctr 1954; Pulmonary Disease, VA Med Ctr 1956; **Fac Appt:** Prof Med, Mount Sinai Sch Med

Thomashow, Byron MD (Pul) - **Spec Exp:** Emphysema; Asthma; Respiratory Failure; Chronic Obstructive Lung Disease (COPD); **Hospital:** NY-Presby Hosp/Columbia (page 104); **Address:** 161 Fort Washington Ave, rm 311, New York, NY 10032; **Phone:** 212-305-5261; **Board Cert:** Internal Medicine 1977; Pulmonary Disease 1980; **Med School:** Columbia P&S 1974; **Resid:** Internal Medicine, Roosevelt Hosp 1977; Pulmonary Disease, Roosevelt Hosp 1978; **Fellow:** Pulmonary Disease, Harlem Hosp Ctr 1979; **Fac Appt:** Clin Prof Med, Columbia P&S

Villamena, Patricia C MD (Pul) - **Spec Exp:** Lung Cancer; Chronic Obstructive Lung Disease (COPD); Critical Care; **Hospital:** Beth Israel Med Ctr - Petrie Division (page 94); **Address:** 1st Ave & 16th St, Dazian Bldg, 7th Fl, Pulmonary Div, New York, NY 10003; **Phone:** 212-420-2377; **Board Cert:** Internal Medicine 1989; Pulmonary Disease 2006; **Med School:** NY Med Coll 1977; **Resid:** Internal Medicine, Metropolitan Hosp 1980; **Fellow:** Pulmonary Disease, Beth Israel Med Ctr 1986; **Fac Appt:** Asst Prof Med, Albert Einstein Coll Med

Volcovici, Guido MD (Pul) - **Spec Exp:** Asthma; Emphysema; **Hospital:** Saint Joseph's Med Ctr - Yonkers; **Address:** 4915 Broadway, Ste 1J, New York, NY 10034-3119; **Phone:** 212-567-2323; **Board Cert:** Internal Medicine 1985; Pulmonary Disease 1988; **Med School:** Romania 1962; **Resid:** Internal Medicine, Jewish Hosp 1974; **Fellow:** Pulmonary Disease, VA Med Ctr 1976

Yip, Chun MD (Pul) - **Spec Exp:** Asthma; Emphysema; Chronic Obstructive Lung Disease (COPD); **Hospital:** NY-Presby Hosp/Columbia (page 104); **Address:** 161 Fort Washington Ave, rm 311, New York, NY 10032-3713; **Phone:** 212-305-8548; **Board Cert:** Internal Medicine 1979; Pulmonary Disease 1984; **Med School:** Albert Einstein Coll Med 1976; **Resid:** Internal Medicine, Columbia-Presby Med Ctr 1979; **Fellow:** Pulmonary Disease, Bellevue Hosp Ctr 1981; **Fac Appt:** Clin Prof Med, Columbia P&S

Radiation Oncology

Ennis, Ronald D MD (RadRO) - **Spec Exp:** Prostate Cancer; Brachytherapy; Gynecologic Cancer; **Hospital:** St Luke's - Roosevelt Hosp Ctr - Roosevelt Div (page 94), Beth Israel Med Ctr - Petrie Division (page 94); **Address:** St Luke's Roosevelt Hosp, Dept Rad Oncol, 1000 10th Ave, Lower Level, New York, NY 10019; **Phone:** 212-523-7165; **Board Cert:** Radiation Oncology 2005; **Med School:** Yale Univ 1990; **Resid:** Therapeutic Radiology, Yale-New Haven Hosp 1994

Formenti, Silvia C MD (RadRO) - **Spec Exp:** Breast Cancer; Chemo-Radiation Combined Therapy; **Hospital:** NYU Langone Med Ctr (page 106); **Address:** NYU Med Ctr, Dept Radiation Oncology, 160 E 34th St, New York, NY 10016; **Phone:** 212-263-2601; **Board Cert:** Radiation Oncology 1991; **Med School:** Italy 1980; **Resid:** Internal Medicine, San Carlo Borromeo Hosp 1983; Medical Oncology, Univ of Pavia Med Ctr 1985; **Fellow:** Radiation Oncology, USC Med Ctr 1990; **Fac Appt:** Asst Prof RadRO, NYU Sch Med

Harrison, Louis B MD (RadRO) - **Spec Exp:** Brachytherapy; Head & Neck Cancer; Radiation Therapy-Intraoperative; **Hospital:** Beth Israel Med Ctr - Petrie Division (page 94), St Luke's - Roosevelt Hosp Ctr - Roosevelt Div (page 94); **Address:** Beth Israel Med Ctr, Dept Rad Onc, 10 Union Square East, Ste 4G, New York, NY 10003-3314; **Phone:** 212-844-8087; **Board Cert:** Therapeutic Radiology 1986; **Med School:** SUNY Downstate 1982; **Resid:** Therapeutic Radiology, Yale-New Haven Hosp 1986; **Fac Appt:** Prof RadRO, Albert Einstein Coll Med

Hayes, Mary Katherine MD (RadRO) - **Spec Exp:** Breast Cancer; **Hospital:** NY-Presby Hosp/Weill Cornell (page 104); **Address:** 525 E 68th St, Box 575, New York, NY 10065; **Phone:** 212-746-3679; **Board Cert:** Radiation Oncology 1988; **Med School:** Dominica 1984; **Resid:** Radiation Oncology, Meml Sloan Kettering Cancer Ctr 1988

Isaacson, Steven R MD (RadRO) - **Spec Exp:** Brain Tumors; Neuro-Oncology; Stereotactic Radiosurgery; Arteriovenous Malformations; **Hospital:** NY-Presby Hosp/Columbia (page 104); **Address:** Columbia Presby Med Ctr, Dept Radiation Oncology, 622 W 168th St BHN Bldg - rm B-11, New York, NY 10032-3720; **Phone:** 212-305-2611; **Board Cert:** Radiation Oncology 1988; Otolaryngology 1978; **Med School:** Jefferson Med Coll 1973; **Resid:** Otolaryngology, Hosp Univ Penn 1978; Radiation Oncology, SUNY Hlth Sci Ctr 1988; **Fac Appt:** Clin Prof RadRO, Columbia P&S

Lee, Nancy MD (RadRO) - **Spec Exp:** Intensity Modulated Radiotherapy (IMRT); Head & Neck Cancer; Skin Cancer; **Hospital:** Meml Sloan-Kettering Cancer Ctr (page 112); **Address:** Meml Sloan Kettering Cancer Ctr, Dept Rad Onc, 1275 York Ave, New York, NY 10021; **Phone:** 800-525-2225; **Board Cert:** Radiation Oncology 2000; **Med School:** UMDNJ-NJ Med Sch, Newark 1995; **Resid:** Radiation Oncology, NY-Presby/Columbia 2001

McCormick, Beryl MD (RadRO) - **Spec Exp:** Breast Cancer; Eye Tumors/Cancer; **Hospital:** Meml Sloan-Kettering Cancer Ctr (page 112), NY-Presby Hosp/Weill Cornell (page 104); **Address:** 1275 York Avenue, New York, NY 10065; **Phone:** 800-525-2225; **Board Cert:** Therapeutic Radiology 1977; **Med School:** UMDNJ-NJ Med Sch, Newark 1973; **Resid:** Therapeutic Radiology, Meml Sloan Kettering Cancer Ctr 1977; **Fac Appt:** Prof RadRO, Cornell Univ-Weill Med Coll

Ng, John Paul Tracy MD (RadRO) - **Spec Exp:** Prostate Cancer; Head & Neck Cancer; **Address:** 325 W 15th St, New York, NY 10011-5903; **Phone:** 212-604-6083; **Board Cert:** Radiation Oncology 1993; **Med School:** Albert Einstein Coll Med 1988; **Resid:** Radiation Oncology, Meml Sloan Kettering Cancer Ctr 1992; **Fac Appt:** Asst Prof RadRO, NY Med Coll

Nori, Dattatreyudu MD (RadRO) - **Spec Exp:** Prostate Cancer; Brachytherapy; Lung Cancer; Breast Cancer; **Hospital:** NY-Presby Hosp/Weill Cornell (page 104), NY Hosp Queens; **Address:** 525 E 68th St, Box 575, New York, NY 10065; **Phone:** 212-746-3679; **Board Cert:** Therapeutic Radiology 1979; **Med School:** India 1970; **Resid:** Radiation Oncology, Meml Sloan Kettering Cancer Ctr 1975; **Fellow:** Radiation Oncology, Meml Sloan Kettering Cancer Ctr 1978; **Fac Appt:** Prof RadRO, Cornell Univ-Weill Med Coll

Rosenbaum, Alfred MD (RadRO) - **Spec Exp:** Breast Cancer; Prostate Cancer; Intensity Modulated Radiotherapy (IMRT); **Hospital:** Mount Sinai Med Ctr (page 102), Lenox Hill Hosp; **Address:** 1421 Third Ave, New York, NY 10028; **Phone:** 212-744-5538; **Board Cert:** Diagnostic Radiology 1973; **Med School:** Germany 1966; **Resid:** Diagnostic Radiology, Maimonides Med Ctr 1970; Radiation Oncology, Mount Sinai Hosp 1972; **Fellow:** Diagnostic Radiology, Montefiore Med Ctr 1973; **Fac Appt:** Asst Clin Prof, Mount Sinai Sch Med

Schiff, Peter B MD/PhD (RadRO) - **Spec Exp:** Prostate Cancer; Gynecologic Cancer; Breast Cancer; **Hospital:** NYU Langone Med Ctr (page 106); **Address:** NYU Clinical Cancer Ctr, 160 E 34th St Fl 1, New York, NY 10016; **Phone:** 212-731-5003; **Board Cert:** Radiation Oncology 1990; **Med School:** Albert Einstein Coll Med 1984; **Resid:** Radiation Oncology, Meml Sloan Kettering Cancer Ctr 1988; **Fac Appt:** Prof RadRO, NYU Sch Med

Stock, Richard MD (RadRO) - **Spec Exp:** Prostate Cancer; **Hospital:** Mount Sinai Med Ctr (page 102); **Address:** Dept Radiation Oncology, 1184 5th Ave, Box 1236, New York, NY 10029; **Phone:** 212-241-7502; **Board Cert:** Radiation Oncology 1993; **Med School:** Mount Sinai Sch Med 1988; **Resid:** Radiation Oncology, Meml Sloan Kettering Cancer Ctr 1992; **Fac Appt:** Prof RadRO, Mount Sinai Sch Med

Yahalom, Joachim MD (RadRO) - **Spec Exp:** Lymphoma; Hodgkin's Disease; Multiple Myeloma; **Hospital:** Meml Sloan-Kettering Cancer Ctr (page 112); **Address:** 1275 York Ave, SM03, Dept Radiation Onc, New York, NY 10065; **Phone:** 212-639-5999; **Board Cert:** Radiation Oncology 1988; **Med School:** Israel 1976; **Resid:** Internal Medicine, Hadassah Hosp 1979; Radiation Oncology, Hadassah Hosp 1984; **Fellow:** Radiation Oncology, Meml Sloan Kettering Canc Ctr 1986; **Fac Appt:** Prof RadRO, Cornell Univ-Weill Med Coll

Zelefsky, Michael J MD (RadRO) - **Spec Exp:** Prostate Cancer; Brachytherapy; Head & Neck Cancer; **Hospital:** Meml Sloan-Kettering Cancer Ctr (page 112); **Address:** 1275 York Avenue, New York, NY 10065; **Phone:** 800-525-2225; **Board Cert:** Radiation Oncology 1991; **Med School:** Albert Einstein Coll Med 1986; **Resid:** Radiation Oncology, Meml Sloan Kettering Cancer Ctr 1990; **Fac Appt:** Prof RadRO, Cornell Univ-Weill Med Coll

Reproductive Endocrinology

Chang, Peter L MD (RE) - **Spec Exp:** Infertility-IVF; Polycystic Ovarian Syndrome; **Hospital:** Beth Israel Med Ctr - Petrie Division (page 94); **Address:** 10 Union Square E, Ste 2E, New York, NY 10003; **Phone:** 212-844-8587; **Board Cert:** Obstetrics & Gynecology 2009; Reproductive Endocrinology/Infertility 2009; **Med School:** Univ Tex, San Antonio 1992; **Resid:** Obstetrics & Gynecology, Univ TX Hlth Sci Ctr 1996; **Fellow:** Reproductive Endocrinology, Columbia P&S 1998; **Fac Appt:** Asst Prof ObG, Albert Einstein Coll Med

Cholst, Ina N MD (RE) - **Spec Exp:** Gynecologic Surgery-Laparoscopic; Infertility-IVF; Menopause Problems; **Hospital:** NY-Presby Hosp/Weill Cornell (page 104); **Address:** Ctr for Reproductive Med & Infertility, 1305 York Ave Fl 6, New York, NY 10021; **Phone:** 646-962-3025; **Board Cert:** Obstetrics & Gynecology 1984; Reproductive Endocrinology 1985; **Med School:** NYU Sch Med 1977; **Resid:** Obstetrics & Gynecology, Yale-New Haven Hosp 1981; **Fellow:** Reproductive Endocrinology, Columbia-Presby Med Ctr 1983; **Fac Appt:** Assoc Prof ObG, Cornell Univ-Weill Med Coll

Copperman, Alan B MD (RE) - **Spec Exp:** Infertility-IVF; Endometriosis; Laparoscopic Surgery; Hysteroscopic Surgery; **Hospital:** Mount Sinai Med Ctr (page 102); **Address:** 635 Madison Ave Fl 10, New York, NY 10022; **Phone:** 212-756-5777; **Board Cert:** Obstetrics & Gynecology 2008; Reproductive Endocrinology 2008; **Med School:** NY Med Coll 1989; **Resid:** Obstetrics & Gynecology, Yale-New Haven Hosp 1993; **Fellow:** Reproductive Endocrinology, Mt Sinai Med Ctr 1995; **Fac Appt:** Clin Prof ObG, Mount Sinai Sch Med

David, Sami MD (RE) - **Spec Exp:** Infertility; Miscarriage-Recurrent; Endometriosis; Uterine Fibroids; **Hospital:** Mount Sinai Med Ctr (page 102); **Address:** 1045 Fifth Ave, Ste 1A, New York, NY 10028-1002; **Phone:** 212-831-0430; **Board Cert:** Obstetrics & Gynecology 1980; **Med School:** Columbia P&S 1971; **Resid:** Obstetrics & Gynecology, New York Hosp 1976; **Fellow:** Reproductive Endocrinology, Hosp Univ Penn 1978; **Fac Appt:** Prof ObG, Mount Sinai Sch Med

Davis, Owen K MD (RE) - **Spec Exp:** Infertility-IVF; Reproductive Surgery; **Hospital:** NY-Presby Hosp/Weill Cornell (page 104); **Address:** 1305 York Ave Fl 6, New York, NY 10021-4872; **Phone:** 646-962-3765; **Board Cert:** Obstetrics & Gynecology 2008; Reproductive Endocrinology/Infertility 2008; **Med School:** Wake Forest Univ 1982; **Resid:** Obstetrics & Gynecology, NY Hosp 1986; **Fellow:** Reproductive Endocrinology, Brigham & Women's Hosp 1988; **Fac Appt:** Assoc Prof ObG, Cornell Univ-Weill Med Coll

Fateh, Majid MD (RE) - **Spec Exp:** Endometriosis; Laparoscopic Surgery; Infertility; **Hospital:** Lenox Hill Hosp; **Address:** 1016 5th Ave, New York, NY 10028-0132; **Phone:** 212-734-5555; **Board Cert:** Obstetrics & Gynecology 2009; **Med School:** West Indies 1980; **Resid:** Obstetrics & Gynecology, Lenox Hill Hosp 1984; **Fellow:** Reproductive Endocrinology, Univ Penn 1986

Grifo, James A MD/PhD (RE) - **Spec Exp:** Infertility-IVF; Prenatal Genetic Diagnosis; Hysteroscopic Surgery; Laparoscopic Surgery; **Hospital:** NYU Langone Med Ctr (page 106); **Address:** 660 1st Ave Fl 5, New York, NY 10016; **Phone:** 212-263-7978; **Board Cert:** Obstetrics & Gynecology 2009; Reproductive Endocrinology 2009; **Med School:** Case West Res Univ 1984; **Resid:** Obstetrics & Gynecology, NY Hosp-Cornell Med Ctr 1988; **Fellow:** Reproductive Endocrinology, Yale-New Haven Hosp 1990; **Fac Appt:** Prof ObG, NYU Sch Med

Grunfeld, Lawrence MD (RE) - **Spec Exp:** Infertility-IVF; Hysteroscopic Surgery; Laparoscopic Surgery; **Hospital:** Mount Sinai Med Ctr (page 102), Lenox Hill Hosp; **Address:** 635 Madison Ave Fl 10, New York, NY 10022-1009; **Phone:** 212-756-5777; **Board Cert:** Obstetrics & Gynecology 2009; Reproductive Endocrinology 2009; **Med School:** Mount Sinai Sch Med 1979; **Resid:** Obstetrics & Gynecology, Montefiore Med Ctr 1984; **Fellow:** Reproductive Endocrinology, Montefiore Med Ctr 1987; **Fac Appt:** Assoc Clin Prof ObG, Mount Sinai Sch Med

Keefe, David Lawrence MD (RE) - **Spec Exp:** Infertility-IVF; Infertility-Advanced Maternal Age; **Hospital:** NYU Langone Med Ctr (page 106); **Address:** 660 First Ave Fl 5, New York, NY 10016; **Phone:** 212-263-3360; **Board Cert:** Obstetrics & Gynecology 2009; Reproductive Endocrinology 2009; **Med School:** Georgetown Univ 1980; **Resid:** Psychiatry, Harvard Psych Srv/Camb Hosp 1983; Obstetrics & Gynecology, Yale New Haven Hosp 1989; **Fellow:** Psychiatry, Univ Chicago Hosp & Clins 1985; Reproductive Endocrinology, Yale New Haven Hosp 1991; **Fac Appt:** Prof ObG, Univ S Fla Coll Med

Licciardi, Frederick L MD (RE) - **Spec Exp:** Infertility-IVF; Infertility; Fertility Preservation in Cancer; **Hospital:** NYU Langone Med Ctr (page 106); **Address:** NYU Medical Ctr, 660 First Ave, 5th Fl, New York, NY 10016; **Phone:** 212-263-7754; **Board Cert:** Obstetrics & Gynecology 2007; Reproductive Endocrinology 2007; **Med School:** UMDNJ-Rutgers Med Sch 1986; **Resid:** Obstetrics & Gynecology, St Barnabas Med Ctr 1990; **Fellow:** Reproductive Endocrinology, NY Hosp-Cornell Med Ctr 1992; **Fac Appt:** Assoc Prof ObG, NYU Sch Med

Matera, Cristina MD (RE) - **Spec Exp:** Infertility; Laparoscopic Surgery; Menopause Problems; **Hospital:** NY-Presby Hosp/Columbia (page 104); **Address:** 50 E 77th St, New York, NY 10021; **Phone:** 212-639-9122; **Board Cert:** Obstetrics & Gynecology 2009; Reproductive Endocrinology 2009; **Med School:** NYU Sch Med 1986; **Resid:** Obstetrics & Gynecology, Columbia-Presby Hosp 1990; **Fellow:** Reproductive Endocrinology, Columbia-Presby Hosp 1992; **Fac Appt:** Assoc Prof ObG, Columbia P&S

Mukherjee, Tanmoy MD (RE) - **Spec Exp:** Infertility-IVF; Endometriosis; Uterine Fibroids; **Hospital:** Mount Sinai Med Ctr (page 102); **Address:** 635 Madison Ave Fl 10, New York, NY 10022; **Phone:** 212-756-5777; **Board Cert:** Obstetrics & Gynecology 2009; Reproductive Endocrinology 2009; **Med School:** Albert Einstein Coll Med 1990; **Resid:** Obstetrics & Gynecology, Montefiore Med Ctr 1994; **Fellow:** Reproductive Endocrinology, Mt Sinai Hosp 1996

Noyes, Nicole MD (RE) - **Spec Exp:** Infertility-IVF; Fertility Preservation in Cancer; Reproductive Surgery; **Hospital:** NYU Langone Med Ctr (page 106); **Address:** NYU Med Ctr, 660 First Ave, 5th FL, New York, NY 10016; **Phone:** 212-263-7981; **Board Cert:** Obstetrics & Gynecology 2007; Reproductive Endocrinology 2007; **Med School:** Univ VT Coll Med 1986; **Resid:** Obstetrics & Gynecology, NY Hosp-Cornell Med Ctr 1990; **Fellow:** Reproductive Endocrinology, NY Hosp-Cornell Med Ctr 1992; **Fac Appt:** Assoc Prof ObG, NYU Sch Med

Quagliarello, John MD (RE) - **Spec Exp:** Infertility; Gynecologic Surgery; Uterine Fibroids; Endometriosis; **Hospital:** NYU Langone Med Ctr (page 106), Bellevue Hosp Ctr; **Address:** 530 1st Ave SKB Bldg Fl 10 - Ste Q, New York, NY 10016-6402; **Phone:** 212-263-6358; **Board Cert:** Obstetrics & Gynecology 1979; Reproductive Endocrinology 1981; **Med School:** McGill Univ 1970; **Resid:** Obstetrics & Gynecology, NYU Med Ctr 1977; **Fellow:** Reproductive Endocrinology, NYU Med Ctr 1979; **Fac Appt:** Assoc Prof ObG, NYU Sch Med

Rosenwaks, Zev MD (RE) - **Spec Exp:** Infertility-IVF; Genetic Disorders; Fertility Preservation in Cancer; **Hospital:** NY-Presby Hosp/Weill Cornell (page 104); **Address:** Ctr For Reproductive Medicine & Infertility, 1305 York Ave Fl 6, New York, NY 10021-4872; **Phone:** 646-962-3743; **Board Cert:** Obstetrics & Gynecology 1978; Reproductive Endocrinology 1981; **Med School:** SUNY Downstate 1972; **Resid:** Obstetrics & Gynecology, LI Jewish Med Ctr 1976; **Fellow:** Reproductive Endocrinology, Johns Hopkins Hosp 1978; **Fac Appt:** Prof ObG, Cornell Univ-Weill Med Coll

Sandler, Benjamin MD (RE) - **Spec Exp:** Infertility-IVF; Reproductive Surgery; **Hospital:** Mount Sinai Med Ctr (page 102); **Address:** 635 Madison Ave Fl 10, New York, NY 10022-1009; **Phone:** 212-756-5777; **Board Cert:** Obstetrics & Gynecology 2008; **Med School:** Mexico 1982; **Resid:** Obstetrics & Gynecology, Michael Reese Hosp 1987; **Fellow:** Reproductive Endocrinology, Mt Sinai Hosp 1989; **Fac Appt:** Asst Clin Prof ObG, Mount Sinai Sch Med

Sauer, Mark MD (RE) - **Spec Exp:** Infertility-IVF; **Hospital:** NY-Presby Hosp/Columbia (page 104); **Address:** 1790 Broadway Fl 2, New York, NY 10019; **Phone:** 646-756-8282; **Board Cert:** Obstetrics & Gynecology 2009; Reproductive Endocrinology 2009; **Med School:** Univ IL Coll Med 1980; **Resid:** Obstetrics & Gynecology, Univ Illinois Med Ctr 1984; **Fellow:** Reproductive Endocrinology, Harbor-UCLA Med Ctr 1986; **Fac Appt:** Prof ObG, Columbia P&S

Schattman, Glenn L MD (RE) - **Spec Exp:** Infertility; Robotic Assisted Laparoscopic Surgery; Minimally Invasive Surgery; Congenital Anomalies-Gynecologic; **Hospital:** NY-Presby Hosp/Weill Cornell (page 104); **Address:** New York Hosp Cornell Med Ctr, Center for Reproductive Medicine, 1305 York Ave, New York, NY 10021; **Phone:** 646-962-3836; **Board Cert:** Obstetrics & Gynecology 2008; Reproductive Endocrinology 2008; **Med School:** SUNY Downstate 1987; **Resid:** Obstetrics & Gynecology, Geo Wash Univ Med Ctr 1991; **Fellow:** Reproductive Endocrinology, New York Hosp/Cornell 1993; **Fac Appt:** Assoc Prof ObG, Cornell Univ-Weill Med Coll

Schmidt-Sarosi, Cecilia MD (RE) - **Spec Exp:** Infertility-IVF; Menopause Problems; Polycystic Ovarian Syndrome; Uterine Fibroids; **Hospital:** NYU Langone Med Ctr (page 106); **Address:** 51 E 67th St, New York, NY 10021-5949; **Phone:** 212-535-5350; **Board Cert:** Obstetrics & Gynecology 2009; Reproductive Endocrinology 2009; **Med School:** NYU Sch Med 1976; **Resid:** Obstetrics & Gynecology, NYU Med Ctr 1980; **Fellow:** Reproductive Endocrinology, NYU Med Ctr 1982; **Fac Appt:** Prof ObG, NYU Sch Med

Spandorfer, Steven MD (RE) - **Spec Exp:** Infertility-IVF; **Hospital:** NY-Presby Hosp/Weill Cornell (page 104); **Address:** 1305 York Ave Fl 6, New York, NY 10021; **Phone:** 646-962-3638; **Board Cert:** Obstetrics & Gynecology 2007; Reproductive Endocrinology 2007; **Med School:** Emory Univ 1988; **Resid:** Obstetrics & Gynecology, Univ Penn Med Ctr 1996; **Fellow:** Reproductive Endocrinology, NY Hosp 1998; **Fac Appt:** Asst Prof ObG, Cornell Univ-Weill Med Coll

Sultan, Khalid M MD (RE) - **Spec Exp:** Infertility-IVF; Laparoscopic Surgery; **Hospital:** Lenox Hill Hosp; **Address:** 1016 5th Ave, New York, NY 10028-0132; **Phone:** 212-734-5555; **Board Cert:** Obstetrics & Gynecology 2009; Reproductive Endocrinology 2009; **Med School:** NY Med Coll 1988; **Resid:** Obstetrics & Gynecology, Lenox Hill Hosp 1992; **Fellow:** Reproductive Endocrinology, New York Hosp 1994; **Fac Appt:** Asst Clin Prof ObG, NYU Sch Med

Warren, Michelle MD (RE) - **Spec Exp:** Menopause Problems; Infertility; Menstrual Disorders; Women's Health; **Hospital:** NY-Presby Hosp/Columbia (page 104); **Address:** 134 E 73rd St, New York, NY 10021; **Phone:** 212-737-4664; **Board Cert:** Internal Medicine 1972; Endocrinology 1973; **Med School:** Cornell Univ-Weill Med Coll 1965; **Resid:** Internal Medicine, Bellevue Hosp Ctr 1968; Internal Medicine, Meml Sloan Kettering Canc Ctr 1968; **Fellow:** Endocrinology, Columbia Presby Med Ctr 1971; **Fac Appt:** Prof ObG, Columbia P&S

Rheumatology

Abramson, Steven B MD (Rhu) - **Spec Exp:** Arthritis; Inflammatory Muscle Disease; Osteoarthritis; **Hospital:** NYU Hosp For Joint Diseases (page 106), NYU Langone Med Ctr (page 106); **Address:** Hosp for Joint Diseases, 301 E 17th St, rm 1410, New York, NY 10003; **Phone:** 212-598-6110; **Board Cert:** Internal Medicine 1977; Rheumatology 1980; **Med School:** Harvard Med Sch 1974; **Resid:** Internal Medicine, Bellevue Hosp/NYU Med Ctr 1978; **Fellow:** Rheumatology, Bellevue Hosp/NYU Med Ctr 1983; **Fac Appt:** Prof Med, NYU Sch Med

Adlersberg, Jay B MD (Rhu) - **Spec Exp:** Rheumatoid Arthritis; Osteoarthritis; Psoriatic Arthritis; Sports Medicine; **Hospital:** Lenox Hill Hosp, NYU Hosp For Joint Diseases (page 106); **Address:** 220 E 69th St, Ground Fl, New York, NY 10021-5737; **Phone:** 212-570-1800; **Board Cert:** Internal Medicine 1972; Rheumatology 1980; **Med School:** Univ Pennsylvania 1969; **Resid:** Internal Medicine, Bellevue Hosp 1972; **Fellow:** Rheumatology, Bellevue Hosp 1974; **Fac Appt:** Asst Prof Med, Mount Sinai Sch Med

Agus, Bertrand MD (Rhu) - **Spec Exp:** Lupus/SLE; Rheumatoid Arthritis; Sarcoidosis; Gout; **Hospital:** NYU Langone Med Ctr (page 106); **Address:** 251 E 33rd St, Fl 4, New York, NY 10016-4804; **Phone:** 212-779-8421; **Board Cert:** Internal Medicine 1972; Rheumatology 1972; **Med School:** NYU Sch Med 1965; **Resid:** Internal Medicine, NYU Med Ctr 1970; **Fellow:** Rheumatology, NYU Med Ctr 1972; **Fac Appt:** Assoc Clin Prof Med, NYU Sch Med

Bauer, Bertha A MD (Rhu) - **Spec Exp:** Fibromyalgia; Osteoporosis; **Hospital:** NY-Presby Hosp/Columbia (page 104); **Address:** 1185 Park Ave, Ste 1L, New York, NY 10128-6217; **Phone:** 212-828-7933; **Board Cert:** Internal Medicine 1980; **Med School:** Columbia P&S 1977; **Resid:** Internal Medicine, New England Deaconess Hosp 1980; **Fellow:** Rheumatology, Yale-New Haven Hosp 1982; **Fac Appt:** Asst Clin Prof Med, NYU Sch Med

Belmont, H Michael MD (Rhu) - **Spec Exp:** Lupus/SLE; Antiphospholipid Syndrome (APS); Wegener's Granulomatosis; Rheumatoid Arthritis; **Hospital:** NYU Hosp For Joint Diseases (page 106), NYU Langone Med Ctr (page 106); **Address:** 305 2nd Ave, Ste 16, New York, NY 10003-2739; **Phone:** 212-598-6516; **Board Cert:** Internal Medicine 1983; Rheumatology 1986; **Med School:** Univ Pittsburgh 1980; **Resid:** Internal Medicine, Mt Sinai Hosp 1983; **Fellow:** Rheumatology, NYU/Bellevue Hosp 1985; **Fac Appt:** Assoc Prof Med, NYU Sch Med

Blume, Ralph S MD (Rhu) - **Spec Exp:** Vasculitis; Lupus/SLE; Rheumatoid Arthritis; **Hospital:** NY-Presby Hosp/Columbia (page 104); **Address:** 161 Fort Washington Ave, Ste 537, New York, NY 10032-3713; **Phone:** 212-305-5512; **Board Cert:** Internal Medicine 1972; Rheumatology 1974; **Med School:** Columbia P&S 1964; **Resid:** Internal Medicine, Columbia-Presby Med Ctr 1968; **Fellow:** Rheumatology, Columbia-Presby Med Ctr 1970; **Fac Appt:** Clin Prof Med, Columbia P&S

Buyon, Jill P MD (Rhu) - **Spec Exp:** Lupus/SLE in Pregnancy; Lupus/SLE in Menopause; **Hospital:** NYU Hosp For Joint Diseases (page 106), NYU Langone Med Ctr (page 106); **Address:** 246 E 20th St, New York, NY 10003; **Phone:** 646-356-9400; **Board Cert:** Internal Medicine 1981; Rheumatology 1984; **Med School:** Albert Einstein Coll Med 1978; **Resid:** Internal Medicine, Montefiore Med Ctr 1981; **Fellow:** Rheumatology, NYU Med Ctr 1983; **Fac Appt:** Prof Med, NYU Sch Med

Crane, Richard MD (Rhu) - **Spec Exp:** Rheumatoid Arthritis; Gout; Osteoarthritis; Arthritis; **Hospital:** Mount Sinai Med Ctr (page 102); **Address:** 1088 Park Ave, New York, NY 10128-1132; **Phone:** 212-860-4000; **Board Cert:** Internal Medicine 1984; Rheumatology 1986; **Med School:** Mount Sinai Sch Med 1981; **Resid:** Internal Medicine, Mt Sinai Hosp 1984; **Fellow:** Rheumatology, Mt Sinai Hosp 1986

Faller, Jason MD (Rhu) - **Spec Exp:** Lyme Disease; Rheumatoid Arthritis; Gout; Lupus/SLE; **Hospital:** St Luke's - Roosevelt Hosp Ctr - Roosevelt Div (page 94), Lenox Hill Hosp; **Address:** 333 W 57th St, Ste 104, New York, NY 10019-3115; **Phone:** 212-307-6880; **Board Cert:** Internal Medicine 1980; Rheumatology 1982; **Med School:** Univ Pennsylvania 1977; **Resid:** Internal Medicine, Rush Presby St Lukes Hosp 1980; **Fellow:** Rheumatology, Univ Mich 1982; **Fac Appt:** Asst Clin Prof Med, Columbia P&S

Fields, Theodore R MD (Rhu) - **Spec Exp:** Gout; Rheumatoid Arthritis; Osteoarthritis; **Hospital:** Hosp For Special Surgery (page 111), NY-Presby Hosp/Weill Cornell (page 104); **Address:** Hosp Special Surg-Faculty Practice, 535 E 70th St Fl 7 - Ste 719, New York, NY 10021-4872; **Phone:** 212-606-1286; **Board Cert:** Internal Medicine 1979; Rheumatology 1982; **Med School:** SUNY Downstate 1976; **Resid:** Internal Medicine, Nassau Co Med Ctr 1979; **Fellow:** Rheumatology, Univ Hosp 1982; **Fac Appt:** Clin Prof Med, Cornell Univ-Weill Med Coll

Fischer, Harry MD (Rhu) - **Spec Exp:** Lupus/SLE; Rheumatoid Arthritis; Vasculitis; **Hospital:** Beth Israel Med Ctr - Petrie Division (page 94); **Address:** 10 Union Square East, Ste 3D, New York, NY 10003-3314; **Phone:** 212-844-8101; **Board Cert:** Internal Medicine 1983; Rheumatology 2000; **Med School:** Mount Sinai Sch Med 1979; **Resid:** Internal Medicine, Beth Israel Med Ctr 1983; **Fellow:** Rheumatology, Hosp Joint Diseases 1985; **Fac Appt:** Assoc Clin Prof Med, Albert Einstein Coll Med

Gibofsky, Allan MD (Rhu) - **Spec Exp:** Rheumatic Fever; Rheumatoid Arthritis; Inflammatory Arthritis; Behcet's Syndrome; **Hospital:** Hosp For Special Surgery (page 111), NY-Presby Hosp/Weill Cornell (page 104); **Address:** Hospital for Special Surgery, 535 E 70th St, New York, NY 10021-4872; **Phone:** 212-606-1423; **Board Cert:** Internal Medicine 1977; Rheumatology 1980; **Med School:** Cornell Univ-Weill Med Coll 1973; **Resid:** Pathology, NY-Cornell Med Ctr 1974; Internal Medicine, NY-Cornell Med Ctr 1977; **Fellow:** Rheumatology/Immunology, Hosp for Special Surgery 1979; **Fac Appt:** Prof Med, Cornell Univ-Weill Med Coll

Goodman, Susan M MD (Rhu) - **Spec Exp:** Lupus Nephritis; Rheumatoid Arthritis; Psoriatic Arthritis; **Hospital:** Hosp For Special Surgery (page 111), NY-Presby Hosp/Weill Cornell (page 104); **Address:** 535 E 70th St, New York, NY 10021; **Phone:** 212-606-1163; **Board Cert:** Internal Medicine 1980; Rheumatology 1982; **Med School:** Univ Cincinnati 1977; **Resid:** Internal Medicine, Lenox Hill Hosp 1980; **Fellow:** Rheumatology, Columbia Presby Hosp 1983; **Fac Appt:** Asst Clin Prof Med, Cornell Univ-Weill Med Coll

Gorevic, Peter D MD (Rhu) - **Spec Exp:** Autoimmune Disease; Amyloidosis/Joint Disease; Cryoglobulinemia; **Hospital:** Mount Sinai Med Ctr (page 102), Huntington Hosp; **Address:** Mount Sinai Medical Ctr, 1 Gustave L Levy Pl, New York, NY 10029; **Phone:** 212-241-1671; **Board Cert:** Allergy & Immunology 1977; Rheumatology 1976; Diagnostic Lab Immunology 1986; Internal Medicine 1973; **Med School:** NYU Sch Med 1970; **Resid:** Internal Medicine, NYU Med Ctr 1974; **Fellow:** Rheumatology, NYU Med Ctr 1976; Allergy & Immunology, NYU Med Ctr 1977; **Fac Appt:** Prof Med, Mount Sinai Sch Med

Greisman, Stewart G MD (Rhu) - **Spec Exp:** Lupus/SLE; Rheumatoid Arthritis; **Hospital:** St Luke's - Roosevelt Hosp Ctr - Roosevelt Div (page 94), Hosp For Special Surgery (page 111); **Address:** 457 W 57th St, Ste 106, New York, NY 10019-1701; **Phone:** 212-265-1471; **Board Cert:** Rheumatology 1986; Internal Medicine 1984; **Med School:** Yale Univ 1981; **Resid:** Internal Medicine, Yale-New Haven Hosp 1984; **Fellow:** Rheumatology, Hosp Special Surg 1986; **Fac Appt:** Assoc Clin Prof Med, Columbia P&S

Honig, Stephen MD (Rhu) - **Spec Exp:** Osteoporosis; Rheumatoid Arthritis; Osteoarthritis; Lupus/SLE; **Hospital:** NYU Hosp For Joint Diseases (page 106), NYU Langone Med Ctr (page 106); **Address:** 301 E 17th St, Ste 1101, New York, NY 10003-3804; **Phone:** 212-598-6367; **Board Cert:** Internal Medicine 1975; Rheumatology 1978; **Med School:** Univ Tenn Coll Med, Memphis 1972; **Resid:** Internal Medicine, St Vincent's Hosp Med Ctr 1975; **Fellow:** Rheumatology, NYU Med Ctr 1977; **Fac Appt:** Assoc Clin Prof Med, NYU Sch Med

Horowitz, Mark D MD (Rhu) - **Spec Exp:** Lupus/SLE; Rheumatoid Arthritis; Fibromyalgia; **Hospital:** Mount Sinai Med Ctr (page 102); **Address:** 21 E 90th St, Ground Fl, New York, NY 10128-0654; **Phone:** 212-860-3077; **Board Cert:** Internal Medicine 1986; Rheumatology 2000; **Med School:** NE Ohio Univ 1983; **Resid:** Internal Medicine, Mt Sinai Med Ctr 1986; **Fellow:** Rheumatology, Mt Sinai Med Ctr 1989

Kerr, Leslie D MD (Rhu) - **Spec Exp:** Rheumatoid Arthritis; Scleroderma; Lupus/SLE; Geriatric Rheumatology; **Hospital:** Mount Sinai Med Ctr (page 102); **Address:** Mount Sinai Med Ctr, 1 Gustave Levy Pl, Box 1244, New York, NY 10029; **Phone:** 212-241-1671; **Board Cert:** Internal Medicine 1983; Rheumatology 1986; **Med School:** Columbia P&S 1980; **Resid:** Internal Medicine, Mt Sinai Hospital 1983; **Fellow:** Rheumatology, Mt Sinai Hospital 1985; **Fac Appt:** Assoc Prof Med, Mount Sinai Sch Med

Lee, Sicy H MD (Rhu) - **Spec Exp:** Rheumatoid Arthritis; Psoriatic Arthritis; Lupus/SLE; **Hospital:** NYU Hosp For Joint Diseases (page 106), NYU Langone Med Ctr (page 106); **Address:** 305 2nd Ave, rm 16, New York, NY 10003; **Phone:** 212-598-6516; **Board Cert:** Internal Medicine 1982; Rheumatology 1984; **Med School:** Univ Cincinnati 1979; **Resid:** Internal Medicine, Good Samaritan 1982; **Fellow:** Rheumatology, Hosp for Joint Diseases 1984; **Fac Appt:** Asst Clin Prof Med, NYU Sch Med

Lockshin, Michael D MD (Rhu) - **Spec Exp:** Lupus/SLE in Women; Antiphospholipid Syndrome (APS); Pregnancy & Rheumatic Disease; Lupus/SLE in Pregnancy; **Hospital:** Hosp For Special Surgery (page 111), NY-Presby Hosp/Weill Cornell (page 104); **Address:** 535 E 70th St, rm 661, New York, NY 10021-4872; **Phone:** 212-606-1461; **Board Cert:** Internal Medicine 1969; Rheumatology 1972; **Med School:** Harvard Med Sch 1963; **Resid:** Internal Medicine, Bellevue Hosp 1968; **Fellow:** Rheumatology, Columbia-Presby Hosp 1970; **Fac Appt:** Prof Med, Cornell Univ-Weill Med Coll

Magid, Steven K MD (Rhu) - **Spec Exp:** Rheumatoid Arthritis; Osteoarthritis; Lyme Disease; Polymyalgia Rheumatica; **Hospital:** Hosp For Special Surgery (page 111), NY-Presby Hosp/Weill Cornell (page 104); **Address:** 535 E 70th St West Bldg Fl 7 - rm 778, New York, NY 10021; **Phone:** 212-606-1060; **Board Cert:** Internal Medicine 1979; Rheumatology 1984; **Med School:** Cornell Univ-Weill Med Coll 1976; **Resid:** Internal Medicine, New York Hosp 1979; **Fellow:** Rheumatology, Hosp For Special Surgery 1981; **Fac Appt:** Clin Prof Med, Cornell Univ-Weill Med Coll

Markenson, Joseph A MD (Rhu) - **Spec Exp:** Rheumatoid Arthritis; Lupus/SLE; Osteoarthritis; **Hospital:** Hosp For Special Surgery (page 111), NY-Presby Hosp/Weill Cornell (page 104); **Address:** Hosp for Special Surgery, 535 E 70th St, Ste 659W, New York, NY 10021-4892; **Phone:** 212-606-1261; **Board Cert:** Internal Medicine 1976; Rheumatology 1978; **Med School:** SUNY Downstate 1970; **Resid:** Internal Medicine, New York Hosp 1975; **Fellow:** Rheumatology, Hosp For Special Surg 1976; **Fac Appt:** Clin Prof Med, Cornell Univ-Weill Med Coll

Meed, Steven D MD (Rhu) - **Spec Exp:** Lyme Disease; Chronic Fatigue Syndrome; Acupuncture; Fibromyalgia; **Hospital:** Lenox Hill Hosp, St Luke's - Roosevelt Hosp Ctr - Roosevelt Div (page 94); **Address:** 150 E 58th St Fl 18, New York, NY 10155; **Phone:** 212-583-2960; **Board Cert:** Internal Medicine 1979; Rheumatology 1986; **Med School:** NYU Sch Med 1975; **Resid:** Internal Medicine, Brookdale Hosp 1977; **Fellow:** Rheumatology, Barnes Hosp-Wash Univ 1979; **Fac Appt:** Asst Clin Prof Med, NYU Sch Med

Mitnick, Hal J MD (Rhu) - **Spec Exp:** Rheumatoid Arthritis; Psoriatic Arthritis; Osteoporosis; Dermatomyositis; **Hospital:** NYU Langone Med Ctr (page 106); **Address:** 333 E 34th St, Ste 1C, New York, NY 10016-4977; **Phone:** 212-889-7217; **Board Cert:** Internal Medicine 1976; Rheumatology 1978; **Med School:** NYU Sch Med 1972; **Resid:** Internal Medicine, Bellevue Hosp 1976; **Fellow:** Rheumatology, NYU Med Ctr 1978; **Fac Appt:** Clin Prof Med, NYU Sch Med

Nickerson, Katherine G MD (Rhu) - **Hospital:** NY-Presby Hosp/Columbia (page 104); **Address:** 161 Fort Washington Ave, Irving Bldg, rm 221, New York, NY 10032-3713; **Phone:** 212-305-8039; **Board Cert:** Internal Medicine 1984; Rheumatology 1986; **Med School:** UCSF 1981; **Resid:** Internal Medicine, Beth Israel Hosp 1984; **Fellow:** Rheumatology, Columbia-Presby Med Ctr 1986; **Fac Appt:** Assoc Prof Med, Columbia P&S

Paget, Stephen MD (Rhu) - **Spec Exp:** Rheumatoid Arthritis; Lupus/SLE; Vasculitis; Connective Tissue Disorders; **Hospital:** Hosp For Special Surgery (page 111), NY-Presby Hosp/Weill Cornell (page 104); **Address:** 535 E 70th St, rm 721 West, New York, NY 10021; **Phone:** 212-606-1845; **Board Cert:** Internal Medicine 1974; Rheumatology 1976; **Med School:** SUNY Downstate 1971; **Resid:** Internal Medicine, Johns Hopkins Hosp 1973; **Fellow:** Rheumatology, Hosp Special Surg 1975; **Fac Appt:** Prof Med, Cornell Univ-Weill Med Coll

Parrish, Edward MD (Rhu) - **Spec Exp:** Immune Deficiency; **Hospital:** Hosp For Special Surgery (page 111), NY-Presby Hosp/Weill Cornell (page 104); **Address:** 535 E 70th St Fl 6, New York, NY 10021; **Phone:** 212-606-1743; **Board Cert:** Internal Medicine 1983; Rheumatology 1986; **Med School:** Wake Forest Univ 1980; **Resid:** Internal Medicine, Columbia-Presby Med Ctr 1983; **Fellow:** Rheumatology/Immunology, Columbia-Presby Med Ctr 1985

Rackoff, Paula MD (Rhu) - **Spec Exp:** Osteoporosis; Sjogren's Syndrome; Arthritis; **Hospital:** Beth Israel Med Ctr - Petrie Division (page 94); **Address:** 10 Union Square East, Ste 3D, New York, NY 10003-3314; **Phone:** 212-844-8101; **Board Cert:** Internal Medicine 1989; Rheumatology 2004; **Med School:** Yale Univ 1986; **Resid:** Internal Medicine, Yale-New Haven Hosp 1989; **Fellow:** Rheumatology, Yale-New Haven Hosp 1992; **Fac Appt:** Asst Prof Med, Albert Einstein Coll Med

Radin, Allen R MD (Rhu) - **Spec Exp:** Rheumatoid Arthritis; Lupus/SLE; Osteoarthritis; Scleroderma; **Hospital:** Lenox Hill Hosp, NY-Presby Hosp/Weill Cornell (page 104); **Address:** 50 E 81st St, Ste 1, New York, NY 10028; **Phone:** 212-289-6855; **Board Cert:** Internal Medicine 1980; Rheumatology 1982; **Med School:** NYU Sch Med 1977; **Resid:** Internal Medicine, Univ Hosp 1980; **Fellow:** Rheumatology, NYU Med Ctr 1982

Salmon, Jane E MD (Rhu) - **Spec Exp:** Lupus/SLE; Rheumatoid Arthritis; Antiphospholipid Syndrome (APS); **Hospital:** Hosp For Special Surgery (page 111), NY-Presby Hosp/Weill Cornell (page 104); **Address:** 535 E 70th St, New York, NY 10021-4872; **Phone:** 212-606-1671; **Board Cert:** Internal Medicine 1981; Rheumatology 1984; **Med School:** Columbia P&S 1978; **Resid:** Internal Medicine, New York Hosp 1981; **Fellow:** Rheumatology, Hosp Spec Surg 1983; **Fac Appt:** Prof Med, Cornell Univ-Weill Med Coll

Schwartzman, Sergio MD (Rhu) - **Spec Exp:** Lupus/SLE; Raynaud's Disease; Uveitis; Vasculitis; **Hospital:** Hosp For Special Surgery (page 111); **Address:** Hosp for Special Surgery, 535 E 70th St, New York, NY 10021-4892; **Phone:** 212-606-1557; **Board Cert:** Internal Medicine 1985; Rheumatology 1988; **Med School:** Mount Sinai Sch Med 1982; **Resid:** Internal Medicine, LI Jewish Med Ctr 1985; **Fellow:** Rheumatology, Hosp Special Surgery 1987; **Fac Appt:** Assoc Prof Med, Cornell Univ-Weill Med Coll

Smiles, Stephen MD (Rhu) - **Spec Exp:** Arthritis; Osteoporosis; Lupus/SLE; Gout; **Hospital:** NYU Langone Med Ctr (page 106); **Address:** Ctr for Arthritis & Autoimmunity, 305 Second Ave, Ste 16, New York, NY 10003; **Phone:** 212-473-3280; **Board Cert:** Internal Medicine 1977; Rheumatology 1980; **Med School:** SUNY Buffalo 1973; **Resid:** Internal Medicine, Bellevue Hosp Ctr 1977; **Fellow:** Rheumatology, Bellevue Hosp Ctr 1979; **Fac Appt:** Asst Clin Prof Med, NYU Sch Med

Solitar, Bruce M MD (Rhu) - **Spec Exp:** Arthritis; Fibromyalgia; Reiter's Syndrome; Retroperitoneal Fibrosis; **Hospital:** NYU Langone Med Ctr (page 106), NYU Hosp For Joint Diseases (page 106); **Address:** 333 E 34th St, New York, NY 10016; **Phone:** 212-889-7217; **Board Cert:** Internal Medicine 2001; Rheumatology 2004; **Med School:** NYU Sch Med 1988; **Resid:** Internal Medicine, NYU/Bellevue Med Ctr 1992; **Fellow:** Rheumatology, NYU/Bellevue Med Ctr 1994; **Fac Appt:** Assoc Clin Prof Med, NYU Sch Med

Solomon, Gary MD (Rhu) - **Spec Exp:** Psoriatic Arthritis; Rheumatoid Arthritis; Autoimmune Disease; **Hospital:** NYU Hosp For Joint Diseases (page 106), NYU Langone Med Ctr (page 106); **Address:** Hosp Joint Diseases, Dept Rheumatology, 305 2nd Ave, Ste 16, New York, NY 10003-2747; **Phone:** 212-598-6516; **Board Cert:** Internal Medicine 1980; Rheumatology 1982; **Med School:** Mount Sinai Sch Med 1977; **Resid:** Internal Medicine, Mt Sinai Med Ctr 1980; **Fellow:** Rheumatology, Montefiore Med Ctr 1982; **Fac Appt:** Assoc Clin Prof Med, NYU Sch Med

Spiera, Harry MD (Rhu) - **Spec Exp:** Lupus/SLE; Scleroderma; Vasculitis; Behcet's Syndrome; **Hospital:** Mount Sinai Med Ctr (page 102), NY-Presby Hosp/Weill Cornell (page 104); **Address:** 1088 Park Ave, New York, NY 10128-1132; **Phone:** 212-860-4000 x36; **Board Cert:** Internal Medicine 1965; Rheumatology 1972; **Med School:** NYU Sch Med 1958; **Resid:** Internal Medicine, VA Med Ctr 1960; Internal Medicine, Mt Sinai Hosp 1961; **Fellow:** Rheumatology, Columbia-Presby Med Ctr 1963; **Fac Appt:** Clin Prof Med, Mount Sinai Sch Med

Spiera, Robert MD (Rhu) - **Spec Exp:** Vasculitis; Lupus/SLE; Scleroderma; **Hospital:** Hosp For Special Surgery (page 111), Mount Sinai Med Ctr (page 102); **Address:** 1088 Park Ave, New York, NY 10128-1132; **Phone:** 212-860-2100; **Board Cert:** Internal Medicine 2002; Rheumatology 2004; **Med School:** Yale Univ 1989; **Resid:** Internal Medicine, New York Hosp 1992; **Fellow:** Rheumatology, Hosp Special Surg 1995; **Fac Appt:** Assoc Clin Prof Med, Cornell Univ-Weill Med Coll

Stern, Richard MD (Rhu) - **Spec Exp:** Rheumatoid Arthritis; Osteoporosis; Osteoarthritis; Polymyalgia Rheumatica; **Hospital:** Hosp For Special Surgery (page 111), NY-Presby Hosp/Weill Cornell (page 104); **Address:** 475 E 72nd St, New York, NY 10021-4458; **Phone:** 212-879-2282; **Board Cert:** Internal Medicine 1973; Rheumatology 1976; **Med School:** Tufts Univ 1970; **Resid:** Internal Medicine, NY Hosp 1973; **Fellow:** Immunology, Rockefeller Univ Hosp 1975; Rheumatology, Hosp Special Surgery 1975; **Fac Appt:** Assoc Clin Prof Med, Cornell Univ-Weill Med Coll

Yee, Arthur M F MD/PhD (Rhu) - **Spec Exp:** Sarcoidosis; Gout; Rheumatoid Arthritis; Psoriatic Arthritis; **Hospital:** Hosp For Special Surgery (page 111), NY-Presby Hosp/Weill Cornell (page 104); **Address:** Hosp for Special Surgery, 535 E 70th St, New York, NY 10021; **Phone:** 212-606-1171; **Board Cert:** Internal Medicine 2004; Rheumatology 2006; **Med School:** NYU Sch Med 1991; **Resid:** Internal Medicine, NY Hosp-Cornell Med Ctr 1993; **Fellow:** Rheumatology, NY Hosp-Cornell Med Ctr 1995; **Fac Appt:** Asst Prof Med, Cornell Univ-Weill Med Coll

Sports Medicine

Altchek, David MD (SM) - **Spec Exp:** Shoulder Surgery; Elbow Surgery; Knee Surgery; Arthroscopic Surgery; **Hospital:** Hosp For Special Surgery (page 111), NY-Presby Hosp/Weill Cornell (page 104); **Address:** Hospital for Special Surgery, 535 E 70th St, New York, NY 10021; **Phone:** 212-606-1909; **Board Cert:** Orthopaedic Surgery 2001; **Med School:** Cornell Univ-Weill Med Coll 1982; **Resid:** Orthopaedic Surgery, Hosp for Special Surg 1987; **Fellow:** Sports Medicine, Hosp for Special Surg 1988; **Fac Appt:** Assoc Prof OrS, Cornell Univ-Weill Med Coll

Callahan, Lisa MD (SM) - **Spec Exp:** Primary Care Sports Medicine; Sports Medicine-Women; Fractures-Stress; **Hospital:** Hosp For Special Surgery (page 111), NY-Presby Hosp/Weill Cornell (page 104); **Address:** Hospital for Special Surgery, 535 E 70th St, New York, NY 10021; **Phone:** 212-606-1532; **Board Cert:** Family Medicine 2004; Sports Medicine 2003; **Med School:** E Carolina Univ 1987; **Resid:** Family Medicine, San Jose Med Ctr 1990; **Fellow:** Sports Medicine, Stanford Univ 1991; **Fac Appt:** Assoc Prof FMed, Cornell Univ-Weill Med Coll

Halpern, Brian MD (SM) - **Spec Exp:** Primary Care Sports Medicine; Knee Injuries; Shoulder Injuries; **Hospital:** Hosp For Special Surgery (page 111); **Address:** 535 E 70th St, New York, NY 10021; **Phone:** 212-606-1329; **Board Cert:** Family Medicine 2008; Sports Medicine 2004; **Med School:** Cornell Univ-Weill Med Coll 1981; **Resid:** Family Medicine, Univ Md Med Ctr 1984; **Fellow:** Sports Medicine, Hughston Ortho Clinic 1985; **Fac Appt:** Asst Clin Prof Med, Cornell Univ-Weill Med Coll

Hamner, Daniel MD (SM) - **Spec Exp:** Running Injuries; Acupuncture; Primary Care Sports Medicine; **Address:** 80 E 11th St, Ste 619, New York, NY 10003; **Phone:** 212-260-5999; **Board Cert:** Physical Medicine & Rehabilitation 1986; **Med School:** NY Med Coll 1976; **Resid:** Physical Medicine & Rehabilitation, New York Hosp-Cornell Med Ctr 1979; **Fellow:** Cardiac Rehabilitation, Emory Med Ctr 1980

Levine, William MD (SM) - **Spec Exp:** Arthroscopic Surgery; Shoulder & Elbow Surgery; Knee Injuries; **Hospital:** NY-Presby Hosp/Columbia (page 104); **Address:** 622 W 168th St Fl PH-11, New York, NY 10032; **Phone:** 212-305-0762; **Board Cert:** Orthopaedic Surgery 2010; Orthopaedic Sports Medicine 2008; **Med School:** Case West Res Univ 1990; **Resid:** Surgery, Beth Israel Hosp 1991; Orthopaedic Surgery, New Eng Med Ctr Hosps 1995; **Fellow:** Shoulder Surgery, Columbia-Presby Med Ctr 1996; Sports Medicine, Univ MD Med Ctr 1998; **Fac Appt:** Clin Prof OrS, Columbia P&S

Maharam, Lewis G MD (SM) - **Spec Exp:** Primary Care Sports Medicine; Running Injuries; Pain-Back; Pain-Back; **Hospital:** NYU Hosp For Joint Diseases (page 106), NYU Langone Med Ctr (page 106); **Address:** 24 W 57th St, Ste 509, New York, NY 10019-3918; **Phone:** 212-765-5763; **Board Cert:** Sports Medicine 1991; **Med School:** Emory Univ 1985; **Resid:** Internal Medicine, Danbury Hosp 1987; Internal Medicine, NY Infirm/Beekman Downtown 1989; **Fellow:** Sports Medicine, Pascack Valley Hosp 1990; **Fac Appt:** Asst Clin Prof OrS, NYU Sch Med

Metzl, Jordan D MD (SM) - **Spec Exp:** Adolescent Sports Medicine; Running Injuries; Dance/Ballet Injuries; **Hospital:** Hosp For Special Surgery (page 111); **Address:** Hospital for Special Surgery, Sports Med, 535 E 70 St, New York, NY 10021-4872; **Phone:** 212-606-1678; **Board Cert:** Sports Medicine 2001; **Med School:** Univ MO-Columbia Sch Med 1993; **Resid:** Pediatrics, New Eng Med Ctr 1996; **Fellow:** Sports Medicine, Vanderbilt Univ Med Ctr 1996; Sports Medicine, Hosp Special Surgery 1997; **Fac Appt:** Asst Prof Ped, Cornell Univ-Weill Med Coll

Nisonson, Barton MD (SM) - **Spec Exp:** Shoulder & Knee Surgery; Arthroscopic Surgery; Knee Replacement; **Hospital:** Lenox Hill Hosp; **Address:** 130 E 77th St, New York, NY 10021-1851; **Phone:** 212-570-9120; **Board Cert:** Orthopaedic Surgery 1974; **Med School:** Columbia P&S 1966; **Resid:** Surgery, Columbia-Presby Med Ctr 1968; Orthopaedic Surgery, Columbia-Presby Med Ctr 1973

Plancher, Kevin D MD (SM) - **Spec Exp:** Shoulder Surgery; Elbow Surgery; Cartilage Damage & Transplant; Shoulder Replacement; **Hospital:** Beth Israel Med Ctr - Petrie Division (page 94), Lenox Hill Hosp; **Address:** 1160 Park Ave, New York, NY 10128; **Phone:** 212-876-5200; **Board Cert:** Orthopaedic Surgery 2007; Hand Surgery 2008; Orthopaedic Sports Medicine 2009; **Med School:** Georgetown Univ 1986; **Resid:** Orthopaedic Surgery, Mass Genl Hosp/Brigham & Womens Hosp 1991; **Fellow:** Hand Surgery, Indiana Hand Ctr 1993; Sports Medicine, Steadman-Hawkins Clinic 1994; **Fac Appt:** Assoc Clin Prof OrS, Albert Einstein Coll Med

Rodeo, Scott A MD (SM) - **Spec Exp:** Knee Injuries; Cartilage Damage; **Hospital:** Hosp For Special Surgery (page 111); **Address:** Hosp for Special Surgery, 525 E 71st St, New York, NY 10021; **Phone:** 212-606-1513; **Board Cert:** Orthopaedic Surgery 1998; **Med School:** Cornell Univ-Weill Med Coll 1989; **Resid:** Orthopaedic Surgery, Hosp Special Surgery 1994; **Fellow:** Sports Medicine, Hosp Special Surgery 1996; **Fac Appt:** Assoc Clin Prof OrS, Cornell Univ-Weill Med Coll

Roth, Neil S MD (SM) - **Hospital:** Lenox Hill Hosp, White Plains Hosp Ctr; **Address:** Lenox Hill Hospital, 130 E 77th St, Black Hall Fl 8, New York, NY 10021; **Phone:** 212-861-2300; **Board Cert:** Orthopaedic Surgery 2001; Orthopaedic Sports Medicine 2008; **Med School:** Duke Univ 1991; **Resid:** Orthopaedic Surgery, Columbia Presby Med Ctr 1997; **Fellow:** Sports Medicine, Kerlan-Jobe Orth Clin 1999

Surgery

Amory, Spencer E MD (S) - **Spec Exp:** Laparoscopic Surgery; Gastrointestinal Surgery; Hernia; **Hospital:** NY-Presby Hosp/The Allen Hosp (page 104); **Address:** 5141 Broadway, Ste 3-178, New York, NY 10034; **Phone:** 212-305-5221; **Board Cert:** Surgery 2000; **Med School:** Johns Hopkins Univ 1983; **Resid:** Surgery, Columbia Presby Med Ctr 1989; **Fellow:** Emergency Medicine, Peninsula Hosp 1990; **Fac Appt:** Assoc Clin Prof S, Columbia P&S

Attiyeh, Fadi F MD (S) - **Spec Exp:** Colon & Rectal Cancer; Hepatobiliary Surgery; Pancreatic Surgery; **Hospital:** St Luke's - Roosevelt Hosp Ctr - Roosevelt Div (page 94); **Address:** 425 W 59th St, Ste 8B-1, New York, NY 10019; **Phone:** 212-307-1144; **Board Cert:** Surgery 1975; Colon & Rectal Surgery 1982; **Med School:** Amer Univ Beirut 1969; **Resid:** Surgery, Amer Univ Hosp 1973; **Fellow:** Surgical Oncology, Meml Sloan Kettering Canc Ctr 1976; **Fac Appt:** Assoc Clin Prof S, Columbia P&S

Axelrod, Deborah MD (S) - **Spec Exp:** Breast Cancer; Breast Disease; **Hospital:** NYU Langone Med Ctr (page 106); **Address:** NYU Clinical Cancer Ctr, 160 E 34th St, New York, NY 10016; **Phone:** 212-731-5366; **Board Cert:** Surgery 2008; **Med School:** Israel 1982; **Resid:** Surgery, Beth Israel Med Ctr 1988; **Fellow:** Surgical Oncology, Meml Sloan Kettering Cancer Ctr 1986; **Fac Appt:** Assoc Prof S, NYU Sch Med

Barie, Philip MD (S) - **Spec Exp:** Trauma; Critical Care; Hernia; Sepsis; **Hospital:** NY-Presby Hosp/Weill Cornell (page 104), Hosp For Special Surgery (page 111); **Address:** Weill Med College-Cornell Univ, 525 E 68th St, Ste P713A, New York, NY 10021-4873; **Phone:** 212-746-5401; **Board Cert:** Surgery 2004; Surgical Critical Care 2005; **Med School:** Boston Univ 1977; **Resid:** Surgery, NY Hosp-Cornell Med Ctr 1984; **Fellow:** Trauma, Albany Med Coll 1981; **Fac Appt:** Prof S, Cornell Univ-Weill Med Coll

Berman, Russell MD (S) - **Spec Exp:** Melanoma; **Hospital:** NYU Langone Med Ctr (page 106); **Address:** NYU Clinical Cancer Ctr, 160 E 34th St Fl 3, New York, NY 10016; **Phone:** 212-731-5415; **Board Cert:** Surgery 2007; **Med School:** NYU Sch Med 1990; **Resid:** Surgery, NYU Med Ctr/Bellevue Hosp 1997; **Fellow:** Surgical Oncology, Meml Sloan Kettering Cancer Ctr 1994; Surgical Oncology, UT MD Anderson Cancer Ctr 2000; **Fac Appt:** Asst Prof S, NYU Sch Med

Bernik, Stephanie F MD (S) - **Spec Exp:** Breast Cancer & Surgery; Breast Disease; Phyllodes Tumors; Angiosarcoma; **Hospital:** Lenox Hill Hosp; **Address:** Lenox Hill Hosp, 100 E 77th St Fl 3rd, New York, NY 10075; **Phone:** 212-434-6900; **Board Cert:** Surgery 2001; **Med School:** Yale Univ 1993; **Resid:** Surgery, St Vincents Hosp 1999; **Fellow:** Breast Surgery, Meml Sloan Kettering Cancer Ctr 2000

Bessey, Palmer Q MD (S) - **Spec Exp:** Burn Care; Wound Healing/Care; Nutrition; **Hospital:** NY-Presby Hosp/Weill Cornell (page 104); **Address:** 525 E 68th St, Box 137, New York, NY 10065; **Phone:** 212-746-0242; **Board Cert:** Surgery 2000; Surgical Critical Care 2005; **Med School:** Univ VT Coll Med 1975; **Resid:** Surgery, Univ Alabama Hosp 1981; **Fellow:** Metabolism, Brigham & Women's Hosp 1983; **Fac Appt:** Prof S, Cornell Univ-Weill Med Coll

Bessler, Marc MD (S) - **Spec Exp:** Obesity/Bariatric Surgery; Laparoscopic Surgery; Gastrointestinal Metabolic Surgery; **Hospital:** NY-Presby Hosp/Columbia (page 104); **Address:** NY Presby Med Ctr, Dept of Surgery, 161 Fort Washington Ave, rm 612, New York, NY 10032; **Phone:** 212-305-9506; **Board Cert:** Surgery 2007; **Med School:** NYU Sch Med 1989; **Resid:** Surgery, Columbia Presby Med Ctr 1995; **Fac Appt:** Assoc Prof S, Columbia P&S

Bloom, Norman MD (S) - **Spec Exp:** Breast Cancer; Sarcoma; Cancer Surgery; **Hospital:** Beth Israel Med Ctr - Petrie Division (page 94), NYU Langone Med Ctr (page 106); **Address:** The Gramercy, 61 Irving Pl @ 18th St, New York, NY 10003; **Phone:** 212-505-6167; **Board Cert:** Surgery 1999; **Med School:** SUNY Downstate 1974; **Resid:** Surgery, Maimonides Med Ctr 1978; **Fellow:** Surgical Oncology, Meml Sloan Kettering Canc Ctr 1979; **Fac Appt:** Clin Prof S, NYU Sch Med

Brem, Harold MD (S) - **Spec Exp:** Wound Healing/Care; Lower Limb Ulcers; **Hospital:** NYU Langone Med Ctr (page 106); **Address:** Wound Ctr; Hosp for Joint Diseases, 301 E 17th St, New York, NY 10003; **Phone:** 212-263-7187; **Board Cert:** Surgery 2007; **Med School:** McGill Univ 1987; **Resid:** Surgery, Ohio State Univ Hosp 1989; **Fellow:** Surgical Research, Harvard Med Sch 1992; **Fac Appt:** Assoc Prof S, NYU Sch Med

Brennan, Murray F MD (S) - **Spec Exp:** Sarcoma; Pancreatic Cancer; Stomach Cancer; Endocrine Cancers; **Hospital:** Meml Sloan-Kettering Cancer Ctr (page 112); **Address:** 1275 York Avenue, New York, NY 10065; **Phone:** 800-525-2225; **Board Cert:** Surgery 1975; **Med School:** New Zealand 1964; **Resid:** Surgery, Univ Otago Hosp 1969; **Fellow:** Surgery, Harvard Med Sch 1972; Surgery, Peter Bent Brigham Hosp 1975; **Fac Appt:** Prof S, Cornell Univ-Weill Med Coll

Cassell, Lauren S MD (S) - **Spec Exp:** Breast Surgery; Breast Cancer; **Hospital:** Lenox Hill Hosp; **Address:** 114A E 78th St, New York, NY 10075; **Phone:** 212-535-4040; **Board Cert:** Surgery 2003; **Med School:** NY Med Coll 1977; **Resid:** Surgery, Lenox Hill Hosp 1982

Chabot, John A MD (S) - **Spec Exp:** Liver & Biliary Surgery; Pancreatic Cancer; Pancreatic Surgery; Thyroid & Parathyroid Surgery; **Hospital:** NY-Presby Hosp/Columbia (page 104); **Address:** NY Presby-Columbia Medical Ctr, 161 Ft Washington Ave Fl 8 - Ste 819, New York, NY 10032; **Phone:** 212-305-9468; **Board Cert:** Surgery 2000; **Med School:** Dartmouth Med Sch 1983; **Resid:** Surgery, Columbia-Presby Med Ctr 1990; **Fac Appt:** Prof S, Columbia P&S

Cioroiu, Michael G MD (S) - **Spec Exp:** Breast Disease; Wound Healing/Care; Endoscopy; **Hospital:** Mount Sinai Hosp of Queens (page 102); **Address:** 247 3rd Ave, Ste L 3, New York, NY 10010-7453; **Phone:** 212-995-8099; **Board Cert:** Surgery 2004; **Med School:** Romania 1971; **Resid:** Surgery, Cabrini Med Ctr 1985; **Fac Appt:** Assoc Clin Prof S, Mount Sinai Sch Med

Coit, Daniel G MD (S) - **Spec Exp:** Melanoma; Pancreatic Cancer; Stomach Cancer; **Hospital:** Meml Sloan-Kettering Cancer Ctr (page 112); **Address:** 1275 York Avenue, New York, NY 10065; **Phone:** 800-525-2225; **Board Cert:** Surgery 2004; **Med School:** Univ Cincinnati 1976; **Resid:** Internal Medicine, New Eng Deaconess Hosp 1978; Surgery, New Eng Deaconess Hosp 1983; **Fellow:** Surgical Oncology, Meml Sloan Kettering Canc Ctr 1985; **Fac Appt:** Prof S, Cornell Univ-Weill Med Coll

Edye, Michael MD (S) - **Spec Exp:** Laparoscopic Abdominal Surgery; Colon Cancer; Diverticulitis; Obesity/Bariatric Surgery; **Hospital:** Mount Sinai Med Ctr (page 102), Westchester Med Ctr; **Address:** 1060 Fifth Ave, New York, NY 10128; **Phone:** 212-241-0872; **Med School:** Australia 1977; **Resid:** Surgery, St Vincents Hosp 1980; Surgery, Royal N Shore Hosp 1984; **Fellow:** Laparoscopic Surgery, Univ Bordeaux 1992; **Fac Appt:** Assoc Clin Prof S, Mount Sinai Sch Med

El-Tamer, Mahmoud B MD (S) - **Spec Exp:** Breast Cancer; **Hospital:** Meml Sloan-Kettering Cancer Ctr (page 112); **Address:** Meml Sloan Kettering Cancer Ctr, 300 E 66th St, New York, NY 10032; **Phone:** 646-888-4753; **Board Cert:** Surgery 2001; **Med School:** Lebanon 1981; **Resid:** Surgery, American Univ Hosp 1985; Surgery, SUNY Hlth Sci Ctr 1992; **Fellow:** Surgical Oncology, Meml Sloan Kettering Cancer Ctr 1989; **Fac Appt:** Assoc Prof S, Columbia P&S

Emond, Jean C MD (S) - **Spec Exp:** Transplant-Liver; Liver Cancer; Liver & Biliary Cancer; Hepatobiliary Surgery; **Hospital:** NY-Presby Hosp/Columbia (page 104), Holy Name Med Ctr (page 657); **Address:** 622 W 168th St, PH - Fl 14, New York, NY 10032; **Phone:** 212-305-9691; **Board Cert:** Surgery 2006; **Med School:** Univ Chicago-Pritzker Sch Med 1979; **Resid:** Surgery, Cook Cty Hosp 1984; **Fellow:** Surgery, Hopital P Brousse/Univ de Paris Sud 1985; Transplant Surgery, Univ Chicago Hosps 1987; **Fac Appt:** Prof S, Columbia P&S

Eng, Kenneth MD (S) - **Spec Exp:** Colon & Rectal Cancer & Surgery; Pancreatic Cancer; Inflammatory Bowel Disease; **Hospital:** NYU Langone Med Ctr (page 106); **Address:** 530 1st Ave, Ste 6B, New York, NY 10016-6402; **Phone:** 212-263-7301; **Board Cert:** Surgery 1982; **Med School:** NYU Sch Med 1967; **Resid:** Surgery, NYU Med Ctr 1972; **Fac Appt:** Prof S, NYU Sch Med

Estabrook, Alison MD (S) - **Spec Exp:** Breast Cancer; Breast Disease; Breast Cancer-High Risk Women; **Hospital:** St Luke's - Roosevelt Hosp Ctr - Roosevelt Div (page 94); **Address:** 425 W 59th St, Ste 7A, New York, NY 10019-1104; **Phone:** 212-523-7500; **Board Cert:** Surgery 2004; **Med School:** NYU Sch Med 1978; **Resid:** Surgery, Columbia Presby Med Ctr 1984; **Fellow:** Surgical Oncology, Columbia Presby Med Ctr 1982; **Fac Appt:** Prof S, Columbia P&S

Fahey III, Thomas J MD (S) - **Spec Exp:** Endocrine Surgery; Pheochromocytoma; Pancreatic Cancer; Minimally Invasive Surgery; **Hospital:** NY-Presby Hosp/Weill Cornell (page 104); **Address:** NY Presby Cornell Med Ctr, Dept Surgery, 525 E 68 St, rm F2024, Box 249, New York, NY 10065; **Phone:** 212-746-5130; **Board Cert:** Surgery 2002; **Med School:** Cornell Univ-Weill Med Coll 1986; **Resid:** Surgery, New York Hosp 1992; **Fellow:** Endocrine Surgery, Royal North Shore Hosp 1993; **Fac Appt:** Prof S, Cornell Univ-Weill Med Coll

Feldman, Sheldon M MD (S) - **Spec Exp:** Breast Surgery; Breast Cancer; Complementary Medicine; **Hospital:** NY-Presby Hosp/Columbia (page 104); **Address:** NY Presbyterian-Columbia Med Ctr, Div Surgical Oncology, 161 Fort Washington Ave Fl 10 - Ste 1005, New York, NY 10032; **Phone:** 212-305-9676; **Board Cert:** Surgery 2000; **Med School:** NYU Sch Med 1975; **Resid:** Surgery, NYU-Bellevue Med Ctr 1980; **Fellow:** Peripheral Vascular Surgery, Beth Israel Med Ctr 1981; **Fac Appt:** Asst Clin Prof S, Columbia P&S

Fielding, George MD (S) - **Spec Exp:** Obesity/Bariatric Surgery; Hernia; Laparoscopic Surgery; **Hospital:** NYU Langone Med Ctr (page 106); **Address:** 530 First Ave, Ste 10-S, New York, NY 10016; **Phone:** 212-263-3166; **Med School:** Australia 1980; **Resid:** Surgery, Royal Brisbane Hosp 1982; Surgery, Berne 1988; **Fac Appt:** Assoc Prof S, NYU Sch Med

Fong, Yuman MD (S) - **Spec Exp:** Pancreatic Cancer; Liver & Biliary Cancer; Stomach Cancer; **Hospital:** Meml Sloan-Kettering Cancer Ctr (page 112), NY-Presby Hosp/Weill Cornell (page 104); **Address:** 1275 York Ave, rm C887, New York, NY 10065; **Phone:** 800-525-2225; **Board Cert:** Surgery 2002; **Med School:** Cornell Univ-Weill Med Coll 1984; **Resid:** Surgery, NY Hosp-Cornell Med Ctr 1992; **Fellow:** Surgical Oncology, Meml Sloan-Kettering Cancer Ctr 1994; **Fac Appt:** Prof S, Cornell Univ-Weill Med Coll

Geller, Peter MD (S) - **Spec Exp:** Gastrointestinal Surgery; Hernia; Breast Cancer; Sentinel Node Surgery; **Hospital:** NY-Presby Hosp/Columbia (page 104); **Address:** Columbia Eastside, 16 E 60 St, rm 330, New York, NY 10022; **Phone:** 212-305-6657; **Board Cert:** Surgery 2004; **Med School:** Columbia P&S 1980; **Resid:** Surgery, Columbia-Presby Med Ctr 1985; **Fellow:** Vascular Surgery, Columbia-Presby Med Ctr 1986; **Fac Appt:** Assoc Prof S, Columbia P&S

Gouge, Thomas H MD (S) - **Spec Exp:** Esophageal Cancer; Pancreatic Cancer; Gastroesophageal Reflux Disease (GERD); **Hospital:** Bellevue Hosp Ctr; **Address:** 336 Central Park W, New York, NY 10025; **Phone:** 212-951-3366; **Board Cert:** Surgery 2007; **Med School:** Yale Univ 1970; **Resid:** Surgery, NYU Med Ctr 1975; **Fac Appt:** Prof S, NYU Sch Med

Heerdt, Alexandra S MD (S) - **Spec Exp:** Breast Cancer; **Hospital:** Meml Sloan-Kettering Cancer Ctr (page 112); **Address:** 300 E 66th St, New York, NY 10065; **Phone:** 800-525-2225; **Board Cert:** Surgery 2002; **Med School:** Jefferson Med Coll 1987; **Resid:** Surgery, NY Hosp-Cornell Med Ctr 1992; **Fellow:** Surgical Oncology, Meml Sloan Kettering Cancer Ctr 1993

Heller, Keith S MD (S) - **Spec Exp:** Thyroid & Parathyroid Surgery; Minimally Invasive Surgery; Head & Neck Tumors; Endocrine Surgery; **Hospital:** NYU Langone Med Ctr (page 106); **Address:** 530 First Ave, Ste 6H, New York, NY 10016; **Phone:** 212-263-7710; **Board Cert:** Surgery 2006; **Med School:** NYU Sch Med 1971; **Resid:** Surgery, NYU-Bellevue Hosp 1976; **Fellow:** Surgical Oncology, Meml Sloan Kettering Cancer Ctr 1978; **Fac Appt:** Prof S, NYU Sch Med

Herron, Daniel M MD (S) - **Spec Exp:** Obesity/Bariatric Surgery; Laparoscopic Surgery; Endoscopic Surgery; **Hospital:** Mount Sinai Med Ctr (page 102); **Address:** Mt Sinai Med Ctr, 5 E 98th St, Box 1259, New York, NY 10029; **Phone:** 212-241-5339; **Board Cert:** Surgery 2008; **Med School:** Univ Pennsylvania 1992; **Resid:** Surgery, New England Med Ctr 1998; **Fellow:** Laparoscopic Surgery, Oregon U Hlth Sci Ctr 1999; **Fac Appt:** Assoc Prof S, Mount Sinai Sch Med

Inabnet, William B MD (S) - **Spec Exp:** Thyroid Surgery; Adrenal Surgery; Pancreatic Surgery; Minimally Invasive Surgery; **Hospital:** Mount Sinai Med Ctr (page 102); **Address:** 5 E 98th St Fl 15, Box 1259, New York, NY 10029; **Phone:** 212-241-6918; **Board Cert:** Surgery 2007; **Med School:** Univ NC Sch Med 1991; **Resid:** Surgery, Rush Presby-St Lukes Med Ctr 1996; **Fellow:** Endocrine Surgery, Cochin Hosp 1997; **Fac Appt:** Asst Prof S, Columbia P&S

Jarnagin, William MD (S) - **Spec Exp:** Hepatobiliary Surgery; Liver Cancer; Pancreatic Cancer; Gallbladder & Biliary Cancer; **Hospital:** Meml Sloan-Kettering Cancer Ctr (page 112); **Address:** 1275 York Ave, New York, NY 10065; **Phone:** 212-639-7601; **Board Cert:** Surgery 2006; **Med School:** Rush Med Coll 1988; **Resid:** Surgery, Univ Calif San Francisco 1996; **Fellow:** Hepatopancreatobiliary Surgery, Meml Sloan-Kettering Cancer Ctr 1997; **Fac Appt:** Prof S, Cornell Univ

Kapur, Sandip MD (S) - **Spec Exp:** Transplant-Kidney; Pancreatic Islet Cell Transplant; Hepatobiliary Surgery; Transplant-Pancreas; **Hospital:** NY-Presby Hosp/Weill Cornell (page 104), NY-Presby Hosp/Columbia (page 104); **Address:** 520 E 68th St, Ste F1919, New York, NY 10065; **Phone:** 212-746-5330; **Board Cert:** Surgery 2007; **Med School:** Cornell Univ-Weill Med Coll 1990; **Resid:** Surgery, Cornell Univ Med Ctr 1996; **Fellow:** Research, The Rogosin Inst 1994; Transplant Surgery, Thomas E Starzl Transplant Inst 1998; **Fac Appt:** Assoc Prof S, Cornell Univ-Weill Med Coll

Karpeh Jr, Martin S MD (S) - **Spec Exp:** Gastrointestinal Cancer; Esophageal Cancer; Pancreatic Cancer; Liver Cancer; **Hospital:** Beth Israel Med Ctr - Petrie Division (page 94); **Address:** Beth Israel Med Ctr, Philips Ambulatory Ctr, 10 Union Square E, Ste 4D, New York, NY 10003; **Phone:** 212-420-4041; **Board Cert:** Surgery 1998; **Med School:** Penn State Univ-Hershey Med Ctr 1983; **Resid:** Surgery, Hosp Univ Penn 1989; **Fellow:** Surgical Oncology, Meml Sloan Kettering Cancer Ctr 1991; **Fac Appt:** Prof S, Mount Sinai Sch Med

Kato, Tomoaki MD (S) - **Spec Exp:** Transplant-Liver; Transplant Surgery-Pediatric; Transplant-Multi Organ; Transplant-Auto Transplantation; **Hospital:** NY-Presby Hosp/Columbia (page 104); **Address:** Columbia Univ Med Ctr, PH Bldg - rm 14-105, 622 W 168 St, New York, NY 10032; **Phone:** 212-305-5101; **Med School:** Japan 1991; **Resid:** Surgery, Itami City Hospital 1995; **Fellow:** Transplant Surgery, Jackson Meml Hosp 1997; **Fac Appt:** Prof S, Columbia P&S

Kimmelstiel, Fred M MD (S) - **Spec Exp:** Laparoscopic Surgery; Breast Surgery; Cancer Surgery; Hernia; **Hospital:** St Luke's - Roosevelt Hosp Ctr - Roosevelt Div (page 94); **Address:** 225 W 71st St, New York, NY 10023; **Phone:** 212-362-6060; **Board Cert:** Surgery 2006; **Med School:** NY Med Coll 1980; **Resid:** Surgery, St Lukes Roosevelt Hosp Ctr 1985; **Fellow:** Transplant Surgery, Univ Hosp 1986; **Fac Appt:** Asst Clin Prof S, Columbia P&S

Labow, Daniel M MD (S) - **Spec Exp:** Pancreatic Cancer; Gastrointestinal Cancer; Liver Cancer; **Hospital:** Mount Sinai Med Ctr (page 102); **Address:** 1 Gustave L Levy Pl, Box 1259, New York, NY 10029; **Phone:** 212-241-6764; **Board Cert:** Surgery 2003; **Med School:** Brown Univ 1995; **Resid:** Surgery, Univ Chicago Hosps 1997; Research, NY Presby/Cornell Med Ctr 1999; **Fellow:** Surgical Oncology, Sloan Kettering Cancer Ctr 2004; **Fac Appt:** Asst Prof S, Mount Sinai Sch Med

Lee, James A MD (S) - **Spec Exp:** Endocrine Surgery; Thyroid Cancer; **Hospital:** NY-Presby Hosp/Columbia (page 104); **Address:** Columbia University Medical Ctr, Irving Pavilion, 161 Fort Washington Ave, New York, NY 10032; **Phone:** 212-305-0444; **Board Cert:** Surgery 2005; **Med School:** Columbia P&S 1999; **Resid:** Surgery, NY Presby Hosp 2005; Research, NY Presby Hosp 2003; **Fellow:** Endocrine Surgery, UCSF Med Ctr 2006; **Fac Appt:** Asst Prof S, Columbia P&S

Lieberman, Michael D MD (S) - **Spec Exp:** Gastrointestinal Cancer; Colon & Rectal Surgery; Hepatobiliary Surgery; Pancreatic Cancer; **Hospital:** NY-Presby Hosp/Weill Cornell (page 104); **Address:** 1315 York Ave, Box 216, New York, NY 10021; **Phone:** 212-746-5434; **Board Cert:** Surgery 2003; **Med School:** UMDNJ-NJ Med Sch, Newark 1985; **Resid:** Surgery, Hosp Univ Penn 1992; **Fellow:** Surgical Oncology, Hosp Univ Penn 1990; Surgical Oncology, Meml Sloan-Kettering Cancer Ctr 1994; **Fac Appt:** Assoc Prof S, Cornell Univ-Weill Med Coll

Michelassi, Fabrizio MD (S) - **Spec Exp:** Gastrointestinal Cancer; Crohn's Disease; Ulcerative Colitis; Colon Cancer; **Hospital:** NY-Presby Hosp/Weill Cornell (page 104); **Address:** Weill Cornell Med College, Surg Dept, 525 E 68th St, rm F-739, New York, NY 10021; **Phone:** 212-746-6006; **Board Cert:** Surgery 2002; **Med School:** Italy 1975; **Resid:** Surgery, NYU Med Ctr 1981; **Fellow:** Research, Mass Genl Hosp 1983; **Fac Appt:** Prof S, Cornell Univ-Weill Med Coll

Mills, Christopher B MD (S) - **Spec Exp:** Breast Surgery; Cancer Surgery; **Address:** 325 W 15th St, New York, NY 10011; **Phone:** 212-604-6006; **Board Cert:** Surgery 2009; **Med School:** UMDNJ-NJ Med Sch, Newark 1973; **Resid:** Surgery, St Vincent's Hosp & Med Ctr 1978; **Fellow:** Nutrition & Metabolism, Ravenswood Hosp Med Ctr 1979; **Fac Appt:** Asst Prof S, NY Med Coll

Moncrief, Robyn M MD (S) - **Spec Exp:** Breast Surgery; Minimally Invasive Surgery; Breast Cancer; **Address:** St Vincent Comprehensive Cancer Ctr, 325 W 15th St, New York, NY 10011; **Phone:** 212-604-6006; **Board Cert:** Surgery 2006; **Med School:** Univ Tex, San Antonio 1997; **Resid:** Surgery, SUNY Downstate 2000; Surgery, St Vincents Hosp 2003; **Fellow:** Breast Surgery, Northwestern Meml Hosp 2004

Morrissey, Kevin MD (S) - **Spec Exp:** Colon & Rectal Surgery; Gastrointestinal Surgery; **Hospital:** NY-Presby Hosp/Weill Cornell (page 104); **Address:** 50 E 69th St, New York, NY 10021-5016; **Phone:** 212-744-0060; **Board Cert:** Surgery 1972; **Med School:** Cornell Univ-Weill Med Coll 1965; **Resid:** Surgery, NY Hosp 1971; **Fellow:** Gastroenterology, NY Hosp 1973

Morrow, Monica MD (S) - **Spec Exp:** Breast Cancer; **Hospital:** Meml Sloan-Kettering Cancer Ctr (page 112); **Address:** 300 E 66th St, New York, NY 10065; **Phone:** 800-525-2225; **Board Cert:** Surgery 2001; **Med School:** Jefferson Med Coll 1976; **Resid:** Surgery, Med Ctr Hosp Vermont 1981; **Fellow:** Surgical Oncology, Meml Sloan Kettering Cancer Ctr 1983; **Fac Appt:** Prof S, Cornell Univ-Weill Med Coll

Newman, Elliot MD (S) - **Spec Exp:** Gastrointestinal Cancer; Pancreatic Cancer; Liver Cancer; Colon & Rectal Cancer; **Hospital:** NYU Langone Med Ctr (page 106); **Address:** NYU Medical Ctr, 530 1st Ave, Ste 6C, New York, NY 10016-6402; **Phone:** 212-263-7302; **Board Cert:** Surgery 2004; **Med School:** NYU Sch Med 1986; **Resid:** Surgery, NYU Med Ctr 1989; Surgery, NYU Med Ctr 1993; **Fellow:** Research, Meml Sloan Kettering Cancer Ctr 1991; Surgical Oncology, Meml Sloan Kettering Cancer Ctr 1995; **Fac Appt:** Assoc Prof S, NYU Sch Med

Nowak, Eugene MD (S) - **Spec Exp:** Breast Cancer; Hernia; Gastrointestinal Surgery; Sentinel Node Surgery; **Hospital:** NY-Presby Hosp/Weill Cornell (page 104); **Address:** 325 E 79th St, New York, NY 10021-0954; **Phone:** 212-517-6693; **Board Cert:** Surgery 2002; **Med School:** UMDNJ-NJ Med Sch, Newark 1975; **Resid:** Surgery, NY Hosp-Cornell Med Ctr 1980; **Fac Appt:** Assoc Prof S, Cornell Univ-Weill Med Coll

Osborne, Michael P MD (S) - **Spec Exp:** Breast Cancer; Breast Cancer-High Risk Women; Breast Disease; Sentinel Node Surgery; **Hospital:** Beth Israel Med Ctr - Petrie Division (page 94); **Address:** Philip Ambulatory Care Ctr, 10 Union Square E, Ste 4E, New York, NY 10003; **Phone:** 212-844-8770; **Med School:** England, UK 1970; **Resid:** Surgery, Charing Cross Hosp 1977; Surgery, Royal Marsden Hosp 1980; **Fellow:** Surgical Oncology, Meml Sloan-Kettering Canc Ctr 1981; **Fac Appt:** Prof S, Cornell Univ-Weill Med Coll

Pachter, H Leon MD (S) - **Spec Exp:** Adrenal Surgery; Gastrointestinal Surgery; Pancreatic Cancer; Hernia; **Hospital:** NYU Langone Med Ctr (page 106), Bellevue Hosp Ctr; **Address:** 530 1st Ave, Ste 6C, New York, NY 10016; **Phone:** 212-263-7302; **Board Cert:** Surgery 2010; **Med School:** NYU Sch Med 1971; **Resid:** Surgery, NYU Med Ctr 1976; **Fac Appt:** Prof S, NYU Sch Med

Paty, Philip B MD (S) - **Spec Exp:** Colon & Rectal Cancer; Pelvic Tumors; Appendix Cancer; **Hospital:** Meml Sloan-Kettering Cancer Ctr (page 112); **Address:** 1275 York Avenue, New York, NY 10065; **Phone:** 800-525-2225; **Board Cert:** Surgery 2001; **Med School:** Stanford Univ 1983; **Resid:** Surgery, UCSF Med Ctr 1990; **Fellow:** Surgical Oncology, Meml Sloan Kettering Cancer Ctr 1992; **Fac Appt:** Prof S, Cornell Univ-Weill Med Coll

Pomp, Alfons MD (S) - **Spec Exp:** Obesity/Bariatric Surgery; Laparoscopic Abdominal Surgery; Hernia; **Hospital:** NY-Presby Hosp/Weill Cornell (page 104); **Address:** Weill Cornell College of Medicine, 525 E 68th St, Box 294, New York, NY 10021; **Phone:** 212-746-5294; **Board Cert:** Surgery 1999; **Med School:** Univ Sherbrooke 1980; **Resid:** Surgery, Univ Montreal Med Ctr 1985; **Fellow:** Nutrition, Rhode Island Hosp 1988; **Fac Appt:** Prof S, Cornell Univ-Weill Med Coll

Ratner, LLoyd MD (S) - **Spec Exp:** Transplant-Kidney; Transplant-Pancreas; Pancreatic Surgery; **Hospital:** NY-Presby Hosp/Columbia (page 104); **Address:** Columbia University, PH 14, 622 W 168th St, New York, NY 10032; **Phone:** 212-305-6469; **Board Cert:** Surgery 2009; **Med School:** Hahnemann Univ 1983; **Resid:** Surgery, LIJ Med Ctr 1988; **Fellow:** Transplant Surgery, Barnes Jewish Hosp 1990; **Fac Appt:** Assoc Prof S, Columbia P&S

Reader, Robert MD (S) - **Spec Exp:** Breast Surgery; Hernia; Gastrointestinal Surgery; **Hospital:** NYU Langone Med Ctr (page 106); **Address:** 530 First Ave, Ste 6C, New York, NY 10016-6402; **Phone:** 212-263-7302; **Board Cert:** Surgery 2001; **Med School:** Univ Pennsylvania 1975; **Resid:** Surgery, NYU Med Ctr 1980; **Fac Appt:** Asst Clin Prof S, NYU Sch Med

Reiner, Mark MD (S) - **Spec Exp:** Laparoscopic Surgery; Hernia; Esophageal Surgery; Pancreatic Surgery; **Hospital:** Mount Sinai Med Ctr (page 102); **Address:** 1010 5th Ave, New York, NY 10028-0130; **Phone:** 212-879-6677; **Board Cert:** Surgery 2001; **Med School:** SUNY Downstate 1974; **Resid:** Surgery, Mt Sinai Hosp 1979; **Fac Appt:** Clin Prof S, Mount Sinai Sch Med

Ren-Fielding, Christine J MD (S) - **Spec Exp:** Obesity/Bariatric Surgery; Laparoscopic Surgery; **Hospital:** NYU Langone Med Ctr (page 106); **Address:** NYU Med Ctr, 530 First Ave, Ste 10-S, New York, NY 10016; **Phone:** 212-263-3166; **Board Cert:** Surgery 2000; **Med School:** Tufts Univ 1993; **Resid:** Surgery, NYU Med Ctr 1999; **Fellow:** Bariatric Surgery, NYU Med Ctr 2000; **Fac Appt:** Asst Prof S, NYU Sch Med

Rosenberg, Vladimiro MD (S) - **Spec Exp:** Breast Cancer; Melanoma; Thyroid & Parathyroid Surgery; Sarcoma-Soft Tissue; **Hospital:** Mount Sinai Med Ctr (page 102), Lenox Hill Hosp; **Address:** 1440 York Ave, Ste P-10, New York, NY 10075; **Phone:** 212-772-0010; **Med School:** Argentina 1965; **Resid:** Surgery, Mt Sinai Hosp 1977; **Fellow:** Surgical Oncology, MD Anderson Cancer Ctr 1978; **Fac Appt:** Asst Clin Prof S, Mount Sinai Sch Med

Roses, Daniel F MD (S) - **Spec Exp:** Breast Cancer; Melanoma; Thyroid & Parathyroid Surgery; **Hospital:** NYU Langone Med Ctr (page 106); **Address:** 530 First Ave, Ste 6B, New York, NY 10016-6402; **Phone:** 212-263-7329; **Board Cert:** Surgery 1975; **Med School:** NYU Sch Med 1969; **Resid:** Surgery, NYU-Bellevue Hosp 1974; **Fellow:** Surgical Oncology, NYU-Bellevue Hosp 1978; **Fac Appt:** Prof Surg & Onc, NYU Sch Med

Rubino, Francesco MD (S) - **Spec Exp:** Gastrointestinal Metabolic Surgery; Diabetes Surgery-Rubino's Procedure; Obesity/Bariatric Surgery; **Hospital:** NY-Presby Hosp/Weill Cornell (page 104); **Address:** NY Presbyterian Hosp/Weill Cornell, 525 E 68th St, rm P714, New York, NY 10065; **Phone:** 212-746-5925; **Med School:** Italy 1994; **Resid:** Surgery, Catholic Univ/Policlinico Gemelli; **Fellow:** Laparoscopic Surgery, European Inst of Telesurgery; Research, Catholic Univ; **Fac Appt:** Asst Prof S, Cornell Univ-Weill Med Coll

Salky, Barry A MD (S) - **Spec Exp:** Laparoscopic Abdominal Surgery; Gastroesophageal Reflux Disease (GERD); Colon Cancer; Ulcerative Colitis; **Hospital:** Mount Sinai Med Ctr (page 102); **Address:** Mt Sinai Medical Center, Div of Laparoscopic Surgery, 5 E 98th St, Box 1259, New York, NY 10029; **Phone:** 212-241-6156; **Board Cert:** Surgery 1998; **Med School:** Univ Tenn Coll Med, Memphis 1970; **Resid:** Surgery, Mount Sinai Hosp 1973; Surgery, Mount Sinai Hosp 1978; **Fac Appt:** Prof S, Mount Sinai Sch Med

Schnabel, Freya MD (S) - **Spec Exp:** Breast Cancer; Breast Cancer-High Risk Women; **Hospital:** NYU Langone Med Ctr (page 106); **Address:** 160 E 34th St Fl 3, New York, NY 10016; **Phone:** 212-731-5367; **Board Cert:** Surgery 2008; **Med School:** NYU Sch Med 1982; **Resid:** Surgery, NYU Med Ctr 1987; **Fellow:** Research, SUNY Hlth Sci Ctr 1988; **Fac Appt:** Prof S, NYU Sch Med

Schwartz, Myron E MD (S) - **Spec Exp:** Gastrointestinal Cancer; Liver Cancer; Hepatobiliary Surgery; **Hospital:** Mount Sinai Med Ctr (page 102); **Address:** Mount Sinai Med Ctr, Dept Surg, Div Surgical Onc, 19 E 98th St, Box 1104, New York, NY 10029; **Phone:** 212-241-2891; **Board Cert:** Surgery 2009; **Med School:** Jefferson Med Coll 1976; **Resid:** Surgery, Mt Sinai Hosp 1986; Vascular Surgery, Mt Sinai Hosp 1987; **Fac Appt:** Prof S, Mount Sinai Sch Med

Shah, Jatin P MD/PhD (S) - **Spec Exp:** Head & Neck Cancer & Surgery; Thyroid Cancer; Skull Base Tumors; Salivary Gland Tumors & Surgery; **Hospital:** Meml Sloan-Kettering Cancer Ctr (page 112); **Address:** 1275 York Avenue, New York, NY 10065; **Phone:** 800-525-2225; **Board Cert:** Surgery 1975; **Med School:** India 1964; **Resid:** Surgery, SSG Hosp 1967; Surgery, NY Eye & Ear Infirm 1974; **Fellow:** Head & Neck Surgical Oncology, Meml Sloan-Kettering Hosp 1972; **Fac Appt:** Prof S, Cornell Univ-Weill Med Coll

Shah, Paresh C MD (S) - **Spec Exp:** Laparoscopic Surgery; Obesity/Bariatric Surgery; **Hospital:** Lenox Hill Hosp; **Address:** 186 E 76th St, 1st Fl, New York, NY 10021; **Phone:** 212-434-3285; **Board Cert:** Surgery 2000; **Med School:** SUNY Downstate 1991; **Resid:** Surgery, SUNY- Downstate Med Ctr 1993; Surgery, Mass General Hosp 1995; **Fellow:** Laparoscopic Surgery, Lahey Clinic 1999

Shapiro, Richard L MD (S) - **Spec Exp:** Breast Cancer; Melanoma; Thyroid & Parathyroid Surgery; Cancer Surgery; **Hospital:** NYU Langone Med Ctr (page 106); **Address:** NYU Medical Ctr, 160 E 34th St Fl 4, New York, NY 10016; **Phone:** 212-731-5347; **Board Cert:** Surgery 2004; **Med School:** NYU Sch Med 1988; **Resid:** Surgery, NYU Langone Med Ctr 1993; **Fellow:** Surgical Oncology, NYU Langone Med Ctr 1995; **Fac Appt:** Assoc Prof S, NYU Sch Med

Simmons, Rache M MD (S) - **Spec Exp:** Breast Cancer & Surgery; Breast Disease; **Hospital:** NY-Presby Hosp/Weill Cornell (page 104); **Address:** Weill Cornell Breast Ctr, 425 E 61st St Fl 10, New York, NY 10065; **Phone:** 212-821-0853; **Board Cert:** Surgery 2005; **Med School:** Duke Univ 1988; **Resid:** Surgery, Univ NC Hosp 1993; **Fellow:** Surgical Oncology, NY Hosp-Cornell Hosp 1994; **Fac Appt:** Assoc Prof S, Cornell Univ-Weill Med Coll

Singer, Samuel MD (S) - **Spec Exp:** Sarcoma-Soft Tissue; **Hospital:** Meml Sloan-Kettering Cancer Ctr (page 112); **Address:** 1275 York Avenue, New York, NY 10065; **Phone:** 800-525-2225; **Board Cert:** Surgery 1998; **Med School:** Harvard Med Sch 1982; **Resid:** Surgery, Brigham & Women's Hosp 1988; **Fellow:** Surgical Oncology, Dana Farber Cancer Inst 1990; **Fac Appt:** Assoc Prof S, Cornell Univ-Weill Med Coll

Slater, Gary MD (S) - **Spec Exp:** Gastrointestinal Surgery; Laparoscopic Surgery; Hernia; **Hospital:** Mount Sinai Med Ctr (page 102); **Address:** 5 E 98th St Fl 14, Ste C, New York, NY 10029-6501; **Phone:** 212-241-9281; **Board Cert:** Surgery 1975; **Med School:** NYU Sch Med 1968; **Resid:** Surgery, Mount Sinai Hosp 1974; **Fac Appt:** Prof S, Mount Sinai Sch Med

Swistel, Alexander J MD (S) - **Spec Exp:** Breast Cancer; Breast Disease; Sentinel Node Surgery; Nipple Sparing Mastectomy; **Hospital:** NY-Presby Hosp/Weill Cornell (page 104), St Luke's - Roosevelt Hosp Ctr - Roosevelt Div (page 94); **Address:** 425 E 61st St Fl 10, New York, NY 10021; **Phone:** 212-821-0602; **Board Cert:** Surgery 2005; **Med School:** Brown Univ 1975; **Resid:** Surgery, St Luke's Roosevelt Hosp Ctr 1981; **Fellow:** Surgical Oncology, Meml Sloan Kettering Canc Ctr 1983; **Fac Appt:** Asst Prof S, Cornell Univ-Weill Med Coll

Tartter, Paul MD (S) - **Spec Exp:** Breast Cancer; Breast Cancer in Elderly; Sentinel Node Surgery; **Hospital:** St Luke's - Roosevelt Hosp Ctr - Roosevelt Div (page 94), Mount Sinai Med Ctr (page 102); **Address:** 425 W 59th St, Ste 7A, New York, NY 10019-1104; **Phone:** 212-523-7500; **Board Cert:** Surgery 2003; **Med School:** Brown Univ 1977; **Resid:** Surgery, Mt Sinai Hosp 1982; **Fac Appt:** Assoc Prof S, Columbia P&S

Teperman, Lewis W MD (S) - **Spec Exp:** Transplant-Liver; Transplant-Kidney; Liver Cancer; **Hospital:** NYU Langone Med Ctr (page 106); **Address:** 403 E 34th St Fl 3, Transplant Assocs, New York, NY 10016; **Phone:** 212-263-8134; **Board Cert:** Surgery 2007; **Med School:** Mount Sinai Sch Med 1981; **Resid:** Surgery, Columbia Presby Med Ctr 1984; Surgery, LI Jewish Med Ctr 1986; **Fellow:** Transplant Surgery, Univ Pittsburgh 1988; **Fac Appt:** Assoc Prof S, NYU Sch Med

Van Zee, Kimberly J MD (S) - **Spec Exp:** Breast Cancer & Surgery; **Hospital:** Meml Sloan-Kettering Cancer Ctr (page 112); **Address:** Meml Sloan Kettering Cancer Ctr, 300 E 66th St, New York, NY 10065; **Phone:** 800-525-2225; **Board Cert:** Surgery 2003; **Med School:** Harvard Med Sch 1987; **Resid:** Surgery, NY Hosp-Cornell 1990; Surgery, NY Hosp-Cornell 1994; **Fellow:** Research, NY Hosp-Cornell 1993; **Fac Appt:** Prof S, Cornell Univ-Weill Med Coll

Vine, Anthony J MD (S) - **Spec Exp:** Laparoscopic Abdominal Surgery; Gastroesophageal Reflux Disease (GERD); Colon & Rectal Surgery; **Hospital:** Mount Sinai Med Ctr (page 102); **Address:** 1010 5th Ave, New York, NY 10028-0130; **Phone:** 212-879-6677; **Board Cert:** Surgery 2009; **Med School:** Vanderbilt Univ 1989; **Resid:** Surgery, Mt Sinai Med Ctr 1996; **Fellow:** Colon & Rectal Surgery, Mass Genl Hosp 1994; **Fac Appt:** Asst Clin Prof S, Mount Sinai Sch Med

Wallack, Marc MD (S) - **Spec Exp:** Melanoma; Breast Surgery; **Hospital:** Metropolitan Hosp Ctr - NY; **Address:** 1901 1st Ave, rm 12A-1, New York, NY 10029; **Phone:** 212-423-6614; **Board Cert:** Surgery 2001; **Med School:** Univ Pittsburgh 1970; **Resid:** Surgery, Hosp Univ Penn 1977; **Fellow:** Medical Oncology, Wistar Inst Anatomy & Biology 1977; **Fac Appt:** Prof S, NY Med Coll

Wedderburn, Raymond MD (S) - **Hospital:** St Luke's - Roosevelt Hosp Ctr - Roosevelt Div (page 94); **Address:** 1111 Amsterdam Ave, Muhlenber Bldg, Fl 2 - Ste MU208N, New York, NY 10025; **Phone:** 212-523-5295; **Board Cert:** Surgery 2002; Surgical Critical Care 2003; **Med School:** Cornell Univ-Weill Med Coll 1986; **Resid:** Surgery, St Luke's-Roosevelt Hosp Ctr 1991; **Fellow:** Surgical Critical Care, Jackson Meml Hosp 1993; **Fac Appt:** Asst Clin Prof S, Columbia P&S

Thoracic Surgery

Adams, David H MD (TS) - **Spec Exp:** Mitral Valve Surgery; Heart Valve Surgery; Minimally Invasive Cardiac Surgery; Coronary Artery Surgery; **Hospital:** Mount Sinai Med Ctr (page 102); **Address:** Mt Sinai Hosp, Cardiac & Thoracic Surg, 1190 Fifth Ave, Box 1028, New York, NY 10029; **Phone:** 212-659-6820; **Board Cert:** Thoracic Surgery 2003; **Med School:** Duke Univ 1983; **Resid:** Surgery, Brigham & Women's Hosp 1988; Thoracic Surgery, Brigham & Women's Hosp 1990; **Fac Appt:** Prof TS, Mount Sinai Sch Med

Altorki, Nasser MD (TS) - **Spec Exp:** Esophageal Cancer; Lung Cancer; Thoracic Cancers; Vaccine Therapy; **Hospital:** NY-Presby Hosp/Weill Cornell (page 104); **Address:** 525 E 68th St, M-404, New York, NY 10065; **Phone:** 212-746-5156; **Board Cert:** Surgery 2006; Thoracic Surgery 2007; **Med School:** Egypt 1978; **Resid:** Surgery, Univ Chicago Hosps 1985; **Fellow:** Cardiothoracic Surgery, Univ Chicago Hosps 1987; **Fac Appt:** Prof S, Cornell Univ-Weill Med Coll

Argenziano, Michael MD (TS) - **Spec Exp:** Robotic Cardiac Surgery; Coronary Artery Surgery; Maze Procedure for Atrial Fibrillation; **Hospital:** NY-Presby Hosp/Columbia (page 104); **Address:** Columbia Presby Med Ctr, Milstein Bldg, 177 Fort Washington Ave, rm 7-435, New York, NY 10032; **Phone:** 212-305-5888; **Board Cert:** Thoracic Surgery 2002; **Med School:** Columbia P&S 1992; **Resid:** Surgery, Columbia Presby Med Ctr 1998; **Fellow:** Cardiothoracic Surgery, Columbia Presby Med Ctr 1999; **Fac Appt:** Asst Prof S, Columbia P&S

Bacha, Emile A MD (TS) - **Spec Exp:** Pediatric Cardiac Surgery; Heart Valve Surgery; Neonatal Cardiac Surgery; Minimally Invasive Cardiac Surgery; **Hospital:** NY-Presby Hosp/Columbia (page 104); **Address:** Morgan Stanley Chldns Hosp North, Room 274, 3959 Broadway, New York, NY 10032; **Phone:** 212-305-2688; **Board Cert:** Thoracic Surgery 2000; **Med School:** Germany 1989; **Resid:** Thoracic Surgery, Mass Genl Hosp 1993; Surgery, Emory Univ 1995; **Fellow:** Pediatric Cardiac Surgery, Hosp Marie Lanne Longe 1996; Pediatric Cardiac Surgery, Mass Genl Hosp/Harvard 1998

Bains, Manjit MD (TS) - **Spec Exp:** Cardiothoracic Surgery; Esophageal Cancer; Lung Cancer; **Hospital:** Meml Sloan-Kettering Cancer Ctr (page 112); **Address:** 1275 York Ave, rm C681, New York, NY 10065; **Phone:** 800-525-2225; **Board Cert:** Surgery 1971; Thoracic Surgery 1972; **Med School:** India 1963; **Resid:** Surgery, Rochester Genl Hosp 1970; **Fellow:** Thoracic Surgery, Sloan Kettering Cancer Ctr 1972; **Fac Appt:** Clin Prof S, Cornell Univ-Weill Med Coll

Camunas, Jorge L MD (TS) - **Spec Exp:** Pacemakers; Defibrillators; Lung Cancer; Thymoma; **Hospital:** Mount Sinai Med Ctr (page 102), VA Med Ctr - Bronx; **Address:** 16 E 98th St Fl 1, New York, NY 10029; **Phone:** 212-423-5817; **Board Cert:** Thoracic Surgery 2002; **Med School:** Georgetown Univ 1970; **Resid:** Surgery, Harlem Hosp 1976; Cardiothoracic Surgery, Mount Sinai Hosp 1980; **Fellow:** Cardiothoracic Surgery, St Lukes-Roosevelt Med Ctr 1978; **Fac Appt:** Assoc Prof TS, Mount Sinai Sch Med

Chen, Jonathan M MD (TS) - **Spec Exp:** Pediatric Cardiothoracic Surgery; Arrhythmias; Congenital Heart Disease; **Hospital:** NYPresby-Morgan Stanley Children's Hosp (page 104), NY-Presby Hosp/Columbia (page 104); **Address:** NY Presbyterian-Weill Cornell Med Ctr, 525 E 68th St, rm F695B, New York, NY 10021; **Phone:** 212-746-5014; **Board Cert:** Surgery 2001; Thoracic Surgery 2003; **Med School:** Columbia P&S 1994; **Resid:** Surgery, NY Columbia Presby Hosp 2000; **Fellow:** Cardiothoracic Surgery, NY Columbia Presby Hosp 2001; **Fac Appt:** Asst Prof S, Columbia P&S

Connery, Cliff MD (TS) - **Spec Exp:** Thoracic Cancers; Mediastinal Tumors; Minimally Invasive Surgery; Lung Cancer; **Hospital:** St Luke's - Roosevelt Hosp Ctr - Roosevelt Div (page 94), Beth Israel Med Ctr - Petrie Division (page 94); **Address:** 1000 Tenth Ave, Ste 2B-05, New York, NY 10019; **Phone:** 212-523-7475; **Board Cert:** Thoracic Surgery 2003; Critical Care Medicine 2003; Surgery 2000; **Med School:** Eastern VA Med Sch 1984; **Resid:** Surgery, Univ Hosp 1989; Thoracic Surgery, Strong Meml Hosp 1992; **Fac Appt:** Asst Prof S, Columbia P&S

Crawford, Bernard MD (TS) - **Spec Exp:** Lung Cancer; Minimally Invasive Surgery; Esophageal Cancer; **Hospital:** NYU Langone Med Ctr (page 106); **Address:** 160 E 34th St Fl 8, New York, NY 10016; **Phone:** 212-731-5580; **Board Cert:** Thoracic Surgery 2009; **Med School:** Geo Wash Univ 1980; **Resid:** Surgery, NYU Med Ctr 1985; **Fellow:** Cardiothoracic Surgery, NYU Med Ctr 1987; **Fac Appt:** Asst Prof TS, NYU Sch Med

Culliford, Alfred T MD (TS) - **Spec Exp:** Mitral Valve Minimally Invasive Surgery; Coronary Artery Surgery; **Hospital:** NYU Langone Med Ctr (page 106); **Address:** NYU Medical Ctr, 530 1st Ave, Ste 9V, New York, NY 10016; **Phone:** 212-263-7288; **Board Cert:** Thoracic Surgery 2007; Surgery 1975; **Med School:** NY Med Coll 1969; **Resid:** Surgery, NYU Med Ctr 1974; **Fellow:** Thoracic Surgery, NYU Med Ctr 1976; **Fac Appt:** Prof TS, NYU Sch Med

DeAnda Jr, Abelardo MD (TS) - **Spec Exp:** Aneurysm-Aortic; Heart Valve Surgery; Cardiothoracic Surgery; **Hospital:** NYU Langone Med Ctr (page 106); **Address:** NYU Medical Ctr, Cardiothoracic Surgery, 530 First Ave, Ste 9V, New York, NY 10016; **Phone:** 212-263-6516; **Board Cert:** Surgery 1999; Thoracic Surgery 2002; **Med School:** Stanford Univ 1990; **Resid:** Surgery, Stanford Med Ctr 1997; **Fellow:** Thoracic Surgery, Stanford Med Ctr 2000; **Fac Appt:** Assoc Prof TS, NYU Sch Med

Downey, Robert MD (TS) - **Spec Exp:** Lung Cancer; Thoracic Cancers; **Hospital:** Meml Sloan-Kettering Cancer Ctr (page 112); **Address:** 1275 York Avenue, New York, NY 10065; **Phone:** 800-525-2225; **Board Cert:** Surgery 2002; Thoracic Surgery 2005; Thoracic Surgery 2005; **Med School:** Columbia P&S 1985; **Resid:** Surgery, Columbia-Presby Med Ctr 1991; **Fellow:** Thoracic Surgery, Mayo Clinic 1992; Thoracic Surgery, Columbia-Presby Med Ctr 1994

Filsoufi, Farzan MD (TS) - **Spec Exp:** Mitral Valve Surgery; Minimally Invasive Heart Valve Surgery; Heart Valve Surgery; Robotic Cardiac Surgery; **Hospital:** Mount Sinai Med Ctr (page 102), Elmhurst Hosp Ctr; **Address:** Mt Sinai Med Ctr, Dept Cardiothoracic Surg, 1190 5th Ave, Box 1028, New York, NY 10029; **Phone:** 212-659-6813; **Med School:** France 1991; **Resid:** Surgery, Univ Paris Hosps 1994; Thoracic Surgery, Hospital Broussais/U of Paris 1995; **Fellow:** Cardiothoracic Surgery, Hospital Broussais/U of Paris 1996; Heart Valve Surgery, Brigham & Women's Hosp 2000; **Fac Appt:** Asst Prof TS, Mount Sinai Sch Med

Flores, Raja M MD (TS) - **Spec Exp:** Mesothelioma; Lung Cancer; Video Assisted Thoracic Surgery (VATS); Esophageal Cancer; **Hospital:** Meml Sloan-Kettering Cancer Ctr (page 112); **Address:** 1275 York Avenue, New York, NY 10065; **Phone:** 800-525-2225; **Board Cert:** Surgery 1999; Thoracic Surgery 2001; **Med School:** Albert Einstein Coll Med 1992; **Resid:** Surgery, Columbia Presby Med Ctr 1997; **Fellow:** Thoracic Surgery, Brigham & Womens Hosp/Dana Faber Cancer Inst 2000; **Fac Appt:** Assoc Prof TS, Cornell Univ-Weill Med Coll

Galloway, Aubrey MD (TS) - **Spec Exp:** Minimally Invasive Heart Valve Surgery; Coronary Artery Surgery; Aneurysm-Thoracic Aortic; **Hospital:** NYU Langone Med Ctr (page 106), Bellevue Hosp Ctr; **Address:** 530 1st Ave, Ste 9V, New York, NY 10016-6402; **Phone:** 212-263-7185; **Board Cert:** Thoracic Surgery 2006; **Med School:** Tulane Univ 1978; **Resid:** Surgery, Univ Colo Hlth Sci Ctr 1983; Cardiovascular Surgery, NYU Med Ctr 1985; **Fellow:** Research, Boston Chldns Hosp 1981; Cardiothoracic Surgery, NYU Med Ctr 1985; **Fac Appt:** Prof TS, NYU Sch Med

Ginsburg, Mark MD (TS) - **Spec Exp:** Lung Cancer; Transplant-Lung; Emphysema-Lung Volume Reduction; **Hospital:** NY-Presby Hosp/Columbia (page 104), Good Samaritan Hosp - Suffern; **Address:** 161 Ft Washington Ave Fl 3 - rm 301, New York, NY 10032; **Phone:** 212-305-3408; **Board Cert:** Surgery 2006; Thoracic Surgery 2005; **Med School:** Tufts Univ 1980; **Resid:** Surgery, Strong Meml Hosp 1985; **Fellow:** Thoracic Surgery, Strong Meml Hosp 1987; **Fac Appt:** Asst Clin Prof S, Columbia P&S

Girardi, Leonard N MD (TS) - **Spec Exp:** Aneurysm-Aortic; Cardiac Surgery; Marfan's Syndrome; Cardiothoracic Surgery; **Hospital:** NY-Presby Hosp/Weill Cornell (page 104); **Address:** 525 E 68th St, M404, New York, NY 10065; **Phone:** 212-746-5194; **Board Cert:** Surgery 2005; Thoracic Surgery 2007; **Med School:** Cornell Univ-Weill Med Coll 1989; **Resid:** Surgery, NY Presby-Cornell Med Ctr 1994; **Fellow:** Cardiothoracic Surgery, NY Presby Hosp 1996; Cardiothoracic Surgery, Baylor Coll Med 1997; **Fac Appt:** Assoc Prof TS, Cornell Univ-Weill Med Coll

Griepp, Randall B MD (TS) - **Spec Exp:** Aneurysm-Abdominal Aortic; Aneurysm-Thoracic Aortic; **Hospital:** Mount Sinai Med Ctr (page 102); **Address:** Mt Sinai Med Ctr, Dept Cardiothoracic Surgery, 1190 5th Ave, New York, NY 10029; **Phone:** 212-659-9495; **Board Cert:** Thoracic Surgery 2007; **Med School:** Stanford Univ 1967; **Resid:** Surgery, Stanford Univ Hosp 1973; **Fellow:** Cardiothoracic Surgery, Stanford Univ Hosp 1972; **Fac Appt:** Prof TS, Mount Sinai Sch Med

Grossi, Eugene A MD (TS) - **Spec Exp:** Minimally Invasive Cardiac Surgery; Mitral Valve Surgery; Cardiac Tumors, Myxomas; **Hospital:** NYU Langone Med Ctr (page 106); **Address:** NYU Langone Med Ctr, 530 1st Ave, Ste 9V, New York, NY 10016-6402; **Phone:** 212-263-7452; **Board Cert:** Thoracic Surgery 2002; **Med School:** Columbia P&S 1981; **Resid:** Surgery, NYU Med Ctr 1987; Thoracic Surgery, NYU Med Ctr 1991; **Fac Appt:** Prof S, NYU Sch Med

Hoffman, Darryl M MD (TS) - **Spec Exp:** Cardiac Surgery; Maze Procedure for Atrial Fibrillation; Pacemakers/Defibrillators; **Hospital:** Beth Israel Med Ctr - Petrie Division (page 94), St Luke's - Roosevelt Hosp Ctr - Roosevelt Div (page 94); **Address:** Division of Cardiac Surgery, 317 E 17th St, Fierman Hall, 11th Fl, New York, NY 10003; **Phone:** 212-420-2584; **Med School:** South Africa 1983; **Resid:** Surgery 1989Edinburgh Royal Infirm; **Fellow:** Cardiac Surgery, Allegheny Genl Hosp 1993; Cardiac Surgery, Mayo Clinic 1994; **Fac Appt:** Asst Prof S, Albert Einstein Coll Med

Isom, O Wayne MD (TS) - **Spec Exp:** Cardiac Surgery; Coronary Artery Surgery; Heart Valve Surgery; **Hospital:** NY-Presby Hosp/Weill Cornell (page 104), NY Hosp Queens; **Address:** 525 E 68th St, rm M-404, New York, NY 10065; **Phone:** 212-746-5151; **Board Cert:** Surgery 1971; Thoracic Surgery 1972; **Med School:** Univ Tex, Houston 1965; **Resid:** Surgery, Parkland Meml Hosp 1970; **Fellow:** Thoracic Surgery, NYU Med Ctr 1972; **Fac Appt:** Prof TS, Cornell Univ-Weill Med Coll

Krellenstein, Daniel J MD (TS) - **Spec Exp:** Lung Cancer; Minimally Invasive Thoracic Surgery; Asbestos-related Lung Disease; **Hospital:** Mount Sinai Med Ctr (page 102), Lenox Hill Hosp; **Address:** 16 E 98th St, Ste 1F, New York, NY 10029-6545; **Phone:** 212-423-9311; **Board Cert:** Surgery 1974; Thoracic Surgery 2006; **Med School:** SUNY Buffalo 1964; **Resid:** Surgery, SUNY Downstate Med Ctr 1972; **Fac Appt:** Assoc Clin Prof TS, Mount Sinai Sch Med

Krieger, Karl H MD (TS) - **Spec Exp:** Heart Valve Surgery; Coronary Artery Surgery; Cardiac Surgery-Adult; **Hospital:** NY-Presby Hosp/Weill Cornell (page 104), NY Hosp Queens; **Address:** Cardiothoracic Surgery Dept, 525 E 68th St, Ste M404, New York, NY 10021-4873; **Phone:** 212-746-5152; **Board Cert:** Thoracic Surgery 2004; **Med School:** Johns Hopkins Univ 1975; **Resid:** Surgery, Johns Hopkins 1976Bellevue Hosp 1979; **Fellow:** Thoracic Surgery, NYU Med Ctr 1981; **Fac Appt:** Prof S, Cornell Univ-Weill Med Coll

Loulmet, Didier F MD (TS) - **Spec Exp:** Heart Valve Surgery; Robotic Cardiac Surgery; Minimally Invasive Cardiac Surgery; **Hospital:** NYU Langone Med Ctr (page 106); **Address:** NYU Medical Ctr, Cardiothoracic Surgery, 550 1st Ave, Ste 9V, New York, NY 10016; **Phone:** 212-263-2329; **Med School:** France 1984; **Resid:** Cardiothoracic Surgery, Paris Univ Hosp 1990; Cardiothoracic Surgery, Brigham & Women's Hosp 1991; **Fellow:** Pediatric Cardiac Surgery, Children's Hosp 1992

Mosca, Ralph S MD (TS) - **Spec Exp:** Cardiothoracic Surgery; Congenital Heart Disease-Adult & Child; Pediatric Cardiac Surgery; **Hospital:** NYU Langone Med Ctr (page 106); **Address:** 530 1st Ave, Ste 9V, New York, NY 10016; **Phone:** 212-263-5989; **Board Cert:** Thoracic Surgery 2001; **Med School:** SUNY Upstate Med Univ 1985; **Resid:** Surgery, SUNY Hlth Sci Ctr 1990; **Fellow:** Cardiothoracic Surgery, Columbia-Presby Med Ctr 1992; Pediatric Cardiac Surgery, Univ Mich Med Ctr 1993; **Fac Appt:** Prof TS, NYU Sch Med

Naka, Yoshifumi MD/PhD (TS) - **Spec Exp:** Transplant-Heart & Lung; Ventricular Assist Device (LVAD); Heart Failure & Ventricular Containment; Mitral Valve Surgery; **Hospital:** NY-Presby Hosp/Columbia (page 104); **Address:** 177 Fort Washington Ave, MHB 7-435, New York, NY 10032; **Phone:** 212-305-0828; **Med School:** Japan 1984; **Resid:** Surgery, Osaka Police Hosp 1991; **Fellow:** Cardiovascular Surgery, Osaka Police Hosp 1993; Cardiothoracic Surgery, Columbia Univ Med Ctr 1998; **Fac Appt:** Asst Prof S, Columbia P&S

Nguyen, Khanh H MD (TS) - **Spec Exp:** Pediatric Cardiothoracic Surgery; **Hospital:** Mount Sinai Med Ctr (page 102); **Address:** Mount Sinai Med Ctr, 1190 5th Ave, Box 1028, New York, NY 10029; **Phone:** 212-659-9472; **Board Cert:** Thoracic Surgery 2006; **Med School:** UC Irvine 1985; **Resid:** Surgery, Flushing Hosp 1992; Thoracic Surgery, Mt Sinai Med Ctr 1995

Oz, Mehmet C MD (TS) - **Spec Exp:** Transplant-Heart; Heart Valve Surgery; Minimally Invasive Cardiac Surgery; **Hospital:** NY-Presby Hosp/Columbia (page 104); **Address:** NY Presby Hosp, Dept Cardiothoracic Surg, 177 Ft Washington Ave, MHB- Rm 7, GN435, New York, NY 10032; **Phone:** 212-305-4434; **Board Cert:** Thoracic Surgery 2003; **Med School:** Univ Pennsylvania 1986; **Resid:** Surgery, Columbia Presby Med Ctr 1991; **Fellow:** Cardiothoracic Surgery, Columbia Presby Med Ctr 1993; **Fac Appt:** Prof S, Columbia P&S

Pass, Harvey MD (TS) - **Spec Exp:** Lung Cancer; Mesothelioma; Clinical Trials; **Hospital:** NYU Langone Med Ctr (page 106); **Address:** NYU Cancer Ctr, 160 E 34th St Fl 8, New York, NY 10016; **Phone:** 212-731-5414; **Board Cert:** Thoracic Surgery 2001; **Med School:** Duke Univ 1973; **Resid:** Surgery, Duke Univ Med Ctr 1975; Surgery, Univ Miss Med Ctr 1980; **Fellow:** Cardiothoracic Surgery, MUSC Med Ctr 1982; **Fac Appt:** Prof S, NYU Sch Med

Plestis, Konstadinos MD (TS) - **Spec Exp:** Aortic Surgery; Heart Valve Surgery; Aneurysm-Aortic; Aneurysm-Abdominal Aortic; **Hospital:** Lenox Hill Hosp; **Address:** Aortic Wellness Ctr at Lenox Hill, 130 E 77th St Fl 4th, New York, NY 10075; **Phone:** 212-434-6030; **Board Cert:** Surgery 2003; Vascular Surgery 2005; Thoracic Surgery 2008; **Med School:** Greece 1987; **Resid:** Surgery, Brooklyn Hosp Ctr 1993; Vascular Surgery, Baylor Univ Med Ctr 1995; **Fellow:** Cardiothoracic Surgery, Montefiore Med Ctr 1999; **Fac Appt:** Asst Prof S, Mount Sinai Sch Med

Port, Jeffrey L MD (TS) - **Spec Exp:** Cardiothoracic Surgery; Lung Cancer; Esophageal Cancer; **Hospital:** NY-Presby Hosp/Weill Cornell (page 104); **Address:** 525 E 68th St, Box 110, New York, NY 10065; **Phone:** 212-746-5197; **Board Cert:** Surgery 2009; Thoracic Surgery 2009; **Med School:** NYU Sch Med 1991; **Resid:** Surgery, NYU Med Ctr 1998; **Fellow:** Thoracic Surgery, NY Presby Hosp 2000; **Fac Appt:** Assoc Prof TS, Cornell Univ-Weill Med Coll

Smith, Craig R MD (TS) - **Spec Exp:** Mitral Valve Surgery; Transplant-Heart; Minimally Invasive Cardiac Surgery; Robotic Cardiac Surgery; **Hospital:** NY-Presby Hosp/Columbia (page 104); **Address:** Columbia Presbyterian Med Ctr, 177 Fort Washington Ave, Ste 7-435, New York, NY 10032; **Phone:** 212-305-8312; **Board Cert:** Thoracic Surgery 2004; **Med School:** Case West Res Univ 1977; **Resid:** Surgery, Strong Meml Hosp 1982; **Fellow:** Cardiothoracic Surgery, Columbia Presby Med Ctr 1984; **Fac Appt:** Prof S, Columbia P&S

Sonett, Joshua R MD (TS) - **Spec Exp:** Minimally Invasive Thoracic Surgery; Transplant-Lung; Thoracic Cancers; Emphysema-Lung Volume Reduction; **Hospital:** NY-Presby Hosp/Columbia (page 104); **Address:** 161 Fort Washington Ave, Ste 301, New York, NY 10032; **Phone:** 212-305-8086; **Board Cert:** Surgery 2004; Thoracic Surgery 2007; **Med School:** E Carolina Univ 1988; **Resid:** Surgery, Univ Mass Med Ctr 1993; **Fellow:** Cardiothoracic Surgery, Univ Pittsburgh Med Ctr 1994; Thoracic Surgery, Meml Sloan Kettering Cancer Ctr; **Fac Appt:** Assoc Prof S, Columbia P&S

Spotnitz, Henry MD (TS) - **Spec Exp:** Pacemakers/Defibrillators; Heart Valve Surgery; **Hospital:** NY-Presby Hosp/Columbia (page 104); **Address:** 622 W 168th St, Vanderbilt Clinic, rm 1010, New York, NY 10032; **Phone:** 212-305-6191; **Board Cert:** Surgery 1974; Thoracic Surgery 2005; **Med School:** Columbia P&S 1966; **Resid:** Surgery, Columbia-Presby Med Ctr 1973; Thoracic Surgery, Columbia-Presby Med Ctr 1975; **Fellow:** Research, Natl Inst Hlth 1969; **Fac Appt:** Prof S, Columbia P&S

Stelzer, Paul MD (TS) - **Spec Exp:** Heart Valve Surgery; Aneurysm-Thoracic Aortic; Ross Procedure/Aortic Valve Disease; **Hospital:** Mount Sinai Med Ctr (page 102); **Address:** 1190 5th Ave, Box 1028, New York, NY 10029; **Phone:** 212-659-6871; **Board Cert:** Thoracic Surgery 2000; **Med School:** Columbia P&S 1972; **Resid:** Surgery, St Luke's Roosevelt Hosp 1977; Thoracic Surgery, NY Hosp 1981; **Fac Appt:** Assoc Clin Prof TS, Albert Einstein Coll Med

Stewart, Allan MD (TS) - **Spec Exp:** Heart Valve Surgery-Aortic; Aneurysm-Aortic; Aortic Surgery; **Hospital:** NY-Presby Hosp/Columbia (page 104); **Address:** 177 Fort Washington Ave, Milstein Hosp Bldg Fl 7 - rm 435, New York, NY 10010; **Phone:** 212-305-4980; **Board Cert:** Surgery 2003; Thoracic Surgery 2006; **Med School:** UMDNJ-NJ Med Sch, Newark 1995; **Resid:** Surgery, Univ PA Hlth Sys 2002; **Fellow:** Thoracic Surgery, NY Presby Hosp 2004; **Fac Appt:** Asst Prof TS, Columbia P&S

Swistel, Daniel MD (TS) - **Spec Exp:** Coronary Artery Surgery; Minimally Invasive Surgery; Heart Valve Surgery; Hypertrophic Cardiomyopathy; **Hospital:** St Luke's - Roosevelt Hosp Ctr - St Luke's Hosp (page 94); **Address:** 1090 Amsterdam Ave, Ste 8B, New York, NY 10025; **Phone:** 212-523-4088; **Board Cert:** Thoracic Surgery 2006; **Med School:** UMDNJ-RW Johnson Med Sch 1979; **Resid:** Surgery, St Lukes-Roosevelt Hosp 1984; Cardiothoracic Surgery, Montefiore Med Ctr 1986; **Fac Appt:** Assoc Clin Prof TS, Columbia P&S

Tranbaugh, Robert MD (TS) - **Spec Exp:** Coronary Artery Surgery; Heart Valve Surgery; Aneurysm-Thoracic Aortic; **Hospital:** Beth Israel Med Ctr - Petrie Division (page 94); **Address:** 317 E 17th St Fl 11, New York, NY 10003; **Phone:** 212-420-2584; **Board Cert:** Thoracic Surgery 2004; **Med School:** Univ Pennsylvania 1976; **Resid:** Surgery, UCSF Med Ctr 1983; Cardiothoracic Surgery, UCSF Med Ctr 1985; **Fac Appt:** Assoc Prof TS, Albert Einstein Coll Med

Williams, Mathew R MD (TS) - **Spec Exp:** Interventional Cardiology; Heart Valve Surgery; **Hospital:** NY-Presby Hosp/Columbia (page 104); **Address:** Milstein Hospital Bldg Fl 7 - rm 435, 177 Fort Washington Ave, New York, NY 10032; **Phone:** 212-305-4980; **Board Cert:** Thoracic Surgery 2007; **Med School:** Columbia P&S 1996; **Resid:** Surgery, UCLA Med Ctr 1998; Surgery, NY Presby Hosp/Columbia 2003; **Fellow:** Cardiothoracic Surgery, NY Presby Hosp/Columbia 2005; Interventional Cardiology, NY Presby Hosp/Columbia 2006; **Fac Appt:** Asst Prof S, Columbia P&S

Urology

Armenakas, Noel MD (U) - **Spec Exp:** Genitourinary Reconstruction; Erectile Dysfunction; **Hospital:** Lenox Hill Hosp, NY-Presby Hosp/Weill Cornell (page 104); **Address:** 880 5th Ave, New York, NY 10021-4951; **Phone:** 212-535-1950; **Board Cert:** Urology 2003; **Med School:** Greece 1985; **Resid:** Urology, Monmouth Med Ctr 1987; Urology, Lenox Hill Hosp 1991; **Fellow:** Trauma, UCSF Med Ctr 1992; Reconstructive Surgery, UCSF Med Ctr 1992; **Fac Appt:** Assoc Clin Prof U, Cornell Univ-Weill Med Coll

Bar-Chama, Natan MD (U) - **Spec Exp:** Infertility-Male; Erectile Dysfunction; Vasectomy Reversal; Varicocele Microsurgery; **Hospital:** Mount Sinai Med Ctr (page 102); **Address:** Center for Male Reproductive Health, 635 Madison Ave, New York, NY 10022; **Phone:** 212-756-5777; **Board Cert:** Urology 2006; **Med School:** Albert Einstein Coll Med 1987; **Resid:** Urology, Montefiore Med Ctr 1993; **Fellow:** Male Infertility, Baylor Coll Med 1994; **Fac Appt:** Assoc Prof U, Mount Sinai Sch Med

Benson, Mitchell C MD (U) - **Spec Exp:** Prostate Cancer/Robotic Surgery; Bladder Cancer; Kidney Cancer; Continent Urinary Diversions; **Hospital:** NY-Presby Hosp/Columbia (page 104); **Address:** NY Presby Hosp-Columbia, Dept Urology, 161 Ft Washington Ave Fl 11 - rm 1102, New York, NY 10032-3713; **Phone:** 212-305-5201; **Board Cert:** Urology 1984; **Med School:** Columbia P&S 1977; **Resid:** Surgery, Mount Sinai Med Ctr 1979; Urology, Columbia-Presby Hosp 1982; **Fellow:** Oncology, Johns Hopkins Hosp 1984; **Fac Appt:** Prof U, Columbia P&S

Berman, Steven MD (U) - **Spec Exp:** Prostate Cancer; Kidney Stones; **Hospital:** Beth Israel Med Ctr - Petrie Division (page 94); **Address:** 201 E 19th St, New York, NY 10003-6399; **Phone:** 212-673-7300; **Board Cert:** Urology 2006; **Med School:** SUNY Downstate 1981; **Resid:** Surgery, Montefiore Med Ctr 1983; Urology, Montefiore Med Ctr 1986

Birkhoff, John MD (U) - **Spec Exp:** Urologic Cancer; Kidney Stones; **Hospital:** NY-Presby Hosp/Columbia (page 104); **Address:** 161 Fort Washington Ave, rm 347, New York, NY 10032; **Phone:** 212-305-5421; **Board Cert:** Urology 1976; **Med School:** Columbia P&S 1969; **Resid:** Urology, Columbia-Presby 1975; **Fac Appt:** Asst Clin Prof Med, Columbia P&S

Birns, Douglas MD (U) - **Spec Exp:** Prostate Cancer; Kidney Cancer; Bladder Cancer; **Hospital:** Mount Sinai Med Ctr (page 102), Beth Israel Med Ctr - Petrie Division (page 94); **Address:** 157 E 72nd St, Ground Fl, New York, NY 10021-4331; **Phone:** 212-744-8700; **Board Cert:** Urology 2006; **Med School:** SUNY Downstate 1981; **Resid:** Surgery, Mount Sinai Hosp 1982; Urology, Mount Sinai Hosp 1986; **Fac Appt:** Asst Clin Prof U, Mount Sinai Sch Med

Blaivas, Jerry G MD (U) - **Spec Exp:** Uro-Gynecology; Urology-Female; Neurogenic Bladder; Incontinence after Prostate Cancer; **Hospital:** NY-Presby Hosp/Weill Cornell (page 104), Lenox Hill Hosp; **Address:** 445 E 77th St, New York, NY 10075; **Phone:** 212-772-3900; **Board Cert:** Urology 1978; **Med School:** Tufts Univ 1968; **Resid:** Surgery, Boston Med Ctr 1971; Urology, New England Med Ctr 1976; **Fac Appt:** Clin Prof U, Cornell Univ-Weill Med Coll

Bochner, Bernard MD (U) - **Spec Exp:** Bladder Cancer; Urinary Reconstruction; **Hospital:** Meml Sloan-Kettering Cancer Ctr (page 112); **Address:** Meml Sloan Kettering Cancer Ctr, 1275 York Ave, Dept Urology, New York, NY 10065; **Phone:** 646-422-4387; **Board Cert:** Urology 2001; **Med School:** UCLA 1990; **Resid:** Surgery, LAC/USC Med Ctr 1992; Urology, LAC/USC Med Ctr 1996; **Fellow:** Urologic Oncology, USC/Norris Comp Cancer Ctr 1999

Boczko, Stanley MD (U) - **Spec Exp:** Prostate Cancer; Impotence; Prostate Disease; **Hospital:** Montefiore Med Ctr - Div. Moses (page 100), Lenox Hill Hosp; **Address:** 23 E 79th St, New York, NY 10021; **Phone:** 212-628-1800; **Board Cert:** Urology 1981; **Med School:** Albert Einstein Coll Med 1973; **Resid:** Surgery, Montefiore Med Ctr 1975; Urology, Montefiore Med Ctr 1979; **Fellow:** Transplant Surgery, Montefiore Med Ctr 1975; **Fac Appt:** Assoc Prof U, Albert Einstein Coll Med

Brodherson, Michael MD (U) - **Spec Exp:** Urologic Cancer; Kidney Stones; **Hospital:** Lenox Hill Hosp; **Address:** 4 E 76th St, New York, NY 10021-2611; **Phone:** 212-794-2749; **Board Cert:** Urology 1981; **Med School:** SUNY Downstate 1973; **Resid:** Internal Medicine, Lenox Hill Hosp 1976; Urology, Lenox Hill Hosp 1979

DelPizzo, Joseph J MD (U) - **Spec Exp:** Laparoscopic Kidney Surgery; Robotic Surgery; Minimally Invasive Surgery; Kidney Stones; **Hospital:** NY-Presby Hosp/Weill Cornell (page 104); **Address:** NY Presby-Cornell Med Ctr, Dept Urology, 525 E 68th St, Ste Starr 900, New York, NY 10065; **Phone:** 212-746-5250; **Board Cert:** Urology 2003; **Med School:** Albert Einstein Coll Med 1994; **Resid:** Surgery, Mercy Med Ctr 1996; Urology, Univ Maryland Med System 2000; **Fac Appt:** Assoc Prof U, Cornell Univ-Weill Med Coll

Dillon, Robert W MD (U) - **Spec Exp:** Kidney Stones; Urologic Cancer; Urology-Female; **Hospital:** Mount Sinai Med Ctr (page 102), Lenox Hill Hosp; **Address:** 58-A E 79th St, New York, NY 10021-4331; **Phone:** 212-794-9000; **Board Cert:** Urology 1980; **Med School:** NY Med Coll 1973; **Resid:** Surgery, Mt Sinai Hosp 1975; Urology, Mt Sinai Hosp 1978; **Fac Appt:** Asst Clin Prof U, Mount Sinai Sch Med

Droller, Michael J MD (U) - **Spec Exp:** Urologic Cancer; Bladder Cancer; Prostate Cancer; Kidney Cancer; **Hospital:** Mount Sinai Med Ctr (page 102); **Address:** 5 E 98th St Fl 6, Box 1272, New York, NY 10029-6501; **Phone:** 212-241-3868; **Board Cert:** Urology 2001; **Med School:** Harvard Med Sch 1968; **Resid:** Surgery, Peter Bent Brigham Hosp 1970; Urology, Stanford Univ Med Ctr 1976; **Fellow:** Immunology, Univ Stockholm 1977; **Fac Appt:** Prof U, Mount Sinai Sch Med

Eastham, James MD (U) - **Spec Exp:** Prostate Cancer; Prostate Cancer/Robotic Surgery; **Hospital:** Meml Sloan-Kettering Cancer Ctr (page 112); **Address:** 1275 York Avenue, New York, NY 10065; **Phone:** 800-525-2225; **Board Cert:** Urology 2005; **Med School:** USC Sch Med 1987; **Resid:** Urology, USC Med Ctr 1993

Fine, Eugene M MD (U) - **Spec Exp:** Prostate Cancer; Kidney Stones; Erectile Dysfunction; Prostate Disease; **Hospital:** Mount Sinai Med Ctr (page 102), Lenox Hill Hosp; **Address:** 12 E 86th St, New York, NY 10028; **Phone:** 212-517-9555; **Board Cert:** Urology 2005; **Med School:** Mexico 1978; **Resid:** Surgery, Univ Hosp 1981; Urology, Mount Sinai Hosp 1985; **Fac Appt:** Asst Clin Prof U, Mount Sinai Sch Med

Fisch, Harry MD (U) - **Spec Exp:** Infertility-Male; Microsurgery; Vasectomy Reversal; **Hospital:** NY-Presby Hosp/Columbia (page 104), Lenox Hill Hosp; **Address:** 944 Park Ave, Ste 1C, New York, NY 10028; **Phone:** 212-879-0800; **Board Cert:** Urology 1999; **Med School:** Mount Sinai Sch Med 1983; **Resid:** Surgery, Montefiore Med Ctr 1985; Urology, Montefiore Med Ctr 1989; **Fac Appt:** Prof U, Columbia P&S

Fracchia, John MD (U) - **Spec Exp:** Urologic Cancer; **Hospital:** Lenox Hill Hosp, NY-Presby Hosp/Weill Cornell (page 104); **Address:** 245 E 54th St, Ste 2N, New York, NY 10022; **Phone:** 212-570-6800 x185; **Board Cert:** Urology 1981; **Med School:** UMDNJ-NJ Med Sch, Newark 1973; **Resid:** Urology, New York Hosp 1978; **Fac Appt:** Assoc Clin Prof S, Cornell Univ-Weill Med Coll

Glassberg, Kenneth MD (U) - **Spec Exp:** Pediatric Urology; Genital Reconstruction; Varicocele In Adolescents; **Hospital:** NYPresby-Morgan Stanley Children's Hosp (page 104); **Address:** Morgan Stanley Chlds Hosp of NY-Presby, 3959 Broadway, BHN 1118, New York, NY 10032; **Phone:** 212-305-9918; **Board Cert:** Urology 1977; Pediatric Urology 2009; **Med School:** SUNY Downstate 1968; **Resid:** Surgery, Montefiore Hosp Med Ctr 1972; Urology, Univ Hosp 1975; **Fellow:** Pediatric Urology, Adler Hey Chldns Hosp 1976; Pediatric Urology, Hosp For Sick Chldn 1976; **Fac Appt:** Prof U, Columbia P&S

Goldstein, Marc MD (U) - **Spec Exp:** Infertility-Male; Vasectomy Reversal; Varicocele Micro-surgery; Erectile Dysfunction; **Hospital:** NY-Presby Hosp/Weill Cornell (page 104); **Address:** Cornell Inst for Reproductive Med, 525 E 68th St, Box 580, New York, NY 10021-4870; **Phone:** 212-746-5470; **Board Cert:** Urology 1982; **Med School:** SUNY Downstate 1972; **Resid:** Surgery, Columbia-Presby Med Ctr 1974; Urology, SUNY Downstate Med Ctr 1980; **Fellow:** Microsurgery, Rockefeller Univ 1982; **Fac Appt:** Prof U, Cornell Univ-Weill Med Coll

Goluboff, Erik T MD (U) - **Spec Exp:** Robotic Urologic Surgery; Urologic Cancer; Bladder Cancer; Kidney Cancer; **Hospital:** NY-Presby Hosp/Columbia (page 104); **Address:** 5141 Broadway, New York, NY 10034; **Phone:** 212-932-4309; **Board Cert:** Urology 2007; **Med School:** Johns Hopkins Univ 1990; **Resid:** Urology, NY Presy Hosp/Columbia 1996; **Fellow:** Urologic Oncology, NY Presy Hosp/Columbia 1997; **Fac Appt:** Prof U, Columbia P&S

Grasso, Michael MD (U) - **Spec Exp:** Urologic Cancer; Laparoscopic Surgery; Kidney Stones; Testicular Cancer; **Hospital:** Lenox Hill Hosp; **Address:** Lenox Hill Hosp, 100 E 77th St, East Bldg Fl 4th, New York, NY 10075; **Phone:** 212-434-6300; **Board Cert:** Urology 2002; **Med School:** Jefferson Med Coll 1986; **Resid:** Surgery, Jefferson Univ Hosp 1988; Urology, Jefferson Univ Hosp 1992; **Fac Appt:** Prof U, NY Med Coll

Gribetz, Michael MD (U) - **Spec Exp:** Prostate Disease; Urology-Female; Sexual Dysfunction; Kidney Stones; **Hospital:** Mount Sinai Med Ctr (page 102); **Address:** 1155 Park Ave, New York, NY 10128-1209; **Phone:** 212-831-1300; **Board Cert:** Urology 1980; **Med School:** Albert Einstein Coll Med 1973; **Resid:** Surgery, Montefiore Med Ctr 1975; Urology, Mt Sinai Hosp 1978; **Fac Appt:** Asst Clin Prof U, Mount Sinai Sch Med

Hall, Simon J MD (U) - **Spec Exp:** Urologic Cancer; Minimally Invasive Urologic Surgery; Continent Urinary Diversions; Prostate Cancer; **Hospital:** Mount Sinai Med Ctr (page 102); **Address:** Mount Sinai Medical Ctr, 5 98th St, Box 1272, New York, NY 10029; **Phone:** 212-241-4812; **Board Cert:** Urology 2009; **Med School:** Columbia P&S 1988; **Resid:** Surgery, Mt Sinai Med Ctr 1990; Urology, Boston Univ 1994; **Fellow:** Urology, Baylor Coll Med 1996; **Fac Appt:** Assoc Prof U, Mount Sinai Sch Med

Hensle, Terry MD (U) - **Spec Exp:** Pediatric Urology; Hypospadias; Urinary Reconstruction; Wilms' Tumor; **Hospital:** NYPresby-Morgan Stanley Children's Hosp (page 104), Hackensack Univ Med Ctr (page 96); **Address:** Morgan Stanley Chldns Hosp of NY-Presby, 3959 Broadway, Ste 219N, New York, NY 10032; **Phone:** 212-305-8510; **Board Cert:** Urology 1978; **Med School:** Cornell Univ-Weill Med Coll 1968; **Resid:** Surgery, Boston City Hosp 1973; Urology, Mass Genl Hosp 1976; **Fellow:** Pediatric Urology, Mass Genl Hosp 1977; Pediatric Urology, Great Ormond St Hosp 1978; **Fac Appt:** Prof U, Columbia P&S

Herr, Harry W MD (U) - **Spec Exp:** Bladder Cancer; Prostate Cancer; Testicular Cancer; **Hospital:** Meml Sloan-Kettering Cancer Ctr (page 112), NY-Presby Hosp/Weill Cornell (page 104); **Address:** 1275 York Avenue, New York, NY 10065; **Phone:** 800-525-2225; **Board Cert:** Urology 1976; **Med School:** UCSF 1969; **Resid:** Urology, UC Irvine Med Ctr 1974; **Fellow:** Urology, Meml Sloan Kettering Cancer Ctr 1976; **Fac Appt:** Assoc Prof S, Cornell Univ-Weill Med Coll

Kaminetsky, Jed MD (U) - **Spec Exp:** Sexual Dysfunction; Prostate Cancer; Kidney Stones; **Hospital:** NYU Langone Med Ctr (page 106); **Address:** 215 Lexington Ave Fl 20, New York, NY 10016; **Phone:** 212-686-9015; **Board Cert:** Urology 2010; **Med School:** NYU Sch Med 1984; **Resid:** Urology, NYU Med Ctr 1990; **Fac Appt:** Asst Clin Prof U, NYU Sch Med

Kaplan, Steven A MD (U) - **Spec Exp:** Urodynamics; Voiding Dysfunction; Incontinence after Prostate Cancer; Incontinence; **Hospital:** NY-Presby Hosp/Weill Cornell (page 104); **Address:** NY Presbyterian-Weill Cornell Med Ctr, 525 E 68th St, rm F9West, New York, NY 10021-4870; **Phone:** 212-746-4811; **Board Cert:** Urology 2001; **Med School:** Mount Sinai Sch Med 1982; **Resid:** Surgery, Mount Sinai Hosp 1984; Urology, Columbia Presby Med Ctr 1988; **Fellow:** Urology, Columbia Presby Med Ctr 1990; **Fac Appt:** Prof U, Cornell Univ-Weill Med Coll

Katz, Aaron E MD (U) - **Spec Exp:** Prostate Cancer-Cryosurgery; Kidney Cancer-Cryosurgery; Complementary Medicine; Nutrition & Cancer Prevention; **Hospital:** NY-Presby Hosp/Columbia (page 104); **Address:** NY Presby Med Ctr, Herbert Irving Pav, 161 Ft Washington Ave Fl 11, New York, NY 10032; **Phone:** 212-305-6408; **Board Cert:** Urology 2006; **Med School:** NY Med Coll 1986; **Resid:** Urology, Maimonides Med Ctr 1992; **Fellow:** Urologic Oncology, Columbia Presby Med Ctr 1993; **Fac Appt:** Assoc Clin Prof U, Columbia P&S

Kirschenbaum, Alexander M MD (U) - **Spec Exp:** Prostate Cancer; Bladder Cancer; Kidney Cancer; **Hospital:** Mount Sinai Med Ctr (page 102); **Address:** 58A E 79th St, New York, NY 10021; **Phone:** 646-422-0926; **Board Cert:** Urology 2006; **Med School:** Mount Sinai Sch Med 1980; **Resid:** Surgery, Mt Sinai Hosp 1982; Urology, Mt Sinai Hosp 1985; **Fellow:** Urologic Oncology, Mt Sinai Hosp 1987; **Fac Appt:** Assoc Prof U, Mount Sinai Sch Med

Klein, George MD (U) - **Spec Exp:** Kidney Stones; Sexual Dysfunction; Prostate Cancer; **Hospital:** Mount Sinai Med Ctr (page 102), Lenox Hill Hosp; **Address:** 157 E 72nd St, Ground Fl, New York, NY 10021; **Phone:** 212-744-8700; **Board Cert:** Urology 1983; **Med School:** Cornell Univ-Weill Med Coll 1976; **Resid:** Surgery, North Shore Univ Hosp 1978; Urology, Mount Sinai Hosp 1981; **Fac Appt:** Asst Prof U, Mount Sinai Sch Med

Landman, Jaime MD (U) - **Spec Exp:** Minimally Invasive Urologic Surgery; Kidney Stones; Kidney Cancer; **Hospital:** NY-Presby Hosp/Columbia (page 104); **Address:** 161 Fort Washington Ave Fl 11, New York, NY 10032; **Phone:** 212-305-0114; **Board Cert:** Urology 2003; **Med School:** Columbia P&S 1993; **Resid:** Urology, Mount Sinai Hosp 1999; **Fellow:** Urologic Laparoscopic Surg-Endourology, Wash Univ Med Ctr 2001; **Fac Appt:** Assoc Prof U, Columbia P&S

Lepor, Herbert MD (U) - **Spec Exp:** Prostate Cancer; **Hospital:** NYU Langone Med Ctr (page 106); **Address:** 150 E 32nd St Fl 2, New York, NY 10016; **Phone:** 646-825-6327; **Board Cert:** Urology 2006; **Med School:** Johns Hopkins Univ 1975; **Resid:** Urology, Johns Hopkins Hosp 1986; **Fac Appt:** Prof U, NYU Sch Med

Lizza, Eli F MD (U) - **Spec Exp:** Impotence; Infertility-Male; **Hospital:** Lenox Hill Hosp, NY-Presby Hosp/Weill Cornell (page 104); **Address:** New York Urological Assocs, 245 E 54th St, New York, NY 10022; **Phone:** 212-570-6800 x180; **Board Cert:** Urology 2006; **Med School:** UMDNJ-NJ Med Sch, Newark 1979; **Resid:** Surgery, Lenox Hill Hosp 1981; Urology, W VA Med Ctr 1984; **Fellow:** Infertility, Columbia Presby Med Ctr 1985

Loo, Marcus Hsieu-Hong MD (U) - **Spec Exp:** Prostate Disease; Kidney Stones; Voiding Dysfunction; Prostate Cancer; **Hospital:** NY-Presby Hosp/Weill Cornell (page 104); **Address:** 254 Canal St, Ste 3001, New York, NY 10013-3501; **Phone:** 212-925-8388; **Board Cert:** Urology 2008; **Med School:** Cornell Univ-Weill Med Coll 1981; **Resid:** Surgery, NY Hosp-Cornell Med Ctr 1983; Urology, NY Hosp-Cornell Med Ctr 1988; **Fellow:** Urology, NY Hosp-Cornell Med Ctr 1984; **Fac Appt:** Clin Prof U, Cornell Univ-Weill Med Coll

Lowe, Franklin MD (U) - **Spec Exp:** Prostate Disease; Complementary Medicine; Prostate Cancer; **Hospital:** St Luke's - Roosevelt Hosp Ctr - Roosevelt Div (page 94), NY-Presby Hosp/Columbia (page 104); **Address:** 425 W 59th St, Ste 3A, New York, NY 10019-1104; **Phone:** 212-523-7790; **Board Cert:** Urology 2006; **Med School:** Columbia P&S 1979; **Resid:** Surgery, Johns Hopkins Hosp 1981; Urology, Johns Hopkins Hosp 1984; **Fac Appt:** Clin Prof U, Columbia P&S

Marks, Jon O MD (U) - **Spec Exp:** Kidney Stones; Interstitial Cystitis; **Hospital:** Beth Israel Med Ctr - Petrie Division (page 94); **Address:** 201 E 19th St, New York, NY 10003; **Phone:** 212-673-7300; **Board Cert:** Urology 1983; **Med School:** NY Med Coll 1976; **Resid:** Surgery, Lenox Hill Hosp 1978; Urology, Lenox Hill Hosp 1981

McCullough, Andrew R MD (U) - **Spec Exp:** Erectile Dysfunction; Infertility-Male; Prostate Cancer; **Hospital:** NYU Langone Med Ctr (page 106); **Address:** 150 E 32nd St, 2nd Fl, New York, NY 10016; **Phone:** 646-825-6311; **Board Cert:** Urology 2005; **Med School:** Univ MD Sch Med 1978; **Resid:** Urology, Johns Hopkins Hosp 1983; **Fellow:** Urologic Oncology, Johns Hopkins Hosp 1984; **Fac Appt:** Assoc Prof U, NYU Sch Med

McGovern, Thomas P MD (U) - **Spec Exp:** Bladder Cancer; Prostate Cancer; **Hospital:** NY-Presby Hosp/Weill Cornell (page 104), Lenox Hill Hosp; **Address:** 927 5th Ave, New York, NY 10021; **Phone:** 212-772-7411; **Board Cert:** Urology 1983; **Med School:** Cornell Univ-Weill Med Coll 1974; **Resid:** Surgery, Mass Genl Hosp 1976; Urology, New York Hosp 1980; **Fac Appt:** Asst Clin Prof U, Cornell Univ-Weill Med Coll

McKiernan, James M MD (U) - **Spec Exp:** Urologic Cancer; Bladder Cancer; Prostate Cancer; Testicular Cancer; **Hospital:** NY-Presby Hosp/Columbia (page 104); **Address:** Dept Urology, 161 Fort Washington Ave Fl 11, New York, NY 10032; **Phone:** 212-305-0114; **Board Cert:** Urology 2003; **Med School:** Columbia P&S 1993; **Resid:** Surgery, Columbia Presby Med Ctr 1995; Urology, Columbia Presby Med Ctr 1999; **Fellow:** Urologic Oncology, Meml Sloan-Kettering Cancer Ctr 2001; **Fac Appt:** Asst Prof U, Columbia P&S

Mulhall, John P MD (U) - **Spec Exp:** Erectile Dysfunction; Peyronie's Disease; Penile Prostheses; Infertility-Male; **Hospital:** Meml Sloan-Kettering Cancer Ctr (page 112); **Address:** Prostate Ctr at Meml Sloan Kettering, 353 E 68th St Fl 5, New York, NY 10021; **Phone:** 646-422-4359; **Board Cert:** Urology 2008; **Med School:** Ireland 1985; **Resid:** Urology, Univ Conn Health Ctr 1995; **Fellow:** Urology, Boston Univ Med Ctr 1996; **Fac Appt:** Assoc Prof U, Cornell Univ-Weill Med Coll

Nagler, Harris M MD (U) - **Spec Exp:** Vasectomy Reversal; Infertility-Male; Varicocele Microsurgery; Erectile Dysfunction; **Hospital:** Beth Israel Med Ctr - Petrie Division (page 94); **Address:** Beth Israel Med Ctr, Dept Urology, 10 Union Square E, Ste 3A, New York, NY 10003-3314; **Phone:** 212-844-8700; **Board Cert:** Urology 1982; **Med School:** Temple Univ 1975; **Resid:** Urology, Columbia Presby Med Ctr 1980; **Fellow:** Reproductive Medicine, Columbia Presby Med Ctr 1981; **Fac Appt:** Prof U, Albert Einstein Coll Med

Nitti, Victor MD (U) - **Spec Exp:** Urology-Female; Incontinence-Male & Female; Urodynamics; Voiding Dysfunction; **Hospital:** NYU Langone Med Ctr (page 106); **Address:** NYU Urology Assocs, 150 E 32nd St, 2nd Fl, New York, NY 10016; **Phone:** 646-825-6324; **Board Cert:** Urology 2002; **Med School:** UMDNJ-NJ Med Sch, Newark 1985; **Resid:** Surgery, Univ Hosp 1987; Urology, Univ Hosp 1991; **Fellow:** Female Urology, UCLA 1992; **Fac Appt:** Prof U, NYU Sch Med

Palese, Michael MD (U) - **Spec Exp:** Kidney Cancer; Laparoscopic Surgery; Robotic Surgery; Kidney Stones; **Hospital:** Mount Sinai Med Ctr (page 102); **Address:** 5 E 98th St Fl 6, New York, NY 10029; **Phone:** 212-241-3868; **Board Cert:** Urology 2006; **Med School:** Mount Sinai Sch Med 1997; **Resid:** Surgery, Univ MD Med Ctr 1999; Urology, Univ MD Med Ctr 2003; **Fellow:** Urologic Oncology, NY Presby-Cornell Med Ctr 2004; Robotic Surgery, NY Presby-Cornell Med Ctr 2004; **Fac Appt:** Assoc Prof U, Mount Sinai Sch Med

Peng, Benjamin MD (U) - **Spec Exp:** Prostate Disease; Kidney Stones; Urologic Cancer; **Hospital:** NY Downtown Hosp, NYU Langone Med Ctr (page 106); **Address:** 168 Canal St, Ste 510, New York, NY 10013-4503; **Phone:** 212-226-2200; **Board Cert:** Urology 2001; **Med School:** Columbia P&S 1984; **Resid:** Surgery, Mount Sinai Hosp 1986; Urology, Columbia-Presby Hosp 1990; **Fac Appt:** Asst Clin Prof U, NYU Sch Med

Poppas, Dix P MD (U) - **Spec Exp:** Genital Reconstruction-Pediatric; Robotic Surgery-Pediatric; Minimally Invasive Surgery-Pediatric; Pediatric Urology; **Hospital:** NY-Presby Hosp/Weill Cornell (page 104); **Address:** Inst for Pediatric Urology, NY Presby Hosp-Weill Cornell, 525 E 68th St, Box 94, New York, NY 10021-4870; **Phone:** 212-746-5337; **Board Cert:** Urology 1999; Pediatric Urology 2008; **Med School:** Eastern VA Med Sch 1988; **Resid:** Urology, NY Hosp-Cornell Med Ctr 1994; **Fellow:** Pediatric Urology, Chldns Hosp Harvard Med Sch 1996; **Fac Appt:** Prof U, Cornell Univ-Weill Med Coll

Provet, John A MD (U) - **Spec Exp:** Urologic Cancer; Kidney Stones; Prostate Disease; **Hospital:** NYU Langone Med Ctr (page 106); **Address:** 215 Lexington Ave, FL 20, New York, NY 10016; **Phone:** 212-686-9015; **Board Cert:** Urology 2009; **Med School:** NYU Sch Med 1983; **Resid:** Surgery, NYU/VA Med Ctr/Bellevue Hosp 1985; Urology, NYU/VA Med Ctr/Bellevue Hosp 1989; **Fac Appt:** Assoc Clin Prof U, NYU Sch Med

Reckler, Jon M MD (U) - **Hospital:** NY-Presby Hosp/Weill Cornell (page 104), Lenox Hill Hosp; **Address:** 880 5th Ave, New York, NY 10021; **Phone:** 212-535-1950; **Board Cert:** Urology 1976; **Med School:** Harvard Med Sch 1966; **Resid:** Surgery, Univ Hosp 1968; Urology, Peter Bent Brigham Hosp 1974; **Fac Appt:** Assoc Clin Prof U, Cornell Univ-Weill Med Coll

Romas, Nicholas A MD (U) - **Spec Exp:** Prostate Disease; Prostate Cancer; Erectile Dysfunction; **Hospital:** St Luke's - Roosevelt Hosp Ctr - Roosevelt Div (page 94), NY-Presby Hosp/Columbia (page 104); **Address:** 425 W 59th St, Ste 3A, New York, NY 10019-1104; **Phone:** 212-523-7788; **Board Cert:** Urology 1974; **Med School:** Columbia P&S 1962; **Resid:** Surgery, New York Hosp-Cornell 1964; Urology, Columbia-Presby Med Ctr 1968; **Fac Appt:** Clin Prof U, Columbia P&S

Russo, Paul MD (U) - **Spec Exp:** Kidney Cancer; Prostate Cancer; Penile Cancer; **Hospital:** Meml Sloan-Kettering Cancer Ctr (page 112); **Address:** 1275 York Avenue, New York, NY 10065; **Phone:** 800-525-2225; **Board Cert:** Urology 2004; **Med School:** Columbia P&S 1979; **Resid:** Urology, Barnes Hosp-Wash Univ 1984; **Fellow:** Urologic Oncology, Mem Sloan Kettering Cancer Ctr 1988; **Fac Appt:** Assoc Prof U, Cornell Univ-Weill Med Coll

Samadi, David B MD (U) - **Spec Exp:** Prostate Cancer/Robotic Surgery; Kidney Cancer; Bladder Cancer; Urologic Cancer; **Hospital:** Mount Sinai Med Ctr (page 102); **Address:** 625 Madison Ave Fl 2, New York, NY 10022; **Phone:** 212-241-8779; **Board Cert:** Urology 2004; **Med School:** SUNY Stony Brook 1994; **Resid:** Surgery, Montefiore Med Ctr 1996; Urology, Montefiore Med Ctr 2000; **Fellow:** Urologic Oncology, Meml Sloan Kettering Cancer Ctr 2001; Laparoscopic Surgery, Henri Mondor Hosp 2003; **Fac Appt:** Asst Prof U, Mount Sinai Sch Med

Scardino, Peter T MD (U) - **Spec Exp:** Prostate Cancer; Bladder Cancer; Urologic Cancer; Urinary Reconstruction; **Hospital:** Meml Sloan-Kettering Cancer Ctr (page 112); **Address:** 1275 York Avenue, New York, NY 10065; **Phone:** 646-422-4329; **Board Cert:** Urology 1981; **Med School:** Duke Univ 1971; **Resid:** Surgery, Mass Genl Hosp 1973; Urology, UCLA Med Ctr 1979; **Fellow:** Urology, Natl Cancer Inst 1976; **Fac Appt:** Prof U, Cornell Univ-Weill Med Coll

Scherr, Douglas S MD (U) - **Spec Exp:** Prostate Cancer/Robotic Surgery; Bladder Cancer; Robotic Surgery; Testicular Cancer; **Hospital:** NY-Presby Hosp/Weill Cornell (page 104); **Address:** NY Cornell Medical Ctr, Dept Urology, 525 E 68th St Starr 900, New York, NY 10021; **Phone:** 212-746-5788; **Board Cert:** Urology 2003; **Med School:** Geo Wash Univ 1994; **Resid:** Urology, NY Hosp-Cornell Med Ctr 1999; **Fellow:** Urologic Oncology, Meml Sloan-Kettering Canc Ctr 2002; **Fac Appt:** Assoc Prof U, Cornell Univ-Weill Med Coll

Schiff, Howard I MD (U) - **Spec Exp:** Prostate Benign Disease; Infertility-Male; Prostate Cancer; Lupus Cystitis; **Hospital:** Mount Sinai Med Ctr (page 102), NY-Presby Hosp/Weill Cornell (page 104); **Address:** 1120 Park Ave, Ste 1E, New York, NY 10128-1242; **Phone:** 212-996-6660; **Board Cert:** Urology 1982; **Med School:** W VA Univ 1975; **Resid:** Surgery, Montefiore Hosp Med Ctr 1977; Urology, Mount Sinai Hosp 1980; **Fac Appt:** Asst Clin Prof U, Mount Sinai Sch Med

Schlegel, Peter N MD (U) - **Spec Exp:** Prostate Cancer; Infertility-Male; **Hospital:** NY-Presby Hosp/Weill Cornell (page 104); **Address:** 525 E 68th St, Starr 900, New York, NY 10021-4870; **Phone:** 212-746-5491; **Board Cert:** Urology 2001; **Med School:** Univ Mass Sch Med 1983; **Resid:** Surgery, Johns Hopkins Hosp 1985; Urology, Johns Hopkins Hosp 1989; **Fellow:** Medical Oncology, Johns Hopkins Hosp 1987; Male Reproduction, NY Hosp-Cornell Med Ctr 1991; **Fac Appt:** Prof U, Cornell Univ-Weill Med Coll

Schlussel, Richard MD (U) - **Spec Exp:** Pediatric Urology; Hypospadias; Robotic Surgery; Reconstructive Surgery; **Hospital:** NY-Presby Hosp/Columbia (page 104), Englewood Hosp & Med Ctr (page 656); **Address:** 65 E 96th St, New York, NY 10128; **Phone:** 212-305-1114; **Board Cert:** Urology 2006; **Med School:** Albert Einstein Coll Med 1986; **Resid:** Urology, Mt Sinai Med Ctr 1992; **Fellow:** Urology, Harvard Univ/Chldns Hosp 1994; **Fac Appt:** Asst Prof U, Columbia P&S

Shapiro, Ellen MD (U) - **Spec Exp:** Pediatric Urology; **Hospital:** NYU Langone Med Ctr (page 106), Hackensack Univ Med Ctr (page 96); **Address:** 150 E 32nd St Fl 2, New York, NY 10016; **Phone:** 646-825-6326; **Board Cert:** Urology 2006; Pediatric Urology 2008; **Med School:** Univ Nebr Coll Med 1978; **Resid:** Surgery, Johns Hopkins Hosp 1980; Urology, Johns Hopkins Hosp 1986; **Fellow:** Pediatric Urology, Chldns Hosp Michigan 1987; **Fac Appt:** Prof U, NYU Sch Med

Sheinfeld, Joel MD (U) - **Spec Exp:** Testicular Cancer; Bladder Cancer; Fertility Preservation in Cancer; **Hospital:** Meml Sloan-Kettering Cancer Ctr (page 112); **Address:** 1275 York Avenue, New York, NY 10065; **Phone:** 800-525-2225; **Board Cert:** Urology 2009; **Med School:** Univ Fla Coll Med 1981; **Resid:** Urology, Strong Meml Hosp 1986; **Fellow:** Urologic Oncology, Meml Sloan Kettering Cancer Ctr 1989; **Fac Appt:** Assoc Prof U, Cornell Univ-Weill Med Coll

Silva, Jose V MD (U) - **Spec Exp:** Urologic Cancer; **Hospital:** St Luke's - Roosevelt Hosp Ctr - Roosevelt Div (page 94), Montefiore Med Ctr - Div. Moses (page 100); **Address:** 425 W 59th St, Ste 3A, New York, NY 10019; **Phone:** 212-582-3421; **Board Cert:** Urology 1983; **Med School:** India 1970; **Resid:** Surgery, Beth Israel Med Ctr 1978; Urology, St Luke's-Roosevelt Hosp Ctr 1981; **Fellow:** Surgery, Meml Sloan Kettering Cancer Ctr 1982

Sogani, Pramod MD (U) - **Spec Exp:** Prostate Cancer; Testicular Cancer; Bladder Cancer; Kidney Cancer; **Hospital:** Meml Sloan-Kettering Cancer Ctr (page 112); **Address:** 1275 York Avenue, New York, NY 10065; **Phone:** 800-525-2225; **Board Cert:** Urology 1976; **Med School:** India 1960; **Resid:** Urology, NYU Med Ctr 1969; Urology, Geo Wash Univ Med Ctr 1971; **Fellow:** Surgical Oncology, Meml Sloan Kettering Cancer Ctr 1973; **Fac Appt:** Prof U, Cornell Univ-Weill Med Coll

Sosa, R Ernest MD (U) - **Spec Exp:** Kidney Stones; Laparoscopic Surgery; Adrenal Surgery; **Hospital:** Lenox Hill Hosp, NY-Presby Hosp/Weill Cornell (page 104); **Address:** 880 5th Ave, New York, NY 10021; **Phone:** 212-570-6800; **Board Cert:** Urology 2006; **Med School:** Cornell Univ-Weill Med Coll 1978; **Resid:** Surgery, New York Hosp 1980; Urology, New York Hosp 1984; **Fellow:** Renal Physiology, New York Hosp-Cornell 1986; **Fac Appt:** Assoc Clin Prof U, Cornell Univ-Weill Med Coll

Stifelman, Michael D MD (U) - **Spec Exp:** Robotic Surgery; Urologic Cancer; Urinary Reconstruction; Retroperitoneal Fibrosis; **Hospital:** NYU Langone Med Ctr (page 106), Bellevue Hosp Ctr; **Address:** 150 E 32nd St Fl 2, New York, NY 10016-6024; **Phone:** 646-825-6325; **Board Cert:** Urology 2002; **Med School:** Albert Einstein Coll Med 1993; **Resid:** Surgery, Columbia-Presby Med Ctr 1995; Urology, Columbia-Presby Med Ctr 1999; **Fellow:** Laparoscopic Surgery, NY Hosp 2000; **Fac Appt:** Asst Prof U, NYU Sch Med

Taneja, Samir S MD (U) - **Spec Exp:** Kidney Cancer; Prostate Cancer; Bladder Cancer; **Hospital:** NYU Langone Med Ctr (page 106); **Address:** NYU Urology Assocs, 150 E 32nd St Fl 2, New York, NY 10016-6024; **Phone:** 646-825-6321; **Board Cert:** Urology 2009; **Med School:** Northwestern Univ 1990; **Resid:** Urology, UCLA Med Ctr 1996; **Fellow:** Urologic Oncology, NYU Med Ctr 1998; **Fac Appt:** Assoc Prof U, NYU Sch Med

Te, Alexis E MD (U) - **Spec Exp:** Prostate Benign Disease; Prostate Surgery; Incontinence; **Hospital:** NY-Presby Hosp/Weill Cornell (page 104); **Address:** Weill Medical College, Brady Prostate Center, 525 E 68th St Fl 9 - rm F9W, New York, NY 10065; **Phone:** 212-746-4811; **Board Cert:** Urology 2006; **Med School:** Cornell Univ-Weill Med Coll 1988; **Resid:** Urology, NY Presbyterian-Columbia Presby Med Ctr 1994; **Fellow:** Urodynamics, NY Presbyterian-Columbia Presby Med Ctr 1995; **Fac Appt:** Assoc Prof U, Cornell Univ-Weill Med Coll

Tewari, Ashutosh MD (U) - **Spec Exp:** Prostate Cancer/Robotic Surgery; **Hospital:** NY-Presby Hosp/Weill Cornell (page 104); **Address:** Weill Cornell Brady Urologic Health Ct, 525 E 68th St, Starr 900, New York, NY 10021; **Phone:** 212-746-5638; **Board Cert:** Urology 2006; **Med School:** India 1984; **Resid:** Surgery, GSVM Medical College 1990; Urology, Henry Ford Hosp 2003; **Fellow:** Transplant Surgery, Liverpool Univ Med Ctr 1993; Urologic Oncology, Shands Healthcare 1995; **Fac Appt:** Assoc Prof U, Cornell Univ-Weill Med Coll

Vapnek, Jonathan M MD (U) - **Spec Exp:** Incontinence; Urology-Female; Neurogenic Bladder; Urodynamics; **Hospital:** Mount Sinai Med Ctr (page 102); **Address:** 229 E 79th St, Ste 1A, New York, NY 10075; **Phone:** 212-717-9500; **Board Cert:** Urology 2005; **Med School:** UCSD 1986; **Resid:** Surgery, UCSD Med Ctr 1988; Urology, UCSF Med Ctr 1992; **Fellow:** Neurourology, UC Davis Med Ctr 1993; **Fac Appt:** Assoc Clin Prof U, Mount Sinai Sch Med

Williams, John J MD (U) - **Spec Exp:** Genitourinary Cancer; Prostate Disease; Kidney Stones; **Hospital:** NY-Presby Hosp/Weill Cornell (page 104), Lenox Hill Hosp; **Address:** 820 Park Ave, New York, NY 10021-2758; **Phone:** 212-861-1100; **Board Cert:** Urology 1976; **Med School:** Georgetown Univ 1966; **Resid:** Surgery, Strong Meml Hosp 1968; Urology, NY Hosp 1974

Young, George P H MD (U) - **Spec Exp:** Incontinence-Female; Urologic Cancer; Urology-Female; **Hospital:** Lenox Hill Hosp, N Shore Univ Hosp; **Address:** 1060 5th Ave, New York, NY 10128; **Phone:** 212-876-9811; **Board Cert:** Urology 2006; **Med School:** Brazil 1983; **Resid:** Surgery, Staten Island Univ Hosp 1989; Urology, New York Hosp 1993; **Fellow:** Microsurgery, Population Council, Rockefeller Univ 1985; Female Urology, UCLA Med Ctr 1994; **Fac Appt:** Assoc Prof U, Cornell Univ-Weill Med Coll

Vascular & Interventional Radiology

Brown, Karen T MD (VIR) - **Spec Exp:** Liver Cancer; Radiofrequency Tumor Ablation; Interventional Radiology; **Hospital:** Meml Sloan-Kettering Cancer Ctr (page 112); **Address:** 1275 York Avenue, New York, NY 10065; **Phone:** 800-525-2225; **Board Cert:** Diagnostic Radiology 1984; Vascular & Interventional Radiology 2004; **Med School:** Boston Univ 1979; **Resid:** Diagnostic Radiology, Mass Genl Hosp 1984; **Fellow:** Vascular & Interventional Radiology, Mass Genl Hosp 1985; **Fac Appt:** Prof Rad, Cornell Univ-Weill Med Coll

Khilnani, Neil M MD (VIR) - **Spec Exp:** Vein Disorders; Varicose Veins; Uterine Fibroid Embolization; **Hospital:** NY-Presby Hosp/Weill Cornell (page 104); **Address:** Cornell Vascular Assocs, 416 E 55th St, Main Floor, New York, NY 10022; **Phone:** 212-752-7999; **Board Cert:** Diagnostic Radiology 1991; Vascular & Interventional Radiology 2007; **Med School:** Mount Sinai Sch Med 1986; **Resid:** Radiology, Columbia Presby Med Ctr 1991; **Fellow:** Vascular & Interventional Radiology, Columbia Presby Med Ctr 1992; **Fac Appt:** Assoc Prof Rad, Cornell Univ-Weill Med Coll

Rosen, Robert J MD (VIR) - **Spec Exp:** Vascular Malformations; Aneurysm-Aortic; Chemoembolization & Tumor Ablation; **Hospital:** Lenox Hill Hosp; **Address:** Lenox Hill Heart & Vascular Inst, 130 E 77th St Fl 9, New York, NY 10075; **Phone:** 212-434-2606; **Board Cert:** Diagnostic Radiology 1980; **Med School:** Hahnemann Univ 1976; **Resid:** Diagnostic Radiology, Hahnemann Med Coll 1979; **Fellow:** Vascular & Interventional Radiology, Hosp Univ Penn 1980; **Fac Appt:** Assoc Prof Rad, NYU Sch Med

Saboeiro, Gregory R MD (VIR) - **Spec Exp:** Musculoskeletal Imaging; Ultrasound; **Hospital:** Hosp For Special Surgery (page 111); **Address:** Hosp for Special Surgery, 3rd Floor, Radiology, 535 E 70th St, New York, NY 10021; **Phone:** 212-606-1566; **Board Cert:** Diagnostic Radiology 1993; **Med School:** St Louis Univ 1989; **Resid:** Radiology, St Louis Univ Hosp 1993; **Fellow:** Interventional Radiology, Mallinckrodt Inst 1994; Musculoskeletal Imaging, Hosp Special Surgery 2005; **Fac Appt:** Asst Prof Rad, Cornell Univ-Weill Med Coll

Weintraub, Joshua L MD (VIR) - **Spec Exp:** Gastrointestinal Cancer; Chemoembolization & Tumor Ablation; Uterine Fibroid Embolization; Vein Disorders; **Hospital:** Mount Sinai Med Ctr (page 102); **Address:** Mount Sinai Medical Ctr, Dept Radiology, One Gustave L Levy Pl, Box 1234, New York, NY 10029; **Phone:** 212-241-7409; **Board Cert:** Diagnostic Radiology 1996; Vascular & Interventional Radiology 1998; **Med School:** Wayne State Univ 1991; **Resid:** Diagnostic Radiology, Beth Israel Hosp 1996; **Fellow:** Vascular & Interventional Radiology, Hosp Univ Penn 1997; **Fac Appt:** Assoc Prof Rad, Mount Sinai Sch Med

Vascular Surgery

Adelman, Mark MD (VascS) - **Spec Exp:** Carotid Artery Surgery; Aneurysm-Abdominal Aortic; Vein Disorders; Endovascular Surgery; **Hospital:** NYU Langone Med Ctr (page 106), Bellevue Hosp Ctr; **Address:** 530 1st Ave, Ste 6F, New York, NY 10016-6402; **Phone:** 212-263-7311; **Board Cert:** Surgery 1999; Vascular Surgery 2001; **Med School:** NYU Sch Med 1985; **Resid:** Surgery, NYU Med Ctr 1990; **Fellow:** Vascular Surgery, NYU Med Ctr 1991; **Fac Appt:** Prof VascS, NYU Sch Med

Benvenisty, Alan I MD (VascS) - **Spec Exp:** Renovascular Disease; Aneurysm-Aortic; Endovascular Surgery; Minimally Invasive Vascular Surgery; **Hospital:** St Luke's - Roosevelt Hosp Ctr - St Luke's Hosp (page 94), St Luke's - Roosevelt Hosp Ctr - Roosevelt Div (page 94); **Address:** 1090 Amsterdam Ave Fl 12, New York, NY 10025; **Phone:** 212-523-4706; **Board Cert:** Surgery 2004; Vascular Surgery 1999; **Med School:** Columbia P&S 1978; **Resid:** Surgery, Columbia-Presby Med Ctr 1983; **Fellow:** Vascular Surgery, Columbia-Presby Med Ctr 1984; Transplant Surgery, Columbia-Presby Med Ctr 1984; **Fac Appt:** Clin Prof S, Columbia P&S

Bernik, Thomas R MD (VascS) - **Spec Exp:** Carotid Artery Surgery; Aortic Surgery; Peripheral Vascular Disease; Chemoembolization & Tumor Ablation; **Hospital:** Beth Israel Med Ctr - Petrie Division (page 94), Lenox Hill Hosp; **Address:** 20 W 13th St, Ground Level, New York, NY 10011; **Phone:** 212-838-3055; **Board Cert:** Surgery 2001; Vascular Surgery 2005; **Med School:** Geo Wash Univ 1994; **Resid:** Surgery, St Vincents Hosp Med Ctr 2000; **Fellow:** Vascular Surgery, N Shore Univ Hosp 2002; Endovascular Surgery, Strong Memorial Hosp 2002; **Fac Appt:** Asst Prof VascS, NY Med Coll

Chideckel, Norman MD (VascS) - **Spec Exp:** Vein Disorders; Wound Healing/Care; Laser Surgery; **Hospital:** Beth Israel Med Ctr - Petrie Division (page 94); **Address:** 380 2nd Ave, Ste 1004, New York, NY 10010; **Phone:** 212-473-1877; **Board Cert:** Surgery 2007; **Med School:** SUNY Downstate 1979; **Resid:** Surgery, Beth Israel Med Ctr 1984; **Fellow:** Vascular Surgery, Lutheran Med Ctr 1985; **Fac Appt:** Asst Clin Prof S, Albert Einstein Coll Med

Fantini, Gary A MD (VascS) - **Spec Exp:** Spinal Access Surgery; Thoracic Outlet Syndrome; **Hospital:** Hosp For Special Surgery (page 111), NY-Presby Hosp/Weill Cornell (page 104); **Address:** 635 Madison Ave Fl 7, New York, NY 10022; **Phone:** 212-317-4550; **Board Cert:** Surgery 2007; Vascular Surgery 2000; **Med School:** Albert Einstein Coll Med 1983; **Resid:** Surgery, NY Hosp-Cornell Med Ctr 1989; **Fellow:** Vascular Surgery, UCSF Med Ctr 1990; **Fac Appt:** Assoc Prof S, Cornell Univ-Weill Med Coll

Faries, Peter MD (VascS) - **Spec Exp:** Aneurysm-Abdominal Aortic; Peripheral Vascular Disease; Renovascular Disease; Carotid Artery Surgery; **Hospital:** Mount Sinai Med Ctr (page 102); **Address:** 5 E 98th St, Ste 415, New York, NY 10021; **Phone:** 212-241-5386; **Board Cert:** Surgery 1999; Vascular Surgery 2001; **Med School:** Univ Pennsylvania 1992; **Resid:** Surgery, Montefiore Med Ctr 1998; **Fellow:** Vascular Surgery, Beth Israel Deaconess Med Ctr 2000; **Fac Appt:** Prof S, Mount Sinai Sch Med

Green, Richard M MD (VascS) - **Spec Exp:** Aneurysm-Abdominal Aortic; Carotid Artery Surgery; Percutaneous Vascular Interventions; **Hospital:** Lenox Hill Hosp; **Address:** 130 E 77th St Fl 13, New York, NY 10021; **Phone:** 212-434-3420; **Board Cert:** Vascular Surgery 2003; **Med School:** Univ Rochester 1970; **Resid:** Surgery, Strong Meml Hosp 1976

Grossi, Robert J MD (VascS) - **Spec Exp:** Carotid Artery Surgery; Aneurysm-Abdominal Aortic; Wound Healing/Care; **Hospital:** Beth Israel Med Ctr - Petrie Division (page 94), NY Downtown Hosp; **Address:** 20 W 13th St, New York, NY 10011; **Phone:** 212-838-3055; **Board Cert:** Surgery 2006; Vascular Surgery 2008; **Med School:** UMDNJ-NJ Med Sch, Newark 1981; **Resid:** Surgery, St Vincent's Hosp 1986; **Fellow:** Vascular Surgery, Temple Univ Hosp 1987

Harrington, Elizabeth MD (VascS) - **Spec Exp:** Carotid Artery Surgery; Aneurysm-Aortic; Arterial Bypass Surgery-Leg; **Hospital:** Mount Sinai Med Ctr (page 102); **Address:** 2 E 93rd St, New York, NY 10128; **Phone:** 212-876-7400; **Board Cert:** Surgery 1999; Vascular Surgery 2006; **Med School:** NY Med Coll 1975; **Resid:** Surgery, Mt Sinai Hosp 1980; **Fellow:** Vascular Surgery, Mt Sinai Hosp 1981; **Fac Appt:** Assoc Prof VascS, Mount Sinai Sch Med

Harrington, Martin MD (VascS) - **Spec Exp:** Carotid Artery Surgery; Aneurysm-Aortic; Arterial Bypass Surgery-Leg; **Hospital:** Mount Sinai Med Ctr (page 102); **Address:** 2 E 93rd St, New York, NY 10128; **Phone:** 212-876-7400; **Board Cert:** Internal Medicine 1978; Hematology 1980; Surgery 2003; Vascular Surgery 2007; **Med School:** Harvard Med Sch 1975; **Resid:** Internal Medicine, St Luke's Roosevelt Hosp Ctr 1979; Surgery, Mt Sinai Hosp 1984; **Fellow:** Surgical Oncology, Meml Sloan Kettering Cancer Ctr 1986; Vascular Surgery, Mt Sinai Hosp 1989

Jacobowitz, Glenn R MD (VascS) - **Spec Exp:** Vein Disorders; Minimally Invasive Vascular Surgery; Aneurysm-Abdominal Aortic; Carotid Artery Surgery; **Hospital:** NYU Langone Med Ctr (page 106), Bellevue Hosp Ctr; **Address:** Schwartz Health Care Ctr, 530 First Ave, Ste 6F, New York, NY 10016; **Phone:** 212-263-7311; **Board Cert:** Surgery 2006; Vascular Surgery 2005; **Med School:** NYU Sch Med 1989; **Resid:** Surgery, NYU Med Ctr 1995; **Fellow:** Vascular Surgery, NYU Med Ctr 1996; **Fac Appt:** Assoc Prof VascS, NYU Sch Med

Maldonado, Thomas MD (VascS) - **Spec Exp:** Aortic Stent Grafts; Endovascular Surgery; **Hospital:** NYU Langone Med Ctr (page 106), Bellevue Hosp Ctr; **Address:** NYU Medical Center, 530 First Ave, Ste 6F, New York, NY 10016; **Phone:** 212-263-7311; **Board Cert:** Surgery 2003; Vascular Surgery 2005; **Med School:** NYU Sch Med 1995; **Resid:** Surgery, NYU Med Ctr 1998; Surgery, NYU Med Ctr 2002; **Fellow:** Research, NYU Med Ctr 2000; Vascular Surgery, NYU Med Ctr 2003; **Fac Appt:** Assoc Prof S, NYU Sch Med

Marin, Michael L MD (VascS) - **Spec Exp:** Aneurysm-Aortic; Carotid Artery Surgery; Limb Sparing Surgery; Endovascular Surgery; **Hospital:** Mount Sinai Med Ctr (page 102), N Genl Hosp; **Address:** Mount Sinai Medical Ctr, 5 E 98th St, Box 1273, New York, NY 10029; **Phone:** 212-241-5315; **Board Cert:** Surgery 1999; **Med School:** Mount Sinai Sch Med 1984; **Resid:** Surgery, Columbia-Presby Med Ctr 1990; **Fellow:** Transplant Surgery, Columbia-Presby Med Ctr 1988; Vascular Surgery, Montefiore Med Ctr 1992; **Fac Appt:** Prof S, Mount Sinai Sch Med

Mendes, Donna M MD (VascS) - **Spec Exp:** Varicose Veins; Aneurysm-Aortic; Limb Sparing Surgery; **Hospital:** St Luke's - Roosevelt Hosp Ctr - Roosevelt Div (page 94), Lenox Hill Hosp; **Address:** 1090 Amsterdam Ave at 114th St, Ste 7H, New York, NY 10025-1737; **Phone:** 212-636-4990; **Board Cert:** Surgery 2004; Vascular Surgery 1999; **Med School:** Columbia P&S 1977; **Resid:** Surgery, St Luke's-Roosevelt Hosp Ctr 1982; **Fellow:** Vascular Surgery, Englewood Hosp 1984; **Fac Appt:** Asst Clin Prof S, Columbia P&S

Nalbandian, Matthew M MD (VascS) - **Spec Exp:** Spinal Access Surgery; Endovascular Surgery; Varicose Veins; Vein Disorders; **Hospital:** NYU Langone Med Ctr (page 106), Holy Name Med Ctr (page 657); **Address:** 247 Third Ave, Ste L1, New York, NY 10010; **Phone:** 212-254-6882; **Board Cert:** Surgery 2009; Vascular Surgery 2008; **Med School:** UMDNJ-NJ Med Sch, Newark 1993; **Resid:** Surgery, Boston Med Ctr 1998; **Fellow:** Vascular Surgery, NYU Med Ctr 2000; **Fac Appt:** Asst Prof VascS, NYU Sch Med

Nowygrod, Roman MD (VascS) - **Spec Exp:** Aneurysm; Carotid Artery Surgery; Endovascular Surgery; Vein Disorders; **Hospital:** NY-Presby Hosp/Columbia (page 104); **Address:** 161 Ft Washington Ave, Irving Pavilion, New York, NY 10032-3713; **Phone:** 212-305-5374; **Board Cert:** Surgery 2009; Vascular Surgery 2002; **Med School:** Columbia P&S 1970; **Resid:** Surgery, Columbia-Presby Med Ctr 1976; **Fellow:** Vascular Surgery, Columbia-Presby Med Ctr 1978; **Fac Appt:** Prof S, Columbia P&S

Riles, Thomas MD (VascS) - **Spec Exp:** Aneurysm-Abdominal Aortic; Carotid Artery Surgery; **Hospital:** NYU Langone Med Ctr (page 106); **Address:** NYU Med Ctr, Univ Vascular Assoc, 530 1st Ave, HCC-6D, New York, NY 10016; **Phone:** 212-263-6360; **Board Cert:** Vascular Surgery 2003; **Med School:** Baylor Coll Med 1969; **Resid:** Surgery, NYU Med Ctr 1976; **Fellow:** Vascular Surgery, NYU Med Ctr 1977; **Fac Appt:** Prof S, NYU Sch Med

Schneider, Darren B MD (VascS) - **Spec Exp:** Endovascular Surgery; Minimally Invasive Vascular Surgery; Aneurysm-Aortic; Peripheral Vascular Disease; **Hospital:** NY-Presby Hosp/Weill Cornell (page 104); **Address:** Weill Cornell Dept Vascular Surgery, 525 E 68th St, New York, NY 10021; **Phone:** 212-746-5192; **Board Cert:** Surgery 2001; Vascular Surgery 2003; **Med School:** UCSD 1992; **Resid:** Surgery, UCSF Med Ctr 2000; **Fellow:** Interventional Radiology, UCSF 2001; Vascular Surgery, UCSF 2002; **Fac Appt:** Asst Prof S, Cornell Univ-Weill Med Coll

Stein, Jeffrey S MD (VascS) - **Spec Exp:** Aneurysm-Aortic; Arterial Disease; Varicose Veins; **Hospital:** Mount Sinai Med Ctr (page 102), Lenox Hill Hosp; **Address:** 12 E 97th St, Ste 1C, New York, NY 10029; **Phone:** 212-396-0500; **Board Cert:** Surgery 2009; Vascular Surgery 2002; Surgical Critical Care 2001; **Med School:** Washington Univ, St Louis 1982; **Resid:** Surgery, Mt Sinai Hosp 1988; **Fellow:** Surgical Critical Care, Mt Sinai Hosp 1989; Vascular Surgery, Mt Sinai Hosp 1990; **Fac Appt:** Asst Clin Prof S, Mount Sinai Sch Med

Teodorescu, Victoria MD (VascS) - **Spec Exp:** Endovascular Surgery; Aneurysm; Diabetic Leg/Foot; Peripheral Vascular Disease; **Hospital:** Mount Sinai Med Ctr (page 102); **Address:** 5 E 98th St, Fl 15, Box 1259, New York, NY 10029; **Phone:** 212-241-5315; **Board Cert:** Surgery 2000; Vascular Surgery 2003; **Med School:** NYU Sch Med 1985; **Resid:** Surgery, Mt Sinai Hosp 1991; **Fellow:** Vascular Surgery, Mt Sinai Hosp 1992; **Fac Appt:** Assoc Prof S, Mount Sinai Sch Med

Todd, George MD (VascS) - **Spec Exp:** Minimally Invasive Vascular Surgery; Aneurysm-Abdominal Aortic; Carotid Artery Surgery; **Hospital:** St Luke's - Roosevelt Hosp Ctr - Roosevelt Div (page 94); **Address:** St Luke's-Roosevelt Hosp Ctr, Dept Surg, 1000 10th Ave, rm 5G77, New York, NY 10019; **Phone:** 212-523-7481; **Board Cert:** Surgery 2000; **Med School:** Penn State Univ-Hershey Med Ctr 1974; **Resid:** Surgery, Columbia-Presby Med Ctr 1979; **Fellow:** Vascular Surgery, Columbia-Presby Med Ctr 1980; **Fac Appt:** Prof S, Columbia P&S

Bronx

Addiction Psychiatry

Smith, Michael O MD (AdP) - **Spec Exp:** Addiction/Substance Abuse; Acupuncture; **Hospital:** Lincoln Med & Mental Hlth Ctr; **Address:** 349 E 140th St, Bronx, NY 10454; **Phone:** 718-993-3100 x113; **Med School:** UCSF 1968; **Resid:** Psychiatry, Albert Einstein Med Ctr 1972; **Fac Appt:** Assoc Prof Psyc, Cornell Univ-Weill Med Coll

Adolescent Medicine

Alderman, Elizabeth MD (AM) - **Spec Exp:** Adolescent Gynecology; Eating Disorders; Parenting Issues; **Hospital:** Montefiore Med Ctr - Div. Moses (page 100); **Address:** Children's Hospital at Montefiore, Dept Adolescent Medicine, 2415 Bainbridge Rd, Bronx, NY 10467; **Phone:** 718-920-6614; **Board Cert:** Pediatrics 2005; Adolescent Medicine 2002; **Med School:** SUNY Stony Brook 1987; **Resid:** Pediatrics, Montefiore Med Ctr 1990; **Fellow:** Adolescent Medicine, Montefiore Med Ctr 1992; **Fac Appt:** Clin Prof Ped, Albert Einstein Coll Med

Coupey, Susan MD (AM) - **Spec Exp:** Adolescent Gynecology; Menstrual Disorders; Reproductive Endocrinology; Uterine/Vaginal Agenisis; **Hospital:** Montefiore Med Ctr - Div. Moses (page 100); **Address:** Children's Hosp at Montefiore, Dept Adolescent Medicine, 3415 Bainbridge Rd, Bronx, NY 10467; **Phone:** 718-741-2450; **Board Cert:** Pediatrics 1979; Adolescent Medicine 2009; **Med School:** Canada 1975; **Resid:** Pediatrics, Chldns Hosp 1978; **Fellow:** Adolescent Medicine, Montefiore Hosp Med Ctr 1979; **Fac Appt:** Prof Ped, Albert Einstein Coll Med

Allergy & Immunology

Kaufman, Alan MD (A&I) - **Spec Exp:** Asthma; Sinus Disorders; Urticaria; **Hospital:** Montefiore Med Ctr - Div. Moses (page 100), Lawrence Hosp Ctr; **Address:** 3626 E Tremont Ave, Bronx, NY 10465-2030; **Phone:** 718-597-9000; **Board Cert:** Internal Medicine 1988; Allergy & Immunology 2009; **Med School:** West Indies 1984; **Resid:** Internal Medicine, Metropolitan Hosp Ctr 1987; **Fellow:** Allergy & Immunology, Montefiore Med Ctr 1989

Lehach, Joan G MD (A&I) - **Spec Exp:** Asthma; **Hospital:** St Barnabas Hosp - Bronx, Montefiore Med Ctr - Div. Weiler (page 100); **Address:** 1488 Metropolitan Ave, Ste 12, Bronx, NY 10462; **Phone:** 718-918-1991; **Board Cert:** Internal Medicine 2000; **Med School:** Chile 1985; **Resid:** Internal Medicine, St Barnabas Med Ctr 1988; **Fellow:** Allergy & Immunology, Albert Einstein Med Ctr 1990

Rosenstreich, David L MD (A&I) - **Spec Exp:** Urticaria; Sinusitis; Atopic Dermatitis; **Hospital:** Montefiore Med Ctr - Div. Moses (page 100), Jacobi Med Ctr; **Address:** 1515 Blondell Ave, Fl 2 - Ste 220, Bronx, NY 10461; **Phone:** 866-633-8255; **Board Cert:** Internal Medicine 1972; Allergy & Immunology 1975; Clinical & Laboratory Immunology 1990; **Med School:** NYU Sch Med 1967; **Resid:** Internal Medicine, Albert Einstein Med Ctr 1969; **Fellow:** Allergy & Immunology, Natl Inst Hlth 1972; **Fac Appt:** Prof Med, Albert Einstein Coll Med

Rubinstein, Arye MD/PhD (A&I) - **Spec Exp:** Immune Deficiency; Asthma; Allergy; **Hospital:** Montefiore Med Ctr - Div. Moses (page 100), Montefiore Med Ctr - Div. Weiler (page 100); **Address:** 1180 Morris Park Ave, Montefiore, Bronx, NY 10461-1925; **Phone:** 718-863-8465; **Board Cert:** Pediatrics 1976; Allergy & Immunology 1977; **Med School:** Switzerland 1962; **Resid:** Pediatrics, Tel Aviv Univ Hosp 1967; **Fellow:** Allergy & Immunology, Univ Bern 1969; Allergy & Immunology, Harvard Med Sch 1973; **Fac Appt:** Prof Ped, Albert Einstein Coll Med

Cardiac Electrophysiology

Ferrick, Kevin J MD (CE) - **Spec Exp:** Arrhythmias; **Hospital:** Montefiore Med Ctr - Div. Moses (page 100), Bronx Lebanon Hosp Ctr; **Address:** Arrhythmia Service, 111 E 210 St, Bronx, NY 10467; **Phone:** 718-920-4148; **Board Cert:** Internal Medicine 1981; Cardiac Electrophysiology 2002; Cardiovascular Disease 1983; **Med School:** Med Coll Wisc 1977; **Resid:** Internal Medicine, Montefiore Hospital 1980; **Fellow:** Cardiovascular Disease, Columbia-Presby Med Ctr 1981; Cardiac Electrophysiology, Columbia-Presby Med Ctr 1983; **Fac Appt:** Prof Med, Albert Einstein Coll Med

Gross, Jay MD (CE) - **Spec Exp:** Pacemakers; **Hospital:** Montefiore Med Ctr - Div. Weiler (page 100); **Address:** 111 E 210th St, Arrhythmia Service, Bronx, NY 10467-2490; **Phone:** 718-920-4291; **Board Cert:** Internal Medicine 1986; Cardiovascular Disease 1989; Cardiac Electrophysiology 2002; **Med School:** Albert Einstein Coll Med 1983; **Resid:** Internal Medicine, Montefiore Med Ctr 1986; **Fellow:** Cardiovascular Disease, Montrfiore Med Ctr 1988; **Fac Appt:** Prof Med, Albert Einstein Coll Med

Krumerman, Andrew K MD (CE) - **Spec Exp:** Atrial Fibrillation; Arrhythmias; **Hospital:** Montefiore Med Ctr - Div. Moses (page 100); **Address:** Arrhythmia Service, 111 E 210th St Fl 2, Bronx, NY 10467; **Phone:** 718-920-4776; **Board Cert:** Internal Medicine 1999; Cardiovascular Disease 2003; Cardiac Electrophysiology 2004; **Med School:** Israel 1996; **Resid:** Internal Medicine, Montefiore Med Ctr 1999; **Fellow:** Cardiovascular Disease, N Shore Univ Hosp 2001; Cardiac Electrophysiology, Montefiore Med Ctr 2002

Cardiovascular Disease

Greenberg, Mark A MD (Cv) - **Spec Exp:** Interventional Cardiology; Cardiac Catheterization; Heart Valve Disease; **Hospital:** Montefiore Med Ctr - Div. Moses (page 100); **Address:** 111 E 210th St, Division of Cardiology, Bronx, NY 10467; **Phone:** 718-920-4212; **Board Cert:** Internal Medicine 1973; Cardiovascular Disease 1979; Interventional Cardiology 1999; **Med School:** Univ IL Coll Med 1973; **Resid:** Internal Medicine, Montefiore Hosp Med Ctr 1976; **Fellow:** Cardiovascular Disease, Montefiore Hosp Med Ctr 1978; **Fac Appt:** Clin Prof Med, Albert Einstein Coll Med

Kaufman, David B MD (Cv) - **Spec Exp:** Nuclear Cardiology; **Hospital:** Montefiore Med Ctr - Div. Weiler (page 100); **Address:** Riverdale Heart Ctr, 2600 Netherland Ave, Ste 121, Riverdale, NY 10463; **Phone:** 718-548-1590; **Board Cert:** Internal Medicine 1980; Cardiovascular Disease 1983; **Med School:** Cornell Univ-Weill Med Coll 1977; **Resid:** Internal Medicine, Montefiore Med Ctr 1980; **Fellow:** Cardiovascular Disease, Montefiore Med Ctr 1983

Keller, Peter Karl MD (Cv) - **Spec Exp:** Congestive Heart Failure; Coronary Artery Disease; Arrhythmias; **Hospital:** Montefiore Med Ctr - Div. Weiler (page 100), NY Westchester Sq Med Ctr; **Address:** 1578 Williamsbridge Rd, Bronx, NY 10461-6265; **Phone:** 718-892-7817; **Board Cert:** Internal Medicine 1988; Cardiovascular Disease 2000; **Med School:** Mount Sinai Sch Med 1985; **Resid:** Internal Medicine, Bronx Municipal Hosp 1988; **Fellow:** Cardiovascular Disease, Bronx Municipal Hosp 1991; **Fac Appt:** Assoc Clin Prof Med, Albert Einstein Coll Med

Lucariello, Richard MD (Cv) - **Spec Exp:** Congestive Heart Failure; Angina; Hypertension; **Hospital:** Montefiore Med Ctr - Div. North (page 100); **Address:** 600 E 233 St, Bronx, NY 10466; **Phone:** 718-920-9256; **Board Cert:** Internal Medicine 1987; Cardiovascular Disease 2000; **Med School:** NY Med Coll 1984; **Resid:** Internal Medicine, Westchester Med Ctr 1987; **Fellow:** Cardiovascular Disease, St Vincent's Hosp & Med Ctr 1989; Cardiovascular Disease, Westchester Med Ctr 1990; **Fac Appt:** Assoc Clin Prof Med, NY Med Coll

Menegus, Mark MD (Cv) - **Spec Exp:** Acute Coronary Syndromes; Cardiac Catheterization; Interventional Cardiology; Heart Valve Disease; **Hospital:** Montefiore Med Ctr - Div. Moses (page 100), St Barnabas Hosp - Bronx; **Address:** Montefiore Med Ctr, Dept Cardiology, 111 E 210th St, Bronx, NY 10467-2401; **Phone:** 718-920-5528; **Board Cert:** Internal Medicine 1984; Cardiovascular Disease 1987; Interventional Cardiology 1999; **Med School:** UMDNJ-RW Johnson Med Sch 1981; **Resid:** Internal Medicine, Montefiore Med Ctr 1984; **Fellow:** Cardiovascular Disease, Montefiore Med Ctr 1987; **Fac Appt:** Assoc Prof Med, Albert Einstein Coll Med

Monrad, E Scott MD (Cv) - **Spec Exp:** Coronary Artery Disease; Heart Valve Disease; Cardiac Catheterization; **Hospital:** Montefiore Med Ctr - Div. Weiler (page 100), Jacobi Med Ctr; **Address:** 1628 Eastchester Ave, Bronx, NY 10461; **Phone:** 646-670-5120; **Board Cert:** Internal Medicine 1982; Cardiovascular Disease 1985; Interventional Cardiology 1999; **Med School:** McGill Univ 1979; **Resid:** Internal Medicine, New England Med Ctr 1982; **Fellow:** Cardiovascular Disease, Beth Israel Med Ctr 1985; **Fac Appt:** Clin Prof Med, Albert Einstein Coll Med

Neuberg, Gerald W MD (Cv) - **Spec Exp:** Congestive Heart Failure; **Hospital:** NY-Presby Hosp/Columbia (page 104), NY-Presby Hosp/The Allen Hosp (page 104); **Address:** 3765 Riverdale Ave, Ste 6, Bronx, NY 10463; **Phone:** 718-601-8720; **Board Cert:** Internal Medicine 1986; Cardiovascular Disease 1989; **Med School:** Columbia P&S 1983; **Resid:** Internal Medicine, NY Presby Hosp 1986; **Fellow:** Cardiovascular Disease, Westchester Med Ctr 1988; Cardiovascular Disease, Mt Sinai Med Ctr 1989; **Fac Appt:** Assoc Clin Prof Med, Columbia P&S

Phillips, Malcolm C MD (Cv) - **Spec Exp:** Preventive Cardiology; Echocardiography; Cardiac Stress Testing; **Hospital:** St Barnabas Hosp - Bronx; **Address:** 4422 3rd Ave, Bronx, NY 10457-2545; **Phone:** 718-960-6205; **Board Cert:** Internal Medicine 1979; Cardiovascular Disease 1981; **Med School:** Columbia P&S 1976; **Resid:** Internal Medicine, New York Hosp 1978; **Fellow:** Cardiovascular Disease, New York Hosp 1980; **Fac Appt:** Asst Clin Prof Med, Cornell Univ-Weill Med Coll

Sahar, David I MD (Cv) - **Spec Exp:** Arrhythmias; Atrial Fibrillation; Heart Valve Disease; Coronary Artery Disease; **Hospital:** NY-Presby Hosp/Columbia (page 104); **Address:** 2600 Netherland Ave, Ste 106, Bronx, NY 10463-4813; **Phone:** 212-305-4567; **Board Cert:** Internal Medicine 1983; Cardiovascular Disease 1987; **Med School:** Columbia P&S 1980; **Resid:** Internal Medicine, Ohio State Univ 1983; **Fellow:** Cardiovascular Disease, St Lukes Hosp 1985; Cardiac Electrophysiology, Columbia Presby Hosp 1987; **Fac Appt:** Assoc Prof Med, Columbia P&S

Schick, David MD (Cv) - **Hospital:** Montefiore Med Ctr - Div. Moses (page 100); **Address:** 3201 Grand Concourse, Ste 1J, Bronx, NY 10468-1226; **Phone:** 718-933-2244; **Board Cert:** Internal Medicine 1972; Cardiovascular Disease 1975; **Med School:** Albert Einstein Coll Med 1966; **Resid:** Internal Medicine, Montefiore Hosp 1971; Cardiovascular Disease, Montefiore Hosp 1973; **Fac Appt:** Asst Clin Prof Med, Albert Einstein Coll Med

Silverman, Rubin MD (Cv) - **Spec Exp:** Echocardiography; **Hospital:** St Barnabas Hosp - Bronx, Montefiore Med Ctr - Div. Weiler (page 100); **Address:** 1180 Morris Park Ave, FL 2, Bronx, NY 10461-1925; **Phone:** 718-409-3335; **Board Cert:** Internal Medicine 1981; Cardiovascular Disease 1983; **Med School:** Albert Einstein Coll Med 1978; **Resid:** Internal Medicine, Jacobi Med Ctr 1981; **Fellow:** Cardiovascular Disease, Montefiore Med Ctr 1983; **Fac Appt:** Asst Prof Med, Albert Einstein Coll Med

Child & Adolescent Psychiatry

Gerbino-Rosen, Ginny M MD (ChAP) - **Spec Exp:** Child & Adolescent Psychiatry; Aggression Disorders; **Hospital:** Bronx Children's Psych Ctr; **Address:** Bronx Chldn's Psych Ctr, 1000 Waters Pl, House 8, Bronx, NY 10461-2701; **Phone:** 718-239-3699; **Board Cert:** Psychiatry 1981; Child & Adolescent Psychiatry 1987; Forensic Psychiatry 2009; **Med School:** Creighton Univ 1976; **Resid:** Psychiatry, Bellevue-NYU Med Ctr 1979; **Fellow:** Child & Adolescent Psychiatry, Bellevue-NYU Med Ctr 1981; **Fac Appt:** Asst Prof Psyc, Albert Einstein Coll Med

Lomonaco, Salvatore MD (ChAP) - **Hospital:** Montefiore Med Ctr - Div. Moses (page 100); **Address:** Albert Einstein College Med, 1300 Morris Park Ave, Belfer Bldg - rm 405, Bronx, NY 10461; **Phone:** 718-430-2020; **Board Cert:** Psychiatry 1976; **Med School:** SUNY Downstate 1966; **Resid:** Psychiatry, Montefiore Med Ctr 1971; Child Psychiatry, Montefiore Med Ctr 1972; **Fac Appt:** Assoc Prof Psyc, Albert Einstein Coll Med

Child Neurology

Moshe, Solomon L MD (ChiN) - **Spec Exp:** Epilepsy/Seizure Disorders; **Hospital:** Montefiore Med Ctr - Div. Moses (page 100); **Address:** 111 E 210 St, Bronx, NY 10467; **Phone:** 718-920-4378; **Board Cert:** Pediatrics 1978; Child Neurology 1979; Clinical Neurophysiology 2006; **Med School:** Greece 1972; **Resid:** Pediatrics, Univ MD Hosp 1975; Pediatric Neurology, Albert Einstein 1978; **Fellow:** Neurology, Albert Einstein 1979; **Fac Appt:** Prof N, Albert Einstein Coll Med

Shinnar, Shlomo MD/PhD (ChiN) - **Spec Exp:** Epilepsy/Seizure Disorders; Headache; **Hospital:** Montefiore Med Ctr - Div. Moses (page 100); **Address:** Montefiore Med Ctr, Children's Hospital, 111 E 210th St Fl 4, Bronx, NY 10467-2401; **Phone:** 718-920-4378; **Board Cert:** Neurology 1984; Pediatrics 1984; Clinical Neurophysiology 2005; **Med School:** Albert Einstein Coll Med 1978; **Resid:** Pediatrics, Johns Hopkins Hosp 1980; Neurology, Johns Hopkins Hosp 1983; **Fac Appt:** Prof N, Albert Einstein Coll Med

Clinical Genetics

Gross, Susan MD (CG) - **Spec Exp:** Prenatal Diagnosis; Prenatal Ultrasound; Reproductive Genetics; **Hospital:** Montefiore Med Ctr - Div. Moses (page 100), N Central Bronx Hosp; **Address:** Montefiore Med Ctr, Clinical Genetics, 1695 Eastchester Rd, Ste 301, Bronx, NY 10461; **Phone:** 718-918-6310; **Board Cert:** Obstetrics & Gynecology 2009; Clinical Genetics 2010; **Med School:** Univ Toronto 1985; **Resid:** Obstetrics & Gynecology, Univ Toronto Hosp 1991; **Fellow:** Maternal & Fetal Medicine, Univ Toronto 1992; Clinical Genetics, Univ Tenn 1994; **Fac Appt:** Prof ObG, Albert Einstein Coll Med

Marion, Robert W MD (CG) - **Spec Exp:** Spina Bifida; Williams Syndrome; Marfan's Syndrome; Down Syndrome; **Hospital:** Montefiore Med Ctr - Div. Moses (page 100), Blythedale Children's Hosp; **Address:** 3415 Bainbridge Ave, Bronx, NY 10467; **Phone:** 718-741-2323; **Board Cert:** Pediatrics 1985; Clinical Genetics 1987; **Med School:** Albert Einstein Coll Med 1979; **Resid:** Pediatrics, Montefiore Med Ctr 1982; **Fellow:** Clinical Genetics, Montefiore Med Ctr 1984; **Fac Appt:** Prof Ped, Albert Einstein Coll Med

Critical Care Medicine

Siegel, Robert MD (CCM) - **Spec Exp:** Pneumonia; Infectious Disease; **Hospital:** VA Med Ctr - Bronx, Mount Sinai Med Ctr (page 102); **Address:** 130 W Kingsbridge Rd, Ste 8C, Bronx, NY 10468-3992; **Phone:** 718-584-9000 x6723; **Board Cert:** Internal Medicine 1982; Pulmonary Disease 1986; Critical Care Medicine 2009; **Med School:** Columbia P&S 1979; **Resid:** Internal Medicine, St Luke's Hosp 1982; Internal Medicine, Booth Meml Hosp 1983; **Fellow:** Pulmonary Disease, Bronx Municipal Hosp 1985; **Fac Appt:** Assoc Clin Prof Med, Mount Sinai Sch Med

Dermatology

Cohen, Steven R MD (D) - **Spec Exp:** Occupational Dermatology; Contact Dermatitis; Psoriasis; **Hospital:** Montefiore Med Ctr - Div. Moses (page 100); **Address:** 3514 Bainbridge Ave, Bronx, NY 10467; **Phone:** 866-633-8255; **Board Cert:** Dermatology 2009; **Med School:** Univ Pennsylvania 1971; **Resid:** Dermatology, Yale-New Haven Hosp 1977; **Fac Appt:** Prof D, Albert Einstein Coll Med

Katz, Susan MD (D) - **Spec Exp:** Psoriasis; Skin Cancer & Moles; Cutaneous Lymphoma; Cosmetic Dermatology; **Hospital:** Montefiore Med Ctr - Div. Weiler (page 100); **Address:** 1578 Williamsbridge Rd, Bronx, NY 10461-6265; **Phone:** 718-518-8888; **Board Cert:** Dermatology 2009; **Med School:** NYU Sch Med 1977; **Resid:** Internal Medicine, Roosevelt Hosp 1979; Dermatology, Montefiore Med Ctr 1983; **Fac Appt:** Asst Clin Prof D, Albert Einstein Coll Med

Liteplo, Ronald R MD (D) - **Spec Exp:** Melanoma; Skin Diseases-Immunologic; **Hospital:** Montefiore Med Ctr - Div. Moses (page 100); **Address:** 3176 Bainbridge Ave, Bronx, NY 10467-3980; **Phone:** 718-515-0200; **Board Cert:** Internal Medicine 1975; Dermatology 1978; **Med School:** NYU Sch Med 1972; **Resid:** Internal Medicine, Univ Hosp 1975; Dermatology, Univ Hosp 1978; **Fellow:** Immunology, Univ Hosp 1976; **Fac Appt:** Asst Clin Prof Med, Albert Einstein Coll Med

Rosen, Douglas MD (D) - **Spec Exp:** Skin Cancer; Hair Removal-Laser; Acne; **Hospital:** NY Westchester Sq Med Ctr; **Address:** 3620 E Tremont Ave, FL 2, Bronx, NY 10465-2022; **Phone:** 718-792-4700; **Board Cert:** Dermatology 1984; **Med School:** Albert Einstein Coll Med 1980; **Resid:** Dermatology, Montefiore Hosp Med Ctr 1984; **Fac Appt:** Assoc Prof D, Albert Einstein Coll Med

Rudikoff, Donald MD (D) - **Spec Exp:** AIDS Related Skin Disorders; Skin Infections; Smallpox; **Hospital:** Bronx Lebanon Hosp Ctr; **Address:** 2737 3rd Ave, Bronx, NY 10451; **Phone:** 718-838-1016; **Board Cert:** Internal Medicine 1980; Dermatology 2009; **Med School:** NY Med Coll 1973; **Resid:** Internal Medicine, Beth Israel Med Ctr 1980; Dermatology, Mount Sinai Hosp 1982; **Fac Appt:** Assoc Prof D, Mount Sinai Sch Med

Diagnostic Radiology

Amis Jr, E Stephen MD (DR) - **Spec Exp:** Urologic Imaging; **Hospital:** Montefiore Med Ctr - Div. Moses (page 100); **Address:** Montefiore Med Ctr, Dept Radiology, 111 E 210th St, Bronx, NY 10467; **Phone:** 718-920-5113; **Board Cert:** Urology 1975; Diagnostic Radiology 1979; **Med School:** Northwestern Univ 1967; **Resid:** Urology, US Naval Hosp 1972; Diagnostic Radiology, US Naval Hosp 1978; **Fellow:** Urologic Radiology, Mass General Hosp 1981; **Fac Appt:** Prof, Albert Einstein Coll Med

Friedman, Stanley N MD (DR) - **Hospital:** NY Westchester Sq Med Ctr; **Address:** NY Westchester Sq Med Ctr, Dept Rad, 2475 St Raymond Ave, Bronx, NY 10461-3124; **Phone:** 718-430-7321; **Board Cert:** Diagnostic Radiology 1974; **Med School:** NY Med Coll 1968; **Resid:** Diagnostic Radiology, Mt Sinai Hosp 1970; Radiation Oncology, Albert Einstein 1972; **Fellow:** Diagnostic Radiology, Mt Sinai Hosp 1973; **Fac Appt:** Asst Clin Prof, Cornell Univ-Weill Med Coll

Haramati, Linda B MD (DR) - **Spec Exp:** AIDS/HIV; Lung Cancer; **Hospital:** Montefiore Med Ctr - Div. Moses (page 100), Jacobi Med Ctr; **Address:** Montefiore Med Ctr, Dept Radiology, 111 E 210th St, Bronx, NY 10467-2401; **Phone:** 718-920-7458; **Board Cert:** Diagnostic Radiology 1990; **Med School:** Albert Einstein Coll Med 1985; **Resid:** Diagnostic Radiology, Montefiore Med Ctr 1990; **Fellow:** Thoracic Radiology, Columbia-Presby Med Ctr 1991; **Fac Appt:** Prof, Albert Einstein Coll Med

Haramati, Nogah MD (DR) - **Spec Exp:** Orthopaedic Imaging; Rheumatology; Musculoskeletal Imaging; **Hospital:** Montefiore Med Ctr - Div. Moses (page 100), Jacobi Med Ctr; **Address:** 1825 Eastchester Rd, rm 3-006, Bronx, NY 10461; **Phone:** 718-904-2965; **Board Cert:** Diagnostic Radiology 1990; **Med School:** SUNY Hlth Sci Ctr 1985; **Resid:** Diagnostic Radiology, Montefiore Hosp Med Ctr 1990; **Fellow:** Musculoskeletal Imaging, Columbia-Presby Med Ctr 1991; **Fac Appt:** Clin Prof Rad, Albert Einstein Coll Med

Koenigsberg, Mordecai MD (DR) - **Spec Exp:** Ultrasound; **Hospital:** Montefiore Med Ctr - Div. Weiler (page 100); **Address:** Montefiore Med Ctr-Weiler Einstein, 1825 Eastchester Rd, rm 3035, Bronx, NY 10475; **Phone:** 718-904-2322; **Board Cert:** Pediatrics 1970; Nuclear Medicine 1973; Diagnostic Radiology 1974; **Med School:** Albert Einstein Coll Med 1963; **Resid:** Pediatrics, Jacobi Med Ctr 1966; Diagnostic Radiology, Jacobi Med Ctr 1974; **Fac Appt:** Prof Rad, Albert Einstein Coll Med

Laks, Mitchell MD (DR) - **Spec Exp:** MRI; Ultrasound; CT Body Scan; **Hospital:** Montefiore Med Ctr - Div. Moses (page 100); **Address:** Montefiore Med Ctr, Dept Rad, 111 E 210th St, Bronx, NY 10467; **Phone:** 718-920-4396; **Board Cert:** Diagnostic Radiology 1990; **Med School:** Harvard Med Sch 1985; **Resid:** Diagnostic Radiology, Albert Einstein 1990; **Fellow:** Magnetic Resonance Imaging, Brigham Women's Hosp 1991; **Fac Appt:** Asst Prof Rad, Albert Einstein Coll Med

Morehouse, Helen MD (DR) - **Spec Exp:** Genitourinary Imaging; MRI; Ultrasound; **Hospital:** Bronx Lebanon Hosp Ctr; **Address:** Bronx Lebanon Hosp, Dept Radiology, 1650 Grand Concourse, Bronx, NY 10457-7606; **Phone:** 718-518-5272; **Board Cert:** Diagnostic Radiology 1976; **Med School:** Univ KY Coll Med 1971; **Resid:** Diagnostic Radiology, Rochester Genl Hosp 1975; **Fellow:** Diagnostic Radiology, Downstate Med Ctr 1976; **Fac Appt:** Prof, Albert Einstein Coll Med

Rozenblit, Alla MD (DR) - **Spec Exp:** Liver Disease; CT Scan; MRI; **Hospital:** Montefiore Med Ctr - Div. Moses (page 100); **Address:** 111 E 210th St, Bronx, NY 10467-2401; **Phone:** 718-920-4396; **Board Cert:** Diagnostic Radiology 1984; **Med School:** Russia 1971; **Resid:** Diagnostic Radiology, Queens Hosp Ctr 1984; **Fellow:** Ultrasound/CT, LI Jewish Med Ctr 1985; **Fac Appt:** Clin Prof Rad, Albert Einstein Coll Med

Spindola-Franco, Hugo MD (DR) - **Spec Exp:** Cardiac Imaging; Congenital Heart Disease; Thoracic Radiology; **Hospital:** Montefiore Med Ctr - Div. Moses (page 100); **Address:** 111 E 210th St, Bronx, NY 10467-2401; **Phone:** 718-920-4872; **Board Cert:** Diagnostic Radiology 1970; **Med School:** Mexico 1966; **Resid:** Diagnostic Radiology, Montefiore Hosp Med Ctr 1970; **Fellow:** Cardiovascular Radiology, Peter Bent Brigham Hosp/Harvard Med Sch 1971; **Fac Appt:** Prof, Albert Einstein Coll Med

Stern, Harvey MD (DR) - **Spec Exp:** Nuclear Medicine; **Hospital:** Bronx Lebanon Hosp Ctr; **Address:** 1650 Grand Concourse, Bronx, NY 10457-7606; **Phone:** 718-518-5030; **Board Cert:** Diagnostic Radiology 1975; Nuclear Radiology 1978; **Med School:** Albert Einstein Coll Med 1971; **Resid:** Diagnostic Radiology, Bronx Municipal Hosp 1975; **Fac Appt:** Asst Prof Rad, Albert Einstein Coll Med

Swirsky, Michael MD (DR) - **Spec Exp:** Mammography; Gastrointestinal Imaging; CT Scan; Abdominal Imaging; **Hospital:** Montefiore Med Ctr - Div. North (page 100), White Plains Hosp Ctr; **Address:** 600 E 233rd St, Dept Radiology, Bronx, NY 10466; **Phone:** 718-920-9188; **Board Cert:** Diagnostic Radiology 1979; **Med School:** Case West Res Univ 1975; **Resid:** Diagnostic Radiology, Strong Meml Hosp 1979; **Fac Appt:** Assoc Prof Rad, NY Med Coll

Wolf, Ellen L MD (DR) - **Spec Exp:** Gastrointestinal Imaging; Abdominal Imaging; **Hospital:** Montefiore Med Ctr - Div. Moses (page 100); **Address:** 111 E 210th St, Bronx, NY 10467; **Phone:** 718-920-4851; **Board Cert:** Diagnostic Radiology 1976; **Med School:** Mount Sinai Sch Med 1972; **Resid:** Diagnostic Radiology, Columbia-Presby 1974; Diagnostic Radiology, Johns Hopkins 1976; **Fellow:** Pediatric Radiology, Columbia-Presby 1977; **Fac Appt:** Clin Prof Rad, Albert Einstein Coll Med

Endocrinology, Diabetes & Metabolism

Allen, Carol B MD (EDM) - **Spec Exp:** Diabetes; **Hospital:** VA Med Ctr - Bronx; **Address:** 130 W Kingsbridge Rd, Primary Care, Bronx, NY 10468-3904; **Phone:** 718-584-9000 x3777; **Board Cert:** Internal Medicine 1982; **Med School:** Univ Pennsylvania 1979; **Resid:** Internal Medicine, VA Med Ctr 1982; **Fellow:** Endocrinology, Diabetes & Metabolism, VA Med Ctr 1984

Cohen, Charmian MD (EDM) - **Spec Exp:** Diabetes; Thyroid Disorders; Obesity; **Hospital:** Montefiore Med Ctr - Div. Weiler (page 100); **Address:** 1200 Waters Pl, Ste M105, Bronx, NY 10461; **Phone:** 718-892-7033; **Board Cert:** Internal Medicine 1987; Endocrinology, Diabetes & Metabolism 1989; **Med School:** South Africa 1977; **Resid:** Internal Medicine, G Schuer Hosp 1984; **Fellow:** Endocrinology, Diabetes & Metabolism, Albert Einstein 1986; **Fac Appt:** Asst Prof Med, Albert Einstein Coll Med

Grajower, Martin M MD (EDM) - **Spec Exp:** Diabetes; Osteoporosis; **Hospital:** Montefiore Med Ctr - Div. Moses (page 100); **Address:** 3736 Henry Hudson Pkwy E, Riverdale, NY 10463; **Phone:** 718-549-6268; **Board Cert:** Internal Medicine 1987; Endocrinology, Diabetes & Metabolism 1981; **Med School:** Albert Einstein Coll Med 1973; **Resid:** Internal Medicine, Montefiore Hosp Med Ctr 1975; Internal Medicine, Boston Med Ctr 1976; **Fellow:** Endocrinology, Diabetes & Metabolism, Montefiore Hosp Med Ctr 1978; **Fac Appt:** Asst Prof Med, Albert Einstein Coll Med

Guzman, Rodolfo MD (EDM) - **Spec Exp:** Endocrinology; Diabetes; Thyroid Disorders; **Hospital:** Bronx Lebanon Hosp Ctr; **Address:** 860 Grand Concourse, Ste 1K, Bronx, NY 10451; **Phone:** 718-585-5060; **Board Cert:** Internal Medicine 2000; Endocrinology, Diabetes & Metabolism 2000; **Med School:** Dominican Republic 1979; **Resid:** Internal Medicine, Bronx Lebanon Hosp 1990; **Fellow:** Endocrinology, Diabetes & Metabolism, Lincoln Med Ctr 1992

Shamoon, Harry MD (EDM) - **Hospital:** Montefiore Med Ctr - Div. Weiler (page 100); **Address:** 1575 Blondell Ave, Ste 200, Bronx, NY 10461-2601; **Phone:** 718-405-8260; **Board Cert:** Internal Medicine 1977; Endocrinology, Diabetes & Metabolism 1979; **Med School:** Yale Univ 1974; **Resid:** Internal Medicine, Jacobi Med Ctr 1977; **Fellow:** Endocrinology, Diabetes & Metabolism, Yale-New Haven Hosp 1979; **Fac Appt:** Prof Med, Albert Einstein Coll Med

Surks, Martin MD (EDM) - **Spec Exp:** Thyroid Disorders; **Hospital:** Montefiore Med Ctr - Div. Moses (page 100), N Central Bronx Hosp; **Address:** 3400 Bainbridge Ave Fl 2, Bronx, NY 10467; **Phone:** 866-633-8255; **Board Cert:** Internal Medicine 1967; Endocrinology, Diabetes & Metabolism 1977; **Med School:** NYU Sch Med 1960; **Resid:** Internal Medicine, Montefiore Hosp Med Ctr 1962; Internal Medicine, VA Hosp 1964; **Fellow:** Research, Natl Inst Arthritis-Metabolic Disease 1964; **Fac Appt:** Prof Med, Albert Einstein Coll Med

Zonszein, Joel MD (EDM) - **Spec Exp:** Thyroid Disorders; Diabetes; **Hospital:** Montefiore Med Ctr - Div. Moses (page 100); **Address:** 1575 Blondell Ave, Ste 200, Bronx, NY 10461; **Phone:** 718-405-8260; **Board Cert:** Nuclear Medicine 1976; Internal Medicine 1977; Endocrinology 1977; **Med School:** Mexico 1969; **Resid:** Internal Medicine, Maimonides Med Ctr 1972; Internal Medicine, Jacobi Med Ctr 1973; **Fellow:** Endocrinology, Northwestern Univ Med Sch 1974; Endocrinology, Georgetown Univ Hosp 1975; **Fac Appt:** Assoc Prof Med, Albert Einstein Coll Med

Family Medicine

Biagiotti, Wendy MD (FMed) *PCP* - **Hospital:** Montefiore Med Ctr - Div. Moses (page 100); **Address:** 3101 E Tremont Ave, Bronx, NY 10461; **Phone:** 718-863-7925; **Board Cert:** Family Medicine 2009; **Med School:** Mexico 1988; **Resid:** Family Medicine, St Joseph's Hosp&Med Ctr 1994

Coloka-Kump, Rodika DO (FMed) *PCP* - **Spec Exp:** Preventive Medicine; **Hospital:** Saint Joseph's Med Ctr - Yonkers, St John's Riverside Hosp; **Address:** 530 W 236th St, rm #1D, Bronx, NY 10463; **Phone:** 718-548-4560; **Board Cert:** Family Medicine 2004; **Med School:** NY Coll Osteo Med 1988; **Resid:** Family Medicine, NY Methodist Hosp 1989St Joseph's Med Ctr 1991

Cordero, Evelyn MD (FMed) *PCP* - **Hospital:** Montefiore Med Ctr - Div. North (page 100), NY Westchester Sq Med Ctr; **Address:** 941 Castle Hill Ave, Bronx, NY 10473; **Phone:** 718-792-3117; **Board Cert:** Family Medicine 2003; **Med School:** SUNY Hlth Sci Ctr 1979; **Resid:** Family Medicine, St Joseph's Med Ctr 1982

Delaney, Brian MD (FMed) *PCP* - **Spec Exp:** Geriatric Care; **Hospital:** Montefiore Med Ctr - Div. Moses (page 100), St Barnabas Hosp - Bronx; **Address:** 2371 Arthur Ave, Bronx, NY 10458; **Phone:** 718-364-6199; **Board Cert:** Family Medicine 2007; Geriatric Medicine 2002; **Med School:** Albert Einstein Coll Med 1983; **Resid:** Family Medicine, Montefiore Med Ctr 1986; **Fac Appt:** Asst Prof FMed, Albert Einstein Coll Med

Franzetti, Carl J DO (FMed) *PCP* - **Spec Exp:** Diabetes; **Hospital:** Saint Joseph's Med Ctr - Yonkers, NY-Presby Hosp/Columbia (page 104); **Address:** 3125 Tibbett Ave, Bronx, NY 10463-3897; **Phone:** 718-543-2700; **Board Cert:** Family Medicine 2005; **Med School:** NY Coll Osteo Med 1984; **Resid:** Family Medicine, Warren Hosp 1987

Maselli, Frank J MD (FMed) *PCP* - **Spec Exp:** Diving Medicine; Hyperbaric Medicine; **Hospital:** Saint Joseph's Med Ctr - Yonkers, NY-Presby Hosp/Columbia (page 104); **Address:** 3125 Tibbett Ave, Bronx, NY 10463; **Phone:** 718-543-2700; **Board Cert:** Family Medicine 2004; **Med School:** Israel 1983; **Resid:** Family Medicine, Univ Hosp 1986; **Fac Appt:** Asst Prof FMed, SUNY Downstate

Morrow, Robert MD (FMed) *PCP* - **Spec Exp:** Preventive Medicine; Geriatric Medicine; Autism; **Hospital:** Montefiore Med Ctr - Div. Moses (page 100), Saint Joseph's Med Ctr - Yonkers; **Address:** 5997 Riverdale Ave, Bronx, NY 10471-1602; **Phone:** 718-884-9803; **Board Cert:** Geriatric Medicine 1998; Family Medicine 2009; **Med School:** Mount Sinai Sch Med 1974; **Resid:** Family Medicine, Montefiore Med Ctr 1977; **Fac Appt:** Assoc Clin Prof FMed, Albert Einstein Coll Med

Soloway, Bruce H MD (FMed) *PCP* - **Spec Exp:** AIDS/HIV; **Hospital:** Montefiore Med Ctr - Div. Moses (page 100); **Address:** Montefiore Medical Center, 360 E 193 St, Bronx, NY 10458; **Phone:** 718-933-2400; **Board Cert:** Family Medicine 2007; **Med School:** Albert Einstein Coll Med 1985; **Resid:** Family Medicine, Montefiore Med Ctr 1988; **Fac Appt:** Assoc Prof FMed, Albert Einstein Coll Med

Gastroenterology

Abelow, Arthur MD (Ge) - **Spec Exp:** Endoscopy; Nutrition; **Hospital:** Montefiore Med Ctr - Div. Weiler (page 100), NY Westchester Sq Med Ctr; **Address:** 1200 Waters Pl, Ste M100, Bronx, NY 10461; **Phone:** 718-863-7397; **Board Cert:** Internal Medicine 1983; Gastroenterology 1985; **Med School:** Albert Einstein Coll Med 1980; **Resid:** Internal Medicine, Bronx Muni Hosp Ctr 1983; **Fellow:** Gastroenterology, Montefiore Med Ctr 1985; **Fac Appt:** Asst Clin Prof Med, Albert Einstein Coll Med

Antony, Michael MD (Ge) - **Spec Exp:** Colonoscopy; Endoscopy; Liver Disease; **Hospital:** Montefiore Med Ctr - Div. Weiler (page 100), NY Westchester Sq Med Ctr; **Address:** 1842 Williamsbridge Rd, Bronx, NY 10461; **Phone:** 718-828-0100; **Board Cert:** Internal Medicine 1985; Gastroenterology 1989; **Med School:** SUNY Hlth Sci Ctr 1982; **Resid:** Internal Medicine, Bronx Muni Hosp 1985; **Fellow:** Gastroenterology, Montefiore Hosp Med Ctr 1988; **Fac Appt:** Assoc Clin Prof Med, Albert Einstein Coll Med

Brandt, Lawrence MD (Ge) - **Spec Exp:** Inflammatory Bowel Disease; Clostridium Difficile Disease; **Hospital:** Montefiore Med Ctr - Div. Moses (page 100), Montefiore Med Ctr - Div. Weiler (page 100); **Address:** 3400 Bainbridge Ave Fl 2, Bronx, NY 10467-2401; **Phone:** 866-633-8255; **Board Cert:** Internal Medicine 1972; Gastroenterology 2006; **Med School:** SUNY Downstate 1968; **Resid:** Internal Medicine, Mt Sinai Hosp 1972; **Fellow:** Gastroenterology, Mt Sinai Hosp 1972; **Fac Appt:** Prof Med, Albert Einstein Coll Med

Frager, Joseph MD (Ge) - **Spec Exp:** Colon Cancer; Endoscopy; Laser Surgery; **Hospital:** Montefiore Med Ctr - Div. Moses (page 100), NY Hosp Queens; **Address:** 277 Van Cortlandt Ave E, Bronx, NY 10467-3011; **Phone:** 718-798-8867; **Board Cert:** Internal Medicine 1983; Gastroenterology 1985; **Med School:** Univ Pennsylvania 1980; **Resid:** Internal Medicine, Montefiore Med Ctr 1983; **Fellow:** Gastroenterology, Montefiore Med Ctr 1985; **Fac Appt:** Asst Clin Prof Med, Albert Einstein Coll Med

Greenwald, David A MD (Ge) - **Spec Exp:** Endoscopy; Gastroesophageal Reflux Disease (GERD); Peptic Ulcer Disease; **Hospital:** Montefiore Med Ctr - Div. Moses (page 100), Montefiore Med Ctr - Div. Weiler (page 100); **Address:** Montefiore Med Ctr, Div Gastroenterology, 111 E 210th St, Bronx, NY 10467; **Phone:** 718-920-4846; **Board Cert:** Internal Medicine 1989; Gastroenterology 2003; **Med School:** Albert Einstein Coll Med 1986; **Resid:** Internal Medicine, Columbia Presby Med Ctr 1989; **Fellow:** Gastroenterology, Columbia Presby Med Ctr 1993; **Fac Appt:** Assoc Prof Med, Albert Einstein Coll Med

Gupta, Sanjeev MD (Ge) - **Spec Exp:** Hepatitis; Liver Disease; Gastrointestinal Disorders; **Hospital:** Montefiore Med Ctr - Div. Weiler (page 100); **Address:** 1515 Blondell Ave, Ste 220, Bronx, NY 10461-2601; **Phone:** 866-633-8255; **Board Cert:** Internal Medicine 1989; **Med School:** India 1977; **Resid:** Internal Medicine, PGIMER 1981; Internal Medicine, Hammersmith Hosp 1982; **Fellow:** Gastroenterology, Hammersmith Hosp 1985; Hepatology, LAC-USC Med Ctr 1987; **Fac Appt:** Prof Med, Albert Einstein Coll Med

Gutwein, Isadore P MD (Ge) - **Spec Exp:** Pancreatic/Biliary Endoscopy (ERCP); Colonoscopy; Hepatitis; Inflammatory Bowel Disease/Crohn's; **Hospital:** Montefiore Med Ctr - Div. Moses (page 100); **Address:** 3765 Riverdale Ave, Bronx, NY 10463-1845; **Phone:** 718-549-4267; **Board Cert:** Internal Medicine 1976; Gastroenterology 1979; **Med School:** Albert Einstein Coll Med 1973; **Resid:** Internal Medicine, Montefiore Hosp Med Ctr 1976; **Fellow:** Gastroenterology, St Luke's Hosp 1978; **Fac Appt:** Asst Prof Med, Albert Einstein Coll Med

Hertan, Hilary I MD (Ge) - **Spec Exp:** Endoscopic Ultrasound; **Hospital:** Montefiore Med Ctr - Div. North (page 100); **Address:** Dept Gastroenterology, 600 E 233rd St Fl 4, Bronx, NY 10466; **Phone:** 718-920-9887; **Board Cert:** Internal Medicine 1986; Gastroenterology 1989; **Med School:** NY Med Coll 1982; **Resid:** Internal Medicine, North Shore Univ Hosp 1985; **Fellow:** Gastroenterology, Our Lady of Mercy Med Ctr 1990; **Fac Appt:** Asst Prof Med, NY Med Coll

Korsten, Mark A MD (Ge) - **Spec Exp:** Constipation; Gastrointestinal Motility Disorders; Spinal Cord Injury & Colonic Motility; Liver Disease; **Hospital:** Mount Sinai Med Ctr (page 102), VA Med Ctr - Bronx; **Address:** 130 W Kingsbridge Rd, Bronx, NY 10468-3904; **Phone:** 718-584-9000 x6753; **Board Cert:** Internal Medicine 1973; Gastroenterology 1975; **Med School:** Yale Univ 1970; **Resid:** Internal Medicine, Mt Sinai Hosp 1973; **Fellow:** Gastroenterology, Mt Sinai Hosp 1975; **Fac Appt:** Prof Med, Mount Sinai Sch Med

Mehta, Rekha MD (Ge) - **Spec Exp:** Palliative Care; **Hospital:** Calvary Hosp (page 110); **Address:** 1740 Eastchester Rd, Bronx, NY 10461; **Phone:** 718-518-2208; **Board Cert:** Internal Medicine 1984; Gastroenterology 1987; **Med School:** India 1972; **Resid:** Internal Medicine, New Rochelle Med Ctr 1977; **Fellow:** Gastroenterology, Univ of South Carolina 1981; Nutrition, Univ of Pitt Sch of Med 1989; **Fac Appt:** Asst Clin Prof Med, NY Med Coll

Remy, Prospere MD (Ge) - **Spec Exp:** Liver Disease; **Hospital:** Bronx Lebanon Hosp Ctr; **Address:** 860 Grand Concourse, Ste 1A, Bronx, NY 10451-2815; **Phone:** 718-585-5060; **Board Cert:** Internal Medicine 2004; Gastroenterology 2004; **Med School:** Mexico 1984; **Resid:** Internal Medicine, Bronx Lebanon Hosp 1990; **Fellow:** Gastroenterology, Bronx Lebanon Hosp 1992; **Fac Appt:** Asst Prof Med, Albert Einstein Coll Med

Sable, Robert A MD (Ge) - **Spec Exp:** Hepatitis B & C; Gastroesophageal Reflux Disease (GERD); Inflammatory Bowel Disease; Irritable Bowel Syndrome; **Hospital:** Montefiore Med Ctr - Div. Moses (page 100), St Barnabas Hosp - Bronx; **Address:** 3765 Riverdale Ave, Ste 7, Bronx, NY 10463-1845; **Phone:** 718-543-3636; **Board Cert:** Internal Medicine 1987; Gastroenterology 2000; Geriatric Medicine 2000; **Med School:** Albert Einstein Coll Med 1973; **Resid:** Internal Medicine, Montefiore Hosp Med Ctr 1976; **Fellow:** Gastroenterology, NY Med Coll 1978; **Fac Appt:** Asst Prof Med, Albert Einstein Coll Med

Schweitzer, Philip E MD (Ge) - **Spec Exp:** Liver Disease; Gastrointestinal Disorders; Esophageal Disorders; **Hospital:** Montefiore Med Ctr - Div. Moses (page 100), Montefiore Med Ctr - Div. North (page 100); **Address:** 3184 Grand Concourse, Ste 2D, Bronx, NY 10458-1031; **Phone:** 718-584-0404; **Board Cert:** Internal Medicine 1972; Gastroenterology 1977; **Med School:** Cornell Univ-Weill Med Coll 1967; **Resid:** Internal Medicine, St Lukes-Roosevelt Hosp 1972; **Fellow:** Gastroenterology, Mount Sinai Hosp 1974

Sherman, Howard I MD (Ge) - **Spec Exp:** Colonoscopy; Biliary Disease; **Hospital:** Montefiore Med Ctr - Div. Weiler (page 100), NY Westchester Sq Med Ctr; **Address:** 1200 Waters Ave, Ste M100, Bronx, NY 10461-3000; **Phone:** 718-863-7397; **Board Cert:** Internal Medicine 1976; Gastroenterology 1979; **Med School:** Albert Einstein Coll Med 1973; **Resid:** Internal Medicine, Emory Univ Hosp 1976; **Fellow:** Gastroenterology, Emory Univ Hosp 1978; **Fac Appt:** Assoc Clin Prof Med, Albert Einstein Coll Med

Stein, David F MD (Ge) - **Spec Exp:** Liver Disease; Hepatitis B & C; HIV & Hepatitis co-infection; Endoscopy; **Hospital:** Montefiore Med Ctr - Div. Moses (page 100), St Barnabas Hosp - Bronx; **Address:** Riverdale Gastro & Liver Diseases, 3765 Riverdale Ave, Ste 7, Bronx, NY 10463; **Phone:** 718-549-4267; **Board Cert:** Gastroenterology 2008; **Med School:** SUNY Downstate 1990; **Resid:** Internal Medicine, NYU/Bellvue Med Ctr/VA Med Ctr 1994; **Fellow:** Gastroenterology, NYU Med Ctr/Bellvue Med Ctr/VA Med Ctr 1996; **Fac Appt:** Asst Clin Prof Med, Albert Einstein Coll Med

Geriatric Medicine

Dharmarajan, Thiruvinvamvalai MD (Ger) - **Spec Exp:** Kidney Disease; **Hospital:** Montefiore Med Ctr - Div. North (page 100); **Address:** 600 E 233rd St, Bronx, NY 10468; **Phone:** 718-920-9041; **Board Cert:** Internal Medicine 1977; Geriatric Medicine 1998; Nephrology 1980; **Med School:** India 1967; **Resid:** Internal Medicine, Misericordia Hosp 1977; **Fellow:** Nephrology, Misericordia Hosp 1979; **Fac Appt:** Prof Med, NY Med Coll

Goldberg, Roy J MD (Ger) *PCP* - **Spec Exp:** Long Term Care; Medications in the Elderly; Palliative Care; **Hospital:** Montefiore Med Ctr - Div. Weiler (page 100), Sound Shore Med Ctr - Westchester; **Address:** Director-Kings Harbor Multicare Ctr, 2000 E Gunhill Rd, Bronx, NY 10469; **Phone:** 718-405-3535; **Board Cert:** Internal Medicine 1985; Geriatric Medicine 2002; **Med School:** Albert Einstein Coll Med 1982; **Resid:** Internal Medicine, Montefiore Med Ctr 1985; **Fac Appt:** Assoc Clin Prof Med, Albert Einstein Coll Med

Jacobs, Laurie MD (Ger) *PCP* - **Spec Exp:** Stroke; Vein Disorders; **Hospital:** Montefiore Med Ctr - Div. Moses (page 100); **Address:** Montefiore Med Ctr, Dept Geriatrics, 3400 Bainbridge Ave, Bronx, NY 10467; **Phone:** 866-633-8255; **Board Cert:** Internal Medicine 1988; Geriatric Medicine 2002; **Med School:** Columbia P&S 1985; **Resid:** Internal Medicine, Montefiore Med Ctr 1988; **Fellow:** Geriatric Medicine, Montefiore Med Ctr 1990; **Fac Appt:** Clin Prof Med, Albert Einstein Coll Med

Malik, Rubina MD (Ger) *PCP* - **Spec Exp:** Osteoporosis; **Hospital:** Montefiore Med Ctr - Div. Moses (page 100); **Address:** MMC Greene Med Arts, Pavilion, 3400 Bainbridge Ave, Bronx, NY 10467; **Phone:** 866-633-8255; **Board Cert:** Internal Medicine 2006; Geriatric Medicine 2009; **Med School:** SUNY Stony Brook 1992; **Resid:** Internal Medicine, Univ Hosp 1993; Gastroenterology, Univ Hosp 1996; **Fac Appt:** , Albert Einstein Coll Med

Russell, Robin MD (Ger) - **Spec Exp:** Kidney Failure; Kidney Disease; Geriatric Dialysis; **Hospital:** Montefiore Med Ctr - Div. North (page 100); **Address:** 4234 Bronx Blvd, Medical Village Geriatrics, Bronx, NY 10466; **Phone:** 347-341-9340; **Board Cert:** Internal Medicine 1974; Nephrology 1980; Geriatric Medicine 2002; **Med School:** Univ New Mexico 1971; **Resid:** Internal Medicine, Harlem Hosp 1974; **Fellow:** Nephrology, Harlem Hosp 1976; **Fac Appt:** Asst Prof Med, NY Med Coll

Geriatric Psychiatry

Kennedy, Gary MD (GerPsy) - **Spec Exp:** Alzheimer's Disease; Dementia; Depression; **Hospital:** Montefiore Med Ctr - Div. Moses (page 100); **Address:** Dept Psyc & Behav Science, Montefiore Medical Center, 111 E 210th St, Bronx, NY 10467; **Phone:** 718-920-4236; **Board Cert:** Psychiatry 1980; Geriatric Psychiatry 2000; Psychosomatic Medicine 2005; **Med School:** Univ Tex, San Antonio 1975; **Resid:** Psychiatry, VA Hosp-Univ Texas 1979; **Fellow:** Geriatric Psychiatry, Montefiore Med Ctr 1981; Psychosomatic Medicine, Montefiore Med Ctr 1983; **Fac Appt:** Prof Psyc, Albert Einstein Coll Med

Gynecologic Oncology

Smith, Harriet O MD (GO) - **Spec Exp:** Uterine Cancer; Pelvic Reconstruction; Ovarian Cancer; **Hospital:** Montefiore Med Ctr - Div. Moses (page 100), Jacobi Med Ctr; **Address:** 1695 Eastchester Rd, Ste 601, Bronx, NY 10461; **Phone:** 718-405-8082; **Board Cert:** Obstetrics & Gynecology 2009; Gynecologic Oncology 2009; **Med School:** Med Coll GA 1981; **Resid:** Obstetrics & Gynecology, Med Coll Georgia 1985; Gynecologic Oncology, MD Anderson Cancer Ctr 1988; **Fellow:** Reconstructive Pelvic Surgery, Emory Univ Hosp 1989; Gynecologic Oncology, Montefiore Med Ctr 1990

Smotkin, David MD (GO) - **Spec Exp:** Gynecologic Cancer; Gynecologic Cancer-Rare; **Hospital:** Montefiore Med Ctr - Div. Moses (page 100); **Address:** Montefiore Women's Ctr, 3332 Rochambeau Ave, Bronx, NY 10467; **Phone:** 718-920-5157; **Board Cert:** Obstetrics & Gynecology 2009; Gynecologic Oncology 2009; **Med School:** Yale Univ 1980; **Resid:** Obstetrics & Gynecology, Univ Colorado Hosp 1984; **Fellow:** Gynecologic Oncology, UCLA Med Ctr 1987; **Fac Appt:** Asst Prof ObG, Albert Einstein Coll Med

Hand Surgery

Kulick, Roy G MD (HS) - **Spec Exp:** Carpal Tunnel Syndrome; Arthritis; Tendon Surgery; Hand & Upper Extremity Surgery; **Hospital:** Montefiore Med Ctr - Div. Weiler (page 100); **Address:** The Tower at Montefiore Medical Park, 1695 Eastchester Rd Fl 2, Bronx, NY 10461; **Phone:** 718-920-2060; **Board Cert:** Orthopaedic Surgery 1980; Hand Surgery 2001; **Med School:** Cornell Univ-Weill Med Coll 1973; **Resid:** Surgery, St Lukes-Roosevelt Hosp 1975; Orthopaedic Surgery, Columbia-Presby ed tr 1978; **Fellow:** Hand Surgery, Hosp for Special Surgery 1979; **Fac Appt:** Assoc Prof OrS, Albert Einstein Coll Med

Hematology

Billett, Henny H MD (Hem) - **Spec Exp:** Bleeding/Coagulation Disorders; Thrombotic Disorders; Platelet Disorders; Sickle Cell Disease; **Hospital:** Montefiore Med Ctr - Div. Weiler (page 100), Montefiore Med Ctr - Div. Moses (page 100); **Address:** 1515 Blondell Ave, Ste 220, Bronx, NY 10461-2601; **Phone:** 718-405-8323; **Board Cert:** Internal Medicine 1979; Hematology 1982; **Med School:** Mount Sinai Sch Med 1974; **Resid:** Internal Medicine, Montefiore Hosp Med Ctr 1979; **Fellow:** Tropical Medicine, London Sch Hygiene/Trop Med 1977; Hematology, Montefiore Hosp Med Ctr 1981; **Fac Appt:** Prof Med, Albert Einstein Coll Med

Landau, Leon MD (Hem) - **Hospital:** Montefiore Med Ctr - Div. Moses (page 100), Comm Hosp - Dobbs Ferry; **Address:** 75 E Gun Hill Rd, Bronx, NY 10467-2103; **Phone:** 718-655-3932; **Board Cert:** Internal Medicine 1977; Hematology 1978; Medical Oncology 1981; **Med School:** Albert Einstein Coll Med 1971; **Resid:** Internal Medicine, Montefiore Med Ctr 1973; Internal Medicine, Metropolitan Hosp Ctr 1974; **Fellow:** Hematology, Montefiore Med Ctr 1978; Medical Oncology, Montefiore Med Ctr 1978; **Fac Appt:** Asst Prof Med, Albert Einstein Coll Med

Rand, Jacob H MD (Hem) - **Spec Exp:** Bleeding/Coagulation Disorders; Pregnancy & Hematologic Abnormalities; Thrombotic Disorders; **Hospital:** Montefiore Med Ctr - Div. Moses (page 100); **Address:** Montefiore Medical Ctr, 111 E 210th St, Foreman 8, Bronx, NY 10467-2401; **Phone:** 718-920-5991; **Board Cert:** Internal Medicine 1977; Hematology 1978; **Med School:** Albert Einstein Coll Med 1973; **Resid:** Pathology, Montefiore Med Ctr 1974; Internal Medicine, Mount Sinai Hosp 1975; **Fellow:** Hematology, Montefiore Med Ctr 1978; Research, Montefiore Med Ctr 1983; **Fac Appt:** Prof Med, Albert Einstein Coll Med

Infectious Disease

Berger, Judith MD (Inf) - **Spec Exp:** AIDS/HIV; Travel Medicine; **Hospital:** St Barnabas Hosp - Bronx; **Address:** 4422 Third Ave, Bronx, NY 10457; **Phone:** 718-960-6205; **Board Cert:** Internal Medicine 1984; Infectious Disease 1986; **Med School:** Mount Sinai Sch Med 1980; **Resid:** Internal Medicine, Brookdale Hosp 1984; **Fellow:** Infectious Disease, Downstate Med Ctr 1986; **Fac Appt:** Asst Clin Prof Med, Cornell Univ-Weill Med Coll

Corpuz, Marilou MD (Inf) - **Spec Exp:** Hospital Acquired Infections; **Hospital:** Montefiore Med Ctr - Div. North (page 100); **Address:** Montefiore North Division, 4234 Bronx Blvd, Bronx, NY 10466-2604; **Phone:** 347-341-4340; **Board Cert:** Internal Medicine 1988; Infectious Disease 2002; **Med School:** Philippines 1985; **Resid:** Internal Medicine, Griffin Hosp 1988; **Fellow:** Infectious Disease, LI Jewish Med Ctr 1991; **Fac Appt:** Assoc Prof Med, NY Med Coll

Robbins, Noah MD (Inf) - **Spec Exp:** AIDS/HIV; Sexually Transmitted Diseases; **Hospital:** Montefiore Med Ctr - Div. Moses (page 100); **Address:** 3400 Bainbridge Ave Fl 8, Bronx, NY 10467-2490; **Phone:** 718-920-8888; **Board Cert:** Internal Medicine 1974; Infectious Disease 1980; **Med School:** McGill Univ 1969; **Resid:** Internal Medicine, Albany Med Ctr 1975; **Fellow:** Infectious Disease, Montefiore Hosp Med Ctr 1976; **Fac Appt:** Clin Prof Med, Albert Einstein Coll Med

Saltzman, Simone MD (Inf) - **Hospital:** Montefiore Med Ctr - Div. Weiler (page 100); **Address:** 1575 Blondell Ave, Ste 200, Bronx, NY 10461-1915; **Phone:** 866-633-8255; **Board Cert:** Internal Medicine 1977; Infectious Disease 1980; **Med School:** SUNY Downstate 1973; **Resid:** Internal Medicine, Montefiore Hosp Med Ctr 1976; **Fellow:** Infectious Disease, Montefiore Hosp Med Ctr 1979; **Fac Appt:** Asst Prof Med, Albert Einstein Coll Med

Tanowitz, Herbert B MD (Inf) - **Spec Exp:** Parasitic Infections; Tropical Diseases; **Hospital:** Montefiore Med Ctr - Div. Weiler (page 100), Jacobi Med Ctr; **Address:** 1300 Morris Park Ave Bldg F - rm 504, Bronx, NY 10461-1926; **Phone:** 718-430-3342; **Board Cert:** Internal Medicine 1974; Infectious Disease 1976; **Med School:** Albert Einstein Coll Med 1967; **Resid:** Internal Medicine, Lincoln Hosp 1971; **Fellow:** Infectious Disease, Albert Einstein 1973; **Fac Appt:** Prof Med, Albert Einstein Coll Med

Telzak, Edward E MD (Inf) - **Spec Exp:** AIDS/HIV; Tuberculosis; Infections-Opportunistic; **Hospital:** Bronx Lebanon Hosp Ctr; **Address:** 1650 Selwyn Ave, Milstein Bldg - Ste 10C, Bronx, NY 10457-7606; **Phone:** 718-960-1212; **Board Cert:** Internal Medicine 1983; Infectious Disease 1988; **Med School:** Albert Einstein Coll Med 1980; **Resid:** Internal Medicine, New England Med Ctr 1983; **Fellow:** Infectious Disease, Brigham & Women's Hosp 1985; Tropical Medicine, New England Med Ctr 1986; **Fac Appt:** Prof Med, Albert Einstein Coll Med

Weiss, Louis MD (Inf) - **Spec Exp:** Parasitic Infections; AIDS/HIV; **Hospital:** Montefiore Med Ctr - Div. Weiler (page 100); **Address:** 1575 Blondell Ave, Ste 200, Bronx, NY 10461; **Phone:** 718-405-8311; **Board Cert:** Internal Medicine 1985; Infectious Disease 1988; **Med School:** Johns Hopkins Univ 1982; **Resid:** Internal Medicine, Univ Chicago 1985; **Fellow:** Infectious Disease, Montefiore Med Ctr 1989; **Fac Appt:** Prof Med, Albert Einstein Coll Med

Internal Medicine

Buatti, Elizabeth MD (IM) *PCP* - **Hospital:** Montefiore Med Ctr - Div. Moses (page 100); **Address:** 3444 Kossuth, Bronx, NY 10467; **Phone:** 718-920-2273; **Board Cert:** Internal Medicine 1981; **Med School:** Georgetown Univ 1978; **Resid:** Internal Medicine, St Vincent's Hosp 1981; **Fac Appt:** Asst Prof Med, Albert Einstein Coll Med

Ernst, Jerome MD (IM) *PCP* - **Spec Exp:** AIDS/HIV; **Hospital:** Bronx Lebanon Hosp Ctr; **Address:** 1770 Grand Concourse Fl 2, Avalon Medical, Bronx, NY 10457; **Phone:** 718-518-5581; **Board Cert:** Internal Medicine 1978; Pulmonary Disease 1982; **Med School:** Israel 1969; **Resid:** Internal Medicine, Montefiore Hosp Med Ctr 1972; **Fellow:** Pulmonary Disease, Montefiore Hosp Med Ctr 1977; **Fac Appt:** Assoc Prof Med, Albert Einstein Coll Med

Fojas, Antonio MD (IM) *PCP* - **Hospital:** Montefiore Med Ctr - Div. North (page 100); **Address:** 4234 Bronx Blvd, Bronx, NY 10466; **Phone:** 347-341-4300; **Board Cert:** Internal Medicine 2003; **Med School:** Philippines 1984; **Resid:** Internal Medicine, Our Lady of Mercy Med Ctr 1987; **Fellow:** Internal Medicine, Our Lady of Mercy Med Ctr 1988; **Fac Appt:** Asst Prof Med, NY Med Coll

Mojtabai, Shaparak MD (IM) *PCP* - **Spec Exp:** Women's Health-Geriatric; Diabetes; Hypertension; **Hospital:** St Barnabas Hosp - Bronx; **Address:** 2016 Bronxdale Ave, Ste 302, Bronx, NY 10462-3389; **Phone:** 718-822-1515; **Board Cert:** Internal Medicine 1989; Geriatric Medicine 2004; **Med School:** Iran 1982; **Resid:** Internal Medicine, St Barnabas Hosp-Cornell 1988; **Fellow:** Internal Medicine, St Barnabas Hosp-Cornell 1989

Sander, Norbert MD (IM) *PCP* - **Spec Exp:** Preventive Medicine; Sports Medicine; **Hospital:** Sound Shore Med Ctr - Westchester; **Address:** 340 City Island Ave, Bronx, NY 10464; **Phone:** 718-885-0333; **Board Cert:** Internal Medicine 1981; **Med School:** Albert Einstein Coll Med 1971; **Resid:** Internal Medicine, Metropolitan Hosp Ctr 1974

Selwyn, Peter MD (IM) - **Spec Exp:** AIDS/HIV; Palliative Care; Addiction/Substance Abuse; **Hospital:** Montefiore Med Ctr - Div. Moses (page 100); **Address:** Montfiore Family Health Ctr, 860 E 93rd St, Bronx, NY 10458; **Phone:** 718-933-2400; **Board Cert:** Family Medicine 2005; Hospice & Palliative Medicine 2006; **Med School:** Harvard Med Sch 1981; **Resid:** Family Medicine, Montefiore Med Ctr 1984; **Fac Appt:** Prof Med, Albert Einstein Coll Med

Swiderski, Deborah M MD (IM) *PCP* - **Hospital:** Montefiore Med Ctr - Div. Moses (page 100); **Address:** MMG-Comprehensive Heath Care Ctr, 305 E 161 St, Bronx, NY 10451; **Phone:** 718-579-2500; **Board Cert:** Internal Medicine 1986; **Med School:** Columbia P&S 1980; **Resid:** Internal Medicine, Montefiore Hosp 1983; **Fac Appt:** Asst Prof Med, Albert Einstein Coll Med

Teffera, Fassil MD (IM) *PCP* - **Spec Exp:** Diabetes; Hypertension; Preventive Medicine; **Hospital:** Montefiore Med Ctr - Div. North (page 100), Montefiore Med Ctr - Div. Moses (page 100); **Address:** 2426 Eastchester Rd, Bronx, NY 10469; **Phone:** 718-708-4726; **Board Cert:** Internal Medicine 2003; **Med School:** Ethiopia 1976; **Resid:** Internal Medicine, Our Lady of Mercy Med Ctr 1993; **Fac Appt:** Asst Clin Prof Med, NY Med Coll

Maternal & Fetal Medicine

Chazotte, Cynthia MD (MF) - **Spec Exp:** Pregnancy-High Risk; Asthma in Pregnancy; **Hospital:** Montefiore Med Ctr - Div. Weiler (page 100); **Address:** 1695 Eastchester Rd, Ste L2, Bronx, NY 10461; **Phone:** 718-405-8200; **Board Cert:** Obstetrics & Gynecology 2009; Maternal & Fetal Medicine 2009; **Med School:** NY Med Coll 1981; **Resid:** Obstetrics & Gynecology, Montefiore Med Ctr 1985; **Fellow:** Maternal & Fetal Medicine, Montefiore Med Ctr 1987; **Fac Appt:** Prof ObG, Albert Einstein Coll Med

Henderson, Cassandra E MD (MF) - **Spec Exp:** Pregnancy-High Risk; **Hospital:** Montefiore Med Ctr - Div. North (page 100); **Address:** 600 E 233rd St, Bronx, NY 10466; **Phone:** 718-920-9600; **Board Cert:** Obstetrics & Gynecology 2009; Maternal & Fetal Medicine 2009; **Med School:** Loyola Univ-Stritch Sch Med 1980; **Resid:** Obstetrics & Gynecology, Univ Chicago Hosp 1984; **Fellow:** Maternal & Fetal Medicine, Albert Einstein 1986; **Fac Appt:** Assoc Prof ObG, Albert Einstein Coll Med

Medical Oncology

Camacho, Fernando J MD (Onc) - **Spec Exp:** Breast Cancer; Lymphoma; Bladder Cancer; **Hospital:** Montefiore Med Ctr - Div. Moses (page 100), Saint Joseph's Med Ctr - Yonkers; **Address:** 60 E 208th St, Bronx, NY 10467-2702; **Phone:** 718-405-1700; **Board Cert:** Internal Medicine 1976; Hematology 1978; Medical Oncology 1981; **Med School:** SUNY Buffalo 1973; **Resid:** Internal Medicine, Montefiore Med Ctr 1976; Hematology, Montefiore Med Ctr 1977; **Fellow:** Medical Oncology, Sloan-Kettering Cancer Ctr 1979; **Fac Appt:** Asst Clin Prof Med, Albert Einstein Coll Med

Dutcher, Janice P MD (Onc) - **Spec Exp:** Kidney Cancer; Melanoma; Breast Cancer; Lymphoma; **Hospital:** Montefiore Med Ctr - Div. North (page 100), Montefiore Med Ctr - Div. Moses (page 100); **Address:** Oncology Division, 600 E 233rd St, Bronx, NY 10466-2697; **Phone:** 718-304-7219; **Board Cert:** Internal Medicine 1978; Medical Oncology 1983; **Med School:** UC Davis 1975; **Resid:** Internal Medicine, Rush Presbyterian Med Ctr 1978; **Fellow:** Medical Oncology, National Cancer Inst 1981; **Fac Appt:** Prof Med, NY Med Coll

Fuks, Joachim MD (Onc) - **Spec Exp:** Lung Cancer; Breast Cancer; Colon Cancer; **Hospital:** NY Westchester Sq Med Ctr, Montefiore Med Ctr - Div. Weiler (page 100); **Address:** 1578 Williamsbridge Rd Fl 2, Bronx, NY 10461-6265; **Phone:** 718-931-2290; **Board Cert:** Internal Medicine 1981; Medical Oncology 1983; **Med School:** Spain 1975; **Resid:** Internal Medicine, Mt Sinai Hosp 1978; **Fellow:** Medical Oncology, Natl Cancer Ctr 1981

Madajewicz, Stefan MD/PhD (Onc) - **Spec Exp:** Gastrointestinal Cancer; Brain Tumors; Breast Cancer; **Hospital:** Montefiore Med Ctr - Div. North (page 100); **Address:** 600 E 233 St Fl 6S, Bronx, NY 10466; **Phone:** 718-304-7200; **Board Cert:** Internal Medicine 1981; Medical Oncology 1983; **Med School:** Poland 1963; **Resid:** Internal Medicine, NY Med Coll 1974; Internal Medicine, SUNY-Buffalo Med Ctr 1979; **Fellow:** Medical Oncology, Roswell Park Cancer Inst 1978; **Fac Appt:** Prof Med, SUNY Stony Brook

Perez-Soler, Roman MD (Onc) - **Spec Exp:** Lung Cancer; Mesothelioma; Drug Development; **Hospital:** Montefiore Med Ctr - Div. Weiler (page 100), Montefiore Med Ctr - Div. Moses (page 100); **Address:** Montefiore Med Ctr, Dept Oncology, 111 E 210th St, Hoffheimer Main-Rm 100, Bronx, NY 10467; **Phone:** 718-920-4001; **Board Cert:** Internal Medicine 1987; Medical Oncology 1989; **Med School:** Spain 1977; **Resid:** Internal Medicine, Univ Autonoma Med Ctr 1982; **Fellow:** Medical Oncology, MD Anderson Hosp 1985; **Fac Appt:** Prof Med, Albert Einstein Coll Med

Ramirez, Mark A MD (Onc) - **Spec Exp:** Lymphoma, Non-Hodgkin's; Breast Cancer; Lung Cancer; **Hospital:** Montefiore Med Ctr - Div. Moses (page 100), Saint Joseph's Med Ctr - Yonkers; **Address:** 60 E 208th St, Bronx, NY 10467; **Phone:** 718-405-1700; **Board Cert:** Internal Medicine 1985; Medical Oncology 1989; Hematology 2005; **Med School:** Cornell Univ-Weill Med Coll 1982; **Resid:** Internal Medicine, Montefiore Med Ctr 1985; **Fellow:** Hematology & Oncology, Montefiore Med Ctr 1988; **Fac Appt:** Asst Clin Prof Med, Albert Einstein Coll Med

Reed, Mary K MD (Onc) - **Spec Exp:** Breast Cancer; AIDS/HIV; Pain-Cancer; **Hospital:** Bronx Lebanon Hosp Ctr; **Address:** 1650 Selwyn Ave Fl 2, Bronx, NY 10457; **Phone:** 718-239-8359; **Board Cert:** Internal Medicine 1984; Medical Oncology 2000; Hematology 2004; **Med School:** Boston Univ 1980; **Resid:** Internal Medicine, Henry Ford Hosp 1983; **Fellow:** Hematology & Oncology, LI Jewish Med Ctr 1988; **Fac Appt:** Asst Prof Med, Albert Einstein Coll Med

Sparano, Joseph A MD (Onc) - **Spec Exp:** Breast Cancer; Lymphoma; **Hospital:** Montefiore Med Ctr - Div. Weiler (page 100); **Address:** 1825 Eastchester Rd Fl 2 - Ste 2S-48, Bronx, NY 10461; **Phone:** 718-904-2555; **Board Cert:** Internal Medicine 1986; Medical Oncology 1989; **Med School:** NY Med Coll 1982; **Resid:** Internal Medicine, St Vincents Hosp 1986; **Fellow:** Medical Oncology, Montefiore Med Ctr 1988; **Fac Appt:** Prof Med, Albert Einstein Coll Med

Stein, Cy A MD/PhD (Onc) - **Spec Exp:** Prostate Cancer; Bladder Cancer; **Hospital:** Montefiore Med Ctr - Div. Moses (page 100); **Address:** Montefiore Med Ctr, Dept Oncology, 111 E 210 St, Hofheimer 100, Bronx, NY 10467; **Phone:** 718-920-8980; **Board Cert:** Internal Medicine 1986; Medical Oncology 1987; **Med School:** Albert Einstein Coll Med 1982; **Resid:** Internal Medicine, NY Hosp-Cornell Med Ctr 1985; **Fellow:** Medical Oncology, Natl Cancer Inst 1988; **Fac Appt:** Prof Med, Albert Einstein Coll Med

Vogl, Steven E MD (Onc) - **Spec Exp:** Breast Cancer; Lung Cancer; **Hospital:** Montefiore Med Ctr - Div. Weiler (page 100), White Plains Hosp Ctr; **Address:** 2220 Tiemann Ave, Bronx, NY 10469; **Phone:** 718-519-7774; **Board Cert:** Internal Medicine 1975; Medical Oncology 1975; **Med School:** Cornell Univ-Weill Med Coll 1970; **Resid:** Internal Medicine, Jacobi Med Ctr 1972; **Fellow:** Medical Oncology, Mt Sinai Med Ctr 1975

Neonatal-Perinatal Medicine

Campbell, Deborah MD (NP) - **Spec Exp:** Prematurity/Low Birth Weight Infants; Neurodevelopmental Disabilities; **Hospital:** Montefiore Med Ctr - Div. Weiler (page 100); **Address:** 1825 Eastchester Rd, Ste 725, Bronx, NY 10461-2301; **Phone:** 718-904-4105; **Board Cert:** Pediatrics 1983; Neonatal-Perinatal Medicine 1985; **Med School:** SUNY Buffalo 1978; **Resid:** Pediatrics, Montefiore Med Ctr 1981; **Fellow:** Neonatal-Perinatal Medicine, Montefiore Med Ctr 1983; **Fac Appt:** Clin Prof Ped, Albert Einstein Coll Med

Katzenstein, Martin S MD (NP) - **Spec Exp:** Neonatal Nutrition; Ethics; Neonatal Respiratory Care; **Hospital:** Montefiore Med Ctr - Div. North (page 100), Westchester Med Ctr; **Address:** 600 E 233rd St, Bronx, NY 10466-2604; **Phone:** 718-920-9541; **Board Cert:** Pediatrics 2004; **Med School:** NY Med Coll 1978; **Resid:** Pediatrics, New York Hosp 1981; **Fellow:** Neonatal-Perinatal Medicine, New York Hosp-Cornell 1982; Neonatal-Perinatal Medicine, Westchester Co Med Ctr 1984; **Fac Appt:** Assoc Clin Prof Ped, NY Med Coll

Nephrology

Charytan, Chaim MD (Nep) - **Spec Exp:** Hypertension; Diabetic Kidney Disease; Kidney Stones; **Hospital:** NY Hosp Queens, Montefiore Med Ctr - Div. Weiler (page 100); **Address:** 1874 Pelham Pkwy South, Bronx, NY 10461-3733; **Phone:** 718-931-5800; **Board Cert:** Internal Medicine 1969; Nephrology 1974; **Med School:** Albert Einstein Coll Med 1964; **Resid:** Internal Medicine, Bronx Municipal Hosp 1967; **Fellow:** Nephrology, Boston Univ Hosp 1968; **Fac Appt:** Clin Prof Med, Cornell Univ-Weill Med Coll

Coco, Maria MD (Nep) - **Spec Exp:** Hypertension; Kidney Disease; **Hospital:** Montefiore Med Ctr - Div. Moses (page 100); **Address:** 3332 E Rochambeau Ave Fl 4, Bronx, NY 10467-2401; **Phone:** 718-920-4136; **Board Cert:** Internal Medicine 1985; Nephrology 1988; **Med School:** Italy 1982; **Resid:** Internal Medicine, Bronx Lebanon Hosp 1985; **Fellow:** Nephrology, Montefiore Hosp Med Ctr 1988; **Fac Appt:** Prof Med, Albert Einstein Coll Med

Croll, James MD (Nep) - **Spec Exp:** Dialysis Care; Hypertension; Kidney Failure-Chronic; **Hospital:** St Barnabas Hosp - Bronx; **Address:** 4422 3rd Ave, Bronx, NY 10457; **Phone:** 718-960-6295; **Board Cert:** Internal Medicine 1978; Nephrology 1982; **Med School:** Belgium 1975; **Resid:** Internal Medicine, Genesee Hosp 1978; **Fellow:** Nephrology, VA Med Ctr 1981

Gorkin, Janet U MD (Nep) - **Spec Exp:** Hypertension; Diabetic Kidney Disease; Kidney Failure; **Hospital:** Montefiore Med Ctr - Div. Moses (page 100); **Address:** 3327 Bainbridge Ave, Bronx, NY 10467; **Phone:** 718-881-5100; **Board Cert:** Internal Medicine 1976; Nephrology 1980; **Med School:** Mount Sinai Sch Med 1973; **Resid:** Internal Medicine, Mt Sinai Hosp 1976; **Fellow:** Nephrology, Mt Sinai Hosp 1978; **Fac Appt:** Prof Med, Albert Einstein Coll Med

Laitman, Robert MD (Nep) - **Spec Exp:** Diabetic Kidney Disease; Cholesterol/Lipid Disorders; **Hospital:** Montefiore Med Ctr - Div. Weiler (page 100); **Address:** 1521 Jarett Pl, Bronx, NY 10461-2606; **Phone:** 718-518-1276; **Board Cert:** Internal Medicine 1986; Nephrology 1988; Geriatric Medicine 2000; **Med School:** Washington Univ, St Louis 1983; **Resid:** Internal Medicine, Jacobi Med Ctr 1986; **Fellow:** Nephrology, Montefiore Hosp Med Ctr 1988

Lynn, Robert I MD (Nep) - **Spec Exp:** Hypertension; Dialysis Care; **Hospital:** Montefiore Med Ctr - Div. Weiler (page 100), Sound Shore Med Ctr - Westchester; **Address:** 1200 Waters Pl, Ste M104, Bronx, NY 10461; **Phone:** 718-794-1200; **Board Cert:** Internal Medicine 1977; Nephrology 1980; **Med School:** Columbia P&S 1974; **Resid:** Internal Medicine, Columbia-Presby Med Ctr 1977; **Fellow:** Nephrology, Yale-New Haven Hosp 1979; **Fac Appt:** Assoc Prof Med, Albert Einstein Coll Med

Uday, Kalpana MD (Nep) - **Spec Exp:** Hypertension; **Hospital:** Bronx Lebanon Hosp Ctr; **Address:** 1650 Grand Concourse Fl 10, Bronx, NY 10457-7606; **Phone:** 718-992-7669; **Board Cert:** Internal Medicine 1989; Nephrology 2003; **Med School:** India 1980; **Resid:** Internal Medicine, Jamaica Med Ctr 1989; **Fellow:** Nephrology, Montefiore Med Ctr 1991; **Fac Appt:** Asst Prof Med, Albert Einstein Coll Med

Yoo, Jinil MD (Nep) - **Spec Exp:** Kidney Disease; Hypertension; Diabetes; **Hospital:** Montefiore Med Ctr - Div. North (page 100); **Address:** 233 E 233rd St, Bronx, NY 10468; **Phone:** 718-920-9041; **Board Cert:** Internal Medicine 1974; Nephrology 1976; **Med School:** South Korea 1967; **Resid:** Internal Medicine, Joslin Diabetes Center 1973; Internal Medicine, Metropolitan Hosp Ctr 1974; **Fellow:** Nephrology, NY Med Coll/Metro Hosp 1976; **Fac Appt:** Prof Med, NY Med Coll

Neurological Surgery

Flamm, Eugene S MD (NS) - **Spec Exp:** Aneurysm-Cerebral; Brain Tumors; Cerebrovascular Neurosurgery; **Hospital:** Montefiore Med Ctr - Div. Moses (page 100); **Address:** Montefiore Med Ctr, Dept Neurosurgery, 3316 Rochambeau Ave, Bronx, NY 10467-2841; **Phone:** 718-920-2339; **Board Cert:** Neurological Surgery 1973; **Med School:** SUNY Buffalo 1962; **Resid:** Surgery, New York Hosp 1964; Neurological Surgery, NYU Med Ctr 1970; **Fellow:** Neurological Surgery, Univ Zurich 1971; **Fac Appt:** Prof NS, Albert Einstein Coll Med

LaSala, Patrick MD (NS) - **Spec Exp:** Brain Tumors; Epilepsy; Stereotactic Radiosurgery; **Hospital:** Montefiore Med Ctr - Div. Moses (page 100); **Address:** Dept Neurosurgery, 3316 Rochambeau Ave, Bronx, NY 10467-2803; **Phone:** 718-920-7466; **Board Cert:** Neurological Surgery 1991; **Med School:** Columbia P&S 1980; **Resid:** Neurological Surgery, Columbia-Presby Med Ctr 1987; **Fac Appt:** Assoc Prof NS, Albert Einstein Coll Med

Neurology

Cohen, Joel S MD (N) - **Spec Exp:** Epilepsy; Headache; Stroke; Parkinson's Disease; **Hospital:** Montefiore Med Ctr - Div. Moses (page 100), Montefiore Med Ctr - Div. Weiler (page 100); **Address:** 1610 Williamsbridge Rd Fl 2, Bronx, NY 10461-2601; **Phone:** 718-597-8000; **Board Cert:** Neurology 1992; **Med School:** Albert Einstein Coll Med 1983; **Resid:** Neurology, Montefiore Med Ctr 1987; **Fellow:** Neurology, Montefiore Med Ctr 1988; **Fac Appt:** Assoc Prof N, Albert Einstein Coll Med

Freddo, Lorenza MD (N) - **Spec Exp:** Pain Management; Multiple Sclerosis; Peripheral Neuropathy; **Hospital:** St Barnabas Hosp - Bronx; **Address:** 2371 Arthur Ave, Bronx, NY 10458-8113; **Phone:** 718-364-6199; **Board Cert:** Neurology 1992; **Med School:** Italy 1980; **Resid:** Neurology, Italy 1984; Neurology, Columbia Presby Hosp 1990; **Fellow:** Columbia Presby Hosp 1986

Grenell, Steven L MD (N) - **Spec Exp:** Pain Management; Headache; **Hospital:** Montefiore Med Ctr - Div. Moses (page 100), Lawrence Hosp Ctr; **Address:** 3975 Sedgewick Ave, Ste 1-F, Bronx, NY 10463; **Phone:** 718-796-6055; **Board Cert:** Neurology 1989; **Med School:** UMDNJ-Rutgers Med Sch 1977; **Resid:** Internal Medicine, Montefiore Hosp 1979; Neurology, Montefiore Hosp 1982; **Fellow:** Internal Medicine, Montefiore Hosp 1682; **Fac Appt:** Asst Prof N, Albert Einstein Coll Med

Herskovitz, Steven MD (N) - **Spec Exp:** Electromyography; Neuromuscular Disorders; Peripheral Neuropathy; **Hospital:** Montefiore Med Ctr - Div. Moses (page 100); **Address:** 111 E 210th St, Bronx, NY 10467-2401; **Phone:** 718-920-4930; **Board Cert:** Internal Medicine 1983; Neurology 1987; Neuromuscular Medicine 2008; **Med School:** Cornell Univ-Weill Med Coll 1980; **Resid:** Internal Medicine, Montefiore Med Ctr 1983; Neurology, Montefiore Med Ctr 1986; **Fellow:** Electromyography, Montefiore Med Ctr 1987; **Fac Appt:** Prof N, Albert Einstein Coll Med

Kaufman, David Myland MD (N) - **Spec Exp:** Movement Disorders; **Hospital:** Montefiore Med Ctr - Div. Moses (page 100); **Address:** 3400 Bainbridge Ave, Main Fl, Bronx, NY 10467; **Phone:** 718-920-4730; **Board Cert:** Internal Medicine 1972; Neurology 1976; **Med School:** Univ Chicago-Pritzker Sch Med 1968; **Resid:** Internal Medicine, Montefiore Med Ctr 1971; Neurology, Montefiore Med Ctr 1974; **Fac Appt:** Prof N, Albert Einstein Coll Med

Lipton, Richard MD (N) - **Spec Exp:** Headache; Clinical Trials; **Hospital:** Montefiore Med Ctr - Div. Weiler (page 100); **Address:** Montefiore Headache Center, 1575 Blondell Ave, Ste 225, Bronx, NY 10461-2662; **Phone:** 718-405-8360; **Board Cert:** Neurology 1985; **Med School:** Univ Chicago-Pritzker Sch Med 1980; **Resid:** Neurology, Montefiore Med Ctr 1984; **Fellow:** Neurological Physiology, Montefiore Med Ctr 1985; NeuroEpidemiology, Columbia Univ 1990; **Fac Appt:** Prof N, Albert Einstein Coll Med

Sparr, Steven MD (N) - **Spec Exp:** Stroke; **Hospital:** Montefiore Med Ctr - Div. Moses (page 100); **Address:** Montefiore Med Ctr, 111 E 210th St, Bronx, NY 10467; **Phone:** 718-920-6402; **Board Cert:** Internal Medicine 1984; Neurology 1987; Vascular Neurology 2009; **Med School:** SUNY Buffalo 1980; **Resid:** Internal Medicine, Boston City Hosp 1983; Neurology, Albert Einstein 1986; **Fellow:** Neurological Rehabilitation, Burke Rehabilitation Hosp 1987; **Fac Appt:** Assoc Prof N, Albert Einstein Coll Med

Swerdlow, Michael L MD (N) - **Spec Exp:** Myasthenia Gravis; Spinal Disorders; Multiple Sclerosis; **Hospital:** Montefiore Med Ctr - Div. Moses (page 100); **Address:** 3400 Bainbridge Ave, Bronx, NY 10467-2401; **Phone:** 718-920-4178; **Board Cert:** Neurology 1975; **Med School:** Univ Pennsylvania 1967; **Resid:** Internal Medicine, Mount Sinai Hosp 1969; Neurology, Montefiore Med Ctr 1972; **Fellow:** Neurology, Natl Inst Hlth 1974; **Fac Appt:** Prof N, Albert Einstein Coll Med

Neuroradiology

Bello, Jacqueline A MD (NRad) - **Spec Exp:** Aneurysm-Cerebral; Pain-Back; **Hospital:** Montefiore Med Ctr - Div. Moses (page 100); **Address:** Montefiore Med Ctr, 111 E 210th St, Red Zone, Bronx, NY 10467; **Phone:** 718-920-4030; **Board Cert:** Diagnostic Radiology 1984; **Med School:** Columbia P&S 1980; **Resid:** Diagnostic Radiology, Columbia-PresbyMed Ctr 1984; **Fellow:** Neuroradiology, Neuro Inst/Columbia-Presby Med Ctr 1986; **Fac Appt:** Prof Rad, Albert Einstein Coll Med

Nuclear Medicine

Freeman, Leonard M MD (NuM) - **Spec Exp:** Nuclear Oncology; Gastrointestinal Disorders; PET Imaging; CT Scan; **Hospital:** Montefiore Med Ctr - Div. Moses (page 100); **Address:** 111 E 210th St, Bronx, NY 10467-2401; **Phone:** 718-920-6060; **Board Cert:** Diagnostic Radiology 1966; Nuclear Medicine 1972; Nuclear Radiology 1974; **Med School:** Ros Franklin Univ/Chicago Med Sch 1961; **Resid:** Diagnostic Radiology, Bronx Municipal Hosp 1965; **Fac Appt:** Prof NuM, Albert Einstein Coll Med

Milstein, David M MD (NuM) - **Hospital:** Montefiore Med Ctr - Div. Weiler (page 100), Montefiore Med Ctr - Div. Moses (page 100); **Address:** 1825 Eastchester Rd, Bronx, NY 10461; **Phone:** 718-904-4058; **Board Cert:** Nuclear Medicine 1972; Diagnostic Radiology 1972; **Med School:** Albert Einstein Coll Med 1967; **Resid:** Diagnostic Radiology, Bronx Muni Hosp Ctr 1972; **Fellow:** Diagnostic Radiology, Bronx Muni Hosp Ctr 1972; **Fac Appt:** Prof NuM, Albert Einstein Coll Med

Obstetrics & Gynecology

Duvivier, Roger MD (ObG) *PCP* - **Spec Exp:** Ultrasound; Preventive Medicine; Laparoscopy/Hysteroscopy; Women's Health; **Hospital:** Montefiore Med Ctr - Div. Weiler (page 100); **Address:** 305 E 161 St, Bronx, NY 10451; **Phone:** 718-579-2500; **Board Cert:** Obstetrics & Gynecology 2006; **Med School:** Albert Einstein Coll Med 1974; **Resid:** Obstetrics & Gynecology, Bronx Muni Hosp-Albert Einstein 1978; **Fac Appt:** Assoc Prof ObG, Albert Einstein Coll Med

Reilly, Kevin D MD (ObG) *PCP* - **Spec Exp:** Menopause Problems; **Hospital:** Montefiore Med Ctr - Div. North (page 100); **Address:** 600 E 233rd St, Bronx, NY 10466-2604; **Phone:** 718-920-9647; **Board Cert:** Obstetrics & Gynecology 1976; **Med School:** Univ Mich Med Sch 1969; **Resid:** Obstetrics & Gynecology, St Vincent's Hosp & Med Ctr 1974; **Fac Appt:** Assoc Prof ObG, NY Med Coll

Young, Constance MD (ObG) - **Spec Exp:** Gynecology Only; Pelvic Surgery; Menopause Problems; **Hospital:** Bronx Lebanon Hosp Ctr; **Address:** 1650 Grand Concourse, Bronx, NY 10457; **Phone:** 718-294-7100; **Board Cert:** Obstetrics & Gynecology 2009; **Med School:** Cornell Univ-Weill Med Coll 1983; **Resid:** Obstetrics & Gynecology, North Shore Univ Hosp 1987

Ophthalmology

Chess, Jeremy MD (Oph) - **Spec Exp:** Retina/Vitreous Surgery; **Hospital:** Montefiore Med Ctr - Div. Moses (page 100); **Address:** 2221 Boston Rd, Bronx, NY 10467; **Phone:** 718-798-3030; **Board Cert:** Ophthalmology 1977; **Med School:** Boston Univ 1970; **Resid:** Ophthalmology, Boston Univ Med Ctr 1974; **Fellow:** Vitreoretinal Surgery, Boston Univ Med Ctr 1983; **Fac Appt:** Assoc Clin Prof Oph, Albert Einstein Coll Med

Gurland, Judith E MD (Oph) - **Spec Exp:** Pediatric Ophthalmology; Eye Muscle Disorders; **Hospital:** Montefiore Med Ctr - Div. Moses (page 100), Bronx Lebanon Hosp Ctr; **Address:** 3400 Bainbridge Ave, Bronx, NY 10467-2404; **Phone:** 718-920-2020; **Board Cert:** Ophthalmology 1974; **Med School:** SUNY Downstate 1968; **Resid:** Ophthalmology, SUNY Downstate 1972; **Fellow:** Neuro-Ophthalmology, Kingsbrook Jewish Med Ctr 1973; Pediatric Ophthalmology, Columbia-Presby Hosp 1973; **Fac Appt:** Assoc Prof Oph, Albert Einstein Coll Med

Hayworth, Robin S MD (Oph) - **Spec Exp:** Cataract Surgery; Glaucoma; **Hospital:** Lenox Hill Hosp (Manh Eye, Ear & Throat Hosp), Montefiore Med Ctr - Div. Weiler (page 100); **Address:** 787 Lydig Ave, Bronx, NY 10462-2144; **Phone:** 718-863-7774; **Board Cert:** Ophthalmology 1985; **Med School:** Cornell Univ-Weill Med Coll 1978; **Resid:** Surgery, NY Hosp 1980; Ophthalmology, Manhattan EET Hosp 1983

Maher, Elizabeth MD (Oph) - **Spec Exp:** Orbital Surgery; Oculoplastic Surgery; **Hospital:** New York Eye & Ear Infirm (page 113); **Address:** 2135 Colonial Ave, Bronx, NY 10461; **Phone:** 212-979-4575; **Board Cert:** Ophthalmology 1989; **Med School:** Harvard Med Sch 1984; **Resid:** Ophthalmology, Manhattan EE&T Hosp 1988; **Fellow:** Ophthalmic Plastic & Reconstructive Surgery, Manhattan EE&T Hosp 1990

Mayers, Martin MD (Oph) - **Spec Exp:** Cataract Surgery; Cornea Transplant; Eye Infections; **Hospital:** Bronx Lebanon Hosp Ctr, Montefiore Med Ctr - Div. North (page 100); **Address:** Bronx Lebanon Hosp Ctr, Dept Ophth, 1650 Selwyn Ave Fl ground, Bronx, NY 10457; **Phone:** 718-518-8008; **Board Cert:** Ophthalmology 1985; **Med School:** Albert Einstein Coll Med 1979; **Resid:** Ophthalmology, SUNY Downstate Med Ctr 1983; **Fellow:** Cornea, Proctor Fdn-UCSF 1984; **Fac Appt:** Assoc Prof Oph, Albert Einstein Coll Med

Rosenbaum, Pearl MD (Oph) - **Spec Exp:** Cataract Surgery; Oculoplastic & Orbital Surgery; Ophthalmic Pathology; Glaucoma; **Hospital:** Montefiore Med Ctr - Div. Moses (page 100), Bronx Lebanon Hosp Ctr; **Address:** 1250 Waters Pl, Ste 502, Bronx, NY 10467; **Phone:** 718-518-0060; **Board Cert:** Ophthalmology 1988; **Med School:** Albert Einstein Coll Med 1982; **Resid:** Ophthalmology, Albert Einstein 1986; **Fellow:** Ophthalmic Pathology, Baylor Coll of Med 1987; Ophthalmic Oncololgy, Baylor Coll of Med 1988; **Fac Appt:** Prof Oph, Albert Einstein Coll Med

Slamovits, Thomas L MD (Oph) - **Spec Exp:** Neuro-Ophthalmology; Optic Nerve Disorders; Vision Loss-Unexplained Loss; Diabetic Eye Disease/Retinopathy; **Hospital:** Montefiore Med Ctr - Div. Moses (page 100), Hackensack Univ Med Ctr (page 96); **Address:** 1250 Pelham Pkwy S, Bronx, NY 10461; **Phone:** 718-794-1500; **Board Cert:** Ophthalmology 1980; **Med School:** Ohio State Univ 1975; **Resid:** Ophthalmology, Univ Pitts Eye & Ear 1979; **Fellow:** Neuro-Ophthalmology, Washington Univ-Barnes Hosp 1980; **Fac Appt:** Clin Prof Oph, Albert Einstein Coll Med

Tiwari, Ram MD (Oph) - **Spec Exp:** Diabetic Eye Disease/Retinopathy; Glaucoma; Cataract Surgery; **Hospital:** Montefiore Med Ctr - Div. North (page 100), NY-Presby Hosp/Columbia (page 104); **Address:** 1739 Williamsbridge Rd, Bronx, NY 10461-6203; **Phone:** 718-824-1560; **Board Cert:** Ophthalmology 1977; **Med School:** India 1966; **Resid:** Ophthalmology, Maulana Azad Med Coll 1971; **Fellow:** Retina, Columbia-Presby Med Ctr 1978; **Fac Appt:** Asst Clin Prof Oph, Columbia P&S

Wolf, Kenneth J MD (Oph) - **Spec Exp:** Diabetic Eye Disease/Retinopathy; Cataract Surgery; **Hospital:** Montefiore Med Ctr - Div. Weiler (page 100); **Address:** 1180 Morris Park Ave Fl 2, Bronx, NY 10461-1925; **Phone:** 718-892-6110; **Board Cert:** Ophthalmology 1980; **Med School:** Albert Einstein Coll Med 1974; **Resid:** Ophthalmology, Montefiore Hosp Med Ctr 1978; **Fac Appt:** Asst Clin Prof Oph, Albert Einstein Coll Med

Orthopaedic Surgery

Cobelli, Neil MD (OrS) - **Spec Exp:** Knee Replacement; Hip Replacement; **Hospital:** Montefiore Med Ctr - Div. Weiler (page 100); **Address:** Montefiore Med Ctr, Dept Orthopaedics, 1695 Eastchester Rd Fl 2, Bronx, NY 10461; **Phone:** 718-920-2060; **Board Cert:** Orthopaedic Surgery 1985; **Med School:** Dartmouth Med Sch 1976; **Resid:** Orthopaedic Surgery, Montefiore Med Ctr 1983; **Fac Appt:** Assoc Prof OrS, Albert Einstein Coll Med

Kirschenbaum, Ira H MD (OrS) - **Spec Exp:** Hip & Knee Replacement; Arthroscopic Surgery; Joint Reconstruction; Trauma; **Hospital:** Bronx Lebanon Hosp Ctr, NYU Hosp For Joint Diseases (page 106); **Address:** Bronx Lebanon Hosp, Dept Orthopaedics, 1650 Grand Concourse, Bronx, NY 10457; **Phone:** 718-518-5814; **Board Cert:** Orthopaedic Surgery 2004; **Med School:** Albert Einstein Coll Med 1984; **Resid:** Orthopaedic Surgery, Montefiore Med Ctr 1990; **Fellow:** Joint Replacement Surgery, Rothman Inst-Penn Hosp-Thonas Jefferson 1991; **Fac Appt:** Asst Clin Prof OrS, NYU Sch Med

Kleinman, Paul MD (OrS) - **Spec Exp:** Pediatric Orthopaedic Surgery; Hand Surgery; Trauma; Sports Medicine; **Hospital:** St Barnabas Hosp - Bronx; **Address:** 2016 Bronxdale Ave, Ste 202, Bronx, NY 10462-3365; **Phone:** 718-863-8695; **Board Cert:** Orthopaedic Surgery 2009; **Med School:** Stanford Univ 1979; **Resid:** Surgery, St Luke's Hosp 1981; Orthopaedic Surgery, Columbia-Presby Hosp 1985; **Fellow:** Hand Surgery, Allegheny Genl Hosp; Pediatric Orthopaedic Surgery, Hosp Joint Dis 1990

Kulsakdinun, Chaiyaporn MD (OrS) - **Spec Exp:** Foot & Ankle Surgery; Fractures; Sports Injuries; **Hospital:** Montefiore Med Ctr - Div. Weiler (page 100); **Address:** 1695 Eastchester Rd Fl 2, Bronx, NY 10461; **Phone:** 718-920-2060; **Board Cert:** Orthopaedic Surgery 2003; **Med School:** Yale Univ 1993; **Resid:** Orthopaedic Surgery, Yale-New Haven Hosp 1998; **Fellow:** Foot & Ankle Surgery, Hosp Special Surgery 1999; **Fac Appt:** Asst Prof OrS, Albert Einstein Coll Med

Levy, I Martin MD (OrS) - **Spec Exp:** Sports Medicine; Arthroscopic Surgery; **Hospital:** Montefiore Med Ctr - Div. Weiler (page 100); **Address:** Montefiore Med Ctr, Dept Orthopaedics, 1695 Eastchester Rd Fl 2, Bronx, NY 10461; **Phone:** 718-405-8132; **Board Cert:** Orthopaedic Surgery 1982; **Med School:** NY Med Coll 1976; **Resid:** Orthopaedic Surgery, Bronx Municipal Hosps 1980; **Fellow:** Sports Medicine, Hosp for Special Surg 1981

Olsewski, John M MD (OrS) - **Spec Exp:** Spinal Reconstructive Surgery; Scoliosis; Spinal Surgery-Neck; Cervical Myelopathy; **Hospital:** Montefiore Med Ctr - Div. Weiler (page 100), Sound Shore Med Ctr - Westchester; **Address:** 2157 Tomlinson Ave, Bronx, NY 10461; **Phone:** 718-794-2501; **Board Cert:** Orthopaedic Surgery 2007; **Med School:** SUNY Buffalo 1986; **Resid:** Orthopaedic Surgery, SUNY Buffalo 1992; **Fellow:** Spinal Surgery, Twin Cities Scoliosis/Spine Ctr 1994; **Fac Appt:** Assoc Clin Prof OrS, Albert Einstein Coll Med

Wilson, Arnold B MD (OrS) - **Spec Exp:** Hip Replacement; Knee Replacement; Knee Injuries/Ligament Surgery; Sports Medicine; **Hospital:** Montefiore Med Ctr - Div. Moses (page 100), NYU Hosp For Joint Diseases (page 106); **Address:** Wilson Orthopaedics, 75 E Gun Hill Rd, Bronx, NY 10467-2103; **Phone:** 718-798-1000; **Board Cert:** Orthopaedic Surgery 2007; **Med School:** UMDNJ-Univ Med Dent NJ 1987; **Resid:** Orthopaedic Surgery, Catholic Med Ctr of Brooklyn & Queens 1993; **Fellow:** Sports Medicine/Knee Surgery, Beth Israel Med Ctr 1994

Otolaryngology

Feghali, Joseph G MD (Oto) - **Spec Exp:** Ear Disorders/Surgery; Acoustic Neuroma; Hearing Disorders; Neuro-Otology; **Hospital:** Montefiore Med Ctr - Div. Moses (page 100); **Address:** 182 E 210th St, Bronx, NY 10467; **Phone:** 718-881-3277; **Board Cert:** Otolaryngology 1990; **Med School:** Lebanon 1978; **Resid:** Otolaryngology, American Univ Beirut 1982; Otolaryngology, Montefiore Med Ctr 1990; **Fellow:** Otology & Neurotology, House Ear Inst 1983; Neurological Surgery, Meml Sloan Kettering Cancer Ctr 1984; **Fac Appt:** Clin Prof Oto, Albert Einstein Coll Med

Fried, Marvin P MD (Oto) - **Spec Exp:** Endoscopic Sinus Surgery; Head & Neck Tumors; Laryngeal & Voice Disorders; Sinus Disorders/Surgery; **Hospital:** Montefiore Med Ctr - Div. Moses (page 100), Montefiore Med Ctr - Div. Weiler (page 100); **Address:** 3400 Bainbridge Ave Fl 3, Bronx, NY 10467; **Phone:** 718-920-4646; **Board Cert:** Otolaryngology 1975; **Med School:** Tufts Univ 1969; **Resid:** Surgery, Jewish Hosp 1971; Otolaryngology, Barnes Hosp 1975; **Fellow:** Stroke, Washington Univ 1976; **Fac Appt:** Prof Oto, Albert Einstein Coll Med

Goldstein, Steven I MD (Oto) - **Spec Exp:** Sinus Surgery; Nasal Surgery; **Hospital:** NY Westchester Sq Med Ctr, St John's Riverside Hosp; **Address:** 1200 Waters Pl, Bronx, NY 10461; **Phone:** 718-863-4366; **Board Cert:** Otolaryngology 1987; **Med School:** SUNY Buffalo 1982; **Resid:** Surgery, NYU Med Ctr 1984; Otolaryngology, NYU Med Ctr 1987; **Fellow:** Facial Plastic Surgery, Mt Sinai Hosp 1988

Smith, Richard V MD (Oto) - **Spec Exp:** Head & Neck Cancer; Thyroid & Parathyroid Surgery; Salivary Gland Tumors; **Hospital:** Montefiore Med Ctr - Div. Moses (page 100), Montefiore Med Ctr - Div. Weiler (page 100); **Address:** 3400 Bainbridge Ave, MAP Bldg Fl 3, Bronx, NY 10467; **Phone:** 718-920-4646; **Board Cert:** Otolaryngology 1996; **Med School:** Univ VT Coll Med 1990; **Resid:** Otolaryngology, Georgetown Univ Hosp 1995; **Fac Appt:** Assoc Clin Prof Oto, Albert Einstein Coll Med

Yankelowitz, Stanley M MD (Oto) - **Spec Exp:** Nasal & Sinus Surgery; Pediatric Otolaryngology; **Hospital:** Montefiore Med Ctr - Div. Moses (page 100), NY Westchester Sq Med Ctr; **Address:** 1200 Waters Pl, Ste 110, Bronx, NY 10461; **Phone:** 718-863-4366; **Med School:** South Africa 1974; **Resid:** Otolaryngology, Univ Stellenbosch 1985; Otolaryngology, Univ Cape Town 1987; **Fellow:** Pediatric Otolaryngology, Montefiore Med Ctr-Weiler Div 1988

Pediatric Allergy & Immunology

Wiznia, Andrew A MD (PA&I) - **Spec Exp:** AIDS/HIV; **Hospital:** Jacobi Med Ctr, N Central Bronx Hosp; **Address:** Jacobi Medical Ctr, Bldg 1, 1400 Pelham Pkwy S, rm 1W5-8, Bronx, NY 10461; **Phone:** 718-918-4903; **Board Cert:** Pediatrics 1986; **Med School:** Columbia P&S 1980; **Resid:** Pediatrics, Bronx Muni Hosp Ctr 1983; Pediatrics, Bronx-Lebanon Hosp Ctr 1984; **Fellow:** Allergy & Immunology, Montefiore-Weiler Einstein Div 1986; **Fac Appt:** Prof Ped, Albert Einstein Coll Med

Pediatric Cardiology

Hsu, Daphne MD (PCd) - **Spec Exp:** Interventional Cardiology; Heart Failure; Transplant Medicine-Heart; **Hospital:** Montefiore Med Ctr - Div. Moses (page 100); **Address:** Chldn's Hosp at Montefiore, 3415 Bainbridge Ave, Bronx, NY 10467; **Phone:** 718-741-2315; **Board Cert:** Pediatrics 1988; Pediatric Cardiology 2003; **Med School:** Yale Univ 1982; **Resid:** Pediatrics, Columbia Babies & Chldn's Hosp 1985; **Fellow:** Pediatric Cardiology, Columbia Babies & Chldn's Hosp 1988; **Fac Appt:** Prof Ped, Albert Einstein Coll Med

Schiller, Myles S MD (PCd) - **Spec Exp:** Congenital Heart Disease & Acquired; Exercise Physiology; **Hospital:** Montefiore Med Ctr - Div. Moses (page 100), St Barnabas Hosp - Bronx; **Address:** Children's Hosp Montefiore, 3415 Bainbridge Ave, Bronx, NY 10457; **Phone:** 718-741-2343; **Board Cert:** Pediatrics 1978; Pediatric Cardiology 1979; **Med School:** Ros Franklin Univ/Chicago Med Sch 1973; **Resid:** Pediatrics, New York Hosp-Cornell 1975; **Fellow:** Pediatric Cardiology, New York Hosp-Cornell 1977; **Fac Appt:** Assoc Clin Prof Ped, Albert Einstein Coll Med

Shenoy, Rajesh U MD (PCd) - **Spec Exp:** Echocardiography; Fetal Echocardiography; Congenital Heart Disease; **Hospital:** Montefiore Med Ctr - Div. Moses (page 100), St Barnabas Hosp - Bronx; **Address:** Chldn's Hosp at Montefiore, 3415 Bainbridge Ave, Bronx, NY 10467; **Phone:** 718-741-2370; **Board Cert:** Pediatrics 2006; Pediatric Cardiology 2008; **Med School:** India 1995; **Resid:** Pediatrics, Univ Illinois Affil Hosp 1996; **Fellow:** Pediatric Cardiology, N Shore Hosp 2000; **Fac Appt:** Asst Prof Ped, Albert Einstein Coll Med

Walsh, Christine A MD (PCd) - **Spec Exp:** Arrhythmias; Congenital Heart Disease; Sudden Infant Death Syndrome (SIDS); **Hospital:** Montefiore Med Ctr - Div. Moses (page 100), Montefiore Med Ctr - Div. Weiler (page 100); **Address:** 3415 Bainbridge Ave, Bronx, NY 10467-2401; **Phone:** 718-741-2343; **Board Cert:** Pediatrics 1978; Pediatric Cardiology 1983; Pediatric Critical Care Medicine 2003; **Med School:** Yale Univ 1973; **Resid:** Pediatrics, Columbia-Presby Med Ctr 1976; **Fellow:** Pediatric Cardiology, Columbia-Presby Med Ctr 1978; Cardiac Electrophysiology, Columbia P&S 1980; **Fac Appt:** Prof Ped, Albert Einstein Coll Med

Pediatric Critical Care Medicine

Singer, Lewis MD (PCCM) - **Spec Exp:** Respiratory Failure; Airway Disorders; **Hospital:** Montefiore Med Ctr - Div. Moses (page 100); **Address:** The Chldns Hosp at Montefiore, 111 E 210th St, Bronx, NY 10467-2401; **Phone:** 718-741-2477; **Board Cert:** Pediatrics 1981; Neonatal-Perinatal Medicine 1983; Pediatric Critical Care Medicine 2005; **Med School:** UMDNJ-NJ Med Sch, Newark 1977; **Resid:** Pediatrics, Montefiore Hosp Med Ctr 1981; **Fellow:** Neonatology, Montefiore Hosp Med Ctr 1983; **Fac Appt:** Prof Ped, Albert Einstein Coll Med

Ushay, H Michael MD/PhD (PCCM) - **Spec Exp:** Respiratory Failure; Sepsis & Septic Shock; Cardiac Critical Care; **Hospital:** Montefiore Med Ctr - Div. Moses (page 100); **Address:** CHAM, Div Critical Care Med, 3415 Bainbridge Ave, Bronx, NY 10467; **Phone:** 718-741-2440; **Board Cert:** Pediatrics 2005; Pediatric Critical Care Medicine 2009; **Med School:** UMDNJ-NJ Med Sch, Newark 1986; **Resid:** Pediatrics, Montefiore/Bronx Muni Hosp 1990; **Fellow:** Pediatric Pulmonology, Montefiore Med Ctr 1991; Pediatric Critical Care Medicine, NY Hosp-Cornell Univ Med Ctr 1993; **Fac Appt:** Assoc Clin Prof Ped, Albert Einstein Coll Med

Weingarten, Jacqueline MD (PCCM) - **Spec Exp:** Heart Disease; Lung Disease; Nutrition; **Hospital:** Montefiore Med Ctr - Div. Moses (page 100); **Address:** Rosenthal 4/Chlds Hosp @ Montefiore, 111 E 210th St, Bronx, NY 10467; **Phone:** 718-741-2440; **Board Cert:** Pediatrics 2004; Pediatric Critical Care Medicine 2004; **Med School:** Cornell Univ-Weill Med Coll 1986; **Resid:** Pediatrics, Columbia-Presbyterian 1989; Pediatrics, Columbia-Presbyterian 1990; **Fellow:** Pediatric Critical Care Medicine, Cornell0New York Hospital 1996; **Fac Appt:** Assoc Prof Ped, Albert Einstein Coll Med

Pediatric Hematology-Oncology

Dasgupta, Indira K MD (PHO) - **Spec Exp:** Sickle Cell Disease; Anemia; **Hospital:** Montefiore Med Ctr - Div. North (page 100); **Address:** 600 E 233rd St, Fl 4, Bronx, NY 10466-2697; **Phone:** 718-920-9014; **Board Cert:** Pediatrics 1981; Pediatric Hematology-Oncology 1984; **Med School:** India 1967; **Resid:** Pediatrics, New York Methodist Hosp 1974; **Fellow:** Pediatric Hematology-Oncology, Meml Sloan Kettering Cancer Ctr 1979; Pediatric Hematology-Oncology, Mount Sinai Hosp 1980; **Fac Appt:** Assoc Clin Prof Ped, NY Med Coll

Gorlick, Richard MD (PHO) - **Spec Exp:** Bone Tumors; Sarcoma; Solid Tumors; **Hospital:** Montefiore Med Ctr - Div. Moses (page 100); **Address:** 111 E 210th St, Rosenthal 3, Bronx, NY 10467-2940; **Phone:** 718-741-2342; **Board Cert:** Pediatrics 2008; Pediatric Hematology-Oncology 2004; **Med School:** SUNY Downstate 1990; **Resid:** Pediatrics, Columbia-Presby Med Ctr 1993; **Fellow:** Pediatric Hematology-Oncology, Meml Sloan Kettering Cancer Ctr 1995

Levy, Adam S MD (PHO) - **Spec Exp:** Brain Tumors; Neuro-Oncology; **Hospital:** Montefiore Med Ctr - Div. Moses (page 100); **Address:** Chldns Hosp at Montefiore, 3415 Bainbridge Ave, Bronx, NY 10467; **Phone:** 718-741-2342; **Board Cert:** Pediatrics 2005; Pediatric Hematology-Oncology 2002; **Med School:** NYU Sch Med 1994; **Resid:** Pediatrics, Mt Sinai Hosp 1998; **Fellow:** Pediatric Hematology-Oncology, Meml Sloan Kettering Cancer Ctr 2001; **Fac Appt:** Assoc Prof Ped, Albert Einstein Coll Med

Moulton, Thomas MD (PHO) - **Spec Exp:** Sickle Cell Disease; **Hospital:** Bronx Lebanon Hosp Ctr; **Address:** Bronx Lebanon Hosp Ctr, 1650 Grand Concourse, Bronx, NY 10457; **Phone:** 718-518-5131; **Board Cert:** Pediatric Hematology-Oncology 2005; **Med School:** Loyola Univ-Stritch Sch Med 1984; **Resid:** Pediatrics, Rainbow-Babies Chldns Hosp 1987; **Fellow:** Pediatric Hematology-Oncology, Babies Hosp 1990; **Fac Appt:** Asst Prof Ped, Albert Einstein Coll Med

Pediatric Infectious Disease

Herold, Betsy C MD (PInf) - **Hospital:** Montefiore Med Ctr - Div. Weiler (page 100); **Address:** 1300 Morris Park Ave, Forchheimer Bldg, Ste 702, Bronx, NY 10461; **Phone:** 718-430-4222; **Board Cert:** Pediatrics 1986; Pediatric Infectious Disease 2005; **Med School:** Univ Pennsylvania 1982; **Resid:** Pediatrics, Northwestern Meml Hosp 1985; **Fellow:** Infectious Disease, Northwestern Meml Hosp 1989; **Fac Appt:** Prof Ped, Albert Einstein Coll Med

Litman, Nathan MD (PInf) - **Spec Exp:** Infections in Immunocompromised Patients; Hospital Acquired Infections; **Hospital:** Montefiore Med Ctr - Div. Moses (page 100); **Address:** Montefiore Med Ctr, Div Ped Infectious Disease, 111 E 210th St Fl 4, Bronx, NY 10467-2401; **Phone:** 718-741-2470; **Board Cert:** Pediatrics 1978; Pediatric Infectious Disease 2009; **Med School:** Albert Einstein Coll Med 1971; **Resid:** Pediatrics, Montefiore Med Ctr 1974; **Fellow:** Infectious Disease, Montefiore Med Ctr 1978; **Fac Appt:** Prof Ped, Albert Einstein Coll Med

Pediatric Nephrology

Kaskel, Frederick J MD/PhD (PNep) - **Spec Exp:** Transplant Medicine-Kidney; Nephrotic Syndrome; Kidney Disease-Chronic; Dialysis Care; **Hospital:** Montefiore Med Ctr - Div. Moses (page 100), Bronx Lebanon Hosp Ctr; **Address:** Children's Hosp at Montefiore, 111 E 210th St, Bronx, NY 10467-2401; **Phone:** 718-741-2450; **Board Cert:** Pediatrics 1980; Pediatric Nephrology 1982; **Med School:** Univ Cincinnati 1975; **Resid:** Pediatrics, Montefiore Med Ctr 1977; **Fellow:** Pediatric Nephrology, Montefiore Med Ctr 1981; **Fac Appt:** Prof Ped, Albert Einstein Coll Med

Pediatric Otolaryngology

Bent, John P MD (PO) - **Spec Exp:** Airway Reconstruction; Sinus Disorders/Surgery; Hearing Loss; **Hospital:** Montefiore Med Ctr - Div. Moses (page 100); **Address:** Children's Hospital at Montefiore, Dept Otolaryngology, Head & Neck Surgery, 3400 Bainbridge Ave Fl 3, Bronx, NY 10467-2490; **Phone:** 718-920-4646; **Board Cert:** Otolaryngology 1995; **Med School:** Wake Forest Univ 1989; **Resid:** Otolaryngology, Med Coll Georgia 1994; **Fellow:** Pediatric Otolaryngology, Univ Iowa Hosp & Clins 1995; **Fac Appt:** Assoc Prof Oto, Albert Einstein Coll Med

Parikh, Sanjay R MD (PO) - **Spec Exp:** Airway Disorders; Cochlear Implants; **Hospital:** Montefiore Med Ctr - Div. Moses (page 100); **Address:** Chldns Hosp at Montefiore, 3400 Bainbridge Ave Fl 3, Bronx, NY 10467; **Phone:** 718-920-4646; **Board Cert:** Otolaryngology 2000; **Med School:** Rush Med Coll 1994; **Resid:** Surgery, Harbor UCLA Med Ctr 1996; Otolaryngology, Univ Toronto 1999; **Fellow:** Pediatric Otolaryngology, Chldns Hosp 2001; **Fac Appt:** Asst Prof Oto, Albert Einstein Coll Med

Pediatric Pulmonology

Arens, Raanan MD (PPul) - **Spec Exp:** Sleep Disorders/Apnea; **Hospital:** Montefiore Med Ctr - Div. Weiler (page 100); **Address:** Chldns Hosp at Montefiore, Respiratory & Sleep Medicine, 3415 Bainbridge Ave, Bronx, NY 10467; **Phone:** 718-515-2330 x225; **Board Cert:** Pediatrics 2003; Pediatric Pulmonology 2004; **Med School:** Israel 1986; **Resid:** Pediatrics, Shera Med Ctr 1990; Pediatrics, Chldns Hosp 1995; **Fellow:** Pediatric Pulmonology, Chldns Hosp 1994; **Fac Appt:** Assoc Prof Ped, Albert Einstein Coll Med

Pediatric Rheumatology

Ilowite, Norman T MD (PRhu) - **Spec Exp:** Juvenile Arthritis; Lyme Disease; Lupus/SLE; Dermatomyositis; **Hospital:** Montefiore Med Ctr - Div. Moses (page 100), Jacobi Med Ctr; **Address:** Chldns Hosp-Montefiore, Rheumatology, 3415 Bainbridge Ave, Bronx, NY 10467; **Phone:** 718-741-2456; **Board Cert:** Pediatrics 1985; Clinical & Laboratory Immunology 1990; Pediatric Rheumatology 2007; **Med School:** SUNY Downstate 1979; **Resid:** Pediatrics, Chldns Hosp Natl Med Ctr 1982; **Fellow:** Pediatric Rheumatology, Univ WA Med Ctr 1984; **Fac Appt:** Prof Ped, Albert Einstein Coll Med

Pediatric Surgery

Weinberg, Gerard MD (PS) - **Spec Exp:** Abdominal Wall Reconstruction; Trauma; Neonatal Surgery; **Hospital:** Montefiore Med Ctr - Div. Moses (page 100); **Address:** 3355 Bainbridge Ave, Bronx, NY 10467; **Phone:** 718-920-7200; **Board Cert:** Surgery 2009; Pediatric Surgery 2009; **Med School:** Albert Einstein Coll Med 1973; **Resid:** Surgery, Albert Einstein Affil Hosps 1976; Pediatric Surgery, Childrens Hosp 1977; **Fellow:** Pediatric Surgery, Univ of Miami Hosps 1979; **Fac Appt:** Prof S, Albert Einstein Coll Med

Pediatrics

Adam, Henry M MD (Ped) *PCP* - **Spec Exp:** AIDS/HIV; Chronic Illness; **Hospital:** Montefiore Med Ctr - Div. Weiler (page 100); **Address:** Chldns Hosp- Montefiore Med Ctr, 3415 Bainbridge Ave, Bronx, NY 10467; **Phone:** 718-920-2605; **Board Cert:** Pediatrics 1984; **Med School:** SUNY Upstate Med Univ 1979; **Resid:** Pediatrics, Mt Sinai Med Ctr 1982; **Fellow:** Ambulatory Pediatrics, Albert Einstein Affil Hosp 1983; **Fac Appt:** Prof Ped, Albert Einstein Coll Med

Andrade, Joseph MD (Ped) *PCP* - **Spec Exp:** Asthma; **Hospital:** Montefiore Med Ctr - Div. North (page 100); **Address:** 1163 Manor Ave, Bronx, NY 10472; **Phone:** 718-589-3501; **Board Cert:** Pediatrics 2007; Internal Medicine 2001; **Med School:** Ecuador 1981; **Resid:** Pediatrics, Our Lady of Mercy Med Ctr 1986; Internal Medicine, Our Lady of Mercy Med Ctr 1988

Arnstein, Ellis MD (Ped) *PCP* - **Spec Exp:** Developmental Disorders; **Hospital:** Bronx Lebanon Hosp Ctr; **Address:** Bronx Lebanon Hosp Ctr, 1650 Selwyn Ave, Ste 6D, Bronx, NY 10457; **Phone:** 718-579-7337; **Board Cert:** Pediatrics 1975; Neurodevelopmental Disabilities 2001; **Med School:** SUNY Downstate 1969; **Resid:** Pediatrics, Univ Wash Med Ctr 1973; **Fellow:** Child & Adolescent Psychiatry, Tufts-New England Med Ctr 1974; **Fac Appt:** Asst Prof Ped, NY Med Coll

Balk, Sophie J MD (Ped) *PCP* - **Spec Exp:** Environmental Medicine; **Hospital:** Montefiore Med Ctr - Div. Moses (page 100), Montefiore Med Ctr - Div. Weiler (page 100); **Address:** 1621 Eastchester Road, Bronx, NY 10461-2604; **Phone:** 718-405-8090; **Board Cert:** Pediatrics 1979; **Med School:** Albert Einstein Coll Med 1974; **Resid:** Pediatrics, Montefiore Hosp Med Ctr 1977; **Fac Appt:** Assoc Prof Ped, Albert Einstein Coll Med

Belamarich, Peter F MD (Ped) - **Spec Exp:** Cholesterol/Lipid Disorders; **Hospital:** Montefiore Med Ctr - Div. Weiler (page 100); **Address:** Children's Hospital, 3415 Bainbridge Ave Fl Cham 4, Bronx, NY 10467; **Phone:** 718-696-6060; **Board Cert:** Pediatrics 1987; **Med School:** Boston Univ 1983; **Resid:** Pediatrics, Brookdale Hosp 1986; **Fellow:** Pediatric Gastroenterology, Columbia Presby Hosp 1989

Bloomfield, Diane MD (Ped) *PCP* - **Hospital:** Montefiore Med Ctr - Div. Moses (page 100); **Address:** 3444 Kossuth Ave, DTC Bldg, FL 1B, Bronx, NY 10467-2461; **Phone:** 718-920-5873; **Board Cert:** Pediatrics 1987; **Med School:** Cornell Univ-Weill Med Coll 1982; **Resid:** Pediatrics, NY Hosp 1985; **Fellow:** Ambulatory Pediatrics, NY Hosp 1986; **Fac Appt:** Asst Prof Ped, Cornell Univ-Weill Med Coll

Cahill, Linda T MD (Ped) - **Spec Exp:** Child Abuse; **Hospital:** Montefiore Med Ctr - Div. Moses (page 100); **Address:** Butler Child Advocacy Ctr, Chldns Hosp-Montefiore, 3314 Steuben Ave, Bronx, NY 10467; **Phone:** 718-920-5833; **Board Cert:** Pediatrics 1975; **Med School:** Med Coll PA 1969; **Resid:** Pediatrics, Beth Israel Med Ctr 1972; **Fellow:** Pediatric Infectious Disease, Mt Sinai Hosp 1974; **Fac Appt:** Assoc Prof Ped, Albert Einstein Coll Med

Easton, Lon MD (Ped) *PCP* - **Spec Exp:** Sports Medicine; **Hospital:** Montefiore Med Ctr - Div. Moses (page 100), Montefiore Med Ctr - Div. Weiler (page 100); **Address:** 3594 E Tremont Ave, Bronx, NY 10465-2032; **Phone:** 718-863-1050; **Board Cert:** Pediatrics 1983; **Med School:** NY Med Coll 1978; **Resid:** Pediatrics, Metropolitan Hosp 1981; **Fac Appt:** Asst Clin Prof Ped, Albert Einstein Coll Med

Esteban-Cruciani, Nora MD (Ped) *PCP* - **Spec Exp:** Chronic Illness; Nutrition; Metabolic Disorders; **Hospital:** Montefiore Med Ctr - Div. Moses (page 100), Montefiore Med Ctr - Div. Weiler (page 100); **Address:** 111 E 210th St, Pediatrics, Rosenthal-4, Bronx, NY 10467; **Phone:** 718-741-2257; **Board Cert:** Pediatrics 2008; **Med School:** Argentina 1980; **Resid:** Pediatrics, Italian Hosp 1983; Pediatrics, Albert Einstein Coll Med 1993; **Fellow:** Research, Nat Inst Hlth 1991; Research, Albert Einstein Coll Med 2005; **Fac Appt:** Assoc Prof Ped, Albert Einstein Coll Med

Haber, Patricia MD (Ped) *PCP* - **Hospital:** Montefiore Med Ctr - Div. Moses (page 100); **Address:** 1500 Astor Ave Fl 2, Bronx, NY 10469-5900; **Phone:** 718-881-0100; **Board Cert:** Pediatrics 1981; Pediatric Rheumatology 2004; **Med School:** Johns Hopkins Univ 1976; **Resid:** Pediatrics, Johns Hopkins Hosp 1979; **Fellow:** Immunology, Univ Alabama Hosp 1982; Pediatric Rheumatology, Univ Alabama Hosp 1984; **Fac Appt:** Asst Prof Ped, Albert Einstein Coll Med

Hirschman, Alan MD (Ped) *PCP* - **Spec Exp:** Asthma; **Hospital:** Montefiore Med Ctr - Div. Moses (page 100); **Address:** 3765 Riverdale Ave, Ste 4, Bronx, NY 10463-1845; **Phone:** 718-548-7300; **Board Cert:** Pediatrics 1981; **Med School:** UMDNJ-NJ Med Sch, Newark 1976; **Resid:** Pediatrics, Montefiore Med Ctr 1980; **Fac Appt:** Asst Clin Prof, Albert Einstein Coll Med

Igel, Gerard MD (Ped) *PCP* - **Spec Exp:** Chronic Illness; Behavioral Disorders; Developmental Disorders; Foster Care; **Hospital:** Montefiore Med Ctr - Div. Moses (page 100), Jacobi Med Ctr; **Address:** 1613 Tenbroeck Ave, Bronx, NY 10461-2007; **Phone:** 718-828-9060; **Board Cert:** Pediatrics 1986; **Med School:** Israel 1981; **Resid:** Pediatrics, Jacobi Med Ctr 1984; **Fac Appt:** Asst Clin Prof Ped, Albert Einstein Coll Med

Kaminer, Ruth MD (Ped) - **Spec Exp:** Developmental & Behavioral Disorders; **Hospital:** Montefiore Med Ctr - Div. Moses (page 100); **Address:** Rose F Kennedy Ctr, 1410 Pelham Pkwy S, rm 108, Bronx, NY 10461-1101; **Phone:** 718-430-2445; **Board Cert:** Pediatrics 1971; Neurodevelopmental Disabilities 2001; Developmental-Behavioral Pediatrics 2002; **Med School:** NYU Sch Med 1962; **Resid:** Pediatrics, Chldn's Hops 1964Bronx Munipal Hosp 1968; **Fellow:** Developmental-Behavioral Pediatrics, Albert Einstein Affil Hosp 1974; **Fac Appt:** Clin Prof Ped, Albert Einstein Coll Med

London, Ronald MD (Ped) *PCP* - **Hospital:** Montefiore Med Ctr - Div. Moses (page 100), Montefiore Med Ctr - Div. Weiler (page 100); **Address:** 3594 E Tremont Ave, Lower Level, Bronx, NY 10456; **Phone:** 347-515-2130; **Board Cert:** Pediatrics 2003; **Med School:** Israel 1984; **Resid:** Pediatrics, Montefiore Hosp Med Ctr 1987; **Fellow:** Child Development, Albert Einstein 1988

Mayers, Marguerite MD (Ped) *PCP* - **Spec Exp:** Tuberculosis; AIDS/HIV; Travel Medicine; **Hospital:** Montefiore Med Ctr - Div. Moses (page 100); **Address:** 111 E 210th St, Bronx, NY 10467-2401; **Phone:** 718-920-5871; **Board Cert:** Pediatrics 1977; Pediatric Infectious Disease 2009; **Med School:** Albert Einstein Coll Med 1971; **Resid:** Pediatrics, Montefiore Hosp Med Ctr 1974; **Fellow:** Infectious Disease, Montefiore Hosp Med Ctr 1976; **Fac Appt:** Clin Prof Ped, Albert Einstein Coll Med

Okun, Alexander MD (Ped) *PCP* - **Spec Exp:** Chronic Illness; Palliative Care; **Hospital:** Montefiore Med Ctr - Div. Moses (page 100); **Address:** 1621 Eastchester Rd, Ste 115, Bronx, NY 10461-2604; **Phone:** 718-405-8040; **Board Cert:** Pediatrics 2009; Developmental-Behavioral Pediatrics 2002; **Med School:** Columbia P&S 1983; **Resid:** Pediatrics, Columbia-Presby Med Ctr 1986; **Fellow:** Child & Adolescent Psychiatry, Jacobi Med Ctr-Albert Einstein Coll Med 1990; **Fac Appt:** Assoc Clin Prof Ped, Albert Einstein Coll Med

Oppedisano, Carlyn MD (Ped) *PCP* - **Spec Exp:** Parenting Issues; **Hospital:** NYPresby-Morgan Stanley Children's Hosp (page 104); **Address:** 2600 Netherland Ave, Ste 120, Riverdale, NY 10463-4813; **Phone:** 718-796-3580; **Board Cert:** Pediatrics 2009; **Med School:** Columbia P&S 1981; **Resid:** Pediatrics, Babies Hosp 1985; **Fac Appt:** Assoc Clin Prof Ped, Columbia P&S

Schechter, Miriam MD (Ped) *PCP* - **Spec Exp:** Asthma; Vaccines; **Hospital:** Montefiore Med Ctr - Div. Moses (page 100); **Address:** 1621 Eastchester Rd, Ste 115, Bronx, NY 10461-2604; **Phone:** 718-405-8040; **Board Cert:** Pediatrics 2007; **Med School:** NYU Sch Med 1989; **Resid:** Pediatrics, Mount Sinai 1992; Pediatrics, Mount Sinai 1993; **Fac Appt:** Asst Prof Ped, Albert Einstein Coll Med

Stein, Ruth E K MD (Ped) *PCP* - **Spec Exp:** Chronic Illness; Developmental & Behavioral Disorders; **Hospital:** Montefiore Med Ctr - Div. Moses (page 100); **Address:** 111 E 210th St, Bronx, NY 10467-2401; **Phone:** 718-920-7932; **Board Cert:** Pediatrics 1971; Developmental-Behavioral Pediatrics 2004; **Med School:** Albert Einstein Coll Med 1966; **Resid:** Pediatrics, Bronx Muni Hosp 1968; Pediatrics, Chldns Hosp Natl Med Ctr 1969; **Fellow:** Community Medicine, Chldns Hosp Natl Med Ctr 1969; **Fac Appt:** Prof Ped, Albert Einstein Coll Med

Strassberg, Barbara E MD (Ped) *PCP* - **Spec Exp:** Developmental Disorders; **Hospital:** NYPresby-Morgan Stanley Children's Hosp (page 104); **Address:** Riverdale Pediatrics, 2600 Netherland Ave, Ste 120, Bronx, NY 10463-4813; **Phone:** 718-796-3580; **Board Cert:** Pediatrics 2009; **Med School:** SUNY Upstate Med Univ 1981; **Resid:** Pediatrics, Columbia-Presby Hosp 1984; **Fac Appt:** Assoc Clin Prof Ped, Columbia P&S

Tolchin, Sara D MD (Ped) *PCP* - **Spec Exp:** Preventive Medicine; **Hospital:** Montefiore Med Ctr - Div. Moses (page 100), Montefiore Med Ctr - Div. Weiler (page 100); **Address:** 1500 Astor Ave Fl 2, Bronx, NY 10469-5900; **Phone:** 718-881-0100; **Board Cert:** Pediatrics 2002; **Med School:** SUNY Hlth Sci Ctr 1971; **Resid:** Pediatrics, Kings County Hospital 1967; Pediatrics, Jacobi Med Ctr 1969; **Fac Appt:** Clin Prof Ped, Albert Einstein Coll Med

Weiner, Richard L MD (Ped) *PCP* - **Spec Exp:** Adolescent Medicine; **Hospital:** Montefiore Med Ctr - Div. Moses (page 100), Montefiore Med Ctr - Div. Weiler (page 100); **Address:** 1500 Astor Ave, Bronx, NY 10469-5938; **Phone:** 718-881-0100; **Board Cert:** Pediatrics 1991; **Med School:** Albert Einstein Coll Med 1975; **Resid:** Pediatrics, Jacobi Med Ctr 1978; **Fac Appt:** Assoc Prof Ped, Albert Einstein Coll Med

Wong, Martha S MD (Ped) *PCP* - **Spec Exp:** Sickle Cell Disease; Hemophilia; **Hospital:** Bronx Lebanon Hosp Ctr; **Address:** 1770 Grand Concourse, Ste 2A, Bronx, NY 10457; **Phone:** 718-901-8109; **Board Cert:** Pediatrics 1972; Pediatric Hematology-Oncology 1978; **Med School:** Taiwan 1966; **Resid:** Pediatrics, Kings County Hosp 1970; **Fellow:** Pediatric Hematology-Oncology, Montefiore Med Ctr 1972

Zoltan, Irving MD (Ped) *PCP* - **Spec Exp:** Diagnostic Problems; Asthma; Infectious Disease; **Hospital:** Montefiore Med Ctr - Div. Moses (page 100), Montefiore Med Ctr - Div. Weiler (page 100); **Address:** 1613 Tenbroeck Ave, Bronx, NY 10461; **Phone:** 718-828-9060; **Board Cert:** Pediatrics 1979; **Med School:** Albert Einstein Coll Med 1974; **Resid:** Pediatrics, Jacobi Med Ctr 1978; **Fac Appt:** Asst Prof Ped, Albert Einstein Coll Med

Physical Medicine & Rehabilitation

DeAraujo, Maria MD (PMR) - **Spec Exp:** Arthritis; Pain-Low Back; Electromyography; Pain-Musculoskeletal; **Hospital:** Montefiore Med Ctr - Div. North (page 100); **Address:** Dept of Phy Med & Rehab, 600 E 233rd St, Bronx, NY 10466-2604; **Phone:** 718-920-9171; **Board Cert:** Physical Medicine & Rehabilitation 1989; **Med School:** Brazil 1972; **Resid:** Physical Medicine & Rehabilitation, St Vincent's Hosp & Med Ctr 1981; **Fellow:** Physical Medicine & Rehabilitation, Westchester Med Ctr 1989; **Fac Appt:** Clin Prof PMR, NY Med Coll

Fast, Avital MD (PMR) - **Spec Exp:** Pain-Back; **Hospital:** Montefiore Med Ctr - Div. Moses (page 100), Montefiore Med Ctr - Div. Weiler (page 100); **Address:** 150 E 210th St, Bronx, NY 10467; **Phone:** 718-920-2751; **Board Cert:** Physical Medicine & Rehabilitation 1978; **Med School:** Israel 1972; **Resid:** Physical Medicine & Rehabilitation, Montefiore Med Ctr 1976

Levin, Sheryl MD (PMR) - **Spec Exp:** Neuro-Rehabilitation; Pain-Musculoskeletal; Arthritis; **Hospital:** Montefiore Med Ctr - Div. Moses (page 100); **Address:** 3435 Dekalb Ave, Bronx, NY 10467-2301; **Phone:** 718-547-8899; **Board Cert:** Physical Medicine & Rehabilitation 1989; **Med School:** Cornell Univ-Weill Med Coll 1984; **Resid:** Physical Medicine & Rehabilitation, New York Hosp 1988; **Fac Appt:** Assoc Clin Prof PMR, Albert Einstein Coll Med

Thomas, Mark A MD (PMR) - **Hospital:** Montefiore Med Ctr - Div. Moses (page 100); **Address:** 150 E 210th St Fl 2, Bronx, NY 10467; **Phone:** 718-920-2753; **Board Cert:** Physical Medicine & Rehabilitation 1988; **Med School:** Mexico 1982; **Resid:** Physical Medicine & Rehabilitation, Nassau Co Med Ctr 1986; **Fac Appt:** Assoc Prof PMR, Albert Einstein Coll Med

Plastic Surgery

Goldstein, Robert MD (PlS) - **Spec Exp:** Breast Surgery; Nasal Surgery; Abdominoplasty; **Hospital:** Montefiore Med Ctr - Div. Weiler (page 100), Montefiore Med Ctr - Div. Moses (page 100); **Address:** 2425 Eastchester Rd, Bronx, NY 10469; **Phone:** 718-405-7500; **Board Cert:** Plastic Surgery 1985; **Med School:** Penn State Univ-Hershey Med Ctr 1977; **Resid:** Surgery, Montefiore Med Ctr 1981; Plastic Surgery, Montefiore Med Ctr 1984; **Fellow:** Hand Surgery, Montefiore Med Ctr-Einstein Div 1982; **Fac Appt:** Assoc Clin Prof PlS, Albert Einstein Coll Med

Greenstein, Bruce MD (PlS) - **Spec Exp:** Burn Care; Burns-Reconstructive Plastic Surgery; **Hospital:** Jacobi Med Ctr, N Central Bronx Hosp; **Address:** Jacobi Med Ctr, Dept Plastic Surgery, 1400 Pelham Pkwy S, rm 209, Bronx, NY 10461; **Phone:** 718-918-5970; **Board Cert:** Plastic Surgery 1984; **Med School:** SUNY Upstate Med Univ 1975; **Resid:** Surgery, Montefiore Hosp Med Ctr 1980; Plastic Surgery, Montefiore Hosp Med Ctr 1982; **Fellow:** Hand Surgery, Montefiore Hosp Med Ctr 1983; **Fac Appt:** Assoc Clin Prof PlS, Albert Einstein Coll Med

Liebling, Ralph W MD (PlS) - **Spec Exp:** Reconstructive Surgery; Microsurgery; Hand Surgery; Burn Care; **Hospital:** Jacobi Med Ctr, N Central Bronx Hosp; **Address:** Jacobi Med Ctr, Dept Plastic Recons Surg, 1400 Pelham Parkway South, Bronx, NY 10461; **Phone:** 718-918-7000; **Board Cert:** Plastic Surgery 1988; **Med School:** Albert Einstein Coll Med 1977; **Resid:** Surgery, Montefiore Med Ctr 1981; Plastic Surgery, Montefiore Med Ctr 1983; **Fellow:** Reconstructive Microsurgery, NYU/Bellevue Hosp Ctr 1984; **Fac Appt:** Assoc Prof S, Albert Einstein Coll Med

Staffenberg, David A MD (PlS) - **Spec Exp:** Craniofacial Surgery/Reconstruction; Pediatric Plastic Surgery; Ear Reconstruction/Microtia; Cosmetic Surgery-Face; **Hospital:** Montefiore Med Ctr - Div. Moses (page 100); **Address:** 1625 Poplar St, Bronx, NY 10467; **Phone:** 718-405-8337; **Board Cert:** Plastic Surgery 2009; **Med School:** NY Med Coll 1989; **Resid:** Surgery, Maimonides Med Ctr 1995; Plastic Surgery, Emory Univ Med Ctr 1997; **Fellow:** Craniofacial Surgery, UCLA Med Ctr 1998; **Fac Appt:** Assoc Prof PlS, Albert Einstein Coll Med

Psychiatry

Asnis, Gregory M MD (Psyc) - **Spec Exp:** Psychopharmacology; Mood Disorders; Anxiety Disorders; Depression; **Hospital:** Montefiore Med Ctr - Div. Moses (page 100), Phelps Meml Hosp Ctr (page 592); **Address:** 111 E 210th St, Bronx, NY 10467-2401; **Phone:** 718-920-4287; **Board Cert:** Psychiatry 1978; **Med School:** Hahnemann Univ 1972; **Resid:** Psychiatry, Mt Sinai Hosp 1976; **Fellow:** Psychiatry, Columbia-Presby Med Ctr 1981; **Fac Appt:** Prof Psyc, Albert Einstein Coll Med

Gelfand, Janice MD (Psyc) - **Spec Exp:** Depression; Anxiety Disorders; Psychosomatic Disorders; Personality Disorders; **Hospital:** NY-Presby Hosp/Columbia (page 104); **Address:** 3765 Riverdale Ave, Bronx, NY 10463-1845; **Phone:** 718-361-3482; **Board Cert:** Psychiatry 1990; **Med School:** NYU Sch Med 1985; **Resid:** Psychiatry, NYU Med Ctr 1989; **Fellow:** Psychiatry, Beth Israel Med Ctr 1991; **Fac Appt:** Asst Prof Psyc, Columbia P&S

Heiman, Peter L MD (Psyc) - **Spec Exp:** Medical Illness in Psychiatry; **Hospital:** Montefiore Med Ctr - Div. Moses (page 100); **Address:** 4491 Manhattan College Pkwy, Bronx, NY 10471; **Phone:** 212-472-8885; **Board Cert:** Psychiatry 1975; **Med School:** Albert Einstein Coll Med 1968; **Resid:** Psychiatry, Montefiore Hosp Med Ctr 1972; **Fac Appt:** Asst Clin Prof Psyc, Albert Einstein Coll Med

Lebinger, Martin B MD (Psyc) - **Spec Exp:** Depression; Anxiety Disorders; Panic Disorder; **Hospital:** Bronx Psych Ctr; **Address:** 1540 Pelham Pkwy S, Ste 1A, Bronx, NY 10461-1130; **Phone:** 718-518-0222; **Board Cert:** Psychiatry 1980; **Med School:** Albert Einstein Coll Med 1976; **Resid:** Psychiatry, Montefiore Hosp Med Ctr 1979; **Fellow:** Psychiatry, LI Jewish-Hillside Med Ctr 1981; **Fac Appt:** Asst Clin Prof Psyc, Albert Einstein Coll Med

Osei-Tutu, John MD (Psyc) - **Spec Exp:** Anxiety & Depression; Addiction/Substance Abuse; **Hospital:** Bronx Lebanon Hosp Ctr, Brunswick Hall Psych Hosp; **Address:** 1276 Fulton Ave, Bronx, NY 10456; **Phone:** 718-901-6133; **Board Cert:** Psychiatry 1990; Addiction Psychiatry 2003; **Med School:** Ghana 1976; **Resid:** Psychiatry, Bronx Lebanon Hosp 1983; **Fac Appt:** Asst Prof Psyc, Albert Einstein Coll Med

Schwartz, Bruce J MD (Psyc) - **Spec Exp:** Depression; Bipolar/Mood Disorders; Schizophrenia; Anxiety & Depression; **Hospital:** Montefiore Med Ctr - Div. Moses (page 100); **Address:** Montefiore Medical Ctr, Dept Psychiatry, 111 E 210th St, Bronx, NY 10467-2490; **Phone:** 718-920-4040; **Board Cert:** Psychiatry 1980; **Med School:** SUNY Downstate 1975; **Resid:** Psychiatry, Bronx Muni Hosp 1979; **Fac Appt:** Prof Psyc, Albert Einstein Coll Med

Wyszynski, Bernard MD (Psyc) - **Hospital:** Montefiore Med Ctr - Div. Moses (page 100); **Address:** Montefore Medical Ctr, KLAU 2, 111 E 210th St, Bronx, NY 10467; **Phone:** 718-920-4737; **Board Cert:** Neurology 1987; **Med School:** Univ Pennsylvania 1980; **Resid:** Neurology, Mount Sinai Med Ctr 1984; Psychiatry, Mount Sinai Med Ctr 1987; **Fac Appt:** Assoc Prof Psyc, Albert Einstein Coll Med

Pulmonary Disease

Aldrich, Thomas K MD (Pul) - **Spec Exp:** Asthma; Chronic Obstructive Lung Disease (COPD); Sickle Cell Disease-Lung; **Hospital:** Montefiore Med Ctr - Div. Moses (page 100); **Address:** Montefiore Med Ctr, Pulmonary Div, 111 E 210th St, Bronx, NY 10467-2401; **Phone:** 718-920-6087; **Board Cert:** Critical Care Medicine 2001; Pulmonary Disease 1980; Internal Medicine 1978; **Med School:** Univ Minn 1975; **Resid:** Internal Medicine, UC Irvine Med Ctr 1978; **Fellow:** Pulmonary Disease, Univ Virginia Med Ctr 1980; Physiology, Univ Penn 1982; **Fac Appt:** Prof Med, Albert Einstein Coll Med

Appel, David MD (Pul) - **Spec Exp:** Sleep Disorders/Apnea; Asthma; Smoking Cessation; **Hospital:** Montefiore Med Ctr - Div. Moses (page 100); **Address:** 111 E 210th St, Pulmonary Div, Bronx, NY 10467; **Phone:** 718-920-6055; **Board Cert:** Internal Medicine 1976; Sleep Medicine 2002; **Med School:** Albert Einstein Coll Med 1973; **Resid:** Internal Medicine, Bronx Municipal Hosp 1976; **Fellow:** Pulmonary Disease, Bronx Municipal Hosp 1978; **Fac Appt:** Assoc Prof Med, Albert Einstein Coll Med

Casper, Theodore MD (Pul) - **Spec Exp:** Critical Care Medicine; **Hospital:** NY Westchester Sq Med Ctr, Montefiore Med Ctr - Div. Weiler (page 100); **Address:** 1250 Waters Pl, Ste 506, Bronx, NY 10461; **Phone:** 718-892-1200; **Board Cert:** Internal Medicine 1983; Pulmonary Disease 1986; **Med School:** Columbia P&S 1980; **Resid:** Internal Medicine, St Luke's Hosp 1983; **Fellow:** Pulmonary Disease, St Luke's Hosp 1985

Karetzky, Monroe MD (Pul) - **Spec Exp:** Asthma; Sleep Disorders; **Hospital:** Hackensack Univ Med Ctr (page 96), Englewood Hosp & Med Ctr (page 656); **Address:** 441 E Tremont Ave, Bronx, NY 10457; **Phone:** 718-583-9240; **Board Cert:** Pain Medicine 1974; Critical Care Medicine 1999; Geriatric Medicine 2002; Internal Medicine 1971; **Med School:** Cornell Univ-Weill Med Coll 1963; **Resid:** Internal Medicine, Mary I Bassett Hosp 1966; **Fellow:** Cardiopulmonary Disease, Mary I Bassett Hosp 1967; **Fac Appt:** Assoc Clin Prof Med, UMDNJ-NJ Med Sch, Newark

Klapper, Philip MD (Pul) - **Spec Exp:** Asthma; Emphysema; Chronic Obstructive Lung Disease (COPD); **Hospital:** Montefiore Med Ctr - Div. Moses (page 100), Lawrence Hosp Ctr; **Address:** 3322 Bainbridge Ave, Bronx, NY 10467; **Phone:** 718-884-2000; **Board Cert:** Internal Medicine 1986; Pulmonary Disease 2000; Critical Care Medicine 2003; **Med School:** Albert Einstein Coll Med 1983; **Resid:** Internal Medicine, Montefiore Hosp Med Ctr 1986; **Fellow:** Pulmonary Disease, SUNY Downstate Med Ctr 1990; Critical Care Medicine, Montefiore Hosp Med Ctr 1991; **Fac Appt:** Asst Clin Prof Med, Albert Einstein Coll Med

Marino, William MD (Pul) - **Spec Exp:** Respiratory Failure; Asthma; Bronchoscopy; **Hospital:** Montefiore Med Ctr - Div. North (page 100); **Address:** 4234 Bronx Blvd Fl 2, Bronx, NY 10466; **Phone:** 347-341-4340; **Board Cert:** Internal Medicine 1980; Pulmonary Disease 1984; Critical Care Medicine 2007; **Med School:** Albert Einstein Coll Med 1977; **Resid:** Internal Medicine, Montefiore Hosp Med Ctr 1980; **Fellow:** Pulmonary Disease, Columbia-Presby Med ctr 1982; **Fac Appt:** Assoc Clin Prof Med, NY Med Coll

Menon, Latha MD (Pul) - **Spec Exp:** Asthma; Critical Care; Breathing Disorders; **Hospital:** Bronx Lebanon Hosp Ctr; **Address:** 1770 Grand Concourse, Ste 2G, Bronx, NY 10457-5528; **Phone:** 718-518-5581; **Board Cert:** Internal Medicine 1978; Pulmonary Disease 1980; Critical Care Medicine 2002; **Med School:** India 1972; **Resid:** Internal Medicine, Flushing Hosp 1978; **Fellow:** Pulmonary Disease, Montefiore Med Ctr 1981; **Fac Appt:** Assoc Prof Med, Albert Einstein Coll Med

Pinsker, Kenneth MD (Pul) - **Spec Exp:** Asthma; Lung Cancer; Sarcoidosis; **Hospital:** Montefiore Med Ctr - Div. Moses (page 100); **Address:** 111 E 210th St, Bronx, NY 10467-2490; **Phone:** 718-920-6095; **Board Cert:** Internal Medicine 1972; Pulmonary Disease 1976; **Med School:** Ros Franklin Univ/Chicago Med Sch 1968; **Resid:** Internal Medicine, Montefiore Hosp Med Ctr 1970; Internal Medicine, Jacobi Med Ctr 1971; **Fellow:** Pulmonary Disease, Montefiore Hosp Med Ctr 1972; Pulmonary Disease, Montefiore Hosp Med Ctr 1975; **Fac Appt:** Prof Med, Albert Einstein Coll Med

Prezant, David MD (Pul) - **Spec Exp:** Asthma; **Hospital:** Montefiore Med Ctr - Div. Moses (page 100); **Address:** 111 E 210th St, Bronx, NY 10467-2401; **Phone:** 718-920-6095; **Board Cert:** Internal Medicine 1984; Pulmonary Disease 1986; **Med School:** Albert Einstein Coll Med 1981; **Resid:** Internal Medicine, Harlem Hosp 1984; **Fellow:** Pulmonary Disease, Montefiore Hosp Med Ctr 1986; **Fac Appt:** Assoc Prof Med, Albert Einstein Coll Med

Sender, Joel MD (Pul) - **Spec Exp:** Asthma; Sarcoidosis; **Hospital:** St Barnabas Hosp - Bronx; **Address:** 2016 Bronxdale Ave, Ste 301, Bronx, NY 10462-3300; **Phone:** 718-409-2222; **Board Cert:** Internal Medicine 1978; Pulmonary Disease 1980; Geriatric Medicine 2005; **Med School:** Albany Med Coll 1975; **Resid:** Internal Medicine, Mount Sinai Hosp 1978; **Fellow:** Pulmonary Disease, Mount Sinai Hosp 1980

Radiation Oncology

Bodner, William R MD (RadRO) - **Spec Exp:** Brachytherapy; **Hospital:** Montefiore Med Ctr - Div. North (page 100); **Address:** MMC Medical Park, 1625 Poplar St, Ste 101, Bronx, NY 10461; **Phone:** 718-405-8550; **Board Cert:** Radiation Oncology 2005; **Med School:** Wake Forest Univ 1987; **Resid:** Radiation Oncology, NY Med Coll Affil Hosp 1995; **Fac Appt:** Assoc Prof, NY Med Coll

Rheumatology

Fomberstein, Barry MD (Rhu) - **Spec Exp:** Rheumatoid Arthritis; Gout; **Hospital:** Montefiore Med Ctr - Div. North (page 100); **Address:** Montefiore Med Ctr-North Div, 600 E 233rd St, Bronx, NY 10466-2697; **Phone:** 718-920-9168; **Board Cert:** Internal Medicine 1979; Rheumatology 1982; **Med School:** Albert Einstein Coll Med 1976; **Resid:** Internal Medicine, LIJ Med Ctr 1979; **Fellow:** Rheumatology, LIJ Med Ctr 1981; **Fac Appt:** Assoc Clin Prof Med, NY Med Coll

Keiser, Harold D MD (Rhu) - **Spec Exp:** Rheumatoid Arthritis; Lupus/SLE; **Hospital:** Montefiore Med Ctr - Div. Weiler (page 100), Jacobi Med Ctr; **Address:** 1515 Blondell Ave, Ste 220, Bronx, NY 10461-2662; **Phone:** 866-633-8255; **Board Cert:** Internal Medicine 1972; Rheumatology 1972; **Med School:** NYU Sch Med 1964; **Resid:** Internal Medicine, Clevelnd Metro Genl Hosp 1968; **Fellow:** Rheumatology, Albert Einstein Coll Med 1972; **Fac Appt:** Prof Med, Albert Einstein Coll Med

Weinstein, Joshua W MD (Rhu) - **Spec Exp:** Lupus/SLE; Rheumatoid Arthritis; Gout; **Hospital:** Montefiore Med Ctr - Div. Weiler (page 100), NY Hosp Queens; **Address:** 1554 Astor Ave, Bronx, NY 10469; **Phone:** 718-994-8900; **Board Cert:** Internal Medicine 1975; Rheumatology 1978; **Med School:** SUNY Downstate 1972; **Resid:** Internal Medicine, Maimonides Med Ctr 1975; **Fellow:** Rheumatology, Montefiore Med Ctr 1977; **Fac Appt:** Asst Prof Med, Albert Einstein Coll Med

Surgery

Agarwal, Nanakram MD (S) - **Spec Exp:** Breast Surgery; Colon & Rectal Surgery; **Hospital:** Montefiore Med Ctr - Div. North (page 100), Westchester Med Ctr; **Address:** 600 E 233rd St Fl 4, Bronx, NY 10466; **Phone:** 718-920-9143; **Board Cert:** Surgery 2001; Critical Care Medicine 2005; **Med School:** India 1973; **Resid:** Surgery, Our Lady of Mercy Med Ctr 1981; **Fellow:** Critical Care Medicine, Westchester Co Med Ctr 1982; **Fac Appt:** Prof S, NY Med Coll

Bellemare, Sarah MD (S) - **Spec Exp:** Hepatobiliary Surgery; Transplant-Liver; Robotic Surgery; Laparoscopic Surgery; **Hospital:** Montefiore Med Ctr - Div. Weiler (page 100), Montefiore Med Ctr - Div. Moses (page 100); **Address:** Montefiore Med Ctr - Weiler Div, 111 E 210th St, Rosenfeld 2, Bronx, NY 10467; **Phone:** 718-904-2047; **Board Cert:** Surgery 2001; **Med School:** Canada 1996; **Resid:** Surgery, Montreal Univ Med Ctr 2001; **Fellow:** Hepatobiliary Surgery, NY Presby-Columbia Med Ctr 2003; Transplant Surgery, NY Presby-Columbia Med Ctr 2004; **Fac Appt:** Asst Clin Prof S, Albert Einstein Coll Med

Cosgrove, John M MD (S) - **Spec Exp:** Laparoscopic Surgery; Endoscopy; Biliary Surgery; Gastrointestinal Surgery; **Hospital:** Bronx Lebanon Hosp Ctr, N Shore Univ Hosp; **Address:** 1650 Selwyn Ave, Ste 4A, Bronx, NY 10457; **Phone:** 718-960-1227; **Board Cert:** Surgery 2008; **Med School:** NY Med Coll 1983; **Resid:** Surgery, Beth Israel Med Ctr 1988; **Fac Appt:** Assoc Prof S, Albert Einstein Coll Med

Greenstein, Stuart MD (S) - **Spec Exp:** Laparoscopic Surgery; Dialysis Access Surgery; Transplant-Kidney; **Hospital:** Montefiore Med Ctr - Div. Moses (page 100); **Address:** 111 E 210th St, Bronx, NY 10467; **Phone:** 877-287-3536; **Board Cert:** Surgery 2003; **Med School:** Harvard Med Sch 1979; **Resid:** Surgery, UMDNJ Med Ctr 1984; **Fellow:** Vascular Surgery, Hosp Univ Penn 1985; Transplant Surgery, SUNY Downstate 1986; **Fac Appt:** Prof S, Albert Einstein Coll Med

Hodgson, W John B MD (S) - **Spec Exp:** Proctology; Hemorrhoids; Anal Disorders & Reconstruction; **Hospital:** Montefiore Med Ctr - Div. Weiler (page 100), Montefiore Med Ctr - Div. North (page 100); **Address:** 1575 Blondell Ave, Ste 125, Montefiore Med Ctr, Dept of Surgery, Bronx, NY 10461; **Phone:** 718-405-8239; **Board Cert:** Surgery 1975; **Med School:** England, UK 1964; **Resid:** Surgery, Univ of London Hosps 1972; **Fellow:** Colon & Rectal Surgery, Mount Sinai Med Ctr 1974; **Fac Appt:** Prof S, Albert Einstein Coll Med

Kennedy, Timothy J MD (S) - **Spec Exp:** Laparoscopic Surgery; Pancreatic Surgery; **Hospital:** Montefiore Med Ctr - Div. Weiler (page 100), Montefiore Med Ctr - Div. Moses (page 100); **Address:** Montefiore-Weiler Einstein Hosp, 1575 Blondell Ave, Bronx, NY 10461; **Phone:** 718-405-8244; **Board Cert:** Surgery 2007; **Med School:** Georgetown Univ 1999; **Resid:** Surgery, Northwestern Meml Hosp 2006; **Fellow:** Surgical Oncology, Meml Sloan Kettering Cancer Ctr 2008

Kinkhabwala, Milan M MD (S) - **Spec Exp:** Transplant-Liver; Hepatobiliary Surgery; Liver & Biliary Surgery; **Hospital:** Montefiore Med Ctr - Div. Moses (page 100), Montefiore Med Ctr - Div. Weiler (page 100); **Address:** 111 E 210th St, Bronx, NY 10467; **Phone:** 888-795-4837; **Board Cert:** Surgery 2004; **Med School:** Cornell Univ-Weill Med Coll 1989; **Resid:** Surgery, NY Presby/Weil Cornell 1994; **Fellow:** Hepatobiliary Surgery, UCLA Med Ctr; **Fac Appt:** Prof S, Albert Einstein Coll Med

Libutti, Steven K MD (S) - **Spec Exp:** Liver Cancer; Pancreatic Cancer; Neuroendocrine Tumors; Von Hippel-Lindau Disease; **Hospital:** Montefiore Med Ctr - Div. Weiler (page 100), Montefiore Med Ctr - Div. Moses (page 100); **Address:** 3400 Bainbridge Ave Fl 4th, Bronx, NY 10467; **Phone:** 718-920-4231; **Board Cert:** Surgery 2004; **Med School:** Columbia P&S 1990; **Resid:** Surgery, Columbia Presby Med Ctr 1995; **Fellow:** Surgical Oncology, Natl Cancer Inst 1996; **Fac Appt:** Prof S, Albert Einstein Coll Med

Sas, Norman S MD (S) - **Spec Exp:** Breast Cancer; Laparoscopic Surgery; Hernia; **Hospital:** Montefiore Med Ctr - Div. Moses (page 100), Lawrence Hosp Ctr; **Address:** 3220 Fairfield Ave, Riverdale, NY 10463-3240; **Phone:** 718-549-0700; **Board Cert:** Surgery 2009; **Med School:** NY Med Coll 1974; **Resid:** Surgery, Montefiore Med Ctr 1978; **Fac Appt:** Asst Clin Prof S, Albert Einstein Coll Med

Schechner, Richard MD (S) - **Spec Exp:** Transplant-Kidney; Laparoscopic Surgery; Breast Surgery; **Hospital:** Montefiore Med Ctr - Div. Moses (page 100), Montefiore Med Ctr - Div. Weiler (page 100); **Address:** Transplant Surgery Department, 111 E 210th St Fl 2, Bronx, NY 10467-2401; **Phone:** 877-287-3536; **Board Cert:** Surgery 2001; **Med School:** NY Med Coll 1983; **Resid:** Surgery, Montefiore Hosp Med Ctr 1988; **Fellow:** Pancreas & Intestinal Transplant, University Hosp 1989; **Fac Appt:** Asst Prof S, Albert Einstein Coll Med

Thoracic Surgery

DeRose Jr, Joseph J MD (TS) - **Spec Exp:** Robotic Cardiac Surgery; Minimally Invasive Cardiac Surgery; Mitral Valve Surgery; **Hospital:** Montefiore Med Ctr - Div. Weiler (page 100), Montefiore Med Ctr - Div. Moses (page 100); **Address:** Montefiore-Weiler Medical Ctr, Dept Cardiothoracic Surgery, 1575 Blondell Ave, Ste 125, Bronx, NY 10461; **Phone:** 718-405-8371; **Board Cert:** Surgery 2000; Thoracic Surgery 2002; **Med School:** Columbia P&S 1993; **Resid:** Surgery, Columbia Presby Med Ctr 1995; **Fellow:** Cardiothoracic Surgery, Columbia Presby Med Ctr 1999; **Fac Appt:** Assoc Prof TS, Albert Einstein Coll Med

Keller, Steven M MD (TS) - **Spec Exp:** Lung Cancer; Esophageal Cancer; Mediastinal Tumors; Hyperhidrosis-Palmar; **Hospital:** Montefiore Med Ctr - Div. Moses (page 100), Montefiore Med Ctr - Div. Weiler (page 100); **Address:** 1575 Blondell St, Ste 125, Bronx, NY 10461; **Phone:** 718-405-8378; **Board Cert:** Thoracic Surgery 2007; **Med School:** Albany Med Coll 1977; **Resid:** Surgery, Mount Sinai Hosp 1985; Thoracic Surgery, Mem Sloan Kettering Cancer Ctr 1987; **Fellow:** Surgical Oncology, NIH/National Cancer Inst 1983; **Fac Appt:** Prof TS, Albert Einstein Coll Med

Michler, Robert E MD (TS) - **Spec Exp:** Heart Valve Surgery; Coronary Artery Surgery; Minimally Invasive Surgery; Atrial Fibrillation; **Hospital:** Montefiore Med Ctr - Div. Moses (page 100), Montefiore Med Ctr - Div. Weiler (page 100); **Address:** Montefiore, Dept Cardiothoracic Surgery, 3400 Bainbridge Ave Fl 5, Bronx, NY 10467; **Phone:** 718-920-2100; **Board Cert:** Surgery 1990; Thoracic Surgery 2000; **Med School:** Dartmouth Med Sch 1981; **Resid:** Surgery, Columbia Presby Med Ctr 1987; **Fellow:** Cardiothoracic Surgery, Columbia Presby Med Ctr 1989; Pediatric Surgery, Boston Children's Hosp 1990; **Fac Appt:** Prof S, Albert Einstein Coll Med

Weinstein, Samuel MD (TS) - **Spec Exp:** Pediatric Cardiac Surgery; Congenital Heart Disease-Adult; Transplant-Heart; **Hospital:** Montefiore Med Ctr - Div. Moses (page 100), Montefiore Med Ctr - Div. Weiler (page 100); **Address:** Montefiore Med Ctr, Moses Div, Dept Cardiothoracic Surgery, 3400 Bainbridge Ave Fl 5 - Ste 5A, Bronx, NY 10467; **Phone:** 718-920-7745; **Board Cert:** Surgery 2004; Thoracic Surgery 2007; **Med School:** SUNY Stony Brook 1989; **Resid:** Surgery, Columbia Presby Med Ctr 1996; Cardiothoracic Surgery, Columbia Presby Med Ctr 1998; **Fellow:** Pediatric Cardiothoracic Surgery, Chldns Hosp 1999; **Fac Appt:** Assoc Prof TS, Albert Einstein Coll Med

Urology

Geisler, Edward MD (U) - **Spec Exp:** Urologic Cancer; Impotence; **Hospital:** Bronx Lebanon Hosp Ctr; **Address:** 1770 Grand Concourse, Ste 1F, Bronx, NY 10457-5524; **Phone:** 718-901-8173; **Board Cert:** Urology 2005; **Med School:** Jefferson Med Coll 1978; **Resid:** Surgery, Beth Israel 1980; Urology, NYU Med Ctr 1984; **Fac Appt:** Asst Prof U, Albert Einstein Coll Med

Ghavamian, Reza MD (U) - **Spec Exp:** Urologic Cancer; Prostate Cancer/Robotic Surgery; Minimally Invasive Surgery; **Hospital:** Montefiore Med Ctr - Div. Moses (page 100); **Address:** MMC Medical Arts Pavilion, 3400 Bainbridge Ave, Bronx, NY 10467; **Phone:** 718-920-8475; **Board Cert:** Urology 2008; **Med School:** Boston Univ 1991; **Resid:** Urology, Univ Mass Med Ctr 1997; **Fellow:** Urologic Oncology, Mayo Clinic 1998; **Fac Appt:** Clin Prof U, Albert Einstein Coll Med

Stein, Mark MD (U) - **Spec Exp:** Incontinence; Impotence; **Hospital:** Beth Israel Med Ctr - Petrie Division (page 94), NY Westchester Sq Med Ctr; **Address:** 3594 E Tremont Ave, Ste 320, Bronx, NY 10465; **Phone:** 718-518-9300; **Board Cert:** Urology 2000; **Med School:** Yale Univ 1984; **Resid:** Surgery, Montefiore Med Ctr 1985; Urology, Montefiore Med Ctr 1990; **Fac Appt:** Asst Prof U, NY Med Coll

Stone, Peter L MD (U) - **Spec Exp:** Prostate Cancer; Kidney Stones; Erectile Dysfunction; **Hospital:** Montefiore Med Ctr - Div. Weiler (page 100), NY Westchester Sq Med Ctr; **Address:** 2510 Westchester Ave, Ste A, Bronx, NY 10461-6268; **Phone:** 718-892-2100; **Board Cert:** Urology 2006; **Med School:** NY Med Coll 1979; **Resid:** Surgery, Montefiore Med Ctr 1981; Urology, Montefiore Med Ctr 1984; **Fac Appt:** Asst Clin Prof U, Albert Einstein Coll Med

Vascular & Interventional Radiology

Cynamon, Jacob MD (VIR) - **Spec Exp:** Peripheral Vascular Disease; Uterine Fibroids; Liver Cancer; Dialysis Access; **Hospital:** Montefiore Med Ctr - Div. Moses (page 100); **Address:** Montefiore Med Ctr, Dept Interventional Radiology, 111 E 210th St, Bronx, NY 10467; **Phone:** 718-920-5729; **Board Cert:** Diagnostic Radiology 1987; Vascular & Interventional Radiology 2004; **Med School:** Albert Einstein Coll Med 1983; **Resid:** Surgery, Montefiore Hosp Med Ctr 1984; Diagnostic Radiology, Montefiore Hosp Med Ctr 1987; **Fellow:** Vascular & Interventional Radiology, New York Hosp-Cornell 1988; **Fac Appt:** Clin Prof Rad, Albert Einstein Coll Med

Vascular Surgery

Lipsitz, Evan C MD (VascS) - **Spec Exp:** Aneurysm-Abdominal Aortic; Aneurysm-Thoracic Aortic; Carotid Artery Surgery; Endovascular Surgery; **Hospital:** Montefiore Med Ctr - Div. Moses (page 100), Montefiore Med Ctr - Div. Weiler (page 100); **Address:** 3400 Brainbridge Ave - MAP 4, Bronx, NY 10467; **Phone:** 718-920-2016; **Board Cert:** Surgery 1998; Vascular Surgery 2008; **Med School:** Columbia P&S 1990; **Resid:** Surgery, Columbia Presby Hosp 1996; **Fellow:** Vascular Surgery, Montefiore Med Ctr 1999; **Fac Appt:** Assoc Prof S, Albert Einstein Coll Med

Suggs, William D MD (VascS) - **Spec Exp:** Vein Disorders; Wound Healing/Care; Carotid Artery Surgery; **Hospital:** Montefiore Med Ctr - Div. Moses (page 100); **Address:** 111 E 210th St, Bronx, NY 10467; **Phone:** 718-920-6338; **Board Cert:** Vascular Surgery 2002; **Med School:** Wake Forest Univ 1983; **Resid:** Surgery, Geo Wash Univ Med Ctr 1989; **Fellow:** Vascular Surgery, Emory Univ Hosp 1991; **Fac Appt:** Assoc Prof VascS, Albert Einstein Coll Med

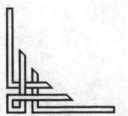
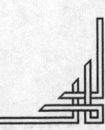

The Best in American Medicine
www.CastleConnolly.com

Kings (Brooklyn)

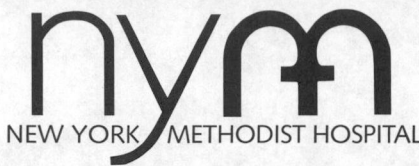

NEW YORK METHODIST HOSPITAL

506 Sixth Street, Brooklyn, N.Y. 11215
Phone (718) 780-3000, Fax (718) 780-3770
http://www.nym.org

Sponsorship	Voluntary, Not-for-Profit
Beds	591; 60 bassinets
Accreditation	Joint Commission on Accreditation of Healthcare Organizations (JCAHO), Council on Graduate Medical Education

GENERAL DESCRIPTION

New York Methodist Hospital (NYM), a member of the NewYork-Presbyterian Healthcare System, has served the neighborhoods of Brooklyn for over 125 years. NYM's medical programs have recently expanded significantly and the hospital's campus facilities in Park Slope have been extensively renovated. In addition, New York Methodist maintains satellite outpatient health centers throughout Brooklyn.

MEDICAL STAFF

NYM has over 1,000 physicians on staff; 90 percent are board certified or board eligible. Many physicians at NYM are known for the impressive and outstanding work they have done in their individual fields. New York Methodist Hospital offers medical residency programs in internal medicine, surgery, pediatrics, obstetrics/gynecology, radiation oncology, nuclear medicine, anesthesiology, emergency medicine, podiatry and dentistry. The Hospital also offers fellowships in several medical subspecialties.

SPECIAL PROGRAMS

Emergency Medicine: A recently renovated, expanded Emergency Department houses a pediatric emergency room and private rooms for obstetrics/gynecology patients. The Hospital is a State-designated Stroke Center, an AHA Heart Center and EMS 911 Receiving Hospital. 718 780-3148.

Institute for Advanced and Minimally Invasive Surgery: 866 DOCS-14U.

Institute for Asthma and Lung Diseases: See Centers of Excellence Section. 866 ASK-LUNG.

Institute for Cancer Care: 866-411-ONCO.

Institute for Cardiology and Cardiac Surgery: See Centers of Excellence Section. 866 84-HEART.

Institute for Diabetes and Other Endocrine Disorders: 866-4-GLAND-2.

Institute for Digestive and Liver Disorders: See Centers of Excellence Section.866 DIGEST-1.

Institute for Family Care: 866 432-CARE.

Institute for Neurosciences: See Centers of Excellence Section. 866 DO-NEURO.

Institute for Orthopedic Medicine and Surgery: See Centers of Excellence Section. 866 ORTHO-11.

Institute for Vascular Medicine and Surgery: 866 438-VEIN.

Institute for Women's Health: 877 41-WOMAN.

Birthing Center: Spacious, beautifully appointed rooms allow women to experience a "home-like" birth with the reassurance that high-tech medical equipment and specialists are instantly accessible if needed. Full-time lactation services are available for new mothers.

Physician Referral: The Hospital has a free seven-day, 24-hour telephone and computer on-line physician referral service. To find a doctor in any specialty with a convenient office location, area of specialization and insurance and billing policies, call 718 499-CARE or go to http://www.nym.org.

Adolescent Medicine

Browner-Elhanan, Karen MD (AM) - **Hospital:** New York Methodist Hosp (page 404); **Address:** Park Slope Pediatrics, 1 Prospect Park W, Ste A, Brooklyn, NY 11215; **Phone:** 718-636-3960; **Board Cert:** Pediatrics 2003; Adolescent Medicine 2005; **Med School:** Israel 1988; **Resid:** Pediatrics, Montefiore Med Ctr 1996; **Fellow:** Adolescent Medicine, Maimonides Med Ctr 2003; **Fac Appt:** Asst Clin Prof Ped, Cornell Univ-Weill Med Coll

Hayes, Leslie Allyson MD (AM) - **Spec Exp:** Nutrition; Adolescent Gynecology; **Hospital:** Brooklyn Hosp Ctr-Downtown; **Address:** The Brooklyn Hospital Ctr, 121 DeKalb Ave, Brooklyn, NY 11201; **Phone:** 718-250-6594; **Board Cert:** Addiction Medicine 2005; **Med School:** Mount Sinai Sch Med 1986; **Resid:** Pediatrics, Chldn's Hosp Natl Med Ctr 1989; **Fellow:** Adolescent Medicine, UMDNJ Med Ctr 1991

Allergy & Immunology

Greeley, Norman H MD (A&I) - **Spec Exp:** Asthma; **Hospital:** Long Island Coll Hosp (page 94); **Address:** 140 Clinton St Fl 1, Brooklyn, NY 11201-4701; **Phone:** 718-624-4465; **Board Cert:** Internal Medicine 1985; Allergy & Immunology 1987; Clinical & Laboratory Immunology 1988; **Med School:** Mexico 1980; **Resid:** Internal Medicine, Long Island Coll Hosp 1985; **Fellow:** Allergy & Immunology, Downstate Med Ctr 1987

Klein, Norman MD (A&I) - **Spec Exp:** Asthma; Food Allergy; Hay Fever; Immune Deficiency; **Hospital:** Brookdale Univ Hosp Med Ctr, Brooklyn Hosp Ctr-Downtown; **Address:** 1648 E 14th St, Brooklyn, NY 11229-1175; **Phone:** 718-627-0183; **Board Cert:** Pediatrics 1981; Allergy & Immunology 1983; **Med School:** SUNY Hlth Sci Ctr 1976; **Resid:** Pediatrics, Brookdale Univ Hosp 1979; **Fellow:** Allergy & Immunology, Montefiore Med Ctr 1980; **Fac Appt:** Asst Prof Ped, SUNY Hlth Sci Ctr

Rao, Yalamanchi K MD (A&I) - **Spec Exp:** Pediatric Allergy & Immunology; **Hospital:** New York Methodist Hosp (page 404); **Address:** 565 Bay Ridge Pkwy, Brooklyn, NY 11209; **Phone:** 718-748-7551; **Board Cert:** Pediatrics 1978; Allergy & Immunology 1989; **Med School:** India 1968; **Resid:** Pediatrics, Long Island Coll Hosp 1977; Allergy & Immunology, Long Island Coll Hosp 1979

Schneider, Arlene T MD (A&I) - **Spec Exp:** Asthma; Sinusitis; Food Allergy; **Hospital:** Long Island Coll Hosp (page 94); **Address:** Allergy & Asthma Care Ctr, 159 Clinton St, Brooklyn, NY 11201-4601; **Phone:** 718-624-6495; **Board Cert:** Pediatrics 1974; Allergy & Immunology 1975; **Med School:** SUNY Downstate 1968; **Resid:** Pediatrics, LI Coll Hosp 1972; **Fellow:** Allergy & Immunology, LI Coll Hosp 1974; **Fac Appt:** Asst Clin Prof Ped, SUNY Hlth Sci Ctr

Silverman, Bernard A MD (A&I) - **Spec Exp:** Asthma & Allergy; Food Allergy; Urticaria; Atopic Dermatitis; **Hospital:** Mount Sinai Med Ctr (page 102), Long Island Coll Hosp (page 94); **Address:** 2044 Ocean Ave, Ste A7, Brooklyn, NY 11230; **Phone:** 718-998-5556; **Board Cert:** Pediatrics 1984; Allergy & Immunology 1985; **Med School:** Wayne State Univ 1979; **Resid:** Pediatrics, Brookdale Hosp Med Ctr 1982; **Fellow:** Allergy & Immunology, Montefiore-Weiler Einstein Div 1984; **Fac Appt:** Asst Clin Prof Ped, Mount Sinai Sch Med

Cardiac Electrophysiology

Turitto, Gioia MD (CE) - **Spec Exp:** Pacemakers; Defibrillators; Arrhythmias; **Hospital:** New York Methodist Hosp (page 404); **Address:** NY Methodist Hosp, Div Cardiology, 506 Sixth St Fl 2, Brooklyn, NY 11215; **Phone:** 718-780-3626; **Board Cert:** Internal Medicine 2002; Cardiovascular Disease 2003; Cardiac Electrophysiology 2004; **Med School:** Italy 1981; **Resid:** Internal Medicine, SUNY Downstate Med Ctr 1992; **Fellow:** Cardiovascular Disease, SUNY Downstate Med Ctr 1987; **Fac Appt:** Assoc Prof Med, SUNY Downstate

Wilbur, Sabrina L MD (CE) - **Spec Exp:** Arrhythmias; Pacemakers/Defibrillators; **Hospital:** Long Island Coll Hosp (page 94), New York Methodist Hosp (page 404); **Address:** 185 Montague St Fl 3, Brooklyn, NY 11201; **Phone:** 718-855-7223; **Board Cert:** Cardiovascular Disease 2005; Cardiac Electrophysiology 1999; **Med School:** Dominican Republic 1987; **Resid:** Internal Medicine, Episcopal Hosp 1991; **Fellow:** Cardiovascular Disease, Episcopal Hosp 1994; Cardiac Electrophysiology, Hosp Univ Penn 1995

Cardiovascular Disease

Borer, Jeffrey S MD (Cv) - **Spec Exp:** Heart Valve Disease; Heart Failure; Nuclear Cardiology; **Hospital:** SUNY Downstate Med Ctr (page 405), NY-Presby Hosp/Weill Cornell (page 104); **Address:** SUNY Downstate Med Ctr, Div Cardiology, 445 Lenox Rd, Brooklyn, NY 11226; **Phone:** 212-289-7777; **Board Cert:** Internal Medicine 1973; Cardiovascular Disease 1975; **Med School:** Cornell Univ-Weill Med Coll 1969; **Resid:** Internal Medicine, Mass Genl Hosp 1971; **Fellow:** Cardiovascular Disease, Natl Heart, Lung & Blood Inst 1974; Cardiovascular Disease, Guy's Hosp 1975; **Fac Appt:** Prof Med, SUNY Downstate

Charnoff, Judah A MD (Cv) - **Spec Exp:** Coronary Artery Disease; Congestive Heart Failure; Cholesterol/Lipid Disorders; **Hospital:** Maimonides Med Ctr (page 98), Beth Israel Med Ctr- Kings Hwy Div (page 94); **Address:** 1262 Ocean Pkwy, Brooklyn, NY 11230-5102; **Phone:** 718-859-5843; **Board Cert:** Internal Medicine 1987; Cardiovascular Disease 2005; **Med School:** NYU Sch Med 1984; **Resid:** Internal Medicine, Brookdale Hosp 1987; **Fellow:** Cardiovascular Disease, Maimonides Med Ctr 1989; **Fac Appt:** Asst Prof Med, SUNY Downstate

Feit, Alan MD (Cv) - **Spec Exp:** Interventional Cardiology; **Hospital:** SUNY Downstate Med Ctr (page 405); **Address:** SUNY, Dept Cardiology, 450 Clarkson Ave, Box 1199, Brooklyn, NY 11203-2012; **Phone:** 718-270-2631; **Board Cert:** Internal Medicine 1978; Cardiovascular Disease 1981; Interventional Cardiology 1999; **Med School:** Columbia P&S 1975; **Resid:** Internal Medicine, Roosevelt Hosp 1978; **Fellow:** Cardiovascular Disease, Roosevelt Hosp Ctr 1980; **Fac Appt:** Prof Med, SUNY Downstate

Gelbfish, Joseph S MD (Cv) - **Spec Exp:** Preventive Cardiology; Heart Valve Disease; **Hospital:** New York Methodist Hosp (page 404), NY-Presby Hosp/Columbia (page 104); **Address:** 3031 Bedford Ave, Brooklyn, NY 11210; **Phone:** 718-951-0100; **Board Cert:** Internal Medicine 1986; Cardiovascular Disease 1989; **Med School:** NYU Sch Med 1980; **Resid:** Surgery, Maimonides Medical Ctr 1984; Internal Medicine, Maimonides Medical Ctr 1985; **Fellow:** Cardiovascular Disease, Maimonides Medical Ctr 1988; Cardiovascular Disease, Beth Israel 1989

Gelles, Jeremiah MD (Cv) - **Spec Exp:** Heart Failure; Hypertension; Arrhythmias; Preventive Cardiology; **Hospital:** New York Methodist Hosp (page 404), Maimonides Med Ctr (page 98); **Address:** 263 7th Ave, Ste 5H, Brooklyn, NY 11215-3690; **Phone:** 718-832-1818; **Board Cert:** Internal Medicine 1972; Cardiovascular Disease 1975; **Med School:** NYU Sch Med 1966; **Resid:** Internal Medicine, Mount Sinai Hosp 1970; **Fellow:** Cardiovascular Disease, Mount Sinai Hosp 1971; Cardiac Electrophysiology, Columbia Presby Med Ctr 1973; **Fac Appt:** Asst Clin Prof Med, Cornell Univ-Weill Med Coll

Greengart, Alvin MD (Cv) - **Spec Exp:** Echocardiography; Non-Invasive Cardiology; **Hospital:** Maimonides Med Ctr (page 98); **Address:** Maimonides Medical Ctr, Dept Cardiology, 4802 Tenth Ave, Brooklyn, NY 11219; **Phone:** 718-283-7489; **Board Cert:** Internal Medicine 1977; Cardiovascular Disease 1979; **Med School:** Mount Sinai Sch Med 1974; **Resid:** Internal Medicine, Brookdale Med Ctr 1977; **Fellow:** Cardiovascular Disease, Brookdale Med Ctr 1979

Gupta, Prem MD (Cv) - **Spec Exp:** Heart Valve Disease; Congestive Heart Failure; Atrial Fibrillation; **Hospital:** Maimonides Med Ctr (page 98); **Address:** 4709 Fort Hamilton Pkwy, Brooklyn, NY 11219-2927; **Phone:** 718-633-4244; **Board Cert:** Internal Medicine 1971; Cardiovascular Disease 1973; **Med School:** India 1964; **Resid:** Internal Medicine, VA Med Ctr 1968; Internal Medicine, VA Med Ctr 1969; **Fellow:** Cardiovascular Disease, VA Med Ctr 1971; **Fac Appt:** Clin Prof Med, Mount Sinai Sch Med

Hanley, Gerard MD (Cv) - **Hospital:** Beth Israel Med Ctr- Kings Hwy Div (page 94), New York Methodist Hosp (page 404); **Address:** 3131 Kings Hwy, Ste B1, Brooklyn, NY 11234; **Phone:** 718-421-1212; **Board Cert:** Internal Medicine 1989; Cardiovascular Disease 2001; **Med School:** SUNY Stony Brook 1984; **Resid:** Internal Medicine, Univ Hosp 1987; **Fellow:** Cardiovascular Disease, Univ Hosp 1990; Cardiovascular Disease, Westchester Co Med Ctr 1991

Heitner, John F MD (Cv) - **Spec Exp:** Nuclear Cardiology; Cardiac MRI; **Hospital:** New York Methodist Hosp (page 404); **Address:** Div Cardiology, 506 Sixth St, Brooklyn, NY 11215; **Phone:** 718-780-5037; **Board Cert:** Internal Medicine 2000; Cardiovascular Disease 2004; **Med School:** Albert Einstein Coll Med 1997; **Resid:** Internal Medicine, Duke Univ Hosps 2000; **Fellow:** Cardiovascular Disease, Emory Univ Hosp 2002; Cardiovascular Disease, Duke Univ Hosps 2004

Hollander, Gerald MD (Cv) - **Spec Exp:** Coronary Artery Disease; Heart Failure; **Hospital:** Maimonides Med Ctr (page 98); **Address:** 4802 10th Ave, Professional Bldg, Div Cardiology, Brooklyn, NY 11219-2844; **Phone:** 718-283-7643; **Board Cert:** Internal Medicine 1976; Cardiovascular Disease 1979; **Med School:** SUNY Downstate 1973; **Resid:** Internal Medicine, Brookdale Hosp 1976; **Fellow:** Cardiovascular Disease, Brookdale Hosp 1978; **Fac Appt:** Clin Prof Med, SUNY Hlth Sci Ctr

Kang, Pritpal S MD (Cv) - **Hospital:** Lutheran Med Ctr - Brooklyn, Maimonides Med Ctr (page 98); **Address:** 705 86th St, Brooklyn, NY 11228-3625; **Phone:** 718-836-0600; **Board Cert:** Internal Medicine 1979; Cardiovascular Disease 1981; **Med School:** India 1972; **Resid:** Internal Medicine, Methodist Hosp-SUNY Downstate 1978; **Fellow:** Cardiovascular Disease, VA Med Ctr 1980

Kantrowitz, Niki E MD (Cv) - **Spec Exp:** Interventional Cardiology; Congestive Heart Failure; **Hospital:** Long Island Coll Hosp (page 94), Beth Israel Med Ctr - Petrie Division (page 94); **Address:** 339 Hicks St, Brooklyn, NY 11201; **Phone:** 718-780-4626; **Board Cert:** Internal Medicine 1981; Cardiovascular Disease 1987; Interventional Cardiology 2009; **Med School:** Wayne State Univ 1977; **Resid:** Internal Medicine, Columbia-Presby Med Ctr 1980; **Fellow:** Cardiovascular Disease, Stanford Univ Med Ctr 1983; **Fac Appt:** Assoc Clin Prof Med, NY Med Coll

Kerstein, Joshua MD (Cv) - **Spec Exp:** Atrial Fibrillation; Coronary Artery Disease; Brugada Syndrome; Long QT Syndrome; **Hospital:** Maimonides Med Ctr (page 98); **Address:** Maimonides Medical Ctr, Div Cardiology, 4802 10th Ave Fl 4, Brooklyn, NY 11219; **Phone:** 718-283-8614; **Board Cert:** Cardiovascular Disease 2005; Nuclear Cardiology 2002; **Med School:** SUNY Downstate 1989; **Resid:** Internal Medicine, Maimonides Med Ctr 1992; **Fellow:** Cardiovascular Disease, Maimonides Med Ctr 1995; **Fac Appt:** Asst Prof Med, SUNY Downstate

Kleeman, Harris J MD (Cv) - **Spec Exp:** Hypertension; Coronary Artery Disease; **Hospital:** Maimonides Med Ctr (page 98); **Address:** 1660 E 14th St, Brooklyn, NY 11229-1171; **Phone:** 718-375-6969; **Board Cert:** Internal Medicine 1982; Cardiovascular Disease 1985; **Med School:** SUNY Hlth Sci Ctr 1979; **Resid:** Internal Medicine, Staten Island Hosp 1983; **Fellow:** Cardiovascular Disease, Maimonides Med Ctr 1985

Leff, Sanford MD (Cv) - **Spec Exp:** Heart Failure; Hypertension; Coronary Artery Disease; **Hospital:** New York Methodist Hosp (page 404), Interfaith Med Ctr - St John's Episcopal Hosp; **Address:** 47 Plaza St W, Brooklyn, NY 11217; **Phone:** 718-789-4332; **Board Cert:** Internal Medicine 1974; Cardiovascular Disease 1979; **Med School:** SUNY Buffalo 1968; **Resid:** Internal Medicine, USPHS Hosp 1971; Internal Medicine, Lincoln Hosp 1974; **Fellow:** Cardiovascular Disease, Roosevelt Hosp 1976; **Fac Appt:** Clin Prof Med, SUNY Downstate

Moskovits, Norbert MD (Cv) - **Spec Exp:** Heart Failure; Coronary Artery Disease; Cardiac Catheterization; Cholesterol/Lipid Disorders; **Hospital:** Maimonides Med Ctr (page 98); **Address:** Maimonides Medical Ctr, Div Cardiology, 4802 10th Ave, Brooklyn, NY 11219-2916; **Phone:** 718-283-7948; **Board Cert:** Internal Medicine 2002; Cardiovascular Disease 2005; **Med School:** Germany 1986; **Resid:** Internal Medicine, Maimonides Med Ctr 1992; **Fellow:** Cardiovascular Disease, Beth Israel Med Ctr 1995; **Fac Appt:** Asst Prof Med, Mount Sinai Sch Med

Paiusco, A Dino MD (Cv) - **Spec Exp:** Preventive Cardiology; **Hospital:** Beth Israel Med Ctr- Kings Hwy Div (page 94), New York Methodist Hosp (page 404); **Address:** Univ Heart Associates, 3131 Kings Hwy, Ste A7, Brooklyn, NY 11234; **Phone:** 718-998-2323; **Board Cert:** Internal Medicine 1989; **Med School:** Mexico 1984; **Resid:** Internal Medicine, Univ Hosp 1989; **Fellow:** Cardiovascular Disease, SUNY HLth Sci Ctr 1992

Prabhu, H Sudhakar MD (Cv) - **Spec Exp:** Echocardiography; Nuclear Cardiology; **Hospital:** Long Island Coll Hosp (page 94), Lutheran Med Ctr - Brooklyn; **Address:** 9920 4th Ave, Ste 315, Brooklyn, NY 11209; **Phone:** 718-833-2620; **Board Cert:** Internal Medicine 1978; Cardiovascular Disease 1981; Nuclear Cardiology 2006; Echocardiography 2008; **Med School:** India 1971; **Resid:** Internal Medicine, LI Coll Hosp 1976; **Fellow:** Cardiovascular Disease, LI Coll Hosp 1978; **Fac Appt:** Clin Prof Med, SUNY Downstate

Traube, Charles MD (Cv) - **Hospital:** Beth Israel Med Ctr- Kings Hwy Div (page 94), Brookdale Univ Hosp Med Ctr; **Address:** 2270 Kimball St, Ste 210, Brooklyn, NY 11234; **Phone:** 718-692-2700; **Board Cert:** Internal Medicine 1978; Cardiovascular Disease 1981; **Med School:** Albert Einstein Coll Med 1975; **Resid:** Internal Medicine, Brookdale Hosp 1978; **Fellow:** Cardiovascular Disease, Brookdale Hosp 1980; **Fac Appt:** Asst Clin Prof Med, Albert Einstein Coll Med

Wein, Paul MD (Cv) - **Spec Exp:** Preventive Cardiology; Hypertension; Cholesterol/Lipid Disorders; Coronary Artery Disease; **Hospital:** Beth Israel Med Ctr- Kings Hwy Div (page 94), Long Island Jewish Med Ctr; **Address:** 3131 Kings Hwy, Ste D6, Brooklyn, NY 11234-2642; **Phone:** 718-338-2283; **Board Cert:** Internal Medicine 1979; Cardiovascular Disease 1983; **Med School:** SUNY Hlth Sci Ctr 1976; **Resid:** Internal Medicine, Norwalk Hosp 1979; **Fellow:** Cardiovascular Disease, LI Jewish Medical Ctr 1981

Zaloom, Robert MD (Cv) - **Spec Exp:** Cardiac Catheterization; Angiography-Coronary; Nutrition; **Hospital:** Lutheran Med Ctr - Brooklyn, Lenox Hill Hosp; **Address:** 217 Ovington Ave, Brooklyn, NY 11209-1204; **Phone:** 718-238-0098; **Board Cert:** Internal Medicine 1986; Cardiovascular Disease 1989; **Med School:** France 1983; **Resid:** Internal Medicine, Lutheran Med Ctr 1986; **Fellow:** Cardiovascular Disease, Univ Hosp 1988

Child & Adolescent Psychiatry

Engel, Lenore MD (ChAP) - **Hospital:** Kings County Hosp Ctr, SUNY Downstate Med Ctr (page 405); **Address:** 115 Henry St, Ste 1G, Brooklyn, NY 11201-2562; **Phone:** 718-855-8911; **Board Cert:** Psychiatry 1983; Child & Adolescent Psychiatry 1985; Forensic Psychiatry 2008; **Med School:** SUNY Downstate 1978; **Resid:** Psychiatry, Kings Co Hosp 1982; **Fellow:** Child & Adolescent Psychiatry, SUNY Downstate 1984; **Fac Appt:** Asst Clin Prof Psyc, SUNY Downstate

Shabry, Fryderyka MD (ChAP) - **Spec Exp:** ADD/ADHD; Anxiety Disorders; Depression; **Hospital:** Coney Island Hosp; **Address:** 2601 Pkwy, Brooklyn, NY 11210; **Phone:** 718-616-5383; **Board Cert:** Pediatrics 1970; Psychiatry 1983; Child & Adolescent Psychiatry 1986; **Med School:** Poland 1963; **Resid:** Pediatrics, Brookdale Hosp Med Ctr 1968; Psychiatry, Brookdale Hosp Med Ctr 1981; **Fellow:** Child & Adolescent Psychiatry, Brookdale Hosp Med Ctr 1979; **Fac Appt:** Asst Clin Prof Psyc, SUNY Downstate

Vera, Reinaldo MD (ChAP) - **Hospital:** Maimonides Med Ctr (page 98); **Address:** Community Mental Health Center, 920 48th St Fl 1, Brooklyn, NY 11219-3133; **Phone:** 718-283-8128; **Board Cert:** Psychiatry 1980; Child & Adolescent Psychiatry 1987; **Med School:** Ecuador 1967; **Resid:** Psychiatry, Maimonides Med Ctr 1972; **Fellow:** Child & Adolescent Psychiatry, Maimonides Med Ctr 1974

Child Neurology

Cracco, Joan B MD (ChiN) - **Spec Exp:** Spina Bifida; Epilepsy; Neurophysiology; **Hospital:** SUNY Downstate Med Ctr (page 405), Kings County Hosp Ctr; **Address:** SUNY Downstate Med Ctr, 450 Clarkson Ave, Box 118, Brooklyn, NY 11203-2056; **Phone:** 718-270-2042; **Board Cert:** Pediatrics 1968; Neurology 1972; Clinical Neurophysiology 2001; **Med School:** UMDNJ-NJ Med Sch, Newark 1963; **Resid:** Pediatrics, Mayo Clinic 1966; Neurology, Thomas Jefferson Univ Hosp 1969; **Fac Appt:** Prof N, SUNY Hlth Sci Ctr

Pavlakis, Steven G MD (ChiN) - **Spec Exp:** Cerebrovascular Disease-Pediatric; Stroke; ADD/ADHD; Neurogenetics; **Hospital:** Maimonides Med Ctr (page 98), Mount Sinai Med Ctr (page 102); **Address:** Pediatric Faculty Practice- Neurology, 977 48th St, Brooklyn, NY 11219; **Phone:** 718-283-8260; **Board Cert:** Pediatrics 1985; Child Neurology 1987; Neurodevelopmental Disabilities 2001; **Med School:** Brown Univ 1979; **Resid:** Pediatrics, Columbia-Presby Med Ctr 1981; **Fellow:** Pediatric Neurology, Columbia-Presby Med Ctr 1984; **Fac Appt:** Prof N, Mount Sinai Sch Med

Schubert, Romaine MD (ChiN) - **Spec Exp:** Epilepsy/Seizure Disorders; Developmental Disorders; Tourette's Syndrome; **Hospital:** New York Methodist Hosp (page 404); **Address:** 263 7th Ave, Ste 4A, Brooklyn, NY 11215; **Phone:** 718-246-8590; **Board Cert:** Child Neurology 1991; Pediatrics 2003; Clinical Neurophysiology 1999; Neurodevelopmental Disabilities 2002; **Med School:** Germany 1984; **Resid:** Pediatrics, SUNY Downstate/Kings Co Med Ctr 1987; **Fellow:** Child Neurology, SUNY Downstate/Kings Co Med Ctr 1990; **Fac Appt:** Asst Clin Prof Ped, Cornell Univ-Weill Med Coll

Colon & Rectal Surgery

Asarian, Armand P MD (CRS) - **Spec Exp:** Colon Cancer; Breast Cancer; **Hospital:** Brooklyn Hosp Ctr-Downtown; **Address:** 121 Dekalb Ave, Dept Surgery, Brooklyn, NY 11201; **Phone:** 718-250-6088; **Board Cert:** Surgery 2005; Colon & Rectal Surgery 2009; **Med School:** SUNY Downstate 1991; **Resid:** Surgery, Brooklyn Hosp Ctr 1996; **Fellow:** Colon & Rectal Surgery, Baylor Univ Med Ctr 1997; **Fac Appt:** Asst Clin Prof S, Cornell Univ-Weill Med Coll

Fleischer, Marian MD (CRS) - **Spec Exp:** Colonoscopy; Colon & Rectal Cancer; Pelvic & Perineal Surgery; Pelvic Organ Prolapse Repair; **Hospital:** Maimonides Med Ctr (page 98), St John's Riverside Hosp; **Address:** 9707 4th Ave, Brooklyn, NY 11209-8129; **Phone:** 718-836-3603; **Board Cert:** Colon & Rectal Surgery 1984; **Med School:** Italy 1972; **Resid:** Surgery, Maimonides Med Ctr 1981; Colon & Rectal Surgery, Baltimore Med Ctr 1982

Lacqua, Frank MD (CRS) - **Spec Exp:** Colonoscopy; Colon Cancer; Anal Disorders & Reconstruction; **Hospital:** Lutheran Med Ctr - Brooklyn; **Address:** 7513 Ft Hamilton Pkwy, Brooklyn, NY 11228; **Phone:** 718-680-6604; **Board Cert:** Colon & Rectal Surgery 2003; Surgery 2009; **Med School:** SUNY Buffalo 1985; **Resid:** Surgery, St Lukes-Roosevelt Hosp 1990; **Fellow:** Colon & Rectal Surgery, Univ Tex Hlth Sci Ctr 1991

Dermatology

Baldwin, Hilary MD (D) - **Spec Exp:** Acne & Rosacea; Cosmetic Dermatology; **Hospital:** SUNY Downstate Med Ctr (page 405), Kings County Hosp Ctr; **Address:** 142 Joralemon St, Brooklyn, NY 11201; **Phone:** 718-797-3340; **Board Cert:** Dermatology 1988; **Med School:** Boston Univ 1984; **Resid:** Dermatology, NYU Med Ctr 1988; **Fac Appt:** Assoc Prof D, SUNY Downstate

Berry, Richard MD (D) - **Spec Exp:** Skin Cancer; Hair Removal-Laser; Botox Therapy; **Hospital:** SUNY Downstate Med Ctr (page 405); **Address:** 2820 Ocean Pkwy, Brooklyn, NY 11235-7958; **Phone:** 718-996-3000; **Board Cert:** Dermatology 1978; **Med School:** SUNY Hlth Sci Ctr 1974; **Resid:** Internal Medicine, Roosevelt Hosp 1975; Dermatology, SUNY Downstate Med Ctr 1978; **Fac Appt:** Asst Clin Prof D, SUNY Hlth Sci Ctr

Biro, David MD/PhD (D) - **Spec Exp:** Mohs' Surgery; Skin Laser Surgery; Cosmetic Dermatology; **Hospital:** Lutheran Med Ctr - Brooklyn, SUNY Downstate Med Ctr (page 405); **Address:** 9921 4th Ave Fl 1, Brooklyn, NY 11209-8347; **Phone:** 718-833-7616; **Board Cert:** Dermatology 2004; **Med School:** Columbia P&S 1991; **Resid:** Dermatology, SUNY Hlth Sci Ctr 1995; **Fac Appt:** Asst Clin Prof D, SUNY Hlth Sci Ctr

Brancaccio, Ronald R MD (D) - **Spec Exp:** Contact Dermatitis; Skin Laser Surgery; Cosmetic Dermatology; **Hospital:** Lutheran Med Ctr - Brooklyn, NYU Langone Med Ctr (page 106); **Address:** 7901 4th Ave, Brooklyn, NY 11209-3957; **Phone:** 718-491-5800; **Board Cert:** Dermatology 1977; **Med School:** Geo Wash Univ 1972; **Resid:** Dermatology, Univ Oregon Hlth Sci Ctr 1976; **Fellow:** Tropical Medicine, Univ Sao Paulo 1976; **Fac Appt:** Clin Prof D, NYU Sch Med

Danziger, Stephen MD (D) - **Spec Exp:** Skin Cancer & Moles; Acne & Rosacea; Psoriasis/Eczema; Warts; **Hospital:** New York Methodist Hosp (page 404), Long Island Coll Hosp (page 94); **Address:** 20 Plaza St E, Ste A17, Brooklyn, NY 11238; **Phone:** 718-638-3640; **Board Cert:** Dermatology 1975; **Med School:** SUNY Downstate 1968; **Resid:** Dermatology, SUNY Hlth Sci Ctr 1974; **Fac Appt:** Asst Clin Prof D, SUNY Downstate

Deitz, Marcia MD (D) - **Spec Exp:** Acne; Psoriasis; Warts; Eczema; **Hospital:** Coney Island Hosp; **Address:** 1486 Ocean Pkwy, Brooklyn, NY 11230-6453; **Phone:** 718-627-3024; **Board Cert:** Dermatology 1984; **Med School:** SUNY Downstate 1980; **Resid:** Internal Medicine, Brookdale Hosp 1981; Dermatology, NY Med Coll Affil Hosp 1984; **Fac Appt:** Asst Clin Prof Med, NY Coll Osteo Med

Feldman, Philip MD (D) - **Spec Exp:** Acne; Eczema; Skin Tumors; **Hospital:** Long Island Coll Hosp (page 94); **Address:** 142 Joralemon St, Ste 4B, Brooklyn, NY 11201-4709; **Phone:** 718-237-0404; **Board Cert:** Dermatology 1970; **Med School:** Switzerland 1963; **Resid:** Dermatology, NY Presby Hosp/Columbia 1967; **Fac Appt:** Asst Clin Prof D, SUNY Downstate

Simon, Steven I MD (D) - **Spec Exp:** Skin Cancer; Botox Therapy; Hair Removal-Laser; **Hospital:** SUNY Downstate Med Ctr (page 405), Franklin Hosp; **Address:** 2270 Kimball St, Brooklyn, NY 11234-5139; **Phone:** 718-253-4550; **Board Cert:** Dermatology 1981; **Med School:** Mexico 1975; **Resid:** Internal Medicine, Brookdale Hosp 1978; Dermatology, Downstate Med Ctr 1981; **Fac Appt:** Assoc Clin Prof D, SUNY Hlth Sci Ctr

Diagnostic Radiology

Amodio, John B MD (DR) - **Spec Exp:** Pediatric Radiology; **Hospital:** Kings County Hosp Ctr, SUNY Downstate Med Ctr (page 405); **Address:** Kings County Hosp, Div Radiology, 451 Clarkson Ave, rm S2N50, Brooklyn, NY 11203; **Phone:** 718-245-5103; **Board Cert:** Diagnostic Radiology 1984; Pediatric Radiology 2005; **Med School:** NY Med Coll 1980; **Resid:** Diagnostic Radiology, Montefiore Med Ctr 1984; **Fellow:** Pediatric Radiology, Columbia-Presby Med Ctr 1985

Garner, Steven MD (DR) - **Spec Exp:** Trauma Radiology; **Hospital:** New York Methodist Hosp (page 404); **Address:** NY Methodist Hosp, Dept Radiology, 506 6th St, Brooklyn, NY 11215; **Phone:** 718-780-5870; **Board Cert:** Diagnostic Radiology 1984; Emergency Medicine 1998; **Med School:** Ros Franklin Univ/Chicago Med Sch 1976; **Resid:** Diagnostic Radiology, Mt Sinai Hosp 1983; **Fac Appt:** Asst Prof Rad, NY Med Coll

Lerman, Jay E MD (DR) - **Spec Exp:** Urologic Imaging; Musculoskeletal Imaging; **Address:** Lerman Diagnostic Imaging, 6511 Fort Hamilton Pkwy, Brooklyn, NY 11219; **Phone:** 718-491-4545; **Board Cert:** Diagnostic Radiology 1991; **Med School:** Albert Einstein Coll Med 1986; **Resid:** Diagnostic Radiology, Montefiore Med Ctr 1991; **Fellow:** Cross Sectional Imaging, Thom Jefferson Hosp 1992

Ramanathan, Kumudha MD (DR) - **Spec Exp:** Mammography; Women's Imaging; **Address:** Professional Radiology Services, 161 Atlantic Ave, Brooklyn, NY 11201; **Phone:** 718-624-2222; **Board Cert:** Diag Rad with Spec Comp in Nuc Rad 1982; **Med School:** India 1976; **Resid:** Diagnostic Radiology, LI Coll Hosp 1983

Reede, Deborah MD (DR) - **Spec Exp:** Head & Neck Imaging; Chest Radiology; **Hospital:** Long Island Coll Hosp (page 94); **Address:** 339 Hicks St, Brooklyn, NY 11201; **Phone:** 718-780-1793; **Board Cert:** Diagnostic Radiology 1980; **Med School:** SUNY Upstate Med Univ 1976; **Resid:** Diagnostic Radiology, SUNY Upstate Med Ctr 1979; Diagnostic Radiology, NYU Med Ctr 1980; **Fellow:** Head & Neck Radiology, NYU Med Ctr 1981

Endocrinology, Diabetes & Metabolism

Brickman, Alan MD (EDM) - **Spec Exp:** Diabetes; Thyroid Disorders; Cholesterol/Lipid Disorders; Calcium Disorders; **Hospital:** Maimonides Med Ctr (page 98); **Address:** 1318 52nd St, Brooklyn, NY 11219-3802; **Phone:** 718-436-9898; **Board Cert:** Internal Medicine 1979; Endocrinology, Diabetes & Metabolism 1981; **Med School:** Albert Einstein Coll Med 1976; **Resid:** Internal Medicine, Maimonides Med Ctr 1979; **Fellow:** Endocrinology, Diabetes & Metabolism, Yale-New Haven Hosp 1981

Giegerich, Edmund W MD (EDM) - **Spec Exp:** Thyroid Disorders; **Hospital:** Coney Island Hosp; **Address:** 2601 Ocean Pkwy, Brooklyn, NY 11235; **Phone:** 718-616-4803; **Board Cert:** Internal Medicine 1980; Endocrinology, Diabetes & Metabolism 1983; **Med School:** SUNY Downstate 1977; **Resid:** Internal Medicine, Rhode Island Hosp 1980; **Fellow:** Endocrinology, Diabetes & Metabolism, Mount Sinai Hosp 1982; **Fac Appt:** Assoc Clin Prof Med, SUNY Hlth Sci Ctr

Goldman, Joel M MD (EDM) - **Spec Exp:** Thyroid Disorders; Diabetes; Calcium Disorders; **Hospital:** Brookdale Univ Hosp Med Ctr, Beth Israel Med Ctr- Kings Hwy Div (page 94); **Address:** 555 Rockaway Pkwy, rm 101a SBSI, Brooklyn, NY 11212-3132; **Phone:** 718-240-5378; **Board Cert:** Internal Medicine 1976; Endocrinology, Diabetes & Metabolism 1979; **Med School:** Univ Ariz Coll Med 1973; **Resid:** Internal Medicine, UMDNJ-Newark Affil Hosps 1975; Internal Medicine, Albert Einstein Coll of Med 1976; **Fellow:** Endocrinology, Diabetes & Metabolism, NIAMDD-Natl Inst Hlth 1979; **Fac Appt:** Assoc Prof Med, SUNY Downstate

Mann, David MD (EDM) - **Spec Exp:** Endocrinology; Thyroid Disorders; **Hospital:** Long Island Coll Hosp (page 94); **Address:** 142 Joralemon St, Ste 11D, Brooklyn, NY 11201-4709; **Phone:** 718-855-8860; **Board Cert:** Internal Medicine 1980; Endocrinology, Diabetes & Metabolism 1983; **Med School:** Cornell Univ-Weill Med Coll 1977; **Resid:** Internal Medicine, Beth Israel Med Ctr 1980; **Fellow:** Endocrinology, Diabetes & Metabolism, Montefiore Hosp Med Ctr 1983; **Fac Appt:** Asst Prof Med, SUNY Hlth Sci Ctr

Schmidt, Philip MD (EDM) - **Spec Exp:** Diabetes; Thyroid Disorders; Osteoporosis; Parathyroid Disorders; **Hospital:** Beth Israel Med Ctr- Kings Hwy Div (page 94), New York Methodist Hosp (page 404); **Address:** 3043 Ocean Ave, Ste 102, Brooklyn, NY 11235-3400; **Phone:** 718-648-9200; **Board Cert:** Internal Medicine 1977; Endocrinology, Diabetes & Metabolism 1998; **Med School:** Albert Einstein Coll Med 1960; **Resid:** Internal Medicine, Jewish Hosp 1962; Internal Medicine, Jewish Hosp 1965; **Fellow:** Endocrinology, Diabetes & Metabolism, Jewish Hosp 1966; **Fac Appt:** Asst Clin Prof Med, SUNY Downstate

Silverberg, Arnold MD (EDM) - **Spec Exp:** Thyroid Disorders; Osteoporosis; Diabetes; **Hospital:** Maimonides Med Ctr (page 98); **Address:** 908 48th St Fl 1, Brooklyn, NY 11219-2918; **Phone:** 718-283-6200; **Board Cert:** Internal Medicine 1968; Endocrinology 1977; **Med School:** Albert Einstein Coll Med 1961; **Resid:** Internal Medicine, Montefiore Hosp Med Ctr 1965; Internal Medicine, Mount Sinai Hosp 1964; **Fellow:** Endocrinology, Diabetes & Metabolism, Mount Sinai Hosp 1968; **Fac Appt:** Assoc Clin Prof Med, Mount Sinai Sch Med

Spergel, Gabriel MD (EDM) - **Spec Exp:** Diabetes; Thyroid Disorders; **Hospital:** New York Comm Hosp; **Address:** 1806 Ditmas Ave, Brooklyn, NY 11226; **Phone:** 718-853-3702; **Med School:** Albert Einstein Coll Med 1961; **Resid:** Internal Medicine, Kings Co Hosp 1964; **Fellow:** Endocrinology, Diabetes & Metabolism, Kings County Hosp 1965; Endocrinology, Diabetes & Metabolism, Jewish Med Ctr 1967; **Fac Appt:** Assoc Clin Prof Med, Cornell Univ-Weill Med Coll

Warman, Jacob MD (EDM) - **Spec Exp:** Pituitary Disorders; Calcium Disorders; Thyroid Disorders; **Hospital:** Brooklyn Hosp Ctr-Downtown; **Address:** 121 Dekalb Ave, Brooklyn, NY 11201; **Phone:** 718-250-8995; **Board Cert:** Internal Medicine 1976; Endocrinology, Diabetes & Metabolism 1979; **Med School:** SUNY Downstate 1973; **Resid:** Internal Medicine, Maimonides Med Ctr 1976; **Fellow:** Endocrinology, Diabetes & Metabolism, Jewish Hosp 1978; **Fac Appt:** Asst Prof Med, SUNY Downstate

Family Medicine

Athanail, Steven MD (FMed) *PCP* - **Spec Exp:** Sports Medicine; **Hospital:** Lutheran Med Ctr - Brooklyn; **Address:** 268 Bay Ridge Pkwy, Apartment 1B, Brooklyn, NY 11209; **Phone:** 718-748-7272; **Board Cert:** Family Medicine 2008; **Med School:** Howard Univ 1979; **Resid:** Family Medicine, Montefiore Hosp Med Ctr 1983

Krotowski, Mark MD (FMed) *PCP* - **Spec Exp:** Caribbean Health Care; Hypertension; Diabetes; **Hospital:** Brookdale Univ Hosp Med Ctr, SUNY Downstate Med Ctr (page 405); **Address:** Brookdale Hosp, Dept Family Medicine, 8923 Avenue A, Brooklyn, NY 11236-1206; **Phone:** 718-385-8181; **Board Cert:** Family Medicine 2008; **Med School:** Israel 1976; **Resid:** Pediatrics, Brookdale Univ Hosp 1977; Family Medicine, Brookdale Univ Hosp 1979; **Fac Appt:** Assoc Clin Prof FMed, SUNY Downstate

Lopez, Clark MD (FMed) *PCP* - **Spec Exp:** Geriatric Care; **Hospital:** New York Methodist Hosp (page 404), Lutheran Med Ctr - Brooklyn; **Address:** 60 Plaza St E, Brooklyn, NY 11238; **Phone:** 718-783-3919; **Board Cert:** Family Medicine 2003; **Med School:** SUNY Downstate 1972; **Resid:** Family Medicine, Kings County Hosp 1976; **Fellow:** Family Medicine, Kings County Hosp 1977; **Fac Appt:** Asst Prof FMed, SUNY Downstate

Moskowitz, George MD (FMed) *PCP* - **Spec Exp:** Geriatric Medicine; Obesity; Preventive Medicine; **Hospital:** Maimonides Med Ctr (page 98), Beth Israel Med Ctr- Kings Hwy Div (page 94); **Address:** 1318 42nd St, Brooklyn, NY 11219-1405; **Phone:** 718-436-2496; **Board Cert:** Family Medicine 2005; **Med School:** Belgium 1973; **Resid:** Family Medicine, St Vincents Hosp 1976; Family Medicine, Med Coll S Carolina 1978

Sadovsky, Richard MD (FMed) *PCP* - **Spec Exp:** Preventive Medicine; Diabetes; Hepatitis; Thyroid Disorders; **Hospital:** SUNY Downstate Med Ctr (page 405); **Address:** 450 Clarkson Ave, Box 67, Brooklyn, NY 11203-2012; **Phone:** 718-270-2697; **Board Cert:** Family Medicine 2008; **Med School:** SUNY Hlth Sci Ctr 1974; **Resid:** Family Medicine, SUNY Hosp 1977; **Fac Appt:** Assoc Prof FMed, SUNY Hlth Sci Ctr

Schiowitz, Emanuel DO (FMed) *PCP* - **Hospital:** Maimonides Med Ctr (page 98); **Address:** 1701 59th St, Brooklyn, NY 11204-2254; **Phone:** 718-259-0222; **Board Cert:** Family Medicine 1968; **Med School:** Philadelphia Coll Osteo Med 1963; **Resid:** Family Medicine, Interboro Med Ctr 1964; **Fac Appt:** Asst Clin Prof FMed, NY Coll Osteo Med

Sheridan, Bernadette L MD (FMed) *PCP* - **Spec Exp:** Geriatric Cardiology; Women's Health; Adolescent Medicine; **Hospital:** Brookdale Univ Hosp Med Ctr, New York Methodist Hosp (page 404); **Address:** 1222 East 96 St Fl 2, Brooklyn, NY 11236; **Phone:** 718-257-3355; **Board Cert:** Family Medicine 2004; **Med School:** SUNY Buffalo 1979; **Resid:** Family Medicine, Brookdale Hosp Med Ctr 1982

Vincent, Miriam MD/PhD (FMed) *PCP* - **Spec Exp:** Diabetes; Arthritis; Preventive Medicine; Osteoporosis; **Hospital:** SUNY Downstate Med Ctr (page 405), Kings County Hosp Ctr; **Address:** 470 Clarkson Ave, Box 67, Brooklyn, NY 11203-2012; **Phone:** 718-270-2697; **Board Cert:** Family Medicine 2008; **Med School:** SUNY Hlth Sci Ctr 1985; **Resid:** Family Medicine, Univ Hosp 1988; **Fac Appt:** Prof FMed, SUNY Hlth Sci Ctr

Gastroenterology

Erber, William MD (Ge) - **Spec Exp:** Endoscopy; Inflammatory Bowel Disease/Crohn's; Gastrointestinal Cancer; Capsule Endoscopy; **Hospital:** Maimonides Med Ctr (page 98), Beth Israel Med Ctr - Petrie Division (page 94); **Address:** 591 Ocean Pkwy, Brooklyn, NY 11218-5913; **Phone:** 718-972-8500; **Board Cert:** Internal Medicine 1975; Gastroenterology 1979; **Med School:** Ros Franklin Univ/Chicago Med Sch 1967; **Resid:** Internal Medicine, Maimonides Med Ctr 1969; Internal Medicine, Maimonides Med Ctr 1973; **Fellow:** Research, Hadassah Hosp 1972; Gastroenterology, Albert Einstein Coll Med 1975; **Fac Appt:** Asst Clin Prof Med, SUNY Downstate

Gamss, Jeffrey S MD (Ge) - **Spec Exp:** Colonoscopy; **Hospital:** Beth Israel Med Ctr- Kings Hwy Div (page 94); **Address:** 1630 E 14th St, Brooklyn, NY 11229; **Phone:** 718-692-1198; **Board Cert:** Internal Medicine 1986; Gastroenterology 1989; **Med School:** SUNY Downstate 1983; **Resid:** Internal Medicine, Brookdale Hosp 1986; **Fellow:** Gastroenterology, SUNY Downstate 1988

Gettenberg, Gary S MD (Ge) - **Spec Exp:** Gastrointestinal Cancer; Colon Cancer Screening; Gastroesophageal Reflux Disease (GERD); Celiac Disease; **Hospital:** Maimonides Med Ctr (page 98), New York Methodist Hosp (page 404); **Address:** 1630 E 14th St, Brooklyn, NY 11229-1104; **Phone:** 718-339-0391; **Board Cert:** Internal Medicine 1987; Gastroenterology 1989; **Med School:** NY Med Coll 1983; **Resid:** Internal Medicine, Maimonides Med Ctr 1986; **Fellow:** Gastroenterology, Maimonides Med Ctr 1988

Gress, Frank G MD (Ge) - **Spec Exp:** Endoscopy; Gastrointestinal Disorders; Pancreatic Disease; Barrett's Esophagus; **Hospital:** SUNY Downstate Med Ctr (page 405), Kings County Hosp Ctr; **Address:** SUNY Downstate Medical Center, Digestive Disease Center, 760 Parkside Ave, Brooklyn, NY 11226; **Phone:** 718-282-7234; **Board Cert:** Gastroenterology 2001; **Med School:** Mount Sinai Sch Med 1988; **Resid:** Internal Medicine, Montefiore Med Ctr 1991; **Fellow:** Gastroenterology, SUNY Brooklyn & Meth Hosp 1993; Advanced Endoscopy, Indiana Univ Med Ctr 1994; **Fac Appt:** Prof Med, SUNY Downstate

Grosman, Irwin MD (Ge) - **Spec Exp:** Colon Cancer Screening; Irritable Bowel Syndrome; Liver Disease; **Hospital:** Long Island Coll Hosp (page 94); **Address:** 339 Hicks St, Brooklyn, NY 11201-5514; **Phone:** 718-780-1468; **Board Cert:** Internal Medicine 1987; Gastroenterology 1989; **Med School:** SUNY Stony Brook 1984; **Resid:** Internal Medicine, Montefiore Hosp Med Ctr 1987; **Fellow:** Gastroenterology, Montefiore Hosp Med Ctr 1989; **Fac Appt:** Asst Prof Med, SUNY Hlth Sci Ctr

Gupta, Jagdish MD (Ge) - **Spec Exp:** Colon Cancer; Hepatitis; Peptic Ulcer Disease; **Hospital:** Long Island Coll Hosp (page 94); **Address:** 207 Berkeley Pl, Brooklyn, NY 11217; **Phone:** 718-638-3150; **Board Cert:** Internal Medicine 1975; Gastroenterology 1977; **Med School:** India 1970; **Resid:** Internal Medicine, LI Coll Hosp 1975; **Fellow:** Gastroenterology, LI Coll Hosp 1977; **Fac Appt:** Asst Clin Prof Med, SUNY Downstate

Gusset, George MD (Ge) - **Spec Exp:** Colonoscopy; Gastroscopy; Liver Disease; **Hospital:** Beth Israel Med Ctr- Kings Hwy Div (page 94), New York Comm Hosp; **Address:** 2815 Ocean Pkwy, Brooklyn, NY 11235-7839; **Phone:** 718-769-9595; **Board Cert:** Internal Medicine 1975; Gastroenterology 1979; **Med School:** Univ Louisville Sch Med 1960; **Resid:** Internal Medicine, VA Med Ctr 1962; Internal Medicine, Brooklyn Jewish Hosp & Med Ctr 1963; **Fellow:** Gastroenterology, Brooklyn Jewish Hosp & Med Ctr 1964

Iswara, Kadirawel MD (Ge) - **Spec Exp:** Pancreatic/Biliary Endoscopy (ERCP); Colonoscopy; Endoscopy; Hepatitis; **Hospital:** Maimonides Med Ctr (page 98), Coney Island Hosp; **Address:** 2511 Ocean Ave, Ste 104, Brooklyn, NY 11225; **Phone:** 718-615-0400; **Board Cert:** Internal Medicine 1980; Gastroenterology 1975; **Med School:** Sri Lanka 1968; **Resid:** Internal Medicine, Coney Island Hosp 1972; Internal Medicine, Bronx VA Hosp 1973; **Fellow:** Gastroenterology, Maimonides Med Ctr 1976; **Fac Appt:** Asst Clin Prof Med, Mount Sinai Sch Med

Leb, Alvin D MD (Ge) - **Spec Exp:** Endoscopy; **Hospital:** Beth Israel Med Ctr- Kings Hwy Div (page 94), Brookdale Univ Hosp Med Ctr; **Address:** 2985 Quentin Rd, Brooklyn, NY 11229; **Phone:** 718-336-2218; **Board Cert:** Internal Medicine 1985; Gastroenterology 1989; **Med School:** SUNY Downstate 1982; **Resid:** Internal Medicine, Brookdale Univ Hosp 1985; **Fellow:** Gastroenterology, Brookdale Univ Hosp 1988

Maizel, Barry MD (Ge) - **Spec Exp:** Endoscopy; Inflammatory Bowel Disease; Liver Disease; **Hospital:** New York Methodist Hosp (page 404), NY Hosp Queens; **Address:** 90 8th Ave, Brooklyn, NY 11215-1553; **Phone:** 718-622-8255; **Board Cert:** Internal Medicine 1979; Gastroenterology 1981; **Med School:** Italy 1975; **Resid:** Internal Medicine, Jewish Hosp 1978; **Fellow:** Gastroenterology, NY Med Coll-Metropolitan Hosp 1980

Mayer, Ira E MD (Ge) - **Spec Exp:** Inflammatory Bowel Disease/Crohn's; Gastroesophageal Reflux Disease (GERD); Gastrointestinal Motility Disorders; **Hospital:** Maimonides Med Ctr (page 98); **Address:** 575 Kings Hwy, Brooklyn, NY 11223-2046; **Phone:** 718-891-0100; **Board Cert:** Internal Medicine 1978; Gastroenterology 1981; **Med School:** NY Med Coll 1975; **Resid:** Internal Medicine, Metropolitan Hosp Ctr 1978; **Fellow:** Gastroenterology, Emory Univ Hosp 1980; **Fac Appt:** Asst Clin Prof Med, Mount Sinai Sch Med

Notar-Francesco, Vincent J MD (Ge) - **Hospital:** New York Methodist Hosp (page 404); **Address:** 263 7th Ave, Ste 5A, Brooklyn, NY 11215; **Phone:** 718-246-8600; **Board Cert:** Internal Medicine 1989; Gastroenterology 2001; **Med School:** Mount Sinai Sch Med 1986; **Resid:** Internal Medicine, Stony Brook Univ Hosp 1989; **Fellow:** Gastroenterology, SUNY Downstate Med Ctr 1991

Piccione, Paul MD (Ge) - **Hospital:** Lutheran Med Ctr - Brooklyn; **Address:** 560 Bay Ridge Pkwy, Brooklyn, NY 11209-2702; **Phone:** 718-748-5219; **Board Cert:** Internal Medicine 1985; Gastroenterology 1987; **Med School:** Italy 1981; **Resid:** Internal Medicine, Lutheran Med Ctr 1985; **Fellow:** Gastroenterology, St Luke's-Roosevelt Hosp 1986

Sohn, Won MD (Ge) - **Spec Exp:** Endoscopy; Pancreatic/Biliary Endoscopy (ERCP); **Hospital:** New York Methodist Hosp (page 404); **Address:** 263 7th Ave, Ste 5A, Brooklyn, NY 11215; **Phone:** 718-246-8600; **Board Cert:** Gastroenterology 2000; **Med School:** SUNY Downstate 1994; **Resid:** Internal Medicine, Yale New Haven Hosp 1997; Gastroenterology

Sorra, Toomas MD (Ge) - **Spec Exp:** Colon & Rectal Cancer; Hepatitis; Gastroesophageal Reflux Disease (GERD); **Hospital:** Long Island Coll Hosp (page 94); **Address:** 166 Clinton St, Brooklyn, NY 11201-4618; **Phone:** 718-834-0100; **Board Cert:** Internal Medicine 1981; Gastroenterology 1983; **Med School:** Mexico 1975; **Resid:** Internal Medicine, LI Coll Hosp 1980; **Fellow:** Gastroenterology, LI Coll Hosp 1982; **Fac Appt:** Asst Prof Med, SUNY Downstate

Zimbalist, Eliot MD (Ge) - **Spec Exp:** Colon Cancer Screening; Hepatitis C; Irritable Bowel Syndrome; Inflammatory Bowel Disease; **Hospital:** Maimonides Med Ctr (page 98), Lutheran Med Ctr - Brooklyn; **Address:** 452 77th St, Brooklyn, NY 11209-3206; **Phone:** 718-921-5548; **Board Cert:** Internal Medicine 1983; Gastroenterology 1985; **Med School:** Mount Sinai Sch Med 1980; **Resid:** Internal Medicine, Maimonides Med Ctr 1983; **Fellow:** Gastroenterology, Meml Sloan Kettering Cancer Ctr 1985; **Fac Appt:** Assoc Prof Med, Mount Sinai Sch Med

Geriatric Medicine

Baccash, Emil MD (Ger) *PCP* - **Hospital:** New York Methodist Hosp (page 404); **Address:** 20 8th Ave, Brooklyn, NY 11217-3766; **Phone:** 718-622-7000; **Board Cert:** Internal Medicine 1981; Geriatric Medicine 2005; **Med School:** Italy 1978; **Resid:** Internal Medicine, NY Methodist Hosp 1981

Paris, Barbara E MD (Ger) - **Spec Exp:** Preventive Medicine; Frail Elderly; **Hospital:** Maimonides Med Ctr (page 98), Mount Sinai Med Ctr (page 102); **Address:** Maimonides Med Ctr, Div Geriatrics, 4802 10th Ave, Brooklyn, NY 11219; **Phone:** 718-283-7071; **Board Cert:** Internal Medicine 1982; Geriatric Medicine 2008; Hospice & Palliative Medicine 2007; **Med School:** SUNY Downstate 1977; **Resid:** Internal Medicine, St Vincents Hosp 1980; **Fellow:** Geriatric Medicine, Mt Sinai Hosp 1986; **Fac Appt:** Clin Prof Med, Mount Sinai Sch Med

Geriatric Psychiatry

Amin, Ravindra MD (GerPsy) - **Spec Exp:** Alzheimer's Disease; Anxiety Disorders; Depression; Memory Disorders; **Hospital:** Long Island Coll Hosp (page 94); **Address:** 161 Atlantic Ave, Brooklyn, NY 11201; **Phone:** 718-313-2994; **Board Cert:** Psychiatry 1993; Geriatric Psychiatry 1994; Addiction Psychiatry 1996; **Med School:** India 1985; **Resid:** Psychiatry, Elmhurst Hosp 1992; **Fellow:** Geriatric Psychiatry, Mt Sinai Med Ctr 1994

Cohen, Carl MD (GerPsy) - **Spec Exp:** Alzheimer's Disease; Schizophrenia; Depression in the Elderly; **Hospital:** SUNY Downstate Med Ctr (page 405); **Address:** SUNY Health Science Center Assocs, 370 Lenox Rd, Brooklyn, NY 11226-2206; **Phone:** 718-287-4806; **Board Cert:** Psychiatry 1977; Geriatric Psychiatry 2009; **Med School:** SUNY Buffalo 1971; **Resid:** Psychiatry, NYU Med Ctr 1974; **Fellow:** Community Psychiatry, NYU Med Ctr 1975; **Fac Appt:** Prof Psyc, SUNY Hlth Sci Ctr

Rosen, Evelyn MD (GerPsy) - **Hospital:** New York Methodist Hosp (page 404); **Address:** 583 5th St, Brooklyn, NY 11215-3503; **Phone:** 212-813-9410; **Board Cert:** Psychiatry 1992; **Med School:** Mexico 1986; **Resid:** Psychiatry, Univ Hosp 1991; **Fellow:** Geriatric Psychiatry, Univ Hosp 1992

Gynecologic Oncology

Chambers, Joseph MD/PhD (GO) - **Spec Exp:** Uterine Cancer; Pelvic Surgery; **Hospital:** Long Island Coll Hosp (page 94); **Address:** 97 Amity St, rm H320, Brooklyn, NY 11201-5509; **Phone:** 718-780-2984; **Board Cert:** Obstetrics & Gynecology 2009; Gynecologic Oncology 2009; **Med School:** Georgetown Univ 1977; **Resid:** Obstetrics & Gynecology, Univ Virginia Hosp 1981; **Fellow:** Gynecologic Oncology, Yale-New Haven Hosp 1984; **Fac Appt:** Clin Prof ObG, SUNY Downstate

Economos, Katherine MD (GO) - **Spec Exp:** Ovarian Cancer; Cervical Cancer; Uterine Cancer; Vulvar & Vaginal Cancer; **Hospital:** New York Methodist Hosp (page 404); **Address:** New York Methodist Hosp, East Pavilion, 506 6th St Fl 1, Brooklyn, NY 11215; **Phone:** 718-780-3090; **Board Cert:** Gynecologic Oncology 2008; Obstetrics & Gynecology 2008; **Med School:** SUNY Downstate 1986; **Resid:** Obstetrics & Gynecology, Maimonides Med Ctr 1990; **Fellow:** Gynecologic Oncology, Univ Texas SW Med Ctr 1993; **Fac Appt:** Assoc Clin Prof ObG, Cornell Univ-Weill Med Coll

Khulpateea, Neekianund MD (GO) - **Spec Exp:** Hysterectomy Alternatives; Gynecologic Cancer; **Hospital:** Maimonides Med Ctr (page 98), Coney Island Hosp; **Address:** Maimonides Med Ctr, Div Gyn, 953 49th St, Brooklyn, NY 11219-2923; **Phone:** 718-283-7370; **Board Cert:** Obstetrics & Gynecology 1981; **Med School:** Israel 1972; **Resid:** Obstetrics & Gynecology, Meth Hosp 1976; **Fellow:** Gynecologic Oncology, Univ Hosp Downstate 1978; **Fac Appt:** Asst Clin Prof ObG, SUNY Downstate

Serur, Eli MD (GO) - **Spec Exp:** Nutrition & Cancer; Laparoscopic Surgery; Gynecologic Cancer; Minimally Invasive Surgery; **Hospital:** Brooklyn Hosp Ctr-Downtown, Richmond Univ Med Ctr; **Address:** Brooklyn Hospital, 121 DeKalb Ave, Brooklyn, NY 11201; **Phone:** 718-250-8106; **Board Cert:** Obstetrics & Gynecology 2009; Gynecologic Oncology 2009; **Med School:** NYU Sch Med 1985; **Resid:** Obstetrics & Gynecology, Kings County Hosp 1989; **Fellow:** Gynecologic Oncology, Kings County Hosp 1991; **Fac Appt:** Asst Clin Prof ObG, Cornell Univ-Weill Med Coll

Hand Surgery

Caligiuri, Daniel A MD (HS) - **Spec Exp:** Hand & Wrist Surgery; Nerve & Tendon Reconstruction; **Hospital:** Long Island Coll Hosp (page 94); **Address:** Long Island Coll Hosp, 97 Amity St, Brooklyn, NY 11201; **Phone:** 718-780-4700; **Board Cert:** Orthopaedic Surgery 2005; Hand Surgery 2005; **Med School:** SUNY Downstate 1986; **Resid:** Orthopaedic Surgery, SUNY Downstate 1991; **Fellow:** Hand Surgery, Thomas Jefferson Univ Hosp 1992; **Fac Appt:** Asst Clin Prof OrS, SUNY Downstate

Monsanto, Enrique MD (HS) - **Spec Exp:** Nerve Disorders; Arthritis; Rotator Cuff Surgery; **Hospital:** New York Methodist Hosp (page 404); **Address:** 263 7th Ave, Fl 2, Brooklyn, NY 11215; **Phone:** 718-771-1765; **Board Cert:** Orthopaedic Surgery 2009; **Med School:** Columbia P&S 1978; **Resid:** Orthopaedic Surgery, Columbia-Presby Hosp 1983; **Fellow:** Hand Surgery, Columbia-Presby Hosp 1984; **Fac Appt:** Assoc Prof OrS, SUNY Downstate

Solomon, Ronald MD (HS) - **Hospital:** Long Island Coll Hosp (page 94), Brooklyn Hosp Ctr-Downtown; **Address:** 142 Joralemon St, Ste 12A, Brooklyn, NY 11201-4742; **Phone:** 718-625-4975; **Board Cert:** Hand Surgery 2004; **Med School:** Univ Rochester 1977; **Resid:** Surgery, NY Med Coll/Metropolitan Hosp 1982; **Fellow:** Hand Surgery, NY Med Coll/ Metropolitan Hosp 1983

Hematology

Dosik, Harvey MD (Hem) - **Spec Exp:** Leukemia & Lymphoma; Anemia; Multiple Myeloma; **Hospital:** New York Methodist Hosp (page 404); **Address:** 506 6th St, Brooklyn, NY 11215-3609; **Phone:** 718-780-5240; **Board Cert:** Internal Medicine 1970; Hematology 1976; **Med School:** NYU Sch Med 1963; **Resid:** Internal Medicine, Kings County Hosp 1967; **Fellow:** Hematology, Maimonides Med Ctr 1969; **Fac Appt:** Prof Med, Cornell Univ-Weill Med Coll

Hyde, Phyllis MD (Hem) - **Hospital:** Long Island Coll Hosp (page 94); **Address:** 46 Livingston St, Brooklyn, NY 11201; **Phone:** 718-855-1124; **Board Cert:** Internal Medicine 1983; Hematology 1986; Medical Oncology 1987; **Med School:** SUNY Downstate 1980; **Resid:** Internal Medicine, Columbia-Presby 1983; **Fellow:** Hematology & Oncology, NYU Med Ctr 1986

Kopel, Samuel MD (Hem) - **Spec Exp:** Hematologic Malignancies; Solid Tumors; **Hospital:** Maimonides Med Ctr (page 98); **Address:** MMC Hematology/Oncology, 6300 8th Ave, Brooklyn, NY 11220; **Phone:** 718-765-2600; **Board Cert:** Internal Medicine 1975; Hematology 1978; Medical Oncology 1979; **Med School:** Italy 1972; **Resid:** Internal Medicine, Jewish Hosp 1975; **Fellow:** Hematology & Oncology, Mt Sinai Med Ctr 1978; **Fac Appt:** Asst Prof Med, SUNY Downstate

Infectious Disease

Asnis, Deborah S MD (Inf) - **Spec Exp:** West Nile Virus; AIDS/HIV; Meningitis; **Hospital:** Flushing Hosp Med Ctr, NY Hosp Queens; **Address:** 90 Brighton 11th St, Brooklyn, NY 11235; **Phone:** 718-332-7770; **Board Cert:** Internal Medicine 1985; Infectious Disease 1988; **Med School:** Northwestern Univ 1981; **Resid:** Ophthalmology, LI Jewish Hosp 1983; Internal Medicine, LI Jewish Hosp 1985; **Fellow:** Infectious Disease, LI Jewish Hosp 1987; **Fac Appt:** Asst Clin Prof Med, Cornell Univ-Weill Med Coll

Berkowitz, Leonard B MD (Inf) - **Spec Exp:** AIDS/HIV; **Hospital:** Brooklyn Hosp Ctr-Downtown; **Address:** 121 DeKalb Ave, rm 5H, Brooklyn, NY 11201-5425; **Phone:** 718-250-6922; **Board Cert:** Internal Medicine 1980; Infectious Disease 1984; **Med School:** SUNY Downstate 1977; **Resid:** Internal Medicine, Kings Co Med Ctr 1981; **Fellow:** Infectious Disease, Kings Co Med Ctr 1983; **Fac Appt:** Asst Clin Prof Med, SUNY Hlth Sci Ctr

Chapnick, Edward MD (Inf) - **Spec Exp:** AIDS/HIV; Travel Medicine; Antibiotic Resistance; **Hospital:** Maimonides Med Ctr (page 98); **Address:** Maimonides Med Ctr, Infectious Disease, 4802 10th Ave, Brooklyn, NY 11219-2844; **Phone:** 718-283-7492; **Board Cert:** Internal Medicine 1988; Infectious Disease 2002; **Med School:** SUNY Downstate 1985; **Resid:** Internal Medicine, Maimonides Med Ctr 1989; **Fellow:** Infectious Disease, Maimonides Med Ctr 1991; **Fac Appt:** Assoc Prof Med, Mount Sinai Sch Med

Cofsky, Richard MD (Inf) - **Hospital:** Brookdale Univ Hosp Med Ctr; **Address:** Brookdale Univ Hospital, 1 Brookdale Plaza Fl 5 - rm 598, Brooklyn, NY 11212-3139; **Phone:** 718-240-5096; **Board Cert:** Internal Medicine 1981; Infectious Disease 1984; **Med School:** Univ MD Sch Med 1978; **Resid:** Internal Medicine, Maimonides Med Ctr 1981; **Fellow:** Infectious Disease, Downstate Med Ctr 1984

Landesman, Sheldon MD (Inf) - **Hospital:** SUNY Downstate Med Ctr (page 405); **Address:** SUNY Downstate, 450 Clarkson Ave, Box 97, Brooklyn, NY 11203; **Phone:** 718-270-3034; **Board Cert:** Internal Medicine 1976; **Med School:** SUNY Downstate 1972; **Resid:** Interventional Cardiology, Tufts-New England Med Ctr 1976; **Fellow:** Research, Baltimore Cancer Rsrch Inst/NCI 1975; Infectious Disease, Tufts-New England Med Ctr 1977

Lutwick, Larry I MD (Inf) - **Spec Exp:** Hepatitis; Infectious Mononucleosis; Epstein-Barr Virus; **Hospital:** VA Med Ctr - Bklyn, Maimonides Med Ctr (page 98); **Address:** Brooklyn VA Medical Ctr, 800 Poli Pl, rm 12-125, Brooklyn, NY 11209; **Phone:** 718-765-4979; **Board Cert:** Internal Medicine 1975; Infectious Disease 1976; **Med School:** SUNY Downstate 1972; **Resid:** Internal Medicine, Barnes Hosp-Washington Univ 1974; **Fellow:** Infectious Disease, Barnes Hosp-Washington Univ 1976; **Fac Appt:** Prof Med, SUNY Downstate

McCormack, William M MD (Inf) - **Spec Exp:** Vaginal Disease; Vulvar Disease; Sexually Transmitted Diseases; Vulvar Pain(Vestibulodynia); **Hospital:** SUNY Downstate Med Ctr (page 405); **Address:** 450 Clarkson Ave, Box 56, Brooklyn, NY 11203; **Phone:** 718-270-1432; **Board Cert:** Internal Medicine 1971; Infectious Disease 1972; **Med School:** SUNY Downstate 1963; **Resid:** Internal Medicine, Columbia-Presby Hosp 1965; Internal Medicine, Mass Genl Hosp 1969; **Fellow:** Infectious Disease, Boston City Hosp 1971; **Fac Appt:** Prof Med, SUNY Downstate

Pujol-Morato, Fernando MD (Inf) - **Spec Exp:** AIDS/HIV; **Hospital:** New York Methodist Hosp (page 404); **Address:** 460 13th St, Brooklyn, NY 11215; **Phone:** 718-636-7400; **Board Cert:** Internal Medicine 1986; Infectious Disease 1988; **Med School:** Dominican Republic 1979; **Resid:** Internal Medicine, LI College Hosp 1985; **Fellow:** Infectious Disease, LI College Hosp 1987; **Fac Appt:** Asst Prof Med, Cornell Univ-Weill Med Coll

Sepkowitz, Douglas MD (Inf) - **Spec Exp:** AIDS/HIV; Tuberculosis; **Hospital:** Long Island Coll Hosp (page 94); **Address:** 339 Hicks St, Brooklyn, NY 11201; **Phone:** 718-780-1435; **Board Cert:** Internal Medicine 1982; Infectious Disease 1986; **Med School:** Univ Okla Coll Med 1979; **Resid:** Internal Medicine, Maimonides Medical Ctr 1982; **Fellow:** Infectious Disease, Long Island Coll Hosp 1986

Stein, Alan J MD (Inf) - **Spec Exp:** AIDS/HIV; Travel Medicine; **Hospital:** New York Methodist Hosp (page 404), Brooklyn Hosp Ctr-Downtown; **Address:** 348 13th St, Ste 201, Brooklyn, NY 11215; **Phone:** 718-369-4850; **Board Cert:** Internal Medicine 1976; Infectious Disease 1978; **Med School:** NY Med Coll 1972; **Resid:** Internal Medicine, Lenox Hill Hosp 1974; Internal Medicine, Metro Hosp Ctr 1976; **Fellow:** Infectious Disease, NYU Med Ctr 1978; **Fac Appt:** Assoc Clin Prof Med, NYU Sch Med

Internal Medicine

Behm, Dutsi MD (IM) *PCP* - **Hospital:** New York Methodist Hosp (page 404), Maimonides Med Ctr (page 98); **Address:** 421 Ocean Pkwy, Ste 2A, Brooklyn, NY 11218-2408; **Phone:** 718-438-8585; **Med School:** Ukraine 1973; **Resid:** Internal Medicine, NY Methodist Hosp 1983

Berman, Sandra MD (IM) *PCP* - **Hospital:** Long Island Coll Hosp (page 94); **Address:** 96 Joraleman St, Brooklyn, NY 11201; **Phone:** 718-797-5339; **Board Cert:** Internal Medicine 2006; **Med School:** Mexico 1979; **Resid:** Internal Medicine, LI Jewish Med Ctr 1996

Bharathan, Thayyullathil MD (IM) *PCP* - **Spec Exp:** Alzheimer's Disease; Dementia; Palliative Care; Pain Management; **Hospital:** New York Methodist Hosp (page 404); **Address:** 263 7th Ave, Ste 5A, Brooklyn, NY 11215-3691; **Phone:** 718-246-8600; **Board Cert:** Internal Medicine 1976; **Med School:** India 1962; **Resid:** Internal Medicine, New York Methodist Hosp 1972; **Fac Appt:** Asst Clin Prof Med, Cornell Univ-Weill Med Coll

Butt, Ahmar A MD (IM) *PCP* - **Spec Exp:** Stroke; Hypertension; Congestive Heart Failure; **Hospital:** Brooklyn Hosp Ctr-Downtown; **Address:** 121 Dekalb Ave, Brooklyn, NY 11201-5465; **Phone:** 718-250-6120; **Board Cert:** Internal Medicine 2005; **Med School:** Pakistan 1983; **Resid:** Internal Medicine, Brooklyn Hospital 1994; **Fac Appt:** Asst Clin Prof Med, Cornell Univ-Weill Med Coll

Cohen, Barry A MD (IM) *PCP* - **Hospital:** Beth Israel Med Ctr- Kings Hwy Div (page 94); **Address:** 151A West End Ave, Brooklyn, NY 11235-4808; **Phone:** 718-934-1222; **Board Cert:** Internal Medicine 1986; **Med School:** Dominican Republic 1982; **Resid:** Internal Medicine, Elmhurst Hosp/Mt Sinai 1986

Cohn, Steven MD (IM) *PCP* - **Spec Exp:** Perioperative Medical Care; Hypertension; Thromboembolic Disorders; **Hospital:** SUNY Downstate Med Ctr (page 405), Kings County Hosp Ctr; **Address:** 470 Clarkson Ave, Ste A, Box 68, Brooklyn, NY 11203-2012; **Phone:** 718-270-1531; **Board Cert:** Internal Medicine 1983; **Med School:** Mexico 1978; **Resid:** Internal Medicine, SUNY Downstate-Kings Co Hosp 1982; **Fac Appt:** Clin Prof Med, SUNY Downstate

Ditchek, Alan MD (IM) *PCP* - **Spec Exp:** Chronic Fatigue Syndrome; Diabetes; Lyme Disease; Hypertension; **Hospital:** Beth Israel Med Ctr- Kings Hwy Div (page 94), New York Methodist Hosp (page 404); **Address:** 2516 Ocean Ave, Brooklyn, NY 11229-3916; **Phone:** 718-769-0444; **Board Cert:** Internal Medicine 1986, Infectious Disease 2007; **Med School:** Mexico 1981; **Resid:** Internal Medicine, Luthern Med Ctr 1985; **Fellow:** Infectious Disease, Nassau Co Med Ctr 1986; Infectious Disease, SUNY Downstate 1995; **Fac Appt:** Asst Clin Prof Med, SUNY Hlth Sci Ctr

Ellis, Earl A MD (IM) *PCP* - **Spec Exp:** Geriatric Rehabilitation; **Hospital:** Brooklyn Hosp Ctr-Downtown, SUNY Downstate Med Ctr (page 405); **Address:** 66 Rutland Rd, Brooklyn, NY 11225-5313; **Phone:** 718-282-4412; **Board Cert:** Internal Medicine 1984; Geriatric Medicine 2000; **Med School:** Howard Univ 1980; **Resid:** Internal Medicine, Elmhurst Hosp 1983

Gambarin, Boris L MD/PhD (IM) *PCP* - **Spec Exp:** Cardiovascular Disease; Diabetes; **Hospital:** New York Methodist Hosp (page 404); **Address:** 506 6th St, Brooklyn, NY 11215; **Phone:** 718-259-6122; **Board Cert:** Internal Medicine 2005; **Med School:** Russia 1969; **Resid:** Internal Medicine, Interfaith Med Ctr 1995; **Fac Appt:** Asst Prof Med, Cornell Univ-Weill Med Coll

Grunzweig, Milton J MD (IM) *PCP* - **Hospital:** Brookdale Univ Hosp Med Ctr, Beth Israel Med Ctr - Petrie Division (page 94); **Address:** 2000 Ocean Ave, Brooklyn, NY 11230; **Phone:** 718-769-7900; **Board Cert:** Internal Medicine 1989; **Med School:** SUNY Hlth Sci Ctr 1986; **Resid:** Internal Medicine, Brookdale Hosp 1989

Hsuih, Terence CH MD (IM) *PCP* - **Hospital:** Lutheran Med Ctr - Brooklyn; **Address:** 775 57th St, Brooklyn, NY 11220; **Phone:** 718-439-6163; **Board Cert:** Internal Medicine 2008; **Med School:** Mount Sinai Sch Med 1995; **Resid:** Internal Medicine, New York Hosp 1998

Hyman, Jeffrey S MD (IM) *PCP* - **Hospital:** Staten Island Univ Hosp - North; **Address:** 8012 3rd Ave, Brooklyn, NY 11209; **Phone:** 718-745-5600; **Board Cert:** Internal Medicine 2007; **Med School:** Mexico 1980; **Resid:** Internal Medicine, Maimonides Med Ctr 1984

Joy, Mark MD (IM) *PCP* - **Spec Exp:** Diabetes; Thyroid Disorders; **Hospital:** VA Med Ctr - Bklyn; **Address:** 800 Poly Pl, Dept of Medicine, Brooklyn, NY 11209; **Phone:** 718-630-3766; **Board Cert:** Internal Medicine 1983; **Med School:** W VA Univ 1979; **Resid:** Internal Medicine, Mercy Hosp 1982; **Fac Appt:** Asst Clin Prof Med, NY Med Coll

Kaiser, Stephen MD (IM) *PCP* - **Spec Exp:** Diabetes; Hypertension; **Hospital:** Maimonides Med Ctr (page 98); **Address:** 1335 Ocean Pkwy, Brooklyn, NY 11218-5152; **Phone:** 718-382-8900; **Board Cert:** Internal Medicine 1972; **Med School:** SUNY Buffalo 1964; **Resid:** Internal Medicine, Kings County Hosp 1967; **Fellow:** Hematology, Maimonides Med Ctr 1969

Katzenelenbogen, Moshe MD (IM) *PCP* - **Hospital:** Beth Israel Med Ctr- Kings Hwy Div (page 94); **Address:** 3901 Nostrand Ave, Brooklyn, NY 11235; **Phone:** 718-646-1422; **Board Cert:** Internal Medicine 1984; **Med School:** Romania 1980; **Resid:** Internal Medicine, Coney Island Hosp 1984

Kazdin, Hal J MD (IM) *PCP* - **Spec Exp:** Osteoarthritis; Rheumatoid Arthritis; Pain Management; **Hospital:** New York Comm Hosp, Beth Israel Med Ctr- Kings Hwy Div (page 94); **Address:** 90 Brighton 11th St, Brooklyn, NY 11235-5304; **Phone:** 718-332-7770; **Board Cert:** Internal Medicine 1982; **Med School:** Philippines 1977; **Resid:** Internal Medicine, Elmhurst Hosp 1981; **Fellow:** Rheumatology, LI Jewish Hosp 1983

Konka, Sudarsanam MD (IM) - **Hospital:** Long Island Coll Hosp (page 94), Long Island Jewish Med Ctr; **Address:** 100 Clinton St, Brooklyn, NY 11201; **Phone:** 718-935-9837; **Board Cert:** Internal Medicine 1974; Cardiovascular Disease 1977; **Med School:** India 1970; **Resid:** Internal Medicine, Long Island Coll Hosp 1974; **Fellow:** Cardiovascular Disease, Nassau County Med Ctr 1975; Cardiovascular Disease, Long Island Coll Hosp 1976

Levey, Robert MD (IM) *PCP* - **Spec Exp:** Chronic Obstructive Lung Disease (COPD); Alzheimer's Disease; **Hospital:** Long Island Coll Hosp (page 94); **Address:** 339 Hicks St Fl 6th, Brooklyn, NY 11201; **Phone:** 718-780-2838; **Board Cert:** Internal Medicine 1977; **Med School:** Univ Mich Med Sch 1970; **Resid:** Internal Medicine, Long Island Coll Hosp 1977

Lu, Bing MD/PhD (IM) *PCP* - **Spec Exp:** Chinese Community Health; Acupuncture; Sinusitis; Irritable Bowel Syndrome; **Hospital:** Maimonides Med Ctr (page 98), SUNY Downstate Med Ctr (page 405); **Address:** Universal Medical Service, 4506 8th Ave, Brooklyn, NY 11220; **Phone:** 718-972-1233; **Board Cert:** Internal Medicine 2007; **Med School:** China 1982; **Resid:** Internal Medicine, Miriam Hosp 1997; **Fac Appt:** Asst Prof Med, SUNY Hlth Sci Ctr

Malik, Asim R MD (IM) *PCP* - **Spec Exp:** Peptic Acid Disorders; **Hospital:** New York Methodist Hosp (page 404); **Address:** 1224 8th Ave, Brooklyn, NY 11215; **Phone:** 718-788-5588; **Board Cert:** Internal Medicine 2004; Gastroenterology 2007; **Med School:** Pakistan 1976; **Resid:** Surgery, New York Methodist Hosp 1978; Internal Medicine, New York Methodist Hosp 1981; **Fellow:** Gastroenterology, Wayne Cnty Genl Hosp 1983

Marush, Arthur MD (IM) *PCP* - **Hospital:** Beth Israel Med Ctr- Kings Hwy Div (page 94); **Address:** 2270 Kimball St, Ste 210, Brooklyn, NY 11234-5139; **Phone:** 718-692-2700; **Board Cert:** Internal Medicine 1981; **Med School:** Albert Einstein Coll Med 1978; **Resid:** Internal Medicine, Brookdale

Sherman, Frederic MD (IM) *PCP* - **Spec Exp:** Cardiovascular Disease; Alzheimer's Disease; **Hospital:** Long Island Coll Hosp (page 94), Lutheran Med Ctr - Brooklyn; **Address:** 8672 Bay Pkwy, Brooklyn, NY 11214-4102; **Phone:** 718-372-2234; **Board Cert:** Internal Medicine 1976; **Med School:** NY Med Coll 1972; **Resid:** Internal Medicine, Mount Sinai HospLong Island Coll Hosp 1976; **Fellow:** Cardiovascular Disease, Long Island Coll Hosp 1977

Simon, Todd L MD (IM) *PCP* - **Spec Exp:** Preventive Medicine; Asthma; **Hospital:** New York Methodist Hosp (page 404); **Address:** 263 7th Ave, Ste 5F, Brooklyn, NY 11215; **Phone:** 718-246-8600; **Board Cert:** Internal Medicine 2006; **Med School:** NYU Sch Med 1991; **Resid:** Internal Medicine, Mt Sinai Hosp 1994; **Fac Appt:** Assoc Prof Med, Cornell Univ-Weill Med Coll

Tal, Avraham MD (IM) *PCP* - **Spec Exp:** Hypertension; Cholesterol/Lipid Disorders; Diabetes; **Hospital:** Coney Island Hosp; **Address:** 2601 Ocean Pkwy, Ste 4N38, Brooklyn, NY 11235-7745; **Phone:** 718-616-3774; **Board Cert:** Internal Medicine 1983; **Med School:** Italy 1975; **Resid:** Internal Medicine, Kingsbrook Jewish Med Ctr 1979; Internal Medicine, Long Island Coll Hosp 1977

Vieira, Jeffrey MD (IM) *PCP* - **Spec Exp:** Infectious Disease; AIDS/HIV; Chronic Fatigue Syndrome; **Hospital:** Long Island Coll Hosp (page 94), New York Methodist Hosp (page 404); **Address:** 349 Henry St, Brooklyn, NY 11201; **Phone:** 718-857-3237; **Board Cert:** Internal Medicine 1980; **Med School:** NY Med Coll 1977; **Resid:** Internal Medicine, St Elizabeth's Med Ctr 1980; **Fellow:** Infectious Disease, Univ Hosp 1982; **Fac Appt:** Assoc Prof Med, SUNY Downstate

Ziemba, David MD (IM) *PCP* - **Hospital:** Long Island Coll Hosp (page 94); **Address:** 1458 47th St, Brooklyn, NY 11219-2634; **Phone:** 718-438-0600; **Board Cert:** Internal Medicine 1983; **Med School:** SUNY Downstate 1979; **Resid:** Internal Medicine, Coney Island Hosp 1983

Interventional Cardiology

Brener, Sorin MD (IC) - **Spec Exp:** Angioplasty & Stent Placement; **Hospital:** New York Methodist Hosp (page 404); **Address:** New York Methodist Hosp, 506 6th St, Brooklyn, NY 11215; **Phone:** 718-780-7830; **Board Cert:** Internal Medicine 2002; Cardiovascular Disease 2005; Interventional Cardiology 2009; **Med School:** Israel 1984; **Resid:** Internal Medicine, Cleveland Clinic 1992; **Fellow:** Cardiovascular Disease, Cleveland Clinic 1996

Sacchi, Terrence J MD (IC) - **Spec Exp:** Arrhythmias; Cardiac Catheterization; Coronary Angioplasty/Stents; Percutaneous Coronary Intervention; **Hospital:** New York Methodist Hosp (page 404); **Address:** NY Methodist Hospital, Buckley 2, 506 6th St, Brooklyn, NY 11215; **Phone:** 718-780-7830; **Board Cert:** Internal Medicine 1979; Cardiovascular Disease 1981; Interventional Cardiology 1999; **Med School:** Albany Med Coll 1976; **Resid:** Internal Medicine, St Vincents Hosp 1979; **Fellow:** Cardiovascular Disease, Georgetown Univ Hosp 1981; Interventional Cardiology, Mercy Hosp 1987; **Fac Appt:** Assoc Clin Prof Med, SUNY Downstate

Shani, Jacob MD (IC) - Spec Exp: Cardiac Catheterization; Angioplasty & Stent Placement; Percutaneous Valve Repair; **Hospital:** Maimonides Med Ctr (page 98); **Address:** Maimonides Med Ctr, Cardiac Cath Lab, 4802 10th Ave, Brooklyn, NY 11219-2844; **Phone:** 718-283-7480; **Board Cert:** Internal Medicine 1981; Cardiovascular Disease 1983; Interventional Cardiology 2009; **Med School:** Israel 1977; **Resid:** Internal Medicine, Maimonides Med Ctr 1981; **Fellow:** Cardiovascular Disease, Beth Israel Hosp 1983; **Fac Appt:** Prof Med, SUNY Downstate

Maternal & Fetal Medicine

Bush, Jacqueline MD (MF) - Spec Exp: Pregnancy-High Risk; Diabetes in Pregnancy; **Hospital:** New York Methodist Hosp (page 404); **Address:** 263 7th Ave, Ste 3A, Brooklyn, NY 11215; **Phone:** 718-246-8500; **Board Cert:** Obstetrics & Gynecology 2007; **Med School:** SUNY Stony Brook 1989; **Resid:** Obstetrics & Gynecology, Univ Hosp-SUNY Hlth Scis Ctr; Obstetrics & Gynecology, Kings Co Hosp Ctr

Chandra, Prasanta C MD (MF) - Spec Exp: Pregnancy-High Risk; Premature Labor; Pregnancy-Teenage; **Hospital:** Wyckoff Heights Med Ctr; **Address:** 220 Saint Nicholas Ave, Brooklyn, NY 11237; **Phone:** 718-418-8745; **Board Cert:** Obstetrics & Gynecology 1979; Maternal & Fetal Medicine 1980; **Med School:** India 1969; **Resid:** Surgery, Bronx Muni Hosp-Albert Einstein Med Ctr 1972; Obstetrics & Gynecology, Bronx Muni Hosp-Albert Einstein Med Ctr 1976; **Fellow:** Maternal & Fetal Medicine, Bronx Muni Hosp-Albert Einstein Med Ctr 1978

Medical Oncology

Ahmed, Fakhiuddin MD (Onc) - Spec Exp: Breast Cancer; Lung Cancer; Colon Cancer; **Hospital:** Brookdale Univ Hosp Med Ctr, New York Methodist Hosp (page 404); **Address:** 2558 E 18th St, Brooklyn, NY 11235; **Phone:** 718-616-0801; **Board Cert:** Internal Medicine 1972; Hematology 1974; Medical Oncology 1975; **Med School:** India 1966; **Resid:** Internal Medicine, Brookdale Univ Hosp 1970; **Fellow:** Hematology & Oncology, Brookdale Univ Hosp 1973; **Fac Appt:** Assoc Prof Med, SUNY Hlth Sci Ctr

Astrow, Alan MD (Onc) - Spec Exp: Ovarian Cancer; Breast Cancer; Lymphoma; **Hospital:** Maimonides Med Ctr (page 98); **Address:** MMC Hematology/Oncology, 6300 8th Ave, Brooklyn, NY 11220; **Phone:** 718-765-2653; **Board Cert:** Internal Medicine 1983; Hematology 1986; Medical Oncology 1987; **Med School:** Yale Univ 1980; **Resid:** Internal Medicine, Boston City Hosp 1983; **Fellow:** Hematology & Oncology, NYU Med Ctr 1986; **Fac Appt:** Assoc Clin Prof Med, NY Med Coll

Bashevkin, Michael MD (Onc) - Spec Exp: Solid Tumors; Bleeding/Coagulation Disorders; Hematologic Malignancies; **Hospital:** Maimonides Med Ctr (page 98); **Address:** 1660 E 14st St, Ste 501, Brooklyn, NY 11229; **Phone:** 718-382-8500 x501; **Board Cert:** Internal Medicine 1976; Hematology 1978; Medical Oncology 1979; **Med School:** SUNY Downstate 1973; **Resid:** Internal Medicine, VA Med Ctr 1976; Hematology & Oncology, Maimonides Med Ctr 1979

Chandra, Pradeep MD (Onc) - Spec Exp: Gastrointestinal Cancer; Colon Cancer; Breast Cancer; **Hospital:** Wyckoff Heights Med Ctr, New York Methodist Hosp (page 404); **Address:** Wycoff Heights Med Ctr, Dept Medicine, 374 Stockholm St, Brooklyn, NY 11237-4006; **Phone:** 718-963-7585; **Board Cert:** Internal Medicine 1980; Hematology 1974; Medical Oncology 1983; **Med School:** India 1966; **Resid:** Internal Medicine, Wyckoff Heights Hosp 1969; Internal Medicine, Bronx Lebanon Hosp 1971; **Fellow:** Hematology, LIJ Med Ctr 1973; **Fac Appt:** Prof Med, Cornell Univ-Weill Med Coll

Dosik, David MD (Onc) - **Spec Exp:** Breast Cancer; Lung Cancer; Colon Cancer; **Hospital:** New York Methodist Hosp (page 404), New York Comm Hosp; **Address:** NY Methodist Hosp - Dept Medicine, 506 6th St, Brooklyn, NY 11215; **Phone:** 718-780-5240; **Board Cert:** Hematology 2006; Medical Oncology 2007; **Med School:** SUNY Downstate 1990; **Resid:** Internal Medicine, Staten Island Univ Hosp 1993; **Fellow:** Hematology & Oncology, NYU Med Ctr 1996

Geraghty, Michael MD (Onc) - **Hospital:** Long Island Coll Hosp (page 94); **Address:** 339 Hicks St, rm 709A, Brooklyn, NY 11201; **Phone:** 718-833-0215; **Board Cert:** Internal Medicine 1972; Hematology 1974; Medical Oncology 2009; **Med School:** Georgetown Univ 1966; **Resid:** Internal Medicine, Bellevue Hosp 1971; **Fellow:** Hematology, Bellevue Hosp 1973; **Fac Appt:** Asst Clin Prof Med, SUNY Hlth Sci Ctr

Lebowicz, Joseph MD (Onc) - **Spec Exp:** Lung Cancer; Breast Cancer; Gastrointestinal Cancer; **Hospital:** Maimonides Med Ctr (page 98); **Address:** 1660 E 14th St, Ste 501, Brooklyn, NY 11229-1173; **Phone:** 718-382-8500; **Board Cert:** Internal Medicine 1978; Hematology 1980; Medical Oncology 1981; **Med School:** Albert Einstein Coll Med 1975; **Resid:** Internal Medicine, Maimonides Med Ctr 1978; **Fellow:** Hematology & Oncology, Maimonides Med Ctr 1981

Lichter, Stephen M MD (Onc) - **Spec Exp:** Breast Cancer; Lung Cancer; Gastrointestinal Cancer; **Hospital:** Beth Israel Med Ctr- Kings Hwy Div (page 94), Brookdale Univ Hosp Med Ctr; **Address:** 2558 E 18th St, Brooklyn, NY 11235; **Phone:** 718-616-0801; **Board Cert:** Internal Medicine 1978; Medical Oncology 1981; **Med School:** Ros Franklin Univ/Chicago Med Sch 1975; **Resid:** Internal Medicine, Brookdale Hosp 1978; **Fellow:** Medical Oncology, Brookdale Hosp 1980; **Fac Appt:** Asst Clin Prof Med, SUNY Hlth Sci Ctr

Solomon, William B MD (Onc) - **Spec Exp:** Lung Cancer; Urologic Cancer; Clinical Trials; **Hospital:** Maimonides Med Ctr (page 98); **Address:** Maimonides Med Ctr, Hem/Onc Dept, 6300 8th Ave Fl 2, Brooklyn, NY 11220; **Phone:** 718-765-2624; **Board Cert:** Internal Medicine 1978; Hematology 1982; Medical Oncology 1985; **Med School:** Columbia P&S 1975; **Resid:** Internal Medicine, Montefiore Hosp Med Ctr 1978; **Fellow:** Hematology, Beth Israel Hosp 1981; Molecular Biology, Mass Inst Tech; **Fac Appt:** Prof Med, SUNY Downstate

Neonatal-Perinatal Medicine

Gudavalli, Madhu R MD (NP) - **Spec Exp:** Prematurity/Low Birth Weight Infants; **Hospital:** New York Methodist Hosp (page 404); **Address:** New York Methodist Hosp, Dept Pediatrics, 506 6th St, Brooklyn, NY 11215; **Phone:** 718-780-3727; **Board Cert:** Pediatrics 1980; Neonatal-Perinatal Medicine 2009; **Med School:** India 1972; **Resid:** Pediatrics, NY Infirm 1976; Pediatrics, Booth Meml Hosp 1977; **Fellow:** Neonatal-Perinatal Medicine, Bellevue Hosp 1979

Koenig, Eli MD (NP) - **Hospital:** Long Island Coll Hosp (page 94); **Address:** 339 Hicks St, Brooklyn, NY 11201-5509; **Phone:** 718-780-1025; **Board Cert:** Pediatrics 1986; Neonatal-Perinatal Medicine 2007; **Med School:** Italy 1979; **Resid:** Pediatrics, Beth Israel Med Ctr 1982; **Fellow:** Neonatal-Perinatal Medicine, Babies Hosp 1984; **Fac Appt:** Asst Prof Ped, SUNY Downstate

Siracuse, Jeffrey F MD (NP) - **Spec Exp:** Necrotizing Enterocolitis; Respiratory Distress Syndrome; Neonatology; **Hospital:** Long Island Coll Hosp (page 94); **Address:** 339 Hicks St Polak Bldg, Brooklyn, NY 11201; **Phone:** 718-780-1832; **Board Cert:** Pediatrics 1985; Neonatal-Perinatal Medicine 1985; **Med School:** Italy 1977; **Resid:** Pediatrics, St Vincents Hosp 1980; **Fellow:** Neonatal-Perinatal Medicine, Columbia-Presby Med Ctr 1982; **Fac Appt:** Asst Prof Ped, NY Med Coll

Sokal, Myron MD (NP) - **Spec Exp:** Neonatal Care; **Hospital:** Brookdale Univ Hosp Med Ctr; **Address:** 1 Brookdale Plaza, Brooklyn, NY 11212; **Phone:** 718-240-5629; **Board Cert:** Pediatrics 1972; Neonatal-Perinatal Medicine 1975; **Med School:** Albert Einstein Coll Med 1967; **Resid:** Pediatrics, Yale-New Haven Hosp 1969; **Fellow:** Neonatal-Perinatal Medicine, Columbia-Presby Med Ctr 1971; **Fac Appt:** Prof Ped, SUNY Hlth Sci Ctr

Nephrology

Chou, Shyan-Yih MD (Nep) - **Spec Exp:** Kidney Disease; Hypertension; Dialysis Care; **Hospital:** Brookdale Univ Hosp Med Ctr; **Address:** 1 Brookdale Plaza, Ste 169CHC, Brooklyn, NY 11212-3139; **Phone:** 718-240-5615; **Board Cert:** Internal Medicine 1972; Nephrology 1974; **Med School:** Taiwan 1966; **Resid:** Internal Medicine, Brookdale Hosp Med Ctr 1970; Internal Medicine, Brookdale Hosp Med Ctr 1970; **Fellow:** Nephrology, Brookdale Hosp Med Ctr 1973; **Fac Appt:** Prof Med, SUNY Downstate

Delano, Barbara MD (Nep) - **Spec Exp:** Dialysis Care; Kidney Failure-Chronic; **Hospital:** SUNY Downstate Med Ctr (page 405); **Address:** 450 Clarkson Ave, Box 52, Brooklyn, NY 11203-2056; **Phone:** 718-270-1584; **Board Cert:** Internal Medicine 2000; **Med School:** SUNY Hlth Sci Ctr 1965; **Resid:** Internal Medicine, SUNY Downstate Med Ctr 1967; **Fellow:** Nephrology, SUNY Downstate Med Ctr 1969; **Fac Appt:** Prof Med, SUNY Downstate

Lipner, Henry I MD (Nep) - **Spec Exp:** Kidney Disease; Hypertension; Dialysis Care; **Hospital:** Maimonides Med Ctr (page 98), Beth Israel Med Ctr- Kings Hwy Div (page 94); **Address:** 1435 86th St, Brooklyn, NY 11228; **Phone:** 718-648-0101; **Board Cert:** Internal Medicine 1974; Nephrology 1976; **Med School:** NYU Sch Med 1968; **Resid:** Internal Medicine, Jewish Hosp 1971; **Fellow:** Nephrology, Montefiore Hosp Med Ctr 1972

Markell, Mariana S MD (Nep) - **Spec Exp:** Transplant Medicine-Kidney; Complementary Medicine; **Hospital:** SUNY Downstate Med Ctr (page 405), Kings County Hosp Ctr; **Address:** 450 Clarkson Ave, Box 52, Brooklyn, NY 11203; **Phone:** 718-270-1584; **Board Cert:** Internal Medicine 1984; Nephrology 1986; **Med School:** NY Med Coll 1981; **Resid:** Internal Medicine, Columbia-Presby 1984; **Fellow:** Nephrology, Columbia-Presby 1985UCLA Med Ctr 1986; **Fac Appt:** Assoc Prof Med, SUNY Downstate

Mittman, Neal MD (Nep) - **Spec Exp:** Lupus Nephritis; Dialysis Care; Hypertension; **Hospital:** Long Island Coll Hosp (page 94); **Address:** 115 Remsen St, Brooklyn, NY 11201-4212; **Phone:** 718-852-4949; **Board Cert:** Internal Medicine 1980; Nephrology 1982; **Med School:** NY Med Coll 1977; **Resid:** Internal Medicine, Metropolitan Hosp Ctr 1980; **Fellow:** Nephrology, Albert Einstein Coll Med 1982; **Fac Appt:** Assoc Prof Med, SUNY Hlth Sci Ctr

Neelakantappa, Kotresha H MD (Nep) - **Spec Exp:** Kidney Disease; Hypertension; **Hospital:** New York Methodist Hosp (page 404); **Address:** 9920 4th Ave, Ste 309, Brooklyn, NY 11209; **Phone:** 718-745-3079; **Board Cert:** Internal Medicine 1977; Nephrology 1978; **Med School:** India 1969; **Resid:** Internal Medicine, NY Methodist Hosp 1974; **Fellow:** Nephrology, NYU Med Ctr 1976; **Fac Appt:** Asst Prof Med, NYU Sch Med

Pannone, John MD (Nep) - **Spec Exp:** Dialysis Care; Kidney Disease-Chronic; Hypertension; **Hospital:** Lutheran Med Ctr - Brooklyn; **Address:** 61 Oliver St, Ste PR-1, Brooklyn, NY 11209; **Phone:** 718-238-4980; **Board Cert:** Internal Medicine 1978; Nephrology 1980; **Med School:** Italy 1974; **Resid:** Internal Medicine, Lutheran Med Ctr 1977; **Fellow:** Nephrology, Brookdale Hosp Med Ctr 1979; Nephrology, New York Hosp-Cornell Med Ctr 1980

Parnes, Eliezer MD (Nep) - **Spec Exp:** Hypertension; Dialysis Care; Diabetic Kidney Disease; **Hospital:** Beth Israel Med Ctr- Kings Hwy Div (page 94); **Address:** 3131 Kings Hwy, rm D-5, Brooklyn, NY 11234-2643; **Phone:** 718-338-2283; **Board Cert:** Internal Medicine 1989; Nephrology 2003; **Med School:** SUNY Downstate 1986; **Resid:** Internal Medicine, Brookdale Hosp Med Ctr 1989; **Fellow:** Nephrology, Brookdale Hosp Med Ctr 1992

Salifu, Moro MD (Nep) - **Spec Exp:** Kidney Disease; **Hospital:** SUNY Downstate Med Ctr (page 405); **Address:** SUNY Downstate, 450 Clarkson Ave, Box 52, Brooklyn, NY 11203; **Phone:** 718-270-3174; **Board Cert:** Internal Medicine 2009; Nephrology 2000; **Med School:** Turkey 1994; **Resid:** Internal Medicine, SUNY Hlth Sci Ctr 1998; **Fellow:** Nephrology, SUNY Hlth Sci Ctr 2001

Shapiro, Warren B MD (Nep) - **Spec Exp:** Kidney Failure-Chronic; Kidney Failure; Hypertension; Dialysis Care; **Hospital:** Brookdale Univ Hosp Med Ctr; **Address:** 1 Brookdale Plaza, rm 169, Brooklyn, NY 11212-3139; **Phone:** 718-240-5615; **Board Cert:** Internal Medicine 1972; Nephrology 1974; **Med School:** Ros Franklin Univ/Chicago Med Sch 1966; **Resid:** Internal Medicine, UCSF Med Ctr 1967; Internal Medicine, NY Med Coll 1970; **Fellow:** Nephrology, NY Med Coll 1971; **Fac Appt:** Assoc Clin Prof Med, SUNY Downstate

Shein, Leon MD (Nep) - **Spec Exp:** Hypertension; Diabetic Kidney Disease; Electrolyte Disorders; Nutrition; **Hospital:** New York Methodist Hosp (page 404), Interfaith Med Ctr - Bklyn Jewish Div; **Address:** NY Methodist Hosp, 446 McDonald Ave, Brooklyn, NY 11218; **Phone:** 718-972-4200; **Board Cert:** Internal Medicine 1989; Nephrology 2003; **Med School:** Philippines 1983; **Resid:** Internal Medicine, Woodhull Med Ctr 1986; **Fellow:** Nephrology, Brookdale Hosp 1988

Spitalewitz, Samuel MD (Nep) - **Spec Exp:** Diabetic Kidney Disease; Hypertension; **Hospital:** Brookdale Univ Hosp Med Ctr; **Address:** 1 Brookdale Plaza, Ste 169-CHC, Brooklyn, NY 11212-3139; **Phone:** 718-240-5615; **Board Cert:** Internal Medicine 1978; Nephrology 1980; **Med School:** NYU Sch Med 1975; **Resid:** Internal Medicine, Brookdale Hosp 1978; **Fellow:** Nephrology, Brookdale Hosp 1981; **Fac Appt:** Assoc Clin Prof Med, SUNY Downstate

Stam, Lawrence MD (Nep) - **Spec Exp:** Dialysis Care; Plasmapheresis; **Hospital:** New York Methodist Hosp (page 404); **Address:** 506 6th St, Ste 5A, Brooklyn, NY 11215-3609; **Phone:** 718-830-7109; **Board Cert:** Internal Medicine 1981; Nephrology 1984; **Med School:** SUNY Stony Brook 1978; **Resid:** Internal Medicine, St Elizabeth Hosp 1981; **Fellow:** Nephrology, Jewish Hosp 1982; **Fac Appt:** Asst Clin Prof Med, Cornell Univ-Weill Med Coll

Neurological Surgery

Anant, Ashok MD (NS) - **Spec Exp:** Spinal Surgery-Minimally Invasive; Brain Tumors; Spinal Disorders-Degenerative; **Hospital:** Lutheran Med Ctr - Brooklyn; **Address:** 8413 13th Ave, Brooklyn, NY 11228-3325; **Phone:** 718-234-0979; **Board Cert:** Neurological Surgery 1984; **Med School:** India 1973; **Resid:** Surgery, Maimonides Med Ctr 1977; Neurological Surgery, Univ Hosp 1982; **Fac Appt:** Assoc Clin Prof NS, SUNY Downstate

Benardete, Ethan A MD/PhD (NS) - **Spec Exp:** Brain Tumors; Vascular Neurosurgery; Epilepsy; Pediatric Neurosurgery; **Hospital:** SUNY Downstate Med Ctr (page 405), Long Island Coll Hosp (page 94); **Address:** 450 Clarkson Ave, Brooklyn, NY 11203; **Phone:** 718-270-4335; **Board Cert:** Neurological Surgery 2005; **Med School:** Cornell Univ-Weill Med Coll 1995; **Resid:** Neurological Surgery, NYU Med Ctr Bellevue 2002; **Fellow:** Pediatric Neurological Surgery, Boston Chldns Hosp 2003; **Fac Appt:** Asst Prof NS, SUNY Downstate

Cardoso, Erico R MD (NS) - **Spec Exp:** Pituitary Tumors; Spinal Cord Disorders; Hydrocephalus; **Hospital:** Wyckoff Heights Med Ctr; **Address:** 374 Stockholm St, Ste 4-09, Brooklyn, NY 11237; **Phone:** 718-963-7266; **Board Cert:** Neurological Surgery 1994; **Med School:** Brazil 1973; **Resid:** Surgery, Ottawa Civic Hosp 1976; Neurological Surgery, Ottawa Civic Hosp 1980; **Fellow:** Neurological Surgery, Clin Rsch Fellowship Univ Hosp 1981; Neurological Surgery, Inst Neurol Scis 1982; **Fac Appt:** Assoc Prof NS, SUNY Downstate

Onesti, Stephen T MD (NS) - **Spec Exp:** Spinal Surgery; Minimally Invasive Spinal Surgery; Spinal Disorders-Degenerative; Pain-Chronic; **Hospital:** SUNY Downstate Med Ctr (page 405); **Address:** SUNY Downstate Med Ctr, Dept Neurosurgery, 450 Clarkson Ave, Box I189, Brooklyn, NY 11203; **Phone:** 718-270-2111; **Board Cert:** Neurological Surgery 1995; **Med School:** Harvard Med Sch 1986; **Resid:** Neurological Surgery, Columbia-Presby Med Ctr 1993; **Fac Appt:** Prof NS, SUNY Downstate

Schwartz, Amit Y MD (NS) - **Hospital:** Maimonides Med Ctr (page 98), Mount Sinai Med Ctr (page 102); **Address:** Maimonides Medical Ctr, 948 48th St Fl 2 - rm 228, Brooklyn, NY 11219; **Phone:** 718-283-7219; **Board Cert:** Neurological Surgery 2005; **Med School:** Mount Sinai Sch Med 1995; **Resid:** Neurological Surgery, Mt Sinai Med Ctr 2001; **Fellow:** Skull Base Surgery, Jackson Meml Hosp 2002; **Fac Appt:** Asst Clin Prof NS, Mount Sinai Sch Med

Zonenshayn, Martin MD (NS) - **Spec Exp:** Parkinson's Disease; Stereotactic Radiosurgery; Carpal Tunnel Syndrome; Trigeminal Neuralgia; **Hospital:** New York Methodist Hosp (page 404); **Address:** NY Methodist Dept Neurosurgery, 263 Seventh Ave, Ste 4B, Brooklyn, NY 11215; **Phone:** 718-246-8660; **Board Cert:** Neurological Surgery 2008; **Med School:** NYU Sch Med 1996; **Resid:** Neurological Surgery, NY Presby Cornell Med Ctr/MSKCC 2002; **Fellow:** Stereo Neurological Surgery, NYU Hosp Joint Diseases 2003; **Fac Appt:** Assoc Clin Prof NS, Cornell Univ-Weill Med Coll

Neurology

Azhar, Salman MD (N) - **Spec Exp:** Stroke; Headache; Neuro-Rehabilitation; Spasticity Management; **Hospital:** Lutheran Med Ctr - Brooklyn; **Address:** Lutheran Med Ctr, Stroke Ctr, 150 55th St, Ste 3-31, Brooklyn, NY 11220; **Phone:** 718-630-7316; **Board Cert:** Neurology 2008; Vascular Neurology 2008; **Med School:** Med Coll VA 1993; **Resid:** Neurology, Med Coll Va Hosp 1995; Neurology, Mt Sinai Med Ctr 1997; **Fellow:** Research, NINDS/NIH 1999; **Fac Appt:** Asst Prof N, SUNY Downstate

Bodis-Wollner, Ivan MD (N) - **Spec Exp:** Parkinson's Disease; Neuro-Ophthalmology; **Hospital:** SUNY Downstate Med Ctr (page 405), Kings County Hosp Ctr; **Address:** 450 Clarkson Ave, Box 35, Brooklyn, NY 11203; **Phone:** 718-270-2502; **Board Cert:** Neurology 1977; **Med School:** Austria 1965; **Resid:** Neurology, Mount Sinai Hosp 1974; **Fellow:** Clinical Neurophysiology, Mass Genl Hosp 1974; **Fac Appt:** Prof N, SUNY Downstate

Buckner, Cary D MD (N) - **Spec Exp:** Neuromuscular Disorders; Clinical Neurophysiology; **Hospital:** New York Methodist Hosp (page 404); **Address:** NYMH Division of Neurology, 263 7th Ave, Ste 5C, Brooklyn, NY 11215; **Phone:** 718-246-8614; **Board Cert:** Neurology 2009; Clinical Neurophysiology 2001; **Med School:** Georgetown Univ 1994; **Resid:** Neurology, Columbia Presby Med Ctr 1998; **Fellow:** Neuromuscular Disease, Columbia Presby Med Ctr 1999

Crystal, Howard MD (N) - **Spec Exp:** Alzheimer's Disease; Dementia; **Hospital:** SUNY Downstate Med Ctr (page 405), Kings County Hosp Ctr; **Address:** 450 Clarkson Ave, Box 1275, Brooklyn, NY 11203-2056; **Phone:** 718-270-6388; **Board Cert:** Neurology 1981; **Med School:** Univ Pennsylvania 1976; **Resid:** Neurology, Montefiore Med Ctr 1980; **Fellow:** Neurological Pathology, Montefiore Med Ctr 1982; **Fac Appt:** Prof N, SUNY Downstate

Degenhardt, Alexandra MD (N) - **Spec Exp:** Multiple Sclerosis; **Hospital:** New York Methodist Hosp (page 404); **Address:** 263 7th Ave, Ste 5C, Brooklyn, NY 11215; **Phone:** 718-246-8614; **Board Cert:** Neurology 2005; **Med School:** Cornell Univ-Weill Med Coll 1999; **Resid:** Neurology, Beth Israel Deaconess Med Ctr 2003; **Fellow:** Multiple Sclerosis, Beth Israel Deaconess Med Ctr 2005; Multiple Sclerosis, Radcliffe Infirmary 2006; **Fac Appt:** Asst Prof N, Cornell Univ-Weill Med Coll

Drexler, Ellen MD (N) - **Spec Exp:** Headache; **Hospital:** Maimonides Med Ctr (page 98); **Address:** 883 65th St, Brooklyn, NY 11210-4737; **Phone:** 718-283-7470; **Board Cert:** Neurology 1983; Headache Medicine 2006; **Med School:** SUNY Downstate 1978; **Resid:** Neurology, Montefiore Med Ctr 1982; **Fac Appt:** Assoc Prof N, Mount Sinai Sch Med

Gropen, Toby I MD (N) - **Spec Exp:** Stroke; **Hospital:** Long Island Coll Hosp (page 94); **Address:** Dept Neurology, 339 Hicks St, Brooklyn, NY 11201; **Phone:** 718-780-1124; **Board Cert:** Neurology 1993; Vascular Neurology 2008; **Med School:** Univ Tex, San Antonio 1987; **Resid:** Neurology, Neuro Inst/Columbia-Presby Med Ctr 1991; **Fellow:** Neurology, Neuro Inst/Columbia-Presby Med Ctr 1993; **Fac Appt:** Assoc Prof N, SUNY Hlth Sci Ctr

Kay, Arthur D MD (N) - **Spec Exp:** Alzheimer's Disease; Parkinson's Disease; Dementia; Stroke; **Hospital:** Brookdale Univ Hosp Med Ctr, Flushing Hosp Med Ctr; **Address:** 1 Brookdale Plaza, Ste 422, Brooklyn, NY 11212-3139; **Phone:** 718-240-5622; **Board Cert:** Neurology 1983; **Med School:** SUNY Downstate 1978; **Resid:** Internal Medicine, Brookdale Hosp 1979; Neurology, Mount Sinai Hosp 1982; **Fellow:** Natl Inst Hlth 1984; **Fac Appt:** Assoc Prof N, SUNY Downstate

Keilson, Marshall MD (N) - **Spec Exp:** Alzheimer's Disease; Epilepsy; **Hospital:** Maimonides Med Ctr (page 98); **Address:** 883 65th St, Brooklyn, NY 11220; **Phone:** 718-283-7470; **Board Cert:** Neurology 1982; **Med School:** Albert Einstein Coll Med 1977; **Resid:** Internal Medicine, Montefiore Hosp Med Ctr 1978; Neurology, Albert Einstein 1981; **Fellow:** Clinical Neurophysiology, Univ Hosp 1983

Maccabee, Paul J MD (N) - **Spec Exp:** Neuromuscular Disorders; Electromyography; Peripheral Neuropathy; **Hospital:** SUNY Downstate Med Ctr (page 405); **Address:** SUNY Downstate Med Ctr, 450 Clarkson Ave, Box 35, Brooklyn, NY 11203; **Phone:** 718-270-2502; **Board Cert:** Neurology 1977; Clinical Neurophysiology 2003; **Med School:** Boston Univ 1970; **Resid:** Neurology, Boston Univ Med Ctr 1976; **Fellow:** Clinical Neurophysiology, Mass Genl Hosp 1978; Clinical Neurophysiology, Mt Sinai Hosp 1979; **Fac Appt:** Prof N, SUNY Hlth Sci Ctr

Maniscalco, Anthony MD (N) - **Spec Exp:** Movement Disorders; Cerebrovascular Disease; Neuromuscular Disorders; **Hospital:** Maimonides Med Ctr (page 98), Lutheran Med Ctr - Brooklyn; **Address:** Brooklyn Neurology, 117 70th St, Brooklyn, NY 11209-1113; **Phone:** 718-836-8800; **Board Cert:** Internal Medicine 1982; Neurology 1988; **Med School:** Italy 1978; **Resid:** Internal Medicine, Maimonides Medical Ctr 1981; Neurology, St Vincent's Hosp & Med Ctr 1984; **Fac Appt:** Assoc Clin Prof N, SUNY Downstate

Nouri, Shahin MD (N) - **Spec Exp:** Epilepsy/Seizure Disorders; **Hospital:** New York Methodist Hosp (page 404); **Address:** NY Methodist Hosp, Dept Neurology, 263 7th Ave, Ste 5C, Brooklyn, NY 11215; **Phone:** 718-246-8614; **Board Cert:** Neurology 2004; Clinical Neurophysiology 2005; **Med School:** Germany 1994; **Resid:** Internal Medicine, Staten Island Univ Hosp 1998; Neurology, Georgetown Univ Med Ctr 2001; **Fellow:** Clinical Neurophysiology, NYU Med Ctr 2002

Roohi, Fereydoon MD (N) - **Spec Exp:** Electromyography; Neuromuscular Disorders; **Hospital:** Long Island Coll Hosp (page 94); **Address:** Long Island Coll Hosp, Dept Neurology, 339 Hicks St, Brooklyn, NY 11201-5509; **Phone:** 718-780-1124; **Board Cert:** Neurology 1980; **Med School:** Iran 1967; **Resid:** Neurology, Kings Co Hosp 1975; **Fellow:** Neuromuscular Medicine, NY Presby Hosp 1976; **Fac Appt:** Assoc Prof N, SUNY Downstate

Rosenbaum, Daniel MD (N) - **Spec Exp:** Stroke; **Hospital:** SUNY Downstate Med Ctr (page 405), Kings County Hosp Ctr; **Address:** SUNY Downstate, Dept Neurology, 450 Clarkson Ave, Box 1213, Brooklyn, NY 11203; **Phone:** 718-270-2051; **Board Cert:** Neurology 1988; Vascular Neurology 2005; **Med School:** Albert Einstein Coll Med 1982; **Resid:** Internal Medicine, Brookdale Hosp 1983; Neurology, Albert Einstein 1986; **Fellow:** Stroke, Univ Tex Med Sch 1988; **Fac Appt:** Prof N, SUNY Downstate

Rudolph, Steven H MD (N) - **Spec Exp:** Stroke; Neuro-Ophthalmology; **Hospital:** Maimonides Med Ctr (page 98), Mount Sinai Med Ctr (page 102); **Address:** 948 48th St, Brooklyn, NY 11219; **Phone:** 718-283-7670; **Board Cert:** Neurology 1981; Vascular Neurology 2005; **Med School:** SUNY Hlth Sci Ctr 1976; **Resid:** Neurology, Mt Sinai Hosp 1980; **Fellow:** Neuro-Ophthalmology, Mt Sinai Hosp 1982; **Fac Appt:** Asst Clin Prof N, Mount Sinai Sch Med

Salgado, Miran W MD (N) - **Spec Exp:** Movement Disorders; Parkinson's Disease; Botox Therapy; Headache; **Hospital:** New York Methodist Hosp (page 404); **Address:** Center for Neurology, 263 7th Ave, Ste 5C, Brooklyn, NY 11215; **Phone:** 718-246-8614; **Board Cert:** Neurology 2004; Vascular Neurology 2006; **Med School:** Sri Lanka 1990; **Resid:** Neurology, SUNY Downstate Med Ctr 1994; **Fellow:** Movement Disorders, Columbia Presby Med Ctr 1995

Sobol, Norman J MD (N) - **Spec Exp:** Headache; Stroke; Parkinson's Disease; **Hospital:** Beth Israel Med Ctr- Kings Hwy Div (page 94), Maimonides Med Ctr (page 98); **Address:** 3131 Kings Hwy, Ste C7, Brooklyn, NY 11234-2642; **Phone:** 718-677-0009; **Board Cert:** Neurology 1980; Internal Medicine 1977; **Med School:** Univ Chicago-Pritzker Sch Med 1974; **Resid:** Internal Medicine, Kings County Hosp 1976; Neurology, Kings County Hosp 1978; **Fellow:** Clinical Neurophysiology, Kings County Hosp 1980; **Fac Appt:** Asst Prof N, SUNY Downstate

Vas, George A MD (N) - **Spec Exp:** Stroke; Multiple Sclerosis; **Hospital:** SUNY Downstate Med Ctr (page 405), Kings County Hosp Ctr; **Address:** 450 Clarkson Ave, Ste A, Brooklyn, NY 11203-2056; **Phone:** 718-270-2502; **Board Cert:** Internal Medicine 1973; Neurology 1977; Clinical Neurophysiology 2002; **Med School:** Univ Pittsburgh 1970; **Resid:** Internal Medicine, New York Hosp 1972; Neurology, New York Hosp 1975; **Fac Appt:** Prof N, SUNY Downstate

Yellin, Joseph C DO (N) - **Spec Exp:** Headache; Memory Disorders; Dementia; **Hospital:** New York Comm Hosp, Lenox Hill Hosp; **Address:** 2502 Kings Hwy, Brooklyn, NY 11229; **Phone:** 718-377-2223; **Med School:** Univ Osteo Med & Hlth Sci, Des Moines 1978; **Resid:** Neurology, Kings Co Hosp 1982

Nuclear Medicine

Gerard, Perry S MD (NuM) - **Spec Exp:** PET Imaging; CT Scan; Nuclear Imaging; Nuclear Oncology; **Hospital:** Westchester Med Ctr; **Address:** 4802 10th Ave, Brooklyn, NY 11219; **Phone:** 718-283-8355; **Board Cert:** Diagnostic Radiology 1987; Nuclear Radiology 1989; Nuclear Cardiology 2008; **Med School:** Dominica 1980; **Resid:** Diagnostic Radiology, Maimonides Med Ctr 1984; **Fellow:** Diagnostic Imaging, Maimonides Med Ctr 1985; **Fac Appt:** Asst Clin Prof Rad, Mount Sinai Sch Med

Strashun, Arnold M MD (NuM) - **Spec Exp:** Neurologic Imaging; Nuclear Cardiology; Thyroid Disorders; PET Imaging-Brain; **Hospital:** SUNY Downstate Med Ctr (page 405), Kings County Hosp Ctr; **Address:** SUNY Downstate Med Ctr, Dept Radiology, 450 Clarkson Ave, Box 1198, Brooklyn, NY 11203; **Phone:** 718-270-1603; **Board Cert:** Internal Medicine 1977; Nuclear Medicine 1979; **Med School:** Baylor Coll Med 1974; **Resid:** Internal Medicine, Baylor Med Ctr 1975; Internal Medicine, Texas Med Ctr 1977; **Fellow:** Nuclear Medicine, VA Med Ctr 1978; Nuclear Medicine, Mount Sinai Hosp 1979; **Fac Appt:** Prof NuM, SUNY Downstate

Obstetrics & Gynecology

Barzegar, Hooshang MD (ObG) *PCP* - **Spec Exp:** Gynecology Only; **Hospital:** Brookdale Univ Hosp Med Ctr; **Address:** 1636 E 14th St, Ste 124, Brooklyn, NY 11229-1100; **Phone:** 718-998-3500; **Board Cert:** Obstetrics & Gynecology 1999; **Med School:** Iran 1960; **Resid:** Obstetrics & Gynecology, Brooklyn Cumberland Hosp 1968; Obstetrics & Gynecology, Montefiore Hosp Med Ctr 1970; **Fac Appt:** Asst Clin Prof ObG, SUNY Downstate

Comrie, Millicent MD (ObG) *PCP* - **Spec Exp:** Menopause Problems; Uterine Fibroids; **Hospital:** Long Island Coll Hosp (page 94); **Address:** 148 Pierrepont St, Brooklyn, NY 11201; **Phone:** 718-852-9180; **Board Cert:** Obstetrics & Gynecology 1983; **Med School:** SUNY Hlth Sci Ctr 1976; **Resid:** Obstetrics & Gynecology, Long Island Coll Hosp 1980; **Fellow:** Public Health, Columbia Univ 1981; **Fac Appt:** Asst Clin Prof ObG, SUNY Hlth Sci Ctr

Dor, Nathan MD (ObG) - **Spec Exp:** Pregnancy-High Risk; **Hospital:** Maimonides Med Ctr (page 98); **Address:** 943 48th St, Brooklyn, NY 11219-2919; **Phone:** 718-853-1535; **Board Cert:** Obstetrics & Gynecology 2007; Maternal & Fetal Medicine 2007; **Med School:** Israel 1973; **Resid:** Obstetrics & Gynecology, Montefiore Med Ctr 1977; **Fellow:** Perinatal Medicine, Westchester Co Med Ctr 1979; **Fac Appt:** Asst Prof ObG, SUNY Downstate

Haratz-Rubinstein, Natan MD (ObG) - **Spec Exp:** Obstetric Ultrasound; Pregnancy-High Risk; **Hospital:** New York Methodist Hosp (page 404); **Address:** NY Methodist Hosp, Dept Ob/Gyn, 506 6th St Fl 4, Brooklyn, NY 11215; **Phone:** 718-780-5799; **Board Cert:** Obstetrics & Gynecology 2009; **Med School:** Venezuela 1989; **Resid:** Obstetrics & Gynecology, Conception Palacio Maternity Hosp 1994; Obstetrics & Gynecology, NY Presby-Columbia Med Ctr 1997; **Fac Appt:** Asst Prof ObG, SUNY Downstate

Lederman, Sanford MD (ObG) - **Spec Exp:** Pregnancy-High Risk; Ultrasound; Prenatal Diagnosis; **Hospital:** New York Methodist Hosp (page 404); **Address:** 506 6th St, Brooklyn, NY 11215; **Phone:** 718-780-3272; **Board Cert:** Obstetrics & Gynecology 1982; **Med School:** Mexico 1974; **Resid:** Obstetrics & Gynecology, Long Island Coll Hosp 1979; **Fellow:** Maternal & Fetal Medicine, UC-Irvine Mem Hosp 1981; **Fac Appt:** Assoc Clin Prof ObG, SUNY Downstate

Minkoff, Howard L MD (ObG) - **Spec Exp:** AIDS/HIV in Pregnancy-Consultation; Pregnancy-High Risk, Consultation; **Hospital:** Maimonides Med Ctr (page 98), SUNY Downstate Med Ctr (page 405); **Address:** Maimonides Med Ctr, Dept Ob-Gyn, 4802 Tenth Ave, Brooklyn, NY 11219; **Phone:** 718-283-7973; **Board Cert:** Obstetrics & Gynecology 1995; Maternal & Fetal Medicine 1995; **Med School:** Penn State Univ-Hershey Med Ctr 1975; **Resid:** Obstetrics & Gynecology, Kings Co Hosp Ctr 1979; Obstetrics & Gynecology, SUNY Hlth Sci Ctr 1981; **Fellow:** Maternal & Fetal Medicine, Kings Co Hosp Ctr 1981; **Fac Appt:** Prof ObG, SUNY Hlth Sci Ctr

Reizis, Igal MD (ObG) - **Spec Exp:** Gynecology Only; **Hospital:** Maimonides Med Ctr (page 98); **Address:** 5925 15th Ave, Brooklyn, NY 11219-5009; **Phone:** 718-972-2700; **Board Cert:** Obstetrics & Gynecology 1984; **Med School:** Israel 1977; **Resid:** Obstetrics & Gynecology, Maimonides Med Ctr

Ophthalmology

Ackerman, Jacob L MD (Oph) - **Spec Exp:** Glaucoma; Cataract Surgery-Lens Implant; Eyelid Cosmetic Surgery; **Hospital:** Brookdale Univ Hosp Med Ctr, New York Methodist Hosp (page 404); **Address:** 1987 Utica Ave Fl 1, Brooklyn, NY 11234-3213; **Phone:** 718-968-8700; **Board Cert:** Ophthalmology 1976; **Med School:** Albert Einstein Coll Med 1971; **Resid:** Ophthalmology, LI Jewish Hillside Med Ctr 1975; **Fac Appt:** Asst Prof Oph, SUNY Hlth Sci Ctr

Berman, David H MD (Oph) - **Spec Exp:** Retinal Detachment; Diabetic Eye Disease/Retinopathy; Macular Degeneration; **Hospital:** Long Island Coll Hosp (page 94), Brooklyn Hosp Ctr-Downtown; **Address:** 185 Montague St, Ste PH, Brooklyn, NY 11201; **Phone:** 718-222-3050; **Board Cert:** Ophthalmology 1989; **Med School:** SUNY Downstate 1982; **Resid:** Internal Medicine, Kings Co Hosp 1984; Ophthalmology, Kings Co Hosp 1987; **Fellow:** Ophthalmology, Kings Co Hosp 1988; Retina/Vitreous, Hermann Eye Ctr 1989; **Fac Appt:** Assoc Clin Prof Oph, SUNY Downstate

Brecher, Rubin MD (Oph) - **Spec Exp:** Diabetic Eye Disease/Retinopathy; Macular Degeneration; **Hospital:** Maimonides Med Ctr (page 98), Kingsbrook Jewish Med Ctr; **Address:** 736 Ocean Pkwy, Brooklyn, NY 11230-1116; **Phone:** 718-851-1186; **Board Cert:** Ophthalmology 1991; **Med School:** Albert Einstein Coll Med 1984; **Resid:** Ophthalmology, Montefiore Med Ctr 1988; **Fellow:** Medical Retina, Moorefields Eye Hosp 1989

Deutsch, James A MD (Oph) - **Spec Exp:** Strabismus; Cataract Surgery; **Hospital:** Long Island Coll Hosp (page 94); **Address:** 110 Remsen St, Ste 1B, Brooklyn, NY 11201-4261; **Phone:** 718-855-8700; **Board Cert:** Ophthalmology 1989; **Med School:** NYU Sch Med 1984; **Resid:** Ophthalmology, Mt Sinai Hosp 1988; **Fellow:** Pediatric Ophthalmology, Wills Eye Hosp 1989; **Fac Appt:** Asst Clin Prof Oph, Mount Sinai Sch Med

Douros, Stella MD (Oph) - **Spec Exp:** Diabetic Eye Disease/Retinopathy; Retina/Vitreous Surgery; Macular Degeneration; **Hospital:** New York Eye & Ear Infirm (page 113), Lenox Hill Hosp (Manh Eye, Ear & Throat Hosp); **Address:** 7501 6th Ave, Brooklyn, NY 11209; **Phone:** 718-238-2336; **Board Cert:** Ophthalmology 2009; **Med School:** Albert Einstein Coll Med 1991; **Resid:** Ophthalmology, Lenox Hill Hosp 1995; **Fellow:** Vitreoretinal Surgery, Joslin Diabetes Ctr 1998

Dweck, Monica MD (Oph) - **Spec Exp:** Eyelid Surgery; Tear Duct Problems; Orbital Diseases; Tear Duct Problems; **Hospital:** SUNY Downstate Med Ctr (page 405), Long Island Coll Hosp (page 94); **Address:** Dept of Ophthalmology, 339 Hicks St, Brooklyn, NY 11201; **Phone:** 718-780-1530; **Board Cert:** Ophthalmology 2008; **Med School:** SUNY Downstate 1986; **Resid:** Ophthalmology, NY Eye & Ear Infirm 1990; **Fellow:** Oculoplastic Surgery, The Cleveland Clinic 1991; **Fac Appt:** Asst Prof Oph, SUNY Hlth Sci Ctr

Feinstein, Neil C MD (Oph) - **Spec Exp:** Cataract Surgery; Glaucoma; Diabetic Eye Disease/Retinopathy; Macular Degeneration; **Hospital:** Maimonides Med Ctr (page 98), Lenox Hill Hosp (Manh Eye, Ear & Throat Hosp); **Address:** 919 48th St, Brooklyn, NY 11219-2919; **Phone:** 718-435-1800; **Board Cert:** Ophthalmology 1979; **Med School:** Albert Einstein Coll Med 1974; **Resid:** Ophthalmology, SUNY Downstate Med Ctr 1978

Freedman, Jeffrey MD/PhD (Oph) - **Spec Exp:** Glaucoma; Uveitis; Cornea Transplant; **Hospital:** Long Island Coll Hosp (page 94), Interfaith Med Ctr - Bklyn Jewish Div; **Address:** 161 Atlantic Ave, Ste 203, Brooklyn, NY 11201-6720; **Phone:** 718-596-9086; **Board Cert:** Ophthalmology 1975; **Med School:** South Africa 1964; **Resid:** Internal Medicine, Baragwanat Genl Hosp 1966; Ophthalmology, Transvaal General Hosp 1967; **Fellow:** Ophthalmology, SUNY Downstate Med Ctr 1970; **Fac Appt:** Prof Oph, SUNY Downstate

Hyman, George F MD (Oph) - **Spec Exp:** Laser Vision Surgery; Corneal Disease; Cornea & Cataract Surgery; **Hospital:** Brookdale Univ Hosp Med Ctr; **Address:** 2460 Flatbush Ave, Ste 4, Brooklyn, NY 11234-5000; **Phone:** 718-252-1200; **Board Cert:** Ophthalmology 1976; **Med School:** Univ MD Sch Med 1968; **Resid:** Ophthalmology, Univ Hosp/Downstate Med Ctr 1974; **Fellow:** Anterior Segment - External Disease, Univ Witwatersrand 1975; **Fac Appt:** Asst Prof Oph, SUNY Hlth Sci Ctr

Jaffe, Herbert MD (Oph) - **Spec Exp:** Cataract Surgery; Glaucoma; **Hospital:** Beth Israel Med Ctr- Kings Hwy Div (page 94); **Address:** 2128 Ocean Ave, Brooklyn, NY 11229-1406; **Phone:** 718-339-7469; **Board Cert:** Ophthalmology 1983; **Med School:** Belgium 1968; **Resid:** Ophthalmology, SUNY Downstate Med Ctr 1972

Lebowitz, Mark A MD (Oph) - **Spec Exp:** LASIK-Refractive Surgery; Cataract Surgery; Corneal Disease & Surgery; **Hospital:** Lenox Hill Hosp (Manh Eye, Ear & Throat Hosp); **Address:** 1301 Avenue J, Brooklyn, NY 11230-3605; **Phone:** 718-284-1921; **Board Cert:** Ophthalmology 2006; **Med School:** NYU Sch Med 1982; **Resid:** Ophthalmology, SUNY Downstate Med Ctr 1986; **Fellow:** Cornea & Ext Eye Disease, Manhattan EET Hosp 1987

Lieberman, David M MD (Oph) - **Spec Exp:** Contact Lenses; Corneal Disease; **Hospital:** New York Methodist Hosp (page 404); **Address:** 9 Prospect Park West, Ste 1-B, Brooklyn, NY 11215; **Phone:** 718-622-8900; **Board Cert:** Ophthalmology 1973; **Med School:** SUNY Downstate 1965; **Resid:** Ophthalmology, Univ Hosp 1970

Lombardo, James MD (Oph) - **Spec Exp:** Diabetic Eye Disease/Retinopathy; Glaucoma; **Hospital:** New York Eye & Ear Infirm (page 113); **Address:** 7801 4th Ave, Brooklyn, NY 11209-3701; **Phone:** 718-836-6661; **Board Cert:** Ophthalmology 1982; **Med School:** NYU Sch Med 1976; **Resid:** Internal Medicine, St Vincent's Hosp & Med Ctr 1977; Ophthalmology, NY Eye & Ear Infirmary 1980

Mogil, Laurey G MD (Oph) - **Spec Exp:** Glaucoma; **Hospital:** Mount Sinai Med Ctr (page 102); **Address:** KLM Ophthalmology, 1301 Avenue J, Brooklyn, NY 11230-3605; **Phone:** 718-645-0600; **Board Cert:** Ophthalmology 2006; **Med School:** Albert Einstein Coll Med 1980; **Resid:** Ophthalmology, Mt Sinai Med Ctr 1984; **Fellow:** Glaucoma, Mt Sinai Med Ctr 1985; **Fac Appt:** Asst Clin Prof Oph, Mount Sinai Sch Med

Pearlstein, Eric MD (Oph) - **Spec Exp:** Cataract Surgery; Corneal Disease; **Hospital:** Long Island Coll Hosp (page 94); **Address:** 430 Bay Ridge Pkwy, Brooklyn, NY 11209; **Phone:** 718-680-0600; **Board Cert:** Ophthalmology 1988; **Med School:** SUNY Hlth Sci Ctr 1983; **Resid:** Ophthalmology, LI Jewish Med Ctr 1987; **Fellow:** Cornea & Ext Eye Disease, Univ Minn-Duluth Sch Med 1988

Reich, Raymond MD (Oph) - **Spec Exp:** Cataract Surgery; Ophthalmic Plastic Surgery; Laser Refractive Surgery; **Hospital:** Long Island Coll Hosp (page 94), Maimonides Med Ctr (page 98); **Address:** 118 West End Ave, Brooklyn, NY 11235; **Phone:** 718-332-6200; **Board Cert:** Ophthalmology 1978; **Med School:** Albert Einstein Coll Med 1973; **Resid:** Ophthalmology, Univ Hosp 1977; **Fellow:** Ophthalmic Plastic Surgery, Harvard-Mass EE Infirm 1978; **Fac Appt:** Asst Prof Oph, SUNY Hlth Sci Ctr

Saffra, Norman MD (Oph) - **Spec Exp:** Microsurgery; Retinal Disorders; Cataract Surgery; **Hospital:** Maimonides Med Ctr (page 98), New York Eye & Ear Infirm (page 113); **Address:** 902 49th St, Brooklyn, NY 11219-2922; **Phone:** 718-283-8000; **Board Cert:** Ophthalmology 2005; **Med School:** Albert Einstein Coll Med 1988; **Resid:** Ophthalmology, Montefiore Med Ctr 1992; **Fellow:** Retina, SUNY Hlth Sci Ctr 1993; Neuro-Ophthalmology, Kingsbrook Jewish Med Ctr; **Fac Appt:** Clin Prof Oph, Mount Sinai Sch Med

Sciortino, Patrick MD (Oph) - **Spec Exp:** LASIK-Refractive Surgery; Cataract Surgery; **Hospital:** New York Comm Hosp, Long Island Coll Hosp (page 94); **Address:** 914 Bay Ridge Pkwy, Brooklyn, NY 11228-2302; **Phone:** 718-748-5700; **Board Cert:** Ophthalmology 2009; **Med School:** NY Med Coll 1978; **Resid:** Ophthalmology, St Vincents Hosp 1980; Ophthalmology, Catholic Med Ctr; **Fellow:** Ophthalmology, Univ Hosp 1984

Seidman, Mitchell DO (Oph) - **Spec Exp:** Cataract Surgery; **Hospital:** New York Methodist Hosp (page 404); **Address:** 2989 Ocean Pkwy, Brooklyn, NY 11235; **Phone:** 718-332-2020; **Board Cert:** Ophthalmology 1979; **Med School:** Philadelphia Coll Osteo Med 1974; **Resid:** Ophthalmology, Temple Univ Hosp 1978; **Fellow:** Anterior Segment - External Disease 1979

Sherman, Steven I DO (Oph) - **Spec Exp:** Cataract Surgery; Glaucoma; **Hospital:** New York Methodist Hosp (page 404), Interfaith Med Ctr - St John's Episcopal Hosp; **Address:** 2303 Avenue Z, Brooklyn, NY 11235-2805; **Phone:** 718-934-6600; **Board Cert:** Ophthalmology 1989; **Med School:** Univ Osteo Med & Hlth Sci, Des Moines 1977; **Resid:** Internal Medicine, Coney Island Hosp 1979; Ophthalmology, UHPHS Hosp 1982; **Fellow:** Glaucoma, SUNY Downstate Med Ctr 1983; **Fac Appt:** Asst Clin Prof Oph, Touro Coll Osteopathic Med-NY

Silberman, Deborah MD (Oph) - **Spec Exp:** Laser Vision Surgery; Cataract Surgery; **Hospital:** Brookdale Univ Hosp Med Ctr, Maimonides Med Ctr (page 98); **Address:** 1335 Linden Blvd, Brooklyn, NY 11212-4751; **Phone:** 718-240-5557; **Board Cert:** Ophthalmology 1990; **Med School:** SUNY Buffalo 1984; **Resid:** Internal Medicine, St Luke's-Roosevelt Hosp Ctr 1985; Ophthalmology, Brookdale Hosp Med Ctr 1988

Smith, Edward MD (Oph) - **Spec Exp:** Cataract Surgery; Neuro-Ophthalmology; **Hospital:** SUNY Downstate Med Ctr (page 405), Kingsbrook Jewish Med Ctr; **Address:** Downstate Ophthalmology Assocs, 11 Plaza St West, Brooklyn, NY 11217; **Phone:** 718-638-2020; **Board Cert:** Ophthalmology 1989; **Med School:** SUNY Downstate 1984; **Resid:** Ophthalmology, Univ Hosp 1988; **Fellow:** Neuro-Ophthalmology, Univ Hosp 1989; **Fac Appt:** Assoc Prof Oph, SUNY Downstate

Stein, Arnold MD (Oph) - **Spec Exp:** Retinal Disorders; Glaucoma; Cataract Surgery; Laser Surgery; **Hospital:** Beth Israel Med Ctr- Kings Hwy Div (page 94), Long Island Jewish Med Ctr; **Address:** 1226 Ocean Pkwy, Lobby Lvl, Ste 1, Brooklyn, NY 11230; **Phone:** 718-692-0400; **Board Cert:** Ophthalmology 1987; **Med School:** SUNY Downstate 1982; **Resid:** Brookdale 1983; Ophthalmology, LI Jewish Med Ctr 1986; **Fac Appt:** Asst Clin Prof Oph, Albert Einstein Coll Med

Unterricht, Sam MD (Oph) - **Spec Exp:** Macular Disease/Degeneration; Retinal Disorders; Optic Nerve Disorders; Neuro-Ophthalmology; **Hospital:** New York Methodist Hosp (page 404), Kingsbrook Jewish Med Ctr; **Address:** 20 Plaza St, Brooklyn, NY 11238; **Phone:** 718-622-5800; **Board Cert:** Ophthalmology 1982; **Med School:** SUNY Downstate 1976; **Resid:** Ophthalmology, Univ Hosp 1980; **Fellow:** Neuro-Ophthalmology, Kingsbrook Jewish MC 1981; Retina/Vitreous, Univ Hosp 1982; **Fac Appt:** Asst Clin Prof Oph, SUNY Hlth Sci Ctr

Wolintz, Arthur H MD (Oph) - **Spec Exp:** Neuro-Ophthalmology; Headache; Vision Loss-Unexplained Loss; **Hospital:** Kingsbrook Jewish Med Ctr, SUNY Downstate Med Ctr (page 405); **Address:** 100 Ocean Pkwy, Ste 4H, Brooklyn, NY 11218-1755; **Phone:** 718-854-7360; **Board Cert:** Neurology 1970; Ophthalmology 1973; **Med School:** SUNY Downstate 1962; **Resid:** Neurology, Natl Inst Hlth 1966; Ophthalmology, SUNY Downstate Med Ctr 1971; **Fellow:** Neuropathology, Columbia-Presby Hosp 1968; **Fac Appt:** Prof Oph, SUNY Downstate

Zellner, James H MD (Oph) - **Spec Exp:** Laser Refractive Surgery; Cataract Surgery; **Hospital:** New York Eye & Ear Infirm (page 113); **Address:** 7817 5th Ave, Brooklyn, NY 11209-2702; **Phone:** 718-748-2020; **Board Cert:** Ophthalmology 1982; **Med School:** Albert Einstein Coll Med 1977; **Resid:** Ophthalmology, Kings County Hosp Ctr 1981

Orthopaedic Surgery

Mani, John Vijay MD (OrS) - **Spec Exp:** Hip Replacement; Knee Replacement; **Hospital:** Long Island Coll Hosp (page 94); **Address:** 161 Atlantic Ave, Brooklyn, NY 11201-6720; **Phone:** 718-855-0088; **Board Cert:** Orthopaedic Surgery 1977; **Med School:** India 1970; **Resid:** Orthopaedic Surgery, Brookdale Hosp 1976; **Fellow:** Orthopaedic Surgery, Hosp for Special Surgery 1978; **Fac Appt:** Assoc Clin Prof OrS, SUNY Hlth Sci Ctr

Menezes, Placido MD (OrS) - **Spec Exp:** Hip Replacement; Knee Replacement; Fractures; **Hospital:** New York Methodist Hosp (page 404), Brooklyn Hosp Ctr-Downtown; **Address:** 543 2nd St, Brooklyn, NY 11215-2607; **Phone:** 718-788-7600; **Board Cert:** Orthopaedic Surgery 1980; **Med School:** India 1970; **Resid:** Surgery, NY Methodist Hosp 1975; Orthopaedic Surgery, Brooklyn Jewish Hosp & Med Ctr 1978; **Fac Appt:** Asst Clin Prof OrS, SUNY Downstate

Merola, Andrew A MD (OrS) - **Spec Exp:** Spinal Surgery; Scoliosis; **Hospital:** New York Methodist Hosp (page 404), NYU Langone Med Ctr (page 106); **Address:** 142 Prospect Park W, Brooklyn, NY 11215; **Phone:** 718-783-5542; **Board Cert:** Orthopaedic Surgery 2009; **Med School:** Howard Univ 1990; **Resid:** Orthopaedic Surgery, Kings Co Hosp/SUNY Downstate 1995; **Fellow:** Spinal Surgery, Univ Colorado Med Ctr 1996; **Fac Appt:** Assoc Prof OrS, SUNY Downstate

Morgan, Daniel J MD (OrS) - **Spec Exp:** Sports Medicine; Joint Replacement; Arthroscopic Surgery; Shoulder Surgery; **Hospital:** Beth Israel Med Ctr- Kings Hwy Div (page 94); **Address:** 3131 Kings Highway, Ste C11, Brooklyn, NY 11234; **Phone:** 718-258-2588; **Board Cert:** Orthopaedic Surgery 2011; **Med School:** Univ MD Sch Med 1985; **Resid:** Surgery, Washington Hosp Ctr 1986; Orthopaedic Surgery, Kingsbrook Jewish Med Ctr 1997

Scott, Claude MD/PhD (OrS) - **Spec Exp:** Pediatric Orthopaedic Surgery; Fractures-Pediatric; Hip Disorders-Pediatric; Foot Deformities; **Hospital:** SUNY Downstate Med Ctr (page 405), Kings County Hosp Ctr; **Address:** 450 Clarkson Ave, Box 30, Brooklyn, NY 11203; **Phone:** 718-270-2055; **Board Cert:** Orthopaedic Surgery 2004; **Med School:** SUNY Downstate 1995; **Resid:** Orthopaedic Surgery, SUNY Hlth Sci Ctr 2000; **Fellow:** Pediatric Orthopaedic Surgery, Al duPont Hosp for Chldn 2004; **Fac Appt:** Asst Prof OrS, SUNY Downstate

Soifer, Todd MD (OrS) - **Spec Exp:** Arthritis; Knee Injuries; Arthroscopic Surgery; Rotator Cuff Surgery; **Hospital:** Beth Israel Med Ctr- Kings Hwy Div (page 94); **Address:** 3131 Kings Highway, Ste C11, Brooklyn, NY 11234-2643; **Phone:** 718-258-2588 x0; **Board Cert:** Orthopaedic Surgery 2007; **Med School:** Mount Sinai Sch Med 1989; **Resid:** Orthopaedic Surgery, Beth Israel Med Ctr/Kingsbrook Jewish Med Ctr 1994

Spero, Charles R MD (OrS) - **Spec Exp:** Pediatric Orthopaedic Surgery; **Hospital:** SUNY Downstate Med Ctr (page 405), Kings County Hosp Ctr; **Address:** SUNY Downstate Medical Center, 450 Clarkson Ave, Box 30, Brooklyn, NY 11203; **Phone:** 718-270-2055; **Board Cert:** Orthopaedic Surgery 1981; **Med School:** Geo Wash Univ 1973; **Resid:** Orthopaedic Surgery, Lenox Hill Hosp 1978; **Fellow:** Pediatric Orthopaedic Surgery, Hosp for Special Surgery 1979; **Fac Appt:** Assoc Prof OrS, SUNY Downstate

Splain, Shepard H DO (OrS) - **Spec Exp:** Arthroscopic Surgery; Shoulder & Knee Reconstruction; Sports Medicine; Joint Replacement; **Hospital:** Brookdale Univ Hosp Med Ctr; **Address:** Linden Blvd & Rockaway Pkwy, Brooklyn, NY 11212; **Phone:** 718-240-5888; **Board Cert:** Orthopaedic Surgery 1980; **Med School:** Mich State Univ Coll Osteo Med 1973; **Resid:** Orthopaedic Surgery, Brookdale Hosp 1978; **Fellow:** Sports Medicine, Oklahoma Hlth Scis Ctr 1979; **Fac Appt:** Assoc Clin Prof OrS, SUNY Downstate

Tepler, Melvin MD (OrS) - **Spec Exp:** Fractures; **Hospital:** Maimonides Med Ctr (page 98); **Address:** 1252 E 9th St, Brooklyn, NY 11230-5180; **Phone:** 718-677-6000; **Board Cert:** Orthopaedic Surgery 2009; **Med School:** NY Med Coll 1980; **Resid:** Surgery, Maimonides Med Ctr 1981; Orthopaedic Surgery, Maimonides Med Ctr 1985

Tischler, Henry M MD (OrS) - **Spec Exp:** Hip Replacement; Knee Replacement; **Hospital:** New York Methodist Hosp (page 404); **Address:** Brooklyn Spine & Arthritis Ctr, 263 7th Ave, Ste 2B, Brooklyn, NY 11215; **Phone:** 718-246-8700; **Board Cert:** Orthopaedic Surgery 2006; **Med School:** SUNY Downstate 1985; **Resid:** Orthopaedic Surgery, SUNY Downstate Med Ctr 1990; **Fellow:** Orthopaedic Surgery, Tampa Gen Hosp/Fla Osteo Inst 1991; **Fac Appt:** Asst Prof OrS, SUNY Hlth Sci Ctr

Urban, William P MD (OrS) - **Spec Exp:** Sports Medicine; **Hospital:** SUNY Downstate Med Ctr (page 405); **Address:** SUNY Downstate Medical Ctr, Dept Orthopaedics & Rahab Medicine, 450 Clarkson Ave, Box 30, Brooklyn, NY 11203; **Phone:** 718-270-2045; **Board Cert:** Orthopaedic Surgery 2009; **Med School:** SUNY Downstate 1990; **Resid:** Orthopaedic Surgery, SUNY Downstate Medical Ctr 1994; **Fellow:** Sports Medicine, Univ Kentucky Med Ctr 1995; **Fac Appt:** Assoc Prof OrS, SUNY Downstate

Walsh, Raymond B MD (OrS) - **Hospital:** Lutheran Med Ctr - Brooklyn, Maimonides Med Ctr (page 98); **Address:** 6900 4th Ave, Brooklyn, NY 11209-1453; **Phone:** 718-238-6400; **Board Cert:** Orthopaedic Surgery 1981; **Med School:** England, UK 1974; **Resid:** Surgery, Maimonides Med Ctr 1976; Orthopaedic Surgery, Maimonides Med Ctr 1979

Wert, Sanford MD (OrS) - **Hospital:** New York Comm Hosp; **Address:** 3075 Brighton 13th St, Brooklyn, NY 11235-5607; **Phone:** 718-332-4747; **Board Cert:** Orthopaedic Surgery 1985; **Med School:** Mexico 1974; **Resid:** Orthopaedic Surgery, Maimonides Med Ctr 1975; Orthopaedic Surgery, LIJ Hosp 1979

Otolaryngology

Chaudhry, M Rashid MD (Oto) - **Spec Exp:** Cosmetic Surgery-Face; Sinus Surgery; **Hospital:** Brookdale Univ Hosp Med Ctr; **Address:** 1 Brookdale Plaza, Ste 157 CHC, Brooklyn, NY 11212; **Phone:** 718-240-6366; **Board Cert:** Otolaryngology 1978; **Med School:** Pakistan 1969; **Resid:** Otolaryngology, Univ Hosp 1978; **Fac Appt:** Asst Prof Oto, SUNY Downstate

Habib, Mohsen A MD (Oto) - **Spec Exp:** Head & Neck Surgery; Facial Plastic & Reconstructive Surgery; Sleep Disorders/Apnea; **Hospital:** New York Methodist Hosp (page 404), Lutheran Med Ctr - Brooklyn; **Address:** 7333 6th Ave, Brooklyn, NY 11209-2607; **Phone:** 718-833-0515; **Board Cert:** Otolaryngology 1983; **Med School:** Egypt 1969; **Resid:** Otolaryngology, NY Eye & Ear Infirm 1980; **Fellow:** Head and Neck Surgery, Lenox Hill Hosp 1980; **Fac Appt:** Assoc Prof Oto, NY Med Coll

Hanson, Matthew B MD (Oto) - **Spec Exp:** Otology; **Hospital:** SUNY Downstate Med Ctr (page 405), Long Island Coll Hosp (page 94); **Address:** 450 Clarkson Ave, Box 126, Brooklyn, NY 11203; **Phone:** 718-270-4701; **Board Cert:** Otolaryngology 1997; Neurotology 2008; **Med School:** Univ Iowa Coll Med 1989; **Resid:** Otolaryngology, Columbia-Presby Med Ctr 1995; **Fellow:** Neurotology, Baptist Hosp 1997; **Fac Appt:** Asst Prof Oto, SUNY Downstate

Lagmay, Victor MD (Oto) - **Spec Exp:** Thyroid & Parathyroid Surgery; Head & Neck Cancer & Surgery; Endoscopic Sinus Surgery; **Hospital:** Maimonides Med Ctr (page 98); **Address:** 919 49th St, Brooklyn, NY 11219; **Phone:** 718-283-6260; **Board Cert:** Otolaryngology 1999; **Med School:** NYU Sch Med 1992; **Resid:** Otolaryngology, NYU Med Ctr 1998; **Fellow:** Head and Neck Surgery, Beth Israel Med Ctr 1999; **Fac Appt:** Asst Clin Prof S, SUNY Downstate

Sperling, Neil M MD (Oto) - **Spec Exp:** Otosclerosis; Hearing Loss; Meniere's Disease; **Hospital:** Long Island Coll Hosp (page 94), New York Eye & Ear Infirm (page 113); **Address:** New York Otolaryngology Group, 134 Atlantic Ave, Brooklyn, NY 11201; **Phone:** 718-780-1498; **Board Cert:** Otolaryngology 1990; **Med School:** NY Med Coll 1985; **Resid:** Surgery, Beth Israel Med Ctr 1986; Otolaryngology, NY Eye & Ear Infirm 1990; **Fellow:** Otology, Minnesota Ear Clinic 1991; **Fac Appt:** Assoc Prof Oto, SUNY Downstate

Vastola, A Paul MD (Oto) - **Spec Exp:** Throat Disorders; **Hospital:** Maimonides Med Ctr (page 98); **Address:** 919 49th St, Brooklyn, NY 11219-2916; **Phone:** 718-283-6260; **Board Cert:** Otolaryngology 1995; **Med School:** Boston Univ 1988; **Resid:** Otolaryngology, Manhattan Eye, Ear & Throat Hospital 1993; **Fellow:** Pediatric Otolaryngology, Texas Chldn's Hosp 1994; **Fac Appt:** Asst Clin Prof Oto, SUNY Hlth Sci Ctr

Pain Medicine

Lefkowitz, Mathew MD (PM) - **Spec Exp:** Pain-Low Back; Pain-after Spinal Intervention; Sciatica; Pain-Back & Neck; **Hospital:** Long Island Coll Hosp (page 94); **Address:** 185 Montague St Fl 6, Brooklyn, NY 11201; **Phone:** 718-625-4244; **Board Cert:** Anesthesiology 1993; Pain Medicine 2005; **Med School:** Belgium 1983; **Resid:** Anesthesiology, Mount Sinai Hosp 1986; **Fellow:** Pain Medicine, Mount Sinai Hosp 1987

Pathology

Mirra, Suzanne S MD (Path) - **Spec Exp:** Neuropathology; Alzheimer's Disease; **Hospital:** SUNY Downstate Med Ctr (page 405), Kings County Hosp Ctr; **Address:** SUNY Health Science Ctr, Dept Pathology, 450 Clarkson Ave, Box 25, Brooklyn, NY 11203; **Phone:** 718-270-4599; **Board Cert:** Anatomic Pathology 1973; Neuropathology 1973; **Med School:** SUNY Downstate 1967; **Resid:** Anatomic Pathology, Kings Co Hosp 1970; Neuropathology, Montefiore Med Ctr 1971; **Fellow:** Neuropathology, Yale Univ 1973; **Fac Appt:** Prof Path, SUNY Downstate

Vigorita, Vincent J MD (Path) - **Spec Exp:** Bone Pathology; Surgical Pathology; **Hospital:** Maimonides Med Ctr (page 98), SUNY Downstate Med Ctr (page 405); **Address:** 4802 Tenth Ave, Brooklyn, NY 11219; **Phone:** 718-283-7025; **Board Cert:** Anatomic Pathology 1980; **Med School:** NY Med Coll 1976; **Resid:** Pathology, Johns Hopkins Hosp 1978; **Fellow:** Pathology, Meml Sloan Kettering Cancer Ctr 1979; **Fac Appt:** Prof Path, SUNY Downstate

Pediatric Cardiology

Kaplovitz, Harry S MD (PCd) - **Spec Exp:** Syncope; Echocardiography; Heart Failure; **Hospital:** Maimonides Med Ctr (page 98); **Address:** Maimonides Med Ctr, 4802 Tenth Ave, Ste K-106, Brooklyn, NY 11219; **Phone:** 718-283-7501; **Board Cert:** Pediatrics 1988; Pediatric Cardiology 2007; **Med School:** Albert Einstein Coll Med 1981; **Resid:** Pediatrics, North Shore Univ Hosp 1984; **Fellow:** Pediatric Cardiology, NYU Med Ctr 1986

Presti, Salvatore MD (PCd) - **Spec Exp:** Fetal Echocardiography; Congenital Heart Disease; Kawasaki Disease; **Hospital:** Lenox Hill Hosp, NYU Langone Med Ctr (page 106); **Address:** 25 Schermerhorn St, Brooklyn, NY 11201-4824; **Phone:** 718-923-1123; **Board Cert:** Pediatrics 1984; Pediatric Cardiology 2003; **Med School:** Italy 1978; **Resid:** Pediatrics, Lenox Hill Hosp 1982; **Fellow:** Pediatric Cardiology, NYU Med Ctr 1984; **Fac Appt:** Assoc Clin Prof Ped, NYU Sch Med

Ramaswamy, Prema MD (PCd) - **Spec Exp:** Fetal Echocardiography; Congenital Heart Disease; **Hospital:** Maimonides Med Ctr (page 98); **Address:** 4802 10th Ave, rm K106, Brooklyn, NY 11219-2844; **Phone:** 718-283-7501; **Board Cert:** Pediatrics 2009; Pediatric Cardiology 2004; **Med School:** India 1986; **Resid:** Pediatrics, M Y Hosp 1990; Pediatrics, Montefiore Med Ctr 1993; **Fellow:** Pediatric Cardiology, NY Hosp-Cornell 1996; **Fac Appt:** Asst Prof Ped, Mount Sinai Sch Med

Pediatric Endocrinology

Agdere, Levon MD (PEn) - **Spec Exp:** Diabetes; Short Stature in Children; Thyroid Disorders; **Hospital:** New York Methodist Hosp (page 404); **Address:** 263 7th Ave, Ste 3B, Brooklyn, NY 11215; **Phone:** 718-246-8540; **Board Cert:** Pediatric Endocrinology 2006; **Med School:** Turkey 1981; **Resid:** Pediatrics, Lutheran Med Ctr 1986; **Fellow:** Pediatric Endocrinology, NY Hosp-Cornell Med Ctr 1989

Avruskin, Theodore W MD (PEn) - **Spec Exp:** Growth Disorders; Diabetes; Thyroid Disorders; **Hospital:** Brookdale Univ Hosp Med Ctr, SUNY Downstate Med Ctr (page 405); **Address:** 1 Brookdale Plaza, Aaron Bldg, Ste 222, Brooklyn, NY 11212; **Phone:** 718-240-5960; **Board Cert:** Pediatrics 1965; **Med School:** Univ Toronto 1960; **Resid:** Pediatrics, Montreal Chldns Hosp 1962; Pediatrics, Chldns Hosp Med Ctr 1964; **Fellow:** Pediatric Endocrinology, Chldns Hosp Med Ctr 1968; **Fac Appt:** Prof Ped, SUNY Downstate

Pediatric Gastroenterology

Jelin, Abraham MD (PGe) - **Spec Exp:** Nutrition; Breast Feeding Problems; Gastroesophageal Reflux Disease (GERD); Constipation; **Hospital:** Brooklyn Hosp Ctr-Downtown, New York Methodist Hosp (page 404); **Address:** Bklyn Hosp Ctr, Dept Peds, 121 Dekalb Ave, Brooklyn, NY 11201-5425; **Phone:** 718-250-6277; **Board Cert:** Pediatrics 1977; Pediatric Gastroenterology 2005; **Med School:** NYU Sch Med 1972; **Resid:** Pediatrics, Grady Mem'l Hosp 1973; Pediatrics, Montefiore Hosp Med Ctr 1974; **Fellow:** Pediatric Gastroenterology, Emory Univ Hosp 1977; **Fac Appt:** Asst Clin Prof Ped, NYU Sch Med

McFarlane-Ferreira, Yvonne B MD (PGe) - **Spec Exp:** Pain-Abdominal Recurrent; Failure to Thrive; Constipation; Inflammatory Bowel Disease; **Hospital:** New York Methodist Hosp (page 404), Brooklyn Hosp Ctr-Downtown; **Address:** Park Slope Pediatrics, 263 7th Ave, Ste 3B, Brooklyn, NY 11215; **Phone:** 718-246-8515; **Board Cert:** Pediatrics 2005; Pediatric Gastroenterology 2003; **Med School:** West Indies 1983; **Resid:** Anesthesiology, Princess Margaret Hosp 1986; Pediatrics, Brooklyn Hosp 1989; **Fellow:** Pediatric Gastroenterology, Mt Sinai Hosp 1992; **Fac Appt:** Asst Clin Prof Ped, Cornell Univ-Weill Med Coll

Narwal, Shivinder MD (PGe) - **Spec Exp:** Nutrition; **Hospital:** Maimonides Med Ctr (page 98); **Address:** 948 48th St, Brooklyn, NY 11219; **Phone:** 718-283-8260; **Board Cert:** Pediatrics 2004; Pediatric Gastroenterology 2007; **Med School:** India 1983; **Resid:** Pediatrics, Kings Co Hosp Ctr 1993; **Fellow:** Pediatric Gastroenterology, Babies Hosp 1996; **Fac Appt:** Asst Prof Ped, SUNY Hlth Sci Ctr

Schwarz, Steven M MD (PGe) - **Spec Exp:** Gastroesophageal Reflux Disease (GERD); Nutrition; Endoscopy; Inflammatory Bowel Disease; **Hospital:** SUNY Downstate Med Ctr (page 405), Beth Israel Med Ctr - Petrie Division (page 94); **Address:** Children's Hosp at SUNY Downstate, 445 Lenox Rd, Box 49, Brooklyn, NY 11203; **Phone:** 718-270-4714; **Board Cert:** Pediatrics 1979; Pediatric Gastroenterology 2005; **Med School:** Columbia P&S 1974; **Resid:** Pediatrics, Columbia-Presby Med Ctr 1977; **Fellow:** Pediatric Gastroenterology, Stanford Univ Med Ctr 1978; Pediatric Gastroenterology, Columbia-Presby Med Ctr 1980; **Fac Appt:** Prof Ped, SUNY Downstate

Wetzler, Graciela MD (PGe) - **Spec Exp:** Peptic Ulcer Disease; Gastroesophageal Reflux Disease (GERD); Irritable Bowel Syndrome; Crohn's Disease; **Hospital:** Maimonides Med Ctr (page 98); **Address:** Maimonides Med Ctr, Dept Peds GE, 977 48th St, Brooklyn, NY 11219; **Phone:** 718-283-8260; **Board Cert:** Pediatric Gastroenterology 2003; **Med School:** Argentina 1984; **Resid:** Pediatrics, Montefiore Med Ctr 1992; **Fellow:** Pediatric Gastroenterology, NY Hosp-Cornell Med Ctr 1995; **Fac Appt:** Asst Clin Prof Ped, Mount Sinai Sch Med

Pediatric Hematology-Oncology

Guarini, Ludovico MD (PHO) - **Spec Exp:** Leukemia; Solid Tumors; Sickle Cell Disease; **Hospital:** Maimonides Med Ctr (page 98); **Address:** 4802 10th Ave, Dept of Pediatrics, Brooklyn, NY 11219; **Phone:** 718-765-2671; **Board Cert:** Pediatrics 1984; Pediatric Hematology-Oncology 2007; **Med School:** Italy 1974; **Resid:** Pediatrics, Beth Israel Hosp 1981; **Fellow:** Pediatric Hematology-Oncology, Columbia-Presby Med Ctr 1984; **Fac Appt:** Assoc Prof Ped, Mount Sinai Sch Med

Kulpa, Jolanta MD (PHO) - **Spec Exp:** Sickle Cell Disease; Leukemia; Thalassemia; Bleeding/Coagulation Disorders; **Hospital:** Long Island Coll Hosp (page 94), Beth Israel Med Ctr - Petrie Division (page 94); **Address:** Pediatric Private Practice, 339 Hicks St Fl 2, Brooklyn, NY 11201-5514; **Phone:** 718-780-1025; **Board Cert:** Pediatrics 1983; Pediatric Hematology-Oncology 1984; **Med School:** Med Coll PA 1972; **Resid:** Pediatrics, Lenox Hill Hosp 1975; **Fellow:** Blood Banking Transfusion Medicine, NY Blood Center 1977; Pediatric Hematology-Oncology, NY Hosp/Cornell/Sloan Kettering 1979; **Fac Appt:** Asst Clin Prof Ped, SUNY Hlth Sci Ctr

Miller, Scott T MD (PHO) - **Spec Exp:** Sickle Cell Disease; Transfusion Medicine; **Hospital:** SUNY Downstate Med Ctr (page 405), Kings County Hosp Ctr; **Address:** Univ Hosp Brooklyn, 450 Clarkson Ave, Box 49, Brooklyn, NY 11203-2056; **Phone:** 718-270-4714; **Board Cert:** Pediatrics 1981; Pediatric Hematology-Oncology 1982; **Med School:** Albert Einstein Coll Med 1976; **Resid:** Pediatrics, Montefiore Med Ctr 1979; **Fellow:** Pediatric Hematology-Oncology, Cornell/Meml Sloan Kettering 1981; **Fac Appt:** Prof Ped, SUNY Downstate

Sadanandan, Swayam MD (PHO) - **Spec Exp:** Sickle Cell Disease; Bleeding/Coagulation Disorders; Anemia; Pediatric Cancers; **Hospital:** Brooklyn Hosp Ctr-Downtown; **Address:** 121 Dekalb Ave, Brooklyn, NY 11201; **Phone:** 718-250-6074; **Board Cert:** Pediatrics 1980; Pediatric Hematology-Oncology 1984; **Med School:** India 1972; **Resid:** Pediatrics, St Vincent's Hosp & Med Ctr 1979; **Fellow:** Pediatric Hematology-Oncology, NYU Med Ctr 1981; **Fac Appt:** Asst Clin Prof Ped, NYU Sch Med

Sundaram, Revathy MD (PHO) - **Spec Exp:** Thalassemia; Sickle Cell Disease; Leukemia; **Hospital:** Long Island Coll Hosp (page 94), New York Methodist Hosp (page 404); **Address:** 502 8th Ave, Brooklyn, NY 11218; **Phone:** 718-780-3066; **Board Cert:** Pediatrics 1980; Pediatric Hematology-Oncology 1984; **Med School:** India 1973; **Resid:** Pediatrics, Rutgers Univ Hosp 1978; Pediatrics, Long Island Hosp 1980; **Fellow:** Pediatric Hematology-Oncology, Long Island Hosp 1983; **Fac Appt:** Asst Prof Ped, SUNY Hlth Sci Ctr

Viswanathan, Kusum MD (PHO) - **Spec Exp:** Sickle Cell Disease; Pediatric Cancers; Anemia; **Hospital:** Brookdale Univ Hosp Med Ctr; **Address:** 1 Brookdale Plaza CHC Bldg - rm 346, Brooklyn, NY 11212-3139; **Phone:** 718-240-5904; **Board Cert:** Pediatrics 1986; Pediatric Hematology-Oncology 1987; **Med School:** India 1980; **Resid:** Pediatrics, LI Coll Hosp 1984; **Fellow:** Pediatric Hematology-Oncology, LI Coll Hosp 1986; **Fac Appt:** Assoc Clin Prof Ped, SUNY Hlth Sci Ctr

Pediatric Infectious Disease

Gesner, Matthew J MD (PInf) - **Spec Exp:** AIDS/HIV; Kawasaki Disease; **Hospital:** Kings County Hosp Ctr, SUNY Downstate Med Ctr (page 405); **Address:** Kings County Hosp, 451 Clarkson Ave, Box 294, Brooklyn, NY 11203; **Phone:** 718-245-2562; **Board Cert:** Pediatrics 2006; Pediatric Infectious Disease 2009; **Med School:** SUNY Downstate 1988; **Resid:** Pediatrics, Chldns Hosp 1991; **Fellow:** Pediatric Infectious Disease, Bellevue Hosp Ctr 1994; **Fac Appt:** Asst Prof Ped, SUNY Downstate

Pediatric Nephrology

Kaplan, Matthew MD (PNep) - **Spec Exp:** Hypertension; Glomerulonephritis; **Hospital:** Long Island Coll Hosp (page 94), Coney Island Hosp; **Address:** 339 Hicks St, Brooklyn, NY 11201; **Phone:** 718-780-1025; **Board Cert:** Pediatrics 1974; Pediatric Nephrology 1976; **Med School:** SUNY Downstate 1968; **Resid:** Pediatrics, NY Hosp-Cornell Med Ctr 1972; **Fellow:** Pediatric Nephrology, NY Hosp-Cornell Med Ctr 1976; **Fac Appt:** Assoc Clin Prof Ped, SUNY Downstate

Schoeneman, Morris J MD (PNep) - **Spec Exp:** Hypertension; Kidney Failure-Chronic; Urinary Tract Infections; Dialysis Care; **Hospital:** SUNY Downstate Med Ctr (page 405), Richmond Univ Med Ctr; **Address:** SUNY Downstate Med Ctr, 445 Lenox Rd, Box 49, Brooklyn, NY 11203; **Phone:** 718-270-4714; **Board Cert:** Pediatrics 1974; Pediatric Nephrology 1974; **Med School:** Georgetown Univ 1969; **Resid:** Pediatrics, Univ NC Hosp 1970; Pediatrics, Univ MD Hosp 1972; **Fellow:** Pediatric Nephrology, Montefiore Med Ctr 1975; **Fac Appt:** Prof Ped, SUNY Hlth Sci Ctr

Pediatric Otolaryngology

Goldsmith, Ari J MD (PO) - **Spec Exp:** Voice Disorders; Airway Disorders; Hearing Loss; Sleep Apnea; **Hospital:** Long Island Coll Hosp (page 94); **Address:** LICH-Dept Otolaryngology, 134 Atlantic Ave, Brooklyn, NY 11201-5502; **Phone:** 718-780-1498; **Board Cert:** Otolaryngology 1994; **Med School:** Albert Einstein Coll Med 1988; **Resid:** Otolaryngology, LI Jewish Hosp 1993; **Fellow:** Pediatric Otolaryngology, Chldns Hosp 1994; **Fac Appt:** Assoc Prof Oto, SUNY Hlth Sci Ctr

Rosenfeld, Richard M MD (PO) - **Spec Exp:** Sinus Disorders/Surgery; Head & Neck Surgery; Ear Disorders/Surgery; **Hospital:** Long Island Coll Hosp (page 94), SUNY Downstate Med Ctr (page 405); **Address:** Univ Otolaryngologists, 134 Atlantic Ave, Brooklyn, NY 11201; **Phone:** 718-780-1498; **Board Cert:** Otolaryngology 1989; **Med School:** SUNY Buffalo 1984; **Resid:** Otolaryngology, Mount Sinai Med Ctr 1989; **Fellow:** Pediatric Otolaryngology, Chldn's Hosp 1991; **Fac Appt:** Prof Oto, SUNY Downstate

Pediatric Pulmonology

Giusti, Robert J MD (PPul) - **Spec Exp:** Cystic Fibrosis; Asthma; Cough-Chronic; **Hospital:** NYU Langone Med Ctr (page 106); **Address:** NYU Pediatric Pulmonology, 160 E 32nd St, L-3 Medical, New York, NY 10016; **Phone:** 212-263-5940; **Board Cert:** Pediatrics 1987; Pediatric Pulmonology 2004; **Med School:** SUNY Downstate 1981; **Resid:** Pediatrics, Bellevue Hosp 1985; **Fac Appt:** Asst Prof Ped, NYU Sch Med

Lee, Haesoon MD (PPul) - **Spec Exp:** Asthma; Lung Injuries - RSV Related; Sleep Apnea; Tuberculosis; **Hospital:** SUNY Downstate Med Ctr (page 405), Kings County Hosp Ctr; **Address:** SUNY-Downstate Med Ctr, Dept Pediatrics, 450 Clarkson Ave, Box 49, Brooklyn, NY 11203-2056; **Phone:** 718-221-5316; **Board Cert:** Pediatrics 1979; Pediatric Pulmonology 2004; **Med School:** South Korea 1972; **Resid:** Pediatrics, St Francis Hosp 1975; **Fellow:** Pediatric Pulmonology, Albert Einstein Affil Hosp 1977; **Fac Appt:** Assoc Prof Ped, SUNY Downstate

Marcus, Michael MD (PPul) - **Spec Exp:** Asthma; Sleep Apnea; Chronic Lung Disease; Gastroesophageal Reflux Disease (GERD); **Hospital:** Maimonides Med Ctr (page 98), Richmond Univ Med Ctr; **Address:** 4802 10th Ave, brooklyn, NY 11219; **Phone:** 718-980-5864; **Board Cert:** Pediatrics 1984; Allergy & Immunology 1987; Pediatric Pulmonology 2009; **Med School:** SUNY Stony Brook 1980; **Resid:** Pediatrics, Nassau County Med Ctr 1983; **Fellow:** Pediatric Pulmonology, Chldn's Hosp 1985; Allergy & Immunology, Chldn's Hosp 1985; **Fac Appt:** Asst Prof Ped, Mount Sinai Sch Med

Narula, Pramod MD (PPul) - **Spec Exp:** Asthma; Chronic Lung Disease; **Hospital:** New York Methodist Hosp (page 404); **Address:** 502 8th Ave, Brooklyn, NY 11215-3609; **Phone:** 718-780-3066; **Board Cert:** Pediatrics 2005; Pediatric Pulmonology 2009; **Med School:** India 1977; **Resid:** Pediatrics, Winthrop Univ Hosp 1989; **Fellow:** Pediatric Pulmonology, Columbia-Presby Med Ctr 1994; **Fac Appt:** Assoc Clin Prof Ped, Cornell Univ-Weill Med Coll

Pediatrics

Ajl, Stephen MD (Ped) *PCP* - **Hospital:** Brooklyn Hosp Ctr-Downtown; **Address:** 121 Dekalb Ave, Brooklyn, NY 11201; **Phone:** 718-250-8764; **Board Cert:** Pediatrics 1980; **Med School:** Temple Univ 1975; **Resid:** Pediatrics, NY Presby Hosp/Cornell 1978; **Fellow:** Ambulatory Pediatrics, Mount Sinai Hosp 1979; **Fac Appt:** Assoc Clin Prof Ped, SUNY Downstate

Fernandes, David R MD (Ped) *PCP* - **Hospital:** New York Methodist Hosp (page 404); **Address:** 126 95th St, Brooklyn, NY 11209-7203; **Phone:** 718-238-7842; **Board Cert:** Pediatrics 1980; **Med School:** SUNY Downstate 1972; **Resid:** Pediatrics, Kings County Hosp 1974; Pediatrics, N Shore Univ Hosp 1976; **Fellow:** Ambulatory Pediatrics, NYU-Bellevue Hosp 1977; **Fac Appt:** Asst Clin Prof Ped, SUNY Downstate

Gately, Adrian C MD (Ped) *PCP* - **Hospital:** New York Methodist Hosp (page 404); **Address:** 300 Park Pl, Brooklyn, NY 11238; **Phone:** 718-622-0469; **Board Cert:** Pediatrics 1983; **Med School:** Albert Einstein Coll Med 1975; **Resid:** Pediatrics, Jacobi Med Ctr 1978

Glaser, Amy MD (Ped) *PCP* - **Hospital:** Long Island Coll Hosp (page 94), NYU Langone Med Ctr (page 106); **Address:** 60 8th Ave, Brooklyn, NY 11217-3902; **Phone:** 718-636-0999; **Board Cert:** Pediatrics 1985; **Med School:** Mount Sinai Sch Med 1979; **Resid:** Pediatrics, Montefiore Hosp Med Ctr 1982; **Fellow:** Adolescent Medicine, Mt Sinai Hosp 1983

Hes, Dyan MD (Ped) - **Spec Exp:** Obesity; Weight Management; **Hospital:** New York Methodist Hosp (page 404); **Address:** Park Slope Pediatrics, 1 Prospect Park W, Ste A, Brooklyn, NY 11215; **Phone:** 718-636-3960; **Board Cert:** Pediatrics 2009; **Med School:** Israel 1997; **Resid:** Pediatrics, Montefiore Med Ctr 2000; **Fac Appt:** Asst Clin Prof Ped, Cornell Univ-Weill Med Coll

Jackson, Rosemary M MD (Ped) *PCP* - **Spec Exp:** Diabetes; Obesity; **Hospital:** SUNY Downstate Med Ctr (page 405), Long Island Coll Hosp (page 94); **Address:** 86 E 49th St, Ste G, Brooklyn, NY 11203; **Phone:** 718-363-6646; **Board Cert:** Pediatrics 2008; **Med School:** SUNY Upstate Med Univ 1985; **Resid:** Pediatrics, Downstate Med Ctr 1988; **Fac Appt:** Asst Clin Prof Ped, SUNY Downstate

Krieger, Ben Zion MD (Ped) *PCP* - **Spec Exp:** Allergy & Immunology; **Hospital:** Maimonides Med Ctr (page 98); **Address:** 1312 38th St, Brooklyn, NY 11218; **Phone:** 718-686-6700; **Board Cert:** Pediatrics 1986; **Med School:** Italy 1978; **Resid:** Pediatrics, Maimonides Med Ctr 1983; **Fellow:** Allergy & Immunology, Montefiore Med Ctr 1985; **Fac Appt:** Assoc Clin Prof Ped, Mount Sinai Sch Med

Mezey, Andrew MD (Ped) *PCP* - **Spec Exp:** Special Health Care Needs; Behavioral Disorders; **Hospital:** Maimonides Med Ctr (page 98); **Address:** 1301 57th St, Brooklyn, NY 11219; **Phone:** 718-283-3650; **Board Cert:** Pediatrics 1966; **Med School:** NYU Sch Med 1960; **Resid:** Pediatrics, Jacobi Med Ctr 1964; **Fac Appt:** Prof Ped, Albert Einstein Coll Med

Oghia, Hady MD (Ped) *PCP* - **Spec Exp:** Newborn Care; **Hospital:** Richmond Univ Med Ctr; **Address:** 7506 16th Ave, Brooklyn, NY 11214-1064; **Phone:** 718-331-3166; **Med School:** Mexico 1979; **Resid:** Pediatrics, St Vincent's Hosp & Med Ctr 1983

Oppenheim, J Aviva MD (Ped) *PCP* - **Spec Exp:** Special Health Care Needs; **Hospital:** NYU Langone Med Ctr (page 106); **Address:** Pediatric Assocs NYC, 20 Plaza St E, Ste A7, Brooklyn, NY 11238; **Phone:** 718-857-5500; **Board Cert:** Pediatrics 2007; **Med School:** Cornell Univ 1996; **Resid:** Pediatrics, Bellevue Hosp/NYU Med Ctr 1999

Preis, Oded MD (Ped) *PCP* - **Spec Exp:** Prematurity/Low Birth Weight Infants; **Hospital:** Maimonides Med Ctr (page 98), New York Methodist Hosp (page 404); **Address:** 1729 E 12th St, Brooklyn, NY 11229; **Phone:** 718-339-4919; **Board Cert:** Pediatrics 1978; Neonatal-Perinatal Medicine 1981; **Med School:** Israel 1971; **Resid:** Pediatrics, Maimonides Med Ctr 1975; **Fellow:** Neonatal-Perinatal Medicine, SUNY - Downstate Med Ctr 1977; **Fac Appt:** Assoc Clin Prof Ped, SUNY Downstate

Schaeffer, Henry MD (Ped) *PCP* - **Hospital:** Maimonides Med Ctr (page 98), Coney Island Hosp; **Address:** Maimonides Medical Ctr, Dept Pediatrics, 4802 10th Ave, Brooklyn, NY 11219-2844; **Phone:** 718-283-8918; **Board Cert:** Pediatrics 1969; **Med School:** NYU Sch Med 1963; **Resid:** Pediatrics, Bellevue Hosp/NYU Med Ctr 1966; **Fac Appt:** Clin Prof Ped, SUNY Downstate

Sergiou, Harry G MD (Ped) *PCP* - **Hospital:** Long Island Coll Hosp (page 94); **Address:** 554 Henry St, Brooklyn, NY 11231; **Phone:** 718-625-5591; **Board Cert:** Pediatrics 2004; **Med School:** Greece 1979; **Resid:** Pediatrics, Long Island Coll Hosp 1985

Wu, Jason J MD/PhD (Ped) *PCP* - **Spec Exp:** Chinese Community Health; **Hospital:** Maimonides Med Ctr (page 98); **Address:** 781 47th St, Brooklyn, NY 11220; **Phone:** 718-435-5980; **Board Cert:** Pediatrics 2002; **Med School:** China 1982; **Resid:** Pediatrics, Maimonides Med Ctr 2001; **Fac Appt:** Asst Clin Prof Ped, Mount Sinai Sch Med

Physical Medicine & Rehabilitation

Atakent, Pinar E MD (PMR) - **Spec Exp:** Pain Management; Stroke Rehabilitation; Electrodiagnosis; Acupuncture; **Hospital:** Long Island Coll Hosp (page 94); **Address:** LI Coll Hosp, 339 Hicks St, Brooklyn, NY 11201-5509; **Phone:** 718-780-4685; **Board Cert:** Physical Medicine & Rehabilitation 1982; **Med School:** Turkey 1971; **Resid:** Physical Medicine & Rehabilitation, Jacobi Med Ctr 1981

Gifford, Irina MD (PMR) - **Spec Exp:** Musculoskeletal Disorders; Neurologic Rehabilitation; Pediatric Rehabilitation; **Hospital:** Kingsbrook Jewish Med Ctr; **Address:** 585 Schenectady Ave, Ste 333, Brooklyn, NY 11203-1822; **Phone:** 718-604-5369; **Board Cert:** Physical Medicine & Rehabilitation 1990; **Med School:** Romania 1960; **Resid:** Physical Medicine & Rehabilitation, Mount Sinai Hosp 1989; **Fellow:** Pediatric Rehabilitation Medicine, Albert Einstein Med Sch 1990

Ross, Marc MD (PMR) - **Spec Exp:** Sports Medicine; Pain-Back; Gait Disorders; **Hospital:** Kingsbrook Jewish Med Ctr, Mount Sinai Med Ctr (page 102); **Address:** Kingsbrook Jewish Med Ctr, Dept Physical Med & Rehab, 585 Schenectady Ave, Brooklyn, NY 11203; **Phone:** 718-604-5341; **Board Cert:** Physical Medicine & Rehabilitation 2004; **Med School:** NY Med Coll 1989; **Resid:** Physical Medicine & Rehabilitation, Mt Sinai Med Ctr 1993; **Fac Appt:** Asst Prof PMR, Mount Sinai Sch Med

Stein, Perry MD (PMR) - **Spec Exp:** Pain Management; **Hospital:** Mercy Med Ctr - Rockville Centre, Maimonides Med Ctr (page 98); **Address:** 383 Ocean Pkwy, Brooklyn, NY 11218; **Phone:** 718-941-6000; **Board Cert:** Physical Medicine & Rehabilitation 1991; **Med School:** Mexico 1985; **Resid:** Physical Medicine & Rehabilitation, Univ Hosp 1990

Vallarino, Ramon MD (PMR) - **Spec Exp:** Pain Management; Functional Ability Loss; Electromyography; Musculoskeletal Disorders; **Hospital:** New York Methodist Hosp (page 404); **Address:** 816 8th Ave, Brooklyn, NY 11215; **Phone:** 718-788-5762; **Board Cert:** Physical Medicine & Rehabilitation 1977; **Med School:** Peru 1966; **Resid:** Physical Medicine & Rehabilitation, Mount Sinai Hosp 1968; **Fellow:** Rheumatology, Mount Sinai Hosp 1968; **Fac Appt:** Asst Clin Prof PMR, SUNY Hlth Sci Ctr

Plastic Surgery

Feldman, David L MD (PlS) - **Spec Exp:** Cosmetic Surgery; Laser Surgery; **Hospital:** Maimonides Med Ctr (page 98), Lutheran Med Ctr - Brooklyn; **Address:** 925 49th St, Brooklyn, NY 11219; **Phone:** 718-283-7022; **Board Cert:** Plastic Surgery 1994; **Med School:** Duke Univ 1984; **Resid:** Surgery, St Luke's/Roosevelt 1989; Plastic/Reconstructive Surgery, Duke Univ Med Ctr 1992; **Fellow:** Hand Surgery, Kleinert Inst for Hand/Microsurg 1991; **Fac Appt:** Asst Prof PlS, Mount Sinai Sch Med

Roth, Malcolm Z MD (PlS) - **Spec Exp:** Breast Reconstruction; Cosmetic Surgery-Breast; Cosmetic Surgery-Face & Eyelid; Body Contouring after Weight Loss; **Hospital:** Maimonides Med Ctr (page 98), Beth Israel Med Ctr - Petrie Division (page 94); **Address:** 925 49th St, Brooklyn, NY 11219; **Phone:** 718-283-7022; **Board Cert:** Plastic Surgery 1991; Hand Surgery 2003; **Med School:** NY Med Coll 1982; **Resid:** Surgery, Beth Israel Med Ctr 1985; Plastic Surgery, NY Hosp-Cornell 1987; **Fellow:** Hand Surgery, Hosp Special Surgery 1988; **Fac Appt:** Asst Clin Prof PlS, SUNY Hlth Sci Ctr

Psychiatry

Berkowitz, Howard MD (Psyc) - **Spec Exp:** Anxiety Disorders; Depression; Geriatric Psychiatry; **Hospital:** Maimonides Med Ctr (page 98); **Address:** 4715 Fort Hamilton Pkwy, Brooklyn, NY 11219-2927; **Phone:** 718-633-2025; **Board Cert:** Psychiatry 1977; Geriatric Psychiatry 2004; **Med School:** Albert Einstein Coll Med 1972; **Resid:** Internal Medicine, Beth Israel Hosp 1973; Psychiatry, Kings County Hosp 1976; **Fellow:** Consultation Psychiatry, Kings County Hosp 1977; **Fac Appt:** Assoc Clin Prof Psyc, SUNY Downstate

Coplan, Jeremy MD (Psyc) - **Spec Exp:** Anxiety Disorders; Psychosomatic Disorders; Bipolar/Mood Disorders; **Hospital:** SUNY Downstate Med Ctr (page 405); **Address:** 450 Clarkson Ave, Box 1203, Brooklyn, NY 11203; **Phone:** 718-270-2023; **Board Cert:** Psychiatry 1990; **Med School:** South Africa 1983; **Resid:** Psychiatry, SUNY-Downstate Med Ctr 1989; **Fellow:** Biological Psychiatry, Columbia-Presby Med Ctr; **Fac Appt:** Prof Psyc, SUNY Downstate

Eitan, Noam MD (Psyc) - **Spec Exp:** Anxiety Disorders; Depression; Gay & Lesbian Issues; **Hospital:** Woodhull Med & Mental Hlth Ctr; **Address:** 760 Broadway, Brooklyn, NY 11206; **Phone:** 718-963-5793; **Board Cert:** Psychiatry 2008; **Med School:** Israel 1986; **Resid:** Psychiatry, Shalvata Hosp 1991; **Fellow:** Psychoanalysis, Sackler Sch Med 1995

Goldberg, Jeffrey DO (Psyc) - **Spec Exp:** Geriatric Psychiatry; Anxiety & Depression; Mood Disorders; **Hospital:** Coney Island Hosp; **Address:** 5025 Ft Hamilton Pkwy, Brooklyn, NY 11219; **Phone:** 718-633-8183; **Board Cert:** Psychiatry 1986; Geriatric Psychiatry 2006; **Med School:** NY Coll Osteo Med 1981; **Resid:** Psychiatry, Maimonides Med Ctr 1985; **Fac Appt:** Asst Clin Prof Psyc, SUNY Downstate

Heisman, Alexander MD (Psyc) - **Spec Exp:** Addiction/Substance Abuse; Liaison Psychiatry; Pain-Chronic; **Hospital:** Beth Israel Med Ctr- Kings Hwy Div (page 94), New York Methodist Hosp (page 404); **Address:** 2520 Kings Highway, Brooklyn, NY 11229; **Phone:** 718-449-1705; **Board Cert:** Psychiatry 2007; Addiction Medicine 2008; **Med School:** Russia 1976; **Resid:** Psychiatry, Montefiore Med Ctr 1996

Idupuganti, Sudharam MD (Psyc) - **Spec Exp:** Depression; Electroconvulsive Therapy (ECT); Panic Disorder; **Hospital:** Maimonides Med Ctr (page 98); **Address:** 585 Bayridge Pkwy, Brooklyn, NY 11209-3309; **Phone:** 718-921-1001; **Board Cert:** Psychiatry 1981; **Med School:** India 1974; **Resid:** Psychiatry, Maimonides Med Ctr 1979; **Fac Appt:** Asst Prof Psyc, SUNY Downstate

Licht, Arnold MD (Psyc) - **Spec Exp:** Geriatric Psychiatry; Mood Disorders; **Hospital:** Long Island Coll Hosp (page 94); **Address:** Brooklyn Psychiatric Associates, 161 Atlantic Ave, Brooklyn, NY 11201; **Phone:** 718-935-0986; **Board Cert:** Psychiatry 1975; Geriatric Psychiatry 2001; **Med School:** SUNY Hlth Sci Ctr 1969; **Resid:** Psychiatry, Albert Einstein 1973; **Fac Appt:** Asst Prof Psyc, SUNY Downstate

Viswanathan, Ramaswamy MD (Psyc) - **Spec Exp:** Depression; Anxiety Disorders; **Hospital:** SUNY Downstate Med Ctr (page 405), Kings County Hosp Ctr; **Address:** 450 Clarkson Ave, Ste A3-474, Brooklyn, NY 11203-2098; **Phone:** 718-270-2352; **Board Cert:** Psychiatry 1978; Internal Medicine 1989; Addiction Psychiatry 2003; Geriatric Psychiatry 2002; **Med School:** India 1972; **Resid:** Internal Medicine, Queens Hosp Ctr 1974; Psychiatry, SUNY Hlth Sci Ctr 1977; **Fellow:** Psychiatry, SUNY Hlth Sci Ctr 1978; **Fac Appt:** Assoc Clin Prof Psyc, SUNY Hlth Sci Ctr

Pulmonary Disease

Abott, Michael L MD (Pul) - **Spec Exp:** Asthma; Emphysema; **Hospital:** New York Methodist Hosp (page 404), Lutheran Med Ctr - Brooklyn; **Address:** 7124 18th Ave, Brooklyn, NY 11204-5203; **Phone:** 718-234-3333; **Board Cert:** Internal Medicine 1983; Pulmonary Disease 1986; **Med School:** Mexico 1978; **Resid:** Internal Medicine, Coney Island Hosp 1982; **Fellow:** Pulmonary Disease, Montefiore Med Ctr 1984

Amin, Hossam H MD (Pul) - **Spec Exp:** Asthma & Allergy; Critical Care; **Hospital:** Metropolitan Hosp Ctr - NY, New York Methodist Hosp (page 404); **Address:** 6903 4th Ave, Brooklyn, NY 11209; **Phone:** 718-238-6161; **Board Cert:** Internal Medicine 2006; Pulmonary Disease 2008; Critical Care Medicine 2009; **Med School:** Egypt 1988; **Resid:** Internal Medicine, Interfaith Med Ctr 1996; **Fellow:** Pulmonary Disease, Interfaith Med Ctr 1998; Critical Care Medicine, Mt Sinai Med Ctr 1999; **Fac Appt:** Assoc Prof Med, NY Med Coll

Bergman, Michael I MD (Pul) - **Spec Exp:** Asthma; Bronchitis; Respiratory Failure; Pneumonia; **Hospital:** Long Island Coll Hosp (page 94); **Address:** 339 Hicks St, Brooklyn, NY 11201; **Phone:** 718-780-1416; **Board Cert:** Internal Medicine 1981; Pulmonary Disease 1984; Critical Care Medicine 2007; **Med School:** Albert Einstein Coll Med 1978; **Resid:** Internal Medicine, Brookdale Hosp 1981; **Fellow:** Pulmonary Disease, Mount Sinai Hosp 1984; **Fac Appt:** Asst Prof Med, SUNY Hlth Sci Ctr

Bernstein, Chaim MD (Pul) - **Spec Exp:** Asthma; Emphysema; Lung Cancer; **Hospital:** Beth Israel Med Ctr- Kings Hwy Div (page 94); **Address:** 3131 Kings Hwy, Ste D10, Brooklyn, NY 11234-2643; **Phone:** 718-252-3590; **Board Cert:** Internal Medicine 1977; Pulmonary Disease 1982; Critical Care Medicine 2007; **Med School:** NYU Sch Med 1974; **Resid:** Internal Medicine, Brookdale Med Ctr 1977; Pulmonary Disease, Manhattan VA Hosp; **Fellow:** Pulmonary Disease, Bellevue Hosp-NYU 1979

Bondi, Elliott MD (Pul) - **Spec Exp:** Asthma; Tuberculosis; Pneumonia; **Hospital:** Brookdale Univ Hosp Med Ctr; **Address:** Brookdale Hospital, Pulmonary Medicine, 1 Brookdale Plaza, rm A107, Brooklyn, NY 11212; **Phone:** 718-240-5236; **Board Cert:** Internal Medicine 1987; Pulmonary Disease 1982; **Med School:** Univ MD Sch Med 1971; **Resid:** Internal Medicine, Maimonides Medical Ctr 1973; Internal Medicine, Bronx Muni Hosp 1974; **Fellow:** Pulmonary Disease, Bronx Muni Hosp 1976; **Fac Appt:** Assoc Clin Prof Med, SUNY Downstate

Demetis, Spiro MD (Pul) - **Spec Exp:** Sarcoidosis; Lung Cancer; Asthma & Emphysema; Pulmonary Hypertension; **Hospital:** SUNY Downstate Med Ctr (page 405), Lutheran Med Ctr - Brooklyn; **Address:** 450 Clarkson Ave, Box 19, Brooklyn, NY 11203; **Phone:** 718-270-1821; **Board Cert:** Internal Medicine 1989; Pulmonary Disease 2005; Critical Care Medicine 2005; **Med School:** Mexico 1983; **Resid:** Internal Medicine, Univ Hosp 1988; **Fellow:** Pulmonary Disease, Univ Hosp 1990; Critical Care Medicine, Univ Hosp 1991; **Fac Appt:** Assoc Prof Med, SUNY Hlth Sci Ctr

George, Liziamma MD (Pul) - **Spec Exp:** Sleep Disorders; Smoking Cessation; **Hospital:** New York Methodist Hosp (page 404); **Address:** 501 Sixth St, Brooklyn, NY 11215; **Phone:** 718-246-8600; **Board Cert:** Internal Medicine 1987; Critical Care Medicine 1999; Pulmonary Disease 1999; Sleep Medicine 2009; **Med School:** India 1980; **Resid:** Internal Medicine, St Joseph's Med Ctr 1987; **Fellow:** Pulmonary Disease, St Joseph's Med Ctr 1989; **Fac Appt:** Assoc Clin Prof Med, Cornell Univ-Weill Med Coll

Groopman, Jacob MD (Pul) - **Spec Exp:** Asthma; Emphysema; **Hospital:** Maimonides Med Ctr (page 98); **Address:** Pulmonary & Critical Care Medicine, 953 49th St Fl 5 - rm 511, Brooklyn, NY 11219-2923; **Phone:** 718-283-8380; **Board Cert:** Internal Medicine 1979; Pulmonary Disease 1980; **Med School:** SUNY Hlth Sci Ctr 1974; **Resid:** Internal Medicine, Maimonides Med Ctr 1978; **Fellow:** Pulmonary Disease, NYU Med Ctr 1980; **Fac Appt:** Asst Prof Med, Mount Sinai Sch Med

Gulrajani, Ramesh MD (Pul) - **Spec Exp:** Asthma; Sarcoidosis; Lung Cancer; **Hospital:** Brooklyn Hosp Ctr-Downtown; **Address:** 121 Dekalb Ave, Ste 7F, Brooklyn, NY 11201-5425; **Phone:** 718-250-6950; **Board Cert:** Internal Medicine 1979; Pulmonary Disease 1984; **Med School:** India 1974; **Resid:** Internal Medicine, Brooklyn Cumberland Med Ctr 1979; **Fellow:** Pulmonary Disease, Brooklyn Cumberland Med Ctr 1981; **Fac Appt:** Assoc Clin Prof Med, Cornell Univ-Weill Med Coll

Hammer, Arthur MD (Pul) - **Spec Exp:** Asthma; Sleep Disorders; Pulmonary Fibrosis; **Hospital:** Beth Israel Med Ctr- Kings Hwy Div (page 94); **Address:** 3131 Kings Hwy, Ste D10, Brooklyn, NY 11234-2643; **Phone:** 718-252-3590; **Board Cert:** Pulmonary Disease 2009; Internal Medicine 2006; **Med School:** Mexico 1970; **Resid:** Internal Medicine, Brookdale Hosp 1974; **Fellow:** Pulmonary Disease, NYU Med Sch 1976

Kupfer, Yizhak MD (Pul) - **Spec Exp:** Sleep & Snoring Disorders; Cough; Mechanical Ventilation; **Hospital:** Maimonides Med Ctr (page 98); **Address:** Div Pulmonary & Critical Care Medicine, 953 49th St Fl 5 - Ste 511, Brooklyn, NY 11219-2923; **Phone:** 718-283-8380; **Board Cert:** Internal Medicine 1989; Pulmonary Disease 2000; Critical Care Medicine 2000; **Med School:** SUNY Downstate 1986; **Resid:** Internal Medicine, Maimonides Med Ctr 1989; **Fellow:** Pulmonary Disease, Maimonides Med Ctr 1991; Critical Care Medicine, Maimonides Med Ctr 1992; **Fac Appt:** Assoc Clin Prof Med, SUNY Downstate

Lombardo, Gerard T MD (Pul) - **Spec Exp:** Sleep Apnea; Sleep & Snoring Disorders; **Hospital:** New York Methodist Hosp (page 404); **Address:** 9101 4th Ave, Brooklyn, NY 11209; **Phone:** 718-745-1156; **Board Cert:** Internal Medicine 1984; Pulmonary Disease 1986; **Med School:** Grenada 1981; **Resid:** Internal Medicine, NY Methodist Hosp 1984; **Fellow:** Pulmonary Disease, NY Methodist Hosp 1986; **Fac Appt:** Asst Clin Prof Med, Cornell Univ-Weill Med Coll

Miarrostami, Rameen M MD (Pul) - **Spec Exp:** Asthma; Chronic Obstructive Lung Disease (COPD); Emphysema; Cough; **Hospital:** New York Methodist Hosp (page 404), Lutheran Med Ctr - Brooklyn; **Address:** 7124 18th Ave Fl 2, Brooklyn, NY 11204-5203; **Phone:** 718-234-3333; **Board Cert:** Internal Medicine 2001; Pulmonary Disease 2004; **Med School:** Dominican Republic 1985; **Resid:** Internal Medicine, Lincoln Med Ctr 1991; **Fellow:** Pulmonary Disease, LI Coll Hosp 1993

Raoof, Suhail MD (Pul) - **Spec Exp:** Critical Care Medicine; Chronic Obstructive Lung Disease (COPD); Mechanical Ventilation; Lung Disease; **Hospital:** New York Methodist Hosp (page 404); **Address:** Div, Pulmonary & Critical Care, 506 6th St, Brooklyn, NY 11215; **Phone:** 718-780-5835; **Board Cert:** Internal Medicine 2002; Pulmonary Disease 2003; Critical Care Medicine 2004; **Med School:** India 1982; **Resid:** Internal Medicine, LIJ Med Ctr 1989; Internal Medicine, Nassau County Med Ctr 1991; **Fellow:** Pulmonary Critical Care Medicine, Stony Brook Affil Hosps 1992; **Fac Appt:** Prof Med, Cornell Univ-Weill Med Coll

Saleh, Anthony MD (Pul) - **Spec Exp:** Asthma; Interstitial Lung Disease; Lung Cancer; **Hospital:** New York Methodist Hosp (page 404); **Address:** 7206 7th Ave, Brooklyn, NY 11209; **Phone:** 718-745-1200; **Board Cert:** Internal Medicine 1988; Pulmonary Disease 2000; **Med School:** Grenada 1985; **Resid:** Internal Medicine, NY Methodist Hosp 1988; **Fellow:** Pulmonary Disease, NY Methodist Hosp 1990; **Fac Appt:** Asst Clin Prof Med, Cornell Univ-Weill Med Coll

Smith, Peter R MD (Pul) - **Spec Exp:** Chronic Obstructive Lung Disease (COPD); Smoking Cessation; Sarcoidosis; Wegener's Granolomatosis; **Hospital:** Long Island Coll Hosp (page 94); **Address:** Long Island Coll Hosp, Div Pulmonology, 339 Hicks St, Brooklyn, NY 11201-5509; **Phone:** 718-780-2905; **Board Cert:** Internal Medicine 1973; Pulmonary Disease 1974; Critical Care Medicine 2009; **Med School:** Columbia P&S 1968; **Resid:** Internal Medicine, Downstate Med Ctr 1970; Internal Medicine, Jacobi Med Ctr 1971; **Fellow:** Pulmonary Disease, Downstate Med Ctr 1974; **Fac Appt:** Clin Prof Med, SUNY Hlth Sci Ctr

Tessler, Sidney MD (Pul) - **Spec Exp:** Cough; Asthma; Mechanical Ventilation; **Hospital:** Maimonides Med Ctr (page 98); **Address:** 953 49th St Fl 5 - rm 511, Div Pul & Critical Care Med, Brooklyn, NY 11219-2923; **Phone:** 718-283-8380; **Board Cert:** Internal Medicine 1977; Pulmonary Disease 1980; Critical Care Medicine 2007; **Med School:** SUNY Hlth Sci Ctr 1970; **Resid:** Internal Medicine, Coney Island Hosp 1972; Internal Medicine, Maimonides Med Ctr 1976; **Fellow:** Pulmonary Disease, Maimonides Med Ctr 1977; **Fac Appt:** Clin Prof Med, SUNY Hlth Sci Ctr

Radiation Oncology

Ashamalla, Hani MD (RadRO) - **Spec Exp:** Brachytherapy; Prostate Cancer; Gastrointestinal Cancer; Breast Cancer; **Hospital:** New York Methodist Hosp (page 404), Wyckoff Heights Med Ctr; **Address:** NY Methodist Hosp, Dept Rad Oncology, 506 6th St, Brooklyn, NY 11215; **Phone:** 718-780-3677; **Board Cert:** Radiation Oncology 2004; **Med School:** Egypt 1983; **Resid:** Radiation Oncology, NY Methodist Hosp 1994; **Fellow:** Radiation Oncology, NY Methodist Hosp 1995; Radiation Oncology, Chldns Hosp 1995; **Fac Appt:** Assoc Clin Prof RadRO, Cornell Univ-Weill Med Coll

Cooper, Jay MD (RadRO) - **Spec Exp:** Head & Neck Cancer; Skin Cancer; Chemo-Radiation Combined Therapy; **Hospital:** Maimonides Med Ctr (page 98); **Address:** Maimonides Cancer Ctr, 6300 8th Ave, Lower Level, Brooklyn, NY 11220; **Phone:** 718-765-2700; **Board Cert:** Therapeutic Radiology 1977; **Med School:** NYU Sch Med 1973; **Resid:** Radiation Oncology, NYU Med Ctr 1977; **Fac Appt:** Prof RadRO, Albert Einstein Coll Med

Donahue, Bernadine R MD (RadRO) - **Spec Exp:** Brain Tumors; Gastrointestinal Cancer; Pediatric Cancers; Solid Tumors; **Hospital:** Maimonides Med Ctr (page 98); **Address:** Maimonides Med Ctr, Dept Radiation Oncology, 6300 8th Ave, Lower Level, Brooklyn, NY 11220; **Phone:** 718-765-2700; **Board Cert:** Internal Medicine 1987; Radiation Oncology 1991; **Med School:** Boston Univ 1984; **Resid:** Internal Medicine, Boston Univ Med Ctr 1987; **Fellow:** Radiation Oncology, NYU Med Ctr 1990

Gliedman, Paul R MD (RadRO) - **Spec Exp:** Breast Cancer; Prostate Cancer; Brain Tumors; **Hospital:** St Luke's - Roosevelt Hosp Ctr - Roosevelt Div (page 94), Beth Israel Med Ctr - Petrie Division (page 94); **Address:** Brooklyn Radiation Oncology, 2101 Avenue X, Brooklyn, NY 11235; **Phone:** 718-512-2160; **Board Cert:** Radiation Oncology 1987; **Med School:** Columbia P&S 1983; **Resid:** Radiation Oncology, NYU Med Ctr 1987

Reproductive Endocrinology

Grazi, Richard MD (RE) - **Spec Exp:** Infertility-IVF; Preimplantation Genetic Diagnosis; Fertility Preservation in Cancer; **Hospital:** Maimonides Med Ctr (page 98), Richmond Univ Med Ctr; **Address:** 1355 84th St, Brooklyn, NY 11228-3030; **Phone:** 718-283-8600; **Board Cert:** Obstetrics & Gynecology 2006; Reproductive Endocrinology 2006; **Med School:** SUNY Buffalo 1981; **Resid:** Obstetrics & Gynecology, NYU Med Ctr 1985; **Fellow:** Reproductive Endocrinology, UMDNJ Med Ctr 1987; **Fac Appt:** Assoc Clin Prof ObG, Mount Sinai Sch Med

Kofinas, George MD (RE) - **Spec Exp:** Infertility-IVF; Laparoscopic Surgery; Uterine Fibroids; Congenital Anomalies-Gynecologic; **Hospital:** New York Methodist Hosp (page 404); **Address:** Fertility Inst, New York Meth Hosp, 506 6th St Fl WP4, Brooklyn, NY 11215-3609; **Phone:** 718-780-5065; **Board Cert:** Obstetrics & Gynecology 2010; Reproductive Endocrinology 2010; **Med School:** Greece 1975; **Resid:** Obstetrics & Gynecology, NY Methodist Hosp 1982; Obstetrics & Gynecology, Brooklyn Hosp 1984; **Fellow:** Reproductive Endocrinology, Univ Hosp 1986; **Fac Appt:** Asst Prof ObG, SUNY Hlth Sci Ctr

Seifer, David B MD (RE) - **Spec Exp:** Infertility-IVF; Infertility-Advanced Maternal Age; Fertility Preservation in Cancer; **Hospital:** Maimonides Med Ctr (page 98), Richmond Univ Med Ctr; **Address:** 1355 84th St, Brooklyn, NY 11228; **Phone:** 718-283-8600; **Board Cert:** Obstetrics & Gynecology 2010; Reproductive Endocrinology/Infertility 2010; **Med School:** Univ IL Coll Med 1981; **Resid:** Obstetrics & Gynecology, Stanford Univ Hosp 1985; **Fellow:** Reproductive Endocrinology, Yale-New Haven Hosp 1991; **Fac Appt:** Prof ObG, Mount Sinai Sch Med

Rheumatology

Bernstein, Lawrence J MD (Rhu) - **Spec Exp:** Rheumatoid Arthritis; Polymyositis; Scleroderma; **Hospital:** Brookdale Univ Hosp Med Ctr; **Address:** Dept Rehab Medicine, 1 Brookdale Plaza, rm 344 CHC, Brooklyn, NY 11212; **Phone:** 718-240-6126; **Board Cert:** Internal Medicine 1965; Physical Medicine & Rehabilitation 1968; Rheumatology 1972; **Med School:** NYU Sch Med 1958; **Resid:** Internal Medicine, Bellevue Hosp 1961; **Fellow:** Rheumatology, New York Univ Med Ctr 1962

Bienenstock, Harry MD (Rhu) - **Spec Exp:** Rheumatoid Arthritis; Musculoskeletal Disorders; **Hospital:** Hosp For Special Surgery (page 111), Long Island Coll Hosp (page 94); **Address:** 4015 Avenue U, Brooklyn, NY 11234-5117; **Phone:** 718-252-8181; **Board Cert:** Internal Medicine 1965; Rheumatology 1972; **Med School:** Ros Franklin Univ/Chicago Med Sch 1957; **Resid:** Internal Medicine, VA Med Ctr 1960; **Fellow:** Rheumatology, Hosp For Special Surgery 1962; **Fac Appt:** Assoc Clin Prof Med, Cornell Univ-Weill Med Coll

Garner, Bruce MD (Rhu) - **Spec Exp:** Rheumatoid Arthritis; Osteoporosis; Osteoarthritis; Lupus/SLE; **Hospital:** Lutheran Med Ctr - Brooklyn; **Address:** 7901 4th Ave, Ste A5, Brooklyn, NY 11209-3915; **Phone:** 718-921-5239; **Board Cert:** Internal Medicine 1987; Rheumatology 1988; **Med School:** Mexico 1981; **Resid:** Internal Medicine, Lutheran Med Ctr 1985; **Fellow:** Rheumatology, Washington Hosp Ctr 1987; **Fac Appt:** Asst Clin Prof Med, SUNY Downstate

Green, Stuart MD (Rhu) - **Spec Exp:** Rheumatoid Arthritis; Osteoporosis; Lupus/SLE; **Hospital:** Brooklyn Hosp Ctr-Downtown; **Address:** 121 Dekalb Ave Fl 7, Brooklyn, NY 11201-5425; **Phone:** 718-250-6921; **Board Cert:** Internal Medicine 1982; Rheumatology 1986; **Med School:** Georgetown Univ 1979; **Resid:** Internal Medicine, St Luke's/Roosevelt Hosp Ctr 1982; **Fellow:** Rheumatology, SUNY Downstate Med Ctr 1985; **Fac Appt:** Asst Clin Prof Med, NYU Sch Med

Lesser, Robert S MD (Rhu) - **Spec Exp:** Polymyalgia Rheumatica; Rheumatoid Arthritis; Lupus/SLE; **Hospital:** Beth Israel Med Ctr- Kings Hwy Div (page 94); **Address:** 4015 Avenue U, Brooklyn, NY 11234-5117; **Phone:** 718-252-5151; **Board Cert:** Internal Medicine 1985; Rheumatology 1988; **Med School:** Ros Franklin Univ/Chicago Med Sch 1982; **Resid:** Internal Medicine, Hahnemann Univ Hosp 1985; **Fellow:** Rheumatology, Hahnemann Univ Hosp 1987; **Fac Appt:** Assoc Clin Prof Med, SUNY Hlth Sci Ctr

Patel, Jitendra K MD (Rhu) - **Spec Exp:** Arthritis; Fibromyalgia; Pain-Back; **Hospital:** Kingsbrook Jewish Med Ctr, Beth Israel Med Ctr- Kings Hwy Div (page 94); **Address:** 3420 Ave N, Brooklyn, NY 11234-2607; **Phone:** 718-258-7019; **Board Cert:** Internal Medicine 1979; Rheumatology 1982; **Med School:** India 1975; **Resid:** Internal Medicine, Mem U Newfoundland 1979; **Fellow:** Rheumatology, Georgetown Univ Hosp 1982

Schiff, Carl F MD (Rhu) - **Spec Exp:** Rheumatoid Arthritis; Osteoporosis; **Hospital:** Maimonides Med Ctr (page 98); **Address:** Maimonides Med Ctr, 4802 10th Ave, Ste 352, Brooklyn, NY 11219-2916; **Phone:** 718-283-8519; **Board Cert:** Internal Medicine 1983; Rheumatology 1986; **Med School:** Yale Univ 1980; **Resid:** Internal Medicine, Mt Sinai Hosp 1983; **Fellow:** Rheumatology, Columbia-Presby Med Ctr 1986; **Fac Appt:** Asst Clin Prof Med, SUNY Hlth Sci Ctr

Surgery

Adler, Harry MD (S) - **Spec Exp:** Biliary Surgery; Laparoscopic Surgery; Hernia; Colon Surgery; **Hospital:** Maimonides Med Ctr (page 98); **Address:** 948 48th St Fl 3, Brooklyn, NY 11219; **Phone:** 718-283-7952; **Board Cert:** Surgery 2005; Surgical Critical Care 2008; **Med School:** NYU Sch Med 1980; **Resid:** Surgery, Bellevue Hosp/NYU Med Ctr 1985; **Fellow:** Surgical Critical Care, Maimonides Med Ctr 1986; **Fac Appt:** Asst Clin Prof S, SUNY Downstate

Alfonso, Antonio E MD (S) - **Spec Exp:** Breast Cancer; Head & Neck Surgery; Thyroid Cancer; **Hospital:** Long Island Coll Hosp (page 94), SUNY Downstate Med Ctr (page 405); **Address:** Long Island Coll Hosp, 339 Hicks St, Brooklyn, NY 11201; **Phone:** 718-875-3244; **Board Cert:** Surgery 1973; **Med School:** Philippines 1968; **Resid:** Surgery, Temple Univ Hosp 1972; **Fellow:** Surgical Oncology, Meml Sloan Kettering Cancer Ctr 1974; **Fac Appt:** Prof S, SUNY Downstate

Bernstein, Michael O MD (S) - **Spec Exp:** Hernia; Biliary Surgery; Breast Disease; **Hospital:** Long Island Coll Hosp (page 94); **Address:** 350 Henry St, Brooklyn, NY 11201; **Phone:** 718-780-1563; **Board Cert:** Surgery 2007; Surgical Critical Care 1998; **Med School:** Penn State Univ-Hershey Med Ctr 1983; **Resid:** Surgery, SUNY-Kings Co Hosp 1988; **Fac Appt:** Asst Prof S, SUNY Downstate

Borgen, Patrick I MD (S) - **Spec Exp:** Breast Cancer; Breast Cancer & Surgery; **Hospital:** Maimonides Med Ctr (page 98); **Address:** Maimonides Breast Ctr, 6300 8th Ave, Brooklyn, NY 11220; **Phone:** 718-765-2570; **Board Cert:** Surgery 2002; **Med School:** Louisiana State U, New Orleans 1984; **Resid:** Surgery, Ochsner Fdn Hosp 1989; **Fellow:** Surgical Oncology, Meml Sloan Kettering Canc Ctr 1990; **Fac Appt:** Prof S, Cornell Univ-Weill Med Coll

Borriello, Raffaele MD (S) - **Spec Exp:** Breast Surgery; Hernia; Gastrointestinal Surgery; **Hospital:** Long Island Coll Hosp (page 94), New York Methodist Hosp (page 404); **Address:** 100 Clinton St, Ste 2, Brooklyn, NY 11201; **Phone:** 718-625-0767; **Board Cert:** Surgery 2005; Surgical Critical Care 1999; **Med School:** SUNY Downstate 1981; **Resid:** Surgery, Kings Co Hosp 1986; **Fac Appt:** Assoc Prof S, SUNY Downstate

Chiariello, Mario MD (S) - **Spec Exp:** Cancer Surgery; **Hospital:** New York Methodist Hosp (page 404), Victory Memorial Hosp - Bklyn; **Address:** 1479 73rd St, Brooklyn, NY 11228-2111; **Phone:** 718-331-4938; **Board Cert:** Surgery 1998; **Med School:** Italy 1978; **Resid:** Surgery, Brooklyn Cumberland Hosp 1984

Dresner, Lisa S MD (S) - **Spec Exp:** Trauma; Critical Care; Breast Surgery; **Hospital:** SUNY Downstate Med Ctr (page 405), Kings County Hosp Ctr; **Address:** SUNY HSC, Dept Surg, 450 Clarkson Ave, Box 40, Brooklyn, NY 11203-2056; **Phone:** 718-270-1421; **Board Cert:** Surgery 2001; Surgical Critical Care 2003; **Med School:** SUNY Downstate 1985; **Resid:** Surgery, Kings Co Hosp Ctr 1992; **Fellow:** Surgical Critical Care, Jackson Meml Hosp 1993; **Fac Appt:** Assoc Prof S, SUNY Downstate

Fahoum, Bashar MD (S) - **Spec Exp:** Laparoscopic Surgery; Critical Care; Trauma; **Hospital:** New York Methodist Hosp (page 404); **Address:** 506 6th St, Brooklyn, NY 11215-3609; **Phone:** 718-780-3288; **Board Cert:** Surgery 2003; Surgical Critical Care 2004; **Med School:** Syria 1987; **Resid:** Surgery, New York Methodist Hosp 1993; **Fellow:** Surgical Critical Care, New York Med Coll 2003; **Fac Appt:** Asst Prof S, Cornell Univ-Weill Med Coll

Fogler, Richard MD (S) - **Spec Exp:** Breast Surgery; Colon & Rectal Surgery; Gastrointestinal Surgery; **Hospital:** Brookdale Univ Hosp Med Ctr; **Address:** 1 Brookdale Plz, Rm 122, Brooklyn, NY 11212-3139; **Phone:** 718-240-5437; **Board Cert:** Surgery 1975; **Med School:** NY Med Coll 1968; **Resid:** Surgery, Brookdale Hosp 1973; **Fac Appt:** Clin Prof S, SUNY Hlth Sci Ctr

Genato, Romulo MD (S) - **Spec Exp:** Breast Surgery; Laparoscopic Surgery; Hernia; **Hospital:** Brooklyn Hosp Ctr-Downtown; **Address:** Brooklyn Hospital Ctr, Dept Surgery, 121 Dekalb Ave, Brooklyn, NY 11201-5425; **Phone:** 718-250-8970; **Board Cert:** Surgery 1999; **Med School:** Philippines 1972; **Resid:** Surgery, Brooklyn Hosp 1979; **Fac Appt:** Asst Clin Prof S, Cornell Univ-Weill Med Coll

Gorecki, Piotr J MD (S) - **Spec Exp:** Laparoscopic Surgery; Obesity/Bariatric Surgery; Gastrointestinal Surgery; Minimally Invasive Surgery; **Hospital:** New York Methodist Hosp (page 404); **Address:** NY Methodist Hospital, Dept Surgery, 506 Sixth St, Brooklyn, NY 11215; **Phone:** 718-246-8600; **Board Cert:** Surgery 2009; **Med School:** Poland 1991; **Resid:** Surgery, NY Methodist Hosp 1998; **Fellow:** Laparoscopic Surgery, Mayo Clinic 1999; **Fac Appt:** Asst Prof S, Cornell Univ-Weill Med Coll

Hong, Joon Ho MD (S) - **Spec Exp:** Vascular Surgery; **Hospital:** SUNY Downstate Med Ctr (page 405); **Address:** SUNY Downstate Med Ctr, 450 Clarkson Ave, Box 40, Brooklyn, NY 11203; **Phone:** 718-270-1898; **Board Cert:** Surgery 2009; **Med School:** South Korea 1967; **Resid:** Surgery, Downstate Med Ctr 1979; **Fac Appt:** Prof S, SUNY Downstate

Lewis, Theophilus MD (S) - **Spec Exp:** Breast Cancer & Surgery; **Hospital:** SUNY Downstate Med Ctr (page 405); **Address:** 450 Clarkson Ave, Box 40, Brooklyn, NY 11203-0040; **Phone:** 718-270-2155; **Board Cert:** Surgery 2003; **Med School:** SUNY Downstate 1978; **Resid:** Surgery, Kings Co Hosp 1983

Lois, William A MD (S) - **Spec Exp:** Dialysis Access Surgery; Vascular Surgery; **Hospital:** Kingsbrook Jewish Med Ctr; **Address:** 5723 Avenue N, Brooklyn, NY 11234-4026; **Phone:** 718-251-1111; **Board Cert:** Surgery 1999; **Med School:** Spain 1982; **Resid:** Surgery, Interfaith Med Ctr 1987

Lutchman, Gordon MD (S) - **Spec Exp:** Wound Healing/Care; Vein Disorders; Laser Surgery; **Hospital:** Coney Island Hosp, Maimonides Med Ctr (page 98); **Address:** Dept of Surgery, 2601 Ocean Pkwy, rm 7N33, Brooklyn, NY 11235; **Phone:** 718-616-3440; **Board Cert:** Surgery 2007; **Med School:** Jamaica 1976; **Resid:** Surgery, Royal United Hosp 1982; Surgery, Maimonides Med Ctr 1987; **Fellow:** Vascular Surgery, Maimonides Med Ctr 1988

Rajpal, Sanjeev MD (S) - **Spec Exp:** Cancer Surgery; Laparoscopic Surgery; Breast Surgery; **Hospital:** Beth Israel Med Ctr- Kings Hwy Div (page 94), Brookdale Univ Hosp Med Ctr; **Address:** 9413 Flatlands Ave, Ste 203E, Brooklyn, NY 11236-5233; **Phone:** 718-251-1212; **Board Cert:** Surgery 2002; **Med School:** India 1975; **Resid:** Surgery, Brookdale Hosp Med Ctr 1980; **Fellow:** Surgical Oncology, Roswell Park Meml Inst 1982; Laparoscopic Surgery, Yale Univ 2001; **Fac Appt:** Asst Prof S, SUNY Downstate

Rao, Addagada MD (S) - **Spec Exp:** Laparoscopic Abdominal Surgery; Breast Surgery; Pancreatic Surgery; Transfusion Free Surgery; **Hospital:** Wyckoff Heights Med Ctr; **Address:** 145 Saint Nicholas Ave, Brooklyn, NY 11237-4439; **Phone:** 718-418-5900; **Board Cert:** Surgery 1974; **Med School:** India 1965; **Resid:** Surgery, Wyckoff Heights Hosp 1972; **Fac Appt:** Asst Clin Prof S, Cornell Univ-Weill Med Coll

Schwartzman, Alexander MD (S) - **Spec Exp:** Breast Cancer; Colon Surgery; Laparoscopic Surgery; Hernia; **Hospital:** SUNY Downstate Med Ctr (page 405); **Address:** 450 Clarkson Ave, Box 40, Brooklyn, NY 11203; **Phone:** 718-270-1791; **Board Cert:** Surgery 1998; **Med School:** Dominican Republic 1983; **Resid:** Surgery, Brooklyn Hosp 1988

Steiner, Henry MD (S) - **Spec Exp:** Breast Surgery; **Hospital:** Maimonides Med Ctr (page 98), Peninsula Hosp Ctr; **Address:** 8105 Bay Pkwy, Brooklyn, NY 11214; **Phone:** 718-331-7314; **Board Cert:** Surgery 2001; **Med School:** SUNY Downstate 1976; **Resid:** Surgery, Maimonides Med Ctr 1980; **Fellow:** Vascular Surgery, Maimonides Med Ctr 1981

Tanchajja, Supoj MD (S) - **Hospital:** Long Island Coll Hosp (page 94); **Address:** 239 82nd St, Brooklyn, NY 11209-3810; **Phone:** 718-748-4603; **Board Cert:** Surgery 2000; **Med School:** Thailand 1972; **Resid:** Surgery, NY Methodist hosp 1977; Surgery, Long Island Coll Hosp 1980

Wright, Albert M MD (S) - **Spec Exp:** Breast Disease; Colon & Rectal Surgery; Thyroid Surgery; **Hospital:** Interfaith Med Ctr - St John's Episcopal Hosp, New York Methodist Hosp (page 404); **Address:** 1 Plaza St, Ste 1B, Brooklyn, NY 11217; **Phone:** 718-638-1971; **Board Cert:** Surgery 1999; **Med School:** England, UK 1970; **Resid:** Surgery, Mt Sinai Hosp 1977; **Fac Appt:** Asst Clin Prof S, Cornell Univ-Weill Med Coll

Zenilman, Michael MD (S) - **Spec Exp:** Pancreatic Surgery; Gastrointestinal Surgery; Laparoscopic Surgery; **Hospital:** SUNY Downstate Med Ctr (page 405), Long Island Coll Hosp (page 94); **Address:** SUNY Downstate Med Ctr, 450 Clarkson Ave, Box 40, Brooklyn, NY 11203-2056; **Phone:** 718-270-1421; **Board Cert:** Surgery 2003; **Med School:** SUNY Downstate 1984; **Resid:** Surgery, Barnes Jewish Hosp 1991; **Fac Appt:** Prof S, SUNY Downstate

Thoracic Surgery

Abrol, Sunil MD (TS) - **Spec Exp:** Cardiac Surgery; Aneurysm-Thoracic Aortic; Heart Valve Surgery; Aortic Surgery; **Hospital:** Maimonides Med Ctr (page 98), Jamaica Hosp Med Ctr; **Address:** Maimonides Med Ctr, Cardiothoracic Surg, 4802 10th Ave, Administration Bldg Fl 4, Brooklyn, NY 11219; **Phone:** 718-283-7686; **Board Cert:** Surgery 1999; Thoracic Surgery 2002; **Med School:** India 1986; **Resid:** Surgery, Maimonides Med Ctr 1998; **Fellow:** Thoracic Surgery, SUNY Hlth Sci Ctr 2001; **Fac Appt:** Asst Prof S, Mount Sinai Sch Med

Burack, Joshua H MD (TS) - **Spec Exp:** Cardiothoracic Surgery; **Hospital:** SUNY Downstate Med Ctr (page 405), Kings County Hosp Ctr; **Address:** SUNY Downstate, Dept Cardiothor Surg, 450 Clarkson Ave, Box 40, Brooklyn, NY 11203; **Phone:** 718-270-1981; **Board Cert:** Surgery 1999; Thoracic Surgery 2009; **Med School:** Albert Einstein Coll Med 1982; **Resid:** Surgery, Montefiore Med Ctr 1987; **Fellow:** Cardiothoracic Surgery, Univ Hosp 1989; **Fac Appt:** Assoc Prof S, SUNY Downstate

Lazzaro, Richard MD (TS) - **Spec Exp:** Minimally Invasive Surgery; Obesity/Bariatric Surgery; Cardiac Surgery; **Hospital:** New York Methodist Hosp (page 404); **Address:** New York Methodist Hospital, 506 Sixth St, Brooklyn, NY 11215; **Phone:** 718-780-7700; **Board Cert:** Surgery 2006; Thoracic Surgery 2007; **Med School:** Albany Med Coll 1988; **Resid:** Surgery, North Shore Univ Hosp 1994; **Fellow:** Cardiothoracic Surgery, SUNY Downstate Med Ctr 1997; Thoracic Surgery, Univ Pittsburgh Med Ctr 1998; **Fac Appt:** Assoc Prof S, SUNY Downstate

Okadigwe, Chukuma MD (TS) - **Spec Exp:** Lung Cancer; Thoracic Surgery; Minimally Invasive Surgery; **Hospital:** New York Methodist Hosp (page 404), Brookdale Univ Hosp Med Ctr; **Address:** 191 Ocean Ave, Brooklyn, NY 11225-4701; **Phone:** 718-287-0505; **Board Cert:** Surgery 1975; **Med School:** Univ Colorado 1968; **Resid:** Surgery, Kings County Hosp 1974; Thoracic Surgery, Univ Hosp-SUNY Downstate 1976; **Fac Appt:** Asst Prof S, SUNY Downstate

Tortolani, Anthony J MD (TS) - **Spec Exp:** Transfusion Free Surgery; Heart Valve Surgery; Coronary Artery Surgery; **Hospital:** New York Methodist Hosp (page 404), NY-Presby Hosp/Weill Cornell (page 104); **Address:** New York Methodist Hosp, Dept Surgery, 506 6th St Fl 6, Brooklyn, NY 11215; **Phone:** 718-780-5990; **Board Cert:** Surgery 1975; Thoracic Surgery 1999; **Med School:** Geo Wash Univ 1969; **Resid:** Surgery, N Shore Univ Hosp 1974; **Fellow:** Cardiothoracic Surgery, NYU Med Ctr 1978; **Fac Appt:** Assoc Prof S, Cornell Univ-Weill Med Coll

Urology

Friedman, Steven C MD (U) - **Spec Exp:** Pediatric Urology; Urinary Tract Infections; Robotic Urologic Surgery; Urinary Reconstruction; **Hospital:** Maimonides Med Ctr (page 98), Steven & Alexandra Cohen Chldn's Med Ctr of NY; **Address:** 909 49th St, Brooklyn, NY 11219; **Phone:** 718-283-7743; **Board Cert:** Urology 2000; **Med School:** SUNY Downstate 1983; **Resid:** Surgery, Beth Israel 1985; Urology, Maimonides Med Ctr 1988; **Fellow:** Pediatric Urology, Chldns Hosp 1991

Grunberger, Ivan MD (U) - **Spec Exp:** Prostate Cancer; Impotence; Minimally Invasive Surgery; Kidney Stones; **Hospital:** New York Methodist Hosp (page 404), Long Island Coll Hosp (page 94); **Address:** One Prospect Park West, Ste C, Brooklyn, NY 11215; **Phone:** 718-230-7788; **Board Cert:** Urology 2007; **Med School:** NYU Sch Med 1980; **Resid:** Surgery, N Shore Univ Hosp 1982; Urology, NYU Med Ctr 1986; **Fac Appt:** Assoc Clin Prof U, SUNY Downstate

Horowitz, Mark MD (U) - **Spec Exp:** Pediatric Urology; **Hospital:** SUNY Downstate Med Ctr (page 405), Staten Island Univ Hosp - North; **Address:** 450 Clarkson Ave, Box 79, Brooklyn, NY 11203; **Phone:** 718-270-1958; **Board Cert:** Urology 2006; **Med School:** NY Med Coll 1986; **Resid:** Urology, SUNY Downstate Med Ctr 1992; **Fellow:** Pediatric Urology, Chldns Hosp & Med Ctr 1994

Irwin, Mark MD (U) - **Spec Exp:** Prostate Disease; Erectile Dysfunction; Kidney Stones; **Hospital:** Long Island Coll Hosp (page 94); **Address:** LI Coll Hosp, Dept Urology, 339 Hicks St Fl 7, Brooklyn, NY 11201; **Phone:** 718-780-1520; **Board Cert:** Urology 1999; **Med School:** Med Coll Wisc 1982; **Resid:** Surgery, Kings County Hosp 1985; Urology, Kings County Hosp 1988; **Fac Appt:** Assoc Clin Prof U, SUNY Downstate

Kim, Hong MD (U) - **Hospital:** Brookdale Univ Hosp Med Ctr; **Address:** Brookdale Hospital, 1 Brookdale Plaza, Ste 5C4, Brooklyn, NY 11212; **Phone:** 718-240-5323; **Board Cert:** Urology 1976; **Med School:** South Korea 1965; **Resid:** Surgery, Brookdale Hosp 1971; Urology, Univ Nebraska Med Ctr 1974; **Fac Appt:** Assoc Clin Prof U, SUNY Downstate

Lindsay, Gaius K MD (U) - **Hospital:** Maimonides Med Ctr (page 98), Coney Island Hosp; **Address:** 3121 Ocean Ave, Sheeps Head Bay, NY 11235; **Phone:** 718-283-7741; **Board Cert:** Urology 1976; **Med School:** India 1967; **Resid:** Surgery, NY Methodist Hosp 1970; Urology, Maimonides Med Ctr 1973; **Fac Appt:** Asst Clin Prof U, SUNY Downstate

Meisenberg, Gene MD (U) - **Spec Exp:** Prostate Disease; Kidney Stones; Impotence; **Hospital:** NY-Presby Hosp/Weill Cornell (page 104), Long Island Coll Hosp (page 94); **Address:** 1523 Voorhies Ave, Brooklyn, NY 11235; **Phone:** 718-743-2200; **Board Cert:** Urology 2001; **Med School:** Russia 1981; **Resid:** Surgery, Beth Israel Hosp 1993; Urology, RW Johnson Univ Hosp 1997

Rosenthal, Sheldon MD (U) - **Spec Exp:** Kidney Stones; Prostate Disease; **Hospital:** Wyckoff Heights Med Ctr, St John's Queens Hosp; **Address:** 359 Stockholm St, Brooklyn, NY 11237; **Phone:** 718-821-3200; **Board Cert:** Urology 1977; **Med School:** Ros Franklin Univ/Chicago Med Sch 1967; **Resid:** Surgery, Albert Einstein 1970; Urology, NY Med Coll 1973

Saada, Simon MD (U) - **Spec Exp:** Kidney Stones; Prostate Cancer; Kidney Cancer; **Hospital:** Richmond Univ Med Ctr, NY-Presby Hosp/Columbia (page 104); **Address:** 705 86th St, Ste M2, Brooklyn, NY 11228-3219; **Phone:** 718-238-1075; **Board Cert:** Urology 1981; **Med School:** Egypt 1970; **Resid:** Surgery, LI Coll Med Ctr 1974; Urology, Charleston Area Med Ctr 1977

Shabsigh, Ridwan MD (U) - **Spec Exp:** Erectile Dysfunction; Hypogonadism; Clinical Trials; **Hospital:** Maimonides Med Ctr (page 98), NY-Presby Hosp/Columbia (page 104); **Address:** 3121 Ocean Ave, Brooklyn, NY 11235; **Phone:** 718-283-7746; **Board Cert:** Urology 2000; **Med School:** Syria 1976; **Resid:** Urology, Seepark Hosp 1983; Urology, Baylor Affil Hsop 1990; **Fellow:** Urology, Baylor Affil Hosp 1987; **Fac Appt:** Clin Prof U, Columbia P&S

Silver, David A MD (U) - **Spec Exp:** Laparoscopic Surgery; Urologic Cancer; Robotic Surgery; Continent Urinary Diversions; **Hospital:** Maimonides Med Ctr (page 98), Lutheran Med Ctr - Brooklyn; **Address:** 6323 7th Ave, Brooklyn, NY 11220; **Phone:** 718-283-7153; **Board Cert:** Urology 2007; **Med School:** Albert Einstein Coll Med 1989; **Resid:** Surgery, Maimonides Med Ctr 1995; **Fellow:** Urology, Meml Sloan-Kettering Canc Ctr 1997

Wainstein, Sasha MD (U) - **Spec Exp:** Impotence; Voiding Dysfunction; Endourology; **Hospital:** Maimonides Med Ctr (page 98); **Address:** 4711 12th Ave, Brooklyn, NY 11219-2500; **Phone:** 718-436-3900; **Board Cert:** Urology 1977; **Med School:** Colombia 1969; **Resid:** Urology, Maimonides Medical Ctr 1975

Vascular & Interventional Radiology

Sclafani, Salvatore MD (VIR) - **Spec Exp:** Uterine Fibroid Embolization; Vascular Malformations; Varicocele Embolization; **Hospital:** SUNY Downstate Med Ctr (page 405), Kings County Hosp Ctr; **Address:** 451 Clarkson Ave, Box S2N50, S Bldg Fl 2, Brooklyn, NY 11206; **Phone:** 718-245-4447; **Board Cert:** Diagnostic Radiology 1976; Vascular & Interventional Radiology 2009; **Med School:** SUNY Upstate Med Univ 1972; **Resid:** Diagnostic Radiology, Univ Hosp-SUNY 1976; **Fac Appt:** Prof Rad, SUNY Downstate

Vascular Surgery

Ascher, Enrico MD (VascS) - **Spec Exp:** Endovascular Surgery; Carotid Artery Surgery; Limb Sparing Surgery; Aneurysm; **Hospital:** Maimonides Med Ctr (page 98), Mount Sinai Med Ctr (page 102); **Address:** 903 49th St, Brooklyn, NY 11219; **Phone:** 718-283-7957; **Board Cert:** Vascular Surgery 2004; **Med School:** Brazil 1974; **Resid:** Surgery, NY Med Coll 1981; **Fellow:** Vascular Surgery, Montefiore Med Ctr 1982; **Fac Appt:** Prof S, SUNY Downstate

D'Ayala, Marcus D MD (VascS) - **Spec Exp:** Endovascular Surgery; Aneurysm-Abdominal Aortic; **Hospital:** New York Methodist Hosp (page 404); **Address:** NY Methodist Hospital, Dept Surgery, 506 Sixth St, Brooklyn, NY 11215; **Phone:** 718-780-3288; **Board Cert:** Surgery 2008; Vascular Surgery 2000; **Med School:** Univ Wisc 1992; **Resid:** Surgery, Montefiore Med Ctr 1997; **Fellow:** Vascular Surgery, Mt Sinai Med Ctr 1998; **Fac Appt:** Asst Prof S, Mount Sinai Sch Med

Flores, Lucio MD (VascS) - **Hospital:** Brookdale Univ Hosp Med Ctr; **Address:** 2035 Ralph Ave, Ste B5, Brooklyn, NY 11234; **Phone:** 718-209-1400; **Board Cert:** Surgery 2007; Vascular Surgery 2008; **Med School:** Peru 1968; **Resid:** Surgery, Jewish Hosp Med Ctr 1975

Weiser, Robert MD (VascS) - **Spec Exp:** Lower Limb Arterial Disease; Carotid Artery Surgery; Lower Limb Ulcers; **Hospital:** Long Island Coll Hosp (page 94), New York Methodist Hosp (page 404); **Address:** 186 Joralemon St Fl 7, Brooklyn, NY 11201-4326; **Phone:** 718-797-1101; **Board Cert:** Surgery 2005; **Med School:** Albert Einstein Coll Med 1977; **Resid:** Surgery, Montefiore Med Ctr 1982; **Fellow:** Vascular Surgery, Montefiore Med Ctr 1983

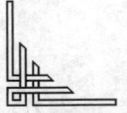
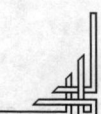

The Best in American Medicine
www.CastleConnolly.com

Queens

Queens

Allergy & Immunology

Bernstein, Larry J MD (A&I) - **Spec Exp:** Asthma; Immune Deficiency; Sinus Disorders; Food Allergy; **Hospital:** Montefiore Med Ctr - Div. Moses (page 100), NY Hosp Queens; **Address:** 72-35 112th St, Ste PR-5, Forest Hills, NY 11375; **Phone:** 718-544-6641; **Board Cert:** Pediatrics 1981; Allergy & Immunology 1985; **Med School:** Albert Einstein Coll Med 1977; **Resid:** Pediatrics, Jacobi Med Ctr 1981; **Fellow:** Allergy & Immunology, Albert Einstein Coll Med 1983; **Fac Appt:** Assoc Clin Prof Ped, Albert Einstein Coll Med

Fine, Stanley MD (A&I) - **Spec Exp:** Asthma; Drug Sensitivity; Latex Allergy; **Hospital:** NY Hosp Queens, Flushing Hosp Med Ctr; **Address:** 37-31 149th St, Flushing, NY 11354-4841; **Phone:** 718-358-5565; **Board Cert:** Internal Medicine 1964; Allergy & Immunology 1972; **Med School:** Columbia P&S 1957; **Resid:** Internal Medicine, Jacobi Med Ctr 1959; Internal Medicine, Montefiore Hosp Med Ctr 1962; **Fellow:** Allergy & Immunology, St Luke's-Roosevelt Hosp Ctr 1963; **Fac Appt:** Asst Clin Prof Med, Cornell Univ-Weill Med Coll

Menchell, David L MD (A&I) - **Spec Exp:** Asthma; Nasal & Sinus Disorders; **Hospital:** NY Hosp Queens; **Address:** 73-03 198th St, Fresh Meadows, NY 11366-1818; **Phone:** 718-465-4100; **Board Cert:** Internal Medicine 1980; Allergy & Immunology 1983; **Med School:** NYU Sch Med 1977; **Resid:** Internal Medicine, NY Hosp Med Ctr 1980; **Fellow:** Allergy & Immunology, NY Hosp Med Ctr 1983

Cardiovascular Disease

Akinboboye, Olakunle MD (Cv) - **Spec Exp:** Diabetes & Heart Disease; Nuclear Stress Testing; Hypertension; Coronary Artery Disease; **Address:** Laurelton Heart Specialists, 243-36 Merrick Blvd, Rosedale, NY 11413; **Phone:** 718-949-9400; **Board Cert:** Internal Medicine 2005; Cardiovascular Disease 2005; Nuclear Cardiology 1996; **Med School:** Nigeria 1984; **Resid:** Internal Medicine, Nassau County Med Ctr 1991; **Fellow:** Cardiovascular Disease, Columbia Presby Med Ctr 1995; Nuclear Cardiology, Columbia Presby Med Ctr 1994; **Fac Appt:** Assoc Prof Med, SUNY Stony Brook

Kirtane, Sanjay MD (Cv) - **Spec Exp:** Coronary Artery Disease; Arrhythmias; Heart Failure; Nuclear Cardiology; **Hospital:** St John's Epis Hosp - S Shore, Peninsula Hosp Ctr; **Address:** 114-12 Beach Channel Drive, Ste 7, Rockaway Park, NY 11694; **Phone:** 718-318-1021; **Board Cert:** Internal Medicine 1980; Cardiovascular Disease 1983; Nuclear Cardiology 2009; **Med School:** India 1974; **Resid:** Internal Medicine, St John's Episcopal Hosp 1980; **Fellow:** Cardiovascular Disease, LI Jewish Med Ctr/St John's Episcopal Hosp 1982

Qadir, Shuja MD (Cv) *PCP* - **Spec Exp:** Heart Failure; Arrhythmias; Coronary Artery Disease; **Hospital:** NY Hosp Queens, N Shore Univ Hosp; **Address:** 85-04 67th Rd, Rego Park, NY 11374; **Phone:** 718-275-6061; **Board Cert:** Internal Medicine 1984; Cardiovascular Disease 1987; **Med School:** Pakistan 1977; **Resid:** Internal Medicine, Catholic Med Ctr 1985; **Fellow:** Cardiovascular Disease, Catholic Med Ctr 1987; **Fac Appt:** Asst Prof Med, NY Med Coll

Robbins, Michael MD (Cv) - **Spec Exp:** Echocardiography; Non-Invasive Cardiology; **Hospital:** Mount Sinai Med Ctr (page 102); **Address:** 94-36 58th Ave, Ste G4, Rego Park, NY 11373-5149; **Phone:** 718-760-0011; **Board Cert:** Internal Medicine 1984; Cardiovascular Disease 1987; **Med School:** Cornell Univ-Weill Med Coll 1981; **Resid:** Internal Medicine, Bronx Muni Hosp Ctr/Albert Einstein 1985; **Fellow:** Cardiovascular Disease, Mt Sinai Hosp 1987; **Fac Appt:** Assoc Prof Med, Mount Sinai Sch Med

Rydzinski, Mayer MD (Cv) - **Spec Exp:** Echocardiography; **Hospital:** NY Hosp Queens, Forest Hills Hosp; **Address:** 70-31 108th St, Ste 7, Forest Hills, NY 11375-4450; **Phone:** 718-268-7633; **Board Cert:** Internal Medicine 1979; Cardiovascular Disease 1981; Echocardiography 2008; **Med School:** Albert Einstein Coll Med 1976; **Resid:** Internal Medicine, Metropolitan Hosp Ctr 1977; Internal Medicine, Montefiore Hosp Med Ctr 1979; **Fellow:** Cardiovascular Disease, LI Jewish Hosp 1981

Siskind, Steven J MD (Cv) - **Spec Exp:** Angina; Heart Failure; Arrhythmias; **Hospital:** NY Hosp Queens, Lenox Hill Hosp; **Address:** 142-42 Booth Memorial Ave, Flushing, NY 11355; **Phone:** 718-353-4004; **Board Cert:** Internal Medicine 1979; Cardiovascular Disease 1981; **Med School:** Albert Einstein Coll Med 1976; **Resid:** Internal Medicine, Jacobi Med Ctr 1979; **Fellow:** Cardiovascular Disease, Albert Einstein 1981; **Fac Appt:** Asst Prof, Cornell Univ-Weill Med Coll

Child & Adolescent Psychiatry

Fornari, Victor MD (ChAP) - **Spec Exp:** Eating Disorders; Trauma Psychiatry; Post Traumatic Stress Disorder; **Hospital:** Zucker Hillside Hosp; **Address:** Zucker Hillside Hospital, Ambulatory Care Pavilion Lower Level, 75-59 263rd St, Glen Oaks, NY 11004; **Phone:** 718-470-3510; **Board Cert:** Psychiatry 1984; Child & Adolescent Psychiatry 1985; **Med School:** SUNY Downstate 1979; **Resid:** Psychiatry, Hosp Univ Penn 1982; **Fellow:** Child & Adolescent Psychiatry, LIJ Med Ctr 1984; **Fac Appt:** Prof Psyc, NYU Sch Med

Kafantaris, Vivian P MD (ChAP) - **Spec Exp:** Bipolar/Mood Disorders; ADD/ADHD; Aggression Disorders; Clinical Trials; **Hospital:** Zucker Hillside Hosp; **Address:** The Zucker Hillside Hospital, Psychiatry Rsch, 75-59 263rd St, Glen Oaks, NY 11004; **Phone:** 718-470-8556; **Board Cert:** Psychiatry 1989; Child & Adolescent Psychiatry 1990; Addiction Psychiatry 2007; **Med School:** Albert Einstein Coll Med 1983; **Resid:** Psychiatry, Albert Einstein Coll Med 1987; **Fellow:** Child & Adolescent Psychiatry, NYU/Bellevue Hosp Ctr 1989; Psychopharmacology, Dr Magda Campbell 1989; **Fac Appt:** Assoc Prof Psyc, Albert Einstein Coll Med

Colon & Rectal Surgery

Tiszenkel, Howard I MD (CRS) - **Spec Exp:** Colon Cancer; **Hospital:** NY Hosp Queens; **Address:** 56-45 Main St Fl 2 - rm WLL300, Flushing, NY 11355-5000; **Phone:** 718-445-0220; **Board Cert:** Surgery 2006; Colon & Rectal Surgery 1988; **Med School:** NY Med Coll 1981; **Resid:** Surgery, St Luke's Hosp 1986; Colon & Rectal Surgery, Carle Clinic 1987

Critical Care Medicine

Efferen, Linda S MD (CCM) - **Spec Exp:** Sarcoidosis; Tuberculosis; **Hospital:** Long Island Jewish Med Ctr, N Shore Univ Hosp; **Address:** 270-05 76th Ave, rm B205, New Hyde Park, NY 11040; **Phone:** 718-470-7717; **Board Cert:** Internal Medicine 1988; Pulmonary Disease 2001; Critical Care Medicine 2001; **Med School:** Israel 1983; **Resid:** Internal Medicine, Kings Co Hosp 1987; **Fellow:** Pulmonary Disease, Albert Einstein 1989; Critical Care Medicine, Albert Einstein 1990; **Fac Appt:** Assoc Clin Prof Med, Albert Einstein Coll Med

Nierman, David M MD (CCM) - **Spec Exp:** Critical Illness-Prolonged; Respiratory Failure; Sepsis; **Hospital:** Mount Sinai Hosp of Queens (page 102), Mount Sinai Med Ctr (page 102); **Address:** 25-10 30th Ave, Astoria, NY 11102; **Phone:** 718-267-4293; **Board Cert:** Internal Medicine 1984; Pulmonary Disease 1988; Critical Care Medicine 2002; **Med School:** Israel 1981; **Resid:** Internal Medicine, LIJ-Hillside Med Ctr 1984; Emergency Medicine, LIJ-Hillside Med Ctr 1986; **Fellow:** Pulmonary Disease, St Lukes-Roosevelt Hosp 1988; **Fac Appt:** Assoc Prof Med, Mount Sinai Sch Med

Dermatology

Beyda, Bernadette A MD (D) - **Hospital:** NY Hosp Queens; **Address:** 141-23 59th Ave, Flushing, NY 11355-5304; **Phone:** 718-445-0566; **Board Cert:** Dermatology 1982; **Med School:** France 1976; **Resid:** Pathology, Booth Meml Med Ctr 1979; Dermatology, NY Hosp 1982

Gladstein, Michael J MD (D) - **Hospital:** Mount Sinai Hosp of Queens (page 102); **Address:** 3062 36th Street, Astoria, NY 11103-4798; **Phone:** 718-728-8979; **Board Cert:** Dermatology 1987; **Med School:** NYU Sch Med 1979; **Resid:** Dermatology, NYU Med Ctr 1985

Pereira, Frederick A MD (D) - **Spec Exp:** Skin Cancer; Geriatric Dermatology; **Hospital:** NY Hosp Queens, Mount Sinai Med Ctr (page 102); **Address:** 51-14 Kissena Blvd, Flushing, NY 11355-4163; **Phone:** 718-359-4425; **Board Cert:** Dermatology 2009; **Med School:** UMDNJ-NJ Med Sch, Newark 1968; **Resid:** Dermatology, Mt Sinai Hosp 1974; Dermatology, Metro Hosp 1975

Diagnostic Radiology

Mollin, Joel MD (DR) - **Spec Exp:** Ultrasound; CT Scan; **Hospital:** Elmhurst Hosp Ctr; **Address:** 79-01 Broadway, E1-18, Radiology, Elmhurst, NY 11373; **Phone:** 718-334-2052; **Board Cert:** Diagnostic Radiology 1985; Psychiatry 1976; **Med School:** SUNY Downstate 1969; **Resid:** Diagnostic Radiology, USPHS Hosp-Staten Island 1981; Diagnostic Radiology, Mt Sinai Hosp 1983; **Fac Appt:** Asst Clin Prof, Mount Sinai Sch Med

Novick, Mark D MD (DR) - **Spec Exp:** Breast Imaging; Mammography; MRI; **Hospital:** St Charles Hosp, Good Samaritan Hosp Med Ctr - West Islip; **Address:** Dynamic Med Imaging, 7336 Grand Ave, Maspeth, NY 11378; **Phone:** 212-744-8000; **Board Cert:** Diagnostic Radiology 1983; **Med School:** Univ Tenn Coll Med, Memphis 1978; **Resid:** Diagnostic Radiology, Univ Tenn Med Ctr 1982; **Fellow:** Magnetic Resonance Imaging, UCSF Med Ctr

Sprecher, Stanley MD (DR) - **Hospital:** Peninsula Hosp Ctr; **Address:** Peninsula Radiology Assocs, 51-15 Beach Channel Drive, Far Rockaway, NY 11691-1042; **Phone:** 718-734-2616; **Board Cert:** Diagnostic Radiology 1982; Nuclear Radiology 1983; **Med School:** Albert Einstein Coll Med 1977; **Resid:** Diagnostic Radiology, Univ Hosp 1979; Nuclear Medicine, St Vincent's Hosp & Med Ctr 1980

Tartell, Jay D MD (DR) - **Hospital:** Mount Sinai Hosp of Queens (page 102); **Address:** Advanced Radiological Imaging, 89-40 56th Ave, Elmhurst, NY 11373-4943; **Phone:** 718-335-5532; **Board Cert:** Diagnostic Radiology 1987; **Med School:** NY Med Coll 1982; **Resid:** Diagnostic Radiology, Bronx Muni Hosp 1986; **Fellow:** Ultrasound/CT/MRI, North Shore Univ Hosp 1987

Youner, Craig J MD (DR) - **Hospital:** Mount Sinai Hosp of Queens (page 102); **Address:** Advanced Radiological Imaging, 29-16 Astoria Blvd, Astoria, NY 11102-1742; **Phone:** 718-204-5800; **Board Cert:** Diagnostic Radiology 1978; **Med School:** Albany Med Coll 1973; **Resid:** Internal Medicine, N Shore Univ Hosp 1975; Diagnostic Radiology, N Shore Univ Hosp 1978; **Fac Appt:** Asst Clin Prof Rad, Cornell Univ-Weill Med Coll

Endocrinology, Diabetes & Metabolism

Kukar, Narinder MD (EDM) - **Spec Exp:** Diabetes; Thyroid Disorders; Osteoporosis; **Hospital:** Wyckoff Heights Med Ctr, Jamaica Hosp Med Ctr; **Address:** 374 Stockholm St, Brooklyn, NY 11237; **Phone:** 718-963-7586; **Board Cert:** Internal Medicine 1977; Endocrinology, Diabetes & Metabolism 1981; **Med School:** India 1960; **Resid:** Internal Medicine, Wycoff Heights Hosp 1969; **Fellow:** Endocrinology, Diabetes & Metabolism, SUNY Downstate Med Ctr 1971; **Fac Appt:** Asst Prof Med, SUNY Hlth Sci Ctr

Lorber, Daniel MD (EDM) - **Spec Exp:** Diabetes; **Hospital:** NY Hosp Queens, Flushing Hosp Med Ctr; **Address:** 59-45 161st St, Flushing, NY 11365-1414; **Phone:** 718-762-3111; **Board Cert:** Internal Medicine 1987; Endocrinology, Diabetes & Metabolism 1977; **Med School:** Albert Einstein Coll Med 1972; **Resid:** Internal Medicine, Jacobi Med Ctr 1975; **Fellow:** Endocrinology, Diabetes & Metabolism, Vanderbilt Univ Hosp 1977; **Fac Appt:** Assoc Clin Prof Med, Cornell Univ-Weill Med Coll

Resta, Christine MD (EDM) - **Spec Exp:** Diabetes; Thyroid Disorders; Osteoporosis; **Hospital:** NY Hosp Queens, Flushing Hosp Med Ctr; **Address:** 59-45 161st St, Flushing, NY 11365; **Phone:** 718-762-3111; **Board Cert:** Internal Medicine 2002; Endocrinology, Diabetes & Metabolism 2005; **Med School:** Albert Einstein Coll Med 1989; **Resid:** Internal Medicine, Montefiore Med Ctr 1992; **Fellow:** Endocrinology, Diabetes & Metabolism, Montefiore Med Ctr 1995; **Fac Appt:** Asst Clin Prof Med, Albert Einstein Coll Med

Rosman, Lawrence D MD (EDM) - **Spec Exp:** Thyroid Disorders; Osteoporosis; Diabetes; Pituitary Disorders; **Hospital:** NY Hosp Queens, NYU Langone Med Ctr (page 106); **Address:** 112-03 Queens Blvd, Ste 207, Forest Hills, NY 11375-5550; **Phone:** 718-263-3718; **Board Cert:** Internal Medicine 1978; Endocrinology 1983; **Med School:** NYU Sch Med 1975; **Resid:** Internal Medicine, NYU Med Ctr 1978; **Fellow:** Endocrinology, Diabetes & Metabolism, NYU Med Ctr 1980; **Fac Appt:** Asst Clin Prof Med, NYU Sch Med

Tibaldi, Joseph M MD (EDM) - **Spec Exp:** Diabetes; Thyroid Disorders; Geriatric Endocrinology; **Hospital:** Flushing Hosp Med Ctr, NY Hosp Queens; **Address:** 59-45 161st St, Flushing, NY 11365-1414; **Phone:** 718-762-3111; **Board Cert:** Internal Medicine 1982; Endocrinology, Diabetes & Metabolism 1985; **Med School:** Mount Sinai Sch Med 1979; **Resid:** Internal Medicine, Mt Sinai Hosp 1982; **Fellow:** Endocrinology, Montefiore Hosp Med Ctr 1984; **Fac Appt:** Asst Clin Prof Med, Albert Einstein Coll Med

Family Medicine

Fisher, George C MD (FMed) *PCP* - **Spec Exp:** Preventive Medicine; Hypertension; Cholesterol/Lipid Disorders; Diabetes; **Hospital:** Mount Sinai Hosp of Queens (page 102), Mount Sinai Med Ctr (page 102); **Address:** 22-33 33rd St, Astoria, NY 11105; **Phone:** 718-726-1000; **Board Cert:** Family Medicine 2008; **Med School:** England, UK 1979; **Resid:** Family Medicine, St Joseph Med Ctr 1993

Istrico, Richard A DO (FMed) *PCP* - **Spec Exp:** Sports Injuries; Nutrition; Preventive Medicine; **Hospital:** Long Island Jewish Med Ctr; **Address:** 158-01 Crossbay Blvd, Jamaica, NY 11414-3137; **Phone:** 718-738-9115; **Board Cert:** Family Medicine 1981; **Med School:** Philadelphia Coll Osteo Med 1978; **Resid:** Family Medicine, Interboro Hosp 1979; Sports Medicine, Baptist Med Ctr 1980

Molnar, Thomas G MD (FMed) *PCP* - **Spec Exp:** Hypertension; Diabetes; **Hospital:** NY Hosp Queens, Flushing Hosp Med Ctr; **Address:** 83-39 Daniels St, Jamaica, NY 11435-1208; **Phone:** 718-291-5151; **Board Cert:** Family Medicine 2007; **Med School:** Hungary 1982; **Resid:** Surgery, Flushing Hosp 1985; Family Medicine, Univ Hosp 1988

Muraca, Glenn DO (FMed) *PCP* - **Spec Exp:** Sports Medicine; Nutrition; **Hospital:** Flushing Hosp Med Ctr, St John's Queens Hosp; **Address:** 104-01 Corona Ave, Corona, NY 11368; **Phone:** 718-271-2020; **Board Cert:** Family Medicine 1994; **Med School:** NY Coll Osteo Med 1990; **Resid:** Family Medicine, Peninsula Hosp 1994

Reddy, Mallikarjuna D MD (FMed) *PCP* - **Spec Exp:** Geriatric Care; **Hospital:** NY Hosp Queens; **Address:** 72-18 164th St, Flushing, NY 11365-4222; **Phone:** 718-969-6640; **Board Cert:** Family Medicine 2009; **Med School:** India 1982; **Resid:** Family Medicine, Catholic Med Ctr 1990

Roth, Alan R DO (FMed) *PCP* - **Spec Exp:** Palliative Care; Diabetes; Hypertension; **Hospital:** Jamaica Hosp Med Ctr, Flushing Hosp Med Ctr; **Address:** 11940 Metropolitan Ave, Kew Gardens, NY 11415; **Phone:** 718-849-0624; **Board Cert:** Family Medicine 2009; Hospice & Palliative Medicine 2008; **Med School:** NY Coll Osteo Med 1986; **Resid:** Family Medicine, Jamaica Hosp Med Ctr 1989; **Fac Appt:** Asst Clin Prof FMed, Albert Einstein Coll Med

Gastroenterology

Esposito, Stephen P MD (Ge) - **Hospital:** NY Hosp Queens, NY-Presby Hosp/Columbia (page 104); **Address:** 26-19 Francis Lewis Blvd, Bayside, NY 11358; **Phone:** 718-224-7186; **Board Cert:** Internal Medicine 1989; Gastroenterology 2002; **Med School:** SUNY Upstate Med Univ 1986; **Resid:** Internal Medicine, LI Jewish Hosp 1989; **Fellow:** Gastroenterology, Booth Meml Hosp 1991

Harooni, Robert MD (Ge) - **Spec Exp:** Colonoscopy; Peptic Ulcer Disease; Capsule Endoscopy; **Hospital:** NY Hosp Queens; **Address:** 55-16 Main St, Lower Level, Flushing, NY 11355; **Phone:** 718-461-6161; **Board Cert:** Internal Medicine 1981; Gastroenterology 1985; **Med School:** Iran 1973; **Resid:** Internal Medicine, Booth Meml Hosp 1982; **Fellow:** Gastroenterology, Booth Meml Hosp 1984; **Fac Appt:** Med, Cornell Univ-Weill Med Coll

Nussbaum, Michel E MD (Ge) - **Spec Exp:** Endoscopy & Colonoscopy; Colon Cancer Screening; Inflammatory Bowel Disease; Peptic Ulcer Disease; **Hospital:** NY Hosp Queens, Flushing Hosp Med Ctr; **Address:** 142-43 Booth Memorial Ave, Flushing, NY 11355-5343; **Phone:** 718-886-1919; **Board Cert:** Internal Medicine 1981; Gastroenterology 1983; **Med School:** Belgium 1977; **Resid:** Internal Medicine, NY Hosp Queens 1980; **Fellow:** Gastroenterology, NY Hosp Queens 1982; **Fac Appt:** Assoc Clin Prof Med, Cornell Univ-Weill Med Coll

Ramgopal, Mekala MD (Ge) - **Spec Exp:** Peptic Acid Disorders; Inflammatory Bowel Disease; Colon & Rectal Cancer Detection; Hepatitis; **Hospital:** St John's Epis Hosp - S Shore, Peninsula Hosp Ctr; **Address:** 21-24 Camp Rd, Far Rockaway, NY 11691; **Phone:** 718-327-0207; **Board Cert:** Internal Medicine 1978; Gastroenterology 1979; **Med School:** India 1974; **Resid:** Internal Medicine, Jersey City Med Ctr 1976; Internal Medicine, VA Med Ctr 1977; **Fellow:** Gastroenterology, Univ of Med/Dentistry 1979

Rand, James A MD (Ge) - **Spec Exp:** Colonoscopy; Endoscopy; **Hospital:** NY Hosp Queens; **Address:** 200-12 44th Ave, Bayside, NY 11361; **Phone:** 718-224-7454; **Board Cert:** Internal Medicine 1978; Gastroenterology 1981; **Med School:** Albert Einstein Coll Med 1975; **Resid:** Internal Medicine, Strong Meml Hosp 1977; Internal Medicine, Columbia-Presby 1978; **Fellow:** Gastroenterology, Montefiore Hosp Med Ctr 1980

Vogelman, Arthur MD (Ge) - **Spec Exp:** Colon Cancer; Peptic Ulcer Disease; Gastroe-sophageal Reflux Disease (GERD); **Hospital:** Forest Hills Hosp, NY Hosp Queens; **Address:** 7146 110th St, Forest Hills, NY 11375-4842; **Phone:** 718-261-2500; **Board Cert:** Internal Medicine 1979; Gastroenterology 1981; **Med School:** Univ Pittsburgh 1975; **Resid:** Internal Medicine, Mt Sinai Hosp 1978; **Fellow:** Gastroenterology, Mt Sinai Hosp 1980

Weg, Arnold MD (Ge) - **Spec Exp:** Endoscopy; Inflammatory Bowel Disease/Crohn's; **Hospital:** NY-Presby Hosp/Weill Cornell (page 104); **Address:** 71-36 110th St, Ste 1G, Forest Hills, NY 11375-4836; **Phone:** 718-520-2210; **Board Cert:** Internal Medicine 1985; Gastroenterology 1987; **Med School:** NYU Sch Med 1982; **Resid:** Internal Medicine, Columbia-Presby 1985; **Fellow:** Gastroenterology, NY Hosp 1986

Geriatric Medicine

Brody, Samuel MD (Ger) - **Spec Exp:** Frail Elderly; **Hospital:** Forest Hills Hosp; **Address:** 69-15 Yellowstone Blvd, Forest Hills, NY 11375; **Phone:** 718-268-4500; **Board Cert:** Internal Medicine 1980; Gastroenterology 1983; Geriatric Medicine 2008; **Med School:** Vanderbilt Univ 1977; **Resid:** Internal Medicine, Vanderbilt Med Ctr 1980; **Fellow:** Gastroenterology, Temple Univ Hosp 1982

Geriatric Psychiatry

Greenwald, Blaine MD (GerPsy) - **Spec Exp:** Depression; Dementia; **Hospital:** Zucker Hillside Hosp, N Shore Univ Hosp; **Address:** Zudker Hillside Hospital, Ambulatory Care Pavilion, 75-59 263rd St, rm 2102, Glen Oaks, NY 11004; **Phone:** 718-470-8159; **Board Cert:** Psychiatry 1983; Geriatric Psychiatry 2000; **Med School:** NY Med Coll 1978; **Resid:** Psychiatry, Mt Sinai Hosp 1982; **Fellow:** Geriatric Psychiatry, Mt Sinai Hosp/Bronx VA Hosp 1983; **Fac Appt:** Assoc Prof Psyc, Albert Einstein Coll Med

Gynecologic Oncology

Welshinger, Marie MD (GO) - **Spec Exp:** Gynecologic Cancer; **Hospital:** NY Hosp Queens; **Address:** 56-45 Main St, West Wing, lower level, rm 100, Fresh Meadows, NY 11355; **Phone:** 718-670-1170; **Board Cert:** Obstetrics & Gynecology 2009; Gynecologic Oncology 2009; **Med School:** Univ Minn 1988; **Resid:** Obstetrics & Gynecology, SUNY Stony Brook Hosp 1992; **Fellow:** Gynecologic Oncology, Meml Sloan Kett Cancer Ctr 1996

Infectious Disease

Masci, Joseph MD (Inf) - **Spec Exp:** AIDS/HIV; Tropical Diseases; Disaster Preparedness; **Hospital:** Elmhurst Hosp Ctr; **Address:** Elmhurst Hosp, Dept Med, 79-01 Broadway, rm C 6-10, Elmhurst, NY 11373; **Phone:** 718-334-3446; **Board Cert:** Internal Medicine 1979; Infectious Disease 1982; **Med School:** NYU Sch Med 1976; **Resid:** Internal Medicine, Boston City Hosp 1979; **Fellow:** Infectious Disease, Mt Sinai Hosp 1982; **Fac Appt:** Prof Med, Mount Sinai Sch Med

Segal-Maurer, Sorana MD (Inf) - **Spec Exp:** AIDS/HIV; **Hospital:** NY Hosp Queens; **Address:** 56-45 Main St, Infectious Disease Section, Flushing, NY 11355-5000; **Phone:** 718-670-1525; **Board Cert:** Internal Medicine 2000; Infectious Disease 2000; **Med School:** Mount Sinai Sch Med 1988; **Resid:** Internal Medicine, Bronx Muni Hosp Ctr 1991; **Fellow:** Infectious Disease, Montefiore Med Ctr 1993

Internal Medicine

Amin, Mahendra MD (IM) *PCP* - **Hospital:** NY Hosp Queens, Long Island Jewish Med Ctr; **Address:** 89-02 Springfield Blvd, Queens Village, NY 11427-2514; **Phone:** 718-776-4444; **Board Cert:** Internal Medicine 1984; **Med School:** India 1978; **Resid:** Internal Medicine, Metro Hosp Ctr 1982; **Fellow:** Internal Medicine, Metro Hosp Ctr 1985

Beyda, Allan E MD (IM) *PCP* - **Spec Exp:** Preventive Medicine; Cholesterol/Lipid Disorders; **Hospital:** NY Hosp Queens; **Address:** 141-23 59th Ave, Flushing, NY 11355-5304; **Phone:** 718-359-7406; **Board Cert:** Internal Medicine 1979; **Med School:** France 1976; **Resid:** Internal Medicine, New York Hosp Med Ctr 1979

Blum, Daniel N MD (IM) *PCP* - **Spec Exp:** Geriatric Care; Hypertension; Diabetes; **Hospital:** NY Hosp Queens; **Address:** 13806 Jewel Ave, Flushing, NY 11367-1933; **Phone:** 718-520-0248; **Board Cert:** Internal Medicine 1984; **Med School:** Albert Einstein Coll Med 1980; **Resid:** Internal Medicine, NY Hosp of Queens 1984

Brewer, Marlon E MD (IM) *PCP* - **Spec Exp:** Diabetes; Hypertension; **Hospital:** Elmhurst Hosp Ctr; **Address:** 79-01 Broadway, rm A116, Elmhurst, NY 11373; **Phone:** 718-334-2920; **Board Cert:** Internal Medicine 2004; **Med School:** Spain 1986; **Resid:** Internal Medicine, Elmhurst Hosp 1992; **Fac Appt:** Asst Clin Prof Med, Mount Sinai Sch Med

Fukilman, Oscar J MD (IM) *PCP* - **Spec Exp:** Preventive Medicine; **Hospital:** Mount Sinai Hosp of Queens (page 102); **Address:** 25-31 30th Road, Ste 1A, Astoria, NY 11102; **Phone:** 718-267-1102; **Board Cert:** Internal Medicine 1979; **Med School:** Argentina 1968; **Resid:** Internal Medicine, Elmhurst Hosp/Mt Sinai Hosp Svc 1972

Joseph, John L MD (IM) *PCP* - **Spec Exp:** Rheumatology; Osteoporosis; Arthritis; **Hospital:** Forest Hills Hosp, NY Hosp Queens; **Address:** 66-20 108th St, Forest Hills, NY 11375; **Phone:** 718-896-8920; **Board Cert:** Internal Medicine 1983; **Med School:** Mexico 1977; **Resid:** Internal Medicine, Coney Island Hosp 1982; **Fellow:** Rheumatology, Long Island Coll Hosp 1984

Messana, Ida MD (IM) *PCP* - **Hospital:** Long Island Jewish Med Ctr, N Shore Univ Hosp; **Address:** 109-33 71st Rd, Ste 2E, Forest Hills, NY 11375; **Phone:** 718-263-4345; **Board Cert:** Internal Medicine 1988; **Med School:** SUNY Stony Brook 1984; **Resid:** Internal Medicine, Montefiore Med Ctr 1987; **Fellow:** Geriatric Medicine, Montefiore Med Ctr 1989

Pasquale, Jack MD (IM) - **Spec Exp:** Nutrition in Cancer Treatment; **Hospital:** NY Hosp Queens, Jamaica Hosp Med Ctr; **Address:** 176-60 Union Tpke, Ste 360, Fresh Meadows, NY 11366; **Phone:** 718-460-2300; **Board Cert:** Internal Medicine 1987; **Med School:** Grenada 1981; **Resid:** Internal Medicine, Millard Fillmore Hosp 1984; **Fellow:** Nutrition, Hosp Univ Penn 1985

Reilly, Thomas MD (IM) *PCP* - **Hospital:** NY Hosp Queens; **Address:** 86-27 Forest Pkwy, Woodhaven, NY 11421-1143; **Phone:** 718-805-2404; **Board Cert:** Internal Medicine 1984; **Med School:** SUNY Hlth Sci Ctr 1979; **Resid:** Internal Medicine, Staten Island Hosp 1982; **Fellow:** Hematology, St Vincent's Hosp & Med Ctr 1985

Somogyi, Anthony MD (IM) *PCP* - **Hospital:** NY Hosp Queens; **Address:** 42-23 Francis Lewis Blvd, Ste 201, Bayside, NY 11361; **Phone:** 718-224-5687; **Board Cert:** Internal Medicine 1979; **Med School:** Belgium 1976; **Resid:** Internal Medicine, NY Hosp Queens 1980

Interventional Cardiology

Papadakos, Stylianos P MD (IC) - **Spec Exp:** Cardiac Catheterization; Percutaneous My-ocardial Revasc (PMR); **Hospital:** Lenox Hill Hosp, NY Hosp Queens; **Address:** CV Assocs NY & Bayside, 44-01 Francis Lewis Blvd, Level 3, Bayside, NY 11361; **Phone:** 718-423-3355; **Board Cert:** Cardiovascular Disease 2004; Interventional Cardiology 1999; **Med School:** Greece 1985; **Resid:** Internal Medicine, Booth Meml Med Ctr 1989; Internal Medicine, Mt Sinai Hosp 1990; **Fellow:** Cardiovascular Disease, Univ Conn Hosp 1994; **Fac Appt:** Asst Clin Prof Med, Cornell Univ-Weill Med Coll

Maternal & Fetal Medicine

Inglis, Steven MD (MF) - **Spec Exp:** Pregnancy-High Risk; Obstetric Ultrasound; Prenatal Diagnosis; **Hospital:** Jamaica Hosp Med Ctr; **Address:** Jamaica Hospital, Dept OB/GYN, 89-06 135th St, Ste 6A, Jamaica, NY 11418; **Phone:** 718-206-7642; **Board Cert:** Obstetrics & Gynecology 2009; Maternal & Fetal Medicine 2009; **Med School:** NY Med Coll 1986; **Resid:** Obstetrics & Gynecology, Albany Med Ctr 1990; **Fellow:** Maternal & Fetal Medicine, New York Hosp 1992; **Fac Appt:** Assoc Prof ObG, Cornell Univ-Weill Med Coll

Skupski, Daniel MD (MF) - **Spec Exp:** Fetal Therapy; Multiple Gestation; **Hospital:** NY Hosp Queens, NY-Presby Hosp/Weill Cornell (page 104); **Address:** 56-45 Main St, Flushing, NY 11355-5060; **Phone:** 718-670-1534; **Board Cert:** Obstetrics & Gynecology 2009; Maternal & Fetal Medicine 2009; **Med School:** Univ Mich Med Sch 1985; **Resid:** Obstetrics & Gynecology, Hurley Med Ctr 1989; **Fellow:** Maternal & Fetal Medicine, NY Hosp Cornell Med Ctr 1994; **Fac Appt:** Assoc Prof ObG, Cornell Univ-Weill Med Coll

Medical Oncology

Abramowitz, Avram L MD (Onc) - **Spec Exp:** Bone Marrow Transplant; **Hospital:** Mount Sinai Hosp of Queens (page 102), Long Island Jewish Med Ctr; **Address:** 176-60 Union Tpke, Ste 360, Fresh Meadows, NY 11366; **Phone:** 718-460-2300; **Board Cert:** Internal Medicine 1987; Hematology 2004; Medical Oncology 2004; **Med School:** NY Med Coll 1984; **Resid:** Internal Medicine, Roosevelt Hosp 1987; **Fellow:** Hematology & Oncology, Roosevelt Hosp 1989; Bone Marrow Transplant, Mount Sinai Med Ctr 1993

Benisovich, Vladimir I MD (Onc) - **Spec Exp:** Breast Cancer; Lung Cancer; Colon Cancer; **Hospital:** Elmhurst Hosp Ctr, Mount Sinai Med Ctr (page 102); **Address:** 79-01 Broadway, Ste H2-04, Elmhurst, NY 11373-1329; **Phone:** 718-334-3723; **Board Cert:** Internal Medicine 1982; Hematology 1984; Medical Oncology 1985; **Med School:** Russia 1966; **Resid:** Internal Medicine, Bronx Lebanon Med Ctr 1980; **Fellow:** Hematology, NYU Med Ctr 1982; Medical Oncology, Mt Sinai Med Ctr 1983

Cortes, Engracio P MD (Onc) - **Spec Exp:** Breast Cancer; Gastrointestinal Cancer; Lung Cancer; Lymphoma; **Hospital:** NY Hosp Queens, Long Island Jewish Med Ctr; **Address:** 200-20 44th Ave, Bayside, NY 11361; **Phone:** 718-279-9101; **Board Cert:** Internal Medicine 1976; Medical Oncology 1977; **Med School:** Philippines 1964; **Resid:** Internal Medicine, Lemuel Shattuck Hosp 1968; **Fellow:** Medical Oncology, Roswell Park Cancer Inst 1971; **Fac Appt:** Assoc Clin Prof Med, Cornell Univ-Weill Med Coll

Daly, Jane E MD (Onc) - **Hospital:** NY Hosp Queens; **Address:** 87-23 Myrtle Ave, Glendale, NY 11385-7431; **Phone:** 718-441-5581; **Board Cert:** Internal Medicine 1978; Hematology 1980; Medical Oncology 1981; **Med School:** NY Med Coll 1975; **Resid:** Internal Medicine, Kings County Hosp 1978; **Fellow:** Hematology, LI Jewish Med Ctr 1980; Medical Oncology, Albert Einstein 1981

Greenberg, Howard J MD (Onc) - **Spec Exp:** Breast Cancer; Colon Cancer; Lymphoma; Co-agulation/Bleeding Disorders; **Hospital:** Mount Sinai Hosp of Queens (page 102), Mount Sinai Med Ctr (page 102); **Address:** 2710 Astoria Blvd, Astoria, NY 11102; **Phone:** 718-278-3569; **Board Cert:** Internal Medicine 1976; Hematology 1978; Medical Oncology 1979; **Med School:** SUNY Downstate 1973; **Resid:** Internal Medicine, Mt Sinai Hosp 1976; **Fellow:** Hematology, Mt Sinai Hosp 1978; Medical Oncology, Meml Sloan Kettering Cancer Ctr 1979; **Fac Appt:** Asst Clin Prof Med, Mount Sinai Sch Med

Shum, Kee Y MD (Onc) - **Spec Exp:** Breast Cancer; Lung Cancer; Colon Cancer; **Hospital:** NY Hosp Queens, Flushing Hosp Med Ctr; **Address:** 136-25 Maple Ave, Ste 205, Flushing, NY 11355-3891; **Phone:** 718-463-2245; **Board Cert:** Internal Medicine 1984; Medical Oncology 1987; **Med School:** Cornell Univ-Weill Med Coll 1981; **Resid:** Internal Medicine, Kings County Hosp 1985; **Fellow:** Medical Oncology, Meml Sloan Kettering Cancer Ctr 1987

Neonatal-Perinatal Medicine

Hand, Ivan L MD (NP) - **Spec Exp:** Respiratory Distress Syndrome; Prematurity/Low Birth Weight Infants; Neonatal Infections; Breast Feeding Problems; **Hospital:** Queens Hosp Ctr - Jamaica, Elmhurst Hosp Ctr; **Address:** 82-68 164 St, Neonatal Intensive Care Unit, Jamaica, NY 11432; **Phone:** 718-883-4517; **Board Cert:** Pediatrics 1986; Neonatal-Perinatal Medicine 2004; **Med School:** Mount Sinai Sch Med 1982; **Resid:** Pediatrics, Montefiore Med Ctr 1985; Pediatrics, Bronx Lebanon Hosp 1986; **Fellow:** Neonatal-Perinatal Medicine, NY Hosp-Cornell Univ 1988; **Fac Appt:** Assoc Prof Ped, Mount Sinai Sch Med

Nephrology

Galler, Marilyn MD (Nep) - **Spec Exp:** Hypertension; Kidney Disease; **Hospital:** NY Hosp Queens, Montefiore Med Ctr - Div. Weiler (page 100); **Address:** 56-45 Main St, rm M201, Flushing, NY 11355; **Phone:** 718-670-1151; **Board Cert:** Internal Medicine 1979; Nephrology 1984; **Med School:** NYU Sch Med 1975; **Resid:** Internal Medicine, Bronx Municipal Hosp 1979; **Fellow:** Nephrology, Montefiore Med Ctr 1981; **Fac Appt:** Asst Clin Prof Med, Cornell Univ-Weill Med Coll

Kostadaras, Ari MD (Nep) - **Spec Exp:** Hypertension; Dialysis Care; Kidney Stones; **Hospital:** Mount Sinai Hosp of Queens (page 102), NY Hosp Queens; **Address:** 23-18 31st St, Astoria, NY 11105; **Phone:** 718-721-4440; **Board Cert:** Nephrology 1998; **Med School:** Grenada 1989; **Resid:** Internal Medicine, LaGuardia Hosp 1992; **Fellow:** Nephrology, Nassau County Med Ctr 1994

Mattoo, Nirmal K MD (Nep) - **Spec Exp:** Kidney Failure; Hypertension; Dialysis Care; **Hospital:** Wyckoff Heights Med Ctr, Forest Hills Hosp; **Address:** 385 Seneca Ave, Ridgewood, NY 11385; **Phone:** 347-312-3041; **Board Cert:** Internal Medicine 1974; Nephrology 1978; **Med School:** India 1967; **Resid:** Internal Medicine, Queens Hosp Ctr 1971; Internal Medicine, Catholic Med Ctr 1972; **Fellow:** Nephrology, Elmhurst Hosp Ctr 1975

Scott III, David MD (Nep) - **Spec Exp:** Hypertension; Kidney Disease; Diabetes; **Hospital:** NY Hosp Queens; **Address:** 134-35 Springfield Blvd, Springfield Gardens, NY 11413; **Phone:** 718-276-4750; **Board Cert:** Internal Medicine 2003; Nephrology 2005; **Med School:** Tufts Univ 1985; **Resid:** Internal Medicine, Harlem Hosp 1988; **Fellow:** Nephrology, Harlem Hosp 1990

Spinowitz, Bruce S MD (Nep) - **Spec Exp:** Kidney Disease-Diabetic; Hypertension; Kidney Stones; **Hospital:** NY Hosp Queens, Montefiore Med Ctr - Div. Weiler (page 100); **Address:** 56-45 Main St, rm M201, Flushing, NY 11355-5045; **Phone:** 718-670-1151; **Board Cert:** Internal Medicine 1976; Nephrology 1978; **Med School:** NYU Sch Med 1973; **Resid:** Internal Medicine, Bellevue Hosp 1976; **Fellow:** Nephrology, Bellevue Hosp 1978; **Fac Appt:** Assoc Clin Prof Med, Cornell Univ-Weill Med Coll

Neurology

Appelbaum, Jeffrey C DO (N) - **Spec Exp:** Multiple Sclerosis; Peripheral Neuropathy; **Hospital:** NY Hosp Queens, Long Island Jewish Med Ctr; **Address:** 59-07 175 Pl, Flushing, NY 11365; **Phone:** 718-939-0800; **Board Cert:** Neurology 1982; **Med School:** Philadelphia Coll Osteo Med 1977; **Resid:** Neurology, Downstate Med Ctr 1981; **Fac Appt:** Assoc Prof N, NY Coll Osteo Med

Casson, Ira MD (N) - **Spec Exp:** Sports Neurology; Headache; Head Injury; **Hospital:** Long Island Jewish Med Ctr; **Address:** 112-03 Queens Blvd, Forest Hills, NY 11375-5550; **Phone:** 718-544-6633; **Board Cert:** Neurology 1980; **Med School:** NYU Sch Med 1975; **Resid:** Neurology, NYU Med Ctr 1979; **Fac Appt:** Asst Prof N, Albert Einstein Coll Med

Obstetrics & Gynecology

Benedicto, Milagros A MD (ObG) - **Hospital:** Wyckoff Heights Med Ctr; **Address:** 68-52 Fresh Pond Rd, Ridgewood, NY 11385; **Phone:** 718-381-7016; **Board Cert:** Obstetrics & Gynecology 2009; **Med School:** Philippines 1964; **Resid:** Obstetrics & Gynecology, Wyckoff Heights Hosp 1969; **Fellow:** Obstetrics & Gynecology, Wyckoff Heights Hosp 1971

Olanescu, Andrea D MD (ObG) - **Spec Exp:** Laparoscopic Surgery; Uterine Fibroids; Pelvic Organ Prolapse Repair; **Hospital:** Mount Sinai Hosp of Queens (page 102), Flushing Hosp Med Ctr; **Address:** 23-22 30th Rd, Ste 1F, Astoria, NY 11102; **Phone:** 718-278-0888; **Board Cert:** Internal Medicine 2001; Obstetrics & Gynecology 2007; **Med School:** Romania 1992; **Resid:** Obstetrics & Gynecology, Jersey City Med Ctr 2002

Ophthalmology

Aharon, Raphael MD (Oph) - **Hospital:** Montefiore Med Ctr - Div. Moses (page 100), NY Hosp Queens; **Address:** 108-37 71st Ave, Forest Hills, NY 11375-4566; **Phone:** 718-268-6120; **Board Cert:** Ophthalmology 1987; **Med School:** Albert Einstein Coll Med 1980; **Resid:** Internal Medicine, Brookdale Hosp 1981; Ophthalmology, Albert Einstein Coll Med 1984; **Fac Appt:** Asst Clin Prof Oph, Albert Einstein Coll Med

Fishman, Allen J MD (Oph) - **Spec Exp:** Cataract Surgery-Lens Implant; LASIK-Refractive Surgery; **Hospital:** Flushing Hosp Med Ctr; **Address:** 92-29 Queens Blvd, Ste 2I, Rego Park, NY 11374; **Phone:** 718-261-7007; **Board Cert:** Ophthalmology 1981; **Med School:** Ros Franklin Univ/Chicago Med Sch 1976; **Resid:** Surgery, Beth Israel Hospital 1977; Ophthalmology, Brookdale Hospital 1980

Grasso, Cono M MD (Oph) - **Spec Exp:** Cataract Surgery; Glaucoma; Oculoplastic Surgery; **Hospital:** Jamaica Hosp Med Ctr, Flushing Hosp Med Ctr; **Address:** 83-05 Grand Ave, Elmhurst, NY 11373-4104; **Phone:** 718-429-0300; **Board Cert:** Ophthalmology 1979; **Med School:** NY Med Coll 1974; **Resid:** Ophthalmology, Wills Eye 1978; **Fac Appt:** Assoc Prof Oph, NY Med Coll

Mackool, Richard J MD (Oph) - **Spec Exp:** Cataract Surgery; LASIK-Refractive Surgery; Lens Implants-Multifocal; Corneal Disease & Surgery; **Hospital:** New York Eye & Ear Infirm (page 113), NYU Langone Med Ctr (page 106); **Address:** 31-27 41st St, Astoria, NY 11103; **Phone:** 718-728-3400; **Board Cert:** Ophthalmology 1975; **Med School:** Boston Univ 1968; **Resid:** Ophthalmology, New York EE Infirm 1973; **Fac Appt:** Clin Prof Oph, NYU Sch Med

Seidenfeld, Andrew MD (Oph) - **Spec Exp:** Cataract Surgery; **Hospital:** New York Eye & Ear Infirm (page 113), Wyckoff Heights Med Ctr; **Address:** 73-09 Myrtle Ave, Glendale, NY 11385-7431; **Phone:** 718-456-9500; **Board Cert:** Ophthalmology 1982; **Med School:** Ros Franklin Univ/Chicago Med Sch 1976; **Resid:** Ophthalmology, NY EE Infirmary 1980

Orthopaedic Surgery

Besser, Walter A MD (OrS) - **Spec Exp:** Joint Replacement; Fractures; **Hospital:** Mount Sinai Hosp of Queens (page 102), NY Hosp Queens; **Address:** 30-71 29th St, Astoria, NY 11102; **Phone:** 718-204-7752; **Board Cert:** Orthopaedic Surgery 1977; **Med School:** Spain 1968; **Resid:** Orthopaedic Surgery, LI Jewish Hosp 1971; Orthopaedic Surgery, Brooklyn Jewish Hosp 1974; **Fellow:** Orthopaedic Surgery, Hosp Special Surg 1977; **Fac Appt:** Asst Clin Prof OrS, NYU Sch Med

Schwartz, Evan MD (OrS) - **Spec Exp:** Sports Medicine; Shoulder Surgery; Knee Surgery; Joint Replacement; **Hospital:** Lenox Hill Hosp; **Address:** 72-41 Grand Ave, Maspeth, NY 11378; **Phone:** 718-558-1975; **Board Cert:** Orthopaedic Surgery 2000; **Med School:** SUNY Buffalo 1981; **Resid:** Orthopaedic Surgery, Montefiore Med Ctr 1986; **Fellow:** Sports Medicine, Hosp Special Surg 1987; **Fac Appt:** Asst Prof OrS, NY Med Coll

Touliopoulos, Steven J MD (OrS) - **Spec Exp:** Sports Medicine; **Hospital:** Mount Sinai Hosp of Queens (page 102); **Address:** 23-18 31st St, Ste 210, Astoria, NY 11105; **Phone:** 718-777-1885; **Board Cert:** Orthopaedic Surgery 2010; Orthopaedic Sports Medicine 2007; **Med School:** SUNY Downstate 1991; **Resid:** Orthopaedic Surgery, SUNY Hlth Sci Ctr 1997; **Fac Appt:** Asst Prof OrS, Mount Sinai Sch Med

Otolaryngology

Huo, Jerry MD (Oto) - **Spec Exp:** Endoscopic Sinus Surgery; Thyroid Surgery; Parotid Surgery; Vocal Cord Disorders; **Hospital:** NY Hosp Queens; **Address:** 136-20 38th Ave, Ste 7J, Flushing, NY 11354; **Phone:** 718-670-0006; **Board Cert:** Otolaryngology 1998; **Med School:** Mount Sinai Sch Med 1991; **Resid:** Surgery, Lenox Hill Hosp 1993; Otolaryngology, Manhattan EE&T Hosp 1997; **Fac Appt:** Asst Clin Prof Oto, Cornell Univ-Weill Med Coll

La Marca, Charles MD (Oto) - **Hospital:** NS-LIJ Hlth Sys; **Address:** 75-06 Eliot Ave, Middle Village, NY 11379-1207; **Phone:** 718-335-2224; **Board Cert:** Otolaryngology 1984; **Med School:** Mexico 1977; **Resid:** Otolaryngology, Downstate Med Ctr 1982

Snyder, Gary M MD (Oto) - **Spec Exp:** Cosmetic Surgery-Face; Endoscopic Sinus Surgery; Voice Disorders; **Hospital:** Flushing Hosp Med Ctr, N Shore Univ Hosp; **Address:** 26-01 Corporal Kennedy St, FL 1, Bayside, NY 11360-2452; **Phone:** 718-423-4091; **Board Cert:** Otolaryngology 1983; **Med School:** NY Med Coll 1979; **Resid:** Surgery, North Shore Univ Hosp 1980; Otolaryngology, Manhattan EET Hosp 1983

Pediatric Cardiology

Rutkovsky, Lisa E MD (PCd) - **Spec Exp:** Congenital Heart Disease; Arrhythmias; **Hospital:** NY Hosp Queens; **Address:** 56-34 Main St, Flushing, NY 11355; **Phone:** 718-670-1945; **Board Cert:** Pediatrics 2007; Pediatric Cardiology 2007; **Med School:** NYU Sch Med 1986; **Resid:** Pediatrics, N Shore Univ Hosp 1989; **Fellow:** Pediatric Cardiology, NYU-Bellevue Hosp 1989; **Fac Appt:** Asst Clin Prof Ped, NYU Sch Med

Pediatric Endocrinology

Speiser, Phyllis W MD (PEn) - **Spec Exp:** Pubertal Disorders; Growth/Development Disorders; Adrenal Disorders; Thyroid Disorders; **Hospital:** Steven & Alexandra Cohen Chldn's Med Ctr of NY, N Shore Univ Hosp; **Address:** Cohen Childrens Med Ctr of NY, Div Ped Endocrinology, 269-01 76th Ave, New Hyde Park, NY 11040-1433; **Phone:** 718-470-3290; **Board Cert:** Pediatrics 1984; Pediatric Endocrinology 2004; **Med School:** Columbia P&S 1979; **Resid:** Pediatrics, Jacobi Med Ctr 1982; **Fellow:** Pediatric Endocrinology, New York Hosp-Cornell 1984; **Fac Appt:** Prof Ped, NYU Sch Med

Pediatrics

Abularrage, Joseph J MD (Ped) *PCP* - **Hospital:** NY Hosp Queens; **Address:** 56-45 Main St, Flushing, NY 11355-5045; **Phone:** 718-670-1033; **Board Cert:** Pediatrics 1981; **Med School:** NYU Sch Med 1975; **Resid:** Pediatrics, NYU-Bellevue Hosp 1979; **Fellow:** Public Health & Genl Preventive Med, Columbia-Presby Med Ctr 1981

Goldstein, Steven J MD (Ped) *PCP* - **Spec Exp:** Nutrition; Asthma; **Hospital:** Long Island Jewish Med Ctr, NY Hosp Queens; **Address:** 141-49 70th Rd, Flushing, NY 11367; **Phone:** 718-268-5282; **Board Cert:** Pediatrics 1983; **Med School:** SUNY Hlth Sci Ctr 1978; **Resid:** Pediatrics, LI Jewish Med Ctr 1981

Yadoo, Moshe MD (Ped) *PCP* - **Hospital:** St Mary's Hosp for Chldn, Long Island Jewish Med Ctr; **Address:** St Mary's Hosp for Children, 29-01 216 St, Bayside, NY 11360; **Phone:** 718-281-8525; **Board Cert:** Pediatrics 1987; **Med School:** SUNY Hlth Sci Ctr 1983; **Resid:** Pediatrics, Brookdale Hosp 1986; **Fellow:** Neonatal-Perinatal Medicine, Schneider Chldns Hosp 1988

Physical Medicine & Rehabilitation

Gasalberti, Richard MD (PMR) - **Spec Exp:** Pain Management; Sports Medicine; Acupuncture; **Hospital:** Forest Hills Hosp, NYU Hosp For Joint Diseases (page 106); **Address:** 111-20 Queens Blvd, Forest Hills, NY 11375-6343; **Phone:** 718-544-7700; **Board Cert:** Physical Medicine & Rehabilitation 2004; **Med School:** West Indies 1984; **Resid:** Physical Medicine & Rehabilitation, Mount Sinai Hosp 1988; Surgery, New York Hosp Med Ctr 1986; **Fellow:** Sports Medicine, Hosp for Joint Diseases 1989

Psychiatry

Brenner, Ronald MD (Psyc) - **Spec Exp:** Depression; Dementia; Panic Disorder; **Hospital:** St John's Epis Hosp - S Shore, Mercy Med Ctr - Rockville Centre; **Address:** 327 Beach 19th St, Far Rockaway, NY 11691; **Phone:** 718-869-7248; **Board Cert:** Psychiatry 1979; Geriatric Psychiatry 2006; **Med School:** Spain 1974; **Resid:** Psychiatry, St Luke's Hosp 1978; **Fellow:** Pharmacology, New York Univ Med Ctr 1979; **Fac Appt:** Clin Prof Psyc, SUNY Hlth Sci Ctr

Kalash, Glenn DO (Psyc) - **Spec Exp:** Psychiatry in Physical Illness; Psychosomatic Disorders; Forensic Psychiatry; Liaison Psychiatry; **Hospital:** Jamaica Hosp Med Ctr, St Francis Hosp - The Heart Ctr (page 115); **Address:** Jamaica Hosp, Dept Psychiatry, 8900 Van Wyck Expressway, Jamaica, NY 11418; **Phone:** 718-206-7167; **Board Cert:** Psychiatry 2008; Forensic Psychiatry 1999; Psychosomatic Medicine 2005; **Med School:** NY Coll Osteo Med 1992; **Resid:** Psychiatry, LIJ Med Ctr 1996; **Fellow:** Liaison Psychiatry, Meml Sloan Kettering Cancer Ctr 1997

Mendelowitz, Alan MD (Psyc) - **Spec Exp:** Schizophrenia; Psychopharmacology; **Hospital:** Zucker Hillside Hosp; **Address:** 75-59 263rd St, rm 208, Glen Oaks, NY 11004; **Phone:** 718-470-8397; **Board Cert:** Psychiatry 1992; **Med School:** UMDNJ-Rutgers Med Sch 1987; **Resid:** Psychiatry, Hillside Hosp-LIJ Med Ctr 1991; **Fac Appt:** Asst Prof Psyc, Albert Einstein Coll Med

Selzer, Jeffrey A MD (Psyc) - **Spec Exp:** Mood Disorders; Depression; **Hospital:** Zucker Hillside Hosp, N Shore Univ Hosp; **Address:** 75-59 263rd St, Glen Oaks, NY 11004-1150; **Phone:** 718-470-8023; **Board Cert:** Psychiatry 1985; Addiction Psychiatry 2003; **Med School:** Univ Mich Med Sch 1979; **Resid:** Psychiatry, UCLA Med Ctr 1983; **Fac Appt:** Assoc Prof Psyc, Albert Einstein Coll Med

Siris, Samuel G MD (Psyc) - **Spec Exp:** Schizophrenia; Depression in Schizophrenia; Panic Disorder in Schizophrenia; **Hospital:** Zucker Hillside Hosp; **Address:** 7559 263rd St, Glen Oaks, NY 11004-1150; **Phone:** 718-470-8138; **Board Cert:** Psychiatry 1976; **Med School:** Columbia P&S 1970; **Resid:** Psychiatry, NY State Psychiatric Inst 1974; **Fellow:** Biological Psychiatry, Nat Inst Mental Hlth 1976; Psychoanalysis, Columbia Univ 1982; **Fac Appt:** Prof Psyc, Albert Einstein Coll Med

Sullivan, Ann Marie MD (Psyc) - **Spec Exp:** Psychotherapy; Psychopharmacology; **Hospital:** Elmhurst Hosp Ctr, Mount Sinai Med Ctr (page 102); **Address:** Elmhurst Hosp, 79-01 Broadway, rm D8, Elmhurst, NY 11369; **Phone:** 718-334-1141; **Board Cert:** Psychiatry 1978; **Med School:** NYU Sch Med 1974; **Resid:** Psychiatry, Bellevue Hosp 1978; **Fac Appt:** Assoc Prof Psyc, Mount Sinai Sch Med

Vivek, Seeth MD (Psyc) - **Spec Exp:** Depression; Panic Disorder; Obsessive-Compulsive Disorder; Liaison Psychiatry; **Hospital:** Jamaica Hosp Med Ctr, Flushing Hosp Med Ctr; **Address:** 75-58 113th St, Ste 1A, Forest Hills, NY 11375-7429; **Phone:** 718-268-9595; **Board Cert:** Psychiatry 1980; Psychosomatic Medicine 2005; **Med School:** India 1972; **Resid:** Psychiatry, Natl Inst Mental Hlth 1976; Psychiatry, Mount Sinai Hosp 1979; **Fellow:** Liaison Psychiatry, Montefiore Hosp 1981; **Fac Appt:** Prof Psyc, NY Coll Osteo Med

Pulmonary Disease

Ankobiah, William MD (Pul) - **Spec Exp:** Chronic Obstructive Lung Disease (COPD); Tuberculosis; Pulmonary Disease; **Hospital:** Franklin Hosp, St John's Epis Hosp - S Shore; **Address:** 253-02 147th Ave, Rosedale, NY 11422-2541; **Phone:** 718-341-3535; **Board Cert:** Internal Medicine 2003; Pulmonary Disease 2002; **Med School:** Ghana 1978; **Resid:** Internal Medicine, Woodhull Med Ctr 1987; **Fellow:** Pulmonary Disease, Univ Hosp 1989; **Fac Appt:** Asst Prof Med, SUNY Downstate

Chadha, Jang B S MD (Pul) - **Spec Exp:** Sleep Disorders; Asthma; Emphysema; Critical Care Medicine; **Hospital:** Flushing Hosp Med Ctr, Forest Hills Hosp; **Address:** 11203 Queens Blvd, Ste 201, Forest Hills, NY 11375; **Phone:** 718-544-6660; **Board Cert:** Internal Medicine 1982; Pulmonary Disease 1984; Critical Care Medicine 2008; Sleep Medicine 2007; **Med School:** India 1976; **Resid:** Internal Medicine, Lincoln Hosp 1982; **Fellow:** Pulmonary Disease, NY Med Coll 1984

Donath, Joseph MD (Pul) - **Spec Exp:** Asthma; Lung Cancer; Critical Care; **Hospital:** NY Hosp Queens, Flushing Hosp Med Ctr; **Address:** 112-41 Queens Blvd, Ste 101A, Forest Hills, NY 11375-5564; **Phone:** 718-380-1553; **Board Cert:** Internal Medicine 1980; Pulmonary Disease 1982; Critical Care Medicine 2009; **Med School:** Hungary 1972; **Resid:** Internal Medicine, VA Med Ctr 1980; **Fellow:** Pulmonary Disease, Mt Sinai Hosp 1982; **Fac Appt:** Asst Clin Prof Med, NY Med Coll

Fleischman, Jean K MD (Pul) - **Hospital:** Queens Hosp Ctr - Jamaica; **Address:** Queens Hosp Ctr, Dept Medicine, 82-68 164th St N Bldg Fl 7, Jamaica, NY 11432-1140; **Phone:** 718-883-4050; **Board Cert:** Internal Medicine 1985; Pulmonary Disease 1988; **Med School:** NYU Sch Med 1982; **Resid:** Internal Medicine, Manhattan VA/NYU Med Ctr 1985; **Fellow:** Pulmonary Disease, NYU Med Ctr 1987; **Fac Appt:** Assoc Clin Prof Med, Mount Sinai Sch Med

Nath, Sunil MD (Pul) - **Spec Exp:** Asthma; Emphysema; Lung Cancer; **Hospital:** NY Hosp Queens; **Address:** 55-14 Main St, Flushing, NY 11355-5044; **Phone:** 718-359-3131; **Board Cert:** Internal Medicine 1980; Pulmonary Disease 1982; **Med School:** India 1976; **Resid:** Internal Medicine, NY Hosp Med Ctr 1980; **Fellow:** Pulmonary Disease, NY Hosp Med Ctr 1982

Silverman, Joel R MD (Pul) - **Spec Exp:** Emphysema; Asthma; Pulmonary Rehabilitation; Sarcoidosis; **Hospital:** Flushing Hosp Med Ctr, N Shore Univ Hosp; **Address:** 111-20 Queens Blvd, Forest Hills, NY 11375-6341; **Phone:** 718-544-4224; **Board Cert:** Internal Medicine 1977; Pulmonary Disease 1980; Critical Care Medicine 2005; **Med School:** Univ Okla Coll Med 1974; **Resid:** Internal Medicine, N Shore Univ Hosp 1977; **Fellow:** Pulmonary Disease, Bellevue Hosp 1979

Radiation Oncology

Dalton, Jack F MD (RadRO) - **Spec Exp:** Brain Tumors; Head & Neck Cancer; Breast Cancer; **Hospital:** Mount Sinai Med Ctr (page 102), Lenox Hill Hosp; **Address:** 106-14 70th Ave, Forest Hills, NY 11375-4253; **Phone:** 718-520-6620; **Board Cert:** Internal Medicine 1974; Hematology 1976; Medical Oncology 1981; Therapeutic Radiology 1983; **Med School:** Univ Pittsburgh 1970; **Resid:** Hematology, Mt Sinai Hosp 1975; Diagnostic Radiology, Mt Sinai Hosp 1981; **Fac Appt:** Asst Clin Prof Med, Mount Sinai Sch Med

Lipsztein, Roberto MD (RadRO) - **Hospital:** Lenox Hill Hosp, Mount Sinai Med Ctr (page 102); **Address:** 106-14 70th Ave, Forest Hills, NY 11375-4253; **Phone:** 718-535-8931; **Board Cert:** Therapeutic Radiology 1982; **Med School:** Brazil 1974; **Resid:** Internal Medicine, Mount Sinai Hosp 1979; **Fellow:** Radiation Oncology, Mount Sinai Hosp 1981

Varsos, George MD (RadRO) - **Spec Exp:** Gynecologic Cancer; Urologic Cancer; **Hospital:** Mount Sinai Hosp of Queens (page 102), Mount Sinai Med Ctr (page 102); **Address:** 23-22 30th Ave, Astoria, NY 11102; **Phone:** 718-267-2763; **Board Cert:** Radiation Oncology 1992; **Med School:** Mount Sinai Sch Med 1985; **Resid:** Surgery, Univ Hosp-SUNY 1987; Radiation Oncology, SUNY Hlth Sci Ctr 1991; **Fellow:** Radiation Oncology, Meml Sloan-Kettering Cancer Ctr 1992; **Fac Appt:** Asst Clin Prof RadRO, Mount Sinai Sch Med

Rheumatology

Sharon, Ezra MD (Rhu) - **Spec Exp:** Rheumatoid Arthritis; Lupus/SLE; Fibromyalgia; Gout; **Hospital:** Mount Sinai Hosp of Queens (page 102), Long Island Jewish Med Ctr; **Address:** 70-31 108 St, Forest Hills, NY 11375; **Phone:** 718-793-6832; **Board Cert:** Internal Medicine 1973; Rheumatology 1974; **Med School:** Israel 1967; **Resid:** Internal Medicine, Mt Sinai Med Ctr 1971; Rheumatology, SUNY Downstate Med Ctr 1973

Sonpal, Girish K M MD (Rhu) - **Spec Exp:** Osteoporosis; Rheumatoid Arthritis; Lupus/SLE; Autoimmune Disease; **Hospital:** NY Hosp Queens, Flushing Hosp Med Ctr; **Address:** 149-65 24th Ave, Flushing, NY 11357-3646; **Phone:** 718-445-0500; **Board Cert:** Internal Medicine 1974; Rheumatology 1976; **Med School:** India 1969; **Resid:** Internal Medicine, Catholic Med Ctr 1974; **Fellow:** Rheumatology, Worcester City Hosp 1975; Rheumatology, Queens Hosp Ctr 1976; **Fac Appt:** Asst Prof Med, Cornell Univ-Weill Med Coll

Surgery

Biviano, Bernard J MD (S) - **Spec Exp:** Critical Care; **Hospital:** Mount Sinai Hosp of Queens (page 102); **Address:** 25-10 30th Ave, Astoria, NY 11102; **Phone:** 718-267-4363; **Board Cert:** Surgery 2006; Surgical Critical Care 2007; **Med School:** UMDNJ-RW Johnson Med Sch 1990; **Resid:** Surgery, Cabrini Med Ctr 1995; **Fellow:** Surgical Critical Care, Metropolitan Hosp 1996; **Fac Appt:** S, Mount Sinai Sch Med

Kemeny, M Margaret MD (S) - **Spec Exp:** Liver Cancer; Pancreatic Cancer; Colon & Rectal Cancer; Cancer Surgery; **Hospital:** Queens Hosp Ctr - Jamaica, N Shore Univ Hosp; **Address:** Queens Cancer Ctr at Queens Hosp, 82-68 164th St, Jamaica, NY 11432-1140; **Phone:** 718-883-4031; **Board Cert:** Surgery 2003; **Med School:** Columbia P&S 1972; **Resid:** Surgery, Columbia-Presby Hosp 1974; Surgery, Univ Colorado Med Ctr 1976; **Fellow:** Surgery, Meml Sloan Kettering Cancer Ctr 1977; Surgical Oncology, National Cancer Inst 1981; **Fac Appt:** Prof S, Mount Sinai Sch Med

Mendoza, Ernesto MD (S) - **Spec Exp:** Parathyroid Surgery; Throat Disorders; Head & Neck Surgery; **Hospital:** New York Methodist Hosp (page 404); **Address:** 40-45 78th St, Elmhurst, NY 11373-1152; **Phone:** 718-397-9058; **Board Cert:** Surgery 2009; **Med School:** Peru 1974; **Resid:** Surgery, Jewish Hosp 1983; **Fellow:** Head and Neck Surgery, Tulane Univ 1985; Surgical Oncology, Roswell Park Meml Inst 1986

Pace, Benjamin W MD (S) - **Spec Exp:** Breast Surgery; Breast Cancer; **Hospital:** Queens Hosp Ctr - Jamaica; **Address:** Queens Hosp, Department of Surgery, 82-68 164th St, rm A-365, Jamaica, NY 11432-1140; **Phone:** 718-883-4640; **Board Cert:** Surgery 2004; **Med School:** Mexico 1977; **Resid:** Surgery, LI Jewish Med Ctr 1983; **Fac Appt:** Assoc Prof S, Mount Sinai Sch Med

Sung, Kap-Jae MD (S) - **Spec Exp:** Breast Cancer; Laparoscopic Surgery; **Hospital:** Forest Hills Hosp, NY Hosp Queens; **Address:** 68-07 Eliot Ave, Middle Village, NY 11379-1130; **Phone:** 718-651-2929; **Board Cert:** Surgery 2005; **Med School:** South Korea 1973; **Resid:** Surgery, Wyckoff Heights Hosp 1986; **Fac Appt:** Asst Prof S, NY Med Coll

Zeitlin, Alan P MD (S) - **Spec Exp:** Vascular Surgery; Breast Cancer; Gastrointestinal Surgery; **Hospital:** Flushing Hosp Med Ctr, Mount Sinai Hosp of Queens (page 102); **Address:** 69-60 108th St, Forest Hills, NY 11375-4323; **Phone:** 718-544-0442; **Board Cert:** Surgery 2002; **Med School:** Univ Miami Sch Med 1974; **Resid:** Surgery, Montefiore Med Ctr 1979; **Fac Appt:** Asst Clin Prof S, Mount Sinai Sch Med

Thoracic Surgery

Graver, L Michael MD (TS) - **Spec Exp:** Heart Valve Surgery-Aortic; Coronary Artery Surgery; Atrial Fibrillation; **Hospital:** Long Island Jewish Med Ctr, N Shore Univ Hosp; **Address:** 270-05 76th Ave, New Hyde Park, NY 11040-1433; **Phone:** 718-470-7460; **Board Cert:** Surgery 2003; Thoracic Surgery 2004; **Med School:** Albany Med Coll 1977; **Resid:** Surgery, St Luke's-Roosevelt Hosp Ctr 1982; Cardiovascular Surgery, Deaconess Hosp 1983; **Fellow:** Cardiovascular Pathology, NY Hosp-Cornell Med Ctr 1985; **Fac Appt:** Prof TS, Albert Einstein Coll Med

Lang, Samuel J MD (TS) - **Spec Exp:** Minimally Invasive Cardiac Surgery; Heart Valve Surgery; Cardiothoracic Surgery; **Hospital:** NY Hosp Queens; **Address:** 56-45 Main St, Cardiac Surgery-3S, Flushing, NY 11355; **Phone:** 718-670-1137; **Board Cert:** Thoracic Surgery 2006; **Med School:** Univ Alabama 1978; **Resid:** Surgery, UCLA Med Ctr 1982; Thoracic Surgery, NYU Med Ctr 1983; **Fellow:** Cardiothoracic Surgery, UCLA Med Ctr 1985; Pediatric Cardiac Surgery, Hosp for Sick Chldn 1986

Lee, Paul C MD (TS) - **Spec Exp:** Lung Cancer; Esophageal Cancer; Gastroesophageal Reflux Disease (GERD); Minimally Invasive Thoracic Surgery; **Hospital:** NY Hosp Queens, NY-Presby Hosp/Weill Cornell (page 104); **Address:** 56-45 Main St, Ste WA-100, Flushing, NY 11355; **Phone:** 718-670-2707; **Board Cert:** Surgery 2002; Thoracic Surgery 2004; **Med School:** Johns Hopkins Univ 1995; **Resid:** Cardiothoracic Surgery, NY Presby Hosp-Cornell 2003; Thoracic Surgery, Meml Sloan Kettering Cancer Ctr 2003; **Fellow:** Minimally Invasive Surgery, Meml SUniv Pittsburgh 2003; **Fac Appt:** Asst Prof S, Cornell Univ-Weill Med Coll

Urology

Farrell, Robert M MD (U) - **Spec Exp:** Endourology; Urologic Cancer; **Hospital:** NY Hosp Queens, Flushing Hosp Med Ctr; **Address:** 58-42 Main St, Flushing, NY 11355; **Phone:** 718-353-3710; **Board Cert:** Urology 1976; **Med School:** Cornell Univ-Weill Med Coll 1966; **Resid:** Surgery, NY Hosp 1968; Urology, NY Hosp 1975

Sandhaus, Jeffrey MD (U) - **Spec Exp:** Prostate Cancer; Minimally Invasive Surgery; Vasectomy-Scalpelless; **Hospital:** Mount Sinai Hosp of Queens (page 102), NY-Presby Hosp/Weill Cornell (page 104); **Address:** 36-01 31st Ave Fl 1, Astoria, NY 11106-1051; **Phone:** 718-932-3535; **Board Cert:** Urology 1976; **Med School:** NY Med Coll 1966; **Resid:** Urology, Univ Hosp 1973; **Fellow:** Nephrology, Univ Hosp 1970; **Fac Appt:** Asst Clin Prof U, Mount Sinai Sch Med

Tarasuk, Albert P MD (U) - **Spec Exp:** Prostate Disease; Bladder Surgery; Kidney Stones; **Hospital:** NY Hosp Queens, Flushing Hosp Med Ctr; **Address:** 58-42 Main St, Flushing, NY 11355-5336; **Phone:** 718-353-3710; **Board Cert:** Urology 1972; **Med School:** Geo Wash Univ 1964; **Resid:** Urology, Beth Israel Med Ctr 1969

Tillem, Steven MD (U) - **Hospital:** Mount Sinai Hosp of Queens (page 102), NY Hosp Queens; **Address:** 36-01 31st Ave Fl 1st, Astoria, NY 11106; **Phone:** 718-932-3535; **Board Cert:** Urology 2009; **Med School:** UMDNJ-NJ Med Sch, Newark 1992; **Resid:** Surgery, LI Jewish Med Ctr 1994; Urology, LI Jewish Med Ctr 1998

Vascular & Interventional Radiology

Rogers, David M MD (VIR) - **Hospital:** NY Hosp Queens, Wyckoff Heights Med Ctr; **Address:** 56-45 Main St, Flushing, NY 11355; **Phone:** 718-670-1050; **Board Cert:** Diagnostic Radiology 1987; **Med School:** Columbia P&S 1981; **Resid:** Diagnostic Radiology, Mt Sinai Med Ctr 1987; **Fellow:** Vascular & Interventional Radiology, NYU Med Ctr 1988

Richmond (Staten Island)

Richmond (Staten Island)

Adolescent Medicine

Lee, April C MD (AM) - **Hospital:** Staten Island Univ Hosp - North, NS-LIJ Hlth Sys; **Address:** Staten Island Univ Hosp, Dept Adol Med, 242 Mason Ave, Staten Island, NY 10305; **Phone:** 718-226-6294; **Board Cert:** Pediatrics 1986; Adolescent Medicine 2009; **Med School:** NYU Sch Med 1980; **Resid:** Pediatrics, NYU Med Ctr 1983; **Fellow:** Adolescent Medicine, Brookdale Hosp 1986; **Fac Appt:** Asst Clin Prof Ped, SUNY Hlth Sci Ctr

Allergy & Immunology

Rao, Yalamanchili A K MD (A&I) - **Hospital:** Staten Island Univ Hosp - North; **Address:** 896 Targee St, Staten Island, NY 10304; **Phone:** 718-816-8200; **Board Cert:** Internal Medicine 1977; Allergy & Immunology 1977; **Med School:** India 1968; **Resid:** Allergy & Immunology, Long Island Coll Hosp 1975; Internal Medicine, Long Island Coll Hosp 1977; **Fac Appt:** Asst Clin Prof Med, SUNY Downstate

Cardiovascular Disease

Besser, Louis M MD (Cv) - **Spec Exp:** Coronary Artery Disease; Arrhythmias; **Hospital:** Richmond Univ Med Ctr, Staten Island Univ Hosp - North; **Address:** 11 Ralph Pl, ste 310, Staten Island, NY 10304-4419; **Phone:** 718-442-1777; **Board Cert:** Internal Medicine 1988; Cardiovascular Disease 1989; **Med School:** Mexico 1981; **Resid:** Internal Medicine, St Vincents Med Ctr 1986; **Fellow:** Cardiovascular Disease, St Vincents Med Ctr 1988; **Fac Appt:** Asst Clin Prof Med, NY Med Coll

Bogin, Marc MD (Cv) - **Spec Exp:** Echocardiography; Cardiac Catheterization; **Hospital:** Staten Island Univ Hosp - North, Richmond Univ Med Ctr; **Address:** Heart, Lung & Surgery Ctr, 501 Seaview Ave, Ste 200, Staten Island, NY 10305; **Phone:** 718-663-6400; **Board Cert:** Internal Medicine 1989; Cardiovascular Disease 2003; **Med School:** Mexico 1985; **Resid:** Internal Medicine, Booth Meml Hosp 1990; **Fellow:** Cardiovascular Disease, St Vincent's Hosp & Med Ctr 1993; **Fac Appt:** Asst Clin Prof Med, NY Med Coll

Grodman, Richard S MD (Cv) - **Spec Exp:** Echocardiography; Cardiac Catheterization; **Hospital:** Richmond Univ Med Ctr; **Address:** Richmond University Medical Center, 355 Bard Ave, Staten Island, NY 10310-1664; **Phone:** 718-818-4642; **Board Cert:** Internal Medicine 1976; Cardiovascular Disease 1979; **Med School:** SUNY Downstate 1973; **Resid:** Internal Medicine, SUNY Downstate 1976; Critical Care Medicine, SUNY Downstate 1977; **Fellow:** Cardiovascular Disease, Rhode Island Hosp-Brown 1979; **Fac Appt:** Assoc Clin Prof Med, NY Med Coll

Lafferty, James MD (Cv) - **Spec Exp:** Electrophysiologic Testing; **Hospital:** Staten Island Univ Hosp - North; **Address:** Staten Island Heart, 501 Seaview Ave, Ste 300, Staten Island, NY 10305; **Phone:** 718-663-7000 x6; **Board Cert:** Internal Medicine 1985; Cardiovascular Disease 1987; Cardiac Electrophysiology 2006; **Med School:** SUNY Hlth Sci Ctr 1982; **Resid:** Internal Medicine, Staten Island Hosp 1985; **Fellow:** Cardiovascular Disease, Univ Hosp 1987; **Fac Appt:** Assoc Prof Med, SUNY Downstate

Schwartz, Charles A MD (Cv) - **Spec Exp:** Cardiac Stress Testing; Cardiac Catheterization; Echocardiography; **Hospital:** Staten Island Univ Hosp - North; **Address:** 501 Seaview Ave, Ste 300, Staten Island, NY 10312-3836; **Phone:** 718-663-7000; **Board Cert:** Internal Medicine 1983; Cardiovascular Disease 1985; Echocardiography 2002; **Med School:** SUNY Downstate 1980; **Resid:** Internal Medicine, Staten Island Hosp 1983; **Fellow:** Cardiovascular Disease, St Vincent's Hosp & Med Ctr 1985; **Fac Appt:** Asst Clin Prof Med, SUNY Downstate

Swamy, Samala R MD (Cv) - **Spec Exp:** Preventive Cardiology; Invasive Cardiology; Interventional Cardiology; Nuclear Cardiology; **Hospital:** Richmond Univ Med Ctr, Staten Island Univ Hosp - South; **Address:** 1366 Victory Blvd, Ste B, Staten Island, NY 10301-3907; **Phone:** 718-442-8351; **Board Cert:** Internal Medicine 1977; Cardiovascular Disease 1979; Interventional Cardiology 2004; **Med School:** India 1972; **Resid:** Internal Medicine, St Vincents Hosp 1977; **Fellow:** Cardiovascular Disease, Cook Co Hosp 1978; Cardiovascular Disease, St Vincents Hosp 1979; **Fac Appt:** Asst Prof Med, NY Med Coll

Vazzana, Thomas MD (Cv) - **Spec Exp:** Invasive Cardiology; Non-Invasive Cardiology; Interventional Cardiology; **Hospital:** Staten Island Univ Hosp - North, Richmond Univ Med Ctr; **Address:** 501 Seaview Ave, Ste 200, Staten Island, NY 10305; **Phone:** 718-447-7899; **Board Cert:** Internal Medicine 1989; Cardiovascular Disease 2001; Interventional Cardiology 2002; **Med School:** Grenada 1985; **Resid:** Internal Medicine, St Joseph's Hosp & Med Ctr 1989; **Fellow:** Cardiovascular Disease, St Vincent's Hosp & Med Ctr 1991; **Fac Appt:** Asst Prof Med, NY Med Coll

Winter, Steven MD (Cv) - **Spec Exp:** Cholesterol/Lipid Disorders; Preventive Cardiology; Non-Invasive Cardiology; **Hospital:** Staten Island Univ Hosp - North, Richmond Univ Med Ctr; **Address:** 2627 Hylan Blvd, Bldg B, Staten Island, NY 10306-4339; **Phone:** 718-351-5600; **Board Cert:** Internal Medicine 1979; Cardiovascular Disease 1981; **Med School:** UMDNJ-NJ Med Sch, Newark 1976; **Resid:** Internal Medicine, N Shore Univ Hosp 1979; Internal Medicine, Meml Sloan Kettering Cancer Ctr 1979; **Fellow:** Cardiovascular Disease, Rhode Island Hosp 1981; **Fac Appt:** Asst Clin Prof Med, SUNY Hlth Sci Ctr

Child Neurology

De Carlo, Regina MD (ChiN) - **Spec Exp:** Autism; Headache; Learning Disorders; ADD/ADHD; **Hospital:** Richmond Univ Med Ctr, NYU Langone Med Ctr (page 106); **Address:** 2550 Victory Blvd, Staten Island, NY 10314-6635; **Phone:** 718-983-0923; **Board Cert:** Pediatrics 1984; Child Neurology 1984; **Med School:** UMDNJ-NJ Med Sch, Newark 1977; **Resid:** Pediatrics, NYU Med Ctr 1979; Neurology, NYU Med Ctr 1981; **Fellow:** Child Neurology, NYU Med Ctr 1982; **Fac Appt:** Asst Clin Prof N, NYU Sch Med

Dermatology

Bernstein, Charles MD (D) - **Hospital:** Staten Island Univ Hosp - North; **Address:** 244 Buel Ave Fl 2, Staten Island, NY 10305; **Phone:** 718-980-5767; **Board Cert:** Internal Medicine 1983; Dermatology 1987; **Med School:** SUNY Downstate 1980; **Resid:** Internal Medicine, Staten Island Hosp 1984; Dermatology, Downstate Med Ctr 1987; **Fac Appt:** Assoc Clin Prof D, SUNY Hlth Sci Ctr

Lederman, Josiane MD (D) - **Spec Exp:** Cosmetic Dermatology; Skin Cancer; Laser Surgery; **Address:** 116 Lamberts Ln, Staten Island, NY 10314-7210; **Phone:** 718-370-0422; **Board Cert:** Dermatology 1986; **Med School:** France 1981; **Resid:** Dermatology, Saint Louis Hosp 1983; **Fellow:** Dermatology, Mass Genl Hosp-Harvard 1986

McCormack, Patricia MD (D) - **Spec Exp:** Psoriasis; Skin Cancer; Skin Laser Surgery; **Hospital:** Richmond Univ Med Ctr; **Address:** 1550 Richmond Ave, Ste 207, Staten Island, NY 10314; **Phone:** 718-698-1616; **Board Cert:** Dermatology 1985; **Med School:** UMDNJ-Rutgers Med Sch 1981; **Resid:** Dermatology, NY Med Coll 1985; **Fac Appt:** Asst Prof D, NY Med Coll

Urbanek, Richard W MD (D) - **Spec Exp:** Liposuction; Laser Surgery; Botox Therapy; **Address:** 1324 Victory Blvd, Staten Island, NY 10301; **Phone:** 718-448-4488; **Board Cert:** Dermatology 1977; **Med School:** Cornell Univ-Weill Med Coll 1972; **Resid:** Dermatology, Temple Univ Hosp 1976; **Fac Appt:** Asst Prof D, NYU Sch Med

Endocrinology, Diabetes & Metabolism

Cohen, Neil MD (EDM) - **Spec Exp:** Diabetes; Thyroid Disorders; Osteoporosis; **Hospital:** Staten Island Univ Hosp - North, Staten Island Univ Hosp - South; **Address:** 1460 Victory Blvd, Staten Island, NY 10301-3914; **Phone:** 718-442-0300; **Board Cert:** Internal Medicine 2003; Endocrinology, Diabetes & Metabolism 2005; **Med School:** Med Coll PA Hahnemann 1990; **Resid:** Internal Medicine, N Shore Univ Hosp 1993; **Fellow:** Endocrinology, Diabetes & Metabolism, Montefiore Med Ctr 1995; **Fac Appt:** Assoc Clin Prof Med, SUNY Downstate

Das, Seshadri MD (EDM) - **Spec Exp:** Diabetes; Thyroid Disorders; **Hospital:** Richmond Univ Med Ctr, Staten Island Univ Hosp - South; **Address:** 45 Little Clove Rd, Staten Island, NY 10301; **Phone:** 718-273-5522; **Board Cert:** Internal Medicine 1983; Endocrinology, Diabetes & Metabolism 2008; **Med School:** India 1968; **Resid:** Internal Medicine, North Middlesex Hosp 1975; Internal Medicine, Whittington Hosp 1976; **Fellow:** Endocrinology, Diabetes & Metabolism, SUNY Downstate 1980

Hoffman, Richard S MD (EDM) - **Spec Exp:** Diabetes; Thyroid Disorders; Parathyroid Disorders; Adrenal Disorders; **Hospital:** Staten Island Univ Hosp - North; **Address:** 1460 Victory Blvd, Staten Island, NY 10301; **Phone:** 718-442-0300; **Board Cert:** Internal Medicine 1971; Endocrinology, Diabetes & Metabolism 1975; **Med School:** SUNY Hlth Sci Ctr 1965; **Resid:** Internal Medicine, Boston City Hosp 1968; Internal Medicine, Long Island Coll Hosp 1967; **Fellow:** Endocrinology, Boston City Hosp 1970; **Fac Appt:** Assoc Clin Prof Med, SUNY Downstate

Rothman, Jeffrey G MD (EDM) - **Spec Exp:** Diabetes; Osteoporosis; Thyroid Disorders; **Hospital:** Staten Island Univ Hosp - North, Staten Island Univ Hosp - South; **Address:** 1460 Victory Blvd, Staten Island, NY 10301-3914; **Phone:** 718-442-0300; **Board Cert:** Internal Medicine 1973; Endocrinology, Diabetes & Metabolism 1977; **Med School:** SUNY Buffalo 1970; **Resid:** Internal Medicine, Hosp Univ Penn 1973; **Fellow:** Endocrinology, Diabetes & Metabolism, Hosp Univ Penn 1977; **Fac Appt:** Asst Clin Prof Med, SUNY Downstate

Family Medicine

Nepola, Neil MD (FMed) *PCP* - **Hospital:** Staten Island Univ Hosp - South; **Address:** 217 Rose Ave, Staten Island, NY 10306-2918; **Phone:** 718-667-6767; **Board Cert:** Family Medicine 2004; **Med School:** Philippines 1979; **Resid:** Family Medicine, UMDNJ-St Peter's Hosp 1983

Gastroenterology

Bruckstein, Alex MD (Ge) - **Spec Exp:** Colonoscopy; Gastroscopy; Gastroesophageal Reflux Disease (GERD); **Hospital:** Richmond Univ Med Ctr, Staten Island Univ Hosp - North; **Address:** 2627 Hylan Blvd, Staten Island, NY 10306-4339; **Phone:** 718-667-3200; **Board Cert:** Internal Medicine 1979; Gastroenterology 1983; **Med School:** Albert Einstein Coll Med 1975; **Resid:** Internal Medicine, Roosevelt Hosp 1977; Internal Medicine, St Luke's Hosp 1978; **Fellow:** Gastroenterology, VA Med Ctr-NYU 1980; **Fac Appt:** Asst Clin Prof Med, SUNY Downstate

Fazio, Richard MD (Ge) - **Spec Exp:** Colonoscopy; Gastroesophageal Reflux Disease (GERD); **Hospital:** Richmond Univ Med Ctr; **Address:** 78 Todt Hill Rd, Ste 203, Staten Island, NY 10314-4528; **Phone:** 718-448-1122; **Board Cert:** Internal Medicine 1982; Gastroenterology 1983; **Med School:** Italy 1978; **Resid:** Internal Medicine, Maimonides Med Ctr 1981; **Fellow:** Gastroenterology, St Vincent's Med Ctr 1983; **Fac Appt:** Prof Med, SUNY Downstate

Wickremesinghe, Prasanna C MD (Ge) - **Spec Exp:** Inflammatory Bowel Disease/Crohn's; Hepatitis; Endoscopy; **Hospital:** Richmond Univ Med Ctr; **Address:** 481 Bard Ave, Staten Island, NY 10310; **Phone:** 718-448-0865; **Board Cert:** Internal Medicine 1980; Gastroenterology 1975; **Med School:** Sri Lanka 1968; **Resid:** Internal Medicine, Coney Ismand Hosp 1972; **Fellow:** Gastroenterology, Maimonides Medical Ctr 1975; **Fac Appt:** Asst Prof Med, NY Med Coll

Geriatric Medicine

Seminara, Donna MD (Ger) - **Hospital:** Staten Island Univ Hosp - North; **Address:** Island Internists, 420 Lyndale Ave, Staten Island, NY 10312-6131; **Phone:** 718-967-5630; **Board Cert:** Internal Medicine 2000; Geriatric Medicine 2000; **Med School:** Mexico 1986; **Resid:** Internal Medicine, Staten Island Univ Hosp 1990

Gynecologic Oncology

Maiman, Mitchell MD (GO) - **Spec Exp:** Cervical Cancer; Ovarian Cancer; Uterine Cancer; **Hospital:** Staten Island Univ Hosp - North; **Address:** 256 Mason Ave, Staten Island, NY 10305-3408; **Phone:** 718-226-6400; **Board Cert:** Obstetrics & Gynecology 2008; Gynecologic Oncology 2008; **Med School:** SUNY Hlth Sci Ctr 1981; **Resid:** Obstetrics & Gynecology, Montefiore Med Ctr 1985; **Fellow:** Gynecologic Oncology, SUNY Downstate Med Ctr 1987; **Fac Appt:** Prof ObG, SUNY Downstate

Infectious Disease

Glaser, Jordan MD (Inf) - **Spec Exp:** AIDS/HIV; **Hospital:** Staten Island Univ Hosp - North, Staten Island Univ Hosp - South; **Address:** 1408 Richmond Rd, Staten Island, NY 10304; **Phone:** 718-816-3362; **Board Cert:** Internal Medicine 1982; Infectious Disease 1984; **Med School:** SUNY Hlth Sci Ctr 1979; **Resid:** Internal Medicine, Staten Island Hosp 1980; Infectious Disease, Staten Island Hosp 1982; **Fellow:** Infectious Disease, Univ Hosp 1984; **Fac Appt:** Assoc Clin Prof Med, SUNY Hlth Sci Ctr

Internal Medicine

Fulop, Robert MD (IM) *PCP* - **Spec Exp:** Diagnostic Problems; Geriatric Medicine; **Hospital:** Richmond Univ Med Ctr, Staten Island Univ Hosp - North; **Address:** 476 Klondike Ave, Staten Island, NY 10314-6216; **Phone:** 718-761-1156; **Board Cert:** Internal Medicine 1982; Geriatric Medicine 2005; **Med School:** SUNY Upstate Med Univ 1978; **Resid:** Internal Medicine, Brookdale Hosp 1981; **Fac Appt:** Asst Clin Prof Med, NY Med Coll

Gazzara, Paul MD (IM) *PCP* - **Spec Exp:** Complementary Medicine; Acupuncture; Addiction/Substance Abuse; **Hospital:** Staten Island Univ Hosp - North; **Address:** 3589 Hylan Blvd, Staten Island, NY 10308-3513; **Phone:** 718-966-3700; **Board Cert:** Internal Medicine 1986; **Med School:** SUNY Downstate 1983; **Resid:** Internal Medicine, Staten Island Hosp 1986; **Fac Appt:** Asst Clin Prof Med, SUNY Hlth Sci Ctr

Hendricks, Judith MD (IM) *PCP* - **Spec Exp:** Hypertension; Cholesterol/Lipid Disorders; **Hospital:** Staten Island Univ Hosp - North; **Address:** 1870 Richmond Rd, Staten Island, NY 10306; **Phone:** 718-667-5400; **Board Cert:** Internal Medicine 1978; **Med School:** Univ Okla Coll Med 1975; **Resid:** Internal Medicine, Staten Island Hosp 1978; **Fac Appt:** Asst Clin Prof Med, SUNY Hlth Sci Ctr

Malach, Barbara MD (IM) *PCP* - **Spec Exp:** Geriatric Medicine; **Hospital:** Staten Island Univ Hosp - North; **Address:** 2627B Hylan Blvd, Staten Island, NY 10306-4339; **Phone:** 718-987-6000; **Board Cert:** Internal Medicine 1983; Geriatric Medicine 2008; **Med School:** SUNY Downstate 1979; **Resid:** Internal Medicine, Staten Island Hosp 1982

Strange, Theodore MD (IM) *PCP* - **Spec Exp:** Geriatric Medicine; **Hospital:** Staten Island Univ Hosp - South, Staten Island Univ Hosp - North; **Address:** 68 Seguine Ave, Staten Island, NY 10309-3723; **Phone:** 718-356-6500; **Board Cert:** Internal Medicine 2001; Geriatric Medicine 2002; **Med School:** SUNY Hlth Sci Ctr 1985; **Resid:** Internal Medicine, Staten Island Univ Hosp 1988; **Fac Appt:** Assoc Clin Prof Med, SUNY Downstate

Interventional Cardiology

Malpeso, James V MD (IC) - **Spec Exp:** Cardiac Catheterization; Angioplasty & Stent Placement; Cardiac CT Angiography; **Hospital:** Staten Island Univ Hosp - North; **Address:** 501 Seaview Ave, Ste 300, Staten Island, NY 10306; **Phone:** 718-663-7000; **Board Cert:** Internal Medicine 1979; Cardiovascular Disease 1981; Interventional Cardiology 2000; Cardiovascular Computed Tomography 2008; **Med School:** Albert Einstein Coll Med 1975; **Resid:** Internal Medicine, Kings County Hosp 1978; **Fellow:** Cardiovascular Disease, St Vincent's Hosp & Med Ctr 1980; **Fac Appt:** Asst Prof Med, SUNY Downstate

Maternal & Fetal Medicine

Moretti, Michael MD (MF) - **Hospital:** Richmond Univ Med Ctr; **Address:** 355 Bard Ave, Ste 208, Staten Island, NY 10310-1664; **Phone:** 718-818-3287; **Board Cert:** Obstetrics & Gynecology 2007; Maternal & Fetal Medicine 2007; **Med School:** Mexico 1981; **Resid:** Obstetrics & Gynecology, Staten Island Hosp 1986; **Fellow:** Maternal & Fetal Medicine, Univ Tenn Hosp 1988

Medical Oncology

Forlenza, Thomas J MD (Onc) - **Spec Exp:** Palliative Care; Bleeding/Coagulation Disorders; Breast Cancer; Lung Cancer; **Hospital:** Richmond Univ Med Ctr; **Address:** 102 Hart Blvd, Staten Island, NY 10301-2615; **Phone:** 718-816-4949; **Board Cert:** Internal Medicine 1981; Hematology 1984; Blood Banking 1984; Medical Oncology 1985; **Med School:** Boston Univ 1977; **Resid:** Internal Medicine, Univ Kentucky Med Ctr 1980; **Fellow:** Hematology, NYU Med Ctr 1982; Medical Oncology, Kings County Hosp 1983; **Fac Appt:** Asst Prof Med, NYU Sch Med

Friscia, Philip MD (Onc) - **Spec Exp:** Lung Cancer; Colon Cancer; Hematology; **Hospital:** Staten Island Univ Hosp - North, Staten Island Univ Hosp - South; **Address:** 256 Mason Ave Bldg C, Nalitt Inst, Staten Island, NY 10305; **Phone:** 718-226-6400; **Board Cert:** Internal Medicine 1978; Medical Oncology 1981; **Med School:** Italy 1972; **Resid:** Internal Medicine, Long Island Coll Hosp 1976; **Fellow:** Hematology & Oncology, Long Island Coll Hosp 1979; **Fac Appt:** Asst Clin Prof Med, SUNY Downstate

Odaimi, Marcel MD (Onc) - **Spec Exp:** Brain Tumors; **Hospital:** Staten Island Univ Hosp - South; **Address:** 256C Mason Ave, Staten Island, NY 10305-3408; **Phone:** 718-226-6400; **Board Cert:** Internal Medicine 1987; Medical Oncology 1989; **Med School:** Amer Univ Beirut 1981; **Resid:** Internal Medicine, Amer Univ Beirut 1983; Internal Medicine, Staten Island Hosp 1987; **Fellow:** Medical Oncology, MD Anderson Hosp 1985

Terjanian, Terenig O MD (Onc) - **Hospital:** Staten Island Univ Hosp - North; **Address:** 256 Mason Ave C Bldg, Nalitt Inst, Staten Island, NY 10305-3408; **Phone:** 718-226-6400; **Board Cert:** Internal Medicine 1984; Medical Oncology 1987; Hematology 1988; **Med School:** France 1978; **Resid:** Anatomic Pathology, Amer Univ Beirut 1981; Internal Medicine, Staten Island Univ Hosp 1984; **Fellow:** Medical Oncology, MD Anderson Cancer Ctr 1986; Hematology, NYU Med Ctr 1988

Neonatal-Perinatal Medicine

Harin, Anantham MD (NP) - **Spec Exp:** Neonatal Care; **Hospital:** Richmond Univ Med Ctr; **Address:** 355 Bard Ave, Staten Island, NY 10310; **Phone:** 718-818-4310; **Board Cert:** Pediatrics 1975; Neonatal-Perinatal Medicine 1977; **Med School:** Sri Lanka 1970; **Resid:** Pediatrics, Kings County Hosp 1973; **Fellow:** Neonatology, N Shore Univ Hosp 1975; **Fac Appt:** Clin Prof Ped, NYU Sch Med

Roth, Philip MD/PhD (NP) - **Spec Exp:** Neonatal Infections/Immunity; Breast Feeding Problems; **Hospital:** Staten Island Univ Hosp - North; **Address:** 475 Seaview Ave Fl 4 East, Staten Island, NY 10305-3436; **Phone:** 718-226-9796; **Board Cert:** Pediatrics 1987; Neonatal-Perinatal Medicine 2004; **Med School:** Columbia P&S 1982; **Resid:** Pediatrics, Chldns Hosp 1986; **Fellow:** Neonatal-Perinatal Medicine, Hosp Univ Penn 1988; **Fac Appt:** Assoc Prof Ped, SUNY Downstate

Nephrology

Grossman, Susan D MD (Nep) - **Hospital:** Richmond Univ Med Ctr; **Address:** Richmond Univ Med Ctr, Dept Med, 355 Bard Ave, Staten Island, NY 10310; **Phone:** 718-818-2416; **Board Cert:** Internal Medicine 1980; Nephrology 1982; **Med School:** UMDNJ-NJ Med Sch, Newark 1977; **Resid:** Internal Medicine, Univ Hosp 1980; **Fellow:** Nephrology, New England Med Ctr 1982

Kleiner, Morton MD (Nep) - **Spec Exp:** Hypertension; Kidney Disease; **Hospital:** Staten Island Univ Hosp - North; **Address:** 347 Edison St, Staten Island, NY 10306-3034; **Phone:** 718-351-1136; **Board Cert:** Internal Medicine 1977; Nephrology 1982; **Med School:** NY Med Coll 1974; **Resid:** Internal Medicine, N Shore Univ Hosp 1977; **Fellow:** Nephrology, NY Hosp-Cornell Med Ctr 1979; **Fac Appt:** Asst Clin Prof Med, SUNY Downstate

Pepe, John M MD (Nep) - **Spec Exp:** Transplant Medicine-Kidney; **Hospital:** Richmond Univ Med Ctr, Staten Island Univ Hosp - South; **Address:** 1550 Richmond Ave, Ste 205, Staten Island, NY 10314-1519; **Phone:** 718-982-7800; **Board Cert:** Internal Medicine 1978; Nephrology 1980; **Med School:** Med Coll PA Hahnemann 1975; **Resid:** Internal Medicine, Univ Hosp 1978; **Fellow:** Nephrology, Bronx Muni Hosp/ Einstein 1980; **Fac Appt:** Asst Prof Med, NY Med Coll

Petra, Eugene MD (Nep) - **Hospital:** Staten Island Univ Hosp - South, Richmond Univ Med Ctr; **Address:** Richmond Kidney Ctr, 1366 Victory Blvd, Ste C, Staten Island, NY 10301-3907; **Phone:** 718-273-3400; **Board Cert:** Internal Medicine 1988; Nephrology 2002; **Med School:** Italy 1985; **Resid:** Internal Medicine, Englewood Hosp 1988; **Fellow:** Nephrology, Brookdale Hosp 1990

Neurology

Jutkowitz, Robert S MD (N) - **Spec Exp:** Headache; Seizure Disorders; **Hospital:** Richmond Univ Med Ctr; **Address:** 78 Todt Hill Rd, Ste 205, Staten Island, NY 10314-4528; **Phone:** 718-442-7133; **Board Cert:** Neurology 1976; **Med School:** Univ Louisville Sch Med 1968; **Resid:** Internal Medicine, St Viincents Hosp 1970; Neurology, Mt Sinai Hosp 1974

Najjar, Souhel MD (N) - **Spec Exp:** Epilepsy; Seizure Disorders; **Hospital:** Staten Island Univ Hosp - North, NYU Langone Med Ctr (page 106); **Address:** 501 Seaview Ave, Ste 104, Staten Island, NY 10305; **Phone:** 718-683-3766; **Board Cert:** Neurology 1993; **Med School:** Syria 1983; **Resid:** Pathology, Albany Med Ctr 1988; Neurology, Albany Med Ctr 1992; **Fellow:** Neurological Pathology, NYU Med Ctr 1994; **Fac Appt:** Assoc Clin Prof N, NYU Sch Med

Obstetrics & Gynecology

Ponterio, Jane M MD (ObG) *PCP* - **Spec Exp:** Menopause Problems; Hysterectomy Alternatives; Adolescent Gynecology; **Hospital:** Richmond Univ Med Ctr, Staten Island Univ Hosp - North; **Address:** 1583 Richmond Ave, Staten Island, NY 10314; **Phone:** 718-983-0204; **Board Cert:** Obstetrics & Gynecology 2009; **Med School:** NY Med Coll 1981; **Resid:** Obstetrics & Gynecology, St Luke's-Roosevelt Hosp Ctr 1985; **Fac Appt:** Asst Prof ObG, NY Med Coll

Reilly, James G DO (ObG) - **Spec Exp:** Colposcopy; Gynecologic Surgery-Laparoscopic; Hysterectomy Alternatives; **Hospital:** Richmond Univ Med Ctr, Staten Island Univ Hosp - North; **Address:** 668 Castleton Ave, Staten Island, NY 10301-2044; **Phone:** 718-448-4300; **Board Cert:** Obstetrics & Gynecology 1998; **Med School:** NY Coll Osteo Med 1991; **Resid:** Obstetrics & Gynecology, St Vincent Cath Med Ctr 1995; **Fac Appt:** Asst Clin Prof ObG, NY Coll Osteo Med

Ophthalmology

Derespinis, Patrick MD (Oph) - **Spec Exp:** Eye Muscle Disorders; Pediatric Ophthalmology; Eye Disorders-Congenital; **Hospital:** Staten Island Univ Hosp - South, Univ Hosp-UMDNJ—Newark; **Address:** 2504 Richmond Rd, Staten Island, NY 10306; **Phone:** 718-667-1010; **Board Cert:** Ophthalmology 1989; **Med School:** Mexico 1981; **Resid:** Internal Medicine, Booth Meml Med Ctr 1983; Ophthalmology, UMDNJ 1987; **Fellow:** Pediatric Ophthalmology, Manhattan EE&T Hosp 1988; **Fac Appt:** Assoc Clin Prof Oph, UMDNJ-NJ Med Sch, Newark

Kramer, Philip W MD (Oph) - **Spec Exp:** Diabetic Eye Disease/Retinopathy; Cataract Surgery; Glaucoma; **Hospital:** Staten Island Univ Hosp - South, New York Eye & Ear Infirm (page 113); **Address:** 1460 Victory Blvd, Staten Island, NY 10301-3914; **Phone:** 718-447-0022; **Board Cert:** Ophthalmology 1985; **Med School:** Temple Univ 1980; **Resid:** Ophthalmology, NY Eye & Ear Infirmary 1984

Zerykier, Abraham MD (Oph) - **Spec Exp:** Cataract Surgery; Diabetic Eye Disease/Retinopathy; Glaucoma; **Hospital:** Staten Island Univ Hosp - South, Beth Israel Med Ctr-Kings Hwy Div (page 94); **Address:** 16 Ross Ave, Staten Island, NY 10306-2216; **Phone:** 718-667-4444; **Board Cert:** Ophthalmology 1980; **Med School:** Hahnemann Univ 1975; **Resid:** Internal Medicine, Brookdale Hosp 1976; Ophthalmology, Jewish Hosp 1979; **Fac Appt:** Asst Clin Prof Oph, SUNY Downstate

Orthopaedic Surgery

Accettola, Albert MD (OrS) - **Hospital:** Staten Island Univ Hosp - North, Staten Island Univ Hosp - South; **Address:** 3311 Hylan Blvd, Staten Island, NY 10306; **Phone:** 718-667-7500; **Board Cert:** Orthopaedic Surgery 1982; **Med School:** Belgium 1974; **Resid:** Surgery, Staten Island Hosp 1976; Orthopaedic Surgery, Bellevue Hosp Ctr-NYU 1979

Drucker, David MD (OrS) - **Spec Exp:** Hip & Knee Replacement; **Hospital:** Staten Island Univ Hosp - North, Beth Israel Med Ctr- Kings Hwy Div (page 94); **Address:** 11th Ralph Pl, Ste 103A, Staten Island, NY 10304; **Phone:** 718-727-6945; **Board Cert:** Orthopaedic Surgery 2004; **Med School:** Univ Chicago-Pritzker Sch Med 1983; **Resid:** Orthopaedic Surgery, UNDMJ Univ Hosp 1989; **Fellow:** Hip & Knee Surgery, Indiana Univ 1990; **Fac Appt:** Asst Clin Prof OrS, UMDNJ-NJ Med Sch, Newark

Flynn, Maryirene MD (OrS) - **Spec Exp:** Arthroscopic Surgery; Sports Medicine; **Hospital:** Richmond Univ Med Ctr, Staten Island Univ Hosp - North; **Address:** 2052 Richmond Rd, Staten Island, NY 10304-2313; **Phone:** 718-351-6500; **Board Cert:** Orthopaedic Surgery 2005; **Med School:** Albert Einstein Coll Med 1986; **Resid:** Orthopaedic Surgery, Montefiore Hosp Med Ctr 1991; **Fellow:** Sports Medicine, Staten Island Hosp 1992

Jayaram, Nadubeethi MD (OrS) - **Spec Exp:** Hand Surgery; **Hospital:** Richmond Univ Med Ctr; **Address:** 11 Ralph Pl, Ste 102, Staten Island, NY 10304; **Phone:** 718-447-6545; **Board Cert:** Orthopaedic Surgery 2003; **Med School:** India 1973; **Resid:** Surgery, Univ Hosp 1981; Orthopaedic Surgery, Univ Hosp 1985; **Fellow:** Vascular Surgery, Lutheran Med Ctr 1982; Hand Surgery, Univ Alabama Hosp 1988

Reilly, John P MD (OrS) - **Spec Exp:** Sports Medicine; Trauma; **Hospital:** Staten Island Univ Hosp - North; **Address:** 3311 Hylan Blvd, Staten Island, NY 10308; **Phone:** 718-667-7500; **Board Cert:** Orthopaedic Surgery 2010; **Med School:** SUNY Downstate 1981; **Resid:** Orthopaedic Surgery, Lenox Hill Hosp 1986; Orthopaedic Surgery, Chldns Hosp; **Fellow:** Orthopaedic Surgery, Univ MD Hosp 1987

Sherman, Mark F MD (OrS) - **Spec Exp:** Sports Medicine; Knee Injuries; **Hospital:** Richmond Univ Med Ctr, Staten Island Univ Hosp - North; **Address:** 2052 Richmond Rd, Staten Island, NY 10304; **Phone:** 718-351-6500; **Board Cert:** Orthopaedic Surgery 1981; **Med School:** NYU Sch Med 1975; **Resid:** Surgery, Bellevue Hosp 1976; Orthopaedic Surgery, Bellevue Hosp 1979; **Fellow:** Sports Medicine, Hosp for Special Surgery 1980

Otolaryngology

Castellano, Bartolomeo MD (Oto) - **Hospital:** Mount Sinai Med Ctr (page 102); **Address:** 78 Todt Hill Rd, Ste 204, Staten Island, NY 10314-4528; **Phone:** 718-273-2626; **Board Cert:** Otolaryngology 1985; **Med School:** Mexico 1979; **Resid:** Otolaryngology, NYU Med Ctr 1984; **Fellow:** Plastic Surgery, Mt Sinai Med Ctr 1985; **Fac Appt:** Asst Prof Oto, NYU Sch Med

Sinnreich, Abraham MD (Oto) - **Spec Exp:** Sinus Disorders; Sleep Disorders/Apnea; **Hospital:** Long Island Coll Hosp (page 94), Mount Sinai Med Ctr (page 102); **Address:** 1887 Richmond Ave, Ste 5, Staten Island, NY 10314; **Phone:** 718-370-0072; **Board Cert:** Otolaryngology 1984; **Med School:** Albert Einstein Coll Med 1979; **Resid:** Otolaryngology, Mount Sinai Hosp 1983; **Fac Appt:** Asst Clin Prof Oto, SUNY Downstate

Pain Medicine

Stilwell, Anne Marie MD (PM) - **Spec Exp:** Pain-Spine; Pain-after Spinal Intervention; **Hospital:** Richmond Univ Med Ctr; **Address:** 45 McLean Ave, Staten Island, NY 10305; **Phone:** 718-448-6373; **Board Cert:** Anesthesiology 1995; Pain Medicine 2007; **Med School:** Univ Rochester 1990; **Resid:** Anesthesiology, NY Hosp-Cornell Med Ctr 1994; **Fellow:** Pain Management, NY Hosp-Cornell Med Ctr 1996

Pediatric Endocrinology

Torrado-Jule, Carmen MD (PEn) - **Spec Exp:** Diabetes; Thyroid Disorders; Growth Disorders; Obesity; **Hospital:** Staten Island Univ Hosp - North, N Shore Univ Hosp; **Address:** 584 Forest Ave, Staten Island, NY 10310-2512; **Phone:** 718-226-5619; **Board Cert:** Pediatrics 2008; Pediatric Endocrinology 2005; **Med School:** Dominican Republic 1983; **Resid:** Pediatrics, Kings County Hosp 1987; **Fellow:** Pediatric Endocrinology, Kings County Hosp 1990; **Fac Appt:** Asst Prof Ped, SUNY Hlth Sci Ctr

Pediatric Gastroenterology

Rabinowitz, Simon S MD/PhD (PGe) - **Spec Exp:** Inflammatory Bowel Disease; Hepatitis; Gastroesophageal Reflux Disease (GERD); Gastrointestinal Disorders; **Hospital:** Richmond Univ Med Ctr; **Address:** 800 Castleton Ave, Staten Island, NY 10310; **Phone:** 718-818-4636; **Board Cert:** Pediatrics 2009; Pediatric Gastroenterology 2007; **Med School:** Univ Miami Sch Med 1983; **Resid:** Pediatrics, Mount Sinai Hosp 1985; **Fellow:** Pediatric Gastroenterology, Mount Sinai Hosp 1987; **Fac Appt:** Assoc Clin Prof Ped, NY Med Coll

Pediatric Hematology-Oncology

Potaznik, Daniel MD (PHO) - **Spec Exp:** Hematology; **Hospital:** Staten Island Univ Hosp - North; **Address:** 256 Mason Ave C Bldg, Staten Island, NY 10305; **Phone:** 718-226-6474; **Board Cert:** Pediatrics 1987; Pediatric Hematology-Oncology 1987; **Med School:** Belgium 1970; **Resid:** Pediatrics, Sheba Med Ctr 1975; **Fellow:** Pediatric Hematology-Oncology, Meml Sloan Kettering Cancer Ctr 1983; **Fac Appt:** Clin Prof Ped, NYU Sch Med

Pediatrics

Bastawros, Mary N MD (Ped) *PCP* - **Hospital:** Richmond Univ Med Ctr, Staten Island Univ Hosp - North; **Address:** 314 Seaview Ave, Staten Island, NY 10305; **Phone:** 718-668-3417; **Board Cert:** Pediatrics 1985; **Med School:** Egypt 1966; **Resid:** Pediatrics, Methodist Hosp 1974

Duchnowska, Alicja B MD (Ped) *PCP* - **Hospital:** Staten Island Univ Hosp - North; **Address:** 934 Ionia Ave, Staten Island, NY 10309-2308; **Phone:** 718-984-5255; **Board Cert:** Pediatrics 1985; **Med School:** Poland 1965; **Resid:** Pediatrics, National Inst of Mother & Child 1970; Pediatrics, Staten Island Hosp 1982; **Fellow:** Pediatrics, Staten Island Hosp 1984

Short, Joan MD (Ped) *PCP* - **Hospital:** Richmond Univ Med Ctr, Staten Island Univ Hosp - North; **Address:** 32 2nd St, Staten Island, NY 10306; **Phone:** 718-979-7472; **Board Cert:** Pediatrics 1982; **Med School:** Univ Tenn Coll Med, Memphis 1966; **Resid:** Pediatrics, City of Memphis Hosp; **Fellow:** Pediatric Oncology, St Jude Chldns Hosp

Visconti, Ernest MD (Ped) *PCP* - **Spec Exp:** Infectious Disease; **Hospital:** Lutheran Med Ctr - Brooklyn, Richmond Univ Med Ctr; **Address:** 314 Seaview Ave, Staten Island, NY 10305-2246; **Phone:** 718-668-3417; **Board Cert:** Pediatrics 1992; Pediatric Infectious Disease 2009; **Med School:** SUNY Upstate Med Univ 1971; **Resid:** Pediatrics, New York Hosp 1974; **Fellow:** Infectious Disease, Rhode Island Hosp 1978

Physical Medicine & Rehabilitation

Weinberg, Jeffrey B MD (PMR) - **Spec Exp:** Geriatric Rehabilitation; Musculoskeletal Injuries; **Hospital:** Staten Island Univ Hosp - North; **Address:** Staten Island Univ Hosp, Dept Rehab Med, 475 Seaview Ave, Staten Island, NY 10314; **Phone:** 718-226-6362; **Board Cert:** Physical Medicine & Rehabilitation 1985; **Med School:** NY Med Coll 1980; **Resid:** Physical Medicine & Rehabilitation, NYU Med Ctr 1983; **Fellow:** Geriatric Medicine, NYU Med Ctr 1986; **Fac Appt:** Asst Clin Prof PMR, SUNY Downstate

Plastic Surgery

Cherofsky, Alan MD (PlS) - **Spec Exp:** Breast Surgery; Pediatric Plastic Surgery; Cosmetic Surgery-Body; **Hospital:** Staten Island Univ Hosp - South, Richmond Univ Med Ctr; **Address:** 4546 Hylan Blvd, Staten Island, NY 10312-6400; **Phone:** 718-967-3300; **Board Cert:** Plastic Surgery 1993; **Med School:** SUNY Hlth Sci Ctr 1982; **Resid:** Surgery, Staten Island Univ Hosp 1987; Plastic Surgery, Univ Missouri Hosp 1989

Cutolo Jr, Louis C MD (PlS) - **Spec Exp:** Breast Augmentation; Liposuction; Eyelid Surgery; Cosmetic Surgery-Face & Neck; **Hospital:** Staten Island Univ Hosp - North, Long Island Coll Hosp (page 94); **Address:** 1557 Victory Blvd, Staten Island, NY 10314; **Phone:** 718-720-9400; **Board Cert:** Plastic Surgery 2003; **Med School:** SUNY Downstate 1985; **Resid:** Surgery, Staten Island Hosp 1990; **Fellow:** Plastic Surgery, Univ Florida/Shands Hosp 1992

Psychiatry

Di Buono, Mark MD (Psyc) - **Spec Exp:** Geriatric Psychiatry; Depression; Autism; **Address:** Richmond Behavioral Assocs, 4349 Hylan Blvd, Staten Island, NY 10312; **Phone:** 718-227-1897; **Board Cert:** Psychiatry 1990; Geriatric Psychiatry 2008; **Med School:** Mexico 1981; **Resid:** Psychiatry, Stony Brook Univ Hosp 1986; **Fac Appt:** Asst Clin Prof Psyc, SUNY Downstate

Pulmonary Disease

Castellano, Michael A MD (Pul) - **Spec Exp:** Asthma; Emphysema; **Hospital:** Staten Island Univ Hosp - North; **Address:** 501 Seaview Ave, Ste 102, Staten Island, NY 10305; **Phone:** 718-980-5700; **Board Cert:** Internal Medicine 1974; Pulmonary Disease 1978; Critical Care Medicine 2007; Geriatric Medicine 2004; **Med School:** Italy 1968; **Resid:** Internal Medicine, Staten Island Hosp 1972; **Fellow:** Pulmonary Disease, NYU-Bellvue Hosp 1974; **Fac Appt:** Asst Prof Med, SUNY Downstate

Maniatis, Theodore MD (Pul) - **Spec Exp:** Asthma; Lung Cancer; Chronic Obstructive Lung Disease (COPD); Interstitial Lung Disease; **Hospital:** Staten Island Univ Hosp - North, Staten Island Univ Hosp - South; **Address:** 501 Seaview Ave, Ste 102, Staten Island, NY 10305; **Phone:** 718-980-5700; **Board Cert:** Internal Medicine 1983; Pulmonary Disease 1986; Critical Care Medicine 2007; **Med School:** SUNY Hlth Sci Ctr 1980; **Resid:** Internal Medicine, Staten Island Univ Hosp 1983; **Fellow:** Pulmonary Disease, UMDNJ Med Ctr 1985; **Fac Appt:** Asst Clin Prof Med, SUNY Downstate

Martins, Publius MD (Pul) - **Spec Exp:** Asthma; Emphysema; **Hospital:** Richmond Univ Med Ctr; **Address:** 283 Bard Ave, Staten Island, NY 10310-1664; **Phone:** 718-816-8068; **Board Cert:** Internal Medicine 1984; **Med School:** Portugal 1975; **Resid:** Internal Medicine, St Vincent's Hosp 1981; **Fellow:** Pulmonary Disease, Meml Hosp 1983; **Fac Appt:** Assoc Clin Prof Med, NY Med Coll

Sasso, Louis MD (Pul) - **Spec Exp:** Asthma; Chronic Obstructive Lung Disease (COPD); Interstitial Lung Disease; **Hospital:** Staten Island Univ Hosp - North; **Address:** 501 Seaview Ave, Staten Island, NY 10305-3400; **Phone:** 718-980-5700; **Board Cert:** Internal Medicine 1976; Pulmonary Disease 1978; Critical Care Medicine 2005; Geriatric Medicine 2009; **Med School:** UMDNJ-NJ Med Sch, Newark 1972; **Resid:** Internal Medicine, St Vincent's Hosp & Med Ctr 1974; Internal Medicine, CMDNJ-Martland Hosp 1975; **Fellow:** Pulmonary Disease, Bellevue Hosp/NYU Med Ctr 1977; **Fac Appt:** Asst Clin Prof Med, SUNY Downstate

Radiation Oncology

Adams, Marc MD (RadRO) - **Spec Exp:** Prostate Cancer; Breast Cancer; Lung Cancer; Brain Tumors; **Hospital:** Richmond Univ Med Ctr; **Address:** 360 Bard Ave, Staten Island, NY 10310; **Phone:** 718-876-2023; **Board Cert:** Radiation Oncology 1990; **Med School:** Univ Alabama 1985; **Resid:** Radiation Oncology, St Barnabas Hosp 1989; **Fac Appt:** Asst Prof RadRO, NY Med Coll

Rheumatology

Goldstein, Mark A MD (Rhu) - **Spec Exp:** Rheumatoid Arthritis; Osteoporosis; Lupus/SLE; **Hospital:** Staten Island Univ Hosp - South, Richmond Univ Med Ctr; **Address:** 1534 Victory Blvd, Staten Island, NY 10314; **Phone:** 718-447-0055; **Board Cert:** Internal Medicine 1982; Rheumatology 1988; **Med School:** NY Med Coll 1979; **Resid:** Internal Medicine, Montefiore Med Ctr 1980; Internal Medicine, Montefiore Med Ctr 1982; **Fellow:** Critical Care Medicine, Montefiore Med Ctr 1983; Rheumatology, Montefiore Med Ctr 1987

Jarrett, Mark MD (Rhu) - **Spec Exp:** Lupus/SLE; Osteoporosis; Rheumatoid Arthritis; **Hospital:** Staten Island Univ Hosp - North; **Address:** 500 Seaview Ave, Ste 110, Staten Island, NY 10305; **Phone:** 718-447-0055; **Board Cert:** Internal Medicine 1978; Rheumatology 1980; Geriatric Medicine 2008; **Med School:** NYU Sch Med 1975; **Resid:** Internal Medicine, Montefiore Med Ctr 1978; **Fellow:** Rheumatology, Montefiore Med Ctr 1980; **Fac Appt:** Asst Clin Prof Med, SUNY Downstate

Surgery

D'Anna, John MD (S) - **Spec Exp:** Vascular Surgery; **Hospital:** Staten Island Univ Hosp - North, Staten Island Univ Hosp - South; **Address:** 256 Mason Ave B Bldg, Staten Island, NY 10305; **Phone:** 718-226-6398; **Board Cert:** Surgery 2002; **Med School:** Georgetown Univ 1977; **Resid:** Surgery, St Vincent's Hosp Med Ctr 1982; **Fellow:** Vascular Surgery, St Vincent's Hosp Med Ctr 1983; **Fac Appt:** Assoc Clin Prof S, SUNY Downstate

Hornyak, Stephen W MD (S) - **Spec Exp:** Breast Surgery; Laparoscopic Surgery; Gastrointestinal Surgery; **Hospital:** Staten Island Univ Hosp - North, Richmond Univ Med Ctr; **Address:** 1130 Victory Blvd, Staten Island, NY 10301; **Phone:** 718-442-3400; **Board Cert:** Surgery 1999; **Med School:** SUNY Hlth Sci Ctr 1974; **Resid:** Surgery, Kings County Hosp 1979; **Fellow:** Research, Meml Sloan Kettering Cancer Ctr 1980; **Fac Appt:** Asst Clin Prof S, SUNY Downstate

Pahuja, Murlidhar MD (S) - **Spec Exp:** Breast Cancer; Laparoscopic Surgery; Wound Healing/Care; **Hospital:** Staten Island Univ Hosp - North, Staten Island Univ Hosp - South; **Address:** 4287 Richmond Ave, Staten Island, NY 10312; **Phone:** 718-967-6230; **Board Cert:** Surgery 2004; **Med School:** Pakistan 1971; **Resid:** Surgery, Stamford Hosp 1978; Surgery, Staten Island Hosp 1982; **Fellow:** Burn Surgery, NY Hosp 1980

Thoracic Surgery

Harris, Loren MD (TS) - **Spec Exp:** Thoracic Cancers; Esophageal Cancer; **Hospital:** Richmond Univ Med Ctr; **Address:** 355 Bard Ave, Staten Island, NY 10310; **Phone:** 718-818-2420; **Board Cert:** Thoracic Surgery 2006; **Med School:** NYU Sch Med 1987; **Resid:** Surgery, NYU Med Ctr 1994; **Fellow:** Cardiovascular Surgery, NYU Med Ctr 1996; **Fac Appt:** Asst Prof S, Albert Einstein Coll Med

McGinn Jr, Joseph MD (TS) - **Spec Exp:** Cardiothoracic Surgery; **Hospital:** Staten Island Univ Hosp - North, Richmond Univ Med Ctr; **Address:** 501 Seaview Ave, Ste 202, Staten Island, NY 10305; **Phone:** 718-226-1612; **Board Cert:** Surgery 2009; Thoracic Surgery 2009; Surgical Critical Care 2003; **Med School:** SUNY Downstate 1981; **Resid:** Surgery, Downstate Med Ctr 1985; Thoracic Surgery, LIJ Med Ctr 1987; **Fellow:** Cardiothoracic Surgery, LIJ Med Ctr 1988; **Fac Appt:** Asst Clin Prof S, SUNY Downstate

Rosell, Frank M MD (TS) - **Hospital:** Staten Island Univ Hosp - North; **Address:** 501 Seaview Ave, Ste 202, Staten Island, NY 10305; **Phone:** 718-226-6210; **Board Cert:** Thoracic Surgery 2001; Surgery 2006; **Med School:** NYU Sch Med 1992; **Resid:** Surgery, NY Med Coll 1997; **Fellow:** Thoracic Surgery, Long Island Jewish Med Ctr 2000

Urology

Lessing, Jeffrey MD (U) - **Spec Exp:** Prostate Disease; Impotence; Kidney Stones; Infertility-Male; **Hospital:** Staten Island Univ Hosp - North, Staten Island Univ Hosp - South; **Address:** 78 Todt Hill Rd, Ste 112, Staten Island, NY 10312; **Phone:** 718-448-3880; **Board Cert:** Urology 1982; **Med School:** NYU Sch Med 1975; **Resid:** Surgery, New York Univ Med Ctr 1977; Urology, Mount Sinai Hosp 1980

Raboy, Adley MD (U) - **Spec Exp:** Prostate Disease; Kidney Stones; Minimally Invasive Surgery; **Hospital:** Staten Island Univ Hosp - North, Staten Island Univ Hosp - South; **Address:** 1460 Victory Blvd, Staten Island, NY 10301-3914; **Phone:** 718-273-8100; **Board Cert:** Urology 2002; **Med School:** SUNY Downstate 1984; **Resid:** Surgery, Staten Island Hosp 1986; **Fellow:** Urology, Univ Hosp 1990; **Fac Appt:** Asst Clin Prof U, SUNY Downstate

Savino, Michael MD (U) - **Spec Exp:** Robotic Surgery; Prostate Cancer; Kidney Stones; Laparoscopic Surgery; **Hospital:** Staten Island Univ Hosp - North, Maimonides Med Ctr (page 98); **Address:** 78 Todt Hill Rd, Ste 112, Staten Island, NY 10314-4528; **Phone:** 718-448-3880; **Board Cert:** Urology 2007; **Med School:** Mexico 1979; **Resid:** Surgery, Maimonides Med Ctr 1982; Urology, Maimonides Med Ctr 1985

Vascular Surgery

Deitch, Jonathan MD (VascS) - **Spec Exp:** Aneurysm-Aortic; Carotid Artery Surgery; Endovascular Surgery; **Hospital:** Staten Island Univ Hosp - North; **Address:** 256 Mason Ave B Bldg Fl 2, Staten Island, NY 10305; **Phone:** 718-226-6800; **Board Cert:** Vascular Surgery 2000; Surgery 1998; **Med School:** NY Med Coll 1991; **Resid:** Surgery, Montefiore Med Ctr 1996; **Fellow:** Vascular Surgery, Wake Forest Univ 1998; Endovascular Surgery, UMDNJ 1998

Rodino, William MD (VascS) - **Hospital:** New York Methodist Hosp (page 404); **Address:** 8120 15th Ave, Brooklyn, NY 11228; **Phone:** 718-259-3436; **Board Cert:** Surgery 2006; Vascular Surgery 2007; **Med School:** SUNY Downstate 1990; **Resid:** Surgery, SUNY Hlth Sci Ctr 1995; **Fellow:** Vascular Surgery, SUNY Hlth Sci Ctr 1997

Nassau

Adolescent Medicine

Arden, Martha MD (AM) - **Spec Exp:** Adolescent Gynecology; Nutrition; Eating Disorders; **Hospital:** Steven & Alexandra Cohen Chldn's Med Ctr of NY, N Shore Univ Hosp; **Address:** 2001 Marcus Ave, Ste N204, New Hyde Park, NY 11040; **Phone:** 347-882-1321; **Board Cert:** Pediatrics 2003; Adolescent Medicine 2009; **Med School:** Yale Univ 1984; **Resid:** Pediatrics, Babies Hosp 1987; **Fellow:** Adolescent Medicine, Schneider Chldn's Hosp 1990; **Fac Appt:** Assoc Clin Prof Ped, Albert Einstein Coll Med

Fisher, Martin M MD (AM) - **Spec Exp:** Eating Disorders; Chronic Fatigue Syndrome; **Hospital:** Steven & Alexandra Cohen Chldn's Med Ctr of NY, N Shore Univ Hosp; **Address:** 410 Lakeville Rd, Ste 108, New Hyde Park, NY 11040; **Phone:** 516-465-3270; **Board Cert:** Pediatrics 1979; Adolescent Medicine 2009; **Med School:** Albert Einstein Coll Med 1975; **Resid:** Pediatrics, LIJ Med Ctr 1978; **Fellow:** Adolescent Medicine, LIJ Med Ctr 1980; **Fac Appt:** Prof Ped, NYU Sch Med

Jacobson, Marc S MD (AM) - **Spec Exp:** Cholesterol/Lipid Disorders; Obesity; Preventive Cardiology; **Address:** 1300 Union Turnpike, Ste 301, New Hyde Park, NY 11040; **Phone:** 516-829-8600; **Board Cert:** Pediatrics 1983; Adolescent Medicine 2009; **Med School:** Univ Kans 1973; **Resid:** Pediatrics, Univ Kansas Med Ctr 1976; **Fellow:** Adolescent Medicine, Univ Maryland Hosp 1979; **Fac Appt:** Prof Ped, Albert Einstein Coll Med

Levin Carmine, Linda MD (AM) - **Spec Exp:** AIDS/HIV in Adolescents; **Hospital:** Steven & Alexandra Cohen Chldn's Med Ctr of NY; **Address:** Steven Alexandra Cohen Chldns Med Ctr, Adolescent Med, 410 Lakeville Rd, Ste 108, New Hyde Park, NY 11042; **Phone:** 516-465-3270; **Board Cert:** Pediatrics 1987; Adolescent Medicine 2009; **Med School:** NYU Sch Med 1982; **Resid:** Pediatrics, Montefiore Hosp Med Ctr 1985; **Fellow:** Adolescent Medicine, Montefiore Hosp Med Ctr 1986

Allergy & Immunology

Boxer, Mitchell MD (A&I) - **Spec Exp:** Asthma; Drug Sensitivity; Allergic Aspergillosis; Churg-Strauss Vasculitis; **Hospital:** Long Island Jewish Med Ctr; **Address:** 2001 Marcus Ave, rm N220, Lake Success, NY 11042; **Phone:** 516-482-0910; **Board Cert:** Internal Medicine 1984; Allergy & Immunology 1987; **Med School:** NY Med Coll 1981; **Resid:** Internal Medicine, LI Jewish Med Ctr 1984; **Fellow:** Allergy & Immunology, Northwestern Meml Med Ctr 1987; **Fac Appt:** Asst Clin Prof Med, Albert Einstein Coll Med

Corriel, Robert N MD (A&I) - **Spec Exp:** Asthma & Allergy; Sinus Disorders; Rhinitis; Food Allergy; **Hospital:** N Shore Univ Hosp, Long Island Jewish Med Ctr; **Address:** 1129 Northern Blvd, Manhasset, NY 11030-3527; **Phone:** 516-365-6077; **Board Cert:** Pediatrics 1983; Allergy & Immunology 1985; **Med School:** Wake Forest Univ 1976; **Resid:** Pediatrics, N Shore Univ Hosp 1979; **Fellow:** Allergy & Immunology, Univ Tex Hlth Sci Ctr 1981; **Fac Appt:** Asst Clin Prof Ped, NYU Sch Med

Edwards, Bruce L MD (A&I) - **Spec Exp:** Asthma; Sinus Disorders; Food Allergy; **Hospital:** Long Island Jewish Med Ctr, Plainview Hosp; **Address:** 700 Old Country Rd, Ste 105, Plainview, NY 11803-4932; **Phone:** 516-933-1125; **Board Cert:** Allergy & Immunology 2009; **Med School:** Case West Res Univ 1984; **Resid:** Pediatrics, Babies Hosp/Columbia Presby 1987; **Fellow:** Allergy & Immunology, Schneider Chldns Hosp-LIJ 1989

Fonacier, Luz MD (A&I) - **Spec Exp:** Drug Sensitivity; Skin Allergies; Asthma & Allergy; **Hospital:** Winthrop - Univ Hosp; **Address:** 120 Mineola Blvd, Ste 410, Mineola, NY 11501; **Phone:** 516-663-2097; **Board Cert:** Internal Medicine 1989; Allergy & Immunology 2001; **Med School:** Philippines 1978; **Resid:** Dermatology, Univ Philippines 1983; Internal Medicine, Lutheran Med Ctr 1989; **Fellow:** Dermatology, NYU Med Ctr 1986; Allergy & Immunology, NY Hosp-Cornell Med Ctr 1991; **Fac Appt:** Assoc Prof A&I, SUNY Stony Brook

Frieri, Marianne MD/PhD (A&I) - **Spec Exp:** Asthma; Food Allergy; Immune Deficiency; Rhinitis; **Hospital:** N Shore Univ Hosp, Nassau Univ Med Ctr; **Address:** 566 Broadway, Massapequa, NY 11758; **Phone:** 516-541-6262; **Board Cert:** Internal Medicine 1984; Allergy & Immunology 1985; Clinical & Laboratory Immunology 1990; **Med School:** Loyola Univ-Stritch Sch Med 1978; **Resid:** Internal Medicine, St Josephs Hosp 1980; **Fellow:** Allergy & Immunology, NIH/NIAID 1983; **Fac Appt:** Prof Med, SUNY Stony Brook

Goldstein, Stanley MD (A&I) - **Spec Exp:** Asthma; Pulmonary Disease; **Hospital:** Long Island Jewish Med Ctr, Mercy Med Ctr - Rockville Centre; **Address:** 242 Merrick Rd, Ste 401, Rockville Centre, NY 11570; **Phone:** 516-536-7336; **Board Cert:** Pediatrics 1979; Allergy & Immunology 1981; Pediatric Pulmonology 2004; **Med School:** NY Med Coll 1975; **Resid:** Pediatrics, LI Jewish Med Ctr 1978; **Fellow:** Allergy & Immunology, Chldns Hosp 1982

Lang, Paul MD (A&I) - **Spec Exp:** Asthma; Food Allergy; Insect Allergies; **Hospital:** N Shore Univ Hosp, Winthrop - Univ Hosp; **Address:** One Hollow Lane, Ste 110, New Hyde Park, NY 11042; **Phone:** 516-365-6666; **Board Cert:** Pediatrics 1978; Allergy & Immunology 1979; **Med School:** Cornell Univ-Weill Med Coll 1973; **Resid:** Pediatrics, USC Med Ctr 1975; Allergy & Immunology, Roosevelt Hosp 1977; **Fac Appt:** Assoc Clin Prof Ped, NYU Sch Med

Markovics, Sharon B MD (A&I) - **Spec Exp:** Allergy; Asthma; Rhinitis; Sinus Disorders; **Hospital:** N Shore Univ Hosp, Long Island Jewish Med Ctr; **Address:** 1129 Northern Blvd, Ste 300, Manhasset, NY 11030-3527; **Phone:** 516-365-6077; **Board Cert:** Pediatrics 1979; Allergy & Immunology 1981; **Med School:** Albert Einstein Coll Med 1975; **Resid:** Pediatrics, Bellevue Hosp 1977; **Fellow:** Allergy & Immunology, Montreal Chldns Hosp 1979; **Fac Appt:** Asst Clin Prof Ped, NYU Sch Med

Novick, Brian MD (A&I) - **Spec Exp:** Asthma-Adult & Pediatric; Sinus Disorders; Food Allergy; Hives; **Hospital:** Montefiore Med Ctr - Div. Moses (page 100), Lenox Hill Hosp; **Address:** 30 Newbridge Rd, Ste 101, East Meadow, NY 11554; **Phone:** 516-731-5740; **Board Cert:** Pediatrics 1984; Allergy & Immunology 1999; **Med School:** Mexico 1978; **Resid:** Pediatrics, Albert Einstein Coll Med 1982; **Fellow:** Allergy & Immunology, Albert Einstein Coll Med 1984; **Fac Appt:** Asst Clin Prof A&I, Albert Einstein Coll Med

Sicklick, Marc MD (A&I) - **Spec Exp:** Asthma; Allergy; Immune Deficiency; **Hospital:** N Shore Univ Hosp, Long Island Jewish Med Ctr; **Address:** 123 Grove Ave, Ste 110, Cedarhurst, NY 11516-2302; **Phone:** 516-569-5550; **Board Cert:** Pediatrics 1979; Allergy & Immunology 1987; **Med School:** Albert Einstein Coll Med 1974; **Resid:** Pediatrics, Bronx Muni Hosp Ctr 1977; **Fellow:** Allergy & Immunology, Montefiore Med Ctr 1979; **Fac Appt:** Assoc Clin Prof Ped, Albert Einstein Coll Med

Weinstock, Gary A MD (A&I) - **Spec Exp:** Asthma; Allergy; Hives; **Hospital:** N Shore Univ Hosp, Glen Cove Hosp; **Address:** 310 E Shore Rd, Ste 207, Great Neck, NY 11023-2432; **Phone:** 516-487-1073; **Board Cert:** Internal Medicine 1982; Pulmonary Disease 1984; Allergy & Immunology 1985; **Med School:** Albany Med Coll 1979; **Resid:** Internal Medicine, North Shore Univ/Meml Sloan Kettering Cancer Ctr 1982; **Fellow:** Pulmonary Disease, SUNY-Stony Brook 1983; Allergy & Immunology, SUNY-Stony Brook 1986; **Fac Appt:** Asst Clin Prof Med, NYU Sch Med

Cardiac Electrophysiology

Jadonath, Ram L MD (CE) - **Spec Exp:** Arrhythmias; Atrial Fibrillation; Pacemakers; Defibrillators; **Hospital:** N Shore Univ Hosp; **Address:** 300 Community Drive, Manhasset, NY 11030; **Phone:** 516-562-2300; **Board Cert:** Internal Medicine 1989; Cardiovascular Disease 2006; Cardiac Electrophysiology 2006; **Med School:** Columbia P&S 1986; **Resid:** Internal Medicine, St Lukes Hosp 1989; **Fellow:** Cardiovascular Disease, St Lukes/Roosevelt Hosps 1992; Cardiac Electrophysiology, /Philadelphia Heart Inst 1993; **Fac Appt:** Assoc Prof Med, Albert Einstein Coll Med

Levine, Joseph H MD (CE) - **Spec Exp:** Arrhythmias; Sudden Death Prevention; Atrial Fibrillation; Pacemakers; **Hospital:** St Francis Hosp - The Heart Ctr (page 115); **Address:** 100 Port Washington Blvd, Roslyn, NY 11576; **Phone:** 516-622-1011; **Board Cert:** Internal Medicine 1983; Cardiovascular Disease 1987; Cardiac Electrophysiology 2003; **Med School:** Univ Rochester 1980; **Resid:** Internal Medicine, Yale-New Haven Hosp 1983; **Fellow:** Cardiovascular Disease, Johns Hopkins Hosp 1986; Cardiac Electrophysiology, Hosp Univ Penn 1986

Cardiovascular Disease

Anto, Maliakal Joseph MD (Cv) - **Spec Exp:** Hypertension; Coronary Artery Disease; Non-Invasive Cardiology; Congestive Heart Failure; **Hospital:** Syosset Hosp, Plainview Hosp; **Address:** 8 Greenfield Rd, Syosset, NY 11791; **Phone:** 516-496-7900; **Board Cert:** Internal Medicine 1980; Cardiovascular Disease 1989; **Med School:** India 1974; **Resid:** Internal Medicine, Our Lady of Mercy Med Ctr 1979; **Fellow:** Cardiovascular Disease, Nassau County Med Ctr 1981

Breen, William J MD (Cv) - **Spec Exp:** Echocardiography; **Hospital:** Plainview Hosp; **Address:** 43 Crossways Park Dr, Woodbury, NY 11797; **Phone:** 516-938-3000; **Board Cert:** Internal Medicine 1980; Cardiovascular Disease 1983; **Med School:** NY Med Coll 1977; **Resid:** Internal Medicine, North Shore Univ Hosp 1980; **Fellow:** Cardiovascular Disease, North Shore Univ Hosp 1982; **Fac Appt:** Assoc Prof Med, NYU Sch Med

Chadda, Kul MD (Cv) - **Hospital:** South Nassau Comm Hosp, Wyckoff Heights Med Ctr; **Address:** South Nassau Comm Hosp, Electrophysiology Svcs, 1 Healthy Way, Oceanside, NY 11572; **Phone:** 516-632-3418; **Board Cert:** Internal Medicine 1974; Cardiovascular Disease 1977; **Med School:** India 1966; **Resid:** Internal Medicine, Elmhurst City Hosp 1972; Cardiovascular Disease, Prebyterian Hosp 1973; **Fac Appt:** Clin Prof Med, SUNY Stony Brook

Chesner, Michael D MD (Cv) - **Spec Exp:** Preventive Cardiology; Cholesterol/Lipid Disorders; Cardiac Stress Testing; **Hospital:** Long Beach Med Ctr; **Address:** 325 W Park Ave, Long Beach, NY 11561-3223; **Phone:** 516-432-2004; **Board Cert:** Internal Medicine 2004; Cardiovascular Disease 2007; **Med School:** Albert Einstein Coll Med 1987; **Resid:** Internal Medicine, Bronx Municipal Hosp 1990; **Fellow:** Cardiovascular Disease, LI Jewish Hosp 1993; **Fac Appt:** Assoc Prof Med, NY Coll Osteo Med

Cramer, Marvin MD (Cv) - **Spec Exp:** Coronary Artery Disease; Echocardiography; Stress Echocardiography; **Hospital:** N Shore Univ Hosp, St Francis Hosp - The Heart Ctr (page 115); **Address:** 225 Community Drive, Ste 130, Great Neck, NY 11021; **Phone:** 516-504-0474; **Board Cert:** Internal Medicine 1974; Cardiovascular Disease 1977; Nuclear Cardiology 2005; Echocardiography 2007; **Med School:** Jefferson Med Coll 1969; **Resid:** Internal Medicine, St Lukes Med Ctr 1973; **Fellow:** Cardiovascular Disease, Columbia-Presby Med Ctr 1976; **Fac Appt:** Assoc Clin Prof Med, NYU Sch Med

D'Agostino, Ronald DO (Cv) - **Spec Exp:** Hypertension; Cholesterol/Lipid Disorders; Mitral Valve Disease; **Hospital:** Long Island Jewish Med Ctr, N Shore Univ Hosp; **Address:** 1129 Northern Blvd, Ste 408, Manhasset, NY 11030-3022; **Phone:** 516-627-2121; **Board Cert:** Internal Medicine 2000; Cardiovascular Disease 2000; **Med School:** NY Coll Osteo Med 1985; **Resid:** Internal Medicine, Long Island Jewish Hosp 1989; Internal Medicine, Long Island Jewish Hosp 1993; **Fellow:** Cardiovascular Disease, Long Island Jewish Hosp 1992; **Fac Appt:** Asst Prof Med, NY Coll Osteo Med

Davison, Edward MD (Cv) - **Spec Exp:** Geriatric Cardiology; **Hospital:** Franklin Hosp, St Francis Hosp - The Heart Ctr (page 115); **Address:** 300 Franklin Ave, Valley Stream, NY 11580; **Phone:** 516-599-8280; **Board Cert:** Internal Medicine 1966; Cardiovascular Disease 1977; **Med School:** Bowman Gray 1959; **Resid:** Internal Medicine, Maimonides Med Ctr 1963; **Fellow:** Cardiovascular Disease, Mt Sinai Hosp 1965

Dresdale, Robert J MD (Cv) - **Spec Exp:** Heart Disease in Women; Pulmonary Hypertension; **Hospital:** N Shore Univ Hosp, St Francis Hosp - The Heart Ctr (page 115); **Address:** 225 Community Drive, Ste 130, Great Neck, NY 11021-5506; **Phone:** 516-504-0474; **Board Cert:** Internal Medicine 1975; Cardiovascular Disease 1977; **Med School:** Columbia P&S 1972; **Resid:** Internal Medicine, Columbia-Presby Med Ctr 1974; **Fellow:** Cardiovascular Disease, Columbia-Presby Med Ctr 1976; **Fac Appt:** Assoc Clin Prof Med, NYU Sch Med

Ezratty, Ari M MD (Cv) - **Spec Exp:** Interventional Cardiology; **Hospital:** St Francis Hosp - The Heart Ctr (page 115); **Address:** 100 Port Washington Blvd, Roslyn, NY 11576; **Phone:** 516-570-6907; **Board Cert:** Internal Medicine 1988; Cardiovascular Disease 2002; **Med School:** Mount Sinai Sch Med 1985; **Resid:** Internal Medicine, Mt Sinai Hosp 1989; **Fellow:** Cardiovascular Disease, Brigham & Womens Hosp 1992; Interventional Cardiology, Mt Sinai Hosp 1994

Fein, Frederick S MD (Cv) - **Spec Exp:** Heart Disease; **Hospital:** Winthrop - Univ Hosp; **Address:** 120 Mineola Blvd, Ste 500, Mineola, NY 11501; **Phone:** 516-663-4480; **Board Cert:** Internal Medicine 1975; Cardiovascular Disease 1977; **Med School:** NYU Sch Med 1972; **Resid:** Internal Medicine, Montefiore Hosp Med Ctr 1975; **Fellow:** Cardiovascular Disease, Montefiore Hosp Med Ctr 1977; **Fac Appt:** Assoc Prof Med, Albert Einstein Coll Med

Gindea, Aaron MD (Cv) - **Spec Exp:** Heart Valve Disease; Congestive Heart Failure; Congenital Heart Disease; **Hospital:** St Francis Hosp - The Heart Ctr (page 115), N Shore Univ Hosp; **Address:** 800 Community Drive, Manhasset, NY 11030-3803; **Phone:** 516-627-6622; **Board Cert:** Internal Medicine 1985; Cardiovascular Disease 1989; **Med School:** NYU Sch Med 1982; **Resid:** Internal Medicine, Bellevue Hosp 1985; **Fellow:** Cardiovascular Disease, Bellevue Hosp 1987; **Fac Appt:** Assoc Clin Prof Med, NYU Sch Med

Gleckel, Louis W MD (Cv) - **Spec Exp:** Preventive Cardiology; Cardiac Stress Testing; Cholesterol/Lipid Disorders; Hypertension; **Hospital:** Long Island Jewish Med Ctr, Forest Hills Hosp; **Address:** 2 Ohio Drive, Lake Success, NY 11042-1052; **Phone:** 516-622-6060; **Board Cert:** Internal Medicine 1986; **Med School:** SUNY Hlth Sci Ctr 1983; **Resid:** Internal Medicine, LI Jewish Hosp 1986; **Fellow:** Cardiovascular Disease, LI Jewish Hosp 1988; **Fac Appt:** Asst Prof Med, Albert Einstein Coll Med

Goldberg, Steven Mark MD (Cv) - **Spec Exp:** Cholesterol/Lipid Disorders; Preventive Cardiology; **Hospital:** N Shore Univ Hosp; **Address:** 1010 Northern Blvd, Ste 110, Great Neck, NY 11021-5306; **Phone:** 516-390-2430; **Board Cert:** Internal Medicine 1982; Cardiovascular Disease 1985; **Med School:** Univ Pennsylvania 1979; **Resid:** Internal Medicine, N Shore Univ Hosp 1982; **Fellow:** Cardiovascular Disease, N Shore Univ Hosp 1984; **Fac Appt:** Assoc Prof Med, NYU Sch Med

Goodman, Mark A MD (Cv) - **Spec Exp:** Cholesterol/Lipid Disorders; Pacemakers/Defibrillators; Coronary Artery Disease; Congestive Heart Failure; **Hospital:** Winthrop - Univ Hosp, N Shore Univ Hosp; **Address:** 975 Stewart Ave, Garden City, NY 11530-4816; **Phone:** 516-222-8610; **Board Cert:** Internal Medicine 1972; Cardiovascular Disease 1973; **Med School:** SUNY Upstate Med Univ 1967; **Resid:** Internal Medicine, Montefiore Med Ctr 1969; Internal Medicine, Mt Sinai Hosp 1970; **Fellow:** Cardiovascular Disease, Montefiore Med Ctr 1972; **Fac Appt:** Assoc Clin Prof Med, SUNY Stony Brook

Green, Stephen J MD (Cv) - **Spec Exp:** Heart Attack; Angioplasty; Cholesterol/Lipid Disorders; Interventional Cardiology; **Hospital:** N Shore Univ Hosp, Long Island Jewish Med Ctr; **Address:** Dept Cardiology, 300 Community Drive, Manhasset, NY 11030; **Phone:** 516-562-4100; **Board Cert:** Internal Medicine 1983; Cardiovascular Disease 1985; Interventional Cardiology 1999; **Med School:** Tufts Univ 1980; **Resid:** Internal Medicine, N Shore Univ Hosp 1983; **Fellow:** Cardiovascular Disease, N Shore Univ Hosp 1985

Greenberg, Steven M MD (Cv) - **Spec Exp:** Pacemakers/Defibrillators; Arrhythmias; Congestive Heart Failure; **Hospital:** St Francis Hosp - The Heart Ctr (page 115); **Address:** 100 Port Washington Blvd, Arrhythmia Center, Roslyn, NY 11576-1353; **Phone:** 516-562-6672; **Board Cert:** Internal Medicine 1986; Cardiovascular Disease 1989; **Med School:** Albany Med Coll 1983; **Resid:** Internal Medicine, Bronx Muni Hosp Ctr 1987; **Fellow:** Cardiovascular Disease, Mt Sinai Med Ctr 1990

Hershman, Ronnie MD (Cv) - **Spec Exp:** Invasive Cardiology; **Hospital:** St Francis Hosp - The Heart Ctr (page 115); **Address:** 1 Hollow Ln, Ste 103, Lake Success, NY 11042; **Phone:** 516-869-5400; **Board Cert:** Internal Medicine 1985; Cardiovascular Disease 1987; **Med School:** Mount Sinai Sch Med 1982; **Resid:** Internal Medicine, Mt Sinai Med Ctr 1985; **Fellow:** Cardiovascular Disease, Mt Sinai Med Ctr 1989

Jelveh, Mansoor MD (Cv) - **Hospital:** N Shore Univ Hosp, St Joseph's Hosp-Nassau; **Address:** 875 Old Country Rd, Ste 102, Plainview, NY 11803; **Phone:** 516-935-8877; **Board Cert:** Internal Medicine 1975; Cardiovascular Disease 1977; **Med School:** Iran 1968; **Resid:** Internal Medicine, Nassau County Med Ctr 1975; **Fellow:** Cardiovascular Disease, Beth Israel 1977

Kobren, Steven M MD (Cv) - **Spec Exp:** Heart Failure; Mitral Valve Prolapse; Nuclear Stress Testing; **Hospital:** Long Island Jewish Med Ctr, St Francis Hosp - The Heart Ctr (page 115); **Address:** Great Neck Med Group, 488 Great Neck Rd, Great Neck, NY 11021-4308; **Phone:** 516-482-6747; **Board Cert:** Internal Medicine 1986; Cardiovascular Disease 1989; Critical Care Medicine 2001; Echocardiography 2007; **Med School:** SUNY Downstate 1983; **Resid:** Internal Medicine, LIJ Medical Ctr 1987; **Fellow:** Cardiovascular Disease, LIJ Medical Ctr 1990; **Fac Appt:** Asst Prof Med, Albert Einstein Coll Med

Koss, Jerome MD (Cv) - **Spec Exp:** Interventional Cardiology; Heart Valve Disease; Nuclear Cardiology; Atrial Fibrillation; **Hospital:** Long Island Jewish Med Ctr, St Francis Hosp - The Heart Ctr (page 115); **Address:** 3003 New Hyde Park Rd, Ste 406, New Hyde Park, NY 11042; **Phone:** 516-358-5401; **Board Cert:** Internal Medicine 1977; Cardiovascular Disease 1981; Interventional Cardiology 1999; **Med School:** Albert Einstein Coll Med 1974; **Resid:** Internal Medicine, Jacobi Med Ctr 1978; **Fellow:** Cardiovascular Disease, Montefiore Med Ctr 1980; **Fac Appt:** Asst Prof Med, Albert Einstein Coll Med

Lachmann, Justine S MD (Cv) - **Spec Exp:** Heart Failure; Pulmonary Hypertension; **Hospital:** Winthrop - Univ Hosp; **Address:** 120 Mineola Blvd, Ste 500, Mineola, NY 11501; **Phone:** 516-663-4481; **Board Cert:** Cardiovascular Disease 2001; **Med School:** UMDNJ-RW Johnson Med Sch 1995; **Resid:** Internal Medicine, NYU Med Ctr 1998; **Fellow:** Cardiovascular Disease, Montifiere Med Ctr 1998

Mintz, Guy L MD (Cv) - **Spec Exp:** Preventive Cardiology; Cholesterol/Lipid Disorders; Coronary Artery Disease; Hypertension; **Hospital:** N Shore Univ Hosp, St Francis Hosp - The Heart Ctr (page 115); **Address:** 287 Northern Blvd, Ste 211, Great Neck, NY 11021; **Phone:** 516-482-3401; **Board Cert:** Internal Medicine 1987; Cardiovascular Disease 2003; **Med School:** Boston Univ 1984; **Resid:** Internal Medicine, N Shore Univ Hosp 1987; **Fellow:** Cardiovascular Disease, N Shore Univ Hosp 1989; **Fac Appt:** Assoc Prof Med, NYU Sch Med

Nicosia, Thomas A MD (Cv) - **Spec Exp:** Coronary Artery Disease; Congestive Heart Failure; **Hospital:** St Francis Hosp - The Heart Ctr (page 115), N Shore Univ Hosp; **Address:** 1615 Northern Blvd, Ste 301, Manhasset, NY 11030; **Phone:** 516-627-9355; **Board Cert:** Internal Medicine 1979; Cardiovascular Disease 1981; **Med School:** Univ Cincinnati 1974; **Resid:** Internal Medicine, University Hosp 1978; **Fellow:** Cardiovascular Disease, Bellevue Hosp 1980

Pappas, Thomas W MD (Cv) - **Spec Exp:** Interventional Cardiology; Coronary Angioplasty/Stents; Angiography-Coronary; Cardiac Imaging; **Hospital:** St Francis Hosp - The Heart Ctr (page 115); **Address:** 100 Port Washington Blvd, Ste 105, Roslyn, NY 11576-1353; **Phone:** 516-390-9640; **Board Cert:** Internal Medicine 1986; Cardiovascular Disease 1989; Interventional Cardiology 2000; **Med School:** Cornell Univ-Weill Med Coll 1983; **Resid:** Internal Medicine, New York Hosp 1986; **Fellow:** Cardiovascular Disease, New York Hosp-Cornell 1988; Interventional Cardiology, NYU Med Ctr 1990

Ragno, Philip D MD (Cv) - **Spec Exp:** Cholesterol/Lipid Disorders; Congestive Heart Failure; **Hospital:** Winthrop - Univ Hosp, N Shore Univ Hosp; **Address:** 1300 Franklin Ave, Ste ML6, Garden City, NY 11501; **Phone:** 516-877-2626; **Board Cert:** Internal Medicine 1987; Cardiovascular Disease 1989; **Med School:** SUNY Stony Brook 1984; **Resid:** Internal Medicine, Winthrop Univ Hosp 1987; **Fellow:** Cardiovascular Disease, Winthrop Univ Hosp 1989

Rutkovsky, Edward V MD (Cv) - **Spec Exp:** Nuclear Stress Testing; Echocardiography; **Hospital:** N Shore Univ Hosp, St Francis Hosp - The Heart Ctr (page 115); **Address:** 2035 Lakeville Rd, Ste 101, New Hyde Park, NY 11040-1661; **Phone:** 516-328-9797; **Board Cert:** Internal Medicine 1987; Cardiovascular Disease 1989; **Med School:** NYU Sch Med 1984; **Resid:** Internal Medicine, NYU Med Ctr 1987; **Fellow:** Cardiovascular Disease, N Shore Univ Hosp 1989; **Fac Appt:** Asst Clin Prof Med, NYU Sch Med

Schreiber, Carl MD (Cv) - **Spec Exp:** Coronary Artery Disease; Nuclear Cardiology; Non-Invasive Cardiology; **Hospital:** Glen Cove Hosp, N Shore Univ Hosp; **Address:** 70 Glen St, Glen Cove, NY 11542-2853; **Phone:** 516-484-7893; **Board Cert:** Internal Medicine 1982; Cardiovascular Disease 1985; **Med School:** Med Coll GA 1979; **Resid:** Internal Medicine, Columbia-Presby Med Ctr 1982; **Fellow:** Cardiovascular Disease, Westchester Med Ctr 1984

Shlofmitz, Richard A MD (Cv) - **Spec Exp:** Interventional Cardiology; Cardiac Catheterization; **Hospital:** St Francis Hosp - The Heart Ctr (page 115); **Address:** 100 Port Washington Blvd, Ste 105, Roslyn, NY 11576; **Phone:** 516-390-9640; **Board Cert:** Internal Medicine 1984; Cardiovascular Disease 1987; **Med School:** NYU Sch Med 1980; **Resid:** Internal Medicine, North Shore Univ Hosp 1984; **Fellow:** Cardiovascular Disease, Columbia Presby Med Ctr 1987

Sokol, Sergio MD (Cv) - **Spec Exp:** Echocardiography; **Hospital:** St John's Epis Hosp - S Shore; **Address:** Five Towns Heart Imaging, 650 Central Ave, Ste K, Cedarhurst, NY 11516; **Phone:** 516-804-8590; **Board Cert:** Internal Medicine 2001; Cardiovascular Disease 2004; **Med School:** Israel 1994; **Resid:** Internal Medicine, Montefiore Med Ctr 1998; **Fellow:** Cardiovascular Disease, N Shore Univ Hosp 2001

Spadaro, Louise A MD (Cv) - **Spec Exp:** Preventive Cardiology; Heart Disease in Women; Cardiac Imaging; **Hospital:** St Francis Hosp - The Heart Ctr (page 115); **Address:** St Francis Hosp, 100 Port Washington Blvd, VIZZA Bldg - rm 101, Roslyn, NY 11576; **Phone:** 516-562-6653; **Board Cert:** Internal Medicine 1987; Cardiovascular Disease 1989; **Med School:** NYU Sch Med 1984; **Resid:** Internal Medicine, Bellevue Hosp 1987; **Fellow:** Cardiovascular Disease, Bellevue Hosp/NYU Med Ctr 1989

Tenet, William MD (Cv) - **Spec Exp:** Congestive Heart Failure; Coronary Artery Disease; **Hospital:** N Shore Univ Hosp, Lenox Hill Hosp; **Address:** 1155 Northern Blvd, Ste 330, Manhasset, NY 11030; **Phone:** 516-627-4330; **Board Cert:** Internal Medicine 1983; Cardiovascular Disease 1987; **Med School:** Italy 1980; **Resid:** Internal Medicine, Booth Meml Med Ctr 1984; **Fellow:** Cardiovascular Disease, Univ Conn Hlth Ctr 1986; **Fac Appt:** Asst Clin Prof Med, Cornell Univ-Weill Med Coll

Weg, Ira L MD (Cv) - **Spec Exp:** Congestive Heart Failure; Coronary Artery Disease; **Hospital:** South Nassau Comm Hosp; **Address:** 158 Hempstead Ave, Lynbrook, NY 11563; **Phone:** 516-593-3541; **Board Cert:** Internal Medicine 1979; Cardiovascular Disease 1981; Nuclear Cardiology 2000; **Med School:** SUNY Hlth Sci Ctr 1976; **Resid:** Internal Medicine, Kings County Hosp 1979; **Fellow:** Cardiovascular Disease, Montefiore Med Ctr 1981; **Fac Appt:** Asst Prof Med, Albert Einstein Coll Med

Zeldis, Steven M MD (Cv) - **Spec Exp:** Echocardiography; Cardiac Stress Testing; Cardiac Imaging; **Hospital:** Winthrop - Univ Hosp; **Address:** 200 Old Country Rd, Ste 278, Mineola, NY 11501-4298; **Phone:** 516-877-0977; **Board Cert:** Internal Medicine 1975; Cardiovascular Disease 1977; **Med School:** Yale Univ 1972; **Resid:** Internal Medicine, Yale Med Ctr 1975; **Fellow:** Cardiovascular Disease, Hosp Univ Penn 1977; **Fac Appt:** Assoc Prof Med, SUNY Stony Brook

Child & Adolescent Psychiatry

Foley, Carmel A MD (ChAP) - **Spec Exp:** Mood Disorders; **Hospital:** Steven & Alexandra Cohen Chldn's Med Ctr of NY; **Address:** 420 Lakeville Rd, 1st Floor, New Hyde Park, NY 11040; **Phone:** 718-470-3550; **Board Cert:** Psychiatry 1979; Child & Adolescent Psychiatry 1981; Forensic Psychiatry 1999; Psychosomatic Medicine 2009; **Med School:** Ireland 1972; **Resid:** Psychiatry, St Patrick's Hosp 1976; Psychiatry, Lafayette Clinic 1977; **Fellow:** Child & Adolescent Psychiatry, Lafayette Clinic 1979; **Fac Appt:** Assoc Prof Psyc, Albert Einstein Coll Med

Perlmutter, Ilisse R MD (ChAP) - **Spec Exp:** Disaster Psychiatry; Post Traumatic Stress Disorder; Depression in Adolescents; **Hospital:** Nassau Univ Med Ctr; **Address:** Nassau Univ Med Ctr, Dept Child & Adolescent Psychiatry, 2201 Hempstead Turnpike, East Meadow, NY 11554; **Phone:** 516-572-6511; **Board Cert:** Psychiatry 1989; Child & Adolescent Psychiatry 1991; **Med School:** Geo Wash Univ 1984; **Resid:** Psychiatry, Mt Sinai Med Ctr 1987; **Fellow:** Child & Adolescent Psychiatry, Columbia-Presby Med Ctr 1989

Williams, Daniel T MD (ChAP) - **Spec Exp:** Neuro-Psychiatry; Psychopharmacology; Psychosomatic Disorders; **Hospital:** NYPresby-Morgan Stanley Children's Hosp (page 104), Long Island Jewish Med Ctr; **Address:** 3003 New Hyde Park Rd, Ste 204, New Hyde Park, NY 11042; **Phone:** 516-488-3636; **Board Cert:** Psychiatry 1975; Child & Adolescent Psychiatry 1976; **Med School:** Cornell Univ-Weill Med Coll 1969; **Resid:** Psychiatry, Mount Sinai Hosp 1972; **Fellow:** Child & Adolescent Psychiatry, Columbia-Presby Hosp 1974

Child Neurology

Bergtraum, Marcia MD (ChiN) - **Hospital:** Long Island Jewish Med Ctr; **Address:** 3003 New Hyde Park Rd, Ste 204, New Hyde Park, NY 11042-1214; **Phone:** 516-488-2323; **Board Cert:** Pediatrics 1981; Child Neurology 1988; **Med School:** Georgetown Univ 1974; **Resid:** Pediatric Hematology-Oncology, LI Jewish Hosp 1978; Pediatric Neurology, LI Jewish Hosp 1982; **Fellow:** Child Neurology, Neur Inst/Columbia-Presby 1983

Eviatar, Lydia MD (ChiN) - **Spec Exp:** Balance Disorders; Tourette's Syndrome; Headache; Cerebral Palsy; **Hospital:** Steven & Alexandra Cohen Chldn's Med Ctr of NY; **Address:** 410 Lakeville Rd, Ste 105, New Hyde Park, NY 11042-1433; **Phone:** 516-465-5255; **Board Cert:** Pediatrics 1969; Child Neurology 1977; **Med School:** Israel 1961; **Resid:** Pediatrics, Tel Hashomer Hosp 1966; Neurology, Montefiore Med Ctr 1977; **Fellow:** Developmental-Behavioral Pediatrics, UCLA Med Ctr 1967; Pediatric Neurology, UCLA Med Ctr 1969; **Fac Appt:** Prof N, Albert Einstein Coll Med

Maytal, Joseph MD (ChiN) - **Spec Exp:** Epilepsy/Seizure Disorders; Migraine; **Hospital:** Steven & Alexandra Cohen Chldn's Med Ctr of NY; **Address:** Dept Pediatric Neurology, 410 Lakeville Rd, Ste 105, New Hyde Park, NY 11042; **Phone:** 516-465-5255; **Board Cert:** Pediatrics 1986; Child Neurology 1988; **Med School:** Israel 1979; **Resid:** Pediatrics, Brookdale Hosp 1983; Child Neurology, Montefiore Med Ctr 1986; **Fellow:** Neurological Physiology, Albert Einstein Med Coll 1987; **Fac Appt:** Clin Prof N, Albert Einstein Coll Med

Clinical Genetics

Bialer, Martin G MD/PhD (CG) - **Spec Exp:** Marfan's Syndrome; Neurofibromatosis; Metabolic Genetic Disorders; Cancer Genetics; **Hospital:** Steven & Alexandra Cohen Chldn's Med Ctr of NY, NS-LIJ Hlth Sys; **Address:** 1554 Northern Blvd, Ste 204, Manhasset, NY 11030; **Phone:** 516-365-3996; **Board Cert:** Pediatrics 1987; Clinical Biochemical Genetics 1990; Clinical Genetics 1990; **Med School:** Med Univ SC 1983; **Resid:** Pediatrics, N Shore Univ Hosp 1986; **Fellow:** Clinical Genetics, Univ VA Hlth Sci Ctr 1989; **Fac Appt:** Clin Prof Ped, NYU Sch Med

Fox, Joyce MD (CG) - **Hospital:** Long Island Jewish Med Ctr, Steven & Alexandra Cohen Chldn's Med Ctr of NY; **Address:** 1554 Northern Blvd, Ste 204, Manhasset, NY 11030; **Phone:** 516-365-3996; **Board Cert:** Pediatrics 1986; Clinical Genetics 1987; **Med School:** Columbia P&S 1980; **Resid:** Pediatrics, Case Western Univ Hosp 1983; **Fellow:** Clinical Genetics, Yale-New Haven Hosp 1986; **Fac Appt:** , Albert Einstein Coll Med

Colon & Rectal Surgery

Greenwald, Marc MD (CRS) - **Spec Exp:** Laparoscopic Surgery; Colonoscopy; Anorectal Disorders; Colon & Rectal Cancer; **Hospital:** N Shore Univ Hosp, St Francis Hosp - The Heart Ctr (page 115); **Address:** 310 E Shore Rd, Ste 203, Great Neck, NY 11023-2432; **Phone:** 516-482-8657; **Board Cert:** Surgery 2000; Colon & Rectal Surgery 2003; **Med School:** Albert Einstein Coll Med 1985; **Resid:** Surgery, Montefiore Hosp Med Ctr 1990; **Fellow:** Colon & Rectal Surgery, St Francis Hosp 1991

Kalafatic, Alfredo MD (CRS) - **Spec Exp:** Colonoscopy; Anorectal Disorders; **Hospital:** St Joseph's Hosp-Nassau, Plainview Hosp; **Address:** 4277 Hempstead Tpke, Ste 203, Bethpage, NY 11714-5706; **Phone:** 516-735-3001; **Board Cert:** Colon & Rectal Surgery 1983; **Med School:** Italy 1970; **Resid:** Surgery, LI Jewish Med Ctr 1979; **Fellow:** Colon & Rectal Surgery, New-Island Hosp 1981

Moseson, Michael MD (CRS) - **Spec Exp:** Anorectal Disorders; Colonoscopy/Polypectomy; **Hospital:** St Francis Hosp - The Heart Ctr (page 115), N Shore Univ Hosp; **Address:** 60 Cuttermill Rd, Ste 507, Great Neck, NY 11021; **Phone:** 516-487-8738; **Board Cert:** Colon & Rectal Surgery 1982; Surgery 2002; **Med School:** Spain 1975; **Resid:** Surgery, North Shore Univ Hosp 1980; Colon & Rectal Surgery, UMDNJ-RWJohnson Med Ctr 1981; **Fac Appt:** Asst Clin Prof S, Cornell Univ-Weill Med Coll

Procaccino Jr, John A MD (CRS) - **Spec Exp:** Inflammatory Bowel Disease/Crohn's; Colon & Rectal Cancer; Anorectal Disorders; Colon & Rectal Cancer-Familial Polyposis; **Hospital:** N Shore Univ Hosp, Long Island Jewish Med Ctr; **Address:** Chief, Division of Colon & Rectal Surg, 900 Northern Blvd, Ste 100, Great Neck, NY 11021; **Phone:** 516-730-2100; **Board Cert:** Colon & Rectal Surgery 2003; Surgery 1998; **Med School:** NYU Sch Med 1984; **Resid:** Surgery, N Shore Univ Hosp 1989; **Fellow:** Colon & Rectal Surgery, Cleveland Clin 1990; **Fac Appt:** Asst Clin Prof S, Cornell Univ-Weill Med Coll

Sullivan III, James D MD (CRS) - **Spec Exp:** Cancer Surgery; Colon & Rectal Cancer & Surgery; **Hospital:** N Shore Univ Hosp, St Francis Hosp - The Heart Ctr (page 115); **Address:** North Shore Oncology Associates, 600 Northern Blvd, Ste 111, Great Neck, NY 11021; **Phone:** 516-487-9454; **Board Cert:** Surgery 2004; Colon & Rectal Surgery 2005; **Med School:** NY Med Coll 1987; **Resid:** Surgery, N Shore Univ Hosp 1992; **Fellow:** Colon & Rectal Surgery, Cleveland Clinic 1993

Dermatology

Aprile, Georgette MD (D) - **Spec Exp:** Acne; Atopic Dermatitis; **Hospital:** Glen Cove Hosp; **Address:** 8 Med Plaza, Lower Level, Ste 103, Glen Cove, NY 11542; **Phone:** 516-759-9200; **Board Cert:** Dermatology 1978; **Med School:** NY Med Coll 1974; **Resid:** Dermatology, New York Hosp 1978

Bruckstein, Robert MD (D) - **Spec Exp:** Acne; Skin Cancer; Cosmetic Dermatology; Skin Laser Surgery; **Hospital:** St John's Epis Hosp - S Shore, Peninsula Hosp Ctr; **Address:** 290 Central Ave, Ste 206, Lawrence, NY 11559-8507; **Phone:** 516-239-2332; **Board Cert:** Dermatology 1977; **Med School:** NYU Sch Med 1972; **Resid:** Dermatology, Bellevue Hosp Ctr-NYU 1975; **Fac Appt:** Asst Clin Prof D, NYU Sch Med

De Pietro, William MD (D) - **Spec Exp:** Skin Laser Surgery; Dermatologic Surgery; **Hospital:** Glen Cove Hosp; **Address:** 10 Medical Plaza, Ste 102, Glen Cove, NY 11542; **Phone:** 516-671-1780; **Board Cert:** Dermatology 1980; **Med School:** Georgetown Univ 1976; **Resid:** Dermatology, St Luke's Hosp 1980

Demento, Frank MD (D) - **Spec Exp:** Dermatologic Surgery; Skin Cancer; **Hospital:** Winthrop - Univ Hosp, NY-Presby Hosp/Columbia (page 104); **Address:** 520 Franklin Ave, Ste 229, Garden City, NY 11530; **Phone:** 516-746-1227; **Board Cert:** Dermatology 1969; **Med School:** UMDNJ-NJ Med Sch, Newark 1964; **Resid:** Dermatology, USPHS Hosp 1966; **Fellow:** Dermatology, Columbia-Presby Hosp 1968

Dolitsky, Charisse MD (D) - **Spec Exp:** Acne; Skin Cancer; Botox Therapy; Facial Rejuvenation; **Hospital:** Long Beach Med Ctr; **Address:** 604 E Park Ave, Long Beach, NY 11561; **Phone:** 516-432-0011; **Board Cert:** Dermatology 1989; **Med School:** SUNY Downstate 1985; **Resid:** Dermatology, Univ Hosp 1989

Falcon, Ronald MD (D) - **Spec Exp:** Skin Cancer; Acne; Psoriasis; **Hospital:** Long Beach Med Ctr; **Address:** 604 E Park Ave, Long Beach, NY 11561-2505; **Phone:** 516-432-0011; **Board Cert:** Dermatology 1989; **Med School:** SUNY Downstate 1985; **Resid:** Dermatology, SUNY Downstate 1989

Franck, Jeanne M MD (D) - **Spec Exp:** Mohs' Surgery; **Hospital:** Winthrop - Univ Hosp, NY-Presby Hosp/Columbia (page 104); **Address:** 520 Franklin Ave, Ste 207, Garden City, NY 11530; **Phone:** 516-741-1055; **Board Cert:** Dermatology 2004; **Med School:** Columbia P&S 1991; **Resid:** Dermatology, Columbia Presby Med Ctr 1995; **Fellow:** Mohs Surgery, Univ Minn Med Ctr

Hefter, Harold MD (D) - **Spec Exp:** Cosmetic Dermatology; Dermatologic Surgery; Acne; **Hospital:** Franklin Hosp, Jacobi Med Ctr; **Address:** 135 Rockaway Tpke, Ste 100, Lawrence, NY 11559-1033; **Phone:** 516-371-1600; **Board Cert:** Dermatology 1985; **Med School:** Albert Einstein Coll Med 1981; **Resid:** Dermatology, Albert Einstein 1985; **Fac Appt:** Asst Prof D, Albert Einstein Coll Med

Hisler, Barbara M MD (D) - **Spec Exp:** Skin Cancer; Acne; Psoriasis; **Hospital:** Long Island Jewish Med Ctr; **Address:** 1300 Union Tpke, Ste 303, New Hyde Park, NY 11040-1759; **Phone:** 516-326-0333; **Board Cert:** Internal Medicine 1986; Dermatology 1989; **Med School:** NY Med Coll 1983; **Resid:** Internal Medicine, LI Jewish Med Ctr 1985; Dermatology, Detroit Med Ctr 1988; **Fac Appt:** Asst Prof Med, Albert Einstein Coll Med

Kristal, Leonard MD (D) - **Spec Exp:** Pediatric Dermatology; **Hospital:** Steven & Alexandra Cohen Chldn's Med Ctr of NY, Stony Brook Univ Med Ctr; **Address:** 2001 Marcus Ave, Ste S40, Lake Success, NY 11042; **Phone:** 516-352-6151; **Board Cert:** Pediatrics 2004; Dermatology 2001; Pediatric Dermatology 2004; **Med School:** Ros Franklin Univ/Chicago Med Sch 1986; **Resid:** Pediatrics, Chldns Hosp 1989; Dermatology, Univ Hosp-SUNY 1993; **Fellow:** Dermatology, Chldns Hosp 1994; **Fac Appt:** Asst Clin Prof Ped, SUNY Stony Brook

Krivo, James MD (D) - **Spec Exp:** Skin Cancer; **Hospital:** Franklin Hosp; **Address:** 54 New Hyde Park Rd, Garden City, NY 11530; **Phone:** 516-481-4920; **Board Cert:** Dermatology 1973; **Med School:** Univ Chicago-Pritzker Sch Med 1966; **Resid:** Dermatology, Univ Chicago Hosp 1968; Dermatology, NY Med Coll Affil Hosp 1972; **Fac Appt:** D, SUNY Stony Brook

Levine, Laurie J MD (D) - **Spec Exp:** Skin Laser Surgery; Botox Therapy; Cosmetic Dermatology; **Hospital:** Winthrop - Univ Hosp; **Address:** 200 Old Country Rd, Ste 140, Mineola, NY 11501-4237; **Phone:** 516-742-6136; **Board Cert:** Dermatology 1988; **Med School:** SUNY Stony Brook 1984; **Resid:** Dermatology, T Jefferson Univ Hosp 1988; **Fellow:** Dermatologic Surgery, T Jefferson Univ Hosp 1989; **Fac Appt:** Asst Clin Prof D, SUNY Stony Brook

Paltzik, Robert L MD (D) - **Spec Exp:** Pediatric Dermatology; Dermatologic Surgery; **Hospital:** N Shore Univ Hosp, Winthrop - Univ Hosp; **Address:** 2 Hillside Ave, Ste G, Williston Park, NY 11596-2335; **Phone:** 516-747-2230; **Board Cert:** Dermatology 1977; Pediatrics 1976; **Med School:** NYU Sch Med 1971; **Resid:** Pediatrics, Yale-New Haven Hosp 1973; Dermatology, SUNY Downstate Med Ctr 1977; **Fac Appt:** Asst Prof D, NYU Sch Med

Sarnoff, Deborah S MD (D) - **Spec Exp:** Skin Laser Surgery; Cosmetic Dermatology; Mohs' Surgery; Skin Cancer; **Hospital:** NYU Langone Med Ctr (page 106); **Address:** 31 Northern Blvd, Greenvale, NY 11548; **Phone:** 516-484-9000; **Board Cert:** Dermatology 1984; **Med School:** Geo Wash Univ 1980; **Resid:** Dermatology, NYU Med Ctr 1984; **Fellow:** Dermatologic Surgery, NYU Med Ctr 1986; **Fac Appt:** Clin Prof D, NYU Sch Med

Sklar, Jeffrey MD (D) - **Spec Exp:** Liposuction; Cosmetic Dermatology; Botox Therapy; **Hospital:** NY-Presby Hosp/Columbia (page 104), Syosset Hosp; **Address:** 800 Woodbury Rd, Ste A, Woodbury, NY 11797-2503; **Phone:** 516-496-9400; **Board Cert:** Dermatology 1986; **Med School:** Columbia P&S 1982; **Resid:** Dermatology, Columbia Presby Hosp 1986; **Fac Appt:** Asst Clin Prof D, Columbia P&S

Spinowitz, Alan MD (D) - **Spec Exp:** Skin Cancer; Mohs' Surgery; **Hospital:** Franklin Hosp; **Address:** 877 Stewart Ave, Ste 27, Garden City, NY 11530-4803; **Phone:** 516-745-0606; **Board Cert:** Dermatology 1985; **Med School:** SUNY Hlth Sci Ctr 1981; **Resid:** Dermatology, Univ Illinois Med Ctr 1985; **Fellow:** Dermatologic Surgery, Univ Illinois Med Ctr 1987

Walczyk, John MD (D) - **Hospital:** NY-Presby Hosp/Columbia (page 104), Plainview Hosp; **Address:** 1165 Northern Blvd, Ste 405, Manhasset, NY 11030; **Phone:** 516-365-8030; **Board Cert:** Dermatology 2003; **Med School:** Columbia P&S 1990; **Resid:** Internal Medicine, N Shore Univ Hosp 1991; Dermatology, Columbia Presby Hosp 1994

Diagnostic Radiology

Goodman, Kenneth J MD (DR) - **Spec Exp:** Urologic Imaging; Ultrasound; CT Scan; **Hospital:** St Francis Hosp - The Heart Ctr (page 115); **Address:** 100 Port Washington Blvd, Roslyn, NY 11576-1353; **Phone:** 516-562-6500; **Board Cert:** Diagnostic Radiology 1977; **Med School:** Univ Tex, San Antonio 1972; **Resid:** Diagnostic Radiology, Cornell Med Ctr 1977; **Fellow:** Diagnostic Radiology, Cornell Med Ctr 1978

Hammel, Jay D MD (DR) - **Spec Exp:** MRI; **Hospital:** N Shore Univ Hosp, Syosset Hosp; **Address:** 4277 Hempstead Tpke, Bethpage, NY 11714; **Phone:** 516-796-4340; **Board Cert:** Diagnostic Radiology 1989; **Med School:** SUNY Upstate Med Univ 1984; **Resid:** Diagnostic Radiology, St Vincent's Med Ctr 1989

Hoffman, Janet C MD (DR) - **Hospital:** Long Island Jewish Med Ctr; **Address:** 270-05 76th Ave, rm C-204, New Hyde Park, NY 11040; **Phone:** 718-470-4177; **Board Cert:** Diagnostic Radiology 1978; **Med School:** SUNY Downstate 1974; **Resid:** Diagnostic Radiology, Colum Presby Hosp 1978; **Fellow:** Ultrasound, NY Hosp-Cornell Med Ctr 1979

Khan, Arfa MD (DR) - **Spec Exp:** Thoracic Radiology; **Hospital:** Long Island Jewish Med Ctr; **Address:** 270-05 76th Ave, rm C204, New Hyde Park, NY 11040; **Phone:** 718-470-3456; **Board Cert:** Diagnostic Radiology 1971; **Med School:** India 1964; **Resid:** Diagnostic Radiology, Queens Hosp 1970; **Fellow:** Diagnostic Radiology, LI Jewish Med Ctr 1971; **Fac Appt:** Assoc Prof Rad, Albert Einstein Coll Med

Port, Abraham MD (DR) - **Spec Exp:** Breast Cancer; Mammography; **Hospital:** South Nassau Comm Hosp; **Address:** Complete Women's Imaging, 44 Merrick Rd, Oceanside, NY 11572; **Phone:** 516-222-4873; **Board Cert:** Diagnostic Radiology 1985; **Med School:** Albert Einstein Coll Med 1981; **Resid:** Diagnostic Radiology, Montefiore Med Ctr 1985; **Fellow:** Body Imaging, NY Presby-Cornell Med Ctr 1996

Rossi, Dennis R MD (DR) - **Spec Exp:** MRI; **Hospital:** Long Beach Med Ctr, St. John's Episcopal Hosp-Queens; **Address:** Elmont MRI, 545 Elmont Rd, Elmont, NY 11003; **Phone:** 516-328-7200; **Board Cert:** Diagnostic Radiology 1973; **Med School:** SUNY Downstate 1968; **Resid:** Diagnostic Radiology, Montefiore Hosp Med Ctr 1972; **Fac Appt:** Assoc Clin Prof, SUNY Stony Brook

Sherman, Scott J MD (DR) - **Spec Exp:** CT Scan; PET Imaging; **Hospital:** St Francis Hosp - The Heart Ctr (page 115); **Address:** 40 The Birches, Roslyn, NY 11576; **Phone:** 516-562-6511; **Board Cert:** Diagnostic Radiology 1983; Nuclear Medicine 1984; **Med School:** Northwestern Univ 1979; **Resid:** Diagnostic Radiology, NY Hosp 1983; Nuclear Medicine, NY Hosp 1984; **Fellow:** Ultrasound, NY Hosp 1985

Weck, Steven MD (DR) - **Spec Exp:** Interventional Radiology; **Hospital:** Glen Cove Hosp; **Address:** Dept Radiology, Glen Cove Hospital, 101 St Andrew's Ln, Glen Cove, NY 11542; **Phone:** 516-674-7540; **Board Cert:** Diagnostic Radiology 1977; **Med School:** NYU Sch Med 1973; **Resid:** Diagnostic Radiology, NYU Med Ctr 1977

Yoon, Sydney S MD (DR) - **Spec Exp:** MRI; CT Scan; Neuroradiology; Neuroradiology; **Hospital:** South Nassau Comm Hosp; **Address:** 1 Healthy Way, Oceanside, NY 11572; **Phone:** 516-632-4660; **Board Cert:** Internal Medicine 1989; Diagnostic Radiology 1993; Vascular & Interventional Radiology 1998; Neuroradiology 2006; **Med School:** Univ Chicago-Pritzker Sch Med 1986; **Resid:** Internal Medicine, Johns Hopkins Hosp 1989; Diagnostic Radiology, UCLA Med Ctr 1993; **Fellow:** Neuroradiology, Columbia Presby Med Ctr 1995; Vascular & Interventional Radiology, UCLA Med Ctr 1997

Endocrinology, Diabetes & Metabolism

Aloia, John MD (EDM) - **Spec Exp:** Osteoporosis; **Hospital:** Winthrop - Univ Hosp; **Address:** 222 Station Plaza North, Ste 350, Mineola, NY 11501; **Phone:** 516-663-3511; **Board Cert:** Internal Medicine 1969; Endocrinology 1972; **Med School:** Creighton Univ 1962; **Resid:** Internal Medicine, Meadowbrook Hosp 1966; Internal Medicine, Harrisburg Hosp 1967; **Fellow:** Endocrinology, Diabetes & Metabolism, Jefferson Univ Med Ctr 1969; **Fac Appt:** Prof Med, SUNY Stony Brook

Bhatt, Anjani A MD (EDM) - **Spec Exp:** Thyroid Disorders; Diabetes; **Hospital:** Long Beach Med Ctr; **Address:** 871 E Park Ave, Long Beach, NY 11561; **Phone:** 516-889-8853; **Board Cert:** Internal Medicine 1983; Endocrinology, Diabetes & Metabolism 1985; **Med School:** India 1976; **Resid:** Internal Medicine, Brooklyn Hosp 1981; **Fellow:** Endocrinology, Brooklyn Hosp 1984

Bitton, Rachelle N MD (EDM) - **Spec Exp:** Osteoporosis; Thyroid Disorders; Diabetes; Pituitary Disorders; **Hospital:** Long Island Jewish Med Ctr, N Shore Univ Hosp; **Address:** 2 Pro Health Plaza Fl 2, Lake Success, NY 11042; **Phone:** 516-390-5760; **Board Cert:** Internal Medicine 1981; Endocrinology, Diabetes & Metabolism 1985; **Med School:** SUNY Downstate 1978; **Resid:** Internal Medicine, Brookdale Hosp 1981; **Fellow:** Endocrinology, Diabetes & Metabolism, Univ Hosp 1984

Friedman, Seth G MD (EDM) - **Spec Exp:** Thyroid Disorders; Pituitary Disorders; Diabetes; Osteoporosis; **Hospital:** N Shore Univ Hosp, Long Island Jewish Med Ctr; **Address:** 560 Northern Blvd, Ste 207, Great Neck, NY 11021; **Phone:** 516-466-6165; **Board Cert:** Internal Medicine 2002; Endocrinology, Diabetes & Metabolism 2003; **Med School:** Mount Sinai Sch Med 1988; **Resid:** Internal Medicine, LI Jewish Med Ctr 1991; **Fellow:** Endocrinology, Diabetes & Metabolism, Albert Einstein 1993

Gordon, Jeffrey H MD (EDM) - **Spec Exp:** Diabetes; Thyroid Disorders; Pituitary Disorders; **Hospital:** St Francis Hosp - The Heart Ctr (page 115), N Shore Univ Hosp; **Address:** 3 School St, Ste 306, Glen Cove, NY 11542-2548; **Phone:** 516-759-2420; **Board Cert:** Internal Medicine 1972; Endocrinology, Diabetes & Metabolism 1973; **Med School:** Cornell Univ-Weill Med Coll 1965; **Resid:** Internal Medicine, Bellevue Hosp 1967; **Fellow:** Endocrinology, Duke Univ Med Ctr 1970; Endocrinology, VA Hosp 1972; **Fac Appt:** Asst Clin Prof Med, NYU Sch Med

Greenfield, Martin MD (EDM) - **Spec Exp:** Diabetes; Thyroid Disorders; Osteoporosis; Adrenal Disorders; **Hospital:** Long Island Jewish Med Ctr, N Shore Univ Hosp; **Address:** 2 ProHealth Plaza, Lake Success, NY 11042; **Phone:** 516-608-6823; **Board Cert:** Internal Medicine 1987; Endocrinology, Diabetes & Metabolism 1979; **Med School:** SUNY Downstate 1968; **Resid:** Internal Medicine, Ll Jewish Med Ctr 1971; **Fellow:** Endocrinology, Diabetes & Metabolism, Brigham & Womens Hosp 1975; **Fac Appt:** Asst Clin Prof Med, Albert Einstein Coll Med

Hupart, Kenneth H MD (EDM) - **Spec Exp:** Thyroid Disorders; Osteoporosis; Diabetes; Cholesterol/Lipid Disorders; **Hospital:** Nassau Univ Med Ctr; **Address:** Nu Hlth, Nassau Univ Med Ctr, Div Endocrinology, Diabetes, & Metabolism, 2201 Heampstead Tpke, East Meadow, NY 11554; **Phone:** 516-572-4848; **Board Cert:** Internal Medicine 1985; Endocrinology 1989; **Med School:** SUNY Stony Brook 1982; **Resid:** Internal Medicine, Montefiore Hosp Med Ctr 1986; **Fellow:** Endocrinology, Diabetes & Metabolism, Montefiore Hosp Med Ctr 1988; **Fac Appt:** Assoc Clin Prof Med, Albert Einstein Coll Med

Klein, Irwin MD (EDM) - **Spec Exp:** Thyroid Disorders; Thyroid Cancer; **Hospital:** N Shore Univ Hosp; **Address:** 2800 Marcus Ave, Ste 200, Lake Success, NY 11042; **Phone:** 516-708-2540; **Board Cert:** Internal Medicine 1978; Endocrinology 1985; **Med School:** NYU Sch Med 1973; **Resid:** Internal Medicine, Hosp Univ Penn 1975; **Fellow:** Endocrinology, Diabetes & Metabolism, Natl Cancer Inst/NIH 1977; Endocrinology, Diabetes & Metabolism, Univ Miami Hosps 1979; **Fac Appt:** Prof Med, NYU Sch Med

Lomasky, Steven MD (EDM) - **Spec Exp:** Diabetes; Cholesterol/Lipid Disorders; Thyroid Disorders; **Hospital:** South Nassau Comm Hosp, Long Island Jewish Med Ctr; **Address:** 242 Merrick Rd, rm 403, Rockville Ctr, NY 11570; **Phone:** 516-536-3700; **Board Cert:** Endocrinology, Diabetes & Metabolism 1989; Internal Medicine 1985; **Med School:** Israel 1982; **Resid:** Internal Medicine, Montefiore Med Ctr 1986; **Fellow:** Endocrinology, Diabetes & Metabolism, Montefiore Med Ctr 1987; **Fac Appt:** Asst Clin Prof Med, Albert Einstein Coll Med

Margulies, Paul MD (EDM) - **Spec Exp:** Thyroid Disorders; Adrenal Disorders; Pituitary Disorders; Addison's Disease; **Hospital:** N Shore Univ Hosp; **Address:** 444 Community, Ste 312, Manhasset, NY 11030-3820; **Phone:** 516-627-1366; **Board Cert:** Internal Medicine 1975; Endocrinology, Diabetes & Metabolism 1977; **Med School:** Univ Chicago-Pritzker Sch Med 1970; **Resid:** Internal Medicine, New York Hosp 1975; **Fellow:** Endocrinology, Diabetes & Metabolism, New York Hosp 1976; **Fac Appt:** Assoc Prof Med, NYU Sch Med

Rosenthal, David S MD (EDM) - **Spec Exp:** Thyroid Disorders; Pituitary Disorders; Adrenal Disorders; **Hospital:** Nassau Univ Med Ctr; **Address:** Nassau Univ Med Ctr, Div Endocrinology, 2201 Hempstead Tpke, East Meadow, NY 11554; **Phone:** 516-572-4848; **Board Cert:** Internal Medicine 1969; Endocrinology, Diabetes & Metabolism 1972; **Med School:** NYU Sch Med 1963; **Resid:** Internal Medicine, Wilford Hall USAF Med Ctr 1967; **Fellow:** Endocrinology, Diabetes & Metabolism, Boston Univ Med Ctr 1972; Nuclear Medicine, Boston Univ Med Ctr 1972; **Fac Appt:** Asst Prof Med, SUNY Stony Brook

Shapiro, Lawrence E MD (EDM) - **Spec Exp:** Thyroid Disorders; Diabetes; **Hospital:** Winthrop - Univ Hosp; **Address:** 222 Station Plaza N, Ste 350, Mineola, NY 11501; **Phone:** 516-663-3511; **Board Cert:** Internal Medicine 1975; Endocrinology 1977; **Med School:** SUNY Downstate 1971; **Resid:** Internal Medicine, Bellevue Hosp 1974; **Fellow:** Endocrinology, Diabetes & Metabolism, NYU Med Ctr 1975; **Fac Appt:** Prof Med, SUNY Stony Brook

Vaswani, Ashok N MD (EDM) - **Spec Exp:** Osteoporosis; Obesity; **Hospital:** Winthrop - Univ Hosp; **Address:** 901 Stewart Ave, Ste 204, Garden City, NY 11530; **Phone:** 516-739-0414; **Board Cert:** Internal Medicine 1977; Endocrinology, Diabetes & Metabolism 1983; **Med School:** India 1970; **Resid:** Internal Medicine, Nassau County Med Ctr 1974; **Fac Appt:** Asst Prof Med, SUNY Stony Brook

Weinerman, Stuart MD (EDM) - **Spec Exp:** Osteoporosis; Calcium Disorders; Paget's Disease of Bone; **Hospital:** N Shore Univ Hosp, Long Island Jewish Med Ctr; **Address:** 2800 Marcus Ave, Ste 200, Lake Success, NY 11021-5310; **Phone:** 516-708-2540; **Board Cert:** Internal Medicine 1987; Endocrinology, Diabetes & Metabolism 1989; **Med School:** Albert Einstein Coll Med 1984; **Resid:** Internal Medicine, N Shore Univ Hosp 1987; **Fellow:** Endocrinology, Diabetes & Metabolism, NY Hosp/Meml Sloan Kettering Cancer Ctr 1989; **Fac Appt:** Asst Prof Med, NYU Sch Med

Family Medicine

Arcati, Anthony T MD (FMed) *PCP* - **Hospital:** Winthrop - Univ Hosp; **Address:** 530 Hicksville Rd, Bethpage, NY 11714; **Phone:** 516-937-5000; **Board Cert:** Family Medicine 2003; **Med School:** Mexico 1975; **Resid:** Family Medicine, Nassau Co Med Ctr 1979

Arcati, Robert J MD (FMed) *PCP* - **Hospital:** Winthrop - Univ Hosp; **Address:** 530 Hicksville Rd, Bethpage, NY 11714; **Phone:** 516-931-4285; **Board Cert:** Family Medicine 2008; **Med School:** Mount Sinai Sch Med 1986; **Resid:** Family Medicine, Somerset Med Ctr 1989

Capobianco, Luigi MD (FMed) *PCP* - **Spec Exp:** Geriatric Care; **Hospital:** Glen Cove Hosp; **Address:** One School St, Ste 203, Glen Cove, NY 11542; **Phone:** 516-671-9800; **Board Cert:** Family Medicine 2007; Geriatric Medicine 2008; **Med School:** Italy 1984; **Resid:** Family Medicine, N Shore Univ Hosp 1988

Edelstein, Martin P MD (FMed) *PCP* - **Spec Exp:** Preventive Medicine; **Hospital:** N Shore Univ Hosp; **Address:** 11 Beverly Rd, Great Neck, NY 11021-1320; **Phone:** 516-487-1614; **Board Cert:** Family Medicine 2008; **Med School:** McGill Univ 1971; **Resid:** Family Medicine, Jewish Genl Hosp 1973; **Fac Appt:** Asst Clin Prof FMed, NYU Sch Med

Klein, Steven E MD (FMed) *PCP* - **Spec Exp:** Diabetes; Cardiovascular Disease; Geriatric Medicine; Asthma; **Hospital:** Southside Hosp; **Address:** 99 Grand Ave, Massapequa, NY 11758; **Phone:** 516-541-9700; **Board Cert:** Family Medicine 2003; **Med School:** Univ VT Coll Med 1983; **Resid:** Family Medicine, Southside Hosp 1986

Moynihan, Brian T DO (FMed) *PCP* - **Spec Exp:** Hypertension; Diabetes; Skin Diseases; **Hospital:** St Joseph's Hosp-Nassau, N Shore Univ Hosp; **Address:** 2840 Jerusalem Ave, Wantagh, NY 11793-2017; **Phone:** 516-781-1141; **Med School:** NY Coll Osteo Med 1983; **Resid:** Family Medicine, Massapequa Genl Hosp 1984; Family Medicine, Kennedy Meml Hosp 1985; **Fac Appt:** Asst Prof FMed, NY Coll Osteo Med

Rechter, Lesley MD (FMed) *PCP* - **Spec Exp:** Women's Health; **Hospital:** Stony Brook Univ Med Ctr; **Address:** 54 Birchwood Park Dr, Jericho, NY 11753-2202; **Phone:** 516-933-6850; **Board Cert:** Family Medicine 2003; **Med School:** NY Med Coll 1976; **Resid:** Family Medicine, Nassau County Med Ctr 1979; **Fac Appt:** Assoc Clin Prof FMed, SUNY Stony Brook

Soskel, Neil DO (FMed) *PCP* - **Spec Exp:** Sports Medicine; **Hospital:** South Nassau Comm Hosp; **Address:** 185 Merrick Rd, Ste 1B, Lynbrook, NY 11563; **Phone:** 516-887-0077; **Board Cert:** Family Medicine 2008; **Med School:** NY Coll Osteo Med 1986; **Resid:** Family Medicine, S Nassau Comm Hosp 1989; **Fac Appt:** Assoc Prof FMed, NY Coll Osteo Med

Gastroenterology

Bartolomeo, Robert S MD (Ge) - **Spec Exp:** Colonoscopy; Inflammatory Bowel Disease; Gastroesophageal Reflux Disease (GERD); Colon Cancer Screening; **Hospital:** Winthrop - Univ Hosp; **Address:** 1103 Stewart Ave, Ste 300, Garden City, NY 11530; **Phone:** 516-248-3737; **Board Cert:** Internal Medicine 1974; Gastroenterology 1977; **Med School:** NY Med Coll 1971; **Resid:** Internal Medicine, Metropolitan Hosp Ctr 1973; Internal Medicine, Beth Israel Hosp 1974; **Fellow:** Gastroenterology, Bridgeport Hosp 1976

Bernstein, David E MD (Ge) - **Spec Exp:** Liver Disease; Hepatitis; Colonoscopy; **Hospital:** N Shore Univ Hosp; **Address:** North Shore Univ Hosp, Div Gastroenterology, 300 Community Drive, Manhasset, NY 11030-3816; **Phone:** 516-562-4281; **Board Cert:** Internal Medicine 2000; Gastroenterology 2003; **Med School:** SUNY Stony Brook 1988; **Resid:** Internal Medicine, Montefiore Med Ctr 1991; **Fellow:** Gastroenterology, Jackson Meml Hosp 1993; **Fac Appt:** Assoc Prof Med, NYU Sch Med

Blumstein, Meyer MD (Ge) - **Spec Exp:** Endoscopy; Gastroesophageal Reflux Disease (GERD); Inflammatory Bowel Disease; **Hospital:** Long Island Jewish Med Ctr, South Nassau Comm Hosp; **Address:** 158 Hempstead Ave, Lynnbrook, NY 11563-1605; **Phone:** 516-593-3541; **Board Cert:** Internal Medicine 1989; Gastroenterology 2001; **Med School:** SUNY Hlth Sci Ctr 1986; **Resid:** Internal Medicine, LI Jewish Med Ctr 1989; **Fellow:** Gastroenterology, LI Jewish Med Ctr 1991; **Fac Appt:** Asst Prof Med, Albert Einstein Coll Med

Caccese, William MD (Ge) - **Spec Exp:** Endoscopy; Colon Cancer; **Hospital:** Plainview Hosp; **Address:** 700 Old Country Rd, Ste 206, Plainview, NY 11803-4932; **Phone:** 516-681-1200; **Board Cert:** Internal Medicine 1981; Gastroenterology 1983; **Med School:** SUNY Hlth Sci Ctr 1978; **Resid:** Internal Medicine, N Shore Univ Hosp 1981; **Fellow:** Gastroenterology, N Shore Univ Hosp 1983

Cerulli, Maurice A MD (Ge) - **Spec Exp:** Liver Disease; Gastroesophageal Reflux Disease (GERD); Nutrition; Hepatitis B & C; **Hospital:** Long Island Jewish Med Ctr, N Shore Univ Hosp; **Address:** 270-05 76th Ave, New Hyde Park, NY 11040; **Phone:** 718-470-7281; **Board Cert:** Internal Medicine 1975; Gastroenterology 1977; **Med School:** SUNY Hlth Sci Ctr 1972; **Resid:** Internal Medicine, Kings County Hosp 1975; **Fellow:** Gastroenterology, Johns Hopkins Hosp 1977; **Fac Appt:** Assoc Prof Med, Albert Einstein Coll Med

Cohen, Jacob L MD (Ge) - **Hospital:** Mercy Med Ctr - Rockville Centre; **Address:** 2 Lincoln Ave, Ste 201, Rockville Centre, NY 11570; **Phone:** 516-536-0600; **Board Cert:** Internal Medicine 1968; Gastroenterology 1972; **Med School:** SUNY Upstate Med Univ 1961; **Resid:** Internal Medicine, Maimonides Med Ctr 1963; Internal Medicine, SUNY Upstate 1966; **Fellow:** Gastroenterology, Maimonides Med Ctr 1968

DeVito, Bethany S MD (Ge) - **Spec Exp:** Women's Health; Capsule Endoscopy; **Hospital:** N Shore Univ Hosp, Long Island Jewish Med Ctr; **Address:** N Shore Univ Hospital, 4 Levitt Pavilion, 300 Community Drive, Manhasset, NY 11030; **Phone:** 516-562-4281; **Board Cert:** Gastroenterology 2007; **Med School:** SUNY Upstate Med Univ 1992; **Resid:** Internal Medicine, St Vincents Hosp 1995; **Fellow:** Gastroenterology, NY Hosp 1997

Eskreis, David MD (Ge) - **Spec Exp:** Ulcerative Colitis/Crohn's; **Hospital:** NS-LIJ Hlth Sys; **Address:** 2001 Marcus Ave, Ste W85, Lake Success, NY 11042; **Phone:** 516-326-2700; **Board Cert:** Internal Medicine 1986; Gastroenterology 1987; **Med School:** Geo Wash Univ 1982; **Resid:** Internal Medicine, Bronx Muni Hosp Ctr 1985; **Fellow:** Gastroenterology, Bronx Muni Hosp Ctr 1987

Farber, Charles MD (Ge) - **Spec Exp:** Colon Cancer; Gastroesophageal Reflux Disease (GERD); **Hospital:** Plainview Hosp; **Address:** 146A Manetto Hill Rd, Ste 205, Plainview, NY 11803; **Phone:** 516-822-4404; **Board Cert:** Gastroenterology 1983; Internal Medicine 1981; **Med School:** SUNY Hlth Sci Ctr 1978; **Resid:** Internal Medicine, N Shore Univ Hosp 1981; **Fellow:** Gastroenterology, Albert Einstein 1983

Goldblum, Lester DO (Ge) - **Spec Exp:** Endoscopy; Colon Cancer; Capsule Endoscopy; **Hospital:** St Joseph's Hosp-Nassau, N Shore Univ Hosp; **Address:** 850 Hicksville Rd, Ste 100, Seaford, NY 11783; **Phone:** 516-796-9000; **Board Cert:** Internal Medicine 1983; Gastroenterology 2001; **Med School:** Univ Osteo Med & Hlth Sci, Des Moines 1979; **Resid:** Internal Medicine, Nassau County Med Ctr 1983; **Fellow:** Gastroenterology, Nassau County Med Ctr 1985; **Fac Appt:** Asst Clin Prof Med, NY Coll Osteo Med

Goldman, Ira S MD (Ge) - **Spec Exp:** Endoscopy & Colonoscopy; Colon Cancer Screening; **Hospital:** N Shore Univ Hosp, St Francis Hosp - The Heart Ctr (page 115); **Address:** 310 E Shore Rd, Ste 206, Great Neck, NY 11023-2432; **Phone:** 516-487-7677; **Board Cert:** Internal Medicine 1980; Gastroenterology 1983; **Med School:** Columbia P&S 1977; **Resid:** Internal Medicine, Columbia-Presby Med Ctr 1980; **Fellow:** Gastroenterology, UCSF Med Ctr 1983; **Fac Appt:** Assoc Prof Med, NYU Sch Med

Gould, Perry M MD (Ge) - **Spec Exp:** Ulcerative Colitis; Colon & Rectal Cancer; Gastroesophageal Reflux Disease (GERD); Capsule Endoscopy; **Hospital:** Winthrop - Univ Hosp; **Address:** 1103 Stewart Ave, Garden City, NY 11530; **Phone:** 516-248-3737; **Board Cert:** Internal Medicine 1980; Gastroenterology 1983; **Med School:** NY Med Coll 1977; **Resid:** Internal Medicine, LI Jewish Hosp 1980; **Fellow:** Gastroenterology, NY Med Coll 1983; **Fac Appt:** Asst Clin Prof Med, SUNY Stony Brook

Greenberg, Ronald MD (Ge) - **Spec Exp:** Inflammatory Bowel Disease; Peptic Acid Disorders; **Hospital:** Long Island Jewish Med Ctr; **Address:** 270-05 76th Ave, rm B 202, New Hyde Park, NY 11040; **Phone:** 718-470-7281; **Board Cert:** Internal Medicine 1982; Gastroenterology 1985; **Med School:** Hahnemann Univ 1979; **Resid:** Internal Medicine, Albany Med Ctr 1982; **Fellow:** Gastroenterology, St Luke's Hosp 1985; **Fac Appt:** Assoc Clin Prof Med, Albert Einstein Coll Med

Grendell, James H MD (Ge) - **Spec Exp:** Pancreatic Disease; Nutrition; Liver Disease; **Hospital:** Winthrop - Univ Hosp; **Address:** 222 Station Plaza N, Ste 428, Mineola, NY 11501-3819; **Phone:** 516-663-2066; **Board Cert:** Internal Medicine 1978; Gastroenterology 1981; **Med School:** Ohio State Univ 1975; **Resid:** Internal Medicine, Beth Israel Hosp 1978; **Fellow:** Gastroenterology, UCSF Med Ctr 1981; **Fac Appt:** Prof Med, SUNY Stony Brook

Katz, Seymour MD (Ge) - **Spec Exp:** Inflammatory Bowel Disease; Colonoscopy; Endoscopy; **Hospital:** N Shore Univ Hosp, Long Island Jewish Med Ctr; **Address:** 1000 Northern Blvd, Ste 140, Great Neck, NY 11021; **Phone:** 516-466-2340; **Board Cert:** Internal Medicine 1971; Gastroenterology 1972; **Med School:** NYU Sch Med 1964; **Resid:** Internal Medicine, Albert Einstein Sch Med 1966; Internal Medicine, Jacobi Med Ctr 1969; **Fellow:** Gastroenterology, NY Hosp 1971; **Fac Appt:** Asst Clin Prof Med, Cornell Univ-Weill Med Coll

McKinley, Matthew MD (Ge) - **Spec Exp:** Gastroesophageal Reflux Disease (GERD); Barrett's Esophagus; Biliary Disease; **Hospital:** N Shore Univ Hosp; **Address:** 2800 Marcus Ave, Ste 201, Lake Success, NY 11042; **Phone:** 516-622-6076; **Board Cert:** Internal Medicine 1978; Gastroenterology 1981; **Med School:** Creighton Univ 1975; **Resid:** Internal Medicine, N Shore Univ Hosp 1978; Internal Medicine, Meml Sloan Kettering Cancer Ctr 1978; **Fellow:** Gastroenterology, Yale-New Haven Hosp 1980; **Fac Appt:** Assoc Prof Med, NYU Sch Med

Miller, Seth MD (Ge) - **Hospital:** Long Beach Med Ctr, South Nassau Comm Hosp; **Address:** 206 West Park Ave, Long Beach, NY 11561; **Phone:** 516-432-8021; **Board Cert:** Internal Medicine 1983; Gastroenterology 1987; **Med School:** Mount Sinai Sch Med 1980; **Resid:** Internal Medicine, Beth Israel Med Ctr 1983; **Fellow:** Gastroenterology, Beth Israel Med Ctr 1985

Milman, Perry J MD (Ge) - **Spec Exp:** Gastroesophageal Reflux Disease (GERD); Colon Cancer; Inflammatory Bowel Disease; Endoscopy; **Hospital:** Long Island Jewish Med Ctr, N Shore Univ Hosp; **Address:** 2001 Marcus Ave, Ste N18, Lake Success, NY 11042-1011; **Phone:** 516-775-7770; **Board Cert:** Internal Medicine 1976; Gastroenterology 1979; **Med School:** SUNY Downstate 1973; **Resid:** Internal Medicine, LI Jewish Med Ctr 1976; **Fellow:** Gastroenterology, VA Hosp/NYU 1978; **Fac Appt:** Asst Clin Prof Med, Albert Einstein Coll Med

Palmer, Melissa MD (Ge) - **Spec Exp:** Liver Disease; Hepatitis C; **Hospital:** Plainview Hosp, NYU Langone Med Ctr (page 106); **Address:** Hepatology Assocs, 1097 Old Country Rd, Ste 104, Plainview, NY 11803-6505; **Phone:** 516-939-2626; **Board Cert:** Internal Medicine 1988; Gastroenterology 2010; **Med School:** Mount Sinai Sch Med 1985; **Resid:** Internal Medicine, Beth Israel Medical Ctr 1988; **Fellow:** Hepatology, Stony Brook Univ Hosp 1989; Gastroenterology, Mt Sinai Med Ctr 1991; **Fac Appt:** Clin Prof Med, NYU Sch Med

Schwartz, Gary MD (Ge) - **Spec Exp:** Colon Cancer Screening; Gastroesophageal Reflux Disease (GERD); **Hospital:** Winthrop - Univ Hosp; **Address:** 1103 Stewart Ave, Garden City, NY 11530; **Phone:** 516-248-3737; **Board Cert:** Internal Medicine 1985; Gastroenterology 1987; **Med School:** Mexico 1979; **Resid:** Internal Medicine, Winthrop Univ Hosp 1983; **Fellow:** Gastroenterology, Univ Hosp 1986

Talansky, Arthur L MD (Ge) - **Spec Exp:** Crohn's Disease; Ulcerative Colitis; Colonoscopy; **Hospital:** N Shore Univ Hosp, St Francis Hosp - The Heart Ctr (page 115); **Address:** 233 E Shore Rd, Ste 101, Great Neck, NY 11023-2433; **Phone:** 516-487-2444; **Board Cert:** Internal Medicine 1980; Gastroenterology 1983; **Med School:** Mount Sinai Sch Med 1977; **Resid:** Internal Medicine, Meml Sloan Kettering Cancer Ctr 1980; **Fellow:** Gastroenterology, Mount Sinai Hosp 1982; **Fac Appt:** Asst Clin Prof Med, NYU Sch Med

Weissman, Gary MD (Ge) - **Spec Exp:** Gastrointestinal Cancer; Inflammatory Bowel Disease; Esophageal Disorders; **Hospital:** N Shore Univ Hosp; **Address:** 2800 Marcus Ave, Ste 201, Lake Success, NY 11042; **Phone:** 516-622-6076; **Board Cert:** Internal Medicine 1980; Gastroenterology 1983; **Med School:** NY Med Coll 1976; **Resid:** Internal Medicine, North Shore Univ Hosp 1980; **Fellow:** Gastroenterology, Meml Sloan Kettering Cancer Ctr 1982; **Fac Appt:** Assoc Clin Prof Med, NYU Sch Med

Geriatric Medicine

Gomolin, Irving MD (Ger) - **Spec Exp:** Medications in the Elderly; Dementia; **Hospital:** Winthrop - Univ Hosp; **Address:** 222 Station Plaza N Fl 5 - Ste 518, Mineola, NY 11501; **Phone:** 516-663-2588; **Board Cert:** Internal Medicine 1979; Geriatric Medicine 2008; **Med School:** McGill Univ 1976; **Resid:** Internal Medicine, Jewish Genl Hosp-McGill Univ 1978; Internal Medicine, Beth Israel/Harvard 1981; **Fellow:** Clinical Pharmacology, Harvard Med Sch 1980; **Fac Appt:** Clin Prof Med, SUNY Stony Brook

Lanman, Geraldine MD (Ger) *PCP* - **Spec Exp:** Geriatric Medicine; **Hospital:** Long Island Jewish Med Ctr; **Address:** 1 Delaware Drive, Ste 48, New Hyde Park, NY 11042; **Phone:** 516-326-5320; **Board Cert:** Internal Medicine 1983; **Med School:** Univ Calgary 1980; **Resid:** Internal Medicine, LIJ Med Ctr 1986; **Fellow:** Geriatric Medicine, LIJ Med Ctr 1988; **Fac Appt:** Asst Clin Prof Med, Albert Einstein Coll Med

Macina, Lucy MD (Ger) *PCP* - **Spec Exp:** Frail Elderly; Dementia; **Hospital:** Winthrop - Univ Hosp; **Address:** 222 Station Plaza N, Ste 518, Mineola, NY 11501-3893; **Phone:** 516-663-2588; **Board Cert:** Internal Medicine 1982; Geriatric Medicine 2002; **Med School:** Loyola Univ-Stritch Sch Med 1978; **Resid:** Internal Medicine, VA Hosp 1980; Internal Medicine, Loyola U-Stritch Sch Med 1982; **Fellow:** Geriatric Medicine, Roger Williams Hosp 1985; **Fac Appt:** Asst Clin Prof Med, SUNY Stony Brook

Wolf-Klein, Gisele MD (Ger) *PCP* - **Spec Exp:** Dementia; Falls in the Elderly; Alzheimer's Disease; **Hospital:** Long Island Jewish Med Ctr; **Address:** 2800 Marcus Ave, Lake Success, NY 11042; **Phone:** 516-708-2520; **Board Cert:** Internal Medicine 1984; **Med School:** Switzerland 1975; **Resid:** Internal Medicine, Long Island Hosp 1978; **Fellow:** Geriatric Medicine, LI Jewish Med Ctr 1979

Gynecologic Oncology

Lovecchio, John L MD (GO) - **Spec Exp:** Ovarian Cancer; Uterine Cancer; Cervical Cancer; Vulvar Disease/Cancer; **Hospital:** N Shore Univ Hosp, Long Island Jewish Med Ctr; **Address:** North Shore Hospital, 10 Monti, 300 Community Drive, Manhasset, NY 11030-3816; **Phone:** 516-562-4438; **Board Cert:** Obstetrics & Gynecology 2005; Gynecologic Oncology 2005; **Med School:** SUNY Buffalo 1975; **Resid:** Obstetrics & Gynecology, Univ Hosp Case West Res 1979; **Fellow:** Gynecologic Oncology, Jackson Meml Hosp 1982; **Fac Appt:** Prof ObG, NYU Sch Med

Menzin, Andrew MD (GO) - **Spec Exp:** Uterine Cancer; Ovarian Cancer; Cervical Cancer; **Hospital:** N Shore Univ Hosp, Long Island Jewish Med Ctr; **Address:** North Shore Univ Hosp, Div Gyn Oncology, 300 Community Drive, 10 Monti, Manhasset, NY 11030-3816; **Phone:** 516-562-4438; **Board Cert:** Obstetrics & Gynecology 2009; Gynecologic Oncology 2009; **Med School:** NYU Sch Med 1989; **Resid:** Obstetrics & Gynecology, Hosp Univ Penn 1993; **Fellow:** Gynecologic Oncology, Hosp Univ Penn 1995; **Fac Appt:** Assoc Clin Prof ObG, NYU Sch Med

Hand Surgery

Kamler, Kenneth MD (HS) - **Spec Exp:** Carpal Tunnel Syndrome; Arthritis; Fractures; **Hospital:** N Shore Univ Hosp; **Address:** 410 Lakeville Rd, Ste 303, New Hyde Park, NY 11042; **Phone:** 516-326-2266; **Med School:** France 1975; **Resid:** Orthopaedic Surgery, LI Jewish Med Ctr 1979; **Fellow:** Hand Surgery, Columbia-Presby Med Ctr 1981

Lane, Lewis B MD (HS) - **Spec Exp:** Carpal Tunnel Syndrome; Arthritis; Sports Injuries; Hand Reconstruction; **Hospital:** N Shore Univ Hosp, St Francis Hosp - The Heart Ctr (page 115); **Address:** 600 Northern Blvd, Ste 300, Great Neck, NY 11021; **Phone:** 516-627-8717; **Board Cert:** Orthopaedic Surgery 1981; Hand Surgery 2000; **Med School:** Columbia P&S 1974; **Resid:** Surgery, NY Hosp 1975; Orthopaedic Surgery, Hosp for Special Surg 1979; **Fellow:** Research, Hosp for Special Surg 1976; Hand Surgery, St Luke's-Roosevelt Hosp Ctr 1980; **Fac Appt:** Assoc Clin Prof OrS, Albany Med Coll

Palmieri, Thomas J MD (HS) - **Spec Exp:** Arthritis; Carpal Tunnel Syndrome; Nerve Compression; Hand Rehabilitation; **Hospital:** Long Island Jewish Med Ctr, N Shore Univ Hosp; **Address:** 1901 New Hyde Park Rd, New Hyde Park, NY 11040; **Phone:** 516-822-4843; **Board Cert:** Surgery 1971; Hand Surgery 1996; **Med School:** SUNY Hlth Sci Ctr 1964; **Resid:** Internal Medicine, St Luke's-Roosevelt Hosp Ctr 1966; Surgery, LI Jewish Med Ctr 1970; **Fellow:** Hand Surgery, Hosp Joint Diseases; Hand Surgery, Columbia Presby Med Ctr; **Fac Appt:** Assoc Clin Prof S, Albert Einstein Coll Med

Teplitz, Glenn A MD (HS) - **Spec Exp:** Carpal Tunnel Syndrome; Fractures; Sports Injuries; Wrist/Hand Injuries; **Hospital:** Winthrop - Univ Hosp; **Address:** Winthrop Orthopaedic Assocs, 1300 Franklin Ave, Ste UL-3A, Garden City, NY 11530; **Phone:** 516-747-8900; **Board Cert:** Orthopaedic Surgery 2007; **Med School:** Tulane Univ 1987; **Resid:** Orthopaedic Surgery, UMDNJ Med Ctr 1993; **Fellow:** Hand Surgery, Hosp for Special Surgery 1994; **Fac Appt:** Asst Clin Prof OrS, SUNY Stony Brook

Hematology

Allen, Steven MD (Hem) - **Spec Exp:** Bleeding/Coagulation Disorders; Leukemia & Lymphoma; Multiple Myeloma; Gaucher Disease; **Hospital:** N Shore Univ Hosp, Long Island Jewish Med Ctr; **Address:** Monter Cancer Ctr, 450 Lakeville Rd, Lake Success, NY 11042; **Phone:** 516-734-8959; **Board Cert:** Internal Medicine 1980; Hematology 1982; Medical Oncology 1983; **Med School:** Johns Hopkins Univ 1977; **Resid:** Internal Medicine, NY Hosp-Cornell 1980; **Fellow:** Hematology & Oncology, NY Hosp-Cornell 1983; **Fac Appt:** Prof Med, Albert Einstein Coll Med

Kolitz, Jonathan E MD (Hem) - **Spec Exp:** Leukemia & Lymphoma; Hodgkin's Disease; Multiple Myeloma; Myelodysplastic Syndromes; **Hospital:** N Shore Univ Hosp; **Address:** 450 Lakeville Rd, Lake Success, NY 11042; **Phone:** 516-734-8970; **Board Cert:** Internal Medicine 1982; Medical Oncology 1985; Hematology 1988; **Med School:** Yale Univ 1979; **Resid:** Internal Medicine, N Shore Univ Hosp 1982; **Fellow:** Hematology & Oncology, Meml Sloan Kettering Cancer Ctr 1985; **Fac Appt:** Assoc Prof Med, NYU Sch Med

Rai, Kanti MD (Hem) - **Spec Exp:** Leukemia; Lymphoma; Multiple Myeloma; **Hospital:** Long Island Jewish Med Ctr; **Address:** 410 Lakeville Rd, Ste 212, New Hyde Park, NY 10042; **Phone:** 718-470-4050; **Board Cert:** Pediatrics 1959; **Med School:** India 1955; **Resid:** Pediatrics, Lincoln Hosp 1958; Pediatrics, North Shore Univ Hosp 1959; **Fellow:** Hematology, LI Jewish Med Ctr 1960; **Fac Appt:** Prof Med, Albert Einstein Coll Med

Staszewski, Harry MD (Hem) - **Spec Exp:** Hematologic Malignancies; **Hospital:** Winthrop - Univ Hosp; **Address:** 200 Old Country Rd, Ste 450, Mineola, NY 11501; **Phone:** 516-663-9500; **Board Cert:** Internal Medicine 1981; Medical Oncology 1983; Hematology 1984; **Med School:** Yale Univ 1978; **Resid:** Internal Medicine, N Shore Univ Hosp 1981; **Fellow:** Medical Oncology, Meml Sloan Kettering Cancer Ctr 1983; Hematology, LI Jewish Hosp 1984; **Fac Appt:** Asst Prof Med, SUNY Stony Brook

Infectious Disease

Cervia, Joseph S MD (Inf) - **Spec Exp:** AIDS/HIV; Travel Medicine; Pediatric Infections; Immune Deficiency; **Hospital:** N Shore Univ Hosp, Steven & Alexandra Cohen Chldn's Med Ctr of NY; **Address:** North Shore-LIJ Health System, 300 Community Drive, Manhasset, NY 11030; **Phone:** 516-562-4280; **Board Cert:** Internal Medicine 1989; Pediatrics 2003; Infectious Disease 1998; Pediatric Infectious Disease 2009; **Med School:** NY Med Coll 1984; **Resid:** Internal Medicine & Pediatrics, Brookdale Hosp 1988; **Fellow:** Infectious Disease, New York Hosp/Cornell 1990; **Fac Appt:** Clin Prof Med, Albert Einstein Coll Med

Cunha, Burke A MD (Inf) - **Spec Exp:** Infections in Immunocompromised Patients; Fevers of Unknown Origin; Pneumonia; Chronic Fatigue Syndrome; **Hospital:** Winthrop - Univ Hosp; **Address:** 222 Station Plz N, Ste 432, Mineola, NY 11501; **Phone:** 516-663-2507; **Board Cert:** Internal Medicine 1977; Infectious Disease 1978; **Med School:** Penn State Univ-Hershey Med Ctr 1972; **Resid:** Internal Medicine, Hartford Hosp 1975; **Fellow:** Infectious Disease, Hartford Hosp 1977; **Fac Appt:** Prof Med, SUNY Stony Brook

Farber, Bruce MD (Inf) - **Hospital:** N Shore Univ Hosp; **Address:** N Shore Univ Hosp, Div Infectious Dis, 300 Community Drive Fl 4, Manhasset, NY 11030; **Phone:** 516-562-4280; **Board Cert:** Internal Medicine 1979; Infectious Disease 1984; **Med School:** Northwestern Univ 1976; **Resid:** Internal Medicine, Univ Va Hosp 1979; **Fellow:** Infectious Disease, Mass Genl Hosp 1982

Greenspan, Joel MD (Inf) - **Spec Exp:** Infective Endocarditis; Infections-CNS; **Hospital:** N Shore Univ Hosp, Long Island Jewish Med Ctr; **Address:** 44 S Bayles Ave, Ste 216, Port Washington, NY 11050; **Phone:** 516-767-7771; **Board Cert:** Infectious Disease 1978; Internal Medicine 1973; **Med School:** SUNY Upstate Med Univ 1969; **Resid:** Internal Medicine, Bellevue Hosp 1972; Internal Medicine, Bellevue Hosp 1973; **Fellow:** Infectious Disease, Bellevue Hosp 1977; **Fac Appt:** Asst Clin Prof Med, NYU Sch Med

Johnson, Diane H MD (Inf) - **Spec Exp:** AIDS/HIV; Sexually Transmitted Diseases; Travel Medicine; **Hospital:** Winthrop - Univ Hosp; **Address:** 222 Station Plaza N, Ste 432, Mineola, NY 11501; **Phone:** 516-663-2507; **Board Cert:** Internal Medicine 2004; Infectious Disease 2004; **Med School:** Univ VT Coll Med 1989; **Resid:** Internal Medicine, Winthrop Univ Hosp 1992; **Fellow:** Infectious Disease, Winthrop Univ Hosp 1994; **Fac Appt:** Asst Prof Med, SUNY Stony Brook

Klein, Natalie MD (Inf) - **Hospital:** Winthrop - Univ Hosp; **Address:** 222 Station Plaza N, Ste 432, Mineola, NY 11501-3957; **Phone:** 516-663-2507; **Board Cert:** Internal Medicine 1982; Infectious Disease 1984; **Med School:** Jefferson Med Coll 1979; **Resid:** Internal Medicine, Mount Sinai Hosp 1982; **Fellow:** Infectious Disease, Mount Sinai Hosp 1984; **Fac Appt:** Assoc Prof Med, SUNY Stony Brook

McGowan, Joseph MD (Inf) - **Spec Exp:** AIDS/HIV; HIV in Pregnancy; HIV/Hepatitis Co-Infection; AIDS/HIV in Elderly; **Hospital:** NS-LIJ Hlth Sys; **Address:** 400 Community Drive, Manhasset, NY 11030; **Phone:** 516-562-4280; **Board Cert:** Internal Medicine 2002; Infectious Disease 2002; **Med School:** Mount Sinai Sch Med 1987; **Resid:** Internal Medicine, Montefiore Med Ctr 1990; **Fellow:** Infectious Disease, Montefiore Med Ctr 1993

Scheer, Max MD (Inf) - **Spec Exp:** Skin/Soft Tissue Infection; Infections-Respiratory; Sexually Transmitted Diseases; **Hospital:** N Shore Univ Hosp; **Address:** 15 Irving Pl, Woodmere, NY 11598-1229; **Phone:** 516-374-6750; **Board Cert:** Internal Medicine 1979; Infectious Disease 1982; **Med School:** SUNY Downstate 1975; **Resid:** Family Medicine, Kings Co Hosp-SUNY 1978; Internal Medicine, Morristown Meml Hosp 1979; **Fellow:** Infectious Disease, Mt Sinai Hosp 1981; **Fac Appt:** Asst Clin Prof Med, NYU Sch Med

Singer, Carol F MD (Inf) - **Spec Exp:** Infections in Immunocompromised Patients; Travel Medicine; **Hospital:** Long Island Jewish Med Ctr; **Address:** 270-05 76th Ave, Staff House, Ste 226, New Hyde Park, NY 11040-1433; **Phone:** 718-470-7290; **Board Cert:** Internal Medicine 1973; Infectious Disease 1978; **Med School:** Cornell Univ-Weill Med Coll 1970; **Resid:** Internal Medicine, Univ Michigan Med Ctr 1972; Internal Medicine, NY Hosp 1973; **Fellow:** Infectious Disease, Meml Hosp 1975; **Fac Appt:** Prof Med, Albert Einstein Coll Med

Internal Medicine

Ammazzalorso, Michael MD (IM) *PCP* - **Spec Exp:** Hypertension; Diabetes; **Hospital:** Winthrop - Univ Hosp; **Address:** 222 Station Plz N, Ste 310, Mineola, NY 11501-3893; **Phone:** 516-663-2051; **Board Cert:** Internal Medicine 1999; Geriatric Medicine 1999; **Med School:** SUNY Downstate 1987; **Resid:** Internal Medicine, Staten Island Hosp 1991; **Fac Appt:** Asst Prof Med, SUNY Stony Brook

Berbari, Nicholas E MD (IM) *PCP* - **Hospital:** Winthrop - Univ Hosp; **Address:** 222 Station Plaza N, Ste 310, Mineola, NY 11501; **Phone:** 516-663-2051; **Board Cert:** Internal Medicine 2006; **Med School:** SUNY Stony Brook 1993; **Resid:** Internal Medicine, Winthrop Univ Hosp 1997; **Fac Appt:** Asst Prof Med, SUNY Stony Brook

Berger, Jeffrey MD (IM) *PCP* - **Spec Exp:** Ethics; Palliative Care; Geriatric Care; **Hospital:** Winthrop - Univ Hosp; **Address:** 222 Station Plaza North, Ste 518, Mineola, NY 11501-3893; **Phone:** 516-663-2588; **Board Cert:** Internal Medicine 2001; Hospice & Palliative Medicine 2008; **Med School:** SUNY Stony Brook 1988; **Resid:** Internal Medicine, Winthrop Univ Hosp 1991; **Fac Appt:** Assoc Prof Med, SUNY Stony Brook

Corapi, Mark MD (IM) *PCP* - **Hospital:** Winthrop - Univ Hosp; **Address:** 222 Station Plaza N, Ste 310, Mineola, NY 11501; **Phone:** 516-663-2051; **Board Cert:** Internal Medicine 1985; **Med School:** SUNY Downstate 1982; **Resid:** Internal Medicine, Long Island Jewish Med Ctr 1985; **Fellow:** Internal Medicine, Long Island Jewish Med Ctr 1986; **Fac Appt:** Assoc Prof Med, SUNY Stony Brook

Cusumano, Stephen MD (IM) *PCP* - **Spec Exp:** Hypertension; Asthma; **Hospital:** St Joseph's Hosp-Nassau, Winthrop - Univ Hosp; **Address:** 850 Hicksville Rd, Ste 110, Seaford, NY 11783; **Phone:** 516-735-5454; **Board Cert:** Internal Medicine 1988; **Med School:** Ros Franklin Univ/Chicago Med Sch 1985; **Resid:** Internal Medicine, Winthrop Univ Hosp 1988

Federbush, Richard MD (IM) *PCP* - **Spec Exp:** Hypertension; Cholesterol/Lipid Disorders; Diabetes; **Hospital:** Plainview Hosp, Syosset Hosp; **Address:** 175 Jericho Tpke, Ste 216, Syosset, NY 11791; **Phone:** 516-364-9800; **Board Cert:** Internal Medicine 2001; **Med School:** Mexico 1985; **Resid:** Internal Medicine, Univ Hosp-SUNY 1989

Gelberg, Burt MD (IM) *PCP* - **Spec Exp:** Preventive Medicine; Colonoscopy; Gastroscopy; **Hospital:** Franklin Hosp; **Address:** 401 Franklin Ave, Franklin Square, NY 11010-1227; **Phone:** 516-326-2255; **Board Cert:** Internal Medicine 1975; **Med School:** SUNY Hlth Sci Ctr 1972; **Resid:** Internal Medicine, Lenox Hill Hosp 1975; **Fellow:** Gastroenterology, Lenox Hill Hosp 1977

Goodman, Michael MD (IM) - **Hospital:** South Nassau Comm Hosp; **Address:** 2495 Newbridge Rd, Bellmore, NY 11710; **Phone:** 516-826-1200; **Board Cert:** Internal Medicine 1980; **Med School:** Italy 1975; **Resid:** Internal Medicine, Nassau County Med Ctr 1978

Gorski, Lydia E MD (IM) *PCP* - **Spec Exp:** Women's Health; Geriatric Medicine; Preventive Medicine; **Hospital:** Winthrop - Univ Hosp, N Shore Univ Hosp; **Address:** 820 Jericho Tpke, New Hyde Park, NY 11040-4514; **Phone:** 516-352-0430; **Board Cert:** Internal Medicine 1988; **Med School:** Poland 1982; **Resid:** Internal Medicine, St Vincent's Catholic Med Ctrs 1987

Gottridge, Joanne MD (IM) *PCP* - **Hospital:** N Shore Univ Hosp; **Address:** 865 Northern Blvd, Ste 102, Great Neck, NY 11021; **Phone:** 516-622-5001; **Board Cert:** Internal Medicine 1983; **Med School:** Case West Res Univ 1980; **Resid:** Internal Medicine, N Shore Univ Hosp 1983; **Fac Appt:** Prof Med, NYU Sch Med

Hotchkiss, Edward MD (IM) *PCP* - **Hospital:** Long Island Jewish Med Ctr, South Nassau Comm Hosp; **Address:** 158 Hempstead Ave, Lynbrook, NY 11563-1605; **Phone:** 516-593-3541; **Board Cert:** Internal Medicine 1972; **Med School:** SUNY Hlth Sci Ctr 1965; **Resid:** Internal Medicine, Ll Jewish Med Ctr 1972; **Fellow:** Psychiatry, Univ Hosp 1971; **Fac Appt:** Assoc Prof Med, Albert Einstein Coll Med

Leong, Pauline MD (IM) *PCP* - **Hospital:** N Shore Univ Hosp; **Address:** 865 Northern Blvd, Ste 102, Great Neck, NY 11021-5310; **Phone:** 516-622-5000; **Board Cert:** Internal Medicine 1988; **Med School:** NYU Sch Med 1983; **Resid:** Internal Medicine, New York Hosp 1988

Pollak, Harvey MD (IM) *PCP* - **Spec Exp:** Hypertension; Heart Disease; Cholesterol/Lipid Disorders; **Hospital:** N Shore Univ Hosp; **Address:** 2 Prohealth Plaza Fl 1st - Ste 101, Lake Success, NY 11042; **Phone:** 516-622-6020; **Board Cert:** Internal Medicine 1974; **Med School:** Ros Franklin Univ/Chicago Med Sch 1971; **Resid:** Internal Medicine, Meml Sloan Kettering Cancer Ctr 1973; Internal Medicine, N Shore Univ Hosp 1975; **Fac Appt:** Clin Prof Med, NYU Sch Med

Rakowitz, Frederic MD (IM) *PCP* - **Spec Exp:** Preventive Medicine; **Hospital:** N Shore Univ Hosp; **Address:** 295 Northern Blvd, Ste 208, Great Neck, NY 11021-4701; **Phone:** 516-482-4940; **Board Cert:** Internal Medicine 1981; **Med School:** Albany Med Coll 1978; **Resid:** Internal Medicine, North Shore Univ Hosp 1981

Rubenstein, Jack MD (IM) *PCP* - **Spec Exp:** Complex Diagnosis; Kidney Failure-Chronic; Geriatric Care; Dialysis Care; **Hospital:** Franklin Hosp, N Shore Univ Hosp; **Address:** 70 Glen Cove Rd, Ste 301, Roslyn Heights, NY 11577-1731; **Phone:** 516-621-1502; **Board Cert:** Internal Medicine 2008; Nephrology 2009; Geriatric Medicine 2008; **Med School:** NY Med Coll 1976; **Resid:** Internal Medicine, North Shore Univ Hosp 1979; Nephrology, North Shore Univ Hosp 1980; **Fellow:** Nephrology, NYU Med Ctr 1982; **Fac Appt:** Assoc Clin Prof Med, NYU Sch Med

Rucker, Steve MD (IM) *PCP* - **Spec Exp:** Hypertension; Kidney Disease; Kidney Stones; **Hospital:** St Francis Hosp - The Heart Ctr (page 115), Long Island Jewish Med Ctr; **Address:** 1999 Marcus Ave, Lake Success, NY 11042; **Phone:** 516-775-4545; **Board Cert:** Internal Medicine 1986; Nephrology 1988; **Med School:** Univ Pittsburgh 1983; **Resid:** Internal Medicine, LI Jewish Med Ctr 1986; **Fellow:** Nephrology, Mount Sinai Med Ctr 1988

Taubman, Lowell MD (IM) *PCP* - **Spec Exp:** Dementia; Alzheimer's Disease; **Hospital:** Long Beach Med Ctr; **Address:** 206 Riverside Blvd, Long Beach, NY 11561; **Phone:** 516-432-5670; **Board Cert:** Internal Medicine 1988; **Med School:** Mexico 1980; **Resid:** Internal Medicine, Montefiore Hosp 1983; Internal Medicine, St Clares Hosp 1984; **Fellow:** Geriatric Medicine, Jewish Inst Geriatric Care 1986

Timpone, Leonard MD (IM) *PCP* - **Spec Exp:** Geriatric Medicine; Headache; **Hospital:** Franklin Hosp, Mercy Med Ctr - Rockville Centre; **Address:** 1051 Adams Ave, Franklin Square, NY 11010-2251; **Phone:** 516-354-4858; **Board Cert:** Internal Medicine 2004; **Med School:** France 1984; **Resid:** Internal Medicine, NY Downtown Hosp 1988

Weinstein, Mark J MD (IM) *PCP* - **Spec Exp:** Hypertension; Diabetes; Cholesterol/Lipid Disorders; **Hospital:** Plainview Hosp, St Joseph's Hosp-Nassau; **Address:** 4045 Hempstead Tpke Fl 3, Bethpage, NY 11714-5706; **Phone:** 516-731-7770; **Board Cert:** Internal Medicine 1978; Infectious Disease 1980; **Med School:** Harvard Med Sch 1975; **Resid:** Internal Medicine, Univ Hosp 1978; **Fellow:** Infectious Disease, Univ Hosp 1980

Interventional Cardiology

Abittan, Meyer H MD (IC) - **Spec Exp:** Angiography-Coronary; Preventive Cardiology; **Hospital:** St Francis Hosp - The Heart Ctr (page 115); **Address:** St Francis Hosp, The Heart Ctr, 100 Port Washington Blvd, Ste G-03, Roslyn, NY 11576; **Phone:** 516-627-1155; **Board Cert:** Internal Medicine 1989; Interventional Cardiology 1999; **Med School:** Mount Sinai Sch Med 1986; **Resid:** Internal Medicine, Brookdale Univ Hosp Med Ctr 1989; **Fellow:** Cardiovascular Disease, Mt Sinai Med Ctr 1990

Berke, Andrew D MD (IC) - **Hospital:** St Francis Hosp - The Heart Ctr (page 115), South Nassau Comm Hosp; **Address:** 100 Port Washington Blvd, Roslyn, NY 11576; **Phone:** 516-365-2211; **Board Cert:** Internal Medicine 1982; Cardiovascular Disease 1985; Interventional Cardiology 2009; **Med School:** Brown Univ 1979; **Resid:** Internal Medicine, Columbia-Presby Med Ctr 1982; **Fellow:** Cardiovascular Disease, Columbia-Presby Med Ctr 1985; **Fac Appt:** Asst Clin Prof Med, Columbia P&S

Lituchy, Andrew MD (IC) - **Spec Exp:** Coronary Artery Disease; Angioplasty & Stent Placement; Peripheral Vascular Disease; Interventional Cardiology; **Hospital:** St Francis Hosp - The Heart Ctr (page 115), South Nassau Comm Hosp; **Address:** 100 Port Washington Blvd Fl G - Ste 05, Roslyn, NY 11576-1353; **Phone:** 516-365-4888; **Board Cert:** Cardiovascular Disease 2005; Interventional Cardiology 2000; **Med School:** Hahnemann Univ 1988; **Resid:** Internal Medicine, Bronx Muni/Albert Einstein Med Ctr 1991; **Fellow:** Cardiovascular Disease, NY-Cornell Med Ctr 1994; Interventional Cardiology, NY-Cornell Med Ctr 1995

Ong, Lawrence MD (IC) - **Spec Exp:** Angioplasty & Stent Placement; **Hospital:** N Shore Univ Hosp; **Address:** N Shore Univ Hosp, Dept Cardiology, 300 Community Drive, Manhasset, NY 11030; **Phone:** 516-562-4100; **Board Cert:** Internal Medicine 1979; Cardiovascular Disease 1981; Interventional Cardiology 2009; **Med School:** UCSF 1976; **Resid:** Internal Medicine, N Shore Univ Hosp 1979; **Fellow:** Cardiovascular Disease, N Shore Univ Hosp 1981; **Fac Appt:** Assoc Prof Med, NYU Sch Med

Petrossian, George A MD (IC) - **Spec Exp:** Carotid Artery Stent Placement; Peripheral Vascular Disease; Coronary Angioplasty/Stents; Renovascular Disease; **Hospital:** St Francis Hosp - The Heart Ctr (page 115), South Nassau Comm Hosp; **Address:** New York Cardiology Group, 1405 Old Northern Blvd Fl 1st, Roslyn, NY 11576-1353; **Phone:** 516-484-6777; **Board Cert:** Internal Medicine 1986; Cardiovascular Disease 1989; Interventional Cardiology 2000; **Med School:** Mount Sinai Sch Med 1983; **Resid:** Internal Medicine, Columbia-Presby Med Ctr 1987; **Fellow:** Cardiovascular Disease, Columbia -Presby Med Ctr 1989; Interventional Cardiology, Mass Genl Hosp 1990

Maternal & Fetal Medicine

Fleischer, Adiel MD (MF) - **Spec Exp:** Pregnancy-High Risk; Maternal & Fetal Medicine; **Hospital:** Long Island Jewish Med Ctr, N Shore Univ Hosp; **Address:** LIJ Med Ctr, Dept ObGyn, 270-05 76th Ave, rm 471, New Hyde Park, NY 11040-1433; **Phone:** 718-470-7636; **Board Cert:** Obstetrics & Gynecology 1999; Maternal & Fetal Medicine 1999; **Med School:** Romania 1972; **Resid:** Obstetrics & Gynecology, Maimonides Med Ctr 1975; **Fellow:** Maternal & Fetal Medicine, Montefiore Med Ctr 1976; **Fac Appt:** Assoc Prof ObG, Albert Einstein Coll Med

Klein, Victor R MD (MF) - **Spec Exp:** Multiple Gestation; Pregnancy-High Risk; Genetic Disorders; **Hospital:** N Shore Univ Hosp, Long Island Jewish Med Ctr; **Address:** 825 Northern Blvd, Ste 301, Great Neck, NY 11021-5302; **Phone:** 516-472-5700; **Board Cert:** Obstetrics & Gynecology 2009; Maternal & Fetal Medicine 2009; Clinical Genetics 2004; **Med School:** SUNY Downstate 1980; **Resid:** Internal Medicine, Kings Co Hosp Ctr 1981; Obstetrics & Gynecology, Johns Hopkins Hosp 1985; **Fellow:** Clinical Genetics, Univ Texas SW Med Ctr 1987; Maternal & Fetal Medicine, Univ Texas SW Med Ctr 1987; **Fac Appt:** Assoc Clin Prof ObG, NYU Sch Med

Meirowitz, Natalie MD (MF) - **Spec Exp:** Prenatal Diagnosis; Pregnancy Loss; Pregnancy-High Risk; **Hospital:** NS-LIJ Hlth Sys; **Address:** LIJ Med Ctr, Dept Ob/Gyn, 270-05 76th Ave, rm 471, New Hyde Park, NY 11040; **Phone:** 516-470-7636; **Board Cert:** Obstetrics & Gynecology 2009; Maternal & Fetal Medicine 2009; **Med School:** Harvard Med Sch 1993; **Resid:** Obstetrics & Gynecology, North Shore Univ Med Ctr 1997; **Fellow:** Maternal & Fetal Medicine, UMDNJ Med Ctr 2000; **Fac Appt:** Asst Prof ObG, Albert Einstein Coll Med

Rochelson, Burton L MD (MF) - **Spec Exp:** Pregnancy-High Risk; Ultrasound; Prenatal Diagnosis; **Hospital:** N Shore Univ Hosp; **Address:** N Shore Univ Hosp, Dept Maternal/Fetal Med, 300 Community Drive, Manhasset, NY 11030-3876; **Phone:** 516-562-4458; **Board Cert:** Obstetrics & Gynecology 2008; Maternal & Fetal Medicine 2008; **Med School:** Univ Mich Med Sch 1978; **Resid:** Obstetrics & Gynecology, LI Jewish Med Ctr 1982; **Fellow:** Maternal & Fetal Medicine, Univ Hosp 1986; **Fac Appt:** Assoc Clin Prof ObG, NYU Sch Med

Vintzileos, Anthony M MD (MF) - **Spec Exp:** Ultrasound; Fetal Therapy; **Hospital:** Winthrop - Univ Hosp; **Address:** Winthrop Univ Hosp, Dept Ob/Gyn, 259 First St, Mineola, NY 11501; **Phone:** 516-663-8657; **Board Cert:** Obstetrics & Gynecology 1999; Maternal & Fetal Medicine 1999; **Med School:** Greece 1975; **Resid:** Obstetrics & Gynecology, St Josephs Hosp Med Ctr 1981; **Fellow:** Maternal & Fetal Medicine, Univ Conn Hlth Ctr 1983; **Fac Appt:** Prof ObG, UMDNJ-RW Johnson Med Sch

Medical Oncology

Arena, Francis P MD (Onc) - **Spec Exp:** Breast Cancer; **Hospital:** NS-LIJ Hlth Sys; **Address:** 1999 Marcus Ave, Ste 120, Lake Success, NY 11042; **Phone:** 516-466-6611; **Board Cert:** Internal Medicine 1978; Medical Oncology 2006; **Med School:** Cornell Univ-Weill Med Coll 1975; **Resid:** Internal Medicine, NY Hosp-Cornell Med Ctr 1979; **Fellow:** Hematology & Oncology, Meml Sloan Kettering Cancer Ctr 1980; **Fac Appt:** Assoc Clin Prof Med, Cornell Univ-Weill Med Coll

Bradley, Thomas P MD (Onc) - **Spec Exp:** Bladder Cancer; Prostate Cancer; Kidney Cancer; **Hospital:** N Shore Univ Hosp; **Address:** Monter Cancer Center, 450 Lakeville Rd, Lake Success, NY 11042; **Phone:** 516-734-8900; **Board Cert:** Internal Medicine 1987; Medical Oncology 2001; Hematology 2002; **Med School:** Mexico 1982; **Resid:** Internal Medicine, Univ Hosp-SUNY Downstate 1988; **Fellow:** Hematology & Oncology, Univ Hosp-SUNY Downstate 1991; **Fac Appt:** Assoc Prof Med, Albert Einstein Coll Med

Budman, Daniel MD (Onc) - **Spec Exp:** Breast Cancer; Lymphoma; Drug Discovery & Development; Psychopharmacology; **Hospital:** N Shore Univ Hosp; **Address:** Monter Cancer Ctr, 450 Lakeville Rd, Lake Success, NY 11042; **Phone:** 516-734-8900; **Board Cert:** Internal Medicine 1975; Hematology 1978; Medical Oncology 1979; **Med School:** Albert Einstein Coll Med 1972; **Resid:** Internal Medicine, Hosp Univ Penn 1974; Hematology, Natl Inst Hlth 1976; **Fellow:** Medical Oncology, Sloan Kettering Cancer Ctr 1977; Hematology, NYU Med Ctr 1978; **Fac Appt:** Prof Med, NYU Sch Med

Citron, Marc L MD (Onc) - **Spec Exp:** Breast Cancer; Lung Cancer; **Hospital:** Long Island Jewish Med Ctr; **Address:** Pro Hlthcare Assoc, Div Oncology, 2800 Marcus Ave, Ste 205, Lake Success, NY 11042-1008; **Phone:** 516-622-6150; **Board Cert:** Internal Medicine 1977; Medical Oncology 1979; **Med School:** Wayne State Univ 1974; **Resid:** Internal Medicine, Georgetown Univ Hosp 1977; **Fellow:** Medical Oncology, Georgetown Univ Hosp 1979; **Fac Appt:** Clin Prof Med, Albert Einstein Coll Med

Gralla, Richard J MD (Onc) - **Spec Exp:** Lung Cancer; **Hospital:** NS-LIJ Hlth Sys; **Address:** Monter Cancer Ctr, 450 Lakeville Rd, Lake Success, NY 11042; **Phone:** 516-734-8966; **Board Cert:** Internal Medicine 1975; Medical Oncology 1977; **Med School:** Univ VA Sch Med 1972; **Resid:** Internal Medicine, St Lukes Hosp Ctr 1974; **Fellow:** Cancer Research, Meml Sloan Kettering Canc Ctr 1975; Medical Oncology, Meml Sloan Kettering Cancer Med Ctr 1977; **Fac Appt:** Prof Med, Columbia P&S

Hindenburg, Alexander A MD (Onc) - **Spec Exp:** Pancreatic Cancer; Breast Cancer; Gynecologic Cancer; Myelodysplastic Syndromes; **Hospital:** Winthrop - Univ Hosp; **Address:** Winthrop Oncology/Hematology Assocs, 200 Old Country Rd, Ste 450, Mineola, NY 11501; **Phone:** 516-663-9500; **Board Cert:** Internal Medicine 1981; Medical Oncology 1983; Hematology 1988; **Med School:** UMDNJ-RW Johnson Med Sch 1978; **Resid:** Internal Medicine, Mt Sinai Hosp 1981; **Fellow:** Hematology & Oncology, Columbia-Presby Med Ctr 1984; **Fac Appt:** Asst Prof Med, SUNY Stony Brook

Kappel, Bruce I MD (Onc) - **Spec Exp:** Breast Cancer; Colon Cancer; **Hospital:** Plainview Hosp, St Joseph's Hosp-Nassau; **Address:** 40 Crossways Park Drive, Ste 103, Woodbury, NY 11791; **Phone:** 516-921-5533; **Board Cert:** Internal Medicine 1985; Medical Oncology 1987; Hematology 1988; **Med School:** Emory Univ 1982; **Resid:** Internal Medicine, Emory Univ Hosp 1985; **Fellow:** Medical Oncology, Columbia-Presby Med Ctr 1988

Kessler, Leonard MD (Onc) - **Hospital:** South Nassau Comm Hosp, Mercy Med Ctr - Rockville Centre; **Address:** 242 Merrick Rd, Ste 301, Rockville Centre, NY 11570; **Phone:** 516-536-1455; **Board Cert:** Internal Medicine 1979; Medical Oncology 1981; Hematology 1982; **Med School:** Albert Einstein Coll Med 1975; **Resid:** Internal Medicine, Montefiore Hosp Med Ctr 1977; **Fellow:** Hematology, Montefiore Hosp Med Ctr 1981; Medical Oncology, Meml Sloan Kettering Cancer Ctr 1980

Marino, John S MD (Onc) - **Spec Exp:** Breast Cancer; Colon Cancer; Lung Cancer; **Hospital:** N Shore Univ Hosp, St Francis Hosp - The Heart Ctr (page 115); **Address:** 2001 Marcus Ave, Lake Success, NY 11042; **Phone:** 516-883-0122; **Board Cert:** Internal Medicine 1982; Medical Oncology 1985; **Med School:** NY Med Coll 1979; **Resid:** Internal Medicine, N Shore Univ Hosp 1982; **Fellow:** Medical Oncology, Jacobi Med Ctr 1983; Medical Oncology, N Shore Univ Hosp 1984; **Fac Appt:** Asst Clin Prof Med, NYU Sch Med

Mehrotra, Bhoomi MD (Onc) - **Spec Exp:** Lung Cancer; Head & Neck Cancer; Gastrointestinal Cancer; **Hospital:** Long Island Jewish Med Ctr; **Address:** Long Island Jewish Medical, 270-05 76th Ave, New Hyde Park, NY 11040; **Phone:** 718-470-8934; **Board Cert:** Internal Medicine 2000; Medical Oncology 2003; Hematology 2004; **Med School:** India 1986; **Resid:** Internal Medicine, LI Jewish Medical Ctr 1990; **Fellow:** Hematology & Oncology, UCSD Med Ctr 1993; **Fac Appt:** Assoc Clin Prof Med, Albert Einstein Coll Med

Rothman, Ivan K MD (Onc) - **Hospital:** South Nassau Comm Hosp, Mercy Med Ctr - Rockville Centre; **Address:** 242 Merrick Rd, Ste 301, Rockville Centre, NY 11570; **Phone:** 516-536-1455; **Board Cert:** Medical Oncology 1977; Hematology 1976; Internal Medicine 1974; **Med School:** NYU Sch Med 1971; **Resid:** Internal Medicine, NC Meml Hosp- UNC 1973; **Fellow:** Hematology, NYU Hosp 1977; **Fac Appt:** Asst Clin Prof Med, SUNY Stony Brook

Schwartz, Paula R MD (Onc) - **Spec Exp:** Breast Cancer; Colon Cancer; **Hospital:** N Shore Univ Hosp, Long Island Jewish Med Ctr; **Address:** 3003 New Hyde Park Rd, Ste 401, New Hyde Park, NY 11042; **Phone:** 516-354-5700; **Board Cert:** Internal Medicine 1986; Hematology 1988; **Med School:** SUNY Downstate 1980; **Resid:** Internal Medicine, LI Jewish Med Ctr 1981; Internal Medicine, LI Jewish Med Ctr 1983; **Fellow:** Hematology, Mt Sinai Hosp 1985; Hematology, N Shore Univ Hosp 1989

Tomao, Frank A MD (Onc) - **Spec Exp:** Lung Cancer; Breast Cancer; **Hospital:** NS-LIJ Hlth Sys, St Francis Hosp - The Heart Ctr (page 115); **Address:** 44 S Bayles Ave, Ste 218, Port Washington, NY 11050-3765; **Phone:** 516-883-0122; **Board Cert:** Internal Medicine 1974; Medical Oncology 1975; **Med School:** Cornell Univ-Weill Med Coll 1965; **Resid:** Medical Oncology, Meml Sloan Kettering Cancer Ctr 1967; Medical Oncology, Bellevue Hosp 1968; **Fellow:** Medical Oncology, Meml Sloan Kettering Cancer Ctr 1969

Vinciguerra, Vincent P MD (Onc) - **Spec Exp:** Breast Cancer; Gastrointestinal Cancer; Lung Cancer; Cancer Prevention; **Hospital:** N Shore Univ Hosp; **Address:** 450 Lakeville Rd, Montra Cancer Ctr, Lake Success, NY 11042; **Phone:** 516-734-8954; **Board Cert:** Internal Medicine 1971; Hematology 1974; Medical Oncology 1975; **Med School:** Georgetown Univ 1966; **Resid:** Internal Medicine, NY Hosp-Cornell 1969; Internal Medicine, N Shore Univ Hosp 1971; **Fellow:** Hematology & Oncology, NY Hosp-Cornell 1970; Hematology & Oncology, N Shore Univ Hosp 1974; **Fac Appt:** Prof Med, NYU Sch Med

Wang, Jen Chin MD (Onc) - **Hospital:** Long Beach Med Ctr, N Shore Univ Hosp; **Address:** 5 E Walnut St, Long Beach, NY 11561; **Phone:** 516-889-7447; **Board Cert:** Internal Medicine 1976; Medical Oncology 1977; Hematology 1978; **Med School:** Taiwan 1969; **Resid:** Internal Medicine, Brookdale Hosp 1974; Hematology & Oncology, Brookdale Hosp 1976; **Fellow:** Hematology & Oncology, Brookdale Hosp 1976; **Fac Appt:** Assoc Prof Med, Mount Sinai Sch Med

Weiselberg, Lora MD (Onc) - **Spec Exp:** Breast Cancer; **Hospital:** N Shore Univ Hosp, Long Island Jewish Med Ctr; **Address:** Monter Cancer Center, 450 Lakeville Rd, Lake Success, NY 11042; **Phone:** 516-734-8900; **Board Cert:** Internal Medicine 1978; Medical Oncology 1981; Hematology 1982; **Med School:** NY Med Coll 1975; **Resid:** Internal Medicine, Stamford Hosp 1978; **Fellow:** Medical Oncology, N Shore Univ Hosp 1980; Hematology, N Shore Univ Hosp 1980; **Fac Appt:** Assoc Prof Med, NYU Sch Med

Weiss, Rita MD/PhD (Onc) - **Hospital:** St Francis Hosp - The Heart Ctr (page 115), N Shore Univ Hosp; **Address:** 107 Northern Blvd, Ste 306, Great Neck, NY 11021-4309; **Phone:** 516-482-0080; **Board Cert:** Internal Medicine 1984; Medical Oncology 1989; **Med School:** Mexico 1977; **Resid:** Internal Medicine, Winthrop Univ Hosp 1980; **Fellow:** Medical Oncology, Mount Sinai 1982; **Fac Appt:** Asst Clin Prof Med, NYU Sch Med

Neonatal-Perinatal Medicine

Boxer, Harriet MD (NP) - **Spec Exp:** Prematurity/Low Birth Weight Infants; Chronic Obstructive Lung Disease (COPD); **Hospital:** Nassau Univ Med Ctr; **Address:** Nassau Univ Med Ctr, Div Neonatology, 2201 Hempstead Tpke, Box 30, East Meadow, NY 11554; **Phone:** 516-572-3319; **Board Cert:** Pediatrics 1977; Neonatal-Perinatal Medicine 1977; **Med School:** SUNY Downstate 1972; **Resid:** Pediatrics, Babies Hosp 1974; Pediatrics, Children's Hosp 1975; **Fellow:** Neonatal-Perinatal Medicine, LI Jewish-Hillside Med Ctr 1977; **Fac Appt:** Asst Prof Ped, SUNY Stony Brook

Davidson, Dennis MD (NP) - **Spec Exp:** Lung Disease in Newborns; **Hospital:** Steven & Alexandra Cohen Chldn's Med Ctr of NY; **Address:** Cohen Childrens Med Ctr, Neonatal Div, 269-01 76th Ave, Ste 344, New Hyde Park, NY 11040; **Phone:** 718-470-3440; **Board Cert:** Pediatrics 1980; Neonatal-Perinatal Medicine 2009; **Med School:** Loyola Univ-Stritch Sch Med 1974; **Resid:** Pediatrics, Babies Hosp-Columbia Univ 1978; **Fellow:** Neonatal-Perinatal Medicine, Babies Hosp-Columbia Univ 1981; **Fac Appt:** Clin Prof Ped, Albert Einstein Coll Med

Schanler, Richard MD (NP) - **Spec Exp:** Nutrition; Breast Feeding Problems; **Hospital:** N Shore Univ Hosp, Steven & Alexandra Cohen Chldn's Med Ctr of NY; **Address:** North Shore Univ Hosp, Chief, Neonatal-Perinatal Medicine, 300 Community Drive, Manhasset, NY 11030; **Phone:** 516-562-4665; **Board Cert:** Pediatrics 1979; Neonatal-Perinatal Medicine 1981; **Med School:** UMDNJ-NJ Med Sch, Newark 1974; **Resid:** Pediatrics, Univ Colorado Hlth Sci Ctr 1977; **Fellow:** Neonatology, Brown Univ 1980; **Fac Appt:** Prof Ped, Albert Einstein Coll Med

Steele, Andrew M MD (NP) - **Spec Exp:** Lung Disease in Newborns; Sudden Infant Death Syndrome (SIDS); **Hospital:** Steven & Alexandra Cohen Chldn's Med Ctr of NY, N Shore Univ Hosp; **Address:** Steven & Alexandra Cohen Chldn's Hosp, 269-01 76th Ave, New Hyde Park, NY 11040-1433; **Phone:** 718-470-3440; **Board Cert:** Pediatrics 1981; Neonatal-Perinatal Medicine 1981; **Med School:** SUNY Hlth Sci Ctr 1976; **Resid:** Pediatrics, LI Jewish Med Ctr 1978; **Fellow:** Neonatal-Perinatal Medicine, LI Jewish Med Ctr 1980; **Fac Appt:** Assoc Prof Ped, Albert Einstein Coll Med

Nephrology

Bellucci, Alessandro G MD (Nep) - **Spec Exp:** Hypertension; Kidney Stones; Kidney Disease; Kidney Failure; **Hospital:** N Shore Univ Hosp; **Address:** North Shore Univ Hosp, Dept Nephrology, 300 Community Drive, Manhasset, NY 11030; **Phone:** 516-562-4312; **Board Cert:** Internal Medicine 1979; Nephrology 1982; **Med School:** Italy 1975; **Resid:** Internal Medicine, Cabrini Med Ctr 1979; **Fellow:** Nephrology, N Shore Univ Hosp 1982; **Fac Appt:** Assoc Prof Med, NYU Sch Med

Bourla, Steven L MD (Nep) - **Spec Exp:** Kidney Disease; **Hospital:** Plainview Hosp, St Joseph's Hosp-Nassau; **Address:** 789 Old Country Rd, Plainview, NY 11803; **Phone:** 516-433-3600; **Board Cert:** Internal Medicine 1979; Nephrology 1982; **Med School:** NY Med Coll 1975; **Resid:** Internal Medicine, LI Jewish Med Ctr 1978; **Fellow:** Nephrology, NYU Med Ctr 1981

Fishbane, Steven MD (Nep) - **Spec Exp:** Kidney Disease-Chronic; Dialysis Care; **Hospital:** Winthrop - Univ Hosp; **Address:** 200 Old Country Rd, Ste 135, Mineola, NY 11501; **Phone:** 516-663-2169; **Board Cert:** Internal Medicine 2001; Nephrology 2004; **Med School:** Albert Einstein Coll Med 1988; **Resid:** Internal Medicine, Montefiore Med Ctr 1991; **Fellow:** Nephrology, Montefiore-Weiler Einstein Med Ctr 1993

Mailloux, Lionel U MD (Nep) - **Spec Exp:** Hypertension; Dialysis Care; **Hospital:** N Shore Univ Hosp, Glen Cove Hosp; **Address:** 50 Seaview Blvd, Port Washington, NY 11050; **Phone:** 516-484-6093; **Board Cert:** Internal Medicine 1977; Nephrology 1972; **Med School:** Hahnemann Univ 1962; **Resid:** Internal Medicine, Hartford Hosp 1965; **Fellow:** Nephrology, Hahnemann Hosp 1966; **Fac Appt:** Assoc Prof Med, NYU Sch Med

Mattana, Joseph MD (Nep) - **Spec Exp:** Diabetic Kidney Disease; Hypertension; Glomerulonephritis; **Hospital:** Long Island Jewish Med Ctr, N Shore Univ Hosp; **Address:** 100 Community Drive Fl 2nd, Great Neck, NY 11021; **Phone:** 516-465-3010; **Board Cert:** Internal Medicine 2000; Nephrology 2004; **Med School:** SUNY Hlth Sci Ctr 1987; **Resid:** Internal Medicine, LI Jewish Hosp 1990; **Fellow:** Nephrology, LI Jewish Hosp 1993; **Fac Appt:** Prof Med, Albert Einstein Coll Med

Singhal, Pravin C MD (Nep) - **Spec Exp:** Hypertension; Diabetic Kidney Disease; **Hospital:** Long Island Jewish Med Ctr, N Shore Univ Hosp; **Address:** 100 Community Drive, Great Neck, NY 11021; **Phone:** 516-465-3010; **Board Cert:** Internal Medicine 1983; Nephrology 1986; **Med School:** India 1970; **Resid:** Internal Medicine, Postgrad Inst Med Ed. 1972; Internal Medicine, Brigham Womens Hosp 1983; **Fellow:** Nephrology, Montefiore Med Ctr 1985; **Fac Appt:** Prof Med, Albert Einstein Coll Med

Wagner, John D MD (Nep) - **Spec Exp:** Hypertension; Dialysis Care; Kidney Failure-Chronic; **Hospital:** Long Island Jewish Med Ctr, N Shore Univ Hosp; **Address:** 410 Lakeville Rd, Ste 107, New Hyde Park, NY 11042-1102; **Phone:** 516-465-3010; **Board Cert:** Internal Medicine 1981; Nephrology 1984; **Med School:** Yale Univ 1978; **Resid:** Internal Medicine, Bellevue-NYU 1982; **Fellow:** Nephrology, Bellevue-NYU-VAMC 1984; **Fac Appt:** Assoc Clin Prof Med, Albert Einstein Coll Med

Neurological Surgery

Brown, Jeffrey A MD (NS) - **Spec Exp:** Trigeminal Neuralgia; Pain-Chronic; **Hospital:** Winthrop - Univ Hosp, N Shore Univ Hosp; **Address:** 600 Northern Blvd, Ste 118, Great Neck, NY 11021-5200; **Phone:** 516-478-0008; **Board Cert:** Neurological Surgery 1986; **Med School:** Univ Chicago-Pritzker Sch Med 1976; **Resid:** Surgery, Univ Chicago Hosps 1977; Neurological Surgery, Univ Chicago Hosps 1982; **Fac Appt:** Prof NS, Wayne State Univ

Eisenberg, Mark MD (NS) - **Spec Exp:** Skull Base Surgery; Spinal Surgery-Minimally Invasive; Pituitary Tumors; Brain Tumors; **Hospital:** Long Island Jewish Med Ctr; **Address:** 900 Northern Blvd, Ste 260, Great Neck, NY 11021; **Phone:** 516-773-7737; **Board Cert:** Neurological Surgery 2010; **Med School:** Univ Miami Sch Med 1988; **Resid:** Neurological Surgery, Mount Sinai Med Ctr 1994; **Fellow:** Skull Base Surgery, Univ Arkansas Med Ctr 1995; **Fac Appt:** Asst Clin Prof NS, NYU Sch Med

Epstein, Nancy E MD (NS) - **Spec Exp:** Spinal Surgery; Spinal Surgery-Neck; Transfusion Free Surgery; **Hospital:** Winthrop - Univ Hosp; **Address:** 410 Lakeville Rd, Ste 204, New Hyde Park, NY 11042-1199; **Phone:** 516-354-3401; **Board Cert:** Neurological Surgery 1984; **Med School:** Columbia P&S 1976; **Resid:** Neurological Surgery, Bellevue Hosp Ctr-NYU 1981; **Fac Appt:** Clin Prof NS, Albert Einstein Coll Med

Langer, David J MD (NS) - **Spec Exp:** Neurovascular Surgery; Arteriovenous Malformations; Aneurysm-Cerebral; Carotid Artery Surgery; **Hospital:** N Shore Univ Hosp; **Address:** 300 Community Drive, Tower 9, Manhasset, NY 11030; **Phone:** 516-562-3023; **Board Cert:** Neurological Surgery 2003; **Med School:** Univ Pennsylvania 1991; **Resid:** Neurological Surgery, Hosp Univ Penn 1998; **Fellow:** Neurological Vascular Surgery, Beth Israel Med Ctr 1999; **Fac Appt:** Asst Prof NS, Albert Einstein Coll Med

Levine, Mitchell E MD (NS) - **Spec Exp:** Brain Tumors; **Hospital:** N Shore Univ Hosp; **Address:** 900 Northern Blvd, Ste 260, Great Neck, NY 11021; **Phone:** 516-773-7737; **Board Cert:** Neurological Surgery 1987; **Med School:** Mount Sinai Sch Med 1977; **Resid:** Surgery, Mt Sinai Hosp 1978; Neurological Surgery, Mt Sinai Hosp 1983

Mittler, Mark A MD (NS) - **Spec Exp:** Pediatric Neurosurgery; Brain & Spinal Cord Tumors; Vascular Malformations; Hydrocephalus; **Hospital:** Steven & Alexandra Cohen Chldn's Med Ctr of NY; **Address:** LI Neurosurgical Assocs, 410 Lakeville Rd, Ste 204, New Hyde Park, NY 11042; **Phone:** 516-354-3401; **Board Cert:** Neurological Surgery 2001; Pediatric Neurological Surgery 2001; **Med School:** Univ Rochester 1991; **Resid:** Neurological Surgery, RI Hosp 1998; **Fellow:** Pediatric Neurological Surgery, Children's Hosp 1999; **Fac Appt:** Asst Clin Prof NS, NYU Sch Med

Schulder, Michael MD (NS) - **Spec Exp:** Brain Tumors; Movement Disorders; Skull Base Surgery; **Hospital:** N Shore Univ Hosp, Long Island Jewish Med Ctr; **Address:** North Shore University Hospital, 300 Community Drive, Tower 9, Manhasset, NY 11030; **Phone:** 516-562-3062; **Board Cert:** Neurological Surgery 1991; **Med School:** Columbia P&S 1982; **Resid:** Neurological Surgery, Montefiore Hosp Med Ctr/Albert Einstein 1988; **Fac Appt:** , UMDNJ-NJ Med Sch, Newark

Neurology

Blanck, Richard H MD (N) - **Spec Exp:** Multiple Sclerosis; Pain-Back; **Hospital:** N Shore Univ Hosp, St Francis Hosp - The Heart Ctr (page 115); **Address:** 1991 Marcus Ave, Ste 110, Lake Success, NY 11042; **Phone:** 516-466-4700; **Board Cert:** Internal Medicine 1976; Neurology 1980; **Med School:** UMDNJ-NJ Med Sch, Newark 1973; **Resid:** Internal Medicine, N Shore Univ Hosp 1975; Neurology, N Shore Univ Hosp 1977; **Fac Appt:** Assoc Clin Prof N, NYU Sch Med

Ettinger, Alan MD (N) - **Spec Exp:** Epilepsy; Seizure Disorders; **Hospital:** Winthrop - Univ Hosp, Huntington Hosp; **Address:** Neurological Surgery, PC, 1991 Marcus Ave, Ste 108, Lake Success, NY 11042; **Phone:** 516-442-2250; **Board Cert:** Neurology 1989; **Med School:** Boston Univ 1983; **Resid:** Internal Medicine, Hartford Hosp 1985; Neurology, Montefiore Med Ctr 1988; **Fellow:** Epilepsy, Montefiore Med Ctr 1989; **Fac Appt:** Prof N, Albert Einstein Coll Med

Gordon, Marc L MD (N) - **Spec Exp:** Dementia; Headache; Multiple Sclerosis; Alzheimer's Disease; **Hospital:** Long Island Jewish Med Ctr; **Address:** LI Jewish Med Ctr, Dept Neurology, 270-05 76th Ave, Ste 222, New Hyde Park, NY 11040-1433; **Phone:** 718-470-7366; **Board Cert:** Neurology 1990; **Med School:** Columbia P&S 1985; **Resid:** Neurology, Albert Einstein 1989; **Fellow:** Neuropsychopharmacology, Albert Einstein Coll Med 1990; **Fac Appt:** Assoc Clin Prof N, Albert Einstein Coll Med

Haimovic, Itzhak C MD (N) - **Spec Exp:** Spinal Disorders; Epilepsy; Headache; **Hospital:** N Shore Univ Hosp, Long Island Jewish Med Ctr; **Address:** 170 Great Neck Rd, Great Neck, NY 11021; **Phone:** 516-487-4464; **Board Cert:** Neurology 1981; **Med School:** NY Med Coll 1975; **Resid:** Neurology, N Shore Univ Hosp 1977; Neurology, NY Hosp-Cornell Univ 1980; **Fellow:** Neurological Physiology, Columbia-Presby 1981; **Fac Appt:** Assoc Clin Prof N, NYU Sch Med

Hainline, Brian MD (N) - **Spec Exp:** Pain-Chronic; Spinal Disorders; Reflex Sympathetic Dystrophy (RSD); **Hospital:** N Shore Univ Hosp; **Address:** 3 Delaware Drive, Lake Success, NY 11042; **Phone:** 516-622-6088; **Board Cert:** Neurology 1987; Pain Medicine 2001; **Med School:** Univ Chicago-Pritzker Sch Med 1982; **Resid:** Neurology, NY Hosp 1986; **Fac Appt:** Assoc Clin Prof N, NYU Sch Med

Kanner, Ronald MD (N) - **Spec Exp:** Headache; Pain-Chronic; **Hospital:** Long Island Jewish Med Ctr; **Address:** 270-05 76th Ave, rm 222, New Hyde Park, NY 11040; **Phone:** 718-470-7311; **Board Cert:** Neurology 1980; **Med School:** Spain 1975; **Resid:** Internal Medicine, Philadelphia Genl Hosp 1976; Neurology, Montefiore Med Ctr 1979; **Fellow:** Neurology, Meml Sloan Kettering Cancer Ctr 1981; **Fac Appt:** Prof N, Albert Einstein Coll Med

Kelemen, John MD (N) - **Spec Exp:** Electromyography; Neuromuscular Disorders; Botox for Muscle Overactivity; Dystonia; **Hospital:** Plainview Hosp; **Address:** 824 Old Country Rd, Plainview, NY 11803-4935; **Phone:** 516-822-2230; **Board Cert:** Neurology 1979; **Med School:** Georgetown Univ 1974; **Resid:** Internal Medicine, Nassau County Med Ctr 1978; **Fellow:** Neuromuscular Medicine, New England Med Ctr 1980

Kessler, Jeffrey T MD (N) - **Spec Exp:** Parkinson's Disease; Dementia; Pain-Facial; **Hospital:** N Shore Univ Hosp, St Francis Hosp - The Heart Ctr (page 115); **Address:** 1991 Marcus Ave, Ste 110, Lake Success, NY 11042; **Phone:** 516-466-4700; **Board Cert:** Internal Medicine 1974; Neurology 1976; **Med School:** Cornell Univ-Weill Med Coll 1969; **Resid:** Internal Medicine, New York Hosp-Cornell Med Ctr 1971; **Fellow:** Neurology, New York Hosp-Cornell Med Ctr 1974; **Fac Appt:** Assoc Clin Prof N, NYU Sch Med

Kula, Roger W MD (N) - **Spec Exp:** Neuromuscular Disorders; Myasthenia Gravis; Syringomyelia & Spinal Cord Diseases; Chiari's Deformity; **Hospital:** N Shore Univ Hosp, Steven & Alexandra Cohen Chldn's Med Ctr of NY; **Address:** 865 Northern Blvd, Ste 302, Great Neck, NY 11021; **Phone:** 516-570-4400; **Board Cert:** Internal Medicine 1975; Neurology 1977; Neuromuscular Medicine 2008; **Med School:** Johns Hopkins Univ 1970; **Resid:** Internal Medicine, New York Hosp 1972; Neurology, UCSF Med Ctr 1974; **Fellow:** Neuromuscular Medicine, Natl Inst Hlth 1977; **Fac Appt:** Assoc Prof N, SUNY Hlth Sci Ctr

Levy, Lewis MD (N) - **Spec Exp:** Tourette's Syndrome; Parkinson's Disease; **Hospital:** South Nassau Comm Hosp; **Address:** 777 Sunrise Hwy, Ste 200, Lynbrook, NY 11563; **Phone:** 516-887-3516; **Board Cert:** Neurology 1979; **Med School:** SUNY Downstate 1973; **Resid:** Neurology, Albert Einstein 1977; **Fac Appt:** Asst Clin Prof N, Albert Einstein Coll Med

Libman, Richard MD (N) - **Spec Exp:** Stroke; **Hospital:** Long Island Jewish Med Ctr; **Address:** 270-05 76th Ave, rm 222, New Hyde Park, NY 11040-1433; **Phone:** 718-470-7311; **Board Cert:** Neurology 1991; Vascular Neurology 2005; **Med School:** McGill Univ 1986; **Resid:** Neurology, Montefiore Med Ctr 1990; **Fellow:** Stroke, Columbia-Presby Med Ctr 1993; **Fac Appt:** Assoc Prof N, Albert Einstein Coll Med

Newman, Stephen M MD (N) - **Spec Exp:** Multiple Sclerosis; Migraine; **Hospital:** Plainview Hosp; **Address:** 824 Old Country Rd, Plainview, NY 11803; **Phone:** 516-822-2230; **Board Cert:** Neurology 1978; **Med School:** SUNY Buffalo 1972; **Resid:** Neurology, Nassau County Med Ctr 1976

Ragone, Philip MD (N) - **Spec Exp:** Electromyography; **Hospital:** St Francis Hosp - The Heart Ctr (page 115), N Shore Univ Hosp; **Address:** 1010 Northern Blvd, Ste 136, Great Neck, NY 11021; **Phone:** 516-482-4100; **Board Cert:** Internal Medicine 1985; Neurology 1989; Electrodiagnostic Medicine 1990; **Med School:** NY Med Coll 1982; **Resid:** Internal Medicine, Lenox Hill Hosp 1985; Neurology, Albert Einstein 1988; **Fellow:** Electromyography, Albert Einstein 1989

Schaul, Neil S MD (N) - **Spec Exp:** Epilepsy/Seizure Disorders; Electrodiagnosis; **Hospital:** NY Hosp Queens; **Address:** 1575 Hillside Ave, New Hyde Park, NY 11040; **Phone:** 718-670-2900; **Board Cert:** Neurology 1976; **Med School:** SUNY Hlth Sci Ctr 1966; **Resid:** Internal Medicine, DC General Hosp 1968; Neurology, Montreal Neur Inst 1974; **Fellow:** Neurological Physiology, Montreal Neur Inst 1977; **Fac Appt:** Assoc Prof Med, Cornell Univ-Weill Med Coll

Turner, Ira MD (N) - **Spec Exp:** Headache; **Hospital:** Plainview Hosp; **Address:** 824 Old Country Rd, Plainview, NY 11803; **Phone:** 516-822-2230; **Board Cert:** Neurology 1978; Headache Medicine 2007; **Med School:** SUNY Downstate 1972; **Resid:** Neurology, Nassau Co Med Ctr 1976

Neuroradiology

Ortiz, Orlando MD (NRad) - **Spec Exp:** Interventional Neuroradiology; Spine Imaging & Intervention; **Hospital:** Winthrop - Univ Hosp; **Address:** 120 Mineola Blvd, Ste 650, Mineola, NY 11501; **Phone:** 516-663-2123; **Board Cert:** Diagnostic Radiology 1990; Neuroradiology 2006; **Med School:** Harvard Med Sch 1985; **Resid:** Diagnostic Radiology, LIJ Med Ctr 1990; **Fellow:** Neurological Radiology, NY Presby-Columbia Med Ctr 1992

Pile-Spellman, John MD (NRad) - **Spec Exp:** Interventional Neuroradiology; Cerebrovascular Disease; Aneurysm; Arteriovenous Malformations; **Hospital:** Winthrop - Univ Hosp; **Address:** Neurological Surgery, PC, 1991 Marcus Ave, Ste 108, Lake Success, NY 11042; **Phone:** 516-442-2250; **Board Cert:** Diagnostic Radiology 1984; **Med School:** Tufts Univ 1978; **Resid:** Neurological Surgery, New England Med Ctr 1981; Neurological Radiology, Mass Genl Hosp 1984; **Fellow:** Interventional Neuroradiology, NYU Med Ctr 1986; **Fac Appt:** Prof Rad, Columbia P&S

Setton, Avi MD (NRad) - **Spec Exp:** Cerebrovascular Disease; **Hospital:** N Shore Univ Hosp; **Address:** N Shore Univ Hospital, 300 Community Drive, 9 Tower, Manhasset, NY 11030; **Phone:** 516-562-3021; **Med School:** Israel 1978; **Resid:** Diagnostic Radiology, Bellevue Med Ctr 1991; **Fellow:** Neurological Radiology, NYU Med Ctr 1992

Nuclear Medicine

Palestro, Christopher MD (NuM) - **Spec Exp:** Pain after Joint Replacement; Diabetic Leg/Foot Infections; AIDS Related Infections; **Hospital:** Long Island Jewish Med Ctr, N Shore Univ Hosp; **Address:** Nuclear Medicine, 270-05 76th Ave, New Hyde Park, NY 11040-1402; **Phone:** 718-470-7080; **Board Cert:** Nuclear Medicine 1982; **Med School:** Mexico 1975; **Resid:** Diagnostic Radiology, Roosevelt Hosp 1980; **Fellow:** Nuclear Medicine, Meml Sloan Kettering Cancer Ctr 1982; **Fac Appt:** Prof NuM, Albert Einstein Coll Med

Yung, Elizabeth MD (NuM) - **Spec Exp:** PET Imaging; **Hospital:** Winthrop - Univ Hosp; **Address:** 259 First St, Mineola, NY 11501; **Phone:** 516-663-2778; **Board Cert:** Diagnostic Radiology 1984; Nuclear Radiology 1991; **Med School:** Tufts Univ 1980; **Resid:** Diagnostic Radiology, St Vincent's Hosp & Med Ctr 1984; **Fellow:** Nuclear Medicine, Yale-New Haven Hosp 1991

Obstetrics & Gynecology

Barbaccia, Ann MD (ObG) - **Spec Exp:** Menopause Problems; Gynecologic Surgery; **Hospital:** Mercy Med Ctr - Rockville Centre; **Address:** 2000 N Village Ave, Ste 104, Rockville Centre, NY 11570; **Phone:** 516-678-4222; **Board Cert:** Obstetrics & Gynecology 1980; **Med School:** NY Med Coll 1972; **Resid:** Obstetrics & Gynecology, Nassau County Med Ctr 1978

Benedict, Leonard A MD (ObG) - **Spec Exp:** Pregnancy-High Risk; Gynecologic Surgery; **Hospital:** NS-LIJ Hlth Sys; **Address:** 433 Uniondale Ave, Uniondale, NY 11553; **Phone:** 516-483-8798; **Board Cert:** Obstetrics & Gynecology 1981; **Med School:** Scotland, UK 1972; **Resid:** Obstetrics & Gynecology, Brooklyn Jewish Hosp 1978; **Fac Appt:** Asst Clin Prof ObG, NYU Sch Med

Haselkorn, Joan MD (ObG) *PCP* - **Spec Exp:** Laparoscopic Surgery; Hysteroscopic Surgery; Uterine Fibroids; **Hospital:** South Nassau Comm Hosp, Long Island Jewish Med Ctr; **Address:** 556 Merrick Rd, Rockville Centre, NY 11570; **Phone:** 516-255-2044; **Board Cert:** Obstetrics & Gynecology 1998; **Med School:** Israel 1982; **Resid:** Obstetrics & Gynecology, NYU Med Ctr 1986

Jacob, Jessica MD (ObG) *PCP* - **Hospital:** N Shore Univ Hosp; **Address:** 3003 New Hyde Park Rd, Ste 407, New Hyde Park, NY 11042-1214; **Phone:** 516-488-8145; **Board Cert:** Obstetrics & Gynecology 1999; **Med School:** NYU Sch Med 1983; **Resid:** Obstetrics & Gynecology, N Shore Univ Hosp 1987; **Fac Appt:** Asst Clin Prof ObG, NYU Sch Med

Krim, Eileen MD (ObG) - **Spec Exp:** Menopause Problems; Adolescent Gynecology; Osteoporosis; Laparoscopic Surgery; **Hospital:** N Shore Univ Hosp; **Address:** 3111 New Hyde Park Rd, North Hills, NY 11040-3500; **Phone:** 516-365-6100; **Board Cert:** Obstetrics & Gynecology 1982; **Med School:** NY Med Coll 1975; **Resid:** Obstetrics & Gynecology, Beth Israel 1979; **Fellow:** Maternal & Fetal Medicine, N Shore Univ Hosp 1981; **Fac Appt:** Assoc Clin Prof ObG, NYU Sch Med

Mack, Laurence F MD (ObG) *PCP* - **Spec Exp:** Infertility; Pregnancy-High Risk; Autoimmune Disease in Pregnancy; Pap Smear Abnormalities; **Hospital:** Plainview Hosp, Mercy Med Ctr - Rockville Centre; **Address:** 1130 N Broadway, PO Box 1550, N Massapequa, NY 11758-0910; **Phone:** 516-799-3462; **Board Cert:** Obstetrics & Gynecology 2009; **Med School:** Univ Hlth Scis, Chicago Med Sch 1985; **Resid:** Obstetrics & Gynecology, Brookdale Hosp 1989

Nimaroff, Michael MD (ObG) *PCP* - **Spec Exp:** Laparoscopic Surgery; Hysterectomy Alternatives; Hysteroscopic Surgery; **Hospital:** N Shore Univ Hosp, Long Island Jewish Med Ctr; **Address:** 825 Northern Blvd Fl 3 - Ste 301, Great Neck, NY 11021; **Phone:** 516-472-5700; **Board Cert:** Obstetrics & Gynecology 2009; **Med School:** UMDNJ-NJ Med Sch, Newark 1987; **Resid:** Obstetrics & Gynecology, N Shore Univ Hosp 1991; **Fac Appt:** Asst Clin Prof ObG, NYU Sch Med

Rothbaum, David MD (ObG) *PCP* - **Spec Exp:** Osteoporosis; Menopause Problems; Uterine Fibroids; **Hospital:** N Shore Univ Hosp; **Address:** 233 E Shore Rd, Ste 109, Great Neck, NY 11023-2433; **Phone:** 516-487-3498; **Board Cert:** Obstetrics & Gynecology 2009; **Med School:** Boston Univ 1982; **Resid:** Obstetrics & Gynecology, North Shore Univ Hosp 1986

Toles, Allen W MD (ObG) *PCP* - **Spec Exp:** Pregnancy-High Risk; **Hospital:** Long Island Jewish Med Ctr, N Shore Univ Hosp; **Address:** 1554 Northern Blvd Fl 5, Manhasset, NY 11030; **Phone:** 516-390-9242; **Board Cert:** Obstetrics & Gynecology 2009; **Med School:** Meharry Med Coll 1986; **Resid:** Obstetrics & Gynecology, Howard Univ Hosp 1990; **Fac Appt:** Asst Prof ObG, Albert Einstein Coll Med

Vasudeva, Kusum MD (ObG) - **Spec Exp:** Pregnancy-High Risk; Menopause Problems; **Hospital:** N Shore Univ Hosp; **Address:** 2 Pro Health Plaza, Lake Success, NY 11042; **Phone:** 516-608-6800; **Board Cert:** Obstetrics & Gynecology 1975; **Med School:** India 1968; **Resid:** Obstetrics & Gynecology, N Shore Univ Hosp 1974; **Fellow:** Maternal & Fetal Medicine, N Shore Univ Hosp 1976

Veloso Jr, Manuel A MD (ObG) - **Spec Exp:** Gynecology Only; Gynecologic Ultrasound; Hysteroscopic Surgery; HPV-Human Papillomavirus; **Hospital:** Long Beach Med Ctr; **Address:** 303 E Park Ave, Long Beach, NY 11561; **Phone:** 516-431-2828; **Board Cert:** Obstetrics & Gynecology 1979; **Med School:** Philippines 1966; **Resid:** Obstetrics & Gynecology, Kings Co Hosp 1972

Occupational Medicine

Mendelsohn, Sara L MD (OM) - **Spec Exp:** Travel Medicine; Occupational Disease & Injury; Preventive Medicine; **Address:** 800 Woodbury Rd, Ste K, Woodbury, NY 11797; **Phone:** 516-682-9142; **Board Cert:** Occupational Medicine 1993; **Med School:** Boston Univ 1988; **Resid:** Occupational Medicine, Univ of Illinois Med Ctr 1991; **Fac Appt:** Asst Clin Prof Med, SUNY Stony Brook

Ophthalmology

Berke, Stanley J MD (Oph) - **Spec Exp:** Glaucoma; Cataract Surgery-Lens Implant; Laser Surgery; **Hospital:** Mercy Med Ctr - Rockville Centre; **Address:** 360 Merrick Rd, Lynbrook, NY 11563-1610; **Phone:** 516-593-7709; **Board Cert:** Ophthalmology 1987; **Med School:** SUNY Buffalo 1981; **Resid:** Ophthalmology, Nassau Med Ctr 1985; **Fellow:** Anterior Segment - External Disease, Mass Eye & Ear Infirmary 1986; **Fac Appt:** Assoc Clin Prof Oph, Albert Einstein Coll Med

Boniuk, Vivien MD (Oph) - **Spec Exp:** Diagnostic Problems; **Hospital:** Long Island Jewish Med Ctr, Queens Hosp Ctr - Jamaica; **Address:** 600 Northern Blvd, Great Neck, NY 11021; **Phone:** 516-470-2020; **Board Cert:** Ophthalmology 1969; **Med School:** Dalhousie Univ 1964; **Resid:** Ophthalmology, Barnes Hosp-Washington Univ 1967; **Fellow:** Ophthalmological Pathology, Baylor Coll Affil Hosp 1968; **Fac Appt:** Assoc Prof Oph, Albert Einstein Coll Med

Broderick, Robert MD (Oph) - **Spec Exp:** LASIK-Refractive Surgery; Cataract Surgery; Glaucoma; **Hospital:** St Francis Hosp - The Heart Ctr (page 115), N Shore Univ Hosp; **Address:** 585 Plandome Rd, Ste 104, Manhasset, NY 11030-1971; **Phone:** 516-627-3232; **Board Cert:** Ophthalmology 1983; **Med School:** NY Med Coll 1977; **Resid:** Ophthalmology, St Vincent's Hosp & Med Ctr 1981; **Fellow:** Ophthalmology, Holy Cross Hosp 1983

Cook, Jack MD (Oph) - **Spec Exp:** Glaucoma; **Hospital:** Long Island Jewish Med Ctr; **Address:** 305 Hillside Ave, Williston Park, NY 11596; **Phone:** 516-747-4011; **Board Cert:** Ophthalmology 1980; **Med School:** Albert Einstein Coll Med 1975; **Resid:** Ophthalmology, LI Jewish Med Ctr 1979

D'Aversa, Gerard MD (Oph) - **Spec Exp:** Cataract Surgery; Laser-Refractive Surgery; Cornea Transplant; **Hospital:** Long Island Jewish Med Ctr, Mercy Med Ctr - Rockville Centre; **Address:** 65 Roosevelt Ave, rm 204, Valley Stream, NY 11580-1106; **Phone:** 516-374-4199; **Board Cert:** Ophthalmology 2006; **Med School:** Albert Einstein Coll Med 1989; **Resid:** Ophthalmology, LI Jewish Med Ctr 1993; **Fellow:** Univ Florida 1994; **Fac Appt:** Asst Prof Oph, Albert Einstein Coll Med

Fastenberg, David M MD (Oph) - **Spec Exp:** Retina/Vitreous Surgery; Macular Degeneration; Diabetic Eye Disease/Retinopathy; **Hospital:** Syosset Hosp, Long Island Jewish Med Ctr; **Address:** 600 Northern Blvd, rm 216, Great Neck, NY 11021; **Phone:** 516-466-0390; **Board Cert:** Ophthalmology 1981; **Med School:** NY Med Coll 1976; **Resid:** Ophthalmology, Northwestern Univ Med Ctr 1980; **Fellow:** Retina, USC-Doheny Eye Inst 1982; **Fac Appt:** Assoc Clin Prof Oph, Albert Einstein Coll Med

Ferrone, Philip J MD (Oph) - **Spec Exp:** Retinal Disorders; **Hospital:** Syosset Hosp, Long Island Jewish Med Ctr; **Address:** 600 Northern Blvd, Ste 216, Great Neck, NY 11021; **Phone:** 516-466-0390; **Board Cert:** Ophthalmology 2006; **Med School:** Harvard Med Sch 1989; **Resid:** Ophthalmology, Duke Univ Med Ctr 1993; **Fellow:** Vitreoretinal Surgery, Associated Retinal Consultants 1995

Garber, Perry MD (Oph) - **Spec Exp:** Ophthalmic Plastic Surgery; Blepharoplasty; Lacrimal Gland Disorders; Tear Duct Problems; **Hospital:** Long Island Jewish Med Ctr, St Francis Hosp - The Heart Ctr (page 115); **Address:** 800 Community Drive, Manhasset, NY 11030; **Phone:** 516-627-6630; **Board Cert:** Ophthalmology 1976; **Med School:** SUNY Downstate 1968; **Resid:** Surgery, Mount Sinai Hosp 1970; Ophthalmology, Bellevue Hosp 1975; **Fellow:** Ophthalmic Plastic Surgery, NY Eye & Ear Infirmary 1976; **Fac Appt:** Assoc Clin Prof Oph, Albert Einstein Coll Med

Girardi, Anthony MD (Oph) - **Spec Exp:** Cataract Surgery; Glaucoma; **Hospital:** Glen Cove Hosp; **Address:** 8 Medical Plaza Bldg 8, Glen Cove, NY 11542; **Phone:** 516-676-4596; **Board Cert:** Ophthalmology 1985; **Med School:** SUNY Stony Brook 1980; **Resid:** Ophthalmology, Kings Co Hosp 1984; **Fac Appt:** Asst Clin Prof Oph, SUNY Downstate

Goldberg, Leslie P MD (Oph) - **Spec Exp:** Cataract Surgery; LASIK-Refractive Surgery; Eyelid Cosmetic Surgery; **Hospital:** St Francis Hosp - The Heart Ctr (page 115), N Shore Univ Hosp; **Address:** 2110 Northern Blvd, Ste 208, Manhasset, NY 11030-3500; **Phone:** 516-627-5113; **Board Cert:** Ophthalmology 1977; **Med School:** Ros Franklin Univ/Chicago Med Sch 1970; **Resid:** Ophthalmology, NYU Med Ctr 1976; **Fac Appt:** Asst Clin Prof Oph, NYU Sch Med

Hatsis, Alexander MD (Oph) - **Spec Exp:** LASIK-Refractive Surgery; Cataract Surgery; Corneal Disease & Surgery; Keratoconus; **Hospital:** South Nassau Comm Hosp, Nassau Univ Med Ctr; **Address:** 2 Lincoln Ave, Ste 401, Rockville Centre, NY 11570; **Phone:** 516-763-4106; **Board Cert:** Ophthalmology 2003; **Med School:** Italy 1978; **Resid:** Surgery, Nassau County Med Ctr 1980; Ophthalmology, Nassau County Med Ctr 1981; **Fellow:** Ophthalmology, Nassau County Med Ctr 1983

Kasper, William S MD (Oph) - **Spec Exp:** Cataract Surgery; Glaucoma; Cornea & External Eye Disease; **Hospital:** Winthrop - Univ Hosp, Mercy Med Ctr - Rockville Centre; **Address:** 520 Franklin Ave, Ste L9, Garden City, NY 11530; **Phone:** 516-742-3937; **Board Cert:** Ophthalmology 1974; **Med School:** Belgium 1967; **Resid:** Ophthalmology, Nassau Co Med Ctr 1971

Malik, Sajid MD (Oph) - **Spec Exp:** Cataract Surgery; Lens Implants-Multifocal; **Hospital:** Winthrop - Univ Hosp; **Address:** Woodbury Optical, 185 Woodbury Rd, Hicksville, NY 11801; **Phone:** 516-681-3937; **Board Cert:** Ophthalmology 2010; **Med School:** SUNY Stony Brook 1989; **Resid:** Ophthalmology, Harlem Hosp 1994

Marks, Alan B MD (Oph) - **Spec Exp:** Cataract Surgery; Laser-Refractive Surgery; Eyelid Cosmetic Surgery; **Hospital:** St Francis Hosp - The Heart Ctr (page 115), Syosset Hosp; **Address:** 2110 Northern Blvd, Ste 208, Manhasset, NY 11030; **Phone:** 516-627-5113; **Board Cert:** Ophthalmology 1983; **Med School:** NY Med Coll 1978; **Resid:** Ophthalmology, N Shore Univ Hosp 1982

Nelson, David B MD (Oph) - **Spec Exp:** Cataract Surgery; Glaucoma; **Hospital:** Mercy Med Ctr - Rockville Centre; **Address:** 2000 N Village Ave, Ste 402, Oceanside, NY 11570-1001; **Phone:** 516-766-2519; **Board Cert:** Ophthalmology 1977; **Med School:** SUNY Hlth Sci Ctr 1972; **Resid:** Ophthalmology, NY Eye & Ear Infirmary 1976; **Fac Appt:** Asst Prof Oph, SUNY Stony Brook

Packer, Samuel MD (Oph) - **Spec Exp:** Ethics; **Hospital:** N Shore Univ Hosp, Long Island Jewish Med Ctr; **Address:** 600 Northern Blvd, Ste 214, Great Neck, NY 11021; **Phone:** 516-465-8400; **Board Cert:** Ophthalmology 1973; **Med School:** SUNY Hlth Sci Ctr 1966; **Resid:** Ophthalmology, Yale-New Haven Hosp 1971; **Fac Appt:** Prof Oph, NYU Sch Med

Perry, Henry MD (Oph) - **Spec Exp:** Laser-Refractive Surgery; Cornea Transplant; Cataract Surgery; Eyelid/Tear Duct Disorders; **Hospital:** Mercy Med Ctr - Rockville Centre, Syosset Hosp; **Address:** 2000 N Village Ave, Ste 402, Rockville Centre, NY 11570-1001; **Phone:** 516-766-2519; **Board Cert:** Ophthalmology 1977; **Med School:** Univ Cincinnati 1971; **Resid:** Ophthalmology, Nassau County Med Ctr 1975; Ophthalmology, Hosp Univ Penn 1974; **Fellow:** Cornea, Mass Eye & Ear Infirmary 1977; Ophthalmic Pathology, Armed Forces Inst of Pathology 1976; **Fac Appt:** Assoc Clin Prof Oph, Cornell Univ-Weill Med Coll

Prywes, Arnold MD (Oph) - **Spec Exp:** Glaucoma; Cataract Surgery; **Hospital:** St Joseph's Hosp-Nassau, Syosset Hosp; **Address:** 4212 Hempstead Tpke, Bethpage, NY 11714-5709; **Phone:** 516-731-4800; **Board Cert:** Ophthalmology 1978; **Med School:** Mount Sinai Sch Med 1972; **Resid:** Ophthalmology, Mount Sinai 1977; **Fellow:** Ophthalmology, Mount Sinai 1974; **Fac Appt:** Asst Clin Prof Oph, Albert Einstein Coll Med

Rosenthal, Kenneth J MD (Oph) - **Spec Exp:** Corneal Disease; Cataract Surgery; **Hospital:** St Francis Hosp - The Heart Ctr (page 115), Syosset Hosp; **Address:** 310 E Shore Rd, rm 102, Great Neck, NY 11023; **Phone:** 516-466-8989; **Board Cert:** Ophthalmology 1986; **Med School:** Albany Med Coll 1978; **Resid:** Ophthalmology, N Shore Univ Hosp 1983

Rubin, Laurence MD (Oph) - **Spec Exp:** Cataract Surgery; Intraocular Lenses; Glaucoma; **Hospital:** St Joseph's Hosp-Nassau, Syosset Hosp; **Address:** 4277 Hempstead Tpke, Ste 109, Bethpage, NY 11714-5706; **Phone:** 516-796-4030; **Board Cert:** Ophthalmology 1987; **Med School:** NY Med Coll 1980; **Resid:** Ophthalmology, New York Eye & Ear Infirm 1984

Rubin, Steven E MD (Oph) - **Spec Exp:** Strabismus; Pediatric Ophthalmology; Amblyopia; **Hospital:** N Shore Univ Hosp, Long Island Jewish Med Ctr; **Address:** 600 Northern Blvd, Ste 220, Great Neck, NY 11021-5200; **Phone:** 516-465-8444; **Board Cert:** Ophthalmology 1983; **Med School:** SUNY Downstate 1978; **Resid:** Ophthalmology, Univ Penn-Scheie Eye Inst 1982; **Fellow:** Pediatric Ophthalmology, Wills Eye Hosp 1983; **Fac Appt:** Prof Oph, NYU Sch Med

Sturm, Richard T MD (Oph) - **Spec Exp:** Glaucoma; Cataract Surgery; **Hospital:** Mercy Med Ctr - Rockville Centre, Long Island Jewish Med Ctr; **Address:** 360 Merrick Rd Fl 3, Lynbrook, NY 11563; **Phone:** 516-593-7709; **Board Cert:** Ophthalmology 1989; **Med School:** NY Med Coll 1983; **Resid:** Ophthalmology, St Luke's-Roosevelt Hosp Ctr 1987; **Fellow:** Glaucoma, Mass Eye & Ear Infirm 1988

Svitra, Paul MD (Oph) - **Spec Exp:** Diabetic Eye Disease/Retinopathy; Macular Degeneration; **Hospital:** N Shore Univ Hosp; **Address:** 3003 New Hyde Park Rd, Ste 203, New Hyde Park, NY 11042; **Phone:** 516-327-0505; **Board Cert:** Ophthalmology 1990; **Med School:** Cornell Univ-Weill Med Coll 1984; **Resid:** Ophthalmology, Mass Eye & Ear Infirmary 1989; **Fellow:** Retina/Vitreous, Duke Eye Ctr 1990; **Fac Appt:** Asst Prof Oph, Cornell Univ-Weill Med Coll

Udell, Ira J MD (Oph) - **Spec Exp:** Cornea Transplant; Corneal Disease; Tear Duct Problems; **Hospital:** Long Island Jewish Med Ctr, N Shore Univ Hosp; **Address:** Ll Jewish Med Ctr, Dept Ophthamololgy, 600 Northern Blvd, Ste 214, Great Neck, NY 11021-5200; **Phone:** 516-470-2020; **Board Cert:** Ophthalmology 1980; **Med School:** Tulane Univ 1974; **Resid:** Ophthalmology, Ll Jewish Med Ctr 1979; **Fellow:** Cornea, Mass Eye & Ear Infirm 1981; **Fac Appt:** Prof Oph, Albert Einstein Coll Med

Weinstein, Joseph MD (Oph) - **Spec Exp:** Cataract Surgery; Refractive Surgery; Contact Lenses; **Hospital:** N Shore Univ Hosp, Syosset Hosp; **Address:** 4212 Hempstead Tpke, Eye Care Assoc, Bethpage, NY 11714-5712; **Phone:** 516-731-4800; **Board Cert:** Ophthalmology 1982; **Med School:** Albert Einstein Coll Med 1977; **Resid:** Ophthalmology, Long Island Jewish Med Ctr 1981

Orthopaedic Surgery

Asnis, Stanley MD (OrS) - **Spec Exp:** Hip Replacement; Knee Replacement; **Hospital:** N Shore Univ Hosp, St Francis Hosp - The Heart Ctr (page 115); **Address:** 600 Northern Blvd, Great Neck, NY 11021; **Phone:** 516-627-8717; **Board Cert:** Orthopaedic Surgery 1976; **Med School:** Washington Univ, St Louis 1968; **Resid:** Surgery, NY Hosp 1971; Orthopaedic Surgery, Hosp for Special Surg 1975; **Fellow:** Research, Hosp for Special Surg 1972; **Fac Appt:** Assoc Clin Prof OrS, Albert Einstein Coll Med

Capozzi, James MD (OrS) - **Spec Exp:** Joint Replacement; Fractures in the Elderly; Arthroscopic Surgery; **Hospital:** Winthrop - Univ Hosp; **Address:** 1300 Franklin Ave, Ste UL3A, Garden City, NY 11530; **Phone:** 516-747-8900; **Board Cert:** Orthopaedic Surgery 2010; **Med School:** Mount Sinai Sch Med 1981; **Resid:** Orthopaedic Surgery, Mount Sinai Hosp 1986; **Fellow:** Joint Replacement Surgery, New England Baptist Hosp 1987; **Fac Appt:** Assoc Clin Prof OrS, Mount Sinai Sch Med

D'Agostino, Richard J MD (OrS) - **Spec Exp:** Sports Medicine; Knee Surgery; Shoulder Surgery; **Hospital:** St Francis Hosp - The Heart Ctr (page 115), N Shore Univ Hosp; **Address:** 600 Northern Blvd, Great Neck, NY 11021; **Phone:** 516-627-8717; **Board Cert:** Orthopaedic Surgery 2001; **Med School:** Mount Sinai Sch Med 1982; **Resid:** Orthopaedic Surgery, Mt Sinai Med Ctr 1987; **Fellow:** Sports Medicine, New Eng Baptist Hosp 1988; **Fac Appt:** Asst Prof OrS, Cornell Univ-Weill Med Coll

Dines, David M MD (OrS) - **Spec Exp:** Shoulder Surgery; Sports Medicine; Shoulder Replacement; **Hospital:** Long Island Jewish Med Ctr, Hosp For Special Surgery (page 111); **Address:** 935 Northern Blvd, Ste 303, Great Neck, NY 11021-5309; **Phone:** 516-482-1037; **Board Cert:** Orthopaedic Surgery 1980; **Med School:** UMDNJ-NJ Med Sch, Newark 1974; **Resid:** Surgery, NY Hosp-Cornell Med Ctr 1976; Orthopaedic Surgery, Hosp Special Surg 1979; **Fac Appt:** Clin Prof OrS, Albert Einstein Coll Med

Kenan, Samuel MD (OrS) - **Spec Exp:** Bone Tumors; Hip Replacement; Knee Replacement; **Hospital:** NYU Hosp For Joint Diseases (page 106), NYU Langone Med Ctr (page 106); **Address:** 300 Old Country Rd, Ste 221, Mineola, NY 11501; **Phone:** 516-280-3733; **Med School:** Israel 1976; **Resid:** Orthopaedic Surgery, Hadassah Univ Hosp 1984; **Fellow:** Orthopaedic Pathology, Hosp for Joint Diseases 1987; **Fac Appt:** Prof OrS, NYU Sch Med

Levitz, Craig L MD (OrS) - **Spec Exp:** Sports Medicine; Shoulder Surgery; Knee Injuries/ACL; Cartilage Damage & Transplant; **Hospital:** South Nassau Comm Hosp, NS-LIJ Hlth Sys; **Address:** 36 Lincoln Ave Fl 3, Rockville Centre, NY 11570; **Phone:** 516-536-2800; **Board Cert:** Orthopaedic Surgery 2011; Orthopaedic Sports Medicine 2007; **Med School:** Univ Pennsylvania 1992; **Resid:** Orthopaedic Surgery, Hosp Univ Penn 1997; **Fellow:** Sports Medicine, Amer Sports Med Inst 1998

Lewis, Ronald MD (OrS) - **Spec Exp:** Pediatric Orthopaedic Surgery; Arthroscopic Surgery; Sports Medicine; Trauma; **Hospital:** Winthrop - Univ Hosp, NS-LIJ Hlth Sys; **Address:** Pediatric Orthopaedics of LI, 598 Jericho Turnpike, Syosset, NY 11791; **Phone:** 516-762-4040; **Board Cert:** Orthopaedic Surgery 2001; **Med School:** SUNY Stony Brook 1993; **Resid:** Orthopaedic Surgery, SUNY Stony Brook 1998; **Fellow:** Pediatric Orthopaedic Surgery, Chldns Hosp Med Ctr 1999

Mauri, Thomas MD (OrS) - **Spec Exp:** Spinal Surgery; **Hospital:** N Shore Univ Hosp; **Address:** 865 Northern Blvd Fl 2 - Ste 203, Great Neck, NY 11021; **Phone:** 516-918-6300; **Board Cert:** Orthopaedic Surgery 2009; **Med School:** Albany Med Coll 1980; **Resid:** Neurological Surgery, North Shore Univ Hosp 1982; Orthopaedic Surgery, Hosp for Special Surgery 1985; **Fellow:** Spinal Surgery, Rancho Los Amigos Natl Rehab Ctr 1986

Montero, Carlos F MD (OrS) - **Spec Exp:** Hand Surgery; **Hospital:** St Joseph's Hosp-Nassau, Plainview Hosp; **Address:** 2920 Hempstead Tpke, Levittown, NY 11756; **Phone:** 516-735-4048; **Board Cert:** Orthopaedic Surgery 1974; **Med School:** Argentina 1968; **Resid:** Surgery, Bronx VA Hosp 1970; Orthopaedic Surgery, Nassau County Med Ctr 1973; **Fellow:** Hand Surgery, Nassau County Med Ctr 1974; **Fac Appt:** Asst Clin Prof OrS, SUNY Stony Brook

Rich, Daniel MD (OrS) - **Spec Exp:** Hip Replacement; Knee Replacement; **Hospital:** St Francis Hosp - The Heart Ctr (page 115), Hosp For Special Surgery (page 111); **Address:** 585 Plandome Rd, Ste 103, Manhasset, NY 11030-1971; **Phone:** 516-627-1525; **Board Cert:** Orthopaedic Surgery 1984; **Med School:** Harvard Med Sch 1977; **Resid:** Surgery, St Luke's-Roosevelt Hosp Ctr 1979; Orthopaedic Surgery, Hosp for Special Surgery 1982; **Fac Appt:** Asst Clin Prof OrS, Cornell Univ-Weill Med Coll

Sgaglione, Nicholas MD (OrS) - **Spec Exp:** Sports Medicine; **Hospital:** N Shore Univ Hosp; **Address:** 600 Northern Blvd, Ste 300, Great Neck, NY 11021; **Phone:** 516-627-8717; **Board Cert:** Orthopaedic Surgery 2002; **Med School:** Mount Sinai Sch Med 1983; **Resid:** Orthopaedic Surgery, Hosp Special Surg 1988; **Fellow:** Sports Medicine, Southern Cal Ortho Inst 1989; **Fac Appt:** Assoc Clin Prof OrS, Albert Einstein Coll Med

Shebairo, Raymond MD (OrS) - **Spec Exp:** Arthroscopic Surgery; Shoulder & Knee Surgery; Joint Replacement; **Hospital:** Long Island Jewish Med Ctr; **Address:** 1575 Hillside Ave, Ste 303, New Hyde Park, NY 11040; **Phone:** 516-437-5500; **Board Cert:** Orthopaedic Surgery 1982; **Med School:** Med Coll Wisc 1973; **Resid:** Orthopaedic Surgery, LIJ Med Ctr 1977

Simonson, Barry G MD (OrS) - **Spec Exp:** Sports Medicine; Arthroscopic Surgery; Hip & Knee Reconstruction; Hip & Knee Replacement; **Hospital:** Glen Cove Hosp; **Address:** 825 Northern Blvd, Ste 201, Great Neck, NY 11021-5323; **Phone:** 516-773-7500; **Board Cert:** Orthopaedic Surgery 2004; **Med School:** Mount Sinai Sch Med 1984; **Resid:** Orthopaedic Surgery, LI Jewish Med Ctr 1990; **Fellow:** Sports Medicine, New York Univ Med Ctr 1991

Ticker, Jonathan MD (OrS) - **Spec Exp:** Shoulder Surgery; Rotator Cuff Surgery; Shoulder Arthroscopic Surgery; Sports Medicine; **Hospital:** N Shore Univ Hosp, St Joseph's Hosp-Nassau; **Address:** Island Orthopaedics & Sports Medicine, 660 Broadway, Massapequa, NY 11758; **Phone:** 516-798-0111; **Board Cert:** Orthopaedic Surgery 2008; **Med School:** UMDNJ-NJ Med Sch, Newark 1988; **Resid:** Orthopaedic Surgery, NY Presby-Columbia Med Ctr 1994; **Fellow:** Shoulder Surgery, NY Presby-Columbia Med Ctr 1991; Sports Medicine & Shoulder Surgery, Univ Pittsburgh 1995; **Fac Appt:** Asst Prof OrS, Columbia P&S

Otolaryngology

Draizin, Dennis L MD (Oto) - **Spec Exp:** Hearing Disorders; Nasal & Sinus Disorders; Voice Disorders; **Hospital:** South Nassau Comm Hosp, Winthrop - Univ Hosp; **Address:** 195 N Village Ave, Ste 1, Rockville Centre, NY 11570-3814; **Phone:** 516-536-7777; **Board Cert:** Otolaryngology 1980; **Med School:** Univ VA Sch Med 1975; **Resid:** Surgery, Northshore Univ Hosp 1977; Otolaryngology, Mt Sinai Sch Med 1980

Durante, Anthony J MD (Oto) - **Hospital:** Winthrop - Univ Hosp; **Address:** 134 Mineola Blvd, Ste 201, Mineola, NY 11501; **Phone:** 516-294-9363; **Board Cert:** Otolaryngology 1975; **Med School:** Italy 1967; **Resid:** Surgery, Nassau Hosp 1970; Otolaryngology, Albert Einstein Coll Med 1975; **Fac Appt:** Asst Clin Prof S, SUNY Stony Brook

Frank, Douglas K MD (Oto) - **Spec Exp:** Head & Neck Cancer & Surgery; Thyroid & Parathyroid Surgery; Salivary Gland Tumors & Surgery; Skull Base Surgery; **Hospital:** Long Island Jewish Med Ctr, N Shore Univ Hosp; **Address:** 430 Lakeville Rd, New Hyde Park, NY 11042; **Phone:** 718-470-7552; **Board Cert:** Otolaryngology 1997; **Med School:** Univ Pennsylvania 1990; **Resid:** Surgery, St Vincent Hosp 1992; Otolaryngology, NY Ear & Ear Infirm 1996; **Fellow:** Head and Neck Surgery, UT MD Anderson Cancer Ctr 1999; **Fac Appt:** Assoc Prof Oto, Albert Einstein Coll Med

Gordon, Michael A MD (Oto) - **Spec Exp:** Balance Disorders; Hearing Disorders; Otosclerosis; Ear Surgery; **Hospital:** Long Island Jewish Med Ctr; **Address:** 901 Stewart Ave, Ste 270, Garden City, NY 11530; **Phone:** 516-222-1881; **Board Cert:** Otolaryngology 1993; **Med School:** Albert Einstein Coll Med 1986; **Resid:** Otolaryngology, Montrfiore Hosp Med Ctr 1992; **Fellow:** Otology & Neurotology, Ear Research Foundation 1993; **Fac Appt:** Asst Prof Oto, Albert Einstein Coll Med

Grosso, John MD (Oto) - **Spec Exp:** Pediatric Otolaryngology; Otology; **Hospital:** Plainview Hosp, Syosset Hosp; **Address:** 875 Old Country Rd, Ste 200, Plainview, NY 11803-4934; **Phone:** 516-931-5552; **Board Cert:** Otolaryngology 1993; **Med School:** SUNY Upstate Med Univ 1986; **Resid:** Otolaryngology, Univ Hosp 1992

Mattucci, Kenneth MD (Oto) - **Spec Exp:** Otology; Neuro-Otology; Nasal & Sinus Disorders; **Hospital:** St Francis Hosp - The Heart Ctr (page 115), N Shore Univ Hosp; **Address:** 29 Barstow Rd, Ste 203, Manhasset, NY 11021; **Phone:** 516-482-7960; **Board Cert:** Otolaryngology 1970; **Med School:** Wake Forest Univ 1964; **Resid:** Surgery, New York Hosp 1966; Otolaryngology, NY Eye & Ear Infirm 1969; **Fellow:** Otolaryngology, New York Hosp 1970; **Fac Appt:** Clin Prof Oto, NY Med Coll

Mendelsohn, Michael MD (Oto) - **Spec Exp:** Pediatric Otolaryngology; **Hospital:** Long Island Jewish Med Ctr; **Address:** 901 Stewart Ave, Ste 270, Garden City, NY 11530; **Phone:** 516-222-1881; **Board Cert:** Otolaryngology 1999; **Med School:** Boston Univ 1990; **Resid:** Otolaryngology, LI Jewish Med Ctr 1995; **Fellow:** Pediatric Otolaryngology, Univ Virginia Med Ctr 1996; **Fac Appt:** Asst Prof Oto, SUNY Downstate

Moisa, Idel MD (Oto) - **Spec Exp:** Thyroid Surgery; Sinusitis; Snoring/Sleep Apnea; Endoscopic Sinus Surgery; **Hospital:** Glen Cove Hosp, Winthrop - Univ Hosp; **Address:** 3 School St, Rm 304, Glen Cove, NY 11542-2548; **Phone:** 516-671-0085; **Board Cert:** Otolaryngology 1988; **Med School:** Albert Einstein Coll Med 1983; **Resid:** Otolaryngology, Montefiore Med Ctr 1988; **Fellow:** Head and Neck Surgery, Montefiore Med Ctr 1990; **Fac Appt:** Asst Clin Prof Oto, NYU Sch Med

Perlman, Philip W MD (Oto) - **Spec Exp:** Pediatric & Adult Otolaryngology; Endoscopic Sinus Surgery; Head & Neck Surgery; Snoring/Sleep Apnea; **Hospital:** St Francis Hosp - The Heart Ctr (page 115), N Shore Univ Hosp; **Address:** Progressive Ear, Nose & Throat Assocs, 333 E Shore Rd, Manhasset, NY 11030-2911; **Phone:** 516-466-5100; **Board Cert:** Otolaryngology 1988; Facial Plastic & Reconstr Surgery 1993; **Med School:** SUNY Downstate 1983; **Resid:** Surgery, Staten Island Hosp 1985; Otolaryngology, Albany Meml Hosp 1988; **Fellow:** Facial Plastic & Reconstr Surgery, AAFPRS 1989

Rosner, Louis M MD (Oto) - **Spec Exp:** Rhinoplasty; Endoscopic Sinus Surgery; Head & Neck Cancer; **Hospital:** South Nassau Comm Hosp, Mercy Med Ctr - Rockville Centre; **Address:** 176 N Village Ave, Ste 1A, Rockville Centre, NY 11570-3800; **Phone:** 516-678-0303; **Board Cert:** Otolaryngology 1982; **Med School:** Ros Franklin Univ/Chicago Med Sch 1978; **Resid:** Otolaryngology, NY Eye & Ear Infirm 1982

Setzen, Michael MD (Oto) - **Spec Exp:** Nasal & Sinus Surgery; Rhinoplasty; Sleep Disorders/Apnea; Snoring/Sleep Apnea; **Hospital:** N Shore Univ Hosp, St Francis Hosp - The Heart Ctr (page 115); **Address:** 600 Northern Blvd, Ste 312, Great Neck, NY 11021-5200; **Phone:** 516-829-0045; **Board Cert:** Otolaryngology 1982; **Med School:** South Africa 1974; **Resid:** Surgery, Cleveland Clinic Fdn 1978; Otolaryngology, Barnes Jewish Hosp 1982; **Fac Appt:** Assoc Clin Prof Oto, NYU Sch Med

Shikowitz, Mark J MD (Oto) - **Hospital:** Long Island Jewish Med Ctr, Steven & Alexandra Cohen Chldn's Med Ctr of NY; **Address:** Hearing & Speech Bldg, 430 Lakeville Rd, New Hyde Park, NY 11042; **Phone:** 718-470-7550; **Board Cert:** Otolaryngology 1987; **Med School:** Dominica 1981; **Resid:** Otolaryngology, LI Jewish Med Ctr 1986; **Fac Appt:** Assoc Prof Oto, Albert Einstein Coll Med

Soletic, Raymond MD (Oto) - **Spec Exp:** Endoscopic Sinus Surgery; Cosmetic Surgery-Face; **Hospital:** St Francis Hosp - The Heart Ctr (page 115); **Address:** 1615 Northern Blvd, Ste 201, Manhasset, NY 11030; **Phone:** 516-365-7952; **Board Cert:** Otolaryngology 1990; **Med School:** Mexico 1982; **Resid:** Surgery, Baystate/Tufts 1985; Otolaryngology, Manhattan EE&T Hosp 1989

Tawfik, Bernard MD (Oto) - **Spec Exp:** Thyroid Disorders; Sinus Disorders; Snoring/Sleep Apnea; Sleep Disorders/Apnea; **Hospital:** Glen Cove Hosp, Winthrop - Univ Hosp; **Address:** 3 School St, Ste 304, Glen Cove, NY 11542; **Phone:** 516-671-0085; **Board Cert:** Otolaryngology 1977; **Med School:** Johns Hopkins Univ 1971; **Resid:** Otolaryngology, Manhattan Eye & Ear 1977

Turk, Jon B MD (Oto) - **Hospital:** Lenox Hill Hosp (Manh Eye, Ear & Throat Hosp); **Address:** 173 Froehlich Farm Blvd, Woodbury, NY 11797; **Phone:** 516-921-8989; **Board Cert:** Otolaryngology 1995; Facial Plastic & Reconstr Surgery 1996; **Med School:** SUNY Downstate 1988; **Resid:** Surgery, Mt Sinai Hosp 1990; Otolaryngology, Mt Sinai Hosp 1993; **Fellow:** Facial Plastic Surgery, Inselspital-Bern 1994

Vambutas, Andrea MD (Oto) - **Spec Exp:** Hearing & Balance Disorders; Pediatric Otolaryngology; Cochlear Implants; **Hospital:** Long Island Jewish Med Ctr; **Address:** Hearing and Speech Ctr, 430 Lakeville Rd, New Hyde Park, NY 11042; **Phone:** 516-470-7955; **Board Cert:** Otolaryngology 1998; **Med School:** Albert Einstein Coll Med 1992; **Resid:** Otolaryngology, LIJ Med Ctr 1998; **Fellow:** Otology, Fairview Univ Med Ctr 1999; **Fac Appt:** Asst Prof Oto, Albert Einstein Coll Med

Youngerman, Jay MD (Oto) - **Spec Exp:** Head & Neck Surgery; Sleep & Snoring Disorders; Ear Disorders/Surgery; Pediatric Otolaryngology; **Hospital:** Plainview Hosp, Syosset Hosp; **Address:** 875 Old Country Rd, Ste 200, Plainview, NY 11803-4934; **Phone:** 516-931-5552; **Board Cert:** Otolaryngology 1984; **Med School:** Med Coll VA 1979; **Resid:** Otolaryngology, LI Jewish Med Ctr 1983

Zahtz, Gerald MD (Oto) - **Spec Exp:** Sinus Disorders/Surgery; Pediatric Otolaryngology; **Hospital:** Long Island Jewish Med Ctr; **Address:** 430 Lakeville Rd, New Hyde Park, NY 11042; **Phone:** 718-470-7554; **Board Cert:** Otolaryngology 1981; **Med School:** St Louis Univ 1977; **Resid:** Surgery, LIJ-Hillside Med Ctr 1978; Otolaryngology, LIJ-Hillside Med Ctr 1981; **Fac Appt:** Assoc Prof Oto, Albert Einstein Coll Med

Zelman, Warren H MD (Oto) - **Spec Exp:** Head & Neck Surgery; Sinus Disorders/Surgery; Pediatric & Adult Otolaryngology; **Hospital:** Winthrop - Univ Hosp; **Address:** 975 Franklin Ave Fl 2 - Ste 203B, Garden City, NY 11530; **Phone:** 516-739-3999; **Board Cert:** Otolaryngology 1987; **Med School:** Ros Franklin Univ/Chicago Med Sch 1982; **Resid:** Surgery, Univ Hosp-SUNY 1984; Otolaryngology, Manhattan EE&T Hosp 1987

Pain Medicine

Pinsky, Steven MD (PM) - **Hospital:** Mercy Med Ctr - Rockville Centre; **Address:** 176 N Village Ave, Ste 2D, Rockville Centre, NY 11570; **Phone:** 516-764-4875; **Board Cert:** Anesthesiology 1994; Pain Medicine 2007; **Med School:** Albert Einstein Coll Med 1989; **Resid:** Anesthesiology, SUNY Downstate 1993; **Fellow:** Pain Medicine, St Lukes Roosevelt Med Ctr 1994

Pathology

Crawford, James M MD/PhD (Path) - **Spec Exp:** Liver Pathology; Gastrointestinal Pathology; Gastrointestinal Cancer; **Hospital:** N Shore Univ Hosp, Long Island Jewish Med Ctr; **Address:** N Shore-LI Jewish Laboratories, 10 Nevada Drive, Lake Success, NY 11042-1114; **Phone:** 516-719-1060; **Board Cert:** Anatomic Pathology 1987; **Med School:** Duke Univ 1982; **Resid:** Pathology, Brigham & Women's Hosp 1984; **Fellow:** Gastrointestinal Pathology, Brigham & Women's Hosp 1987; Pathology, Royal Free hosp 1989

Kahn, Leonard B MD (Path) - **Spec Exp:** Bone Pathology; Head & Neck Pathology; Soft Tissue Tumors; **Hospital:** Long Island Jewish Med Ctr, N Shore Univ Hosp; **Address:** 270-05 76th Ave, rm B67, New Hyde Park, NY 11040-1433; **Phone:** 718-470-7491; **Board Cert:** Anatomic Pathology 1980; **Med School:** South Africa 1960; **Resid:** Pathology, Univ Cape Town 1966; **Fellow:** Pathology, Washington Univ 1969; **Fac Appt:** Prof Path, Albert Einstein Coll Med

Wasserman, Patricia G MD (Path) - **Spec Exp:** Cervical Cancer; Thyroid Cancer; **Hospital:** Long Island Jewish Med Ctr, N Shore Univ Hosp; **Address:** North Shore LIJ Hlth System, 6 Ohio Drive, Ste 202, Lake Success, NY 11042; **Phone:** 718-470-7490; **Board Cert:** Anatomic & Clinical Pathology 1990; Cytopathology 1994; **Med School:** Argentina 1983; **Resid:** Pathology, Mt Sinai Med Ctr 1989; **Fellow:** Cytopathology, Mt Sinai Med Ctr 1990; **Fac Appt:** Asst Prof Path, Albert Einstein Coll Med

Pediatric Allergy & Immunology

Bonagura, Vincent R MD (PA&I) - **Spec Exp:** AIDS/HIV; **Hospital:** Steven & Alexandra Cohen Chldn's Med Ctr of NY, Long Island Jewish Med Ctr; **Address:** 865 Northern Blvd, Ste 101, Great Neck, NY 11021; **Phone:** 516-622-5070; **Board Cert:** Pediatrics 1979; Allergy & Immunology 1981; Clinical & Laboratory Immunology 1986; **Med School:** Columbia P&S 1975; **Resid:** Pediatrics, Columbia Presby Hosp 1978; **Fellow:** Allergy & Immunology, Columbia Presby Hosp 1983; **Fac Appt:** Prof Ped, Albert Einstein Coll Med

Fagin, James MD (PA&I) - **Spec Exp:** Asthma; Ear Infections; Sinus Disorders; Immunodeficiency Disorders; **Hospital:** Steven & Alexandra Cohen Chldn's Med Ctr of NY, N Shore Univ Hosp; **Address:** Steven & Alexandra Cohen Chldn's Med Ctr, Div of Allergy/Immunology, 865 Northern Blvd, Ste 101, Great Neck, NY 11021-5303; **Phone:** 516-622-5070; **Board Cert:** Pediatrics 1980; Allergy & Immunology 1983; **Med School:** Belgium 1976; **Resid:** Pediatrics, N Shore Univ Hosp 1979; **Fellow:** Allergy & Immunology, Chldns Hosp of Pittsburgh 1981; **Fac Appt:** Asst Prof Ped, NYU Sch Med

Pediatric Cardiology

Better, Donna J MD (PCd) - **Spec Exp:** Echocardiography; Fetal Echocardiography; **Hospital:** Winthrop - Univ Hosp, NYPresby-Morgan Stanley Children's Hosp (page 104); **Address:** 120 Mineola Blvd, Ste 210, Mineola, NY 11501; **Phone:** 516-663-4600; **Board Cert:** Pediatric Cardiology 2004; **Med School:** Albert Einstein Coll Med 1989; **Resid:** Pediatrics, Mt Sinai Hosp 1992; **Fellow:** Pediatric Cardiology, Columbia-Presby Med Ctr 1995

Bierman, Fredrick MD (PCd) - **Spec Exp:** Fetal Echocardiography; Kawasaki Disease; Congenital Heart Disease; Echocardiography; **Hospital:** Steven & Alexandra Cohen Chldn's Med Ctr of NY; **Address:** Chldns Heart Ctr, Schneider Chldns Hosp, 269-01 76th Ave, rm 139, New Hyde Park, NY 11040; **Phone:** 718-470-7350; **Board Cert:** Pediatrics 1978; Pediatric Cardiology 1981; **Med School:** SUNY Downstate 1973; **Resid:** Pediatrics, Mount Sinai Med Ctr 1976; **Fellow:** Pediatric Cardiology, Harvard Chldns Hosp 1979; **Fac Appt:** Prof Ped, Albert Einstein Coll Med

Cooper, Rubin MD (PCd) - **Spec Exp:** Congenital Heart Disease; Rheumatic Heart Disease; Kawasaki Disease; **Hospital:** Steven & Alexandra Cohen Chldn's Med Ctr of NY; **Address:** Steven & Alexandra Cohen Children's Hosp, 269-01 76th Ave, New Hyde Park, NY 11040; **Phone:** 718-470-3661; **Board Cert:** Pediatrics 1976; Pediatric Cardiology 1979; **Med School:** NY Med Coll 1971; **Resid:** Pediatrics, Strong Meml Hosp 1973; **Fellow:** Pediatric Cardiology, Strong Meml Hosp 1975; **Fac Appt:** Prof Ped, Cornell Univ-Weill Med Coll

Levchuck, Sean G MD (PCd) - **Spec Exp:** Interventional Cardiology; Congenital Heart Disease; Atrial Septal Defect; **Hospital:** St Francis Hosp - The Heart Ctr (page 115), Steven & Alexandra Cohen Chldn's Med Ctr of NY; **Address:** 100 Port Washington Blvd, Roslyn, NY 11576-1353; **Phone:** 516-365-3340; **Board Cert:** Pediatrics 2008; Pediatric Cardiology 2004; **Med School:** West Indies 1989; **Resid:** Pediatrics, Winthrop Univ Hosp 1992; **Fellow:** Pediatric Cardiology, St Christophers Hosp 1995

Reitman, Milton J MD (PCd) - **Spec Exp:** Interventional Cardiology; **Hospital:** St Francis Hosp - The Heart Ctr (page 115), Steven & Alexandra Cohen Chldn's Med Ctr of NY; **Address:** 100 Port Washington Blvd, Roslyn, NY 11576; **Phone:** 516-365-3340; **Board Cert:** Pediatrics 1974; Pediatric Cardiology 1978; **Med School:** NY Med Coll 1969; **Resid:** Pediatrics, Flower Fifth Ave Hosp 1971; **Fellow:** Pediatric Cardiology, Texas Chldns Hosp 1974

Romano, Angela MD (PCd) - **Spec Exp:** Echocardiography; Marfan's Syndrome; Kawasaki Disease; **Hospital:** Steven & Alexandra Cohen Chldn's Med Ctr of NY; **Address:** Dept Pediatric Cardiology, 26901 76th Ave Fl 1 - rm 139, New Hyde Park, NY 11040; **Phone:** 718-470-7350; **Board Cert:** Pediatrics 1984; Pediatric Cardiology 2003; **Med School:** Columbia P&S 1980; **Resid:** Pediatrics, Babies Hosp/Columbia Univ Med Ctr 1984; **Fellow:** Pediatric Cardiology, Children's Hosp 1987; **Fac Appt:** Asst Prof Ped, Albert Einstein Coll Med

Schiff, Russell J MD (PCd) - **Spec Exp:** Echocardiography; Fetal Echocardiography; **Hospital:** Winthrop - Univ Hosp; **Address:** 120 Mineola Blvd, Ste 210, Mineola, NY 11501; **Phone:** 516-663-4600; **Board Cert:** Pediatrics 1986; Pediatric Cardiology 2003; **Med School:** SUNY Stony Brook 1981; **Resid:** Pediatrics, Schneider Chldns Hosp 1984; **Fellow:** Pediatric Cardiology, Schneider Chldns Hosp 1986; **Fac Appt:** Asst Prof Ped, NYU Sch Med

Shapir, Yehuda MD (PCd) - **Spec Exp:** Congenital Heart Disease & Acquired; Echocardiography; Fetal Echocardiography; **Hospital:** Steven & Alexandra Cohen Chldn's Med Ctr of NY; **Address:** Cohen Chldn's Med Ctr, 269-01 76th Ave, New Hyde Park, NY 11040-1433; **Phone:** 718-470-7350; **Board Cert:** Pediatric Cardiology 2006; **Med School:** Israel 1977; **Resid:** Pediatrics, Rambam Med Ctr 1981; **Fellow:** Pediatric Cardiology, UCLA Med Ctr 1985; **Fac Appt:** Assoc Prof Ped, Albert Einstein Coll Med

Vallone, Ambrose M MD (PCd) - **Spec Exp:** Cardiac Catheterization; Syncope; Fetal Echocardiography; **Hospital:** St Francis Hosp - The Heart Ctr (page 115), NS-LIJ Hlth Sys; **Address:** 100 Port Washington Blvd, Ste 108, Roslyn, NY 11576-1353; **Phone:** 516-365-3340; **Board Cert:** Pediatrics 1983; Pediatric Cardiology 2003; **Med School:** Johns Hopkins Univ 1977; **Resid:** Pediatrics, Johns Hopkins Hosp 1980; **Fellow:** Pediatric Cardiology, Yale-New Haven Hosp 1983; Pediatric Critical Care Medicine, Yale-New Haven Hosp 1983

Pediatric Critical Care Medicine

Sagy, Mayer MD (PCCM) - **Spec Exp:** Critical Care; **Hospital:** Long Island Jewish Med Ctr; **Address:** Schneider Children's Hospital, 269-01 76th Ave, New Hyde Park, NY 11040; **Phone:** 718-470-3330; **Board Cert:** Pediatrics 2007; Pediatric Critical Care Medicine 2007; **Med School:** Israel 1972; **Resid:** Pediatrics, Chaim Sheba Med Ctr 1982; **Fellow:** Pediatric Critical Care Medicine, Children's Hosp 1984

Pediatric Endocrinology

Carey, Dennis MD (PEn) - **Spec Exp:** Diabetes; Calcium Disorders; Growth Disorders; Thyroid Disorders; **Hospital:** Steven & Alexandra Cohen Chldn's Med Ctr of NY; **Address:** Pediatric Endocrinology, 400 Lakeville Rd, Ste 180, New Hyde Park, NY 11042; **Phone:** 718-470-3290; **Board Cert:** Pediatrics 1979; Pediatric Endocrinology 1983; **Med School:** SUNY Downstate 1973; **Resid:** Pediatric Surgery, LI Jewish Med Ctr 1979; **Fellow:** Pediatric Endocrinology, UCSD Med Ctr 1980; **Fac Appt:** Assoc Prof Ped, Albert Einstein Coll Med

Castro-Magana, Mariano MD (PEn) - **Spec Exp:** Growth/Development Disorders; Adrenal Disorders; Sexual Development Problems; **Hospital:** Winthrop - Univ Hosp; **Address:** Winthrop Univ Hosp, Div Ped Endo, 120 Mineola Blvd, Ste 210, Mineola, NY 11501; **Phone:** 516-663-3069; **Board Cert:** Pediatrics 1983; Pediatric Endocrinology 1983; **Med School:** El Salvador 1974; **Resid:** Pediatrics, Nassau County Med Ctr 1980; **Fellow:** Pediatric Endocrinology, Nassau County Med Ctr 1982; **Fac Appt:** Prof Ped, NYU Sch Med

Fort, Pavel MD (PEn) - **Spec Exp:** Diabetes; Growth/Development Disorders; Thyroid Disorders; **Hospital:** Steven & Alexandra Cohen Chldn's Med Ctr of NY; **Address:** Schneider Chldn's Hosp, Peds Endo, 400 Lakeville Rd, Ste 180, New Hyde Park, NY 11042; **Phone:** 718-470-3290; **Board Cert:** Pediatrics 1976; Pediatric Endocrinology 1978; **Med School:** Czech Republic 1969; **Resid:** Pediatrics, N Shore Univ Hosp 1974; **Fellow:** Pediatric Endocrinology, N Shore Univ Hosp 1976; **Fac Appt:** Assoc Clin Prof Ped, NYU Sch Med

Frank, Graeme MD (PEn) - **Spec Exp:** Pubertal Disorders; Growth/Development Disorders; Diabetes; Thyroid Disorders; **Hospital:** Steven & Alexandra Cohen Chldn's Med Ctr of NY; **Address:** Schneider Chldn's Hosp, Peds Endo, 400 Lakeville Rd, Ste 180, New Hyde Park, NY 11040; **Phone:** 718-470-3290; **Board Cert:** Pediatrics 2005; Pediatric Endocrinology 2003; **Med School:** South Africa 1982; **Resid:** Pediatrics, LIJ-Schneider Chldns Hosp 1991; **Fellow:** Pediatric Endocrinology, Children's Hosp 1994; **Fac Appt:** Assoc Clin Prof Ped, Albert Einstein Coll Med

Kreitzer, Paula MD (PEn) - **Spec Exp:** Diabetes; Growth/Development Disorders; **Hospital:** Steven & Alexandra Cohen Chldn's Med Ctr of NY, Long Island Jewish Med Ctr; **Address:** Schneider Chldn's Hosp, Dept Ped En, 400 Lakeville Rd, Ste 180, New Hyde Park, NY 11040; **Phone:** 718-470-3290; **Board Cert:** Pediatrics 1987; Pediatric Endocrinology 2004; **Med School:** Univ NC Sch Med 1982; **Resid:** Pediatrics, LIJ-Schneider Chldns Hosp; Pediatric Endocrinology, LIJ-Schneider Chldns Hosp

Pediatric Gastroenterology

Daum, Fredric MD (PGe) - **Spec Exp:** Inflammatory Bowel Disease; Liver Disease; Incontinence-Fecal; **Hospital:** Winthrop - Univ Hosp; **Address:** 120 Mineola Blvd, Ste 210, Mineola, NY 11501; **Phone:** 516-663-8534; **Board Cert:** Pediatrics 1972; Pediatric Gastroenterology 2005; **Med School:** Tufts Univ 1967; **Resid:** Pediatrics, Jacobi Med Ctr 1969; **Fellow:** Adolescent Medicine, Montefiore Med Ctr 1972

Levine, Jeremiah MD (PGe) - **Spec Exp:** Inflammatory Bowel Disease; Crohn's Disease; Liver Disease; **Hospital:** Steven & Alexandra Cohen Chldn's Med Ctr of NY; **Address:** Dept GI & Nutrition, 269-01 76th Ave, rm 161, New Hyde Park, NY 11040-1433; **Phone:** 718-470-3430; **Board Cert:** Pediatrics 1985; Pediatric Gastroenterology 2005; **Med School:** Harvard Med Sch 1980; **Resid:** Pediatrics, Albert Einstein Coll Med Ctr 1983; **Fellow:** Pediatric Gastroenterology, Children's Hosp 1985; **Fac Appt:** Prof Ped, Albert Einstein Coll Med

Markowitz, James MD (PGe) - **Spec Exp:** Inflammatory Bowel Disease/Crohn's; Gastroesophageal Reflux Disease (GERD); **Hospital:** Steven & Alexandra Cohen Chldn's Med Ctr of NY; **Address:** 269-01 76th Ave Fl 2 - rm 234, New Hyde Park, NY 11030; **Phone:** 718-470-3430; **Board Cert:** Pediatrics 1981; Pediatric Gastroenterology 2005; **Med School:** Cornell Univ-Weill Med Coll 1977; **Resid:** Pediatrics, NY Hosp 1980; **Fellow:** Pediatric Gastroenterology, N Shore Univ Hosp 1983; **Fac Appt:** Assoc Prof Ped, NYU Sch Med

Pettei, Michael J MD/PhD (PGe) - **Spec Exp:** Cholesterol/Lipid Disorders; Nutrition; Celiac Disease; **Hospital:** Steven & Alexandra Cohen Chldn's Med Ctr of NY, N Shore Univ Hosp; **Address:** Schneider Children's Hospital, 269-01 76th Ave, rm 234, New Hyde Park, NY 11040-1433; **Phone:** 718-470-3430; **Board Cert:** Pediatrics 1986; Pediatric Gastroenterology 2005; **Med School:** Univ Miami Sch Med 1980; **Resid:** Pediatrics, Mt Sinai Med Ctr 1982; **Fellow:** Pediatric Gastroenterology, Columbia-Presby Med Ctr 1984; **Fac Appt:** Assoc Prof Ped, Albert Einstein Coll Med

Weinstein, Toba MD (PGe) - **Spec Exp:** Inflammatory Bowel Disease/Crohn's; Gastroesophageal Reflux Disease (GERD); Irritable Bowel Syndrome; Constipation; **Hospital:** Steven & Alexandra Cohen Chldn's Med Ctr of NY, Long Island Jewish Med Ctr; **Address:** 269-01 76th Ave, New Hyde Park, NY 11040-1433; **Phone:** 718-470-3430; **Board Cert:** Pediatrics 2007; Pediatric Gastroenterology 2007; **Med School:** Columbia P&S 1986; **Resid:** Pediatrics, Children's Hosp Natl MC 1989; **Fellow:** Pediatric Gastroenterology, Schneider Children's Hosp-LIJ 1991; **Fac Appt:** Assoc Prof Ped, Albert Einstein Coll Med

Pediatric Hematology-Oncology

Lipton, Jeffrey M MD/PhD (PHO) - **Spec Exp:** Bone Marrow Failure Disorders; Stem Cell Transplant; Bone Marrow Transplant; **Hospital:** Steven & Alexandra Cohen Chldn's Med Ctr of NY; **Address:** Div Hem-Onc & Stem Cell Transplant, 269-01 76th Ave, rm 255, MC-07670, New Hyde Park, NY 11040-1433; **Phone:** 718-470-3460; **Board Cert:** Pediatrics 1981; **Med School:** St Louis Univ 1975; **Resid:** Pediatrics, Boston Chldns Hosp 1977; **Fellow:** Pediatric Hematology-Oncology, Boston Chldns Hosp/Dana Farber Cancer Inst 1979; **Fac Appt:** Prof Ped, Albert Einstein Coll Med

Redner, Arlene MD (PHO) - **Spec Exp:** Leukemia; Brain Tumors; Solid Tumors; Neuro-Oncology; **Hospital:** Steven & Alexandra Cohen Chldn's Med Ctr of NY; **Address:** 269-01 76th Ave, rm 255, New Hyde Park, NY 11040-1434; **Phone:** 718-470-3460; **Board Cert:** Pediatrics 1982; Pediatric Hematology-Oncology 1984; **Med School:** Univ Pennsylvania 1977; **Resid:** Pediatrics, Boston Floating Hosp 1980; **Fellow:** Pediatric Hematology-Oncology, Meml Sloan Kettering Hosp 1985; **Fac Appt:** Assoc Clin Prof Ped, Albert Einstein Coll Med

Sabatino, Dominick P MD (PHO) - **Spec Exp:** Cooley's Anemia; Thalassemia; Sickle Cell Disease; **Hospital:** Nassau Univ Med Ctr; **Address:** Nassau Univ Med Ctr, Dept Peds, 2201 Hempstead Tpke, East Meadow, NY 11554; **Phone:** 516-572-6177; **Board Cert:** Pediatrics 1975; Pediatric Hematology-Oncology 1982; **Med School:** Italy 1968; **Resid:** Pediatrics, LI College Hosp 1974; **Fellow:** Pediatric Hematology-Oncology, LI College Hosp 1975; **Fac Appt:** Clin Prof Ped, SUNY Stony Brook

Weinblatt, Mark E MD (PHO) - **Spec Exp:** Leukemia & Lymphoma; Sickle Cell Disease; Bleeding/Coagulation Disorders; Thalassemia; **Hospital:** Winthrop - Univ Hosp; **Address:** Winthrop Univ Hosp, 120 Mineola Blvd, Ste 460, Mineola, NY 11501; **Phone:** 516-663-9400; **Board Cert:** Pediatrics 1980; Pediatric Hematology-Oncology 1982; **Med School:** Albert Einstein Coll Med 1976; **Resid:** Pediatrics, Jacobi Med Ctr 1979; **Fellow:** Pediatric Hematology-Oncology, Children's Hosp 1981; **Fac Appt:** Prof Ped, SUNY Stony Brook

Wolfe, Lawrence C MD (PHO) - **Spec Exp:** Palliative Care; Transfusion Medicine; Neuroblastoma; Adrenal Cancer; **Hospital:** Long Island Jewish Med Ctr; **Address:** LIJ Medical Ctr, Div Pediatric Hematology/Oncology, 269-01 76th Ave, New Hyde Park, NY 11040; **Phone:** 718-470-3460; **Board Cert:** Pediatrics 1981; Pediatric Hematology-Oncology 1987; **Med School:** Harvard Med Sch 1976; **Resid:** Pediatrics, Chldns Hosp 1978; **Fellow:** Pediatric Hematology-Oncology, Chldns Hosp 1991

Pediatric Infectious Disease

Krilov, Leonard MD (PInf) - **Spec Exp:** Infections-Respiratory; Infections in Int'l Adopted Children; Chronic Fatigue Syndrome; Lyme Disease; **Hospital:** Winthrop - Univ Hosp; **Address:** 120 Mineola Blvd, Ste 210, Mineola, NY 11501; **Phone:** 516-663-9570; **Board Cert:** Pediatrics 1983; Pediatric Infectious Disease 2009; **Med School:** Columbia P&S 1978; **Resid:** Pediatrics, Johns Hopkins Hosp 1981; **Fellow:** Pediatric Infectious Disease, Chldns Hosp 1984; **Fac Appt:** Prof Ped, SUNY Stony Brook

Rubin, Lorry MD (PInf) - **Spec Exp:** Kawasaki Disease; Tuberculosis; Fevers of Unknown Origin; **Hospital:** Steven & Alexandra Cohen Chldn's Med Ctr of NY, N Shore Univ Hosp; **Address:** 269-01 76th Ave, Ste 365, New Hyde Park, NY 11040-1433; **Phone:** 718-470-3480; **Board Cert:** Pediatrics 1983; Pediatric Infectious Disease 2009; **Med School:** Rush Med Coll 1978; **Resid:** Pediatrics, Children's Hosp 1980; **Fellow:** Pediatric Infectious Disease, Johns Hopkins Hosp 1982; **Fac Appt:** Prof Ped, Albert Einstein Coll Med

Sood, Sunil K MD (PInf) - **Spec Exp:** Fevers of Unknown Origin; Tuberculosis; Lyme Disease; **Hospital:** N Shore Univ Hosp, Steven & Alexandra Cohen Chldn's Med Ctr of NY; **Address:** 269-01 76th Ave, New Hyde Park, NY 11040-1433; **Phone:** 718-470-3480; **Board Cert:** Pediatrics 1987; Pediatric Infectious Disease 2009; **Med School:** India 1976; **Resid:** Pediatrics, Baltimore City Hosp 1983; Pediatrics, Georgetown Univ Hosp 1985; **Fellow:** Infectious Disease, Tulane Univ 1988; **Fac Appt:** Assoc Prof Ped, Albert Einstein Coll Med

Pediatric Nephrology

Trachtman, Howard MD (PNep) - **Spec Exp:** Electrolyte Disorders; Hypertension; Hemolytic Uremic Syndrome; Nephrotic Syndrome; **Hospital:** Steven & Alexandra Cohen Chldn's Med Ctr of NY, Long Island Jewish Med Ctr; **Address:** 269-01 76th Ave, rm 365, New Hyde Park, NY 11040-1433; **Phone:** 718-470-3491; **Board Cert:** Pediatrics 1983; Nephrology 2003; **Med School:** Univ Pennsylvania 1978; **Resid:** Pediatrics, New England Med Ctr 1980; Pediatrics, Bronx Muni Hosp Ctr 1981; **Fellow:** Pediatric Nephrology, Albert Einstein 1983; **Fac Appt:** Prof Ped, Albert Einstein Coll Med

Pediatric Pulmonology

Schaeffer, Janis MD (PPul) - **Spec Exp:** Asthma; Cough-Chronic; Lung Disorders-Congenital; **Hospital:** Steven & Alexandra Cohen Chldn's Med Ctr of NY, N Shore Univ Hosp; **Address:** 3003 New Hyde Park Rd, Ste 204, New Hyde Park, NY 11042-1214; **Phone:** 516-488-7575; **Board Cert:** Pediatrics 1984; Pediatric Pulmonology 2004; **Med School:** SUNY Downstate 1979; **Resid:** Pediatrics, LI Jewish Med Ctr 1982; **Fellow:** Pediatric Pulmonology, Columbia-Presby Med Ctr 1985; **Fac Appt:** Asst Prof Ped, Albert Einstein Coll Med

Pediatric Rheumatology

Gottlieb, Beth Susan MD (PRhu) - **Hospital:** Steven & Alexandra Cohen Chldn's Med Ctr of NY; **Address:** Div Pediatric Rheumatology, 269-01 76th Ave, New Hyde Park, NY 11040; **Phone:** 718-470-3530; **Board Cert:** Pediatrics 2003; Pediatric Rheumatology 2006; **Med School:** Israel 1992; **Resid:** Pediatrics, Schneider Children's Hosp 1995; **Fellow:** Pediatric Rheumatology, Schneider Children's Hosp 1998; **Fac Appt:** Asst Prof Ped, Albert Einstein Coll Med

Pediatric Surgery

Coren, Charles V MD (PS) - **Hospital:** Winthrop - Univ Hosp, NY Hosp Queens; **Address:** 320 Post Ave, Ste 101, Westbury, NY 11590; **Phone:** 516-997-1199; **Board Cert:** Pediatric Surgery 2005; **Med School:** Univ Cincinnati 1978; **Resid:** Surgery, NYU Med Ctr 1983; **Fellow:** Pediatric Surgery, Univ Hosp 1985; **Fac Appt:** Asst Prof S, SUNY Hlth Sci Ctr

Dolgin, Stephen MD (PS) - **Spec Exp:** Neonatal Surgery; Ulcerative Colitis; Inflammatory Bowel Disease/Crohn's; Ovarian Masses in Children/Adolescents; **Hospital:** Steven & Alexandra Cohen Chldn's Med Ctr of NY, N Shore Univ Hosp; **Address:** Cohen Chldn's Med Ctr, Pediatric Surgery, 269-01 76th Ave, New Hyde Park, NY 11040; **Phone:** 718-470-3636; **Board Cert:** Surgery 2000; Pediatric Surgery 2003; Surgical Critical Care 2000; **Med School:** NYU Sch Med 1977; **Resid:** Surgery, Peter Bent Brigham Hosp 1982; **Fellow:** Pediatric Surgery, Chldns Meml Hosp 1984; **Fac Appt:** Prof S, Albert Einstein Coll Med

Hong, Andrew MD (PS) - **Spec Exp:** Neonatal Surgery; Minimally Invasive Surgery; Chest Wall Deformities; **Hospital:** Steven & Alexandra Cohen Chldn's Med Ctr of NY, N Shore Univ Hosp; **Address:** Schneider Children's Hospital, 269-01 76th Ave, New Hyde Park, NY 11040; **Phone:** 718-470-3636; **Board Cert:** Surgery 2002; **Med School:** Univ Wisc 1985; **Resid:** Surgery, Med Ctr Hosp 1990; **Fellow:** Pediatric Surgery, Montreal Chldns Hosp 1992; **Fac Appt:** Asst Prof S, Albert Einstein Coll Med

Kessler, Edmund MD (PS) - **Spec Exp:** Neck Masses; Tumor Surgery; Gallbladder Surgery-Pediatric; Neonatal Surgery; **Hospital:** Steven & Alexandra Cohen Chldn's Med Ctr of NY, New York Methodist Hosp (page 404); **Address:** 1000 Northern Blvd, Ste 250, Great Neck, NY 11021; **Phone:** 516-498-9000; **Med School:** South Africa 1968; **Resid:** Surgery, Univ Witwatersrand 1970; **Fellow:** Pediatric Surgery, Univ Witwatersrand 1977; **Fac Appt:** Asst Clin Prof S, Columbia P&S

Parnell, Vincent MD (PS) - **Spec Exp:** Pediatric Cardiothoracic Surgery; Congenital Heart Disease; **Hospital:** Steven & Alexandra Cohen Chldn's Med Ctr of NY, N Shore Univ Hosp; **Address:** Schneider Chldns Hosp, Ped Cardiothoracic Surgery, 26901 76th Ave, New Hyde Park, NY 11040; **Phone:** 718-470-3580; **Board Cert:** Surgery 2000; Thoracic Surgery 2002; **Med School:** SUNY Downstate 1976; **Resid:** Surgery, N Shore Univ Hosp 1981; Thoracic Surgery, Harper Hosp 1983; **Fellow:** Pediatric Cardiac Surgery, Chldns Hosp 1984

Pediatrics

Adesman, Andrew MD (Ped) - **Spec Exp:** Autism; Asperger's Syndrome; Developmental Disorders; Tourette's Syndrome; **Hospital:** Steven & Alexandra Cohen Chldn's Med Ctr of NY; **Address:** 1983 Marcus Ave, Ste 130, Lake Success, NY 11042; **Phone:** 516-802-6100; **Board Cert:** Pediatrics 1987; Neurodevelopmental Disabilities 2001; Developmental-Behavioral Pediatrics 2002; **Med School:** Univ Pennsylvania 1981; **Resid:** Pediatrics, Chldn's Hosp Natl Med Ctr 1984; **Fellow:** Developmental-Behavioral Pediatrics, Chldn's Hosp 1986; **Fac Appt:** Assoc Prof Ped, Albert Einstein Coll Med

Chianese, Maurice MD (Ped) *PCP* - **Spec Exp:** Pediatric Sports Medicine; Asthma; Behavioral Disorders; **Hospital:** N Shore Univ Hosp, Steven & Alexandra Cohen Chldn's Med Ctr of NY; **Address:** Dept Pediatrics, 12 Nevada Drive, Lake Success, NY 11042; **Phone:** 516-622-7337; **Board Cert:** Pediatrics 2004; **Med School:** NY Med Coll 1986; **Resid:** Pediatrics, North Shore Univ Hosp 1990; **Fac Appt:** Asst Prof Ped, NYU Sch Med

Cooper, Seymour M MD (Ped) *PCP* - **Hospital:** Winthrop - Univ Hosp, Steven & Alexandra Cohen Chldn's Med Ctr of NY; **Address:** 1101 Stewart Ave, Ste 306, Garden City, NY 11530; **Phone:** 516-746-2299; **Board Cert:** Pediatrics 1977; **Med School:** NY Med Coll 1972; **Resid:** Pediatrics, Montefiore Hosp Med Ctr 1975

Friedman, Eugene B MD (Ped) *PCP* - **Hospital:** Steven & Alexandra Cohen Chldn's Med Ctr of NY, Winthrop - Univ Hosp; **Address:** 271 Jericho Tpke, Floral Park, NY 11002; **Phone:** 516-354-7575; **Board Cert:** Pediatrics 1973; **Med School:** NY Med Coll 1968; **Resid:** Pediatrics, Metropolitan Hosp Ctr 1971; **Fac Appt:** Asst Clin Prof Ped, Albert Einstein Coll Med

Galinkin, Lawrence MD (Ped) *PCP* - **Hospital:** N Shore Univ Hosp, Long Island Jewish Med Ctr; **Address:** 700 Old Bethpage Rd, Old Bethpage, NY 11804; **Phone:** 516-293-0666; **Board Cert:** Pediatrics 1976; **Med School:** Tulane Univ 1971; **Resid:** Pediatrics, Bronx Muni Hosp 1974

Gerberg Jr, Lynda Frances MD (Ped) - **Spec Exp:** Sports Medicine; Obesity; **Hospital:** Long Island Jewish Med Ctr; **Address:** 200 Middle Neck Rd, Ste 108, Great Neck, NY 110 458; **Phone:** 516-466-3311; **Board Cert:** Pediatrics 2009; **Med School:** Mexico 1987; **Resid:** Pediatrics, Schneider Chldns Hosp 1993; **Fellow:** Pediatrics, Children's Hosp 1994; **Fac Appt:** Asst Prof Ped, Albert Einstein Coll Med

Glatt, Hershel H MD (Ped) *PCP* - **Spec Exp:** Asthma; Obesity; **Hospital:** South Nassau Comm Hosp, Winthrop - Univ Hosp; **Address:** 3051 Long Beach Rd, Ste 1, Oceanside, NY 11572; **Phone:** 516-536-2000; **Board Cert:** Pediatrics 1977; **Med School:** Belgium 1969; **Resid:** Pediatrics, Maimonides Medical Ctr 1972; **Fellow:** Pediatric Cardiology, Maimonides Medical Ctr 1972; **Fac Appt:** Asst Clin Prof Ped, SUNY Stony Brook

Gould, Eric MD (Ped) *PCP* - **Spec Exp:** Developmental Disorders; **Hospital:** Long Island Jewish Med Ctr, N Shore Univ Hosp; **Address:** 225 Community Drive, Ste 105, Great Neck, NY 11021-2229; **Phone:** 516-829-9409; **Board Cert:** Pediatrics 1976; **Med School:** NY Med Coll 1970; **Resid:** Pediatrics, Bellevue Hosp Ctr/NYU 1974; **Fellow:** Child Development, Montefiore Med Ctr 1976

Green, Abraham I MD (Ped) *PCP* - **Spec Exp:** Asthma; Nutrition; ADD/ADHD; **Hospital:** Long Island Jewish Med Ctr, Winthrop - Univ Hosp; **Address:** 115 Franklin Pl, Woodmere, NY 11598; **Phone:** 516-295-1200; **Board Cert:** Pediatrics 1984; **Med School:** Albert Einstein Coll Med 1979; **Resid:** Pediatrics, Jacobi Med Ctr 1983

Grijnsztein, Jacob MD (Ped) *PCP* - **Spec Exp:** Allergy; **Hospital:** Long Island Jewish Med Ctr, N Shore Univ Hosp; **Address:** 107 Northern Blvd, Ste 201, Great Neck, NY 11021; **Phone:** 516-487-6565; **Board Cert:** Pediatrics 1979; **Med School:** NYU Sch Med 1973; **Resid:** Pediatrics, Bellevue Hosp 1976

Hankin, Dorie MD (Ped) - **Spec Exp:** Developmental Disorders; Behavioral Disorders; **Hospital:** Winthrop - Univ Hosp, Steven & Alexandra Cohen Chldn's Med Ctr of NY; **Address:** 173 Mineola Blvd, Ste 301B, Mineola, NY 11501; **Phone:** 516-739-1936; **Board Cert:** Pediatrics 1980; Neurodevelopmental Disabilities 2001; Developmental-Behavioral Pediatrics 2002; **Med School:** Albert Einstein Coll Med 1974; **Resid:** Pediatrics, Montefiore Med Ctr 1978; **Fellow:** Child Development, Montefiore-Einstein Med Ctr 1980; **Fac Appt:** Asst Clin Prof Ped, Albert Einstein Coll Med

Leavens-Maurer, Jill MD (Ped) *PCP* - **Hospital:** Winthrop - Univ Hosp; **Address:** Winthrop Pediatrics Assocs, 222 Station Plaza N, Ste 611, Mineola, NY 11501-3893; **Phone:** 516-663-2532; **Board Cert:** Pediatrics 2004; **Med School:** SUNY Upstate Med Univ 1984; **Resid:** Pediatrics, NY Hosp-Cornell Med Ctr 1987

Levy, Morton G MD (Ped) *PCP* - **Hospital:** N Shore Univ Hosp, Steven & Alexandra Cohen Chldn's Med Ctr of NY; **Address:** 133 Andover Rd, Roslyn Heights, NY 11577-1009; **Phone:** 516-621-9360; **Board Cert:** Pediatrics 1966; **Med School:** SUNY Downstate 1961; **Resid:** Pediatrics, Mount Sinai 1964; **Fac Appt:** Asst Clin Prof Ped, NYU Sch Med

Marino, Ronald DO (Ped) *PCP* - **Spec Exp:** Developmental & Behavioral Disorders; **Hospital:** Winthrop - Univ Hosp, Good Samaritan Hosp Med Ctr - West Islip; **Address:** 222 Station Plaza N, Ste 611, Mineola, NY 11501-3808; **Phone:** 516-663-2532; **Board Cert:** Pediatrics 1985; **Med School:** Mich State Univ 1978; **Resid:** Pediatrics, Doctors Hosp 1981; **Fellow:** Behavioral Pediatrics, Univ Maryland Med Ctr 1985; **Fac Appt:** Prof Ped, NY Coll Osteo Med

Nerwen, Clifford MD (Ped) *PCP* - **Hospital:** Steven & Alexandra Cohen Chldn's Med Ctr of NY, N Shore Univ Hosp; **Address:** Schneider Chldns Hosp, Genl Peds Div, 410 Lakeville Rd, Ste 108, New Hyde Park, NY 11040; **Phone:** 516-465-4377; **Board Cert:** Pediatrics 2003; **Med School:** Univ Conn 1991; **Resid:** Pediatrics, Schneider Chldns Hosp 1994

Rabinowicz, Morris MD (Ped) *PCP* - **Hospital:** Plainview Hosp, Steven & Alexandra Cohen Chldn's Med Ctr of NY; **Address:** 995 Old Country Rd, Plainview, NY 11803; **Phone:** 516-935-7333; **Board Cert:** Pediatrics 1985; **Med School:** SUNY Downstate 1978; **Resid:** Surgery, LI Jewish Med Ctr 1982; Pediatrics, Brookdale Hosp 1983

Resmovits, Marvin MD (Ped) *PCP* - **Hospital:** Steven & Alexandra Cohen Chldn's Med Ctr of NY, N Shore Univ Hosp; **Address:** 107 NE Northern Blvd Fl s - Ste 201, Great Neck, NY 11021-4309; **Phone:** 516-487-6565; **Board Cert:** Pediatrics 1984; **Med School:** SUNY Buffalo 1979; **Resid:** Pediatrics, LI Jewish Hosp 1982

Physical Medicine & Rehabilitation

Lipetz, Jason S MD (PMR) - **Spec Exp:** Spinal Rehabilitation; Pain-Spine; **Hospital:** N Shore Univ Hosp; **Address:** LI Spine Rehab Medicine, 801 Merrick Ave, East Meadow, NY 11554; **Phone:** 516-393-8941; **Board Cert:** Physical Medicine & Rehabilitation 1999; Pain Medicine 2001; Electrodiagnostic Medicine ; **Med School:** Columbia P&S 1994; **Resid:** Physical Medicine & Rehabilitation, Kessler Inst-UMDNJ 1998; **Fellow:** Interventional Spine Medicine, Univ Penn Affil Hosp 1999; **Fac Appt:** Asst Prof PMR, Albert Einstein Coll Med

Root, Barry C MD (PMR) - **Spec Exp:** Spinal Cord Injury; Electromyography; Spinal Rehabilitation; **Hospital:** N Shore Univ Hosp, St Francis Hosp - The Heart Ctr (page 115); **Address:** Dept Physical Med & Rehab, 101 St Andrews Ln Fl 1, Glen Cove, NY 11542-2254; **Phone:** 516-674-7501; **Board Cert:** Physical Medicine & Rehabilitation 1988; Spinal Cord Injury Medicine 2003; **Med School:** Ohio State Univ 1984; **Resid:** Physical Medicine & Rehabilitation, Nassau County Med Ctr 1987; **Fac Appt:** Asst Clin Prof PMR, Cornell Univ-Weill Med Coll

Stein, Adam B MD (PMR) - **Spec Exp:** Spinal Cord Injury; Multiple Sclerosis; Stroke Rehabilitation; **Hospital:** NS-LIJ Hlth Sys, Glen Cove Hosp; **Address:** 825 Northern Blvd Fl 1, Great Neck, NY 11021; **Phone:** 516-465-8609; **Board Cert:** Physical Medicine & Rehabilitation 1992; Spinal Cord Injury Medicine 2003; **Med School:** NYU Sch Med 1987; **Resid:** Physical Medicine & Rehabilitation, Rusk Inst-NYU Med Ctr 1991

Plastic Surgery

Alizadeh, Kaveh MD (PlS) - **Spec Exp:** Breast Cosmetic & Reconstructive Surgery; Facial Plastic & Reconstructive Surgery; Liposuction & Body Contouring; Blepharoplasty; **Hospital:** Winthrop - Univ Hosp, Lenox Hill Hosp; **Address:** 999 Franklin Ave, Garden City, NY 11530; **Phone:** 516-742-3404; **Board Cert:** Plastic Surgery 2001; **Med School:** Cornell Univ 1993; **Resid:** Plastic Surgery, Univ Chicago Hosps 1999; **Fellow:** Meml Sloan Kettering Cancer Ctr 2000; Cosmetic Plastic Surgery, Manhattan Eye, Ear, & Throat Hosp 2000

Breitbart, Arnold MD (PlS) - **Spec Exp:** Cosmetic Surgery-Face & Body; Liposuction; Breast Reconstruction; Cosmetic Surgery-Breast; **Hospital:** N Shore Univ Hosp, NY-Presby Hosp/Weill Cornell (page 104); **Address:** 1155 Northern Blvd, Ste 110, Manhasset, NY 11030; **Phone:** 516-365-3511; **Board Cert:** Surgery 2003; Plastic Surgery 2004; **Med School:** NYU Sch Med 1985; **Resid:** Surgery, NYU Med Ctr 1991; Plastic Surgery, NYU Med Ctr 1993; **Fellow:** Craniofacial Surgery, NYU Med Ctr 1994; Microsurgery, Meml Sloan Kettering Cancer Ctr 1995; **Fac Appt:** Asst Prof S, Cornell Univ-Weill Med Coll

DeVita, Gregory MD (PlS) - **Spec Exp:** Rhinoplasty; Rhinoplasty Revision; Cosmetic Surgery-Face; Cosmetic Surgery-Breast; **Hospital:** St Francis Hosp - The Heart Ctr (page 115), N Shore Univ Hosp; **Address:** 650 Northern Blvd, Great Neck, NY 11021-5204; **Phone:** 516-466-7000; **Board Cert:** Plastic Surgery 1989; **Med School:** SUNY Downstate 1980; **Resid:** Surgery, St Luke's Hosp 1982; Surgery, Jersey City Med Ctr 1983; **Fellow:** Plastic Surgery, New York Methodist Hosp 1984; Plastic Surgery, SUNY Downstate Med Ctr 1986

DiGregorio, Vincent R MD (PlS) - **Spec Exp:** Rhinoplasty Revision; Cosmetic Surgery-Face; Breast Reconstruction & Augmentation; **Hospital:** Winthrop - Univ Hosp, Mercy Med Ctr - Rockville Centre; **Address:** 999 Franklin Ave Fl 4, Garden City, NY 11530; **Phone:** 516-742-3404; **Board Cert:** Plastic Surgery 1978; **Med School:** Albany Med Coll 1968; **Resid:** Surgery, Thomas Jefferson Univ Hosp 1974; Plastic Surgery, Nassau County Med Ctr 1976; **Fac Appt:** Assoc Prof PlS, SUNY Stony Brook

Doctor, Naishad MD (PlS) - **Hospital:** Mercy Med Ctr - Rockville Centre, Winthrop - Univ Hosp; **Address:** 2000 N Village Ave, Ste 103, Rockville Centre, NY 11570-1001; **Phone:** 516-678-2517; **Board Cert:** Plastic Surgery 1993; **Med School:** India 1974; **Resid:** Surgery, Univ Hosp 1987; Plastic Surgery, Univ Utah Hosp 1990; **Fellow:** Burn Surgery, Univ Hosp 1988

Dubner, Sanford MD (PlS) - **Spec Exp:** Head & Neck Tumors; Melanoma; Reconstructive Plastic Surgery; **Hospital:** Long Island Jewish Med Ctr, N Shore Univ Hosp; **Address:** Long Island Surgical Specialists, 410 Lakeville Rd, Ste 310, Lake Success, NY 11042; **Phone:** 516-437-1111; **Board Cert:** Surgery 2006; Plastic Surgery 1992; **Med School:** SUNY Stony Brook 1982; **Resid:** Surgery, Booth Meml Med Ctr 1987; Plastic Surgery, Montefiore Med Ctr 1989; **Fellow:** Head and Neck Surgery, Meml Sloan Kettering Cancer Ctr 1990; **Fac Appt:** Clin Prof S, Albert Einstein Coll Med

Elkowitz, Marc J MD (PlS) - **Spec Exp:** Cosmetic Surgery; Reconstructive Surgery; **Hospital:** Long Island Jewish Med Ctr, N Shore Univ Hosp; **Address:** 107 Northern Blvd, Ste 203, Great Neck, NY 11021; **Phone:** 516-773-9200; **Board Cert:** Surgery 2007; Plastic Surgery 2002; **Med School:** Albany Med Coll 1993; **Resid:** Surgery, NY Med Coll 1998; **Fellow:** Plastic Surgery, Montefiore Med Ctr 2000; **Fac Appt:** Asst Clin Prof PlS, Albert Einstein Coll Med

Feinberg, Joseph MD (PlS) - **Spec Exp:** Cosmetic Surgery-Face & Eyes; Breast Augmentation; Abdominoplasty; **Hospital:** St Francis Hosp - The Heart Ctr (page 115), N Shore Univ Hosp; **Address:** 1201 Northern Blvd, Ste 202, Manhasset, NY 11030; **Phone:** 516-869-6200; **Board Cert:** Plastic Surgery 1980; **Med School:** Cornell Univ-Weill Med Coll 1973; **Resid:** Surgery, NY Hosp 1976; Plastic Surgery, NY Hosp 1978; **Fellow:** Facial Plastic & Reconstr Surgery, Meml Sloan Kettering Cancer Ctr; **Fac Appt:** Asst Clin Prof S, Cornell Univ-Weill Med Coll

Funt, David MD (PlS) - **Spec Exp:** Cosmetic Surgery-Face & Body; Liposuction; Botox Therapy; Facial Rejuvenation; **Hospital:** South Nassau Comm Hosp, N Shore Univ Hosp; **Address:** 19 Irving Pl, Woodmere, NY 11598; **Phone:** 516-295-0404; **Board Cert:** Plastic Surgery 1987; **Med School:** Geo Wash Univ 1979; **Resid:** Surgery, Montefiore Med Ctr 1983; Plastic Surgery, Montefiore Med Ctr 1985; **Fac Appt:** Asst Clin Prof PlS, Albert Einstein Coll Med

Gallagher, Pamela M MD (PlS) - **Spec Exp:** Abdominoplasty; Body Contouring; Facial Rejuvenation; Breast Augmentation; **Hospital:** Winthrop - Univ Hosp, N Shore Univ Hosp; **Address:** 190 E Jericho Tpke, Mineola, NY 11501; **Phone:** 516-977-9922; **Board Cert:** Plastic Surgery 1980; **Med School:** Univ Chicago-Pritzker Sch Med 1974; **Resid:** Surgery, NY Hosp 1977; Plastic Surgery, NY Hosp 1979

Gold, Alan H MD (PlS) - **Spec Exp:** Cosmetic Surgery-Face & Eyes; Cosmetic Surgery-Breast; Cosmetic Surgery-Body; Nasal Surgery; **Hospital:** N Shore Univ Hosp, Long Island Jewish Med Ctr; **Address:** 833 Northern Blvd, Ste 240, Great Neck, NY 11021-5322; **Phone:** 516-498-2800; **Board Cert:** Plastic Surgery 1979; **Med School:** SUNY Downstate 1971; **Resid:** Surgery, N Shore Univ Hosp 1975; Plastic Surgery, Kings County-Suny Med Ctr 1978; **Fellow:** Hand Surgery, Nassau County Med Ctr 1976

Gotkin, Robert MD (PlS) - **Spec Exp:** Cosmetic Surgery-Face & Breast; Liposuction; Skin Laser Surgery; **Address:** 31 Northern Blvd, Greenvale, NY 11548; **Phone:** 516-484-9000; **Board Cert:** Plastic Surgery 1990; **Med School:** Howard Univ 1980; **Resid:** Surgery, SUNY Stony Brook 1985; Plastic Surgery, Georgetown Univ 1988; **Fellow:** Surgical Critical Care, SUNY Stony Brook 1986

Groeger, William E MD (PlS) - **Spec Exp:** Skin Cancer; **Hospital:** Long Beach Med Ctr, South Nassau Comm Hosp; **Address:** 1490 Broadway Fl 2, Hewlett, NY 11557-1645; **Phone:** 516-887-5502; **Board Cert:** Plastic Surgery 1982; **Med School:** SUNY Downstate 1972; **Resid:** Surgery, Beth Israel Hosp 1977; Plastic Surgery, Univ Hosp 1979

Israeli, Ron MD (PlS) - **Spec Exp:** Plastic & Reconstructive Surgery; Breast Reconstruction; Microsurgery; **Hospital:** N Shore Univ Hosp, St Francis Hosp - The Heart Ctr (page 115); **Address:** 833 Northern Blvd, Ste 160, Great Neck, NY 11021; **Phone:** 516-498-8400; **Board Cert:** Plastic Surgery 2009; **Med School:** Boston Univ 1990; **Resid:** Surgery, Mt Sinai Hosp 1995; Plastic Surgery, Mass Genl Hosp 1997; **Fellow:** Microsurgery, Mt Sinai Hosp 1992

Kasabian, Armen K MD (PlS) - **Spec Exp:** Hand Reconstruction; Plastic & Reconstructive Surgery; Microsurgery; **Hospital:** NS-LIJ Hlth Sys; **Address:** Dept of Surgery, 1999 Marcus Ave, Lake Success, NY 11042; **Phone:** 516-233-3659; **Board Cert:** Plastic Surgery 1992; Hand Surgery 2004; **Med School:** Cornell Univ-Weill Med Coll 1982; **Resid:** Surgery, NYU Med Ctr 1987; Plastic Surgery, NYU Med Ctr 1989; **Fellow:** Microsurgery, NYU Med Ctr 1990; **Fac Appt:** Asst Prof PlS, NYU Sch Med

Keller, Alex J MD (PlS) - **Spec Exp:** Breast Reconstruction; Poland Syndrome; **Hospital:** Long Island Jewish Med Ctr, Huntington Hosp; **Address:** 900 Northern Blvd, Ste 130, Great Neck, NY 11021; **Phone:** 516-482-1100; **Board Cert:** Plastic Surgery 1984; **Med School:** NYU Sch Med 1975; **Resid:** Surgery, NYU Med Ctr 1978; Surgery, LI Jewish Hosp 1980; **Fellow:** Plastic Surgery, NYU Med Ctr 1982; Microsurgery, NYU Med Ctr 1983; **Fac Appt:** Asst Clin Prof PlS, NYU Sch Med

Kessler, Martin E MD (PlS) - **Spec Exp:** Cosmetic Surgery-Face & Body; Reconstructive Surgery-Face; Breast Reconstruction; Hand Surgery; **Hospital:** South Nassau Comm Hosp, N Shore Univ Hosp; **Address:** 242 Merrick Rd, Ste 302, Rockville Centre, NY 11570-5254; **Phone:** 516-536-5858; **Board Cert:** Plastic Surgery 1987; **Med School:** Cornell Univ-Weill Med Coll 1980; **Resid:** Surgery, NY Hosp 1983; Plastic Surgery, NY Hosp 1985; **Fellow:** Hand Surgery, Cleveland Clinic 1986; Microsurgery, Univ Louisville Hlth Ctr 1986; **Fac Appt:** Assoc Clin Prof PlS, Cornell Univ-Weill Med Coll

Leipziger, Lyle S MD (PlS) - **Spec Exp:** Cosmetic Surgery-Face & Eyes; Cosmetic Surgery-Breast; Breast Reconstruction; Liposuction & Body Contouring; **Hospital:** N Shore Univ Hosp, Long Island Jewish Med Ctr; **Address:** 825 Northern Blvd Fl 3, Great Neck, NY 11021; **Phone:** 516-465-8787; **Board Cert:** Plastic Surgery 1994; **Med School:** Cornell Univ-Weill Med Coll 1985; **Resid:** Plastic Surgery, New York Hosp 1990; **Fellow:** Craniofacial Surgery, Johns Hopkins Hosp 1991; **Fac Appt:** Asst Prof S, Albert Einstein Coll Med

Lukash, Frederick MD (PlS) - **Spec Exp:** Pediatric Plastic Surgery; Cosmetic Surgery-Face; Breast Cosmetic & Reconstructive Surgery; Rhinoplasty; **Hospital:** Long Island Jewish Med Ctr, Steven & Alexandra Cohen Chldn's Med Ctr of NY; **Address:** 1129 Northern Blvd, Ste 403, Manhasset, NY 11030-3022; **Phone:** 516-365-1040; **Board Cert:** Plastic Surgery 1982; **Med School:** Tulane Univ 1973; **Resid:** Surgery, Emory Univ Hosp 1975; Surgery, Univ Hosp 1980; **Fellow:** Plastic Surgery, Mass Genl Hosp 1981; **Fac Appt:** Asst Prof S, Albert Einstein Coll Med

Silberman, Mark I MD (PlS) - **Spec Exp:** Cosmetic Surgery-Face; Breast Cosmetic & Reconstructive Surgery; Facial Rejuvenation; Body Contouring; **Hospital:** N Shore Univ Hosp, St Francis Hosp - The Heart Ctr (page 115); **Address:** 650 Northern Blvd, Great Neck, NY 11021-5204; **Phone:** 516-466-7000; **Board Cert:** Plastic Surgery 1988; **Med School:** SUNY Downstate 1980; **Resid:** Surgery, Beth Israel Med Ctr 1983; Plastic Surgery, SUNY Downstate Med Ctr 1985

Simpson, Roger MD (PlS) - **Spec Exp:** Eyelid Surgery; Liposuction & Body Contouring; Cosmetic Surgery-Face & Breast; Burn Care; **Hospital:** Winthrop - Univ Hosp, Mercy Med Ctr - Rockville Centre; **Address:** 999 Franklin Ave, Garden City, NY 11530; **Phone:** 516-742-3404; **Board Cert:** Plastic Surgery 1981; **Med School:** Belgium 1974; **Resid:** Surgery, Nassau Co Med Ctr 1978; Plastic Surgery, Nassau Co Med Ctr 1980; **Fellow:** Hand Surgery, St Luke's-Roosevelt Hosp Ctr 1981; **Fac Appt:** Asst Clin Prof S, SUNY Stony Brook

Sklansky, B Donald MD (PlS) - **Spec Exp:** Cosmetic Surgery; Breast Reconstruction; Skin Cancer; **Hospital:** N Shore Univ Hosp, NY-Presby Hosp/Weill Cornell (page 104); **Address:** 833 Northern Blvd, Ste 115, Great Neck, NY 11021-5308; **Phone:** 516-504-1800; **Board Cert:** Plastic Surgery 1979; Otolaryngology 1976; **Med School:** SUNY Downstate 1969; **Resid:** Otolaryngology, Mass Genl Hosp 1976; **Fellow:** Facial Plastic & Reconstr Surgery, New York Presby/Weill Cornell 1978; Facial Plastic & Reconstr Surgery, Meml Sloan Kettering Cancer Ctr 1978; **Fac Appt:** Asst Clin Prof S, Cornell Univ-Weill Med Coll

Psychiatry

Bailine, Samuel MD (Psyc) - **Spec Exp:** Depression; Psychopharmacology; Electroconvulsive Therapy (ECT); **Hospital:** Long Island Jewish Med Ctr; **Address:** 5 Ridgeway Rd, Port Washington, NY 11050-2729; **Phone:** 516-883-3304; **Board Cert:** Psychiatry 1970; **Med School:** NYU Sch Med 1964; **Resid:** Psychiatry, Tulane Univ Med Ctr 1968; **Fac Appt:** Asst Prof Psyc, Albert Einstein Coll Med

Behr, Raymond MD (Psyc) - **Spec Exp:** Depression; Bipolar/Mood Disorders; Addiction/Substance Abuse; **Hospital:** Long Island Jewish Med Ctr; **Address:** 81-A Arleigh Rd, Great Neck, NY 11021-1442; **Phone:** 516-482-1980; **Board Cert:** Psychiatry 1981; Child & Adolescent Psychiatry 1982; **Med School:** South Africa 1973; **Resid:** Psychiatry, LI Jewish Med Ctr 1978; **Fellow:** Child & Adolescent Psychiatry, LI Jewish Med Ctr 1980; **Fac Appt:** Asst Clin Prof Psyc, Albert Einstein Coll Med

Benjamin, John MD (Psyc) - **Spec Exp:** Depression; Anxiety Disorders; Schizophrenia; **Hospital:** N Shore Univ Hosp; **Address:** 1983 Marcus Ave, Ste E132, Lake Success, NY 11042; **Phone:** 516-216-1780; **Board Cert:** Psychiatry 1983; **Med School:** India 1969; **Resid:** Psychiatry, N Shore Univ Hosp 1981; **Fac Appt:** Asst Clin Prof Psyc, NYU Sch Med

Berman, Sheldon S MD (Psyc) - **Spec Exp:** Psychodynamic Psychotherapy; Psychopharmacology; Palliative Care; **Address:** 8 Payne Circle, Hewlett Harbor, NY 11557; **Phone:** 516-374-4417; **Board Cert:** Psychiatry 1979; **Med School:** Ros Franklin Univ/Chicago Med Sch 1969; **Resid:** Psychiatry, Brookdale Hosp 1973; **Fac Appt:** Asst Clin Prof Psyc, SUNY Downstate

Bhatt, Ashok MD (Psyc) - **Spec Exp:** Depression; Psychopharmacology; **Hospital:** Long Beach Med Ctr; **Address:** 871 E Park Ave, Long Beach, NY 11561; **Phone:** 516-889-8844; **Board Cert:** Psychiatry 1985; **Med School:** India 1976; **Resid:** Psychiatry, LI Jewish Med Ctr 1981; **Fellow:** Psychiatry, LI Jewish Med Ctr 1983

Budman, Cathy L MD (Psyc) - **Spec Exp:** Tourette's Syndrome; ADD/ADHD; Obsessive-Compulsive Disorder; Neuro-Psychiatry; **Hospital:** N Shore Univ Hosp, Long Island Jewish Med Ctr; **Address:** North Shore-LIJ Health System, Dept Psychiatry & Neurology, 400 Community Drive, Manhasset, NY 11030; **Phone:** 516-562-3223; **Board Cert:** Psychiatry 1991; **Med School:** SUNY Buffalo 1984; **Resid:** Psychiatry, Langley Porter Psych Inst/UCSF 1986; Psychiatry, N Shore Univ Hosp 1990; **Fellow:** Family Medicine, Sydney Univ-Royal Price Albert Hosp 1988; Neuropsychiatry, N Shore Univ Hosp 1991; **Fac Appt:** Assoc Prof Psyc, NYU Sch Med

Carone, Patrick F MD (Psyc) - **Spec Exp:** Geriatric Psychiatry; Depression; Anxiety Disorders; **Hospital:** Mercy Med Ctr - Rockville Centre; **Address:** 2000 N Village Ave, Ste 305, Rockville Centre, NY 11570-1001; **Phone:** 516-766-2871; **Board Cert:** Psychiatry 1977; **Med School:** Johns Hopkins Univ 1970; **Resid:** Psychiatry, Yale-New Haven Hosp 1976; Public Health & Genl Preventive Med, Yale-New Haven Hosp 1977; **Fac Appt:** Asst Clin Prof Psyc, SUNY Stony Brook

Crasta, Jovita M MD (Psyc) - **Spec Exp:** Anxiety Disorders; Depression; Bipolar/Mood Disorders; Women's Health-Mental Health; **Hospital:** South Nassau Comm Hosp; **Address:** 2277 Grand Ave, Baldwin, NY 11510-3148; **Phone:** 516-377-5400; **Board Cert:** Psychiatry 1991; **Med School:** India 1981; **Resid:** Psychiatry, Nassau County Med Ctr 1987; **Fac Appt:** Asst Prof Psyc, NY Coll Osteo Med

Frogel, Marvin P MD (Psyc) - **Spec Exp:** Marital/Family Therapy; Psychotherapy; Psychopharmacology; **Hospital:** St Francis Hosp - The Heart Ctr (page 115), N Shore Univ Hosp; **Address:** 78 Oxford Blvd, Great Neck, NY 11023-2329; **Phone:** 516-482-5377; **Board Cert:** Psychiatry 1972; **Med School:** Switzerland 1963; **Resid:** Psychiatry, Hillside Hosp 1967; **Fac Appt:** Asst Clin Prof Psyc, NYU Sch Med

Gurevich, Michael I MD (Psyc) - **Spec Exp:** Psychotherapy & Psychopharmacology; Complementary Medicine; Addiction/Substance Abuse; Psychiatry in Physical Illness; **Hospital:** Glen Cove Hosp; **Address:** 997 Glen Cove Avenue, Glen Head, NY 11545-1584; **Phone:** 516-674-9489; **Board Cert:** Psychiatry 1989; **Med School:** Lithuania 1974; **Resid:** Psychiatry, Elmhurst Hosp Ctr 1987; **Fellow:** Child Psychiatry, Elmhurst Hosp Ctr 1989

Katus, Eli MD (Psyc) - **Spec Exp:** Psychopharmacology; Psychotherapy; Child & Adolescent Psychiatry; **Hospital:** N Shore Univ Hosp, Winthrop - Univ Hosp; **Address:** 1035 Route 106, East Norwich, NY 11732-1005; **Phone:** 516-922-5607; **Board Cert:** Psychiatry 1990; Child & Adolescent Psychiatry 1991; **Med School:** Germany 1982; **Resid:** Psychiatry, N Shore Univ Hosp 1986; **Fellow:** Child & Adolescent Psychiatry, N Shore Univ Hosp 1988

Katz, Jack L MD (Psyc) - **Spec Exp:** Eating Disorders; Mood Disorders; Anxiety Disorders; **Hospital:** N Shore Univ Hosp, Long Island Jewish Med Ctr; **Address:** 1010 Northern Blvd, Ste 208, Great Neck, NY 11021; **Phone:** 516-336-2565; **Board Cert:** Psychiatry 1968; **Med School:** Albert Einstein Coll Med 1960; **Resid:** Psychiatry, Montefiore Med Ctr 1966; **Fellow:** Psychiatry, Montefiore Med Ctr-Einstein 1968; **Fac Appt:** Prof Psyc, NYU Sch Med

Sami, Sherif F MD (Psyc) - **Spec Exp:** Depression; Anxiety & Mood Disorders; Geriatric Psychiatry; **Hospital:** Winthrop - Univ Hosp, N Shore Univ Hosp; **Address:** 7 Bond St, Great Neck, NY 11021; **Phone:** 516-487-9191; **Board Cert:** Psychiatry 1973; **Med School:** Egypt 1961; **Resid:** Psychiatry, Cairo Univ Hosp 1966; Psychiatry, Elmhurst Hosp 1969; **Fellow:** Community Psychiatry, Albert Einstein Coll of Med

Pulmonary Disease

Blum, Alan I MD (Pul) - **Spec Exp:** Cough-Chronic; Asthma; Sleep Disorders; **Hospital:** South Nassau Comm Hosp, Franklin Hosp; **Address:** 444 Merrick Rd Fl Lower Level 1, Lynbrook, NY 11563-2400; **Phone:** 516-593-9500; **Board Cert:** Internal Medicine 1981; Pulmonary Disease 1984; **Med School:** Mexico 1977; **Resid:** Internal Medicine, Mt Sinai Hosp Ctr 1981; **Fellow:** Pulmonary Disease, Mt Sinai Hosp Ctr 1983

Breidbart, David M MD (Pul) - **Spec Exp:** Asthma; Chronic Obstructive Lung Disease (COPD); Sarcoidosis; **Hospital:** N Shore Univ Hosp, St Francis Hosp - The Heart Ctr (page 115); **Address:** 6 Ohio Drive, Ste 201, LSQ Medical Bldg, Lake Success, NY 11042-1129; **Phone:** 516-328-8700; **Board Cert:** Internal Medicine 1982; Pulmonary Disease 1984; **Med School:** SUNY Downstate 1979; **Resid:** Internal Medicine, North Shore Univ Hosp 1982; **Fellow:** Pulmonary Disease, Meml Sloan-Kettering Hosp 1983; Pulmonary Disease, Montefiore-Albert Einstein Med Ctr 1985; **Fac Appt:** Asst Clin Prof Med, NYU Sch Med

Cohen, Michael L MD (Pul) - **Spec Exp:** Asthma; Bronchitis; Emphysema; **Hospital:** N Shore Univ Hosp; **Address:** N Shore Internal Med Assocs, 560 Northern Blvd, Ste 203, Great Neck, NY 11021-5100; **Phone:** 516-482-0600; **Board Cert:** Internal Medicine 1972; Pulmonary Disease 1974; **Med School:** SUNY Upstate Med Univ 1967; **Resid:** Internal Medicine, Montefiore Hosp Med Ctr 1970; **Fellow:** Pulmonary Disease, Montefiore Hosp Med Ctr 1971; Pulmonary Disease, LI Jewish Med Ctr 1974; **Fac Appt:** Asst Clin Prof Med, NYU Sch Med

Fein, Alan MD (Pul) - **Spec Exp:** Chronic Obstructive Lung Disease (COPD); Asthma; Pneumonia; **Hospital:** N Shore Univ Hosp, Long Island Jewish Med Ctr; **Address:** 2800 Marcus Ave, Dept Pulmonary Med, Lake Success, NY 11042; **Phone:** 516-608-2890; **Board Cert:** Pulmonary Disease 1999; Critical Care Medicine 2008; **Med School:** SUNY Downstate 1973; **Resid:** Internal Medicine, Albert Einstein Affil Hosp 1976; **Fellow:** Pulmonary Disease, UC San Francisco Med Ctr 1978

Gordon, Richard Eric MD (Pul) - **Spec Exp:** Emphysema; Sleep Disorders; Asthma; **Hospital:** St Joseph's Hosp-Nassau, Plainview Hosp; **Address:** Island Pulmonary Associates, 4271 Hempstead Tpke, Ste 1, Bethpage, NY 11714-5718; **Phone:** 516-796-3700; **Board Cert:** Internal Medicine 1984; Pulmonary Disease 1986; **Med School:** Mount Sinai Sch Med 1980; **Resid:** Internal Medicine, Beth Israel Med Ctr 1983; **Fellow:** Pulmonary Disease, Queens Hosp Ctr 1985

Greenberg, Harly MD (Pul) - **Spec Exp:** Sleep Disorders/Apnea; Lung Disease; Critical Care; **Hospital:** Long Island Jewish Med Ctr, N Shore Univ Hosp; **Address:** North Shore LIJ Sleep Disorders Ctr, 410 Lakeville Rd, Ste 107, New Hyde Park, NY 11040; **Phone:** 516-465-3899; **Board Cert:** Internal Medicine 1985; Pulmonary Disease 1988; **Med School:** NYU Sch Med 1982; **Resid:** Internal Medicine, North Shore Univ Hosp 1985; **Fellow:** Pulmonary Disease, NYU-Bellevue Hosp Ctr 1987; **Fac Appt:** Assoc Prof Med, Albert Einstein Coll Med

Leeman, Benjamin J MD (Pul) - **Spec Exp:** Asthma; Pneumonia; Pulmonary Infectious Disease; **Hospital:** Franklin Hosp, South Nassau Comm Hosp; **Address:** 20 W Lincoln Ave, Ste 306, North Valley Stream, NY 11580; **Phone:** 516-599-8787; **Board Cert:** Internal Medicine 2006; Pulmonary Disease 2007; **Med School:** SUNY Stony Brook 1988; **Resid:** Internal Medicine, Montefiore Med Ctr 1991; **Fellow:** Pulmonary Disease, NY Presby-Columbia Med Ctr 1993

Mensch, Alan MD (Pul) - **Spec Exp:** Asthma; Chronic Obstructive Lung Disease (COPD); **Hospital:** Plainview Hosp, Syosset Hosp; **Address:** 453 S Oyster Bay Rd, Plainview, NY 11803-3311; **Phone:** 516-433-2922; **Board Cert:** Internal Medicine 1976; Pulmonary Disease 1978; **Med School:** Ros Franklin Univ/Chicago Med Sch 1973; **Resid:** Internal Medicine, Nassau Co Med Ctr 1976; **Fellow:** Pulmonary Disease, Nassau Co Med Ctr 1978; **Fac Appt:** Asst Clin Prof Med, SUNY Stony Brook

Mermelstein, Steve A MD (Pul) - **Spec Exp:** Asthma; Chronic Obstructive Lung Disease (COPD); Cough-Chronic; **Hospital:** South Nassau Comm Hosp, Franklin Hosp; **Address:** 444 Merrick Rd, Lower Level 1, Lynbrook, NY 11563-2456; **Phone:** 516-593-9500; **Board Cert:** Internal Medicine 1980; Pulmonary Disease 1982; **Med School:** Albert Einstein Coll Med 1977; **Resid:** Internal Medicine, Metropolitan Hosp Ctr 1980; **Fellow:** Pulmonary Disease, St Luke's-Roosevelt Hosp Ctr 1982

Multz, Alan S MD (Pul) - **Spec Exp:** Sepsis; Respiratory Distress Syndrome; Critical Care; **Hospital:** Nassau Univ Med Ctr, N Shore Univ Hosp; **Address:** 2201 Hemptstead Tpke, East Meadow, NY 11554; **Phone:** 516-572-6262; **Board Cert:** Internal Medicine 1988; Pulmonary Disease 2000; Critical Care Medicine 2000; **Med School:** Boston Univ 1985; **Resid:** Internal Medicine, Montefiore Hosp Med Ctr 1988; **Fellow:** Pulmonary Disease, Montefiore Hosp Med Ctr 1990; Critical Care Medicine, Montefiore Hosp Med Ctr 1991; **Fac Appt:** Assoc Prof Med, Albert Einstein Coll Med

Newmark, Ian H MD (Pul) - **Spec Exp:** Critical Care; Asthma; Lung Cancer; **Hospital:** Plainview Hosp, Syosset Hosp; **Address:** 8 Greenfield Rd, Syosset, NY 11791-4831; **Phone:** 516-496-3001; **Board Cert:** Internal Medicine 1982; Pulmonary Disease 1986; Critical Care Medicine 2000; **Med School:** SUNY Hlth Sci Ctr 1979; **Resid:** Internal Medicine, Nassau Co Med Ctr 1982; **Fellow:** Pulmonary Intensive Care, Nassau Co Med Ctr 1984; **Fac Appt:** Asst Clin Prof Med, SUNY Stony Brook

Niederman, Michael S MD (Pul) - **Spec Exp:** Infections-Respiratory; Emphysema; Respiratory Failure; Pneumonia; **Hospital:** Winthrop - Univ Hosp; **Address:** 222 Station Plaza N, Ste 400, Mineola, NY 11501-3893; **Phone:** 516-663-2834; **Board Cert:** Internal Medicine 1980; Pulmonary Disease 1982; Critical Care Medicine 2007; **Med School:** Boston Univ 1977; **Resid:** Internal Medicine, Northwestern Univ Med Ctr 1980; **Fellow:** Pulmonary Disease, Yale-New Haven Hosp 1983; **Fac Appt:** Prof Med, SUNY Stony Brook

Rosen, Mark J MD (Pul) - **Spec Exp:** Chronic Obstructive Lung Disease (COPD); Asthma; Sepsis; **Hospital:** Long Island Jewish Med Ctr, N Shore Univ Hosp; **Address:** 410 Lakeville Rd, Ste 107, New Hyde Park, NY 11040; **Phone:** 516-465-5400; **Board Cert:** Internal Medicine 1978; Critical Care Medicine 2007; **Med School:** Brown Univ 1975; **Resid:** Internal Medicine, Mt Sinai Hosp 1978; **Fellow:** Pulmonary Disease, Mt Sinai Hosp 1980; Critical Care Medicine, St Vincent's Med Ctr 1980; **Fac Appt:** Prof Med, Albert Einstein Coll Med

Schulster, Rita B MD (Pul) - **Spec Exp:** Asthma; Bronchitis; **Hospital:** Long Beach Med Ctr, South Nassau Comm Hosp; **Address:** 442 E Waukena Ave, Oceanside, NY 11572; **Phone:** 516-599-8234; **Board Cert:** Pulmonary Disease 1977; Internal Medicine 1978; **Med School:** Albert Einstein Coll Med 1970; **Resid:** Internal Medicine, Beth Israel Med Ctr 1973; Internal Medicine, Beth Israel Med Ctr 1974; **Fellow:** Pulmonary Disease, LI Jewish Med Ctr 1975; Pulmonary Disease, Beth Israel Med Ctr 1976

Steinberg, Harry MD (Pul) - **Spec Exp:** Asthma; Emphysema; Lung Cancer; **Hospital:** Long Island Jewish Med Ctr, N Shore Univ Hosp; **Address:** LI Jewish Med Ctr, Dept Med, 270-05 76th Ave, New Hyde Park, NY 11040-1433; **Phone:** 516-465-5400; **Med School:** Temple Univ 1966; **Resid:** Internal Medicine, LI Jewish Med Ctr 1969; Pulmonary Critical Care Medicine, LI Jewish Med Ctr 1970; **Fellow:** Pulmonary Disease, Hosp Univ Penn 1974; **Fac Appt:** Clin Prof Med, Albert Einstein Coll Med

Wyner, Perry A MD (Pul) - **Spec Exp:** Asthma; Cough-Chronic; Emphysema; Preventive Medicine; **Hospital:** Mercy Med Ctr - Rockville Centre, Winthrop - Univ Hosp; **Address:** 2 Lincoln Ave, Ste 201, Rockville Centre, NY 11570-5775; **Phone:** 516-536-4960; **Board Cert:** Internal Medicine 1980; Pulmonary Disease 1982; **Med School:** Cornell Univ-Weill Med Coll 1977; **Resid:** Internal Medicine, Med Coll Virginia Hosps 1980; **Fellow:** Pulmonary Disease, Bellevue Hosp 1982

Zupnick, Henry MD (Pul) - **Spec Exp:** Asthma; Bronchitis; Cough; **Hospital:** South Nassau Comm Hosp; **Address:** 158 Hempstead Ave, Lynbrook, NY 11563; **Phone:** 516-593-3541; **Board Cert:** Internal Medicine 1983; Pulmonary Disease 1988; Critical Care Medicine 1998; **Med School:** Albert Einstein Coll Med 1980; **Resid:** Internal Medicine, Brookdale Hosp Med Ctr 1983; **Fellow:** Pulmonary Disease, Columbia-Presby Med Ctr 1985; Critical Care Medicine, Mount Sinai Hosp 1987; **Fac Appt:** Asst Clin Prof Med, SUNY Downstate

Radiation Oncology

Bosworth, Jay L MD (RadRO) - **Spec Exp:** Breast Cancer; Prostate Cancer; Lymphoma; **Hospital:** St Francis Hosp - The Heart Ctr (page 115), N Shore Univ Hosp; **Address:** 6 Ohio Drive, Lake Success, NY 11042; **Phone:** 516-365-6544; **Board Cert:** Therapeutic Radiology 1974; **Med School:** Albert Einstein Coll Med 1970; **Resid:** Radiation Oncology, Bronx Muni Hosp Ctr 1974

Diamond, Ezriel MD (RadRO) - **Hospital:** Plainview Hosp, St Joseph's Hosp-Nassau; **Address:** 688 Old Country Rd, Plainview, NY 11803; **Phone:** 516-932-6007; **Board Cert:** Therapeutic Radiology 1982; **Med School:** NYU Sch Med 1978; **Resid:** Radiation Oncology, NYU Med Ctr 1981; **Fellow:** Radiation Oncology, NY Methodist Hosp 1982

Gewanter, Richard M MD (RadRO) - **Hospital:** Meml Sloan-Kettering Cancer Ctr (page 112); **Address:** MSKCC Long Island, 1000 N Village Ave, Rockville Center, NY 11570; **Phone:** 516-256-3600; **Board Cert:** Radiation Oncology 2002; **Med School:** Albert Einstein Coll Med 1995; **Resid:** Radiation Oncology, NY Presby-Columbia Med Ctr 2002

Haas, Jonathan A MD (RadRO) - **Spec Exp:** Brachytherapy; Prostate Cancer; Lung Cancer; Gynecologic Cancer; **Hospital:** Winthrop - Univ Hosp; **Address:** Winthrop Univ Hosp, Radiation Onc, 259 1st St, Mineola, NY 11501; **Phone:** 516-663-2501; **Board Cert:** Radiation Oncology 2008; **Med School:** Washington Univ, St Louis 1993; **Resid:** Radiation Oncology, Hosp Univ Penn 1997; **Fac Appt:** Asst Clin Prof RadRO, SUNY Stony Brook

Marin, Lorraine A MD (RadRO) - **Spec Exp:** Breast Cancer; Gynecologic Cancer; Pediatric Cancers; Lymphoma; **Address:** HealthCare Partners, 1225 Franklin Ave, Garden City, NY 11530; **Phone:** 516-515-8820; **Board Cert:** Internal Medicine 1980; Medical Oncology 1983; Therapeutic Radiology 1986; **Med School:** UC Davis 1977; **Resid:** Internal Medicine, UC Davis Med Ctr 1980; **Fellow:** Medical Oncology, Natl Cancer Inst/NIH 1983; Radiation Oncology, Natl Cancer Inst/NIH 1985; **Fac Appt:** Asst Clin Prof RadRO, Albert Einstein Coll Med

Mullen, Edward E MD (RadRO) - **Spec Exp:** Brain Tumors; Breast Cancer; Stereotactic Radiosurgery; **Hospital:** South Nassau Comm Hosp; **Address:** South Nassau Comm Hosp, One Healthy Way, Oceanside, NY 11572; **Phone:** 516-632-3330; **Board Cert:** Radiation Oncology 1991; **Med School:** Univ VA Sch Med 1986; **Resid:** Radiation Oncology, Columbia-Presby Med Ctr 1990

Pollack, Jed MD (RadRO) - **Spec Exp:** Head & Neck Cancer; Prostate Cancer; Brain Tumors; **Hospital:** N Shore Univ Hosp, St Francis Hosp - The Heart Ctr (page 115); **Address:** Long Island Radiation Therapy, 6 Ohio Drive, Ste 103, Lake Success, NY 11042; **Phone:** 516-394-8100; **Board Cert:** Therapeutic Radiology 1985; **Med School:** Univ New Mexico 1981; **Resid:** Therapeutic Radiology, Meml Sloan-Kettering Cancer Ctr 1985; **Fac Appt:** Asst Clin Prof RadRO, Albert Einstein Coll Med

Potters, Louis MD (RadRO) - **Spec Exp:** Prostate Cancer; Intensity Modulated Radiotherapy (IMRT); Brachytherapy; **Hospital:** Long Island Jewish Med Ctr, N Shore Univ Hosp; **Address:** LIJ Med Ctr, Dept Radiation Oncology, 270-05 76th Ave, New Hyde Park, NY 11040; **Phone:** 718-470-7190; **Board Cert:** Internal Medicine 1988; Radiation Oncology 1999; **Med School:** UMDNJ-NJ Med Sch, Newark 1985; **Resid:** Internal Medicine, Beth Israel Med Ctr 1988; Radiation Oncology, SUNY Downstate Med Ctr 1991; **Fac Appt:** Prof RadRO, Hungary

Reproductive Endocrinology

Brenner, Steven H MD (RE) - **Spec Exp:** Infertility-IVF; Polycystic Ovarian Syndrome; **Hospital:** Long Island Jewish Med Ctr, John T Mather Meml Hosp; **Address:** 2001 Marcus Ave, Ste N213, Lake Success, NY 11042; **Phone:** 516-358-6363; **Board Cert:** Obstetrics & Gynecology 1985; Reproductive Endocrinology 1987; **Med School:** SUNY Downstate 1978; **Resid:** Obstetrics & Gynecology, Beth Israel Med Ctr 1982; **Fellow:** Reproductive Endocrinology, NYU Med Ctr 1984; **Fac Appt:** Assoc Clin Prof ObG, Albert Einstein Coll Med

Rosenfeld, David L MD (RE) - **Spec Exp:** Infertility-IVF; Endometriosis; Uterine Fibroids; **Hospital:** N Shore Univ Hosp; **Address:** Div Human Reproduction, 300 Community Drive Ambulatory Bldg, Manhasset, NY 11030-3816; **Phone:** 516-562-2229; **Board Cert:** Obstetrics & Gynecology 1976; Reproductive Endocrinology 1980; **Med School:** Univ Pennsylvania 1970; **Resid:** Obstetrics & Gynecology, Hosp Univ Penn 1974; **Fellow:** Reproductive Endocrinology, Hosp Univ Penn 1976; **Fac Appt:** Prof ObG, NYU Sch Med

Rheumatology

Belilos, Elise MD (Rhu) - **Spec Exp:** Polymyalgia Rheumatica; Giant Cell Arteritis; Rheumatoid Arthritis; **Hospital:** Winthrop - Univ Hosp; **Address:** Winthrop Univ Hosp, Div Rheum, 120 Mineola Blvd, Ste 410, Mineola, NY 11501; **Phone:** 516-663-2097; **Board Cert:** Internal Medicine 1989; Rheumatology 2004; **Med School:** SUNY Stony Brook 1986; **Resid:** Internal Medicine, Winthrop Univ Hosp 1990; **Fellow:** Rheumatology, Winthrop UnivHosp 1993; **Fac Appt:** Asst Clin Prof Med, SUNY Stony Brook

Blau, Sheldon P MD (Rhu) - **Spec Exp:** Lupus/SLE; Scleroderma; Rheumatoid Arthritis; Osteoporosis; **Hospital:** Winthrop - Univ Hosp; **Address:** 566 Broadway, Massapequa, NY 11758-5017; **Phone:** 516-541-6262; **Board Cert:** Internal Medicine 1969; Rheumatology 1972; **Med School:** Albert Einstein Coll Med 1961; **Resid:** Internal Medicine, Montefiore Med Ctr 1964; **Fellow:** Rheumatology, Albert Einstein Coll Med 1965; **Fac Appt:** Clin Prof Med, SUNY Stony Brook

Carsons, Steven MD (Rhu) - **Spec Exp:** Rheumatoid Arthritis; Sjogren's Syndrome; **Hospital:** Winthrop - Univ Hosp; **Address:** Div Rheumatology & Allergy, 120 Mineola Blvd, Ste 410, Mineola, NY 11501; **Phone:** 516-663-2097; **Board Cert:** Internal Medicine 1978; Rheumatology 1980; Clinical & Laboratory Immunology 1988; **Med School:** NY Med Coll 1975; **Resid:** Internal Medicine, Maimonides Med Ctr 1978; **Fellow:** Rheumatology, SUNY Brooklyn Med Ctr 1980; **Fac Appt:** Prof Med, SUNY Hlth Sci Ctr

Cohen, Daniel H MD (Rhu) - **Spec Exp:** Osteoporosis; Arthritis; **Hospital:** South Nassau Comm Hosp, St John's Epis Hosp - S Shore; **Address:** 1157 Broadway, Hewlett, NY 11557; **Phone:** 516-295-4481; **Board Cert:** Rheumatology 1984; Internal Medicine 1981; **Med School:** NYU Sch Med 1978; **Resid:** Internal Medicine, Columbia-Presby Med Ctr 1981; **Fellow:** Rheumatology, NYU Med Ctr 1983

Furie, Richard A MD (Rhu) - **Spec Exp:** Lupus/SLE; Antiphospholipid Syndrome (APS); Rheumatoid Arthritis; **Hospital:** N Shore Univ Hosp, Long Island Jewish Med Ctr; **Address:** N Shore Long Island Jewish Hlth System, 2800 Marcus Ave, Ste 200, Lake Success, NY 11042; **Phone:** 516-708-2550; **Board Cert:** Internal Medicine 1982; Rheumatology 1984; **Med School:** Cornell Univ-Weill Med Coll 1979; **Resid:** Internal Medicine, NY Hosp 1982; **Fellow:** Rheumatology, Hosp Spec Surg 1984; **Fac Appt:** Prof Med, Albert Einstein Coll Med

Greenwald, Robert MD (Rhu) - **Spec Exp:** Rheumatoid Arthritis; Psoriatic Arthritis; Osteoarthritis; **Hospital:** Long Island Jewish Med Ctr; **Address:** 2 ProHealth Plaza, Lake Success, NY 11042; **Phone:** 516-622-6090; **Board Cert:** Internal Medicine 1973; Rheumatology 1974; **Med School:** Johns Hopkins Univ 1967; **Resid:** Internal Medicine, LI Jewish-Hillside Med Ctr 1970; **Fellow:** Rheumatology, SUNY Brooklyn Med Ctr 1972; **Fac Appt:** Prof Med, Albert Einstein Coll Med

Hoffman, Michael L MD (Rhu) - **Spec Exp:** Lupus/SLE; Rheumatoid Arthritis; Osteoarthritis; Osteoporosis; **Hospital:** Long Island Jewish Med Ctr, N Shore Univ Hosp; **Address:** 277 Northern Blvd, Ste 312, Great Neck, NY 11021; **Phone:** 516-498-3500; **Board Cert:** Internal Medicine 1971; **Med School:** SUNY Downstate 1965; **Resid:** Internal Medicine, Maimonides Med Ctr 1967; Internal Medicine, Jacobi Med Ctr 1968; **Fellow:** Rheumatology, Hosp for Special Surg 1970; **Fac Appt:** Assoc Clin Prof Med, Albert Einstein Coll Med

Lipstein-Kresch, Esther MD (Rhu) - **Spec Exp:** Rheumatoid Arthritis; Osteoarthritis; Osteoporosis; Fibromyalgia; **Hospital:** Long Island Jewish Med Ctr, N Shore Univ Hosp; **Address:** 2 Pro Health Plaza, Ste 200-A, Lake Success, NY 11042-1111; **Phone:** 516-622-6090; **Board Cert:** Internal Medicine 1982; Rheumatology 1984; **Med School:** SUNY Hlth Sci Ctr 1979; **Resid:** Internal Medicine, LI Jewish Med Ctr 1982; **Fellow:** Rheumatology, LI Jewish Med Ctr 1984; **Fac Appt:** Asst Prof Med, Mount Sinai Sch Med

Meredith, Gary MD (Rhu) - **Spec Exp:** Gout; Lupus/SLE; Rheumatoid Arthritis; **Hospital:** Mercy Med Ctr - Rockville Centre, South Nassau Comm Hosp; **Address:** 242 Merrick Rd, Ste 303, Rockville Centre, NY 11570-5254; **Phone:** 516-536-9424; **Board Cert:** Internal Medicine 1984; Rheumatology 1986; **Med School:** NYU Sch Med 1981; **Resid:** Internal Medicine, Bellevue Hosp 1984; **Fellow:** Rheumatology, NYU Med Ctr 1986; **Fac Appt:** Asst Clin Prof Med, NYU Sch Med

Porges, Andrew J MD (Rhu) - **Spec Exp:** Osteoporosis; **Hospital:** N Shore Univ Hosp, Glen Cove Hosp; **Address:** 1044 Northern Blvd, Ste 104, Roslyn, NY 11576; **Phone:** 516-484-6880; **Board Cert:** Internal Medicine 1989; Rheumatology 2002; **Med School:** Cornell Univ-Weill Med Coll 1986; **Resid:** Internal Medicine, NY Hosp 1989; **Fellow:** Rheumatology, Hosp Special Surg 1992; **Fac Appt:** Asst Prof Med, Cornell Univ-Weill Med Coll

Sullivan, James M MD (Rhu) - **Spec Exp:** Rheumatoid Arthritis; Lupus/SLE; Osteoarthritis; **Hospital:** Winthrop - Univ Hosp; **Address:** 975 Stewart Ave, Garden City, NY 11530; **Phone:** 516-222-8654; **Board Cert:** Internal Medicine 1977; Rheumatology 1980; **Med School:** SUNY Upstate Med Univ 1974; **Resid:** Internal Medicine, Univ Michigan Med Ctr 1977; **Fellow:** Rheumatology, Univ Michigan Med Ctr 1979

Tiger, Louis MD (Rhu) - **Spec Exp:** Rheumatoid Arthritis; Lupus/SLE; Osteoarthritis; **Hospital:** Winthrop - Univ Hosp; **Address:** 566 Broadway, Massapequa, NY 11758-5017; **Phone:** 516-541-6262; **Board Cert:** Internal Medicine 1975; Rheumatology 1976; **Med School:** Univ Louisville Sch Med 1967; **Resid:** Internal Medicine, Maimonides Medical Ctr 1970; **Fellow:** Rheumatology, Albert Einstein Med Ctr 1974; **Fac Appt:** Asst Clin Prof Med, SUNY Stony Brook

Surgery

Auguste, Louis J MD (S) - **Spec Exp:** Breast Disease; Melanoma; Thyroid & Parathyroid Surgery; Hernia; **Hospital:** Long Island Jewish Med Ctr, N Shore Univ Hosp; **Address:** 2035 Lakeville Rd, Ste 206, New Hyde Park, NY 11042-1102; **Phone:** 516-775-2070; **Board Cert:** Surgery 2000; **Med School:** Haiti 1973; **Resid:** Surgery, LI Jewish Med Ctr 1980; **Fellow:** Surgical Oncology, Roswell Park Meml Inst 1982; **Fac Appt:** Assoc Clin Prof S, Albert Einstein Coll Med

Conte, Charles C MD (S) - **Spec Exp:** Cancer Surgery; Breast Cancer; Pancreatic Cancer; **Hospital:** N Shore Univ Hosp, Flushing Hosp Med Ctr; **Address:** 600 Northern Blvd, Ste 111, Great Neck, NY 11021; **Phone:** 516-487-9454; **Board Cert:** Surgery 2005; **Med School:** Dartmouth Med Sch 1981; **Resid:** Surgery, Hartford Hosp 1986; **Fellow:** Surgical Oncology, Roswell Park Cancer Inst 1988

Coppa, Gene F MD (S) - **Spec Exp:** Minimally Invasive Surgery; Hepatobiliary Surgery; Gastrointestinal Surgery; Pancreatic Surgery; **Hospital:** NS-LIJ Hlth Sys; **Address:** 1999 Marcus Ave, Lake Success, NY 11042; **Phone:** 516-562-2870; **Board Cert:** Surgery 2000; **Med School:** NYU Sch Med 1974; **Resid:** Surgery, NYU/Bellevue Med Ctr 1979; **Fac Appt:** Prof S, SUNY Downstate

Datta, Rajiv V MD (S) - **Spec Exp:** Breast Cancer; Colon & Rectal Cancer; Gastrointestinal Cancer; Head & Neck Cancer; **Hospital:** South Nassau Comm Hosp; **Address:** South Nassau Cancer Ctr, Surg Oncology, 1 Healthy Way, Oceanside, NY 11572; **Phone:** 516-632-3350; **Board Cert:** Surgery 1999; **Med School:** India 1984; **Resid:** Surgery, Maimonides Med Ctr 1998; **Fellow:** Surgical Oncology, Roswell Park Cancer Inst 1999; Head and Neck Surgery, Roswell Park Cancer Inst 2000; **Fac Appt:** Assoc Clin Prof S, NY Coll Osteo Med

Denoto, George MD (S) - **Spec Exp:** Laparoscopic Surgery; Hernia; **Hospital:** N Shore Univ Hosp; **Address:** 1999 Marcus Ave, Ste 106C, Lake Success, NY 11042; **Phone:** 516-233-3600; **Board Cert:** Surgery 2006; **Med School:** SUNY Stony Brook 1988; **Resid:** Surgery, Mt Sinai Hosp 1993

Gecelter, Gary MD (S) - **Spec Exp:** Pancreatic Cancer; Esophageal Surgery; Laparoscopic Surgery; Biliary Surgery; **Hospital:** St Francis Hosp - The Heart Ctr (page 115); **Address:** 139 Plandome Rd, Manhasset, NY 11030; **Phone:** 516-627-5262; **Med School:** South Africa 1981; **Resid:** Surgery, Johannesburg Hosp 1990; **Fellow:** Gastroenterology, Johannesburg Hosp 1992

Grieco, Michael B MD (S) - **Spec Exp:** Breast Surgery; Laparoscopic Abdominal Surgery; Hernia; Laparoscopic Cholecystectomy; **Hospital:** Glen Cove Hosp, St Francis Hosp - The Heart Ctr (page 115); **Address:** 10 Medical Plaza, Glen Cove, NY 11542; **Phone:** 516-676-1060; **Board Cert:** Surgery 2001; Colon & Rectal Surgery 1982; **Med School:** Albany Med Coll 1974; **Resid:** Surgery, N Shore Univ Hosp 1979; **Fellow:** Surgery, Lahey Clinic 1980; Colon & Rectal Surgery, Greater Baltimore Med Ctr 1981; **Fac Appt:** Asst Clin Prof S, SUNY Stony Brook

Khalife, Michael E MD (S) - **Spec Exp:** Laparoscopic Surgery; Breast Surgery; **Hospital:** Winthrop - Univ Hosp, N Shore Univ Hosp; **Address:** 300 Old Country Rd, Ste 101, Mineola, NY 11501; **Phone:** 516-741-4138; **Board Cert:** Surgery 2003; **Med School:** France 1978; **Resid:** Surgery, Univ Hosp 1984; **Fac Appt:** Asst Clin Prof S, SUNY Stony Brook

Kurtz, Lewis MD (S) - **Spec Exp:** Breast Surgery; Gallbladder Surgery; Hernia; **Hospital:** St Francis Hosp - The Heart Ctr (page 115), Long Island Jewish Med Ctr; **Address:** 310 E Shore Rd, Ste 203, Great Neck, NY 11023; **Phone:** 516-482-8657; **Board Cert:** Surgery 2000; **Med School:** Italy 1972; **Resid:** Surgery, Long Island Jewish-Hillside Med Ctr 1977; **Fellow:** Research, Long Island Jewish-Hillside Med Ctr 1978

Mansouri, Hormoz MD (S) - **Spec Exp:** Varicose Veins; **Hospital:** St Joseph's Hosp-Nassau, Plainview Hosp; **Address:** 175 Jericho Tpke, Ste 201, Syosset, NY 11791; **Phone:** 516-682-4800; **Board Cert:** Surgery 1980; **Med School:** Iran 1964; **Resid:** Surgery, Henry Ford Hosp 1969; Surgery, Nassau Co Med Ctr 1971; **Fac Appt:** Asst Prof S, SUNY Stony Brook

Reed Jr, William P MD (S) - **Spec Exp:** Breast Cancer; Stomach Cancer; **Hospital:** Winthrop - Univ Hosp; **Address:** Winthrop Surgical Assoc, 120 Mineola Blvd, Ste 320, Mineola, NY 11501; **Phone:** 516-663-3300; **Board Cert:** Surgery 2008; **Med School:** Harvard Med Sch 1968; **Resid:** Surgery, Stanford Univ 1976; **Fellow:** Surgical Oncology, Inst Gustave-Roussy 1977; **Fac Appt:** Prof S, SUNY Stony Brook

Reiner, Dan MD (S) - **Spec Exp:** Laparoscopic Surgery; Hernia; Gastrointestinal Surgery; **Hospital:** N Shore Univ Hosp, Syosset Hosp; **Address:** 2800 Marcus Ave, Ste 204, Lake Success, NY 11042-1008; **Phone:** 516-622-6120; **Board Cert:** Surgery 2005; Surgical Critical Care 2007; **Med School:** St Louis Univ 1980; **Resid:** Surgery, St Louis Univ-Group Hosps 1985; **Fellow:** Surgical Critical Care, UMDNJ-NJ Hosp 1986; **Fac Appt:** Assoc Clin Prof S, NYU Sch Med

Romero, Carlos MD (S) - **Spec Exp:** Laparoscopic Surgery; Head & Neck Surgery; Breast Surgery; **Hospital:** Winthrop - Univ Hosp; **Address:** 173 Mineola Blvd, Ste 401, Mineola, NY 11501-2555; **Phone:** 516-741-6464; **Board Cert:** Surgery 2007; **Med School:** Argentina 1969; **Resid:** Surgery, Winthrop Univ Hosp 1975; **Fellow:** Surgical Oncology, Med Coll Virginia Affil Hosp 1977; **Fac Appt:** Assoc Prof S, SUNY Stony Brook

Vitale, Gerard F MD (S) - **Spec Exp:** Aneurysm; Carotid Artery Surgery; Varicose Veins; Arterial Bypass Surgery; **Hospital:** Glen Cove Hosp; **Address:** 10 Medical Plaza, Ste 305, Glen Cove, NY 11542; **Phone:** 516-759-5559; **Board Cert:** Surgery 1997; **Med School:** SUNY Buffalo 1982; **Resid:** Surgery, N Shore Univ Hosp 1987; **Fellow:** Vascular Surgery, St Vincents Hosp 1988

Thoracic Surgery

Andaz, Shahriyour MD (TS) - **Spec Exp:** Thoracic Cancer; Lung Cancer; **Hospital:** South Nassau Comm Hosp, Franklin Hosp; **Address:** 444 Merrick Rd, Ste 380, Lynbrook, NY 11563; **Phone:** 516-255-5010; **Board Cert:** Surgery 1999; Thoracic Surgery 2002; **Med School:** India 1983; **Resid:** Surgery, Bronx Lebanon Hosp; **Fellow:** Thoracic Surgery, SUNY Hlth Sci Ctr

Esposito, Rick A MD (TS) - **Spec Exp:** Cardiac Surgery; Coronary Artery Surgery; Mitral Valve Minimally Invasive Surgery; **Hospital:** N Shore Univ Hosp; **Address:** N Shore Univ Hospital, Dept Cardiothoracic Surgery, 300 Community Drive, Manhasset, NY 11030; **Phone:** 516-562-4970; **Board Cert:** Thoracic Surgery 2006; **Med School:** Univ Chicago-Pritzker Sch Med 1979; **Resid:** Surgery, NYU Med Ctr 1984; **Fellow:** Thoracic Surgery, NYU Med Ctr 1986; **Fac Appt:** Assoc Clin Prof S, NYU Sch Med

Fernandez, Harold A MD (TS) - **Spec Exp:** Cardiac Surgery-High Risk; Minimally Invasive Heart Valve Surgery; Ventricular Assist Device (LVAD); Atrial Fibrillation; **Hospital:** St Francis Hosp - The Heart Ctr (page 115); **Address:** 100 Port Washington Blvd, Ste G01, Roslyn, NY 11576; **Phone:** 516-627-2173; **Board Cert:** Surgery 2003; Thoracic Surgery 2005; **Med School:** Harvard Med Sch 1993; **Resid:** Surgery, NYU Med Ctr 1999; **Fellow:** Thoracic Surgery, NYU Med Ctr 2001

Fox, Stewart MD (TS) - **Spec Exp:** Minimally Invasive Thoracic Surgery; Pacemakers; Hyperhidrosis-Palmar; **Hospital:** South Nassau Comm Hosp, Mercy Med Ctr - Rockville Centre; **Address:** 444 Merrick Rd, Ste 380, Lynbrook, NY 11563-2465; **Phone:** 516-255-5010; **Board Cert:** Thoracic Surgery 2000; **Med School:** Med Coll VA 1972; **Resid:** Surgery, Yale-New Haven Hosp 1977; **Fellow:** Thoracic Surgery, MS Hershey Med Ctr 1979

Glassman, Lawrence R MD (TS) - **Spec Exp:** Lung Cancer; Esophageal Cancer; Emphysema; Tracheal Surgery; **Hospital:** N Shore Univ Hosp; **Address:** 225 Community Drive, Ste 110, GReat Neck, NY 11021; **Phone:** 516-918-4388; **Board Cert:** Thoracic Surgery 2000; **Med School:** NYU Sch Med 1981; **Resid:** Surgery, U Minnesota Hosps 1983; Surgery, NYU Med Ctr 1987; **Fellow:** Thoracic Surgery, Meml Sloan Kettering 1988; Thoracic Surgery, NYU Med Ctr 1990

Hartman, Alan R MD (TS) - **Spec Exp:** Cardiothoracic Surgery; Minimally Invasive Heart Valve Surgery; Aneurysm-Thoracic Aortic; Coronary Artery Surgery; **Hospital:** N Shore Univ Hosp, Long Island Jewish Med Ctr; **Address:** N Shore Univ Hosp, Div Cardiothoracic Surg, 300 Community Drive, Manhasset, NY 11030; **Phone:** 516-562-4970; **Board Cert:** Surgery 2004; Thoracic Surgery 2005; Surgical Critical Care 2000; **Med School:** Mount Sinai Sch Med 1979; **Resid:** Surgery, Bellevue Hosp/NYU Med Ctr 1984; **Fellow:** Cardiothoracic Surgery, Bellevue Hosp/NYU Med Ctr 1986; **Fac Appt:** Assoc Prof S, NYU Sch Med

Kline, Gary M MD (TS) - **Spec Exp:** Thoracic Surgery; Lung Cancer; Emphysema; Mediastinal Tumors; **Hospital:** Winthrop - Univ Hosp; **Address:** Summit Thoracic Institute, 410 Lakeville Rd, Ste 310, New Hyde Park, NY 11042; **Phone:** 516-233-1952; **Board Cert:** Surgery 2004; Thoracic Surgery 2005; **Med School:** Wayne State Univ 1986; **Resid:** Surgery, Detroit Med Ctr 1991; **Fellow:** Thoracic Surgery, Hosp Univ Penn 1994; **Fac Appt:** Asst Prof S, Albert Einstein Coll Med

Robinson, Newell B MD (TS) - **Spec Exp:** Minimally Invasive Cardiac Surgery; Maze Procedure for Atrial Fibrillation; **Hospital:** St Francis Hosp - The Heart Ctr (page 115); **Address:** 100 Port Washington Blvd, Vizza Bldg - rm G-01, Roslyn, NY 11576; **Phone:** 516-627-2173; **Board Cert:** Surgery 2005; Thoracic Surgery 2006; **Med School:** Univ Miss 1973; **Resid:** Surgery, NY-Cornell Med Ctr 1984; Surgery, Meml Sloan Kettering Cancer Ctr 1984; **Fellow:** Trauma, Univ Washington Med Ctr 1981; Cardiothoracic Surgery, NY-Cornell Med Ctr 1986

Saha, Chanchal MD (TS) - **Spec Exp:** Lung Cancer; Pacemakers; Esophageal Cancer; Mediastinal Tumors; **Hospital:** Plainview Hosp, St Joseph's Hosp-Nassau; **Address:** 754 Old Country Rd, Plainview, NY 11803; **Phone:** 516-931-0182; **Board Cert:** Thoracic Surgery 2000; **Med School:** India 1964; **Resid:** Surgery, Hosp for Joint Diseases 1973; Thoracic Surgery, Mt Sinai Hosp 1976; **Fellow:** Cardiothoracic Surgery, Mt Sinai Hosp 1977; **Fac Appt:** Assoc Prof S, Cornell Univ-Weill Med Coll

Schubach, Scott L MD (TS) - **Spec Exp:** Cardiac Surgery; Coronary Artery Surgery; Heart Valve Surgery; Minimally Invasive Surgery; **Hospital:** Winthrop - Univ Hosp; **Address:** 120 Mineola Blvd, Ste 300, Mineola, NY 11501; **Phone:** 516-663-4400; **Board Cert:** Surgery 2007; Thoracic Surgery 2000; Surgical Critical Care 2000; **Med School:** Baylor Coll Med 1983; **Resid:** Surgery, Dartmouth Hitchcock Med Ctr Ctr. 1988; Cardiothoracic Surgery, Univ of Pittsburgh Med Ctr 1991

Taylor Jr, James R MD (TS) - **Spec Exp:** Thoracic Aortic Surgery; Aneurysm-Aortic; **Hospital:** St Francis Hosp - The Heart Ctr (page 115); **Address:** St Francis Hospital-The Heart Center, 100 Port Washington Blvd, Ste GO1, Roslyn, NY 11576; **Phone:** 516-627-2173; **Board Cert:** Surgery 2008; Thoracic Surgery 2001; **Med School:** Med Univ SC 1984; **Resid:** Surgery, NY Hosp-Cornell Med Ctr 1989; **Fellow:** Cardiothoracic Surgery, NY Hosp-Cornell Med Ctr 1991

Zeltsman, Vadim MD (TS) - **Spec Exp:** Thoracic Cancers; Video Assisted Thoracic Surgery (VATS); **Hospital:** Long Island Jewish Med Ctr, N Shore Univ Hosp; **Address:** 225 Community Drive, Ste 110, Great Neck, NY 11040; **Phone:** 516-918-4388; **Board Cert:** Surgery 1999; Thoracic Surgery 2002; **Med School:** Russia 1986; **Resid:** Surgery, Mercy Catholic Med Ctr 1997; **Fellow:** Cardiothoracic Surgery, UMDNJ Affil Hosp 2000; Cardiothoracic Surgery, Univ Pennsylvania 2001

Urology

Ashley, Richard N MD (U) - **Hospital:** N Shore Univ Hosp; **Address:** 233 7th St, Ste 203, Garden City, NY 11530; **Phone:** 516-294-7666; **Board Cert:** Urology 1980; **Med School:** NY Med Coll 1972; **Resid:** Surgery, St Vincents Hosp 1975; Urology, SUNY Downstate 1978; **Fac Appt:** Asst Clin Prof U, SUNY Stony Brook

Bruno, Anthony MD (U) - **Spec Exp:** Prostate Cancer; Kidney Stones; Voiding Dysfunction; **Hospital:** Winthrop - Univ Hosp; **Address:** 1305 Franklin Ave, Ste 100, Garden City, NY 11530; **Phone:** 516-746-5550; **Board Cert:** Urology 1977; **Med School:** Italy 1968; **Resid:** Surgery, Nassau Hosp 1972; Urology, Bellevue Hosp Ctr 1975; **Fac Appt:** Asst Prof U, SUNY Stony Brook

Girardi, Sarah K MD (U) - **Spec Exp:** Infertility-Male; Incontinence-Female; **Hospital:** N Shore Univ Hosp, St Francis Hosp - The Heart Ctr (page 115); **Address:** 535 Plandome Rd, Manhasset, NY 11030; **Phone:** 516-627-6188; **Board Cert:** Urology 2006; **Med School:** Univ NC Sch Med 1989; **Resid:** Urology, Cornell Univ Med Ctr 1995; **Fellow:** Urology, Yale Univ 1996

Hanna, Moneer K MD (U) - **Spec Exp:** Pediatric Urology; Hydronephrosis; Hypospadias; Bladder Surgery; **Hospital:** Steven & Alexandra Cohen Chldn's Med Ctr of NY, NY-Presby Hosp/Weill Cornell (page 104); **Address:** 935 Northern Blvd, Ste 303, Great Neck, NY 11021; **Phone:** 516-466-6950; **Board Cert:** Urology 1978; **Med School:** Egypt 1963; **Resid:** Urology, Univ Affiliated Hosp 1972; Urology, Univ West Ont Affil Hosps 1976; **Fellow:** Pediatric Urology, Hosp For Sick Chldn 1975; **Fac Appt:** Clin Prof U, Cornell Univ-Weill Med Coll

Harris, Steven M MD (U) - **Spec Exp:** Impotence; Prostate Disease; Kidney Stones; **Hospital:** Long Beach Med Ctr, South Nassau Comm Hosp; **Address:** 309 W Park Ave, Ste 5, Long Beach, NY 11561-3241; **Phone:** 516-431-9800; **Board Cert:** Urology 1984; **Med School:** Albert Einstein Coll Med 1976; **Resid:** Urology, Mount Sinai Med Ctr 1981; **Fac Appt:** Asst Prof U, NY Coll Osteo Med

Kavoussi, Louis R MD (U) - **Spec Exp:** Laparoscopic Surgery; Urologic Cancer; Prostate Cancer; Kidney Cancer; **Hospital:** Long Island Jewish Med Ctr, N Shore Univ Hosp; **Address:** 450 Lakeville Rd, Ste M-41, New Hyde Park, NY 11040; **Phone:** 516-734-8558; **Board Cert:** Urology 2009; **Med School:** SUNY Buffalo 1983; **Resid:** Surgery, Barnes Jewish Hosp 1985; Urology, Barnes Jewish Hosp 1989; **Fac Appt:** Prof U, NYU Sch Med

Layne, Jeffrey MD (U) - **Spec Exp:** Kidney Stones; Incontinence; Impotence; **Hospital:** Plainview Hosp, Syosset Hosp; **Address:** 1181 Old Country Rd, Ste 1, Plainview, NY 11803-5018; **Phone:** 516-933-6060; **Board Cert:** Urology 2007; **Med School:** SUNY Stony Brook 1989; **Resid:** Surgery, New England Med Ctr 1991; Urology, New England Med Ctr 1995

Leventhal, Arnold MD (U) - **Spec Exp:** Prostate Cancer; Kidney Stones; **Hospital:** Franklin Hosp; **Address:** 1800 Rockaway Ave, Ste 212, Hewlett, NY 11557-1677; **Phone:** 516-593-1838; **Board Cert:** Urology 2000; **Med School:** NYU Sch Med 1984; **Resid:** Surgery, Bellevue Hosp 1986; Urology, Bellevue Hosp 1990

Lieberman, Elliott MD (U) - **Spec Exp:** Urologic Cancer; Interstitial Cystitis; Prostate Disease; **Hospital:** Plainview Hosp; **Address:** 875 Old Country Road Rd, Ste 301, Plainview, NY 11803-4934; **Phone:** 516-931-1710; **Board Cert:** Urology 1983; **Med School:** SUNY Downstate 1976; **Resid:** Surgery, Mount Sinai 1978; Urology, SUNY-Downstate 1981

Mellinger, Brett MD (U) - **Spec Exp:** Infertility-Male; Impotence; Peyronie's Disease; Andrology; **Hospital:** Winthrop - Univ Hosp, N Shore Univ Hosp; **Address:** Mellinger Urology, 100 Garden City Plaza, Ste 101, Garden City, NY 11530; **Phone:** 516-873-5353; **Board Cert:** Urology 1999; **Med School:** Indiana Univ 1981; **Resid:** Urology, Downstate Med Ctr 1985; Urology, New York Hosp-Cornell 1986; **Fellow:** Male Infertility, New York Hosp-Cornell 1988; **Fac Appt:** Assoc Clin Prof U, SUNY Stony Brook

Moldwin, Robert MD (U) - **Spec Exp:** Interstitial Cystitis; Prostate Benign Disease; Urinary Tract Infections; **Hospital:** NS-LIJ Hlth Sys; **Address:** 450 Lakeville Rd, Ste M41, New Hyde Park, NY 11040-1433; **Phone:** 516-734-8500; **Board Cert:** Urology 2003; **Med School:** Univ Chicago-Pritzker Sch Med 1984; **Resid:** Urology, LI Jewish Med Ctr 1990; **Fellow:** Infectious Disease, Thomas Jefferson Univ Hosp 1991; **Fac Appt:** Assoc Clin Prof U, Albert Einstein Coll Med

Shepard, Barry R MD (U) - **Spec Exp:** Kidney Stones; Urologic Cancer; **Hospital:** Winthrop - Univ Hosp, N Shore Univ Hosp; **Address:** 601 Franklin Ave, Ste 300, Garden City, NY 11530; **Phone:** 516-742-3200; **Board Cert:** Urology 2006; **Med School:** SUNY Downstate 1979; **Resid:** Surgery, LIJ Med Ctr 1981; Urology, Columbia-Presby Med Ctr 1984

Sunshine, Robert D MD (U) - **Spec Exp:** Vasectomy-Scalpelless; Prostate Disease; **Hospital:** St Joseph's Hosp-Nassau, Plainview Hosp; **Address:** 4230 Hempstead Tpke, Ste 200, Bethpage, NY 11714-5700; **Phone:** 516-796-2222; **Board Cert:** Urology 2005; **Med School:** Mexico 1977; **Resid:** Surgery, Long Island Jewish Hosp 1981; Urology, Mount Sinai Med Ctr 1985

Ziegelbaum, Michael M MD (U) - **Spec Exp:** Incontinence-Male & Female; Prostate Disease; Laparoscopic Surgery; Kidney Stones; **Hospital:** Long Island Jewish Med Ctr, St Francis Hosp - The Heart Ctr (page 115); **Address:** 2001 Marcus Ave, Lake Success, NY 11042; **Phone:** 516-437-4228; **Board Cert:** Urology 2009; **Med School:** Cornell Univ-Weill Med Coll 1982; **Resid:** Urology, Cleveland Clinic 1988; **Fellow:** Stone Disease, Univ Hosp 1989; **Fac Appt:** Asst Clin Prof S, Albert Einstein Coll Med

Vascular & Interventional Radiology

Crystal, Kenneth MD (VIR) - **Spec Exp:** Interventional Radiology; Angioplasty; Uterine Fibroid Embolization; **Hospital:** St Francis Hosp - The Heart Ctr (page 115); **Address:** 100 Port Washington Blvd, Roslyn, NY 11576; **Phone:** 516-562-6509; **Board Cert:** Diagnostic Radiology 1986; **Med School:** Univ Rochester 1981; **Resid:** Internal Medicine, Beth Israel Med Ctr 1982; Diagnostic Radiology, NYU Med Ctr 1986; **Fellow:** Vascular & Interventional Radiology, NYU Med Ctr 1986; **Fac Appt:** Asst Prof Rad, NYU Sch Med

Vascular Surgery

Chaudhry, Saqib S MD (VascS) - **Spec Exp:** Aneurysm-Aortic; Carotid Artery Surgery; Dialysis Access Surgery; Limb Sparing Surgery; **Hospital:** Forest Hills Hosp, N Shore Univ Hosp; **Address:** 2001 Marcus Ave, Ste South, Box 50, Lake Success, NY 11042; **Phone:** 516-328-9800; **Board Cert:** Thoracic Surgery 2000; Vascular Surgery 2009; **Med School:** Iraq 1972; **Resid:** Surgery, Flushing Hosp 1974; Thoracic Surgery, Wayne State Univ 1980

Faust, Glenn MD (VascS) - **Spec Exp:** Carotid Artery Surgery; Diabetic Leg/Foot; Aneurysm-Abdominal Aortic; Vein Disorders; **Hospital:** Nassau Univ Med Ctr; **Address:** 2201 Hempstead Tpke, East Meadow, NY 11554; **Phone:** 516-572-4848; **Board Cert:** Vascular Surgery 2004; **Med School:** Yale Univ 1986; **Resid:** Surgery, LI Jewish Med Ctr 1991; **Fellow:** Vascular Surgery, LI Jewish Med Ctr 1992; **Fac Appt:** Asst Prof S, Albert Einstein Coll Med

Purtill, William A MD (VascS) - **Spec Exp:** Carotid Artery Surgery; Endovascular Surgery; Lower Limb Arterial Disease; Aneurysm-Aortic; **Hospital:** N Shore Univ Hosp, St Francis Hosp - The Heart Ctr (page 115); **Address:** 900 Northern Blvd, Ste 140, Great Neck, NY 11021; **Phone:** 516-466-0485; **Board Cert:** Surgery 2007; Vascular Surgery 2007; **Med School:** Ireland 1989; **Resid:** Surgery, SUNY Stony Brook Med Ctr 1996; Surgery, John Hopkins Hosp 1993; **Fellow:** Vascular Surgery, Univ Maryland Med Ctr 1997; **Fac Appt:** Asst Prof S, SUNY Stony Brook

Rockland

Rockland

Allergy & Immunology

Bosso, John MD (A&I) - **Spec Exp:** Asthma; Contact Dermatitis; Food Allergy; Drug Sensitivity; **Hospital:** Nyack Hosp, Valley Hosp (page 658); **Address:** 2 Crossfield Ave, Ste 406, West Nyack, NY 10994-2212; **Phone:** 845-353-9600; **Board Cert:** Internal Medicine 1988; Allergy & Immunology 2001; **Med School:** SUNY Buffalo 1985; **Resid:** Internal Medicine, Staten Island Univ Hosp 1988; **Fellow:** Allergy & Immunology, Scripps Clinic Reseach Fdn 1990

Lo Galbo, Peter MD (A&I) - **Spec Exp:** Asthma; Food Allergy; **Hospital:** Nyack Hosp, Good Samaritan Hosp - Suffern; **Address:** 1 Crossfield Ave, Ste 201, West Nyack, NY 10994; **Phone:** 845-727-1370; **Board Cert:** Pediatrics 1983; Allergy & Immunology 1983; Pediatric Rheumatology 2002; **Med School:** SUNY Stony Brook 1978; **Resid:** Pediatrics, Mount Sinai Med Ctr 1980; **Fellow:** Allergy & Immunology, Duke Univ Med Ctr 1982; **Fac Appt:** Asst Clin Prof Ped, Albert Einstein Coll Med

Cardiovascular Disease

Beniaminovitz, Ainat MD (Cv) - **Spec Exp:** Heart Failure; **Hospital:** Good Samaritan Hosp - Suffern; **Address:** Hudson Heart Associates, 222 Rte 59, Ste 302, Suffern, NY 10901; **Phone:** 845-368-0100; **Board Cert:** Internal Medicine 2003; Cardiovascular Disease 1997; **Med School:** Columbia P&S 1990; **Resid:** Internal Medicine, CPMC/Columbia Presby Hosp 1994; **Fellow:** Cardiovascular Disease, CPMC/Columbia Presby Hosp 1997

Roth, Richard MD (Cv) - **Spec Exp:** Cholesterol/Lipid Disorders; Non-Invasive Cardiology; **Hospital:** Good Samaritan Hosp - Suffern, Nyack Hosp; **Address:** 222 Route 59, Ste 302, Suffern, NY 10901; **Phone:** 845-368-0100; **Board Cert:** Internal Medicine 1978; Cardiovascular Disease 1981; **Med School:** Yale Univ 1975; **Resid:** Internal Medicine, Boston Med Ctr 1978; **Fellow:** Cardiovascular Disease, Boston Med Ctr 1980; **Fac Appt:** Asst Clin Prof Med, Columbia P&S

Southren, David MD (Cv) - **Spec Exp:** Cholesterol/Lipid Disorders; Non-Invasive Cardiology; Preventive Cardiology; **Hospital:** Nyack Hosp, Englewood Hosp & Med Ctr (page 656); **Address:** Cardiovascular Care Ctr, 206 Route 303, Valley Cottage, NY 10989-2019; **Phone:** 845-268-0880; **Board Cert:** Internal Medicine 1984; Cardiovascular Disease 1987; **Med School:** NY Med Coll 1981; **Resid:** Internal Medicine, Barnes Jewish Hosp 1984; **Fellow:** Cardiovascular Disease, Emory Univ Hosp 1985; Cardiovascular Disease, Westchester Med Ctr 1986

Colon & Rectal Surgery

Ozuner, Gokhan MD (CRS) - **Spec Exp:** Inflammatory Bowel Disease; Colon & Rectal Cancer; Rectal Prolapse; Laparoscopic Surgery; **Hospital:** Good Samaritan Hosp - Suffern, Nyack Hosp; **Address:** 100 Route 59, Ste 101, Suffern, NY 10901; **Phone:** 845-357-8800; **Board Cert:** Surgery 2002; Colon & Rectal Surgery 2006; **Med School:** Turkey 1984; **Resid:** Surgery, Staten Island Univ Hosp 1993; **Fellow:** Colon & Rectal Surgery, Cleveland Clin Fdn 1995

Dermatology

Waldorf, Donald MD (D) - **Spec Exp:** Skin Cancer; Acne; Psoriasis; Cosmetic Dermatology; **Hospital:** Rockland Psych Ctr; **Address:** 57 N Middletown Rd, Nanuet, NY 10954-2312; **Phone:** 845-623-7077; **Board Cert:** Dermatology 1967; **Med School:** Univ Pennsylvania 1962; **Resid:** Dermatology, Hosp Univ Penn 1964; Dermatology, NYU Medical Center 1967; **Fellow:** Dermatology, Natl Cancer Inst 1966

Waldorf, Heidi A MD (D) - **Spec Exp:** Cosmetic Dermatology; Skin Laser Surgery; Skin Cancer; Mohs' Surgery; **Hospital:** Mount Sinai Med Ctr (page 102); **Address:** 57 N Middletown Rd, Nanuet, NY 10954; **Phone:** 845-623-7077; **Board Cert:** Dermatology 2001; **Med School:** Univ Pennsylvania 1990; **Resid:** Internal Medicine, Hosp Univ Penn 1991; Dermatology, Mass Genl Hosp 1994; **Fellow:** Mohs Surgery, Laser & Skin Surg Ctr 1995; **Fac Appt:** Assoc Clin Prof D, Mount Sinai Sch Med

Diagnostic Radiology

Bobroff, Lewis M MD (DR) - **Spec Exp:** Mammography; Nuclear Medicine; PET Imaging; **Hospital:** Good Samaritan Hosp - Suffern; **Address:** 255 Lafayette Ave, Dept Radiology, Suffern, NY 10901-5103; **Phone:** 845-368-5196; **Board Cert:** Diagnostic Radiology 1974; **Med School:** Harvard Med Sch 1969; **Resid:** Diagnostic Radiology, Montefiore Hosp Med Ctr 1973; **Fellow:** Interventional Radiology, Montefiore Hosp Med Ctr 1973

Geller, Mark E MD (DR) - **Spec Exp:** MRI; Ultrasound; Nuclear Medicine; **Hospital:** Nyack Hosp; **Address:** 18 Squadron Blvd, New City, NY 10956; **Phone:** 845-634-9729; **Board Cert:** Diagnostic Radiology 1989; **Med School:** SUNY Downstate 1985; **Resid:** Diagnostic Radiology, Westchester Co Med Ctr 1989; **Fac Appt:** Asst Clin Prof Rad, NY Med Coll

Endocrinology, Diabetes & Metabolism

Cosman, Felicia MD (EDM) - **Spec Exp:** Osteoporosis; Bone Densitometry; **Hospital:** Helen Hayes Hosp, NY-Presby Hosp/Columbia (page 104); **Address:** Helen Hayes Hosp, Reg Bone Ctr, Route 9W, West Haverstraw, NY 10993-1195; **Phone:** 845-786-4318; **Board Cert:** Internal Medicine 1986; Endocrinology, Diabetes & Metabolism 1989; **Med School:** SUNY Stony Brook 1983; **Resid:** Internal Medicine, Columbia Presby Med Ctr 1986; **Fellow:** Endocrinology, Columbia Presby Med Ctr 1988; **Fac Appt:** Prof Med, Columbia P&S

Family Medicine

Ibelli, Vincent MD (FMed) *PCP* - **Spec Exp:** Asthma; Hypertension; Osteoporosis; Gastroesophageal Reflux Disease (GERD); **Hospital:** Nyack Hosp; **Address:** 97 Route 303, Tappan, NY 10983-2514; **Phone:** 845-359-5005; **Board Cert:** Family Medicine 2007; **Med School:** Italy 1983; **Resid:** Family Medicine, JFK Med Ctr 1986

Ingrassia, Joseph T MD (FMed) *PCP* - **Hospital:** Good Samaritan Hosp - Suffern, Nyack Hosp; **Address:** 36 College Ave, Nanuet, NY 10954-3093; **Phone:** 845-623-2456; **Board Cert:** Family Medicine 2003; **Med School:** Mexico 1974; **Resid:** Family Medicine, Nassau Co Hosp 1978

Gastroenterology

May, Louis MD (Ge) - **Spec Exp:** Hepatitis; Endoscopy; Pancreatic/Biliary Endoscopy (ERCP); **Hospital:** Good Samaritan Hosp - Suffern, Nyack Hosp; **Address:** 500 New Hempstead Rd, New City, NY 10956; **Phone:** 845-362-3200; **Board Cert:** Internal Medicine 1981; Gastroenterology 1983; **Med School:** Univ Miami Sch Med 1978; **Resid:** Internal Medicine, Univ Utah Med Ctr 1981; **Fellow:** Gastroenterology, Univ Utah Med Ctr 1983

Internal Medicine

Glassman, Charles F MD (IM) *PCP* - **Spec Exp:** Concierge Medicine; Preventive Medicine; Complementary Medicine; **Hospital:** Good Samaritan Hosp - Suffern, Nyack Hosp; **Address:** 7 Medical Park Drive, Ste C, Pomona, NY 10970; **Phone:** 845-362-1110; **Board Cert:** Internal Medicine 1989; **Med School:** NY Med Coll 1985; **Resid:** Internal Medicine, Westchester Co Med Ctr 1988; **Fac Appt:** Asst Clin Prof Med, NY Med Coll

Handelsman, Richard E DO (IM) - **Spec Exp:** Concierge Medicine; Preventive Medicine; **Hospital:** Nyack Hosp, Good Samaritan Hosp - Suffern; **Address:** 7 Medical Park Drive, Ste C, Pomona, NY 10970-3562; **Phone:** 845-362-1169; **Board Cert:** Internal Medicine 1981; **Med School:** Univ Osteo Med & Hlth Sci, Des Moines 1976; **Resid:** Internal Medicine, UMDNJ Med Ctr 1978; Internal Medicine, Norwalk Hosp 1980; **Fac Appt:** Asst Clin Prof Med, NY Med Coll

Leahy, Mary MD (IM) *PCP* - **Spec Exp:** Preventive Medicine; **Hospital:** Nyack Hosp, Good Samaritan Hosp - Suffern; **Address:** 2 Crossfield Ave, Ste 318, West Nyack, NY 10994; **Phone:** 845-353-5600; **Board Cert:** Internal Medicine 1988; **Med School:** Italy 1983; **Resid:** Internal Medicine, Misericordia Hosp 1986; **Fellow:** Nephrology, Westchester Co Med Ctr 1988

Interventional Cardiology

Innerfield, Michael MD (IC) - **Spec Exp:** Coronary Artery Disease; Preventive Cardiology; **Hospital:** Hackensack Univ Med Ctr (page 96), Good Samaritan Hosp - Suffern; **Address:** 2 Executive Blvd, Ste 406, Suffern, NY 10901; **Phone:** 845-368-0048; **Board Cert:** Internal Medicine 1984; Cardiovascular Disease 1987; Interventional Cardiology 1999; Nuclear Cardiology 2008; **Med School:** NY Med Coll 1981; **Resid:** Internal Medicine, Bronx Muni Hosp 1984; **Fellow:** Cardiovascular Disease, Montefiore Hosp Med Ctr 1986; Cardiovascular Disease, Cooper Hosp 1987; **Fac Appt:** Asst Prof S, Mount Sinai Sch Med

Medical Oncology

Goldberg, Robert MD (Onc) - **Spec Exp:** Brain Tumors; **Hospital:** Good Samaritan Hosp - Suffern, Nyack Hosp; **Address:** 10 Esquire Rd, Ste 6, New City, NY 10956; **Phone:** 845-634-2727; **Board Cert:** Internal Medicine 1982; Medical Oncology 1985; Hematology 1984; **Med School:** Mount Sinai Sch Med 1979; **Resid:** Internal Medicine, Beth Israel Med Ctr 1982; **Fellow:** Hematology & Oncology, Univ Minnesota Hosp 1985

Lonberg, Mathew MD (Onc) - **Spec Exp:** Lung Cancer; Breast Cancer; Lymphoma; Melanoma; **Hospital:** Nyack Hosp, NY-Presby Hosp/Columbia (page 104); **Address:** 255 5th Ave, Nyack, NY 10960; **Phone:** 845-362-1750; **Board Cert:** Internal Medicine 1984; Medical Oncology 1987; Hematology 1988; **Med School:** Univ VA Sch Med 1981; **Resid:** Internal Medicine, Bellevue Hosp Ctr 1982; **Fellow:** Hematology & Oncology, Meml Sloan-Kettering Cancer Ctr 1985; **Fac Appt:** Asst Clin Prof Med, Columbia P&S

Zimmerman, Marc MD (Onc) - **Hospital:** Nyack Hosp, Good Samaritan Hosp - Suffern; **Address:** 974 Rte 45, Ste 1200, Pomonoa, NY 10970; **Phone:** 845-362-3970; **Board Cert:** Internal Medicine 1980; Medical Oncology 1981; Hematology 1984; **Med School:** Albany Med Coll 1977; **Resid:** Internal Medicine, Albany Med Ctr 1979; **Fellow:** Medical Oncology, Albany Med Ctr 1982

Neonatal-Perinatal Medicine

Mendoza, Glenn MD (NP) - **Hospital:** Good Samaritan Hosp - Suffern, Children's & Women's Phys.of Westchester; **Address:** Good Samaritan Hosp, Dept Neonatology, 255 Lafayette Ave, Suffern, NY 10901; **Phone:** 845-368-5104; **Board Cert:** Pediatrics 1985; **Med School:** Philippines 1976; **Resid:** Family Medicine, Elyria Meml Hosp 1980; Pediatrics, Brooklyn Jewish Hosp & Med Ctr 1983; **Fellow:** Neonatal-Perinatal Medicine, Mt Sinai Hosp 1985; **Fac Appt:** Asst Prof Ped, Columbia P&S

Nephrology

Kozin, Arthur MD (Nep) - **Spec Exp:** Hypertension; Kidney Failure-Chronic; Diabetic Kidney Disease; **Hospital:** Nyack Hosp, Good Samaritan Hosp - Suffern; **Address:** 2 Crossfield Ave, Ste 312, West Nyack, NY 10994-2212; **Phone:** 845-358-2400; **Board Cert:** Internal Medicine 1985; Nephrology 1988; Critical Care Medicine 2002; **Med School:** Albert Einstein Coll Med 1982; **Resid:** Internal Medicine, Montefiore Hosp Med Ctr 1985; **Fellow:** Nephrology, Bellevue Hosp 1987

Shapiro, Kenneth S MD (Nep) - **Spec Exp:** Hypertension; Kidney Disease-Diabetic; Transplant Medicine-Kidney; **Hospital:** Nyack Hosp, Good Samaritan Hosp - Suffern; **Address:** 2 Crossfield Ave, Ste 312, West Nyack, NY 10994-2220; **Phone:** 845-358-2400; **Board Cert:** Internal Medicine 1978; Nephrology 1980; **Med School:** Rush Med Coll 1975; **Resid:** Internal Medicine, Albany Meml Hosp 1978; **Fellow:** Nephrology, New England Med Ctr 1980; **Fac Appt:** Asst Clin Prof Med, NY Med Coll

Yablon, Steven MD (Nep) - **Spec Exp:** Hypertension; Kidney Failure; Dialysis Care; **Hospital:** Nyack Hosp, Good Samaritan Hosp - Suffern; **Address:** 2 Crosfield Ave, Ste 312, West Nyack, NY 10994-2220; **Phone:** 845-358-2400; **Board Cert:** Internal Medicine 1976; Nephrology 1978; **Med School:** UMDNJ-NJ Med Sch, Newark 1973; **Resid:** Internal Medicine, Tufts New England Med Ctr 1975; **Fellow:** Nephrology, Hosp Univ Penn 1977

Neurological Surgery

Oppenheim, Jeffrey MD (NS) - **Spec Exp:** Spinal Disorders-Degenerative; Brain Tumors; Spinal Surgery; Microsurgery; **Hospital:** Nyack Hosp, Good Samaritan Hosp - Suffern; **Address:** Hudson Valley Neurosurgical Assocs, 222 Route 59, Ste 205, Suffern, NY 10901-5206; **Phone:** 845-368-0286; **Board Cert:** Neurological Surgery 1996; **Med School:** Cornell Univ-Weill Med Coll 1988; **Resid:** Neurological Surgery, Mount Sinai Hosp 1994

Spitzer, Daniel MD (NS) - **Spec Exp:** Brain Tumors; Spinal Surgery; Stereotactic Radiosurgery; **Hospital:** Nyack Hosp, Good Samaritan Hosp - Suffern; **Address:** 222 Route 59, Ste 205, Suffern, NY 10901-5206; **Phone:** 845-368-0286; **Board Cert:** Neurological Surgery 1992; **Med School:** NYU Sch Med 1983; **Resid:** Neurological Surgery, Montefiore Med Ctr 1989; **Fac Appt:** Asst Clin Prof NS, Columbia P&S

Neurology

Ober, David T MD (N) - **Spec Exp:** Neuromuscular Disorders; Botox Therapy; **Hospital:** Nyack Hosp; **Address:** 2 Crossfield Ave, Ste 202, West Nyack, NY 10994; **Phone:** 845-353-4344; **Board Cert:** Neurology 2009; Electrodiagnostic Medicine 2001; **Med School:** Albany Med Coll 1994; **Resid:** Neurology, Mt Sinai Hosp 1998; **Fellow:** Neurological Physiology, St Elizabeth's Med Ctr 1999

Seliger, Glenn MD (N) - **Spec Exp:** Brain Injury; **Hospital:** Helen Hayes Hosp; **Address:** Helen Hayes Hospital, Dept Neurology, Route 9W, West Haverstraw, NY 10993; **Phone:** 845-786-4459; **Board Cert:** Neurology 1988; **Med School:** SUNY Downstate 1983; **Resid:** Neurology, Neurological Inst 1987; **Fellow:** Neurological Rehabilitation, Braintree Hosp 1988; **Fac Appt:** Assoc Clin Prof N, Columbia P&S

Neuroradiology

Schwartz, Joel M MD (NRad) - **Spec Exp:** Head & Neck Imaging; **Hospital:** Nyack Hosp; **Address:** 18 Squaron Blvd, New City, NY 10956; **Phone:** 845-634-9729; **Board Cert:** Diagnostic Radiology 1990; Neuroradiology 2006; **Med School:** SUNY Upstate Med Univ 1985; **Resid:** Diagnostic Radiology, NYU Med Ctr 1990; **Fellow:** Neuroradiology, NYU Med Ctr 1991

Ophthalmology

Weingarten, Phyllis MD (Oph) - **Spec Exp:** Pediatric Ophthalmology; Strabismus; **Hospital:** Good Samaritan Hosp - Suffern, Beth Israel Med Ctr - Petrie Division (page 94); **Address:** 4A Medical Park Drive, Pomona, NY 10970-3516; **Phone:** 845-354-6225; **Board Cert:** Ophthalmology 1991; **Med School:** NY Med Coll 1986; **Resid:** Ophthalmology, Brookdale Hosp Med Ctr 1990; **Fellow:** Strabismus, Downstate Med Ctr 1991; Pediatric Ophthalmology, Johns Hopkins Hosp 1992

Orthopaedic Surgery

Austin, Kenneth S MD (OrS) - **Spec Exp:** Shoulder Injuries; Knee Injuries; Sports Medicine; **Hospital:** Good Samaritan Hosp - Suffern; **Address:** Rockland Orthopaedics & Sports Med, 327 Route 59, Airmont, NY 10952; **Phone:** 845-356-2900; **Board Cert:** Orthopaedic Surgery 2007; **Med School:** NYU Sch Med 1988; **Resid:** Orthopaedic Surgery, Bellvue Hosp-NYU Sch Med 1993; **Fellow:** Sports Medicine, Mass Genl Hosp 1994

Kraushaar, Barry S MD (OrS) - **Spec Exp:** Shoulder Arthroscopic Surgery; Rotator Cuff Surgery; Hip & Knee Replacement; Knee Injuries/Ligament Surgery; **Hospital:** Nyack Hosp, Good Samaritan Hosp - Suffern; **Address:** 2 Perlman Drive, Ste 204, Spring Valley, NY 10977; **Phone:** 845-425-0555; **Board Cert:** Orthopaedic Surgery 2009; Orthopaedic Sports Medicine 2007; **Med School:** Albert Einstein Coll Med 1990; **Resid:** Orthopaedic Surgery, Bronx Lebanon Hosp 1995; **Fellow:** Sports Medicine, Arlington Hosp/Georgetown Univ 1996

Medici, Mark MD (OrS) - **Spec Exp:** Sports Medicine; Joint Replacement; Trauma; **Hospital:** Nyack Hosp, Good Samaritan Hosp - Suffern; **Address:** 2 Crosfield Ave, Ste 422, West Nyack, NY 10994; **Phone:** 845-358-1000; **Board Cert:** Orthopaedic Surgery 2001; **Med School:** NY Med Coll 1993; **Resid:** Orthopaedic Surgery, NY Med Coll 1995; Orthopaedic Surgery, Montefiore Med Ctr 1998; **Fellow:** Sports Medicine, Staten Is Ortho & Sports Med 1999

Rubin, Cheryl J MD (OrS) - **Spec Exp:** Shoulder Arthroscopic Surgery; Knee Surgery; **Hospital:** Good Samaritan Hosp - Suffern; **Address:** 327 Route 59, Rockland Orthopedic, Airmont, NY 10901-5204; **Phone:** 845-356-2900; **Board Cert:** Orthopaedic Surgery 2003; **Med School:** Mount Sinai Sch Med 1983; **Resid:** Orthopaedic Surgery, Montefiore Med Ctr 1988; **Fellow:** Arthroscopic Surgery, Ortho Research Of Virginia

Pain Medicine

Burns, Paul MD (PM) - **Hospital:** Good Samaritan Hosp - Suffern; **Address:** Ramapo Anesthesiologists, 133 Lafayette Ave, Suffern, NY 10901-5614; **Phone:** 845-368-5000 x5039; **Board Cert:** Anesthesiology 1984; Pain Medicine 2007; **Med School:** SUNY Buffalo 1978; **Resid:** Anesthesiology, NY Hosp 1981

Pediatrics

Bernstein, William H MD (Ped) *PCP* - **Hospital:** Nyack Hosp; **Address:** 67 N Main St, New City, NY 10956; **Phone:** 845-634-8911; **Board Cert:** Pediatrics 1966; **Med School:** Vanderbilt Univ 1960; **Resid:** Pediatrics, Bellevue Hosp 1962; Pediatrics, Mt Sinai Hosp 1965; **Fellow:** Neonatology, Mt Sinai Hosp 1966

Diamant, Esther MD (Ped) *PCP* - ; **Address:** Refauh Hlth Ctr, 728 N Main St, Spring Valley, NY 10977-1960; **Phone:** 845-354-9300; **Board Cert:** Pediatrics 2005; **Med School:** Mount Sinai Sch Med 1987; **Resid:** Pediatrics, Mt Sinai Hosp 1991; **Fellow:** Pediatrics, Mt Sinai Hosp 1993

Puder, Douglas R MD (Ped) *PCP* - **Spec Exp:** Asthma; Developmental Disorders; **Hospital:** Nyack Hosp; **Address:** 35 Smith St, Nanuet, NY 10954; **Phone:** 845-623-7100; **Board Cert:** Pediatrics 1987; **Med School:** NYU Sch Med 1982; **Resid:** Pediatrics, NYU/Bellevue Hosp 1985; **Fellow:** Ambulatory Pediatrics, NYU Med Ctr 1987; **Fac Appt:** Assoc Clin Prof Ped, Columbia P&S

Siegal, Elliot MD (Ped) *PCP* - **Spec Exp:** Thyroid Disorders; Growth Disorders; Diabetes; **Hospital:** Nyack Hosp; **Address:** Clarkstown Pediatrics, 200 E Eckerson Rd, New City, NY 10956-7169; **Phone:** 845-352-5511; **Board Cert:** Pediatrics 1973; Pediatric Endocrinology 1978; **Med School:** Univ Pennsylvania 1968; **Resid:** Pediatrics, NY Hosp 1971; **Fellow:** Pediatric Endocrinology, NY Hosp 1972

Physical Medicine & Rehabilitation

Brief, Rochelle MD (PMR) - **Spec Exp:** Electrodiagnosis; **Hospital:** Nyack Hosp; **Address:** 175 Route 304, Bardonia, NY 10954-2042; **Phone:** 845-623-7949; **Board Cert:** Physical Medicine & Rehabilitation 2003; **Med School:** Albert Einstein Coll Med 1987; **Resid:** Physical Medicine & Rehabilitation, Montefiore Med Ctr 1992

Guarracini, Mary MD (PMR) - **Spec Exp:** Pain Management; **Hospital:** Helen Hayes Hosp; **Address:** Helen Hayes Hosp, Route 9W, West Haverstraw, NY 10993; **Phone:** 845-786-4410; **Board Cert:** Physical Medicine & Rehabilitation 1986; **Med School:** St Louis Univ 1982; **Resid:** Physical Medicine & Rehabilitation, Northwestern Univ Med Ctr 1985

Robinson, Michael MD (PMR) - **Spec Exp:** Pain-Neuropathic; Pain-Back & Neck; Musculoskeletal Disorders; **Hospital:** Good Samaritan Hosp - Suffern; **Address:** Rockland Orthopedic & Sports Med, 327 Rte 59, Airmont, NY 10952; **Phone:** 845-356-2900; **Board Cert:** Physical Medicine & Rehabilitation 2003; Pain Medicine 2000; Electrodiagnostic Medicine 2000; **Med School:** Tufts Univ 1988; **Resid:** Rehabilitation, Walter Reed Army Med Ctr 1992

Psychiatry

Levy, Michael I MD (Psyc) - **Spec Exp:** Psychopharmacology; Geriatric Psychiatry; **Hospital:** Nyack Hosp; **Address:** 160 N Midland Ave, Nyack, NY 10960-2505; **Phone:** 845-348-2116; **Board Cert:** Psychiatry 1982; Geriatric Psychiatry 2001; **Med School:** Albert Einstein Coll Med 1977; **Resid:** Psychiatry, Mount Sinai Hosp 1981; **Fac Appt:** Asst Clin Prof Psyc, NY Med Coll

Schroeder, Karl MD (Psyc) - **Spec Exp:** Addiction/Substance Abuse; Psychiatry in Physical Illness; Post Traumatic Stress Disorder; **Address:** 104 Montebello Rd, Suffern, NY 10901; **Phone:** 845-357-9367; **Board Cert:** Psychiatry 1980; **Med School:** Columbia P&S 1974; **Resid:** Psychiatry, Columbia-Presby Hosp 1977; **Fac Appt:** Asst Clin Prof Med, Columbia P&S

Pulmonary Disease

Harris, Leon MD (Pul) - **Hospital:** Good Samaritan Hosp - Suffern; **Address:** 2 Crossfield Ave, Ste 318, West Nyack, NY 10994-2212; **Phone:** 845-353-5600; **Board Cert:** Internal Medicine 1979; Pulmonary Disease 1982; Critical Care Medicine 2004; **Med School:** Mount Sinai Sch Med 1976; **Resid:** Internal Medicine, Mt Sinai Hosp 1979; **Fellow:** Pulmonary Disease, Mass Genl Hosp 1981

Hodes, David L MD (Pul) - **Hospital:** Nyack Hosp, Good Samaritan Hosp - Suffern; **Address:** 2 Med Park Drive, Ste 3, West Nyack, NY 10994; **Phone:** 845-727-7733; **Board Cert:** Internal Medicine 1976; Pulmonary Disease 1978; Critical Care Medicine 2001; **Med School:** NYU Sch Med 1973; **Resid:** Internal Medicine, St Luke's Hosp 1976; **Fellow:** Pulmonary Disease, Bellevue Hosp/NYU 1978

Menitove, Stephen MD (Pul) - **Hospital:** Nyack Hosp; **Address:** Rockland Pulmonary & Medical Assocs, 2 Crosfield Ave, Ste 318, West Nyack, NY 10994-2212; **Phone:** 845-353-5600; **Board Cert:** Internal Medicine 1980; Pulmonary Disease 1982; **Med School:** Mount Sinai Sch Med 1977; **Resid:** Internal Medicine, Mount Sinai Hospital 1983; **Fellow:** Pulmonary Disease, Bellevue/NYU Med Ctr 1982; **Fac Appt:** Med, Mount Sinai Sch Med

Osei, Clement MD (Pul) - **Spec Exp:** Asthma; Emphysema; Lung Cancer; **Hospital:** Good Samaritan Hosp - Suffern, Nyack Hosp; **Address:** 2 Crossfield Ave, Ste 318, West Nyack, NY 10994; **Phone:** 845-353-5600; **Board Cert:** Internal Medicine 1975; Pulmonary Disease 1978; **Med School:** Germany 1970; **Resid:** Internal Medicine, Elmhurst Hosp Ctr/Mt Sinai 1975; **Fellow:** Pulmonary Disease, Elmhurst Hosp Ctr/Mt Sinai 1977

Pellicone, John MD (Pul) - **Spec Exp:** Critical Care; **Hospital:** Helen Hayes Hosp, Nyack Hosp; **Address:** Helen Hayes Hosp, Route 9W, West Haverstraw, NY 10993; **Phone:** 845-786-4410; **Board Cert:** Internal Medicine 1984; Critical Care Medicine 2000; Pulmonary Disease 2000; **Med School:** Columbia P&S 1981; **Resid:** Internal Medicine, Montefiore Med Ctr 1984; **Fellow:** Pulmonary Disease, NYU-Bellevue Med Ctr 1986

Rheumatology

Becker, Alfred MD (Rhu) - **Hospital:** Good Samaritan Hosp - Suffern, Nyack Hosp; **Address:** 222 Rte 59, Ste 204, Suffern, NY 10901; **Phone:** 845-357-6464; **Board Cert:** Internal Medicine 1969; Rheumatology 1972; **Med School:** Albert Einstein Coll Med 1962; **Resid:** Internal Medicine, Pittsburgh Hlth Ctr 1967; **Fellow:** Rheumatology, Montefiore Med Ctr 1968; **Fac Appt:** Asst Clin Prof Med, Columbia P&S

Sports Medicine

Berezin, Marc A MD (SM) - **Spec Exp:** Arthroscopic Surgery; Knee Surgery; **Hospital:** Nyack Hosp, Good Samaritan Hosp - Suffern; **Address:** 99 Dutch Hill Rd, Orangeburg, NY 10962-2106; **Phone:** 845-359-1877; **Board Cert:** Orthopaedic Surgery 2004; **Med School:** NY Med Coll 1985; **Resid:** Orthopaedic Surgery, NY Med Coll 1990; **Fellow:** Sports Medicine, Arthoscopy Assoc Ortho 1991

Surgery

Fleischer, Lee S MD (S) - **Spec Exp:** Breast Disease; Laparoscopic Surgery; Gastrointestinal Surgery; **Hospital:** Good Samaritan Hosp - Suffern, Nyack Hosp; **Address:** 100 Route 59, Ste 101, Suffern, NY 10901-4927; **Phone:** 845-357-8800; **Board Cert:** Surgery 2002; **Med School:** McGill Univ 1987; **Resid:** Surgery, Beth Israel Med Ctr 1992

Joseph, Patricia K MD (S) - **Spec Exp:** Breast Cancer; **Hospital:** Nyack Hosp; **Address:** Nyack Breast & Women's Health Ctr, 160 N Midland Ave, Nyack, NY 10960; **Phone:** 845-348-8507; **Board Cert:** Surgery 2005; **Med School:** Univ Fla Coll Med 1979; **Resid:** Surgery, Montefiore Med Ctr 1984

Simon, Lawrence MD (S) - **Spec Exp:** Breast Surgery; Hernia; Gallbladder Surgery; **Hospital:** Nyack Hosp, Good Samaritan Hosp - Suffern; **Address:** 11 Med Park, Ste 203, Pomona, NY 10970-3559; **Phone:** 845-354-2241; **Board Cert:** Surgery 1971; **Med School:** SUNY Upstate Med Univ 1965; **Resid:** Surgery, St Lukes Hosp 1970

Thoracic Surgery

Gorenstein, Lyall MD (TS) - **Spec Exp:** Thoracic Cancers; Esophageal Surgery; Minimally Invasive Thoracic Surgery; Hyperhidrosis-Palmar; **Hospital:** Good Samaritan Hosp - Suffern, NY-Presby Hosp/Columbia (page 104); **Address:** 5A Medical Park Drive, Pomona, NY 10970-3565; **Phone:** 845-362-0075; **Board Cert:** Surgery 2009; Thoracic Surgery 2001; **Med School:** Canada 1983; **Resid:** Radiation Therapy, Univ Toronto 1988; Thoracic Surgery, Univ Toronto 1992; **Fellow:** Thoracic Surgery, MD Anderson Cancer Ctr 1990; **Fac Appt:** Asst Clin Prof S, Columbia P&S

Lundy, Edward MD/PhD (TS) - **Spec Exp:** Cardiothoracic Surgery; **Hospital:** Good Samaritan Hosp - Suffern; **Address:** 257 Lafayette Ave, Suffern, NY 10901; **Phone:** 845-368-8800; **Board Cert:** Surgery 1999; Thoracic Surgery 2009; **Med School:** Univ Mich Med Sch 1981; **Resid:** Surgery, Univ Mich Med Ctr 1987; **Fellow:** Thoracic Surgery, Univ Mich Med Ctr 1989

Urology

Giella, John G MD (U) - **Spec Exp:** Kidney Stones; Prostate Cancer; Hypospadias; **Hospital:** Nyack Hosp, Good Samaritan Hosp - Suffern; **Address:** 2 Medical Park Drive, Ste 10, West Nyack, NY 10994; **Phone:** 845-354-5000; **Board Cert:** Urology 2002; **Med School:** Harvard Med Sch 1986; **Resid:** Surgery, St Vincent's Hosp 1988; Urology, Columbia-Presby Med Ctr 1992

Rudin, Leonard MD (U) - **Spec Exp:** Urologic Cancer; Kidney Stones; **Hospital:** Good Samaritan Hosp - Suffern, Nyack Hosp; **Address:** 2 Medical Park Drive, West Nyack, NY 10994; **Phone:** 845-354-5000; **Board Cert:** Urology 1976; **Med School:** SUNY Upstate Med Univ 1966; **Resid:** Surgery, St Luke's-Roosevelt Hosp 1968; Urology, Columbia-Presby Med Ctr 1974

Suffolk

Suffolk

Allergy & Immunology

Cancellieri, Russell P MD (A&I) - **Spec Exp:** Asthma; **Hospital:** Southampton Hosp; **Address:** 596 Hampton Rd, Southampton, NY 11968; **Phone:** 631-283-3300; **Board Cert:** Pediatrics 1979; Allergy & Immunology 1981; **Med School:** Georgetown Univ 1974; **Resid:** Pediatrics, Georgetown Univ Hosp 1977; Allergy & Immunology, St Luke's-Roosevelt Hosp Ctr 1979

Guida Jr, Louis E MD (A&I) - **Spec Exp:** Allergy; Urticaria; Asthma; Cystic Fibrosis; **Hospital:** Good Samaritan Hosp Med Ctr - West Islip, St Charles Hosp; **Address:** Bay Shore Allergy/Asthma, 649 Montauk Hwy, Bay Shore, NY 11706-8542; **Phone:** 631-665-2700; **Board Cert:** Pediatrics 2004; **Med School:** Grenada 1984; **Resid:** Pediatrics, Monmouth Med Ctr 1987; Allergy & Immunology, Nassau Co Med Ctr 1993; **Fellow:** Pediatric Pulmonology, Hahnemann Univ Hosp 1990

Lusman, Paul A MD (A&I) - **Spec Exp:** Asthma; Sinus Disorders; Hives; **Hospital:** John T Mather Meml Hosp, St Charles Hosp; **Address:** 120 N Country Rd, Port Jefferson, NY 11777; **Phone:** 631-928-4990; **Board Cert:** Pediatrics 1971; Allergy & Immunology 1974; **Med School:** Albert Einstein Coll Med 1965; **Resid:** Pediatrics, Bellevue Hosp 1968; **Fellow:** Allergy & Immunology, Duke Univ Med Ctr 1972; **Fac Appt:** Asst Clin Prof Med, SUNY Stony Brook

Mayer, Daniel L MD (A&I) - **Spec Exp:** Asthma; Allergic Rhinitis; Food Allergy; Sinusitis; **Hospital:** Stony Brook Univ Med Ctr, St Catherine's of Siena Med Ctr; **Address:** 263 E Main St, Smithtown, NY 11787; **Phone:** 631-366-5252; **Board Cert:** Pediatrics 1983; **Med School:** Italy 1978; **Resid:** Pediatrics, Albany Med Ctr 1985; **Fellow:** Allergy & Immunology, Long Island Hosp 1987; **Fac Appt:** Asst Prof A&I, SUNY Stony Brook

Richheimer, Michael MD (A&I) - **Spec Exp:** Asthma; Skin Allergies; Sinus Disorders; Immunodeficiency Disorders; **Hospital:** Stony Brook Univ Med Ctr, South Nassau Comm Hosp; **Address:** 1855 Union Blvd, Bay Shore, NY 11706; **Phone:** 631-665-6363; **Board Cert:** Allergy & Immunology 2006; **Med School:** Grenada 1985; **Resid:** Internal Medicine, St Joseph's Hosp-Seton Hall Univ 1988; **Fellow:** Allergy & Immunology, SUNY Stony Brook Med Ctr 1990; **Fac Appt:** Assoc Clin Prof A&I, SUNY Stony Brook

Satnick, Steven MD (A&I) - **Spec Exp:** Asthma; Urticaria; **Hospital:** Stony Brook Univ Med Ctr; **Address:** 900 Main St, Ste 102, Holbrook, NY 11741-1813; **Phone:** 631-588-4486; **Board Cert:** Internal Medicine 1983; Allergy & Immunology 1987; **Med School:** SUNY Downstate 1980; **Resid:** Internal Medicine, Univ Hosp 1984; **Fellow:** Allergy & Immunology, Univ Hosp 1987

Cardiac Electrophysiology

Rashba, Eric J MD (CE) - **Spec Exp:** Arrhythmias; Pacemakers; Syncope; Atrial Fibrillation; **Hospital:** Stony Brook Univ Med Ctr; **Address:** Stony Brook Univ Med Ctr, Cardiology, HSC Bldg Fl 16 - rm 080, Stony Brook, NY 11794-8167; **Phone:** 631-444-3575; **Board Cert:** Internal Medicine 2006; Cardiovascular Disease 2008; Cardiac Electrophysiology 2009; **Med School:** Yale Univ 1992; **Resid:** Internal Medicine, Strong Meml Hosp 1995; **Fellow:** Cardiovascular Disease, New England Med Ctr 1999; Cardiac Electrophysiology, New England Med Ctr 1999; **Fac Appt:** Prof Med, SUNY Stony Brook

Cardiovascular Disease

Altschul, Larry MD (Cv) - **Spec Exp:** Non-Invasive Cardiology; Echocardiography; Nuclear Cardiology; **Hospital:** Good Samaritan Hosp Med Ctr - West Islip, Southside Hosp; **Address:** 540 Union Blvd, West Islip, NY 11795; **Phone:** 631-669-2555; **Board Cert:** Internal Medicine 1980; Cardiovascular Disease 1983; **Med School:** SUNY Buffalo 1977; **Resid:** Internal Medicine, Nassau County Med Ctr 1980; **Fellow:** Cardiovascular Disease, Nassau County Med Ctr 1982

Borek, Mark G MD (Cv) - **Spec Exp:** Nuclear Cardiology; Echocardiography; Cardiac Catheterization; **Hospital:** St Catherine's of Siena Med Ctr, John T Mather Meml Hosp; **Address:** 496 Smithtown Bypass, Ste 101, Smithtown, NY 11787; **Phone:** 631-979-8880; **Board Cert:** Internal Medicine 1985; Cardiovascular Disease 1987; **Med School:** SUNY Downstate 1981; **Resid:** Internal Medicine, Nassau Co Med Ctr 1984; **Fellow:** Cardiovascular Disease, Long Island Coll Hosp 1987

Brown, David L MD (Cv) - **Spec Exp:** Percutaneous ASD/PFO closure; Critical Care Medicine; Preventive Cardiology; Heart Valve Disease; **Hospital:** Stony Brook Univ Med Ctr; **Address:** SUNY Stony Brook Sch Med, Div Cardiology, Health Sci Ctr T16-080, Stony Brook, NY 11794; **Phone:** 631-444-3699; **Board Cert:** Internal Medicine 1986; Cardiovascular Disease 2005; Interventional Cardiology 2001; **Med School:** Baylor Coll Med 1982; **Resid:** Internal Medicine, Baylor Coll Med 1986; Cardiovascular Disease, UCSF Med Ctr 1990; **Fellow:** Interventional Cardiology, Cleveland Clinic 1993; Hematology, USCF Med Ctr 1988; **Fac Appt:** Prof Med, SUNY Stony Brook

Chengot, Mathew T MD (Cv) - **Spec Exp:** Nuclear Cardiology; Interventional Cardiology; Heart Failure; Echocardiography; **Hospital:** Good Samaritan Hosp Med Ctr - West Islip, St Joseph's Hosp-Nassau; **Address:** Amityville Heart Ctr, 129 Broadway, Amityville, NY 11701-2729; **Phone:** 631-598-3434; **Board Cert:** Internal Medicine 1983; Cardiovascular Disease 1985; **Med School:** India 1976; **Resid:** Internal Medicine, Lincoln Med Ctr 1982; **Fellow:** Cardiovascular Disease, Mt Sinai Hosp 1984

Dervan, John MD (Cv) - **Spec Exp:** Interventional Cardiology; Cholesterol/Lipid Disorders; Heart Failure; **Hospital:** Stony Brook Univ Med Ctr, St Catherine's of Siena Med Ctr; **Address:** 220 Belle Mead Rd, Ste A, East Setauket, NY 11733; **Phone:** 631-941-2273; **Board Cert:** Internal Medicine 1979; Cardiovascular Disease 1985; Interventional Cardiology 2009; **Med School:** St Louis Univ 1976; **Resid:** Internal Medicine, Faulkner Hosp 1980; **Fellow:** Cardiovascular Disease, Beth Israel Hosp 1983; **Fac Appt:** Assoc Clin Prof Med, SUNY Stony Brook

Falco, Thomas MD (Cv) - **Hospital:** Peconic Bay Med Ctr, Eastern Long Island Hosp; **Address:** 1279 E Main St, Riverhead, NY 11901; **Phone:** 631-727-2100; **Board Cert:** Internal Medicine 1985; Cardiovascular Disease 1987; **Med School:** Mexico 1980; **Resid:** Internal Medicine, Winthrop Univ Hosp 1984; Cardiovascular Disease, Winthrop Univ Hosp 1985; **Fellow:** Cardiovascular Disease, Albany Med Ctr 1987

Jeremias, Allen MD (Cv) - **Spec Exp:** Interventional Cardiology; Peripheral Vascular Disease; Percutaneous Vascular Interventions; Vascular Disease; **Hospital:** Stony Brook Univ Med Ctr; **Address:** Stony Brook Univ Med Ctr, Hlth Sci Ctr T16-080, Stony Brook, NY 11794; **Phone:** 631-444-1069; **Board Cert:** Internal Medicine 2002; Cardiovascular Disease 2005; Interventional Cardiology 2006; Vascular Medicine 2006; **Med School:** Germany 1995; **Resid:** Internal Medicine, Cleveland Clinic Hosp 2002; **Fellow:** Cardiovascular Disease, Beth Israel-Deaconess Med Ctr 2004; Interventional Cardiology, Beth Israel-Deaconess Med Ctr 2005; **Fac Appt:** Asst Prof Med, SUNY Stony Brook

Lense, Lloyd MD (Cv) - **Spec Exp:** Cholesterol/Lipid Disorders; Hypertension; Coronary Artery Disease; **Hospital:** Stony Brook Univ Med Ctr, John T Mather Meml Hosp; **Address:** 210 Belle Mead Rd, East Setauket, NY 11733; **Phone:** 631-689-1400; **Board Cert:** Internal Medicine 1980; Cardiovascular Disease 1983; **Med School:** NYU Sch Med 1977; **Resid:** Internal Medicine, Mt Sinai Hosp 1980; **Fellow:** Cardiovascular Disease, Montefiore Med Ctr 1983; **Fac Appt:** Assoc Clin Prof Med, SUNY Stony Brook

Masciello, Michael A MD (Cv) - **Spec Exp:** Coronary Artery Disease; Congestive Heart Failure; **Hospital:** Southside Hosp, Good Samaritan Hosp Med Ctr - West Islip; **Address:** 540 Union Blvd, West Islip, NY 11795; **Phone:** 631-669-2555 x107; **Board Cert:** Internal Medicine 1983; Cardiovascular Disease 1985; Critical Care Medicine 2003; **Med School:** Univ Miami Sch Med 1980; **Resid:** Cardiovascular Disease, Nassau County Med Ctr 1985

Matilsky, Michael A MD (Cv) - **Spec Exp:** Cholesterol/Lipid Disorders; Hypertension; Coronary Artery Disease; Atrial Fibrillation; **Hospital:** St Charles Hosp, John T Mather Meml Hosp; **Address:** Three Village Cardiology, 210 Belle Mead Rd, East Setauket, NY 11733-3327; **Phone:** 631-689-1400; **Board Cert:** Internal Medicine 1985; Cardiovascular Disease 1987; **Med School:** SUNY Stony Brook 1982; **Resid:** Internal Medicine, Mt Sinai Hosp 1985; **Fellow:** Cardiovascular Disease, NY Hosp Cornell Med Ctr 1988; **Fac Appt:** Asst Clin Prof Med, SUNY Stony Brook

Poon, Michael MD (Cv) - **Spec Exp:** Coronary Artery Disease; Pulmonary Hypertension; Cardiac CT Angiography; Cardiac Imaging; **Hospital:** Stony Brook Univ Med Ctr, Mount Sinai Med Ctr (page 102); **Address:** Stony Brook Health Science Ctr, Level 4, rm 120, Stony Brook, NY 11794; **Phone:** 631-444-5400; **Board Cert:** Cardiovascular Disease 2007; **Med School:** Mount Sinai Sch Med 1987; **Resid:** Internal Medicine, Mount Sinai Med Ctr 1991; **Fellow:** Cardiovascular Disease, Mount Sinai Med Ctr 1993; **Fac Appt:** Prof Med, SUNY Stony Brook

Skopicki, Hal A MD/PhD (Cv) - **Spec Exp:** Congestive Heart Failure; **Hospital:** Stony Brook Univ Med Ctr; **Address:** University Physicians at Stony Brook, 3001 Expressway Drive N, Ste 200B, Islandia, NY 11749; **Phone:** 631-444-9600; **Board Cert:** Internal Medicine 2003; Cardiovascular Disease 2007; **Med School:** Ros Franklin Univ/Chicago Med Sch 1990; **Resid:** Internal Medicine, Yale-New Haven Hosp 1993; **Fellow:** Cardiovascular Disease, Mass Genl Hosp 1994; **Fac Appt:** Asst Prof Med, SUNY Stony Brook

Weinberg, Marc MD (Cv) - **Hospital:** Huntington Hosp; **Address:** West Carver Med Assocs, 200 W Carver St, Ste 8, Huntington, NY 11743-3303; **Phone:** 631-421-0020; **Board Cert:** Internal Medicine 1976; Cardiovascular Disease 1979; Critical Care Medicine 2007; **Med School:** Yale Univ 1973; **Resid:** Internal Medicine, New Haven Hosp 1977; **Fellow:** Cardiovascular Disease, New Haven Hosp 1979

Child & Adolescent Psychiatry

Carlson, Gabrielle A MD (ChAP) - **Spec Exp:** Child Psychiatry; Bipolar/Mood Disorders; ADD/ADHD; **Hospital:** Stony Brook Univ Med Ctr; **Address:** Putnam Hall, South Campus, SUNY-Stony Brook, Child & Adol Psych, Stony Brook, NY 11794-8790; **Phone:** 631-632-8840; **Board Cert:** Child & Adolescent Psychiatry 1978; Psychiatry 1975; **Med School:** Cornell Univ-Weill Med Coll 1968; **Resid:** Psychiatry, Barnes Hosp-Washington Univ 1970; Psychiatry, Nat Inst Mental Hlth 1972; **Fellow:** Child & Adolescent Psychiatry, UCLA Med Ctr 1978; **Fac Appt:** Prof Psyc, SUNY Stony Brook

Gandhi, Lajpat R MD (ChAP) - **Spec Exp:** Anxiety & Mood Disorders; ADD/ADHD; **Hospital:** Huntington Hosp; **Address:** 110 E Main St, Ste 5, Huntington, NY 11743; **Phone:** 631-427-6411; **Board Cert:** Psychiatry 1981; Child & Adolescent Psychiatry 1985; **Med School:** India 1975; **Resid:** Psychiatry, Metropolitan Hosp 1979; **Fellow:** Psychiatry, Elmhurst Hosp-Mt Sinai 1980; Child & Adolescent Psychiatry, LI Jewish-Hillside Med Ctr 1981

Greenberg, Judith J MD (ChAP) - **Hospital:** Long Island Jewish Med Ctr, N Shore Univ Hosp; **Address:** 775 Park Ave, Ste 155, Huntington, NY 11743; **Phone:** 631-629-4790; **Board Cert:** Psychiatry 1990; Pediatrics 1985; Child & Adolescent Psychiatry 1990; **Med School:** SUNY Downstate 1980; **Resid:** Pediatrics, Chldns Meml Hosp 1983; Psychiatry, N Shore Univ Hosp 1987; **Fellow:** Child Psychiatry, Univ Illinois Hosp 1984; Child Psychiatry, N Shore Univ Hosp 1985

Pomeroy, John C MD (ChAP) - **Spec Exp:** Autism; Mental Retardation; Developmental Disorders; **Hospital:** Stony Brook Univ Med Ctr; **Address:** The Cody Center for Autism, 5 Medical Drive, Port Jefferson Stn, NY 11776; **Phone:** 631-632-3070; **Board Cert:** Psychiatry 1984; Child & Adolescent Psychiatry 1988; **Med School:** England, UK 1973; **Resid:** Psychiatry, St Mary's Hosp 1979; **Fellow:** Child & Adolescent Psychiatry, Univ Iowa Hosps 1981; **Fac Appt:** Assoc Prof Psyc, SUNY Stony Brook

Weisbrot, Deborah M MD (ChAP) - **Spec Exp:** Anxiety & Mood Disorders; Neuro-Psychiatry; **Hospital:** Stony Brook Univ Med Ctr; **Address:** SUNY Stony Brook, Div Child & Adolescent Psych, Putnam Hall, South Campus, Stony Brook, NY 11794-8790; **Phone:** 631-632-8840; **Board Cert:** Psychiatry 1985; Child & Adolescent Psychiatry 1991; **Med School:** SUNY Buffalo 1979; **Resid:** Psychiatry, Yale-New Haven Hosp 1983; **Fellow:** Child Psychiatry, NY Hosp-Payne Whitney Clin 1986; **Fac Appt:** Assoc Clin Prof Psyc, SUNY Stony Brook

Child Neurology

Andriola, Mary R MD (ChiN) - **Spec Exp:** Epilepsy; ADD/ADHD; Headache; Developmental Disorders; **Hospital:** Stony Brook Univ Med Ctr; **Address:** SUNY-Stony Brook, Dept Neurology, HSC T12-020, Stony Brook, NY 11794-0001; **Phone:** 631-444-2599; **Board Cert:** Pediatrics 1970; Child Neurology 1972; Clinical Neurophysiology 2002; Neurodevelopmental Disabilities 2005; **Med School:** Duke Univ 1965; **Resid:** Pediatrics, Univ Fla Shands Hosp 1967; **Fellow:** Neurology, Univ Fla Shands Hosp 1970; **Fac Appt:** Prof N, SUNY Stony Brook

Clinical Genetics

Hyman, David B MD (CG) - **Spec Exp:** Prenatal Diagnosis; Genetic Disorders; Cancer Risk Assessment; Metabolic Genetic Disorders; **Hospital:** Stony Brook Univ Med Ctr, St Catherine's of Siena Med Ctr; **Address:** 48 Route 25-A, Ste 205, Smithtown, NY 11787-1448; **Phone:** 631-862-3620; **Board Cert:** Pediatrics 1983; Clinical Genetics 1984; Clinical Biochemical Genetics 1990; Clinical Molecular Genetics 1990; **Med School:** Univ IL Coll Med 1978; **Resid:** Pediatrics, Yale Univ Sch Med 1980; **Fellow:** Clinical Genetics, Yale Univ Sch Med 1983

McGovern, Margaret MD/PhD (CG) - **Hospital:** Stony Brook Univ Med Ctr; **Address:** Stony Brook Univ Med Ctr, Pediatrics Fl 11, Nicolls Rd, Stony Brook, NY 11794; **Phone:** 631-444-5437; **Board Cert:** Pediatrics 2005; Clinical Genetics 1990; **Med School:** Mount Sinai Sch Med 1986; **Resid:** Pediatrics, Mt Sinai Hosp 1988; **Fellow:** Genetics, Mt Sinai Hosp 1990; **Fac Appt:** Prof Ped, SUNY Stony Brook

Colon & Rectal Surgery

Leiboff, Arnold R MD (CRS) - **Hospital:** John T Mather Meml Hosp, St Charles Hosp; **Address:** 3400 Nesconset Hwy, Ste 100, East Setauket, NY 11733; **Phone:** 631-689-2600; **Board Cert:** Surgery 2007; Colon & Rectal Surgery 2001; **Med School:** NY Med Coll 1978; **Resid:** Surgery, SUNY at Stony Brook 1985; **Fellow:** Colon & Rectal Surgery, Carle Foundation Hosp-Univ Ill 1989

Smithy, William B MD (CRS) - **Spec Exp:** Colon & Rectal Cancer; Anorectal Disorders; Colonoscopy; **Hospital:** Stony Brook Univ Med Ctr, St Catherine's of Siena Med Ctr; **Address:** 222 Middle Country Rd, Ste 209, Smithtown, NY 11787; **Phone:** 631-638-2800; **Board Cert:** Surgery 1997; Colon & Rectal Surgery 1989; **Med School:** Columbia P&S 1981; **Resid:** Surgery, Roosevelt Hosp 1987; **Fellow:** Colon & Rectal Surgery, RWJ Univ Hosp 1988; **Fac Appt:** Asst Clin Prof S, SUNY Stony Brook

Dermatology

Basuk, Pamela MD (D) - **Spec Exp:** Cosmetic Dermatology; Melanoma; Skin Laser Surgery; Skin Cancer; **Hospital:** Southside Hosp; **Address:** 2011 Union Blvd, Ste 1, Bayshore, NY 11706; **Phone:** 631-666-2900; **Board Cert:** Dermatology 1988; **Med School:** NYU Sch Med 1984; **Resid:** Dermatology, Brown Univ Hosp 1988

Berger, Bernard MD (D) - **Hospital:** Southampton Hosp, Stony Brook Univ Med Ctr; **Address:** 319 Hampton Rd, Southampton, NY 11968-5029; **Phone:** 631-283-7722; **Board Cert:** Dermatology 1975; **Med School:** UC Irvine 1963; **Resid:** Dermatology, Mount Sinai Hosp 1971

Clark, Richard MD (D) - **Spec Exp:** Eczema; Contact Dermatitis; Skin Cancer; **Hospital:** Stony Brook Univ Med Ctr; **Address:** 181 N Belle Meade Rd, Ste 6, East Setauket, NY 11733; **Phone:** 631-444-4270; **Board Cert:** Internal Medicine 1974; Allergy & Immunology 1977; Dermatology 1980; **Med School:** Univ Rochester 1971; **Resid:** Internal Medicine, Strong Meml Hosp 1973; **Fellow:** Allergy & Immunology, Nat Inst Health 1976; Dermatology, Mass Genl Hosp 1980; **Fac Appt:** Prof D, SUNY Stony Brook

Huh, Julie MD (D) - **Spec Exp:** Acne; Skin Cancer; Eczema; **Hospital:** Good Samaritan Hosp Med Ctr - West Islip, Southside Hosp; **Address:** 332 E Main St, Bayshore, NY 11706-8404; **Phone:** 631-666-0500; **Board Cert:** Dermatology 2005; **Med School:** Columbia P&S 1991; **Resid:** Dermatology, Columbia-Presby Med Ctr 1995

Marghoob, Ashfaq A MD (D) - **Spec Exp:** Skin Cancer; Melanoma; **Hospital:** Meml Sloan-Kettering Cancer Ctr (page 112); **Address:** Meml Sloan Kettering Cancer Ctr, 800 Veterans Meml Hwy Fl 2, Hauppage, NY 11788; **Phone:** 212-610-0780; **Board Cert:** Dermatology 2005; **Med School:** SUNY Stony Brook 1987; **Resid:** Family Medicine, SUNY Stony Brook Med Ctr 1990; **Fellow:** Dermatology, NYU Sch Med Hosp 1995

Moynihan, Gavan D MD (D) - **Spec Exp:** Melanoma; Skin Cancer; **Hospital:** Good Samaritan Hosp Med Ctr - West Islip; **Address:** 332 E Main St, Bay Shore, NY 11706-8404; **Phone:** 631-666-0500; **Board Cert:** Dermatology 1977; **Med School:** Howard Univ 1973; **Resid:** Dermatology, USPHS Hosp-Staten Island NY & USPHS Hosp 1976; **Fellow:** Dermatology, Columbia-Presby Med Ctr 1977; **Fac Appt:** Asst Prof D, SUNY Stony Brook

Notaro, Antoinette MD (D) - **Spec Exp:** Skin Cancer; Botox Therapy; Psoriasis; Acne; **Hospital:** Eastern Long Island Hosp, Peconic Bay Med Ctr; **Address:** 13405 Main Rd, Box 93, Mattituck, NY 11952-0093; **Phone:** 631-298-1122; **Board Cert:** Dermatology 1982; **Med School:** SUNY Downstate 1978; **Resid:** Dermatology, Albert Einstein 1982; **Fac Appt:** Asst Clin Prof D, SUNY Stony Brook

Siegel, Daniel M MD (D) - **Spec Exp:** Mohs' Surgery; Dermatologic Surgery; Skin Cancer; **Hospital:** St Catherine's of Siena Med Ctr, Eastern Long Island Hosp; **Address:** 994 Jericho Tpke, Ste 103, Smithtown, NY 11787; **Phone:** 631-864-6647; **Board Cert:** Dermatology 2009; **Med School:** Albany Med Coll 1981; **Resid:** Dermatology, Parkland Univ Texas SW Med Ctr 1985; **Fellow:** Mohs Surgery, Baylor Coll Med 1986; **Fac Appt:** Clin Prof D, SUNY Downstate

Skrokov, Robert MD (D) - **Spec Exp:** Vascular Malformations/Birthmarks; Psoriasis; Skin Cancer; **Hospital:** Good Samaritan Hosp Med Ctr - West Islip, Southside Hosp; **Address:** 332 E Main St, Bay Shore, NY 11706-8404; **Phone:** 631-666-0500; **Board Cert:** Dermatology 2009; **Med School:** SUNY Downstate 1982; **Resid:** Dermatology, SUNY-Downstate Med Ctr 1986; **Fac Appt:** Asst Clin Prof D, SUNY Stony Brook

Tom, Jack MD (D) - **Spec Exp:** Acne; Geriatric Dermatology; **Hospital:** Mount Sinai Med Ctr (page 102); **Address:** 207 Hallock Rd, Ste 211, Stony Brook, NY 11790-3076; **Phone:** 631-444-0004; **Board Cert:** Dermatology 1986; **Med School:** NYU Sch Med 1982; **Resid:** Internal Medicine, NYU Med Ctr 1983; Dermatology, Mount Sinai Med Ctr 1986; **Fac Appt:** Asst Clin Prof D, Mount Sinai Sch Med

Diagnostic Radiology

Brancaccio, William R MD (DR) - **Spec Exp:** Abdominal Imaging; Mammography; **Hospital:** Southampton Hosp, Eastern Long Island Hosp; **Address:** 240 Meeting House Ln, Radiology Dept, Southampton, NY 11968; **Phone:** 631-726-8411; **Board Cert:** Diagnostic Radiology 1981; **Med School:** Geo Wash Univ 1975; **Resid:** Diagnostic Radiology, Univ Hosp 1979; **Fellow:** Diagnostic Radiology, NYU Med Ctr 1980

Kirshy, David MD (DR) - **Spec Exp:** CT Scan; MRI; PET Imaging; **Hospital:** Southampton Hosp; **Address:** Southampton Hospital, Dept Radiology, 240 Meeting House Ln, Southampton, NY 11968; **Phone:** 631-727-2755; **Board Cert:** Diagnostic Radiology 1993; **Med School:** SUNY Downstate 1988; **Resid:** Diagnostic Radiology, SUNY Hlth Sci Ctr 1993

Laucella, Michael MD (DR) - ; **Address:** 375 E Main St, Bay Shore, NY 11706; **Phone:** 631-665-2261; **Board Cert:** Diagnostic Radiology 1984; Neuroradiology 2006; **Med School:** Univ Chicago-Pritzker Sch Med 1980; **Resid:** Diagnostic Radiology, Tufts-New Eng Med Ctr 1984; **Fellow:** Neurological Radiology, Tufts-New Eng Med Ctr 1986

Mankes, Seth MD (DR) - **Hospital:** Stony Brook Univ Med Ctr; **Address:** Radiology Dept, HSC/Level 4/rm 120, Stony Brook, NY 11794-8460; **Phone:** 631-444-7224; **Board Cert:** Diagnostic Radiology 1981; **Med School:** NYU Sch Med 1976; **Resid:** Diagnostic Radiology, NYU Med Ctr 1981; **Fellow:** Ultrasound, NYU Med Ctr 1982

Rifkin, Matthew MD (DR) - **Spec Exp:** Ultrasound; Cardiac CT Angiography; **Hospital:** Good Samaritan Hosp Med Ctr - West Islip, St Catherine's of Siena Med Ctr; **Address:** 1000 Montauk Hwy, West Islip, NY 11795; **Phone:** 631-376-4027; **Board Cert:** Diagnostic Radiology 1978; **Med School:** Albert Einstein Coll Med 1974; **Resid:** Diagnostic Radiology, Montefiore Hosp 1978; **Fellow:** Ultrasound/CT, Johns Hopkins Hosp 1979; **Fac Appt:** Prof Rad, SUNY Stony Brook

Endocrinology, Diabetes & Metabolism

Balkin, Michael MD (EDM) - **Spec Exp:** Diabetes; Thyroid Disorders; Hirsutism (Excessive Body Hair); Osteoporosis; **Hospital:** Huntington Hosp, Nassau Univ Med Ctr; **Address:** 191 E Main St, Huntington, NY 11743-2921; **Phone:** 631-549-2525; **Board Cert:** Internal Medicine 1976; Endocrinology 1977; **Med School:** Mount Sinai Sch Med 1972; **Resid:** Internal Medicine, Kings County Med Ctr 1975; **Fellow:** Endocrinology, Diabetes & Metabolism, Mt Sinai Med Ctr 1977; Endocrinology, Diabetes & Metabolism, Meml Sloan Kettering Cancer Ctr 1980; **Fac Appt:** Asst Clin Prof Med, SUNY Stony Brook

Brand, Howard A MD (EDM) - **Spec Exp:** Thyroid Disorders; Pituitary Disorders; Diabetes; Cholesterol/Lipid Disorders; **Hospital:** St Charles Hosp, John T Mather Meml Hosp; **Address:** 2500 Nesconset Hwy 3C Bldg, Stony Brook, NY 11790; **Phone:** 631-751-2400; **Board Cert:** Internal Medicine 1987; Endocrinology, Diabetes & Metabolism 2001; **Med School:** UMDNJ-RW Johnson Med Sch 1984; **Resid:** Internal Medicine, Mt Sinai Hosp 1987; Internal Medicine, Bronx VA Med Ctr 1988; **Fellow:** Endocrinology, Diabetes & Metabolism, NYU Med Ctr 1990

Carlson, Harold E MD (EDM) - **Spec Exp:** Thyroid Disorders; Pituitary Disorders; Gynecomastia; **Hospital:** Stony Brook Univ Med Ctr; **Address:** Stony Brook Univ Hosp, Dept Medicine, Div Endocrinology & Metabolism, 26 Research Way, East Setauket, NY 11733-3453; **Phone:** 631-444-0580; **Board Cert:** Internal Medicine 1974; Endocrinology, Diabetes & Metabolism 1975; **Med School:** Cornell Univ-Weill Med Coll 1968; **Resid:** Internal Medicine, Barnes-Jewish Hosp 1970; Internal Medicine, Natl Inst Hlth 1972; **Fellow:** Endocrinology, Washington Univ 1974; **Fac Appt:** Prof Med, SUNY Stony Brook

Gelato, Marie MD (EDM) - **Spec Exp:** Thyroid Disorders; Pituitary Disorders; Adrenal Disorders; Polycystic Ovarian Syndrome; **Hospital:** Stony Brook Univ Med Ctr; **Address:** 26 Research Way, East Setauket, NY 11733; **Phone:** 631-444-0580; **Board Cert:** Internal Medicine 1982; Endocrinology 1985; **Med School:** Mich State Univ 1979; **Resid:** Internal Medicine, Dartmouth Med Ctr 1982; **Fellow:** Endocrinology, Natl Inst Hlth 1985; **Fac Appt:** Prof Med, SUNY Stony Brook

Gioia, Leonard V MD (EDM) - **Spec Exp:** Diabetes; Thyroid Disorders; **Hospital:** Southside Hosp, Good Samaritan Hosp Med Ctr - West Islip; **Address:** 53 Brentwood Rd, Ste E, Bay Shore, NY 11706; **Phone:** 631-666-6275; **Board Cert:** Internal Medicine 1979; Endocrinology, Diabetes & Metabolism 1981; **Med School:** SUNY Downstate 1976; **Resid:** Internal Medicine, St Vincent's Hosp & Med Ctr 1979; **Fellow:** Endocrinology, Diabetes & Metabolism, Boston Univ Med Ctr 1981

Goldenberg, Alan MD (EDM) - **Spec Exp:** Diabetes; Thyroid Disorders; Hormonal Disorders; Addison's Disease; **Hospital:** Southampton Hosp, Peconic Bay Med Ctr; **Address:** East End Endocine Associates, 189 Main Rd, Riverhead, NY 11901; **Phone:** 631-288-7120; **Board Cert:** Internal Medicine 2008; Endocrinology, Diabetes & Metabolism 2008; **Med School:** SUNY Stony Brook 1993; **Resid:** Internal Medicine, Winthrop Univ Hosp 1996; **Fellow:** Endocrinology, Diabetes & Metabolism, Winthrop Univ Hosp 1998

Wexler, Craig B MD (EDM) - **Spec Exp:** Diabetes; Thyroid Disorders; Hormonal Disorders; Cholesterol/Lipid Disorders; **Hospital:** Brookhaven Meml Hosp & Med Ctr; **Address:** 285 Sills Rd, Bldg 15 - Ste D, East Patchogue, NY 11772-8810; **Phone:** 631-758-5858; **Board Cert:** Internal Medicine 1981; Endocrinology, Diabetes & Metabolism 1989; **Med School:** Ros Franklin Univ/Chicago Med Sch 1978; **Resid:** Internal Medicine, LIJ-Hillside Med Ctr 1981; **Fellow:** Endocrinology, Diabetes & Metabolism, LIJ-Hillside Med Ctr 1989

Family Medicine

Aponte, Alex M MD (FMed) *PCP* - **Spec Exp:** Preventive Medicine; **Hospital:** Southampton Hosp; **Address:** Westhampton Primary Care, 80 Old Riverhead Rd, Westhampton Beach, NY 11978; **Phone:** 631-288-7746; **Board Cert:** Family Medicine 2002; **Med School:** SUNY Buffalo 1992; **Resid:** Family Medicine, Overlook Hosp 1995

Blyskal, Stanley MD (FMed) *PCP* - **Spec Exp:** Preventive Cardiology; Depression; Osteoporosis; Bipolar/Mood Disorders; **Hospital:** Southside Hosp; **Address:** 126 E Main St, Ste I, East Islip, NY 11730-2600; **Phone:** 631-581-0090; **Board Cert:** Family Medicine 2004; **Med School:** Albany Med Coll 1974; **Resid:** Family Medicine, Southside Hosp 1977; **Fac Appt:** Asst Clin Prof FMed, SUNY Stony Brook

Fishkin, Michael DO (FMed) *PCP* - **Hospital:** John T Mather Meml Hosp, St Charles Hosp; **Address:** 2500 Nesconset Hwy 7D Bldg, Stony Brook, NY 11790-2566; **Phone:** 631-751-3322; **Board Cert:** Family Medicine 2006; **Med School:** Univ Osteo Med & Hlth Sci, Des Moines 1973; **Resid:** Family Medicine, Nassau County Med Ctr 1976; **Fac Appt:** Assoc Prof FMed, SUNY Stony Brook

Franco, John MD (FMed) *PCP* - **Spec Exp:** Geriatric Care; **Hospital:** St Catherine's of Siena Med Ctr; **Address:** 9 Brooksite Dr, Smithtown, NY 11787; **Phone:** 631-724-1331; **Board Cert:** Family Medicine 2002; **Med School:** Mexico 1974; **Resid:** Family Medicine, Nassau County Med Ctr 1978

Giugliano, James E DO (FMed) *PCP* - **Spec Exp:** Lyme Disease; **Hospital:** Southampton Hosp; **Address:** 290 N Sea Rd, Southampton, NY 11968; **Phone:** 631-283-5900; **Board Cert:** Family Medicine 2005; **Med School:** NY Coll Osteo Med 1988; **Resid:** Family Medicine, Southside Hosp 1991

Greenblatt, Louis DO (FMed) *PCP* - **Spec Exp:** Preventive Medicine; Geriatric Medicine; **Hospital:** St Catherine's of Siena Med Ctr, Stony Brook Univ Med Ctr; **Address:** 533 Rte 111, Hauppauge, NY 11788; **Phone:** 631-366-1788; **Board Cert:** Family Medicine 2007; Geriatric Medicine 2006; **Med School:** NY Coll Osteo Med 1983; **Resid:** Family Medicine, Univ Hosp 1986; **Fac Appt:** Asst Clin Prof FMed, SUNY Stony Brook

Levites, Kenneth MD (FMed) *PCP* - **Spec Exp:** Asthma; Occupational Medicine; Hypertension; Diabetes; **Hospital:** Southside Hosp, Good Samaritan Hosp Med Ctr - West Islip; **Address:** 213 Montauk Hwy, West Sayville, NY 11796-1800; **Phone:** 631-563-6205; **Board Cert:** Family Medicine 2003; **Med School:** Albany Med Coll 1974; **Resid:** Family Medicine, Southside Hosp 1977

Schwinn, Hans Dieter MD (FMed) *PCP* - **Hospital:** Southampton Hosp; **Address:** 80 Old Riverhead Rd, Westhampton Beach, NY 11978-1401; **Phone:** 631-288-7746; **Board Cert:** Family Medicine 2007; **Med School:** Germany 1978; **Resid:** Family Medicine, Community Hosp 1981

Gastroenterology

Cohn, William J MD (Ge) - **Spec Exp:** Liver Disease; **Hospital:** John T Mather Meml Hosp, St Charles Hosp; **Address:** 3400 Nesconset Hwy, Ste 101, Setauket, NY 11733-3327; **Phone:** 631-751-8700; **Board Cert:** Internal Medicine 1975; Gastroenterology 1979; **Med School:** Med Coll VA 1972; **Resid:** Internal Medicine, Med Coll Virginia Affil Hosp 1975; **Fellow:** Gastroenterology, Albert Einstein Med Ctr 1978; **Fac Appt:** Asst Clin Prof Med, SUNY Stony Brook

Duva, Joseph M MD (Ge) - **Spec Exp:** Endoscopy & Colonoscopy; Gastroesophageal Reflux Disease (GERD); Irritable Bowel Syndrome; Colonoscopy/Polypectomy; **Hospital:** Peconic Bay Med Ctr; **Address:** 887 Old Country Rd, Ste A, Riverhead, NY 11901-2115; **Phone:** 631-727-6122; **Board Cert:** Internal Medicine 1981; Gastroenterology 2007; **Med School:** Mount Sinai Sch Med 1978; **Resid:** Internal Medicine, Nassau County Med Ctr 1980; **Fellow:** Gastroenterology, Nassau County Med Ctr 1983

Glanzman, Barry MD (Ge) - **Spec Exp:** Colonoscopy; Gastroesophageal Reflux Disease (GERD); Liver Disease; **Hospital:** Huntington Hosp; **Address:** 152 E Main St, Ste C, Huntington, NY 11743; **Phone:** 631-421-2185; **Board Cert:** Gastroenterology 1989; Internal Medicine 1984; **Med School:** SUNY Downstate 1980; **Resid:** Internal Medicine, LI Jewish hosp 1981; Internal Medicine, LI Jewish Hosp 1983; **Fellow:** Gastroenterology, Med Coll of VA 1986

Harrison, Aaron R MD (Ge) - **Spec Exp:** Gastroesophageal Reflux Disease (GERD); Colon Cancer; Crohn's Disease; **Hospital:** Southside Hosp, Good Samaritan Hosp Med Ctr - West Islip; **Address:** 375 E Main St, Ste 21, Bay Shore, NY 11706; **Phone:** 631-968-8288; **Board Cert:** Internal Medicine 1977; Gastroenterology 1979; **Med School:** Albert Einstein Coll Med 1974; **Resid:** Internal Medicine, Jacobi Med Ctr 1977; **Fellow:** Gastroenterology, UCLA Med Ctr 1979; **Fac Appt:** Asst Clin Prof Med, SUNY Stony Brook

Lazar, Robert MD (Ge) - **Hospital:** St Catherine's of Siena Med Ctr; **Address:** 48 Route 25A, Ste 107, Smithtown, NY 11787-1431; **Phone:** 631-862-3680; **Board Cert:** Internal Medicine 1986; Gastroenterology 2000; **Med School:** Mexico 1982

Spielberg, Alan MD (Ge) - **Spec Exp:** Inflammatory Bowel Disease; Colitis; Colonoscopy; **Hospital:** St Catherine's of Siena Med Ctr; **Address:** 48 Route 25A, Ste 203, Smithtown, NY 11787-1448; **Phone:** 631-724-1178; **Board Cert:** Internal Medicine 1977; Gastroenterology 1979; **Med School:** Belgium 1974; **Resid:** Internal Medicine, Albany Med Ctr 1977; **Fellow:** Gastroenterology, Albany Med Ctr 1979

Gynecologic Oncology

Pearl, Michael L MD (GO) - **Spec Exp:** Gynecologic Cancer; Gynecologic Surgery-Complex; **Hospital:** Stony Brook Univ Med Ctr; **Address:** 3 Edmund D Pellegrino Drive, Stony Brook, NY 11794-9456; **Phone:** 631-444-2989; **Board Cert:** Obstetrics & Gynecology 2008; Gynecologic Oncology 2008; **Med School:** UCSF 1986; **Resid:** Obstetrics & Gynecology, UCSF Med Ctr 1990; **Fellow:** Gynecologic Oncology, Univ Michigan 1994; **Fac Appt:** Prof ObG, SUNY Stony Brook

Hand Surgery

Hurst, Lawrence C MD (HS) - **Spec Exp:** Microvascular Surgery; Nerve Disorders; Dupuytren's Contracture; **Hospital:** Stony Brook Univ Med Ctr; **Address:** 14 Technology Drive, Ste 11, E Setauket, NY 11733-3464; **Phone:** 631-444-3145; **Board Cert:** Orthopaedic Surgery 1980; Hand Surgery 2010; **Med School:** Univ VT Coll Med 1973; **Resid:** Orthopaedic Surgery, N Carolina Meml Hosp 1978; **Fellow:** Hand Surgery, Columbia-Presby Med Ctr 1979; **Fac Appt:** Prof OrS, SUNY Stony Brook

Hematology

Avvento, Louis MD (Hem) - **Spec Exp:** Breast Cancer; Lymphoma; **Hospital:** Peconic Bay Med Ctr, Southampton Hosp; **Address:** 1333 E Main St, Riverhead, NY 11901; **Phone:** 631-727-8500; **Board Cert:** Internal Medicine 1985; Medical Oncology 1987; Hematology 2004; **Med School:** Italy 1981; **Resid:** Internal Medicine, Jamaica Med Ctr 1985; **Fellow:** Hematology, Univ Hosp-SUNY 1988

Buchholtz, Michael MD (Hem) - **Spec Exp:** Hematologic Malignancies; Breast Cancer; **Hospital:** Huntington Hosp; **Address:** 270 Pulaski Rd, Ste D, Greenlawn, NY 11740; **Phone:** 631-427-6060; **Board Cert:** Medical Oncology 1999; **Med School:** Italy 1983; **Resid:** Internal Medicine, Mt Sinai Sch Med/Bronx VAMC 1986; **Fellow:** Medical Oncology, North Shore Univ Hosp 1989

Schulman, Philip MD (Hem) - **Spec Exp:** Leukemia; Lymphoma; Multiple Myeloma; Myelodysplastic Syndromes; **Hospital:** Meml Sloan-Kettering Cancer Ctr (page 112), St Catherine's of Siena Med Ctr; **Address:** Meml Sloan Kettering at Suffolk, 650 Commack Rd, Commack, NY 11725; **Phone:** 631-623-4100; **Board Cert:** Internal Medicine 1977; Medical Oncology 1979; Hematology 1980; **Med School:** SUNY Upstate Med Univ 1974; **Resid:** Internal Medicine, N Shore Univ Hosp 1976; Medical Oncology, Meml Sloan-Kettering 1977; **Fellow:** Medical Oncology, Meml Sloan-Kettering 1978; Hematology, N Shore Univ Hosp 1979; **Fac Appt:** Prof Med, Cornell Univ-Weill Med Coll

Schuster, Michael W MD (Hem) - **Spec Exp:** Bone Marrow Transplant; **Hospital:** Stony Brook Univ Med Ctr, NY-Presby Hosp/Weill Cornell (page 104); **Address:** Stony Brook University, SUNY-7099, 100 Nichols Rd, Stony Brook, NY 11794-7909; **Phone:** 631-444-3577; **Board Cert:** Internal Medicine 1984; Hematology 1986; **Med School:** Dartmouth Med Sch 1980; **Resid:** Internal Medicine, New Eng Deaconess Hosp 1983; **Fellow:** Hematology & Oncology, Beth Israel Med Ctr 1987; **Fac Appt:** Assoc Prof Med, Cornell Univ-Weill Med Coll

Infectious Disease

Nash, Bernard J MD (Inf) - **Hospital:** Good Samaritan Hosp Med Ctr - West Islip, Southside Hosp; **Address:** 500 Montauk Hwy, Ste S, West Islip, NY 11795; **Phone:** 631-587-7733; **Board Cert:** Internal Medicine 1978; Infectious Disease 1982; **Med School:** Georgetown Univ 1975; **Resid:** Internal Medicine, St Elizabeth Hosp 1978; **Fellow:** Infectious Disease, Boston Univ Med Ctr 1981

Sacks-Berg, Anne C MD (Inf) - **Spec Exp:** Travel Medicine; **Hospital:** Huntington Hosp; **Address:** 120 New York Ave, Ste 5W, Huntington, NY 11743-2743; **Phone:** 631-423-9809; **Board Cert:** Internal Medicine 1986; Infectious Disease 1988; **Med School:** SUNY Hlth Sci Ctr 1983; **Resid:** Internal Medicine, Winthrop Univ Hosp 1986; **Fellow:** Infectious Disease, Winthrop Univ Hosp 1988

Samuels, Steven MD (Inf) - **Spec Exp:** Lyme Disease; AIDS/HIV; **Hospital:** Good Samaritan Hosp Med Ctr - West Islip, Southside Hosp; **Address:** 500 Montauk Hwy, Ste S, West Islip, NY 11795; **Phone:** 631-587-7733; **Board Cert:** Internal Medicine 1977; Infectious Disease 1982; **Med School:** NY Med Coll 1974; **Resid:** Internal Medicine, Nassau County Med Ctr 1977; **Fellow:** Immunopathology, UC Irvine Med Ctr 1979; **Fac Appt:** Asst Prof Med, SUNY Stony Brook

Internal Medicine

Balot, Barry DO (IM) *PCP* - **Spec Exp:** Geriatric Medicine; **Hospital:** Good Samaritan Hosp Med Ctr - West Islip, Southside Hosp; **Address:** 150 E Sunrise Hwy, Lindenhurst, NY 11757; **Phone:** 631-225-6200; **Board Cert:** Internal Medicine 1989; **Med School:** NY Coll Osteo Med 1985; **Resid:** Internal Medicine, Univ Hosp 1987; Internal Medicine, Overlook Hosp 1989

Bernard, Robert MD (IM) *PCP* - **Spec Exp:** Heart Disease; Skin Diseases; **Hospital:** Peconic Bay Med Ctr; **Address:** 6144 Rte 25-A C Bldg - Ste 10, Wading River, NY 11792; **Phone:** 631-929-5900; **Board Cert:** Internal Medicine 1989; **Med School:** Grenada 1986; **Resid:** Internal Medicine, St Joseph's Hosp & Med Ctr 1989

Covey, Alexander J MD (IM) - **Spec Exp:** Aging Skin; **Hospital:** Peconic Bay Med Ctr; **Address:** 445 Main St, Center Moriches, NY 11934; **Phone:** 631-878-9200; **Board Cert:** Internal Medicine 1988; **Med School:** Ros Franklin Univ/Chicago Med Sch 1985; **Resid:** Internal Medicine, Winthrop Univ Hosp 1988

Delman, Michael MD (IM) *PCP* - **Spec Exp:** Addiction/Substance Abuse; Gastroenterology; **Hospital:** Southside Hosp; **Address:** 301 E Main St, Bayshore, NY 11706; **Phone:** 631-968-3322; **Board Cert:** Internal Medicine 1972; Gastroenterology 1975; Addiction Medicine 1991; **Med School:** NY Med Coll 1968; **Resid:** Internal Medicine, NY Med-Metro Hosp Ctr 1971; Gastroenterology, NY Med-Metro Hosp Ctr 1972; **Fellow:** Gastroenterology, NY Med-Metro Hosp Ctr 1973; **Fac Appt:** Asst Clin Prof Med, SUNY Stony Brook

Friedling, Steven MD (IM) *PCP* - **Spec Exp:** Preventive Medicine; Chronic Illness; **Hospital:** St Catherine's of Siena Med Ctr, Stony Brook Univ Med Ctr; **Address:** 267 E Main St A Bldg, Smithtown, NY 11787-2580; **Phone:** 631-724-8348; **Board Cert:** Internal Medicine 1973; Infectious Disease 1980; **Med School:** SUNY Downstate 1968; **Resid:** Medical Oncology, Natl Cancer Inst 1971; Internal Medicine, Barnes Hosp 1973; **Fellow:** Infectious Disease, Barnes Hosp 1974; **Fac Appt:** Asst Prof Med, SUNY Stony Brook

German, Harold MD (IM) *PCP* - **Spec Exp:** Hematology; **Hospital:** Huntington Hosp; **Address:** 150 Main St, Huntington, NY 11743-6908; **Phone:** 631-271-8700; **Board Cert:** Internal Medicine 1973; Hematology 1978; **Med School:** Columbia P&S 1967; **Resid:** Internal Medicine, Lenox Hill Hosp 1968; Internal Medicine, Columbia Presby Hosp 1972; **Fellow:** Hematology, Columbia Presby Hosp 1973

Goldfarb, Steven MD (IM) *PCP* - **Spec Exp:** Lyme Disease; Preventive Medicine; Concierge Medicine; **Hospital:** Southampton Hosp; **Address:** 365 County Rd 39-A, Ste 12, Southampton, NY 11968; **Phone:** 631-283-5542; **Board Cert:** Internal Medicine 1989; **Med School:** Italy 1983; **Resid:** Internal Medicine, Berkshire Med Ctr-Univ Mass 1986

Hallal, Edward J MD (IM) *PCP* - **Hospital:** Southside Hosp, Good Samaritan Hosp Med Ctr - West Islip; **Address:** 180 E Main St, Bay Shore, NY 11706; **Phone:** 631-665-0027; **Board Cert:** Internal Medicine 1987; **Med School:** Grenada 1984; **Resid:** Internal Medicine, NY Methodist Hosp 1987

Lalli, Corradino MD (IM) *PCP* - **Spec Exp:** Geriatric Medicine; **Hospital:** St Catherine's of Siena Med Ctr; **Address:** 363 Route 111, Ste 106, Smithtown, NY 11787-4739; **Phone:** 631-366-0404; **Board Cert:** Internal Medicine 1979; Geriatric Medicine 1998; **Med School:** Albert Einstein Coll Med 1976; **Resid:** Internal Medicine, Nassau County Med Ctr 1979; **Fellow:** Pulmonary Disease, Nassau County Med Ctr 1980; **Fac Appt:** Asst Clin Prof Med, SUNY Stony Brook

Oppenheimer, John MD (IM) *PCP* - **Spec Exp:** Geriatric Medicine; AIDS/HIV; **Hospital:** Southampton Hosp; **Address:** PO Box 3137, Sag Harbor, NY 11963; **Phone:** 631-725-4600; **Board Cert:** Internal Medicine 1984; Geriatric Medicine 2009; **Med School:** Tulane Univ 1981; **Resid:** Internal Medicine, Tulane Univ Hosp 1982; Internal Medicine, Harlem Hosp 1983; **Fac Appt:** Asst Clin Prof Med, SUNY Stony Brook

Romano, Rosario MD (IM) *PCP* - **Spec Exp:** Geriatric Care; Cholesterol/Lipid Disorders; **Hospital:** John T Mather Meml Hosp, St Charles Hosp; **Address:** 5225-15 Rte 347, Port Jefferson Station, NY 11776-2054; **Phone:** 631-331-1000; **Board Cert:** Internal Medicine 1977; **Med School:** NY Med Coll 1973; **Resid:** Internal Medicine, Lenox Hill Hosp 1977; **Fac Appt:** Asst Clin Prof Med, SUNY Stony Brook

Simon, Lloyd MD (IM) *PCP* - **Spec Exp:** Addiction/Substance Abuse; **Hospital:** Eastern Long Island Hosp; **Address:** 44210C County Rd 48, Box 1341, Southold, NY 11971; **Phone:** 631-765-4150; **Board Cert:** Internal Medicine 1983; **Med School:** SUNY Buffalo 1980; **Resid:** Internal Medicine, Univ Mass Med Ctr 1983

Maternal & Fetal Medicine

Monheit, Alan G MD (MF) - **Spec Exp:** Pregnancy-High Risk; Preconception Planning; **Hospital:** Stony Brook Univ Med Ctr; **Address:** 6 Technology Drive, East Setauket, NY 11733; **Phone:** 631-444-4686; **Board Cert:** Obstetrics & Gynecology 1982; Maternal & Fetal Medicine 1983; **Med School:** Univ Pennsylvania 1975; **Resid:** Obstetrics & Gynecology, UCSD Med Ctr 1979; **Fellow:** Maternal & Fetal Medicine, UCSD Med Ctr 1981; **Fac Appt:** Assoc Clin Prof ObG, SUNY Stony Brook

Medical Oncology

Akhund, Birjis G MD (Onc) - **Spec Exp:** Breast Cancer; Lymphoma; Lung Cancer; **Hospital:** Huntington Hosp, N Shore Univ Hosp; **Address:** Huntington Medical Group, 180 East Pulaski Rd, Huntington Sta, NY 11746; **Phone:** 631-425-2280; **Board Cert:** Internal Medicine 1989; Medical Oncology 2003; Hematology 2004; **Med School:** Lebanon 1986; **Resid:** Internal Medicine, Beth Israel Med Ctr 1990; **Fellow:** Hematology & Oncology, NYU Med Ctr 1992; Hematology Research, NYU Med Ctr 1993

Caruso, Rocco MD (Onc) - **Spec Exp:** Lymphoma; **Hospital:** Stony Brook Univ Med Ctr, St Catherine's of Siena Med Ctr; **Address:** 2500 Nesconset Hway 26B Bldg, Stony Brook, NY 11790; **Phone:** 631-751-8305; **Board Cert:** Internal Medicine 1982; Hematology 1984; Medical Oncology 2005; **Med School:** Univ Pennsylvania 1979; **Resid:** Internal Medicine, St Luke's-Roosevelt Hosp Ctr 1982; **Fellow:** Hematology, NYU Med Ctr 1985; Medical Oncology, LI Jewish Med Ctr 1994; **Fac Appt:** Asst Prof Med, SUNY Stony Brook

Fiore, John J MD (Onc) - **Spec Exp:** Lung Cancer; **Hospital:** St Catherine's of Siena Med Ctr; **Address:** Meml Sloan Kettering at Suffolk, 650 Commack Rd, Commack, NY 11725; **Phone:** 631-623-4100; **Board Cert:** Internal Medicine 1978; Hematology 1982; Medical Oncology 1983; **Med School:** Tufts Univ 1975; **Resid:** Internal Medicine, VA Med Ctr 1979; **Fellow:** Hematology, VA Med Ctr 1981; Medical Oncology, Meml Sloan Kettering Cancer Ctr 1984

Ostrow, Stanley MD (Onc) - **Spec Exp:** Lymphoma; Breast Cancer; Leukemia; Carcinoid Tumors; **Hospital:** John T Mather Meml Hosp, Brookhaven Meml Hosp & Med Ctr; **Address:** 235 N Belle Mead Rd, East Setauket, NY 11733; **Phone:** 631-751-5151; **Board Cert:** Internal Medicine 1978; Medical Oncology 1979; Hematology 1982; **Med School:** SUNY Downstate 1974; **Resid:** Internal Medicine, Jewish Meml Hosp 1976; **Fellow:** Hematology & Oncology, Natl Cancer Inst 1980; **Fac Appt:** Asst Prof Med, SUNY Stony Brook

Rizvi, Hasan A MD (Onc) - **Hospital:** Good Samaritan Hosp Med Ctr - West Islip, Southside Hosp; **Address:** 180 E Main St, Bay Shore, NY 11706-8427; **Phone:** 631-666-0262; **Board Cert:** Medical Oncology 1999; Hematology 2002; **Med School:** Pakistan 1975; **Resid:** Clinical Pathology, Ellis Hosp 1978; Internal Medicine, Mt Sinai Sch Med 1981; **Fellow:** Hematology & Oncology, Winthrop Univ Hosp 1983; Hematology & Oncology, St Elizabeth Hosp 1984

Strauss, Barry MD (Onc) - **Spec Exp:** Lung Cancer; Breast Cancer; Colon Cancer; **Hospital:** Southampton Hosp; **Address:** 353 Meeting House Ln, Southampton, NY 11968-5051; **Phone:** 631-283-6611; **Board Cert:** Internal Medicine 1975; Medical Oncology 1975; **Med School:** Geo Wash Univ 1971; **Resid:** Internal Medicine, Beth Israel Hosp 1973; **Fellow:** Medical Oncology, National Cancer Inst 1975

Neonatal-Perinatal Medicine

Parekh, Aruna MD (NP) - **Hospital:** Stony Brook Univ Med Ctr, Long Island Coll Hosp (page 94); **Address:** Stony Brook Univ Med Ctr, Dept of Pediatrics, Level 11-060, Stony Brook, NY 11794; **Phone:** 631-444-5437; **Board Cert:** Pediatrics 1976; Neonatal-Perinatal Medicine 1985; **Med School:** India 1970; **Resid:** Pediatrics, LI Coll Hosp 1974; **Fellow:** Neonatal-Perinatal Medicine, N Shore Univ Hosp 1977

Nephrology

Schwarz, Richard B MD (Nep) - **Spec Exp:** Hypertension; Kidney Disease; **Hospital:** Huntington Hosp; **Address:** 325 Park Ave, Huntington, NY 11743-2798; **Phone:** 631-351-3784; **Board Cert:** Internal Medicine 1983; Geriatric Medicine 2000; Nephrology 2000; **Med School:** NYU Sch Med 1979; **Resid:** Internal Medicine, LAC-USC Med Ctr 1981; Internal Medicine, Kaiser Fdn Hosp 1982; **Fellow:** Nephrology, Kaiser Fdn Hosp 1984; **Fac Appt:** Assoc Clin Prof Med, SUNY Stony Brook

Neurological Surgery

Davis, Raphael P MD (NS) - **Spec Exp:** Acoustic Neuroma; Skull Base Surgery; Spinal Disc Replacement; Brain & Spinal Surgery; **Hospital:** Stony Brook Univ Med Ctr, St Charles Hosp; **Address:** 24 Research Way, East Setauket, NY 11733; **Phone:** 631-444-1213; **Board Cert:** Neurological Surgery 1990; **Med School:** Mount Sinai Sch Med 1981; **Resid:** Neurological Surgery, Mt Sinai Med Ctr 1987; **Fac Appt:** Prof NS, SUNY Stony Brook

Woo, Henry H MD (NS) - **Spec Exp:** Brain Tumors; Aneurysm-Cerebral; Cerebrovascular Surgery; Stroke; **Hospital:** Stony Brook Univ Med Ctr; **Address:** 24 Research Way, Ste 200, East Setauket, NY 11733; **Phone:** 631-444-1213; **Board Cert:** Neurological Surgery 2008; **Med School:** NYU Sch Med 1995; **Resid:** Neurological Surgery, NYU Med Ctr 2000; **Fellow:** Neuroradiology, NYU Med Ctr; **Fac Appt:** Assoc Prof NS, SUNY Stony Brook

Neurology

Cohen, Daniel H MD/PhD (N) - **Spec Exp:** Stroke; Neuromuscular Disorders; Multiple Sclerosis; Dementia; **Hospital:** Good Samaritan Hosp Med Ctr - West Islip, Southside Hosp; **Address:** 370 E Main St, Ste 1, Bay Shore, NY 11706; **Phone:** 631-666-4767; **Board Cert:** Neurology 1986; Clinical Neurophysiology 1985; **Med School:** Univ Miami Sch Med 1980; **Resid:** Neurology, Jackson Meml Hosp 1984

Coyle, Patricia K MD (N) - **Spec Exp:** Multiple Sclerosis; Neuro-Immunology; Lyme Disease; Infections-Neurologic; **Hospital:** Stony Brook Univ Med Ctr; **Address:** Dept Neurology, HSC T-12, rm 020, Stonybrook Univ Med Ctr, Stony Brook, NY 11794-8121; **Phone:** 631-444-2599; **Board Cert:** Neurology 2004; **Med School:** Johns Hopkins Univ 1974; **Resid:** Neurology, Johns Hopkins Hosp 1978; **Fellow:** Neurological Immunology, Johns Hopkins Hosp 1980; **Fac Appt:** Prof N, SUNY Stony Brook

Gerber, Oded MD (N) - **Spec Exp:** Stroke; Parkinson's Disease; Neuromuscular Disorders; **Hospital:** Stony Brook Univ Med Ctr; **Address:** SUNY-Stony Brook, Dept Neurology, HSC Bldg Fl 12 - rm 020, Stony Brook, NY 11794-8121; **Phone:** 631-444-2599; **Board Cert:** Neurology 1979; **Med School:** SUNY Downstate 1972; **Resid:** Internal Medicine, Kings County Hosp 1974; Neurology, Mt Sinai Hosp 1977; **Fac Appt:** Asst Clin Prof N, Mount Sinai Sch Med

Moreta, Henry G MD (N) - **Hospital:** Peconic Bay Med Ctr; **Address:** 811 E Main St, Ste 106, Riverhead, NY 11901; **Phone:** 631-727-0660; **Board Cert:** Neurology 1987; **Med School:** Harvard Med Sch 1977; **Resid:** Neurology, New York Hosp 1981

Neuroradiology

Fiorella, David J MD (NRad) - **Spec Exp:** Stroke; Endovascular Surgery; Arteriovenous Malformations; Interventional Neuroradiology; **Hospital:** Stony Brook Univ Med Ctr; **Address:** 24 Research Way, Ste 200, East Setauket, NY 11733; **Phone:** 631-444-1213; **Board Cert:** Diagnostic Radiology 2001; Neuroradiology 2004; **Med School:** SUNY Buffalo 1986; **Resid:** Diagnostic Radiology, Duke Univ Med Ctr 2001; **Fellow:** Neurological Radiology, Barrow Neuro Inst 2003

Obstetrics & Gynecology

Baker, David A MD (ObG) - **Spec Exp:** Infectious Disease; Premature Labor; Vulvar Disease; Vaginal Disease; **Hospital:** Stony Brook Univ Med Ctr; **Address:** Dept Ob/Gyn HSCT9030, Stony Brooke Univ Med Ctr, Nicolls Rd, Stony Brook, NY 11794-8091; **Phone:** 631-444-4686; **Board Cert:** Obstetrics & Gynecology 1979; Maternal & Fetal Medicine 1981; **Med School:** SUNY Hlth Sci Ctr 1973; **Resid:** Obstetrics & Gynecology, Hosp Univ Penn 1977; **Fellow:** Maternal & Fetal Medicine, Med Ctr Hosp 1979; **Fac Appt:** Prof ObG, SUNY Stony Brook

Davenport, Deborah M MD (ObG) - **Spec Exp:** Menopause Problems; **Hospital:** Stony Brook Univ Med Ctr; **Address:** 100-16 S Jersey Ave, East Setauket, NY 11733-2036; **Phone:** 631-689-6400; **Board Cert:** Obstetrics & Gynecology 2009; **Med School:** Univ Pennsylvania 1975; **Resid:** Obstetrics & Gynecology, Univ Hosp 1983; **Fac Appt:** Asst Clin Prof ObG, SUNY Stony Brook

Gentilesco, Michael MD (ObG) *PCP* - **Hospital:** St Catherine's of Siena Med Ctr, Stony Brook Univ Med Ctr; **Address:** 48 Route 25A, Ste 207, Smithtown, NY 11787; **Phone:** 631-862-3800; **Board Cert:** Obstetrics & Gynecology 2009; **Med School:** Albert Einstein Coll Med 1980; **Resid:** Obstetrics & Gynecology, Columbia-Presby Med Ctr 1984

Hirt, Paula MD (ObG) - **Hospital:** Good Samaritan Hosp Med Ctr - West Islip; **Address:** 83 W Main St, East Islip, NY 11730; **Phone:** 631-277-5800; **Board Cert:** Obstetrics & Gynecology 1985; **Med School:** NYU Sch Med 1979; **Resid:** Obstetrics & Gynecology, NYU Med Ctr 1983

Kramer, Mitchell MD (ObG) - **Spec Exp:** Gynecologic Surgery-Complex; Menopause Problems; Minimally Invasive Surgery; Cervical Disease; **Hospital:** Huntington Hosp, N Shore Univ Hosp; **Address:** 180 E Pulaski Rd, Huntington Station, NY 11746; **Phone:** 631-425-2218; **Board Cert:** Obstetrics & Gynecology 2008; **Med School:** NY Med Coll 1985; **Resid:** Obstetrics & Gynecology, LI Jewish Med Ctr 1989; **Fac Appt:** Asst Clin Prof ObG, NYU Sch Med

Lee, Douglas S MD (ObG) *PCP* - **Spec Exp:** Gynecology Only; Menopause Problems; Cervical Disease; **Hospital:** John T Mather Meml Hosp, St Charles Hosp; **Address:** Suffolk Ob/Gyn, 118 N Country Rd, Port Jefferson, NY 11776; **Phone:** 631-475-4404; **Board Cert:** Obstetrics & Gynecology 1979; **Med School:** NYU Sch Med 1973; **Resid:** Obstetrics & Gynecology, Bronx Muni Hosp 1977; **Fac Appt:** Asst Clin Prof ObG, SUNY Stony Brook

Mann, Charles T MD (ObG) *PCP* - **Hospital:** St Catherine's of Siena Med Ctr, Stony Brook Univ Med Ctr; **Address:** 48 Route 25-A, Ste 207, Smithtown, NY 11787; **Phone:** 631-862-3800; **Board Cert:** Obstetrics & Gynecology 1979; **Med School:** Creighton Univ 1974; **Resid:** Obstetrics & Gynecology, Barnes Hosp 1977

Matalon, Martin MD (ObG) - **Hospital:** Southside Hosp, Good Samaritan Hosp Med Ctr - West Islip; **Address:** 375 E Main St, Ste 4, Bay Shore, NY 11706-8418; **Phone:** 631-665-8226; **Board Cert:** Obstetrics & Gynecology 1973; **Med School:** Univ Cincinnati 1966; **Resid:** Obstetrics & Gynecology, Brookdale Univ Med Ctr 1971

Ott, Allen MD (ObG) - **Spec Exp:** Infertility; Colposcopy; Gynecology Only; **Hospital:** Southampton Hosp; **Address:** 595 Hampton Rd, Southampton, NY 11968-3021; **Phone:** 631-283-0918; **Board Cert:** Obstetrics & Gynecology 1979; **Med School:** Boston Univ 1972; **Resid:** Obstetrics & Gynecology, Hosp Univ Penn 1976

San Roman, Gerardo A MD (ObG) - **Spec Exp:** Minimally Invasive Surgery; **Hospital:** St Charles Hosp, John T Mather Meml Hosp; **Address:** 118 N Country Rd, Port Jefferson, NY 11777; **Phone:** 631-473-7171; **Board Cert:** Obstetrics & Gynecology 2009; **Med School:** Johns Hopkins Univ 1981; **Resid:** Obstetrics & Gynecology, NY Hosp 1985

Ophthalmology

Aries, Philip MD (Oph) - **Hospital:** Southside Hosp, Good Samaritan Hosp Med Ctr - West Islip; **Address:** 375 E Main St, rm 24, Bay Shore, NY 11706; **Phone:** 631-665-1330; **Board Cert:** Ophthalmology 1975; **Med School:** NY Med Coll 1967; **Resid:** Ophthalmology, Nassau Co Med Ctr 1973

Bogaty, Stanley MD (Oph) - **Spec Exp:** Glaucoma; **Hospital:** St Charles Hosp, John T Mather Meml Hosp; **Address:** 251 E Oakland Ave, Port Jefferson, NY 11777-2170; **Phone:** 631-473-5329; **Board Cert:** Ophthalmology 1974; **Med School:** Ros Franklin Univ/Chicago Med Sch 1966; **Resid:** Ophthalmology, Beth Israel Hosp 1972

Cossari Jr, Alfred J MD (Oph) - **Spec Exp:** Pediatric Ophthalmology; Strabismus; **Hospital:** John T Mather Meml Hosp, St Charles Hosp; **Address:** 311 Barnum Ave, Port Jefferson, NY 11777-1682; **Phone:** 631-928-6400; **Board Cert:** Ophthalmology 1976; **Med School:** Italy 1969; **Resid:** Ophthalmology, Nassau County Med Ctr 1974; **Fellow:** Retina, Johns Hopkins Hosp 1974; Pediatric Ophthalmology, Chldns Natl Med Ctr 1975

Di Leo, Frank MD (Oph) - **Spec Exp:** Oculoplastic Surgery; **Hospital:** Southampton Hosp, St Luke's - Roosevelt Hosp Ctr - Roosevelt Div (page 94); **Address:** 365 County Road 39A, Ste 2, Southampton, NY 11968-5243; **Phone:** 631-283-3677; **Board Cert:** Ophthalmology 1987; **Med School:** Albert Einstein Coll Med 1981; **Resid:** Ophthalmology, St Luke's-Roosevelt Hosp Ctr 1985

Elbaba, Fadi MD (Oph) - **Spec Exp:** Retina/Vitreous Surgery; Diabetic Eye Disease/Retinopathy; Macular Degeneration; HIV Retinitis; **Hospital:** Stony Brook Univ Med Ctr; **Address:** 33 Research Way, Ste 13, East Setauket, NY 11733; **Phone:** 631-444-4090; **Board Cert:** Ophthalmology 2003; **Med School:** Amer Univ Beirut 1982; **Resid:** Ophthalmology, Amer Univ Beirut 1987; Ophthalmology, Doheny Eye Inst/USC Med Ctr 1991; **Fellow:** Eye Pathology, Wilmer Eye Inst/Johns Hopkins 1986; Retina, Oregon Lions Sight & Hearing Inst 1987; **Fac Appt:** Assoc Prof Oph, SUNY Stony Brook

Martin, Jeffrey MD (Oph) - **Spec Exp:** Cataract Surgery; Laser Vision Surgery; **Hospital:** St Catherine's of Siena Med Ctr, Stony Brook Univ Med Ctr; **Address:** 260 Middle Country Rd, Ste 201, Smithtown, NY 11787; **Phone:** 631-265-8780; **Board Cert:** Ophthalmology 1999; **Med School:** SUNY Stony Brook 1994; **Resid:** Ophthalmology, Nassau Co Med Ctr 1998; **Fac Appt:** Asst Clin Prof Oph, SUNY Stony Brook

Michalos, Peter MD (Oph) - **Spec Exp:** Cataract Surgery; Reconstructive Surgery; Eyelid Tumors/Cancer; Oculoplastic Surgery; **Hospital:** Southampton Hosp, NY-Presby Hosp/Columbia (page 104); **Address:** 365 County Road 39-A, Ste 14, Southampton, NY 11968-5243; **Phone:** 631-283-8604; **Board Cert:** Ophthalmology 1991; **Med School:** SUNY Downstate 1986; **Resid:** Ophthalmology, St Luke's-Roosevelt Hosp Ctr 1990; **Fellow:** Ophthalmic Plastic & Reconstructive Surgery, Columbia-Presby Med Ctr 1991; **Fac Appt:** Assoc Clin Prof Oph, Columbia P&S

Morris, Robert P MD (Oph) - **Hospital:** St Catherine's of Siena Med Ctr; **Address:** 222 E Main St, Ste 330, Smithtown, NY 11787; **Phone:** 631-724-4488; **Board Cert:** Ophthalmology 1974; **Med School:** SUNY Upstate Med Univ 1966; **Resid:** Ophthalmology, SUNY Downstate Med Ctr 1972

Nattis, Richard J MD (Oph) - **Spec Exp:** Cataract Surgery; Laser Vision Surgery; **Hospital:** Good Samaritan Hosp Med Ctr - West Islip, Southside Hosp; **Address:** 150 East Sunrise Hwy, Ste 105, Lindenhurst, NY 11757; **Phone:** 631-957-3355; **Board Cert:** Ophthalmology 1985; **Med School:** NY Med Coll 1980; **Resid:** Ophthalmology, St Vincent's Hosp 1984; **Fac Appt:** Asst Clin Prof Oph, NY Coll Osteo Med

O'Malley, Grace M MD (Oph) - **Spec Exp:** Cataract Surgery; LASIK-Refractive Surgery; **Hospital:** Southampton Hosp; **Address:** 186 Old Towne Rd, Southampton, NY 11968; **Phone:** 631-283-3533; **Board Cert:** Ophthalmology 1987; **Med School:** NY Med Coll 1981; **Resid:** Ophthalmology, NY Med Coll 1985

Pizzarello, Louis MD (Oph) - **Spec Exp:** Diabetic Eye Disease/Retinopathy; Oculoplastic Surgery; **Hospital:** Southampton Hosp, Eastern Long Island Hosp; **Address:** 137 Hampton Rd, Southampton, NY 11968; **Phone:** 631-283-5152; **Board Cert:** Ophthalmology 1980; **Med School:** Univ VA Sch Med 1975; **Resid:** Ophthalmology, Columbia-Presby Med Ctr 1979

Romanelli, John MD (Oph) - **Spec Exp:** Cataract Surgery; Glaucoma; **Hospital:** St Catherine's of Siena Med Ctr, Stony Brook Univ Med Ctr; **Address:** 222 E Main St, Ste 330, Smithtown, NY 11787-2814; **Phone:** 631-724-4488; **Board Cert:** Ophthalmology 2003; **Med School:** Harvard Med Sch 1987; **Resid:** Ophthalmology, Manhattan EET Hosp 1991; **Fac Appt:** Clin Prof Oph, SUNY Stony Brook

Rothberg, Charles MD (Oph) - **Spec Exp:** Cataract Surgery; Glaucoma; LASIK-Refractive Surgery; **Hospital:** Brookhaven Meml Hosp & Med Ctr; **Address:** 331 East Main Street, Patchogue, NY 11772-3114; **Phone:** 631-758-5300; **Board Cert:** Ophthalmology 1989; **Med School:** SUNY Downstate 1983; **Resid:** Ophthalmology, Univ Hosp 1987

Schneck, Gideon MD (Oph) - **Spec Exp:** Eyelid Cosmetic Surgery; Thyroid Eye Disease; Orbital Surgery; **Hospital:** Stony Brook Univ Med Ctr, St Charles Hosp; **Address:** 2500 Rt 347 17B, Stony Brook, NY 11790; **Phone:** 631-246-9140; **Board Cert:** Ophthalmology 1991; **Med School:** Boston Univ 1986; **Resid:** Ophthalmology, Northwestern Univ Med Sch 1990; **Fellow:** Oculoplastic Surgery, IL Eye & Ear Infirmary 1991; **Fac Appt:** Asst Clin Prof Oph, SUNY Stony Brook

Sibony, Patrick A MD (Oph) - **Spec Exp:** Neuro-Ophthalmology; Orbital Diseases; **Hospital:** Stony Brook Univ Med Ctr; **Address:** Stony Brook Ophthalmology, 33 Research Way, East Setauket, NY 11733; **Phone:** 631-444-4090; **Board Cert:** Ophthalmology 1982; **Med School:** Boston Univ 1977; **Resid:** Ophthalmology, Boston Univ Med Ctr 1981; **Fellow:** Ophthalmology, Eye & Ear Hosp 1982; **Fac Appt:** Prof Oph, SUNY Stony Brook

Stoller, Gerald MD (Oph) - **Spec Exp:** Retinal Disorders; **Hospital:** St Charles Hosp, John T Mather Meml Hosp; **Address:** 251 E Oakland Ave, Port Jefferson, NY 11777-2170; **Phone:** 631-473-5329; **Board Cert:** Ophthalmology 1973; **Med School:** Temple Univ 1966; **Resid:** Ophthalmology, Bronx Municipal Hosp 1971

Weber, Pamela MD (Oph) - **Spec Exp:** Retinal Disorders; Macular Degeneration; Diabetic Eye Disease/Retinopathy; **Hospital:** Stony Brook Univ Med Ctr, St Charles Hosp; **Address:** 1500 William Floyd Pkwy, Ste 304, Shirley, NY 11967; **Phone:** 631-924-4300; **Board Cert:** Ophthalmology 1989; **Med School:** Columbia P&S 1984; **Resid:** Ophthalmology, New York Eye & Ear Infirm 1988; **Fellow:** Vitreoretinal Surgery, Retina Assoc 1990; **Fac Appt:** Asst Prof Oph, SUNY Stony Brook

Zweibel, Lawrence MD (Oph) - **Spec Exp:** LASIK-Refractive Surgery; Cataract Surgery; Glaucoma; **Hospital:** St Catherine's of Siena Med Ctr; **Address:** 260 Middle Country Rd, Ste 201, Smithtown, NY 11787-2982; **Phone:** 631-265-8780; **Board Cert:** Ophthalmology 1977; **Med School:** Albany Med Coll 1972; **Resid:** Ophthalmology, French-Polyclinic Hosp 1976

Orthopaedic Surgery

Alpert, Scott W MD (OrS) - **Spec Exp:** Shoulder & Elbow Surgery; Hip Surgery; Knee Surgery; Sports Medicine; **Hospital:** Huntington Hosp, Hosp For Special Surgery (page 111); **Address:** 379 Oakwood Rd, Huntington Station, NY 11746-3627; **Phone:** 631-423-4090; **Board Cert:** Orthopaedic Surgery 2008; **Med School:** Harvard Med Sch 1989; **Resid:** Orthopaedic Surgery, Hosp Joint Diseases 1994; **Fellow:** Sports Medicine, Kerlan-Jobe Orth Clinic 1995

Dowling, Thomas MD (OrS) - **Spec Exp:** Spinal Surgery; Spinal Deformity; **Hospital:** St Catherine's of Siena Med Ctr, Huntington Hosp; **Address:** 763 Larkfield Rd Fl 2, Commack, NY 11725-2900; **Phone:** 631-462-2225; **Board Cert:** Orthopaedic Surgery 2000; **Med School:** Boston Univ 1981; **Resid:** Surgery, North Shore Univ Hosp 1983; Orthopaedic Surgery, SUNY Univ Hosp 1987; **Fellow:** Spinal Surgery, North Shore Univ Hosp 1983; Spinal Surgery, Univ Toronto 1988

Tabershaw, Richard MD (OrS) - **Spec Exp:** Shoulder Surgery; Sports Medicine; Reconstructive Surgery; Arthroscopic Surgery; **Hospital:** Southside Hosp, St Joseph's Hosp-Nassau; **Address:** 375 E Main St, Ste 1, Bay Shore, NY 11706-8418; **Phone:** 631-665-8790; **Board Cert:** Orthopaedic Surgery 2009; **Med School:** Georgetown Univ 1980; **Resid:** Surgery, St Vincent Med Ctr 1983; Orthopaedic Surgery, Columbia-Presby Hosp 1986

Otolaryngology

Chitkara, Dev MD (Oto) - **Spec Exp:** Hearing Disorders; Balance Disorders; **Hospital:** St Catherine's of Siena Med Ctr; **Address:** 29 Manor Rd, Smithtown, NY 11787-2714; **Phone:** 631-979-0311; **Board Cert:** Otolaryngology 1967; **Med School:** India 1961; **Resid:** Surgery, LI Coll Hosp 1964; Otolaryngology, Boston Med Ctr 1967; **Fellow:** Otolaryngology, Georgetown Univ Hosp 1970; **Fac Appt:** Asst Clin Prof Oto, SUNY Stony Brook

Gargano, Robert M MD (Oto) - **Hospital:** Southside Hosp; **Address:** 375 E Main St, rm 17, Bay Shore, NY 11706; **Phone:** 631-665-2430; **Board Cert:** Otolaryngology 1989; **Med School:** Tufts Univ 1984; **Resid:** Otolaryngology, New England Med Ctr 1989

Litman, Richard MD (Oto) - **Spec Exp:** Pediatric Otolaryngology; Head & Neck Surgery; Otology; Sinus Surgery; **Hospital:** John T Mather Meml Hosp, St Charles Hosp; **Address:** 251 E Oakland Ave, Port Jefferson, NY 11777; **Phone:** 631-928-0188; **Board Cert:** Otolaryngology 1976; **Med School:** Wake Forest Univ 1971; **Resid:** Surgery, LIJ Med Ctr 1973; **Fellow:** Otolaryngology, Bronx Muni Hosp 1976; **Fac Appt:** Asst Clin Prof Oto, SUNY Stony Brook

Pain Medicine

Agin, Carole MD (PM) - **Spec Exp:** Acupuncture; Complex Regional Pain Syndrome; Pain-Neuropathic; Pain-Back; **Hospital:** Stony Brook Univ Med Ctr; **Address:** Pain Management Ctr, Stony Brook Univ Hosp, 3 Edmund D. Pellegrino Rd, Stony Brook, NY 11794-9464; **Phone:** 631-638-0800; **Board Cert:** Anesthesiology 1991; Pain Medicine 2004; **Med School:** Ros Franklin Univ/Chicago Med Sch 1986; **Resid:** Anesthesiology, Beth Israel Med Ctr 1990; **Fellow:** Pain Medicine, Meml Sloan Kettering Cancer Ctr 1991; **Fac Appt:** Assoc Prof Anes, SUNY Stony Brook

Gargiulo, Juan MD (PM) - **Spec Exp:** Pain-Chronic; Pain-Back; Pain-Cancer; **Hospital:** Southampton Hosp, Peconic Bay Med Ctr; **Address:** 365 County Rd 39A, Ste 15-16, Southampton, NY 11968; **Phone:** 631-702-2300; **Board Cert:** Anesthesiology 1993; Pain Medicine 2009; **Med School:** Uruguay 1984; **Resid:** Anesthesiology, Westchester Med Ctr 1991; Pain Medicine, Westchester Med Ctr 1991

Litman, Steven J MD (PM) - **Spec Exp:** Pain-Back & Neck; Pain-after Spinal Intervention; **Hospital:** Good Samaritan Hosp Med Ctr - West Islip, St Charles Hosp; **Address:** All Island Pain Consultants, 387 E Main St, Ste 104, Bayshore, NY 11706; **Phone:** 631-665-0075; **Board Cert:** Anesthesiology 2003; Pain Medicine 2007; **Med School:** NY Med Coll 1987; **Resid:** Anesthesiology, Westchester Co Med Ctr 1991; **Fac Appt:** Asst Clin Prof Anes, SUNY Stony Brook

Vaillancourt, Philippe D MD (PM) - **Spec Exp:** Headache; Pain-Chronic; **Hospital:** Southampton Hosp, Peconic Bay Med Ctr; **Address:** 877 E Main St, Ste 106, Riverhead, NY 11901; **Phone:** 631-727-0660; **Board Cert:** Neurology 1986; Pain Medicine 2000; **Med School:** McGill Univ 1978; **Resid:** Neurology, Mount Sinai Med Ctr 1983; **Fac Appt:** Assoc Prof N, SUNY Stony Brook

Pathology

Tornos, Carmen MD (Path) - **Spec Exp:** Gynecologic Cancer; Breast Cancer; Ovarian Cancer; **Hospital:** Stony Brook Univ Med Ctr; **Address:** Stony Brook Univ Hosp, Dept Pathology, Level 2, rm 766, Stony Brook, NY 11794; **Phone:** 631-444-2222; **Board Cert:** Anatomic & Clinical Pathology 1989; **Med School:** Spain 1977; **Resid:** Hematology, Ciudad Sanitaria Valle de Hebron 1982; Anatomic & Clinical Pathology, Univ Texas HSC 1989; **Fellow:** Surgical Pathology, MD Anderson Cancer Ctr 1990; **Fac Appt:** Prof Path, SUNY Stony Brook

Pediatric Cardiology

Biancaniello, Thomas MD (PCd) - **Spec Exp:** Congenital Heart Disease; Fetal Echocardiography; Interventional Cardiology; Cardiac Catheterization; **Hospital:** Stony Brook Univ Med Ctr, Steven & Alexandra Cohen Chldn's Med Ctr of NY; **Address:** Stony Brook Univ Hosp, Dept Pediatrics, HSC T11, 040, Stony Brook, NY 11794-8111; **Phone:** 631-444-5437; **Board Cert:** Pediatrics 1979; Pediatric Cardiology 1981; **Med School:** NY Med Coll 1975; **Resid:** Pediatrics, North Shore Univ Hosp 1977; **Fellow:** Pediatric Cardiology, Cincinnati Chldns Hosp 1980; **Fac Appt:** Prof Ped, SUNY Stony Brook

Pediatric Endocrinology

Wilson, Thomas MD (PEn) - **Spec Exp:** Growth Disorders; Adrenal Disorders; Sexual Differentiation Disorders; Thyroid Disorders; **Hospital:** Stony Brook Univ Med Ctr; **Address:** SUNY Stony Brook, Dept Pediatric Endocrinology, HSC T11, rm 080, Stony Brook, NY 11794-8111; **Phone:** 631-444-5437; **Board Cert:** Pediatrics 1983; **Med School:** Univ Pennsylvania 1973; **Resid:** Pediatrics, Chldns Hosp 1976; **Fellow:** Pediatric Endocrinology, Univ Virginia Med Ctr 1982; **Fac Appt:** Prof Ped, SUNY Stony Brook

Pediatric Gastroenterology

Chawla, Anupama MD (PGe) - **Spec Exp:** Gastroesophageal Reflux Disease (GERD); Crohn's Disease; Inflammatory Bowel Disease; **Hospital:** Stony Brook Univ Med Ctr; **Address:** University Med Ctr, Level 5, Nicholls Road, Stony Brook, NY 11790; **Phone:** 631-444-5437; **Board Cert:** Pediatrics 2008; Pediatric Gastroenterology 2007; **Med School:** India 1980; **Resid:** Pediatrics, Stony Brook Med Ctr 1987; **Fellow:** Pediatric Gastroenterology, N Shore Univ Hosp 1987; **Fac Appt:** Asst Prof Ped, SUNY Stony Brook

Gold, David MD (PGe) - **Spec Exp:** Gastroesophageal Reflux Disease (GERD); Irritable Bowel Syndrome; Ulcerative Colitis/Crohn's; **Hospital:** Good Samaritan Hosp Med Ctr - West Islip; **Address:** 655 Deer Park Ave, Babylon, NY 11702; **Phone:** 631-321-2190; **Board Cert:** Pediatric Gastroenterology 2003; **Med School:** Albert Einstein Coll Med 1987; **Resid:** Pediatrics, LI Jewish Med Ctr 1990; **Fellow:** Pediatric Gastroenterology, LI Jewish Med Ctr 1993

Kessler, Bradley MD (PGe) - **Spec Exp:** Inflammatory Bowel Disease/Crohn's; Liver Disease; Malabsorption; **Hospital:** Good Samaritan Hosp Med Ctr - West Islip, Mercy Med Ctr - Rockville Centre; **Address:** 655 Deer Park Ave Fl 3, Babylon, NY 11702; **Phone:** 631-321-2190; **Board Cert:** Pediatrics 1988; Pediatric Gastroenterology 2005; **Med School:** SUNY Downstate 1982; **Resid:** Pediatrics, N Shore Univ Hosp 1985; **Fellow:** Pediatric Gastroenterology, Baylor-Tex Chldns Hosp 1987; **Fac Appt:** Assoc Prof Ped, NY Coll Osteo Med

Pediatric Hematology-Oncology

Parker, Robert MD (PHO) - **Spec Exp:** Pediatric Cancers; Bleeding/Coagulation Disorders; Platelet Disorders; Lymphoma; **Hospital:** Stony Brook Univ Med Ctr; **Address:** Stony Brook Univ Hosp, Dept Peds, HSC T-11, Rm 029, Stony Brook, NY 11794-8111; **Phone:** 631-444-7720; **Board Cert:** Pediatrics 1983; Pediatric Hematology-Oncology 1984; **Med School:** Brown Univ 1976; **Resid:** Internal Medicine, Roger Williams Med Ctr 1977; Pediatrics, Rhode Island Hosp 1979; **Fellow:** Pediatric Hematology-Oncology, Natl Cancer Inst 1981; Hematology, Natl Cancer Inst 1984; **Fac Appt:** Prof Ped, SUNY Stony Brook

Pediatric Infectious Disease

Nachman, Sharon MD (PInf) - **Spec Exp:** Lyme Disease; AIDS/HIV; **Hospital:** Stony Brook Univ Med Ctr; **Address:** SUNY at Stony Brook, Dept of Pediatrics, T 11, rm 031, Stony Brook, NY 11794-8111; **Phone:** 631-444-7692; **Board Cert:** Pediatrics 1987; Pediatric Infectious Disease 2009; **Med School:** SUNY Stony Brook 1983; **Resid:** Pediatrics, Schneiders Chldns Hosp 1986; **Fellow:** Pediatric Infectious Disease, NY Med Coll 1987Rockefeller Univ 1989; **Fac Appt:** Prof Ped, SUNY Stony Brook

Pediatric Nephrology

Whyte, Dilys A MD (PNep) - **Spec Exp:** Kidney Disease; **Hospital:** Stony Brook Univ Med Ctr; **Address:** 37 Research Way, Setauket, NY 11733; **Phone:** 631-444-5437; **Med School:** SUNY Buffalo 1991; **Resid:** Pediatrics, Kaleida Hlth Chldn Hosp 1994; **Fellow:** Pediatric Nephrology, Yale-New Haven Hosp 1998

Pediatric Surgery

Kutin, Neil MD (PS) - **Spec Exp:** Hernia; Gastrointestinal Surgery; Undescended Testis; **Hospital:** Good Samaritan Hosp Med Ctr - West Islip; **Address:** 655 Deer Park Ave, Babylon, NY 11702; **Phone:** 631-321-2220; **Board Cert:** Pediatric Surgery 2007; **Med School:** NYU Sch Med 1970; **Resid:** Surgery, Bellevue-NYU Med Ctr 1975; **Fellow:** Pediatric Surgery, Children's Hosp 1979; **Fac Appt:** Asst Prof S, NYU Sch Med

Lee, Thomas Kang-Ming MD (PS) - **Spec Exp:** Hernia; Cancer Surgery; Minimally Invasive Surgery; **Hospital:** Stony Brook Univ Med Ctr; **Address:** 37 Research Way, E Setauket, NY 11733; **Phone:** 631-444-4538; **Board Cert:** Surgery 2005; Pediatric Surgery 2007; **Med School:** Univ Chicago-Pritzker Sch Med 1988; **Resid:** Surgery, NY Hosp-Cornell Med Ctr 1995; **Fellow:** Surgery, Hosps Univ Pittsburgh 1992; Pediatric Surgery, Cardinal Glennon Chldns Hosp/St Louis Univ 1997; **Fac Appt:** Assoc Prof S, SUNY Stony Brook

Pediatrics

Bernstein, Harvey E MD (Ped) *PCP* - **Hospital:** St Catherine's of Siena Med Ctr, Stony Brook Univ Med Ctr; **Address:** Smithtown Pediatric Group, 260 Middle Country Rd, Ste 107, Smithtown, NY 11787; **Phone:** 631-979-7222; **Board Cert:** Pediatrics 2009; **Med School:** Univ Pennsylvania 1973; **Resid:** Pediatrics, Bronx Muni Hosp 1976; **Fac Appt:** Assoc Clin Prof Ped, SUNY Stony Brook

Chernobilsky, Lev MD (Ped) *PCP* - **Spec Exp:** Asthma; **Hospital:** Stony Brook Univ Med Ctr, St Catherine's of Siena Med Ctr; **Address:** 269-D E Main St, Smithtown, NY 11787; **Phone:** 631-361-2121; **Board Cert:** Pediatrics 1987; **Med School:** Russia 1974; **Resid:** Pediatrics, SUNY Med Ctr 1985; **Fac Appt:** Assoc Clin Prof Ped, SUNY Stony Brook

Cusumano, Barbara MD (Ped) *PCP* - **Hospital:** Southampton Hosp; **Address:** 325 Meeting House Ln, Southampton, NY 11968-5087; **Phone:** 631-283-7733; **Board Cert:** Pediatrics 2009; **Med School:** Ros Franklin Univ/Chicago Med Sch 1984; **Resid:** Pediatrics, New York Hosp 1987

Festa, Robert S MD (Ped) *PCP* - **Hospital:** St Charles Hosp, Stony Brook Univ Med Ctr; **Address:** 911 Montauk Hwy, Shirley, NY 11967; **Phone:** 631-281-2525; **Board Cert:** Pediatrics 1978; Pediatric Hematology-Oncology 1980; **Med School:** SUNY Downstate 1972; **Resid:** Pediatrics, Montefiore Med Ctr 1975; **Fellow:** Pediatric Hematology-Oncology, Chldns Hosp 1978

Kaplan, Martin MD (Ped) *PCP* - **Spec Exp:** Asthma; Developmental Disorders; ADD/ADHD; **Hospital:** St Charles Hosp, Stony Brook Univ Med Ctr; **Address:** 12 Medical Drive, Port Jefferson Station, NY 11776-1588; **Phone:** 631-331-1710; **Board Cert:** Pediatrics 1977; **Med School:** NYU Sch Med 1972; **Resid:** Pediatrics, Bellevue Hosp 1974; Pediatrics, Duke Univ Med Ctr 1975; **Fac Appt:** Asst Clin Prof Ped, SUNY Stony Brook

Kolker, Harvey A MD (Ped) *PCP* - **Hospital:** St Charles Hosp, Stony Brook Univ Med Ctr; **Address:** 111 Sylvan Ave, Miller Place, NY 11764-2420; **Phone:** 631-928-4888; **Board Cert:** Pediatrics 1971; **Med School:** SUNY Downstate 1966; **Resid:** Pediatrics, Madigan Genl Hosp 1969; **Fac Appt:** Assoc Clin Prof Ped, SUNY Stony Brook

Kurfist, Lee A MD (Ped) *PCP* - **Spec Exp:** Adolescent Medicine; **Hospital:** Huntington Hosp; **Address:** 205 E Main St, Ste 2-8, Huntington, NY 11743; **Phone:** 631-424-1741; **Board Cert:** Pediatrics 2007; **Med School:** Italy 1985; **Resid:** Pediatrics, Nassau County Med Ctr 1988; **Fellow:** Pediatric Gastroenterology, Mt Sinai Hosp 1990

Manners, Richard MD (Ped) *PCP* - **Hospital:** St Charles Hosp, Stony Brook Univ Med Ctr; **Address:** Mid-Suffolk Pediatrics, 1770 Motor Pkwy, Islandia, NY 11749; **Phone:** 631-434-1770; **Board Cert:** Pediatrics 1980; **Med School:** Albert Einstein Coll Med 1975; **Resid:** Pediatrics, Univ MN Med Ctr 1978

Musiker, Seymour B MD (Ped) *PCP* - **Spec Exp:** Breast Feeding Problems; **Hospital:** Stony Brook Univ Med Ctr, St Charles Hosp; **Address:** 2233 Nesconset Hwy, Ste 106, Lake Grove, NY 11755-1000; **Phone:** 631-585-4440; **Board Cert:** Pediatrics 1966; **Med School:** Ros Franklin Univ/Chicago Med Sch 1961; **Resid:** Pediatrics, Bronx Muni Hosp Ctr 1964; **Fac Appt:** Assoc Clin Prof Ped, SUNY Stony Brook

Parles, James G MD (Ped) *PCP* - **Hospital:** Stony Brook Univ Med Ctr, St Catherine's of Siena Med Ctr; **Address:** 260 Middle Country Rd, Smithtown, NY 11787; **Phone:** 631-979-7222; **Board Cert:** Pediatrics 2009; **Med School:** NYU Sch Med 1985; **Resid:** Pediatrics, Mount Sinai Hospital 1988; **Fac Appt:** Asst Clin Prof Ped, SUNY Upstate Med Univ

Quinn, Joseph B MD (Ped) *PCP* - **Spec Exp:** ADD/ADHD; **Hospital:** Southampton Hosp; **Address:** 325 Meeting House Ln Bldg 2, Southampton, NY 11968; **Phone:** 631-283-7733; **Board Cert:** Pediatrics 1987; **Med School:** Univ VT Coll Med 1981; **Resid:** Pediatrics, New York Hosp 1984

Sosulski, Richard MD (Ped) *PCP* - **Spec Exp:** Lung Disease in Newborns; Neonatal Critical Care; Neonatology; **Hospital:** Stony Brook Univ Med Ctr, St Catherine's of Siena Med Ctr; **Address:** 269 E Main St, Ste D, Smithtown, NY 11787-2807; **Phone:** 631-361-2121; **Board Cert:** Pediatrics 1982; Neonatal-Perinatal Medicine 1983; **Med School:** SUNY Downstate 1977; **Resid:** Pediatrics, LI Jewish Med Ctr 1980; **Fellow:** Neonatal-Perinatal Medicine, Chldns Hosp 1982; **Fac Appt:** Assoc Clin Prof Ped, SUNY Stony Brook

Physical Medicine & Rehabilitation

Rosenberg, Craig H MD (PMR) - **Spec Exp:** Repetitive Strain Injuries; Pain-Back & Neck; Neuro-Rehabilitation; Spasticity Management; **Hospital:** Southside Hosp, Stony Brook Univ Med Ctr; **Address:** Southside Hospital - Health Institute, 301 E Main St, Bay Shore, NY 11706; **Phone:** 631-675-4550; **Board Cert:** Physical Medicine & Rehabilitation 1987; **Med School:** Mexico 1981; **Resid:** Physical Medicine & Rehabilitation, NYU Med Ctr/Rusk Inst 1985; **Fac Appt:** Asst Clin Prof PMR, SUNY Stony Brook

Plastic Surgery

Anton, John R MD (PIS) - **Spec Exp:** Cosmetic Surgery-Face; Eyelid Surgery; Liposuction; **Hospital:** Southampton Hosp, Peconic Bay Med Ctr; **Address:** 138 Old Town Rd, Southampton, NY 11968-5011; **Phone:** 631-283-9100; **Board Cert:** Plastic Surgery 1992; **Med School:** Univ VT Coll Med 1981; **Resid:** Surgery, Mass Genl Hosp 1986; Plastic Surgery, Wayne State Univ Med Ctr 1987; **Fellow:** Surgery, Mass Genl Hosp 1986; Plastic Surgery, Nassau County Med Ctr 1988

Dagum, Alexander B MD (PIS) - **Spec Exp:** Reconstructive Plastic Surgery; Cleft Palate/Lip; Hand Surgery; Microsurgery; **Hospital:** Stony Brook Univ Med Ctr; **Address:** SUNY Health Science Ctr, T19-060, Box 8191, Stony Brook, NY 11794-8191; **Phone:** 631-444-8210; **Board Cert:** Plastic Surgery 2003; Hand Surgery 2004; **Med School:** Canada 1987; **Resid:** Surgery, Univ Ottawa Civic Hosp 1988; Plastic Surgery, Univ Toronto Med Ctr 1993; **Fellow:** Microsurgery, Univ Toronto Med Ctr 1984; Hand Surgery, Stony Brook Univ Hosp 1995; **Fac Appt:** Prof S, SUNY Stony Brook

Duboys, Elliot B MD (PIS) - **Spec Exp:** Cosmetic & Reconstructive Surgery; Pediatric Plastic Surgery; Breast Surgery; Birth Defects; **Hospital:** Plainview Hosp, Stony Brook Univ Med Ctr; **Address:** 864 W Jericho Tpke, West Hills, NY 11743-6037; **Phone:** 631-423-1000; **Board Cert:** Plastic Surgery 1985; **Med School:** Belgium 1977; **Resid:** Surgery, SUNY - Stony Brook Univ Hosp 1982; Plastic Surgery, Nassau County Med Ctr 1984

Psychiatry

Aronson, Thomas MD (Psyc) - **Spec Exp:** Depression; Bipolar/Mood Disorders; **Hospital:** St Catherine's of Siena Med Ctr; **Address:** 2 Brooksite, Ste 220, Smithtown, NY 11787-3400; **Phone:** 631-265-0909; **Board Cert:** Psychiatry 1985; **Med School:** Washington Univ, St Louis 1980; **Resid:** Psychiatry, Hosp Univ Penn 1984; **Fac Appt:** Assoc Clin Prof Psyc, SUNY Stony Brook

Koreen, Amy R MD (Psyc) - ; **Address:** 28 Elm St, Huntington, NY 11743; **Phone:** 631-423-8368; **Board Cert:** Psychiatry 1993; **Med School:** Mount Sinai Sch Med 1988; **Resid:** Psychiatry, Univ Maryland Med Ctr 1991; Psychiatry, LIJ Med Ctr 1992; **Fellow:** Neuropsychopharmacology, LIJ Med Ctr 1993

Lee, Kwang Soo MD (Psyc) - ; **Address:** 221 Broadway, Ste 303, Amityville, NY 11701-2726; **Phone:** 631-789-7448; **Board Cert:** Psychiatry 1979; **Med School:** South Korea 1965; **Resid:** Internal Medicine, Booth Meml Hosp 1967; Psychiatry, Bellevue Hosp 1969; **Fellow:** Psychiatry, Amer Inst Psychoanalysis 1969

Liang, Vera MD (Psyc) - **Spec Exp:** Women's Health-Mental Health; Depression; Anxiety Disorders; **Hospital:** Long Island Jewish Med Ctr; **Address:** 221 Broadway, Ste 201, Amityville, NY 11701-2700; **Phone:** 631-598-7396; **Board Cert:** Psychiatry 1977; Child & Adolescent Psychiatry 1981; **Med School:** Hong Kong 1969; **Resid:** Psychiatry, LI Jewish Med Ctr 1973; **Fellow:** Child & Adolescent Psychiatry, Albert Einstein Coll Med 1975

Nass, Jack MD (Psyc) - **Spec Exp:** Geriatric Rehabilitation; Bipolar/Mood Disorders; Depression; Neuro-Psychiatry; **Hospital:** S Oaks Hosp, Good Samaritan Hosp Med Ctr - West Islip; **Address:** 580 Sunrise Hwy, West Babylon, NY 11704; **Phone:** 631-321-7697; **Board Cert:** Psychiatry 1980; **Med School:** Belgium 1975; **Resid:** Psychiatry, LI Jewish Med Ctr 1979

Rosen, Bruce I MD (Psyc) - **Spec Exp:** Depression; Anxiety Disorders; Bipolar/Mood Disorders; Psychopharmacology; **Hospital:** St Catherine's of Siena Med Ctr, Stony Brook Univ Med Ctr; **Address:** 222 E Middle Country Rd, Ste 210, Smithtown, NY 11787-2814; **Phone:** 631-265-6868; **Board Cert:** Psychiatry 1976; **Med School:** Loyola Univ-Stritch Sch Med 1971; **Resid:** Psychiatry, LI Jewish-Hillside Med Ctr 1974; **Fellow:** Psychiatry, LI Jewish-Hillside Med Ctr 1975; **Fac Appt:** Assoc Clin Prof Psyc, SUNY Stony Brook

Schwartz, Michael MD (Psyc) - **Spec Exp:** Forensic Psychiatry; Psychotherapy & Psychopharmacology; Mood Disorders; Anxiety Disorders; **Hospital:** Stony Brook Univ Med Ctr; **Address:** 33 Walt Whitman Rd, Ste 202, Huntington Station, NY 11746; **Phone:** 631-385-3313; **Board Cert:** Psychiatry 1984; Geriatric Psychiatry 2001; Forensic Psychiatry 1999; **Med School:** Univ Miami Sch Med 1977; **Resid:** Internal Medicine, Mount Sinai Hosp 1978; Psychiatry, Mount Sinai Hosp 1981; **Fellow:** Research, Natl Inst Aging 1983; **Fac Appt:** Assoc Prof Psyc, SUNY Stony Brook

Upadhyay, Yogendra MD (Psyc) - **Spec Exp:** Child & Adolescent Psychiatry; Bipolar/Mood Disorders; Depression; **Hospital:** S Oaks Hosp; **Address:** 400 Sunrise Hwy, Amityville, NY 11701-2508; **Phone:** 631-608-5212; **Board Cert:** Pediatrics 1967; Psychiatry 1977; Child & Adolescent Psychiatry 1978; **Med School:** India 1962; **Resid:** Psychiatry, Albert Einstein Coll Med 1974; **Fellow:** Child & Adolescent Psychiatry, Johns Hopkins 1972; Child & Adolescent Psychiatry, Albert Einstein Coll Med 1975

Pulmonary Disease

Baram, Daniel MD (Pul) - **Spec Exp:** Critical Care Medicine; Lung Cancer; **Hospital:** John T Mather Meml Hosp; **Address:** 640 Belle Terre Rd, Bldg D, Ste 2, Port Jefferson, NY 11777; **Phone:** 631-473-0037; **Board Cert:** Internal Medicine 2004; Critical Care Medicine 2007; Pulmonary Disease 2008; **Med School:** Jefferson Med Coll 1990; **Resid:** Internal Medicine, New York Hosp 1993; **Fellow:** Critical Care Medicine, Natl Inst of Health 1996; Pulmonary Disease, NYU/Bellevue Hosps 1998

Bernardini, Dennis L MD (Pul) - **Spec Exp:** Asthma; Emphysema; Bronchitis; **Hospital:** Huntington Hosp; **Address:** 175 E Main St, Huntington, NY 11743-2939; **Phone:** 631-424-3787; **Board Cert:** Internal Medicine 1983; Pulmonary Disease 1986; Critical Care Medicine 2002; **Med School:** Johns Hopkins Univ 1980; **Resid:** Internal Medicine, St Luke's Hosp 1983; **Fellow:** Pulmonary Disease, Univ Hospital 1985; Critical Care Medicine, Univ Hospital 1985

Glaser, Morton L MD (Pul) - **Hospital:** John T Mather Meml Hosp, St Charles Hosp; **Address:** 60 N Country Rd, Ste 203, Port Jefferson, NY 11777; **Phone:** 631-509-1888; **Board Cert:** Internal Medicine 1980; Pulmonary Disease 1984; Critical Care Medicine 1999; Undersea & Hyperbaric Medicine 2005; **Med School:** Med Coll Wisc 1976; **Resid:** Internal Medicine, Roger Williams Med Ctr 1979; **Fellow:** Pulmonary Disease, Univ Hosp 1981

Sklarek, Howard MD (Pul) - **Spec Exp:** Asthma; Cough; Chronic Obstructive Lung Disease (COPD); Interstitial Lung Disease; **Hospital:** Southampton Hosp; **Address:** 325 Meeting House Ln Bldg 1 - Ste K, Southampton, NY 11968; **Phone:** 631-283-8008; **Board Cert:** Internal Medicine 1984; Pulmonary Disease 1986; Critical Care Medicine 1998; **Med School:** SUNY Buffalo 1981; **Resid:** Internal Medicine, Winthrop Univ Hosp 1984; **Fellow:** Pulmonary Critical Care Medicine, Winthrop Univ Hosp 1986

Walser, Lawrence A MD (Pul) - **Hospital:** Peconic Bay Med Ctr, Eastern Long Island Hosp; **Address:** 185 Old Country Rd, Ste 3, Riverhead, NY 11901; **Phone:** 631-727-2523; **Board Cert:** Internal Medicine 1982; Pulmonary Disease 2007; Critical Care Medicine 2007; **Med School:** SUNY Downstate 1979; **Resid:** Internal Medicine, Berkshire Med Ctr 1982; **Fellow:** Pulmonary Disease, SUNY/Univ Hosp 1984

Wohlberg, Gary MD (Pul) - **Spec Exp:** Sleep Disorders/Apnea; **Hospital:** Southside Hosp, Good Samaritan Hosp Med Ctr - West Islip; **Address:** 370 E Main St, Ste 5, Bay Shore, NY 11706-8405; **Phone:** 631-666-5864; **Board Cert:** Internal Medicine 1985; Pulmonary Disease 1986; Critical Care Medicine 1999; Sleep Medicine 2007; **Med School:** SUNY Hlth Sci Ctr 1981; **Resid:** Internal Medicine, Long Island Hosp 1984; **Fellow:** Pulmonary Disease, Montefiore Hosp Med Ctr 1986

Radiation Oncology

Katz, Alan J MD (RadRO) - **Spec Exp:** Brachytherapy; Prostate Cancer; Intensity Modulated Radiotherapy (IMRT); **Address:** North Shore Radiation Therapy, 270 Pulaski Rd, Greenlawn, NY 11740; **Phone:** 631-427-2273; **Board Cert:** Therapeutic Radiology 1981; **Med School:** NYU Sch Med 1977; **Resid:** Therapeutic Radiology, NYU Med Ctr 1981

Meek, Allen G MD (RadRO) - **Spec Exp:** Breast Cancer; Prostate Cancer; Stereotactic Radiosurgery; Head & Neck Cancer; **Hospital:** Stony Brook Univ Med Ctr, John T Mather Meml Hosp; **Address:** Stony Brook Univ Hosp, Dept Rad Onc - L2, 100 Nicholls Rd, Stony Brook, NY 11794-7028; **Phone:** 631-444-2327; **Board Cert:** Internal Medicine 1979; Therapeutic Radiology 1983; **Med School:** Johns Hopkins Univ 1974; **Resid:** Internal Medicine, Johns Hopkins Hosp 1979; Radiation Oncology, Johns Hopkins Hosp 1982; **Fellow:** Medical Oncology, Johns Hopkins Hosp 1980; **Fac Appt:** Prof RadRO, SUNY Stony Brook

Park, Tae L MD (RadRO) - **Spec Exp:** Prostate Cancer; Breast Cancer; Gynecologic Cancer; **Hospital:** Stony Brook Univ Med Ctr; **Address:** Stony Brook Univ Hosp, Fl Level 2 - rm 664, Stony Brook, NY 11794-7028; **Phone:** 631-444-2210; **Board Cert:** Therapeutic Radiology 1984; **Med School:** South Korea 1976; **Resid:** Radiation Oncology, Kings Co Downstate Med Ctr. 1984; **Fellow:** Radiation Oncology, MD Anderson Cancer Ctr 1985; **Fac Appt:** Assoc Clin Prof RadRO, SUNY Stony Brook

Reproductive Endocrinology

Bronson, Richard A MD (RE) - **Spec Exp:** Infertility-IVF; Pregnancy Loss-Recurrent; Reproductive Immunology; **Hospital:** Stony Brook Univ Med Ctr; **Address:** State Univ of NY at Stony Brook, Div of Reproductive Endocrinology, Health Sci Ctr, T9-080, Stony Brook, NY 11794-8091; **Phone:** 631-246-9100; **Board Cert:** Obstetrics & Gynecology 1976; Reproductive Endocrinology 1976; **Med School:** NYU Sch Med 1966; **Resid:** Surgery, NYU Med Ctr 1971; Obstetrics & Gynecology, Hosp Univ Penn 1974; **Fellow:** Reproductive Endocrinology, Pennsylvania Hosp 1976; **Fac Appt:** Prof ObG, SUNY Stony Brook

Kenigsberg, Daniel J MD (RE) - **Spec Exp:** Infertility-IVF; Uterine Fibroids; Endometriosis; Reproductive Surgery; **Hospital:** John T Mather Meml Hosp, Stony Brook Univ Med Ctr; **Address:** 2500 Nesconset Highway, Bldg 19A, Stony Brook, NY 11790; **Phone:** 631-331-7575; **Board Cert:** Obstetrics & Gynecology 1995; Reproductive Endocrinology 1995; **Med School:** NY Med Coll 1978; **Resid:** Obstetrics & Gynecology, Johns Hopkins Hosp 1982; **Fellow:** Reproductive Endocrinology, Natl Inst Hlth 1984; **Fac Appt:** Assoc Clin Prof ObG, SUNY Stony Brook

Lydic, Michael L MD (RE) - **Spec Exp:** Polycystic Ovarian Syndrome; Pregnancy Loss-Recurrent; Infertility; Infertility-IVF; **Hospital:** Stony Brook Univ Med Ctr; **Address:** Reproductive Specialists of NY, 2500 Nesonset Hwy Bldg 23, Stony Brook, NY 11790; **Phone:** 631-246-9100; **Board Cert:** Obstetrics & Gynecology 2007; Reproductive Endocrinology 2007; **Med School:** Hahnemann Univ 1989; **Resid:** Obstetrics & Gynecology, Hahnemann Univ Hosp 1993; **Fellow:** Reproductive Endocrinology, Univ of Cincinnati Hosp 1995; **Fac Appt:** Asst Clin Prof ObG, SUNY Stony Brook

Rheumatology

Hamburger, Max MD (Rhu) - **Spec Exp:** Rheumatoid Arthritis; Psoriatic Arthritis; Osteoarthritis; Vasculitis; **Hospital:** St Catherine's of Siena Med Ctr, John T Mather Meml Hosp; **Address:** 1895 Walt Whitman Rd, Melville, NY 11747; **Phone:** 631-249-9525; **Board Cert:** Internal Medicine 1977; Rheumatology 1980; **Med School:** Albert Einstein Coll Med 1973; **Resid:** Internal Medicine, Bellevue Hosp 1976; **Fellow:** Allergy & Immunology, Nat Inst Health 1979; **Fac Appt:** Asst Clin Prof Med, SUNY Stony Brook

Kaell, Alan MD (Rhu) - **Spec Exp:** Geriatric Rheumatology; Vasculitis; Connective Tissue Disorders; Osteoporosis; **Hospital:** St Charles Hosp, John T Mather Meml Hosp; **Address:** 315 Middle Country Rd, Ste 6, Smithtown, NY 11787-2817; **Phone:** 631-360-7778; **Board Cert:** Internal Medicine 1981; Rheumatology 1984; Geriatric Medicine 2000; **Med School:** Brown Univ 1978; **Resid:** Internal Medicine, Strong Meml Hosp 1981; **Fellow:** Rheumatology, Hosp For Special Surgery/Cornell 1983; **Fac Appt:** Clin Prof Med, SUNY Stony Brook

Repice, Michael MD (Rhu) - **Spec Exp:** Arthritis; Connective Tissue Disorders; **Hospital:** Huntington Hosp; **Address:** 5 E Main St, Huntington, NY 11743-2812; **Phone:** 631-271-1640; **Board Cert:** Internal Medicine 1976; Rheumatology 1980; **Med School:** Georgetown Univ 1973; **Resid:** Internal Medicine, Worcester City Hosp 1977; **Fellow:** Rheumatology, Northwestern Univ Hosp 1979; **Fac Appt:** Asst Prof Med, SUNY Stony Brook

Tan, Mark MD (Rhu) - **Spec Exp:** Lupus/SLE; Rheumatoid Arthritis; **Hospital:** St Catherine's of Siena Med Ctr, St Charles Hosp; **Address:** 222 Middle Country Rd Fl 3 - Ste 312, Smithtown, NY 11787; **Phone:** 631-724-8900; **Board Cert:** Internal Medicine 1989; Rheumatology 2004; **Med School:** SUNY Buffalo 1983; **Resid:** Internal Medicine, Univ Hosp 1986; **Fellow:** Rheumatology, Johns Hopkins Univ 1989

Sports Medicine

Kottmeier, Stephen A MD (SM) - **Spec Exp:** Trauma; Sports Injuries; **Hospital:** Stony Brook Univ Med Ctr; **Address:** 14 Technology Drive, Ste 11, East Setauket, NY 11733; **Phone:** 631-444-4233; **Board Cert:** Orthopaedic Surgery 2004; **Med School:** SUNY Downstate 1984; **Resid:** Orthopaedic Surgery, SUNY Downstate Med Ctr 1989; **Fellow:** Sports Medicine, Penn State Univ-Hershey Med Ctr 1990; Orthopaedic Trauma Surgery, Southern NJ Regl Trauma Ctr 1990; **Fac Appt:** Asst Prof OrS, SUNY Stony Brook

Putterman, Eric A MD (SM) - **Spec Exp:** Arthroscopic Surgery; **Address:** 1800 Walt Whitman Rd, Ste 120, Melville, NY 11747; **Phone:** 631-293-9540; **Board Cert:** Orthopaedic Surgery 2009; **Med School:** Mount Sinai Sch Med 1980; **Resid:** Orthopaedic Surgery, NYU-Bellevue Med Ctr 1985; **Fellow:** Sports Medicine, NYU-Bellevue Med Ctr 1985

Surgery

Busch-Devereaux, Erna MD (S) - **Spec Exp:** Breast Cancer; Breast Surgery; **Hospital:** Huntington Hosp, N Shore Univ Hosp; **Address:** 270 Pulaski Rd, Ste A, Greenlawn, NY 11740; **Phone:** 631-423-1414; **Board Cert:** Surgery 2000; **Med School:** UMDNJ-NJ Med Sch, Newark 1985; **Resid:** Surgery, St Vincents Hosp 1990; **Fellow:** Surgical Oncology, Roswell Park Cancer 1993; **Fac Appt:** Asst Prof S, NYU Sch Med

Cohen, Bradley D MD (S) - Spec Exp: Breast Disease; Cancer Surgery; Laparoscopic Surgery; Sentinel Node Surgery; **Hospital:** Good Samaritan Hosp Med Ctr - West Islip, Southside Hosp; **Address:** 15 Park Ave, Bay Shore, NY 11706; **Phone:** 631-581-4400; **Board Cert:** Surgery 2009; **Med School:** Mount Sinai Sch Med 1983; **Resid:** Surgery, Lenox Hill Hosp 1988; **Fellow:** Surgical Oncology, Meml Sloan Kettering Cancer Ctr 1989

Francfort, John MD (S) - Spec Exp: Breast Surgery; Gastrointestinal Surgery; Vascular Surgery; **Hospital:** Good Samaritan Hosp Med Ctr - West Islip, Southside Hosp; **Address:** 580 Union Blvd, West Islip, NY 11795-3105; **Phone:** 631-321-6801; **Board Cert:** Surgery 2005; Vascular Surgery 2006; **Med School:** UMDNJ-NJ Med Sch, Newark 1980; **Resid:** Surgery, Hosp Univ Penn 1986; **Fellow:** Vascular Surgery, Northwesten Univ 1987; **Fac Appt:** Asst Clin Prof S, SUNY Stony Brook

Klausner, Stanley MD (S) - Spec Exp: Breast Surgery; **Hospital:** Brookhaven Meml Hosp & Med Ctr; **Address:** 100 Hospital Rd, Ste 106, Patchogue, NY 11772; **Phone:** 631-475-8846; **Board Cert:** Surgery 1975; **Med School:** NYU Sch Med 1967; **Resid:** Surgery, Bronx Muni Hosp 1973

O'Hea, Brian J MD (S) - Spec Exp: Breast Cancer; Sentinel Node Surgery; **Hospital:** Stony Brook Univ Med Ctr; **Address:** SUNY Stony Brook, Dept Surgery, HSC T-18, Rm 060, Stony Brook, NY 11794-8191; **Phone:** 631-444-1795; **Board Cert:** Surgery 2002; **Med School:** Georgetown Univ 1986; **Resid:** Surgery, St Vincent's Hosp 1991; **Fellow:** Breast Disease, Meml Sloan-Kettering Cancer Ctr 1996; **Fac Appt:** Asst Prof S, SUNY Stony Brook

Sclafani, Lisa MD (S) - Spec Exp: Breast Surgery; Breast Cancer; **Hospital:** Meml Sloan-Kettering Cancer Ctr (page 112); **Address:** 650 Commack Rd, Commack, NY 11725; **Phone:** 800-525-2225; **Board Cert:** Surgery 2007; **Med School:** NYU Sch Med 1982; **Resid:** Surgery, Albert Einstein Coll Med 1987; **Fellow:** Surgical Oncology, Meml Sloan Kettering Cancer Ctr 1989; **Fac Appt:** Assoc Clin Prof S, Cornell Univ-Weill Med Coll

Shapiro, Marc MD (S) - Spec Exp: Laparoscopic Surgery; Gastrointestinal Surgery; Burn Care; Trauma; **Hospital:** Stony Brook Univ Med Ctr; **Address:** Stony Brook Univ Hosp, Nicolls Rd HSC T-18 Bldg - rm 040, Stony Brook, NY 11794-8191; **Phone:** 631-444-1045; **Board Cert:** Surgery 2004; Surgical Critical Care 2005; **Med School:** Univ Mich Med Sch 1979; **Resid:** Surgery, Henry Ford Hosp 1984; **Fellow:** Critical Care Medicine, Univ Pittsburgh Hosp 1985; **Fac Appt:** Prof S, SUNY Stony Brook

Zingale, Robert MD (S) - Spec Exp: Laparoscopic Surgery; Colon & Rectal Cancer; Gastrointestinal Surgery; Breast Disease; **Hospital:** Huntington Hosp; **Address:** 158 E Main St, Ste 7, Huntington, NY 11743-2988; **Phone:** 631-271-1822; **Board Cert:** Surgery 2007; Surgical Critical Care 1999; **Med School:** SUNY Downstate 1983; **Resid:** Surgery, Maimonides Med Ctr 1988; **Fellow:** Trauma, Coney Island Hosp 1989; **Fac Appt:** Assoc Clin Prof S, NY Med Coll

Thoracic Surgery

Bilfinger, Thomas MD (TS) - Spec Exp: Cardiac Surgery-Adult; Lung Cancer; **Hospital:** Stony Brook Univ Med Ctr; **Address:** Stony Brook Univ Med Ctr, Dept Surgery, HSC Bldg Fl 19 - rm 080, Stony Brook, NY 11794-8191; **Phone:** 631-444-1820; **Board Cert:** Surgery 2006; Thoracic Surgery 2008; Surgical Critical Care 2000; **Med School:** Switzerland 1978; **Resid:** Surgery, Univ Chicago 1982; Surgery, Univ TX Med Branch Hosp 1986; **Fellow:** Thoracic Surgery, Univ TX Med Branch Hosp 1988; **Fac Appt:** Prof S, SUNY Stony Brook

Palatt, Terry MD (TS) - **Spec Exp:** Lung Cancer; Video Assisted Thoracic Surgery (VATS); **Hospital:** Good Samaritan Hosp Med Ctr - West Islip, Southside Hosp; **Address:** 15 Park Ave, Bay Shore, NY 11706; **Phone:** 631-581-4400; **Board Cert:** Thoracic Surgery 2008; **Med School:** Grenada 1981; **Resid:** Surgery, Maimonides Med Ctr 1986; Thoracic Surgery, Maimonides Med Ctr 1988

Rosengart, Todd MD (TS) - **Spec Exp:** Transfusion Free Surgery; Gene Therapy-Cardiac Angiogenesis; Minimally Invasive Surgery; Cardiac Surgery; **Hospital:** Stony Brook Univ Med Ctr; **Address:** Stonybrook Univ Hosp, Health Sci Ctr, Cardiothoracic Surgery, HSC-T19, rm 020, Stonybrook, NY 11794-0001; **Phone:** 631-444-7875; **Board Cert:** Surgery 1999; Thoracic Surgery 2001; **Med School:** Northwestern Univ 1983; **Resid:** Surgery, NYU Med Ctr 1985; Surgery, NYU Med Ctr 1989; **Fellow:** Thoracic Surgery, Natl Inst Hlth 1987; Cardiothoracic Surgery, NY-Cornell Med Ctr 1991; **Fac Appt:** Prof S, SUNY Stony Brook

Urology

Beccia, David J MD (U) - **Spec Exp:** Prostate Cancer; Erectile Dysfunction; **Hospital:** Southside Hosp, Good Samaritan Hosp Med Ctr - West Islip; **Address:** 332 E Main St, Bay Shore, NY 11706-8404; **Phone:** 631-665-3737; **Board Cert:** Urology 1979; **Med School:** NY Med Coll 1970; **Resid:** Surgery, Hartford Hosp 1973; Urology, Boston Univ Med Ctr 1977

Mills, Carl MD (U) - **Spec Exp:** Urologic Cancer; **Hospital:** Brookhaven Meml Hosp & Med Ctr, St Charles Hosp; **Address:** 250 Yaphank Rd, Ste 15, East Patchogue, NY 11772-4863; **Phone:** 631-475-5051; **Board Cert:** Urology 1984; **Med School:** Geo Wash Univ 1975; **Resid:** Surgery, New York Hosp 1978; Urology, New York Hosp 1982

Wasnick, Robert MD (U) - **Spec Exp:** Undescended Testis; Pediatric Urology; Hydronephrosis; Hypospadias; **Hospital:** Stony Brook Univ Med Ctr, St Charles Hosp; **Address:** Stony Brook Medical Park, 24 Research Way, Ste 500, East Setauket, NY 11733; **Phone:** 631-444-6270; **Board Cert:** Urology 1982; Pediatric Urology 2008; **Med School:** Jefferson Med Coll 1974; **Resid:** Surgery, St Vincents Hosp Med Ctr 1977; Urology, Downstate Med Ctr 1980; **Fellow:** Pediatric Urology, Alder Hey Chldns Hosp 1981; **Fac Appt:** Clin Prof U, SUNY Stony Brook

Vascular Surgery

Arnold, Thomas E MD (VascS) - **Spec Exp:** Carotid Artery Surgery; Aneurysm-Abdominal Aortic; Varicose Veins; Dialysis Access Surgery; **Hospital:** John T Mather Meml Hosp, St Charles Hosp; **Address:** 1110 Hallock Ave, Port Jefferson, NY 11776; **Phone:** 631-476-9100; **Board Cert:** Surgery 2003; Vascular Surgery 2003; **Med School:** SUNY Downstate 1985; **Resid:** Surgery, Presbyterian Med Ctr/Univ Penn 1987; Surgery, Medical Coll Penn 1991

Pollina, Robert M MD (VascS) - **Spec Exp:** Varicose Veins; Aneurysm; Carotid Artery Surgery; Dialysis Access Surgery; **Hospital:** John T Mather Meml Hosp, St Charles Hosp; **Address:** 1110 Hallock Ave, Port Jefferson Station, NY 11776; **Phone:** 631-476-9100; **Board Cert:** Vascular Surgery 2007; **Med School:** SUNY Hlth Sci Ctr 1988; **Resid:** Surgery, Kings County Hosp 1993; **Fellow:** Vascular Surgery, Maimonides Medical Ctr 1995

Tassiopoulos, Apostolos K MD (VascS) - **Hospital:** Stony Brook Univ Med Ctr; **Address:** Stony Brook Univ Medical Ctr, HSC Bldg Fl 19 - rm 090, Stony Brook, NY 11794; **Phone:** 631-444-4545; **Board Cert:** Surgery 2001; Vascular Surgery 2002; **Med School:** Greece 1989; **Resid:** Surgery, SUNY Upstate Med Ctr 1999; Vascular Surgery, Loyola Univ Med Ctr 2001; **Fac Appt:** Assoc Prof S, SUNY Stony Brook

Westchester

PHELPS
MEMORIAL HOSPITAL CENTER

701 N. Broadway • Sleepy Hollow, NY 10591 • (914) 366-3000 • www.phelpshospital.org

Sponsorship: Not-for-Profit   Beds: 238
Accreditations: The Joint Commission, College of American Pathologists, the American College of Radiology, and NYS Office of Alcoholism and Substance Abuse Services (OASAS)

A 238-bed acute care community hospital with 475 medical staff members, Phelps Memorial Hospital Center offers a broader range of services than any other community hospital in the region. Its Emergency Department has 32 private rooms. Phelps is the exclusive Westchester location for Memorial Sloan-Kettering Cancer Center. Services include:

Advanced Endoscopy and Gastroenterology: Tertiary-level therapies and groundbreaking techniques to diagnose and treat Barrett's esophagus, intestinal bleeding/ unexplained anemia, abdominal pain, non-cardiac chest pain, swallowing disorders including Zenker's diverticulum, polyps, small pancreatic cancers and other cancerous and precancerous lesions in the digestive tract.

Diabetes and Metabolism Center: Offers adult patients convenient access in one location to a complete range of diabetes and specialty care.

Geriatrics: The Senior Health Consultation Service and Memory Loss Program offer older adults comprehensive health and memory assessments.

Hyperbaric Medicine Center: Therapy for non-healing wounds, post-radiation tissue damage, carbon monoxide poisoning; chronic osteomyelitis, and decompression sickness. The comfortable 12-seat chamber is the largest in the northeast. A hyperbaric nurse or technician accompanies patients and with a primary physician present throughout treatment.

Infusion Center: Patients are administered "biologics," the most advanced class of medications to treat inflammatory diseases and chronic illnesses, including rheumatoid arthritis, psoriatic arthritis, ankylosing spondylitis, juvenile arthritis, psoriasis, and Crohn's disease. One of only a few programs of its kind in the region.

Mental Health:
Inpatient – General psychiatric care is available as well as treatment for mentally ill, chemically addicted adults.
Outpatient – Alcohol and chemical dependency programs, counseling services, continuing day treatment, and supportive case management are offered at the Hospital and in the community.

Orthopedics/Joint Replacement: Over 4,000 total joint replacements performed at Phelps, including the northeast's first anterior approach hip replacement, a minimally invasive operation with less pain and quicker recovery.

Pain Center: Medical specialists from many disciplines use a comprehensive approach to provide diagnostic and therapeutic treatment for acute and chronic pain disorders.

Physical Medicine & Rehabilitation:
Inpatient – Surgical care and acute rehabilitation from a single, integrated team.
Outpatient – physical and occupational therapy with specialists in hand injuries, incontinence, lymphedema, vestibular (dizziness), and aquatherapy in a spacious new facility that includes a therapeutic pool.

Stroke Center: A NYS DOH-designated center. Received the silver performance achievement award from the American Heart Association for outstanding stroke care.

Thoracic Center: Advanced and minimally invasive chest surgery to treat malignant and benign diseases affecting the lungs and other organs inside the chest cavity, except the heart. Quick diagnosis and treatment and full-time care by the Center's director, a renowned cardiothoracic surgeon.

Voice & Swallowing Disorders Institute and the Donald R. Reed Speech & Hearing Center: Comprehensive diagnosis and advanced treatment.

Wound Healing Institute: State-of-the-art outpatient wound care for patients with difficult wounds from diabetes, vascular problems, chronic infections or traumas.

Allergy & Immunology

Geraci-Ciardullo, Kira MD (A&I) - **Spec Exp:** Asthma; Sinus Disorders; Food Allergy; Insect Allergies; **Hospital:** White Plains Hosp Ctr, NY-Presby Hosp/Westchester Div (page 104); **Address:** 1600 Harrison Ave, Ste 304, Rockledge Plaza, Mamaroneck, NY 10543-3145; **Phone:** 914-777-1179; **Board Cert:** Pediatrics 1984; Allergy & Immunology 2008; **Med School:** Columbia P&S 1980; **Resid:** Pediatrics, NY-Cornell Hosp 1983; **Fellow:** Allergy & Immunology, NY-Cornell Hosp 1985

Goldman, Neil C MD (A&I) - **Spec Exp:** Asthma; Drug Sensitivity; Sinusitis; **Hospital:** Hudson Valley Hosp Ctr, Phelps Meml Hosp Ctr (page 592); **Address:** 35 S Riverside Ave, Ste 106, Croton On Hudson, NY 10520-2653; **Phone:** 914-271-0001; **Board Cert:** Allergy & Immunology 1977; **Med School:** NY Med Coll 1966; **Resid:** Internal Medicine, Beth Israel Hosp 1968; Internal Medicine, Metropolitan Hosp Ctr 1969; **Fellow:** Allergy & Immunology, Jewish Hosp 1970

Pollowitz, James MD (A&I) - **Spec Exp:** Asthma; Food Allergy; Hives; Drug Sensitivity; **Hospital:** White Plains Hosp Ctr, Lawrence Hosp Ctr; **Address:** 281 Garth Rd, Ste A, Scarsdale, NY 10583-4034; **Phone:** 914-472-3833; **Board Cert:** Pediatrics 1978; Allergy & Immunology 1979; **Med School:** NYU Sch Med 1973; **Resid:** Pediatrics, Bronx Muni Hosp Ctr 1976; **Fellow:** Allergy & Immunology, St Vincent Med Ctr 1978; **Fac Appt:** Asst Clin Prof Ped, NY Med Coll

Tuerk-Mendelsohn, Lois MD (A&I) - **Spec Exp:** Asthma; Hay Fever; Food Allergy; Eczema; **Hospital:** Northern Westchester Hosp; **Address:** 103 S Bedford Rd, Ste 208, Mt Kisco, NY 10549; **Phone:** 914-666-7171; **Board Cert:** Internal Medicine 1989; Allergy & Immunology 2001; **Med School:** NY Med Coll 1986; **Resid:** Internal Medicine, Lenox Hill Hosp 1989; **Fellow:** Allergy & Immunology, Mt Sinai Hosp 1991

Cardiac Electrophysiology

Cohen, Martin B MD (CE) - **Spec Exp:** Interventional Cardiology; Pacemakers; Defibrillators; Coronary Angioplasty/Stents; **Hospital:** Westchester Med Ctr, White Plains Hosp Ctr; **Address:** 19 Bradhurst Ave, Ste 700, Hawthorne, NY 10532-2140; **Phone:** 914-593-7800; **Board Cert:** Internal Medicine 1983; Cardiovascular Disease 1985; Cardiac Electrophysiology 2006; Interventional Cardiology 2004; **Med School:** SUNY Downstate 1980; **Resid:** Internal Medicine, Univ Hosp 1983; **Fellow:** Cardiovascular Disease, Univ Hosp 1985; Interventional Cardiology, Westchester Co Med Ctr 1986; **Fac Appt:** Assoc Clin Prof Med, NY Med Coll

Rubin, David A MD (CE) - **Spec Exp:** Arrhythmias; Radiofrequency Ablation; Pacemakers/Defibrillators; **Hospital:** NY-Presby Hosp/Columbia (page 104), White Plains Hosp Ctr; **Address:** 222 Westchester Ave, White Plains, NY 10604-2906; **Phone:** 914-428-3888; **Board Cert:** Internal Medicine 1978; Cardiovascular Disease 1981; Cardiac Electrophysiology 2002; **Med School:** Columbia P&S 1975; **Resid:** Internal Medicine, Columbia-Presby Hosp 1978; **Fellow:** Cardiovascular Disease, Mount Sinai Hosp 1980; **Fac Appt:** Clin Prof Med, Columbia P&S

Cardiovascular Disease

Bleiberg, Melvyn S MD (Cv) - **Hospital:** Saint Joseph's Med Ctr - Yonkers; **Address:** 127 S Broadway Fl 4th - Ste 409, Yonkers, NY 10701; **Phone:** 914-965-6060; **Board Cert:** Internal Medicine 1978; Cardiovascular Disease 1981; **Med School:** Albert Einstein Coll Med 1974; **Resid:** Internal Medicine, Brookdale Hosp 1977; **Fellow:** Cardiovascular Disease, Brookdale Hosp 1979

Catanese, James W MD (Cv) - **Spec Exp:** Coronary Artery Disease; Congestive Heart Failure; Heart Valve Disease; **Hospital:** Northern Westchester Hosp, Westchester Med Ctr; **Address:** Westchester Health- Cardiology, 105 S Bedford Rd, Ste 320, Mt Kisco, NY 10549; **Phone:** 914-242-9400; **Board Cert:** Cardiovascular Disease 2005; **Med School:** Albany Med Coll 1988; **Resid:** Internal Medicine, Montefiore Med Ctr 1991; **Fellow:** Cardiovascular Disease, Montefiore Med Ctr 1992

Charney, Richard MD (Cv) - **Spec Exp:** Interventional Cardiology; **Hospital:** Sound Shore Med Ctr - Westchester, NY-Presby Hosp/Weill Cornell (page 104); **Address:** Sound Shore Cardiology, 175 Memorial Hwy, New Rochelle, NY 10801; **Phone:** 914-235-3535; **Board Cert:** Internal Medicine 2009; Cardiovascular Disease 2009; Interventional Cardiology 2000; **Med School:** Mount Sinai Sch Med 1986; **Resid:** Internal Medicine, Mt Sinai Hosp 1989; **Fellow:** Cardiovascular Disease, Montefiore Med Ctr 1992; Interventional Cardiology, Montefiore Med Ctr 1993; **Fac Appt:** Asst Prof Med, Cornell Univ-Weill Med Coll

Cooper, Jerome MD (Cv) - **Spec Exp:** Coronary Artery Disease; Hypertension; Heart Valve Disease; **Hospital:** Sound Shore Med Ctr - Westchester, NY-Presby Hosp/Columbia (page 104); **Address:** 150 Lockwood Ave, Ste 28, New Rochelle, NY 10801; **Phone:** 914-633-7870; **Board Cert:** Internal Medicine 1968; Cardiovascular Disease 1973; **Med School:** SUNY Hlth Sci Ctr 1961; **Resid:** Internal Medicine, Baltimore City Hosps 1963; Cardiovascular Disease, Montefiore Hosp Med Ctr 1964; **Fellow:** Cardiovascular Disease, Johns Hopkins Univ Hosp 1966; Cardiovascular Disease, Johns Hopkins Univ Hosp 1967; **Fac Appt:** Assoc Clin Prof Med, Columbia P&S

Cziner, David MD (Cv) - **Hospital:** White Plains Hosp Ctr, Greenwich Hosp (page 862); **Address:** Westchester Medical Group, 33 Davis Ave, White Plains, NY 10605; **Phone:** 914-948-3630; **Board Cert:** Internal Medicine 1989; Cardiovascular Disease 2001; **Med School:** NYU Sch Med 1986; **Resid:** Internal Medicine, Bellevue/NYU Med Ctr 1989; **Fellow:** Cardiovascular Disease, Bellevue/NYU Med Ctr 1992

Fass, Arthur MD (Cv) - **Spec Exp:** Preventive Cardiology; Coronary Artery Disease; Hypertension; Cholesterol/Lipid Disorders; **Hospital:** Phelps Meml Hosp Ctr (page 592), Westchester Med Ctr; **Address:** 465 N State Rd, Briarcliff Manor, NY 10510; **Phone:** 914-762-5810; **Board Cert:** Internal Medicine 1979; Cardiovascular Disease 1981; **Med School:** NY Med Coll 1976; **Resid:** Internal Medicine, Metropolitan Hosp 1979; **Fellow:** Cardiovascular Disease, Westchester Med Ctr 1981; **Fac Appt:** Assoc Clin Prof Med, NY Med Coll

Feld, Michael MD (Cv) - **Spec Exp:** Pacemakers; Coronary Artery Disease; Congestive Heart Failure; **Hospital:** Phelps Meml Hosp Ctr (page 592), Comm Hosp - Dobbs Ferry; **Address:** 200 S Broadway, Tarrytown, NY 10591-4500; **Phone:** 914-631-2895; **Board Cert:** Internal Medicine 1980; Cardiovascular Disease 1983; **Med School:** Penn State Univ-Hershey Med Ctr 1977; **Resid:** Internal Medicine, Montefiore Med Ctr 1981; **Fellow:** Cardiovascular Disease, Montefiore Med Ctr 1983; **Fac Appt:** Asst Clin Prof Med, Albert Einstein Coll Med

Fishbach, Mitchell MD (Cv) - **Spec Exp:** Non-Invasive Cardiology; Sports Medicine; **Hospital:** Lawrence Hosp Ctr, NY-Presby Hosp/Columbia (page 104); **Address:** 688 White Plains Rd, Ste 201, Scarsdale, NY 10583; **Phone:** 914-722-6300; **Board Cert:** Internal Medicine 1980; Cardiovascular Disease 1983; **Med School:** Albert Einstein Coll Med 1977; **Resid:** Internal Medicine, Montefiore Hosp Med Ctr 1980; **Fellow:** Cardiovascular Disease, Montefiore Hosp Med Ctr 1982

Frishman, William MD (Cv) - **Spec Exp:** Coronary Artery Disease; Preventive Cardiology; Hypertension; Heart Failure; **Hospital:** Westchester Med Ctr; **Address:** NY Med Coll, Dept Med, Munger Pavilion, rm 263, Valhalla, NY 10595; **Phone:** 914-594-4383; **Board Cert:** Internal Medicine 1997; Cardiovascular Disease 1997; Geriatric Medicine 2002; **Med School:** Boston Univ 1969; **Resid:** Internal Medicine, Montefiore Med Ctr 1971; Internal Medicine, Bronx Muni Hosp 1972; **Fellow:** Cardiovascular Disease, NY Hosp 1974; **Fac Appt:** Prof Med, NY Med Coll

Gabelman, Gary S MD (Cv) - **Spec Exp:** Non-Invasive Cardiology; Echocardiography; Nuclear Cardiology; Preventive Cardiology; **Hospital:** Lawrence Hosp Ctr, NY-Presby Hosp/Columbia (page 104); **Address:** 688 White Plains Rd, Scarsdale, NY 10583; **Phone:** 914-722-6300; **Board Cert:** Internal Medicine 1988; Cardiovascular Disease 2001; **Med School:** Mount Sinai Sch Med 1985; **Resid:** Internal Medicine, Montefiore Med Ctr 1989; **Fellow:** Cardiovascular Disease, Montefiore Med Ctr 1991; **Fac Appt:** Assoc Clin Prof Med, Columbia P&S

Gitler, Bernard MD (Cv) - **Spec Exp:** Hypertension; Heart Valve Disease; Congestive Heart Failure; Cholesterol/Lipid Disorders; **Hospital:** Sound Shore Med Ctr - Westchester, NY-Presby Hosp/Columbia (page 104); **Address:** 150 Lockwood Ave, Ste 28, New Rochelle, NY 10801-4913; **Phone:** 914-633-7870; **Board Cert:** Internal Medicine 2009; Cardiovascular Disease 2009; Critical Care Medicine 2010; Echocardiography 2009; **Med School:** Cornell Univ-Weill Med Coll 1976; **Resid:** Internal Medicine, Jacobi Med Ctr 1979; **Fellow:** Cardiovascular Disease, Montefiore Hosp Med Ctr 1981; **Fac Appt:** Assoc Clin Prof Med, Albert Einstein Coll Med

Golier, Francis MD (Cv) - **Spec Exp:** Transesophageal Echocardiography; Stress Echocardiography; **Hospital:** Phelps Meml Hosp Ctr (page 592), Montefiore Med Ctr - Div. Moses (page 100); **Address:** 200 S Broadway, Tarrytown, NY 10591-4500; **Phone:** 914-631-2895; **Board Cert:** Internal Medicine 1972; Cardiovascular Disease 1979; **Med School:** Med Coll Wisc 1969; **Resid:** Internal Medicine, Lenox Hill Hosp 1972; **Fellow:** Cardiovascular Disease, Montefiore Hosp Med Ctr 1974; **Fac Appt:** Asst Clin Prof Med, Albert Einstein Coll Med

Greif, Richard H MD (Cv) - **Hospital:** Saint Joseph's Med Ctr - Yonkers; **Address:** 127 S Broadway Fl 4th - Ste 409, Yonkers, NY 10701; **Phone:** 914-965-6060; **Board Cert:** Internal Medicine 1978; Cardiovascular Disease 1981; **Med School:** NY Med Coll 1975; **Resid:** Internal Medicine, Metropolitan Hosp 1978; **Fellow:** Cardiovascular Disease, St Vincents Hosp 1981; **Fac Appt:** Assoc Clin Prof Med, NY Med Coll

Kaplan, Kenneth C MD (Cv) - **Hospital:** Phelps Meml Hosp Ctr (page 592); **Address:** 160 N State Rd, Briarcliff Manor, NY 10510; **Phone:** 914-762-3821; **Board Cert:** Internal Medicine 1970; Cardiovascular Disease 1975; Echocardiography 1996; **Med School:** NYU Sch Med 1962; **Resid:** Internal Medicine, Bellevue Hosp 1966; **Fellow:** Cardiovascular Disease, Bellevue Hosp/NYU 1969; **Fac Appt:** Asst Clin Prof Med, NY Med Coll

Kay, Richard H MD (Cv) - **Spec Exp:** Preventive Cardiology; Congestive Heart Failure; Non-Invasive Cardiology; **Hospital:** Westchester Med Ctr; **Address:** 19 Bradhurst Ave, Ste 700, Hawthorne, NY 10532-2140; **Phone:** 914-593-7800; **Board Cert:** Internal Medicine 1979; Cardiovascular Disease 1981; **Med School:** Johns Hopkins Univ 1976; **Resid:** Internal Medicine, Columbia-Presby Med Ctr 1979; **Fellow:** Cardiovascular Disease, Mount Sinai Hosp 1981; **Fac Appt:** Assoc Prof Med, NY Med Coll

Keltz, Theodore MD (Cv) - **Spec Exp:** Echocardiography; Nuclear Cardiology; Coronary Artery Disease; Preventive Cardiology; **Hospital:** Sound Shore Med Ctr - Westchester, NY-Presby Hosp/Columbia (page 104); **Address:** 150 Lockwood Ave, Ste 28, New Rochelle, NY 10801-4913; **Phone:** 914-633-7870; **Board Cert:** Internal Medicine 1983; Cardiovascular Disease 1985; Echocardiography 2006; Nuclear Cardiology 1996; **Med School:** Albany Med Coll 1980; **Resid:** Internal Medicine, Mt Sinai Med Ctr 1983; **Fellow:** Cardiovascular Disease, Montefiore Med Ctr 1985; **Fac Appt:** Assoc Clin Prof Med, Albert Einstein Coll Med

Levine, Evan MD (Cv) - **Spec Exp:** Cardiac Stress Testing; **Hospital:** Montefiore Med Ctr - Div. Moses (page 100), St John's Riverside Hosp; **Address:** Riverside Cardiology, 955 Yonkers Ave, Ste 200, Yonkers, NY 10704; **Phone:** 914-237-1332; **Board Cert:** Internal Medicine 1988; Cardiovascular Disease 2000; **Med School:** Mount Sinai Sch Med 1985; **Resid:** Internal Medicine, Montefiore Med Ctr 1988; **Fellow:** Cardiovascular Disease, Montefiore Med Ctr 1990; **Fac Appt:** Asst Clin Prof Med, Albert Einstein Coll Med

Lieb, Mark MD (Cv) - **Hospital:** Northern Westchester Hosp; **Address:** 110 S Bedford Rd Fl 2, Mt Kisco, NY 10549-3412; **Phone:** 914-241-1050; **Board Cert:** Cardiovascular Disease 2006; **Med School:** Boston Univ 1988; **Resid:** Internal Medicine, Mt Sinai Med Ctr 1991; **Fellow:** Cardiovascular Disease, Mt Sinai Med Ctr 1995

Matos, Marshall MD (Cv) - **Spec Exp:** Coronary Artery Disease; Preventive Cardiology; Arrhythmias; Cholesterol/Lipid Disorders; **Hospital:** Sound Shore Med Ctr - Westchester, Lenox Hill Hosp; **Address:** 140 Lockwood Ave, Ste 310, New Rochelle, NY 10801-4909; **Phone:** 914-576-7171; **Board Cert:** Internal Medicine 1980; Cardiovascular Disease 1985; **Med School:** Albert Einstein Coll Med 1977; **Resid:** Internal Medicine, Bronx Muni Hosp 1981; **Fellow:** Cardiovascular Disease, Albert Einstein Coll Med 1983; **Fac Appt:** Asst Prof Med, NYU Sch Med

McClung, John A MD (Cv) - **Spec Exp:** Echocardiography; **Hospital:** Westchester Med Ctr; **Address:** 19 Bradhurst Ave, Ste 700, Hawthorne, NY 10532; **Phone:** 914-593-7800; **Board Cert:** Internal Medicine 1980; Cardiovascular Disease 1983; **Med School:** NY Med Coll 1975; **Resid:** Internal Medicine, Lincoln Med Ctr 1979; **Fellow:** Cardiovascular Disease, Westchester Med Ctr 1982; **Fac Appt:** Assoc Prof Med, NY Med Coll

Medina, Emma MD (Cv) - **Spec Exp:** Non-Invasive Cardiology; **Hospital:** Sound Shore Med Ctr - Westchester, Montefiore Med Ctr - Div. Weiler (page 100); **Address:** 140 Lockwood Ave, Ste 310, New Rochelle, NY 10801-4909; **Phone:** 914-632-1600; **Board Cert:** Internal Medicine 1982; Cardiovascular Disease 1985; **Med School:** NYU Sch Med 1979; **Resid:** Internal Medicine, Jacobi Med Ctr 1982; **Fellow:** Cardiovascular Disease, Jacobi Med Ctr 1984; **Fac Appt:** Asst Clin Prof Med, Albert Einstein Coll Med

Mercando, Anthony MD (Cv) - **Spec Exp:** Cholesterol/Lipid Disorders; Pacemakers/Defibrillators; Preventive Cardiology; **Hospital:** Lawrence Hosp Ctr, NY-Presby Hosp/Columbia (page 104); **Address:** 688 White Plains Rd, Ste 201, Scarsdale, NY 10583; **Phone:** 914-722-6300; **Board Cert:** Internal Medicine 1983; Cardiovascular Disease 1987; **Med School:** Harvard Med Sch 1980; **Resid:** Internal Medicine, Montefiore Med Ctr 1984; **Fellow:** Cardiovascular Disease, Montefiore Med Ctr 1986; **Fac Appt:** Clin Prof Med, Albert Einstein Coll Med

Perry-Bottinger, Lynne V MD (Cv) - **Spec Exp:** Cardiac Catheterization; Coronary Angioplasty/Stents; Heart Disease in Women; Heart Disease in African Americans; **Hospital:** NY-Presby Hosp/Columbia (page 104), Sound Shore Med Ctr - Westchester; **Address:** Clinical & Interventional Cardiology, 140A Lockwood Ave, New Rochelle, NY 10801; **Phone:** 914-576-7577; **Board Cert:** Cardiovascular Disease 1997; **Med School:** Yale Univ 1986; **Resid:** Internal Medicine, Yale-New Haven Hosp 1990; **Fellow:** Cardiovascular Disease, Johns Hopkins Hosp 1993; Interventional Cardiology, Johns Hopkins Hosp 1994; **Fac Appt:** Asst Clin Prof Med, Columbia P&S

Price Jr, Thomas J MD (Cv) - **Hospital:** Mount Vernon Hosp, Sound Shore Med Ctr - Westchester; **Address:** 105 Stevens Ave, Ste 603, Mt Vernon, NY 10550; **Phone:** 914-664-4052; **Board Cert:** Internal Medicine 1984; Cardiovascular Disease 1987; **Med School:** Univ Cincinnati 1975; **Resid:** Internal Medicine, Harlem Hosp 1979; **Fellow:** Cardiovascular Disease, Harlem Hosp 1983; **Fac Appt:** Asst Clin Prof Med, Columbia P&S

Pucillo, Anthony MD (Cv) - **Spec Exp:** Coronary Angioplasty/Stents; Peripheral Vascular Disease; Cardiac Catheterization; Interventional Cardiology; **Hospital:** Westchester Med Ctr; **Address:** 19 Bradhurst Ave, Ste 700, Hawthorne, NY 10532; **Phone:** 914-593-7800; **Board Cert:** Internal Medicine 1981; Cardiovascular Disease 1983; Interventional Cardiology 2000; **Med School:** Mount Sinai Sch Med 1978; **Resid:** Internal Medicine, Columbia-Presby Med Ctr 1981; **Fellow:** Cardiovascular Disease, Columbia-Presby Med Ctr 1984; **Fac Appt:** Assoc Prof Med, NY Med Coll

Sheikh, Shahid MD (Cv) - **Hospital:** St John's Riverside Hosp, Montefiore Med Ctr - Div. North (page 100); **Address:** 970 N Broadway, Ste 210, Yonkers, NY 10701-1311; **Phone:** 914-963-0111; **Board Cert:** Internal Medicine 1977; Cardiovascular Disease 1979; **Med School:** Pakistan 1971; **Resid:** Internal Medicine, Lady of Mercy Med Ctr 1976

Silver, Michael M MD (Cv) - **Spec Exp:** Hypertension; Cholesterol/Lipid Disorders; Coronary Artery Disease; **Hospital:** White Plains Hosp Ctr, Greenwich Hosp (page 862); **Address:** Westchester Medical Group, 33 Davis Ave, White Plains, NY 10605-1030; **Phone:** 914-948-3630; **Board Cert:** Internal Medicine 1980; Cardiovascular Disease 1983; **Med School:** SUNY Downstate 1977; **Resid:** Internal Medicine, Thomas Jefferson Univ Hosp 1980; **Fellow:** Cardiovascular Disease, Presby-Hosp Univ Penn 1982

Sorbera, Carmine A MD (Cv) - **Spec Exp:** Arrhythmias; Cardiac Catheterization; **Hospital:** Westchester Med Ctr, Kingston Hosp; **Address:** 19 Bradhurst Ave, Ste 700, Hawthorne, NY 10532; **Phone:** 914-593-7823; **Board Cert:** Internal Medicine 1987; Cardiovascular Disease 1989; Cardiac Electrophysiology 2004; **Med School:** NY Med Coll 1983; **Resid:** Internal Medicine, Westchester Med Ctr 1987; **Fellow:** Cardiovascular Disease, Westchester Med Ctr 1989; Interventional Cardiology, Westchester Med Ctr 1990

Tartaglia, Joseph J MD (Cv) - **Spec Exp:** Angina; Congestive Heart Failure; Arrhythmias; **Hospital:** White Plains Hosp Ctr, Greenwich Hosp (page 862); **Address:** 311 North St, Ste 402, White Plains, NY 10605-2232; **Phone:** 914-946-3388; **Board Cert:** Internal Medicine 1988; Cardiovascular Disease 2001; Geriatric Medicine 2004; **Med School:** Italy 1984; **Resid:** Internal Medicine, Our Lady of Mercy Med Ctr 1988; **Fellow:** Cardiovascular Disease, N Shore Univ Hosp 1990; **Fac Appt:** Asst Clin Prof Med, NY Med Coll

Weiss, Melvin MD (Cv) - **Spec Exp:** Cardiac Imaging; Congestive Heart Failure; Diabetes & Heart Disease; Coronary Artery Disease; **Hospital:** Westchester Med Ctr; **Address:** 19 Bradhurst Ave, Ste 700, Hawthorne, NY 10532-2140; **Phone:** 914-593-7800; **Board Cert:** Internal Medicine 1972; Cardiovascular Disease 1975; Interventional Cardiology 1999; **Med School:** SUNY Hlth Sci Ctr 1967; **Resid:** Internal Medicine, NY Hosp 1971; **Fellow:** Cardiovascular Disease, NY Presby Med Ctr 1972; **Fac Appt:** Prof Med, NY Med Coll

Weissman, Ronald MD (Cv) - **Spec Exp:** Coronary Artery Disease; Congestive Heart Failure; Arrhythmias; Hypertrophic Cardiomyopathy; **Hospital:** White Plains Hosp Ctr, Westchester Med Ctr; **Address:** 15 N Broadway Fl 2, White Plains, NY 10601; **Phone:** 914-428-6000; **Board Cert:** Internal Medicine 1980; Cardiovascular Disease 1983; **Med School:** NY Med Coll 1977; **Resid:** Internal Medicine, LI Jewish Hosp 1980; **Fellow:** Cardiovascular Disease, LI Jewish Hosp 1982; **Fac Appt:** Assoc Clin Prof Med, NY Med Coll

Zimmerman, Franklin (Bud) MD (Cv) - **Spec Exp:** Preventive Cardiology; Sports Medicine Cardiology; Cholesterol/Lipid Disorders; **Hospital:** Phelps Meml Hosp Ctr (page 592), Westchester Med Ctr; **Address:** 465 N State Rd, Briarcliff Manor, NY 10510-1468; **Phone:** 914-762-5810; **Board Cert:** Internal Medicine 1983; Cardiovascular Disease 1987; Critical Care Medicine 2006; **Med School:** Brown Univ 1980; **Resid:** Internal Medicine, St Lukes-Roosevelt Hosp Ctr 1983; **Fellow:** Cardiovascular Disease, St Lukes-Roosevelt Hosp Ctr 1988; **Fac Appt:** Asst Prof Med, Columbia P&S

Child & Adolescent Psychiatry

Cohen, Lee Steven MD (ChAP) - **Spec Exp:** Anxiety & Mood Disorders; Psychopharmacology; ADD/ADHD; Autism; **Hospital:** NY-Presby Hosp/Columbia (page 104), St Luke's - Roosevelt Hosp Ctr - Roosevelt Div (page 94); **Address:** 623 Warburton Ave, Hastings On Hudson, NY 10706-1523; **Phone:** 914-478-1330; **Board Cert:** Psychiatry 1987; Child & Adolescent Psychiatry 1988; **Med School:** SUNY Stony Brook 1982; **Resid:** Psychiatry, Mt Sinai Med Ctr 1985; Pediatrics, Mt Sinai Med Ctr 1983; **Fellow:** Child & Adolescent Psychiatry, Columbia-Presby Med Ctr 1987; **Fac Appt:** Asst Clin Prof Psyc, Columbia P&S

Hyler, Irene MD (ChAP) - **Spec Exp:** Psychotherapy; Psychoanalysis; **Hospital:** NY-Presby Hosp/Weill Cornell (page 104); **Address:** 2A Berkeley Rd, Scarsdale, NY 10583-1102; **Phone:** 914-472-8447; **Board Cert:** Psychiatry 1984; Child & Adolescent Psychiatry 1986; **Med School:** Albert Einstein Coll Med 1979; **Resid:** Psychiatry, Albert Einstein Coll Med 1982; **Fellow:** Child & Adolescent Psychiatry, Bronx Muni Hosp 1984; **Fac Appt:** Asst Clin Prof Psyc, Cornell Univ-Weill Med Coll

Kalikow, Kevin T MD (ChAP) - ; **Address:** 39 Smith Ave, Mt Kisco, NY 10549; **Phone:** 914-666-3000; **Board Cert:** Psychiatry 1984; Child & Adolescent Psychiatry 1986; **Med School:** Tulane Univ 1979; **Resid:** Psychiatry, NY Hosp-Westchester Div 1983; **Fellow:** Child & Adolescent Psychiatry, NY State Psych Inst 1985; **Fac Appt:** Asst Clin Prof Psyc, NY Med Coll

Rubinstein, Boris MD (ChAP) - **Spec Exp:** Psychopharmacology; Neuro-Psychiatry; Mood Disorders; Developmental Disorders; **Hospital:** NYPresby-Morgan Stanley Children's Hosp (page 104); **Address:** 623 Warburton Ave, Hastings On Hudson, NY 10706; **Phone:** 914-478-1330; **Board Cert:** Pediatrics 1976; Psychiatry 1979; Child & Adolescent Psychiatry 1981; **Med School:** Mexico 1970; **Resid:** Pediatrics, Chldns Hosp 1974; Psychiatry, Jacobi Med Ctr 1976; **Fellow:** Child & Adolescent Psychiatry, Jacobi Med Ctr 1978; Public Health & Genl Preventive Med, Harvard Sch Pub Hlth 1974

Schreiber, Klaus MD (ChAP) - **Spec Exp:** Developmental Disorders; **Address:** 1 Neperan Rd, Tarrytown, NY 10591; **Phone:** 914-332-0270; **Board Cert:** Psychiatry 1976; Child & Adolescent Psychiatry 1986; **Med School:** Germany 1966; **Resid:** Psychiatry, Elmhurst City Hosp Ctr 1971; Psychiatry, Westchester Med Ctr 1972; **Fellow:** Child & Adolescent Psychiatry, Westchester Med Ctr 1973; Child & Adolescent Psychiatry, Albert Einstein Coll Med 1982; **Fac Appt:** Asst Prof Psyc, NY Med Coll

Seaver, Robert MD (ChAP) - **Spec Exp:** Forensic Psychiatry; Art & Creativity; Psychopharmacology; **Address:** 83 S Bedford Ave Fl 2nd, Mt Kisco, NY 10549; **Phone:** 914-241-8979; **Board Cert:** Pediatrics 1978; Psychiatry 1984; Child & Adolescent Psychiatry 1986; **Med School:** Mount Sinai Sch Med 1973; **Resid:** Pediatrics, Mt Sinai Hosp 1975; Pediatrics, St Luke's-Roosevelt Hosp 1976; **Fellow:** Psychiatry, NY Hosp-Westchester Div 1984; Child & Adolescent Psychiatry, Jacobi Med Ctr 1985

Slater, Jonathan MD (ChAP) - **Spec Exp:** Psychopharmacology; Medical Illness in Psychiatry; **Hospital:** NYPresby-Morgan Stanley Children's Hosp (page 104); **Address:** 1 Bridge St, Ste 24, Irvington, NY 10533; **Phone:** 914-591-4135; **Board Cert:** Psychiatry 1991; Child & Adolescent Psychiatry 1993; Psychosomatic Medicine 2006; **Med School:** Columbia P&S 1985; **Resid:** Psychiatry, Columbia-Presby Med Ctr 1990; **Fellow:** Research, NY State Psychiatric Inst 1986; Child & Adolescent Psychiatry, Columbia-Presby Med Ctr 1992; **Fac Appt:** Clin Prof Psyc, Columbia P&S

Child Neurology

Jacobson, Ronald I MD (ChiN) - **Spec Exp:** Epilepsy; Headache; ADD/ADHD; Autism; **Hospital:** Westchester Med Ctr, Children's & Women's Phys.of Westchester; **Address:** Pediatric Neurology Assocs, 755 N Broadway, Medical Services Bldg, Ste 540, Sleepy Hollow, NY 10591; **Phone:** 914-358-0190; **Board Cert:** Pediatrics 1981; Child Neurology 1984; **Med School:** Albert Einstein Coll Med 1975; **Resid:** Pediatrics, Yale-New Haven Hosp 1979; **Fellow:** Pediatric Neurology, Univ Minn Med Ctr 1982; **Fac Appt:** Assoc Clin Prof N, NY Med Coll

Kang, Harriet MD (ChiN) - **Spec Exp:** Epilepsy/Seizure Disorders; **Hospital:** Beth Israel Med Ctr - Petrie Division (page 94); **Address:** 141 S Central Park Ave, Hartsdale, NY 10530; **Phone:** 914-428-0529; **Board Cert:** Pediatrics 1979; Child Neurology 1981; Clinical Neurophysiology 2006; **Med School:** Johns Hopkins Univ 1974; **Resid:** Pediatrics, Johns Hopkins Hosp 1976; Child Neurology, Univ Minn Med Ctr 1979; **Fellow:** Clinical Neurophysiology, Univ Minn Med Ctr 1980; **Fac Appt:** Assoc Prof N, Albert Einstein Coll Med

Kutscher, Martin MD (ChiN) - **Spec Exp:** ADD/ADHD; Asperger's Syndrome; Autism; **Hospital:** Westchester Med Ctr; **Address:** 800 Westchester Ave, Ste N641, Rye Brook, NY 10573; **Phone:** 914-232-1810; **Board Cert:** Pediatrics 1986; Child Neurology 1989; **Med School:** Columbia P&S 1981; **Resid:** Pediatrics, St Christopher's Hosp 1984; Neurology, Montefiore Med Ctr 1987; **Fellow:** Child Neurology, Montefiore Med Ctr 1989; **Fac Appt:** Asst Clin Prof Ped, NY Med Coll

Clinical Genetics

Kronn, David F MD (CG) - **Spec Exp:** Bone Disorders-Metabolic; Bone Disorders-Inherited; **Hospital:** Westchester Med Ctr, Children's & Women's Phys.of Westchester; **Address:** Regional Med Genetics Ctr, Children/Women's Physicians of Westchester, 503 Grasslands Rd, Ste 200, Valhalla, NY 10595; **Phone:** 914-304-5300; **Board Cert:** Clinical Genetics 2007; Pediatrics 2002; Clinical Biochemical Genetics 1999; **Med School:** Ireland 1989; **Resid:** Pediatrics, NYU Med Ctr 1996; **Fellow:** Clinical Genetics, NYU Med Ctr 1996; **Fac Appt:** CG, NY Med Coll

Shapiro, Lawrence R MD (CG) - **Spec Exp:** Dysmorphology; Prenatal Diagnosis; Hereditary Cancer; Developmental Disorders; **Hospital:** Westchester Med Ctr, Nyack Hosp; **Address:** Regional Med Genetics Ctr, Children/Women's Physicians of Westchester, 503 Grasslands Ave, Ste 200, Valhalla, NY 10595; **Phone:** 914-304-5300; **Board Cert:** Pediatrics 1967; Clinical Genetics 1982; Clinical Cytogenetics 1982; **Med School:** NYU Sch Med 1962; **Resid:** Pediatrics, Chldns Hosp 1964; Pediatrics, Bellevue Hosp 1965; **Fellow:** Clinical Genetics, Mount Sinai Med Ctr 1968; **Fac Appt:** Prof Ped, NY Med Coll

Colon & Rectal Surgery

Krakovitz, Evan K MD (CRS) - **Spec Exp:** Colon & Rectal Cancer & Surgery; Hemorrhoids; Laparoscopic Surgery; **Hospital:** Greenwich Hosp (page 862), White Plains Hosp Ctr; **Address:** Westmed Grp, 210 Westchester Ave, White Plains, NY 10604; **Phone:** 914-682-6557; **Board Cert:** Surgery 2005; Colon & Rectal Surgery 2007; **Med School:** Hahnemann Univ 1989; **Resid:** Surgery, Graduate Hospital 1994; **Fellow:** Colon & Rectal Surgery, RWJ Univ Hosp 1995

Wishner, Jerald D MD (CRS) - **Spec Exp:** Colon & Rectal Cancer; Laparoscopic Surgery; **Hospital:** Northern Westchester Hosp; **Address:** Mount Kisco Med Grp, 110 S Bedford Rd, Mount Kisco, NY 10549; **Phone:** 914-241-1050; **Board Cert:** Surgery 2004; Colon & Rectal Surgery 2006; **Med School:** Northwestern Univ 1988; **Resid:** Surgery, St Luke's-Roosevelt Hosp Ctr 1993; Colon & Rectal Surgery, Grtr Baltimore Med Ctr 1994; **Fellow:** Minimally Invasive Surgery, Eastern Va Med Sch 1995; **Fac Appt:** Asst Prof S, Columbia P&S

Dermatology

Bank, David MD (D) - **Spec Exp:** Liposuction; Skin Laser Surgery; Botox Therapy; **Hospital:** NY-Presby Hosp/Columbia (page 104), Northern Westchester Hosp; **Address:** 359 E Main St, Ste 4G, Mt Kisco, NY 10549-3035; **Phone:** 914-241-3003; **Board Cert:** Dermatology 1989; **Med School:** Columbia P&S 1985; **Resid:** Dermatology, Columbia-Presby Med Ctr 1989; **Fac Appt:** Assoc Clin Prof D, Columbia P&S

Berkowitz, Rhonda K MD (D) - **Spec Exp:** Melanoma; Skin Cancer; **Hospital:** NY-Presby Hosp/Columbia (page 104); **Address:** 325 S Highland Ave, Briarcliff Manor, NY 10510-2031; **Phone:** 914-941-5769; **Board Cert:** Dermatology 1986; **Med School:** NYU Sch Med 1982; **Resid:** Internal Medicine, N Shore Univ Hosp 1983; Dermatology, Columbia-Presby Med Ctr 1986

Bronin, Andrew MD (D) - **Spec Exp:** Melanoma; Skin Cancer; Complex Diagnosis; **Hospital:** Greenwich Hosp (page 862), Yale-New Haven Hosp; **Address:** 4 Rye Ridge Plaza, Rye Brook, NY 10573-2820; **Phone:** 914-253-8080; **Board Cert:** Dermatology 1981; **Med School:** NY Med Coll 1975; **Resid:** Dermatology, New York Hosp 1979; **Fac Appt:** Assoc Clin Prof D, Yale Univ

Davis, Ira C MD (D) - **Spec Exp:** Mohs' Surgery; Skin Cancer; Laser Surgery; Cosmetic Dermatology; **Hospital:** Westchester Med Ctr, Richmond Univ Med Ctr; **Address:** 280 N Central Park Ave, Ste 114, Hartsdale, NY 10530; **Phone:** 914-288-0500; **Board Cert:** Dermatology 1990; **Med School:** NYU Sch Med 1986; **Resid:** Dermatology, Duke Univ Med Ctr 1990; **Fellow:** Dermatologic Pharmacology, NYU Med Ctr 1991; Mohs Surgery, Wake Forest Univ Med Ctr 1994; **Fac Appt:** Asst Clin Prof D, NY Med Coll

Felsenstein, Jerome M MD (D) - **Hospital:** Phelps Meml Hosp Ctr (page 592), NYU Langone Med Ctr (page 106); **Address:** 100 S Highland Ave, Ossining, NY 10562; **Phone:** 914-941-5770; **Board Cert:** Dermatology 1976; **Med School:** NYU Sch Med 1971; **Resid:** Dermatology, Kings County Hosp 1975

Goldberg, Neil S MD (D) - **Spec Exp:** Pediatric Dermatology; Acne; **Hospital:** White Plains Hosp Ctr, Lawrence Hosp Ctr; **Address:** 222 Westchester Ave, Ste 203, White Plains, NY 10604-2926; **Phone:** 914-761-8140; **Board Cert:** Dermatology 1986; **Med School:** Northwestern Univ 1982; **Resid:** Dermatology, Northwestern Meml Hosp 1986

Grossman, Marc E MD (D) - **Spec Exp:** Skin Diseases in Transplants/Cancer; Psoriasis; Rare Skin Disorders; Cutaneous Lymphoma; **Hospital:** NY-Presby Hosp/Columbia (page 104), White Plains Hosp Ctr; **Address:** 12 Greenridge Ave, White Plains, NY 10605-1238; **Phone:** 914-946-1101; **Board Cert:** Internal Medicine 1977; Dermatology 2009; **Med School:** Univ Pennsylvania 1974; **Resid:** Internal Medicine, Hosp Univ Penn 1976; **Fellow:** Dermatology, Columbia-Presby Med Ctr 1979; **Fac Appt:** Prof D, Columbia P&S

Hurwitz, Diana S MD (D) - **Hospital:** White Plains Hosp Ctr; **Address:** Westchester Medical Group, 1 Theall Rd, Rye, NY 10580; **Phone:** 914-848-8840; **Board Cert:** Dermatology 2005; **Med School:** Mount Sinai Sch Med 1992; **Resid:** Dermatology, Mt Sinai Med Ctr 1996

Kaplan, Sherri MD (D) - **Hospital:** Comm Hosp - Dobbs Ferry, St John's Riverside Hosp; **Address:** 1055 Saw Mill River Rd, Ste 208, Ardsley, NY 10502-1046; **Phone:** 914-693-7191; **Board Cert:** Dermatology 1987; **Med School:** NY Med Coll 1983; **Resid:** Dermatology, Westchester Co Med Ctr 1987; **Fac Appt:** Asst Clin Prof D, NY Med Coll

Klar, Tobi MD (D) - **Spec Exp:** Skin Cancer; **Hospital:** Sound Shore Med Ctr - Westchester, Montefiore Med Ctr - Div. Weiler (page 100); **Address:** 150 Lockwood Ave, Ste 20, New Rochelle, NY 10801; **Phone:** 914-636-2039; **Board Cert:** Dermatology 1989; **Med School:** SUNY Downstate 1981; **Resid:** Dermatology, Downstate Med Ctr 1986

Lerman, Jay S MD (D) - **Spec Exp:** Acne; Eczema; **Hospital:** White Plains Hosp Ctr, Montefiore Med Ctr - Div. Moses (page 100); **Address:** 280 Dobbs Ferry Rd, Ste 205, White Plains, NY 10607-1912; **Phone:** 914-949-9196; **Board Cert:** Dermatology 1974; **Med School:** SUNY Downstate 1969; **Resid:** Dermatology, Jacobi Med Ctr 1973; **Fac Appt:** Asst Clin Prof D, Albert Einstein Coll Med

Levy, Ross MD (D) - **Spec Exp:** Skin Laser Surgery; Dermatologic Surgery; Skin Cancer; **Hospital:** Northern Westchester Hosp, Montefiore Med Ctr - Div. Moses (page 100); **Address:** Mt Kisco Med Group, 110 S Bedford Rd, Mt Kisco, NY 10549; **Phone:** 914-242-1355; **Board Cert:** Dermatology 1981; **Med School:** Albert Einstein Coll Med 1976; **Resid:** Internal Medicine, Montefiore Med Ctr 1978; **Fellow:** Dermatology, Montefiore Med Ctr 1981; **Fac Appt:** Assoc Clin Prof Med, Albert Einstein Coll Med

Lukash, Barbara MD (D) - **Spec Exp:** Skin Cancer; Acne; Psoriasis; Melanoma; **Hospital:** NY-Presby Hosp/Columbia (page 104); **Address:** 14 Lawton St, New Rochelle, NY 10801; **Phone:** 914-712-2800; **Board Cert:** Dermatology 1980; **Med School:** Tulane Univ 1976; **Resid:** Dermatology, Univ Chicago Hosps 1980; **Fellow:** Dermatology, Univ of Chicago Hosps 1980; **Fac Appt:** Assoc Clin Prof D, Columbia P&S

Mackler, Karen MD (D) - **Spec Exp:** Pediatric Dermatology; Skin Cancer; **Hospital:** Sound Shore Med Ctr - Westchester, Montefiore Med Ctr - Div. Moses (page 100); **Address:** 150 Lockwood Ave, Ste 34, New Rochelle, NY 10801-4914; **Phone:** 914-576-7070; **Board Cert:** Pediatrics 1978; Dermatology 1983; **Med School:** NYU Sch Med 1973; **Resid:** Pediatrics, NY Hosp 1976; Dermatology, Montefiore Hosp Med Ctr 1983; **Fac Appt:** Asst Prof D, Albert Einstein Coll Med

Mattison, Timothy D MD (D) - **Hospital:** Northern Westchester Hosp; **Address:** Mt Kisco Medical Group, 90 S Bedford Rd, Mt Kisco, NY 10549-3412; **Phone:** 914-242-1355; **Board Cert:** Dermatology 1980; **Med School:** Dartmouth Med Sch 1976; **Resid:** Dermatology, NYU Med Ctr 1980

Mermelstein, Harold MD (D) - **Spec Exp:** Cosmetic Dermatology; Aging Skin; Sclerotherapy; Laser Surgery; **Hospital:** NYU Langone Med Ctr (page 106), Lawrence Hosp Ctr; **Address:** 559 Gramatan Ave, Ste 205, Mt Vernon, NY 10552-3234; **Phone:** 914-667-2242; **Board Cert:** Dermatology 1979; **Med School:** NY Med Coll 1975; **Resid:** Dermatology, NYU Med Ctr 1979; **Fellow:** Dermatologic Surgery, NYU Med Ctr 1980; **Fac Appt:** Assoc Clin Prof D, NYU Sch Med

Narins, Rhoda MD (D) - **Spec Exp:** Liposuction; Cosmetic Dermatology; Botox Therapy; Facial Rejuvenation; **Hospital:** NYU Langone Med Ctr (page 106), White Plains Hosp Ctr; **Address:** 222 Westchester Ave, Ste 300, White Plains, NY 10604-2925; **Phone:** 914-684-1000; **Board Cert:** Dermatology 1970; **Med School:** NYU Sch Med 1965; **Resid:** Dermatology, NYU Med Ctr 1969; **Fac Appt:** Clin Prof D, NYU Sch Med

Newburger, Amy E MD (D) - **Spec Exp:** Contact Dermatitis; Cosmetic Dermatology; **Hospital:** White Plains Hosp Ctr; **Address:** 2 Overhill Rd, Ste 330, Scarsdale, NY 10583; **Phone:** 914-725-1800; **Board Cert:** Dermatology 1979; **Med School:** NYU Sch Med 1974; **Resid:** Dermatology, Univ Miami Hosps 1978

Rosenthal, Elizabeth R MD (D) - **Spec Exp:** Acne; Atopic Dermatitis; **Hospital:** Jacobi Med Ctr; **Address:** 1600 Harrison Ave, Ste 303, Mamaroneck, NY 10543-3151; **Phone:** 914-698-2190; **Board Cert:** Dermatology 1975; **Med School:** NYU Sch Med 1967; **Resid:** Dermatology, Henry Ford Hosp 1969; Dermatology, Roosevelt Hosp 1970; **Fellow:** Dermatology, Boston Univ Med Ctr 1974; **Fac Appt:** Asst Clin Prof D, Albert Einstein Coll Med

Schliftman, Alan B MD (D) - **Spec Exp:** Laser Surgery; Skin Cancer; **Hospital:** Westchester Med Ctr, White Plains Hosp Ctr; **Address:** 244 Westchester Ave, Ste 211, White Plains, NY 10604-2926; **Phone:** 914-761-1400; **Board Cert:** Dermatology 1981; **Med School:** Geo Wash Univ 1977; **Resid:** Dermatology, Montefiore Med Ctr 1981

Stillman, Michael MD (D) - **Spec Exp:** Skin Cancer; Acne; Eczema; **Hospital:** Northern Westchester Hosp; **Address:** Mt Kisco Medical Group, 111 Bedford Rd, Katonah, NY 10536; **Phone:** 914-232-3135; **Board Cert:** Dermatology 1973; **Med School:** SUNY Downstate 1967; **Resid:** Dermatology, NYU Med Ctr 1973; **Fellow:** Dermatology, Letterman Army Inst Rsch 1970

Sturza, Jeffrey MD (D) - **Spec Exp:** Psoriasis; Laser Surgery; Cosmetic Dermatology; **Hospital:** Phelps Meml Hosp Ctr (page 592), Jacobi Med Ctr; **Address:** 150 White Plains Rd, Ste 210, Tarrytown, NY 10591; **Phone:** 914-631-4666; **Board Cert:** Dermatology 1988; **Med School:** SUNY Hlth Sci Ctr 1984; **Resid:** Dermatology, Cook Co Hosp 1988

Treiber, Ruth K MD (D) - **Spec Exp:** Botox Therapy; Acne; Facial Rejuvenation; Skin Cancer; **Hospital:** NY-Presby Hosp/Columbia (page 104); **Address:** 175 Purchase St, Rye, NY 10580; **Phone:** 914-967-2153; **Board Cert:** Dermatology 1983; **Med School:** Cornell Univ-Weill Med Coll 1978; **Resid:** Internal Medicine, New York Hosp 1980; Dermatology, Columbia-Presby Med Ctr 1983; **Fac Appt:** Assoc Clin Prof D, Columbia P&S

Zweibel, Stuart M MD/PhD (D) - **Spec Exp:** Mohs' Surgery; Skin Cancer; Skin Laser Surgery; Cosmetic Dermatology; **Hospital:** Northern Westchester Hosp; **Address:** 185 Kisco Ave, Ste 3, Mt Kisco, NY 10549; **Phone:** 914-242-2020; **Board Cert:** Dermatology 2009; **Med School:** Mount Sinai Sch Med 1985; **Resid:** Dermatology, Rhode Island Hosp 1989; **Fellow:** Mohs Surgery, Univ of Wisconsin Hosp 1991

Diagnostic Radiology

Hertz, Marc MD (DR) - **Spec Exp:** CT Scan; MRI; **Address:** Mt Kisco Medical Group, 90 S Bedford Rd, Mount Kisco, NY 10549; **Phone:** 914-242-1395; **Board Cert:** Diagnostic Radiology 1985; **Med School:** Howard Univ 1979; **Resid:** Pathology, Lenox Hill Hospital 1981; Diagnostic Radiology, Montefiore Hospital 1984; **Fellow:** Ultrasound/CT, North Shore Univ Hosp 1985

Khoury, Paul MD (DR) - **Hospital:** White Plains Hosp Ctr; **Address:** White Plains Hosp Ctr, Dept Radiology, 41 E Post Rd, White Plains, NY 10601; **Phone:** 914-681-1219; **Board Cert:** Diagnostic Radiology 1979; Nuclear Radiology 1980; **Med School:** Lebanon 1973; **Resid:** Diagnostic Radiology, Hotel Dieu de France Hosp 1975; Diagnostic Radiology, St Luke's-Roosevelt Hosp Ctr 1978

Kutcher, Rosalyn MD (DR) - **Spec Exp:** Mammography; Ultrasound; Women's Imaging; **Hospital:** White Plains Hosp Ctr; **Address:** 90 S Ridge St, Women's Imaging Ctr, Rye Brook, NY 10573; **Phone:** 914-935-0011; **Board Cert:** Diagnostic Radiology 1975; **Med School:** SUNY Hlth Sci Ctr 1970; **Resid:** Diagnostic Radiology, Montefiore Med Ctr 1974; **Fac Appt:** Prof Rad, Albert Einstein Coll Med

Lefkovitz, Zvi MD (DR) - **Spec Exp:** Chest Radiology; **Hospital:** Westchester Med Ctr; **Address:** WMC Advanced Physician Services, 100 Woods Rd, Valhalla, NY 10595; **Phone:** 914-493-2500; **Board Cert:** Diagnostic Radiology 1986; **Med School:** Ros Franklin Univ/Chicago Med Sch 1982; **Resid:** Diagnostic Radiology, Maimonides Med Ctr 1986; **Fellow:** Interventional Radiology, Univ Hosp 1987

Leslie, Denise MD (DR) - **Spec Exp:** Neuroradiology; **Hospital:** Good Samaritan Hosp - Suffern, St John's Riverside Hosp; **Address:** East Westchester Radiology, 503 Grasslands Rd, Ste 100, Valhalla, NY 10595; **Phone:** 914-345-0376; **Board Cert:** Diagnostic Radiology 1985; **Med School:** SUNY Buffalo 1981; **Resid:** Diagnostic Radiology, Westchester Co Med Ctr 1985; **Fellow:** Neuroradiology, Westchester Co Med Ctr 1987

LoRusso, Diane MD (DR) - **Spec Exp:** Breast Imaging; Women's Health; Ultrasound; MRI; **Address:** Rye Radiology Assoc, 30 Rye Ridge Plaza, Rye Brook, NY 10573-2830; **Phone:** 914-253-9200; **Board Cert:** Diagnostic Radiology 1974; **Med School:** SUNY Upstate Med Univ 1969; **Resid:** Diagnostic Radiology, Montefiore Med Ctr 1974

Poplausky, Maurice R MD (DR) - **Spec Exp:** Interventional Radiology; **Hospital:** Hudson Valley Hosp Ctr, Westchester Med Ctr; **Address:** Hudson Valley Hospital, Dept Radiology, 1980 Crompound Rd, Cortland Manor, NY 10567; **Phone:** 914-734-3680; **Board Cert:** Diagnostic Radiology 1995; Vascular & Interventional Radiology 2008; **Med School:** SUNY Buffalo 1990; **Resid:** Diagnostic Radiology, SUNY Downstate Med Ctr 1995; **Fellow:** Vascular & Interventional Radiology, Mass Genl Hosp 1996; **Fac Appt:** Assoc Prof Rad, NY Med Coll

Endocrinology, Diabetes & Metabolism

Albin, Joan MD (EDM) - **Spec Exp:** Diabetes; Thyroid Disorders; Polycystic Ovarian Syndrome; **Hospital:** Sound Shore Med Ctr - Westchester, Lawrence Hosp Ctr; **Address:** 140 Lockwood Ave, Ste 212, New Rochelle, NY 10801-4908; **Phone:** 914-235-8503; **Board Cert:** Internal Medicine 1972; Endocrinology, Diabetes & Metabolism 1973; **Med School:** NY Med Coll 1967; **Resid:** Internal Medicine, Metropolitan Hosp 1969; Internal Medicine, Montefiore Hosp Med Ctr 1970; **Fellow:** Endocrinology, Diabetes & Metabolism, Mount Sinai Hosp 1971; Endocrinology, Diabetes & Metabolism, New York Med Coll 1972; **Fac Appt:** Assoc Clin Prof Med, Albert Einstein Coll Med

Bloomgarden, David K MD (EDM) - **Spec Exp:** Diabetes; Osteoporosis; Thyroid Disorders; **Hospital:** White Plains Hosp Ctr; **Address:** Scarsdale Medical Group, LLP, 550 Mamaroneck Ave, Ste 101, Harrison, NY 10528; **Phone:** 914-723-8100 x302; **Board Cert:** Internal Medicine 1980; Endocrinology, Diabetes & Metabolism 1983; **Med School:** NYU Sch Med 1977; **Resid:** Internal Medicine, Jacobi Med Ctr 1980; **Fellow:** Endocrinology, Diabetes & Metabolism, Albert Einstein 1982

Blum, David MD (EDM) - **Spec Exp:** Diabetes; Osteoporosis; Thyroid Disorders; **Hospital:** Sound Shore Med Ctr - Westchester; **Address:** Director Diabetes Center, Sound Shore Med Ctr, 16 Guion Pl, New Rochelle, NY 10802; **Phone:** 914-633-8680; **Board Cert:** Internal Medicine 1977; Endocrinology, Diabetes & Metabolism 1979; **Med School:** Northwestern Univ 1974; **Resid:** Internal Medicine, Mt Sinai Hosp 1977; **Fellow:** Endocrinology, Mt Sinai Hosp 1979; **Fac Appt:** Asst Clin Prof Med, NY Med Coll

Gitler, Ellen MD (EDM) - **Spec Exp:** Cardiac Rehabilitation; **Hospital:** Burke Rehab Hosp; **Address:** 785 Mamaroneck Ave, White Plains, NY 10605-2523; **Phone:** 914-597-2409; **Board Cert:** Internal Medicine 1980; Endocrinology, Diabetes & Metabolism 1983; **Med School:** Cornell Univ-Weill Med Coll 1977; **Resid:** Internal Medicine, Bronx Municipal Hosp 1980; **Fellow:** Endocrinology, Diabetes & Metabolism, Mt Sinai Hosp 1982

Hellerman, James MD (EDM) - **Spec Exp:** Thyroid Disorders; Diabetes; Calcium Disorders; **Hospital:** Phelps Meml Hosp Ctr (page 592), St Barnabas Hosp - Bronx; **Address:** 200 S Broadway, Ste 100, Tarrytown, NY 10591-4504; **Phone:** 914-631-9300; **Board Cert:** Internal Medicine 1979; Endocrinology 1983; **Med School:** Univ Rochester 1976; **Resid:** Internal Medicine, Montefiore Med Ctr 1980; **Fellow:** Endocrinology, Diabetes & Metabolism, Mass Genl Hosp 1984

Kantor, Alan MD (EDM) - **Spec Exp:** Thyroid Disorders; Osteoporosis; Diabetes; Endocrine Tumors; **Hospital:** Northern Westchester Hosp; **Address:** 1940 Commerce St, Ste 310, Yorktown Heights, NY 10598; **Phone:** 914-245-1111; **Board Cert:** Internal Medicine 1981; Endocrinology, Diabetes & Metabolism 1983; **Med School:** South Africa 1975; **Resid:** Internal Medicine, La Guardia Hosp 1980; Internal Medicine, LI Jewish-Hillside Med Ctr 1981; **Fellow:** Endocrinology, Diabetes & Metabolism, Meml Sloan Kettering Cancer Ctr 1983; **Fac Appt:** Asst Clin Prof Med, NY Med Coll

Leibowitz, Jonas MD (EDM) - **Spec Exp:** Diabetes; Osteoporosis; Thyroid Disorders; Nutrition; **Hospital:** White Plains Hosp Ctr, Lawrence Hosp Ctr; **Address:** 770 B McLean Ave, Yonkers, NY 10704; **Phone:** 914-237-3636; **Board Cert:** Internal Medicine 2005; Endocrinology, Diabetes & Metabolism 2007; **Med School:** SUNY Downstate 1992; **Resid:** Internal Medicine, Mt Sinai Med Ctr 1995; **Fellow:** Endocrinology, Mt Sinai Med Ctr 1997; **Fac Appt:** Asst Clin Prof Med, NY Med Coll

Marshall, Merville MD (EDM) - **Spec Exp:** Thyroid Disorders; Diabetes; Pituitary Disorders; Adrenal Disorders; **Hospital:** Westchester Med Ctr; **Address:** Endocrine Institute, 21 Seymour Pl, White Plains, NY 10605; **Phone:** 914-949-8650; **Board Cert:** Internal Medicine 1977; Endocrinology, Diabetes & Metabolism 1981; **Med School:** Columbia P&S 1974; **Resid:** Internal Medicine, St Luke's-Roosevelt Hosp Ctr 1976; **Fellow:** Endocrinology, Diabetes & Metabolism, Nat Inst Health 1979

Powell, Jeffrey S MD (EDM) - **Hospital:** Northern Westchester Hosp; **Address:** Mount Kisco Med Group, 90 S Bedford Rd, Mount Kisco, NY 10549; **Phone:** 914-241-1050; **Board Cert:** Internal Medicine 2008; Endocrinology, Diabetes & Metabolism 2000; **Med School:** Albert Einstein Coll Med 1995; **Resid:** Internal Medicine, Columbia-Presby Med Ctr 1998; **Fellow:** Endocrinology, Diabetes & Metabolism, Columbia-Presby Med Ctr 2000

Pretto, Zorayda MD (EDM) - **Hospital:** White Plains Hosp Ctr; **Address:** Mid-Westchester Medical Assocs, 33 Davis Ave, White Plains, NY 10605; **Phone:** 914-948-3630; **Board Cert:** Internal Medicine 2005; Endocrinology, Diabetes & Metabolism 2006; **Med School:** Panama 1986; **Resid:** Internal Medicine, St John's Episcopal Hosp 1991; **Fellow:** Endocrinology, Diabetes & Metabolism, Beth Israel Hosp 1993

Rudin, Eric A MD (EDM) - **Spec Exp:** Diabetes; **Hospital:** Northern Westchester Hosp; **Address:** Mt Kisco Medical Group, 111 Bedford Rd, Katonah, NY 10549; **Phone:** 914-232-3135; **Board Cert:** Internal Medicine 2003; Endocrinology, Diabetes & Metabolism 2005; **Med School:** Mount Sinai Sch Med 2000; **Resid:** Internal Medicine, Thomas Jefferson Univ Hosp` 2003; **Fellow:** Endocrinology, Diabetes & Metabolism, Montefiore Med Ctr 2005

Family Medicine

Annabi, Iyad N MD (FMed) *PCP -* **Hospital:** St John's Riverside Hosp; **Address:** 472 Palmer Rd, Yonkers, NY 10701-5207; **Phone:** 914-375-2300; **Board Cert:** Family Medicine 2001; **Med School:** Mexico 1988; **Resid:** Family Medicine, St Joseph Med Ctr 1993

Apuzzo, Thomas MD (FMed) *PCP -* **Hospital:** Saint Joseph's Med Ctr - Yonkers, St John's Riverside Hosp; **Address:** 955 Yonkers Ave, Yonkers, NY 10704; **Phone:** 914-237-0994; **Board Cert:** Family Medicine 2002; **Med School:** Italy 1985; **Resid:** Family Medicine, St Joseph's Med Ctr 1989

Gottesfeld, Peter MD (FMed) *PCP -* **Spec Exp:** Preventive Medicine; Aging; ADD/ADHD; **Hospital:** Northern Westchester Hosp, Hudson Valley Hosp Ctr; **Address:** 101 S Bedford Rd, Ste 412, Mt Kisco, NY 10549-3455; **Phone:** 914-241-7800; **Board Cert:** Family Medicine 2003; **Med School:** UMDNJ-RW Johnson Med Sch 1985; **Resid:** Family Medicine, Thomas Jefferson U Hosp 1988; **Fac Appt:** Assoc Clin Prof FMed, NY Med Coll

Kelly, Stephen P MD (FMed) *PCP -* **Spec Exp:** Tropical Diseases; Smoking Cessation; **Hospital:** Comm Hosp - Dobbs Ferry, St John's Riverside Hosp; **Address:** 18 Ashford Ave, Ste MW, Dobbs Ferry, NY 10522-1800; **Phone:** 914-693-1660; **Board Cert:** Family Medicine 2003; **Med School:** Univ Cincinnati 1975; **Resid:** Family Medicine, John F Kennedy Hosp 1978; **Fac Appt:** Asst Clin Prof FMed, NY Med Coll

Merker, Edward MD (FMed) *PCP -* **Spec Exp:** Geriatric Care; **Hospital:** Phelps Meml Hosp Ctr (page 592); **Address:** 180 Marble Ave, Pleasantville, NY 10570; **Phone:** 914-769-7300 x202; **Board Cert:** Family Medicine 2005; **Med School:** Albert Einstein Coll Med 1981; **Resid:** Family Medicine, Overlook Hosp 1984; **Fac Appt:** Asst Clin Prof FMed, Albert Einstein Coll Med

Miller, Daniel MD (FMed) *PCP -* **Hospital:** Saint Joseph's Med Ctr - Yonkers; **Address:** 503 S Broadway, Yonkers, NY 10703; **Phone:** 914-965-9771; **Board Cert:** Family Medicine 2007; **Med School:** Univ Cincinnati 1984; **Resid:** Family Medicine, Montefiore Hosp Med Ctr 1987; **Fac Appt:** Asst Prof FMed, NY Med Coll

Piccirilli, Dora C MD (FMed) *PCP -* **Hospital:** Phelps Meml Hosp Ctr (page 592); **Address:** 180 Marble Ave, Pleasantville, NY 10570; **Phone:** 914-769-7300; **Board Cert:** Family Medicine 2005; **Med School:** SUNY Hlth Sci Ctr 1988; **Resid:** Family Medicine, Overlook Hosp 1991

Strongwater, Richard F MD (FMed) *PCP -* **Spec Exp:** Travel Medicine; **Hospital:** Phelps Meml Hosp Ctr (page 592); **Address:** North Star Medical, 180 Marble Ave, Pleasantville, NY 10570; **Phone:** 914-769-7300; **Board Cert:** Family Medicine 2005; **Med School:** SUNY Upstate Med Univ 1981; **Resid:** Family Medicine, Overlook Hosp 1984

Sutton, Ira MD (FMed) *PCP -* **Spec Exp:** Preventive Medicine; Skin Diseases; **Hospital:** Sound Shore Med Ctr - Westchester; **Address:** 77 Quaker Ridge Rd, Ste 101, New Rochelle, NY 10804-2820; **Phone:** 914-636-0077; **Board Cert:** Family Medicine 2008; **Med School:** Albert Einstein Coll Med 1980; **Resid:** Family Medicine, Memorial Hosp 1983

Vaidya, Sudhir P MD (FMed) - **Spec Exp:** Primary Care Sports Medicine; Pain Management; Geriatric Rehabilitation; **Hospital:** Burke Rehab Hosp, St Joseph's Hosp; **Address:** Burke Rehab Hospital, 785 Mamaroneck Ave, White Plains, NY 10605; **Phone:** 914-597-2332; **Board Cert:** Family Medicine 2005; Sports Medicine 2001; **Med School:** India 1979; **Resid:** Physical Medicine & Rehabilitation, NHS Hosps-Leicester, Milton Keynes, Bedford 1995; Family Medicine, St Joseph's Hosp 1998; **Fac Appt:** Asst Prof FMed, Cornell Univ-Weill Med Coll

Yudin, Howard MD (FMed) *PCP* - **Hospital:** Greenwich Hosp (page 862), Sound Shore Med Ctr - Westchester; **Address:** 18 Rye Ridge Plaza, Rye Brook, NY 10573-2820; **Phone:** 914-251-1261; **Board Cert:** Family Medicine 2008; **Med School:** Univ Montreal 1974; **Resid:** Family Medicine, Jewish Genl Hosp 1976

Gastroenterology

Abemayor, Elie M MD (Ge) - **Spec Exp:** Inflammatory Bowel Disease; Endoscopy; Irritable Bowel Syndrome; **Hospital:** Northern Westchester Hosp, NYU Langone Med Ctr (page 106); **Address:** 91 Smith Ave, Mt Kisco, NY 10549-2810; **Phone:** 914-241-9026; **Board Cert:** Internal Medicine 1988; Gastroenterology 2005; **Med School:** SUNY Stony Brook 1985; **Resid:** Internal Medicine, NYU-Bellevue Med Ctr 1988; **Fellow:** Gastroenterology, NYU/Manhattan VA Med Ctr 1990; **Fac Appt:** Asst Clin Prof Med, NYU Sch Med

Antonelle, Robert MD (Ge) - **Spec Exp:** Gastroesophageal Reflux Disease (GERD); Liver & Biliary Disease; Colonoscopy; **Hospital:** White Plains Hosp Ctr, Westchester Med Ctr; **Address:** 311 North St, rm 403, White Plains, NY 10605-2232; **Phone:** 914-949-7171; **Board Cert:** Gastroenterology 2006; **Med School:** NY Med Coll 1989; **Resid:** Internal Medicine, Westchester Med Ctr 1990; **Fellow:** Gastroenterology, Westchester Med Ctr 1994; **Fac Appt:** Asst Clin Prof Med, NY Med Coll

Auerbach, Mitchell E MD (Ge) - **Spec Exp:** Colonoscopy; Crohn's Disease; Ulcerative Colitis; **Hospital:** Saint Joseph's Med Ctr - Yonkers, St John's Riverside Hosp; **Address:** 469 N Broadway, Yonkers, NY 10701-1923; **Phone:** 914-969-1115; **Board Cert:** Gastroenterology 2008; **Med School:** Tufts Univ 1991; **Resid:** Internal Medicine, Mt Sinai Hosp 1994; **Fellow:** Gastroenterology, Mt Sinai Hosp 1996

Chinitz, Marvin MD (Ge) - **Spec Exp:** Colonoscopy; Inflammatory Bowel Disease; Liver Disease; Gastroesophageal Reflux Disease (GERD); **Hospital:** Northern Westchester Hosp; **Address:** Mt Kisco Medical Group, 90 S Bedford Rd, Mt Kisco, NY 10549-3422; **Phone:** 914-241-1050; **Board Cert:** Internal Medicine 1981; Gastroenterology 1985; **Med School:** Boston Univ 1978; **Resid:** Internal Medicine, Boston Med Ctr 1981; **Fellow:** Gastroenterology, Montefiore Med Ctr 1984; **Fac Appt:** Assoc Prof Med, Albert Einstein Coll Med

Dworkin, Brad M MD (Ge) - **Spec Exp:** Gastrointestinal Motility Disorders; Endoscopy; Inflammatory Bowel Disease; **Hospital:** Westchester Med Ctr, Greenwich Hosp (page 862); **Address:** NY Medical College, Munger Pavilion, Ste 206, Valhalla, NY 10595; **Phone:** 914-493-7337; **Board Cert:** Internal Medicine 1979; Gastroenterology 1981; **Med School:** Jefferson Med Coll 1976; **Resid:** Internal Medicine, New York Hosp 1979; **Fellow:** Gastroenterology, Meml Sloan Kettering Cancer Ctr 1981; **Fac Appt:** Prof Med, NY Med Coll

Ehrlich, James B MD (Ge) - **Spec Exp:** Ulcerative Colitis; Colonoscopy; Gastroesophageal Reflux Disease (GERD); Gastroscopy; **Hospital:** Lawrence Hosp Ctr; **Address:** 1 Pondfield Rd, Ste 205, Bronxville, NY 10708-3706; **Phone:** 914-779-3333; **Board Cert:** Internal Medicine 1983; Gastroenterology 1985; **Med School:** Univ Hlth Scis, Chicago Med Sch 1980; **Resid:** Internal Medicine, Univ Illinois Med Ctr 1983; **Fellow:** Gastroenterology, Michael Reese Med Ctr 1985

Field, Barry E MD (Ge) - **Spec Exp:** Ulcerative Colitis; Crohn's Disease; **Hospital:** Phelps Meml Hosp Ctr (page 592); **Address:** Westchester Gastroenterology, 777 N Broadway Fl 3 - Ste 305, Sleepy Hollow, NY 10591-1040; **Phone:** 914-366-6120; **Board Cert:** Internal Medicine 1976; Gastroenterology 1979; **Med School:** Albert Einstein Coll Med 1972; **Resid:** Internal Medicine, Metropolitan Hosp Ctr 1976; **Fellow:** Gastroenterology, Harbor Genl Hosp 1978

Geders, Jane MD/PhD (Ge) - **Spec Exp:** Hepatitis C; Nutrition; Colon Cancer Screening; **Hospital:** Northern Westchester Hosp, Putnam Hosp Ctr; **Address:** 90 S Bedford Rd, Mt Kisco, NY 10549; **Phone:** 914-242-1307; **Board Cert:** Internal Medicine 2001; Gastroenterology 2003; **Med School:** Univ S Fla Coll Med 1987; **Resid:** Internal Medicine, Meml Sloan Kettering Cancer Ctr 1988; Internal Medicine, N Shore Univ Hosp 1990; **Fellow:** Gastroenterology, Mt Sinai Med Ctr 1992; Hepatology, Mt Sinai Med Ctr 1993; **Fac Appt:** Asst Prof Med, NYU Sch Med

Genn, David A MD (Ge) - **Spec Exp:** Liver Disease; Colon Cancer; Gastroesophageal Reflux Disease (GERD); Barrett's Esophagus; **Hospital:** Hudson Valley Hosp Ctr; **Address:** 1985 Crompond Road, Bldg D, Cortlandt Manor, NY 10567-4146; **Phone:** 914-739-2400; **Board Cert:** Gastroenterology 2003; **Med School:** Boston Univ 1988; **Resid:** Internal Medicine, Montefiore Med Ctr 1991; **Fellow:** Gastroenterology, Westchester Med Ctr 1993

Goldblatt, Robert MD (Ge) - **Spec Exp:** Liver Disease; Biliary Disease; Endoscopy; Inflammatory Bowel Disease; **Hospital:** White Plains Hosp Ctr, Greenwich Hosp (page 862); **Address:** 18 Rye Ridge Plaza, Rye Brook, NY 10573-2820; **Phone:** 914-253-9252; **Board Cert:** Internal Medicine 1978; Gastroenterology 1979; **Med School:** Geo Wash Univ 1974; **Resid:** Internal Medicine, Univ FL-Shands Hosp 1977; **Fellow:** Gastroenterology, Yale-New Haven Hosp 1979; **Fac Appt:** Asst Prof Med, Cornell Univ-Weill Med Coll

Gould, Richard B MD (Ge) - **Spec Exp:** Colonoscopy; Gastroscopy; **Hospital:** Lawrence Hosp Ctr, Montefiore Med Ctr - Div. Weiler (page 100); **Address:** 1 Pondfield Rd W, Ste 1R, Bronxville, NY 10708; **Phone:** 914-779-6200; **Board Cert:** Internal Medicine 1975; Gastroenterology 1977; **Med School:** SUNY Upstate Med Univ 1972; **Resid:** Internal Medicine, Montefiore Hosp Med Ctr 1975; **Fellow:** Gastroenterology, Montefiore Hosp Med Ctr 1977; **Fac Appt:** Assoc Clin Prof Med, Columbia P&S

Heier, Stephen K MD (Ge) - **Spec Exp:** Colonoscopy/Polypectomy; Gastric & Esophageal Disorders; Pancreatic/Biliary Endoscopy (ERCP); **Hospital:** Phelps Meml Hosp Ctr (page 592); **Address:** Phelps Memorial Hosp, Advanced Endoscopy & Gastroenterology, 755 N Broadway, Ste 530, Sleepy Hollow, NY 10591; **Phone:** 914-366-1190; **Board Cert:** Internal Medicine 1979; Gastroenterology 1981; **Med School:** Albany Med Coll 1976; **Resid:** Internal Medicine, Metro Hosp Ctr 1979; **Fellow:** Gastroenterology, Tufts Univ 1981; **Fac Appt:** Clin Prof Med, NY Med Coll

Jaffe, Alan H MD (Ge) - **Hospital:** White Plains Hosp Ctr, Greenwich Hosp (page 862); **Address:** Westchester Medical Group, 210 Westchester Ave, White Plains, NY 10604; **Phone:** 914-682-6466; **Board Cert:** Internal Medicine 1977; Gastroenterology 1979; **Med School:** Cornell Univ-Weill Med Coll 1974; **Resid:** Internal Medicine, N Shore U Med Ctr 1977; **Fellow:** Gastroenterology, St Raphael Hosp 1979

Kahn, Oren MD (Ge) - **Spec Exp:** Colon Cancer; Inflammatory Bowel Disease; Peptic Ulcer Disease; Gastroesophageal Reflux Disease (GERD); **Hospital:** Northern Westchester Hosp; **Address:** 90 S Bedford Rd, Mount Kisco, NY 10549; **Phone:** 914-241-1050; **Board Cert:** Internal Medicine 2004; Gastroenterology 2007; **Med School:** Albert Einstein Coll Med 1990; **Resid:** Internal Medicine, Mt Sinai Med Ctr 1994; **Fellow:** Gastroenterology, Mt Sinai Med Ctr 1996; **Fac Appt:** Assoc Clin Prof Med, Mount Sinai Sch Med

Katz, Henry J MD (Ge) - **Hospital:** Montefiore Med Ctr - Div. Moses (page 100), St John's Riverside Hosp; **Address:** 1234 Central Park Ave, Yonkers, NY 10704-1068; **Phone:** 914-793-1600; **Board Cert:** Internal Medicine 1983; Gastroenterology 1985; **Med School:** Albany Med Coll 1980; **Resid:** Internal Medicine, Bellevue Hosp 1983; **Fellow:** Gastroenterology, Montefiore Med Ctr 1985

Kozicky, Orest J MD (Ge) - **Spec Exp:** Colitis; Peptic Ulcer Disease; Gastroesophageal Reflux Disease (GERD); **Hospital:** St John's Riverside Hosp; **Address:** Westchester Digestive Dis Grp, 469 N Broadway, Yonkers, NY 10701-1923; **Phone:** 914-969-1115; **Board Cert:** Internal Medicine 1985; Gastroenterology 1987; **Med School:** NY Med Coll 1981; **Resid:** Internal Medicine, Jacobi Med Ctr 1985; **Fellow:** Gastroenterology, Montefiore Hosp Med Ctr 1987; **Fac Appt:** Asst Clin Prof Med, Albert Einstein Coll Med

Kressner, Michael MD (Ge) - **Spec Exp:** Colon Cancer; Inflammatory Bowel Disease; Biliary Disease; **Hospital:** Sound Shore Med Ctr - Westchester, Mount Vernon Hosp; **Address:** 140 Lockwood Ave, Ste 110, New Rochelle, NY 10801-4907; **Phone:** 914-636-5222; **Board Cert:** Internal Medicine 1980; Gastroenterology 1983; **Med School:** SUNY Buffalo 1977; **Resid:** Internal Medicine, Montefiore Med Ctr 1980; **Fellow:** Gastroenterology, Montefiore Med Ctr 1982; **Fac Appt:** Asst Clin Prof Med, NY Med Coll

Landau, Steven R MD (Ge) - **Spec Exp:** Inflammatory Bowel Disease; Colon Cancer; **Hospital:** White Plains Hosp Ctr; **Address:** 30 Greenridge Ave, White Plains, NY 10605; **Phone:** 914-328-8555; **Board Cert:** Internal Medicine 1984; Gastroenterology 1987; **Med School:** NYU Sch Med 1981; **Resid:** Internal Medicine, Jacobi Med Ctr 1982; Internal Medicine, Montefiore Med Ctr 1984; **Fellow:** Gastroenterology, Mount Sinai Hosp 1986; **Fac Appt:** Asst Prof Med, Albert Einstein Coll Med

Lebovics, Edward MD (Ge) - **Spec Exp:** Hepatitis B & C; Pancreatic/Biliary Endoscopy (ERCP); Crohn's Disease; Liver Disease; **Hospital:** Westchester Med Ctr, Greenwich Hosp (page 862); **Address:** NY Med College-Div Gastroenterology, Munger Pavilion, Ste 206, Valhalla, NY 10595; **Phone:** 914-493-7337; **Board Cert:** Internal Medicine 1983; Gastroenterology 1985; **Med School:** NYU Sch Med 1980; **Resid:** Internal Medicine, Jewish Hosp 1983; **Fellow:** Hepatology, Mt Sinai Hosp 1984; Gastroenterology, NY Med Coll 1986; **Fac Appt:** Prof Med, NY Med Coll

Liss, Mark MD (Ge) - **Spec Exp:** Endoscopy; Peptic Acid Disorders; Inflammatory Bowel Disease; **Hospital:** Sound Shore Med Ctr - Westchester, Montefiore Med Ctr - Div. Moses (page 100); **Address:** 140 Lockwood Ave, Ste 318, New Rochelle, NY 10801; **Phone:** 914-633-0888; **Board Cert:** Internal Medicine 1980; Gastroenterology 1983; **Med School:** Mount Sinai Sch Med 1977; **Resid:** Internal Medicine, Mt Sinai Hosp 1980; **Fellow:** Gastroenterology, Montefiore Med Ctr 1982; **Fac Appt:** Asst Clin Prof Med, Albert Einstein Coll Med

Rosemarin, Jack MD (Ge) - **Spec Exp:** Colonoscopy; Peptic Acid Disorders; Nutrition; **Hospital:** White Plains Hosp Ctr; **Address:** 2 Gannett Drive, White Plains, NY 10604; **Phone:** 914-683-1555; **Board Cert:** Internal Medicine 1982; Gastroenterology 1983; **Med School:** NY Med Coll 1978; **Resid:** Internal Medicine, NY Med Coll 1981; **Fellow:** Gastroenterology, Yale Affil Hosps 1983

Roston, Alfred MD (Ge) - **Spec Exp:** Pancreatic/Biliary Endoscopy (ERCP); Barrett's Esophagus; Gastroesophageal Reflux Disease (GERD); Inflammatory Bowel Disease; **Hospital:** White Plains Hosp Ctr; **Address:** 2 Gannett Drive, White Plains, NY 10604; **Phone:** 914-683-1555; **Board Cert:** Gastroenterology 2005; **Med School:** NYU Sch Med 1989; **Resid:** Internal Medicine, Mt Sinai Hosp 1992; **Fellow:** Gastroenterology, NY Hosp-Cornell Univ Med 1994; Endoscopy, Brigham & Women's Hospital 1995

Shapiro, Neil H MD (Ge) - **Spec Exp:** Endoscopy; Liver Disease; Inflammatory Bowel Disease; **Hospital:** White Plains Hosp Ctr, Greenwich Hosp (page 862); **Address:** 18 Rye Ridge Plaza, Rye Brook, NY 10573-2820; **Phone:** 914-253-9252; **Board Cert:** Internal Medicine 1978; Gastroenterology 1981; **Med School:** Wayne State Univ 1975; **Resid:** Internal Medicine, Beth Israel Hosp 1978; Gastroenterology, Montefiore Med Ctr 1980; **Fac Appt:** Asst Clin Prof Med, Cornell Univ-Weill Med Coll

Taffet, Sanford L MD (Ge) - **Spec Exp:** Inflammatory Bowel Disease; Colon Cancer; Liver Disease; **Hospital:** Sound Shore Med Ctr - Westchester, Mount Vernon Hosp; **Address:** 140 Lockwood Ave, Ste 110, New Rochelle, NY 10801-4907; **Phone:** 914-636-5222; **Board Cert:** Internal Medicine 1980; Gastroenterology 1981; **Med School:** NY Med Coll 1976; **Resid:** Internal Medicine, Maimonides Med Ctr 1979; **Fellow:** Gastroenterology, Albert Einstein Med Ctr 1981; **Fac Appt:** Assoc Clin Prof Med, NY Med Coll

Torman, Julie MD (Ge) - **Spec Exp:** Colon Cancer Screening; Swallowing Disorders; **Hospital:** Phelps Meml Hosp Ctr (page 592); **Address:** 2005 Albany Post Rd, Ste 15, Croton-on-Hudson, NY 10520; **Phone:** 914-271-4212; **Board Cert:** Internal Medicine 1983; Gastroenterology 1989; **Med School:** Univ Nevada 1980; **Resid:** Internal Medicine, Brigham & Womens Hosp 1983; **Fellow:** Gastroenterology, Stanford Univ Med Ctr 1985

Wayne, Peter MD (Ge) - **Spec Exp:** Hepatitis; Pancreatic/Biliary Endoscopy (ERCP); Colonoscopy; **Hospital:** Saint Joseph's Med Ctr - Yonkers, St John's Riverside Hosp; **Address:** 469 N Broadway, Yonkers, NY 10701-1923; **Phone:** 914-969-1115; **Board Cert:** Internal Medicine 1979; Gastroenterology 1981; **Med School:** Albert Einstein Coll Med 1976; **Resid:** Internal Medicine, Montefiore Hosp Med Ctr 1979; **Fellow:** Gastroenterology, Mount Sinai Hosp 1981

Wolf, David C MD (Ge) - **Spec Exp:** Liver Failure; Transplant Medicine-Liver; Liver Disease; Endoscopy; **Hospital:** Westchester Med Ctr; **Address:** NY Med Coll, Div Gastroenterology, Munger Pavilion, rm 206, Valhalla, NY 10595; **Phone:** 914-493-7337; **Board Cert:** Internal Medicine 1988; Gastroenterology 2001; Transplant Hepatology 2006; **Med School:** Columbia P&S 1985; **Resid:** Internal Medicine, NY Presby Hosp 1988; **Fellow:** Gastroenterology, Montefiore Med Ctr 1991; **Fac Appt:** Clin Prof Med, NY Med Coll

Geriatric Medicine

Escher, Jeffrey MD (Ger) - **Spec Exp:** Geriatric Care; **Hospital:** Saint Joseph's Med Ctr - Yonkers; **Address:** Geriatric Services, 69 S Broadway, Yonkers, NY 10701; **Phone:** 914-376-5555 x314-376-52; **Med School:** Belgium 1980; **Resid:** Internal Medicine, New Britain Gen Hosp 1983; **Fellow:** Geriatric Medicine, NYU Med Ctr 1985

Kalchthaler, Thomas DO (Ger) *PCP* - **Hospital:** Saint Joseph's Med Ctr - Yonkers, Sound Shore Med Ctr - Westchester; **Address:** 69 S Broadway, Yonkers, NY 10701-4004; **Phone:** 914-376-5555; **Board Cert:** Internal Medicine 1976; **Med School:** Chicago Coll Osteo Med 1971; **Resid:** Internal Medicine, Elmhurst Hosp 1975; **Fellow:** Geriatric Medicine, Elmhurst Hosp 1974; **Fac Appt:** Asst Prof Med, NY Med Coll

Martimucci, William A MD (Ger) - **Spec Exp:** Geriatric Care; **Hospital:** White Plains Hosp Ctr, Greenwich Hosp (page 862); **Address:** Westchester Medical Group, 1 Theall Rd, Rye, NY 10580; **Phone:** 914-848-8700; **Board Cert:** Internal Medicine 1989; Geriatric Medicine 2000; **Med School:** Grenada 1985; **Resid:** Internal Medicine, Caledonian Hosp 1988; **Fellow:** Geriatric Medicine, Mt Sinai Med Ctr 1990

Schor, Joshua D MD (Ger) - **Spec Exp:** Alzheimer's Disease; Stroke; Spinal Cord Injury; **Address:** 65 Circle Drive, Hastings-on-Hudson, NY 10706; **Phone:** 877-209-2041; **Board Cert:** Internal Medicine 1988; Geriatric Medicine 2000; **Med School:** Yale Univ 1985; **Resid:** Internal Medicine, Mass General Hosp 1988; **Fellow:** Geriatric Medicine, Beth Israel Med Ctr 1990

Gynecologic Oncology

Chuang, Linus T MD (GO) - **Spec Exp:** Laparoscopic Surgery; Ovarian Cancer; Uterine Cancer; Cervical Cancer; **Hospital:** White Plains Hosp Ctr, Mount Sinai Med Ctr (page 102); **Address:** 2 Longview Ave, Ste 302, White Plains, NY 10601; **Phone:** 914-761-0900; **Board Cert:** Obstetrics & Gynecology 2009; Gynecologic Oncology 2097; **Med School:** Taiwan 1981; **Resid:** Obstetrics & Gynecology, Flushing Hosp 1990; **Fellow:** Gynecologic Oncology, MD Anderson Cancer Ctr 1994; **Fac Appt:** Assoc Prof ObG, Mount Sinai Sch Med

Hand Surgery

Fragner, Paul D MD (HS) - **Spec Exp:** Hand & Wrist Surgery; **Hospital:** White Plains Hosp Ctr; **Address:** 7 Reservoir Rd, N White Plains, NY 10603; **Phone:** 914-684-0300; **Board Cert:** Orthopaedic Surgery 2006; Hand Surgery 2006; **Med School:** SUNY Upstate Med Univ 1986; **Resid:** Orthopaedic Surgery, SUNY Downstate Med Ctr 1991; **Fellow:** Hand Surgery, Hosp Univ Penn 1992

Magill Jr, Richard M MD (HS) - **Spec Exp:** Hand & Upper Extremity Surgery; Microvascular Surgery; Shoulder Surgery; **Hospital:** Westchester Med Ctr, Phelps Meml Hosp Ctr (page 592); **Address:** University Orthopaedics, 19 Bradhurst Ave, Ste 1300-N, Hawthorne, NY 10532; **Phone:** 914-789-2733; **Board Cert:** Orthopaedic Surgery 2006; Hand Surgery 2006; **Med School:** Temple Univ 1983; **Resid:** Surgery, Temple Univ Hosp 1985; Orthopaedic Surgery, Maimonides Med Ctr 1992; **Fellow:** Hand Surgery, Duke Univ Med Ctr 1993

Schefer, Alan MD (HS) - **Spec Exp:** Hand & Upper Extremity Surgery; **Hospital:** Northern Westchester Hosp; **Address:** Mt Kisco Medical Group, 9 S Bedford Rd, Mount Kisco, NY 10549; **Phone:** 914-241-1050; **Board Cert:** Orthopaedic Surgery 2009; Hand Surgery 2009; **Med School:** Hahnemann Univ 1990; **Resid:** Orthopaedic Surgery, Mt Sinai Med Ctr 1995; **Fellow:** Hand Surgery, Univ Hosp-SUNY Downstate 1996

Hematology

Lester, Thomas J MD (Hem) - **Spec Exp:** Lymphoma; Breast Cancer; **Hospital:** Northern Westchester Hosp; **Address:** Mt Kisco Medical Group, 90 S Bedford Rd, Mt Kisco, NY 10549; **Phone:** 914-242-2991; **Board Cert:** Internal Medicine 1982; Hematology 1984; Medical Oncology 1987; **Med School:** UMDNJ-Rutgers Med Sch 1979; **Resid:** Internal Medicine, Mt Sinai Hosp 1982; **Fellow:** Hematology, Mt Sinai Hosp 1984; Medical Oncology, Meml Sloan Kettering Cancer Ctr 1986

Nelson, John C MD (Hem) - **Hospital:** Westchester Med Ctr; **Address:** Westchester Hem/Onc Group, 19 Bradhurst Ave, Ste 2100, Hawthorne, NY 10532; **Phone:** 914-493-8353; **Board Cert:** Internal Medicine 1974; Hematology 1976; **Med School:** Harvard Med Sch 1971; **Resid:** Internal Medicine, Mt Sinai Med Ctr 1974; **Fellow:** Hematology, Westchester Med Ctr 1976; **Fac Appt:** Assoc Prof Med, NY Med Coll

Infectious Disease

Berkey, Peter MD (Inf) - **Spec Exp:** Immune Deficiency; Tick-borne Diseases; Travel Medicine; **Hospital:** St John's Riverside Hosp, Saint Joseph's Med Ctr - Yonkers; **Address:** 970 N Broadway, Ste 212, Yonkers, NY 10701-1311; **Phone:** 914-376-1543; **Board Cert:** Internal Medicine 1985; Infectious Disease 1988; **Med School:** Univ Puerto Rico 1980; **Resid:** Internal Medicine, Westchester Med Ctr 1984; **Fellow:** Infectious Disease, MD Anderson Cancer Ctr 1988

Lederman, Jeffrey A MD (Inf) - **Spec Exp:** Travel Medicine; **Hospital:** Sound Shore Med Ctr - Westchester; **Address:** Sound Shore Medical Ctr, 16 Guion Pl Fl 2, New Rochelle, NY 10802; **Phone:** 914-637-1657; **Board Cert:** Internal Medicine 2000; Infectious Disease 2000; **Med School:** Jefferson Med Coll 1988; **Resid:** Internal Medicine, Mt Sinai Hosp 1991; **Fellow:** Infectious Disease, Montefiore Med Ctr 1995

Nadelman, Robert MD (Inf) - **Spec Exp:** Tick-borne Diseases; Lyme Disease; **Hospital:** Westchester Med Ctr; **Address:** NY Med Coll, Div Infectious Disease, Munger Pavillion, rm 245, Valhalla, NY 10595; **Phone:** 914-493-8865; **Board Cert:** Internal Medicine 1983; Infectious Disease 1988; **Med School:** Albert Einstein Coll Med 1980; **Resid:** Internal Medicine, Beth Israel Hosp 1983; **Fellow:** Infectious Disease, Beth Israel Hosp 1985; **Fac Appt:** Prof Med, NY Med Coll

Raffalli, John T MD (Inf) - **Hospital:** Northern Westchester Hosp; **Address:** Mt Kisco Medical Group, 90 S Bedford Rd, Mount Kisco, NY 10549; **Phone:** 914-241-1050; **Board Cert:** Internal Medicine 2005; Infectious Disease 2005; **Med School:** SUNY Downstate 1989; **Resid:** Internal Medicine, NYU Med Ctr 1992; **Fellow:** Infectious Disease, Meml Sloan Kettering Cancer Ctr 1992; **Fac Appt:** Assoc Clin Prof Med, NY Med Coll

Rush, Thomas MD (Inf) - **Spec Exp:** AIDS/HIV; Lyme Disease; Travel Medicine; **Hospital:** Phelps Meml Hosp Ctr (page 592), Putnam Hosp Ctr; **Address:** 127 State Woodside Ave, Briarcliff Manor, NY 10510; **Phone:** 914-762-2276; **Board Cert:** Internal Medicine 1981; Infectious Disease 1984; **Med School:** Rush Med Coll 1978; **Resid:** Internal Medicine, Genesee Hosp 1981; **Fellow:** Infectious Disease, Strong Meml Hosp 1983; **Fac Appt:** Asst Clin Prof Med, NY Med Coll

Welch, Peter MD (Inf) - **Spec Exp:** Lyme Disease; Tick-borne Diseases; **Hospital:** Northern Westchester Hosp; **Address:** Westchester Health Assocs, 16 Orchard Drive, Armonk, NY 10504; **Phone:** 914-273-3404; **Board Cert:** Internal Medicine 1977; Infectious Disease 1980; **Med School:** SUNY Buffalo 1974; **Resid:** Internal Medicine, New York Hosp 1977; **Fellow:** Infectious Disease, New York Hosp 1979

Wormser, Gary P MD (Inf) - **Spec Exp:** Lyme Disease; AIDS/HIV; Diagnostic Problems; **Hospital:** Westchester Med Ctr; **Address:** New York Medical College, Munger Pavilion, rm 245, Valhalla, NY 10595; **Phone:** 914-493-8865; **Board Cert:** Internal Medicine 1978; Infectious Disease 1982; **Med School:** Johns Hopkins Univ 1972; **Resid:** Internal Medicine, Mt Sinai Hosp 1975; **Fellow:** Infectious Disease, Mt Sinai Hosp 1977; **Fac Appt:** Prof Med, NY Med Coll

Internal Medicine

Abenavoli, Tancredi J MD (IM) *PCP* - **Hospital:** White Plains Hosp Ctr; **Address:** 446 Westchester Ave, Port Chester, NY 10573; **Phone:** 914-939-1573; **Board Cert:** Internal Medicine 1979; Cardiovascular Disease 1981; **Med School:** NYU Sch Med 1976; **Resid:** Internal Medicine, VA Hosp/NYU Med Ctr 1979; **Fellow:** Cardiovascular Disease, VA Hosp/NYU Med Ctr 1981

Ades, Joseph R MD (IM) *PCP* - **Hospital:** Phelps Meml Hosp Ctr (page 592); **Address:** 150 White Plains Rd, Tarrytown, NY 10591; **Phone:** 914-631-2480; **Board Cert:** Internal Medicine 1985; **Med School:** Albert Einstein Coll Med 1982; **Resid:** Internal Medicine, LAC-USC Med Ctr 1986

Alpert, Barbara MD (IM) *PCP* - **Spec Exp:** Osteoporosis; Lyme Disease; **Hospital:** Northern Westchester Hosp; **Address:** 90 S Bedford Rd, Mt Kisco, NY 10549; **Phone:** 914-241-1050; **Board Cert:** Internal Medicine 1987; **Med School:** Univ Pennsylvania 1984; **Resid:** Internal Medicine, NY-Cornell Hosp 1987

Altholz, Jeffrey D MD (IM) *PCP -* **Spec Exp:** Occupational Medicine; Addiction/Substance Abuse; **Hospital:** Phelps Meml Hosp Ctr (page 592); **Address:** 160 S Central Ave, Elmsford, NY 10523; **Phone:** 914-345-3135; **Board Cert:** Internal Medicine 2003; **Med School:** Albert Einstein Coll Med 1986; **Resid:** Internal Medicine, St Vincents Hosp 1989; **Fellow:** Internal Medicine, St Vincents Hosp 1990

Berman, Daniel MD (IM) *PCP -* **Spec Exp:** Infectious Disease; **Hospital:** White Plains Hosp Ctr, NY Westchester Sq Med Ctr; **Address:** 56 Doyer Ave, Ste 1E, White Plains, NY 10605; **Phone:** 914-524-8138; **Board Cert:** Internal Medicine 1985; Infectious Disease 1988; **Med School:** NYU Sch Med 1982; **Resid:** Internal Medicine, NYU Med Ctr 1985; **Fellow:** Infectious Disease, NYU Med Ctr 1989

Carosella, Christine MD (IM) *PCP -* **Spec Exp:** Hypertension; Asthma; Cholesterol/Lipid Disorders; **Hospital:** Westchester Med Ctr; **Address:** 19 Bradhurst Ave, #3090, Hawthorne, NY 10532; **Phone:** 914-592-2400; **Board Cert:** Internal Medicine 2005; **Med School:** NY Med Coll 1992; **Resid:** Internal Medicine, Westchester Med Ctr 1995; **Fac Appt:** Asst Prof Med, NY Med Coll

Colangelo, Daniel MD (IM) *PCP -* **Hospital:** White Plains Hosp Ctr; **Address:** 1600 Harrison Ave, Ste G 105, Mamaroneck, NY 10543-3149; **Phone:** 914-698-4466; **Board Cert:** Internal Medicine 2004; **Med School:** NYU Sch Med 1980; **Resid:** Internal Medicine, Lenox Hill Hosp 1983

Croen, Kenneth MD (IM) *PCP -* **Spec Exp:** Infectious Disease; Herpes Simplex; **Hospital:** White Plains Hosp Ctr; **Address:** 600 Mamaroneck Ave, Ste 200, Harrison, NY 10528; **Phone:** 914-723-8100; **Board Cert:** Internal Medicine 1984; Infectious Disease 1988; **Med School:** Albert Einstein Coll Med 1980; **Resid:** Internal Medicine, Columbia-Presby Hosp 1983; Internal Medicine, Presby Hosp 1984; **Fellow:** Infectious Disease, Natl Inst Hlth 1989

Dennett, Ronald MD (IM) *PCP -* **Hospital:** Lawrence Hosp Ctr, Montefiore Med Ctr - Div. Moses (page 100); **Address:** 1254 Central Park Ave, Yonkers, NY 10704-1059; **Phone:** 914-831-6840; **Board Cert:** Internal Medicine 1980; **Med School:** Univ VT Coll Med 1977; **Resid:** Internal Medicine, Univ Colorado Hosp 1980; **Fac Appt:** Asst Clin Prof Med, Albert Einstein Coll Med

Fazio, Nelson M MD (IM) *PCP -* **Spec Exp:** Skin Diseases; Hypertension; Obesity; Infectious Disease; **Hospital:** Lawrence Hosp Ctr; **Address:** 133 Montgomery Ave, Scarsdale, NY 10583; **Phone:** 914-713-8517; **Board Cert:** Internal Medicine 1986; **Med School:** NY Med Coll 1981; **Resid:** Internal Medicine, Westchester Co Med Ctr 1984; **Fellow:** Infectious Disease, Montefiore Hosp Med Ctr 1994

Fiorentino, Thomas MD (IM) - **Spec Exp:** Palliative Care; **Hospital:** St John's Riverside Hosp, Mount Sinai Med Ctr (page 102); **Address:** 984 N Broadway, Ste 303, Yonkers, NY 10701; **Phone:** 914-969-0770; **Board Cert:** Internal Medicine 1975; Hospice & Palliative Medicine 2008; **Med School:** NY Med Coll 1972; **Resid:** Internal Medicine, Metropolitan Hosp 1976

Goldman, Jack S MD (IM) *PCP -* **Spec Exp:** Colonoscopy/Polypectomy; Liver Disease; Endoscopy; **Hospital:** Saint Joseph's Med Ctr - Yonkers, Montefiore Med Ctr - Div. Moses (page 100); **Address:** 750 McLean Ave, Yonkers, NY 10704; **Phone:** 914-237-8686; **Board Cert:** Internal Medicine 1975; Gastroenterology 1979; **Med School:** Albert Einstein Coll Med 1961; **Resid:** Internal Medicine, Bronx Lebanon Hosp 1963; Internal Medicine, VA Med Ctr 1966; **Fellow:** Gastroenterology, VA Med Ctr 1965

Herzog, David A MD (IM) *PCP* - **Spec Exp:** Cholesterol/Lipid Disorders; Preventive Medicine; **Hospital:** White Plains Hosp Ctr, Sound Shore Med Ctr - Westchester; **Address:** 1 Theall Rd, Ste 204, Rye, NY 10580; **Phone:** 914-848-8700; **Board Cert:** Internal Medicine 1984; **Med School:** Mount Sinai Sch Med 1981; **Resid:** Internal Medicine, St Luke's Hosp 1984; **Fac Appt:** Asst Clin Prof Med, NY Med Coll

Higgins, William J MD (IM) *PCP* - **Spec Exp:** Alzheimer's Disease; Geriatric Medicine; **Hospital:** Hudson Valley Hosp Ctr; **Address:** Westchester Medical Practice, 2050 Saw Mill River Rd, Ste 1, Yorktown Heights, NY 10598; **Phone:** 914-962-5533; **Board Cert:** Internal Medicine 2002; **Med School:** Geo Wash Univ 1986; **Resid:** Internal Medicine, Lenox Hill Hosp 1989; **Fellow:** Pulmonary Disease, Lenox Hill Hosp 1991; **Fac Appt:** Assoc Clin Prof Med, NY Med Coll

Hopkins, Arthur MD (IM) *PCP* - **Hospital:** Montefiore Med Ctr - Div. Moses (page 100); **Address:** 1010 Central Park Ave, Yonkers, NY 10704; **Phone:** 914-964-4183; **Board Cert:** Internal Medicine 1986; **Med School:** Univ Pennsylvania 1983; **Resid:** Internal Medicine, Hosp Univ Penn 1986; **Fac Appt:** Asst Prof Med, Albert Einstein Coll Med

Isaacs, Ellen S MD (IM) *PCP* - **Spec Exp:** Hypertension; Heart Disease; **Hospital:** St John's Riverside Hosp, Saint Joseph's Med Ctr - Yonkers; **Address:** 1019 Yonkers Ave, Yonkers, NY 10704; **Phone:** 914-963-9493; **Board Cert:** Internal Medicine 1972; Cardiovascular Disease 1981; **Med School:** NYU Sch Med 1969; **Resid:** Internal Medicine, Bellevue Hosp 1972; **Fellow:** Cardiovascular Disease, St Vincents Hosp Med Ctr 1974; **Fac Appt:** Asst Prof Med, NY Med Coll

Kapoor, Satish MD (IM) *PCP* - **Spec Exp:** Asthma; Emphysema; Preventive Medicine; **Hospital:** Phelps Meml Hosp Ctr (page 592); **Address:** 362 N Broadway Fl 2, Sleepy Hollow, NY 10591-1040; **Phone:** 914-631-2070; **Board Cert:** Internal Medicine 1979; **Med School:** India 1972; **Resid:** Internal Medicine, Kingsbrook Jewish MC 1979; **Fellow:** Pulmonary Disease, Queens Hosp 1981

Karmen, Carol L MD (IM) *PCP* - **Spec Exp:** Preventive Medicine; **Hospital:** Westchester Med Ctr; **Address:** 19 Bradhurst Ave, Ste 3090 North, Hawthorne, NY 10532; **Phone:** 914-592-2400; **Board Cert:** Internal Medicine 2007; **Med School:** Albert Einstein Coll Med 1986; **Resid:** Internal Medicine, Westchester Med Ctr 1990; **Fac Appt:** Assoc Prof Med, NY Med Coll

Krieger, Sharon MD (IM) *PCP* - **Hospital:** Northern Westchester Hosp; **Address:** Mt Kisco Medical Group, 90 S Bedford Rd, Mt Kisco, NY 10549-3422; **Phone:** 914-241-1050; **Board Cert:** Internal Medicine 2004; **Med School:** Louisiana State U, New Orleans 1991; **Resid:** Internal Medicine, NY Presby-Cornell Med Ctr 1994

Lebofsky, Martin MD (IM) - **Spec Exp:** Kidney Disease; Hypertension; Dialysis Care; **Hospital:** Lawrence Hosp Ctr, Saint Joseph's Med Ctr - Yonkers; **Address:** 1 Stone Pl, Bronxville, NY 10708-3406; **Phone:** 914-337-9004; **Board Cert:** Internal Medicine 1975; Nephrology 1978; **Med School:** Albert Einstein Coll Med 1972; **Resid:** Internal Medicine, Harlem Hosp 1975; **Fellow:** Nephrology, Montefiore Hosp Med Ctr 1978

Lechner, Michael MD (IM) *PCP* - **Spec Exp:** Geriatric Medicine; Geriatric Rehabilitation; **Hospital:** Phelps Meml Hosp Ctr (page 592); **Address:** 14 Church St, Ste 208, Ossining, NY 10562-4831; **Phone:** 914-762-0722; **Board Cert:** Internal Medicine 1980; **Med School:** Albert Einstein Coll Med 1961; **Resid:** Internal Medicine, Westchester Med Ctr 1964; **Fellow:** Hematology, LI Jewish Med Ctr 1965

Margulis, Steven M MD (IM) *PCP* - **Hospital:** Northern Westchester Hosp; **Address:** Mt Kisco Med Grp, 90 S Bedford Rd, Mt Kisco, NY 10549; **Phone:** 914-241-1050; **Board Cert:** Internal Medicine 2000; **Med School:** Albert Einstein Coll Med 1997; **Resid:** Internal Medicine, Mt Sinai Med Ctr 2000

Melman, Martin MD (IM) *PCP* - **Spec Exp:** Hypertension; Asthma; Geriatric Medicine; **Hospital:** Phelps Meml Hosp Ctr (page 592); **Address:** 87 Grand St, Croton On Hudson, NY 10520-2518; **Phone:** 914-271-4845; **Board Cert:** Internal Medicine 1977; **Med School:** NY Med Coll 1974; **Resid:** Internal Medicine, Metropolitan Hosp Ctr 1977; Internal Medicine, Westchester Med Ctr 1978; **Fac Appt:** Asst Clin Prof Med, NY Med Coll

Pappas, Steven MD (IM) *PCP* - **Spec Exp:** Occupational Medicine; Preventive Medicine; **Hospital:** Sound Shore Med Ctr - Westchester; **Address:** 266 White Plains Rd, Ste 1A, Eastchester, NY 10709; **Phone:** 914-793-1115; **Board Cert:** Internal Medicine 1982; Emergency Medicine 2000; **Med School:** Albert Einstein Coll Med 1978; **Resid:** Internal Medicine, St Luke's Roosevelt Hosp Ctr 1981

Peterson, Stephen J MD (IM) *PCP* - **Spec Exp:** Forensic Medicine; Weight Management; **Hospital:** Westchester Med Ctr; **Address:** NY Med College, Munger Pavilion 256, Valhalla, NY 10595; **Phone:** 914-493-8370; **Board Cert:** Internal Medicine 1985; **Med School:** Philippines 1982; **Resid:** Internal Medicine, Metropolitan Hosp Ctr 1986; **Fac Appt:** Prof Med, NY Med Coll

Plesset, Maxwell B MD (IM) *PCP* - **Hospital:** Northern Westchester Hosp; **Address:** 1825 Commerce Rd, Yorktown Hts, NY 10598; **Phone:** 914-962-5060; **Board Cert:** Internal Medicine 1976; **Med School:** Univ Pittsburgh 1968; **Resid:** Internal Medicine, North Shore Univ Hosp/Cornell 1976

Ridge, Gerald A MD (IM) *PCP* - **Spec Exp:** Geriatric Medicine; **Hospital:** Lawrence Hosp Ctr, NY-Presby Hosp/Columbia (page 104); **Address:** Lawrence Medical Assocs, 685 White Plains Rd, Eastchester, NY 10709; **Phone:** 914-787-4100; **Board Cert:** Internal Medicine 2008; Geriatric Medicine 2008; **Med School:** UCSF 1979; **Resid:** Internal Medicine, Bronx Muni Hosp Ctr 1981; Neurology, Columbia-Presby Med Ctr 1982; **Fellow:** Internal Medicine, New York Hosp 1983; **Fac Appt:** Clin Prof Med, Columbia P&S

Rosch, Elliott MD (IM) *PCP* - **Spec Exp:** Preventive Medicine; Cholesterol/Lipid Disorders; Hypertension; Weight Management; **Hospital:** St John's Riverside Hosp; **Address:** 1010 N Broadway, Yonkers, NY 10701-1303; **Phone:** 914-965-4424; **Board Cert:** Internal Medicine 1981; **Med School:** Univ Pennsylvania 1978; **Resid:** Internal Medicine, Pennsylvania Hosp 1981

Saltzman-Gabelman, Lori MD (IM) *PCP* - **Hospital:** White Plains Hosp Ctr, Greenwich Hosp (page 862); **Address:** 210 Westchester Ave Fl 2, White Plains, NY 10604-2914; **Phone:** 914-682-0700; **Board Cert:** Internal Medicine 1989; **Med School:** NY Med Coll 1986; **Resid:** Internal Medicine, Westchester Med Ctr 1989; **Fac Appt:** , NY Med Coll

Soltren, Rafael MD (IM) *PCP* - **Spec Exp:** Diabetes; Hypertension; **Hospital:** Phelps Meml Hosp Ctr (page 592); **Address:** 100 S Highland Ave, Ossining, NY 10562; **Phone:** 914-941-1277; **Board Cert:** Internal Medicine 1985; **Med School:** Cornell Univ-Weill Med Coll 1981; **Resid:** Internal Medicine, Montefiore Med Ctr 1984

Starke, Charles L MD (IM) *PCP* - **Hospital:** Phelps Meml Hosp Ctr (page 592), Westchester Med Ctr; **Address:** 516 N State Rd, Briarcliff Manor, NY 10510-1526; **Phone:** 914-762-4460; **Board Cert:** Internal Medicine 1978; **Med School:** Albert Einstein Coll Med 1975; **Resid:** Internal Medicine, Georgetown Univ Hosp 1978; **Fac Appt:** Prof Med, Columbia P&S

Turro, James J MD (IM) *PCP* - **Hospital:** Northern Westchester Hosp; **Address:** Mt Kisco Medical Grp, 90 S Bedford Rd, Mt Kisco, NY 10549; **Phone:** 914-241-1050; **Board Cert:** Internal Medicine 1985; **Med School:** Cornell Univ-Weill Med Coll 1982; **Resid:** Internal Medicine, Bronx Muni Hosp 1986

Wolfe, Mary J MD (IM) *PCP* - **Spec Exp:** Women's Health; **Hospital:** Phelps Meml Hosp Ctr (page 592); **Address:** 14 Church St, Ossining, NY 10562; **Phone:** 914-941-1334; **Board Cert:** Internal Medicine 1980; **Med School:** Penn State Univ-Hershey Med Ctr 1976; **Resid:** Internal Medicine, Westchester Med Ctr 1979

Wolfson, Robert A MD (IM) *PCP* - **Hospital:** Northern Westchester Hosp; **Address:** 90 S Bedford Rd, Mount Kisco, NY 10549; **Phone:** 914-241-1050; **Board Cert:** Internal Medicine 1980; **Med School:** SUNY Downstate 1977; **Resid:** Internal Medicine, Kings Co Hosp 1981

Zarowitz, William MD (IM) *PCP* - **Spec Exp:** Occupational Medicine; Preventive Medicine; **Hospital:** White Plains Hosp Ctr; **Address:** 143 Maple Ave, White Plains, NY 10601; **Phone:** 914-683-8610; **Board Cert:** Internal Medicine 1981; **Med School:** NY Med Coll 1978; **Resid:** Internal Medicine, Montefiore Med Ctr 1981; **Fac Appt:** Assoc Clin Prof Med, NY Med Coll

Maternal & Fetal Medicine

Berck, David J MD (MF) - **Spec Exp:** Ultrasound; Pregnancy-High Risk; **Hospital:** Northern Westchester Hosp; **Address:** Mount Kisco Medical Group, 90 S Bedford Rd, Mount Kisco, NY 10549; **Phone:** 914-241-1050; **Board Cert:** Obstetrics & Gynecology 1999; Maternal & Fetal Medicine 2001; **Med School:** Harvard Med Sch 1991; **Resid:** Obstetrics & Gynecology, Mass Genl Hosp 1995; **Fellow:** Maternal & Fetal Medicine, Columbia Presby Med Ctr 1998

Devine, Patricia Ann MD (MF) - **Spec Exp:** Pregnancy-High Risk; Prenatal Diagnosis; Diabetes in Pregnancy; Premature Labor; **Hospital:** Sound Shore Med Ctr - Westchester; **Address:** Sound Shore Antenatal Testing Lab, 16 Guion Place Fl 4, New Rochelle, NY 10802; **Phone:** 914-365-4263; **Board Cert:** Obstetrics & Gynecology 2008; Maternal & Fetal Medicine 2008; **Med School:** Mount Sinai Sch Med 1987; **Resid:** Obstetrics & Gynecology, Beth Israel Med Ctr 1991; **Fellow:** Maternal & Fetal Medicine, Westchester Co Med Ctr 1993; **Fac Appt:** Assoc Clin Prof ObG, NY Med Coll

Kirshenbaum, Nancy MD (MF) - **Spec Exp:** Pregnancy-High Risk; Ultrasound; **Hospital:** Montefiore Med Ctr - Div. Weiler (page 100); **Address:** 700 White Plains Rd, Ste 270, Scarsdale, NY 10583; **Phone:** 914-472-0512; **Board Cert:** Obstetrics & Gynecology 2009; Maternal & Fetal Medicine 2009; **Med School:** Mount Sinai Sch Med 1980; **Resid:** Obstetrics & Gynecology, NYU Med Ctr 1984; **Fellow:** Maternal & Fetal Medicine, NYU Med Ctr 1986; **Fac Appt:** Assoc Clin Prof ObG, Albert Einstein Coll Med

Lescale, Keith B MD (MF) - **Spec Exp:** Pregnancy-High Risk; Prenatal Diagnosis; Fetal Ultrasound/Obstetrical Imaging; **Hospital:** White Plains Hosp Ctr, Greenwich Hosp (page 862); **Address:** Hudson Valley Perinatal Consulting, 600 Mamaroneck Ave, Ste 110, Harrison, NY 10528-1647; **Phone:** 914-670-0500; **Board Cert:** Obstetrics & Gynecology 2008; Maternal & Fetal Medicine 2008; **Med School:** Louisiana State U, New Orleans 1987; **Resid:** Obstetrics & Gynecology, New Orleans/LSU Med Ctr 1991; **Fellow:** Maternal & Fetal Medicine, NY Hosp-Cornell Med Ctr 1994

Mootabar, Hamid MD (MF) - **Spec Exp:** Pregnancy-High Risk; **Hospital:** Lawrence Hosp Ctr, NY-Presby Hosp/Columbia (page 104); **Address:** Amniocentesis & Genetics Ctr, 77 Pondfield Rd, Bronxville, NY 10708; **Phone:** 914-337-2102; **Board Cert:** Obstetrics & Gynecology 1975; Maternal & Fetal Medicine 1983; **Med School:** Iran 1966; **Resid:** Obstetrics & Gynecology, Roosevelt Hosp 1973; **Fellow:** Maternal & Fetal Medicine, Roosevelt Hosp 1979; **Fac Appt:** Assoc Clin Prof ObG, Columbia P&S

Medical Oncology

Ahmed, Tauseef MD (Onc) - **Spec Exp:** Bone Marrow Transplant; Lymphoma; Brain Tumors; Genitourinary Cancer; **Hospital:** Westchester Med Ctr; **Address:** Westchester Oncology/Hematology, 19 Bradhurst Ave, Ste 2100, Hawthorne, NY 10532; **Phone:** 914-493-8353; **Board Cert:** Internal Medicine 1980; Hematology 1982; Medical Oncology 1983; **Med School:** Pakistan 1976; **Resid:** Internal Medicine, Mt Sinai Hosp 1980; **Fellow:** Medical Oncology, Meml Sloan Kettering Cancer Ctr 1983; **Fac Appt:** Prof Med, NY Med Coll

Bernhardt, Bernard MD (Onc) - **Spec Exp:** Lung Cancer; Lymphoma; Leukemia-Chronic Lymphocytic; Anemias & Red Cell Disorders; **Hospital:** Sound Shore Med Ctr - Westchester, Montefiore Med Ctr - Div. Weiler (page 100); **Address:** 50 Guion Pl, New Rochelle, NY 10801-5512; **Phone:** 914-632-5397; **Board Cert:** Internal Medicine 1968; Hematology 1972; Medical Oncology 1973; **Med School:** Northwestern Univ 1961; **Resid:** Internal Medicine, DC Genl Hosp 1963; Internal Medicine, NY Med Coll 1966; **Fellow:** Hematology, Montefiore Hosp Med Ctr 1968; **Fac Appt:** Clin Prof Med, NY Med Coll

Caron, Philip C MD/PhD (Onc) - **Spec Exp:** Lymphoma; Gastrointestinal Cancer; **Hospital:** Meml Sloan-Kettering Cancer Ctr (page 112), Phelps Meml Hosp Ctr (page 592); **Address:** Meml Sloan Kettering at Phelps Meml Hosp, 777 N Broadway, Ste 102, Sleepy Hollow, NY 10591; **Phone:** 800-525-2225; **Board Cert:** Internal Medicine 1989; Medical Oncology 2003; Hematology 2007; **Med School:** NY Med Coll 1986; **Resid:** Internal Medicine, Mt Sinai Hosp 1989; **Fellow:** Hematology & Oncology, Meml Sloan Kettering Cancer Ctr 1992

Feldman, Stuart P MD (Onc) - **Spec Exp:** Breast Cancer; Lymphoma; **Hospital:** White Plains Hosp Ctr, Greenwich Hosp (page 862); **Address:** 210 Westchester Ave, White Plains, NY 10604-2901; **Phone:** 914-681-5200; **Board Cert:** Internal Medicine 1980; Hematology 1982; Medical Oncology 1985; **Med School:** Geo Wash Univ 1977; **Resid:** Internal Medicine, New York Hosp-Cornell 1980; **Fellow:** Hematology & Oncology, Meml Sloan Kettering Cancer Ctr 1983; **Fac Appt:** Asst Clin Prof Med, Cornell Univ-Weill Med Coll

Fialk, Mark A MD (Onc) - **Hospital:** White Plains Hosp Ctr, Westchester Med Ctr; **Address:** 259 Heathcote Rd, Scarsdale, NY 10583; **Phone:** 914-723-8100; **Board Cert:** Internal Medicine 1976; Medical Oncology 1977; Hematology 1978; **Med School:** Tufts Univ 1973; **Resid:** Internal Medicine, NY Hosp-Cornell Med Ctr 1975; Internal Medicine, Meml Sloan-Kettering Cancer Ctr 1976; **Fellow:** Hematology & Oncology, NY Hosp-Cornell Med Ctr 1978; Infectious Disease, Meml Sloan-Kettering Cancer Ctr 1979; **Fac Appt:** Asst Clin Prof Med, NY Med Coll

Goldberg, Jonathan S MD (Onc) - **Spec Exp:** Lymphoma; Breast Cancer; Clinical Trials; Lung Cancer; **Hospital:** Northern Westchester Hosp, Putnam Hosp Ctr; **Address:** Mount Kisco Medical Group, 90 S Bedford Rd, Mount Kisco, NY 10549; **Phone:** 914-241-1050; **Board Cert:** Internal Medicine 2007; Hematology 2001; Medical Oncology 2001; **Med School:** Mount Sinai Sch Med 1994; **Resid:** Internal Medicine, NY Presby Med Ctr 1997; **Fellow:** Hematology & Oncology, NY Presby Med Ctr 1999

Halaas, Jeffrey L MD (Onc) - **Hospital:** Northern Westchester Hosp, Putnam Hosp Ctr; **Address:** Mt Kisco Medical Group, 90 S Bedford Rd, Mt Kisco, NY 10549; **Phone:** 914-241-1050; **Board Cert:** Internal Medicine 2002; Medical Oncology 2005; Hematology 2005; **Med School:** Cornell Univ-Weill Med Coll 1999; **Resid:** Internal Medicine, NY Presby Hosp 2001; **Fellow:** Hematology & Oncology, Meml Sloan Kettering Cancer Ctr 2005

Liu, DeLong MD/PhD (Onc) - **Spec Exp:** Lung Cancer; Leukemia; Bone Marrow Transplant; Lymphoma; **Hospital:** Westchester Med Ctr; **Address:** 19 Bradhurst Ave, Hawthorne, NY 10532; **Phone:** 914-493-8374; **Board Cert:** Internal Medicine 2006; Medical Oncology 1999; Hematology 2002; **Med School:** China 1984; **Resid:** Internal Medicine, Montefiore Med Ctr 1996; **Fellow:** Hematology & Oncology, Meml Sloan Kettering Cancer Ctr 1998; **Fac Appt:** Prof Med, NY Med Coll

Mills, Nancy Ellyn MD (Onc) - **Spec Exp:** Breast Cancer; Gynecologic Cancer; **Hospital:** Phelps Meml Hosp Ctr (page 592), Meml Sloan-Kettering Cancer Ctr (page 112); **Address:** Meml Sloan Kettering @ Sleepy Hollow, 777 N Broadway, Ste 102, Sleepy Hollow, NY 10591; **Phone:** 914-366-0664; **Board Cert:** Internal Medicine 2000; Medical Oncology 2003; Hematology 2004; **Med School:** Mount Sinai Sch Med 1987; **Resid:** Internal Medicine, Mt Sinai Med Ctr 1990; **Fellow:** Hematology & Oncology, NYU Med Ctr 1993; **Fac Appt:** Asst Clin Prof Med, Cornell Univ-Weill Med Coll

Phillips, Elizabeth MD (Onc) - **Spec Exp:** Breast Cancer; Lymphoma; Colon Cancer; Bleeding/Coagulation Disorders; **Hospital:** Sound Shore Med Ctr - Westchester, Montefiore Med Ctr - Div. Moses (page 100); **Address:** Advanced Oncology Assocs, 50 Guion Pl, Ste 32, New Rochelle, NY 10801-4914; **Phone:** 914-632-5397; **Board Cert:** Internal Medicine 1974; Hematology 1976; Medical Oncology 1977; **Med School:** Univ Wash 1969; **Resid:** Internal Medicine, Harlem Hosp 1972; Hematology, Montefiore Med Ctr 1973; **Fellow:** Hematology & Oncology, Mem Sloan Kettering Canc Ctr 1976; **Fac Appt:** Assoc Clin Prof Med, NY Med Coll

Provenzano, Anthony F MD (Onc) - **Spec Exp:** Lung Cancer; Breast Cancer; Cancer Genetics; Gastrointestinal Cancer; **Hospital:** Lawrence Hosp Ctr, Mount Vernon Hosp; **Address:** 1 Pondfield Rd W, Ste 4, Bronxville, NY 10708-2635; **Phone:** 914-961-3421; **Board Cert:** Internal Medicine 1979; Medical Oncology 1981; **Med School:** Cornell Univ-Weill Med Coll 1976; **Resid:** Internal Medicine, Lenox Hill Hosp 1978; **Fellow:** Medical Oncology, St Vincents Hosp 1979; Medical Oncology, Lenox Hill Hosp 1981; **Fac Appt:** Asst Clin Prof Med, NY Med Coll

Puccio, Carmelo A MD (Onc) - **Spec Exp:** Breast Cancer; Lung Cancer; Solid Tumors; Gynecologic Cancer; **Hospital:** Westchester Med Ctr, Sound Shore Med Ctr - Westchester; **Address:** 19 Bradhurst Ave, Ste 2100, Hawthorne, NY 10532; **Phone:** 914-493-8353; **Board Cert:** Internal Medicine 1984; Medical Oncology 1989; **Med School:** Mexico 1979; **Resid:** Internal Medicine, Maimonides Med Ctr 1984; **Fellow:** Medical Oncology, Westchesr Co Med Ctr 1985; **Fac Appt:** Asst Prof Med, NY Med Coll

Rosen, Norman MD (Onc) - **Spec Exp:** Lung Cancer; Breast Cancer; **Hospital:** St John's Riverside Hosp, Montefiore Med Ctr - Div. Moses (page 100); **Address:** 984 N Broadway, Ste 311, Yonkers, NY 10701-1308; **Phone:** 914-965-2060; **Board Cert:** Internal Medicine 1975; Medical Oncology 1977; **Med School:** Tufts Univ 1972; **Resid:** Internal Medicine, Montefiore Med Ctr 1975; **Fellow:** Hematology & Oncology, Montefiore Med Ctr 1977; **Fac Appt:** Asst Clin Prof Med, Albert Einstein Coll Med

Sadan, Sara MD (Onc) - **Spec Exp:** Hematology; **Hospital:** White Plains Hosp Ctr; **Address:** 244 Westchester Ave, Ste 411, White Plains, NY 10604; **Phone:** 914-684-8100; **Board Cert:** Internal Medicine 2002; Medical Oncology 2005; **Med School:** Israel 1984; **Resid:** Internal Medicine, St Luke's-Roosevelt Hosp Ctr 1991; **Fellow:** Hematology & Oncology, Meml Sloan Kettering Cancer Ctr 1994

Saponara, Eduardo M MD (Onc) - **Spec Exp:** Breast Cancer; Lung Cancer; Gastrointestinal Cancer; Lymphoma; **Hospital:** Lawrence Hosp Ctr, Mount Sinai Med Ctr (page 102); **Address:** 77 Pondfield Rd, Bronxville, NY 10708-3809; **Phone:** 914-793-1500; **Board Cert:** Internal Medicine 1977; Hematology 1978; Medical Oncology 1979; **Med School:** Peru 1973; **Resid:** Internal Medicine, Westchester Med Ctr 1976; **Fellow:** Hematology & Oncology, Flower Fifth Ave Hospital/NY Med Coll 1978; Oncology, Mount Sinai Hosp 1979; **Fac Appt:** Asst Clin Prof Med, NY Med Coll

Schneider, Robert Jay MD (Onc) - **Spec Exp:** Breast Cancer; Genitourinary Cancer; **Hospital:** Northern Westchester Hosp, Westchester Med Ctr; **Address:** 101 S Bedford, Ste 202A, Mt Kisco, NY 10549-3456; **Phone:** 914-666-8976; **Board Cert:** Internal Medicine 1979; Medical Oncology 1985; **Med School:** Albert Einstein Coll Med 1975; **Resid:** Internal Medicine, Jacobi Med Ctr 1978; **Fellow:** Medical Oncology, Meml Sloan Kettering Cancer Ctr 1980

Schwartz, Simeon MD (Onc) - **Spec Exp:** Breast Cancer; **Hospital:** White Plains Hosp Ctr, Greenwich Hosp (page 862); **Address:** 210 Westchester Ave, White Plains, NY 10604-2901; **Phone:** 914-681-5200; **Board Cert:** Internal Medicine 1980; Medical Oncology 1983; Hematology 1984; **Med School:** Yale Univ 1977; **Resid:** Internal Medicine, NY Hosp 1980; **Fellow:** Hematology & Oncology, Meml Sloan Kettering Cancer Ctr 1983; **Fac Appt:** Assoc Clin Prof Med, Cornell Univ-Weill Med Coll

Seiter, Karen MD (Onc) - **Spec Exp:** Hematologic Malignancies; Leukemia; Myelodysplastic Syndromes; **Hospital:** Westchester Med Ctr; **Address:** 19 Bradhurst Ave, Ste 2100, Hawthorne, NY 10532; **Phone:** 914-493-8353; **Board Cert:** Internal Medicine 1988; Medical Oncology 2001; Hematology 2002; **Med School:** NY Med Coll 1985; **Resid:** Internal Medicine, Albert Einstein Hosp 1988; **Fellow:** Hematology & Oncology, Memorial Sloan Kettering Med Ctr 1991; **Fac Appt:** Prof Med, NY Med Coll

Neonatal-Perinatal Medicine

Golombek, Sergio G MD (NP) - **Spec Exp:** Prematurity/Low Birth Weight Infants; Pulmonary Disease; **Hospital:** Westchester Med Ctr, Children's & Women's Phys.of Westchester; **Address:** Maria Fareri Chldn's Hosp, Westchester Med Ctr, 100 Woods Rd, Valhalla, NY 10595; **Phone:** 914-493-8488; **Board Cert:** Neonatal-Perinatal Medicine 2005; Pediatrics 2008; **Med School:** Argentina 1983; **Resid:** Pediatrics, Dr Ignacio Pirovano Hosp 1987; Pediatrics, Raymond Blank Meml Hosp Chldn 1991; **Fellow:** Neonatal-Perinatal Medicine, Chldns Mercy Hosp 1996; **Fac Appt:** Prof Ped, NY Med Coll

Jaile-Marti, Jesus MD (NP) - **Spec Exp:** Lung Disease in Newborns; Neonatal Nutrition; **Hospital:** White Plains Hosp Ctr, NYPresby-Morgan Stanley Children's Hosp (page 104); **Address:** White Plains Hosp Ctr, Div Neonatology, Davis Ave at East Post Rd, White Plains, NY 10601; **Phone:** 914-681-2282; **Board Cert:** Pediatrics 2005; Neonatal-Perinatal Medicine 2003; **Med School:** Columbia P&S 1987; **Resid:** Pediatrics, Columbia-Presby Med Ctr 1990; **Fellow:** Neonatology, Columbia-Presby Med Ctr 1993

La Gamma, Edmund F MD (NP) - **Spec Exp:** Neonatal Infections; Prematurity/Low Birth Weight Infants; Necrotizing Enterocolitis; **Hospital:** Westchester Med Ctr, Children's & Women's Phys.of Westchester; **Address:** Maria Fareri Chldns Hosp, Grasslands Rd Fl 2, Valhalla, NY 10595-0001; **Phone:** 914-493-8558; **Board Cert:** Pediatrics 1981; Neonatal-Perinatal Medicine 1981; **Med School:** NY Med Coll 1976; **Resid:** Pediatrics, NY Hosp-Cornell Med Ctr 1978; **Fellow:** Neonatal-Perinatal Medicine, NY Hosp-Cornell Med Ctr 1980; Cardiovascular Disease, UCSF Med Ctr 1981; **Fac Appt:** Prof Ped, NY Med Coll

Nephrology

Adler, Stephen MD (Nep) - **Spec Exp:** Kidney Failure; Glomerulonephritis; Hypertension; Dialysis Care; **Hospital:** Westchester Med Ctr, White Plains Hosp Ctr; **Address:** 19 Bradhurst Ave, Ste 100, Hawthorne, NY 10532-2169; **Phone:** 914-493-7701; **Board Cert:** Internal Medicine 1979; Nephrology 1982; **Med School:** NYU Sch Med 1976; **Resid:** Internal Medicine, Mt Sinai Hosp 1979; **Fellow:** Nephrology, Boston Univ Med Ctr 1982; **Fac Appt:** Prof Med, NY Med Coll

Buzzeo, Louis MD (Nep) - **Spec Exp:** Hypertension; Kidney Disease; **Hospital:** Phelps Meml Hosp Ctr (page 592); **Address:** 777 N Broadway, Ste 203, Sleepy Hollow, NY 10591-1019; **Phone:** 914-332-9100; **Board Cert:** Internal Medicine 1975; Nephrology 1978; **Med School:** Tufts Univ 1972; **Resid:** Internal Medicine, St Vincent's Hosp & Med Ctr 1975; **Fellow:** Nephrology, NYU Med Ctr 1977

Delaney, Veronica MD/PhD (Nep) - **Spec Exp:** Transplant Medicine-Kidney; **Hospital:** Westchester Med Ctr; **Address:** 19 Bradhurst Ave, Ste 200N, Valhalla, NY 10532; **Phone:** 914-493-7701; **Board Cert:** Internal Medicine 1981; Nephrology 1982; **Med School:** England, UK 1973; **Resid:** Internal Medicine, Dublin Univ Hosps; **Fellow:** Nephrology, Univ Pittsburgh Med Ctr 1983; **Fac Appt:** Assoc Prof Med, NY Med Coll

Garrick, Renee MD (Nep) - **Spec Exp:** Hypertension; Dialysis Care; **Hospital:** Westchester Med Ctr; **Address:** Nephrology Assocs of Westchester, 19 Bradhurst Ave, Ste 200N, Hawthorne, NY 10532; **Phone:** 914-493-7701; **Board Cert:** Internal Medicine 1981; Nephrology 1984; **Med School:** Rush Med Coll 1978; **Resid:** Internal Medicine, Jacobi Med Ctr 1981; **Fellow:** Nephrology, Hosp Univ Penn 1984; **Fac Appt:** Clin Prof Med, NY Med Coll

Reda, Dominick MD (Nep) - **Spec Exp:** Hypertension; Kidney Disease; **Hospital:** Saint Joseph's Med Ctr - Yonkers; **Address:** 136 S Broadway, Yonkers, NY 10701; **Phone:** 914-965-0621; **Board Cert:** Internal Medicine 1987; Nephrology 1990; **Med School:** Italy 1983; **Resid:** Internal Medicine, Our Lady of Mercy 1987; **Fellow:** Nephrology, Lincoln Med Ctr 1989

Rie, Jonathan MD (Nep) - **Spec Exp:** Hypertension; Kidney Stones; **Hospital:** White Plains Hosp Ctr, Greenwich Hosp (page 862); **Address:** 33 Davis Ave, White Plains, NY 10605; **Phone:** 914-831-2900; **Board Cert:** Internal Medicine 1988; Nephrology 2000; **Med School:** NY Med Coll 1985; **Resid:** Internal Medicine, Montefiore Hosp Med Ctr 1988; **Fellow:** Nephrology, Montefiore Hosp Med Ctr 1990

Rosen, Michael A MD (Nep) - **Spec Exp:** Kidney Disease-Pediatric & Adult; **Hospital:** Northern Westchester Hosp; **Address:** Mt Kisco Medical Group, 90 S Bedford Rd, Mt Kisco, NY 10549; **Phone:** 914-241-1050; **Board Cert:** Internal Medicine 2004; Pediatrics 2004; Nephrology 2007; **Med School:** Indiana Univ 2000; **Resid:** Internal Medicine & Pediatrics, Mt Sinai Med Ctr 2004; **Fellow:** Nephrology, Nt Sinai Med Ctr 2008

Saltzman, Martin MD (Nep) - **Spec Exp:** Kidney Disease; Hypertension; **Hospital:** Northern Westchester Hosp, Putnam Hosp Ctr; **Address:** 90 S Bedford Rd, Mt Kisco, NY 10549; **Phone:** 914-241-1050; **Board Cert:** Internal Medicine 1977; Nephrology 1978; **Med School:** SUNY Downstate 1972; **Resid:** Internal Medicine, Kings County Hosp 1973; Internal Medicine, Harlem Hosp 1974; **Fellow:** Nephrology, Univ Hosp 1976

Neurological Surgery

de Lotbiniere, Alain MD (NS) - **Spec Exp:** Movement Disorders; Brain Tumors; Pituitary Tumors; Deep Brain Stimulation; **Hospital:** Northern Westchester Hosp, White Plains Hosp Ctr; **Address:** Brain & Spine Surgeons of New York, 244 Westchester Ave, Ste 310, White Plains, NY 10603; **Phone:** 914-948-6688; **Board Cert:** Neurological Surgery 1994; **Med School:** McGill Univ 1981; **Resid:** Surgery, Royal Victoria Hosp 1983; Neurological Surgery, Royal Victoria Hosp 1988; **Fellow:** Neurological Surgery, Univ Cambridge 1989

Kornel, Ezriel MD (NS) - **Spec Exp:** Spinal Surgery-Minimally Invasive; Brain Tumors; Spinal Cord Tumors; **Hospital:** Northern Westchester Hosp, White Plains Hosp Ctr; **Address:** 244 Westchester Ave, Ste 310, White Plains, NY 10604; **Phone:** 914-948-0444; **Board Cert:** Neurological Surgery 1987; **Med School:** Rush Med Coll 1978; **Resid:** Surgery, Washington Hosp Ctr 1979; Neurological Surgery, Geo Wash Univ Hosp 1984; **Fac Appt:** Asst Clin Prof NS, Columbia P&S

Lansen, Thomas A MD (NS) - **Spec Exp:** Stereotactic Radiosurgery; Hydrocephalus; Brain Tumors; **Hospital:** Northern Westchester Hosp, Lawrence Hosp Ctr; **Address:** 244 Westchester Ave, Ste 310, White Plains, NY 10604; **Phone:** 914-948-6688; **Board Cert:** Neurological Surgery 1983; **Med School:** Med Coll Wisc 1973; **Resid:** Surgery, Lenox Hill Hosp 1975; Neurological Surgery, Univ Fla-Shands Hosp 1980; **Fac Appt:** Assoc Prof NS, NY Med Coll

Lee, Thomas T MD (NS) - **Spec Exp:** Spinal Surgery; Minimally Invasive Spinal Surgery; Stereotactic Radiosurgery; **Hospital:** St John's Riverside Hosp, Phelps Meml Hosp Ctr (page 592); **Address:** 150 White Plains Rd, Ste 110, Tarrytown, NY 10591; **Phone:** 914-631-9207; **Board Cert:** Neurological Surgery 2001; **Med School:** UCLA 1993; **Resid:** Neurological Surgery, Jackson Meml Med Ctr 1999; **Fac Appt:** Asst Clin Prof NS, Mount Sinai Sch Med

Murali, Raj MD (NS) - **Spec Exp:** Trigeminal Neuralgia; Skull Base Surgery; Aneurysm-Cerebral; Pituitary Tumors; **Hospital:** Westchester Med Ctr; **Address:** Westchester Med Ctr, Dept Neurosurgery, Munger Pavilion, Ste 329, Valhalla, NY 10595; **Phone:** 914-493-8392; **Board Cert:** Neurological Surgery 1982; **Med School:** India 1968; **Resid:** Neurological Surgery, Royal Infirm-Univ Edinburgh 1974; Neurological Surgery, NYU Med Ctr 1979; **Fac Appt:** Prof NS, NY Med Coll

Rosner, Saran S MD (NS) - **Spec Exp:** Spinal Surgery; Brain & Spinal Cord Tumors; **Hospital:** Phelps Meml Hosp Ctr (page 592), Hudson Valley Hosp Ctr; **Address:** 245 Saw Mill River Rd, Hawthorne, NY 10532; **Phone:** 914-741-2666; **Board Cert:** Neurological Surgery 1986; **Med School:** Columbia P&S 1976; **Resid:** Surgery, Johns Hopkins Hosp 1978; Neurological Surgery, Columbia-Presby Med Ctr 1983

Neurology

Ahluwalia, Brij M Singh MD (N) - **Spec Exp:** Dementia; Cerebrovascular Disease; Multiple Sclerosis; **Hospital:** Westchester Med Ctr; **Address:** 19 Bradhurst Ave, Ste 2850, Hawthorne, NY 10532; **Phone:** 914-345-1313; **Board Cert:** Neurology 1974; **Med School:** India 1961; **Resid:** Internal Medicine, Beekman Downtown Hosp 1969; Neurology, Metropolitan Hosp 1972; **Fac Appt:** Prof N, NY Med Coll

Dickoff, David J MD (N) - **Spec Exp:** Epilepsy/Seizure Disorders; Neuromuscular Disorders; Parkinson's Disease; Trigeminal Neuralgia; **Hospital:** St John's Riverside Hosp, Mount Sinai Med Ctr (page 102); **Address:** 984 N Broadway, Ste 509, Yonkers, NY 10701-1308; **Phone:** 914-968-0620; **Board Cert:** Neurology 1987; Electrodiagnostic Medicine 1989; **Med School:** Albany Med Coll 1982; **Resid:** Neurology, Mt Sinai Hosp 1986; **Fellow:** Neuromuscular Disease, Columbia-Presby Med Ctr 1987; **Fac Appt:** Asst Clin Prof N, Mount Sinai Sch Med

Gross, Elliott MD (N) - **Spec Exp:** Alzheimer's Disease; Parkinson's Disease; Headache; Pain-Back & Neck; **Hospital:** Montefiore Med Ctr - Div. Moses (page 100), NY-Presby Hosp/Columbia (page 104); **Address:** 14 Rye Ridge Plaza, Ste 220, Rye Brook, NY 10573-2828; **Phone:** 914-251-1010; **Board Cert:** Neurology 1969; **Med School:** Albert Einstein Coll Med 1962; **Resid:** Neurology, Jacobi Med Ctr 1966; **Fellow:** Neurology, Albert Einstein Med Coll 1970; **Fac Appt:** Asst Clin Prof N, Albert Einstein Coll Med

Jordan, Barry D MD (N) - **Spec Exp:** Brain Injury; Sports Neurology; Concussion; Memory Disorders; **Hospital:** Burke Rehab Hosp; **Address:** Burke Rehabilitation Hosp, 785 Mamaroneck Ave, White Plains, NY 10605; **Phone:** 914-597-2332; **Board Cert:** Neurology 1989; **Med School:** Harvard Med Sch 1981; **Resid:** Neurology, New York Hosp 1986; **Fellow:** Hosp Spec Surgery 1987UCLA Med Ctr 1998; **Fac Appt:** Assoc Prof N, Cornell Univ-Weill Med Coll

Kranzler, L Stephan MD (N) - **Hospital:** White Plains Hosp Ctr; **Address:** 244 Westchester Ave, Ste 315, White Plains, NY 10604; **Phone:** 914-946-9444; **Board Cert:** Neurology 1990; **Med School:** Univ Pennsylvania 1985; **Resid:** Neurology, Neuro Inst/Columbia-Presby Med Ctr 1989

Marks, Stephen J MD (N) - **Spec Exp:** Stroke; Alzheimer's Disease; Dementia; **Hospital:** Westchester Med Ctr; **Address:** NY Medical College, Dept Neurology, Munger Pavilion, Valhalla, NY 10595; **Phone:** 914-345-1313; **Board Cert:** Neurology 1985; Vascular Neurology 2006; **Med School:** NY Med Coll 1980; **Resid:** Neurology, Mt Sinai Hosp 1984; **Fellow:** Stroke, Duke Univ Med Ctr 1985; **Fac Appt:** Prof N, NY Med Coll

Morris, James R MD/PhD (N) - **Spec Exp:** Stroke; Headache; Epilepsy; Parkinson's Disease; **Hospital:** Greenwich Hosp (page 862); **Address:** Neurologic Care, 3020 Westchester Ave, Ste 305, Purchase, NY 10577; **Phone:** 203-629-8029; **Board Cert:** Neurology 2006; **Med School:** Indiana Univ 1990; **Resid:** Neurology, Columbia-Presby Med Ctr 1994; **Fellow:** Clinical Neurophysiology, Columbia-Presby Med Ctr 1995

Reding, Michael MD (N) - **Spec Exp:** Neuro-Rehabilitation; **Hospital:** Burke Rehab Hosp; **Address:** 785 Mamaroneck Ave, White Plains, NY 10605-2523; **Phone:** 914-597-2470; **Board Cert:** Internal Medicine 1976; Neurology 1981; **Med School:** Univ Kans 1973; **Resid:** Internal Medicine, Univ Nebraska Med Ctr 1976; Neurology, Univ Nebraska Med Ctr 1979; **Fellow:** Neurology, NY Hosp/Cornell 1980; **Fac Appt:** Assoc Prof N, Cornell Univ-Weill Med Coll

Selman, Jay E MD (N) - **Spec Exp:** Pediatric Neurology; Epilepsy/Seizure Disorders; Headache/Migraine; Tourette's Syndrome; **Hospital:** Blythedale Children's Hosp, Bronx Lebanon Hosp Ctr; **Address:** Blythedale Childrens Hosp, 95 Bradhurst Ave, Valhalla, NY 10595; **Phone:** 914-592-7138 x333; **Board Cert:** Pediatrics 1978; Child Neurology 1980; Sleep Medicine 2007; Neurodevelopmental Disabilities 2002; **Med School:** Univ Tex SW, Dallas 1973; **Resid:** Pediatrics, Jacobi Med Ctr 1975; Neurology, Jacobi Med Ctr 1978; **Fellow:** Child Neurology, Jacobi Med Ctr 1977; **Fac Appt:** Assoc Clin Prof N, Columbia P&S

Singh, Avtar MD (N) - **Spec Exp:** Stroke; Epilepsy; Headache; **Hospital:** White Plains Hosp Ctr, Westchester Med Ctr; **Address:** 244 Westchester Ave, Ste 315, White Plains, NY 10604; **Phone:** 914-946-9444; **Board Cert:** Neurology 1978; **Med School:** India 1967; **Resid:** Neurology, Metropolitan Hosp Ctr 1976; **Fac Appt:** Assoc Clin Prof N, NY Med Coll

Szabo, Albert MD (N) - **Hospital:** Northern Westchester Hosp; **Address:** Mt Kisco Medical Group, 90 S Bedford Rd, Mount Kisco, NY 10549; **Phone:** 914-241-1050; **Board Cert:** Neurology 2007; **Med School:** Hungary 1989; **Resid:** Neurology, Mount Sinai Sch Med 1994; **Fellow:** Clinical Neurophysiology, Thos Jefferson U Hosp 1996; Clinical Neurophysiology, SUNY Hlth Sci Ctr 1997

Weintraub, Michael MD (N) - **Spec Exp:** Carpal Tunnel Syndrome; Peripheral Neuropathy; Pain-Back & Neck; Diabetic Neuropathy; **Hospital:** Phelps Meml Hosp Ctr (page 592), Putnam Hosp Ctr; **Address:** 325 S Highland Ave, Briarcliff Manor, NY 10510-2093; **Phone:** 914-941-0788; **Board Cert:** Neurology 1972; Clinical Neurophysiology 1977; **Med School:** SUNY Buffalo 1966; **Resid:** Neurology, EJ Meyer Meml Hosp 1968; **Fellow:** Neurology, Yale-New Haven Hosp 1970; **Fac Appt:** Clin Prof N, NY Med Coll

Neuroradiology

Tenner, Michael MD (NRad) - **Spec Exp:** Stroke; Brain & Spinal Tumors; Carotid Artery Stent Placement; **Hospital:** Westchester Med Ctr; **Address:** NY Med Coll, Dept Radiology, 95 Grasslands Rd, Valhalla, NY 10595; **Phone:** 914-493-8158; **Board Cert:** Diagnostic Radiology 1967; Neuroradiology 2007; **Med School:** Univ MD Sch Med 1960; **Resid:** Diagnostic Radiology, Univ Maryland Hosp 1962; Diagnostic Radiology, Univ Maryland Hosp 1966; **Fellow:** Neuroradiology, Neurological Inst-Columbia Presby 1968; **Fac Appt:** Prof Rad, NY Med Coll

Obstetrics & Gynecology

Armbruster, Robert MD (ObG) - **Spec Exp:** Laparoscopy/Hysteroscopy; Colposcopy; Pregnancy-High Risk; **Hospital:** Lawrence Hosp Ctr; **Address:** 77 Pondfield Rd, Bronxville, NY 10708-3809; **Phone:** 914-337-3229; **Board Cert:** Obstetrics & Gynecology 1984; **Med School:** Washington Univ, St Louis 1977; **Resid:** Obstetrics & Gynecology, UCLA Med Ctr 1979; Obstetrics & Gynecology, NY-Cornell Hosp 1981

Burns, Elisa MD (ObG) *PCP* - **Spec Exp:** Minimally Invasive Surgery; Colposcopy; Pregnancy-High Risk; **Hospital:** Northern Westchester Hosp; **Address:** 90 S Bedford Rd, Mt Kisco Medical Group, Mt Kisco, NY 10549-3433; **Phone:** 914-241-1050; **Board Cert:** Obstetrics & Gynecology 2009; **Med School:** Columbia P&S 1982; **Resid:** Obstetrics & Gynecology, Columbia-Presby Hosp 1986

Eilen, Bonnie MD (ObG) *PCP* - **Hospital:** White Plains Hosp Ctr; **Address:** 170 Maple Ave Fl 3 - rm 309, White Plains, NY 10601; **Phone:** 914-831-6800; **Board Cert:** Obstetrics & Gynecology 2007; **Med School:** Albert Einstein Coll Med 1977; **Resid:** Obstetrics & Gynecology, Bronx Municipal Hosp 1981; **Fac Appt:** Asst Clin Prof ObG, Albert Einstein Coll Med

Florio, Philip L MD (ObG) *PCP* - **Spec Exp:** Pregnancy-High Risk; Laparoscopic Surgery; Gynecologic Cancer; Colposcopy; **Hospital:** St John's Riverside Hosp; **Address:** 1022 N Broadway, Yonkers, NY 10701-1303; **Phone:** 914-963-0284; **Board Cert:** Obstetrics & Gynecology 1981; **Med School:** SUNY Upstate Med Univ 1974; **Resid:** Obstetrics & Gynecology, St Barnabas Med Ctr 1978

Giuffrida, Regina MD (ObG) *PCP* - **Spec Exp:** Menopause Problems; Gynecologic Surgery; **Hospital:** Northern Westchester Hosp; **Address:** Mt Kisco Medical Group, 90 S Bedford Rd, Mt Kisco, NY 10549; **Phone:** 914-241-1050; **Board Cert:** Obstetrics & Gynecology 1996; **Med School:** NY Med Coll 1980; **Resid:** Obstetrics & Gynecology, UCSD Med Ctr 1984

Grano, Vanessa MD (ObG) - **Spec Exp:** Laparoscopic Surgery; Pap Smear Abnormalities; Colposcopy; **Hospital:** Greenwich Hosp (page 862); **Address:** Westchester Medical Grp, 1 Theall Rd, Rye, NY 10580; **Phone:** 914-253-4912; **Board Cert:** Obstetrics & Gynecology 2009; **Med School:** SUNY Downstate 1988; **Resid:** Obstetrics & Gynecology, Columbia-Presby Hosp 1993

Hayworth, Scott D MD (ObG) *PCP* - **Spec Exp:** Minimally Invasive Surgery; Endometriosis; Menopause Problems; **Hospital:** Northern Westchester Hosp; **Address:** 90 S Bedford Rd, Mt Kisco, NY 10549-3412; **Phone:** 914-241-1050; **Board Cert:** Obstetrics & Gynecology 2009; **Med School:** Cornell Univ-Weill Med Coll 1984; **Resid:** Obstetrics & Gynecology, Mount Sinai Med Ctr 1988; **Fac Appt:** Asst Clin Prof ObG, Mount Sinai Sch Med

Keller, Adina MD (ObG) - **Spec Exp:** Adolescent Gynecology; **Hospital:** Northern Westchester Hosp; **Address:** Mt Kisco Medical Group, 90 S Bedford Rd, Mount Kisco, NY 10549; **Phone:** 914-241-1050; **Board Cert:** Obstetrics & Gynecology 2009; **Med School:** Mount Sinai Sch Med 1993; **Resid:** Obstetrics & Gynecology, Mount Sinai Med Ctr 1997

Maloney, Romelle J MD (ObG) - **Hospital:** Greenwich Hosp (page 862), Sound Shore Med Ctr - Westchester; **Address:** 145 Huguenot St, Ste 215, New Rochelle, NY 10801; **Phone:** 914-235-6060; **Board Cert:** Obstetrics & Gynecology 2000; **Med School:** E Tenn State Univ 1986; **Resid:** Obstetrics & Gynecology, Westchester Med Ctr 1990; **Fac Appt:** Asst Clin Prof ObG, NY Med Coll

McGovern, Catherine A MD (ObG) - **Hospital:** White Plains Hosp Ctr; **Address:** 170 Maple Ave Fl 3 - Ste 309, White Plains, NY 10605; **Phone:** 914-831-6800; **Board Cert:** Obstetrics & Gynecology 2009; **Med School:** Albany Med Coll 1985; **Resid:** Obstetrics & Gynecology, Albany Med Ctr 1989

Meacham, Kevin MD (ObG) - **Spec Exp:** Pregnancy-High Risk; Laparoscopic Surgery; Gynecologic Surgery; **Hospital:** Sound Shore Med Ctr - Westchester; **Address:** 2071 Boston Post Rd, Larchmont, NY 10538-3701; **Phone:** 914-833-1000; **Board Cert:** Obstetrics & Gynecology 2009; **Med School:** NY Med Coll 1986; **Resid:** Obstetrics & Gynecology, Long Island Jewish Med Ctr 1990

Mendelowitz, Lawrence G MD (ObG) - **Spec Exp:** Pelvic Reconstruction; Laparoscopic Hysterectomy; Gynecologic Surgery; Pregnancy-High Risk; **Hospital:** Phelps Meml Hosp Ctr (page 592), Westchester Med Ctr; **Address:** 755 N Broadway, Ste 560, Sleepy Hollow, NY 10591; **Phone:** 914-631-0337; **Board Cert:** Obstetrics & Gynecology 2009; **Med School:** NYU Sch Med 1976; **Resid:** Obstetrics & Gynecology, Bellevue Hosp-NYU 1980

Mieszerski, Laura E MD (ObG) - **Spec Exp:** Adolescent Gynecology; **Hospital:** Hudson Valley Hosp Ctr; **Address:** 2241 Crompond Rd, Cortlandt Manor, NY 10567; **Phone:** 914-736-6180; **Board Cert:** Obstetrics & Gynecology 2009; **Med School:** Albany Med Coll 1992; **Resid:** Obstetrics & Gynecology, UTSA Affil Hosp 1996

Nelson, William S MD (ObG) - **Spec Exp:** Menopause Problems; **Hospital:** Greenwich Hosp (page 862); **Address:** Westchester Medical Group, 1 Theall Rd, Rye, NY 10580; **Phone:** 914-253-4912; **Board Cert:** Obstetrics & Gynecology 1981; **Med School:** Albert Einstein Coll Med 1960; **Resid:** Obstetrics & Gynecology, Maimonides Med Ctr 1965; **Fac Appt:** Asst Clin Prof ObG, Albert Einstein Coll Med

Regard, Monique M MD (ObG) - **Spec Exp:** Pediatric Gynecology Only; Birth Defects-Vaginal; Ovarian Masses in Children/Adolescents; **Hospital:** Westchester Med Ctr, Children's & Women's Phys.of Westchester; **Address:** Children's/Women's Physicians of Westchester, 503 Grasslands Rd, Ste 200, Valhalla, NY 10595; **Phone:** 914-304-5300; **Board Cert:** Obstetrics & Gynecology 2007; **Med School:** Baylor Coll Med 1989; **Resid:** Obstetrics & Gynecology, Univ Minn Med Ctr 1993; **Fac Appt:** Asst Clin Prof Ped, NY Med Coll

Ullman, Joel MD (ObG) - **Spec Exp:** Laparoscopic Surgery-Complex; Uro-Gynecology; Vulvar Disease; Vaginal Surgery; **Hospital:** Sound Shore Med Ctr - Westchester; **Address:** 2071 Boston Post Rd, Larchmont, NY 10538-3701; **Phone:** 914-833-1000; **Board Cert:** Obstetrics & Gynecology 1978; **Med School:** NY Med Coll 1963; **Resid:** Obstetrics & Gynecology, Beth Israel Med Ctr 1969; **Fac Appt:** Asst Clin Prof ObG, Albert Einstein Coll Med

Wysoki, Randee S MD (ObG) - **Hospital:** White Plains Hosp Ctr; **Address:** Westchester Gynecologists, 170 Maple Ave, Ste 309, White Plains, NY 10601; **Phone:** 914-831-6800; **Board Cert:** Obstetrics & Gynecology 2009; **Med School:** Georgetown Univ 1982; **Resid:** Obstetrics & Gynecology, Emory Univ Med Ctr 1986

Ophthalmology

Bansal, Rajendra K MD (Oph) - **Spec Exp:** Glaucoma; **Hospital:** Mount Vernon Hosp; **Address:** 105 Stevens Ave, Ste 306, Mt Vernon, NY 10550-2686; **Phone:** 914-664-3168; **Board Cert:** Ophthalmology 1977; **Med School:** India 1967; **Resid:** Ophthalmology, Univ Delhi Hosp 1973; **Fellow:** Glaucoma, Columbia Presby Med Ctr 1979; **Fac Appt:** Asst Clin Prof Oph, Columbia P&S

Biser, Seth A MD (Oph) - **Spec Exp:** Corneal Disease & Surgery; Cataract Surgery; Refractive Surgery; **Hospital:** Lawrence Hosp Ctr; **Address:** 654 Gramatan Ave, Fleetwood, NY 10552; **Phone:** 914-664-2300; **Board Cert:** Ophthalmology 2003; **Med School:** Univ Pennsylvania 1997; **Resid:** Ophthalmology, Wilmer Eye Inst 2001; **Fellow:** Refractive Surgery, North Shore Hosp 2002

Brustein, Harris MD (Oph) - **Hospital:** Sound Shore Med Ctr - Westchester; **Address:** 77 Quaker Ridge Rd, Ste 203, New Rochelle, NY 10804-2821; **Phone:** 914-235-0022; **Board Cert:** Ophthalmology 1976; **Med School:** Albert Einstein Coll Med 1970; **Resid:** Ophthalmology, Montefiore Med Ctr 1974; **Fellow:** Pediatric Ophthalmology, Chldns Hosp 1975

Dieck, William MD (Oph) - **Spec Exp:** Cataract Surgery; Glaucoma; Lens Implants-Multifocal; **Hospital:** Northern Westchester Hosp; **Address:** 185 Kisco Ave, Mt Kisco, NY 10549; **Phone:** 914-666-4939; **Board Cert:** Ophthalmology 1990; **Med School:** NY Med Coll 1983; **Resid:** Internal Medicine, Westchester Co Med Ctr 1985; Ophthalmology, Westchester Co Med Ctr 1988

Fleischman, Jay MD (Oph) - **Spec Exp:** Diabetic Eye Disease/Retinopathy; Macular Degeneration; **Hospital:** Montefiore Med Ctr - Div. Moses (page 100); **Address:** 600 Mamaroneck Ave, Ste 103, Harrison, NY 10528-1613; **Phone:** 914-315-5111; **Board Cert:** Ophthalmology 1980; **Med School:** Columbia P&S 1975; **Resid:** Ophthalmology, Johns Hopkins Hosp 1979; **Fac Appt:** Assoc Prof Oph, Albert Einstein Coll Med

Forman, Scott MD (Oph) - **Spec Exp:** Botox Therapy; Eye Muscle Disorders; Neuro-Ophthalmology; **Hospital:** Westchester Med Ctr; **Address:** Westchester Med Ctr, Dept Ophthalmology, Macy Pavilion, Valhalla, NY 10595; **Phone:** 914-493-7666; **Board Cert:** Ophthalmology 1989; **Med School:** UMDNJ-RW Johnson Med Sch 1981; **Resid:** Ophthalmology, New York Med Coll 1986; **Fellow:** Neuro-Ophthalmology, Columbia-Presby Med Ctr 1987; **Fac Appt:** Assoc Prof Oph, NY Med Coll

Glassman, Morris MD (Oph) - **Spec Exp:** Cataract Surgery; Glaucoma; **Hospital:** Northern Westchester Hosp, Westchester Med Ctr; **Address:** 1940 Commerce St, Yorktown Heights, NY 10598; **Phone:** 914-962-5506; **Board Cert:** Ophthalmology 1975; **Med School:** NYU Sch Med 1968; **Resid:** Ophthalmology, Montefiore Med Ctr 1974; **Fac Appt:** Assoc Clin Prof Oph, Albert Einstein Coll Med

Greenbaum, Allen MD (Oph) - **Spec Exp:** Laser Refractive Surgery; Cataract Surgery; **Hospital:** White Plains Hosp Ctr; **Address:** 170 Maple Ave, Ste 402, White Plains, NY 10601; **Phone:** 914-949-9200; **Board Cert:** Ophthalmology 1985; **Med School:** Mount Sinai Sch Med 1979; **Resid:** Ophthalmology, Mount Sinai Hosp 1983

Greenberg, Steven C MD (Oph) - **Spec Exp:** Pediatric Ophthalmology; **Hospital:** White Plains Hosp Ctr, Greenwich Hosp (page 862); **Address:** 1 Theall Rd, Rye, NY 10580; **Phone:** 914-848-8999; **Board Cert:** Ophthalmology 1987; **Med School:** Univ Conn 1982; **Resid:** Ophthalmology, NYU Med Ctr 1986; **Fellow:** Pediatric Ophthalmology, Manhattan EET Hosp 1987

Horowitz, Marc MD (Oph) - **Spec Exp:** Pediatric Ophthalmology; Strabismus; Retinopathy of Prematurity; **Hospital:** Westchester Med Ctr, White Plains Hosp Ctr; **Address:** 14 Harwood Ct, Ste 209, Scarsdale, NY 10583; **Phone:** 914-723-5511; **Board Cert:** Ophthalmology 1983; **Med School:** Mount Sinai Sch Med 1978; **Resid:** Ophthalmology, St Luke's Roosevelt Hosp Ctr 1982; **Fellow:** Pediatric Ophthalmology, Chldns Hosp 1983; **Fac Appt:** Clin Prof Oph, NY Med Coll

Lederman, Martin E MD (Oph) - **Spec Exp:** Pediatric Ophthalmology; Eye Muscle Disorders; Diagnostic Problems; **Hospital:** White Plains Hosp Ctr, NY-Presby Hosp/Columbia (page 104); **Address:** 3020 Westchester Ave, Ste 402, Purchase, NY 10577; **Phone:** 914-417-6441; **Board Cert:** Ophthalmology 2005; **Med School:** Albert Einstein Coll Med 1964; **Resid:** Ophthalmology, Albert Einstein Affil Hosp 1968; **Fellow:** Pediatric Ophthalmology, Chldns Hosp 1970; **Fac Appt:** Assoc Clin Prof Oph, Columbia P&S

Lippman, Jay MD (Oph) - **Spec Exp:** Cataract Surgery; LASIK-Refractive Surgery; Cornea Transplant; **Hospital:** New York Eye & Ear Infirm (page 113); **Address:** 828 Pelhamdale Ave, New Rochelle, NY 10801; **Phone:** 914-636-3600; **Board Cert:** Ophthalmology 1972; **Med School:** Ros Franklin Univ/Chicago Med Sch 1964; **Resid:** Ophthalmology, Montefiore Med Ctr 1970; **Fac Appt:** Clin Prof Oph, NY Med Coll

McKee, Heather MD (Oph) - **Spec Exp:** Cataract Surgery; Glaucoma; **Hospital:** Comm Hosp - Dobbs Ferry, Westchester Med Ctr; **Address:** 200 S Broadway, Ste 202, Tarrytown, NY 10591-4504; **Phone:** 914-631-7300; **Board Cert:** Ophthalmology 1981; **Med School:** Duke Univ 1976; **Resid:** Ophthalmology, Strong Meml Hosp 1980; **Fac Appt:** Asst Clin Prof Oph, NY Med Coll

Mignone, Biagio MD (Oph) - **Spec Exp:** Cataract Surgery; Glaucoma; **Hospital:** Mount Vernon Hosp, Montefiore Med Ctr - Div. North (page 100); **Address:** 202 Stevens Ave, Mt Vernon, NY 10550-2534; **Phone:** 914-664-6001; **Board Cert:** Ophthalmology 1980; **Med School:** NY Med Coll 1975; **Resid:** Ophthalmology, UMDNJ Med Ctr 1979; **Fac Appt:** Asst Clin Prof Oph, NY Med Coll

Miller, Brian MD (Oph) - **Spec Exp:** Cataract Surgery; Glaucoma; **Hospital:** Sound Shore Med Ctr - Westchester, Montefiore Med Ctr - Div. Weiler (page 100); **Address:** 1600 Harrison Ave, Ste 203, Mamaroneck, NY 10543-3145; **Phone:** 914-698-0670; **Board Cert:** Ophthalmology 1988; **Med School:** Mexico 1977; **Resid:** Internal Medicine, Bronx Lebanon Hosp 1979; Ophthalmology, Bronx Lebanon Hosp 1980; **Fac Appt:** Asst Clin Prof Oph, Albert Einstein Coll Med

Morello, Robert F MD (Oph) - **Spec Exp:** Geriatric Ophthalmology; **Hospital:** Sound Shore Med Ctr - Westchester; **Address:** 120 Warren St, New Rochelle, NY 10801; **Phone:** 914-633-7214; **Board Cert:** Ophthalmology 1985; **Med School:** Mexico 1976; **Resid:** Ophthalmology, Bronx Lebanon Hosp 1981

Most, Richard W MD (Oph) - **Spec Exp:** Pediatric Ophthalmology; Strabismus-Adult & Pediatric; Tear Duct Problems; Retinopathy of Prematurity; **Hospital:** Northern Westchester Hosp, Mount Sinai Med Ctr (page 102); **Address:** 101 S Bedford Rd, Ste 401, Mt Kisco, NY 10549; **Phone:** 914-241-2206; **Board Cert:** Ophthalmology 1977; Pediatric Ophthalmology 1978; **Med School:** Italy 1971; **Resid:** Pathology, Maimonides Med Ctr 1973; Ophthalmology, Lenox Hill Hosp 1976; **Fellow:** Pediatric Ophthalmology, Bellevue Hosp 1977; Pediatric Ophthalmology, Chldns Hosp Natl Med Ctr 1978; **Fac Appt:** Assoc Prof Oph, Mount Sinai Sch Med

Phillips, Howard P MD (Oph) - **Spec Exp:** LASIK-Refractive Surgery; Corneal Disease; **Hospital:** Phelps Meml Hosp Ctr (page 592); **Address:** 24 Saw Mill River Rd, Hawthorne, NY 10532; **Phone:** 914-345-3937; **Board Cert:** Ophthalmology 1982; **Med School:** NYU Sch Med 1977; **Resid:** Ophthalmology, NYU Med Ctr 1981; **Fellow:** Retina, NYU Med Ctr 1982

Ray, Audell MD (Oph) - **Spec Exp:** Cataract Surgery; Glaucoma; **Hospital:** Lawrence Hosp Ctr; **Address:** Bronxville Eye Associates, 77 Pondfield Rd, Bronxville, NY 10708-3809; **Phone:** 914-337-8844; **Board Cert:** Ophthalmology 1979; **Med School:** Columbia P&S 1974; **Resid:** Ophthalmology, Manhattan EET Hosp 1978

Salzman, Jacquelin MD (Oph) - **Spec Exp:** Cataract Surgery; Diabetic Eye Disease; Glaucoma; Laser Surgery; **Hospital:** Phelps Meml Hosp Ctr (page 592); **Address:** 200 S Broadway, Ste 211, Tarrytown, NY 10591-4504; **Phone:** 914-332-5394; **Board Cert:** Ophthalmology 1985; **Med School:** NYU Sch Med 1979; **Resid:** Ophthalmology, Bellevue Hosp 1983; **Fellow:** Retina, Bellevue Hosp 1984

Solomon, Ira MD (Oph) - **Spec Exp:** Glaucoma; Laser Surgery; Microsurgery; **Hospital:** Lawrence Hosp Ctr, Lenox Hill Hosp; **Address:** 700 White Plains Rd, Ste 343, Scarsdale, NY 10583; **Phone:** 914-725-5400; **Board Cert:** Ophthalmology 1989; **Med School:** Jefferson Med Coll 1982; **Resid:** Ophthalmology, Montefiore Med Ctr 1986; **Fellow:** Glaucoma, New York E&E Infirm 1987; **Fac Appt:** Asst Clin Prof Oph, Albert Einstein Coll Med

Solomon, Sherry MD (Oph) - **Spec Exp:** Diabetic Eye Disease/Retinopathy; Macular Degeneration; Retinitis Pigmentosa; **Hospital:** Lawrence Hosp Ctr, Sound Shore Med Ctr - Westchester; **Address:** 700 White Plains Rd, Ste 343, Scarsdale, NY 10583; **Phone:** 914-725-5400; **Board Cert:** Ophthalmology 1991; **Med School:** Albert Einstein Coll Med 1986; **Resid:** Ophthalmology, Montefiore Hosp Med Ctr 1990; **Fellow:** Retina, NYU Med Ctr 1991; **Fac Appt:** Asst Clin Prof Oph, Albert Einstein Coll Med

Stein, Mitchell B MD (Oph) - **Spec Exp:** Cataract Surgery; Cornea & External Eye Disease; **Hospital:** Northern Westchester Hosp; **Address:** 69 S Moger Ave, Mount Kisco, NY 10549-2217; **Phone:** 914-666-2961; **Board Cert:** Internal Medicine 1982; Ophthalmology 2005; **Med School:** Albert Einstein Coll Med 1979; **Resid:** Internal Medicine, Bronx Muni Hosp 1982; Ophthalmology, SUNY-Downstate Med Ctr 1986; **Fellow:** Cornea, Mt Sinai Hosp/Beth Israel Hosp 1987; **Fac Appt:** Asst Clin Prof Med, Albert Einstein Coll Med

Tostanoski, Jean R MD (Oph) - **Hospital:** Phelps Meml Hosp Ctr (page 592); **Address:** 24 Saw Mill River Rd, Ste 202, Hawthorne, NY 10532; **Phone:** 914-345-3937; **Board Cert:** Ophthalmology 2006; **Med School:** Albert Einstein Coll Med 1989; **Resid:** Ophthalmology, Bronx Lebanon Hosp Ctr 1993; Ophthalmology, Manhattan E E & T Hosp 1994

Zaidman, Gerald MD (Oph) - **Spec Exp:** Laser Vision Surgery; Cornea Transplant; Cataract Surgery; Corneal Disease-Pediatric; **Hospital:** Westchester Med Ctr, Montefiore Med Ctr - Div. North (page 100); **Address:** Westchester Med Ctr, Macy Pavilion, Dept Ophthalmology, rm 1100, Valhalla, NY 10595; **Phone:** 914-493-1599; **Board Cert:** Ophthalmology 1981; **Med School:** Albert Einstein Coll Med 1975; **Resid:** Ophthalmology, Beth Abraham Hosp 1977; Ophthalmology, Lenox Hill Hosp 1980; **Fellow:** Cornea & Ext Eye Disease, Univ Pittsburgh 1982; **Fac Appt:** Assoc Prof Oph, NY Med Coll

Orthopaedic Surgery

Asprinio, David E MD (OrS) - **Spec Exp:** Trauma; **Hospital:** Westchester Med Ctr; **Address:** University Orthopaedics, 19 Bradhurst Ave, Ste 1300-N, Hawthorne, NY 10595; **Phone:** 914-789-2734; **Board Cert:** Orthopaedic Surgery 2008; **Med School:** Univ VT Coll Med 1986; **Resid:** Surgery, Rhode Island Hosp 1989; Orthopaedic Surgery, Rhode Island Hosp 1992; **Fellow:** Trauma, Hosp for Special Surg 1993

Burak, George MD (OrS) - **Spec Exp:** Sports Injuries; Arthritis; **Hospital:** Phelps Meml Hosp Ctr (page 592); **Address:** 24 Saw Mill River Rd, Ste 206, Hawthorne, NY 10532-1541; **Phone:** 914-631-7777; **Board Cert:** Orthopaedic Surgery 1971; **Med School:** SUNY Upstate Med Univ 1964; **Resid:** Orthopaedic Surgery, Kings County Hosp 1969; **Fac Appt:** Asst Prof OrS, SUNY Downstate

Cristofaro, Robert MD (OrS) - **Spec Exp:** Pediatric Orthopaedic Surgery; Pediatric Sports Medicine; Foot & Hip Disorders-Complex Pediatric; **Hospital:** Westchester Med Ctr, Greenwich Hosp (page 862); **Address:** 3010 Westchester Ave, Purchase, NY 10577; **Phone:** 914-967-8708; **Board Cert:** Orthopaedic Surgery 1978; **Med School:** SUNY Downstate 1971; **Resid:** Surgery, Montefiore Hosp 1973; Orthopaedic Surgery, Montefiore Hosp 1976; **Fellow:** Pediatric Orthopaedic Surgery, Rancho Los Amigos Med Ctr 1977; **Fac Appt:** Assoc Clin Prof OrS, NY Med Coll

Edelson, Charles MD (OrS) - **Spec Exp:** Reconstructive Surgery; Sports Medicine; Joint Replacement; Knee Replacement; **Hospital:** St John's Riverside Hosp, Saint Joseph's Med Ctr - Yonkers; **Address:** 970 N Broadway, Ste 204, Yonkers, NY 10701-1310; **Phone:** 914-476-4343; **Board Cert:** Orthopaedic Surgery 1979; **Med School:** NY Med Coll 1973; **Resid:** Surgery, Montefiore Med Ctr 1975; Orthopaedic Surgery, Montefiore Med Ctr 1978

Gundy, Edward MD (OrS) - **Spec Exp:** Geriatric Orthopaedic Surgery; Sports Medicine; **Hospital:** White Plains Hosp Ctr, Greenwich Hosp (page 862); **Address:** 1 Theall Rd, Rye, NY 10580; **Phone:** 914-682-6540; **Board Cert:** Orthopaedic Surgery 1983; **Med School:** Cornell Univ-Weill Med Coll 1976; **Resid:** Surgery, Roosevelt Hosp 1978; Orthopaedic Surgery, Hosp Special Surg 1981

Haig, Scott V MD (OrS) - **Spec Exp:** Hip & Knee Surgery; Hip Replacement; Knee Replacement; Arthritis-Hip & Knee; **Hospital:** Lawrence Hosp Ctr; **Address:** 700 White Plains Rd, Scarsdale, NY 10583; **Phone:** 914-723-4244; **Board Cert:** Orthopaedic Surgery 2003; **Med School:** Yale Univ 1984; **Resid:** Surgery, Brigham & Womens Hosp 1986; Orthopaedic Surgery, Columbia-Presby Hosp 1989

Holder, Jonathan L MD (OrS) - **Spec Exp:** Sports Medicine; Foot & Ankle Surgery; Joint Replacement; **Hospital:** White Plains Hosp Ctr, Westchester Med Ctr; **Address:** 170 Maple Ave, Ste 109, White Plains, NY 10601; **Phone:** 914-421-0600; **Board Cert:** Orthopaedic Surgery 2003; **Med School:** NY Med Coll 1985; **Resid:** Orthopaedic Surgery, Metropolitan Hosp Ctr 1990; **Fac Appt:** Asst Clin Prof OrS, NY Med Coll

Karas, Evan H MD (OrS) - **Spec Exp:** Shoulder Surgery; Sports Medicine; **Hospital:** Northern Westchester Hosp; **Address:** 90 S Bedford Rd, Mt Kisco, NY 10549; **Phone:** 914-241-1050; **Board Cert:** Orthopaedic Surgery 2010; **Med School:** NYU Sch Med 1991; **Resid:** Orthopaedic Surgery, Mt Sinai Hosp 1996; **Fellow:** Sports Medicine, Univ Penn 1997

Maddalo, Anthony MD (OrS) - **Spec Exp:** Sports Medicine; Shoulder & Knee Injuries; Rotator Cuff Surgery; **Hospital:** Phelps Meml Hosp Ctr (page 592), Comm Hosp - Dobbs Ferry; **Address:** 24 Saw Mill River Rd, Ste 206, Hawthorne, NY 10532; **Phone:** 914-631-7777; **Board Cert:** Orthopaedic Surgery 2009; **Med School:** NY Med Coll 1981; **Resid:** Orthopaedic Surgery, Lenox Hill Hosp 1986

Mann, Ronald L MD (OrS) - **Spec Exp:** Pediatric Orthopaedic Surgery; Joint Replacement; Sports Medicine; **Hospital:** Northern Westchester Hosp; **Address:** 1888 Commerce St, Yorktown Heights, NY 10598-4431; **Phone:** 914-962-7712; **Board Cert:** Orthopaedic Surgery 2009; **Med School:** Univ Pennsylvania 1980; **Resid:** Surgery, Mount Sinai Hosp 1982; Orthopaedic Surgery, Mount Sinai Hosp 1985; **Fellow:** Pediatric Orthopaedic Surgery, Hosp for Special Surgery 1986

Nelson Jr, John M MD (OrS) - **Spec Exp:** Pediatric Orthopaedic Surgery; Joint Replacement; Sports Medicine; **Hospital:** Sound Shore Med Ctr - Westchester, Westchester Med Ctr; **Address:** 3010 Westchester Ave, Ste 104, Lower Level, rm 7, Purchase, NY 10577; **Phone:** 914-632-4420; **Board Cert:** Orthopaedic Surgery 2008; **Med School:** Mount Sinai Sch Med 1979; **Resid:** Orthopaedic Surgery, Hosp for Joint Diseases 1984; **Fellow:** Pediatric Orthopaedic Surgery, Scottish Rite Chldn's Hosp 1985

Pidoriano, Arthur J MD (OrS) - **Spec Exp:** Sports Medicine; Arthroscopic Surgery; Rotator Cuff Surgery; Knee Ligament Reconstruction; **Hospital:** Hudson Valley Hosp Ctr; **Address:** Community Orthopaedic Assocs, 1985 Crompond Rd, Cortlandt Manor, NY 10567; **Phone:** 914-739-2121; **Board Cert:** Orthopaedic Surgery 2008; **Med School:** NY Med Coll 1989; **Resid:** Orthopaedic Surgery, Westchester Med Ctr 1994; **Fellow:** Sports Medicine, Univ Conn 1996

Schlesinger, Iris E MD (OrS) - **Spec Exp:** Pediatric Orthopaedic Surgery; **Hospital:** Westchester Med Ctr, Phelps Meml Hosp Ctr (page 592); **Address:** 19 Bradhurst Ave, Ste 1300N, Hawthorne, NY 10532; **Phone:** 914-789-2731; **Board Cert:** Orthopaedic Surgery 2002; **Med School:** Albany Med Coll 1983; **Resid:** Orthopaedic Surgery, NYU Med Ctr 1988; **Fellow:** Pediatric Orthopaedic Surgery, Hosp Sick Children 1989; **Fac Appt:** Assoc Prof OrS, NY Med Coll

Seebacher, J Robert MD (OrS) - **Spec Exp:** Hip Replacement; Knee Replacement; **Hospital:** Phelps Meml Hosp Ctr (page 592); **Address:** Hudson Valley Bone & Joint Surgeons, 24 Saw Mill River Rd, Ste 206, Hawthorne, NY 10532; **Phone:** 914-631-7777; **Board Cert:** Orthopaedic Surgery 1984; **Med School:** Georgetown Univ 1976; **Resid:** Surgery, Mount Sinai Hosp 1978; Orthopaedic Surgery, Hosp for Special Surgery 1981; **Fellow:** Pediatric Orthopaedic Surgery, Hosp for Sick Children 1982

Weinstein, Richard N MD (OrS) - **Spec Exp:** Shoulder Surgery; Rotator Cuff Surgery; Sports Medicine; **Hospital:** White Plains Hosp Ctr; **Address:** 7 Reservoir Rd, North White Plains, NY 10603; **Phone:** 914-684-0300; **Board Cert:** Orthopaedic Surgery 2010; Orthopaedic Sports Medicine 2007; **Med School:** NYU Sch Med 1991; **Resid:** Orthopaedic Surgery, Bronx Lebanon Hosp 1996; **Fellow:** Sports Medicine, Univ Conn Hlth Syst 1997; **Fac Appt:** , Albert Einstein Coll Med

Yasgur, David MD (OrS) - **Spec Exp:** Knee Replacement; **Hospital:** Northern Westchester Hosp; **Address:** Mount Kisco Medical Group, 111 Bedford Rd, Katonah, NY 10536; **Phone:** 914-232-3135; **Board Cert:** Orthopaedic Surgery 2010; **Med School:** Cornell Univ 1991; **Resid:** Orthopaedic Surgery, Hosp Joint Diseases 1996; **Fellow:** Beth Israel North Med Ctr 1997

Zelicof, Steven B MD (OrS) - **Spec Exp:** Joint Reconstruction; Arthritis; Sports Medicine; Hip & Knee Replacement; **Hospital:** Sound Shore Med Ctr - Westchester, Westchester Med Ctr; **Address:** 600 Mamaroneck Ave, Harrison, NY 10528; **Phone:** 914-686-0111; **Board Cert:** Orthopaedic Surgery 2003; **Med School:** Univ Pennsylvania 1983; **Resid:** Surgery, Lenox Hill Hosp 1985; Orthopaedic Surgery, Hosp Special Surg 1989; **Fellow:** Orthopaedic Surgery, Brigham & Women's Hosp 1990; **Fac Appt:** Clin Prof OrS, NY Med Coll

Otolaryngology

Fox, Mark MD (Oto) - **Spec Exp:** Thyroid Surgery; Salivary Gland Surgery; Head & Neck Cancer; Sinus Surgery; **Hospital:** Lawrence Hosp Ctr, St John's Riverside Hosp; **Address:** 1 Elm St, Ste 2A, Tuckahoe, NY 10707; **Phone:** 914-961-2515; **Board Cert:** Otolaryngology 1979; **Med School:** NY Med Coll 1973; **Resid:** Surgery, Metropolitan Hosp Ctr 1974; Otolaryngology, Manhattan EET Hosp 1979; **Fac Appt:** Asst Clin Prof Oto, Columbia P&S

Jay, Judith MD (Oto) - **Spec Exp:** Endoscopic Sinus Surgery; Pediatric Otolaryngology; **Hospital:** Phelps Meml Hosp Ctr (page 592), St John's Riverside Hosp; **Address:** 425 N State Rd, Briarcliff Manor, NY 10510-1469; **Phone:** 914-945-0505; **Board Cert:** Otolaryngology 1984; **Med School:** Hahnemann Univ 1979; **Resid:** Surgery, Abington Meml Hosp 1980; Otolaryngology, Mount Sinai Hosp 1984

Kase, Steven B MD (Oto) - **Spec Exp:** Sinus Disorders; Pediatric Otolaryngology; **Hospital:** White Plains Hosp Ctr; **Address:** 75 S Broadway Fl 3, White Plains, NY 10601; **Phone:** 914-681-0300; **Board Cert:** Otolaryngology 1981; **Med School:** Loyola Univ-Stritch Sch Med 1976; **Resid:** Surgery, St Francis Hosp 1977; Otolaryngology, NY E&E Infirmary 1980

Kates, Matthew J MD (Oto) - **Spec Exp:** Sinus Disorders/Surgery; Sleep Disorders/Apnea; Balance Disorders; **Hospital:** Sound Shore Med Ctr - Westchester, Lawrence Hosp Ctr; **Address:** 26 Burling Ln, New Rochelle, NY 10801-4914; **Phone:** 914-636-0104; **Board Cert:** Otolaryngology 1992; **Med School:** Cornell Univ-Weill Med Coll 1986; **Resid:** Surgery, St Vincent's Hosp 1988; Otolaryngology, Manhattan EET Hosp 1991

Meiteles, Lawrence MD (Oto) - **Spec Exp:** Cochlear Implants; Skull Base Surgery; Otology & Neuro-Otology; Balance Disorders; **Hospital:** Westchester Med Ctr; **Address:** Northern Westchester Balance Ctr, 400 E Main St, Mount Kisco, NY 10549; **Phone:** 914-242-8111; **Board Cert:** Otolaryngology 1992; **Med School:** Albert Einstein Coll Med 1986; **Resid:** Surgery, Montefiore Hosp Med Ctr 1987; Otolaryngology, New York Eye & Ear 1991; **Fellow:** Univ Michigan Med Ctr 1993; **Fac Appt:** Asst Prof Oto, NY Med Coll

Moscatello, Augustine L MD (Oto) - **Spec Exp:** Nasal & Sinus Disorders; Head & Neck Surgery; **Hospital:** Westchester Med Ctr; **Address:** 1055 Sawmill River Rd, Ste 101, Ardsley, NY 10502; **Phone:** 914-693-7636; **Board Cert:** Otolaryngology 1987; **Med School:** Mount Sinai Sch Med 1982; **Resid:** Surgery, Mt Sinai Hosp 1987; Otolaryngology, Mt Sinai Hosp 1987; **Fac Appt:** Assoc Prof Oto, NY Med Coll

Ryback, Hyman MD (Oto) - **Spec Exp:** Endoscopic Sinus Surgery; Laryngeal Disorders; Snoring/Sleep Apnea; Reconstructive Surgery; **Hospital:** White Plains Hosp Ctr; **Address:** 75 S Broadway Fl 3, White Plains, NY 10601; **Phone:** 914-949-3888; **Board Cert:** Otolaryngology 1977; **Med School:** McGill Univ 1970; **Resid:** Surgery, Jewish Genl Hosp 1973; Otolaryngology, Mount Sinai Hosp 1977

Shapiro, Barry M MD (Oto) - **Spec Exp:** Endoscopic Sinus Surgery; Sleep Disorders/Apnea; **Hospital:** Phelps Meml Hosp Ctr (page 592), St John's Riverside Hosp; **Address:** 425 N State Rd, Briarcliff Manor, NY 10510-1469; **Phone:** 914-945-0505; **Board Cert:** Otolaryngology 1983; **Med School:** Mount Sinai Sch Med 1978; **Resid:** Surgery, Mount Sinai Med Ctr 1979; Otolaryngology, Mount Sinai Med Ctr 1982; **Fac Appt:** Asst Clin Prof Oto, Mount Sinai Sch Med

Stidham, Katrina MD (Oto) - **Spec Exp:** Balance Disorders; **Hospital:** Westchester Med Ctr; **Address:** 1055 Saw Mill River Rd, Ste 101, Ardsley, NY 10502; **Phone:** 914-693-7636; **Board Cert:** Otolaryngology 1999; **Med School:** Duke Univ 1993; **Resid:** Otolaryngology, Stanford Univ Hosp 1998; **Fellow:** CA Inst 2000

Zalvan, Craig H MD (Oto) - **Spec Exp:** Voice Disorders; Swallowing Disorders; Airway Disorders; Vocal Cord Disorders; **Hospital:** Phelps Meml Hosp Ctr (page 592), Westchester Med Ctr; **Address:** Inst Voice & Swallowing Disorders, Phelps Meml Hosp Ctr, 777 N Broadway, Ste 303, North Tarrytown, NY 10591; **Phone:** 914-366-3636; **Board Cert:** Otolaryngology 2002; **Med School:** Albert Einstein Coll Med 1995; **Resid:** Otolaryngology, Manhattan EE&T 1999; Otolaryngology, Ny Presby Columbia Presbyterian Med Ctr 2001; **Fellow:** Laryngology, St Luke's Roosevelt Med Ctr 2002; **Fac Appt:** Asst Prof Oto, NY Med Coll

Pain Medicine

Epstein, Lawrence J MD (PM) - **Hospital:** St John's Riverside Hosp; **Address:** Pain Medicine Wellness Ctr of New York, 220 Westchester Ave, White Plains, NY 10604; **Phone:** 914-289-1507; **Board Cert:** Anesthesiology 1987; Pain Medicine 2004; **Med School:** Israel 1983; **Resid:** Anesthesiology, SUNY Brooklyn Med Ctr 1986; **Fellow:** Obstetrics & Anesthesiology, SUNY Brooklyn Med Ctr 1987

Gevirtz, Clifford MD (PM) - **Spec Exp:** Opiate Addiction/Detoxification; Herpetic Neuralgia (Shingles); Reflex Sympathetic Dystrophy (RSD); Palliative Care; **Hospital:** Forest Hills Hosp; **Address:** Somnia, 627 West St, Harrison, NY 10528; **Phone:** 914-637-3510; **Board Cert:** Anesthesiology 1997; Pain Medicine 2004; **Med School:** Tulane Univ 1981; **Resid:** Surgery, Montefiore Hosp Med Ctr 1983; Anesthesiology, Jacobi Med Ctr 1985; **Fellow:** Pain Medicine, Mass Genl Hosp 1986

Kizelshteyn, Grigory MD (PM) - **Spec Exp:** Pain-Back & Neck; **Hospital:** St John's Riverside Hosp; **Address:** Pain Medicine Wellness Ctr of New York, 220 Westchester Ave, White Plains, NY 10604; **Phone:** 914-289-1507; **Board Cert:** Anesthesiology 1991; Pain Medicine 2004; **Med School:** Russia 1975; **Resid:** Anesthesiology, Westchester Med Ctr 1986

Malits, Bella M MD (PM) - **Spec Exp:** Pain-Chronic; Reflex Sympathetic Dystrophy (RSD); **Hospital:** Northern Westchester Hosp; **Address:** Mt Kisco Med Grp, 34 S Bedford Rd Bldg 34, Mt Kisco, NY 10549; **Phone:** 914-242-4400; **Board Cert:** Anesthesiology 1995; Pain Medicine 2007; **Med School:** NY Med Coll 1990; **Resid:** Anesthesiology, Mt Sinai Med Ctr 1995; **Fellow:** Pain Management, Mt Sinai Med Ctr 1996

Pediatric Cardiology

Fish, Bernard G MD (PCd) - **Spec Exp:** Cardiac Imaging; Fetal Echocardiography; **Hospital:** Westchester Med Ctr, Children's & Women's Phys.of Westchester; **Address:** NY Med Coll, Ped Cardiology, Munger Pavillion, Ste 618, Valhalla, NY 10595; **Phone:** 914-594-4370; **Board Cert:** Pediatrics 1974; Pediatric Cardiology 1975; **Med School:** Univ Chicago-Pritzker Sch Med 1969; **Resid:** Pediatrics, Montefiore Hosp Med Ctr 1971; Pediatric Cardiology, Montefiore Hosp Med Ctr 1973; **Fellow:** Pediatric Cardiology, Yale-New Haven Hosp 1975; **Fac Appt:** Assoc Prof Ped, NY Med Coll

Friedman, Deborah M MD (PCd) - **Spec Exp:** Fetal Cardiology; Echocardiography; Fetal Echocardiography; Congenital Heart Disease; **Hospital:** Westchester Med Ctr, Children's & Women's Phys.of Westchester; **Address:** New York Med College, Munger Pavillion, rm 509, Valhalla, NY 10595; **Phone:** 914-594-4370; **Board Cert:** Pediatrics 1982; Pediatric Cardiology 1983; Pediatric Critical Care Medicine 2007; **Med School:** Univ Chicago-Pritzker Sch Med 1977; **Resid:** Pediatrics, Bronx Muni Hosp Ctr 1980; **Fellow:** Pediatric Cardiology, NYU Med Ctr 1983; **Fac Appt:** Prof Ped, NY Med Coll

Gewitz, Michael MD (PCd) - **Spec Exp:** Neonatal Cardiology; Kawasaki Disease; Echocardiography; Heart Failure; **Hospital:** Westchester Med Ctr, Children's & Women's Phys.of Westchester; **Address:** Maria Fareri Children's Hospital, Rte 100, Munger Pavillion, Ste 618, Valhalla, NY 10595; **Phone:** 914-594-4370; **Board Cert:** Pediatrics 1979; Pediatric Cardiology 1981; **Med School:** Hahnemann Univ 1974; **Resid:** Pediatrics, Chldns Hosp 1976; Pediatrics, Hosp Sick Chldn 1977; **Fellow:** Pediatric Cardiology, Yale-New Haven Hosp 1979; **Fac Appt:** Prof Ped, NY Med Coll

Issenberg, Henry J MD (PCd) - **Spec Exp:** Fetal Echocardiography; Congenital Heart Disease-Adult & Child; Kawaski Disease; Arrhythmias-Fetal; **Hospital:** Westchester Med Ctr, Children's & Women's Phys.of Westchester; **Address:** NY Med College, Dept Ped Cardiology, Munger Pavilion, rm 618, Valhalla, NY 10595; **Phone:** 914-594-4370; **Board Cert:** Pediatrics 1979; Pediatric Cardiology 1979; **Med School:** Emory Univ 1974; **Resid:** Pediatrics, Jacobi Med Ctr 1977; **Fellow:** Pediatric Cardiology, Childrens Med Ctr 1980; **Fac Appt:** Assoc Prof Ped, NY Med Coll

Pediatric Critical Care Medicine

Goltzman, Carey MD (PCCM) - **Spec Exp:** Respiratory Failure; Sepsis & Septic Shock; **Hospital:** Westchester Med Ctr, Children's & Women's Phys.of Westchester; **Address:** NY Med Coll, Chldns Physicians of Westchester, Maria Fareri Chlds Hosp, PCCM, rm 2237, Valhalla, NY 10595; **Phone:** 914-493-7513; **Board Cert:** Pediatrics 2007; **Med School:** Mexico 1981; **Resid:** Pediatrics, Westchester Med Ctr 1987; **Fellow:** Pediatric Critical Care Medicine, Henry Ford Hosp 1989; **Fac Appt:** Asst Prof Ped, NY Med Coll

Pediatric Endocrinology

Handelsman, Dan MD (PEn) - **Hospital:** Phelps Meml Hosp Ctr (page 592), Children's & Women's Phys.of Westchester; **Address:** 755 N Broadway, Ste 500, Sleepy Hollow, NY 10591; **Phone:** 914-366-0015; **Board Cert:** Pediatrics 1973; **Med School:** Albert Einstein Coll Med 1968; **Resid:** Pediatrics, Montefiore Hosp 1971; **Fellow:** Genetics and Metabolism, Montefiore Hosp 1973; **Fac Appt:** Assoc Clin Prof Ped, NY Med Coll

Noto, Richard MD (PEn) - **Spec Exp:** Growth/Development Disorders; Diabetes; Lead Poisoning; Thyroid Disorders; **Hospital:** Westchester Med Ctr, Children's & Women's Phys.of Westchester; **Address:** 755 N Broadway Fl 4 - Ste 400, Sleepy Hollow, NY 10591; **Phone:** 914-366-3400; **Board Cert:** Pediatrics 1981; Pediatric Endocrinology 1983; **Med School:** Mount Sinai Sch Med 1976; **Resid:** Pediatrics, Beth Israel Med Ctr 1978; **Fellow:** Pediatric Endocrinology, NY Hosp 1979; Pediatric Endocrinology, N Shore Univ Hosp 1981; **Fac Appt:** Asst Prof Ped, NY Med Coll

Romano, Alicia MD (PEn) - **Spec Exp:** Growth/Development Disorders; Diabetes; **Hospital:** Westchester Med Ctr, Children's & Women's Phys.of Westchester; **Address:** Diabetes & Endocrine Ctr, 701 N Broadway, Ste 400, Sleepy Hollow, NY 10591; **Phone:** 914-366-3400; **Board Cert:** Pediatric Endocrinology 2006; **Med School:** SUNY Stony Brook 1985; **Resid:** Pediatrics, Schneider Chlds Hosp 1988; **Fellow:** Pediatric Endocrinology, Schneider Chlds Hosp 1991; **Fac Appt:** Asst Prof Ped, NY Med Coll

Saenger, Paul MD (PEn) - **Spec Exp:** Short Stature in Children; Turner's Syndrome; Sexual Differentiation Disorders; **Address:** 150 Lockwood Ave, New Rochelle, NY 10801; **Phone:** 914-636-5924; **Board Cert:** Pediatrics 1973; Pediatric Endocrinology 1978; **Med School:** Germany 1969; **Resid:** Pediatrics, Montefiore Hosp Med Ctr 1970; Pediatrics, Albert Einstein Coll Med 1971; **Fellow:** Pediatric Endocrinology, Cornell Univ Med Ctr 1975; **Fac Appt:** Prof Ped, Albert Einstein Coll Med

Pediatric Gastroenterology

Berezin, Stuart MD (PGe) - **Hospital:** Westchester Med Ctr, Children's & Women's Phys.of Westchester; **Address:** 503 Grasslands Rd, Valhalla, NY 10595; **Phone:** 914-367-0000; **Board Cert:** Pediatrics 1980; Pediatric Gastroenterology 1990; **Med School:** Hahnemann Univ 1976; **Resid:** Pediatrics, Metrohealth Med Ctr 1979; Gastroenterology, Chldns Hosp; **Fac Appt:** Assoc Prof Ped, NY Med Coll

Birnbaum, Audrey MD (PGe) - **Spec Exp:** Food Allergy; Inflammatory Bowel Disease/Crohn's; **Hospital:** Northern Westchester Hosp; **Address:** 110 S Bedford Rd, Mount Kisco, NY 10549; **Phone:** 914-241-1050; **Board Cert:** Pediatric Gastroenterology 2007; **Med School:** NYU Sch Med 1986; **Resid:** Pediatrics, Mt Sinai Hosp 1989; **Fellow:** Pediatric Gastroenterology, Mt Sinai Hosp 1991

Halata, Michael MD (PGe) - **Spec Exp:** Inflammatory Bowel Disease; Functional Bowel Disorders; Gastroesophageal Reflux Disease (GERD); **Hospital:** Westchester Med Ctr, Children's & Women's Phys.of Westchester; **Address:** 503 Grasslands Rd, Ste 201, Valhalla, NY 10595; **Phone:** 914-367-0000; **Board Cert:** Pediatrics 1980; Pediatric Gastroenterology 2005; **Med School:** UMDNJ-NJ Med Sch, Newark 1974; **Resid:** Pediatrics, Westchester Med Ctr 1977; **Fellow:** Pediatric Gastroenterology, Westchester Med Ctr 1979; **Fac Appt:** Assoc Clin Prof Ped, NY Med Coll

Newman, Leonard MD (PGe) - **Spec Exp:** Inflammatory Bowel Disease; Celiac Disease; **Hospital:** Westchester Med Ctr, Children's & Women's Phys.of Westchester; **Address:** NY Med College, Dept Ped, Munger Pavillion - rm 123, Valhalla, NY 10595; **Phone:** 914-367-0000; **Board Cert:** Pediatrics 1975; Pediatric Gastroenterology 1990; **Med School:** NY Med Coll 1970; **Resid:** Pediatrics, UCSD Med Ctr 1972; Pediatrics, NY Med Coll 1973; **Fellow:** Gastroenterology, Bronx Lebanon Hosp/Einstein 1974; **Fac Appt:** Prof Ped, NY Med Coll

Pediatric Hematology-Oncology

Ozkaynak, M Fevzi MD (PHO) - **Hospital:** Westchester Med Ctr, Children's & Women's Phys.of Westchester; **Address:** 19 Bradhurst Ave, Ste 1400, Hawthorne, NY 10532-2140; **Phone:** 914-493-7997; **Board Cert:** Pediatric Hematology-Oncology 2007; **Med School:** Turkey 1978; **Resid:** Pediatrics, Hacettepe Chldn's Hosp 1982; Pediatrics, Chldn's Hosp 1991; **Fellow:** Hematology & Oncology, Chldn's Hosp 1989; **Fac Appt:** Prof Ped, NY Med Coll

Sandoval, Claudio MD (PHO) - **Hospital:** Westchester Med Ctr, Children's & Women's Phys.of Westchester; **Address:** NY Med Coll, Munger Pavillion, rm 110, Valhalla, NY 10595; **Phone:** 914-493-7997; **Board Cert:** Pediatric Hematology-Oncology 2009; **Med School:** NY Med Coll 1987; **Resid:** Pediatrics, Schneider Chldns Hosp 1990; **Fellow:** Pediatric Hematology-Oncology, St Jude Chldns Rsch Hosp

Tugal, Oya L MD (PHO) - **Spec Exp:** Leukemia & Lymphoma; Brain Tumors; Langerhans Cell Histiocytoma; **Hospital:** Westchester Med Ctr, Children's & Women's Phys.of Westchester; **Address:** NY Med Coll, Munger Pavilion, rm 110, Valhalla, NY 10595; **Phone:** 914-493-7997; **Board Cert:** Pediatrics 1986; Pediatric Hematology-Oncology 1987; **Med School:** Turkey 1974; **Resid:** Pediatrics, Hacettepe Med Ctr 1977; Pediatrics, Westchester Med Ctr 1985; **Fellow:** Allergy & Immunology, Hacettepe Med Ctr 1978; Pediatric Hematology-Oncology, Mount Sinai Hosp 1987; **Fac Appt:** Prof Ped, NY Med Coll

Pediatric Infectious Disease

Munoz, Jose Luis MD (PInf) - **Spec Exp:** Lyme Disease; Immune Deficiency; Tick-borne Diseases; **Hospital:** Westchester Med Ctr, Children's & Women's Phys.of Westchester; **Address:** Pediatric Infectious Disease, 19 Bradhurst Ave, Ste 1400, Hawthorne, NY 10532; **Phone:** 914-493-8333; **Board Cert:** Pediatric Infectious Disease 2009; **Med School:** Yale Univ 1978; **Resid:** Pediatrics, Yale New Haven Hosp 1981; **Fellow:** Pediatric Infectious Disease, Univ Rochester 1984; **Fac Appt:** Assoc Prof Ped, NY Med Coll

Pediatric Nephrology

Weiss, Robert A MD (PNep) - **Spec Exp:** Kidney Failure; Nephrotic Syndrome; **Hospital:** Westchester Med Ctr, Children's & Women's Phys.of Westchester; **Address:** Pediatric Nephrology, NY Med Coll, Munger Pavilion, rm 113, Valhalla, NY 10595; **Phone:** 914-493-7583; **Board Cert:** Pediatrics 1976; Pediatric Nephrology 1979; **Med School:** Georgetown Univ 1971; **Resid:** Pediatrics, Bellevue Hosp Ctr 1974; **Fellow:** Pediatric Nephrology, Montefiore Med Ctr 1978; **Fac Appt:** Prof Ped, NY Med Coll

Pediatric Otolaryngology

Keller, Jeffrey L MD (PO) - **Spec Exp:** Otitis Media; Sinusitis; Sleep Disorders/Apnea; **Hospital:** Northern Westchester Hosp, Mount Sinai Med Ctr (page 102); **Address:** 110 S Bedford Rd, Mount Kisco, NY 10549; **Phone:** 914-242-1355; **Board Cert:** Otolaryngology 1996; **Med School:** Stanford Univ 1990; **Resid:** Otolaryngology, Mt Sinai Hosp 1995; **Fellow:** Pediatric Otolaryngology, Chldns Hosp 1996; **Fac Appt:** Asst Prof Oto, Mount Sinai Sch Med

Merer, David M MD (PO) - **Hospital:** Westchester Med Ctr; **Address:** 1055 Saw Mill River Rd, Ste 101, Ardsley, NY 10502; **Phone:** 914-693-7636; **Board Cert:** Otolaryngology 1996; **Med School:** Albert Einstein Coll Med 1990; **Resid:** Otolaryngology, Montefiore Med Ctr 1995; **Fellow:** Pediatric Otolaryngology, Montefiore Med Ctr 1996; **Fac Appt:** Assoc Prof Oto, NY Med Coll

Pediatric Pulmonology

Amin, Nikhil S MD (PPul) - **Spec Exp:** Cystic Fibrosis; Asthma; Lung Disorders-Congenital; Primary Ciliary Dyskinesia; **Hospital:** Westchester Med Ctr, Children's & Women's Phys.of Westchester; **Address:** Munger Pavilion, rm 106, Dept Ped Div Pul, Valhalla, NY 10595; **Phone:** 914-493-7585; **Board Cert:** Pediatrics 2003; Pediatric Pulmonology 2008; **Med School:** India 1980; **Resid:** Pediatrics, Baroda Med Coll 1984; Pediatrics, NY Med Coll 1988; **Fellow:** Pediatric Pulmonology, NY Med Coll 1994; **Fac Appt:** Assoc Prof Ped, NY Med Coll

Boyer, Joseph MD (PPul) - **Spec Exp:** Asthma; Cystic Fibrosis; **Hospital:** Westchester Med Ctr, Children's & Women's Phys.of Westchester; **Address:** New York Med Coll, Pediatric Pulmonology, Munger Pavilion, rm 106, Valhalla, NY 10595; **Phone:** 914-493-7585; **Board Cert:** Pediatric Pulmonology 2006; **Med School:** SUNY Downstate 1988; **Resid:** Pediatrics, Westchester Co Med Ctr 1991; **Fellow:** Pediatric Pulmonology, Westchester Co Med Ctr 1995

Dozor, Allen J MD (PPul) - **Spec Exp:** Asthma; Cystic Fibrosis; **Hospital:** Westchester Med Ctr, Children's & Women's Phys.of Westchester; **Address:** NY Med College, Munger Pavilion, Pediatric Pulmonology, Ste 106, Valhalla, NY 10595-1600; **Phone:** 914-493-7585; **Board Cert:** Pediatrics 1981; Pediatric Pulmonology 2003; **Med School:** Penn State Univ-Hershey Med Ctr 1977; **Resid:** Pediatrics, St Vincent's Hosp & Med Ctr 1980; **Fellow:** Pediatric Pulmonology, Chldns Hosp 1982; **Fac Appt:** Prof Ped, NY Med Coll

Lowenthal, Diana MD (PPul) - **Spec Exp:** Asthma; Cystic Fibrosis; Cough; Bronchoscopy; **Hospital:** Westchester Med Ctr, Children's & Women's Phys.of Westchester; **Address:** NY Med Coll, Pediatric Pulmology, Munger Pavilion, rm 106, Valhalla, NY 10595; **Phone:** 914-493-7585; **Board Cert:** Pediatric Pulmonology 2007; **Med School:** Albert Einstein Coll Med 1986; **Resid:** Pediatrics, Albert Einstein Coll Med 1989; **Fellow:** Pulmonary Disease, Mount Sinai Hosp 1992; **Fac Appt:** Asst Prof Ped, NY Med Coll

Pediatric Surgery

Liebert, Peter S MD (PS) - **Spec Exp:** Chest Wall Deformities; Gastrointestinal Surgery; Hernia; **Hospital:** White Plains Hosp Ctr, Northern Westchester Hosp; **Address:** 222 Westchester Ave, Ste 403, White Plains, NY 10604; **Phone:** 914-428-3533; **Board Cert:** Surgery 1968; Pediatric Surgery 2007; **Med School:** Harvard Med Sch 1961; **Resid:** Surgery, Peter Bent Brigham Hosp 1964; Surgery, Montefiore Hosp 1966; **Fellow:** Pediatric Surgery, Childrens Hosp 1968; **Fac Appt:** Assoc Clin Prof S, Columbia P&S

Stringel, Gustavo MD (PS) - **Spec Exp:** Minimally Invasive Surgery; Cancer Surgery; Neonatal Surgery; **Hospital:** Westchester Med Ctr; **Address:** New York Med College, Div Ped Surgery, Munger Pavilion, rm 321, Valhalla, NY 10595; **Phone:** 914-493-7620; **Board Cert:** Surgery 2007; Pediatric Surgery 2005; Surgical Critical Care 2007; **Med School:** Mexico 1971; **Resid:** Surgery, Univ Toronto 1977; **Fellow:** Pediatric Surgery, Hosp Sick Chldn 1979; **Fac Appt:** Prof S, NY Med Coll

Zitsman, Jeffrey MD (PS) - **Spec Exp:** Minimally Invasive Surgery; Chest Wall Deformities; Obesity/Bariatric Surgery; **Hospital:** NYPresby-Morgan Stanley Children's Hosp (page 104), White Plains Hosp Ctr; **Address:** 688 White Plains Rd, Ste 223, Scarsdale, NY 10583-5015; **Phone:** 914-722-6737; **Board Cert:** Surgery 2001; Pediatric Surgery 2005; **Med School:** Tufts Univ 1976; **Resid:** Surgery, New England Med Ctr 1981; **Fellow:** Pediatric Surgery, Babies Hosp/Columbia Presby Med Ctr 1985; **Fac Appt:** Assoc Clin Prof S, Columbia P&S

Pediatrics

Acker, Peter J MD (Ped) *PCP* - **Spec Exp:** Pediatric Dermatology; Adolescent Medicine; Learning Disorders; **Hospital:** Greenwich Hosp (page 862), Westchester Med Ctr; **Address:** 26 Rye Ridge Plaza, Rye Brook, NY 10573; **Phone:** 914-251-1100; **Board Cert:** Pediatrics 2009; **Med School:** Israel 1982; **Resid:** Pediatrics, NYU-Bellevue Hosp 1985; **Fellow:** Ambulatory Pediatrics, NYU-Bellevue Hosp 1987

Altman, Robin MD (Ped) *PCP* - **Spec Exp:** Child Abuse; **Hospital:** Westchester Med Ctr, Children's & Women's Phys.of Westchester; **Address:** 19 Bradhurst Ave, Ste 2400, Hawthorne, NY 10532; **Phone:** 914-593-8850; **Board Cert:** Pediatrics 1987; **Med School:** Robert W Johnson Med Sch 1983; **Resid:** Pediatrics, Colum-Presby Med Ctr 1986; **Fac Appt:** Asst Prof Ped, NY Med Coll

Amler, David H MD (Ped) *PCP* - **Spec Exp:** Adolescent Medicine; **Hospital:** White Plains Hosp Ctr; **Address:** 15 N Broadway, White Plains, NY 10601-2214; **Phone:** 914-948-4422; **Board Cert:** Pediatrics 1982; **Med School:** SUNY Buffalo 1969; **Resid:** Pediatrics, NYU Med Ctr 1972

Bailey, Michele L MD (Ped) *PCP* - **Spec Exp:** Asthma; **Hospital:** Montefiore Med Ctr - Div. North (page 100), Lawrence Hosp Ctr; **Address:** 16 North Broadway, Ste LMG, White Plains, NY 10601; **Phone:** 914-686-1848; **Board Cert:** Pediatrics 2009; **Med School:** West Indies 1989; **Resid:** Pediatrics, Lincoln Med Ctr 1994; **Fac Appt:** Asst Clin Prof Ped, NY Med Coll

Baskind, Lawrence J MD (Ped) *PCP* - **Hospital:** Hudson Valley Hosp Ctr; **Address:** 35 S Riverside Ave, Ste 101, Croton-On-Hudson, NY 10520; **Phone:** 914-271-2424; **Board Cert:** Pediatrics 2003; **Med School:** UMDNJ-NJ Med Sch, Newark 1983; **Resid:** Pediatrics, Univ Hosp 1987

Berkowitz, Norman MD (Ped) *PCP* - **Hospital:** Greenwich Hosp (page 862), Westchester Med Ctr; **Address:** 26 Rye Ridge Plaza, Rye Brook, NY 10573-2820; **Phone:** 914-251-1100; **Board Cert:** Pediatrics 1972; **Med School:** SUNY Buffalo 1967; **Resid:** Pediatrics, Mount Sinai Med Ctr 1970; **Fellow:** Pediatrics, St Christopher Hosp Chldn 1973

Berman, Morton MD (Ped) *PCP* - **Spec Exp:** Developmental Disorders; **Hospital:** White Plains Hosp Ctr; **Address:** 244 Westchester Ave, Ste 210, White Plains, NY 10604; **Phone:** 914-948-7016; **Board Cert:** Pediatrics 1981; **Med School:** NYU Sch Med 1966; **Resid:** Pediatrics, Bellevue Hosp 1968; Pediatric Neurology, Bellevue Hosp 1971; **Fac Appt:** Asst Clin Prof Ped, NYU Sch Med

Bomback, Fredric MD (Ped) *PCP* - **Spec Exp:** Infectious Disease; Complex Diagnosis; **Hospital:** White Plains Hosp Ctr, NY-Presby Hosp/Columbia (page 104); **Address:** 99 Fieldstone Drive, Hartsdale, NY 10530; **Phone:** 914-428-2120; **Board Cert:** Pediatrics 1984; **Med School:** NYU Sch Med 1969; **Resid:** Pediatrics, Bronx Muni Hosp 1972; **Fellow:** Genetics and Metabolism, Albert Einstein Coll Med 1976; **Fac Appt:** Clin Prof Ped, Columbia P&S

Bookner, Scott D MD (Ped) *PCP* - **Hospital:** White Plains Hosp Ctr, Westchester Med Ctr; **Address:** Scarsdale Pediatric Assocs, 2 Overhill Rd, Ste 220, Scarsdale, NY 10583; **Phone:** 914-725-0800; **Board Cert:** Pediatrics 2007; **Med School:** SUNY Buffalo 1989; **Resid:** Pediatrics, Chldns Hosp 1992; **Fac Appt:** Asst Clin Prof Ped, NY Med Coll

Brown, Jeffrey L MD (Ped) *PCP* - **Spec Exp:** Diagnostic Problems; Behavioral Disorders; Learning Disorders; **Hospital:** Greenwich Hosp (page 862), Westchester Med Ctr; **Address:** 26 Rye Ridge Plaza, Rye Brook, NY 10573-2855; **Phone:** 914-251-1100; **Board Cert:** Pediatrics 1972; **Med School:** Univ MD Sch Med 1965; **Resid:** Pediatrics, Mt Sinai Hosp 1970; **Fellow:** Neonatal-Perinatal Medicine, NY Hosp-Cornell Med Ctr 1971; **Fac Appt:** Clin Prof Ped, NY Med Coll

Coven, Barbara MD (Ped) *PCP* - **Hospital:** Greenwich Hosp (page 862), White Plains Hosp Ctr; **Address:** Westchester Med Grp, Dept Pediatrics, 210 Westchester Ave Fl 2, White Plains, NY 10604; **Phone:** 914-682-0731; **Board Cert:** Pediatrics 1986; **Med School:** Boston Univ 1980; **Resid:** Pediatrics, Boston City Hosp 1983; **Fellow:** Psychosomatic Medicine, Chldns Hosp Med Ctr 1983

Edis, Gloria MD (Ped) *PCP* - **Hospital:** White Plains Hosp Ctr, Westchester Med Ctr; **Address:** 2 Overhill Rd, Ste 220, Scarsdale, NY 10583-5316; **Phone:** 914-725-0800; **Board Cert:** Pediatrics 1970; **Med School:** NYU Sch Med 1963; **Resid:** Pediatrics, Montefiore Hosp Med Ctr 1964; Pediatrics, Columbia-Presby 1968; **Fac Appt:** Assoc Clin Prof Ped, Cornell Univ-Weill Med Coll

Hartz, Cindi MD (Ped) *PCP* - **Hospital:** Sound Shore Med Ctr - Westchester; **Address:** 1415 Boston Post Rd, Larchmont, NY 10538; **Phone:** 914-833-1502; **Board Cert:** Pediatrics 2004; **Med School:** Mount Sinai Sch Med 1983; **Resid:** Pediatrics, Mt Sinai Hosp 1986; **Fellow:** Hematology & Oncology, Mt Sinai Hosp 1987

Levitt, Miriam MD (Ped) *PCP* - **Spec Exp:** Travel Medicine; **Hospital:** Lawrence Hosp Ctr, Montefiore Med Ctr - Div. Moses (page 100); **Address:** 1 Pondfield Rd, Bronxville, NY 10708-3706; **Phone:** 914-961-3604; **Board Cert:** Pediatrics 1975; **Med School:** Albert Einstein Coll Med 1971; **Resid:** Pediatrics, Montefiore Hosp Med Ctr 1973; **Fac Appt:** Asst Clin Prof Ped, Albert Einstein Coll Med

Lubell, Harry R MD (Ped) *PCP* - **Hospital:** Phelps Meml Hosp Ctr (page 592), Westchester Med Ctr; **Address:** 245 N Broadway, Ste 201, Sleepy Hollow, NY 10591-2657; **Phone:** 914-332-4141; **Board Cert:** Pediatrics 1969; **Med School:** Ros Franklin Univ/Chicago Med Sch 1964; **Resid:** Pediatrics, Montefiore Hosp Med Ctr 1967; **Fellow:** Pediatric Hematology-Oncology, Babies Hosp-Columbia Preby 1970; **Fac Appt:** Assoc Clin Prof Ped, NY Med Coll

Meisler, Susan MD (Ped) *PCP* - **Spec Exp:** Adolescent Medicine; **Hospital:** Stony Lodge Hosp, Sound Shore Med Ctr - Westchester; **Address:** 145 Hugenot St, Ste 200, New Rochelle, NY 10801-5011; **Phone:** 914-235-1400; **Board Cert:** Pediatrics 2004; **Med School:** SUNY Downstate 1984; **Resid:** Pediatrics, Schneider Chldn's Hosp 1987

Richel, Peter MD (Ped) *PCP* - **Spec Exp:** Ambulatory Care; **Hospital:** Northern Westchester Hosp; **Address:** 36 Smith Ave, Mt Kisco, NY 10549; **Phone:** 914-666-6655; **Board Cert:** Pediatrics 2008; **Med School:** Dominican Republic 1983; **Resid:** Pediatrics, Albany Med Ctr 1987; **Fellow:** Ambulatory Pediatrics, St Luke's-Roosevelt Hosp Ctr 1988; **Fac Appt:** Asst Clin Prof Ped, Albert Einstein Coll Med

Versfelt, Mary MD (Ped) *PCP* - **Spec Exp:** Chronic Illness; Newborn Care; Adolescent Medicine; **Hospital:** Greenwich Hosp (page 862), Westchester Med Ctr; **Address:** 26 Rye Ridge Plaza, Rye Brook, NY 10573-2820; **Phone:** 914-251-1100; **Board Cert:** Pediatrics 1983; **Med School:** Columbia P&S 1978; **Resid:** Pediatrics, Columbia Presby Med Ctr 1981; **Fac Appt:** Assoc Clin Prof Ped, Columbia P&S

Wager, Marc MD (Ped) *PCP* - **Spec Exp:** Adolescent Medicine; **Hospital:** Sound Shore Med Ctr - Westchester; **Address:** 140 Lockwood Ave, Ste 115, New Rochelle, NY 10801-4907; **Phone:** 914-235-3800; **Board Cert:** Pediatrics 1986; **Med School:** Albert Einstein Coll Med 1981; **Resid:** Pediatrics, Jacobi Med Ctr 1984; **Fellow:** Adolescent Medicine, Montefiore Med Ctr 1986; **Fac Appt:** Asst Clin Prof Ped, Albert Einstein Coll Med

Physical Medicine & Rehabilitation

Nelson, Mario MD (PMR) - **Spec Exp:** Spinal Cord Injury; Electrodiagnosis; Pain Management; **Hospital:** Westchester Med Ctr, Montefiore Med Ctr - Div. North (page 100); **Address:** 19 Bradhurst Ave, Ste 2540N, Hawthorne, NY 10532; **Phone:** 914-909-4168; **Board Cert:** Physical Medicine & Rehabilitation 1986; **Med School:** Haiti 1978; **Resid:** Surgery, State Univ Hosp 1981; Physical Medicine & Rehabilitation, Westchester Med Ctr 1985; **Fellow:** Spinal Cord Injury Medicine, Westchester Med Ctr 1986; **Fac Appt:** Assoc Clin Prof PMR, NY Med Coll

Pechman, Karen M MD (PMR) - **Spec Exp:** Electrodiagnosis; Musculoskeletal Disorders; Amputee Rehabilitation; Pain Management; **Hospital:** Burke Rehab Hosp, White Plains Hosp Ctr; **Address:** 170 Maple Ave, Ste 510, White Plains, NY 10601; **Phone:** 914-683-0020; **Board Cert:** Physical Medicine & Rehabilitation 1987; Electrodiagnostic Medicine 1989; **Med School:** Boston Univ 1980; **Resid:** Physical Medicine & Rehabilitation, Montefiore-Weiler Einstein Div 1986; **Fellow:** Research, NYU Sch Med 1982; **Fac Appt:** Asst Clin Prof PMR, Cornell Univ-Weill Med Coll

Pici, Ralph A MD (PMR) - **Spec Exp:** Musculoskeletal Disorders; **Hospital:** Lawrence Hosp Ctr; **Address:** Lawrence Hospital, Physical Med & Rehab, 55 Palmer Ave Fl 2, Bronxville, NY 10708; **Phone:** 914-787-3370; **Board Cert:** Physical Medicine & Rehabilitation 1974; **Med School:** Italy 1965; **Resid:** Pediatrics, Grasslands Hosp 1967; Physical Medicine & Rehabilitation, Montefiore-Weiler Einstein Div 1972

Randolph, Audrey L MD (PMR) - **Spec Exp:** Musculoskeletal Disorders; Gait Disorders; **Hospital:** Westchester Med Ctr, Montefiore Med Ctr - Div. North (page 100); **Address:** 19 Bradhurst Ave, Ste 2540N, Hawthorne, NY 10532; **Phone:** 914-909-4168; **Board Cert:** Physical Medicine & Rehabilitation 1970; **Med School:** Med Coll PA Hahnemann 1964; **Resid:** Physical Medicine & Rehabilitation, NYU Med Ctr 1968; **Fac Appt:** Prof PMR, NY Med Coll

Plastic Surgery

Bernard, Robert W MD (PlS) - **Spec Exp:** Cosmetic Surgery-Face; Cosmetic Surgery-Body; Breast Reconstruction; **Hospital:** White Plains Hosp Ctr, Northern Westchester Hosp; **Address:** 10 Chester Ave Fl 3, White Plains, NY 10601-5112; **Phone:** 914-761-8667; **Board Cert:** Surgery 1973; Plastic Surgery 1975; **Med School:** Univ VT Coll Med 1967; **Resid:** Surgery, NYU Med Ctr 1972; Plastic Surgery, NYU Med Ctr 1974

Khoury, F Frederic MD (PlS) - **Spec Exp:** Pediatric Plastic Surgery; Cosmetic Surgery-Breast; Cosmetic Surgery-Face; **Hospital:** White Plains Hosp Ctr, Greenwich Hosp (page 862); **Address:** 22 Rye Ridge Plaza, Rye Brook, NY 10573-2820; **Phone:** 914-253-9300; **Board Cert:** Plastic Surgery 2004; **Med School:** Lebanon 1971; **Resid:** Surgery, St Luke's-Roosevelt Hosp Ctr 1976; Plastic Surgery, St Luke's-Roosevelt Hosp Ctr 1979; **Fellow:** Plastic Surgery, St Louis Hosp 1977

Kim, Tae Ho MD (PlS) - **Spec Exp:** Craniofacial Surgery; Pediatric Craniofacial Surgery; **Hospital:** Westchester Med Ctr, Comm Hosp - Dobbs Ferry; **Address:** 155 White Plains Rd, Ste 109, Tarrytown, NY 10591; **Phone:** 914-366-6139; **Board Cert:** Plastic Surgery 2003; **Med School:** Univ Pittsburgh 1991; **Resid:** Surgery, UC Irvine Med Ctr 1993; Plastic Surgery, U Mass Med Ctr 1999

Kleinman, Andrew MD (PlS) - **Spec Exp:** Cosmetic Surgery; Breast Augmentation; Eyelid Surgery; **Hospital:** Sound Shore Med Ctr - Westchester; **Address:** 800 Westchester Ave, Ste S-512, Rye Brook, NY 10573; **Phone:** 914-253-0700; **Board Cert:** Plastic Surgery 1989; **Med School:** Univ Rochester 1979; **Resid:** Surgery, Harvard Surg Svcs 1982; **Fellow:** Plastic Surgery, Baylor Coll Med 1985

Newman, Scott E MD (PlS) - **Spec Exp:** Breast Augmentation; **Hospital:** St John's Riverside Hosp, Montefiore Med Ctr - Div. Weiler (page 100); **Address:** 1 Odell Plaza, Yonkers, NY 10701; **Phone:** 914-423-9000; **Board Cert:** Plastic Surgery 2004; **Med School:** NY Med Coll 1985; **Resid:** Surgery, Westchester Med Ctr 1990; Plastic Surgery, Mt Sinai Hosp 1993; **Fac Appt:** Asst Clin Prof S, Albert Einstein Coll Med

Palaia, David A MD (PIS) - **Spec Exp:** Cosmetic Surgery-Face; Breast Reconstruction; Rhinoplasty; Reconstructive Surgery; **Hospital:** Northern Westchester Hosp; **Address:** 400 E Main St, North Bldg Fl 2, Mt Kisco, NY 10549; **Phone:** 914-242-7610; **Board Cert:** Plastic Surgery 1993; **Med School:** UMDNJ-NJ Med Sch, Newark 1985; **Resid:** Surgery, Montefiore-Weiler Einstein Div 1989; Plastic Surgery, Montefiore-Weiler Einstein Div 1991

Reiffel, Robert S MD (PIS) - **Spec Exp:** Cosmetic & Reconstructive Surgery; Hand Surgery; **Hospital:** White Plains Hosp Ctr; **Address:** 12 Greenridge Ave, Ste 203, White Plains, NY 10605-1238; **Phone:** 914-683-1400; **Board Cert:** Plastic Surgery 1981; **Med School:** Columbia P&S 1972; **Resid:** Surgery, Roosevelt Hosp 1977; Plastic Surgery, NYU Med Ctr 1979; **Fellow:** Hand Surgery, NYU Med Ctr 1980

Rosenberg, Michael H MD (PIS) - **Spec Exp:** Breast Surgery; **Hospital:** Northern Westchester Hosp, Westchester Med Ctr; **Address:** N Westchester Hosp, Plas Recon Surg, 400 N Main St, Mount Kisco, NY 10549; **Phone:** 914-241-0265; **Board Cert:** Surgery 2006; Plastic Surgery 2008; **Med School:** Columbia P&S 1987; **Resid:** Surgery, Columbia Presby Med Ctr 1992; Plastic/Reconstructive Surgery, Columbia Presby Med Ctr 1994

Roth, Douglas A MD (PIS) - **Spec Exp:** Cosmetic Surgery-Face; Cosmetic Surgery-Breast; Facial Plastic & Reconstructive Surgery; Skin Cancer; **Hospital:** Northern Westchester Hosp, Lenox Hill Hosp (Manh Eye, Ear & Throat Hosp); **Address:** Mount Kisco Medical Grp, Dept Plastic Surgery, 110 S Bedford Rd, Mount Kisco, NY 10549; **Phone:** 914-242-5647; **Board Cert:** Surgery 1997; Plastic Surgery 2000; **Med School:** NYU Sch Med 1990; **Resid:** Surgery, NYU Med Ctr 1996; Plastic Surgery, NYU Med Ctr 1998; **Fellow:** Microvascular Surgery, NYU Med Ctr 1999; **Fac Appt:** Asst Clin Prof S, Mount Sinai Sch Med

Salzberg, C Andrew MD (PIS) - **Spec Exp:** Breast Surgery; Cosmetic Surgery-Face; Laser Surgery; Breast Reconstruction; **Hospital:** Westchester Med Ctr, Comm Hosp - Dobbs Ferry; **Address:** 155 White Plains Rd, Ste 109, Tarrytown, NY 10591; **Phone:** 914-366-6139; **Board Cert:** Plastic Surgery 1989; **Med School:** Univ Fla Coll Med 1981; **Resid:** Surgery, Mount Sinai Med Ctr 1987; **Fellow:** Plastic Surgery, Mount Sinai Med Ctr 1989; **Fac Appt:** Assoc Prof PIS, NY Med Coll

Suzman, Michael S MD (PIS) - **Spec Exp:** Rhinoplasty; Cosmetic Surgery-Breast; Cosmetic Surgery-Face; **Hospital:** White Plains Hosp Ctr, Greenwich Hosp (page 862); **Address:** 1 Theall Rd, Rye, NY 10580-1404; **Phone:** 914-848-8880; **Board Cert:** Plastic Surgery 2003; **Med School:** Cornell Univ 1996; **Resid:** Surgery, NY Presby Hosp 2000; Surgical Oncology, Sloan Kettering Cancer Ctr 2000; **Fellow:** Plastic Surgery, NY Presby Hosp 2002

Psychiatry

Addonizio, Gerard C MD (Psyc) - **Spec Exp:** Psychotherapy; Psychopharmacology; Depression; Anxiety Disorders; **Hospital:** NY-Presby Hosp/Westchester Div (page 104); **Address:** 21 Bloomingdale Rd, White Plains, NY 10605-1504; **Phone:** 914-997-5864; **Board Cert:** Psychiatry 1983; **Med School:** Columbia P&S 1978; **Resid:** Psychiatry, New Haven Hosp 1982; **Fac Appt:** Prof Psyc, Cornell Univ-Weill Med Coll

Badikian, Arthur V MD (Psyc) - **Spec Exp:** Mood Disorders; Aging; Women's Health-Mental Health; Psychiatry in Cancer; **Hospital:** St Vincent Cath Med Ctrs - Westchester; **Address:** 600 Mamaroneck Ave, Ste 106, Harrison, NY 10528; **Phone:** 914-948-4277; **Board Cert:** Psychiatry 1981; **Med School:** Univ Fla Coll Med 1976; **Resid:** Psychiatry, NY Med Coll Affil Hosp 1980; **Fac Appt:** Assoc Prof Psyc, NY Med Coll

Bauman, Jonathan H MD (Psyc) - **Spec Exp:** Mood Disorders; Anxiety Disorders; Personality Disorders; **Hospital:** Four Winds Hosp; **Address:** 800 Cross River Rd, Katonah, NY 10536-3549; **Phone:** 914-763-8151; **Board Cert:** Psychiatry 1978; **Med School:** Georgetown Univ 1974; **Resid:** Psychiatry, Univ Va Med Ctr 1975; Psychiatry, Georgetown Univ Med Ctr 1977; **Fac Appt:** Asst Prof Psyc, Albert Einstein Coll Med

Bemporad, Jules R MD (Psyc) - **Spec Exp:** Child & Adolescent Psychiatry; Psychotherapy; ADD/ADHD; **Hospital:** Westchester Med Ctr; **Address:** 415 Joni Ln, Mamaroneck, NY 10543; **Phone:** 914-698-0038; **Board Cert:** Psychiatry 1969; Child & Adolescent Psychiatry 1969; **Med School:** Univ Fla Coll Med 1962; **Resid:** Psychiatry, NY Med Coll 1966; Child Psychiatry, Columbia-Presby Hosp 1968; **Fac Appt:** Clin Prof Psyc, NY Med Coll

Bogen, Steven MD (Psyc) - **Spec Exp:** Addiction/Substance Abuse; **Hospital:** Phelps Meml Hosp Ctr (page 592); **Address:** Phelps Meml Hosp, Psychiatry, 701 N Broadway, Sleepy Hollow, NY 10591; **Phone:** 914-366-3024; **Board Cert:** Psychiatry 2005; Addiction Psychiatry 2006; **Med School:** SUNY Downstate 1988; **Resid:** Psychiatry, Montefiore Med Ctr 1982

Dulit, Rebecca A MD (Psyc) - **Spec Exp:** Personality Disorders-Borderline; Suicidal Behavior-Consult; Anxiety Disorders; Depression; **Hospital:** NY-Presby Hosp/Westchester Div (page 104); **Address:** 45 Popham Rd, Ste D, Scarsdale, NY 10583; **Phone:** 914-722-0608; **Board Cert:** Psychiatry 1991; **Med School:** Mount Sinai Sch Med 1985; **Resid:** Psychiatry, Payne Whitney Clinic-Cornell 1989; **Fellow:** Research, Payne Whitney Clinic-Cornell 1992; **Fac Appt:** Assoc Clin Prof Psyc, Cornell Univ-Weill Med Coll

Gabel, Richard MD (Psyc) - **Spec Exp:** Psychopharmacology; Psychotherapy; **Hospital:** White Plains Hosp Ctr, St Vincent Cath Med Ctrs - Westchester; **Address:** 12 Greenridge Ave, White Plains, NY 10605; **Phone:** 914-681-0202; **Board Cert:** Psychiatry 1982; **Med School:** NYU Sch Med 1976; **Resid:** Psychiatry, Mass Genl Hosp 1980

Halmi, Katherine MD (Psyc) - **Spec Exp:** Eating Disorders; **Hospital:** NY-Presby Hosp/Westchester Div (page 104); **Address:** NY Presby Hosp - Westchester Div, 21 Bloomingdale Rd, White Plains, NY 10605; **Phone:** 914-997-5875; **Board Cert:** Pediatrics 1970; Psychiatry 1977; **Med School:** Univ Iowa Coll Med 1965; **Resid:** Pediatrics, Univ Iowa Hosp 1968; Psychiatry, Univ Iowa Hosp 1972; **Fellow:** Child Development, Univ Iowa Hosp 1969; **Fac Appt:** Prof Psyc, Cornell Univ-Weill Med Coll

Harlam, Dean MD (Psyc) - **Spec Exp:** Depression; Bipolar/Mood Disorders; Psychopharmacology; Schizophrenia; **Hospital:** St Vincent Cath Med Ctrs - Westchester; **Address:** St Vincent's Hospital, 275 North St, Harrison, NY 10528; **Phone:** 914-925-5490; **Board Cert:** Psychiatry 1979; **Med School:** Albert Einstein Coll Med 1972; **Resid:** Psychiatry, Bronx Municipal Hosp/Einstein 1976; **Fellow:** Psychiatry, NY Hosp-Cornell Med Ctr 1977; **Fac Appt:** Assoc Prof Psyc, NY Med Coll

Klagsbrun, Samuel C MD (Psyc) - **Spec Exp:** Psychiatry in Cancer; Psychiatry in Terminal Illness; **Hospital:** Four Winds Hosp; **Address:** Four Winds Hospital, 800 Cross River Rd, Katonah, NY 10536; **Phone:** 914-763-8151 x2222; **Board Cert:** Psychiatry 1977; **Med School:** Ros Franklin Univ/Chicago Med Sch 1962; **Resid:** Psychiatry, Yale-New Haven Hosp 1966; **Fac Appt:** Clin Prof Psyc, Albert Einstein Coll Med

Levin, Andrew P MD (Psyc) - **Spec Exp:** Post Traumatic Stress Disorder; Forensic Psychiatry; Psychopharmacology; Cognitive Psychotherapy; **Hospital:** NY-Presby Hosp (page 104); **Address:** 141 N Central Ave, Hartsdale, NY 10530-1912; **Phone:** 914-949-7699 x376; **Board Cert:** Psychiatry 1985; Forensic Psychiatry 2006; **Med School:** Univ Pennsylvania 1980; **Resid:** Psychiatry, NYS Psych Inst 1984; **Fellow:** Anxiety Disorder, NYS Psych Inst 1986; **Fac Appt:** Asst Clin Prof Psyc, Columbia P&S

Lew, Arthur MD (Psyc) - **Spec Exp:** Psychoanalysis; Child & Adolescent Psychiatry; Psychotherapy; **Address:** 225 Lyncroft Rd, New Rochelle, NY 10804-4120; **Phone:** 914-632-9679; **Board Cert:** Psychiatry 1974; Child & Adolescent Psychiatry 1979; **Med School:** SUNY Downstate 1968; **Resid:** Psychiatry, SUNY Downstate Med Ctr 1972; **Fellow:** Child & Adolescent Psychiatry, SUNY Downstate Med Ctr 1975; **Fac Appt:** Clin Prof Psyc, NYU Sch Med

Meyers, Barnett MD (Psyc) - **Spec Exp:** Depression; Geriatric Psychiatry; Psychopharmacology; Psychotherapy; **Hospital:** NY-Presby Hosp/Westchester Div (page 104); **Address:** 21 Bloomingdale Rd, White Plains, NY 10605-1504; **Phone:** 914-997-5721; **Board Cert:** Psychiatry 1975; Geriatric Psychiatry 2000; **Med School:** NYU Sch Med 1966; **Resid:** Psychiatry, Bronx Muni Hosp 1972; **Fac Appt:** Prof Psyc, Cornell Univ-Weill Med Coll

Milone, Richard MD (Psyc) - **Spec Exp:** Depression; Psychopharmacology; **Hospital:** St Vincent Cath Med Ctrs - Westchester; **Address:** 120 Forest Ave, Rye, NY 10580; **Phone:** 914-925-5311; **Board Cert:** Psychiatry 1970; **Med School:** Creighton Univ 1963; **Resid:** Psychiatry, St Vincent's Hosp & Med Ctr 1967; **Fac Appt:** Assoc Clin Prof Psyc, NY Med Coll

Neschis, Ronald MD (Psyc) - **Spec Exp:** Geriatric Psychiatry; **Hospital:** Saint Joseph's Med Ctr - Yonkers, Rye Hosp Ctr; **Address:** 18 Linden Ave, Larchmont, NY 10538-4139; **Phone:** 914-834-3470; **Board Cert:** Psychiatry 1972; **Med School:** SUNY Downstate 1963; **Resid:** Psychiatry, Montefiore Hosp Med Ctr 1969

Opler, Lewis A MD (Psyc) - **Spec Exp:** Psychopharmacology; Psychotherapy; **Hospital:** NY-Presby Hosp/Columbia (page 104); **Address:** 765 Gramatan Ave, Mount Vernon, NY 10552; **Phone:** 914-668-4799; **Board Cert:** Psychiatry 1983; **Med School:** Albert Einstein Coll Med 1976; **Resid:** Psychiatry, Jacobi Med Ctr 1979; **Fac Appt:** Prof Psyc, Columbia P&S

Perlman, Barry B MD (Psyc) - **Hospital:** Saint Joseph's Med Ctr - Yonkers; **Address:** St Joseph's Med Ctr-Dept of Psychiatry, 127 S Broadway, Yonkers, NY 10701-4006; **Phone:** 914-378-7342; **Board Cert:** Psychiatry 1977; **Med School:** Yale Univ 1971; **Resid:** Psychiatry, Mount Sinai Hosp 1975; **Fac Appt:** Assoc Clin Prof Psyc, NY Med Coll

Perry, Bradford MD (Psyc) - **Spec Exp:** Anxiety & Mood Disorders; Psychopharmacology; **Hospital:** NY-Presby Hosp/Westchester Div (page 104), White Plains Hosp Ctr; **Address:** 455 Central Park Ave, Ste 214, Scarsdale, NY 10583-1034; **Phone:** 914-472-2167; **Board Cert:** Psychiatry 1989; **Med School:** Univ Miami Sch Med 1984; **Resid:** Psychiatry, NY Hosp 1988; **Fellow:** Psychiatry, Columbia-Presby Med Ctr 1989; **Fac Appt:** Assoc Clin Prof Psyc, Cornell Univ-Weill Med Coll

Russakoff, L Mark MD (Psyc) - **Spec Exp:** Mood Disorders; Anxiety Disorders; **Hospital:** Phelps Meml Hosp Ctr (page 592); **Address:** Phelps Memorial Hospital, 701 N Broadway, Sleepy Hollow, NY 10591-1020; **Phone:** 914-366-3600; **Board Cert:** Psychiatry 1976; **Med School:** SUNY Downstate 1971; **Resid:** Psychiatry, Yale-New Haven Hosp 1975

Stabinsky, Susan MD (Psyc) - **Spec Exp:** Psychotherapy; Psychopharmacology; **Hospital:** VA Hudson Valley-FDR/Montrose; **Address:** 15 Boulder Trail, Armonk, NY 10504-1008; **Phone:** 914-273-6637; **Board Cert:** Psychiatry 1986; Geriatric Psychiatry 2000; Addiction Psychiatry 2004; **Med School:** Mexico 1978; **Resid:** Psychiatry, Montefiore Hosp Med Ctr 1984; **Fellow:** Psychiatry, Montefiore Hosp Med Ctr 1985; **Fac Appt:** Asst Clin Prof Psyc, NY Med Coll

Sullivan, Timothy B MD (Psyc) - **Spec Exp:** Bipolar/Mood Disorders; Psychotherapy & Psychopharmacology; Schizophrenia; **Hospital:** St Vincent Cath Med Ctrs - Westchester; **Address:** 275 North St, Harrison, NY 10528-1524; **Phone:** 914-925-5485; **Board Cert:** Internal Medicine 1981; Psychiatry 1986; **Med School:** Dartmouth Med Sch 1977; **Resid:** Internal Medicine, St Vincent's Hosp 1980; Psychiatry, NY Presby Hosp-Westch Div 1984; **Fellow:** Hematology & Oncology, St Vincents Hosp 1981; **Fac Appt:** Asst Prof Psyc, NY Med Coll

Zolkind, Neil A MD (Psyc) - **Spec Exp:** Depression; Anxiety Disorders; **Hospital:** Westchester Med Ctr; **Address:** Westchester Med Ctr-Behavioral Hlth Ctr, Valhalla, NY 10595; **Phone:** 914-493-1818; **Board Cert:** Psychiatry 1981; **Med School:** Geo Wash Univ 1976; **Resid:** Psychiatry, UCLA Neuropsych Hosp 1980; **Fac Appt:** Asst Prof Psyc, NY Med Coll

Pulmonary Disease

Binder, Ralph E MD (Pul) - **Spec Exp:** Asthma; Chronic Obstructive Lung Disease (COPD); Interstitial Lung Disease; **Hospital:** Lawrence Hosp Ctr; **Address:** 329 Whiteplains Rd, Ste 100, Eastchester, NY 10709; **Phone:** 914-337-1610; **Board Cert:** Internal Medicine 1978; Pulmonary Disease 1980; **Med School:** Yale Univ 1975; **Resid:** Internal Medicine, Bronx Muni Hosp 1978; **Fellow:** Pulmonary Disease, Boston Med Ctr 1980; **Fac Appt:** Asst Prof Med, Columbia P&S

Brill, Joseph MD (Pul) - **Spec Exp:** Sarcoidosis; Chronic Obstructive Lung Disease (COPD); Asthma; **Hospital:** St John's Riverside Hosp, Saint Joseph's Med Ctr - Yonkers; **Address:** 102 Park Ave, Yonkers, NY 10703; **Phone:** 914-968-1611; **Board Cert:** Internal Medicine 1988; Pulmonary Disease 2002; **Med School:** Mexico 1981; **Resid:** Internal Medicine, Mt Sinai/Elmhurst City Hosp 1986; **Fellow:** Pulmonary Disease, Mt Sinai/Elmhurst City Hosp 1988

Casino, Joseph E MD (Pul) - **Spec Exp:** Asthma; Sleep Disorders; **Hospital:** Sound Shore Med Ctr - Westchester; **Address:** 2365 Boston Post Rd, Ste 103, Larchmont, NY 10538; **Phone:** 914-833-2020; **Board Cert:** Internal Medicine 1989; Pulmonary Disease 2000; Critical Care Medicine 2001; **Med School:** Italy 1984; **Resid:** Internal Medicine, New Rochelle Med Ctr 1988; **Fellow:** Pulmonary Critical Care Medicine, RW Johnson Univ Hosp 1991; **Fac Appt:** Asst Clin Prof Med, NY Med Coll

De Matteo, Robert E MD (Pul) - **Spec Exp:** Asthma; Emphysema; Lung Cancer-Early Detection; **Hospital:** St John's Riverside Hosp, Saint Joseph's Med Ctr - Yonkers; **Address:** 970 N Broadway, Ste 209, Yonkers, NY 10701; **Phone:** 914-965-3366; **Board Cert:** Internal Medicine 1988; **Med School:** Mexico 1982; **Resid:** Internal Medicine, Mount Sinai/Bronx VA Hosp 1985; **Fellow:** Pulmonary Disease, Westchester Med Ctr 1988

Delorenzo, Lawrence MD (Pul) - **Spec Exp:** Asthma; Emphysema; **Hospital:** Westchester Med Ctr; **Address:** Westchester Med Ctr, Pulmonary Lab - Macy Pavillion, Valhalla, NY 10595; **Phone:** 914-493-7518; **Board Cert:** Internal Medicine 1979; Pulmonary Disease 1982; Critical Care Medicine 1999; **Med School:** NY Med Coll 1976; **Resid:** Internal Medicine, Metropolitan Hosp Ctr 1979; **Fellow:** Pulmonary Disease, Metropolitan Hosp Ctr 1981; **Fac Appt:** Assoc Clin Prof Med, NY Med Coll

DiCosmo, Bruno F MD (Pul) - **Spec Exp:** Pulmonary Fibrosis; Bronchoscopy; Lung Cancer; **Hospital:** White Plains Hosp Ctr, Greenwich Hosp (page 862); **Address:** 1 Theall Rd, Rye, NY 10580; **Phone:** 914-848-8777; **Board Cert:** Internal Medicine 2001; Pulmonary Disease 2004; Critical Care Medicine 2005; **Med School:** Univ Conn 1988; **Resid:** Internal Medicine, Univ Conn Hlth Ctr 1991; **Fellow:** Pulmonary Disease, Yale-New Haven Hosp 1994; Critical Care Medicine, Yale-New Haven Hosp 1994; **Fac Appt:** Asst Clin Prof Med, Cornell Univ-Weill Med Coll

Frimer, Richard MD (Pul) - **Hospital:** White Plains Hosp Ctr; **Address:** 170 Maple Ave, Ste G1, White Plains, NY 10601-4710; **Phone:** 914-328-0932; **Board Cert:** Internal Medicine 1983; Pulmonary Disease 1986; Critical Care Medicine 2010; **Med School:** SUNY Buffalo 1980; **Resid:** Internal Medicine, Montefiore Med Ctr 1983; **Fellow:** Pulmonary Disease, NYU Med Ctr 1985

Jacobowitz, Marilyn MD (Pul) - **Spec Exp:** Asthma; Cough; **Hospital:** Northern Westchester Hosp; **Address:** 90 S Bedford Rd, Mt Kisco, NY 10549-3412; **Phone:** 914-241-1050; **Board Cert:** Internal Medicine 2002; Pulmonary Disease 2004; Critical Care Medicine 2005; **Med School:** NYU Sch Med 1989; **Resid:** Internal Medicine, Mt Sinai Hosp 1992; **Fellow:** Pulmonary Disease, Mt Sinai Hosp 1995

Klares, Scott M MD (Pul) - **Spec Exp:** Critical Care; Asthma; Cough; **Hospital:** Northern Westchester Hosp; **Address:** Mt Kisco Medical Group, 90 S Bedford Rd, Mt Kisco, NY 10549; **Phone:** 914-241-1050; **Board Cert:** Internal Medicine 2006; Pulmonary Disease 2007; Critical Care Medicine 2008; **Med School:** NY Med Coll 1992; **Resid:** Internal Medicine, New Engl Deaconess Hosp 1995; **Fellow:** Pulmonary Critical Care Medicine, Boston Med Ctr 1998

Lehrman, Gary R MD (Pul) - **Spec Exp:** Sleep Disorders; **Hospital:** Phelps Meml Hosp Ctr (page 592); **Address:** 160 N State Rd, Briarcliff Manor, NY 10510-1443; **Phone:** 914-762-8383; **Board Cert:** Internal Medicine 1982; Pulmonary Disease 1986; Critical Care Medicine 2004; Sleep Medicine 2007; **Med School:** NYU Sch Med 1979; **Resid:** Internal Medicine, LI Jewish Med Ctr 1984; **Fellow:** Pulmonary Disease, LIJ Med Ctr/Queens Hosp Affil 1985

Lehrman, Stuart MD (Pul) - **Spec Exp:** Lung Cancer; Asthma; **Hospital:** Westchester Med Ctr; **Address:** Westchester Med Ctr, Pulmonary Lab, Macy Pavilion, Valhalla, NY 10595; **Phone:** 914-493-7518; **Board Cert:** Internal Medicine 1981; Pulmonary Disease 1984; Critical Care Medicine 2007; Sleep Medicine 2007; **Med School:** SUNY Hlth Sci Ctr 1978; **Resid:** Internal Medicine, Cedars-Sinai Med Ctr 1981; **Fellow:** Pulmonary Disease, Cedars-Sinai Med Ctr 1983; **Fac Appt:** Assoc Clin Prof Med, NY Med Coll

Mandel, Michael MD (Pul) - **Spec Exp:** Sleep Disorders/Apnea; Chronic Obstructive Lung Disease (COPD); Asthma; **Hospital:** Sound Shore Med Ctr - Westchester; **Address:** 2365 Boston Post Rd, Ste 103, Larchmont, NY 10538; **Phone:** 914-833-2020; **Board Cert:** Internal Medicine 1986; Pulmonary Disease 1999; Critical Care Medicine 2001; Sleep Medicine 2009; **Med School:** Columbia P&S 1983; **Resid:** Internal Medicine, St Lukes Roosevelt Hosp 1987; **Fellow:** Pulmonary Critical Care Medicine, UMDNJ Med Ctr 1989; **Fac Appt:** Asst Prof Med, NY Med Coll

Meixler, Steven M MD (Pul) - **Spec Exp:** Asthma; Emphysema; Cough-Chronic; **Hospital:** White Plains Hosp Ctr, Greenwich Hosp (page 862); **Address:** 210 Westchester Ave, White Plains, NY 10604; **Phone:** 914-682-0700; **Board Cert:** Internal Medicine 1987; Pulmonary Disease 2000; Critical Care Medicine 2000; **Med School:** Boston Univ 1984; **Resid:** Internal Medicine, VA Med Ctr 1988; **Fellow:** Pulmonary Disease, Bellevue Hosp/NYU 1990

Novitch, Richard MD (Pul) - **Spec Exp:** Pulmonary Rehabilitation; **Hospital:** Burke Rehab Hosp; **Address:** 785 Mamaroneck Ave, White Plains, NY 10605; **Phone:** 914-597-2226; **Board Cert:** Internal Medicine 1987; **Med School:** Mexico 1983; **Resid:** Internal Medicine, UMDNJ Med Ctr 1987; **Fellow:** Pulmonary Disease, UMDNJ Med Ctr 1989; **Fac Appt:** Asst Clin Prof Med, Cornell Univ-Weill Med Coll

Schreiber, Michael MD (Pul) - **Spec Exp:** Asthma; Emphysema; **Hospital:** St John's Riverside Hosp, Saint Joseph's Med Ctr - Yonkers; **Address:** 970 N Broadway, Ste 209, Yonkers, NY 10701; **Phone:** 914-423-8517; **Board Cert:** Internal Medicine 1976; Pulmonary Disease 1978; **Med School:** Univ Ariz Coll Med 1973; **Resid:** Internal Medicine, Montefiore Med Ctr 1976; **Fellow:** Pulmonary Disease, NYU Med Ctr 1978; **Fac Appt:** Asst Clin Prof Med, NY Med Coll

Sherling, Bruce E MD (Pul) - **Hospital:** White Plains Hosp Ctr, Greenwich Hosp (page 862); **Address:** Westchester Medical Group, 1 Theall Rd, Rye, NY 10580; **Phone:** 914-698-6900; **Board Cert:** Internal Medicine 1976; Pulmonary Disease 1978; **Med School:** NY Med Coll 1973; **Resid:** Internal Medicine, Metropolitan Hosp Ctr 1974; **Fellow:** Pulmonary Disease, Metropolitan Hosp Ctr 1977; Pulmonary Disease, Lenox Hill Hosp 1978

Weinberg, Harlan MD (Pul) - **Spec Exp:** Asthma; Critical Care Medicine; **Hospital:** Northern Westchester Hosp; **Address:** 83 S Bedford Rd, Mt Kisco, NY 10549; **Phone:** 914-241-8356; **Board Cert:** Internal Medicine 1984; Pulmonary Disease 1986; Critical Care Medicine 2002; **Med School:** Univ Conn 1981; **Resid:** Internal Medicine, McGaw Med Ctr-Northwestern 1984; **Fellow:** Pulmonary Disease, Cedars-Sinai Med Ctr 1986

Radiation Oncology

Fass, Daniel E MD (RadRO) - **Spec Exp:** Prostate Cancer; Breast Cancer; Head & Neck Cancer; **Hospital:** Greenwich Hosp (page 862); **Address:** 1 Theall Rd, Ste 107, Rye, NY 10580; **Phone:** 914-848-8950; **Board Cert:** Radiation Oncology 1987; **Med School:** Howard Univ 1983; **Resid:** Radiation Oncology, NYU Med Ctr 1986; **Fellow:** Brachytherapy, Meml Sloan Kettering Cancer Ctr 1987; **Fac Appt:** Asst Prof RadRO, Cornell Univ-Weill Med Coll

Moorthy, Chitti MD (RadRO) - **Spec Exp:** Prostate Cancer; Breast Cancer; Brain Tumors; Mycosis Fungoides; **Hospital:** Westchester Med Ctr, St Francis Hosp - Poughkeepsie; **Address:** Westchester Med Ctr, Dept Radiation Med, Macy Pavilion, rm 1297, Valhalla, NY 10595; **Phone:** 914-493-8561; **Board Cert:** Radiation Oncology 1979; **Med School:** India 1974; **Resid:** Surgery, Michael Reese Hosp 1976; Radiation Oncology, Michael Reese Hosp 1979; **Fellow:** Brachytherapy, Meml Sloan Kettering Cancer Ctr 1980; **Fac Appt:** Prof RadRO, NY Med Coll

Tinger, Alfred MD (RadRO) - **Spec Exp:** Prostate Cancer; Breast Cancer; Brain Tumors; **Hospital:** Northern Westchester Hosp, St John's Riverside Hosp; **Address:** 970 N Broadway, Yonkers, NY 10701; **Phone:** 914-969-1600; **Board Cert:** Radiation Oncology 2007; **Med School:** SUNY Downstate 1992; **Resid:** Radiation Oncology, Washington Univ Med Ctr 1997

Reproductive Endocrinology

Klein, Jeffrey MD (RE) - **Spec Exp:** Infertility-IVF; Infertility; Polycystic Ovarian Syndrome; Endometriosis; **Hospital:** White Plains Hosp Ctr, Hudson Valley Hosp Ctr; **Address:** Reproductive Medical Assocs of New York, 15 N Broadway, Garden Level, Ste G, White Plains, NY 10601; **Phone:** 914-997-6200; **Board Cert:** Obstetrics & Gynecology 2006; Reproductive Endocrinology 2006; **Med School:** Albert Einstein Coll Med 1995; **Resid:** Obstetrics & Gynecology, Geo Wash Univ Med Ctr 1999; **Fellow:** Reproductive Endocrinology, Columbia-Presby Med Ctr 2001

Stangel, John MD (RE) - **Spec Exp:** Infertility-IVF; Endometriosis; Miscarriage-Recurrent; **Hospital:** Northern Westchester Hosp, Phelps Meml Hosp Ctr (page 592); **Address:** 70 Maple Ave, Rye, NY 10580-1568; **Phone:** 914-967-6800; **Board Cert:** Obstetrics & Gynecology 1976; Reproductive Endocrinology 1981; **Med School:** NY Med Coll 1969; **Resid:** Obstetrics & Gynecology, Mount Sinai Med Ctr 1974; **Fellow:** Reproductive Endocrinology, Metropolitan Hosp Ctr 1976

Rheumatology

Barone, Richard P MD (Rhu) - **Spec Exp:** Rheumatoid Arthritis; Lupus/SLE; Psoriatic Arthritis; **Hospital:** Sound Shore Med Ctr - Westchester; **Address:** 421 Huguenot St Fl 4 - Ste 44, New Rochelle, NY 10801-7004; **Phone:** 914-235-3065; **Med School:** Italy 1971; **Resid:** Internal Medicine, Brooklyn Jewish Hosp & Med Ctr 1974; **Fellow:** Rheumatology, Brooklyn Jewish Hosp & Med Ctr 1976; **Fac Appt:** Assoc Clin Prof Med, NY Med Coll

Berger, Jack MD (Rhu) - **Spec Exp:** Rheumatoid Arthritis; Psoriatic Arthritis; Spondylitis; Gout; **Hospital:** White Plains Hosp Ctr; **Address:** 210 Westchester Ave, White Plains, NY 10604; **Phone:** 914-682-6532; **Board Cert:** Internal Medicine 1979; Rheumatology 1982; **Med School:** Albert Einstein Coll Med 1976; **Resid:** Rheumatology, Bellevue Hosp 1979; **Fellow:** Rheumatology, Bellevue Hosp 1981

Burns, Mark MD (Rhu) - **Spec Exp:** Lupus Nephritis; Rheumatoid Arthritis; **Hospital:** Sound Shore Med Ctr - Westchester; **Address:** 421 Huguenot St, Ste 44, New Rochelle, NY 10801-7021; **Phone:** 914-235-3065; **Board Cert:** Internal Medicine 1980; Rheumatology 1984; **Med School:** UCSF 1977; **Resid:** Internal Medicine, Montefiore Med Ctr 1980; **Fellow:** Rheumatology, Montefiore Med Ctr 1983; **Fac Appt:** Asst Clin Prof Med, Albert Einstein Coll Med

Lans, David DO (Rhu) - **Spec Exp:** Rheumatoid Arthritis; Lupus/SLE; Asthma; Osteoporosis; **Hospital:** Sound Shore Med Ctr - Westchester, Lawrence Hosp Ctr; **Address:** 838 Pelhamdale Ave, New Rochelle, NY 10801-1032; **Phone:** 914-235-5577; **Board Cert:** Internal Medicine 1984; Allergy & Immunology 1987; Rheumatology 1988; **Med School:** Univ Osteo Med & Hlth Sci, Des Moines 1981; **Resid:** Internal Medicine, Downstate Univ Hosp 1985; **Fellow:** Allergy & Immunology, New Eng Med Ctr 1987; Rheumatology, Hosp For Special Surgery 1989; **Fac Appt:** Asst Clin Prof Med, NY Med Coll

Lenci, Margaret MD (Rhu) - **Hospital:** Northern Westchester Hosp; **Address:** 90 S Bedford Rd, Mt Kisco, NY 10549-3433; **Phone:** 914-241-1050; **Board Cert:** Internal Medicine 1983; Rheumatology 1988; **Med School:** SUNY Downstate 1980

Mascarenhas, Bento MD (Rhu) - **Spec Exp:** Arthritis; Lupus/SLE; Osteoporosis; **Hospital:** Burke Rehab Hosp, Hosp For Special Surgery (page 111); **Address:** 785 Mamaroneck Ave, White Plains, NY 10605-2523; **Phone:** 914-948-6405; **Board Cert:** Internal Medicine 1972; Rheumatology 1974; **Med School:** India 1961; **Resid:** Internal Medicine, Westchester Med Ctr 1967; **Fellow:** Internal Medicine, Cornell Univ Med Ctr 1970; Rheumatology, Hosp for Special Surg 1970; **Fac Appt:** Clin Prof Med, NY Med Coll

Reinitz, Elizabeth MD (Rhu) - **Spec Exp:** Rheumatoid Arthritis; Lupus/SLE; Osteoarthritis; Gout; **Hospital:** White Plains Hosp Ctr; **Address:** Scarsdale Medical Group, 600 Mamaroneck Ave, Harrison, NY 10528; **Phone:** 914-723-8100; **Board Cert:** Internal Medicine 1979; Rheumatology 1982; **Med School:** Albert Einstein Coll Med 1976; **Resid:** Internal Medicine, Boston City Hosp 1979; **Fellow:** Rheumatology, Montefiore Med Ctr 1981

Sloane, Lori MD (Rhu) - **Spec Exp:** Rheumatoid Arthritis; **Hospital:** Northern Westchester Hosp; **Address:** Westchester Hlth Assocs, 322 Underhill Ave, Yorktown Heights, NY 10598; **Phone:** 914-962-5501; **Board Cert:** Internal Medicine 1989; **Med School:** SUNY Downstate 1986; **Resid:** Internal Medicine, Jacobi Med Ctr 1989; **Fellow:** Rheumatology, Montefiore Hosp Med Ctr 1991; **Fac Appt:** Asst Clin Prof Med, Albert Einstein Coll Med

Yegudin-Ash, Julia MD (Rhu) - **Spec Exp:** Lupus/SLE; Rheumatoid Arthritis; Psoriatic Arthritis; Scleroderma; **Hospital:** Westchester Med Ctr; **Address:** NY Med Coll, Div Rheumatology, Munger Pavilion, rm 149, Valhalla, NY 10595; **Phone:** 914-594-4444; **Board Cert:** Rheumatology 2006; **Med School:** SUNY Stony Brook 1987; **Resid:** Internal Medicine, Winthrop Univ Hosp 1990; **Fellow:** Rheumatology, Mass Genl Hosp 1992; Rheumatology, Hosp Joint Diseases 1993; **Fac Appt:** Asst Prof Med, NY Med Coll

Sports Medicine

Cavaliere, Gregg MD (SM) - **Spec Exp:** Rotator Cuff Surgery; Knee Injuries/Ligament Surgery; Shoulder Instability; **Hospital:** Phelps Meml Hosp Ctr (page 592), Lenox Hill Hosp; **Address:** 24 Saw Mill River Rd, Ste 2, Hawthorne, NY 10532; **Phone:** 914-631-7777; **Board Cert:** Orthopaedic Surgery 2006; **Med School:** NY Med Coll 1987; **Resid:** Orthopaedic Surgery, Lenox Hill Hosp 1992; **Fellow:** Sports Medicine, NYU Med Ctr 1993

Luks, Howard J MD (SM) - **Hospital:** Westchester Med Ctr; **Address:** 19 Bradhurst Ave, Ste 1300N, Hawthorne, NY 10532; **Phone:** 914-789-2735; **Board Cert:** Orthopaedic Surgery 1999; **Med School:** NY Med Coll 1991; **Resid:** Orthopaedic Surgery, LI Jewish Med Ctr 1996

Small, Eric W MD (SM) - **Spec Exp:** Primary Care Sports Medicine; Reflex Sympathetic Dystrophy (RSD); Concussion; Sports Injuries; **Hospital:** Mount Sinai Med Ctr (page 102); **Address:** Family Sports Medicine & Fitness, 666 Lexington Ave, Ste 210, Mt Kisco, NY 10549; **Phone:** 914-666-7900; **Board Cert:** Pediatrics 2002; Sports Medicine 2008; **Med School:** UMDNJ-NJ Med Sch, Newark 1989; **Resid:** Pediatrics, Mentefiore-Weiler Einstein Med Ctr 1992; **Fellow:** Pediatric Sports Medicine, McMaster Univ/Hamilton 1994; Sports Medicine, Boston Children's Hosp 1995; **Fac Appt:** Asst Clin Prof Ped, Mount Sinai Sch Med

Surgery

Ashikari, Andrew Y MD (S) - **Spec Exp:** Breast Cancer; Melanoma; Sarcoma-Soft Tissue; Colon Cancer; **Hospital:** Comm Hosp - Dobbs Ferry, Westchester Med Ctr; **Address:** Ashikari Comprehensive Breast Ctr, Community Hospital, 128 Ashford Ave, Dobbs Ferry, NY 10522; **Phone:** 914-693-5025; **Board Cert:** Surgery 2006; **Med School:** Univ Pittsburgh 1991; **Resid:** Surgery, Montefiore Med Ctr 1996; **Fellow:** Surgical Oncology, Univ Chicago Hosps 1999; **Fac Appt:** Assoc Prof S, NY Med Coll

Cahan, Anthony C MD (S) - **Spec Exp:** Breast Surgery; **Hospital:** Northern Westchester Hosp, Hudson Valley Hosp Ctr; **Address:** 3010 Westchester Ave, Ste 201, Purchase, NY 10507; **Phone:** 914-681-9481; **Board Cert:** Surgery 1998; **Med School:** Cornell Univ-Weill Med Coll 1982; **Resid:** Surgery, New York Hosp 1987; **Fac Appt:** Asst Clin Prof Med, NY Med Coll

Cleary, Joseph B MD (S) - **Spec Exp:** Breast Surgery; Cancer Surgery; **Hospital:** Westchester Med Ctr; **Address:** New York Med College, Munger Pavilion, rm 149, Valhalla, NY 10595; **Phone:** 914-493-0133; **Board Cert:** Surgery 1999; **Med School:** NY Med Coll 1973; **Resid:** Surgery, NY Med Coll Affil Hosps 1978; Hand Surgery, St Luke's Roosevelt Hosp Ctr 1979; **Fellow:** Surgical Oncology, NY Med Coll Affil Hosps 1976; Plastic Surgery, Columbia Presby Med Ctr 1980; **Fac Appt:** Asst Clin Prof S, NY Med Coll

Fou, Adora C MD (S) - **Spec Exp:** Breast Cancer; Breast Disease; **Hospital:** White Plains Hosp Ctr, Greenwich Hosp (page 862); **Address:** Westchester Medical Group, 1 Theall Rd, Rye, NY 10580; **Phone:** 914-848-8960; **Board Cert:** Surgery 2007; **Med School:** Univ Ottawa 2000; **Resid:** Surgery, NY Presby Hosp-Weill Cornell 2005

Gordon, Mark S MD (S) - **Spec Exp:** Breast Cancer; Melanoma; Pancreatic Cancer; Colon Cancer; **Hospital:** White Plains Hosp Ctr, Westchester Med Ctr; **Address:** 2 Longview Ave, Ste 302, White Plains, NY 10601-5012; **Phone:** 914-684-5884; **Board Cert:** Surgery 2006; **Med School:** Northwestern Univ 1982; **Resid:** Surgery, NY Hosp/Cornell Med Ctr 1987; **Fellow:** Surgical Oncology, Meml Sloan Kettering Cancer Ctr 1989; **Fac Appt:** Asst Clin Prof S, NY Med Coll

Josephson, Lynn MD (S) - **Spec Exp:** Breast Cancer & Surgery; **Hospital:** White Plains Hosp Ctr; **Address:** Westchester Medical Group, 1 Theall Rd, Rye, NY 10580; **Phone:** 914-848-8960; **Board Cert:** Surgery 2002; **Med School:** Mount Sinai Sch Med 1977; **Resid:** Surgery, Columbia-Presby Med Ctr 1981

Kaleya, Ronald MD (S) - **Spec Exp:** Pancreatic Cancer; Breast Cancer; Colon & Rectal Cancer; **Hospital:** Westchester Med Ctr; **Address:** 19 Bradhurst Ave, Ste 250 North, Hawthorne, NY 10532; **Phone:** 914-493-2100; **Board Cert:** Surgery 2008; **Med School:** Cornell Univ-Weill Med Coll 1980; **Resid:** Surgery, Albert Einstein Med Ctr 1985; **Fellow:** Surgical Oncology, Meml Sloan Kettering Cancer Ctr 1987; **Fac Appt:** Assoc Prof S, Albert Einstein Coll Med

Kassel, Barry A MD (S) - **Spec Exp:** Breast Surgery; Laparoscopic Surgery; **Hospital:** Northern Westchester Hosp; **Address:** 110 S Bedford Rd, Mount Kisco, NY 10549; **Phone:** 914-241-1050; **Board Cert:** Surgery 1998; **Med School:** SUNY Buffalo 1973; **Resid:** Surgery, Montefiore Med Ctr 1977; Surgery, NYU Med Ctr 1979

Lau, Har Chi MD (S) - **Spec Exp:** Laparoscopic Surgery; **Hospital:** Phelps Meml Hosp Ctr (page 592); **Address:** Hudson Valley Surgical Assocs, 777 N Broadway, Ste 204, Sleepy Hollow, NY 10591; **Phone:** 914-631-3660; **Board Cert:** Surgery 2007; **Med School:** Univ Pennsylvania 1992; **Resid:** Surgery, Allegheny Univ Hosps 1998

Lemercier, Maud L MD (S) - **Spec Exp:** Breast Cancer; **Hospital:** Northern Westchester Hosp; **Address:** Mt Kisco Medical Group, 111 Bedford Rd, Katonah, NY 10536; **Phone:** 914-232-3135; **Board Cert:** Surgery 2006; **Med School:** Temple Univ 1999; **Resid:** Surgery, Univ Conn 2005

Pass, Helen MD (S) - **Spec Exp:** Breast Cancer; Breast Disease; **Hospital:** Lawrence Hosp Ctr; **Address:** Ctr for Advanced Surgery-Lawrence Hosp, 55 W Palmer Ave, Fl 5 W, Bronxville, NY 10708; **Phone:** 914-787-4000; **Board Cert:** Surgery 2003; **Med School:** Univ Mich Med Sch 1987; **Resid:** Surgery, Univ Tex Hlth Sci Ctr/MD Anderson Cancer Ctr 1989; Surgery, Georgetown Univ Hosp 1994; **Fellow:** Surgical Oncology, NCI/NIH 1992; **Fac Appt:** Asst Clin Prof S, Columbia P&S

Policastro, Anthony J MD (S) - **Spec Exp:** Breast Surgery; Hernia; Thyroid Surgery; **Hospital:** Westchester Med Ctr; **Address:** 19 Bradhurst Ave, Ste 1700, Hawthorne, NY 10532; **Phone:** 914-347-0162; **Board Cert:** Surgery 2000; Surgical Critical Care 2002; **Med School:** Creighton Univ 1985; **Resid:** Surgery, Westchester Co Med Ctr 1990; **Fellow:** Surgical Critical Care, Westchester Co Med Ctr 1991; **Fac Appt:** Asst Prof S, NY Med Coll

Rajdeo, Heena MD (S) - **Spec Exp:** Dialysis Access Surgery; Thyroid & Parathyroid Surgery; Laparoscopic Surgery; Adrenal Surgery; **Hospital:** Westchester Med Ctr; **Address:** Northeast Surgical Group, 551 Munger Pavilion, Valhalla, NY 10595; **Phone:** 914-493-7378; **Board Cert:** Surgery 2002; **Med School:** India 1969; **Resid:** Surgery, KEM Hosp 1972; Surgery, Westchester Med Ctr 1982; **Fac Appt:** Asst Prof S, NY Med Coll

Rangraj, Madhu S MD (S) - **Spec Exp:** Laparoscopic Surgery; Obesity/Bariatric Surgery; Hernia; **Hospital:** Sound Shore Med Ctr - Westchester; **Address:** 140 Lockwood Ave, Ste 103, New Rochelle, NY 10801; **Phone:** 914-632-9650; **Board Cert:** Surgery 1998; **Med School:** India 1972; **Resid:** Surgery, New Rochelle Hosp 1978; Surgery, VA Med Ctr 1980

Raniolo, Robert MD (S) - **Spec Exp:** Breast Surgery; Gastrointestinal Surgery; Hernia; **Hospital:** Phelps Meml Hosp Ctr (page 592); **Address:** 777 N Broadway, Ste 204, Sleepy Hollow, NY 10591-1019; **Phone:** 914-631-3660; **Board Cert:** Surgery 2007; **Med School:** Mexico 1981; **Resid:** Surgery, Lincoln Hosp 1988

San Filippo, J Anthony MD (S) - **Spec Exp:** Pediatric Surgery; Neonatal Surgery; Hernia; **Hospital:** Westchester Med Ctr, Montefiore Med Ctr - Div. North (page 100); **Address:** 19 Bradhurst Ave, Ste 2550, Hawthorne, NY 10532; **Phone:** 914-761-5437; **Board Cert:** Surgery 1973; **Med School:** Georgetown Univ 1965; **Resid:** Surgery, Bellevue Hosp 1967; Surgery, N Shore Univ Hosp 1970; **Fellow:** Pediatric Surgery, Children's Hosp 1972; **Fac Appt:** Prof S, NY Med Coll

Savino, John A MD (S) - **Spec Exp:** Critical Care; Trauma; Pancreatic Surgery; **Hospital:** Westchester Med Ctr; **Address:** NY Med Coll, Dept Surgery, Munger Pavillion, Valhalla, NY 10595; **Phone:** 914-594-4352; **Board Cert:** Surgery 1975; Surgical Critical Care 1995; **Med School:** Italy 1968; **Resid:** Surgery, Metropolitan Hosp Ctr 1974; **Fac Appt:** Prof S, NY Med Coll

Wertkin, Martin G MD (S) - **Spec Exp:** Breast Cancer; Breast Surgery; **Hospital:** St John's Riverside Hosp, Phelps Meml Hosp Ctr (page 592); **Address:** 1034 N Broadway, Yonkers, NY 10701; **Phone:** 914-965-2026; **Board Cert:** Surgery 2009; **Med School:** SUNY Hlth Sci Ctr 1972; **Resid:** Surgery, Mt Sinai Med Ctr 1978; **Fac Appt:** Asst Clin Prof S, Mount Sinai Sch Med

Thoracic Surgery

Lafaro, Rocco J MD (TS) - **Spec Exp:** Minimally Invasive Cardiac Surgery; **Hospital:** Westchester Med Ctr; **Address:** 100 Woods Rd, Macy 114W, Valhalla, NY 10595; **Phone:** 914-493-7676; **Board Cert:** Thoracic Surgery 2001; **Med School:** NY Med Coll 1982; **Resid:** Surgery, Metropolitan Hosp Ctr 1984; Surgery, Westchester Med Ctr 1986; **Fellow:** Thoracic Surgery, Bronx Muni Hosp Ctr 1991; Thoracic Surgery, Montefiore Med Ctr 1993

Lansman, Steven L MD/PhD (TS) - **Spec Exp:** Coronary Artery Surgery; Heart Valve Surgery; Ventricular Assist Device (LVAD); Transplant-Heart; **Hospital:** Westchester Med Ctr; **Address:** Westchester Medical Ctr, 100 Woods Rd, Macy Pavilion, rm 114W, Valhalla, NY 10595; **Phone:** 914-493-8793; **Board Cert:** Thoracic Surgery 2004; **Med School:** SUNY Hlth Sci Ctr 1977; **Resid:** Surgery, Montefiore Med Ctr 1982; **Fellow:** Thoracic Surgery, Univ Hosp 1984; **Fac Appt:** Prof S, NY Med Coll

Merav, Avraham MD (TS) - **Spec Exp:** Minimally Invasive Thoracic Surgery; Lung Surgery; Esophageal Surgery; Thoracic Cancers; **Hospital:** Phelps Meml Hosp Ctr (page 592); **Address:** Thoracic Center, 755 N Broadway, Ste 535, Sleepy Hollow, NY 10591; **Phone:** 914-366-2333; **Board Cert:** Surgery 1974; Thoracic Surgery 2004; **Med School:** Switzerland 1964; **Resid:** Surgery, Montefiore Hosp Med Ctr 1973; **Fellow:** Cardiothoracic Surgery, Montefiore Hosp Med Ctr 1975; **Fac Appt:** Assoc Prof TS, Albert Einstein Coll Med

Sett, Suvro S MD (TS) - **Spec Exp:** Pediatric Cardiothoracic Surgery; Congenital Heart Disease; Congenital Heart Disease-Adult; **Hospital:** Westchester Med Ctr; **Address:** Maria Fareri's Chlds Hosp @ Westchester Med Ctr, 155 Grasslands Rd, Valhalla, NY 10595; **Phone:** 914-594-3322; **Med School:** Canada 1983; **Resid:** Surgery, Univ of Saskatchewan 1988; Cardiovascular Surgery, Univ of British Columbia 1991; **Fellow:** Pediatric Cardiac Surgery, The Hosp for Sick Chld 1992

Spielvogel, David MD (TS) - **Spec Exp:** Aneurysm-Aortic; Transplant-Heart; Coronary Artery Surgery; Heart Valve Surgery; **Hospital:** Westchester Med Ctr; **Address:** 100 Woods Rd, Macy 114W, Valhalla, NY 10595; **Phone:** 914-493-7676; **Board Cert:** Thoracic Surgery 2009; **Med School:** SUNY Downstate 1990; **Resid:** Surgery, SUNY Hlth Sci Ctr 1995; Thoracic Surgery, Mt Sinai Med Ctr 1998; **Fellow:** Cardiac Surgery, Harefield Hosp 1999; **Fac Appt:** Assoc Prof S, NY Med Coll

Urology

Axelrod, Sheldon L MD (U) - **Spec Exp:** Prostate Cancer; Prostate Disease; Robotic Surgery; **Hospital:** Northern Westchester Hosp; **Address:** Mt Kisco Medical Group, 111 Bedford Rd, Katonah, NY 10536-2190; **Phone:** 914-232-3135; **Board Cert:** Urology 2003; **Med School:** Albert Einstein Coll Med 1982; **Resid:** Surgery, Montefiore Med Ctr 1984; Urology, NY Presby-Columbia Med Ctr 1988

Blair, Bryan P MD (U) - **Hospital:** White Plains Hosp Ctr; **Address:** Westchester Med Grp, 210 Westchester Ave, White Plains, NY 10604; **Phone:** 914-682-6542; **Board Cert:** Urology 2004; **Med School:** Tulane Univ 1994; **Resid:** Urology, Natl Naval Med Ctr 2001

Boczko, Judd MD (U) - **Spec Exp:** Prostate Cancer/Robotic Surgery; Robotic Urologic Surgery; **Hospital:** White Plains Hosp Ctr, Greenwich Hosp (page 862); **Address:** 210 Westchester Ave, White Plains, NY 10604; **Phone:** 914-682-6470; **Board Cert:** Urology 2008; **Med School:** Albert Einstein Coll Med 1999; **Resid:** Surgery, Montefiore Med Ctr 2001; Urology, Montefiore Med Ctr 2005; **Fellow:** Urologic Surgery, Strong Meml Hosp 2006; **Fac Appt:** Asst Prof U, NY Med Coll

Choudhury, Muhammad MD (U) - **Spec Exp:** Prostate Cancer; Bladder Cancer; Kidney Cancer; Testicular Cancer; **Hospital:** Westchester Med Ctr, Sound Shore Med Ctr - Westchester; **Address:** 19 Bradhurst Ave, Ste 1900, Hawthorne, NY 10532-2144; **Phone:** 914-347-1900; **Board Cert:** Urology 1982; **Med School:** Bangladesh 1972; **Resid:** Urology, Columbia-Presby Med Ctr 1978; Urology, NY Med Coll 1980; **Fellow:** Urologic Oncology, Roswell Park Cancer Inst 1981; **Fac Appt:** Prof U, NY Med Coll

Eshghi, A Majid MD (U) - **Spec Exp:** Kidney Stones; Laparoscopic Surgery; **Hospital:** Westchester Med Ctr; **Address:** 19 Bradhurst Ave, Ste 1900, Hawthorne, NY 10532; **Phone:** 914-347-1900; **Board Cert:** Urology 2005; **Med School:** Iran 1976; **Resid:** Surgery, St Barnabas Med Ctr 1981; Urology, Ll Jewish Med Ctr 1985; **Fac Appt:** Prof U, NY Med Coll

Glassman, Charles N MD (U) - **Spec Exp:** Prostate Cancer; Incontinence; Pediatric Urology; Sexual Dysfunction; **Hospital:** White Plains Hosp Ctr; **Address:** 170 Maple Ave, Ste 104, White Plains, NY 10601-4707; **Phone:** 914-949-7556; **Board Cert:** Urology 1980; **Med School:** Tufts Univ 1973; **Resid:** Surgery, UCSF Med Ctr 1975; Urology, UCSF Med Ctr 1978; **Fellow:** Pediatric Urology, Mayo Clinic 1979

Housman, Arno D MD (U) - **Spec Exp:** Kidney Stones; Prostate Cancer; Incontinence; **Hospital:** Phelps Meml Hosp Ctr (page 592); **Address:** 325 S Highland Ave, Briarcliff Manor, NY 10510-2093; **Phone:** 914-941-0617; **Board Cert:** Urology 1999; **Med School:** SUNY Downstate 1980; **Resid:** Surgery, SUNY-Kings Co Hosp Ctr 1983; Urology, Yale-New Haven Hosp 1986

Lerner, Seth E MD (U) - **Spec Exp:** Prostate Cancer/Robotic Surgery; Robotic Urologic Surgery; **Hospital:** White Plains Hosp Ctr; **Address:** 170 Maple Ave, Ste 104, White Plains, NY 10601; **Phone:** 914-949-7556; **Board Cert:** Urology 2005; **Med School:** SUNY Downstate 1988; **Resid:** Surgery, Montefiore-Weiler Einstein Div 1990; Urology, Montefiore-Weler Einstein Div 1994; **Fellow:** Urologic Oncology, Mayo Clinic 1995; **Fac Appt:** Asst Prof U, Albert Einstein Coll Med

Matthews, Gerald J MD (U) - **Spec Exp:** Infertility-Male; Impotence; **Hospital:** Westchester Med Ctr, Montefiore Med Ctr - Div. North (page 100); **Address:** 19 Bradhurst Ave, Ste 1900, Hawthorne, NY 10532-2144; **Phone:** 914-347-1900; **Board Cert:** Urology 2006; **Med School:** NY Med Coll 1986; **Resid:** Urology, Lenox Hill Hosp 1993; Surgery, St Francis Hosp Med Ctr 1989; **Fellow:** Urology, NY Hosp-Cornell Med Ctr 1995; Urology, Rockefeller Univ Hosp 1995; **Fac Appt:** Assoc Prof U, NY Med Coll

Owens, George F MD (U) - **Spec Exp:** Prostate Disease; Erectile Dysfunction; Incontinence; Minimally Invasive Surgery; **Hospital:** White Plains Hosp Ctr, Westchester Med Ctr; **Address:** 311 North St, Ste 201, White Plains, NY 10605-2232; **Phone:** 914-946-1406; **Board Cert:** Urology 2005; **Med School:** NY Med Coll 1979; **Resid:** Surgery, Montefiore Hosp Med Ctr 1981; Urology, Montefiore Hosp Med Ctr 1984; **Fellow:** Urology, NY Med Coll 1985; **Fac Appt:** Assoc Clin Prof U, NY Med Coll

Putignano, Joseph D MD (U) - **Spec Exp:** Bladder Surgery; Laser Surgery; Kidney Stones; Prostate Surgery; **Hospital:** Lawrence Hosp Ctr, Westchester Med Ctr; **Address:** 26 Pondfield Rd W, Bronxville, NY 10708; **Phone:** 914-793-1200; **Board Cert:** Urology 1975; **Med School:** Canada 1965; **Resid:** Urology, St Lukes-Roosevelt Hosp Ctr 1971; **Fac Appt:** Assoc Prof U, NY Med Coll

Reda, Edward F MD (U) - **Spec Exp:** Pediatric Urology; **Hospital:** Westchester Med Ctr; **Address:** Pediatric Urology Assocs, 150 White Plains Rd, Ste 306, Tarrytown, NY 10591; **Phone:** 914-493-8628; **Board Cert:** Urology 1984; **Med School:** Mexico 1976; **Resid:** Surgery, Bronx Lebanon Hosp 1979; Urology, Montefiore Med Ctr 1982; **Fellow:** Pediatric Urology, Chldns Hosp 1984; **Fac Appt:** Assoc Prof U, NY Med Coll

Riechers, Roger MD (U) - **Spec Exp:** Incontinence-Female; Prostate Cancer; **Hospital:** Northern Westchester Hosp; **Address:** 110 S Bedford Rd Fl 3, Mt Kisco, NY 10549; **Phone:** 914-242-1520; **Board Cert:** Urology 1976; **Med School:** NYU Sch Med 1968; **Resid:** Urology, Mount Sinai Med Ctr 1973

Roberts, Larry P MD (U) - **Spec Exp:** Infertility-Male; Erectile Dysfunction; Incontinence; **Hospital:** Sound Shore Med Ctr - Westchester, Lawrence Hosp Ctr; **Address:** 175 Memorial Hwy, Ste 3-2, New Rochelle, NY 10801-5641; **Phone:** 914-235-2929; **Board Cert:** Urology 1981; **Med School:** Univ Miami Sch Med 1974; **Resid:** Surgery, Univ Miami Hosps 1976; Urology, Montefiore Hosp 1979; **Fac Appt:** Asst Clin Prof U, Albert Einstein Coll Med

Schrager, Alan MD (U) - **Spec Exp:** Prostate Disease; Urology-Female; Urologic Cancer; Voiding Dysfunction; **Hospital:** Greenwich Hosp (page 862), Sound Shore Med Ctr - Westchester; **Address:** 1600 Harrison Ave, Ste G102, Mamaroneck, NY 10543-3124; **Phone:** 914-698-8106; **Board Cert:** Urology 1975; **Med School:** Ros Franklin Univ/Chicago Med Sch 1966; **Resid:** Surgery, Maimonides Med Ctr 1970; Urology, SUNY Downstate Med Ctr 1973

Siegel, Judy F MD (U) - **Spec Exp:** Voiding Dysfunction-Female; Voiding Dysfunction-Pediatric; **Hospital:** St John's Riverside Hosp, Phelps Meml Hosp Ctr (page 592); **Address:** 623 Warburton Ave, Hastings-on-Hudson, NY 10706; **Phone:** 914-478-3001; **Board Cert:** Urology 2009; **Med School:** Univ VT Coll Med 1988; **Resid:** Surgery, LI Jewish Med Ctr 1990; Urology, LI Jewish Med Ctr 1994; **Fellow:** Pediatric Urology, Schneider Chldns Hosp 1996

Vascular Surgery

Babu, Sateesh C MD (VascS) - **Spec Exp:** Carotid Artery Surgery; Aneurysm-Abdominal Aortic; Lower Limb Arterial Disease; Vein Disorders; **Hospital:** Westchester Med Ctr, Northern Westchester Hosp; **Address:** 19 Bradhurst Ave, Medical Arts Atrium/Westchester Med Ctr, Hawthorne, NY 10532-2140; **Phone:** 914-593-1200; **Board Cert:** Vascular Surgery 2001; **Med School:** India 1969; **Resid:** Surgery, Jewish Memorial Hosp 1972; Surgery, Metropolitan Hosp 1975; **Fellow:** Vascular Surgery, Metropolitan Hosp 1977; **Fac Appt:** Prof S, NY Med Coll

Karanfilian, Richard MD (VascS) - **Spec Exp:** Varicose Veins; Carotid Artery Surgery; Endovascular Surgery; **Hospital:** Sound Shore Med Ctr - Westchester; **Address:** 150 Lockwood Ave, Ste 14, New Rochelle, NY 10801-4912; **Phone:** 914-636-1700; **Board Cert:** Surgery 2002; Vascular Surgery 2006; **Med School:** Italy 1977; **Resid:** Surgery, UMDNJ-NJ Med Sch 1983; **Fellow:** Vascular Surgery, UMDNJ-NJ Med Sch 1985; **Fac Appt:** Assoc Clin Prof S, NY Med Coll

Schwartz, Kenneth S MD (VascS) - **Spec Exp:** Arterial Disease; Vein Disorders; Dialysis Access Surgery; **Hospital:** White Plains Hosp Ctr, Greenwich Hosp (page 862); **Address:** 1 Theall Rd, Rye, NY 10580; **Phone:** 914-723-7737; **Board Cert:** Surgery 2001; **Med School:** Albert Einstein Coll Med 1977; **Resid:** Surgery, Montefiore Hosp Med Ctr 1981; **Fellow:** Peripheral Vascular Surgery, USC Med Ctr 1982; **Fac Appt:** Asst Clin Prof S, NY Med Coll

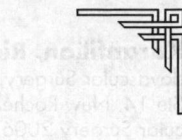

The Best in American Medicine
www.CastleConnolly.com

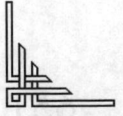
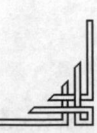

The State of New Jersey

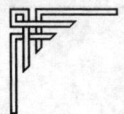

The Best in American Medicine
www.CastleConnolly.com

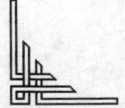
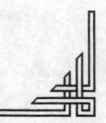

Bergen

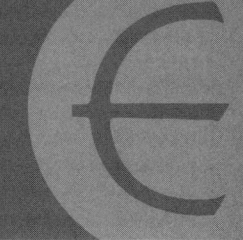

ENGLEWOOD
HOSPITAL AND MEDICAL CENTER℠
AN AFFILIATE OF MOUNT SINAI SCHOOL OF MEDICINE

350 Engle Street, Englewood, New Jersey 07631
Physician Referral: 1.866.980.EHMC
www.englewoodhospital.com

Sponsorship: Voluntary, Not-for-profit
Beds: 520
Accreditation: The Joint Commission

GENERAL OVERVIEW

Englewood Hospital and Medical Center provides patients with the highest level of compassionate care through a broad range of state-of-the-art clinical programs and the most advanced treatments and diagnostic services. Through our affiliation with the Mount Sinai School of Medicine, residents in surgery, pediatrics and pathology, as well as critical care medicine fellows, rotate through our Medical Center. We also maintain a freestanding internal medicine residency program, and offer advanced surgical training through the Herbert Dardik Vascular Fellowship Program.

SELECT NATIONAL PERFORMANCE RECOGNITION

HealthGrades® Maternity Care Excellence Award™: 2009-2011

HealthGrades® 5-star rating: Maternity Care, Coronary Bypass Surgery, Treatment of Heart Attack, Treatment of Pneumonia, and GI Procedures and Surgeries

J.D. Power and Associates Distinguished Hospital Program℠: recognized Englewood Hospital as a provider of "An Outstanding Maternity Experience," "An Outstanding Emergency Experience," "An Outstanding Cardiovascular Experience"

American Nurses Credentialing Center: Magnet Recognition Program® Award Status

American Society for Metabolic and Bariatric Surgery: Bariatric Surgery Center of Excellence®

The Joint Commission: *Accreditation*: Hospital, Home Health and Hospice Care; *Advanced Certification*: Primary Stroke Center; *Certified Programs*: Joint Replacement (Hip & Knee)

SPECIAL PROGRAMS AND SERVICES

World-Class Emergency Care Center: Highlights of our 35,000-square-foot Emergency Care Center include 40 private treatment rooms; fast-track triage and treatment; specialized treatment rooms for pediatric, behavioral health and trauma patients; and a dedicated 24/7 imaging suite.

The Institute for Patient Blood Management and Bloodless Medicine and Surgery: Now in its 15th year, The Institute is a national and international research, education and referral center and a world-recognized leader in patient blood management. At Englewood Hospital, 95% of all elective surgeries are performed transfusion-free. (See Center of Excellence listing under "Surgery.")

The Leslie Simon Breast Care and Cytodiagnosis Center: Our Breast Care Center offers rapid, highly accurate and frequently conclusive diagnoses, usually without surgery. It is one of the only all-digital mammography centers in New Jersey, and is home to an Aurora Dedicated Breast MRI System – the only FDA-cleared MRI system designed specifically for breast imaging. The Center was recently awarded Center of Excellence designation from the American College of Radiology (ACR) and the National Accreditation Program for Breast Centers. (See Center of Excellence listing under "Cancer Care.")

Heart and Vascular Institute of New Jersey: Celebrating a Decade of Cardiac Excellence, our Heart and Vascular Institute offers patients access to world-renowned experts in all areas of heart and cardiovascular care, including cardiac surgery, interventional cardiology, cardiac electrophysiology, and vascular surgery. The New Jersey Department of Health and Senior Services has recognized Englewood Hospital as one of the top New Jersey hospitals for isolated coronary bypass surgery since the program's inception. (See Center of Excellence listing under "Cardiovascular Disease.")

The Orthopedic and Neurosurgical Institute: The Institute brings together a multidisciplinary team of medical professionals who are at the forefront of minimally invasive orthopedic and spine surgeries. Our Knee and Hip Replacement programs have received Disease-Specific Care Certification from The Joint Commission. (See Center of Excellence listing under "Orthopaedic Surgery.")

Radiology and Imaging: Committed to providing the most advanced and comprehensive services, we offer three Spiral CT Scanners, one 64-slice multi-detector CT, three 1.5 Tesla high-field MRI machines, breast MRI, and 4-D ultrasound imaging in our Antepartum Testing Unit. We also offer the latest generation combination PET/CT scanner for the most advanced diagnostic imaging in cancer care.

Referral: For a referral to one of our physicians, call 1.866.980.EHMC

THE VALLEY HOSPITAL

223 North Van Dien Avenue, Ridgewood, NJ 07450
Phone: 201-447-8000 • www.valleyhealth.com

Sponsorship: Voluntary Not-for-Profit   **Beds:** 451 Acute Care Beds
Accredited by The Joint Commission

■ PROFILE

The Valley Hospital is affiliated with the NewYork-Presbyterian Healthcare System. Valley has been recognized seven consecutive times under the J.D. Power and Associates Distinguished Hospital Program and is a two-time recipient of the Magnet Award for Nursing Excellence. Valley is the second busiest hospital in New Jersey based on admissions.

Valley has been recognized for clinical excellence in cardiology, neuroscience and stroke, obstetrics, oncology, orthopedics, and spine surgery.

Valley has earned an impressive 10 Disease-Specific Care Certifications for healthcare quality from the Joint Commission: acute myocardial infarction, heart failure, knee replacement, hip replacement, stroke, colorectal cancer, lung cancer, breast cancer, pancreatic cancer, and prostate cancer.

Valley also prides itself on service excellence and consistently scores above the state and national average on measures of patient satisfaction, including whether patients would recommend the hospital to their friends and family.

■ MEDICAL STAFF

The Valley Hospital has more than 1,000 physicians on its Active Medical Staff, 93 percent of whom are board certified.

■ CARDIOLOGY

In partnership with the NewYork-Presbyterian Healthcare System, The Valley Columbia Heart Center is a leader in the field of cardiology services, including cardiac surgery; coronary angioplasty and other interventional procedures; electrophysiology studies; and cardiac care research. Valley's cardiac surgery program consistently receives a 3-star rating—the highest designation of quality and clinical excellence—from The Society of Thoracic Surgeons, and was recognized by Consumer Reports as one of the top 50 cardiac surgery groups in the nation. The newly established Heart & Vascular Institute combines the expertise of more than 60 board-certified cardiologists and surgeons to provide the highest-quality cardiovascular care.

■ ONCOLOGY

Valley is known for its centers specializing in the diagnosis, care, and treatment of prostate and lung cancer, as well as its surgical oncology gynecologic oncology programs, its comprehensive oncology clinical trials program, and its Department of Radiation Oncology, including Tomotherapy.

■ OBSTETRICS

The hospital is well-known for its maternity services including Maternal-Fetal Medicine, an enhanced Neonatal Intensive Care Unit, a maternal and child health home care program, as well as The Kireker Center for Child Development that offers a full spectrum of services.

■ SURGERY

The Valley Hospital is also known for its comprehensive surgical program, including pioneering advances in surgical oncology, gynecologic oncology, thoracic surgery, and its Center for Minimally Invasive and Robotic Surgery. The hospital has also been designated as a Bariatric Surgery Center of Excellence.

Allergy & Immunology

Falk, Theodore MD (A&I) - **Spec Exp:** Asthma; Immune Deficiency; Chronic Fatigue Syndrome; **Hospital:** Holy Name Med Ctr (page 657), Englewood Hosp & Med Ctr (page 656); **Address:** 63 Grand Ave, Ste 100, River Edge, NJ 07661-1930; **Phone:** 201-487-2900; **Board Cert:** Pediatrics 1982; **Med School:** Belgium 1977; **Resid:** Pediatrics, Long Island Jewish Med Ctr 1980; **Fellow:** Allergy & Immunology, Nassau Co Med Ctr 1982

Goodstein, Carolyn E MD (A&I) - **Spec Exp:** Asthma; Rhinitis; Urticaria; Sinusitis; **Hospital:** Englewood Hosp & Med Ctr (page 656), Hackensack Univ Med Ctr (page 96); **Address:** 180 N Dean St, Englewood, NJ 07631-2534; **Phone:** 201-871-4755; **Board Cert:** Internal Medicine 1974; Allergy & Immunology 1980; **Med School:** SUNY Downstate 1964; **Resid:** Internal Medicine, Montefiore Med Ctr 1967; Allergy & Immunology, Roosevelt Hosp 1971

Harish, Ziv MD (A&I) - **Spec Exp:** Asthma & Sinusitis; Hay Fever; Urticaria; Hives; **Hospital:** Englewood Hosp & Med Ctr (page 656), Hackensack Univ Med Ctr (page 96); **Address:** 200 Engle St, Ste 18, Englewood, NJ 07631; **Phone:** 201-871-7475; **Board Cert:** Allergy & Immunology 2001; **Med School:** Israel 1983; **Resid:** Pediatrics, Montefiore Med Ctr 1989; **Fellow:** Allergy & Immunology, Montefiore Med Ctr 1991; **Fac Appt:** Asst Clin Prof Med, Albert Einstein Coll Med

Michelis, Mary Ann MD (A&I) - **Spec Exp:** Asthma; Immune Deficiency; **Hospital:** Hackensack Univ Med Ctr (page 96); **Address:** Hackensack Univ Medical Ctr, 30 Prospect Ave, rm 3674, Hackensack, NJ 07601-1915; **Phone:** 201-996-2065; **Board Cert:** Internal Medicine 1978; Allergy & Immunology 1981; **Med School:** Univ Pittsburgh 1975; **Resid:** Internal Medicine, Lenox Hill Hosp 1978; **Fellow:** Allergy & Immunology, NY Hosp-Cornell Med Ctr 1978; **Fac Appt:** Assoc Clin Prof Med, UMDNJ-NJ Med Sch, Newark

Minikes, Neil I MD (A&I) - **Spec Exp:** Eczema; Food Allergy; Hay Fever; Asthma; **Hospital:** Hackensack Univ Med Ctr (page 96), NY-Presby Hosp/Columbia (page 104); **Address:** Allergy & Asthma Ctr Northern NJ, 500 Piermont Rd, Ste 304, Closter, NJ 07624; **Phone:** 201-564-7777; **Board Cert:** Pediatrics 1986; Allergy & Immunology 2001; **Med School:** Columbia P&S 1980; **Resid:** Pediatrics, Columbia Presby Med Ctr 1983; **Fellow:** Allergy & Immunology, LI Jewish Med Ctr 1990; **Fac Appt:** Asst Clin Prof Ped, Columbia P&S

Cardiovascular Disease

Blood, David K MD (Cv) - **Spec Exp:** Nuclear Cardiology; Transplant Medicine-Heart; **Hospital:** Englewood Hosp & Med Ctr (page 656), NY-Presby Hosp/Columbia (page 104); **Address:** 163 Engle St, 1C Bldg, Englewood, NJ 07631; **Phone:** 201-569-3313; **Board Cert:** Internal Medicine 1972; Cardiovascular Disease 1975; **Med School:** Columbia P&S 1966; **Resid:** Internal Medicine, Bellevue Hosp 1968; Internal Medicine, Harlem Hosp 1972; **Fellow:** Cardiovascular Disease, Columbia-Presby Med Ctr 1974; **Fac Appt:** Assoc Clin Prof Med, Columbia P&S

Conroy Jr, Daniel P MD (Cv) - **Spec Exp:** Non-Invasive Cardiology; Hypertension; Cholesterol/Lipid Disorders; Diabetes & Heart Disease; **Hospital:** St Mary's Hosp - Passaic, Hackensack Univ Med Ctr (page 96); **Address:** 358 Valley Brook Ave, Lyndhurst, NJ 07071; **Phone:** 201-460-0142; **Board Cert:** Internal Medicine 1979; Cardiovascular Disease 1981; **Med School:** Mexico 1975; **Resid:** Internal Medicine, St Michaels Med Ctr 1978; **Fellow:** Cardiovascular Disease, St Michaels Med Ctr 1980

Eisenberg, Sheldon B MD (Cv) - **Spec Exp:** Nuclear Cardiology; Preventive Cardiology; Coronary Artery Disease; **Hospital:** Valley Hosp (page 658), Hackensack Univ Med Ctr (page 96); **Address:** 333 Old Hook Rd, Ste 200, Westwood, NJ 07675-3200; **Phone:** 201-664-0201; **Board Cert:** Internal Medicine 1979; Cardiovascular Disease 1981; **Med School:** Cornell Univ-Weill Med Coll 1976; **Resid:** Internal Medicine, N Shore Univ Hosp 1979; **Fellow:** Cardiovascular Disease, N Shore Univ Hosp 1981

Gardin, Julius M MD (Cv) - **Spec Exp:** Echocardiography; Geriatric Cardiology; Preventive Cardiology; Cholesterol/Lipid Disorders; **Hospital:** Hackensack Univ Med Ctr (page 96); **Address:** Hackensack Univ Med Ctr, Dept Medicine, 30 Prospect Ave, 1 Main, rm 1647, Hackensack, NJ 07601; **Phone:** 201-996-3500; **Board Cert:** Internal Medicine 1975; Cardiovascular Disease 1977; **Med School:** Univ Mich Med Sch 1972; **Resid:** Internal Medicine, Univ Mich Hosp 1975; **Fellow:** Cardiovascular Disease, Georgetown Univ Hosp 1977; **Fac Appt:** Prof Med, UMDNJ-Univ Med Dent NJ

Goldschmidt, Howard Z MD (Cv) - **Spec Exp:** Cardiac Catheterization; Pacemakers; Heart Valve Disease; Atrial Fibrillation; **Hospital:** Valley Hosp (page 658); **Address:** 1200 E Ridgewood Ave, Ridgewood, NJ 07450; **Phone:** 201-670-8660; **Board Cert:** Internal Medicine 1986; Cardiovascular Disease 1989; **Med School:** Columbia P&S 1983; **Resid:** Internal Medicine, Mt Sinai Hosp 1986; **Fellow:** Cardiovascular Disease, Mt Sinai Hosp 1988

Goldweit, Richard S MD (Cv) - **Spec Exp:** Interventional Cardiology; Sleep Disorders/Cardiac Risk; Peripheral Vascular Disease; Cardiac Catheterization; **Hospital:** Englewood Hosp & Med Ctr (page 656); **Address:** 177 N Dean St, Ste 100, Englewood, NJ 07631; **Phone:** 201-569-4901; **Board Cert:** Internal Medicine 1985; Cardiovascular Disease 1987; Interventional Cardiology 2009; **Med School:** Cornell Univ-Weill Med Coll 1982; **Resid:** Internal Medicine, NY Hosp 1985; **Fellow:** Cardiovascular Disease, NY Hosp-Cornell Med Ctr 1987

Haft, Jacob I MD (Cv) - **Spec Exp:** Coronary Artery Disease; Arrhythmias; Heart Failure; **Hospital:** Saint Michael's Med Ctr, Hackensack Univ Med Ctr (page 96); **Address:** 20 Prospect Ave, Ste 719, Hackensack, NJ 07601; **Phone:** 201-343-8505; **Board Cert:** Internal Medicine 1968; Cardiovascular Disease 1973; **Med School:** Columbia P&S 1962; **Resid:** Internal Medicine, Beth Israel Hosp 1964; Internal Medicine, Bellevue-Columbia P&S 1968; **Fellow:** Cardiovascular Disease, Mt Sinai Hosp 1965; Cardiovascular Disease, Peter Bent Brigham Hosp 1969; **Fac Appt:** Prof Med, Seton Hall Univ Sch Hlth & Med Scis

Hodges, David MD (Cv) - **Spec Exp:** Stress Management; **Hospital:** Englewood Hosp & Med Ctr (page 656), NY-Presby Hosp (page 104); **Address:** 12 Palisade Ave, Engelwood, NJ 07666; **Phone:** 201-816-9266; **Board Cert:** Internal Medicine 1987; Cardiovascular Disease 2003; **Med School:** NYU Sch Med 1984; **Resid:** Internal Medicine, Boston Med Ctr 1987; Internal Medicine, Beth Israel Deaconess Med Ctr 1989; **Fellow:** Cardiopulmonary Disease, Brigham & Women's Hosp 1991; **Fac Appt:** Asst Prof Med, Columbia P&S

Landers, David B MD (Cv) - **Spec Exp:** Cardiac Catheterization; Coronary Angioplasty/Stents; Angioplasty; Interventional Cardiology; **Hospital:** Hackensack Univ Med Ctr (page 96), Holy Name Med Ctr (page 657); **Address:** 222 Cedar Ln, Ste 208, Teaneck, NJ 07666-4312; **Phone:** 201-907-0442; **Board Cert:** Internal Medicine 1983; Cardiovascular Disease 1987; Interventional Cardiology 2010; **Med School:** Georgetown Univ 1979; **Resid:** Internal Medicine, St Vincents Hosp 1982; **Fellow:** Cardiovascular Disease, Westchester Co Med Ctr 1985; **Fac Appt:** Asst Clin Prof Med, UMDNJ-NJ Med Sch, Newark

Landzberg, Joel S MD (Cv) - **Spec Exp:** Preventive Cardiology; Coronary Artery Disease; Heart Failure; Heart Valve Disease; **Hospital:** Hackensack Univ Med Ctr (page 96), Valley Hosp (page 658); **Address:** 333 Old Hook Rd, Ste 200, Westwood, NJ 07675-3200; **Phone:** 201-664-0201; **Board Cert:** Internal Medicine 1986; Cardiovascular Disease 1989; Interventional Cardiology 2002; **Med School:** Columbia P&S 1983; **Resid:** Internal Medicine, Vanderbilt Univ Hosp 1986; **Fellow:** Cardiology Research, Moffit Hosp 1987; Cardiovascular Disease, Brigham & Womens Hosp 1991; **Fac Appt:** Assoc Clin Prof Med, UMDNJ-NJ Med Sch, Newark

Lau, Henry MD (Cv) - **Hospital:** Hackensack Univ Med Ctr (page 96); **Address:** 211 Essex St, Ste 403, Hackensack, NJ 07601; **Phone:** 201-646-0044; **Board Cert:** Internal Medicine 1977; Cardiovascular Disease 1981; **Med School:** Taiwan 1973; **Resid:** Internal Medicine, Hackensack Med Ctr 1977; **Fellow:** Cardiovascular Disease, Hackensack Med Ctr 1980

Pumill, Rick MD (Cv) - **Spec Exp:** Coronary Artery Disease; Hypertension; Congestive Heart Failure; **Hospital:** Hackensack Univ Med Ctr (page 96), Meadowlands Hosp Med Ctr; **Address:** 103 River Rd Fl 2, Edgewater, NJ 07020-1002; **Phone:** 201-941-8100; **Board Cert:** Internal Medicine 1988; Cardiovascular Disease 2001; **Med School:** Dominica 1984; **Resid:** Internal Medicine, Jersey City Med Ctr 1988; **Fellow:** Cardiovascular Disease, Jersey City Med Ctr 1990

Reison, Dennis S MD (Cv) - **Spec Exp:** Interventional Cardiology; **Hospital:** Valley Hosp (page 658); **Address:** 1200 E Ridgewood Ave, Ridgewood, NJ 07450; **Phone:** 201-670-8660; **Board Cert:** Internal Medicine 1978; Cardiovascular Disease 1981; Interventional Cardiology 1999; **Med School:** Stanford Univ 1975; **Resid:** Internal Medicine, Columbia Presby Hosp 1978; **Fellow:** Cardiovascular Disease, Mt Sinai Hosp 1979; Cardiovascular Disease, Columbia Presby Hosp 1981; **Fac Appt:** Asst Clin Prof Med, Columbia P&S

Rossakis, Constantine MD (Cv) - **Spec Exp:** Interventional Cardiology; Nuclear Cardiology; **Hospital:** Hackensack Univ Med Ctr (page 96); **Address:** 357 Prospect Ave, Hackensack, NJ 07601-2505; **Phone:** 201-489-3440; **Board Cert:** Internal Medicine 1986; Cardiovascular Disease 1989; Nuclear Cardiology 2009; **Med School:** NYU Sch Med 1983; **Resid:** Internal Medicine, NY Hosp 1986; **Fellow:** Cardiovascular Disease, NY Hosp-Cornell 1989; **Fac Appt:** Asst Clin Prof Med, Cornell Univ-Weill Med Coll

Rothman, Howard C MD (Cv) - **Spec Exp:** Cholesterol/Lipid Disorders; Angina; Women's Health; **Hospital:** Englewood Hosp & Med Ctr (page 656), Holy Name Med Ctr (page 657); **Address:** Advanced Cardiology Inst, 2200 Fletcher Ave, Fort Lee, NJ 07024-5005; **Phone:** 201-461-6200; **Board Cert:** Internal Medicine 1975; Cardiovascular Disease 1979; **Med School:** Univ Cincinnati 1970; **Resid:** Internal Medicine, NY Hosp-Cornell Med Ctr 1975; **Fellow:** Cardiovascular Disease, NY Hosp-Cornell Med Ctr 1976; **Fac Appt:** Asst Clin Prof Med, Columbia P&S

Salerno, William D MD (Cv) - **Hospital:** Hackensack Univ Med Ctr (page 96); **Address:** Heartcare Center, 38 Mayhill St, Saddle Brook, NJ 07663-5307; **Phone:** 201-843-1019; **Board Cert:** Internal Medicine 1987; Cardiovascular Disease 1989; Critical Care Medicine 2001; **Med School:** Mexico 1982; **Resid:** Internal Medicine, Hackensack Med Ctr 1986; Critical Care Medicine, Norwalk Hosp 1987; **Fellow:** Cardiovascular Disease, Hackensack Med Ctr 1989; Interventional Cardiology, Hackensack Med Ctr 1990; **Fac Appt:** Assoc Clin Prof Med, UMDNJ-NJ Med Sch, Newark

Sotsky, Gerald MD (Cv) - **Hospital:** Valley Hosp (page 658); **Address:** 1200 E Ridgewood Ave, Ridgewood, NJ 07450; **Phone:** 201-670-8660; **Board Cert:** Internal Medicine 1984; Cardiovascular Disease 1987; **Med School:** Mount Sinai Sch Med 1981; **Resid:** Internal Medicine, Mt Sinai Med Ctr 1984; **Fellow:** Cardiovascular Disease, Mt Sinai Med Ctr 1986

Teichholz, Louis E MD (Cv) - **Spec Exp:** Mitral Valve Disease; Complementary Medicine; Echocardiography; Cholesterol/Lipid Disorders; **Hospital:** Hackensack Univ Med Ctr (page 96); **Address:** Hackensack Univ Med Ctr, 30 Prospect Ave, Ste 4655, Hackensack, NJ 07601; **Phone:** 201-996-2314; **Board Cert:** Internal Medicine 1972; Cardiovascular Disease 1975; **Med School:** Harvard Med Sch 1966; **Resid:** Internal Medicine, Peter Bent Brigham Hosp 1968; **Fellow:** Cardiovascular Disease, Peter Bent Brigham Hosp 1972; **Fac Appt:** Prof Med, UMDNJ-NJ Med Sch, Newark

Child & Adolescent Psychiatry

Kotler, Lisa A MD (ChAP) - **Spec Exp:** Eating Disorders; ADD/ADHD; Depression; Anxiety Disorders; **Hospital:** NYU Langone Med Ctr (page 106); **Address:** NYU Child Study Ctr-Hackensack, 411 Hackensack Ave Fl 7, Hackensack, NJ 07601; **Phone:** 201-465-8111; **Board Cert:** Psychiatry 2008; Child & Adolescent Psychiatry 2009; **Med School:** Yale Univ 1993; **Resid:** Psychiatry, Mt Sinai Med Ctr 1996; **Fellow:** Child & Adolescent Psychiatry, Columbia-Presby Med Ctr 1998; Eating Disorders Research, NY State Psyc Inst-Columbia Presby MC 1999; **Fac Appt:** Asst Prof Psyc

Pincus, Emile I MD (ChAP) - **Spec Exp:** Substance Abuse; Suicide; **Hospital:** St Clare's Hosp - Denville; **Address:** 912 Kinderkamack Rd Fl 2, River Edge, NJ 07661; **Phone:** 201-615-1352; **Board Cert:** Psychiatry 1986; Child & Adolescent Psychiatry 2004; **Med School:** Mount Sinai Sch Med 1978; **Resid:** Psychiatry, St Lukes Hosp Ctr 1979; Psychiatry, Mt Sinai Med Ctr 1982; **Fellow:** Child & Adolescent Psychiatry, New York Hosp-Cornell Med Ctr 1984

Clinical Genetics

Wallerstein, Robert MD (CG) - **Spec Exp:** Connective Tissue Disorders; Chromosome Disorders; **Hospital:** Hackensack Univ Med Ctr (page 96); **Address:** Hackensack Univ Med Ctr, 30 Prospect Ave, Ste 258, Hackensack, NJ 07601; **Phone:** 201-996-5264; **Board Cert:** Pediatrics 2009; Clinical Genetics 2010; Clinical Cytogenetics 2010; **Med School:** UMDNJ-RW Johnson Med Sch 1991; **Resid:** Pediatrics, RW Johnson Med Sch 1994; **Fellow:** Clinical Genetics, Jefferson Med Coll 1996; **Fac Appt:** Assoc Prof Ped, UMDNJ-NJ Med Sch, Newark

Colon & Rectal Surgery

Helbraun, Mark E MD (CRS) - **Spec Exp:** Colonoscopy; Rectal Cancer; **Hospital:** Hackensack Univ Med Ctr (page 96); **Address:** 20 Prospect Ave, Ste 811, Hackensack, NJ 07601; **Phone:** 201-525-1660; **Board Cert:** Colon & Rectal Surgery 1978; **Med School:** Wayne State Univ 1972; **Resid:** Surgery, New York Hosp-Cornell 1977; **Fellow:** Colon & Rectal Surgery, Lahey Clinic 1978

Nizin, Joel MD (CRS) - **Spec Exp:** Colon Cancer; Inflammatory Bowel Disease; **Hospital:** Valley Hosp (page 658), Chilton Meml Hosp; **Address:** 414 Saddle River Rd, Fair Lawn, NJ 07410-5632; **Phone:** 201-689-9100; **Board Cert:** Colon & Rectal Surgery 1987; Surgery 2008; **Med School:** Howard Univ 1978; **Resid:** Surgery, St Luke's Hosp 1983; **Fellow:** Colon & Rectal Surgery, Univ Minn Med Ctr 1984

Waxenbaum, Steven MD (CRS) - **Spec Exp:** Laparoscopic Surgery; Hemorrhoids; Colon Cancer; **Hospital:** Valley Hosp (page 658), Englewood Hosp & Med Ctr (page 656); **Address:** 216 Engle St, Englewood, NJ 07631; **Phone:** 201-567-7615; **Board Cert:** Surgery 2003; Colon & Rectal Surgery 2006; **Med School:** UMDNJ-RW Johnson Med Sch 1988; **Resid:** Surgery, Westchester Med Ctr 1993; **Fellow:** Colon & Rectal Surgery, Lehigh Valley Hosp 1994

White, Ronald A MD (CRS) - **Spec Exp:** Hemorrhoids; Colon & Rectal Cancer; Colonoscopy; **Hospital:** Englewood Hosp & Med Ctr (page 656), Valley Hosp (page 658); **Address:** 216 Engle St, Ste 203, Englewood, NJ 07631-2428; **Phone:** 201-567-7615; **Board Cert:** Colon & Rectal Surgery 1988; **Med School:** Boston Univ 1981; **Resid:** Surgery, Montefiore Hosp 1986; **Fellow:** Colon & Rectal Surgery, RW Johnson Med Sch 1987

Critical Care Medicine

Cornell, James S MD/PhD (CCM) - **Spec Exp:** Respiratory Distress Syndrome; Lung Cancer; Chronic Obstructive Lung Disease (COPD); **Hospital:** Valley Hosp (page 658); **Address:** 31-00 Broadway, Fair Lawn, NJ 07410-2305; **Phone:** 201-796-2255; **Board Cert:** Internal Medicine 2002; Pulmonary Disease 1999; **Med School:** Cornell Univ-Weill Med Coll 1988; **Resid:** Internal Medicine, New York Hosp-Cornell 1991; Pulmonary Disease, Meml Sloan Kettering Cancer Ctr 1991; **Fellow:** Pulmonary Critical Care Medicine, New York Hosp-Cornell 1994

Dermatology

Ashinoff, Robin MD (D) - **Spec Exp:** Mohs' Surgery; Laser Surgery; Cosmetic Dermatology; Melanoma; **Hospital:** Hackensack Univ Med Ctr (page 96), NYU Langone Med Ctr (page 106); **Address:** 360 Essex St, Ste 201, Hackensack, NJ 07601; **Phone:** 201-336-8660; **Board Cert:** Dermatology 1989; **Med School:** NYU Sch Med 1985; **Resid:** Dermatology, NYU Med Ctr 1989; **Fellow:** Mohs Surgery, NYU Med Ctr 1991; Laser Surgery, NYU Med Ctr 1991; **Fac Appt:** Assoc Clin Prof D, NYU Sch Med

Brauner, Gary J MD (D) - **Spec Exp:** Skin Laser Surgery; Black/Asian Skin Care; Cosmetic Dermatology; Hair Removal-Laser; **Hospital:** Englewood Hosp & Med Ctr (page 656), Mount Sinai Med Ctr (page 102); **Address:** 1625 Anderson Ave, Fort Lee, NJ 07024; **Phone:** 201-461-5522; **Board Cert:** Dermatology 1972; Dermatopathology 1978; **Med School:** Harvard Med Sch 1967; **Resid:** Dermatology, Jewish Hosp 1968; Dermatology, Mass Genl Hosp 1971; **Fac Appt:** Assoc Clin Prof D, Mount Sinai Sch Med

Corey, Timothy MD (D) - **Spec Exp:** Psoriasis; Skin Cancer; **Hospital:** Valley Hosp (page 658), NY-Presby Hosp/Columbia (page 104); **Address:** 400 Rt 17 S, Ridgewood, NJ 07450; **Phone:** 201-652-4536; **Board Cert:** Dermatology 1979; **Med School:** Columbia P&S 1975; **Resid:** Dermatology, Columbia Presby Med Ctr 1979; **Fac Appt:** Asst Clin Prof D, Columbia P&S

Fishman, Miriam MD (D) - **Spec Exp:** Pediatric Dermatology; Skin Cancer; **Hospital:** Englewood Hosp & Med Ctr (page 656); **Address:** 216 Engle St, Ste 104, Englewood, NJ 07631-2428; **Phone:** 201-569-5678; **Board Cert:** Dermatology 1984; **Med School:** NYU Sch Med 1978; **Resid:** Pediatrics, Montefiore Med Ctr 1981; Dermatology, Montefiore Med Ctr 1984

Fried, Sharon MD (D) - **Spec Exp:** Skin Cancer; Acne; Psoriasis; **Hospital:** Englewood Hosp & Med Ctr (page 656); **Address:** 180 N Dean St, Englewood, NJ 07631-2534; **Phone:** 201-569-9800; **Board Cert:** Internal Medicine 1983; Dermatology 2009; **Med School:** NYU Sch Med 1980; **Resid:** Internal Medicine, NYU Med Ctr 1983; Dermatology, SUNY Downstate HSC 1985

Giardina-Beckett, MarieAnne MD (D) - **Spec Exp:** Acne; Botox Therapy; **Hospital:** Meadowlands Hosp Med Ctr, St Mary's Hosp - Passaic; **Address:** 71 Union Ave, Rutherford, NJ 07070; **Phone:** 201-804-8900; **Board Cert:** Dermatology 2009; **Med School:** NY Med Coll 1986; **Resid:** Dermatology, New York Med Coll 1990

Grodberg, Michele MD (D) - **Spec Exp:** Cosmetic Dermatology; Hair Removal-Laser; Botox Therapy; Facial Rejuvenation; **Hospital:** Englewood Hosp & Med Ctr (page 656); **Address:** 106 Grand Ave Fl 3, Englewood, NJ 07631-3574; **Phone:** 201-567-8884; **Board Cert:** Dermatology 2009; **Med School:** NYU Sch Med 1987; **Resid:** Dermatology, NYU Med Ctr 1991

Heldman, Jay MD (D) - **Spec Exp:** Dermatologic Surgery; **Hospital:** Valley Hosp (page 658); **Address:** 2300 Route 208 S, Fair Lawn, NJ 07410-1559; **Phone:** 201-797-7770; **Board Cert:** Dermatology 1981; **Med School:** Columbia P&S 1977; **Resid:** Internal Medicine, Columbia-Presby Med Ctr 1978; Dermatology, Mt Sinai Med Ctr 1981

Morman, Manuel R MD/PhD (D) - **Spec Exp:** Mohs' Surgery; Skin Cancer; Reconstructive Surgery; **Hospital:** St Mary's Hosp - Passaic; **Address:** 47 Orient Way, Rutherford, NJ 07070-2040; **Phone:** 201-460-0280; **Board Cert:** Dermatology 2009; **Med School:** Jefferson Med Coll 1976; **Resid:** Dermatology, Hosp U Penn 1979; **Fellow:** Chemosurgery, Cleveland Clinic 1980

Possick, Paul MD (D) - **Spec Exp:** Skin Cancer; Contact Dermatitis; Eczema; Psoriasis; **Address:** 390 Old Hook Rd Fl 2, Westwood, NJ 07675-2616; **Phone:** 201-666-9550; **Board Cert:** Dermatology 1969; **Med School:** Tufts Univ 1964; **Resid:** Internal Medicine, Montefiore Hosp 1966; Dermatology, Univ Hosp 1968; **Fac Appt:** Asst Prof D, NYU Sch Med

Rapaport, Jeffrey A MD (D) - **Spec Exp:** Cosmetic Dermatology; Scar Revision; Laser Surgery; Skin Laser Surgery; **Hospital:** Holy Name Med Ctr (page 657), Englewood Hosp & Med Ctr (page 656); **Address:** 333 Sylvan Ave Fl 2nd - Ste 207, Englewood Cliffs, NJ 07632; **Phone:** 201-227-1555; **Board Cert:** Dermatology 1983; **Med School:** Emory Univ 1979; **Resid:** Dermatology, Jefferson Univ Hosp 1982

Scherl, Sharon MD (D) - **Spec Exp:** Acne; Cosmetic Dermatology; Photodynamic Therapy; Tattoo Removal; **Hospital:** Englewood Hosp & Med Ctr (page 656); **Address:** 45 Central Ave, Tenafly, NJ 07670; **Phone:** 201-568-8400; **Board Cert:** Dermatology 1999; **Med School:** NY Med Coll 1988; **Resid:** Dermatology, Metropolitan Hosp Ctr 1992

Sweeney, Eugene MD (D) - **Spec Exp:** Skin Cancer; Pediatric Dermatology; Acne; **Hospital:** Holy Name Med Ctr (page 657), Englewood Hosp & Med Ctr (page 656); **Address:** 757 Teaneck Rd, Teaneck, NJ 07666-4241; **Phone:** 201-837-3939; **Board Cert:** Dermatology 1967; **Med School:** NY Med Coll 1960; **Resid:** Dermatology, Columbia-Presby Med Ctr 1966; **Fac Appt:** Assoc Prof D, Columbia P&S

Weiss, Darryl S MD (D) - **Spec Exp:** Hair Restoration/Transplant; Cosmetic Dermatology; Skin Laser Surgery; **Hospital:** Valley Hosp (page 658); **Address:** 23-00 Route 208 South, Fairlawn, NJ 07410; **Phone:** 201-797-7770; **Board Cert:** Dermatology 1990; **Med School:** Med Coll VA 1986; **Resid:** Dermatology, Jackson Meml Hosp 1990

Diagnostic Radiology

Budin, Joel A MD (DR) - **Spec Exp:** Neuroradiology; **Hospital:** Hackensack Univ Med Ctr (page 96); **Address:** 30 S Newman St, Hackensack, NJ 07601; **Phone:** 201-488-1188; **Board Cert:** Diagnostic Radiology 1975; **Med School:** Columbia P&S 1969; **Resid:** Diagnostic Radiology, Columbia-Presby Med Ctr 1975

Calem-Grunat, Jaclyn A MD (DR) - **Spec Exp:** Breast Imaging; Ultrasound; **Hospital:** Valley Hosp (page 658); **Address:** Radiology Assocs of Ridgewood, 20 Franklin Tpke, Waldwick, NJ 07463; **Phone:** 201-445-8822; **Board Cert:** Diagnostic Radiology 1994; **Med School:** Mount Sinai Sch Med 1988; **Resid:** Internal Medicine, Beeth Israel Med Ctr 1990; Diagnostic Radiology, Harbor-UCLA Med Ctr 1994; **Fellow:** Breast Imaging, UCLA Med Ctr 1995

Goldfischer, Mindy A MD (DR) - **Spec Exp:** Breast Imaging; Ultrasound; **Hospital:** Englewood Hosp & Med Ctr (page 656); **Address:** 350 Engle St, Leslie Simon Cytodiag & Breast Care Ctr, Englewood, NJ 07631; **Phone:** 201-894-3530; **Board Cert:** Diagnostic Radiology 1986; **Med School:** NYU Sch Med 1982; **Resid:** Diagnostic Radiology, Montefiore Med Ctr 1986; **Fellow:** Diagnostic Radiology, Thomas Jefferson Univ Hosp 1987

Gross, Joshua MD (DR) - **Spec Exp:** Breast Imaging; Breast Cancer; **Hospital:** Holy Name Med Ctr (page 657); **Address:** Holy Name Hosp, Breast Imaging, 718 Teaneck Rd, Teaneck, NJ 07666; **Phone:** 201-833-7100; **Board Cert:** Diagnostic Radiology 1984; **Med School:** Albert Einstein Coll Med 1980; **Resid:** Diagnostic Radiology, Einstein/Jacobi Hosp 1984

Krinsky, Glenn MD (DR) - **Spec Exp:** MRI; Musculoskeletal Imaging; Gastrointestinal Imaging; **Hospital:** Valley Hosp (page 658); **Address:** Radiology Assocs of Ridgewood, 20 Franklin Tpke, Waldwick, NJ 07463; **Phone:** 201-445-8822; **Board Cert:** Diagnostic Radiology 1994; **Med School:** NYU Sch Med 1988; **Resid:** Surgical Pathology, Bellevue Hosp 1990; Diagnostic Radiology, Bellevue Hosp 1993; **Fellow:** Magnetic Resonance Imaging, NYU/Bellevue Hosp 1994

Levy, Lauren S MD (DR) - **Spec Exp:** Mammography; Breast MRI; Breast Imaging; **Hospital:** Valley Hosp (page 658); **Address:** Radiology Assocs of Ridgewood, 20 Franklin Tpke, Waldwick, NJ 07463; **Phone:** 201-445-8822; **Board Cert:** Diagnostic Radiology 1996; **Med School:** SUNY Downstate 1991; **Resid:** Diagnostic Radiology, NYU-Bellevue Hosp 1996; **Fellow:** Mammography, NYU-Bellevue Hosp 1997

Liebling, Melissa S MD (DR) - **Spec Exp:** Pediatric Radiology; **Hospital:** Hackensack Univ Med Ctr (page 96); **Address:** Hackensack Radiology Group, 30 Prospect Ave, Hackensack, NJ 07601; **Phone:** 201-996-2254; **Board Cert:** Diagnostic Radiology 1992; Pediatric Radiology 2006; **Med School:** Albany Med Coll 1987; **Resid:** Diagnostic Radiology, Columbia-Presby Med Ctr 1992; **Fellow:** Pediatric Radiology, Columbia-Presby/Babies Hosp 1994

Lubat, Edward MD (DR) - **Spec Exp:** Abdominal Imaging; Thoracic Radiology; Musculoskeletal Imaging; Nuclear Medicine; **Hospital:** Valley Hosp (page 658); **Address:** 20 Franklin Tpke, Waldwick, NJ 07463-1749; **Phone:** 201-445-8822; **Board Cert:** Diagnostic Radiology 1989; Nuclear Medicine 1989; **Med School:** Jefferson Med Coll 1982; **Resid:** Diagnostic Radiology, NYU Med Ctr 1988; **Fellow:** Nuclear Medicine, NYU Med Ctr 1985

Rambler, Louis MD (DR) - **Spec Exp:** Ultrasound; **Hospital:** Valley Hosp (page 658); **Address:** Radiology Assocs of Ridgewood, 20 Franklin Tpke, Waldwick, NJ 07463-1749; **Phone:** 201-445-8822; **Board Cert:** Diagnostic Radiology 1977; **Med School:** Cornell Univ-Weill Med Coll 1971; **Resid:** Diagnostic Radiology, Columbia-Presby Med Ctr 1977

Sorabella, Philip MD (DR) - **Spec Exp:** Nuclear Medicine; Breast Imaging; **Hospital:** Valley Hosp (page 658); **Address:** Radiology Assocs of Ridgewood, 20 Franklin Tpke, Waldwick, NJ 07463-1749; **Phone:** 201-445-8822; **Board Cert:** Diagnostic Radiology 1974; Nuclear Medicine 1974; **Med School:** Columbia P&S 1968; **Resid:** Diagnostic Radiology, Columbia-Presby 1974

Endocrinology, Diabetes & Metabolism

Cobin, Rhoda H MD (EDM) - **Spec Exp:** Thyroid Disorders; Diabetes; Pituitary Disorders; **Hospital:** Valley Hosp (page 658), Mount Sinai Med Ctr (page 102); **Address:** 75 N Maple Ave, Ste 202, Ridgewood, NJ 07450; **Phone:** 201-444-5552; **Board Cert:** Internal Medicine 1972; Endocrinology, Diabetes & Metabolism 1975; **Med School:** Univ Puerto Rico 1969; **Resid:** Internal Medicine, Beth Israel Med Ctr 1972; **Fellow:** Endocrinology, Diabetes & Metabolism, Mt Sinai Hosp 1974; **Fac Appt:** Clin Prof Med, Mount Sinai Sch Med

Goldman, Michael MD (EDM) - **Spec Exp:** Thyroid Disorders; Diabetes; Pituitary Disorders; Cholesterol/Lipid Disorders; **Hospital:** Englewood Hosp & Med Ctr (page 656); **Address:** 600 E Palisade Ave, Ste 1, Englewood Cliffs, NJ 07632-1826; **Phone:** 201-568-1108; **Board Cert:** Internal Medicine 1980; Endocrinology, Diabetes & Metabolism 1981; **Med School:** NY Med Coll 1973; **Resid:** Internal Medicine, Englewood Hosp 1978; **Fellow:** Endocrinology, Diabetes & Metabolism, Columbia-Presby Med Ctr 1980; **Fac Appt:** Asst Prof Med, Mount Sinai Sch Med

Hochstein, Martin MD (EDM) - **Spec Exp:** Thyroid Disorders; Thyroid Cancer; Diabetes; Osteoporosis; **Hospital:** Valley Hosp (page 658), Hackensack Univ Med Ctr (page 96); **Address:** 1 Sears Drive, Paramus, NJ 07652; **Phone:** 201-261-2560; **Board Cert:** Internal Medicine 1973; Endocrinology, Diabetes & Metabolism 1975; **Med School:** Univ Louisville Sch Med 1969; **Resid:** Internal Medicine, Maimoides Med Ctr 1971; Internal Medicine, Jacobi Med Ctr 1972; **Fellow:** Endocrinology, Diabetes & Metabolism, Johns Hopkins Med Ctr 1975; **Fac Appt:** Assoc Clin Prof Med, UMDNJ-RW Johnson Med Sch

Tohme, Jack MD (EDM) - **Spec Exp:** Osteoporosis; Thyroid Disorders; Diabetes; **Hospital:** Valley Hosp (page 658), NY-Presby Hosp/Columbia (page 104); **Address:** 265 Ackerman Ave, Ste 101, Ridgewood, NJ 07450-4203; **Phone:** 201-444-4363; **Board Cert:** Internal Medicine 1978; Endocrinology, Diabetes & Metabolism 1979; **Med School:** Amer Univ Beirut 1974; **Resid:** Internal Medicine, American Univ Hosp 1976; **Fellow:** Endocrinology, Diabetes & Metabolism, Columbia-Presby Med Ctr 1977; Endocrinology, Diabetes & Metabolism, Barnes Hosp/Wash Univ 1978; **Fac Appt:** Assoc Clin Prof Med, Columbia P&S

Wehmann, Robert MD/PhD (EDM) - **Spec Exp:** Diabetes; Thyroid Disorders; Pituitary Disorders; **Hospital:** Valley Hosp (page 658), Hackensack Univ Med Ctr (page 96); **Address:** 400 Old Hook Rd, Ste 1-4, Westwood, NJ 07675-2720; **Phone:** 201-666-1400; **Board Cert:** Internal Medicine 1977; Endocrinology 1979; **Med School:** Albany Med Coll 1974; **Resid:** Internal Medicine, VA Med Ctr 1976; **Fellow:** Endocrinology, Natl Inst Hlth 1979

Wiesen, Mark MD (EDM) - **Spec Exp:** Diabetes; Thyroid Disorders; Osteoporosis; **Hospital:** Hackensack Univ Med Ctr (page 96), Holy Name Med Ctr (page 657); **Address:** 870 Palisade Ave, Ste 203, Teaneck, NJ 07666; **Phone:** 201-836-5655; **Board Cert:** Internal Medicine 1978; Endocrinology, Diabetes & Metabolism 1981; **Med School:** Columbia P&S 1975; **Resid:** Internal Medicine, Brookdale Hosp 1978; **Fellow:** Endocrinology, Diabetes & Metabolism, Mt Sinai Hosp 1981; **Fac Appt:** Asst Clin Prof Med, UMDNJ-NJ Med Sch, Newark

Family Medicine

Bello, Mary MD (FMed) *PCP* - **Spec Exp:** Geriatric Care; **Hospital:** Valley Hosp (page 658); **Address:** 400 Franklin Tpke, Ste 106, Mahwah, NJ 07430-3517; **Phone:** 201-327-3333; **Board Cert:** Family Medicine 2002; **Med School:** West Indies 1984; **Resid:** Family Medicine, St Joseph's Hosp 1987; **Fac Appt:** Asst Clin Prof FMed, UMDNJ-NJ Med Sch, Newark

Gross, Harvey MD (FMed) *PCP* - **Spec Exp:** Geriatric Medicine; Dementia; Myasthenia Gravis; **Hospital:** Englewood Hosp & Med Ctr (page 656), Holy Name Med Ctr (page 657); **Address:** 370 Grand Ave, Ste 102, Englewood, NJ 07631; **Phone:** 201-567-3370; **Board Cert:** Family Medicine 2005; Geriatric Medicine 2000; **Med School:** Boston Univ 1970; **Resid:** Family Medicine, Southside Hosp 1974; **Fac Appt:** Asst Clin Prof Med, Mount Sinai Sch Med

Karatoprak, Ohan MD (FMed) *PCP* - **Spec Exp:** Nutrition; Asthma; Obesity; Geriatric Medicine; **Hospital:** Holy Name Med Ctr (page 657); **Address:** 420 Deerwood Rd, Fort Lee, NJ 07024-1643; **Phone:** 201-886-8877; **Board Cert:** Family Medicine 2005; Geriatric Medicine 2003; **Med School:** Turkey 1977; **Resid:** Surgery, Brookdale Univ Hosp 1983; Family Medicine, Southside Hosp 1986; **Fac Appt:** Asst Clin Prof FMed, UMDNJ-NJ Med Sch, Newark

Leipsner, George MD (FMed) *PCP* - **Hospital:** Hackensack Univ Med Ctr (page 96); **Address:** 57 W Pleasant Ave, Maywood, NJ 07607-1334; **Phone:** 201-488-2111; **Board Cert:** Family Medicine 2001; **Med School:** Italy 1966; **Resid:** Family Medicine, Hackensack Hosp 1968; **Fac Appt:** Asst Clin Prof FMed, Robert W Johnson Med Sch

Gastroenterology

Chessler, Richard K MD (Ge) - **Spec Exp:** Pancreatic Cancer; Endoscopy; Pancreatic/Biliary Endoscopy (ERCP); **Hospital:** Englewood Hosp & Med Ctr (page 656), Hackensack Univ Med Ctr (page 96); **Address:** 1555 Center Ave, Fort Lee, NJ 07024-4612; **Phone:** 201-945-6564 x320; **Board Cert:** Internal Medicine 1972; Gastroenterology 1975; **Med School:** Ros Franklin Univ/Chicago Med Sch 1969; **Resid:** Internal Medicine, NY Med Coll/Flower-Fifth Ave Hosp 1972; **Fellow:** Gastroenterology, NY Med Coll/Flower-Fifth Ave Hosp 1974; **Fac Appt:** Asst Clin Prof Med, Mount Sinai Sch Med

Feit, David MD (Ge) - **Spec Exp:** Hepatitis; **Hospital:** Hackensack Univ Med Ctr (page 96); **Address:** 385 Prospect Ave, Hackensack, NJ 07601-2570; **Phone:** 201-488-3003; **Board Cert:** Internal Medicine 1984; Gastroenterology 1989; **Med School:** Columbia P&S 1981; **Resid:** Internal Medicine, Columbia-Presby Med Ctr 1984; **Fellow:** Gastroenterology, Columbia-Presby Med Ctr 1987

Fried, Harry A MD (Ge) - **Hospital:** Englewood Hosp & Med Ctr (page 656); **Address:** 333 Old Hook Rd, Ste 101, Westwood, NJ 07675; **Phone:** 201-594-0535; **Board Cert:** Internal Medicine 1989; Gastroenterology 2005; **Med School:** SUNY Downstate 1986; **Resid:** Internal Medicine, St Lukes Hosp 1989; **Fellow:** Gastroenterology, Cooper Hosp 1995

Friedrich, Ivan MD (Ge) - **Spec Exp:** Colonoscopy; Pancreatic/Biliary Endoscopy (ERCP); Gallbladder Disease; **Hospital:** Englewood Hosp & Med Ctr (page 656), Holy Name Med Ctr (page 657); **Address:** 420 Grand Ave, Englewood, NJ 07631-4152; **Phone:** 201-569-7044; **Board Cert:** Internal Medicine 1979; Gastroenterology 1981; **Med School:** Albany Med Coll 1976; **Resid:** Internal Medicine, Montefiore Med Ctr 1979; **Fellow:** Gastroenterology, Mt Sinai Med Ctr 1982; **Fac Appt:** Asst Clin Prof Med, Mount Sinai Sch Med

Goldfarb, Joel A MD (Ge) - **Spec Exp:** Colonoscopy/Polypectomy; Colon Cancer; Hepatitis; Liver Disease; **Hospital:** Holy Name Med Ctr (page 657), Englewood Hosp & Med Ctr (page 656); **Address:** 1086 Teaneck Rd, Ste 4C, Teaneck, NJ 07666; **Phone:** 201-837-9449; **Board Cert:** Internal Medicine 1978; Gastroenterology 1981; **Med School:** NYU Sch Med 1975; **Resid:** Internal Medicine, NYU Med Ctr 1978; Hepatology, Yale-New Haven Hosp 1979; **Fellow:** Gastroenterology, Columbia-Presby Med Ctr 1981; **Fac Appt:** Asst Clin Prof Med, Mount Sinai Sch Med

Klein, Walter A MD (Ge) - **Spec Exp:** Esophageal Disorders; Gastroesophageal Reflux Disease (GERD); Colon Polyps & Cancer; **Hospital:** Englewood Hosp & Med Ctr (page 656); **Address:** The Park Medical Group, 274 County Rd, Ste A, Tenafly, NJ 07670; **Phone:** 201-568-0493; **Board Cert:** Internal Medicine 2000; Gastroenterology 2000; **Med School:** Cornell Univ-Weill Med Coll 1987; **Resid:** Internal Medicine, NY Hosp-Cornell Med Ctr 1990; **Fellow:** Gastroenterology, Temple Univ Hosp 1992; **Fac Appt:** Asst Clin Prof Med, Mount Sinai Sch Med

Margulis, Stephen MD (Ge) - **Spec Exp:** Hepatitis; Colonoscopy/Polypectomy; Peptic Ulcer Disease; Inflammatory Bowel Disease; **Hospital:** Valley Hosp (page 658); **Address:** 466 Old Hook Rd, Ste 1, Emerson, NJ 07630-1368; **Phone:** 201-967-8221; **Board Cert:** Internal Medicine 1984; Gastroenterology 1987; **Med School:** Brown Univ 1981; **Resid:** Internal Medicine, New York Hosp-Cornell 1984; **Fellow:** Gastroenterology, New York Hosp-Cornell 1987

Nikias, George A MD (Ge) - **Spec Exp:** Hepatitis; Liver Disease; **Hospital:** Hackensack Univ Med Ctr (page 96); **Address:** 130 Kinderkamack Rd, Ste 301, River Edge, NJ 07661; **Phone:** 201-489-7772; **Board Cert:** Internal Medicine 2002; Gastroenterology 2005; **Med School:** NY Med Coll 1989; **Resid:** Internal Medicine, North Shore Univ Hosp 1992; **Fellow:** Gastroenterology, Meml Sloan Kettering Cancer Ctr 1995; Hepatology, Mayo Clin 1993; **Fac Appt:** Asst Clin Prof Med, UMDNJ-NJ Med Sch, Newark

Panella, Vincent S MD (Ge) - **Spec Exp:** Colon & Rectal Cancer; Hepatitis C; Inflammatory Bowel Disease; Endoscopy; **Hospital:** Englewood Hosp & Med Ctr (page 656), Holy Name Med Ctr (page 657); **Address:** 420 Grand Ave, Englewood, NJ 07631-4141; **Phone:** 201-569-7044; **Board Cert:** Internal Medicine 1985; Gastroenterology 1987; **Med School:** NY Med Coll 1982; **Resid:** Internal Medicine, North Shore Univ Hosp 1985; **Fellow:** Gastroenterology, Mem Sloan-Kettering Cancer Cntr 1987; **Fac Appt:** Asst Clin Prof Med, Mount Sinai Sch Med

Rahmin, Michael G MD (Ge) - **Spec Exp:** Endoscopy; Hepatitis; **Hospital:** Valley Hosp (page 658); **Address:** 140 Chestnut St, Ste 300, Ridgewood, NJ 07452; **Phone:** 201-444-2600; **Board Cert:** Internal Medicine 2002; Gastroenterology 2005; **Med School:** NYU Sch Med 1989; **Resid:** Internal Medicine, Mt Sinai Hosp 1992; **Fellow:** Gastroenterology, New York Hosp 1995; Hepatology, Mt Sinai Hosp 1995

Roth, Joseph MD (Ge) - **Spec Exp:** Endoscopy; Inflammatory Bowel Disease; **Hospital:** St Mary's Hosp - Passaic, St Joseph's Regl Med Ctr - Paterson; **Address:** 71 Union Ave, Rutherford, NJ 07070-1272; **Phone:** 201-842-0020; **Board Cert:** Internal Medicine 1984; Gastroenterology 1987; **Med School:** Univ Pittsburgh 1981; **Resid:** Internal Medicine, Lenox Hill Hosp 1984; **Fellow:** Gastroenterology, Univ Conn Hlth Ctr 1986

Rubin, Kenneth MD (Ge) - **Spec Exp:** Gastroesophageal Reflux Disease (GERD); Endoscopy; Inflammatory Bowel Disease; Colon Cancer; **Hospital:** Englewood Hosp & Med Ctr (page 656), Mount Sinai Med Ctr (page 102); **Address:** 420 Grand Ave, Englewood, NJ 07631-4152; **Phone:** 201-569-7044; **Board Cert:** Internal Medicine 1978; Gastroenterology 1981; **Med School:** UMDNJ-NJ Med Sch, Newark 1975; **Resid:** Internal Medicine, Bronx Municipal Hosp 1979; **Fellow:** Gastroenterology, Mount Sinai Hosp 1981; **Fac Appt:** Asst Clin Prof Med, Mount Sinai Sch Med

Rubinoff, Mitchell J MD (Ge) - **Spec Exp:** Hepatitis; Gastroesophageal Reflux Disease (GERD); **Hospital:** Valley Hosp (page 658); **Address:** 140 Chestnut St, Ste 300, Ridgewood, NJ 07450-2536; **Phone:** 201-444-2600; **Board Cert:** Internal Medicine 1982; Gastroenterology 1985; **Med School:** Mount Sinai Sch Med 1979; **Resid:** Internal Medicine, Columbia-Presby Med Ctr 1982; **Fellow:** Gastroenterology, Columbia-Presby Med Ctr 1985

Zingler, Barry M MD (Ge) - **Spec Exp:** Colon Cancer; Hepatitis; Gastroesophageal Reflux Disease (GERD); **Hospital:** Englewood Hosp & Med Ctr (page 656), Holy Name Med Ctr (page 657); **Address:** 1555 Center Ave, Fort Lee, NJ 07024-4612; **Phone:** 201-945-6564; **Board Cert:** Internal Medicine 1988; Gastroenterology 2001; **Med School:** UMDNJ-Rutgers Med Sch 1985; **Resid:** Internal Medicine, NYU Med Ctr 1988; **Fellow:** Gastroenterology, NYU Med Ctr 1990

Zucker, Ira I MD (Ge) - **Spec Exp:** Colon Cancer; Gastroesophageal Reflux Disease (GERD); Ulcerative Colitis/Crohn's; Hepatitis; **Hospital:** Valley Hosp (page 658), Hackensack Univ Med Ctr (page 96); **Address:** 452 Old Hook Rd, Emerson, NJ 07630; **Phone:** 201-666-3900; **Board Cert:** Internal Medicine 1984; Gastroenterology 1987; **Med School:** Ros Franklin Univ/Chicago Med Sch 1981; **Resid:** Internal Medicine, St Vincents Hosp 1984; **Fellow:** Gastroenterology, St Vincents Hosp 1986

Geriatric Medicine

Leifer, Bennett MD (Ger) *PCP* - **Spec Exp:** Dementia; Alzheimer's Disease; **Hospital:** Valley Hosp (page 658); **Address:** 301 Godwin Ave, Midland Park, NJ 07432-1544; **Phone:** 201-444-4526; **Board Cert:** Internal Medicine 2000; Geriatric Medicine 2000; **Med School:** SUNY Upstate Med Univ 1986; **Resid:** Internal Medicine, Hartford Hosp 1989; **Fellow:** Geriatric Medicine, Mt Sinai Hosp 1991

Gynecologic Oncology

Sommers, Gara M MD (GO) - **Spec Exp:** Gynecologic Cancer; **Hospital:** Hoboken Univ Med Ctr - Hoboken, Christ Hosp; **Address:** 718 Teaneck Rd, Teaneck, NJ 07666; **Phone:** 201-792-9011; **Board Cert:** Obstetrics & Gynecology 2009; Gynecologic Oncology 2009; **Med School:** NYU Sch Med 1981; **Resid:** Obstetrics & Gynecology, NYU Med Ctr 1985; **Fellow:** Gynecologic Oncology, Barnes Jewish Hosp 1988; Research, Beckman Inst-City of Hope 1988; **Fac Appt:** Asst Clin Prof ObG, Albert Einstein Coll Med

Hand Surgery

Fakharzadeh, Frederick MD (HS) - **Hospital:** Hackensack Univ Med Ctr (page 96), Valley Hosp (page 658); **Address:** 22 Madison Ave, FL 3, Paramus, NJ 07652-2721; **Phone:** 201-587-7767; **Board Cert:** Orthopaedic Surgery 2009; Hand Surgery 2009; **Med School:** Columbia P&S 1980; **Resid:** Surgery, Roosevelt Hosp 1982; Orthopaedic Surgery, Columbia-Presby Med Ctr 1985; **Fellow:** Hand Surgery, Thomas Jefferson Univ Hosp 1986

Gurland, Mark MD (HS) - **Spec Exp:** Carpal Tunnel Syndrome; Wrist/Hand Injuries; Arthritis Hand Surgery; **Hospital:** Hackensack Univ Med Ctr (page 96), Englewood Hosp & Med Ctr (page 656); **Address:** 216 Engle St, Englewood, NJ 07631-2448; **Phone:** 201-568-4066; **Board Cert:** Orthopaedic Surgery 2009; Hand Surgery 2009; **Med School:** NYU Sch Med 1979; **Resid:** Surgery, Hosp Univ Penn 1980; Orthopaedic Surgery, Hosp For Joint Disease 1984; **Fellow:** Hand Surgery, Thos Jefferson Univ Hosp

Miller-Breslow, Anne J MD (HS) - **Spec Exp:** Rheumatoid Arthritis; Wrist/Hand Injuries; Arthroscopic Surgery; Fractures; **Hospital:** Englewood Hosp & Med Ctr (page 656), Holy Name Med Ctr (page 657); **Address:** 401A S Van Brunt St Fl 3, Englewood, NJ 07631-2904; **Phone:** 201-569-2770; **Board Cert:** Orthopaedic Surgery 2002; Hand Surgery 2002; **Med School:** Harvard Med Sch 1983; **Resid:** Orthopaedic Surgery, Montefiore Med Ctr 1988; **Fellow:** Hand Surgery, New England Med Ctr 1989

Rosenstein, Roger G MD (HS) - **Spec Exp:** Arthritis Hand Surgery; Nerve Compression; Carpal Tunnel Syndrome; **Hospital:** Hackensack Univ Med Ctr (page 96), Valley Hosp (page 658); **Address:** 22 Madison Ave, Paramus, NJ 07652-5474; **Phone:** 201-587-7767; **Board Cert:** Orthopaedic Surgery 1984; Hand Surgery 2010; **Med School:** Columbia P&S 1975; **Resid:** Surgery, St Luke's Roosevelt Hosp Ctr 1977; Orthopaedic Surgery, Columbia-Presby Med Ctr 1980; **Fellow:** Hand Surgery, Thomas Jefferson Univ Hosp 1981; **Fac Appt:** Assoc Clin Prof OrS, UMDNJ-NJ Med Sch, Newark

Hematology

Fernbach, Barry R MD (Hem) - **Hospital:** Valley Hosp (page 658); **Address:** 1 Valley Health Plaza, Paramus, NJ 07652; **Phone:** 201-634-5353; **Board Cert:** Internal Medicine 1974; Medical Oncology 1977; Hematology 1982; **Med School:** Harvard Med Sch 1971; **Resid:** Internal Medicine, Mt Sinai Hosp 1973; Hematology, Mt Sinai Hosp 1976; **Fellow:** Neoplastic Diseases, Mt Sinai Hosp 1977

Israel, Alan M MD (Hem) - **Hospital:** Valley Hosp (page 658); **Address:** 270 Old Hook Rd, Westwood, NJ 07675-3102; **Phone:** 201-666-4949; **Board Cert:** Internal Medicine 1982; Medical Oncology 1985; Hematology 1986; **Med School:** NYU Sch Med 1979; **Resid:** Internal Medicine, Mt Sinai Hosp 1982; **Fellow:** Hematology & Oncology, Meml Sloan Kettering Cancer Ctr 1984; Hematology, LI Jewish Hosp 1985

Rowley, Scott D MD (Hem) - **Spec Exp:** Stem Cell Transplant; Bone Marrow Transplant; Graft vs Host Disease; **Hospital:** Hackensack Univ Med Ctr (page 96); **Address:** 360 Essex St, Ste 303, Hackensack, NJ 07601; **Phone:** 201-336-8297 x8291; **Board Cert:** Internal Medicine 1981; Medical Oncology 1983; Hematology 1984; **Med School:** Univ Mass Sch Med 1978; **Resid:** Internal Medicine, Rhode Island Hosp 1981; **Fellow:** Hematology & Oncology, Rhode Island Hosp 1984; **Fac Appt:** Assoc Prof Med, UMDNJ-NJ Med Sch, Newark

Vesole, David H MD/PhD (Hem) - **Spec Exp:** Multiple Myeloma; Stem Cell Transplant; Amyloidosis; Waldenstrom's Macroglobulinemia; **Hospital:** Hackensack Univ Med Ctr (page 96); **Address:** 360 Essex St, Ste 302, Hackensack, NJ 07601; **Phone:** 201-336-8704; **Board Cert:** Internal Medicine 1987; Hematology 2000; Medical Oncology 2000; **Med School:** Northwestern Univ 1984; **Resid:** Internal Medicine, Univ Iowa Hosp 1987; **Fellow:** Hematology & Oncology, Univ Iowa Hosp 1990

Infectious Disease

Birch, Thomas MD (Inf) - **Spec Exp:** AIDS/HIV; Lyme Disease; West Nile Virus; Antibiotic Resistance; **Hospital:** Holy Name Med Ctr (page 657), Englewood Hosp & Med Ctr (page 656); **Address:** Birch Tree Medical Assocs, 718 Teaneck Rd, Teaneck, NJ 07666; **Phone:** 201-833-7274; **Board Cert:** Internal Medicine 1986; Infectious Disease 2004; **Med School:** Univ Wisc 1983; **Resid:** Internal Medicine, Montefiore Med Ctr 1986; **Fellow:** Infectious Disease, Montefiore Med Ctr 1993

Cicogna, Cristina E MD (Inf) - **Spec Exp:** Infections in Immunocompromised Patients; Hospital Acquired Infections; **Hospital:** Hackensack Univ Med Ctr (page 96); **Address:** 20 Prospect Ave Fl 5 - Ste 507, Hackensack, NJ 07601; **Phone:** 201-487-4088; **Board Cert:** Internal Medicine 2002; Infectious Disease 2004; **Med School:** Switzerland 1986; **Resid:** Internal Medicine, St Luke's Roosevelt Hosp 1989; **Fellow:** Infectious Disease, Meml Sloan Kettering Cancer Ctr 1991; **Fac Appt:** Asst Prof Med, UMDNJ-RW Johnson Med Sch

Knackmuhs, Gary G MD (Inf) - **Spec Exp:** Travel Medicine; **Hospital:** Valley Hosp (page 658); **Address:** Ridgewood Infectious Disease Assocs, 141 Dayton St, Ste 201, Ridgewood, NJ 07450-4407; **Phone:** 201-447-6468; **Board Cert:** Internal Medicine 1979; Infectious Disease 1982; **Med School:** NY Med Coll 1976; **Resid:** Internal Medicine, Mt Sinai Hosp 1979; **Fellow:** Infectious Disease, Montefiore Med Ctr 1981

Kocher, Jeffrey MD (Inf) - **Spec Exp:** Hepatitis B & C; AIDS/HIV; Fungal Infections; Lyme Disease; **Hospital:** Englewood Hosp & Med Ctr (page 656), Holy Name Med Ctr (page 657); **Address:** 25 Rockwood Pl, Englewood, NJ 07631-4957; **Phone:** 201-568-3335; **Board Cert:** Internal Medicine 1983; Infectious Disease 1986; **Med School:** Cornell Univ-Weill Med Coll 1980; **Resid:** Internal Medicine, New York Hosp 1983; Internal Medicine, St Barnabas Hosp 1984; **Fellow:** Infectious Disease, New York Hosp 1986; **Fac Appt:** Assoc Clin Prof Med, Mount Sinai Sch Med

Levine, Jerome F MD (Inf) - **Spec Exp:** AIDS/HIV; Hospital Acquired Infections; Bone Infections; **Hospital:** Hackensack Univ Med Ctr (page 96); **Address:** 20 Prospect Ave, Ste 507, Hackensack, NJ 07601; **Phone:** 201-487-4088; **Board Cert:** Internal Medicine 1979; Infectious Disease 1982; **Med School:** NYU Sch Med 1976; **Resid:** Internal Medicine, NYU/Manhattan VA Hosp 1980; **Fellow:** Infectious Disease, Manhattan VA Hosp 1982; **Fac Appt:** Assoc Clin Prof Med, UMDNJ-NJ Med Sch, Newark

Weisholtz, Steven J MD (Inf) - **Spec Exp:** AIDS/HIV; Antibiotic Resistance; Travel Medicine; **Hospital:** Englewood Hosp & Med Ctr (page 656); **Address:** 25 Rockwood Pl, Englewood, NJ 07631-4957; **Phone:** 201-568-3335; **Board Cert:** Internal Medicine 1981; Infectious Disease 1984; **Med School:** Univ Pennsylvania 1978; **Resid:** Internal Medicine, New York Hosp 1981; **Fellow:** Infectious Disease, New York Hosp 1983; **Fac Appt:** Asst Clin Prof Med, Mount Sinai Sch Med

Internal Medicine

Brunnquell, Stephen MD (IM) *PCP* - **Hospital:** Englewood Hosp & Med Ctr (page 656); **Address:** 24 Elm St, Harrington Park, NJ 07640-1902; **Phone:** 201-784-0123; **Board Cert:** Internal Medicine 2002; **Med School:** UMDNJ-NJ Med Sch, Newark 1989; **Resid:** Internal Medicine, Montefiore Hosp Med Ctr 1992; **Fac Appt:** Asst Clin Prof Med, Mount Sinai Sch Med

Cacciola, Thomas A MD (IM) - **Spec Exp:** Preventive Medicine; Complementary Medicine; **Hospital:** Hackensack Univ Med Ctr (page 96); **Address:** 403 N Farview Ave, Paramus, NJ 07652-4618; **Phone:** 201-261-8386; **Board Cert:** Internal Medicine 1988; **Med School:** Jefferson Med Coll 1983; **Resid:** Internal Medicine, Hackensack Med Ctr 1986; **Fellow:** US Public Hlth Service 1988

Kushner, Evan G MD (IM) *PCP* - **Spec Exp:** Geriatric Medicine; **Hospital:** Hackensack Univ Med Ctr (page 96), Valley Hosp (page 658); **Address:** Forest Hlthcare Assocs, 277 Forest Ave, Ste 200, Paramus, NJ 07652; **Phone:** 201-986-1881; **Board Cert:** Internal Medicine 1989; Geriatric Medicine 2005; **Med School:** SUNY Upstate Med Univ 1986; **Resid:** Internal Medicine, Univ Hosp 1989

Lan, Vivian E MD (IM) *PCP* - **Spec Exp:** Women's Health; Eating Disorders; **Hospital:** Valley Hosp (page 658); **Address:** 466 Old Hook Rd, Ste 1, Emerson, NJ 07630; **Phone:** 201-967-8221; **Board Cert:** Internal Medicine 2007; **Med School:** Mount Sinai Sch Med 1994; **Resid:** Internal Medicine, Mt Sinai Med Ctr 1997

Lauricella, Joseph MD (IM) *PCP* - **Spec Exp:** Coronary Artery Disease; **Hospital:** Holy Name Med Ctr (page 657), Hackensack Univ Med Ctr (page 96); **Address:** 292 Columbia Ave, Fort Lee, NJ 07024-4124; **Phone:** 201-224-0050; **Board Cert:** Internal Medicine 1985; **Med School:** Mexico 1978; **Resid:** Internal Medicine, Rutgers Univ Med Ctr 1985

Miguel, Eduardo E MD (IM) *PCP* - **Spec Exp:** Rheumatoid Arthritis; **Hospital:** Englewood Hosp & Med Ctr (page 656); **Address:** 12 E Pallisade Ave, Englewood, NJ 07631; **Phone:** 201-871-3280; **Board Cert:** Internal Medicine 1982; **Med School:** Paraguay 1966; **Resid:** Internal Medicine, VA Med Ctr 1969; Internal Medicine, NY Polyclinic Hosp 1972; **Fellow:** Rheumatology, Albert Einstein Med Ctr 1973

Pelavin, Martin MD (IM) *PCP* - **Hospital:** Valley Hosp (page 658), Englewood Hosp & Med Ctr (page 656); **Address:** 215 Old Tappan Rd, Old Tappan, NJ 07675-7428; **Phone:** 201-666-1000; **Board Cert:** Internal Medicine 1976; **Med School:** NYU Sch Med 1973; **Resid:** Internal Medicine, Montefiore Hosp Med Ctr 1976

Scibetta, Maria MD (IM) *PCP* - **Hospital:** Valley Hosp (page 658); **Address:** 42 N Franklin Tpke, Ramsey, NJ 07446-2034; **Phone:** 201-327-8765; **Board Cert:** Internal Medicine 2003; **Med School:** UMDNJ-RW Johnson Med Sch 1990; **Resid:** Internal Medicine, Mount Sinai Hosp 1993

Valinoti, Anne Marie MD (IM) - **Spec Exp:** Women's Health; **Hospital:** Valley Hosp (page 658); **Address:** 301 Godwin Avenue, Midland Park, NJ 07432; **Phone:** 201-444-4526; **Board Cert:** Internal Medicine 2004; **Med School:** Columbia P&S 1991; **Resid:** Internal Medicine, New York Hosp 1994

Volpe, Anthony P MD (IM) *PCP* - **Spec Exp:** Hypertension; **Hospital:** Valley Hosp (page 658), Englewood Hosp & Med Ctr (page 656); **Address:** 466 Old Hook Rd, Ste 14, Emerson, NJ 07630-1368; **Phone:** 201-262-6485; **Board Cert:** Internal Medicine 2005; **Med School:** Mexico 1981; **Resid:** Internal Medicine, Texas Tech Hlth Scis Ctr 1986

Wasserman, Kenneth H MD (IM) *PCP* - **Hospital:** Englewood Hosp & Med Ctr (page 656), Holy Name Med Ctr (page 657); **Address:** 401 S Van Brunt St, Ste 402, Englewood, NJ 07631-4200; **Phone:** 201-567-1140 x10; **Board Cert:** Internal Medicine 1982; **Med School:** Albert Einstein Coll Med 1979; **Resid:** Internal Medicine, Lenox Hill Hosp 1982

Interventional Cardiology

Angeli, Stephen J MD (IC) - **Spec Exp:** Angioplasty & Stent Placement; Cardiac Catheterization; Coronary Artery Disease; **Hospital:** Holy Name Med Ctr (page 657); **Address:** Cardiovascular Assocs of Teaneck, 222 Cedar Lane, Ste 309, Teaneck, NJ 07666-4243; **Phone:** 201-836-1788; **Board Cert:** Internal Medicine 1984; Cardiovascular Disease 1987; Interventional Cardiology 2007; **Med School:** SUNY Downstate 1981; **Resid:** Internal Medicine, Kings Co Hosp 1984; **Fellow:** Cardiovascular Disease, St Michael Med Ctr 1986

Lichtstein, Elliott S MD (IC) - **Spec Exp:** Angioplasty & Stent Placement; Peripheral Vascular Disease; Coronary Artery Disease; Heart Failure; **Hospital:** Hackensack Univ Med Ctr (page 96), Valley Hosp (page 658); **Address:** Westwood Cardiology, 333 Old Hook Rd, Ste 200, Westwood, NJ 07675; **Phone:** 201-664-0201; **Board Cert:** Internal Medicine 1984; Cardiovascular Disease 1987; Interventional Cardiology 2009; **Med School:** Temple Univ 1981; **Resid:** Internal Medicine, Albany Med Ctr Hosp 1984; **Fellow:** Cardiovascular Disease, LI Jewish Med Ctr 1986

Maternal & Fetal Medicine

Alvarez, Manuel MD (MF) - **Spec Exp:** Multiple Gestation; Pregnancy-High Risk; **Hospital:** Hackensack Univ Med Ctr (page 96), NYU Langone Med Ctr (page 106); **Address:** 20 Prospect Ave, Ste 601, Hackensack, NJ 07601; **Phone:** 201-996-2765; **Board Cert:** Obstetrics & Gynecology 2004; Maternal & Fetal Medicine 2004; **Med School:** Dominican Republic 1981; **Resid:** Obstetrics & Gynecology, St Joseph Hosp 1987; **Fellow:** Maternal & Fetal Medicine, Mount Sinai Med Ctr 1989; Critical Care Obstetrics, Mount Sinai Med Ctr 1990

Frieden, Faith MD (MF) - **Spec Exp:** Prenatal Ultrasound; Prenatal Diagnosis; **Hospital:** Englewood Hosp & Med Ctr (page 656); **Address:** 350 Engle St, Englewood, NJ 07631-1808; **Phone:** 201-894-3669; **Board Cert:** Obstetrics & Gynecology 2008; Maternal & Fetal Medicine 2008; **Med School:** Mount Sinai Sch Med 1984; **Resid:** Obstetrics & Gynecology, Beth Israel Med Ctr 1988; **Fellow:** Maternal & Fetal Medicine, Bellevue Hosp 1990; **Fac Appt:** Asst Clin Prof ObG, Mount Sinai Sch Med

Principe, David L MD (MF) - **Spec Exp:** Pregnancy-High Risk; **Hospital:** St Joseph's Regl Med Ctr - Paterson, Palisades Med Ctr; **Address:** St Joseph's Perinatal Ctr, 1 Broadway Route 4, Ste 203, Elmwood Park, NJ 07407; **Phone:** 973-569-6264; **Board Cert:** Obstetrics & Gynecology 2009; Maternal & Fetal Medicine 2009; **Med School:** Grenada 1991; **Resid:** Obstetrics & Gynecology, St Joseph Hosp 1995; **Fellow:** Maternal & Fetal Medicine, Univ Chicago/Chicago Lying in Hosp 1997; Maternal & Fetal Medicine, Yale New Haven Hosp 1998

Medical Oncology

Attas, Lewis MD (Onc) - **Spec Exp:** Breast Cancer; Lymphoma; Bleeding/Coagulation Disorders; Gaucher Disease; **Hospital:** Englewood Hosp & Med Ctr (page 656), Holy Name Med Ctr (page 657); **Address:** 25 Rockwood Pl Fl 1, Englewood, NJ 07631-4957; **Phone:** 201-568-5250; **Board Cert:** Internal Medicine 1985; Medical Oncology 1987; Hematology 1988; **Med School:** Mount Sinai Sch Med 1982; **Resid:** Internal Medicine, Montefiore Hosp Med Ctr 1985; **Fellow:** Hematology & Oncology, North Shore Univ Hosp 1988; **Fac Appt:** Assoc Clin Prof Med, Mount Sinai Sch Med

Forte, Francis A MD (Onc) - **Spec Exp:** Breast Cancer; Hematologic Malignancies; Coagulation/Bleeding Disorders; Solid Tumors; **Hospital:** Englewood Hosp & Med Ctr (page 656), Holy Name Med Ctr (page 657); **Address:** 350 Engle St, Englewood, NJ 07631; **Phone:** 201-568-5250; **Board Cert:** Internal Medicine 1971; Hematology 1972; Medical Oncology 1973; **Med School:** Albert Einstein Coll Med 1964; **Resid:** Internal Medicine, Mount Sinai Hosp 1968; **Fellow:** Hematology, Mount Sinai Hosp 1969; **Fac Appt:** Asst Prof Med, Mount Sinai Sch Med

Goldberg, Stuart L MD (Onc) - **Spec Exp:** Leukemia; Stem Cell Transplant; Myelodysplastic Syndromes; **Hospital:** Hackensack Univ Med Ctr (page 96); **Address:** The Cancer Ctr, Hackensack Univ Med Ctr, 20 Prospect Ave, Ste 615, Hackensack, NJ 07601; **Phone:** 201-996-5900; **Board Cert:** Internal Medicine 1989; **Med School:** Penn State Univ-Hershey Med Ctr 1986; **Resid:** Internal Medicine, George Washington Univ Hosp 1989; **Fellow:** Hematology & Oncology, George Washington Univ Hosp 1991; Bone Marrow Transplant, Mayo Clinic 1992; **Fac Appt:** Assoc Clin Prof Med, UMDNJ-NJ Med Sch, Newark

Goy, Andre MD (Onc) - **Spec Exp:** Lymphoma; Hodgkin's Disease; **Hospital:** Hackensack Univ Med Ctr (page 96); **Address:** 20 Prospect Ave, Ste 400, Hackensack, NJ 07601; **Phone:** 201-996-5900; **Med School:** France 1988; **Resid:** Internal Medicine, Grenoble Univ Med Ctr 1992; **Fellow:** Hematology & Oncology, Grenoble Univ Med Ctr 1993

Harper, Harry MD (Onc) - **Spec Exp:** Lung Cancer; **Hospital:** Hackensack Univ Med Ctr (page 96), Holy Name Med Ctr (page 657); **Address:** 60 2nd St, Hackensack, NJ 07601; **Phone:** 201-996-5900; **Board Cert:** Internal Medicine 1980; Hematology 1982; Medical Oncology 1983; **Med School:** Baylor Coll Med 1977; **Resid:** Internal Medicine, NY-Cornell Med Ctr 1980; **Fellow:** Hematology & Oncology, Meml Sloan Kettering Cancer Ctr 1983

Jennis, Andrew MD (Onc) - **Spec Exp:** Gastrointestinal Cancer; **Hospital:** Hackensack Univ Med Ctr (page 96); **Address:** 20 Prospect Ave, Ste 400, Hackensack, NJ 07601; **Phone:** 201-996-5900; **Board Cert:** Internal Medicine 1988; Hematology 2002; Medical Oncology 2001; **Med School:** Columbia P&S 1985; **Resid:** Internal Medicine, Mount Sinai Hosp 1988; **Fellow:** Hematology & Oncology, Beth Israel Hosp 1992

Krutchik, Allan MD (Onc) - **Spec Exp:** Breast Cancer; **Hospital:** St. Joseph's Wayne Hosp, Chilton Meml Hosp; **Address:** 795 Franklin Ave, Ste 106, Franklin Lakes, NJ 07417; **Phone:** 201-848-8791; **Board Cert:** Internal Medicine 1976; Medical Oncology 2001; **Med School:** Ros Franklin Univ/Chicago Med Sch 1973; **Resid:** Internal Medicine, Beth Israel Hosp 1976; **Fellow:** Medical Oncology, MD Anderson Cancer Ctr 1978; **Fac Appt:** Asst Clin Prof Med, UMDNJ-NJ Med Sch, Newark

Ligresti, Louise G MD (Onc) - **Spec Exp:** Breast Cancer; **Hospital:** Valley Hosp (page 658), Chilton Meml Hosp; **Address:** One Valley Hlth Plaza, Paramus, NJ 07652; **Phone:** 201-634-5353; **Board Cert:** Medical Oncology 2008; Hematology 2008; **Med School:** SUNY Upstate Med Univ 1991; **Resid:** Internal Medicine, NY Hosp-Cornell Med Ctr 1994; **Fellow:** Hematology & Oncology, Meml Sloan Kettering Cancer Ctr 1995

Pascal, Mark MD (Onc) - **Spec Exp:** Lung Cancer; Breast Cancer; Neuro-Oncology; **Hospital:** Hackensack Univ Med Ctr (page 96), Holy Name Med Ctr (page 657); **Address:** 20 Prospect Ave, Fl 4 - Ste 400, Hackensack, NJ 07601-1997; **Phone:** 201-996-5900; **Board Cert:** Internal Medicine 1977; Medical Oncology 1979; **Med School:** Jefferson Med Coll 1973; **Resid:** Pathology, Cornell Univ Med Ctr 1976; Internal Medicine, NY Presby Hosp/ Weil Cornell 1977; **Fellow:** Hematology & Oncology, Meml Sloan Kettering Cancer Ctr 1979

Pecora, Andrew L MD (Onc) - **Spec Exp:** Stem Cell Transplant; Myelodysplastic Syndromes; Melanoma; Immunotherapy; **Hospital:** Hackensack Univ Med Ctr (page 96); **Address:** The Cancer Ctr-Hackensack Univ Med Ctr, 20 Prospect Ave, Ste 400, Hackensack, NJ 07601; **Phone:** 201-996-5900; **Board Cert:** Internal Medicine 1986; Hematology 1988; Medical Oncology 1989; **Med School:** UMDNJ-NJ Med Sch, Newark 1983; **Resid:** Internal Medicine, New York Hosp 1986; **Fellow:** Hematology & Oncology, Meml Sloan Kettering Cancer Ctr 1988; **Fac Appt:** Prof Med, UMDNJ-NJ Med Sch, Newark

Rakowski, Thomas MD (Onc) - **Spec Exp:** Breast Cancer; Lung Cancer; Colon Cancer; **Hospital:** Valley Hosp (page 658); **Address:** 301 Godwin Ave, Midland Park, NJ 07432-4426; **Phone:** 201-444-4526; **Board Cert:** Internal Medicine 1979; Medical Oncology 1981; **Med School:** SUNY Upstate Med Univ 1976; **Resid:** Internal Medicine, SUNY Hlth Sci Ctr 1979; Hematology & Oncology, NY Presby Hosp-Columbia Campus 1981

Schleider, Michael MD (Onc) - **Spec Exp:** Breast Cancer; Colon Cancer; Bleeding/Coagulation Disorders; **Hospital:** Englewood Hosp & Med Ctr (page 656), Holy Name Med Ctr (page 657); **Address:** 350 Engle St Berrie Bldg Fl 1, Englewood, NJ 07631; **Phone:** 201-568-5250; **Board Cert:** Internal Medicine 1974; Hematology 1976; Medical Oncology 1977; **Med School:** Univ Pennsylvania 1969; **Resid:** Internal Medicine, New York Hosp 1974; **Fellow:** Hematology & Oncology, New York Hosp 1977

Waintraub, Stanley MD (Onc) - **Spec Exp:** Breast Cancer; Bleeding/Coagulation Disorders; **Hospital:** Hackensack Univ Med Ctr (page 96); **Address:** Northern NJ Cancer Associates, 20 Prospect Ave, Fl 4, Hackensack, NJ 07601-1997; **Phone:** 201-996-5900; **Board Cert:** Internal Medicine 1980; Hematology 1982; Medical Oncology 1983; **Med School:** NY Med Coll 1977; **Resid:** Internal Medicine, Metropolitan Hosp Ctr 1980; **Fellow:** Hematology, Montefiore Hosp Med Ctr 1982; Medical Oncology, Meml Sloan Kettering Cancer Ctr 1983

Neonatal-Perinatal Medicine

Carlin, Elizabeth B MD (NP) - **Hospital:** Englewood Hosp & Med Ctr (page 656), Mount Sinai Med Ctr (page 102); **Address:** Englewood Hosp & Med Ctr, 305 Engle St, Englewood, NJ 07631-1808; **Phone:** 201-894-3849; **Board Cert:** Neonatal-Perinatal Medicine 2006; **Med School:** Boston Univ 1990; **Resid:** Pediatrics, Boston City Hosp 1993; **Fellow:** Neonatal-Perinatal Medicine, Mt Sinai Med Ctr 1996; **Fac Appt:** Asst Clin Prof Ped, Mount Sinai Sch Med

Manginello, Frank P MD (NP) - **Spec Exp:** Prematurity/Low Birth Weight Infants; Lung Disease in Newborns; Developmental Disorders; **Hospital:** Valley Hosp (page 658); **Address:** The Valley Hosp, 223 N Van Dien Ave, Ridgewood, NJ 07450-2736; **Phone:** 201-447-8388; **Board Cert:** Pediatrics 1978; Neonatal-Perinatal Medicine 1979; **Med School:** Georgetown Univ 1973; **Resid:** Pediatrics, Georgetown Univ Hosp 1974; Pediatrics, Georgetown Univ Hosp 1975; **Fellow:** Perinatal Medicine, NY Hosp-Cornell Med Ctr 1977; **Fac Appt:** Asst Prof Ped, Columbia P&S

Perl, Harold MD (NP) - **Spec Exp:** Pulmonary Disease; Jaundice & Bilirubin Metabolism; Sudden Infant Death Syndrome (SIDS); **Hospital:** Hackensack Univ Med Ctr (page 96); **Address:** Hackensack Univ Med Ctr, Dept Pediatrics, 30 Prospect Ave Bldg Imus - rm 217, Hackensack, NJ 07601-1914; **Phone:** 201-996-5362; **Board Cert:** Pediatrics 1980; Neonatal-Perinatal Medicine 1983; **Med School:** Albert Einstein Coll Med 1975; **Resid:** Pediatrics, Montefiore Med Ctr 1978; **Fellow:** Neonatal-Perinatal Medicine, Montefiore Med Ctr 1980; **Fac Appt:** Asst Clin Prof Ped, UMDNJ-NJ Med Sch, Newark

Sison, Joseph S MD (NP) - **Spec Exp:** Neonatology; **Hospital:** Englewood Hosp & Med Ctr (page 656), Mount Sinai Med Ctr (page 102); **Address:** 350 Engle St, Englewood, NJ 07631-1808; **Phone:** 201-894-3321; **Board Cert:** Pediatrics 2007; Neonatal-Perinatal Medicine 2005; **Med School:** Philippines 1984; **Resid:** Pediatrics, Jersey Shore Med Ctr 1992; Neonatal-Perinatal Medicine, Vanderbilt Univ Hosp 1993; **Fellow:** Neonatal-Perinatal Medicine, New York Hosp 1995; **Fac Appt:** Clin Prof Ped, Mount Sinai Sch Med

Nephrology

Fein, Deborah A MD (Nep) - **Spec Exp:** Hypertension; Kidney Disease; Transplant Medicine-Kidney; Lupus Nephritis; **Hospital:** Englewood Hosp & Med Ctr (page 656), Holy Name Med Ctr (page 657); **Address:** 177 N Dean St, Ste 207, Englewood, NJ 07631-2501; **Phone:** 201-567-0446; **Board Cert:** Internal Medicine 1983; Nephrology 2004; **Med School:** Tufts Univ 1980; **Resid:** Internal Medicine, Roosevelt Hosp 1983; **Fellow:** Nephrology, NY Hosp 1986

Grodstein, Gerald MD (Nep) - **Spec Exp:** Hypertension; Dialysis Care; **Hospital:** Englewood Hosp & Med Ctr (page 656); **Address:** 177 N Dean St, Ste 207, Englewood, NJ 07631-2527; **Phone:** 201-567-0446; **Board Cert:** Internal Medicine 1977; Nephrology 1980; **Med School:** SUNY Downstate 1974; **Resid:** Internal Medicine, Kings County Hosp 1977; **Fellow:** Nephrology, UCLA Med Ctr 1978

Kozlowski, Jeffrey MD (Nep) - **Spec Exp:** Hypertension; Dialysis Care; Diabetic Kidney Disease; **Hospital:** Valley Hosp (page 658), Hackensack Univ Med Ctr (page 96); **Address:** 44 Godwin Ave, Ste 301, Midland Park, NJ 07432; **Phone:** 201-447-0013; **Board Cert:** Internal Medicine 1981; Nephrology 1984; **Med School:** NYU Sch Med 1978; **Resid:** Internal Medicine, VA Med Ctr 1981; **Fellow:** Nephrology, NYU Med Ctr 1984

Levin, David N MD (Nep) - **Spec Exp:** Hypertension; Dialysis Care; **Hospital:** Holy Name Med Ctr (page 657), Hackensack Univ Med Ctr (page 96); **Address:** 870 Palisade Ave, Ste 202, Teaneck, NJ 07666-3419; **Phone:** 201-836-0897; **Board Cert:** Internal Medicine 1979; Nephrology 1982; **Med School:** UMDNJ-NJ Med Sch, Newark 1976; **Resid:** Internal Medicine, Jacobi Medical Center 1979; **Fellow:** Nephrology, Albert Einstein 1981

Pattner, Austin M MD (Nep) - **Spec Exp:** Hypertension; Dialysis Care; Kidney Disease; **Hospital:** Englewood Hosp & Med Ctr (page 656), Hackensack Univ Med Ctr (page 96); **Address:** 177 N Dean St, Ste 207, Englewood, NJ 07631-2527; **Phone:** 201-567-0445; **Board Cert:** Internal Medicine 1974; Nephrology 1976; **Med School:** SUNY Upstate Med Univ 1966; **Resid:** Internal Medicine, Roosevelt Hosp 1969; Internal Medicine, Columbia-Presby Med Ctr 1970; **Fellow:** Nephrology, Columbia-Presby Med Ctr 1972; **Fac Appt:** Asst Prof Med, Mount Sinai Sch Med

Rigolosi, Robert S MD (Nep) - **Spec Exp:** Kidney Disease; Hypertension; Dialysis Care; **Hospital:** Holy Name Med Ctr (page 657), Valley Hosp (page 658); **Address:** Holy Name Hosp, 718 Teaneck Rd, Teaneck, NJ 07666-4281; **Phone:** 201-833-3223; **Med School:** Italy 1963; **Resid:** Internal Medicine, Bronx VA Hosp 1967; **Fellow:** Renal Disease, Georgetown Univ Hosp 1969

Tartini, Albert MD (Nep) - **Spec Exp:** Kidney Disease; Hypertension; Dialysis Care; Anemia; **Hospital:** Valley Hosp (page 658), Holy Name Med Ctr (page 657); **Address:** Holy Name Hosp, 718 Teaneck Rd, Hemodialysis Dept, Teaneck, NJ 07666; **Phone:** 201-833-3223; **Board Cert:** Internal Medicine 1988; Nephrology 2000; **Med School:** Grenada 1984; **Resid:** Internal Medicine, St Joseph Hosp Med Ctr 1988; **Fellow:** Nephrology, Univ Vermont Med Ctr 1990

Weizman, Howard MD (Nep) - **Spec Exp:** Dialysis Care; Hypertension; **Hospital:** Hackensack Univ Med Ctr (page 96), Valley Hosp (page 658); **Address:** Bergen Hypertension, 44 Godwin Ave, Midland Park, NJ 07432-1976; **Phone:** 201-447-0013; **Board Cert:** Internal Medicine 1985; Nephrology 2002; **Med School:** Albert Einstein Coll Med 1982; **Resid:** Internal Medicine, Bronx Muni Hosp 1985; **Fellow:** Nephrology, Mount Sinai Med Ctr 1987

Neurological Surgery

Carpenter, Duncan MD (NS) - **Spec Exp:** Spinal Surgery; Spinal Reconstructive Surgery; **Hospital:** Valley Hosp (page 658); **Address:** 225 Dayton St, Ridgewood, NJ 07450-4407; **Phone:** 201-612-0020; **Board Cert:** Neurological Surgery 1987; **Med School:** Columbia P&S 1978; **Resid:** Surgery, St Lukes Hosp 1980; Neurological Surgery, NY Neuro Inst-Columbia 1985

Fried, Arno H MD (NS) - **Spec Exp:** Epilepsy; Brain Tumors; Head Injury; Pediatric Neurosurgery; **Hospital:** Hackensack Univ Med Ctr (page 96), St Peter's Univ Hosp; **Address:** 20 Prospect Ave, Ste 905, Hackensack, NJ 07601; **Phone:** 201-996-5251; **Board Cert:** Neurological Surgery 1990; Pediatric Neurological Surgery 2007; **Med School:** Meharry Med Coll 1980; **Resid:** Neurological Surgery, Albert Einstein Coll Med 1986; Neurological Surgery, Univ Utah 1987; **Fellow:** Pediatric Surgery, Chldns Hosp 1987; **Fac Appt:** Assoc Prof NS, NY Med Coll

Goulart, Hamilton C MD (NS) - **Spec Exp:** Spinal Surgery; Spinal Reconstructive Surgery; Spinal Disc Replacement; **Hospital:** Valley Hosp (page 658); **Address:** 225 Dayton St, Ridgewood, NJ 07450-4407; **Phone:** 201-612-0020; **Board Cert:** Neurological Surgery 1985; **Med School:** Brazil 1975; **Resid:** Neurological Surgery, Mt Sinai Hosp 1982

Rajaraman, Viswanathan MD (NS) - **Spec Exp:** Neuro-Oncology; Stereotactic Radiosurgery; **Hospital:** Hackensack Univ Med Ctr (page 96); **Address:** NJ Brain & Spine Ctr, 20 Prospect Ave, Ste 907, Hackensack, NJ 07601; **Phone:** 201-342-2550; **Board Cert:** Neurological Surgery 2003; **Med School:** India 1981; **Resid:** Neurological Surgery, UMDNJ-New Jersey Med Sch; **Fellow:** Spinal Surgery, Mayfield Neurological Inst; Neuro-Oncology, Meml-Sloan Kettering Cancer Ctr; **Fac Appt:** Asst Clin Prof NS, UMDNJ-Univ Med Dent NJ

Roth, Patrick A MD (NS) - **Spec Exp:** Spinal Surgery; Brain Tumors; **Hospital:** Hackensack Univ Med Ctr (page 96), Valley Hosp (page 658); **Address:** 680 Kinderkamack Rd, Ste 300, Oradell, NJ 07649; **Phone:** 201-342-2550; **Board Cert:** Neurological Surgery 1997; **Med School:** Albert Einstein Coll Med 1987; **Resid:** Neurological Surgery, New England Med Ctr 1994; **Fac Appt:** Clin Prof NS, UMDNJ-NJ Med Sch, Newark

Vingan, Roy D MD (NS) - **Spec Exp:** Brain Surgery; Spinal Surgery; **Hospital:** Hackensack Univ Med Ctr (page 96), Valley Hosp (page 658); **Address:** 680 Kinderkamack Rd, Ste 300, Oradell, NJ 07649; **Phone:** 201-342-2550; **Board Cert:** Neurological Surgery 1995; **Med School:** SUNY Downstate 1985; **Resid:** Neurological Surgery, SUNY Hlth Sci Ctr 1992; **Fac Appt:** Asst Clin Prof NS, UMDNJ-NJ Med Sch, Newark

Neurology

Alweiss, Gary S MD (N) - **Spec Exp:** Electromyography; Carpal Tunnel Syndrome; Headache; **Hospital:** Englewood Hosp & Med Ctr (page 656); **Address:** 25 Rockwood Pl, Ste 110, Englewood, NJ 07631; **Phone:** 201-894-5805; **Board Cert:** Neurology 1993; **Med School:** Mount Sinai Sch Med 1988; **Resid:** Neurology, Mount Sinai Med Ctr 1992; **Fellow:** Nuclear Medicine, Columbia-Presby Med Ctr 1993

Effron, Charles MD (N) - **Spec Exp:** Peripheral Neuropathy; **Hospital:** Mount Sinai Med Ctr (page 102); **Address:** 365 W Passaic St, Rochelle Park, NJ 07662; **Phone:** 201-845-6500; **Board Cert:** Neurology 1989; **Med School:** Brown Univ 1983; **Resid:** Neurology, Mt Sinai Hosp 1987

Klein, Patricia MD (N) - **Spec Exp:** Headache; Dizziness; Stroke; **Hospital:** Holy Name Med Ctr (page 657), Hackensack Univ Med Ctr (page 96); **Address:** 261 Old Hook Rd, Westwood, NJ 07675; **Phone:** 201-263-0101; **Board Cert:** Neurology 1980; **Med School:** UMDNJ-NJ Med Sch, Newark 1976; **Resid:** Neurology, UMDNJ 1979; **Fac Appt:** Asst Clin Prof N, UMDNJ-NJ Med Sch, Newark

Levin, Kenneth A MD (N) - **Spec Exp:** Stroke; Alzheimer's Disease; Parkinson's Disease; Epilepsy; **Hospital:** Valley Hosp (page 658); **Address:** 1200 E Ridgewood Ave Fl 2, Ridgewood, NJ 07450; **Phone:** 201-444-0868; **Board Cert:** Neurology 1987; **Med School:** Indiana Univ 1982; **Resid:** Neurology, Indiana Univ Med Ctr 1986

Perron, Reed C MD (N) - **Hospital:** Valley Hosp (page 658); **Address:** 1200 E Ridgewood Ave Fl 2 E Wing, Ridgewood, NJ 07450; **Phone:** 201-444-0868; **Board Cert:** Neurology 1974; **Med School:** Univ Rochester 1966; **Resid:** Internal Medicine, Cleveland Clinic 1970; Neurology, Albert Einstein Coll Med 1973

Rabin, Aaron MD/PhD (N) - **Spec Exp:** Parkinson's Disease; Dementia; Peripheral Neuropathy; **Hospital:** Englewood Hosp & Med Ctr (page 656); **Address:** 700 E Palisade Ave, Englewood Cliffs, NJ 07631; **Phone:** 201-568-3412; **Board Cert:** Neurology 1981; **Med School:** Albert Einstein Coll Med 1976; **Resid:** Neurology, Albert Einstein Coll Med 1980; **Fellow:** Neuroelectrophysiology, Neuro Inst-Columbia Presby Hosp 1981; **Fac Appt:** Asst Clin Prof Med, Mount Sinai Sch Med

Van Engel, Daniel R MD (N) - **Spec Exp:** Electromyography; **Hospital:** Valley Hosp (page 658); **Address:** 1200 E Ridgewood Ave, East Wing Fl 2, Ridgewood, NJ 07450-3957; **Phone:** 201-444-0868; **Board Cert:** Neurology 1980; **Med School:** SUNY Upstate Med Univ 1973; **Resid:** Internal Medicine, North Shore Univ Hosp 1975; Neurology, Bronx Muni Hosp 1978

Van Slooten, David D MD (N) - **Spec Exp:** Electromyography; Headache; Dementia; **Hospital:** Holy Name Med Ctr (page 657), Valley Hosp (page 658); **Address:** 680 Kinderkamack Rd, Ste 302, Oradell, NJ 07649-1500; **Phone:** 201-261-6222; **Board Cert:** Neurology 1989; Clinical Neurophysiology 2004; Electrodiagnostic Medicine 2004; **Med School:** UMDNJ-NJ Med Sch, Newark 1984; **Resid:** Neurology, UMDNJ Univ Hosp 1988; **Fellow:** Clinical Neurophysiology, VA Med Ctr 1989

Willner, Joseph H MD (N) - **Spec Exp:** Multiple Sclerosis; Myasthenia Gravis; Peripheral Neuropathy; **Hospital:** Englewood Hosp & Med Ctr (page 656); **Address:** 25 Rockwood Pl, Ste 110, Englewood, NJ 07631-4363; **Phone:** 201-894-5805; **Board Cert:** Neurology 1978; **Med School:** NYU Sch Med 1970; **Resid:** Neurology, Columbia-Presby Hosp 1977; **Fac Appt:** Assoc Clin Prof N, Columbia P&S

Neuroradiology

Lerner, Elliot J MD (NRad) - **Spec Exp:** Brain & Spinal Imaging; Head & Neck Imaging; **Hospital:** Valley Hosp (page 658); **Address:** Radiology Assocs of Ridgewood, 20 Franklin Tpke, Waldwick, NJ 07463-1749; **Phone:** 201-445-8822; **Board Cert:** Diagnostic Radiology 1990; Neuroradiology 2004; **Med School:** Brown Univ 1985; **Resid:** Diagnostic Radiology, Hosp Univ Penn 1989; **Fellow:** Neuroradiology, Hosp Univ Penn 1991

Nuclear Medicine

Agress Jr, Harry MD (NuM) - **Spec Exp:** PET Imaging; Cancer Detection & Staging; Nuclear Oncology; CT Scan; **Hospital:** Hackensack Univ Med Ctr (page 96), NY-Presby Hosp/Columbia (page 104); **Address:** Hackensack Univ Med Ctr, 30 Prospect Ave, Hackensack, NJ 07601; **Phone:** 201-996-2196; **Board Cert:** Nuclear Medicine 1976; Diagnostic Radiology 1978; **Med School:** Tufts Univ 1972; **Resid:** Radiology, Columbia- Presby Med Ctr 1978; **Fellow:** Nuclear Medicine, Natl Inst Hlth 1975; **Fac Appt:** Clin Prof Rad, Columbia P&S

Brunetti, Jacqueline C MD (NuM) - **Spec Exp:** PET Imaging; CT Scan; Tumor Imaging; **Hospital:** Holy Name Med Ctr (page 657); **Address:** Holy Name Hosp, Dept Radiology, 718 Teaneck Rd, Teaneck, NJ 07666-4281; **Phone:** 201-833-3445; **Board Cert:** Diagnostic Radiology 1979; Nuclear Medicine 1980; Nuclear Radiology 1980; **Med School:** SUNY Downstate 1975; **Resid:** Diagnostic Radiology, St Vincents Hosp 1979; Nuclear Radiology, St Vincents Hosp 1980; **Fellow:** Nuclear Medicine, St Vincents Hosp 1980; **Fac Appt:** Assoc Clin Prof, Columbia P&S

Obstetrics & Gynecology

Butler, David G MD (ObG) *PCP* - **Spec Exp:** Gynecologic Surgery; Menopause Problems; **Hospital:** Holy Name Med Ctr (page 657), Englewood Hosp & Med Ctr (page 656); **Address:** 420 Grand Ave, Ste 201, Englewood, NJ 07631-4152; **Phone:** 201-871-4040; **Board Cert:** Obstetrics & Gynecology 1972; **Med School:** SUNY Downstate 1965; **Resid:** Obstetrics & Gynecology, St Vincents Hosp 1970

Cavallaro, Barbara MD (ObG) - **Hospital:** Hackensack Univ Med Ctr (page 96); **Address:** 170 Prospect Ave Bldg 2 - Ste 4, Hackensack, NJ 07601-2255; **Phone:** 201-488-2288; **Board Cert:** Obstetrics & Gynecology 2009; **Med School:** NYU Sch Med 1986; **Resid:** Obstetrics & Gynecology, Mt Sinai Med Ctr 1990

Coven, Roger MD (ObG) - **Spec Exp:** Pregnancy-High Risk; **Hospital:** Valley Hosp (page 658), Hackensack Univ Med Ctr (page 96); **Address:** 581 N Franklin Tpke, Ramsey, NJ 07446; **Phone:** 201-447-2200; **Board Cert:** Obstetrics & Gynecology 2009; **Med School:** UMDNJ-NJ Med Sch, Newark 1980; **Resid:** Obstetrics & Gynecology, Thomas Jefferson Univ Hosp 1984

Englert, Christopher A MD (ObG) - **Spec Exp:** Gynecologic Surgery; Laparoscopic Surgery; Robotic Surgery; Vulvar & Vaginal Disorders; **Hospital:** Holy Name Med Ctr (page 657); **Address:** 420 Grand Ave, Ste 201, Englewood, NJ 07631-4141; **Phone:** 201-871-4040; **Board Cert:** Obstetrics & Gynecology 2009; **Med School:** Univ Cincinnati 1985; **Resid:** Obstetrics & Gynecology, Thomas Jefferson Univ Hosp 1989

Faust, Michael G MD (ObG) - **Spec Exp:** Pregnancy-High Risk; Menopause Problems; Gynecologic Surgery; Minimally Invasive Surgery; **Hospital:** Valley Hosp (page 658); **Address:** Valley Ctr for Womens Health, 581 N Franklin Tpke, Ramsey, NJ 07446; **Phone:** 201-236-2100; **Board Cert:** Obstetrics & Gynecology 2007; **Med School:** Univ Pittsburgh 1983; **Resid:** Obstetrics & Gynecology, Thos Jefferson Univ Hosp 1987

Hurst, Wendy R MD (ObG) - **Spec Exp:** Gynecology Only; Laparoscopic Surgery; Menopause Problems; Adolescent Gynecology; **Hospital:** Englewood Hosp & Med Ctr (page 656), Hackensack Univ Med Ctr (page 96); **Address:** 370 Grand Ave, Ste 202, Englewood, NJ 07631-4109; **Phone:** 201-894-9599; **Board Cert:** Obstetrics & Gynecology 2009; **Med School:** Tufts Univ 1986; **Resid:** Obstetrics & Gynecology, Hosp Univ Penn 1990

Meyer, Monica L MD (ObG) *PCP* - **Spec Exp:** Adolescent Gynecology; Gynecology Only; Menopause Problems; **Hospital:** Valley Hosp (page 658); **Address:** The Women's Group of Ridgewood, 1 W Ridgewood Ave, Ste 211, Paramus, NJ 07652; **Phone:** 201-251-2323; **Board Cert:** Obstetrics & Gynecology 2009; **Med School:** SUNY Downstate 1991; **Resid:** Obstetrics & Gynecology, Lenox Hill Hosp 1995

Rezvani, Fred F MD (ObG) - **Spec Exp:** Pregnancy-High Risk; Minimally Invasive Surgery; Congenital Anomalies-Gynecologic; **Hospital:** Valley Hosp (page 658); **Address:** 119 Prospect St, Ridgewood, NJ 07450; **Phone:** 201-444-1600; **Board Cert:** Obstetrics & Gynecology 2007; **Med School:** West Indies 1983; **Resid:** Obstetrics & Gynecology, Lincoln Hosp 1988

Rubenstein, Andrew F MD (ObG) - **Hospital:** Hackensack Univ Med Ctr (page 96); **Address:** 82 E Allendale Rd, Ste 1A, Saddle River, NJ 07458; **Phone:** 201-934-5050; **Board Cert:** Obstetrics & Gynecology 2009; **Med School:** Hahnemann Univ 1980; **Resid:** Obstetrics & Gynecology, Mt Sinai Med Ctr 1994; **Fac Appt:** Asst Clin Prof ObG, UMDNJ-NJ Med Sch, Newark

Ophthalmology

Burke, Patricia MD (Oph) - **Spec Exp:** Corneal Disease; Cataract Surgery; **Hospital:** Holy Name Med Ctr (page 657); **Address:** One Sears Drive, Paramus, NJ 07652; **Phone:** 201-599-0123; **Board Cert:** Ophthalmology 1991; **Med School:** UMDNJ-NJ Med Sch, Newark 1986; **Resid:** Ophthalmology, Columbia-Presby Med Ctr 1990; **Fellow:** Cornea, Manhattan EET Hosp 1991

Chin, Patrick K MD (Oph) - **Spec Exp:** Laser Vision Surgery; Cataract Surgery; Refractive Surgery; **Hospital:** Valley Hosp (page 658); **Address:** Westwood Ophthalmology Assocs, 300 Fairview Ave, Westwood, NJ 07675; **Phone:** 201-666-4014; **Board Cert:** Ophthalmology 2007; **Med School:** UMDNJ-NJ Med Sch, Newark 1989; **Resid:** Ophthalmology, NYU Med Ctr 1994; **Fellow:** Ophthalmology, Gimbel Eye Ctr 1995

DeLuca, Joseph A MD (Oph) - **Spec Exp:** Cataract Surgery; Laser Refractive Surgery; Anterior Segment Surgery; Trauma; **Hospital:** Clara Maass Med Ctr; **Address:** 20 Park Ave Fl 1, Lyndhurst, NJ 07071-1012; **Phone:** 201-896-0096; **Board Cert:** Ophthalmology 1991; **Med School:** UMDNJ-Rutgers Med Sch 1985; **Resid:** Ophthalmology, United Hosp Med Ctr 1990; **Fac Appt:** Asst Clin Prof Oph, UMDNJ-NJ Med Sch, Newark

Hersh, Peter MD (Oph) - **Spec Exp:** LASIK-Refractive Surgery; Cornea Transplant; Keratoconus; **Hospital:** Robert Wood Johnson Univ Hosp - New Brunswick; **Address:** 300 Frank W Burr Blvd, Ste 71, Teaneck, NJ 07666-6704; **Phone:** 201-883-0505; **Board Cert:** Ophthalmology 1987; **Med School:** Johns Hopkins Univ 1982; **Resid:** Internal Medicine, Lenox Hill Hosp 1983; Ophthalmology, Mass Eye & Ear Infirm 1986; **Fellow:** Cornea & Ext Eye Disease, Mass Eye & Ear Infirm 1987; **Fac Appt:** Prof Oph, UMDNJ-NJ Med Sch, Newark

Liva, Douglas MD (Oph) - **Spec Exp:** LASIK-Refractive Surgery; Cataract Surgery; Glaucoma; **Hospital:** Valley Hosp (page 658); **Address:** 1 W Ridgewood Ave, Ste 101, Paramus, NJ 07652-2350; **Phone:** 201-444-7770; **Board Cert:** Ophthalmology 1987; **Med School:** Univ Miami Sch Med 1981; **Resid:** Ophthalmology, UMDNJ Affil Hosps 1986

Silbert, Glenn MD (Oph) - **Spec Exp:** Cataract Surgery; Lens Implants; **Hospital:** Hackensack Univ Med Ctr (page 96), New York Eye & Ear Infirm (page 113); **Address:** 316 State St, Hackensack, NJ 07601-5529; **Phone:** 201-342-8115; **Board Cert:** Ophthalmology 1985; **Med School:** Columbia P&S 1979; **Resid:** Ophthalmology, NYU Med Ctr 1983; **Fac Appt:** Assoc Prof Oph, NY Med Coll

Solomon, Edward MD (Oph) - **Spec Exp:** Cataract Surgery; Laser Surgery; **Hospital:** Valley Hosp (page 658); **Address:** 85 S Maple Ave, Ridgewood, NJ 07450-4500; **Phone:** 201-444-3010; **Board Cert:** Ophthalmology 1976; **Med School:** Tufts Univ 1968; **Resid:** Ophthalmology, NYU Med Ctr 1974

Stabile, John R MD (Oph) - **Spec Exp:** Cataract Surgery; Oculoplastic Surgery; LASIK-Refractive Surgery; **Hospital:** Englewood Hosp & Med Ctr (page 656), Holy Name Med Ctr (page 657); **Address:** 111 Dean Drive, Tenafly, NJ 07670-2764; **Phone:** 201-567-5995; **Board Cert:** Ophthalmology 1981; **Med School:** NY Med Coll 1976; **Resid:** Ophthalmology, St Lukes-Roosevelt Hosp Ctr 1980; **Fellow:** Oculoplastic Surgery, Columbia-Presby Med Ctr 1981; **Fac Appt:** Clin Prof Oph, Columbia P&S

Topilow, Harvey MD (Oph) - **Spec Exp:** Retinal Disorders; Macular Degeneration; Retinopathy of Prematurity; **Hospital:** New York Eye & Ear Infirm (page 113); **Address:** 301 Brdige Plaza N, Fort Lee, NJ 07024; **Phone:** 212-288-3860; **Board Cert:** Ophthalmology 1980; **Med School:** Columbia P&S 1975; **Resid:** Ophthalmology, Albert Einstein 1979; **Fellow:** Vitreoretinal Surgery, Mass Eye & Ear Infirmary 1981; **Fac Appt:** Assoc Clin Prof Oph, Albert Einstein Coll Med

Weinberg, Martin R MD (Oph) - **Spec Exp:** Neuro-Ophthalmology; Glaucoma; **Hospital:** Englewood Hosp & Med Ctr (page 656), Hackensack Univ Med Ctr (page 96); **Address:** 405 Cedar Ln, Ste 5, Teaneck, NJ 07666-1715; **Phone:** 201-836-8333; **Board Cert:** Ophthalmology 1989; **Med School:** Eastern VA Med Sch 1979; **Resid:** Surgery, Albany Memorial Hosp 1981; Ophthalmology, Kings County Hosp 1986; **Fellow:** Ocular Pathology, Scheie Eye Inst-Univ Penn 1983; Ocular Oncology, Manhattan EET Hosp 1988

Orthopaedic Surgery

Altman, Wayne MD (OrS) - **Spec Exp:** Carpal Tunnel Syndrome; Knee Injuries; Hand & Wrist Injuries; Shoulder Injuries; **Hospital:** Meadowlands Hosp Med Ctr, Mountainside Hosp; **Address:** 85 Orient Way, FL 1, Rutherford, NJ 07070-2045; **Phone:** 201-438-5888; **Board Cert:** Orthopaedic Surgery 2009; **Med School:** UMDNJ-NJ Med Sch, Newark 1978; **Resid:** Orthopaedic Surgery, UMDNJ-Newark 1983; **Fellow:** Hand Surgery, Thomas Jefferson Univ Hosp 1984

Berman, Mark MD (OrS) - **Spec Exp:** Knee Surgery; Shoulder Surgery; Rotator Cuff Surgery; Sports Medicine; **Hospital:** Hackensack Univ Med Ctr (page 96), Holy Name Med Ctr (page 657); **Address:** 211 Essex St, Ste 402, Hackensack, NJ 07601-3246; **Phone:** 201-489-8250; **Board Cert:** Orthopaedic Surgery 2009; **Med School:** Mount Sinai Sch Med 1981; **Resid:** Surgery, Mount Sinai Hosp 1983; Orthopaedic Surgery, Univ Hosp 1986; **Fellow:** Sports Medicine, Lenox Hill Hosp 1987

Doidge, Robert DO (OrS) - **Spec Exp:** Knee Surgery; Shoulder Surgery; Sports Medicine; **Hospital:** Englewood Hosp & Med Ctr (page 656); **Address:** 370 Grand Ave, Ste 100, Englewood, NJ 07631-4109; **Phone:** 201-567-5700; **Med School:** Philadelphia Coll Osteo Med 1986; **Resid:** Orthopaedic Surgery, Oakland Genl Hosp 1991; **Fellow:** Sports Medicine, Michigan State Univ 1992

Esformes, Ira MD (OrS) - **Spec Exp:** Sports Medicine; Arthroscopic Surgery; Joint Replacement; **Hospital:** Valley Hosp (page 658), Hackensack Univ Med Ctr (page 96); **Address:** 440 Old Hook Rd Fl 2, Emerson, NJ 07630-1325; **Phone:** 201-261-3333; **Board Cert:** Orthopaedic Surgery 1985; Orthopaedic Sports Medicine 2009; **Med School:** Albany Med Coll 1977; **Resid:** Surgery, North Shore Univ Hosp 1979; Orthopaedic Surgery, Hosp For Joint Diseases 1983

Gennace, Ronald MD (OrS) - **Hospital:** Clara Maass Med Ctr, Saint Michael's Med Ctr; **Address:** 312 Belleville Tpke, Ste 2A, North Arlington, NJ 07031; **Phone:** 201-997-8777; **Board Cert:** Orthopaedic Surgery 1982; **Med School:** UMDNJ-NJ Med Sch, Newark 1976; **Resid:** Orthopaedic Surgery, St Joseph's Hosp & Med Ctr 1980

Hartzband, Mark A MD (OrS) - **Spec Exp:** Knee Replacement; Hip Replacement; **Hospital:** Hackensack Univ Med Ctr (page 96); **Address:** 10 Forest Ave, Paramus, NJ 07652; **Phone:** 201-291-4040; **Board Cert:** Orthopaedic Surgery 2007; **Med School:** McGill Univ 1978; **Resid:** Surgery, Montefiore Hosp Med Ctr 1981; Orthopaedic Surgery, Montefiore Hosp Med Ctr 1984

Lloyd, J Mervyn MD (OrS) - **Spec Exp:** Joint Replacement; Sports Medicine; **Hospital:** Valley Hosp (page 658); **Address:** 221 Old Hook Rd, Westwood, NJ 07675; **Phone:** 201-666-0013; **Board Cert:** Orthopaedic Surgery 2007; **Med School:** England, UK 1971; **Resid:** Orthopaedic Surgery, St George's Hosp 1981; Orthopaedic Surgery, Mt Carmel Mercy Hosp 1983

McIlveen, Stephen J MD (OrS) - **Spec Exp:** Joint Replacement; Sports Medicine; Shoulder Surgery; Knee Surgery; **Hospital:** Valley Hosp (page 658), Hackensack Univ Med Ctr (page 96); **Address:** 1 W Ridgewood Ave, Ste 307, Paramus, NJ 07652; **Phone:** 201-670-6702; **Board Cert:** Orthopaedic Surgery 1983; **Med School:** NYU Sch Med 1973; **Resid:** Surgery, Columbia Presby Med Ctr 1975; Orthopaedic Surgery, Columbia Presby Med Ctr 1978; **Fellow:** Joint Replacement Surgery, Columbia Presby Med Ctr 1979; Elbow & Shoulder Surgery, Columbia Presby Med Ctr 1979; **Fac Appt:** Asst Prof OrS, Columbia P&S

Pizzurro, Joseph MD (OrS) - **Spec Exp:** Hip & Knee Replacement; Joint Replacement; **Hospital:** Valley Hosp (page 658); **Address:** 85 S Maple Ave Fl 2, Ridgewood, NJ 07450-4561; **Phone:** 201-445-2830; **Board Cert:** Orthopaedic Surgery 1972; **Med School:** St Louis Univ 1963; **Resid:** Surgery, Bronx VA Hosp 1968; Orthopaedic Surgery, Bellevue Hosp Ctr/NYU 1971; **Fellow:** Orthopaedic Surgery, Amer Acad Ortho Surg 1975

Pollock, Roger G MD (OrS) - **Spec Exp:** Rotator Cuff Surgery; Shoulder Arthroscopic Surgery; Shoulder Injuries; **Hospital:** NY-Presby Hosp/Columbia (page 104), Valley Hosp (page 658); **Address:** 1 W Ridgewood Ave, Ste 202, Paramus, NJ 07652; **Phone:** 201-612-9774; **Board Cert:** Orthopaedic Surgery 2005; **Med School:** Columbia P&S 1985; **Resid:** Surgery, St Luke's-Roosevelt 1987; Orthopaedic Surgery, Columbia-Presby Med Ctr 1991; **Fellow:** Shoulder Surgery, Columbia-Presby Med Ctr 1992; **Fac Appt:** Asst Prof OrS, Columbia P&S

Salzer Jr, Richard L MD (OrS) - **Spec Exp:** Hip & Knee Replacement; Knee Surgery; Joint Replacement; Minimally Invasive Surgery; **Hospital:** Englewood Hosp & Med Ctr (page 656), Palisades Med Ctr; **Address:** 401 S Van Brunt St Fl 3rd, Englewood, NJ 07631-4800; **Phone:** 201-569-2770; **Board Cert:** Orthopaedic Surgery 1979; **Med School:** Tufts Univ 1973; **Resid:** Surgery, St Paul's Hosp 1975; Orthopaedic Surgery, Hosp Special Surgery 1978

Otolaryngology

Eisenberg, Lee MD (Oto) - **Spec Exp:** Pediatric Otolaryngology; Thyroid Surgery; Ear Surgery; **Hospital:** Englewood Hosp & Med Ctr (page 656), Hackensack Univ Med Ctr (page 96); **Address:** 177 N Dean St, South Penthouse, Englewood, NJ 07631-2527; **Phone:** 201-567-2771; **Board Cert:** Otolaryngology 1977; **Med School:** SUNY Hlth Sci Ctr 1971; **Resid:** Surgery, Valley Med Ctr 1974; Otolaryngology, UCSF Med Ctr 1977; **Fac Appt:** Assoc Clin Prof Oto, Columbia P&S

Garay, Kenneth MD (Oto) - **Spec Exp:** Nasal & Sinus Disorders; **Hospital:** Meadowlands Hosp Med Ctr; **Address:** 475 Grand Ave, Englewood, NJ 07631-4956; **Phone:** 201-871-4545; **Board Cert:** Otolaryngology 1982; **Med School:** Temple Univ 1978; **Resid:** Surgery, Abington Meml Hosp 1979; Otolaryngology, Columbia-Presby 1982

Henick, David H MD (Oto) - **Spec Exp:** Nasal & Sinus Surgery; Endoscopic Sinus Surgery; Head & Neck Surgery; **Hospital:** Englewood Hosp & Med Ctr (page 656), Hackensack Univ Med Ctr (page 96); **Address:** 301 Bridge Plz N Fl 3, Fort Lee, NJ 07024-5059; **Phone:** 201-592-8200; **Board Cert:** Otolaryngology 1993; **Med School:** SUNY Buffalo 1987; **Resid:** Otolaryngology, Montefiore Med Ctr 1992; **Fellow:** Head and Neck Surgery, Montefiore Med Ctr 1993; Rhinoplasty & Sinus Surgery, Hosp Univ Penn 1994; **Fac Appt:** Asst Clin Prof Oto, UMDNJ-NJ Med Sch, Newark

Ho, Bryan MD (Oto) - **Spec Exp:** Sinus Surgery; Thyroid & Parathyroid Surgery; **Hospital:** Englewood Hosp & Med Ctr (page 656), Holy Name Med Ctr (page 657); **Address:** 216 Engle St, Ste 101, Englewood, NJ 07631-2428; **Phone:** 201-816-9800; **Board Cert:** Otolaryngology 1995; **Med School:** Mount Sinai Sch Med 1989; **Resid:** Surgery, Mt Sinai Med Ctr 1991; Otolaryngology, Mt Sinai Med Ctr 1994

Katz, Harry MD (Oto) - **Spec Exp:** Sinus Disorders; **Hospital:** Valley Hosp (page 658); **Address:** 44 Godwin Ave, Midland Park, NJ 07432-1959; **Phone:** 201-445-2900; **Board Cert:** Otolaryngology 1982; **Med School:** NYU Sch Med 1977; **Resid:** Otolaryngology, NYU Med Ctr-Bellevue 1981

Low, Ronald B MD (Oto) - **Spec Exp:** Head & Neck Surgery; Rhinoplasty; Sinus Surgery; **Hospital:** Hackensack Univ Med Ctr (page 96); **Address:** 20 Prospect Ave, Ste 909, Hackensack, NJ 07601-5013; **Phone:** 201-489-6520; **Board Cert:** Otolaryngology 1974; **Med School:** UMDNJ-NJ Med Sch, Newark 1969; **Resid:** Surgery, Montefiore Hosp 1971; Otolaryngology, NYU-Bellevue Hosp Ctr 1974; **Fac Appt:** Asst Clin Prof Oto

Milgrim, Laurence M MD (Oto) - **Spec Exp:** Facial Plastic Surgery; **Hospital:** Holy Name Med Ctr (page 657), Valley Hosp (page 658); **Address:** New Jersey ENT Assocs, 1 Degraw Ave, Teaneck, NJ 07666; **Phone:** 201-837-2174; **Board Cert:** Otolaryngology 1995; Facial Plastic & Reconstr Surgery 2000; **Med School:** UMDNJ-Rutgers Med Sch 1989; **Resid:** Otolaryngology, Montefiore Med Ctr 1995; **Fellow:** Facial Plastic & Reconstr Surgery, Mt Sinai Med Ctr 1995

Rosen, Arie MD (Oto) - **Spec Exp:** Head & Neck Tumors; Sinus Disorders; Facial Plastic Surgery; Ear Surgery; **Hospital:** Hackensack Univ Med Ctr (page 96), Englewood Hosp & Med Ctr (page 656); **Address:** 2 S Summit Ave, Hackensack, NJ 07601-1117; **Phone:** 201-996-9200; **Board Cert:** Otolaryngology 1995; **Med School:** Israel 1982; **Resid:** Otolaryngology, Univ of Chicago-Pritzker Sch of Medicine 1994; **Fellow:** Otolaryngology, Lenox Hill Hosp 1989

Scherl, Michael MD (Oto) - **Spec Exp:** Hearing Loss/Tinnitus; Nasal & Sinus Disorders; **Hospital:** Englewood Hosp & Med Ctr (page 656); **Address:** 219 Old Hook Rd, Westwood, NJ 07675; **Phone:** 201-666-8787; **Board Cert:** Otolaryngology 1987; **Med School:** Albany Med Coll 1982; **Resid:** Surgery, Mount Sinai 1984; Otolaryngology, Mount Sinai 1987; **Fac Appt:** , Mount Sinai Sch Med

Surow, Jason B MD (Oto) - **Spec Exp:** Pediatric Otolaryngology; Sinus Disorders; Voice Disorders; **Hospital:** Valley Hosp (page 658), Good Samaritan Hosp - Suffern; **Address:** 690 Kinderkamack Rd, Ste 101, Oradell, NJ 07649; **Phone:** 201-722-9850; **Board Cert:** Otolaryngology 1987; **Med School:** Univ Pennsylvania 1982; **Resid:** Surgery, Hosp Univ Penn 1984; Otolaryngology, Hosp Univ Penn 1987

Tobias, Geoffrey W MD (Oto) - **Spec Exp:** Rhinoplasty Revision; Nasal Surgery; Nasal Reconstruction; **Hospital:** Englewood Hosp & Med Ctr (page 656), Mount Sinai Med Ctr (page 102); **Address:** 214 Engle St, Ste 22, Englewood, NJ 07631; **Phone:** 201-567-6770; **Board Cert:** Otolaryngology 1978; **Med School:** Tufts Univ 1973; **Resid:** Otolaryngology, Mt Sinai Med Ctr 1978

Pain Medicine

Ragukonis, Thomas P MD (PM) - ; **Address:** Bergen Pain Management, 30 W Century Rd, Ste 310, Paramus, NJ 07652; **Phone:** 201-634-9000; **Board Cert:** Anesthesiology 1999; Pain Medicine 2000; **Med School:** UMDNJ-NJ Med Sch, Newark 1991; **Resid:** Anesthesiology, Columbia Presby Med Ctr 1995; **Fac Appt:** Asst Clin Prof Anes, UMDNJ-NJ Med Sch, Newark

Pathology

Sanchez, Miguel A MD (Path) - **Spec Exp:** Breast Cancer; Thyroid Cancer; **Hospital:** Englewood Hosp & Med Ctr (page 656); **Address:** Englewood Hosp & Med Ctr, Dept Pathology, 350 Engle St, Englewood, NJ 07631-1898; **Phone:** 201-894-3423; **Board Cert:** Anatomic Pathology 1975; Clinical Pathology 1979; Cytopathology 1991; **Med School:** Spain 1969; **Resid:** Pathology, Englewood Hosp 1972; Pathology, Temple Univ 1973; **Fellow:** Pathology, Meml Sloan Kettering Cancer Ctr 1974; Clinical Pathology, St Vincents Hosp 1975; **Fac Appt:** Assoc Prof Path, Mount Sinai Sch Med

Pediatric Allergy & Immunology

Colenda, Maryann MD (PA&I) - **Spec Exp:** Asthma-Adult & Pediatric; Allergy; **Hospital:** Englewood Hosp & Med Ctr (page 656), Meadowlands Hosp Med Ctr; **Address:** 811 Abbott Blvd, Fort Lee, NJ 07024-4116; **Phone:** 201-224-2256; **Board Cert:** Pediatrics 1976; Allergy & Immunology 1979; **Med School:** NY Med Coll 1971; **Resid:** Pediatrics, Columbia Presby Med Ctr 1974; **Fellow:** Allergy & Immunology, Columbia Presby Med Ctr 1978; **Fac Appt:** Assoc Clin Prof Ped, Columbia P&S

Hicks, Patricia MD (PA&I) - **Spec Exp:** Asthma & Sinusitis; Asthma in Pregnancy; **Hospital:** Valley Hosp (page 658); **Address:** 119 1st St, Hohokus, NJ 07423-1575; **Phone:** 201-444-5277; **Board Cert:** Pediatrics 1978; Allergy & Immunology 2001; **Med School:** Penn State Univ-Hershey Med Ctr 1973; **Resid:** Pediatrics, Columbia-Presby Med Ctr 1976; **Fellow:** Allergy & Immunology, Columbia-Presby Med Ctr 1981

Pediatric Cardiology

Messina, John J MD (PCd) - **Spec Exp:** Critical Care; Interventional Cardiology; Congenital Heart Disease; **Hospital:** St Joseph's Regl Med Ctr - Paterson, Valley Hosp (page 658); **Address:** 1 Broadway, Ste 203, Elmwood Park, NJ 07407-1844; **Phone:** 973-569-6250; **Board Cert:** Pediatrics 2002; Pediatric Cardiology 2009; **Med School:** West Indies 1986; **Resid:** Pediatrics, St Joseph's Hosp 1989; **Fellow:** Pediatric Cardiology, NY Hosp 1992; **Fac Appt:** Asst Prof Ped, Columbia P&S

Tozzi, Robert J MD (PCd) - **Spec Exp:** Hypertrophic Cardiomyopathy; Fetal Echocardiography; Sports Medicine; **Hospital:** Hackensack Univ Med Ctr (page 96); **Address:** 155 Polifly Rd Fl 1 - Ste 106, Hackensack, NJ 07601; **Phone:** 201-487-7617; **Board Cert:** Pediatrics 1987; Pediatric Cardiology 2006; **Med School:** UMDNJ-NJ Med Sch, Newark 1983; **Resid:** Pediatrics, UMDNJ Univ Hosp 1987; **Fellow:** Pediatric Cardiology, NYU Med Ctr 1991

Pediatric Hematology-Oncology

Diamond, Steven MD (PHO) - **Spec Exp:** Pediatric Cancers; Sickle Cell Disease; Hemophilia; **Hospital:** Hackensack Univ Med Ctr (page 96); **Address:** 30 Prospect Ave, Hackensack, NJ 07601-1914; **Phone:** 201-996-5437; **Board Cert:** Pediatrics 1979; Pediatric Hematology-Oncology 1980; **Med School:** Univ Pennsylvania 1974; **Resid:** Pediatrics, Mount Sinai Hosp 1977; **Fellow:** Pediatric Hematology-Oncology, Beth Israel Hosp 1979; **Fac Appt:** Asst Clin Prof Ped, UMDNJ-NJ Med Sch, Newark

Flug, Frances MD (PHO) - **Spec Exp:** Bleeding/Coagulation Disorders; Sickle Cell Disease; Pediatric Cancers; **Hospital:** Hackensack Univ Med Ctr (page 96), Saint Michael's Med Ctr; **Address:** 30 Prospect Ave, FL 1, Hackensack, NJ 07601-2129; **Phone:** 201-996-5437; **Board Cert:** Pediatrics 1984; Pediatric Hematology-Oncology 1984; **Med School:** SUNY Downstate 1979; **Resid:** Pediatrics, Bellevue/NYU Med Ctr 1982; **Fellow:** Pediatric Hematology-Oncology, Bellevue/NYU Med Ctr 1984; **Fac Appt:** Assoc Prof Ped, UMDNJ-NJ Med Sch, Newark

Halpern, Steven MD (PHO) - **Spec Exp:** Leukemia & Lymphoma; Brain Tumors; Hodgkin's Disease; Hemophilia; **Hospital:** Hackensack Univ Med Ctr (page 96); **Address:** 30 Prospect Ave, Ste TCI, Hackensack, NJ 07601; **Phone:** 201-996-5437; **Board Cert:** Pediatrics 1981; Pediatric Hematology-Oncology 1982; **Med School:** Ros Franklin Univ/Chicago Med Sch 1976; **Resid:** Pediatrics, St Christophers Hosp for Children 1979; **Fellow:** Pediatric Hematology-Oncology, Childrens Hosp 1982; **Fac Appt:** Asst Prof Ped, UMDNJ-NJ Med Sch, Newark

Harris, Michael B MD (PHO) - **Spec Exp:** Leukemia & Lymphoma; Bone Tumors; Cancer Survivors-Late Effects of Therapy; **Hospital:** Hackensack Univ Med Ctr (page 96); **Address:** Tomorrows Chldns Inst, JM Sanzari Chldns Hosp, 30 Prospect Ave, Imus 1-TCI, rm PC116, Hackensack, NJ 07601; **Phone:** 201-996-5437; **Board Cert:** Pediatrics 1974; Pediatric Hematology-Oncology 1974; **Med School:** Albert Einstein Coll Med 1969; **Resid:** Pediatrics, Chldns Hosp 1971; **Fellow:** Pediatric Hematology-Oncology, Chldns Hosp 1974; **Fac Appt:** Prof Ped, UMDNJ-NJ Med Sch, Newark

Pediatric Infectious Disease

Boscamp, Jeffrey R MD (PInf) - **Spec Exp:** Fevers of Unknown Origin; Lyme Disease; **Hospital:** Hackensack Univ Med Ctr (page 96); **Address:** 30 Prospect Ave, Don Imus Pediatric Bldg, Hackensack Univ Med Ctr PC 360, Hackensack, NJ 07601; **Phone:** 201-996-5308; **Board Cert:** Pediatrics 1986; Pediatric Infectious Disease 2009; **Med School:** NY Med Coll 1981; **Resid:** Pediatrics, Columbia-Presby Med Ctr 1984; Internal Medicine, Greenwich Hosp 1985; **Fellow:** Infectious Disease, Montefiore Med Ctr 1987; **Fac Appt:** Assoc Prof Ped, UMDNJ-Univ Med Dent NJ

Pediatric Nephrology

Lieberman, Kenneth MD (PNep) - **Spec Exp:** Nephrotic Syndrome; Glomerulonephritis; Dialysis Care; Kidney Failure-Chronic; **Hospital:** Hackensack Univ Med Ctr (page 96); **Address:** The Joseph M Sanzari Chlds Hosp, 30 Prospect Ave, Hackensack, NJ 07601; **Phone:** 201-336-8228; **Board Cert:** Pediatrics 1981; Pediatric Nephrology 1982; **Med School:** Albert Einstein Coll Med 1977; **Resid:** Pediatrics, Mount Sinai Hosp 1979; **Fellow:** Nephrology, New York Hosp-Cornell 1981; **Fac Appt:** Prof Ped, UMDNJ-NJ Med Sch, Newark

Pediatric Otolaryngology

Respler, Don MD (PO) - **Spec Exp:** Airway Disorders; Sinus Disorders; Head & Neck Tumors; Sleep Disorders/Apnea; **Hospital:** Hackensack Univ Med Ctr (page 96), Valley Hosp (page 658); **Address:** 2 South Summit Ave, Hackensack, NJ 07601-1117; **Phone:** 201-996-9200; **Board Cert:** Otolaryngology 1986; **Med School:** Mount Sinai Sch Med 1981; **Resid:** Surgery, Beth Israel Hosp 1983; Otolaryngology, UMDNJ-NJ Med Sch 1986; **Fellow:** Pediatric Otolaryngology, Chldns Hosp 1988; **Fac Appt:** Asst Clin Prof S, UMDNJ-NJ Med Sch, Newark

Pediatric Pulmonology

Kanengiser, Steven MD (PPul) - **Spec Exp:** Asthma; Cough-Chronic; Sleep Disorders; **Hospital:** Valley Hosp (page 658), St Joseph's Regl Med Ctr - Paterson; **Address:** 505 Goffle Rd, Ridgewood, NJ 07450-4027; **Phone:** 201-447-8026; **Board Cert:** Pediatrics 2003; Pediatric Pulmonology 2009; **Med School:** UCSF 1984; **Resid:** Pediatrics, Children's Hosp 1987; **Fellow:** Pediatric Pulmonology, Westchester Med Ctr 1994; **Fac Appt:** Asst Clin Prof Ped, Columbia P&S

Pediatric Rheumatology

Haines, Kathleen A MD (PRhu) - **Spec Exp:** Juvenile Arthritis; Lupus/SLE; Immune Deficiency; Scleroderma; **Hospital:** Hackensack Univ Med Ctr (page 96), NYU Langone Med Ctr (page 106); **Address:** Hackensack Univ Med Ctr, Don Imus Pediatric Ctr, 30 Prospect Ave Fl 3, Hackensack, NJ 07601; **Phone:** 201-996-5306; **Board Cert:** Pediatrics 1980; Allergy & Immunology 1981; Pediatric Rheumatology 2007; **Med School:** Albert Einstein Coll Med 1975; **Resid:** Pediatrics, New York Hosp 1977; **Fellow:** Allergy & Immunology, New York Hosp 1980; Rheumatology, NYU Med Sch 1982; **Fac Appt:** Assoc Prof Ped, UMDNJ-NJ Med Sch, Newark

Kimura, Yukiko MD (PRhu) - **Spec Exp:** Juvenile Arthritis; Lupus/SLE; Dermatomyositis; Vasculitis; **Hospital:** Hackensack Univ Med Ctr (page 96); **Address:** Hackensack Univ Med Ctr, 30 Prospect Ave, Hackensack, NJ 07601-1915; **Phone:** 201-996-5306; **Board Cert:** Pediatrics 1987; Pediatric Rheumatology 2007; **Med School:** Albert Einstein Coll Med 1982; **Resid:** Pediatrics, Babies Hosp/Columbia Presby 1985; **Fellow:** Pediatric Rheumatology, Babies Hosp/Columbia Presby 1991; **Fac Appt:** Assoc Prof Ped, UMDNJ-NJ Med Sch, Newark

Pediatric Surgery

Alexander, Frederick MD (PS) - **Spec Exp:** Inflammatory Bowel Disease; Solid Tumors; Congenital Anomalies-Gastrointestinal; **Hospital:** Hackensack Univ Med Ctr (page 96); **Address:** Joseph M Sanzari Chldns Hosp-HUMC, 30 Prospect Ave, Ste PC311, Hackensack, NJ 07601; **Phone:** 201-996-2921; **Board Cert:** Pediatric Surgery 1999; **Med School:** Columbia P&S 1977; **Resid:** Surgery, Brigham-Womens Hosp 1984; **Fellow:** Pediatric Surgery, Chldns Hosp 1986; **Fac Appt:** Clin Prof S

Friedman, David L MD (PS) - **Spec Exp:** Neonatal Surgery; Gastroesophageal Reflux Disease (GERD); Laparoscopic Surgery; **Hospital:** Valley Hosp (page 658), Hackensack Univ Med Ctr (page 96); **Address:** 30 W Century Rd, Ste 235, Paramus, NJ 07652-1433; **Phone:** 201-225-9440; **Board Cert:** Pediatric Surgery 2009; **Med School:** SUNY Downstate 1971; **Resid:** Surgery, Univ Hosp 1976; **Fellow:** Pediatric Surgery, Univ Hosp 1977; **Fac Appt:** Asst Prof S, Columbia P&S

Gandhi, Rajinder MD (PS) - **Spec Exp:** Gastrointestinal Surgery; Laparoscopic Surgery; Chest Wall Deformities; **Hospital:** Valley Hosp (page 658); **Address:** 30 W Century Rd, Ste 235, Paramus, NJ 07652; **Phone:** 201-225-9440; **Board Cert:** Surgery 1975; Pediatric Surgery 2007; **Med School:** Burma 1966; **Resid:** Surgery, Montefiore Med Ctr-Einstein Div 1974; Pediatric Surgery, Columbia-Presby Med Ctr 1977; **Fellow:** Gastroenterology, Columbia-Presby Med Ctr 1975; **Fac Appt:** Assoc Clin Prof S, Columbia P&S

Valda, Victor MD (PS) - **Spec Exp:** Congenital Anomalies; Cancer Surgery; **Hospital:** Hackensack Univ Med Ctr (page 96); **Address:** 30 W Century Rd, Ste 235, Paramus, NJ 07652; **Phone:** 201-225-9440; **Board Cert:** Surgery 1974; Pediatric Surgery 2007; **Med School:** Bolivia 1962; **Resid:** Surgery, Mt Zion Hosp 1968; Surgery, Maricopa Med Ctr 1972; **Fellow:** Pediatric Surgery, St Christopher's Hosp 1974

Pediatrics

Asnes, Russell MD (Ped) *PCP* - **Spec Exp:** Diagnostic Problems; **Hospital:** Englewood Hosp & Med Ctr (page 656), Hackensack Univ Med Ctr (page 96); **Address:** 32 Franklin St, Tenafly, NJ 07670-2005; **Phone:** 201-569-2400; **Board Cert:** Pediatrics 1969; **Med School:** Tufts Univ 1963; **Resid:** Pediatrics, Johns Hopkins Hosp 1966; Pediatrics, Johns Hopkins Hosp 1969; **Fellow:** Neonatology, Babies Hosp/Columbia 1970; **Fac Appt:** Clin Prof Ped, Columbia P&S

Buchalter, Maury MD (Ped) *PCP* - **Spec Exp:** Asthma; Infectious Disease; ADD/ADHD; **Hospital:** Hackensack Univ Med Ctr (page 96), Englewood Hosp & Med Ctr (page 656); **Address:** 301 Bridge Plaza N, Fort Lee, NJ 07670; **Phone:** 201-592-8787; **Board Cert:** Pediatrics 2003; **Med School:** Mount Sinai Sch Med 1984; **Resid:** Pediatrics, Mt Sinai Hosp 1987; **Fellow:** Infectious Disease, Chldns Hosp 1988

Hages, Harry A MD (Ped) *PCP* - **Hospital:** Englewood Hosp & Med Ctr (page 656), Valley Hosp (page 658); **Address:** 215 Old Tappan Rd, Old Tappan, NJ 07675-7000; **Phone:** 201-666-1001; **Board Cert:** Pediatrics 1973; **Med School:** Univ Pittsburgh 1966; **Resid:** Pediatrics, Chldns Hosp 1968; Pediatrics, New York Hosp 1969

Harlow, Paul MD (Ped) *PCP* - **Spec Exp:** Anemia; Bleeding/Coagulation Disorders; **Hospital:** Hackensack Univ Med Ctr (page 96), Valley Hosp (page 658); **Address:** 90 Prospect Ave, Ste 1A, Hackensack, NJ 07601; **Phone:** 201-342-4001 x104; **Board Cert:** Pediatrics 1979; Pediatric Hematology-Oncology 1980; **Med School:** SUNY Hlth Sci Ctr 1974; **Resid:** Pediatrics, Jacobi Med Ctr 1977; **Fellow:** Pediatric Hematology-Oncology, Children's Hosp 1979

Hyatt, Alexander C MD (Ped) *PCP* - **Hospital:** Englewood Hosp & Med Ctr (page 656), Mount Sinai Med Ctr (page 102); **Address:** Englewood Hosp, Dept Pediatrics, 350 Engle St, Englewood, NJ 07631; **Phone:** 201-894-3158; **Board Cert:** Pediatrics 1980; Infectious Disease 2009; **Med School:** Mount Sinai Sch Med 1975; **Resid:** Pediatrics, Johns Hopkins Hosp 1978; **Fellow:** Infectious Disease, Mount Sinai Med Ctr 1979; Pediatric Pulmonology, Johns Hopkins Hosp 1980; **Fac Appt:** Assoc Prof Ped, Mount Sinai Sch Med

Kanter, Alan MD (Ped) *PCP* - **Spec Exp:** ADD/ADHD; Autism; **Hospital:** Englewood Hosp & Med Ctr (page 656), NYPresby-Morgan Stanley Children's Hosp (page 104); **Address:** 704 Palisade Ave, Teaneck, NJ 07666-3198; **Phone:** 201-836-4301; **Board Cert:** Pediatrics 1977; **Med School:** Albert Einstein Coll Med 1970; **Resid:** Pediatrics, St Christopher's Hosp 1971; Pediatrics, Montefiore Med Ctr 1975; **Fac Appt:** Assoc Clin Prof Ped, Columbia P&S

Kolsky, Neil MD (Ped) *PCP* - **Hospital:** Holy Name Med Ctr (page 657), Hackensack Univ Med Ctr (page 96); **Address:** 870 Palisade Ave, Teaneck, NJ 07666-3419; **Phone:** 201-692-1661; **Board Cert:** Pediatrics 1972; **Med School:** UMDNJ-NJ Med Sch, Newark 1966; **Resid:** Pediatrics, Johns Hopkins Hosp 1969

Kushner, Susan C MD (Ped) *PCP* - **Spec Exp:** Atopic Dermatitis; Allergic Rhinitis; Asthma; Otitis Media; **Hospital:** Hackensack Univ Med Ctr (page 96), Valley Hosp (page 658); **Address:** Forrest Pediatrics, 299 Forrest Ave Fl 3, Paramus, NJ 07652; **Phone:** 201-267-0888; **Board Cert:** Pediatrics 2004; **Med School:** SUNY Upstate Med Univ 1986; **Resid:** Pediatrics, LI Jewish Med Ctr 1989

Namerow, David MD (Ped) *PCP* - **Spec Exp:** Behavioral Disorders; Adolescent Medicine; **Hospital:** Valley Hosp (page 658), St Joseph's Regl Med Ctr - Paterson; **Address:** 2020 Fair Lawn Ave, Fair Lawn, NJ 07410-2319; **Phone:** 201-791-4545; **Board Cert:** Pediatrics 1977; **Med School:** Univ Louisville Sch Med 1972; **Resid:** Pediatrics, Children's Hosp 1975; **Fellow:** Adolescent Medicine, Univ MD Hosp 1977; **Fac Appt:** Asst Clin Prof Ped, NY Med Coll

O'Brien, Daryl H MD (Ped) *PCP* - **Hospital:** Valley Hosp (page 658); **Address:** Broadway Pediatric Assocs, 336 Center Ave, Westwood, NJ 07675; **Phone:** 201-664-7444; **Board Cert:** Pediatrics 1986; **Med School:** Dartmouth Med Sch 1979; **Resid:** Pediatrics, Duke Univ Med Ctr 1982

Schuss, Steven A MD (Ped) *PCP* - **Hospital:** Englewood Hosp & Med Ctr (page 656), Hackensack Univ Med Ctr (page 96); **Address:** 197 Cedar Ln, Teaneck, NJ 07666-4301; **Phone:** 201-836-7171; **Board Cert:** Pediatrics 1986; **Med School:** Albert Einstein Coll Med 1979; **Resid:** Pediatrics, Montefiore Hosp Med Ctr 1983; **Fac Appt:** Asst Clin Prof Ped, Albert Einstein Coll Med

Sugarman, Lynn B MD (Ped) *PCP* - **Hospital:** Englewood Hosp & Med Ctr (page 656), Hackensack Univ Med Ctr (page 96); **Address:** 32 Franklin St, Tenafly, NJ 07670-2005; **Phone:** 201-569-2400; **Board Cert:** Pediatrics 1981; **Med School:** Harvard Med Sch 1977; **Resid:** Pediatrics, Bronx Muni Hosp Ctr 1981; **Fellow:** Pediatric Critical Care Medicine, Bronx Muni Hosp Ctr 1983; **Fac Appt:** Assoc Clin Prof Ped, Columbia P&S

Wisotsky, David H MD (Ped) *PCP* - **Hospital:** Englewood Hosp & Med Ctr (page 656), Hackensack Univ Med Ctr (page 96); **Address:** Tenafly Pediatrics, 32 Franklin St, Tenafly, NJ 07670; **Phone:** 201-569-2400; **Board Cert:** Pediatrics 1986; **Med School:** Albert Einstein Coll Med 1974; **Resid:** Pediatrics, Bronx Muni Hosp Ctr 1978; **Fac Appt:** Asst Clin Prof Ped, Columbia P&S

Physical Medicine & Rehabilitation

Liss, Donald MD (PMR) - **Spec Exp:** Pain-Back; Sports Medicine; Osteoarthritis; **Hospital:** NY-Presby Hosp/Columbia (page 104), Englewood Hosp & Med Ctr (page 656); **Address:** 500 Grand Ave, Englewood, NJ 07631-2920; **Phone:** 201-567-2277; **Board Cert:** Physical Medicine & Rehabilitation 1984; **Med School:** Wayne State Univ 1979; **Resid:** Physical Medicine & Rehabilitation, Columbia-Presby Med Ctr 1982; **Fac Appt:** Assoc Clin Prof PMR, Columbia P&S

Zimmerman, Jerald R MD (PMR) - **Spec Exp:** Post Polio Syndrome/Rehabilitation; Musculoskeletal Disorders; Pain Management; **Hospital:** Englewood Hosp & Med Ctr (page 656); **Address:** 370 Grand Ave, Ste 102, Englewood, NJ 07631; **Phone:** 201-567-3370; **Board Cert:** Physical Medicine & Rehabilitation 1989; **Med School:** Univ IL Coll Med 1982; **Resid:** Orthopaedic Surgery, Univ Minn Med Ctr 1985; **Fellow:** Physical Medicine & Rehabilitation, Columbia-Presby Med Ctr 1988

Plastic Surgery

Bikoff, David J MD (PlS) - **Spec Exp:** Cosmetic Surgery-Breast; Breast Reconstruction; Eyelid Surgery; Hand Surgery; **Hospital:** Hackensack Univ Med Ctr (page 96); **Address:** 146 Rte 17 North Fl 3, Hackensack, NJ 07601; **Phone:** 201-488-8584; **Board Cert:** Plastic Surgery 1980; **Med School:** SUNY Downstate 1973; **Resid:** Surgery, Kings Co Hosp 1977; Plastic Surgery, Kings Co Hosp 1979; **Fellow:** Hand Surgery, Kings Co Hosp 1980

D'Amico, Richard A MD (PlS) - **Spec Exp:** Cosmetic Surgery-Face; Cosmetic Surgery-Liposuction; Breast Augmentation; **Hospital:** Englewood Hosp & Med Ctr (page 656), Holy Name Med Ctr (page 657); **Address:** 180 N Dean St, Ste 3NE, Englewood, NJ 07631-2534; **Phone:** 201-567-9595; **Board Cert:** Plastic Surgery 1986; **Med School:** NYU Sch Med 1976; **Resid:** Surgery, Tulsa Med Ctr 1979; Surgery, Strong Meml Hosp 1981; **Fellow:** Plastic/Reconstructive Surgery, Columbia-Presby Med Ctr 1983; **Fac Appt:** Asst Clin Prof PlS, Mount Sinai Sch Med

Lipson, David E MD (PlS) - **Spec Exp:** Breast Augmentation; Body Contouring; Facial Rejuvenation; **Hospital:** Valley Hosp (page 658); **Address:** 2300 Route 208 South, Fair Lawn, NJ 07410; **Phone:** 201-797-7770; **Board Cert:** Plastic Surgery 1981; **Med School:** Albert Einstein Coll Med 1971; **Resid:** Surgery, Bellevue/NYU Med Ctr 1976; Plastic Surgery, Bellevue/NYU Med Ctr 1978

Ofodile, Ferdinand A MD (PlS) - **Spec Exp:** Liposuction; Rhinoplasty; Breast Surgery; **Hospital:** St Luke's - Roosevelt Hosp Ctr - Roosevelt Div (page 94), Harlem Hosp Ctr; **Address:** 84 Woodmont Drive, Woodcliff Lake, NJ 07677; **Phone:** 201-362-5906; **Board Cert:** Surgery 1974; Plastic Surgery 1976; **Med School:** Northwestern Univ 1968; **Resid:** Surgery, Harlem Hosp/Columbia-Presby Hosp 1973; Plastic Surgery, Harlem Hosp/Columbia Presby Hosp 1975; **Fellow:** Plastic Surgery, Mayo Clinic 1976; **Fac Appt:** Clin Prof S, Columbia P&S

Ponamgi, Suri MD (PlS) - **Spec Exp:** Cosmetic & Reconstructive Surgery; **Hospital:** Palisades Med Ctr, Holy Name Med Ctr (page 657); **Address:** 1101 Palisades Ave, Fort Lee, NJ 07024-6329; **Phone:** 201-224-8831; **Board Cert:** Plastic Surgery 1984; **Med School:** India 1970; **Resid:** Surgery, Bronx Lebonon Hosp 1979; Plastic Surgery, NY Methodist Hosp 1982; **Fellow:** Surgery, Bronx Lebonon Hosp 1980

Sternschein, Michael J MD (PlS) - **Spec Exp:** Cosmetic Surgery-Face & Breast; Liposuction & Body Contouring; Laser Surgery; **Hospital:** Hackensack Univ Med Ctr (page 96), Valley Hosp (page 658); **Address:** 1200 E Ridgewood Ave Fl 2 West Wing, Ridgewood, NJ 07450; **Phone:** 201-444-1188; **Board Cert:** Plastic Surgery 1985; **Med School:** Columbia P&S 1976; **Resid:** Surgery, Columbia-Presby Med Ctr 1980; Plastic Surgery, Columbia-Presby Med Ctr 1982; **Fellow:** Microsurgery, Columbia-Presby Med Ctr 1982

Zubowski, Robert I MD (PlS) - **Spec Exp:** Breast Augmentation; Liposuction & Body Contouring; Cosmetic Surgery-Face; **Hospital:** Valley Hosp (page 658); **Address:** 1 Sears Drive Fl 1, Paramus, NJ 07652; **Phone:** 201-261-7550; **Board Cert:** Plastic Surgery 2003; **Med School:** Mexico 1983; **Resid:** Surgery, Westchester Co Med Ctr 1991; **Fellow:** Plastic Surgery, Cleveland Clinic 1994; **Fac Appt:** Asst Clin Prof S, NY Med Coll

Psychiatry

Chertoff, Harvey R MD (Psyc) - **Spec Exp:** Anxiety & Mood Disorders; Psychoanalysis; **Hospital:** Englewood Hosp & Med Ctr (page 656), NY-Presby Hosp/Columbia (page 104); **Address:** 205 Engle St, Englewood, NJ 07631-2409; **Phone:** 201-567-4970; **Board Cert:** Psychiatry 1978; Forensic Psychiatry 1999; **Med School:** Albert Einstein Coll Med 1966; **Resid:** Psychiatry, Columbia-Presby Med Ctr 1970; **Fellow:** Psychoanalysis, Columbia-Psychoanalytic Ctr 1976; **Fac Appt:** Asst Clin Prof Psyc, Columbia P&S

Farkas, Edward MD (Psyc) - **Spec Exp:** Depression in the Elderly; Psychotherapy-Men's Issues; Panic Disorder; **Hospital:** Holy Name Med Ctr (page 657); **Address:** 175 Cedar Ln, Ste A, Teaneck, NJ 07666-4315; **Phone:** 201-692-8354; **Board Cert:** Psychiatry 1988; **Med School:** Italy 1979; **Resid:** Psychiatry, Bronx Lebanon Hosp 1981; Psychiatry, St Luke's-Roosevelt Hosp Ctr 1983; **Fellow:** Psychiatry, William Allison White Inst 1983

Gurland, Frances Effron MD (Psyc) - **Spec Exp:** Eating Disorders; ADD/ADHD; **Address:** 216 Engle St, Englewood, NJ 07631-2444; **Phone:** 201-568-4066; **Board Cert:** Psychiatry 2005; **Med School:** SUNY Hlth Sci Ctr 1989; **Resid:** Psychiatry, St Lukes-Roosevelt Hosp Ctr 1991; **Fellow:** Child & Adolescent Psychiatry, Mount Sinai Hosp 1994; **Fac Appt:** Asst Clin Prof Psyc, Mount Sinai Sch Med

Narula, Amarjot S MD (Psyc) - **Spec Exp:** Geriatric Psychiatry; Mood Disorders; **Hospital:** Valley Hosp (page 658), Bergen Regl Med Ctr; **Address:** 65 N Maple Ave, Ridgewood, NJ 07450-1600; **Phone:** 201-670-4423; **Board Cert:** Psychiatry 1992; Geriatric Psychiatry 2007; **Med School:** India 1979; **Resid:** Psychiatry, Middletown Psychiatric Ctr 1988; **Fellow:** Psychiatry, Metropolitan Hosp 1989

Rosenfeld, David N MD (Psyc) - **Spec Exp:** Mood Disorders; Anxiety Disorders; Personality Disorders; Geriatric Psychiatry; **Hospital:** Valley Hosp (page 658); **Address:** 265 Ackerman Ave, Ste 202, Ridgewood, NJ 07450-4200; **Phone:** 201-447-5630; **Board Cert:** Psychiatry 2005; **Med School:** UMDNJ-RW Johnson Med Sch 1988; **Resid:** Psychiatry, Mount Sinai Sch Med 1990; Psychiatry, Bergen Pines Co 1994

Samuels, Steven MD (Psyc) - **Spec Exp:** Dementia; Depression; Geriatric Psychiatry; **Hospital:** Englewood Hosp & Med Ctr (page 656); **Address:** Englewood Hosp, Behavioral Hlth Unit, 350 Engle St, Englewood, NJ 07631; **Phone:** 201-681-2915; **Board Cert:** Psychiatry 2004; Geriatric Psychiatry 2006; **Med School:** SUNY Buffalo 1989; **Resid:** Psychiatry, St Vincent's Hosp & Med Ctr 1993; **Fellow:** Geriatric Psychiatry, Hosp Univ Penn 1995; **Fac Appt:** Asst Prof Psyc, Mount Sinai Sch Med

Wagle, Sharad MD (Psyc) - **Spec Exp:** Anxiety Disorders; Forensic Psychiatry; Geriatric Psychiatry; **Hospital:** Holy Name Med Ctr (page 657), Pascack Valley Hosp; **Address:** 718 Teaneck Rd, Teaneck, NJ 07666; **Phone:** 201-833-3291; **Board Cert:** Psychiatry 2006; **Med School:** India 1971; **Resid:** Psychiatry, Hackensack Univ Med Ctr 1976; Psychiatry, Albert Einstein Coll Med 1978; **Fellow:** Child & Adolescent Psychiatry, Psychoanalytic Inst 1978

Pulmonary Disease

Birns, Robert I MD (Pul) - **Spec Exp:** Asthma; Emphysema; **Hospital:** Holy Name Med Ctr (page 657), Englewood Hosp & Med Ctr (page 656); **Address:** 200 Grand Ave, Ste 102, Englewood, NJ 07631-4363; **Phone:** 201-871-3636; **Board Cert:** Internal Medicine 1974; Pulmonary Disease 1976; **Med School:** Washington Univ, St Louis 1970; **Resid:** Internal Medicine, Boston City Hosp 1972; **Fellow:** Pulmonary Disease, Boston City Hosp 1973

Brauntuch, Glenn R MD (Pul) - **Spec Exp:** Chronic Obstructive Lung Disease (COPD); Asthma; Lung Cancer; **Hospital:** Englewood Hosp & Med Ctr (page 656), Holy Name Med Ctr (page 657); **Address:** 180 Engle St, Englewood, NJ 07631-2507; **Phone:** 201-567-2050; **Board Cert:** Internal Medicine 1981; Pulmonary Disease 1984; **Med School:** Columbia P&S 1978; **Resid:** Internal Medicine, St Lukes-Roosevelt Hosp 1981; **Fellow:** Pulmonary Disease, NYU Med Ctr 1984

Bromberg, Assia MD (Pul) *PCP* - **Spec Exp:** Asthma; Emphysema; Women's Health; **Hospital:** Valley Hosp (page 658); **Address:** 19-20 Fair Lawn Ave, Fairlawn, NJ 07410; **Phone:** 201-794-1963; **Board Cert:** Internal Medicine 1989; Pulmonary Disease 2004; **Med School:** Israel 1974; **Resid:** Anesthesiology, Chaim Sheba Med Ctr 1981; Internal Medicine, Englewood Hosp 1989; **Fellow:** Pulmonary Disease, Bellevue-NYU Med Ctr 1992; **Fac Appt:** Asst Prof Med, UMDNJ-Univ Med Dent NJ

DiPasquale, Laurene MD (Pul) - **Spec Exp:** Asthma; Sleep Disorders; **Hospital:** Englewood Hosp & Med Ctr (page 656); **Address:** 440 Old Hook Rd, Ste 1-4, Westwood, NJ 07675-2732; **Phone:** 201-664-8663; **Board Cert:** Internal Medicine 2003; **Med School:** Dominican Republic 1982; **Resid:** Internal Medicine, Mountainside Hosp 1988; **Fellow:** Pulmonary Disease, Bronx Lebanon 1990

Engler, Mitchell S MD (Pul) - **Spec Exp:** Pulmonary Disease; Critical Care; Sleep Disorders; **Hospital:** Holy Name Med Ctr (page 657), Englewood Hosp & Med Ctr (page 656); **Address:** 180 Engle St, Englewood, NJ 07631-2507; **Phone:** 201-568-8010; **Board Cert:** Internal Medicine 1981; Pulmonary Disease 1988; Sleep Medicine 2003; **Med School:** Boston Univ 1978; **Resid:** Internal Medicine, St Lukes Hosp 1981; **Fellow:** Pulmonary Disease, St Lukes Hosp 1983

Levine, Selwyn E MD (Pul) - **Spec Exp:** Chronic Obstructive Lung Disease (COPD); Lung Cancer; Asthma; Pneumonia; **Hospital:** Holy Name Med Ctr (page 657), Englewood Hosp & Med Ctr (page 656); **Address:** Pulmonary Assocs of Northern NJ, 200 Grand Ave, Ste 102, Englewood, NJ 07631; **Phone:** 201-871-3636; **Board Cert:** Internal Medicine 1985; Pulmonary Disease 1988; **Med School:** NYU Sch Med 1982; **Resid:** Internal Medicine, Bellevue Hosp/NYU Med Ctr 1985; **Fellow:** Pulmonary Disease, Albert Einstein Coll Med 1987

Malovany, Robert MD (Pul) - **Spec Exp:** Exercise Physiology; Interventional Pulmonology; **Hospital:** Englewood Hosp & Med Ctr (page 656), Holy Name Med Ctr (page 657); **Address:** 180 Engle St, Englewood, NJ 07631-2507; **Phone:** 201-568-8010; **Board Cert:** Internal Medicine 1973; Pulmonary Disease 1976; **Med School:** Jefferson Med Coll 1970; **Resid:** Internal Medicine, Montefiore Hosp Med Ctr 1973; **Fellow:** Pulmonary Disease, Montefiore Hosp Med Ctr 1975; **Fac Appt:** Asst Clin Prof Med, Mount Sinai Sch Med

Polkow, Melvin MD (Pul) - **Spec Exp:** Asthma; Sarcoidosis; Pulmonary Fibrosis; Lung Cancer; **Hospital:** Hackensack Univ Med Ctr (page 96); **Address:** 211 Essex St, Ste 302, Hackensack, NJ 07601; **Phone:** 201-498-1311; **Board Cert:** Internal Medicine 1980; Pulmonary Disease 1982; Critical Care Medicine 2007; **Med School:** SUNY Downstate 1977; **Resid:** Internal Medicine, Lenox Hill Hosp 1980; **Fellow:** Pulmonary Critical Care Medicine, Univ Hosp 1982; **Fac Appt:** Asst Clin Prof Med, UMDNJ-NJ Med Sch, Newark

Rose, Henry J MD (Pul) - **Spec Exp:** Asthma; Emphysema; Sleep Disorders; Lung Cancer; **Hospital:** St Mary's Hosp - Passaic, Clara Maass Med Ctr; **Address:** 639 Ridge Rd, Lyndhurst, NJ 07071-3219; **Phone:** 201-939-8741; **Board Cert:** Internal Medicine 1982; Pulmonary Disease 1984; Critical Care Medicine 2001; **Med School:** UMDNJ-NJ Med Sch, Newark 1979; **Resid:** Internal Medicine, UMDNJ 1982; **Fellow:** Pulmonary Disease, Bronx Municipal Hosp 1984

Simon, Clifford J MD (Pul) - **Spec Exp:** Asthma; Lung Cancer; **Hospital:** Englewood Hosp & Med Ctr (page 656), Holy Name Med Ctr (page 657); **Address:** 180 Engle St, Englewood, NJ 07631-2507; **Phone:** 201-567-2050; **Board Cert:** Internal Medicine 1976; Pulmonary Disease 1980; **Med School:** Cornell Univ-Weill Med Coll 1973; **Resid:** Internal Medicine, Dartmouth Affil Hosps 1975; **Fellow:** Pulmonary Disease, Bellevue Hosp 1977

Radiation Oncology

Dubin, David MD (RadRO) - **Spec Exp:** Breast Cancer; Brachytherapy; Prostate Cancer; **Hospital:** Englewood Hosp & Med Ctr (page 656); **Address:** Englewood Hosp, Dept Radiation Oncology, 350 Engle St, Englewood, NJ 07631-1808; **Phone:** 201-894-3125; **Board Cert:** Radiation Oncology 1991; **Med School:** Albert Einstein Coll Med 1986; **Resid:** Radiation Oncology, St Barnabas Hosp 1990

Gejerman, Glen MD (RadRO) - **Spec Exp:** Prostate Cancer; Intensity Modulated Radiotherapy (IMRT); Breast Cancer; Brachytherapy; **Hospital:** Hackensack Univ Med Ctr (page 96); **Address:** Hackensack Univ Med Ctr, Radiation Onc, 30 Prospect Ave, Hackensack, NJ 07601; **Phone:** 201-996-2464; **Board Cert:** Radiation Oncology 2006; **Med School:** UMDNJ-NJ Med Sch, Newark 1990; **Resid:** Radiation Oncology, Montefiore Med Ctr 1995; **Fac Appt:** Asst Clin Prof RadRO, Albert Einstein Coll Med

Ingenito, Anthony C MD (RadRO) - **Spec Exp:** Brain Tumors; Head & Neck Cancer; Lymphoma; Gastrointestinal Cancer; **Hospital:** Hackensack Univ Med Ctr (page 96); **Address:** Dept Radiation Oncology, 30 Prospect Ave, Hackensack, NJ 07601; **Phone:** 201-996-2210; **Board Cert:** Radiation Oncology 2007; **Med School:** UMDNJ-NJ Med Sch, Newark 1991; **Resid:** Radiation Oncology, NY Presby Hosp 1996

Vialotti, Charles P MD (RadRO) - **Spec Exp:** Lung Cancer; **Hospital:** Holy Name Med Ctr (page 657), St Mary's Hosp - Passaic; **Address:** Holy Name Hosp, Cancer Ctr, 718 Teaneck Rd, Teaneck, NJ 07666; **Phone:** 201-541-5900; **Board Cert:** Therapeutic Radiology 1975; **Med School:** NY Med Coll 1971; **Resid:** Radiology, NYU Med Ctr 1974; **Fellow:** Therapeutic Radiology, NY Med Ctr 1975

Wesson, Michael F MD (RadRO) - **Spec Exp:** Breast Cancer; Prostate Cancer; Brachytherapy; **Hospital:** Valley Hosp (page 658); **Address:** 1 Valley Health Plaza, Paramus, NJ 07652; **Phone:** 201-634-5403; **Board Cert:** Radiation Oncology 1987; **Med School:** Univ VA Sch Med 1983; **Resid:** Radiation Oncology, Meml Sloan Kettering Cancer Ctr 1987

Reproductive Endocrinology

Lesorgen, Philip R MD (RE) - **Spec Exp:** Infertility; Infertility-IVF; Polycystic Ovarian Syndrome; **Hospital:** Englewood Hosp & Med Ctr (page 656), Hackensack Univ Med Ctr (page 96); **Address:** 106 Grand Ave Fl 4, Englewood, NJ 07631-3570; **Phone:** 201-569-6979; **Board Cert:** Obstetrics & Gynecology 1984; **Med School:** Boston Univ 1977; **Resid:** Obstetrics & Gynecology, LI Jewish Med Ctr 1981; **Fellow:** Reproductive Endocrinology, Thomas Jefferson Univ Hosp 1983; **Fac Appt:** Asst Clin Prof ObG, Seton Hall Univ Sch Hlth & Med Scis

McGovern, Peter G MD (RE) - **Spec Exp:** Infertility-IVF; Fertility Preservation in Cancer; **Hospital:** Univ Hosp-UMDNJ—Newark, Hackensack Univ Med Ctr (page 96); **Address:** Univ Reproductive Assocs, 214 Terrace Ave, Hasbrouck Heights, NJ 07604; **Phone:** 201-288-6330; **Board Cert:** Obstetrics & Gynecology 2008; Reproductive Endocrinology/Infertility 2008; **Med School:** NYU Sch Med 1986; **Resid:** Obstetrics & Gynecology, NYU-Bellevue Hosp Ctr 1990; **Fellow:** Reproductive Endocrinology, UMDNJ-Newark 1992; **Fac Appt:** Assoc Prof ObG, UMDNJ-NJ Med Sch, Newark

Navot, Daniel MD (RE) - **Spec Exp:** Infertility-IVF; **Hospital:** Englewood Hosp & Med Ctr (page 656), Valley Hosp (page 658); **Address:** 400 Old Hook Rd, Fl 2nd - rm 2-3, Westwood, NJ 07675-2732; **Phone:** 201-666-4200; **Board Cert:** Obstetrics & Gynecology 2008; Reproductive Endocrinology 2008; **Med School:** Israel 1978; **Resid:** Obstetrics & Gynecology, Hassadah Hosp 1983; **Fellow:** Reproductive Endocrinology, Jones Inst 1987; **Fac Appt:** Prof ObG, NY Med Coll

Weiss, Gerson MD (RE) - **Spec Exp:** Infertility; Menopause Problems; **Hospital:** Hackensack Univ Med Ctr (page 96), Univ Hosp-UMDNJ—Newark; **Address:** 214 Terrace Ave, Hasbrouck Heights, NJ 07604-1815; **Phone:** 201-288-6330; **Board Cert:** Obstetrics & Gynecology 1993; Reproductive Endocrinology 1974; **Med School:** NYU Sch Med 1964; **Resid:** Obstetrics & Gynecology, Bellevue Hosp Ctr 1969; **Fellow:** Reproductive Endocrinology, Univ Pittsburgh 1973; **Fac Appt:** Prof ObG, UMDNJ-NJ Med Sch, Newark

Rheumatology

Guma, Michael DO (Rhu) - **Spec Exp:** Arthritis; Autoimmune Disease; Inflammatory Muscle Disease; Osteoporosis; **Hospital:** Saint Michael's Med Ctr, Bayonne Med Ctr; **Address:** North Jersey Rheumatology Assocs, 312 Belleville Tpke, North Arlington, NJ 07031; **Phone:** 201-998-2800; **Board Cert:** Internal Medicine 2003; Rheumatology 2004; **Med School:** Kirksville Coll Osteo Med 1989; **Resid:** Internal Medicine, St Michaels Med Ctr 1992; **Fellow:** Rheumatology, St Michaels Med Ctr 1994; **Fac Appt:** Asst Clin Prof Med, Univ New Eng Coll Osteo Med

Kopelman, Rima G MD (Rhu) - **Spec Exp:** Rheumatoid Arthritis; Lupus/SLE; Vasculitis; **Hospital:** Valley Hosp (page 658), NY-Presby Hosp/Columbia (page 104); **Address:** 301 Godwin Ave, Midland Park, NJ 07432-1544; **Phone:** 201-444-4526; **Board Cert:** Internal Medicine 1980; Rheumatology 1984; **Med School:** Columbia P&S 1977; **Resid:** Internal Medicine, Columbia-Presby Med Ctr 1981; **Fellow:** Rheumatology, Columbia-Presby Med Ctr 1983; **Fac Appt:** Asst Prof Med, Columbia P&S

Leibowitz, Evan H MD (Rhu) - **Spec Exp:** Rheumatoid Arthritis; Gout; Lupus/SLE; **Hospital:** Valley Hosp (page 658); **Address:** Prospect Medical Office, 301 Godwin Ave, Midland Park, NJ 07432; **Phone:** 201-444-4526; **Board Cert:** Rheumatology 2001; **Med School:** UMDNJ-NJ Med Sch, Newark 1996; **Resid:** Internal Medicine, New York Hosp 1999; **Fellow:** Rheumatology, Hosp for Special Surg 2001

Marcus, Ralph E MD (Rhu) - **Spec Exp:** Rheumatoid Arthritis; Osteoporosis; Lupus/SLE; **Hospital:** Holy Name Med Ctr (page 657), Hackensack Univ Med Ctr (page 96); **Address:** 1415 Queen Anne Rd, Ste 102, Teaneck, NJ 07666-3521; **Phone:** 201-837-7788; **Board Cert:** Internal Medicine 1975; Rheumatology 1976; **Med School:** Albert Einstein Coll Med 1969; **Resid:** Internal Medicine, Mount Sinai Hosp 1974; **Fellow:** Rheumatology, Nat Inst Hlth 1972; Rheumatology, Hosp Special Surg 1976; **Fac Appt:** Assoc Clin Prof Med, UMDNJ-RW Johnson Med Sch

Salem, Noel MD (Rhu) - **Hospital:** Englewood Hosp & Med Ctr (page 656); **Address:** 285 Engle St, Englewood, NJ 07631-2406; **Phone:** 201-871-0223; **Board Cert:** Internal Medicine 1976; Rheumatology 1998; Geriatric Medicine 2004; **Med School:** SUNY Buffalo 1972; **Resid:** Internal Medicine, USPHS Hosp-Staten Island 1974; **Fellow:** Rheumatology, Columbia-Presby 1976; **Fac Appt:** Asst Prof Med, Mount Sinai Sch Med

Zalkowitz, Alan MD (Rhu) - **Spec Exp:** Lupus/SLE; Rheumatoid Arthritis; Polymyositis; **Hospital:** Valley Hosp (page 658); **Address:** 31-00 Broadway, Fair Lawn, NJ 07410-2331; **Phone:** 201-796-2255; **Board Cert:** Internal Medicine 1977; Rheumatology 1982; **Med School:** Belgium 1970; **Resid:** Internal Medicine, Stamford Hosp 1972; **Fellow:** Rheumatology, Mount Sinai Hosp 1974

Sports Medicine

Gross, Michael L MD (SM) - **Spec Exp:** Shoulder & Knee Injuries; **Hospital:** Hackensack Univ Med Ctr (page 96); **Address:** 25 Prospect Ave, Hackensack, NJ 07601; **Phone:** 201-343-2277; **Board Cert:** Orthopaedic Surgery 2002; Orthopaedic Sports Medicine 2008; **Med School:** NYU Sch Med 1983; **Resid:** Orthopaedic Surgery, Montefiore Med Ctr 1988; **Fellow:** Sports Medicine, UCLA Med Ctr 1989

Kelly, Michael A MD (SM) - **Spec Exp:** Knee Surgery; Knee Replacement; Arthroscopic Surgery; **Hospital:** Hackensack Univ Med Ctr (page 96), Lenox Hill Hosp; **Address:** 360 Essex St, Ste 303, Hackensack, NJ 07601; **Phone:** 201-336-8861; **Board Cert:** Orthopaedic Surgery 2009; **Med School:** Georgetown Univ 1979; **Resid:** Surgery, St Vincents Hosp 1981; Orthopaedic Surgery, Columbia-Presby Hosp 1984; **Fellow:** Knee Surgery, Hosp for Special Surgery 1985

Savatsky, Gary MD (SM) - **Spec Exp:** Shoulder & Knee Injuries; **Hospital:** Hackensack Univ Med Ctr (page 96); **Address:** 2 Forest Ave, Paramus, NJ 07652; **Phone:** 201-587-1111; **Board Cert:** Orthopaedic Surgery 2007; **Med School:** Columbia P&S 1975; **Resid:** Surgery, St Luke's-Roosevelt Hosp Ctr 1978; Orthopaedic Surgery, Hosp for Special Surgery 1983; **Fellow:** Orthopaedic Surgery, Hosp for Special Surgery 1979

Surgery

Ahlborn, Thomas N MD (S) - **Spec Exp:** Breast Surgery; Gastrointestinal Surgery; Hernia; Biliary Surgery; **Hospital:** Valley Hosp (page 658); **Address:** 385 S Maple Ave, Glen Rock, NJ 07452; **Phone:** 201-444-5757; **Board Cert:** Surgery 2005; **Med School:** Columbia P&S 1980; **Resid:** Surgery, Columbia-Presby Hosp 1985; **Fellow:** Vascular Surgery, Columbia-Presby Hosp 1986

Ballantyne, Garth H MD (S) - **Spec Exp:** Laparoscopic Surgery; Gastroesophageal Reflux Disease (GERD); Colon Cancer; Obesity/Bariatric Surgery; **Hospital:** Hackensack Univ Med Ctr (page 96); **Address:** 20 Prospect Ave, Ste 901, Hackensack, NJ 07601-1974; **Phone:** 201-996-2959; **Board Cert:** Surgery 2006; Colon & Rectal Surgery 1985; **Med School:** Columbia P&S 1977; **Resid:** Surgery, UCLA Med Ctr 1980; Surgery, Northwestern Univ 1982; **Fellow:** Colon & Rectal Surgery, Mayo Clinic 1984; **Fac Appt:** Prof S, UMDNJ-NJ Med Sch, Newark

Bufalini, Bruno MD (S) - **Spec Exp:** Laparoscopic Surgery; Minimally Invasive Surgery; **Hospital:** Englewood Hosp & Med Ctr (page 656); **Address:** 200 Grand Ave, Englewood, NJ 07631-4371; **Phone:** 201-871-0303; **Med School:** Italy 1971; **Resid:** Surgery, Englewood Hosp 1976

Christoudias, George MD (S) - **Spec Exp:** Laparoscopic Hernia Repair; Laparoscopic Cholecystectomy; Cancer Surgery; **Hospital:** Holy Name Med Ctr (page 657); **Address:** 741 Teaneck Rd, Teaneck, NJ 07666; **Phone:** 201-833-2888; **Med School:** Greece 1969; **Resid:** Surgery, Downstate-Kings Co Med Ctr 1975; **Fellow:** Surgical Oncology, Downstate-Kings Co Med Ctr 1976

Fried, Kenneth S MD (S) - **Spec Exp:** Carotid Artery Surgery; Laparoscopic Surgery; **Hospital:** Englewood Hosp & Med Ctr (page 656), Holy Name Med Ctr (page 657); **Address:** 180 N Dean St, Ste 2 South, Englewood, NJ 07631-2541; **Phone:** 201-568-8666; **Board Cert:** Surgery 2004; **Med School:** NYU Sch Med 1978; **Resid:** Surgery, NYU Med Ctr 1983; **Fellow:** Vascular Surgery, NYU Med Ctr 1984; **Fac Appt:** Asst Clin Prof S, Mount Sinai Sch Med

Licata Jr, Joseph J MD (S) - **Spec Exp:** Laparoscopic Surgery; Breast Surgery; **Hospital:** Valley Hosp (page 658); **Address:** 245 E Main St, Ramsey, NJ 07446-1942; **Phone:** 201-327-0220; **Board Cert:** Surgery 2002; **Med School:** Mexico 1984; **Resid:** Surgery, New York Med Coll 1991

McCain, Donald MD/PhD (S) - **Spec Exp:** Cancer Surgery; Breast Cancer; Gastrointestinal Cancer; Melanoma; **Hospital:** Hackensack Univ Med Ctr (page 96); **Address:** 20 Prospect Ave, Ste 603, Hackensack, NJ 07601; **Phone:** 201-342-1010; **Board Cert:** Surgery 2000; **Med School:** Albert Einstein Coll Med 1991; **Resid:** Surgery, Mt Sinai Med Ctr 1996; **Fellow:** Surgical Oncology, Meml Sloan Kettering Cancer Ctr 1998; **Fac Appt:** Asst Clin Prof S, UMDNJ-NJ Med Sch, Newark

Pereira, Stephen MD (S) - **Spec Exp:** Laparoscopic Abdominal Surgery; **Hospital:** Hackensack Univ Med Ctr (page 96); **Address:** 90 Prospect Ave, Ste 1D, Hackensack, NJ 07601-1918; **Phone:** 201-343-3433; **Board Cert:** Surgery 2007; **Med School:** UMDNJ-RW Johnson Med Sch 1991; **Resid:** Surgery, Northwestern Univ 1996; **Fellow:** Laparoscopic Surgery, Hackensack Univ Med Ctr; **Fac Appt:** Asst Clin Prof S, UMDNJ-NJ Med Sch, Newark

Schmidt, Hans J MD (S) - **Spec Exp:** Obesity/Bariatric Surgery; Laparoscopic Abdominal Surgery; **Hospital:** Hackensack Univ Med Ctr (page 96); **Address:** East 81, Route 4, Ste 401, Paramus, NJ 07652; **Phone:** 201-646-1121; **Board Cert:** Surgery 2008; **Med School:** UMDNJ-NJ Med Sch, Newark 1991; **Resid:** Surgery, UMDNJ Univ Hosp 1997

Shapiro, Michael E MD (S) - **Spec Exp:** Transplant-Kidney; Transplant-Pancreas; Parathyroid Surgery; Dialysis Access Surgery; **Hospital:** Hackensack Univ Med Ctr (page 96); **Address:** 30 Prospect Ave, Hackensack, NJ 07601-1914; **Phone:** 201-996-2608; **Board Cert:** Surgery 2005; **Med School:** Univ Rochester 1977; **Resid:** Surgery, Beth Israel Med Ctr 1983; **Fac Appt:** Prof S, UMDNJ-NJ Med Sch, Newark

Silvestri, Fred MD (S) - **Spec Exp:** Laparoscopic Surgery; Hyperbaric Medicine; **Hospital:** Englewood Hosp & Med Ctr (page 656); **Address:** 375 Engle St, Englewood, NJ 07631; **Phone:** 201-894-0400; **Board Cert:** Surgery 2000; Surgical Critical Care 2002; **Med School:** SUNY Downstate 1983; **Resid:** Surgery, Staten Island Hosp 1988; **Fellow:** Vascular Surgery, Englewood Hosp 1989; Surgical Critical Care, North Shore Hosp 1990

Sussman, Barry MD (S) - **Spec Exp:** Breast Surgery; Laparoscopic Surgery; **Hospital:** Englewood Hosp & Med Ctr (page 656), Holy Name Med Ctr (page 657); **Address:** 375 Engle St, Englewood, NJ 07631-1823; **Phone:** 201-894-0400; **Board Cert:** Surgery 2008; **Med School:** NYU Sch Med 1973; **Resid:** Surgery, NYU Med Ctr 1978; **Fellow:** Vascular Surgery, Englewood Hosp 1979; **Fac Appt:** Asst Clin Prof S, Mount Sinai Sch Med

Yiengpruksawan, Anusak MD (S) - **Spec Exp:** Liver & Biliary Surgery; Endoscopic Ultrasound; Robotic Surgery; Minimally Invasive Surgery; **Hospital:** Valley Hosp (page 658), Chilton Meml Hosp; **Address:** 1 Valley Health Plaza, Paramus, NJ 07652; **Phone:** 201-493-1005; **Board Cert:** Surgery 2001; **Med School:** Japan 1978; **Resid:** Surgery, Harlem Hosp 1989; **Fellow:** Surgical Oncology, Meml Sloan Kettering Cancer Ctr 1991

Thoracic Surgery

Elmann, Elie M MD (TS) - **Spec Exp:** Robotic Cardiac Surgery; Minimally Invasive Cardiac Surgery; Heart Valve Surgery; Atrial Fibrillation; **Hospital:** Hackensack Univ Med Ctr (page 96), Holy Name Med Ctr (page 657); **Address:** 20 Prospect Ave, Ste 900, Hackensack, NJ 07601; **Phone:** 201-996-2261; **Board Cert:** Surgery 2004; **Med School:** NY Med Coll 1987; **Resid:** Surgery, Cabrini Med Ctr/NY Med Coll 1992; **Fellow:** Cardiothoracic Surgery, SUNY Downstate Med Ctr 1995; **Fac Appt:** Asst Prof S, UMDNJ-NJ Med Sch, Newark

Ergin, M Arisan MD (TS) - **Spec Exp:** Cardiac Surgery; Transfusion Free Surgery; Aneurysm; **Hospital:** Englewood Hosp & Med Ctr (page 656); **Address:** 350 Engle St, Ste 1000, Englewood, NJ 07631-1808; **Phone:** 201-894-3636; **Board Cert:** Thoracic Surgery 2007; **Med School:** Turkey 1968; **Resid:** Surgery, Kings Co Hosp 1973; **Fellow:** Thoracic Surgery, Kings Co Hosp-SUNY 1976; **Fac Appt:** Prof S, Mount Sinai Sch Med

Lee, Leonard Y MD (TS) - **Spec Exp:** Coronary Artery Surgery; Minimally Invasive Cardiac Surgery; Heart Failure; Gene Therapy-Cardiac Angiogenesis; **Hospital:** Hackensack Univ Med Ctr (page 96); **Address:** 20 Prospect Ave, Ste 900, Hackensack, NJ 07601; **Phone:** 201-996-2261; **Board Cert:** Surgery 1999; Thoracic Surgery 2002; **Med School:** UMDNJ-RW Johnson Med Sch 1992; **Resid:** Surgery, St Vincent's Hosp 1997; **Fellow:** Thoracic Surgery, Cornell Med Ctr 2001; **Fac Appt:** Assoc Clin Prof TS, Cornell Univ-Weill Med Coll

Park, Bernard J H MD (TS) - **Spec Exp:** Lung Cancer; Esophageal Cancer; Mediastinal Tumors; Robotic Surgery; **Hospital:** Hackensack Univ Med Ctr (page 96); **Address:** 20 Prospect Ave, Ste 900, Hackensack, NJ 07601; **Phone:** 201-996-2261; **Board Cert:** Surgery 2001; Thoracic Surgery 2003; **Med School:** Univ Pennsylvania 1993; **Resid:** Surgery, New York Hosp 1996; Surgery, New York Hosp 2000; **Fellow:** Cardiothoracic Surgery, NY Presby/Cornell 2002; Thoracic Surgery, Meml Sloan Kettering Cancer Ctr 2002; **Fac Appt:** Asst Prof TS, Cornell Univ-Weill Med Coll

Zairis, Ignatios MD (TS) - **Spec Exp:** Endovascular Surgery; Minimally Invasive Thoracic Surgery; **Hospital:** Englewood Hosp & Med Ctr (page 656), Holy Name Med Ctr (page 657); **Address:** 741 Teaneck Rd, Teaneck, NJ 07666-4243; **Phone:** 201-837-8282; **Board Cert:** Surgery 2000; **Med School:** Greece 1973; **Resid:** Surgery, Downstate Med Ctr 1984; Cardiothoracic Surgery, Downstate Med Ctr 1984

Zapolanski, Alex MD (TS) - **Spec Exp:** Minimally Invasive Heart Valve Surgery; Aortic Surgery; Coronary Artery Surgery; **Hospital:** Valley Hosp (page 658); **Address:** Valley Hospital, 223 N Van Dien Ave, Ridgewood, NJ 07450; **Phone:** 201-447-8377; **Board Cert:** Thoracic Surgery 2004; **Med School:** Argentina 1973; **Resid:** Surgery, Cleveland Clinic 1979; Cardiothoracic Surgery, Toronto Genl Hosp 1981

Urology

Basralian, Kevin R MD (U) - **Spec Exp:** Infertility-Male; Prostate Benign Disease; Minimally Invasive Surgery; **Hospital:** Hackensack Univ Med Ctr (page 96), Holy Name Med Ctr (page 657); **Address:** 20 Prospect Ave, Ste 719, Hackensack, NJ 07601; **Phone:** 201-343-0082; **Board Cert:** Urology 2000; **Med School:** Mexico 1979; **Resid:** Surgery, Lenox Hill Hosp 1982; Urology, Lenox Hill Hosp 1985; **Fellow:** Urology, Univ Edinburgh 1986

Berdini, Jeffrey L MD (U) - **Spec Exp:** Kidney Stones; Prostate Cancer; Vasectomy Reversal; **Hospital:** Valley Hosp (page 658); **Address:** 555 Kinderkamack Rd, Oradell, NJ 07649; **Phone:** 201-834-1890; **Board Cert:** Urology 1980; **Med School:** UMDNJ-NJ Med Sch, Newark 1973; **Resid:** Urology, UNDMJ Affil Hosps 1978

Esposito, Michael P MD (U) - **Spec Exp:** Laparoscopic Kidney Surgery; Prostate Cancer/Robotic Surgery; Minimally Invasive Urologic Surgery; Adrenal Surgery; **Hospital:** Hackensack Univ Med Ctr (page 96), Valley Hosp (page 658); **Address:** 255 W Spring Valley Ave, Ste 101, Maywood, NJ 07607; **Phone:** 201-487-8866; **Board Cert:** Urology 2003; **Med School:** UMDNJ-NJ Med Sch, Newark 1994; **Resid:** Urology, UMDNJ Med Ctr 2000; **Fellow:** Urologic Laparoscopic Surg-Endourology, Royal Infirmary/Western Genl Hosp 2001; **Fac Appt:** Asst Clin Prof S, UMDNJ-NJ Med Sch, Newark

Frey, Howard L MD (U) - **Spec Exp:** Prostate Cancer; Bladder Cancer; Kidney Cancer; **Hospital:** Valley Hosp (page 658); **Address:** 4 Godwin Ave, Midland Park, NJ 07432-1980; **Phone:** 201-444-7070; **Board Cert:** Urology 2003; **Med School:** Johns Hopkins Univ 1977; **Resid:** Surgery, Johns Hopkins Hosp 1979; Urology, UCLA Med Ctr 1983

Hajjar, John H MD (U) - **Spec Exp:** Laparoscopic Surgery; Prostate Surgery; **Hospital:** Valley Hosp (page 658); **Address:** 15-01 Broadway, Route 4 West, Fair Lawn, NJ 07410-6001; **Phone:** 201-791-4544; **Board Cert:** Urology 2001; **Med School:** Georgetown Univ 1981; **Resid:** Surgery, NYU Med Ctr 1983; Urology, NYU-Bellevue/Sloan Ketterin 1987; **Fellow:** Research, NYU Med Ctr 1988

Katz, Steven A MD (U) - **Spec Exp:** Transfusion Free Surgery; Prostate Cancer; Laparoscopic Surgery; **Hospital:** Englewood Hosp & Med Ctr (page 656), Holy Name Med Ctr (page 657); **Address:** 75 S Dean St, Englewood, NJ 07631-3512; **Phone:** 201-816-1900; **Board Cert:** Urology 1978; **Med School:** SUNY Buffalo 1969; **Resid:** Urology, Metropolitan Hosp Ctr 1976

Lanteri, Vincent J MD (U) - **Spec Exp:** Prostate Cancer/Robotic Surgery; Urologic Cancer; Minimally Invasive Urologic Surgery; **Hospital:** Hackensack Univ Med Ctr (page 96), Monmouth Med Ctr; **Address:** 255 W Spring Valley Ave, Ste 101, Maywood, NJ 07607; **Phone:** 201-487-8866; **Board Cert:** Urology 1982; **Med School:** Mexico 1974; **Resid:** Surgery, UMDNJ Med Ctr 1977; Urology, UMDNJ Med Ctr 1980; **Fellow:** Urologic Oncology, Roswell Park Cancer Inst 1981

Munver, Ravi MD (U) - **Spec Exp:** Robotic Surgery; Minimally Invasive Urologic Surgery; Endourology; Kidney Stones; **Hospital:** Hackensack Univ Med Ctr (page 96); **Address:** 360 Essex St, Ste 403, Hackensack, NJ 07601; **Phone:** 201-336-8090; **Board Cert:** Urology 2005; **Med School:** Cornell Univ-Weill Med Coll 1996; **Resid:** Urology, Duke Univ Med Ctr 2002; **Fellow:** Endourology, New York Hosp-Cornell Med Ctr 2003; **Fac Appt:** Assoc Prof U, UMDNJ-Univ Med Dent NJ

Rosenberg, Gene S MD (U) - **Spec Exp:** Minimally Invasive Surgery; Prostate Cancer-Cryosurgery; Kidney Cancer-Cryosurgery; **Hospital:** Hackensack Univ Med Ctr (page 96); **Address:** 20 Prospect Ave, Ste 719, Hackensack, NJ 07601; **Phone:** 201-343-0082; **Board Cert:** Urology 1982; **Med School:** NYU Sch Med 1974; **Resid:** Pathology, Kings Co Hosp 1976; Urology, Bellevue/NYU Med Ctr 1980

Sadeghi-Nejad, Hossein MD (U) - **Spec Exp:** Infertility-Male; Erectile Dysfunction; Penile Prostheses; Peyronie's Disease; **Hospital:** Hackensack Univ Med Ctr (page 96), Univ Hosp-UMDNJ—Newark; **Address:** 20 Prospect Ave, rm 711, Hackensack, NJ 07601; **Phone:** 201-342-7977; **Board Cert:** Urology 2009; **Med School:** McGill Univ 1989; **Resid:** Surgery, UCSF Med Ctr 1991; Urology, Boston Univ Med Ctr 1996; **Fellow:** Microsurgery, Boston Univ Med Ctr 1997; Reproductive Medicine, Boston Univ Med Ctr 1997; **Fac Appt:** Assoc Prof U, UMDNJ-NJ Med Sch, Newark

Sawczuk, Ihor S MD (U) - **Spec Exp:** Bladder Cancer; Kidney Cancer; Prostate Cancer/Robotic Surgery; Bladder Surgery; **Hospital:** Hackensack Univ Med Ctr (page 96), NY-Presby Hosp/Columbia (page 104); **Address:** Hackensack Univ Med Ctr, 360 Essex St, Ste 403, Hackensack, NJ 07601; **Phone:** 201-336-8090; **Board Cert:** Urology 2005; **Med School:** Med Coll PA Hahnemann 1979; **Resid:** Surgery, St Vincents Hosp 1981; Urology, Columbia-Presby Med Ctr 1984; **Fellow:** Urologic Oncology, Columbia-Presby Med Ctr 1986; **Fac Appt:** Prof U, Columbia P&S

Tennenbaum, Steven Y MD (U) - **Hospital:** Holy Name Med Ctr (page 657), Valley Hosp (page 658); **Address:** 699 Teaneck Rd, Teaneck, NJ 07666; **Phone:** 201-692-9550; **Board Cert:** Urology 2003; **Med School:** Albert Einstein Coll Med 1984; **Resid:** Surgery, Montefiore Med Ctr 1986; Urology, Montefiore Med Ctr 1990; **Fellow:** Pediatric Urology, San Diego Chldn's Hosp 1991; **Fac Appt:** Asst Prof U, Columbia P&S

Vitenson, Jack MD (U) - **Spec Exp:** Prostate Cancer; Bladder Cancer; Erectile Dysfunction; **Hospital:** Hackensack Univ Med Ctr (page 96); **Address:** 277 Forest Ave, Ste 206, Paramus, NJ 07652; **Phone:** 201-489-8900; **Board Cert:** Urology 1974; **Med School:** NY Med Coll 1965; **Resid:** Surgery, VA Med Ctr 1967; Urology, Metropolitan Hosp Ctr 1970; **Fac Appt:** Assoc Clin Prof U, UMDNJ-NJ Med Sch, Newark

Wasserman, Gary D MD (U) - **Spec Exp:** Kidney Stones; Prostate Surgery; Incontinence; Voiding Dysfunction; **Hospital:** Englewood Hosp & Med Ctr (page 656), Holy Name Med Ctr (page 657); **Address:** 180 N Dean St Fl 1, Englewood, NJ 07631; **Phone:** 201-503-9100; **Board Cert:** Urology 2001; **Med School:** Tulane Univ 1985; **Resid:** Surgery, Geo Wash Univ Med Ctr 1987; Urology, Tulane Univ Med Ctr 1991

Vascular Surgery

Elias, Steven M MD (VascS) - **Spec Exp:** Vein Disorders; Wound Healing/Care; Minimally Invasive Surgery; Varicose Veins; **Hospital:** Englewood Hosp & Med Ctr (page 656), Mount Sinai Med Ctr (page 102); **Address:** Englewood Hosp & Med Ctr, Ctr Vein Disease, 350 Engle St, Englewood, NJ 07631-2541; **Phone:** 201-894-3252; **Board Cert:** Surgery 2007; **Med School:** SUNY Buffalo 1979; **Resid:** Surgery, Millard Filmore Hosp 1981; **Fellow:** Peripheral Vascular Surgery, Englewood Hosp 1985; **Fac Appt:** Assoc Prof S, Mount Sinai Sch Med

Geuder, James W MD (VascS) - **Spec Exp:** Vein Disorders; Carotid Artery Surgery; Aneurysm-Aortic; Endovascular Surgery; **Hospital:** Hackensack Univ Med Ctr (page 96); **Address:** 680 Kinderkamack Rd, Ste 306, Oradell, NJ 07649; **Phone:** 201-262-8346; **Board Cert:** Surgery 2007; Vascular Surgery 1999; **Med School:** Med Coll Wisc 1981; **Resid:** Surgery, UMDNJ Med Ctr 1986; **Fellow:** Vascular Surgery, NYU Med Ctr 1988

Manno, Joseph MD (VascS) - **Spec Exp:** Arterial Disease; Angioplasty; Limb Sparing Surgery; **Hospital:** Holy Name Med Ctr (page 657), Hackensack Univ Med Ctr (page 96); **Address:** 83 Summit Ave, Hackensack, NJ 07601-1262; **Phone:** 201-646-0010; **Board Cert:** Surgery 2009; Vascular Surgery 2002; **Med School:** Oral Roberts Sch Med 1982; **Resid:** Surgery, UMDNJ Univ Hosp 1987; **Fellow:** Vascular Surgery, UMDNJ 1989

Moss, Charles M MD (VascS) - **Spec Exp:** Wound Healing/Care; **Hospital:** Hackensack Univ Med Ctr (page 96), Holy Name Med Ctr (page 657); **Address:** 20 Prospect Ave, Ste 807, Hackensack, NJ 07601; **Phone:** 201-488-2220; **Board Cert:** Surgery 1973; Vascular Surgery 2003; Undersea & Hyperbaric Medicine 2006; **Med School:** Tulane Univ 1967; **Resid:** Surgery, Montefiore Med Ctr 1972; **Fac Appt:** Assoc Clin Prof S, UMDNJ-NJ Med Sch, Newark

Wolodiger, Fred A MD (VascS) - **Spec Exp:** Arterial Bypass Surgery-Leg; Carotid Artery Surgery; Laparoscopic Surgery; **Hospital:** Englewood Hosp & Med Ctr (page 656), Holy Name Med Ctr (page 657); **Address:** 375 Engle St Fl Ground, Englewood, NJ 07631; **Phone:** 201-894-0400; **Board Cert:** Surgery 2004; Vascular Surgery 2008; **Med School:** SUNY Hlth Sci Ctr 1980; **Resid:** Surgery, North Shore Univ Hosp 1985; **Fellow:** Vascular Surgery, Englewood Hosp 1987

The Best in American Medicine
www.CastleConnolly.com

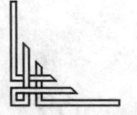
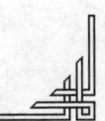

Essex

Essex

Adolescent Medicine

Johnson, Robert L MD (AM) - **Spec Exp:** AIDS/HIV; Abuse/Neglect; Behavioral Disorders; **Hospital:** Univ Hosp-UMDNJ—Newark; **Address:** 185 S Orange Ave, rm C671, Newark, NJ 07101-1709; **Phone:** 973-972-5277; **Board Cert:** Pediatrics 1977; **Med School:** UMDNJ-NJ Med Sch, Newark 1972; **Resid:** Pediatrics, Martland Hosp 1974; **Fellow:** Adolescent Medicine, NYU Med Ctr 1976; **Fac Appt:** Prof Ped, UMDNJ-NJ Med Sch, Newark

Stanford, Paulette D MD (AM) - **Spec Exp:** AIDS/HIV in Adolescents; Adolescent Gynecology; Adolescent Behavior-High Risk; **Hospital:** Univ Hosp-UMDNJ—Newark; **Address:** UMDNJ - Dept Pediatrics, Adolescent Med, 90 Bergen St, Ste 4300, Newark, NJ 07103; **Phone:** 973-972-2100; **Board Cert:** Pediatrics 1984; Adolescent Medicine 2002; **Med School:** UMDNJ-NJ Med Sch, Newark 1975; **Resid:** Pediatrics, UMDNJ-Univ Hosp 1977; **Fellow:** Adolescent Medicine, UMDNJ-Univ Hosp 1979; **Fac Appt:** Prof Ped, UMDNJ-NJ Med Sch, Newark

Allergy & Immunology

Perlman, Donald B MD (A&I) - **Spec Exp:** Asthma; Urticaria; Drug Allergy; **Hospital:** Saint Barnabas Med Ctr, Newark Beth Israel Med Ctr; **Address:** 101 Old Short Hills Rd, Ste 407, West Orange, NJ 07052-1023; **Phone:** 973-736-7722; **Board Cert:** Pediatrics 1978; Allergy & Immunology 1979; **Med School:** Mount Sinai Sch Med 1973; **Resid:** Pediatrics, Mt Sinai Hosp 1976; **Fellow:** Allergy & Immunology, Duke Univ Med Ctr 1978; **Fac Appt:** Asst Clin Prof Ped, UMDNJ-NJ Med Sch, Newark

Weiss, Steven J MD (A&I) - **Spec Exp:** Asthma; Sinus Disorders; **Hospital:** Saint Barnabas Med Ctr; **Address:** 209 S Livingston Ave, Ste 6, Livingston, NJ 07039-4042; **Phone:** 973-992-4171; **Board Cert:** Internal Medicine 1985; Allergy & Immunology 1987; **Med School:** Ros Franklin Univ/Chicago Med Sch 1982; **Resid:** Internal Medicine, St Lukes Roosevelt Hosp Ctr 1985; **Fellow:** Allergy & Immunology, St Lukes Roosevelt Hosp Ctr 1987; **Fac Appt:** Asst Clin Prof Med, Mount Sinai Sch Med

Cardiac Electrophysiology

Correia, Joaquim J MD (CE) - **Spec Exp:** Arrhythmias; Pacemakers; Defibrillators; **Hospital:** Saint Michael's Med Ctr, Univ Hosp-UMDNJ—Newark; **Address:** 243 Chestnut St, Ste 2L, Newark, NJ 07105; **Phone:** 973-589-8668; **Board Cert:** Internal Medicine 1989; Cardiovascular Disease 2001; Cardiac Electrophysiology 2004; **Med School:** NYU Sch Med 1986; **Resid:** Internal Medicine, Columbia-Presby Med Ctr 1989; **Fellow:** Cardiovascular Disease, Columbia-Presby Med Ctr 1992; Cardiac Electrophysiology, Columbia-Presby Med Ctr 1993; **Fac Appt:** Asst Prof Med, UMDNJ-NJ Med Sch, Newark

Costeas, Constantinos A MD (CE) - **Spec Exp:** Arrhythmias; Radiofrequency Ablation; Pacemakers; **Hospital:** Saint Michael's Med Ctr, Saint Barnabas Med Ctr; **Address:** 375 Mount Pleasant Ave, West Orange, NJ 07052; **Phone:** 973-731-9598; **Board Cert:** Cardiac Electrophysiology 2008; Cardiovascular Disease 2008; **Med School:** SUNY Stony Brook 1989; **Resid:** Internal Medicine, Univ Hosp 1992; **Fellow:** Cardiovascular Disease, St Vincent's Hosp 1996; Cardiac Electrophysiology, Columbia-Presby Med Ctr 1998

Roelke, Marc MD (CE) - **Hospital:** Newark Beth Israel Med Ctr, Saint Barnabas Med Ctr; **Address:** Diagnostic & Clinical Cardiology, 375 Mount Pleasant Ave, West Orange, NJ 07052; **Phone:** 973-731-9598; **Board Cert:** Internal Medicine 2000; Cardiovascular Disease 2003; Cardiac Electrophysiology 2006; **Med School:** Columbia P&S 1987; **Resid:** Internal Medicine, Univ Chicago 1990; **Fellow:** Cardiovascular Disease, Mass Genl Hosp 1993; Cardiac Electrophysiology, Mass Genl Hosp 1994

Cardiovascular Disease

Ciccone, John M MD (Cv) - **Spec Exp:** Interventional Cardiology; Complementary Medicine; **Hospital:** Saint Barnabas Med Ctr, Morristown Mem Hosp (page 92); **Address:** 741 Northfield Ave, Ste 205, West Orange, NJ 07052; **Phone:** 973-467-1544; **Board Cert:** Internal Medicine 1982; Cardiovascular Disease 1985; **Med School:** UMDNJ-NJ Med Sch, Newark 1979; **Resid:** Internal Medicine, UMDNJ-Univ Hosp 1982; **Fellow:** Cardiovascular Disease, UMDNJ-Newark Beth Israel Hosp 1984; **Fac Appt:** Asst Clin Prof Med, UMDNJ-NJ Med Sch, Newark

Goldstein, Jonathan E MD (Cv) - **Spec Exp:** Interventional Cardiology; Cardiac Catheterization; **Hospital:** Saint Michael's Med Ctr, Christ Hosp; **Address:** Saint Michael's Med Ctr, Dept Medicine, 111 Central Ave, Newark, NJ 07102; **Phone:** 973-877-5430; **Board Cert:** Internal Medicine 1978; Cardiovascular Disease 1981; Interventional Cardiology 1999; **Med School:** UMDNJ-NJ Med Sch, Newark 1973; **Resid:** Internal Medicine, Jackson Meml Hosp 1976; **Fellow:** Cardiovascular Disease, Boston Med Ctr 1978; **Fac Appt:** Assoc Prof Med, Seton Hall Univ Sch Hlth & Med Scis

Klapholz, Marc MD (Cv) - **Spec Exp:** Congestive Heart Failure; Angioplasty; Interventional Cardiology; Pulmonary Hypertension; **Hospital:** Univ Hosp-UMDNJ—Newark, Mountainside Hosp; **Address:** 185 S Orange Ave Med Sci Bldg, I-538, Newark, NJ 07103-2757; **Phone:** 973-972-4731; **Board Cert:** Internal Medicine 1989; Cardiovascular Disease 2002; Interventional Cardiology 1999; Echocardiography 1997; **Med School:** Albert Einstein Coll Med 1986; **Resid:** Internal Medicine, Bronx Muni Hosp 1989; **Fellow:** Cardiovascular Disease, Bronx Muni Hosp 1992; Interventional Cardiology, Montefiore Med Ctr 1995; **Fac Appt:** Prof Med, UMDNJ-NJ Med Sch, Newark

Rogal, Gary J MD (Cv) - **Spec Exp:** Echocardiography; Coronary Artery Disease; Heart Valve Disease; **Hospital:** Saint Barnabas Med Ctr, Newark Beth Israel Med Ctr; **Address:** 375 Mount Pleasant Ave, W Orange, NJ 07052; **Phone:** 973-731-9442; **Board Cert:** Internal Medicine 1981; Cardiovascular Disease 1983; **Med School:** Geo Wash Univ 1978; **Resid:** Internal Medicine, LI Jewish Med Ctr 1981; **Fellow:** Cardiovascular Disease, Strong Meml Hosp 1984

Saroff, Alan L MD (Cv) - **Spec Exp:** Heart Valve Disease; Cholesterol/Lipid Disorders; Arrhythmias; Preventive Cardiology; **Hospital:** Mountainside Hosp, NY-Presby Hosp/Columbia (page 104); **Address:** Montclair Cardiology Group, 123 Highland Ave, Ste 302, Glen Ridge, NJ 07028-1522; **Phone:** 973-748-9555; **Board Cert:** Internal Medicine 1972; Cardiovascular Disease 1975; **Med School:** SUNY Upstate Med Univ 1965; **Resid:** Internal Medicine, SUNY-Syracuse Med Ctr 1967; Internal Medicine, NY Hosp 1970; **Fellow:** Cardiovascular Disease, Columbia Presby Med Ctr 1972; Cardiac Electrophysiology, Columbia Presby Med Ctr 1973; **Fac Appt:** Assoc Clin Prof Med, Columbia P&S

Shamoon, Fayez E MD (Cv) - **Spec Exp:** Interventional Cardiology; Coronary Artery Disease; Nuclear Cardiology; Angioplasty & Stent Placement; **Hospital:** Saint Michael's Med Ctr, Clara Maass Med Ctr; **Address:** Saint Michael's Med Ctr, Dept Cardiology, 111 Central Ave, Newark, NJ 07102; **Phone:** 973-877-5160; **Board Cert:** Internal Medicine 2006; Cardiovascular Disease 2006; Interventional Cardiology 2009; **Med School:** Jordan 1981; **Resid:** Internal Medicine, Jordan Univ Hosp 1985; Internal Medicine, St Michael's Med Ctr 1992; **Fellow:** Cardiovascular Disease, St Michael's Med Ctr 1995; Interventional Cardiology, St Michael's Med Ctr 1996; **Fac Appt:** Assoc Prof Med, Seton Hall Univ Sch Hlth & Med Scis

Wangenheim, Paul M MD (Cv) - **Spec Exp:** Interventional Cardiology; Complementary Medicine; Echocardiography; **Hospital:** Saint Barnabas Med Ctr, Morristown Mem Hosp (page 92); **Address:** 741 Northfield Ave, Ste 205, West Orange, NJ 07052; **Phone:** 973-467-1544; **Board Cert:** Internal Medicine 1985; Cardiovascular Disease 1987; **Med School:** UMDNJ-NJ Med Sch, Newark 1982; **Resid:** Internal Medicine, UMDNJ-Univ Hosp 1985; **Fellow:** Cardiovascular Disease, Newark Beth Israel Med Ctr 1987

Wu, Chia F MD (Cv) - **Hospital:** Saint Barnabas Med Ctr; **Address:** 35 Park Ave, West Orange, NJ 07052-5526; **Phone:** 973-325-3445; **Board Cert:** Internal Medicine 1972; Cardiovascular Disease 1975; **Med School:** Taiwan 1969; **Resid:** Internal Medicine, Martland Hosp 1972; **Fellow:** Cardiovascular Disease, Martland Hosp 1974; **Fac Appt:** Asst Clin Prof Med, UMDNJ-NJ Med Sch, Newark

Zucker, Mark J MD (Cv) - **Spec Exp:** Transplant Medicine-Heart; Heart Failure; Pulmonary Hypertension; Amyloid Heart Disease; **Hospital:** Newark Beth Israel Med Ctr, Saint Barnabas Med Ctr; **Address:** Heart Failure Trmt & Transplant Program, 201 Lyons Ave, Ste L4, Newark, NJ 07112-2027; **Phone:** 973-926-7205; **Board Cert:** Internal Medicine 1984; Cardiovascular Disease 1987; **Med School:** Northwestern Univ 1981; **Resid:** Internal Medicine, Northwestern Meml Hosp 1984; **Fellow:** Cardiovascular Disease, Northwestern Meml Hosp 1987; **Fac Appt:** Clin Prof Med, UMDNJ-NJ Med Sch, Newark

Child & Adolescent Psychiatry

Bartlett, Jacqueline MD (ChAP) - **Spec Exp:** Stress Management; ADD/ADHD; Mood Disorders; **Hospital:** Univ Hosp-UMDNJ—Newark; **Address:** 183 S Orange Ave, BHSB -rmE1457, Newark, NJ 07103; **Phone:** 973-972-2977; **Board Cert:** Psychiatry 1983; **Med School:** Univ Cincinnati 1971; **Resid:** Pediatrics, Montefiore Hospital 1976; Psychiatry, Columbia-Presby Med Ctr 1981; **Fellow:** Child & Adolescent Psychiatry, Columbia-Presby Med Ctr 1979; **Fac Appt:** Assoc Prof Ped, UMDNJ-NJ Med Sch, Newark

Child Neurology

Pak, Jayoung MD (ChiN) - **Spec Exp:** Epilepsy/Seizure Disorders; **Hospital:** Univ Hosp-UMDNJ—Newark; **Address:** UMDNJ Doctor's Office Ctr, 90 Bergen St, rm 8100, Newark, NJ 07103-2406; **Phone:** 973-972-2922; **Board Cert:** Child Neurology 1993; **Med School:** South Korea 1978; **Resid:** Pediatrics, Ewha Women's Univ 1983; Pediatrics, UMDNJ-Univ Hosp 1988; **Fellow:** Child Neurology, UMDNJ-Univ Hosp 1991; Epilepsy, Columbia-Presby Med Ctr 1993; **Fac Appt:** Assoc Prof N, UMDNJ-NJ Med Sch, Newark

Clinical Genetics

Desposito, Franklin MD (CG) - **Spec Exp:** Birth Defects; Genetic Disorders; **Hospital:** Univ Hosp-UMDNJ—Newark, Saint Barnabas Med Ctr; **Address:** 90 Bergen St, Ste 5400, Newark, NJ 07103; **Phone:** 973-972-3300; **Board Cert:** Pediatrics 1986; Clinical Genetics 1982; Clinical Cytogenetics 1990; Clinical Molecular Genetics 2010; **Med School:** Ros Franklin Univ/Chicago Med Sch 1957; **Resid:** Pediatrics, Long Island Jewish Hosp 1961; **Fellow:** Hematology, Univ Wisc Sch Med 1963; **Fac Appt:** Prof Ped, UMDNJ-NJ Med Sch, Newark

Colon & Rectal Surgery

Gilder, Mark MD (CRS) - **Hospital:** Saint Barnabas Med Ctr, Morristown Mem Hosp (page 92); **Address:** Assocs in Colon & Rectal Diseases, 231 Millburn Ave, Millburn, NJ 07041-1718; **Phone:** 973-467-2277; **Board Cert:** Colon & Rectal Surgery 2006; **Med School:** NY Med Coll 1987; **Resid:** Surgery, North Shore Univ Hosp 1992; **Fellow:** Colon & Rectal Surgery, St Francis Hosp 1993

Rothberg, Robert MD (CRS) - **Spec Exp:** Colon & Rectal Cancer; Colonoscopy; Inflammatory Bowel Disease; **Hospital:** Mountainside Hosp, Clara Maass Med Ctr; **Address:** 39 S Fullerton Ave, Montclair, NJ 07042-6303; **Phone:** 973-744-0550; **Board Cert:** Colon & Rectal Surgery 1978; **Med School:** NYU Sch Med 1972; **Resid:** Surgery, Hackensack Hosp 1977; Colon & Rectal Surgery, Muhlenberg Hosp 1978

Dermatology

Connolly, Adrian L MD (D) - **Spec Exp:** Mohs' Surgery; Skin Cancer; **Hospital:** Saint Barnabas Med Ctr; **Address:** 101 Old Short Hills Rd, Ste 503, West Orange, NJ 07052-1023; **Phone:** 973-731-9131; **Board Cert:** Dermatology 2009; **Med School:** UMDNJ-NJ Med Sch, Newark 1975; **Resid:** Dermatology, NYU Med Ctr 1979; **Fellow:** Mohs Surgery, NYU Med Ctr 1980; **Fac Appt:** Asst Clin Prof D, UMDNJ-NJ Med Sch, Newark

Downie, Jeanine B MD (D) - **Spec Exp:** Cosmetic Dermatology; Botox Therapy; Black/Asian Skin Care; Skin Laser Surgery; **Hospital:** Overlook Hosp (page 92), Mountainside Hosp; **Address:** 51 Park St, Montclair, NJ 07042; **Phone:** 973-509-6900; **Board Cert:** Dermatology 2006; **Med School:** SUNY Downstate 1992; **Resid:** Pediatrics, New York Hosp 1994; Dermatology, Mt Sinai Med Ctr 1997

Liftin, Alan J MD (D) - **Spec Exp:** Cosmetic Dermatology; Botox Therapy; Facial Rejuvenation; Acne & Rosacea; **Hospital:** Saint Barnabas Med Ctr; **Address:** 22 Old Short Hills Rd, Ste 103, Livingston, NJ 07039-5605; **Phone:** 973-535-5800; **Board Cert:** Dermatology 1990; Anatomic Pathology 1987; Dermatopathology 1989; **Med School:** Mount Sinai Sch Med 1987; **Resid:** Pathology, Mt Sinai Hosp 1985; Dermatology, Mt Sinai Hosp 1990; **Fellow:** Dermatopathology, Hosp Univ Penn 1986

Machler, Brian C MD (D) - **Spec Exp:** Contact Dermatitis; Laser Surgery; Skin Cancer; **Hospital:** Saint Barnabas Med Ctr; **Address:** 101 Old Short Hills Rd, West Orange, NJ 07052; **Phone:** 973-736-9535; **Board Cert:** Dermatology 2004; **Med School:** UMDNJ-NJ Med Sch, Newark 1991; **Resid:** Dermatology, Jackson Meml Hosp 1995; **Fac Appt:** Asst Prof D, NYU Sch Med

Rozanski, Reuben MD (D) - **Spec Exp:** Cosmetic Dermatology; Acne; Rosacea; **Hospital:** Mountainside Hosp; **Address:** 200 Highland Ave, Glen Ridge, NJ 07028-1528; **Phone:** 973-748-9474; **Board Cert:** Dermatology 1979; Internal Medicine 1974; **Med School:** Boston Univ 1970; **Resid:** Internal Medicine, Montefiore Med Ctr 1974; Dermatology, Albert Einstein Coll Med 1976

Schwartz, Robert A MD (D) - **Spec Exp:** Skin Cancer; Atopic Dermatitis; Rosacea; **Hospital:** Univ Hosp-UMDNJ—Newark; **Address:** 90 Bergen St, Ste 4400, Newark, NJ 07103-2757; **Phone:** 973-972-1880; **Board Cert:** Dermatology 1978; Clinical & Laboratory Dermatologic Immunology 1985; **Med School:** NY Med Coll 1974; **Resid:** Dermatology, Univ Hosp 1977; Dermatology, Roswell Park Meml Inst 1978; **Fellow:** Dermatopathology, NJ Med Sch Affil Hosps 1990; **Fac Appt:** Prof D, UMDNJ-NJ Med Sch, Newark

Diagnostic Radiology

Byk, Cheryl MD (DR) - **Spec Exp:** Mammography; Nuclear Medicine; **Address:** 61 Main St, Ste 61 A, West Orange, NJ 07052; **Phone:** 973-669-1989; **Board Cert:** Diagnostic Radiology 1976; Nuclear Radiology 1977; **Med School:** UMDNJ-NJ Med Sch, Newark 1972; **Resid:** Diagnostic Radiology, St Vincent's Hosp 1976; **Fellow:** Nuclear Medicine, St Vincent's Hosp 1977; **Fac Appt:** Asst Clin Prof, Mount Sinai Sch Med

Jewel, Kenneth MD (DR) - **Spec Exp:** MRI; CT Scan; **Hospital:** Chilton Meml Hosp; **Address:** 116 Park St, Montclair, NJ 07042-2930; **Phone:** 973-746-2525; **Board Cert:** Diagnostic Radiology 1973; **Med School:** SUNY Buffalo 1968; **Resid:** Diagnostic Radiology, Staten Island USPHS Hosp 1971; **Fellow:** Diagnostic Radiology, Columbia-Presby Hosp 1972

Lee, Huey-Jen MD (DR) - **Spec Exp:** Brain Imaging; Head & Neck Imaging; Spine Neuroradiologic Diagnosis; Brain Tumors; **Hospital:** Univ Hosp-UMDNJ—Newark; **Address:** 150 Bergen St, Ste C320, Dept of Radiology, Newark, NJ 07103; **Phone:** 973-972-4202; **Board Cert:** Diagnostic Radiology 1990; Neuroradiology 2005; **Med School:** Taiwan 1976; **Resid:** Pediatrics, Taipei Jen-Ai Hosp 1979; Diagnostic Radiology, Beth Israel Med Ctr 1988; **Fellow:** Neuroradiology, NY Med Coll 1989; **Fac Appt:** Prof Rad, UMDNJ-NJ Med Sch, Newark

Sanders, Linda M MD (DR) - **Spec Exp:** Breast Imaging; **Hospital:** Saint Barnabas Med Ctr; **Address:** St Barnabas Breast Center, 200 S Orange Ave, Livingston, NJ 07039; **Phone:** 973-322-7804; **Board Cert:** Diagnostic Radiology 1986; **Med School:** Univ Pennsylvania 1982; **Resid:** Diagnostic Radiology, Columbia-Presby Med Ctr 1986; **Fellow:** Mammography, Meml Sloan-Kettering Cancer Ctr 1987

Endocrinology, Diabetes & Metabolism

Baranetsky, Nicholas G MD (EDM) - **Spec Exp:** Thyroid Disorders; Pituitary Disorders; Adrenal Disorders; **Hospital:** Saint Michael's Med Ctr, Clara Maass Med Ctr; **Address:** 111 Central Ave, Newark, NJ 07102; **Phone:** 973-877-5185; **Board Cert:** Internal Medicine 1977; Endocrinology, Diabetes & Metabolism 1981; **Med School:** NY Med Coll 1974; **Resid:** Internal Medicine, Stamford Hosp 1977; **Fellow:** Endocrinology, Diabetes & Metabolism, VA Med Ctr-Wadsworth 1979; **Fac Appt:** Prof Med, Seton Hall Univ Sch Hlth & Med Scis

Dower, Samuel MD (EDM) - **Hospital:** Saint Barnabas Med Ctr; **Address:** 200 S Orange Ave, Ste 219, Livingston, NJ 07039; **Phone:** 973-322-7200; **Board Cert:** Internal Medicine 1984; Endocrinology 1987; **Med School:** NYU Sch Med 1981; **Resid:** Internal Medicine, Bronx Muni Hosp 1984; **Fellow:** Endocrinology, Mount Sinai Hosp 1985

Gewirtz, George MD (EDM) - **Spec Exp:** Diabetes; Thyroid Disorders; Osteoporosis; **Hospital:** Saint Barnabas Med Ctr; **Address:** 200 S Orange Ave, Livingston, NJ 07039; **Phone:** 973-322-7200; **Board Cert:** Internal Medicine 1972; Endocrinology 1975; **Med School:** Harvard Med Sch 1965; **Resid:** Internal Medicine, Bellevue Hosp Ctr-NYU 1967; Internal Medicine, Columbia-Presby Med Ctr 1971; **Fellow:** Endocrinology, Diabetes & Metabolism, Mt Sinai Hosp 1973

Sherry, Stephen H MD (EDM) - **Spec Exp:** Thyroid Disorders; Diabetes; Osteoporosis; **Hospital:** Mountainside Hosp; **Address:** 119 Grove St, Montclair, NJ 07042-2629; **Phone:** 973-744-3733; **Board Cert:** Internal Medicine 1979; Endocrinology, Diabetes & Metabolism 1981; **Med School:** Univ Conn 1976; **Resid:** Internal Medicine, New Eng Deaconess 1979; **Fellow:** Endocrinology, Diabetes & Metabolism, New Eng Deaconess 1981; **Fac Appt:** Asst Clin Prof Med, UMDNJ-NJ Med Sch, Newark

Family Medicine

Cirello, Richard MD (FMed) *PCP* - **Hospital:** Mountainside Hosp; **Address:** 271 Grove Ave, Verona, NJ 07044-1730; **Phone:** 973-239-2600; **Board Cert:** Family Medicine 2004; **Med School:** Mexico 1975; **Resid:** Family Medicine, Mountainside Hosp 1979; **Fac Appt:** Asst Clin Prof FMed, UMDNJ-Rutgers Med Sch

Gorman, Robert T MD (FMed) *PCP* - **Hospital:** Mountainside Hosp, Saint Barnabas Med Ctr; **Address:** 271 Grove Ave, Verona, NJ 07044; **Phone:** 973-239-2600; **Board Cert:** Family Medicine 2005; **Med School:** UMDNJ-NJ Med Sch, Newark 1982; **Resid:** Family Medicine, Mountainside Hosp 1985; **Fac Appt:** Asst Clin Prof FMed, UMDNJ-NJ Med Sch, Newark

Schlam, Everett W MD (FMed) *PCP* - **Spec Exp:** Travel Medicine; **Hospital:** Mountainside Hosp; **Address:** Mountainside Family Practice Assocs, 799 Bloomfield Ave, Box 3201, Verona, NJ 07044; **Phone:** 973-746-7050; **Board Cert:** Family Medicine 2007; Sports Medicine 1999; Adolescent Medicine 2001; **Med School:** UMDNJ-RW Johnson Med Sch 1986; **Resid:** Family Medicine, Mountainside Hosp 1989

Gastroenterology

Finkelstein, Warren MD (Ge) - **Spec Exp:** Crohn's Disease; Ulcerative Colitis; Inflammatory Bowel Disease; **Hospital:** Mountainside Hosp; **Address:** 123 Highland Ave, Ste 103, Glen Ridge, NJ 07028-1522; **Phone:** 973-429-8800; **Board Cert:** Internal Medicine 1975; Gastroenterology 1983; **Med School:** Med Coll VA 1972; **Resid:** Internal Medicine, Boston City Hosp 1974; Internal Medicine, Boston VA Med Ctr 1975; **Fellow:** Gastroenterology, Mass Genl Hosp 1977; **Fac Appt:** Assoc Clin Prof Med, UMDNJ-NJ Med Sch, Newark

Fiske, Steven MD (Ge) - **Spec Exp:** Inflammatory Bowel Disease/Crohn's; Colonoscopy; Peptic Acid Disorders; Gastroesophageal Reflux Disease (GERD); **Hospital:** Saint Barnabas Med Ctr, Clara Maass Med Ctr; **Address:** 741 Northfield Ave, Ste 101, West Orange, NJ 07052-1104; **Phone:** 973-325-5775; **Board Cert:** Internal Medicine 1977; Gastroenterology 1979; **Med School:** NYU Sch Med 1974; **Resid:** Internal Medicine, Bellevue Hosp/NYU Med Ctr 1976; **Fellow:** Gastroenterology, Brigham & Women's Hosp 1978; **Fac Appt:** Assoc Prof Med, Seton Hall Univ Sch Hlth & Med Scis

Kenny, Raymond MD (Ge) - **Spec Exp:** Liver Disease; Hepatitis B & C; Inflammatory Bowel Disease/Crohn's; Ulcerative Colitis; **Hospital:** Mountainside Hosp; **Address:** 123 Highland Ave, Ste 103, Glen Ridge, NJ 07028; **Phone:** 973-429-8800; **Board Cert:** Internal Medicine 1984; Gastroenterology 1987; **Med School:** SUNY Stony Brook 1981; **Resid:** Internal Medicine, Mayo Clinic 1984; **Fellow:** Gastroenterology, Univ Penn Med Ctr 1986; **Fac Appt:** Asst Clin Prof Med, UMDNJ-NJ Med Sch, Newark

Mogan, Glen MD (Ge) - **Spec Exp:** Inflammatory Bowel Disease; Peptic Ulcer Disease; Gastroesophageal Reflux Disease (GERD); **Hospital:** Saint Barnabas Med Ctr; **Address:** 741 N Field Ave, Ste 204, West Orange, NJ 07052-1104; **Phone:** 973-731-8686; **Board Cert:** Internal Medicine 1978; Gastroenterology 1981; **Med School:** SUNY Upstate Med Univ 1975; **Resid:** Internal Medicine, Mount Sinai Hosp 1978; **Fellow:** Gastroenterology, Mount Sinai Hosp 1980; **Fac Appt:** Assoc Clin Prof Med, UMDNJ-Rutgers Med Sch

Schrader, Zalman MD (Ge) - **Spec Exp:** Endoscopy; Colonoscopy; Gastroesophageal Reflux Disease (GERD); Celiac Disease; **Hospital:** Saint Barnabas Med Ctr, Morristown Mem Hosp (page 92); **Address:** 101 Old Short Hills Rd, Ste 217, W Orange, NJ 07052-1023; **Phone:** 973-731-4600; **Board Cert:** Internal Medicine 1968; Gastroenterology 1972; **Med School:** Albert Einstein Coll Med 1961; **Resid:** Internal Medicine, Bronx Municipal Hosp 1967; **Fellow:** Gastroenterology, New York Hosp-Cornell Med Ctr 1969

Sloan, William MD (Ge) - **Spec Exp:** Liver Disease; Inflammatory Bowel Disease; Endoscopy; Hepatitis; **Hospital:** Saint Barnabas Med Ctr, Morristown Mem Hosp (page 92); **Address:** 101 Old Short Hills Rd, Ste 217, West Orange, NJ 07052-1023; **Phone:** 973-731-4600; **Board Cert:** Internal Medicine 1972; Gastroenterology 1972; **Med School:** Univ Pennsylvania 1965; **Resid:** Internal Medicine, Mt Sinai Hosp 1970; **Fellow:** Gastroenterology, Mt Sinai Hosp 1972

Spira, Robert S MD (Ge) - **Spec Exp:** Liver Disease; Inflammatory Bowel Disease; **Hospital:** Saint Michael's Med Ctr, Clara Maass Med Ctr; **Address:** 5 Franklin Ave, Claremont Professional Bldg, Belleville, NJ 07109; **Phone:** 973-759-7240; **Board Cert:** Internal Medicine 1978; Gastroenterology 1981; **Med School:** NYU Sch Med 1975; **Resid:** Internal Medicine, Bellevue Hosp/NYU Med Ctr 1978; **Fellow:** Gastroenterology, VA Med Ctr 1981

Gynecologic Oncology

Cracchiolo, Bernadette M MD (GO) - **Hospital:** Univ Hosp-UMDNJ—Newark; **Address:** UMDNJ-New Jersey Med Sch, Dept OB/Gyn, 185 S Orange Ave, rm E 506, ACC Level C, Newark, NJ 07101; **Phone:** 973-972-5055; **Board Cert:** Obstetrics & Gynecology 2009; Gynecologic Oncology 2008; Hospice & Palliative Medicine 2008; **Med School:** Univ Hlth Scis, Chicago Med Sch 1991; **Resid:** Obstetrics & Gynecology, Columbia Presby Hosp 1995; **Fellow:** Obstetrics & Gynecology, Yale-New Haven Hosp 1997; **Fac Appt:** Asst Prof ObG, UMDNJ-NJ Med Sch, Newark

Denehy, Thad MD (GO) - **Spec Exp:** Uterine Cancer; Ovarian Cancer; Pelvic Organ Prolapse Repair; Laparoscopic Surgery; **Hospital:** Saint Barnabas Med Ctr, Chilton Meml Hosp; **Address:** Gynecologic Cancer & Pelvic Surgery, 101 Old Short Hills Rd, Ste 400, West Orange, NJ 07052; **Phone:** 973-243-9300; **Board Cert:** Obstetrics & Gynecology 2009; Gynecologic Oncology 2009; **Med School:** Wake Forest Univ 1984; **Resid:** Obstetrics & Gynecology, St Barnabas Med Ctr 1988; **Fellow:** Gynecologic Oncology, Strong Meml Hosp 1990

Hematology

Cohen, Alice J MD (Hem) - **Spec Exp:** Bleeding/Coagulation Disorders; **Hospital:** Newark Beth Israel Med Ctr, Saint Barnabas Med Ctr; **Address:** Newark Beth Israel Med Ctr, Div Hem, 201 Lyons Ave at Osborne Terrace, Newark, NJ 07112; **Phone:** 973-926-7230; **Board Cert:** Internal Medicine 1984; Hematology 1986; Medical Oncology 2001; **Med School:** Ros Franklin Univ/Chicago Med Sch 1981; **Resid:** Internal Medicine, NYU-Man VA Med Ctr 1984; **Fellow:** Hematology & Oncology, Geo Wash Univ Med Ctr 1986; Hematology & Oncology, Columbia Presby Med Ctr 1987; **Fac Appt:** Assoc Clin Prof Med, Columbia P&S

Sabnani, Indu MD (Hem) - **Spec Exp:** Lymphoma; **Hospital:** Newark Beth Israel Med Ctr; **Address:** Newark Beth Israel Med Ctr, 2130 Milburn Ave, Ste C11, Maplewood, NJ 07040; **Phone:** 973-762-7676; **Board Cert:** Internal Medicine 1987; Hematology 2001; Medical Oncology 1989; **Med School:** India 1980; **Resid:** Internal Medicine, United Hosp 1987; **Fellow:** Hematology & Oncology, UMDNJ-Newark 1990

Zager, Robert MD (Hem) - **Hospital:** Mountainside Hosp; **Address:** Richard F Harries Ambulatory Care Pav, 1 Bay Ave Fl 2nd - Ste 1, Montclair, NJ 07042; **Phone:** 973-259-3555; **Board Cert:** Internal Medicine 1973; Hematology 1974; Medical Oncology 1975; **Med School:** Cornell Univ-Weill Med Coll 1968; **Resid:** Internal Medicine, New York Hosp 1970; Medical Oncology, Natl Cancer Inst-NIH 1972; **Fellow:** Hematology & Oncology, New York Hosp 1974; **Fac Appt:** Asst Clin Prof Med, UMDNJ-NJ Med Sch, Newark

Zauber, N Peter MD (Hem) - **Hospital:** Saint Barnabas Med Ctr; **Address:** 22 Old Short Hills Rd, Ste 108, Livingston, NJ 07039; **Phone:** 973-533-9299; **Board Cert:** Internal Medicine 1976; Hematology 1978; **Med School:** Johns Hopkins Univ 1971; **Resid:** Internal Medicine, NY-Meml Hosps 1973; Internal Medicine, Baltimore City Hosp 1976; **Fellow:** Hematology & Oncology, Presby Hosp 1978

Infectious Disease

Martinez, Homar MD (Inf) - **Spec Exp:** Travel Medicine; **Hospital:** Clara Maass Med Ctr, Saint Barnabas Med Ctr; **Address:** 50 Newark Ave, Ste 101, Belleville, NJ 07109; **Phone:** 973-759-1221; **Board Cert:** Internal Medicine 2005; Infectious Disease 2007; **Med School:** Mexico 1985; **Resid:** Internal Medicine, St Vincents Hosp 1990; **Fellow:** Infectious Disease, Long Island Coll Hosp 1992

Slim, Jihad MD (Inf) - **Spec Exp:** AIDS/HIV; Hepatitis C; Hospital Acquired Infections; Osteomyelitis; **Hospital:** Saint Michael's Med Ctr, Newark Beth Israel Med Ctr; **Address:** Saint Michael's Med Ctr, 11 Central Ave Blvd, Newark, NJ 07102; **Phone:** 973-877-5644; **Board Cert:** Internal Medicine 1986; Infectious Disease 1988; **Med School:** Lebanon 1980; **Resid:** Internal Medicine, Broussais Hosp 1983; Internal Medicine, Saint Michael's Med Ctr 1986; **Fellow:** Infectious Disease, Saint Michaels Med Ctr 1988; **Fac Appt:** Asst Prof Med, Seton Hall Univ Sch Hlth & Med Scis

Smith, Stephen M MD (Inf) - **Spec Exp:** AIDS/HIV; Diagnostic Problems; **Hospital:** Saint Michael's Med Ctr, Saint Barnabas Med Ctr; **Address:** 111 Central Ave, Saint Michael's Med Ctr, Newark, NJ 07102; **Phone:** 973-877-5482; **Board Cert:** Infectious Disease 2004; **Med School:** Yale Univ 1989; **Resid:** Internal Medicine, Univ VA 1991; **Fellow:** Infectious Disease, Natl Inst Allergy & Inf Dis 1993; **Fac Appt:** Asst Prof Med, Seton Hall Univ Sch Hlth & Med Scis

Soroko, Theresa A MD (Inf) - **Spec Exp:** AIDS/HIV; Lyme Disease; Skin/Soft Tissue Infection; **Hospital:** Mountainside Hosp, Clara Maass Med Ctr; **Address:** 199 Broad St, Ste 2A, Bloomfield, NJ 07003-2635; **Phone:** 973-748-4583; **Board Cert:** Internal Medicine 1988; Infectious Disease 2002; **Med School:** Grenada 1985; **Resid:** Internal Medicine, St Michael's Med Ctr 1988; **Fellow:** Infectious Disease, St Michael's Med Ctr 1990; **Fac Appt:** Asst Clin Prof Med, UMDNJ-NJ Med Sch, Newark

Internal Medicine

Atkin, Suzanne MD (IM) *PCP* - **Hospital:** Univ Hosp-UMDNJ—Newark; **Address:** University Hosp, D217, 150 Bergen St, rm D217, Newark, NJ 07103; **Phone:** 973-972-0440; **Board Cert:** Internal Medicine 1982; Emergency Medicine 2000; **Med School:** UMDNJ-NJ Med Sch, Newark 1979; **Resid:** Internal Medicine, UMDNJ-NJ Med Sch 1982; **Fac Appt:** Assoc Prof Med, UMDNJ-NJ Med Sch, Newark

Bains, Yatinder MD (IM) *PCP* - **Spec Exp:** Liver Disease; Inflammatory Bowel Disease; Gastroesophageal Reflux Disease (GERD); **Hospital:** Clara Maass Med Ctr, Jersey City Med Ctr; **Address:** 116 Millburn Ave, Ste 102, Millburn, NJ 07104; **Phone:** 973-376-2121; **Board Cert:** Internal Medicine 2002; Gastroenterology 2003; **Med School:** UMDNJ-NJ Med Sch, Newark 1987; **Resid:** Internal Medicine, UMDNJ 1990; **Fellow:** Gastroenterology, UMDNJ 1992

Chrisanderson, Donna MD (IM) - **Hospital:** Saint Barnabas Med Ctr; **Address:** 2040 Millburn Ave, Ste 402, Maplewood, NJ 07040; **Phone:** 973-378-9070; **Board Cert:** Internal Medicine 2004; **Med School:** Med Coll GA 1988; **Resid:** Internal Medicine, Greenwich Hosp 1991; **Fellow:** Internal Medicine, Univ Alabama Hosp 1993

De Cosimo, Diana R MD (IM) *PCP* - **Spec Exp:** Women's Health; Geriatric Care; Preventive Medicine; **Hospital:** Univ Hosp-UMDNJ—Newark; **Address:** Doctors Office Ctr, 140 Bergen St, F-Level, Newark, NJ 07103; **Phone:** 973-972-1880; **Board Cert:** Internal Medicine 1977; Cardiovascular Disease 1979; **Med School:** Boston Univ 1974; **Resid:** Internal Medicine, Worcester City Hosp 1977; **Fellow:** Cardiovascular Disease, Univ Mass Med Ctr 1979; **Fac Appt:** Assoc Prof Med, UMDNJ-NJ Med Sch, Newark

Di Giacomo, William A MD (IM) *PCP* - **Hospital:** Saint Michael's Med Ctr, Overlook Hosp (page 92); **Address:** 1072 S Orange Ave, Newark, NJ 07106; **Phone:** 973-623-5309; **Board Cert:** Internal Medicine 1978; **Med School:** Mexico 1974; **Resid:** Internal Medicine, St Michaels Med Ctr 1978; **Fac Appt:** Assoc Prof Med, Seton Hall Univ Sch Hlth & Med Scis

Fortunato, Franklin D MD (IM) *PCP* - **Spec Exp:** Asthma; **Hospital:** Mountainside Hosp, Clara Maass Med Ctr; **Address:** 127 Pine St, Montclair, NJ 07042-4835; **Phone:** 973-744-4075; **Board Cert:** Internal Medicine 1978; Pulmonary Disease 1980; **Med School:** UMDNJ-NJ Med Sch, Newark 1975; **Resid:** Internal Medicine, St Michael's Med Ctr 1977; **Fellow:** Pulmonary Disease, St Michael's Med Ctr 1979

Gribbon, John MD (IM) *PCP* - **Spec Exp:** Hypertension; Diabetes; **Hospital:** Mountainside Hosp; **Address:** 62 S Fullerton Ave, Montclair, NJ 07042-2686; **Phone:** 973-744-3382; **Board Cert:** Internal Medicine 1980; **Med School:** UMDNJ-NJ Med Sch, Newark 1977; **Resid:** Internal Medicine, UMDNJ-NJ Med Schl 1980; **Fac Appt:** Asst Clin Prof Med, UMDNJ-NJ Med Sch, Newark

Haggerty, Mary A MD (IM) *PCP* - **Spec Exp:** Preventive Medicine; Hypertension; **Hospital:** Univ Hosp-UMDNJ—Newark, Newark Beth Israel Med Ctr; **Address:** 90 Bergen St, Newark, NJ 07103; **Phone:** 973-972-1880; **Board Cert:** Internal Medicine 2000; Geriatric Medicine 2000; **Med School:** UMDNJ-NJ Med Sch, Newark 1979; **Resid:** Internal Medicine, UMDNJ-Univ Hosp 1982; **Fac Appt:** Assoc Prof Med, UMDNJ-NJ Med Sch, Newark

Rommer, James A MD (IM) *PCP* - **Spec Exp:** Preventive Medicine; **Hospital:** Saint Barnabas Med Ctr; **Address:** 349 E Northfield Rd, Ste 110, Livingston, NJ 07039-4807; **Phone:** 973-992-2227; **Board Cert:** Internal Medicine 1981; **Med School:** Cornell Univ-Weill Med Coll 1978; **Resid:** Internal Medicine, NY Hosp-Cornell Med Ctr 1981; **Fellow:** Internal Medicine, Johns Hopkins Med Sch 1982; **Fac Appt:** Asst Clin Prof Med, Mount Sinai Sch Med

Russo, John A MD (IM) *PCP* - **Hospital:** Saint Barnabas Med Ctr; **Address:** 1500 Pleasant Valley Way, Ste 201, West Orange, NJ 07052; **Phone:** 973-736-8119; **Board Cert:** Internal Medicine 1988; **Med School:** Mexico 1981; **Resid:** Internal Medicine, UMDNJ Med Ctr 1987

Interventional Cardiology

Cohen, Marc MD (IC) - **Hospital:** Newark Beth Israel Med Ctr; **Address:** Newark Beth Israel Med Ctr, 201 Lyons Ave, Ste C2, Newark, NJ 07112; **Phone:** 973-926-7852; **Board Cert:** Internal Medicine 1980; Cardiovascular Disease 1983; Interventional Cardiology 2009; **Med School:** NYU Sch Med 1977; **Resid:** Internal Medicine, Mt Sinai Hosp 1980; **Fellow:** Cardiovascular Disease, Mt Sinai Hosp 1982; **Fac Appt:** Prof Med, Mount Sinai Sch Med

Miller, Kenneth P MD (IC) - **Spec Exp:** Interventional Cardiology; **Hospital:** Mountainside Hosp, Saint Barnabas Med Ctr; **Address:** 62 S Fullerton Ave, Montclair, NJ 07042-2629; **Phone:** 973-746-8585; **Board Cert:** Internal Medicine 1985; Cardiovascular Disease 1989; Interventional Cardiology 2002; **Med School:** NYU Sch Med 1982; **Resid:** Internal Medicine, Bronx Muni Hosp 1986; **Fellow:** Cardiovascular Disease, Columbia Presby Med Ctr 1989

Maternal & Fetal Medicine

Gimovsky, Martin MD (MF) - **Spec Exp:** Pregnancy-High Risk; **Hospital:** Newark Beth Israel Med Ctr; **Address:** OB/GYN Ultrasound, 201 Lyons Ave, Newark, NJ 07112; **Phone:** 973-926-7342; **Board Cert:** Obstetrics & Gynecology 2009; Maternal & Fetal Medicine 2009; **Med School:** NYU Sch Med 1976; **Resid:** Obstetrics & Gynecology, Sloane Hosp/Columbia Presby hop 1980; **Fellow:** Maternal & Fetal Medicine, USC Med Ctr 1982; **Fac Appt:** Prof ObG, Mount Sinai Sch Med

Smith Jr, Leon G MD (MF) - **Spec Exp:** Ultrasound; Prenatal Diagnosis; Perinatal Infections; Amniocentesis; **Hospital:** Saint Barnabas Med Ctr; **Address:** NJ Perinatal Associates, 94 Old Short Hills Rd, East Wing, Ste 402, Livingston, NJ 07039-5672; **Phone:** 973-322-5287; **Board Cert:** Obstetrics & Gynecology 2009; Maternal & Fetal Medicine 2009; **Med School:** Georgetown Univ 1985; **Resid:** Obstetrics & Gynecology, Tulane Univ Hosp 1989; **Fellow:** Maternal & Fetal Medicine, Baylor Univ Hosp 1991

Warren, Wendy B MD (MF) - **Spec Exp:** Pregnancy-High Risk; **Hospital:** Saint Barnabas Med Ctr; **Address:** NJ Perinatal Associates, 94 Old Short Hills Rd, East Wing, Ste 402, Livingston, NJ 07039; **Phone:** 973-322-5287; **Board Cert:** Obstetrics & Gynecology 2009; Maternal & Fetal Medicine 2008; **Med School:** Cornell Univ 1982; **Resid:** Obstetrics & Gynecology, T Jefferson Univ Hosp 1986; **Fellow:** Maternal & Fetal Medicine, Columbia Presby Hosp 1991

Medical Oncology

Leitner, Stuart P MD (Onc) - **Spec Exp:** Urologic Cancer; Breast Cancer; **Hospital:** Saint Barnabas Med Ctr; **Address:** Medical Oncology Assoc of SBMC, 94 Old Short Hills Rd, SBMC-East Wing, Cancer Ctr, Livington, NJ 07039; **Phone:** 973-322-5200; **Board Cert:** Internal Medicine 1982; Medical Oncology 1985; **Med School:** Mount Sinai Sch Med 1979; **Resid:** Internal Medicine, Univ Tex SW 1982; **Fellow:** Medical Oncology, Meml Sloan Kettering Cancer 1985

Lippman, Alan MD (Onc) - **Hospital:** Clara Maass Med Ctr, Saint Barnabas Med Ctr; **Address:** 36 Newark Ave, Ste 304, Belleville, NJ 07109; **Phone:** 973-751-8880; **Board Cert:** Internal Medicine 1973; Medical Oncology 1975; **Med School:** Hahnemann Univ 1965; **Resid:** Internal Medicine, Newark Beth Israel Med Ctr 1970; **Fellow:** Medical Oncology, Meml Sloan Kettering Canc Hosp 1972; **Fac Appt:** Assoc Clin Prof Med, UMDNJ-NJ Med Sch, Newark

Michaelson, Richard MD (Onc) - **Spec Exp:** Breast Cancer; **Hospital:** Saint Barnabas Med Ctr; **Address:** St Barnabas Med Ctr-East Wing Fl 2, 94 Old Short Hills Rd, Livingston, NJ 07039; **Phone:** 973-322-5362; **Board Cert:** Internal Medicine 1979; Medical Oncology 1981; **Med School:** Univ Pennsylvania 1976; **Resid:** Internal Medicine, Hosp Univ Penn 1979; **Fellow:** Medical Oncology, Meml Sloan Kettering Canc Ctr 1981

Sagorin, Charles MD (Onc) - **Hospital:** Mountainside Hosp; **Address:** 127 Pine St, Ste 6, Montclair, NJ 07042-4868; **Phone:** 973-783-3300; **Board Cert:** Internal Medicine 1981; Medical Oncology 1983; Hematology 1986; **Med School:** SUNY Downstate 1971; **Resid:** Internal Medicine, Bronx Municipal Hosp 1973; **Fellow:** Hematology, Montefiore Med Ctr 1974; Medical Oncology, Montefiore Med Ctr 1978

Scoppetuolo, Michael MD (Onc) - **Spec Exp:** Sarcoma; Palliative Care; Hematologic Malignancies; Lung Cancer; **Hospital:** Saint Barnabas Med Ctr; **Address:** 94 Old Short Hills Rd, Cancer Ctr at St Barnabas Med Ctr, Livingston, NJ 07039; **Phone:** 973-322-5735; **Board Cert:** Internal Medicine 1982; Medical Oncology 1985; **Med School:** Ros Franklin Univ/Chicago Med Sch 1979; **Resid:** Internal Medicine, Univ Hosp UMDNJ 1982; **Fellow:** Hematology & Oncology, Meml Sloan Kettering Cancer Ctr 1984

Neonatal-Perinatal Medicine

Sun, Shyan-chu MD (NP) - **Spec Exp:** Prematurity/Low Birth Weight Infants; Breathing Disorders; Respiratory Distress Syndrome; **Hospital:** Saint Barnabas Med Ctr; **Address:** Dept Neonatology, 94 Old Short Hills Rd, Livingston, NJ 07039; **Phone:** 973-322-5437; **Board Cert:** Pediatrics 1969; Neonatal-Perinatal Medicine 1975; **Med School:** Taiwan 1961; **Resid:** Pediatrics, Univ London 1967; Pediatrics, Harlem Hosp 1970; **Fellow:** Neonatology, LI Jewish Med Ctr 1972; **Fac Appt:** Clin Prof Ped, UMDNJ-NJ Med Sch, Newark

Nephrology

Byrd, Lawrence H MD (Nep) - **Spec Exp:** Hypertension; Kidney Disease; Dialysis Care; **Hospital:** Saint Barnabas Med Ctr, Bayonne Med Ctr; **Address:** 22 Old Short Hills Rd, Ste 212, Livingston, NJ 07039-5605; **Phone:** 973-994-4550; **Board Cert:** Internal Medicine 1977; Nephrology 1978; **Med School:** Med Coll PA 1973; **Resid:** Internal Medicine, UMDNJ-Univ Hosp 1976; **Fellow:** Nephrology, NY Hosp-Cornell 1978; **Fac Appt:** Asst Clin Prof Med, UMDNJ-NJ Med Sch, Newark

Grasso, Michael MD (Nep) - **Spec Exp:** Kidney Disease; Hypertension; Dialysis Care; Transplant Medicine-Kidney; **Hospital:** Newark Beth Israel Med Ctr, Saint Barnabas Med Ctr; **Address:** 111 Northfield Ave, Ste 311, West Orange, NJ 07052-4703; **Phone:** 973-325-2103; **Board Cert:** Internal Medicine 1974; Nephrology 1976; **Med School:** Univ MD Sch Med 1970; **Resid:** Internal Medicine, Univ MD Hosp 1974; **Fellow:** Nephrology, Newark Beth Israel Hosp 1976

Lyman, Neil MD (Nep) - **Spec Exp:** Dialysis Care; Kidney Failure; **Hospital:** Saint Barnabas Med Ctr, Clara Maass Med Ctr; **Address:** 769 Northfield Ave, Ste 200, West Orange, NJ 07052-1106; **Phone:** 973-736-2212; **Board Cert:** Internal Medicine 1976; Nephrology 1980; **Med School:** Albert Einstein Coll Med 1973; **Resid:** Internal Medicine, Mt Sinai Hosp 1976; Nephrology, Mt Sinai Hosp 1979; **Fellow:** Nephrology, Boston Med Ctr 1977; **Fac Appt:** Asst Prof Med, UMDNJ-NJ Med Sch, Newark

Mulgaonkar, Shamkant MD (Nep) - **Spec Exp:** Transplant Medicine-Kidney; **Hospital:** Saint Barnabas Med Ctr, Newark Beth Israel Med Ctr; **Address:** St Barnabas Med Ctr, 94 Old Short Hills Rd, Ste 303, Livingston, NJ 07039; **Phone:** 973-322-8216; **Board Cert:** Internal Medicine 1981; Nephrology 1982; **Med School:** India 1975; **Resid:** Internal Medicine, Morristown Meml Hosp 1980; **Fellow:** Nephrology, St Barnabas Med Ctr 1982; **Fac Appt:** Assoc Prof Med, UMDNJ-NJ Med Sch, Newark

Sipzner, Robert J MD (Nep) - **Spec Exp:** Hypertension; Kidney Failure; **Hospital:** Bayonne Med Ctr, Saint Barnabas Med Ctr; **Address:** 22 Old Short Hills Rd, Ste 212, Livingston, NJ 07039; **Phone:** 973-994-4550; **Board Cert:** Internal Medicine 1985; Nephrology 1988; **Med School:** NYU Sch Med 1982; **Resid:** Internal Medicine, SUNY Downstate Med Ctr 1985; **Fellow:** Nephrology, Univ Tenn Hlth Sci Ctr 1987

Neurological Surgery

Heary, Robert F MD (NS) - **Spec Exp:** Spinal Surgery; Spinal Cord Injury; Spinal Deformity; **Hospital:** Univ Hosp-UMDNJ—Newark, Overlook Hosp (page 92); **Address:** UMDNJ-NJ Med Sch, Div Neurosurg, 90 Bergen St, Ste 8100, Newark, NJ 07103-2499; **Phone:** 973-972-2323; **Board Cert:** Neurological Surgery 2010; **Med School:** Univ Pittsburgh 1986; **Resid:** Surgery, UMDNJ Univ Hosp 1989; Neurological Surgery, UMDNJ Univ Hosp 1994; **Fellow:** Orthopaedic Surgery, Thomas Jefferson Univ Hosp 1995; **Fac Appt:** Prof NS, UMDNJ-NJ Med Sch, Newark

Hubschmann, Otakar R MD (NS) - **Spec Exp:** Spinal Surgery-Complex; Cerebrovascular Neurosurgery; Chiari's Deformity; Brain Tumors; **Hospital:** Saint Barnabas Med Ctr, Newark Beth Israel Med Ctr; **Address:** 101 Old Short Hills Rd, Ste 409, W Orange, NJ 07052; **Phone:** 973-322-6732; **Board Cert:** Neurological Surgery 1978; **Med School:** Czech Republic 1967; **Resid:** Surgery, Montefiore Med Ctr 1970; Neurological Surgery, Montefiore Med Ctr 1976; **Fac Appt:** Prof NS, NY Coll Osteo Med

Neurology

Blady, David MD (N) - **Spec Exp:** Parkinson's Disease; Dementia; Multiple Sclerosis; Stroke; **Hospital:** Mountainside Hosp, Clara Maass Med Ctr; **Address:** 230 Sherman Ave, Ste K, Glen Ridge, NJ 07028-1520; **Phone:** 973-743-9555; **Board Cert:** Neurology 1990; **Med School:** SUNY Downstate 1983; **Resid:** Neurology, Bellevue Hosp/NYU Med Ctr 1987

Cook, Stuart D MD (N) - **Spec Exp:** Multiple Sclerosis; Infectious & Demyelinating Diseases; **Hospital:** Univ Hosp-UMDNJ—Newark; **Address:** 65 Bergen St, rm 1435, Newark, NJ 07101-1709; **Phone:** 973-972-9181; **Board Cert:** Neurology 1970; **Med School:** Univ VT Coll Med 1962; **Resid:** Neurology, Albert Einstein Coll Med 1968; **Fac Appt:** Prof N, UMDNJ-NJ Med Sch, Newark

Fellus, Jonathan L MD (N) - **Spec Exp:** Brain Injury; Neuro-Rehabilitation; Stroke; Dementia; **Hospital:** Kessler Inst for Rehab - W Orange; **Address:** Kessler Inst Rehab, 1199 Pleasant Valley Way, West Orange, NJ 07052; **Phone:** 973-414-4768; **Board Cert:** Neurology 1998; **Med School:** UMDNJ-RW Johnson Med Sch 1992; **Resid:** Neurology, Penn Hosp 1996; **Fellow:** Neurological Rehabilitation, Kernan Hosp-Univ Md Med Ctr 1997; **Fac Appt:** Asst Clin Prof N, UMDNJ-NJ Med Sch, Newark

Geller, Eric B MD (N) - **Spec Exp:** Epilepsy; **Hospital:** Saint Barnabas Med Ctr; **Address:** St Barnabas Inst Neurolgy & Neurosurg, 200 S Orange Ave, Ste 101, Livingston, NJ 07039; **Phone:** 973-322-7580; **Board Cert:** Neurology 2005; Clinical Neurophysiology 2006; **Med School:** Brown Univ 1989; **Resid:** Neurology, Harvard Med Sch Prog 1993; **Fellow:** Clinical Neurophysiology, Cleveland Clinic 1995

Marks, David A MD (N) - **Spec Exp:** Epilepsy/Seizure Disorders; Headache; Migraine; **Hospital:** Univ Hosp-UMDNJ—Newark; **Address:** 90 Bergen St Fl 8th - Ste 8100, Newark, NJ 07103; **Phone:** 973-972-2550; **Board Cert:** Neurology 1989; **Med School:** South Africa 1983; **Resid:** Neurology, Boston Med Ctr 1988; **Fellow:** Neurological Physiology, New England Med Ctr 1989; Epilepsy, Yale-New Haven Hosp 1991; **Fac Appt:** Assoc Prof Med, UMDNJ-NJ Med Sch, Newark

Ruderman, Marvin MD (N) - **Spec Exp:** Neuromuscular Disorders; Peripheral Neuropathy; Myasthenia Gravis; Demyelinating Neuropathy; **Hospital:** Saint Barnabas Med Ctr; **Address:** 1099 Bloomfield Ave, West Caldwell, NJ 07006-7129; **Phone:** 973-439-7000; **Board Cert:** Neurology 1981; **Med School:** Columbia P&S 1976; **Resid:** Neurology, Barnes Hosp 1980; **Fellow:** Neuromuscular Medicine, Columbia-Presby Med Ctr 1981

Nuclear Medicine

Lutzker, Letty G MD (NuM) - **Hospital:** Saint Barnabas Med Ctr; **Address:** St Barnabas Med Ctr, Dept Nuclear Med, 94 Old Short Hills Rd, Livingston, NJ 07039-5672; **Phone:** 973-322-5957; **Board Cert:** Diagnostic Radiology 1973; Nuclear Medicine 1974; Nuclear Radiology 1977; **Med School:** Albert Einstein Coll Med 1968; **Resid:** Diagnostic Radiology, Montefiore Med Ctr 1972; **Fac Appt:** Assoc Clin Prof NuM, Albert Einstein Coll Med

Obstetrics & Gynecology

Apuzzio, Joseph MD (ObG) - **Spec Exp:** Prenatal Diagnosis; Pregnancy-High Risk; Infectious Disease; **Hospital:** Univ Hosp-UMDNJ—Newark, Columbus Hosp; **Address:** UMDNJ Medical School, Dept OB/GYN & Women's Health, 185 S Orange Ave, MSB-rm E506, Newark, NJ 07103-2714; **Phone:** 973-972-5557; **Board Cert:** Obstetrics & Gynecology 2008; Maternal & Fetal Medicine 2008; **Med School:** UMDNJ-NJ Med Sch, Newark 1973; **Resid:** Obstetrics & Gynecology, UMDNJ-Univ Hosp 1976; **Fellow:** Maternal & Fetal Medicine, UMDNJ-Univ Hosp 1982; **Fac Appt:** Prof ObG, UMDNJ-NJ Med Sch, Newark

Cooperman, Alan S MD (ObG) - **Spec Exp:** Laparoscopic Surgery; Pelvic Surgery; Colposcopy; **Hospital:** Overlook Hosp (page 92), Saint Barnabas Med Ctr; **Address:** 235 Millburn Ave, Millburn, NJ 07041-1738; **Phone:** 973-467-9440; **Board Cert:** Obstetrics & Gynecology 1979; **Med School:** Italy 1968; **Resid:** Obstetrics & Gynecology, Newark Beth Israel Med Ctr 1973

Crane, Stephen MD (ObG) - **Hospital:** Saint Barnabas Med Ctr; **Address:** 776 Northfield Ave, Ste 202, West Orange, NJ 07052; **Phone:** 973-731-7707; **Board Cert:** Obstetrics & Gynecology 2001; **Med School:** UMDNJ-NJ Med Sch, Newark 1986; **Resid:** Obstetrics & Gynecology, St Barnabas Med Ctr 1990

Luciani, Richard L MD (ObG) - **Spec Exp:** Laparoscopic Surgery; Pregnancy-High Risk; Endometriosis; **Hospital:** Overlook Hosp (page 92), Saint Barnabas Med Ctr; **Address:** 235 Millburn Ave, Millburn, NJ 07041; **Phone:** 973-467-9440; **Board Cert:** Obstetrics & Gynecology 1982; **Med School:** UMDNJ-NJ Med Sch, Newark 1976; **Resid:** Obstetrics & Gynecology, St Barnabas Hosp 1980

Quartell, Anthony C MD (ObG) - **Spec Exp:** Laparoscopic Surgery-Complex; Pelvic Reconstruction; **Hospital:** Saint Barnabas Med Ctr; **Address:** 316 Eisenhower Pkwy, Ste 202, Livingston, NJ 07039-1718; **Phone:** 973-716-9600; **Board Cert:** Obstetrics & Gynecology 1978; **Med School:** UMDNJ-NJ Med Sch, Newark 1969; **Resid:** Surgery, New Jersey Coll Med 1971; Obstetrics & Gynecology, St Barnabas Med Ctr 1976; **Fac Appt:** Asst Clin Prof ObG, Mount Sinai Sch Med

Sladowski, Catherine F MD (ObG) - **Spec Exp:** Gynecology Only; **Hospital:** Saint Barnabas Med Ctr; **Address:** 22 Old Short Hills Rd, Ste 112, Livingston, NJ 07039; **Phone:** 973-740-1330; **Board Cert:** Obstetrics & Gynecology 1976; **Med School:** Med Coll PA Hahnemann 1970; **Resid:** Obstetrics & Gynecology, St Barnabas Hosp 1974

Ophthalmology

Bhagat, Neelakshi MD (Oph) - **Spec Exp:** Retina/Vitreous Surgery; Trauma; Diabetic Eye Disease/Retinopathy; Macular Degeneration; **Hospital:** Univ Hosp-UMDNJ—Newark; **Address:** NJ Med Sch Dept Ophthalmology, 90 Bergen St Fl DOC 6, Newark, NJ 07103; **Phone:** 973-972-2032; **Board Cert:** Ophthalmology 2009; **Med School:** SUNY Stony Brook 1994; **Resid:** Ophthalmology, UMDNJ-NJ Med School 1997; **Fellow:** Retina, Doheny Eye Inst- USC 1998; **Fac Appt:** Assoc Prof Oph, UMDNJ-NJ Med Sch, Newark

Cangemi, Francis E MD (Oph) - **Spec Exp:** Diabetic Eye Disease/Retinopathy; Macular Degeneration; Retinal Detachment; Retinopathy of Prematurity; **Hospital:** Clara Maass Med Ctr, Valley Hosp (page 658); **Address:** 36 Newark Ave, Ste 212, Belleville, NJ 07109-4121; **Phone:** 973-751-8808; **Board Cert:** Ophthalmology 1976; **Med School:** NY Med Coll 1969; **Resid:** Internal Medicine, Mayo Clinic 1971; Ophthalmology, NY EE Infirm 1975; **Fellow:** Retina/Vitreous, Mass EE Infirm 1972; Vitreoretinal Surgery, Mass EE Infirm 1976; **Fac Appt:** Assoc Clin Prof Oph, UMDNJ-NJ Med Sch, Newark

Caputo, Anthony R MD (Oph) - **Spec Exp:** Pediatric Ophthalmology; Strabismus; **Hospital:** Clara Maass Med Ctr; **Address:** 556 Eagle Rock Ave, Ste 203, Roseland, NJ 07068-1500; **Phone:** 973-228-3111; **Board Cert:** Ophthalmology 1976; **Med School:** Italy 1969; **Resid:** Ophthalmology, UMDNJ-Univ Hosp 1974; **Fellow:** Ophthalmology, Wills Eye Hosp 1975; **Fac Appt:** Prof Oph, UMDNJ-NJ Med Sch, Newark

Cohen, Steven B MD (Oph) - **Spec Exp:** Retina/Vitreous Surgery; Diabetic Eye Disease; Macular Degeneration; **Hospital:** Saint Barnabas Med Ctr, Overlook Hosp (page 92); **Address:** 349 E Northfield Rd, Ste 100, Livingston, NJ 07039-4807; **Phone:** 973-716-0123; **Board Cert:** Ophthalmology 1984; **Med School:** NYU Sch Med 1978; **Resid:** Ophthalmology, LI Jewish Med Ctr 1982; **Fellow:** Vitreoretinal Surgery, Univ Chicago Hosps 1985

Davidson, Lawrence M MD (Oph) - **Spec Exp:** LASIK-Refractive Surgery; Cataract Surgery; Glaucoma; **Hospital:** Mountainside Hosp, Saint Barnabas Med Ctr; **Address:** 825 Bloomfield Ave Fl 1, Verona, NJ 07044-1300; **Phone:** 973-239-4000; **Board Cert:** Ophthalmology 1975; **Med School:** SUNY Downstate 1969; **Resid:** Ophthalmology, Manhattan EE&T Hosp 1973

Eichler, Joel D MD (Oph) - **Spec Exp:** Diabetic Eye Disease/Retinopathy; Macular Degeneration; Retinal Disorders; **Hospital:** Clara Maass Med Ctr; **Address:** Eye Institute of Essex, 5 Franklin Ave, Ste 209, Belleville, NJ 07109; **Phone:** 973-751-6060; **Board Cert:** Ophthalmology 2004; **Med School:** Geo Wash Univ 1988; **Resid:** Ophthalmology, UMDNJ Affil Hosp 1992; **Fellow:** Vitreoretinal Surgery, Touro Infirm-Touro Hosp 1993

Frohman, Larry P MD (Oph) - **Spec Exp:** Neuro-Ophthalmology; Sarcoidosis; Vision Loss-Unexplained Loss; **Hospital:** Univ Hosp-UMDNJ—Newark; **Address:** 90 Bergen St, Ste 6174, Newark, NJ 07103-2425; **Phone:** 973-972-2065; **Board Cert:** Ophthalmology 1985; **Med School:** Univ Pennsylvania 1980; **Resid:** Ophthalmology, Bellevue Hosp 1984; **Fellow:** Neuro-Ophthalmology, Bellevue Hosp/NYU 1985; **Fac Appt:** Prof Oph, UMDNJ-NJ Med Sch, Newark

Glatt, Herbert MD (Oph) - **Spec Exp:** Cataract Surgery-Lens Implant; LASIK-Refractive Surgery; **Hospital:** Mountainside Hosp, Clara Maass Med Ctr; **Address:** 1025 Broad St, Bloomfield, NJ 07003-2844; **Phone:** 973-338-1001; **Board Cert:** Ophthalmology 1991; **Med School:** Mexico 1979; **Resid:** Ophthalmology, UMDNJ-NJ Med Sch 1983; **Fac Appt:** Asst Clin Prof Oph, UMDNJ-NJ Med Sch, Newark

Langer, Paul MD (Oph) - **Spec Exp:** Trauma; Orbital Tumors/Cancer; Thyroid Eye Disease; **Hospital:** Univ Hosp-UMDNJ—Newark; **Address:** 90 Bergen St Fl 6 - Ste 6100, Newark, NJ 07103; **Phone:** 973-972-2065; **Board Cert:** Ophthalmology 2005; **Med School:** Johns Hopkins Univ 1989; **Resid:** Ophthalmology, UCSF Med Ctr 1993; **Fellow:** Ophthalmic Plastic Surgery, Univ Utah Affil Hosp 1995; Orbital Surgery, Moorfields Eye Hosp 1995; **Fac Appt:** Assoc Prof Oph, UMDNJ-NJ Med Sch, Newark

Miller, Philip M MD (Oph) - **Spec Exp:** Laser Refractive Surgery; Cataract Surgery; Glaucoma; **Hospital:** Saint Barnabas Med Ctr; **Address:** 211 Irvington Ave, South Orange, NJ 07079; **Phone:** 973-325-3300; **Board Cert:** Ophthalmology 1967; **Med School:** Northwestern Univ 1961; **Resid:** Ophthalmology, Downstate Univ Med Ctr 1965

Turbin, Roger E MD (Oph) - **Spec Exp:** Neuro-Ophthalmology; Orbital Tumors/Cancer; Oculo-plastic & Orbital Surgery; **Hospital:** Univ Hosp-UMDNJ—Newark, Saint Barnabas Med Ctr; **Address:** 90 Bergen St Fl 6 - Ste 6100, Newark, NJ 07103; **Phone:** 973-972-2065; **Board Cert:** Ophthalmology 1999; **Med School:** Washington Univ, St Louis 1993; **Resid:** Ophthalmology, NYU Med Ctr 1997; **Fellow:** Neuro-Ophthalmology, NYU/NY Eye & Ear/Beth Israel 1998; Oculoplastic Surgery, Allegheny Genl Hosp 1999

Wagner, Rudolph S MD (Oph) - **Spec Exp:** Strabismus; Eye Disorders-Congenital; Botox Therapy; Strabismus; **Hospital:** Clara Maass Med Ctr, Saint Barnabas Med Ctr; **Address:** Childrens Eye Care Ctr New Jersey, 495 N 13th St, Newark, NJ 07107-1317; **Phone:** 973-751-1702; **Board Cert:** Ophthalmology 1983; **Med School:** UMDNJ-NJ Med Sch, Newark 1978; **Resid:** Ophthalmology, NJ Med Sch Affil Hosp 1982; **Fellow:** Pediatric Ophthalmology, Wills Eye Hosp 1983; **Fac Appt:** Assoc Clin Prof Oph, UMDNJ-NJ Med Sch, Newark

Zarbin, Marco A MD/PhD (Oph) - **Spec Exp:** Macular Degeneration; Diabetic Eye Disease/Retinopathy; Eye Trauma; Retinal Detachment; **Hospital:** Univ Hosp-UMDNJ—Newark, Saint Barnabas Med Ctr; **Address:** 90 Bergen St, Bldg DOC - Ste 6156, Newark, NJ 07103-2499; **Phone:** 973-972-2065; **Board Cert:** Ophthalmology 1989; **Med School:** Johns Hopkins Univ 1984; **Resid:** Ophthalmology, Johns Hopkins Hosp 1988; **Fellow:** Vitreoretinal Surgery, Johns Hopkins Hosp 1990; **Fac Appt:** Prof Oph, UMDNJ-NJ Med Sch, Newark

Orthopaedic Surgery

Benevenia, Joseph MD (OrS) - **Spec Exp:** Limb Sparing Surgery; Bone Cancer; Sarcoma-Soft Tissue; **Hospital:** Univ Hosp-UMDNJ—Newark; **Address:** 140 Bergen St, Ste ACC1610, Newark, NJ 07103; **Phone:** 973-972-2153; **Board Cert:** Orthopaedic Surgery 2003; **Med School:** UMDNJ-NJ Med Sch, Newark 1984; **Resid:** Orthopaedic Surgery, UMDNJ-NJ Med Sch Hosp 1988; **Fellow:** Orthopaedic Oncology, Case Western Reserve Univ 1991; **Fac Appt:** Prof OrS, UMDNJ-NJ Med Sch, Newark

Chase, Mark MD (OrS) - **Spec Exp:** Sports Medicine; **Hospital:** Mountainside Hosp; **Address:** 200 Highland Ave, Glen Ridge, NJ 07028-1521; **Phone:** 973-746-2200; **Board Cert:** Orthopaedic Surgery 2002; **Med School:** Boston Univ 1983; **Resid:** Orthopaedic Surgery, Boston Univ Affil Hosps 1988

Decter, Edward MD (OrS) - **Spec Exp:** Knee Reconstruction; Shoulder Reconstruction; **Hospital:** Saint Barnabas Med Ctr; **Address:** 1500 Pleasant Valley Way, Ste 101, West Orange, NJ 07052; **Phone:** 973-669-5600; **Board Cert:** Orthopaedic Surgery 1982; **Med School:** Creighton Univ 1975; **Resid:** Orthopaedic Surgery, Hosp Joint Dis 1980

Mendes, John MD (OrS) - **Spec Exp:** Hip & Knee Replacement; Foot & Ankle Surgery; Spinal Disorders; **Hospital:** Mountainside Hosp, Clara Maass Med Ctr; **Address:** 200 Highland Ave, Glen Ridge, NJ 07028-1521; **Phone:** 973-746-2200; **Board Cert:** Orthopaedic Surgery 1984; **Med School:** Cornell Univ-Weill Med Coll 1976; **Resid:** Surgery, Bryn Mawr Hosp 1978; Orthopaedic Surgery, Hosp Special Surg 1981; **Fellow:** Penn Hosp 1982

Sabharwal, Sanjeev MD (OrS) - **Spec Exp:** Pediatric Orthopaedic Surgery; Limb Lengthening (Ilizarov Procedure); Limb Deformities; **Hospital:** Univ Hosp-UMDNJ—Newark, Overlook Hosp (page 92); **Address:** 90 Bergen St, Ste 7300, Newark, NJ 07103; **Phone:** 973-972-0246; **Board Cert:** Orthopaedic Surgery 2010; **Med School:** India 1986; **Resid:** Surgery, St Elizabeth Hosp 1988; Orthopaedic Surgery, Univ British Columbia 1994; **Fellow:** Pediatric Orthopaedic Surgery, Chldns Hosp/Shriners Hosp 1996; Reconstructive Surgery, Md Ctr for Limb Lengthening & Reconstruction 1996; **Fac Appt:** Assoc Prof OrS, UMDNJ-NJ Med Sch, Newark

Schob, Clifford J MD (OrS) - **Spec Exp:** Sports Medicine; Shoulder & Knee Surgery; **Hospital:** Overlook Hosp (page 92), Saint Barnabas Med Ctr; **Address:** 235 Millburn Ave, Millburn, NJ 07041; **Phone:** 973-258-1177; **Board Cert:** Orthopaedic Surgery 2003; **Med School:** UMDNJ-RW Johnson Med Sch 1982; **Resid:** Surgery, Long Island Jewish Med Ctr 1984; Orthopaedic Surgery, Long Island Jewish Med Ctr 1988; **Fellow:** Sports Medicine, Am Sports Med Inst 1990

Seidenstein, Michael MD (OrS) - **Spec Exp:** Arthroscopic Surgery; Joint Replacement; **Hospital:** Newark Beth Israel Med Ctr; **Address:** 61-C Main St, West Orange, NJ 07052-5338; **Phone:** 973-736-8080; **Board Cert:** Orthopaedic Surgery 1977; **Med School:** NY Med Coll 1970; **Resid:** Orthopaedic Surgery, Hosp for Joint Diseases 1975; **Fellow:** Hip Surgery, Wrightington Hosp Ctr 1975A-O Fellowship 1978; **Fac Appt:** Asst Prof OrS, UMDNJ-NJ Med Sch, Newark

Otolaryngology

Morrow, Todd A MD (Oto) - **Spec Exp:** Cosmetic Surgery-Face; Rhinoplasty; Laser Surgery; Botox Therapy; **Hospital:** Saint Barnabas Med Ctr, Newark Beth Israel Med Ctr; **Address:** 741 Northfield Ave, Ste 104, West Orange, NJ 07052; **Phone:** 973-243-1823; **Board Cert:** Otolaryngology 1992; Facial Plastic & Reconstr Surgery 1995; **Med School:** Jefferson Med Coll 1986; **Resid:** Otolaryngology, UMDNJ-Univ Hosp 1991; **Fellow:** Facial Plastic & Reconstr Surgery, Univ Toronto Med Ctr 1992; **Fac Appt:** Asst Clin Prof Oto, UMDNJ-NJ Med Sch, Newark

Zbar, Lloyd MD (Oto) - **Spec Exp:** Hearing & Balance Disorders; Nasal & Sinus Disorders; Voice Disorders; **Hospital:** Mountainside Hosp, Overlook Hosp (page 92); **Address:** 200 Highland Ave, Glen Ridge, NJ 07028-1528; **Phone:** 973-744-2424; **Board Cert:** Otolaryngology 1970; **Med School:** Queens Univ 1964; **Resid:** Surgery, Beth Israel Hosp 1966; Otolaryngology, NYU-Bellevue Hosp Ctr 1969; **Fellow:** Otolaryngology, NYU-Bellevue Hosp Ctr 1970; **Fac Appt:** Assoc Clin Prof Oto, NYU Sch Med

Pathology

Heller, Debra S MD (Path) - **Spec Exp:** Gynecologic Pathology; Pediatric Pathology; Perinatal Pathology; **Hospital:** Univ Hosp-UMDNJ—Newark; **Address:** UMDNJ-NJ Med Sch Dept Pathology, 185 S Orange Ave, UH/E158, Newark, NJ 07101; **Phone:** 973-972-0751; **Board Cert:** Anatomic Pathology 1988; Obstetrics & Gynecology 2008; Pediatric Pathology 1999; **Med School:** NY Med Coll 1977; **Resid:** Obstetrics & Gynecology, Beth Israel Med Ctr 1981; Anatomic Pathology, Mt Sinai Med Ctr 1988; **Fellow:** Pediatric Pathology, Mt Sinai Med Ctr 1987; Gynecologic Pathology, Mt Sinai Med Ctr 1989; **Fac Appt:** Prof Path, UMDNJ-NJ Med Sch, Newark

Lara, Jonathan F MD (Path) - **Spec Exp:** Breast Cancer; **Hospital:** Saint Barnabas Med Ctr; **Address:** St Barnabas Medical Ctr, Dept Pathology, 94 Old Short Hills Rd, Livingston, NJ 07039-5672; **Phone:** 973-322-5762; **Board Cert:** Anatomic & Clinical Pathology 1988; Cytopathology 1997; **Med School:** Philippines 1984; **Resid:** Pathology, St Barnabas Med Ctr 1988; **Fellow:** Surgical Pathology, Meml Sloan Kettering Cancer Ctr 1989; **Fac Appt:** Asst Clin Prof Path, UMDNJ-NJ Med Sch, Newark

Pediatric Allergy & Immunology

Fost, Arthur MD (PA&I) - **Spec Exp:** Asthma; Sinusitis; Urticaria; **Hospital:** Clara Maass Med Ctr; **Address:** 197 Bloomfield Ave, Verona, NJ 07044-2702; **Phone:** 973-857-0330; **Board Cert:** Pediatrics 1968; Allergy & Immunology 1972; **Med School:** Jefferson Med Coll 1963; **Resid:** Pediatrics, Chldns Hosp 1965; Pediatrics, Hosp Univ Penn 1966; **Fellow:** Allergy & Immunology, St Vincents Hosp 1968; **Fac Appt:** Assoc Clin Prof Ped, UMDNJ-NJ Med Sch, Newark

Morrison, Susan MD (PA&I) - **Spec Exp:** Infectious Disease; Travel Medicine; **Hospital:** Clara Maass Med Ctr; **Address:** 36 Newark Ave, Ste 322, Belleville, NJ 07109; **Phone:** 973-450-0100; **Board Cert:** Pediatrics 1986; Allergy & Immunology 2008; Pediatric Infectious Disease 2009; **Med School:** UMDNJ-NJ Med Sch, Newark 1981; **Resid:** Pediatrics, UMDNJ-Univ Hosp 1985; **Fellow:** Pediatric Allergy & Immunology, UMDNJ-Univ Hosp 1988; Pediatric Infectious Disease, UMDNJ-Univ Hosp 1988; **Fac Appt:** Prof Ped, UMDNJ-NJ Med Sch, Newark

Torre, Arthur J MD (PA&I) - **Spec Exp:** Asthma; Diving Medicine; Rhinitis; Sinusitis; **Hospital:** St Joseph's Regl Med Ctr - Paterson; **Address:** 25 Hollywood Ave, Fairfield, NJ 07004-1113; **Phone:** 973-882-0880; **Board Cert:** Pediatrics 1975; **Med School:** UMDNJ-NJ Med Sch, Newark 1970; **Resid:** Pediatrics, Martland Hosp 1972; **Fellow:** Pediatric Allergy & Immunology, Martland Hosp 1973; **Fac Appt:** Assoc Clin Prof Ped, UMDNJ-NJ Med Sch, Newark

Pediatric Cardiology

Connor, Thomas M MD (PCd) - **Hospital:** Saint Barnabas Med Ctr; **Address:** 101 Old Short Hills Rd, Ste 104, West Orange, NJ 07052; **Phone:** 973-731-5550; **Board Cert:** Pediatrics 1973; Pediatric Cardiology 1977; **Med School:** Italy 1966; **Resid:** Pediatrics, Grasslands Hosp 1970; **Fellow:** Pediatric Cardiology, Yale-New Haven Hosp 1972; **Fac Appt:** Assoc Prof Ped, Columbia P&S

Fernandes, John MD (PCd) *PCP* - **Spec Exp:** Congenital Heart Disease; Fetal Cardiology; **Hospital:** Saint Barnabas Med Ctr, NYPresby-Morgan Stanley Children's Hosp (page 104); **Address:** 349 E Northfield Rd, Ste 201, Livingston, NJ 07039-4086; **Phone:** 973-533-1031; **Board Cert:** Pediatric Cardiology 2006; **Med School:** India 1983; **Resid:** Pediatrics, Hahnemann Univ 1988; **Fellow:** Pediatric Cardiology, NYU Med Ctr 1991; Pediatric Cardiology, Johns Hopkins Hosp 1990; **Fac Appt:** Assoc Clin Prof Ped, Columbia P&S

Langsner, Alan MD (PCd) - **Spec Exp:** Fetal Echocardiography; Congenital Heart Disease-Adult & Child; Preventive Cardiology; **Hospital:** NYU Langone Med Ctr (page 106), Saint Barnabas Med Ctr; **Address:** 405 Northfield Ave, Ste 204, West Orange, NJ 07052-3023; **Phone:** 973-736-9997; **Board Cert:** Pediatrics 1983; Pediatric Cardiology 2006; **Med School:** Mexico 1977; **Resid:** Pediatrics, Metropolitan Hosp Ctr 1981; **Fellow:** Pediatric Cardiology, NYU Med Ctr 1983; **Fac Appt:** Asst Prof Ped, NYU Sch Med

Putman, Donald C MD (PCd) - **Hospital:** Saint Barnabas Med Ctr, Mountainside Hosp; **Address:** MetroPediatric Cardiology Assocs, 349 E Northfield Rd, Ste 105, Livingston, NJ 07039; **Phone:** 973-597-3333; **Board Cert:** Pediatric Cardiology 2004; **Med School:** Grenada 1989; **Resid:** Pediatrics, NYU/Bellevue Hosp 1992; **Fellow:** Pediatric Cardiology, NYU/Bellevue Hosp 1995

Pediatric Critical Care Medicine

Davis, Alan L MD (PCCM) - **Spec Exp:** Sepsis & Septic Shock; Respiratory Failure; Pain Management; **Hospital:** Saint Barnabas Med Ctr; **Address:** 94 Old Short Hills Rd, 4th Fl, West Wing/PICU, St Barnabas Med Ctr, Livingston, NJ 07039; **Phone:** 973-322-5690; **Board Cert:** Pediatrics 1986; Pediatric Critical Care Medicine 2002; **Med School:** Univ Louisville Sch Med 1982; **Resid:** Pediatrics, Chldns Meml Hosp 1985; **Fellow:** Pediatric Critical Care Medicine, Chldns Hosp Natl Med Ctr 1987; **Fac Appt:** Assoc Clin Prof Ped, UMDNJ-NJ Med Sch, Newark

Yeh, Timothy S MD (PCCM) - **Hospital:** Saint Barnabas Med Ctr, Monmouth Med Ctr; **Address:** St Barnabas Med Ctr, 94 Old Short Hills Rd Fl 4th - rm 4134A, Livingston, NJ 07039; **Phone:** 973-322-5691; **Board Cert:** Pediatrics 1982; Pediatric Critical Care Medicine 2003; **Med School:** UC Davis 1976; **Resid:** Pediatrics, UC Davis Med Ctr 1979; **Fellow:** Pediatric Critical Care Medicine, Chldns Hosp Natl Med Ctr 1981

Pediatric Gastroenterology

Sunaryo, Francis MD (PGe) - **Spec Exp:** Inflammatory Bowel Disease; Gastroesophageal Reflux Disease (GERD); **Hospital:** Newark Beth Israel Med Ctr, Saint Barnabas Med Ctr; **Address:** 201 Lyons Ave, Newark, NJ 07112; **Phone:** 973-926-7280; **Board Cert:** Pediatrics 1982; Pediatric Gastroenterology 2005; **Med School:** Indonesia 1973; **Resid:** Pediatrics, North Shore Univ Hosp 1979; **Fellow:** Pediatric Gastroenterology, Chldns Hosp 1982; **Fac Appt:** Asst Prof Ped, UMDNJ-Univ Med Dent NJ

Pediatric Hematology-Oncology

Kamalakar, Peri MD (PHO) - **Spec Exp:** Sickle Cell Disease; Thalassemia; Leukemia; Solid Tumors; **Hospital:** Newark Beth Israel Med Ctr, Monmouth Med Ctr; **Address:** Valerie Fund Children's Ctr, 201 Lyons Ave, Newark, NJ 07112-2027; **Phone:** 973-926-7161; **Board Cert:** Pediatrics 1975; Pediatric Hematology-Oncology 1997; **Med School:** India 1967; **Resid:** Pediatrics, Beth Israel Med Ctr 1973; **Fellow:** Pediatric Hematology-Oncology, Childrens Hosp 1976; **Fac Appt:** Asst Clin Prof Ped, UMDNJ-NJ Med Sch, Newark

Pediatric Infectious Disease

Oleske, James M MD (PInf) - **Spec Exp:** AIDS/HIV; Pediatric Allergy & Immunology; Pain Management; Palliative Care; **Hospital:** Univ Hosp-UMDNJ—Newark; **Address:** UMDNJ Dept Ped, MSB-F 572, 570 S Orange Ave, Newark, NJ 07103; **Phone:** 973-972-5066; **Board Cert:** Pediatrics 1976; Allergy & Immunology 1977; Pediatric Infectious Disease 2002; Hospice & Palliative Medicine 2007; **Med School:** UMDNJ-NJ Med Sch, Newark 1971; **Resid:** Pediatrics, Martland Hosp 1974; **Fellow:** Pediatric Infectious Disease, Grady Meml Hosp 1976; **Fac Appt:** Prof Ped, UMDNJ-NJ Med Sch, Newark

Pediatric Nephrology

Roberti, Isabel M MD/PhD (PNep) - **Spec Exp:** Transplant Medicine-Kidney; Kidney Failure; Hypertension; Kidney Stones; **Hospital:** Saint Barnabas Med Ctr; **Address:** 94 Old Short Hills Rd, Ste 304, Livingston, NJ 07039; **Phone:** 973-322-5264; **Board Cert:** Pediatrics 2003; Pediatric Nephrology 2005; **Med School:** Brazil 1983; **Resid:** Pediatrics, Hosp Sao Paulo 1986; **Fellow:** Pediatric Nephrology, Hosp Sao Paulo 1989; Pediatric Nephrology, Mount Sinai Hosp 1995; **Fac Appt:** Assoc Clin Prof Ped, Mount Sinai Sch Med

Pediatric Pulmonology

Aguila, Helen MD (PPul) - **Spec Exp:** Asthma; Tuberculosis; **Hospital:** Univ Hosp-UMDNJ—Newark, Columbus Hosp; **Address:** UMDNJ-Univ Hosp-Newark, 90 Bergen St Fl 5th - rm 5100, Dept Ped Pulmonology, Newark, NJ 07101; **Phone:** 973-972-5779; **Board Cert:** Pediatrics 1983; Pediatric Pulmonology 2004; **Med School:** Philippines 1974; **Resid:** Pediatrics, Staten Island Hosp 1979; Pediatrics, Kings Co Hosp/Downstate Med Ctr 1980; **Fellow:** Pediatric Pulmonology, Chldns Hosp Michigan 1983; **Fac Appt:** Asst Prof Ped, UMDNJ-NJ Med Sch, Newark

Bisberg, Dorothy S MD (PPul) - **Spec Exp:** Asthma; Cystic Fibrosis; **Hospital:** Saint Barnabas Med Ctr; **Address:** 200 South Orange Ave, Livingston, NJ 07039; **Phone:** 973-322-7600; **Board Cert:** Pediatrics 1977; Pediatric Pulmonology 2007; **Med School:** Cornell Univ-Weill Med Coll 1972; **Resid:** Pediatrics, Montefiore Hosp Med Ctr 1974; Pediatrics, Bronx Lebanon Hosp 1975; **Fac Appt:** Asst Prof Ped, UMDNJ-NJ Med Sch, Newark

Kottler, William MD (PPul) - **Spec Exp:** Asthma; Cystic Fibrosis; **Hospital:** Saint Barnabas Med Ctr, Overlook Hosp (page 92); **Address:** 48 Essex St, Millburn, NJ 07041; **Phone:** 973-218-0900; **Board Cert:** Pediatric Pulmonology 2010; **Med School:** France 1987; **Resid:** Pediatrics, Overlook Hosp 1990; **Fellow:** Pulmonary Disease, Shands Hosp 1993; **Fac Appt:** Asst Prof Ped, UMDNJ-NJ Med Sch, Newark

Pediatric Surgery

Bethel, Colin A MD (PS) - **Spec Exp:** Minimally Invasive Surgery; Neonatal Surgery; **Hospital:** Newark Beth Israel Med Ctr, St Joseph's Regl Med Ctr - Paterson; **Address:** 2130 Millburn Ave, Ste C-1, Maplewood, NJ 07040; **Phone:** 973-313-3115; **Board Cert:** Surgery 2005; Pediatric Surgery 2007; **Med School:** Columbia P&S 1987; **Resid:** Surgery, Yale-New Haven Hosp 1995; **Fellow:** Pediatric Surgery, Chldns Hosp 1997

Pediatrics

Boodish, Wesley MD (Ped) *PCP* - **Hospital:** Saint Barnabas Med Ctr, Overlook Hosp (page 92); **Address:** 159 Millburn Ave, Millburn, NJ 07041-1849; **Phone:** 973-912-0155; **Board Cert:** Pediatrics 1965; **Med School:** Scotland, UK 1960; **Resid:** Pediatrics, US Naval Hosp 1964

Gruenwald, Laurence D MD (Ped) *PCP* - **Spec Exp:** Asthma; Behavioral Disorders; **Hospital:** Saint Barnabas Med Ctr; **Address:** 90 Millburn Ave, Ste 101, Millburn, NJ 07041-1933; **Phone:** 973-378-7990; **Board Cert:** Pediatrics 1981; **Med School:** UMDNJ-NJ Med Sch, Newark 1975; **Resid:** Pediatrics, Chldns Hosp Natl Med Ctr 1978

Marcus, Richard W MD (Ped) *PCP* - **Spec Exp:** ADD/ADHD; **Hospital:** Clara Maass Med Ctr; **Address:** 242 Washington Ave, Ste A, Nutley, NJ 07110-1994; **Phone:** 973-667-6676; **Board Cert:** Pediatrics 1988; **Med School:** UMDNJ-NJ Med Sch, Newark 1982; **Resid:** Pediatrics, UMDNJ-Univ Hosp 1985; **Fac Appt:** Asst Prof Ped, UMDNJ-NJ Med Sch, Newark

Rigtrup, Edward MD (Ped) *PCP* - **Hospital:** Mountainside Hosp, Saint Barnabas Med Ctr; **Address:** 73 Park St, Montclair, NJ 07042-2903; **Phone:** 973-746-7375; **Board Cert:** Pediatrics 1980; **Med School:** NY Med Coll 1975; **Resid:** Pediatrics, Chldns Natl Med Ctr 1978; **Fac Appt:** Assoc Clin Prof Ped, NY Med Coll

Physical Medicine & Rehabilitation

Bach, John MD (PMR) - **Spec Exp:** Neuromuscular Disorders; Amyotrophic Lateral Sclerosis (ALS); Post Polio Syndrome/Rehabilitation; **Hospital:** Univ Hosp-UMDNJ—Newark; **Address:** 150 Bergen St, Ste B403, Newark, NJ 07103; **Phone:** 973-972-7195; **Board Cert:** Physical Medicine & Rehabilitation 1986; **Med School:** UMDNJ-NJ Med Sch, Newark 1976; **Resid:** Physical Medicine & Rehabilitation, NYU Med Ctr 1980; **Fellow:** Neuromuscular Disease, Univ Hosp 1983; **Fac Appt:** Prof PMR, UMDNJ-NJ Med Sch, Newark

Cole, Jeffrey L MD (PMR) - **Spec Exp:** Pain Management; Neuromuscular Disorders; Electromyography; Electrodiagnosis; **Hospital:** Kessler Inst for Rehab - W Orange; **Address:** Kessler Inst for Rehabilitation, 1199 Pleasant Valley Way, West Orange, NJ 07052; **Phone:** 973-243-6943; **Board Cert:** Physical Medicine & Rehabilitation 1983; Pain Medicine 2003; **Med School:** Mexico 1977; **Resid:** Internal Medicine, NY Hosp-Queens Med Ctr 1979; Physical Medicine & Rehabilitation, Montefiore Med Ctr 1982; **Fellow:** Electrodiagnosis, Booth Meml Med Ctr 1983

Francis, Kathleen D MD (PMR) - **Spec Exp:** Lymphedema; **Address:** Lymphedema Physician Services, 200 S Orange Ave, Livingston, NJ 07039; **Phone:** 973-322-7366; **Board Cert:** Physical Medicine & Rehabilitation 2004; **Med School:** UMDNJ-NJ Med Sch, Newark 1989; **Resid:** Physical Medicine & Rehabilitation, UMDNJ-Kessler Inst Rehab 1993; **Fac Appt:** Asst Clin Prof PMR, UMDNJ-NJ Med Sch, Newark

Kirshblum, Steven C MD (PMR) - **Spec Exp:** Spinal Cord Injury; Spasticity Management; **Hospital:** Kessler Inst for Rehab - W Orange, Saint Barnabas Med Ctr; **Address:** Kessley Institute, 1199 Pleasant Valley Way, West Orange, NJ 07052-1424; **Phone:** 973-731-3600 x2258; **Board Cert:** Physical Medicine & Rehabilitation 1991; Spinal Cord Injury Medicine 2008; **Med School:** Univ Hlth Scis, Chicago Med Sch 1986; **Resid:** Physical Medicine & Rehabilitation, Mount Sinai Med Ctr 1990; **Fac Appt:** Prof PMR, UMDNJ-NJ Med Sch, Newark

Plastic Surgery

Ablaza, Valerie MD (PlS) - **Spec Exp:** Breast Reconstruction; **Hospital:** Saint Barnabas Med Ctr, Mountainside Hosp; **Address:** The Plastic Surgery Group, 37 N Fullerton Ave, Montclair, NJ 07003-3014; **Phone:** 973-233-1933; **Board Cert:** Plastic Surgery 2000; **Med School:** Med Coll PA Hahnemann 1989; **Resid:** Surgery, Albert Einstein Med Ctr 1994; Plastic Surgery, NY-Presby/Cornell-Weill 1996; **Fellow:** Breast Surgery, Nashville Plastic Surgery

DiBernardo, Barry E MD (PlS) - **Spec Exp:** Laser Surgery; Hair Restoration/Transplant; Cosmetic Surgery-Face & Body; Body Contouring after Weight Loss; **Hospital:** Mountainside Hosp, Clara Maass Med Ctr; **Address:** 29 Park St, Montclair, NJ 07042; **Phone:** 973-509-2000; **Board Cert:** Plastic Surgery 1994; **Med School:** Cornell Univ-Weill Med Coll 1984; **Resid:** Surgery, Mt Sinai Hosp 1989; Plastic Surgery, Montefiore Med Ctr 1991; **Fac Appt:** Assoc Clin Prof PlS, UMDNJ-NJ Med Sch, Newark

Friedlander, Beverly MD (PlS) - **Spec Exp:** Breast Augmentation; Liposuction & Body Contouring; Cosmetic Surgery-Face & Body; **Hospital:** Overlook Hosp (page 92), Saint Barnabas Med Ctr; **Address:** 636 Morris Tpke, Ste 2G, Short Hills, NJ 07078-2608; **Phone:** 973-912-9120; **Board Cert:** Plastic Surgery 1990; **Med School:** SUNY Downstate 1980; **Resid:** Surgery, Kings Co Hosp 1984; Plastic Surgery, Montefiore Med Ctr 1987

Granick, Mark S MD (PlS) - **Spec Exp:** Reconstructive Surgery; Cosmetic Surgery; Skin Cancer; Liposuction & Body Contouring; **Hospital:** Univ Hosp-UMDNJ—Newark, Newark Beth Israel Med Ctr; **Address:** NJ Medical School Plastic Surgery, 90 Bergen St, Ste 7200, Newark, NJ 07103; **Phone:** 973-972-8092; **Board Cert:** Otolaryngology 1982; Plastic Surgery 1985; **Med School:** Harvard Med Sch 1977; **Resid:** Otolaryngology, Mass E&E Hosp 1982; Plastic Surgery, Univ Pittsburgh Med Ctr 1984; **Fac Appt:** Prof PlS, UMDNJ-NJ Med Sch, Newark

LoVerme, Paul J MD (PlS) - **Spec Exp:** Cosmetic Surgery-Face; Liposuction & Body Contouring; Breast Reconstruction & Augmentation; **Hospital:** Mountainside Hosp, Saint Barnabas Med Ctr; **Address:** 825 Bloomfield Ave, Ste 205, Verona, NJ 07044; **Phone:** 973-857-9499; **Board Cert:** Plastic Surgery 1987; **Med School:** UMDNJ-NJ Med Sch, Newark 1978; **Resid:** Surgery, UMDNJ Univ Hosp 1983; Plastic Surgery, Med Coll Hosp 1985; **Fellow:** Surgical Oncology, UMDNJ Univ Hosp 1982; **Fac Appt:** Assoc Clin Prof PlS, UMDNJ-NJ Med Sch, Newark

Rosen, Allen D MD (PlS) - **Spec Exp:** Cosmetic Surgery-Face & Breast; Breast Reconstruction; Liposuction & Body Contouring; Eyelid Surgery; **Hospital:** Mountainside Hosp, Saint Barnabas Med Ctr; **Address:** 37 N Fullerton Ave, Montclair, NJ 07042; **Phone:** 973-233-1933; **Board Cert:** Plastic Surgery 1991; **Med School:** SUNY Buffalo 1983; **Resid:** Surgery, Columbia Presby Med Ctr 1986; Plastic Surgery, Columbia Presby Med Ctr 1988; **Fellow:** Hand Surgery, Columbia Presby Med Ctr 1987; **Fac Appt:** Asst Clin Prof PlS, UMDNJ-NJ Med Sch, Newark

Psychiatry

Caracci, Giovanni MD (Psyc) - **Spec Exp:** Geriatric Psychiatry; Psychopharmacology; Psychotherapy; Post Traumatic Stress Disorder; **Hospital:** Univ Hosp-UMDNJ—Newark; **Address:** 183 S Orange Ave, rm F1436, Box 1709, Newark, NJ 07101; **Phone:** 973-972-7117; **Board Cert:** Psychiatry 1990; Geriatric Psychiatry 2000; **Med School:** Italy 1977; **Resid:** Psychiatry, Metropolitan Hosp 1983; **Fellow:** Psychiatry, Metropolitan Hosp 1984; **Fac Appt:** Assoc Prof Psyc, UMDNJ-NJ Med Sch, Newark

Faber, Mark P MD (Psyc) - **Spec Exp:** Child Psychiatry; Anxiety Disorders; Depression; ADD/ADHD; **Hospital:** Saint Barnabas Med Ctr; **Address:** 594 Valley Rd, Upper Montclair, NJ 07043-1882; **Phone:** 973-746-6711; **Board Cert:** Psychiatry 1993; Child & Adolescent Psychiatry 2005; **Med School:** Dominica 1988; **Resid:** Psychiatry, CT Valley Hosp-Yale 1991; **Fellow:** Child & Adolescent Psychiatry, UMDNJ-RW Johnson Sch Med 1993; Sleep Medicine, UMDNJ-RW Johnson Sch Med 1996

Kurani, Devendra MD (Psyc) - **Spec Exp:** Depression; Anxiety Disorders; Panic Disorder; **Hospital:** Saint Barnabas Med Ctr, Christ Hosp; **Address:** 50 N Field Ave, West Orange, NJ 07052; **Phone:** 201-656-3116; **Board Cert:** Psychiatry 1986; **Med School:** India 1975; **Resid:** Psychiatry, Warley Hosp 1981; Psychiatry, Harlem Hosp 1983

Nucci, Annamaria MD/PhD (Psyc) - **Spec Exp:** Psychopharmacology; Relationship Problems; Depression; **Address:** 5 Westview Ct, Cedar Grove, NJ 07009-1937; **Phone:** 973-857-2609; **Board Cert:** Psychiatry 1978; **Med School:** Italy 1971; **Resid:** Psychiatry, Manhattan VA Hosp-NYU 1973; Psychiatry, Payne Whitney Clinic 1976; **Fellow:** Child & Adolescent Psychiatry, New York Hosp-Cornell 1976; **Fac Appt:** Asst Clin Prof Psyc, NY Med Coll

Schleifer, Steven J MD (Psyc) - **Spec Exp:** Depression; Psychoneuroimmunology; Anxiety Disorders; **Hospital:** Univ Hosp-UMDNJ—Newark; **Address:** 183 S Orange Ave Bldg BHSB F1430, Newark, NJ 07103; **Phone:** 973-972-5023; **Board Cert:** Psychiatry 1980; **Med School:** Mount Sinai Sch Med 1975; **Resid:** Psychiatry, USC Med Ctr 1976; Psychiatry, Mount Sinai Med Ctr 1979; **Fac Appt:** Prof Psyc, UMDNJ-NJ Med Sch, Newark

Zornitzer, Michael R MD (Psyc) - **Spec Exp:** Psychotherapy; Psychopharmacology; Depression; Panic Disorder; **Hospital:** Saint Barnabas Med Ctr; **Address:** 2 W Northfield Rd, Ste 305, Livingston, NJ 07039-3789; **Phone:** 973-992-6090; **Board Cert:** Psychiatry 1976; **Med School:** SUNY Downstate 1971; **Resid:** Internal Medicine, NYU Med Ctr 1972; Psychiatry, Montefiore Med Ctr 1975; **Fac Appt:** Asst Clin Prof Psyc, NY Coll Osteo Med

Pulmonary Disease

Greenberg, Martin J MD (Pul) - **Spec Exp:** Asthma; Emphysema; **Hospital:** Saint Barnabas Med Ctr; **Address:** 124 East Mt Pleasant Ave, Livingston, NJ 07039; **Phone:** 973-994-4130; **Board Cert:** Internal Medicine 1987; **Med School:** Dominica 1983; **Resid:** Internal Medicine, Univ Hosp UMDNJ 1986; **Fellow:** Pulmonary Disease, Newark Beth Israel 1989

Labissiere, Jean-Claude MD (Pul) - **Spec Exp:** Asthma; **Hospital:** Saint Barnabas Med Ctr; **Address:** Essex Medical Associates, 92 Old Northfield Rd, West Orange, NJ 07052; **Phone:** 973-736-5552; **Board Cert:** Internal Medicine 1988; Pulmonary Disease 2004; Critical Care Medicine 2005; Sleep Medicine 2007; **Med School:** Haiti 1977; **Resid:** Internal Medicine, Lincoln Med Ctr 1984; **Fellow:** Pulmonary Disease, UMDNJ/E Orange VA Hosp 1986

Miller, Richard A MD (Pul) - **Spec Exp:** Sarcoidosis; **Hospital:** Saint Michael's Med Ctr; **Address:** 111 Central Ave, Newark, NJ 07102; **Phone:** 973-877-5493; **Board Cert:** Internal Medicine 1989; Pulmonary Disease 2003; Critical Care Medicine 2005; **Med School:** Mexico 1983; **Resid:** Internal Medicine, St Michaels Med Ctr 1988; **Fellow:** Pulmonary Critical Care Medicine, St Michaels Med Ctr 1991

Reichman, Lee B MD (Pul) - **Spec Exp:** Tuberculosis; Mycobacterial Infections; **Hospital:** Univ Hosp-UMDNJ—Newark; **Address:** 225 Warren St, Box 1709, Newark, NJ 07103-3535; **Phone:** 973-972-3270; **Board Cert:** Internal Medicine 1972; Pulmonary Disease 1972; **Med School:** NYU Sch Med 1964; **Resid:** Internal Medicine, Bellevue Hosp-Colum P&S 1968; Pulmonary Disease, Harlem Hosp-Columbia P&S 1970; **Fac Appt:** Prof Med, UMDNJ-NJ Med Sch, Newark

Safirstein, Benjamin MD (Pul) - **Spec Exp:** Asthma; Sarcoidosis; **Hospital:** Mountainside Hosp, Saint Michael's Med Ctr; **Address:** 62 South Fullerton Ave, Montclair, NJ 07042; **Phone:** 973-744-9125; **Board Cert:** Internal Medicine 1970; Pulmonary Disease 1974; **Med School:** Ros Franklin Univ/Chicago Med Sch 1965; **Resid:** Internal Medicine, Mount Sinai Hosp 1969; **Fellow:** Pulmonary Disease, Inst Dis Chest 1972

Shah, Smita MD (Pul) - **Spec Exp:** Asthma; Chronic Obstructive Lung Disease (COPD); Lung Cancer; Pulmonary Hypertension; **Hospital:** Saint Barnabas Med Ctr, Newark Beth Israel Med Ctr; **Address:** 96 Millburn Ave, Ste 200-A, Millburn, NJ 07040; **Phone:** 973-763-6800; **Board Cert:** Internal Medicine 1986; Pulmonary Disease 2000; Critical Care Medicine 2001; Sleep Medicine 2009; **Med School:** India 1980; **Resid:** Internal Medicine, St Marys Hosp 1986; **Fellow:** Pulmonary Critical Care Medicine, Temple Univ Hosp 1988

Radiation Oncology

Goodman, Robert L MD (RadRO) - **Spec Exp:** Breast Cancer; Lymphoma; Prostate Cancer; Brain Tumors; **Hospital:** Saint Barnabas Med Ctr; **Address:** St Barnabas Med Ctr, Dept Rad Oncology, 94 Old Short Hills Rd, Livingston, NJ 07039; **Phone:** 973-322-5133; **Board Cert:** Internal Medicine 1971; Therapeutic Radiology 1974; Medical Oncology 1975; **Med School:** Columbia P&S 1966; **Resid:** Internal Medicine, Beth Israel Hosp 1970; Radiation Therapy, Harvard Joint Ctr Rad Therapy 1974; **Fellow:** Hematology, NY-Presby Hosp 1969

Wagman, Raquel T MD (RadRO) - **Spec Exp:** Breast Cancer; **Hospital:** Saint Barnabas Med Ctr; **Address:** St Barnabas Med Ctr, 94 Old Short Hills Rd, Livingston, NJ 07039; **Phone:** 973-322-5630; **Board Cert:** Radiation Oncology 2000; **Med School:** Univ Mich Med Sch 1995; **Resid:** Radiation Oncology, Meml Slaon Kettering 2000

Rheumatology

Cannarozzi, Nicholas A MD (Rhu) - **Spec Exp:** Rheumatoid Arthritis; Lupus Nephritis; Osteoporosis; Vasculitis; **Hospital:** Mountainside Hosp; **Address:** 127 Pine St, Montclair, NJ 07042-4835; **Phone:** 973-783-6000; **Board Cert:** Internal Medicine 1980; Rheumatology 1972; **Med School:** Hahnemann Univ 1965; **Resid:** Internal Medicine, Philadelphia Genl Hosp 1967; Internal Medicine, St Michaels Med Ctr 1968; **Fellow:** Rheumatology, Yale-New Haven Hosp 1969; Rheumatology, Yale-New Haven Hosp 1972

Kramer, Neil MD (Rhu) - **Spec Exp:** Rheumatoid Arthritis; Lupus/SLE; Sjogren's Syndrome; Vasculitis; **Hospital:** Saint Barnabas Med Ctr; **Address:** 200 S Orange Ave, Ste 107, Livingston, NJ 07039-5817; **Phone:** 973-322-7400; **Board Cert:** Internal Medicine 1977; Rheumatology 1980; **Med School:** Univ Pennsylvania 1974; **Resid:** Internal Medicine, Manhattan VA Hosp/NYU Med Ctr 1978; **Fellow:** Rheumatology, NYU Med Ctr 1980; **Fac Appt:** Assoc Clin Prof Med, Mount Sinai Sch Med

Lahita, Robert G MD/PhD (Rhu) - **Spec Exp:** Lupus/SLE; Endocrinology & Joint Disorders; Immunodeficiency Disorders; Lupus/SLE; **Hospital:** Newark Beth Israel Med Ctr; **Address:** 201 Lyons Ave, Newark, NJ 07112; **Phone:** 973-926-7472; **Board Cert:** Internal Medicine 2004; Rheumatology 2007; **Med School:** Jefferson Med Coll 1973; **Resid:** Internal Medicine, New York Hosp-Cornell 1976; **Fellow:** Rheumatology, Rockefeller Hosp 1978; **Fac Appt:** Prof Med, Mount Sinai Sch Med

Rosenstein, Elliot D MD (Rhu) - **Spec Exp:** Rheumatoid Arthritis; Lupus/SLE; Sjogren's Syndrome; Behcet's Syndrome; **Hospital:** Saint Barnabas Med Ctr; **Address:** 200 S Orange Ave, Livingston, NJ 07039-5817; **Phone:** 973-322-7400; **Board Cert:** Internal Medicine 1981; Rheumatology 1984; **Med School:** Mount Sinai Sch Med 1978; **Resid:** Internal Medicine, NYU/Bellevue Hosp 1982; **Fellow:** Rheumatology, NYU/Bellevue Hosp 1984; **Fac Appt:** Assoc Clin Prof Med, Mount Sinai Sch Med

Simon, Jonathan M MD (Rhu) - **Hospital:** Mountainside Hosp; **Address:** 1018 Broad St, Bloomfield, NJ 07003-2807; **Phone:** 973-338-3383; **Board Cert:** Internal Medicine 1981; Rheumatology 1984; **Med School:** NYU Sch Med 1978; **Resid:** Internal Medicine, UMDNJ Univ Hosp 1981; **Fellow:** Rheumatology, UMDNJ Univ Hosp 1983

Sports Medicine

Gehrmann, Robin M MD (SM) - **Spec Exp:** Cartilage Damage & Transplant; Knee Ligament Reconstruction; Shoulder Injuries; Arthroscopic Surgery; **Hospital:** Univ Hosp-UMDNJ—Newark; **Address:** North Jersey Orthopaedic Inst, 90 Bergen St, Ste 1200, Newark, NJ 07101; **Phone:** 973-972-8240; **Board Cert:** Orthopaedic Surgery 2004; Orthopaedic Sports Medicine 2007; **Med School:** Hahnemann Univ 1995; **Resid:** Surgery, UMDNJ Med Ctr 1996; Orthopaedic Surgery, UMDNJ Med Ctr 2000; **Fellow:** Orthopaedic Sports Medicine, Pennsylvania Hosp 2001; **Fac Appt:** Asst Prof OrS, UMDNJ-NJ Med Sch, Newark

Levy, Andrew S MD (SM) - **Spec Exp:** Cartilage Damage & Transplant; Ligament Reconstruction; Shoulder Surgery; **Hospital:** Saint Barnabas Med Ctr, Morristown Mem Hosp (page 92); **Address:** 90 Milburn Ave, Ste 204A, Milburn, NJ 07041; **Phone:** 908-598-9199; **Board Cert:** Orthopaedic Surgery 2008; **Med School:** Temple Univ 1987; **Resid:** Orthopaedic Surgery, Albert Einstein Med Ctr 1994; **Fellow:** Sports Medicine, Duke Univ Med Ctr 1995; Shoulder Surgery, Duke Univ Med Ctr 1995; **Fac Appt:** Assoc Clin Prof OrS, UMDNJ-NJ Med Sch, Newark

Surgery

Andrei, Valeriu E MD (S) - **Spec Exp:** Obesity/Bariatric Surgery; Laparoscopic Surgery; **Hospital:** Robert Wood Johnson Univ Hosp - New Brunswick, Saint Barnabas Med Ctr; **Address:** 200 S Orange Ave, Ste 123, Livingston, NJ 07039; **Phone:** 973-322-7265; **Board Cert:** Surgery 1999; **Med School:** Romania 1987; **Resid:** Surgery, Methodist Hosp 1988; **Fellow:** Minimally Invasive Surgery, Mt Sinai Med Ctr 1999

Blackwood, M Michele MD (S) - **Spec Exp:** Breast Cancer; Breast Surgery; Sentinel Node Surgery; Breast Cancer-High Risk Women; **Hospital:** Saint Barnabas Med Ctr; **Address:** Saint Barnabas Ambulatory Care Center, 200 S Orange Ave, Ste 102, Livingston, NJ 07039; **Phone:** 973-322-7020; **Board Cert:** Surgery 2003; **Med School:** Med Univ SC 1988; **Resid:** Surgery, Stamford Hosp 1993; **Fellow:** Surgical Oncology, Meml Sloan Kettering Cancer Ctr 1994; **Fac Appt:** Asst Clin Prof S, Columbia P&S

Chamberlain, Ronald S MD (S) - **Spec Exp:** Liver & Biliary Surgery; Cancer Surgery; Laparoscopic Surgery; Pancreatic Cancer; **Hospital:** Saint Barnabas Med Ctr; **Address:** St Barnabas Med Ctr, Dept Surgery, 94 Old Short Hills Rd, Livingston, NJ 07039; **Phone:** 973-322-5195; **Board Cert:** Surgery 1999; **Med School:** Geo Wash Univ 1991; **Resid:** Surgery, Geo Wash Univ Med Ctr 1997; **Fellow:** Surgical Oncology, Natl Cancer Inst-NIH 1996; Hepatobiliary Surgery, Meml Sloan-Kettering Canc Ctr 1999; **Fac Appt:** Prof S, UMDNJ-NJ Med Sch, Newark

Deitch, Edwin A MD (S) - **Spec Exp:** Trauma; Burn Care; Critical Care; **Hospital:** Univ Hosp-UMDNJ—Newark; **Address:** 185 S Orange Ave, MSB, rm G506, Newark, NJ 07103; **Phone:** 973-972-5045; **Board Cert:** Surgery 1997; Surgical Critical Care 2006; **Med School:** Univ MD Sch Med 1973; **Resid:** Surgery, US Public Hlth Svc Hosp 1976; Surgery, US Public Hlth Svc Hosp 1978; **Fac Appt:** Prof S, UMDNJ-NJ Med Sch, Newark

Huston, Jan A MD (S) - **Spec Exp:** Breast Surgery; Breast Disease; **Hospital:** Saint Michael's Med Ctr, Saint Barnabas Med Ctr; **Address:** 111 Central Ave, Newark, NJ 07102; **Phone:** 908-918-0001; **Board Cert:** Surgery 1998; **Med School:** Mich State Univ 1982; **Resid:** Surgery, St Barnabas Hosp 1987; **Fellow:** Vascular Surgery, Lehigh Valley Hosp 1988

Maheshwari, Vivek MD (S) - **Spec Exp:** Gastrointestinal Cancer; Endocrine Tumors; Melanoma; Breast Cancer; **Hospital:** Saint Barnabas Med Ctr, East Orange Genl Hosp; **Address:** 101 Old Short Hills Rd, Ste 206, West Orange, NJ 07052; **Phone:** 973-731-5005; **Board Cert:** Surgery 2003; **Med School:** India 1992; **Resid:** Surgery, Beth Israel Med Ctr 2002; **Fellow:** Surgical Oncology, Univ Pittsburgh 2004

Mansour, E Hani MD (S) - **Spec Exp:** Burn Care; **Hospital:** Saint Barnabas Med Ctr; **Address:** Burn Surgeons of St Barnabas, 94 Old Short Hills Rd, Livingston, NJ 07039; **Phone:** 973-322-5924; **Board Cert:** Surgery 1999; Surgical Critical Care 1999; **Med School:** Lebanon 1973; **Resid:** Surgery, Union Meml Hosp 1979; **Fellow:** Burn Surgery, Brooke Army Med Ctr

Petrone, Sylvia J MD (S) - **Spec Exp:** Burn Care; Critical Care; **Hospital:** Saint Barnabas Med Ctr; **Address:** Burn Surgeons St Barnabas, 94 Old Short Hills Rd, Livingston, NJ 07039; **Phone:** 973-322-5924; **Board Cert:** Surgery 2001; Surgical Critical Care 2008; **Med School:** Loyola Univ-Stritch Sch Med 1977; **Resid:** Surgery, Boston Univ Med Ctr 1982; **Fellow:** Burn Surgery, New York Hosp-Cornell 1983

Raina, Suresh MD (S) - **Spec Exp:** Endocrine Surgery; Thyroid & Parathyroid Surgery; **Hospital:** Univ Hosp-UMDNJ—Newark, Bayonne Med Ctr; **Address:** 90 Bergen St, DOC 7400, Newark, NJ 07103; **Phone:** 973-972-6294; **Board Cert:** Surgery 2009; **Med School:** India 1971; **Resid:** Surgery, UMDNJ Hosp 1977; **Fellow:** Surgical Oncology, UMDNJ Hosp 1978; Surgical Oncology, Roswell Park Cancer Inst 1979; **Fac Appt:** Assoc Prof S, UMDNJ-NJ Med Sch, Newark

Thoracic Surgery

Burns, Paul G MD (TS) - **Spec Exp:** Cardiac Surgery; **Hospital:** Saint Barnabas Med Ctr; **Address:** St Barnabas Hosp, 94 Old Short Hills Rd, rm 2511, Livingston, NJ 07039; **Phone:** 973-322-2200; **Board Cert:** Thoracic Surgery 2000; Surgery 1998; **Med School:** Columbia P&S 1989; **Resid:** Surgery, Deaconess Hosp/Harvard 1996; **Fellow:** Cardiothoracic Surgery, New York Hosp/Cornell 1998

Camacho, Margarita T MD (TS) - **Spec Exp:** Mechanical Assist Devices; Transplant-Heart; Heart Failure; **Hospital:** Newark Beth Israel Med Ctr; **Address:** Newark Beth Israel Med Ctr, Dept Cardiothoracic Surgery, 201 Lyons Ave, Ste G-5, Newark, NJ 07112; **Phone:** 973-926-6938; **Board Cert:** Thoracic Surgery 2008; **Med School:** NY Med Coll 1984; **Resid:** Surgery, Lenox Hill Hosp 1989; Cardiothoracic Surgery, Albert Einstein Affil Hosp 1991; **Fellow:** Pediatric Cardiothoracic Surgery, LI Jewish Med Ctr 1992; Transplantation/Mechanical Assist Devices, Cleveland Clinic 1994; **Fac Appt:** Assoc Clin Prof TS, Albert Einstein Coll Med

Connolly, Mark W MD (TS) - **Spec Exp:** Minimally Invasive Cardiac Surgery; Coronary Artery Surgery; Cardiac Surgery-Adult; **Hospital:** Saint Michael's Med Ctr; **Address:** St Michael's Med Ctr, 111 Central Ave, Newark, NJ 07102; **Phone:** 973-877-5300; **Board Cert:** Thoracic Surgery 2001; **Med School:** Northwestern Univ 1982; **Resid:** Surgery, Bellevue/NYU Med Ctr 1988; Cardiothoracic Surgery, Emory Univ Hosps 1991; **Fellow:** Surgical Research, Maimonides Med Ctr 1986

Forman, Mark MD (TS) - **Spec Exp:** Lung Cancer; Lung Surgery; Vascular Surgery; Video Assisted Thoracic Surgery (VATS); **Hospital:** Saint Barnabas Med Ctr, Clara Maass Med Ctr; **Address:** 1500 Pleasant Valley Way, Ste 302, West Orange, NJ 07052; **Phone:** 973-324-0988; **Board Cert:** Thoracic Surgery 2007; **Med School:** Tulane Univ 1976; **Resid:** Surgery, LI Jewish Med Ctr 1981; Thoracic Surgery, Montefiore Hosp Med Ctr 1984; **Fellow:** Thoracic Surgery, Montefiore Hosp Med Ctr 1982

Goldenberg, Bruce MD (TS) - **Spec Exp:** Coronary Artery Surgery; Heart Valve Surgery; Minimally Invasive Cardiac Surgery; Arrhythmias; **Hospital:** St Clare's Hosp - Denville, Mountainside Hosp; **Address:** PO Box 377, Short Hills, NJ 07078; **Phone:** 973-365-4722; **Board Cert:** Thoracic Surgery 2003; **Med School:** Northwestern Univ 1976; **Resid:** Surgery, NYU Med Ctr 1981; Thoracic Surgery, NYU Med Ctr 1983; **Fac Appt:** Asst Clin Prof S, UMDNJ-NJ Med Sch, Newark

Saunders, Craig R MD (TS) - **Spec Exp:** Cardiac Surgery; Minimally Invasive Surgery; **Hospital:** Newark Beth Israel Med Ctr, Saint Barnabas Med Ctr; **Address:** 201 Lyons Ave, Ste G5, Newark, NJ 07112; **Phone:** 973-926-7904; **Board Cert:** Thoracic Surgery 2000; **Med School:** Univ Iowa Coll Med 1970; **Resid:** Surgery, Univ Iowa Hosps 1978; Thoracic Surgery, Cleveland Clinic 1980

Syracuse, Donald MD (TS) - **Spec Exp:** Pacemakers; Lung Cancer; Carotid Artery Surgery; **Hospital:** Mountainside Hosp, Clara Maass Med Ctr; **Address:** 5 Franklin Ave, Ste 302, Belleville, NJ 07109-3522; **Phone:** 973-759-9000; **Board Cert:** Thoracic Surgery 2001; **Med School:** Columbia P&S 1973; **Resid:** Surgery, Columbia Presby Hosp 1979; Thoracic Surgery, Columbia Presby Hosp 1981; **Fellow:** Cardiovascular Surgery, Nat Inst Health 1977; **Fac Appt:** Asst Clin Prof S, UMDNJ-NJ Med Sch, Newark

Urology

Boorjian, Peter C MD (U) - **Spec Exp:** Kidney Stones; Prostate Benign Disease; Urinary Tract Infections; Urologic Cancer; **Hospital:** Mountainside Hosp; **Address:** 777 Bloomfield Ave, Glen Ridge, NJ 07028; **Phone:** 973-746-3322; **Board Cert:** Urology 1978; **Med School:** SUNY Downstate 1971; **Resid:** Surgery, Med Coll VA 1973; Urology, SUNY Downstate 1976

Ciccone, Patrick N MD (U) - **Spec Exp:** Prostate Cancer; **Hospital:** Clara Maass Med Ctr, Saint Barnabas Med Ctr; **Address:** 36 Newark Ave, Ste 200, Belleville, NJ 07109; **Phone:** 973-759-6180; **Board Cert:** Urology 1975; **Med School:** Georgetown Univ 1967; **Resid:** Surgery, VA Med Ctr 1969; Urology, VA Med Ctr 1972

Katz, Jeffrey I MD (U) - **Spec Exp:** Prostate Disease; Kidney Stones; Urologic Cancer; **Hospital:** Saint Barnabas Med Ctr; **Address:** 741 Northfield Ave, Ste 206, West Orange, NJ 07052; **Phone:** 973-325-6100; **Board Cert:** Urology 1978; **Med School:** Italy 1970; **Resid:** Surgery, Mt Sinai Hosp 1973; Urology, Albert Einstein 1976

Linsenmeyer, Todd A MD (U) - **Spec Exp:** Infertility-Male in Spinal Cord Injury; Voiding Dysfunction/Spinal Cord Injury; Urodynamics in Spinal Cord Injury; **Hospital:** Kessler Inst for Rehab - W Orange; **Address:** Kessler Inst Rehab, 1199 Pleasant Valley Way, West Orange, NJ 07052; **Phone:** 973-731-3900 x2274; **Board Cert:** Urology 2005; Physical Medicine & Rehabilitation 1990; Spinal Cord Injury Medicine 2002; **Med School:** Univ Hawaii JA Burns Sch Med 1979; **Resid:** Urology, Tripler AMC 1984; **Fellow:** Physical Medicine & Rehabilitation, Stanford Univ Hosp 1989; **Fac Appt:** Assoc Prof S, UMDNJ-NJ Med Sch, Newark

Savatta, Domenico J MD (U) - **Spec Exp:** Robotic Urologic Surgery; Prostate Cancer; Kidney Cancer; Bladder Cancer; **Hospital:** Newark Beth Israel Med Ctr, Saint Barnabas Med Ctr; **Address:** Associates in Urology, 741 Northfield Ave, Ste 206, West Orange, NJ 07052; **Phone:** 973-325-6100; **Board Cert:** Urology 2005; **Med School:** SUNY Stony Brook 1997; **Resid:** Surgery, Indiana Univ Med Ctr 1999; Urologic Surgery, Indiana Univ Med Ctr 2003

Seidman, Barry MD (U) - **Spec Exp:** Sexual Dysfunction; Incontinence; Genitourinary Cancer; **Hospital:** Overlook Hosp (page 92); **Address:** Atlantic Coast Urologic Implant Center, 107 Millburn Ave, Millburn, NJ 07041-1917; **Phone:** 908-219-4479; **Board Cert:** Urology 2004; **Med School:** Mount Sinai Sch Med 1978; **Resid:** Urology, Mt Sinai 1983

Stock, Jeffrey A MD (U) - **Spec Exp:** Pediatric Urology; Robotic Surgery-Pediatric; Minimally Invasive Surgery-Pediatric; **Hospital:** Newark Beth Israel Med Ctr, Saint Barnabas Med Ctr; **Address:** 101 Old Short Hills Rd, Ste 203, West Orange, NJ 07052-1023; **Phone:** 973-325-7188; **Board Cert:** Urology 2004; **Med School:** Mount Sinai Sch Med 1988; **Resid:** Surgery, UMDNJ- Univ Hosp 1990; Urology, UMDNJ- Univ Hosp 1993; **Fellow:** Pediatric Urology, UCSD Med Ctr 1994; **Fac Appt:** Assoc Clin Prof U, UMDNJ-NJ Med Sch, Newark

Strauss, Bernard MD (U) - **Spec Exp:** Kidney Stones; Prostate Disease; Sexual Dysfunction; **Hospital:** Saint Barnabas Med Ctr; **Address:** 741 Northfield Ave, Ste 206, W Orange, NJ 07052; **Phone:** 973-325-6100; **Board Cert:** Urology 1973; **Med School:** Albert Einstein Coll Med 1964; **Resid:** Surgery, Marquette Univ Affil Hosp 1966; **Fellow:** Urology, Bronx Municipal Hosp 1969; **Fac Appt:** Asst Clin Prof S, UMDNJ-NJ Med Sch, Newark

Vascular Surgery

Brener, Bruce J MD (VascS) - **Spec Exp:** Endovascular Surgery; Minimally Invasive Vascular Surgery; Carotid Artery Surgery; Aneurysm-Aortic; **Hospital:** Newark Beth Israel Med Ctr, Saint Barnabas Med Ctr; **Address:** 200 South Orange Ave, Livingston, NJ 07039; **Phone:** 973-322-7233; **Board Cert:** Surgery 1972; Vascular Surgery 2005; **Med School:** Harvard Med Sch 1966; **Resid:** Surgery, Chldns Hosp Med Ctr 1968; Surgery, Peter Bent Brigham Hosp 1972; **Fellow:** Vascular Surgery, Mass Genl Hosp 1973; **Fac Appt:** Assoc Clin Prof S, Columbia P&S

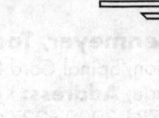

The Best in American Medicine
www.CastleConnolly.com

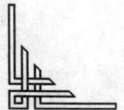
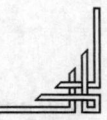

Hudson

Hudson

Cardiovascular Disease

Cruz, Merle C MD (Cv) - **Spec Exp:** Heart Disease; **Hospital:** Christ Hosp; **Address:** 201 St Pauls Ave, Unit 1-D, Jersey City, NJ 07306; **Phone:** 201-653-7533; **Board Cert:** Internal Medicine 1983; Cardiovascular Disease 1985; **Med School:** Philippines 1976; **Resid:** Internal Medicine, Jersey City Med Ctr 1982; **Fellow:** Cardiovascular Disease, Brookdale Hosp Med Ctr 1984

Elkind, Barry M MD (Cv) - **Spec Exp:** Non-Invasive Cardiology; Preventive Cardiology; **Hospital:** Bayonne Med Ctr, Newark Beth Israel Med Ctr; **Address:** 1061 Avenue C, Bayonne, NJ 07002-4726; **Phone:** 201-858-0800; **Board Cert:** Internal Medicine 1979; Cardiovascular Disease 1981; **Med School:** UMDNJ-NJ Med Sch, Newark 1976; **Resid:** Internal Medicine, Boston City Hosp 1979; **Fellow:** Cardiovascular Disease, New England Med Ctr 1982

Moussa, Ghias M MD (Cv) - **Spec Exp:** Heart Valve Disease; Congestive Heart Failure; **Hospital:** Christ Hosp; **Address:** 1815 Kennedy Blvd, Jersey City, NJ 07305; **Phone:** 201-333-3311; **Board Cert:** Internal Medicine 1989; **Med School:** Syria 1979; **Resid:** Internal Medicine, Jersey City Med Ctr 1989; **Fellow:** Cardiovascular Disease, Jersey City Med Ctr 1991; **Fac Appt:** Assoc Prof Med, UMDNJ-NJ Med Sch, Newark

Dermatology

Blank, Ellen MD (D) - **Spec Exp:** Acne; **Hospital:** Mount Sinai Med Ctr (page 102); **Address:** 330 Avenue C, Bayonne, NJ 07002; **Phone:** 201-858-4800; **Board Cert:** Dermatology 1979; **Med School:** Mount Sinai Sch Med 1975; **Resid:** Dermatology, Mount Sinai Hosp 1979

Kopec, Anna V MD (D) - **Spec Exp:** Cosmetic Dermatology; Hair & Nail Disorders; **Hospital:** Bayonne Med Ctr; **Address:** 730 Kennedy Blvd, Bayonne, NJ 07002-1838; **Phone:** 201-858-4300; **Board Cert:** Dermatology 1980; **Med School:** UMDNJ-NJ Med Sch, Newark 1975; **Resid:** Dermatology, Albert Einstein 1979; **Fac Appt:** Assoc Clin Prof D, Albert Einstein Coll Med

Endocrinology, Diabetes & Metabolism

Cam, Jenny R MD (EDM) - **Spec Exp:** Diabetes; Osteoporosis; Obesity; Adrenal Disorders; **Hospital:** Meadowlands Hosp Med Ctr, Christ Hosp; **Address:** 10 Huron Ave, Ste 1P, Jersey City, NJ 07306; **Phone:** 201-656-6003; **Board Cert:** Internal Medicine 1988; Endocrinology, Diabetes & Metabolism 1989; **Med School:** Philippines 1979; **Resid:** Internal Medicine, Interfaith Med Ctr 1987; **Fellow:** Endocrinology, Diabetes & Metabolism, UMDNJ-Univ Hosp 1989

Family Medicine

Levine, Martin S DO (FMed) *PCP* - **Spec Exp:** Primary Care Sports Medicine; Osteopathic Manipulation; **Hospital:** Christ Hosp, Bayonne Med Ctr; **Address:** 789 Avenue C, Bayonne, NJ 07002; **Phone:** 201-339-2620; **Board Cert:** Family Medicine 2007; **Med School:** Kirksville Coll Osteo Med 1980; **Resid:** Family Medicine, Kennedy Meml Hosp 1983; **Fac Appt:** Assoc Clin Prof FMed, Seton Hall Univ Sch Hlth & Med Scis

Sklower, Jay A DO (FMed) *PCP* - **Spec Exp:** Geriatric Medicine; Diabetes; Cholesterol/Lipid Disorders; **Hospital:** Christ Hosp; **Address:** 600 Pavonia Ave, 2nd Fl, Ste AB, Jersey City, NJ 07306-2929; **Phone:** 201-216-3040; **Board Cert:** Family Medicine 2005; **Med School:** SUNY Stony Brook 1971; **Resid:** Family Medicine, Union Meml Hosp 1973; **Fac Appt:** Assoc Prof Ped

Gastroenterology

Hahn, John C MD (Ge) - **Spec Exp:** Colonoscopy; Peptic Acid Disorders; **Hospital:** Bayonne Med Ctr; **Address:** 534 Avenue E, Ste 1C, Bayonne, NJ 07002; **Phone:** 201-823-0450; **Board Cert:** Internal Medicine 1988; Gastroenterology 2000; **Med School:** UMDNJ-NJ Med Sch, Newark 1985; **Resid:** Internal Medicine, Univ Hosp 1988; **Fellow:** Gastroenterology, Univ Hosp 1990

Prakash, Anaka MD (Ge) - **Spec Exp:** Pancreatic/Biliary Endoscopy (ERCP); Capsule Endoscopy; **Hospital:** Bayonne Med Ctr, Jersey City Med Ctr; **Address:** 534 Ave E, Ste 1A, Bayonne, NJ 07002; **Phone:** 201-858-8444; **Board Cert:** Internal Medicine 1976; Gastroenterology 1977; **Med School:** India 1973; **Resid:** Internal Medicine, St Joseph's Hosp 1975; **Fellow:** Gastroenterology, CMDNJ-Newark 1977

Geriatric Medicine

Brown, Mitchell Lee MD (Ger) *PCP* - **Spec Exp:** Alzheimer's Disease; **Hospital:** Bayonne Med Ctr, Jersey City Med Ctr; **Address:** 758 Broadway, Bayonne, NJ 07002; **Phone:** 201-339-2220; **Board Cert:** Internal Medicine 2000; Geriatric Medicine 2002; **Med School:** West Indies 1987; **Resid:** Internal Medicine, St Elizabeth Hosp 1990; **Fellow:** Geriatric Medicine, St Vincent's Hosp & Med Ctr 1992

Reisner, Michelle MD (Ger) *PCP* - **Hospital:** Jersey City Med Ctr; **Address:** 196 Jewitt Ave, Jersey City, NJ 07304; **Phone:** 201-332-3354; **Board Cert:** Internal Medicine 1989; Geriatric Medicine 2005; Hospice & Palliative Medicine 2008; **Med School:** South Africa 1983; **Resid:** Internal Medicine, Jersey City Med Ctr 1989

Geriatric Psychiatry

Greenberg, Robert M MD (GerPsy) - **Spec Exp:** Electroconvulsive Therapy (ECT); Neuro-Psychiatry; **Hospital:** Hoboken Univ Med Ctr - Hoboken, Hackensack Univ Med Ctr (page 96); **Address:** Hoboken Univ Med Ctr, 308 Willow Ave, Hoboken, NJ 07030; **Phone:** 201-418-1893; **Board Cert:** Psychiatry 1986; Geriatric Psychiatry 2001; **Med School:** Mount Sinai Sch Med 1978; **Resid:** Psychiatry, NY Hosp-Westchester Div 1983; **Fac Appt:** Assoc Prof Psyc, Robert W Johnson Med Sch

Internal Medicine

Cardiello, Gary P MD (IM) *PCP* - **Spec Exp:** Diabetes; Hypertension; Hemochromatosis; **Hospital:** Clara Maass Med Ctr, Saint Michael's Med Ctr; **Address:** 744 Broadway, Bayonne, NJ 07002; **Phone:** 201-436-8888; **Board Cert:** Internal Medicine 1986; **Med School:** Italy 1983; **Resid:** Internal Medicine, St Michael's Med Ctr 1986

Condo, Dominick MD (IM) *PCP* - **Spec Exp:** Geriatric Care; **Hospital:** Bayonne Med Ctr, Overlook Hosp (page 92); **Address:** 622 Broadway, Bayonne, NJ 07002; **Phone:** 201-436-2800; **Board Cert:** Internal Medicine 1984; **Med School:** Mexico 1980; **Resid:** Internal Medicine, St Michael's Med Ctr 1984

Dedousis, John T MD (IM) *PCP* - **Hospital:** Bayonne Med Ctr; **Address:** 1166 Kennedy Blvd, Bayonne, NJ 07002-3112; **Phone:** 201-339-1133; **Board Cert:** Internal Medicine 2003; **Med School:** Dominica 1985; **Resid:** Internal Medicine, Univ Hosp 1988

Mutterperl, Mitchell MD (IM) *PCP* - **Spec Exp:** Hypertension; Cholesterol/Lipid Disorders; Cardiovascular Disease; **Hospital:** Bayonne Med Ctr, Jersey City Med Ctr; **Address:** 19 W 33rd St, Bayonne, NJ 07002-3916; **Phone:** 201-858-0090; **Board Cert:** Internal Medicine 1985; **Med School:** Italy 1981; **Resid:** Internal Medicine, UMDNJ-NJ Med Ctr 1985

Nephrology

Thomsen, Stephen MD (Nep) - **Spec Exp:** Diabetes; Hypertension; Kidney Disease; **Hospital:** Christ Hosp, Mountainside Hosp; **Address:** 510 31st St, Union City, NJ 07087; **Phone:** 201-866-3322; **Board Cert:** Internal Medicine 1981; Nephrology 2006; **Med School:** Italy 1977; **Resid:** Internal Medicine, Mountainside Hosp 1980; **Fellow:** Nephrology, UMDNJ-Univ Hosp 1982

Neurology

Anselmi, Gregory D MD (N) - **Spec Exp:** Migraine; Multiple Sclerosis; Stroke; **Hospital:** Bayonne Med Ctr, Hoboken Univ Med Ctr - Hoboken; **Address:** 1222 Kennedy Blvd, Bayonne, NJ 07002-3822; **Phone:** 201-339-6531; **Board Cert:** Neurology 2002; **Med School:** Italy 1988; **Resid:** Internal Medicine, SUNY/Univ Hosp 1989; **Fellow:** Neurology, St Vincent's Hosp & Med Ctr 1992

Charles, James A MD (N) - **Spec Exp:** Headache; Clinical Neurophysiology; **Hospital:** Bayonne Med Ctr, Christ Hosp; **Address:** 956 Kennedy Blvd, Bayonne, NJ 07002; **Phone:** 201-858-2457; **Board Cert:** Neurology 1984; Clinical Neurophysiology 2005; **Med School:** UMDNJ-NJ Med Sch, Newark 1978; **Resid:** Neurology, UMDNJ Med Ctr 1982; **Fac Appt:** Assoc Clin Prof N, UMDNJ-NJ Med Sch, Newark

Sadeghi, Hooshang W MD (N) - **Spec Exp:** Parkinson's Disease; Stroke; Multiple Sclerosis; Dystonia-Cervical; **Hospital:** Bayonne Med Ctr, Jersey City Med Ctr; **Address:** 631 Broadway, FL 3, Bayonne, NJ 07002-3846; **Phone:** 201-823-2888; **Board Cert:** Neurology 1977; **Med School:** Iran 1967; **Resid:** Neurology, UMDNJ Med Ctr 1975; **Fac Appt:** Asst Clin Prof N, UMDNJ-NJ Med Sch, Newark

Obstetrics & Gynecology

Banzon, Manuel MD (ObG) - **Spec Exp:** Laparoscopic Surgery; Vaginal Surgery; Incontinence; **Hospital:** Meadowlands Hosp Med Ctr; **Address:** 1265 Paterson Plank Rd, Ste 3D, Secaucus, NJ 07094; **Phone:** 201-864-4442; **Board Cert:** Obstetrics & Gynecology 1979; **Med School:** Philippines 1962; **Resid:** Obstetrics & Gynecology, Jersey City Med Ctr 1969

Masson, Lalitha MD (ObG) - **Spec Exp:** Infertility; **Hospital:** Christ Hosp; **Address:** 634 Newark Ave, Main Flr, Jersey City, NJ 07306; **Phone:** 201-963-8554; **Board Cert:** Obstetrics & Gynecology 1973; **Med School:** India 1964; **Resid:** Obstetrics & Gynecology, Margaret Hogue Hosp 1969; Obstetrics & Gynecology, St Clares Hosp 1970; **Fellow:** Infertility, UMDNJ-NJ Sch Med 1971

Uy, Vena MD (ObG) *PCP* - **Hospital:** Christ Hosp, Meadowlands Hosp Med Ctr; **Address:** 142 Palisade Ave, Ste 102, Jersey City, NJ 07306; **Phone:** 201-653-0506; **Board Cert:** Obstetrics & Gynecology 1977; **Med School:** Philippines 1968; **Resid:** Obstetrics & Gynecology, Jersey Shore Med Ctr 1973; **Fellow:** Gynecologic Pathology, Magee Womens Hosp 1974

Ophthalmology

Benedetto, Dominick A MD (Oph) - **Spec Exp:** LASIK-Refractive Surgery; Cataract Surgery; **Hospital:** Bayonne Med Ctr, Morristown Mem Hosp (page 92); **Address:** EyeMD Associates, 124 Avenue B, Bayonne, NJ 07002-2033; **Phone:** 201-436-1150; **Board Cert:** Ophthalmology 1982; **Med School:** Univ Fla Coll Med 1975; **Resid:** Ophthalmology, Wills Eye Hosp 1981

Constad, William H MD (Oph) - **Spec Exp:** Cornea Transplant; Cataract Surgery; Refractive Surgery; **Hospital:** Jersey City Med Ctr, Univ Hosp-UMDNJ—Newark; **Address:** 600 Pavonia Ave Fl 6, Jersey City, NJ 07306-2932; **Phone:** 201-963-3937; **Board Cert:** Ophthalmology 1985; **Med School:** Med Coll PA Hahnemann 1980; **Resid:** Ophthalmology, UMDNJ Univ Hosp 1984; **Fellow:** Cornea, NY Eye & Ear Infirm 1985; **Fac Appt:** Clin Prof Oph, UMDNJ-NJ Med Sch, Newark

Orthopaedic Surgery

Granatir, Charles MD (OrS) - **Hospital:** Clara Maass Med Ctr; **Address:** 586 Kearny Ave, Kearny, NJ 07032; **Phone:** 201-997-7667; **Board Cert:** Orthopaedic Surgery 2000; **Med School:** Hahnemann Univ 1979; **Resid:** Orthopaedic Surgery, Montefiore Hosp Med Ctr 1984

Pediatrics

Baker, Azzam A MD (Ped) *PCP* - **Hospital:** Hackensack Univ Med Ctr (page 96), Palisades Med Ctr; **Address:** 714 10th St, Secaucus, NJ 07094-2921; **Phone:** 201-863-3346; **Board Cert:** Pediatrics 2004; **Med School:** Egypt 1972; **Resid:** Pediatrics, Jersey City Med Ctr 1978; **Fellow:** Neonatal-Perinatal Medicine, UMDNJ Univ Hosp 1980

Skripkus, Aldona MD (Ped) *PCP* - **Hospital:** Clara Maass Med Ctr; **Address:** 381 Kearny Ave, Kearny, NJ 07032-2603; **Phone:** 201-991-4824; **Board Cert:** Pediatrics 1971; **Med School:** Med Coll PA Hahnemann 1966; **Resid:** Pediatrics, Chldns Hosp 1969

Physical Medicine & Rehabilitation

Filippone, Mark A MD (PMR) - **Spec Exp:** Electrodiagnosis; Electromyography; Pain Management; **Hospital:** Christ Hosp, Hoboken Univ Med Ctr - Hoboken; **Address:** 2012 John F Kennedy Blvd, Jersey City, NJ 07305-1526; **Phone:** 201-332-6855; **Board Cert:** Physical Medicine & Rehabilitation 1980; **Med School:** Georgetown Univ 1974; **Resid:** Pediatrics, St Vincent's Hosp & Med Ctr 1976; Physical Medicine & Rehabilitation, Bronx Muni Hosp-Einstein 1978; **Fac Appt:** Asst Clin Prof PMR, Albert Einstein Coll Med

Psychiatry

Gewolb, Eric B MD (Psyc) - **Spec Exp:** Anxiety Disorders; Dementia; Bipolar/Mood Disorders; **Hospital:** Bayonne Med Ctr; **Address:** 830 Kennedy Blvd, Bayonne, NJ 07002-2872; **Phone:** 201-339-0200; **Board Cert:** Psychiatry 1979; **Med School:** Tulane Univ 1974; **Resid:** Psychiatry, Mount Sinai Hosp 1978

Jacoby, Jacob H MD/PhD (Psyc) - **Spec Exp:** Psychopharmacology; Mood Disorders; **Hospital:** Bayonne Med Ctr, Saint Barnabas Med Ctr; **Address:** 654 Avenue C, Ste 201, Bayonne, NJ 07002-3899; **Phone:** 201-339-0323; **Board Cert:** Psychiatry 1993; **Med School:** SUNY Buffalo 1980; **Resid:** Psychiatry, Univ Pittsburgh Med Ctr 1981; Psychiatry, Western Psychiatric Inst 1983; **Fellow:** Addiction Psychiatry, Albert Einstein 1983; **Fac Appt:** Assoc Clin Prof Psyc, UMDNJ-NJ Med Sch, Newark

Moraille, Pascale MD (Psyc) - **Spec Exp:** Autism; Developmental Disorders; ADD/ADHD; **Hospital:** Hoboken Univ Med Ctr - Hoboken; **Address:** 506 3rd St, Hoboken, NJ 07030; **Phone:** 201-792-8200; **Board Cert:** Psychiatry 1993; **Med School:** Ponce Med Sch 1988; **Resid:** Psychiatry, UMDNJ-NJ Med Sch 1991; **Fellow:** Child & Adolescent Psychiatry, UMDNJ-NJ Med Sch 1993

Pulmonary Disease

Elamir, Mazhar E MD (Pul) - **Spec Exp:** Sleep Disorders; Allergy; Asthma; **Hospital:** Christ Hosp, Greenville Hosp; **Address:** 192 Harrison Ave, Jersey City, NJ 07304; **Phone:** 201-333-5363; **Board Cert:** Internal Medicine 1987; Pulmonary Disease 2004; **Med School:** Egypt 1982; **Resid:** Internal Medicine, Jersey City Med Ctr 1987; **Fellow:** Pulmonary Disease, Interfaith Med Ctr 1991

Kozel, Joseph M MD (Pul) - **Spec Exp:** Asthma; Chronic Obstructive Lung Disease (COPD); Lung Cancer; Lung Disease in Pregnancy; **Hospital:** Hoboken Univ Med Ctr - Hoboken; **Address:** 331 Grand St, Hoboken, NJ 07030; **Phone:** 201-656-3519; **Board Cert:** Internal Medicine 1984; **Med School:** Mexico 1973; **Resid:** Family Medicine, St Mary Hosp 1979; Internal Medicine, St Michaels Med Ctr 1980; **Fellow:** Pulmonary Disease, St Michaels Med Ctr 1982

Rheumatology

Scarpa, Nicholas P MD (Rhu) - **Spec Exp:** Lupus/SLE in Pregnancy; Rheumatoid Arthritis; Osteoporosis; **Hospital:** Christ Hosp, Univ Hosp-UMDNJ—Newark; **Address:** 600 Pavonia Ave Fl 5 - Ste 1, Jersey City, NJ 07306-2932; **Phone:** 201-216-3050; **Board Cert:** Internal Medicine 1983; Rheumatology 1986; **Med School:** UMDNJ-NJ Med Sch, Newark 1980; **Resid:** Internal Medicine, Hackensack Univ Med Ctr 1983; **Fellow:** Rheumatology, Hosp for Special Surg 1985; **Fac Appt:** Asst Clin Prof Med, UMDNJ-NJ Med Sch, Newark

Surgery

Gildengers, Jaime N MD (S) - **Spec Exp:** Gallbladder Surgery; Colon Surgery; Breast Surgery; **Hospital:** Palisades Med Ctr, Christ Hosp; **Address:** 313 60th St, West New York, NJ 07093; **Phone:** 201-854-0406; **Board Cert:** Surgery 2006; **Med School:** Argentina 1965; **Resid:** Surgery, Mt Sinai Med Ctr 1970; Surgery, St Clares Hosp 1973; **Fellow:** Surgical Research, St Clares Hosp 1974; **Fac Appt:** Asst Clin Prof S, UMDNJ-NJ Med Sch, Newark

McGovern Jr, Patrick J MD (S) - **Spec Exp:** Vascular Surgery; Aneurysm-Aortic; Carotid Artery Surgery; **Hospital:** Christ Hosp, Bayonne Med Ctr; **Address:** Hudson Surgical Grp, 631 Broadway, Bayonne, NJ 07002; **Phone:** 201-858-5705; **Board Cert:** Surgery 2003; Vascular Surgery 2008; **Med School:** UMDNJ-NJ Med Sch, Newark 1978; **Resid:** Surgery, UMDNJ-Univ Hosp 1983; **Fellow:** Vascular Surgery, UMDNJ-RWJ Univ Hosp 1984

Popovich, Joseph F MD (S) - **Spec Exp:** Vascular Surgery; **Hospital:** Christ Hosp, Jersey City Med Ctr; **Address:** 159 Palisade Ave, Jersey City, NJ 07306; **Phone:** 201-217-1110; **Board Cert:** Surgery 2004; **Med School:** UMDNJ-RW Johnson Med Sch 1987; **Resid:** Surgery, Med Ctr Hosp 1993; Surgery, Univ of Med & Dentistry 1991; **Fellow:** Vascular Surgery, St Francis Hosp 1988

Sultan, Ronald H MD (S) - **Spec Exp:** Hernia; Thyroid Cancer; Breast Cancer; **Hospital:** Christ Hosp; **Address:** 2255 John F Kennedy Blvd, Jersey City, NJ 07304-1428; **Phone:** 201-434-3305; **Board Cert:** Surgery 2009; **Med School:** NYU Sch Med 1973; **Resid:** Surgery, Bronx Municipal Hosp 1977; Surgery, Albert Einstein Med Ctr 1980

Thoracic Surgery

McMurtry, Kirk A MD (TS) - **Spec Exp:** Cardiac Surgery-Adult; Thoracic Surgery; Aortic Surgery; Heart Valve Surgery; **Hospital:** Jersey City Med Ctr; **Address:** Liberty Heart Inst, Cardiothor Surg, 355 Grand St, 2E, rm 18, Jersey City, NJ 07302; **Phone:** 201-915-2525; **Board Cert:** Surgery 2001; Thoracic Surgery 2004; **Med School:** Mount Sinai Sch Med 1995; **Resid:** Surgery, Thomas Jefferson Univ Hosp 2000; Cardiothoracic Surgery, Mt Sinai Med Ctr 2003

Urology

Katz, Herbert I MD (U) - **Spec Exp:** Urologic Cancer; Erectile Dysfunction; Kidney Stones; **Hospital:** Bayonne Med Ctr; **Address:** 534 Ave E, Ste 2A, Bayonne, NJ 07002; **Phone:** 201-823-1303; **Board Cert:** Urology 1981; **Med School:** Temple Univ 1974; **Resid:** Surgery, Abington Meml Hosp 1976; Urology, Monterfiore-Weiler Einstein Med Ctr 1979

Shulman, Yale MD (U) - **Spec Exp:** Urologic Cancer; Kidney Stones; Sexual Dysfunction; Incontinence; **Hospital:** Christ Hosp, Englewood Hosp & Med Ctr (page 656); **Address:** 2255 Kennedy Blvd, Jersey City, NJ 07304-1428; **Phone:** 201-433-1057; **Board Cert:** Urology 1984; **Med School:** Albert Einstein Coll Med 1976; **Resid:** Surgery, Montefiore Hosp Med Ctr 1978; Urology, NYU Med Ctr 1982; **Fac Appt:** Assoc Clin Prof U, NYU Sch Med

Steigman, Elliot G MD (U) - **Spec Exp:** Kidney Stones; Prostate Benign Disease; **Hospital:** Christ Hosp; **Address:** 142 Palisade Ave, Ste 211, Jersey City, NJ 07306-1108; **Phone:** 201-435-2244; **Board Cert:** Urology 1982; **Med School:** SUNY Downstate 1975; **Resid:** Surgery, Brookdale Hosp Med Ctr 1977; Urology, SUNY Downstate Med Ctr 1980

Mercer

Mercer

Allergy & Immunology

Ricketti, Anthony J MD (A&I) - **Spec Exp:** Asthma in Pregnancy; Allergic Aspergillosis; Eosinophilic Lung Disorders; **Hospital:** St Francis Med Ctr - Trenton, Robert Wood Johnson Univ Hosp Hamilton; **Address:** Allergy & Pulmonary Assocs, 1542 Kuser Rd, Ste B7, Trenton, NJ 08619-3829; **Phone:** 609-581-1400; **Board Cert:** Internal Medicine 1981; Allergy & Immunology 1983; Pulmonary Disease 1986; Critical Care Medicine 2009; **Med School:** Hahnemann Univ 1978; **Resid:** Internal Medicine, Cleveland Clin Fdn 1981; Allergy & Immunology, Northwestern Univ 1983; **Fellow:** Pulmonary Disease, Northwestern Univ 1984; **Fac Appt:** Asst Clin Prof Med, UMDNJ-RW Johnson Med Sch

Winant Jr, John G MD (A&I) - **Spec Exp:** Asthma; **Hospital:** Univ Med Ctr - Princeton, Capital Hlth Sys - Mercer Campus; **Address:** 8 Quakerbridge Plaza, Bldg 8, Mercerville, NJ 08619-1255; **Phone:** 609-890-8782; **Board Cert:** Pediatrics 1980; Allergy & Immunology 1987; **Med School:** Univ Cincinnati 1975; **Resid:** Pediatrics, Chldns Hosp Med Ctr 1978; **Fellow:** Allergy & Immunology, Chldns Hosp Med Ctr 1980

Cardiovascular Disease

Costin, Andrew MD (Cv) - **Hospital:** Univ Med Ctr - Princeton; **Address:** 419 N Harrison St, Princeton, NJ 08540; **Phone:** 609-924-9300; **Board Cert:** Internal Medicine 1989; Cardiovascular Disease 2003; **Med School:** Yale Univ 1986; **Resid:** Internal Medicine, NY Hosp 1989; **Fellow:** Cardiovascular Disease, Hosp Univ Penn 1993

Hagaman, John F MD (Cv) - **Spec Exp:** Heart Failure; **Hospital:** Univ Med Ctr - Princeton; **Address:** 281 Witherspoon St, Ste 210, Princeton, NJ 08540-3210; **Phone:** 609-921-7456; **Board Cert:** Internal Medicine 1977; Cardiovascular Disease 1981; **Med School:** Columbia P&S 1974; **Resid:** Internal Medicine, Univ Mich Hosp 1977; **Fellow:** Cardiovascular Disease, NC Meml Hosp 1980; **Fac Appt:** Asst Clin Prof Med, Robert W Johnson Med Sch

Mahalingam, Banu MD (Cv) - **Spec Exp:** Heart Disease in Women; Echocardiography; Preventive Cardiology; **Hospital:** Univ Med Ctr - Princeton, Robert Wood Johnson Univ Hosp - New Brunswick; **Address:** Cardiac Associates of Princeton, 281 Witherspoon St, Ste 210, Princeton, NJ 08542; **Phone:** 609-921-7456; **Board Cert:** Internal Medicine 2008; Cardiovascular Disease 2002; **Med School:** India 1995; **Resid:** Internal Medicine, RW Johnson Med Ctr 1998; **Fellow:** Cardiovascular Disease, RW Johnson Med Ctr 2001

Samuel, Steven A MD (Cv) - **Spec Exp:** Congestive Heart Failure; **Hospital:** St Francis Med Ctr - Trenton, Robert Wood Johnson Univ Hosp Hamilton; **Address:** Penn Cardiac Care at Mercer Bucks, 1 Union St, Ste 101, Robbinsville, NJ 08691; **Phone:** 609-890-6677; **Board Cert:** Internal Medicine 1982; Cardiovascular Disease 1985; **Med School:** Albert Einstein Coll Med 1978; **Resid:** Family Medicine, Southside Hosp 1979; Internal Medicine, Univ Hosp 1982; **Fellow:** Cardiovascular Disease, Univ Hosp 1984; **Fac Appt:** Assoc Clin Prof Med, Univ Pennsylvania

Dermatology

Bagel, Jerry MD (D) - **Spec Exp:** Psoriasis; Atopic Dermatitis; Skin Diseases; Exfoliate Erythroderma; **Hospital:** Univ Med Ctr - Princeton; **Address:** 59 One Mile Rd, Ste G, East Windsor, NJ 08520-2505; **Phone:** 609-443-4500; **Board Cert:** Dermatology 1985; **Med School:** Mount Sinai Sch Med 1981; **Resid:** Dermatology, Columbia-Presby Med Ctr 1985; **Fac Appt:** Assoc Clin Prof D, Columbia P&S

Notterman, Robyn MD (D) - **Hospital:** Univ Med Ctr - Princeton; **Address:** 800 Bunn Drive, Ste B 201, Princeton, NJ 08540; **Phone:** 609-924-1033; **Board Cert:** Dermatology 2003; **Med School:** Cornell Univ-Weill Med Coll 1983; **Resid:** Dermatology, NYU Med Ctr 1992

Vine, John E MD (D) - **Spec Exp:** Mohs' Surgery; Cosmetic Dermatology; Hyperhidrosis/Axillary Curettage; **Hospital:** Univ Med Ctr - Princeton, Robert Wood Johnson Univ Hosp - New Brunswick; **Address:** 253 Witherspoon St, Ste L, Princeton, NJ 08540; **Phone:** 609-683-0101; **Board Cert:** Dermatology 2005; **Med School:** Brown Univ 1992; **Resid:** Dermatology, Meml Hermann Hosp 1996; **Fellow:** Mohs Surgery, Scripps Clinic 1997

Diagnostic Radiology

Ford, Robert R MD (DR) - **Spec Exp:** CT Scan; MRI; Nuclear Medicine; Ultrasound; **Hospital:** Univ Med Ctr - Princeton; **Address:** 100 Overlook Ctr, Princeton, NJ 08540; **Phone:** 609-936-2600; **Board Cert:** Diagnostic Radiology 1988; **Med School:** UMDNJ-Rutgers Med Sch 1983; **Resid:** Internal Medicine, R W Johnson Univ Hosp 1985; Diagnostic Radiology, NY Hosp-Cornell 1988

Endocrinology, Diabetes & Metabolism

Feldman, Alan MD (EDM) - **Spec Exp:** Diabetes; **Hospital:** Univ Med Ctr - Princeton; **Address:** Princeton Med Group, 419 N Harrison St, Ste 101, Princeton, NJ 08540-3521; **Phone:** 609-924-9300; **Board Cert:** Internal Medicine 1983; Endocrinology, Diabetes & Metabolism 1985; **Med School:** Univ Pennsylvania 1980; **Resid:** Internal Medicine, Kaiser Fdn Hosp 1983; **Fellow:** Endocrinology, Mt Sinai Hosp 1985

Shelmet, John J MD (EDM) - **Spec Exp:** Diabetes; Metabolic Disorders; **Hospital:** Univ Med Ctr - Princeton; **Address:** 3131 Princeton Pike, Bldg 2B, Ste 104, Lawrenceville, NJ 08648-2526; **Phone:** 609-896-8050; **Board Cert:** Internal Medicine 1984; **Med School:** UMDNJ-RW Johnson Med Sch 1981; **Resid:** Internal Medicine, Middlesex Genl Hosp/Univ Hosp 1984; **Fellow:** Metabolism, Temple Univ 1986; Diabetes, Temple Univ 1986; **Fac Appt:** Clin Prof Med, Robert W Johnson Med Sch

Family Medicine

Lansing, Martha MD (FMed) *PCP* - **Spec Exp:** Chronic Illness; Women's Health; Psychosomatic Disorders; **Hospital:** Capital Health Sys - Fuld Campus, Capital Hlth Sys - Mercer Campus; **Address:** 4056 Quakerbridge Rd, Lawrenceville, NJ 08648; **Phone:** 609-275-0487; **Board Cert:** Family Medicine 2005; **Med School:** Univ Okla Coll Med 1982; **Resid:** Family Medicine, Univ Tenn 1984; Family Medicine, Williamsport Hosp/Univ Penn 1985; **Fac Appt:** Assoc Prof FMed, UMDNJ-RW Johnson Med Sch

Rednor, Jeffrey DO (FMed) *PCP* - **Spec Exp:** Diabetes; Pain-Back; Preventive Cardiology; **Hospital:** Robert Wood Johnson Univ Hosp Hamilton; **Address:** 1 Washington Blvd, Ste A, Robbinsville, NJ 08691; **Phone:** 609-448-4353; **Board Cert:** Family Medicine 1992; **Med School:** UMDNJ Sch Osteo Med 1989; **Resid:** Family Medicine, Kennedy Mem Hosp 1992

Gastroenterology

Afridi, Shariq A MD (Ge) - **Spec Exp:** Liver Disease; **Hospital:** Robert Wood Johnson Univ Hosp Hamilton, St Francis Med Ctr - Trenton; **Address:** 1374 White Horse Square Rd, Yorkshire Bldg Fl 2, Hamilton, NJ 08690; **Phone:** 609-586-1319; **Board Cert:** Internal Medicine 2002; Gastroenterology 2003; **Med School:** Pakistan 1986; **Resid:** Internal Medicine, Bridgeport Hosp 1991; **Fellow:** Gastroenterology, Bridgeport Hosp 1993

De Antonio, Joseph R MD (Ge) - **Spec Exp:** Liver Disease; **Hospital:** Capital Health Sys - Fuld Campus; **Address:** 3100 Princeton Pike Bldg 4 - Ste C, Lawrenceville, NJ 08648; **Phone:** 609-882-2185; **Board Cert:** Internal Medicine 1989; Gastroenterology 2004; **Med School:** St Louis Univ 1982; **Resid:** Internal Medicine, Vet Affairs Med Ctr 1989; **Fellow:** Gastroenterology, Bellevue Hosp Ctr 1991

Marin, Geobel A MD (Ge) - **Spec Exp:** Peptic Ulcer Disease; Colonoscopy; Inflammatory Bowel Disease; **Hospital:** Capital Hlth Sys - Mercer Campus, Robert Wood Johnson Univ Hosp Hamilton; **Address:** 416 Bellevue Ave, Ste 101, Trenton, NJ 08618; **Phone:** 609-394-8844; **Board Cert:** Gastroenterology 1972; Internal Medicine 1977; **Med School:** Columbia P&S 1962; **Resid:** Internal Medicine, Philadelphia Genl Hosp 1966; **Fellow:** Gastroenterology, Philadelphia Genl Hosp 1968

Meirowitz, Robert F MD (Ge) - **Spec Exp:** Inflammatory Bowel Disease; Colon Polyps & Cancer; Colonoscopy; Gastroesophageal Reflux Disease (GERD); **Hospital:** Univ Med Ctr - Princeton; **Address:** 281 Witherspoon St, Ste 230, Princeton, NJ 08540-3210; **Phone:** 609-924-1422; **Board Cert:** Internal Medicine 1987; Gastroenterology 2001; **Med School:** NY Med Coll 1984; **Resid:** Internal Medicine, UMDNJ-RW Johnson Univ Hosp 1988; **Fellow:** Gastroenterology, Univ Maryland 1990; **Fac Appt:** Asst Clin Prof Med, Robert W Johnson Med Sch

Rosner, Bruce P MD (Ge) - **Spec Exp:** Liver Disease; Gastroesophageal Reflux Disease (GERD); Colon Cancer; **Hospital:** St Francis Med Ctr - Trenton; **Address:** 2275 Whitehorse Mercerville Rd, Ste 2, Trenton, NJ 08619-2643; **Phone:** 609-890-0200; **Board Cert:** Internal Medicine 1979; Gastroenterology 1983; **Med School:** Univ Pennsylvania 1976; **Resid:** Internal Medicine, Penn Hosp 1979; **Fellow:** Gastroenterology, Hahnemann Univ 1981

Rubin, Marc R MD (Ge) - **Hospital:** St Francis Med Ctr - Trenton; **Address:** Gastroenterology Associates, 2275 Whitehorse Mercerville Rd, Ste 2, Trenton, NJ 08619-2643; **Phone:** 609-890-0200; **Board Cert:** Internal Medicine 1977; Gastroenterology 1979; **Med School:** Albert Einstein Coll Med 1974; **Resid:** Internal Medicine, Penn Hosp 1977; **Fellow:** Gastroenterology, Univ Hosp 1979

Sachs, Jonathan R MD (Ge) - **Spec Exp:** Colon Cancer Screening; Gastroesophageal Reflux Disease (GERD); Inflammatory Bowel Disease; **Hospital:** Univ Med Ctr - Princeton; **Address:** 281 Witherspoon St, Ste 230, Princeton, NJ 08542-3210; **Phone:** 609-924-1422; **Board Cert:** Internal Medicine 1987; Gastroenterology 1989; **Med School:** Med Coll PA Hahnemann 1984; **Resid:** Internal Medicine, Temple Univ Hosp 1987; **Fellow:** Gastroenterology, Graduate Hosp 1989

Hand Surgery

Ark, Jon Wong Tze-Jen MD (HS) - **Spec Exp:** Hand Surgery; Carpal Tunnel Syndrome; Foot & Ankle Surgery; Arthritis Hand Surgery; **Hospital:** Univ Med Ctr - Princeton; **Address:** 325 Princeton Ave, Princeton, NJ 08540; **Phone:** 609-924-8131; **Board Cert:** Orthopaedic Surgery 2007; Hand Surgery 2007; **Med School:** UMDNJ-RW Johnson Med Sch 1987; **Resid:** Orthopaedic Surgery, Columbia-Presby Med Ctr 1992; **Fellow:** Hand Surgery, Mass Genl Hosp 1993; Foot & Ankle Surgery, Jefferson Hosp 1995

Infectious Disease

Aufiero, Patrick MD (Inf) - **Spec Exp:** AIDS/HIV; Lyme Disease; Osteomyelitis; Skin/Soft Tissue Infection; **Hospital:** Robert Wood Johnson Univ Hosp Hamilton, Capital Hlth Sys - Mercer Campus; **Address:** 2085 Klockner Rd, Trenton, NJ 08690; **Phone:** 609-587-4122; **Board Cert:** Internal Medicine 2005; Infectious Disease 2006; **Med School:** Grenada 1984; **Resid:** Internal Medicine, St Michaels Med Ctr 1989; **Fellow:** Infectious Disease, St Michaels Med Ctr 1991

Cleri, Dennis MD (Inf) - **Spec Exp:** Viral Infections; AIDS/HIV; **Hospital:** St Francis Hosp - Jersey City; **Address:** 601 Hamilton Ave, Outpatient Dept, Trenton, NJ 08629; **Phone:** 609-599-5050; **Board Cert:** Internal Medicine 1976; Infectious Disease 1982; **Med School:** Jefferson Med Coll 1972; **Resid:** Internal Medicine, Coney Island Hosp 1975; **Fellow:** Infectious Disease, Kings Co Hosp Ctr 1980

Gekowski, Kathleen MD (Inf) - **Spec Exp:** Travel Medicine; AIDS/HIV; Lyme Disease; **Hospital:** Capital Hlth Sys - Mercer Campus, Robert Wood Johnson Univ Hosp Hamilton; **Address:** 1450 Parkside Ave, Ste 4, Ewing, NJ 08638; **Phone:** 609-882-3500; **Board Cert:** Internal Medicine 1979; Infectious Disease 1984; **Med School:** Hahnemann Univ 1976; **Resid:** Internal Medicine, Univ Illinois Hosp 1979; **Fellow:** Infectious Disease, Yale Univ 1982; **Fac Appt:** Assoc Clin Prof Med, UMDNJ-RW Johnson Med Sch

Porwancher, Richard B MD (Inf) - **Spec Exp:** Lyme Disease; AIDS/HIV; Disaster Preparedness; **Hospital:** St Francis Med Ctr - Trenton, Robert Wood Johnson Univ Hosp Hamilton; **Address:** 1245 Whitehorse-Mercerville Rd, Ste 411, Mercerville, NJ 08619-3831; **Phone:** 609-581-2000; **Board Cert:** Internal Medicine 1980; Infectious Disease 1982; **Med School:** Northwestern Univ 1977; **Resid:** Internal Medicine, Med Coll Wisconsin Affil Hosps 1980; **Fellow:** Infectious Disease, VA Med Ctr 1982; **Fac Appt:** Assoc Clin Prof Med, Robert W Johnson Med Sch

Internal Medicine

Corazza, Douglas P MD (IM) *PCP* - **Hospital:** Univ Med Ctr - Princeton; **Address:** Montgomery Internal Medicine Group, 727 State Rd, Princeton, NJ 08540; **Phone:** 609-921-6410; **Board Cert:** Internal Medicine 1988; **Med School:** UMDNJ-Rutgers Med Sch 1985; **Resid:** Internal Medicine, RW Johnson Univ Hosp 1988

Murray, Simon D MD (IM) *PCP* - **Spec Exp:** Concierge Medicine; Cholesterol/Lipid Disorders; Nutrition; Preventive Medicine; **Hospital:** Univ Med Ctr - Princeton; **Address:** 727 State Rd, Princeton, NJ 08540; **Phone:** 609-921-7444; **Board Cert:** Internal Medicine 1985; **Med School:** Philippines 1980; **Resid:** Internal Medicine, UMDNJ/RWJ Univ Hosp 1984; **Fac Appt:** Asst Clin Prof Med, UMDNJ-RW Johnson Med Sch

Schaeffer, Mark A MD (IM) - **Hospital:** Univ Med Ctr - Princeton; **Address:** 281 Witherspoon St, Ste 220, Princeton, NJ 08542; **Phone:** 609-921-1680; **Board Cert:** Internal Medicine 1989; **Med School:** NY Med Coll 1984; **Resid:** Internal Medicine, RW Johnson Univ Hosp 1989

Warren, Ronald MD (IM) - **Spec Exp:** Pulmonary Disease; **Hospital:** Capital Health Sys - Fuld Campus; **Address:** Pulmonary & Internal Medicine, 40 Fuld St, Ste 201, Trenton, NJ 08638-5247; **Phone:** 609-695-4422; **Board Cert:** Internal Medicine 1972; Pulmonary Disease 1976; **Med School:** Univ Pennsylvania 1968; **Resid:** Internal Medicine, Presby Hosp 1970; Internal Medicine, Grady Meml Hosp 1971; **Fellow:** Pulmonary Disease, Emory Hosps 1972

Yamane, Michael H MD (IM) *PCP* - **Hospital:** Capital Hlth Sys - Mercer Campus; **Address:** 2480 Pennington Rd, Ste 108, Pennington, NJ 08534-5227; **Phone:** 609-737-6700; **Board Cert:** Internal Medicine 1984; **Med School:** UCSF 1981; **Resid:** Internal Medicine, Univ Hawaii Med Ctr 1984

Interventional Cardiology

Shanahan, Andrew J MD (IC) - **Spec Exp:** Angioplasty; **Hospital:** Univ Med Ctr - Princeton, Robert Wood Johnson Univ Hosp - New Brunswick; **Address:** Cardiology Assocs of Princeton, 281 Witherspoon St, Ste 210, Princeton, NJ 08542; **Phone:** 609-921-7456; **Board Cert:** Internal Medicine 2005; Cardiovascular Disease 2005; Interventional Cardiology 2001; **Med School:** Med Coll Wisc 1989; **Resid:** Internal Medicine, St Lukes-Roosevelt Hosp 1992; **Fellow:** Cardiovascular Disease, St Lukes-Roosevelt Hosp 1995

Medical Oncology

Eleff, Michael MD (Onc) - **Spec Exp:** Colon & Rectal Cancer; Gastrointestinal Cancer; **Hospital:** Robert Wood Johnson Univ Hosp Hamilton; **Address:** Cancer Inst NJ-Hamilton, 2575 Klockner Rd, Hamilton, NJ 08690; **Phone:** 609-631-6960; **Board Cert:** Internal Medicine 1982; Medical Oncology 1985; **Med School:** Case West Res Univ 1979; **Resid:** Internal Medicine, Med Coll Va Hosp 1982; **Fellow:** Medical Oncology, Med Coll Va Hosp 1984; **Fac Appt:** Asst Prof Med, Robert W Johnson Med Sch

Grossman, Bernard MD (Onc) - **Hospital:** Capital Hlth Sys - Mercer Campus, Robert Wood Johnson Univ Hosp Hamilton; **Address:** 2997 Princeton Pike, Lawrenceville, NJ 08648; **Phone:** 609-771-0700; **Board Cert:** Internal Medicine 1977; Medical Oncology 1979; Hematology 1980; **Med School:** Temple Univ 1974; **Resid:** Internal Medicine, Albany Meml Hosp 1977; **Fellow:** Hematology & Oncology, George Wash Univ Hosp 1979; Oncology, Fox Chase Cancer Ctr 1980

Lerma, Pauline M MD (Onc) - **Spec Exp:** Breast Cancer; Hematologic Malignancies; **Hospital:** Robert Wood Johnson Univ Hosp Hamilton; **Address:** Cancer Inst NJ-Hamilton, 2575 Klockner Rd, Hamilton, NJ 08690; **Phone:** 609-631-6960; **Board Cert:** Internal Medicine 2006; Medical Oncology 2009; Hematology 2000; **Med School:** Philippines 1992; **Resid:** Internal Medicine, Abington Meml Hosp 1996; **Fellow:** Hematology & Oncology, Hahnemann Univ Hosp 1999; Bone Marrow Transplant, Hahnemann Univ Hosp 2000; **Fac Appt:** Asst Prof Med, Robert W Johnson Med Sch

Schaebler, David MD (Onc) - **Hospital:** Capital Hlth Sys - Mercer Campus, Robert Wood Johnson Univ Hosp Hamilton; **Address:** Mercer Medical Center, 2997 Princeton Pike, Lawrenceville, NJ 08648; **Phone:** 609-771-0700; **Board Cert:** Internal Medicine 2002; Medical Oncology 2003; **Med School:** Jefferson Med Coll 1988; **Resid:** Internal Medicine, Cooper Univ Med Ctr 1991; **Fellow:** Medical Oncology, Fox Chase 1994

Sierocki, John MD (Onc) - **Spec Exp:** Breast Cancer; Lung Cancer; Lymphoma; Brain Tumors; **Hospital:** Univ Med Ctr - Princeton; **Address:** Princeton Med Grp, 419 N Harrison St, Ste 101, Princeton, NJ 08540-3521; **Phone:** 609-924-9300; **Board Cert:** Internal Medicine 1976; Medical Oncology 1979; **Med School:** Hahnemann Univ 1973; **Resid:** Internal Medicine, Hahnemann Univ Hosp 1976; **Fellow:** Medical Oncology, Meml Sloan-Kettering Cancer Ctr 1978

Yi, Peter I MD (Onc) - **Spec Exp:** Breast Cancer; Lymphoma; Prostate Cancer; Colon Cancer; **Hospital:** Univ Med Ctr - Princeton; **Address:** 419 N Harrison St, Princeton, NJ 08540; **Phone:** 609-924-9300; **Board Cert:** Internal Medicine 1987; Medical Oncology 1989; Hematology 1999; **Med School:** Cornell Univ-Weill Med Coll 1984; **Resid:** Internal Medicine, Brigham & Women's Hosp 1987; **Fellow:** Hematology & Oncology, NY Hosp-Cornell Med Ctr 1990; **Fac Appt:** Asst Clin Prof Med, Robert W Johnson Med Sch

Nephrology

Cohen, Barry H MD (Nep) - **Hospital:** Capital Hlth Sys - Mercer Campus; **Address:** 40 Fuld St, Ste 401, Trenton, NJ 08638-5247; **Phone:** 609-599-1004; **Board Cert:** Internal Medicine 1971; Nephrology 1974; **Med School:** Hahnemann Univ 1965; **Resid:** Internal Medicine, Hahnemann Univ Hosp 1968; **Fellow:** Nephrology, Hahnemann Univ 1969

Ruddy, Michael MD (Nep) - **Spec Exp:** Hypertension; Renovascular Disease; Diabetic Kidney Disease; Pheochromocytoma; **Hospital:** Univ Med Ctr - Princeton, Robert Wood Johnson Univ Hosp - New Brunswick; **Address:** 88 Princeton-Hightstown Rd, Ste 203, Princeton Junction, NJ 08550-1100; **Phone:** 609-750-7330; **Board Cert:** Internal Medicine 1977; Nephrology 1980; **Med School:** UMDNJ-NJ Med Sch, Newark 1974; **Resid:** Internal Medicine, Rutgers Affil Hosps 1977; **Fellow:** Nephrology, NY Hosp-Cornell Med Ctr 1980; **Fac Appt:** Assoc Clin Prof Med, Robert W Johnson Med Sch

Sudhakar, Telechery A MD (Nep) - **Spec Exp:** Kidney Disease; **Hospital:** Capital Hlth Sys - Mercer Campus, Capital Health Sys - Fuld Campus; **Address:** 40 Fuld St, Ste 401, Trenton, NJ 08638; **Phone:** 609-599-1004; **Board Cert:** Internal Medicine 1977; Nephrology 1978; **Med School:** India 1971; **Resid:** Internal Medicine, Helene Fuld Med Ctr 1976; **Fellow:** Nephrology, Washington VA Hosp 1978

Wei, Fong MD (Nep) - **Spec Exp:** Hypertension; Kidney Stones; **Hospital:** Univ Med Ctr - Princeton; **Address:** 419 N Harrison St, Princeton, NJ 08540; **Phone:** 609-924-9300; **Board Cert:** Internal Medicine 1976; Nephrology 1976; **Med School:** Tufts Univ 1967; **Resid:** Internal Medicine, Boston City Hosp 1969; Internal Medicine, Bronx Municipal Hosp 1970; **Fellow:** Nephrology, Univ NC Hosp 1972; **Fac Appt:** Assoc Clin Prof Med, Robert W Johnson Med Sch

Neurological Surgery

Chiurco, Anthony A MD (NS) - **Spec Exp:** Aneurysm-Cerebral; Brain Tumors; Spinal Disc Replacement; **Hospital:** Univ Med Ctr - Princeton, Capital Hlth Sys - Mercer Campus; **Address:** 3131 Princeton Pike Bldg 4 - Ste 201, Lawrenceville, NJ 08648; **Phone:** 609-895-8898; **Board Cert:** Neurological Surgery 1977; **Med School:** Jefferson Med Coll 1967; **Resid:** Surgery, Univ Iowa Coll Med 1971; Neurological Surgery, Univ Iowa Coll Med 1975; **Fellow:** Neurological Surgery, Penn Hosp 1976; **Fac Appt:** Asst Clin Prof NS, Robert W Johnson Med Sch

McLaughlin, Mark R MD (NS) - **Spec Exp:** Spinal Surgery-Complex; Spinal Surgery-Minimally Invasive; Trigeminal Neuralgia; **Hospital:** Univ Med Ctr - Princeton, St Mary Med Ctr -Langhorne, PA; **Address:** Princeton Brain & Spine Care, 713 Executive Drive, Princeton, NJ 08540; **Phone:** 609-921-9001; **Board Cert:** Neurological Surgery 2004; **Med School:** Med Coll VA 1992; **Resid:** Neurological Surgery, Univ Pittsburgh Med Ctr 1999; **Fellow:** Spinal Surgery, Emory Univ Affil Hosp 2000

Neurology

Kaiser, Paul K MD (N) - **Hospital:** Univ Med Ctr - Princeton, Capital Health Sys - Fuld Campus; **Address:** 3131 Princeton Pike 3C Bldg - Ste 202, Lawrenceville, NJ 08648-2526; **Phone:** 609-896-1701; **Board Cert:** Neurology 1993; Clinical Neurophysiology 1999; Vascular Neurology 2009; **Med School:** Jefferson Med Coll 1988; **Resid:** Neurology, Temple Univ Hosp 1992; **Fellow:** Clinical Neurophysiology, Temple Univ Hosp 1993

Kososky, Charles S MD (N) - **Hospital:** St Francis Med Ctr - Trenton; **Address:** St Francis Med Ctr, Neurosci Inst, 601 Hamilton Ave, Trenton, NJ 08629; **Phone:** 609-599-5792; **Board Cert:** Neurology 1981; **Med School:** UMDNJ-NJ Med Sch, Newark 1975; **Resid:** Internal Medicine, Kings Co Hosp 1975; Neurology, UMDNJ-Univ Hosp 1978

Vester, John W MD (N) - **Spec Exp:** Parkinson's Disease; Stroke; Peripheral Neuropathy; Epilepsy/Seizure Disorders; **Hospital:** Univ Med Ctr - Princeton; **Address:** 1000 Herrontown Rd, Princeton, NJ 08540; **Phone:** 609-497-0100; **Board Cert:** Neurology 1979; **Med School:** Georgetown Univ 1973; **Resid:** Internal Medicine, Hartford Hosp 1975; Neurology, Georgetown Univ Hosp 1978

Witte, Arnold S MD (N) - **Spec Exp:** Neuromuscular Disorders; Parkinson's Disease; Electromyography; **Hospital:** Capital Hlth Sys - Mercer Campus, Capital Health Sys - Fuld Campus; **Address:** 2 Princess Rd, Ste 2F, Lawrenceville, NJ 08648; **Phone:** 609-895-9000; **Board Cert:** Internal Medicine 1981; Neurology 1983; **Med School:** Tufts Univ 1977; **Resid:** Internal Medicine, Hosp Univ Penn 1979; Neurology, Hosp Univ Penn 1983

Obstetrics & Gynecology

Brickner, Gary R MD (ObG) *PCP* - **Spec Exp:** Menopause Problems; Gynecology Only; Minimally Invasive Surgery; Weight Management; **Hospital:** Capital Hlth Sys - Mercer Campus; **Address:** Quakerbridge Plaza 1A Bldg, Hamilton, NJ 08619-1241; **Phone:** 609-689-9991; **Board Cert:** Obstetrics & Gynecology 1981; **Med School:** Univ Pittsburgh 1975; **Resid:** Obstetrics & Gynecology, Pennsylvania Hosp 1979

Friedman, Alan L MD (ObG) - **Spec Exp:** Pregnancy-High Risk; Infertility; **Hospital:** Univ Med Ctr - Princeton; **Address:** 253 Witherspoon St, Ste R, Princeton, NJ 08540; **Phone:** 609-683-9292; **Board Cert:** Obstetrics & Gynecology 2007; **Med School:** Univ Chicago-Pritzker Sch Med 1982; **Resid:** Obstetrics & Gynecology, NYU Medical Ctr 1986

Ophthalmology

Matossian, Cynthia MD (Oph) - **Spec Exp:** Cataract Surgery; Glaucoma; **Hospital:** Capital Health Sys - Fuld Campus, Doylestown Hosp; **Address:** 1230 Parkway Ave, Ste 103, Ewing, NJ 08628; **Phone:** 609-882-8833; **Board Cert:** Ophthalmology 1987; **Med School:** Penn State Univ-Hershey Med Ctr 1981; **Resid:** Ophthalmology, Geo Wash Univ Med Ctr 1985

Safran, Steven G MD (Oph) - **Spec Exp:** Cataract Surgery; Laser Vision Surgery; Glaucoma; **Hospital:** Capital Hlth Sys - Mercer Campus, Robert Wood Johnson Univ Hosp Hamilton; **Address:** 132 Franklin Corner Rd, Ste A-1, Lawrenceville, NJ 08648-2523; **Phone:** 609-896-3931; **Board Cert:** Ophthalmology 2003; **Med School:** SUNY Downstate 1987; **Resid:** Ophthalmology, NYU Med Ctr 1991; **Fellow:** Cornea & Ext Eye Disease, Duke Univ Med Ctr 1992

Wasserman, Barry N MD (Oph) - **Spec Exp:** Pediatric Ophthalmology; LASIK-Refractive Surgery; Eyelid Surgery; Botox Therapy; **Hospital:** Robert Wood Johnson Univ Hosp Hamilton, Cooper Univ Hosp; **Address:** 100 Canal Pointe Blvd, Ste 112, Princeton, NJ 08540; **Phone:** 609-243-8711; **Board Cert:** Ophthalmology 2008; **Med School:** UMDNJ-NJ Med Sch, Newark 1992; **Resid:** Ophthalmology, UMDNJ-Univ Hosp 1996; **Fellow:** Pediatric Ophthalmology, Indiana Univ Med Ctr 1997; **Fac Appt:** Asst Clin Prof Oph, UMDNJ-RW Johnson Med Sch

Wong, Michael Y MD (Oph) - **Spec Exp:** LASIK-Refractive Surgery; Cataract Surgery-Lens Implant; Lens Implants-Multifocal; **Hospital:** Wills Eye Hosp, Univ Med Ctr - Princeton; **Address:** 419 N Harrison St, Ste 104, Princeton, NJ 08540-3521; **Phone:** 609-921-9437; **Board Cert:** Ophthalmology 1983; **Med School:** Albany Med Coll 1978; **Resid:** Ophthalmology, Wills Eye Hosp 1982

Wong, Richard H MD (Oph) - **Spec Exp:** Cataract Surgery-Lens Implant; LASIK-Refractive Surgery; **Hospital:** Univ Med Ctr - Princeton; **Address:** 419 N Harrison St, Ste 104, Princeton, NJ 08540-3521; **Phone:** 609-921-9437; **Board Cert:** Internal Medicine 1982; Ophthalmology 1987; **Med School:** UMDNJ-NJ Med Sch, Newark 1979; **Resid:** Internal Medicine, Thomas Jefferson Univ Hosp 1982; Ophthalmology, Wills Eye Hosp 1985

Orthopaedic Surgery

Abrams, Jeffrey S MD (OrS) - **Spec Exp:** Shoulder Surgery; Sports Medicine; Arthroscopic Surgery; Rotator Cuff Surgery; **Hospital:** Univ Med Ctr - Princeton; **Address:** 325 Princeton Ave, Princeton, NJ 08540-1617; **Phone:** 609-924-8131; **Board Cert:** Orthopaedic Surgery 2009; **Med School:** SUNY Upstate Med Univ 1980; **Resid:** Orthopaedic Surgery, Thomas Jefferson Univ Hosp 1985; **Fellow:** Shoulder Surgery, Univ Western Ontario 1986; Sports Medicine, Hughston Sports Med Hosp 1986; **Fac Appt:** Assoc Clin Prof OrS, Seton Hall Univ Sch Hlth & Med Scis

Costa, Leon N MD (OrS) - **Spec Exp:** Arthroscopic Surgery; Joint Replacement; Sports Medicine; **Hospital:** Univ Med Ctr - Princeton, Capital Hlth Sys - Mercer Campus; **Address:** 256 Bunn Dr, Ste 2, Princeton, NJ 08540-2859; **Phone:** 609-924-9229; **Board Cert:** Orthopaedic Surgery 2009; **Med School:** Geo Wash Univ 1980; **Resid:** Surgery, Hosp Univ Penn 1982; Orthopaedic Surgery, NY Ortho Hosp/Colum-Presby 1984; **Fellow:** Sports Medicine, NY Ortho Hosp/Colum-Presby 1985

Glick, Ronald MD (OrS) - **Hospital:** Capital Health Sys - Fuld Campus, Robert Wood Johnson Univ Hosp Hamilton; **Address:** 4065 Quakerbridge Rd, Princeton Junction, NJ 08550; **Phone:** 609-394-3804; **Board Cert:** Orthopaedic Surgery 1977; **Med School:** Univ MD Sch Med 1968; **Resid:** Orthopaedic Surgery, Albert Einstein

Gomez, William MD (OrS) - **Spec Exp:** Sports Medicine; Arthroscopic Surgery; Arthritis; **Hospital:** Robert Wood Johnson Univ Hosp Hamilton, St Francis Med Ctr - Trenton; **Address:** Trenton Orthopaedic Group, 1225 Whitehorse Mercerville Rd, D Bldg - Ste 220, Trenton, NJ 08619-3876; **Phone:** 609-581-2200; **Board Cert:** Orthopaedic Surgery 2010; **Med School:** Columbia P&S 1982; **Resid:** Surgery, St Vincent's Hosp 1984; Orthopaedic Surgery, Columbia-Presby Med Ctr 1987; **Fellow:** Sports Medicine, Univ Pittsburgh Hosp 1988

Grenis, Michael S MD (OrS) - **Spec Exp:** Carpal Tunnel Syndrome; Hand & Wrist Injuries; **Hospital:** Univ Med Ctr - Princeton, Capital Hlth Sys - Mercer Campus; **Address:** 256 Bunn Drive, Ste 2, Princeton, NJ 08540; **Phone:** 609-924-9229; **Board Cert:** Orthopaedic Surgery 2003; **Med School:** NY Med Coll 1984; **Resid:** Surgery, NYU-Bellevue Hosp 1985; Orthopaedic Surgery, NYU-Bellevue Hosp 1989; **Fellow:** Hand Surgery, NYU-Bellevue Hosp 1990

Gutowski III, W Thomas MD (OrS) - **Spec Exp:** Hip Replacement; Knee Replacement; Arthroscopic Surgery; Joint Replacement; **Hospital:** Univ Med Ctr - Princeton; **Address:** Princeton Orthopaedic Assocs, 325 Princeton Ave, Princeton, NJ 08540; **Phone:** 609-924-8131; **Board Cert:** Orthopaedic Surgery 2008; **Med School:** Cornell Univ-Weill Med Coll 1980; **Resid:** Orthopaedic Surgery, Yale-New Haven Hosp 1985

Taitsman, James P MD (OrS) - **Spec Exp:** Sports Medicine; **Hospital:** Capital Hlth Sys - Mercer Campus, Robert Wood Johnson Univ Hosp Hamilton; **Address:** 123 Franklin Corner Rd, Ste 114, Lawrenceville, NJ 08648-2526; **Phone:** 609-896-0707; **Board Cert:** Orthopaedic Surgery 1977; **Med School:** Univ Rochester 1971; **Resid:** Surgery, Yale-New Haven Hosp 1973; Orthopaedic Surgery, Yale-New Haven Hosp 1976

Otolaryngology

Brunner, Eugenie MD (Oto) - **Spec Exp:** Cosmetic Surgery-Face; Rhinoplasty; Skin Laser Surgery; Blepharoplasty; **Hospital:** Univ Med Ctr - Princeton; **Address:** 256 Bunn Drive, Ste 4, Princeton, NJ 08540-2859; **Phone:** 609-921-9497; **Board Cert:** Otolaryngology 1997; Facial Plastic & Reconstr Surgery 2002; **Med School:** UMDNJ-RW Johnson Med Sch 1990; **Resid:** Surgery, NYU Med Ctr 1992; Otolaryngology, NYU Med Ctr 1996; **Fellow:** Facial Plastic & Reconstr Surgery, Univ Toronto 1997

Haroldson, Olaf MD (Oto) - **Spec Exp:** Hearing Disorders; Voice Disorders; **Hospital:** Univ Med Ctr - Princeton; **Address:** Nassau Ear Nose & Throat, 812 Executive Drive, Princeton, NJ 08540-1530; **Phone:** 609-655-3000; **Board Cert:** Otolaryngology 1965; **Med School:** Univ Mich Med Sch 1959; **Resid:** Otolaryngology, Columbia-Presby Med Ctr 1963; Surgery, Columbia-Presby Med Ctr 1964

Li, Ronald MD (Oto) - **Spec Exp:** Cosmetic Surgery-Face; Sinus Disorders; Voice Disorders; **Hospital:** Univ Med Ctr - Princeton; **Address:** 812 Executive Drive, Princeton, NJ 08540; **Phone:** 609-655-3000; **Board Cert:** Otolaryngology 1990; **Med School:** Mount Sinai Sch Med 1984; **Resid:** Otolaryngology, Montefiore Med Ctr 1989

Moses, Brett MD (Oto) - **Hospital:** Robert Wood Johnson Univ Hosp Hamilton; **Address:** 8 Quakerbridge Plaza, Hamilton, NJ 08619-1255; **Phone:** 609-890-7800; **Board Cert:** Otolaryngology 1994; **Med School:** Jefferson Med Coll 1982; **Resid:** Otolaryngology, Johns Hopkins Univ Hosp 1992; **Fellow:** Otolaryngology, Johns Hopkins Univ Hosp 1993

Pain Medicine

Loren, Gary M MD (PM) - **Spec Exp:** Pain-Back; Reflex Sympathetic Dystrophy (RSD); **Hospital:** St Francis Med Ctr - Trenton; **Address:** 1666 Hamilton Ave, Ste 2, Hamilton Township, NJ 08629; **Phone:** 609-584-9080; **Board Cert:** Anesthesiology 1988; Pain Medicine 2002; **Med School:** Univ Pittsburgh 1984; **Resid:** Anesthesiology, LI Jewish Med Ctr 1987; **Fellow:** Pediatrics, LI Jewish Med Ctr 1988

Pediatric Endocrinology

Boim, Marilynn MD (PEn) - **Hospital:** Capital Hlth Sys - Mercer Campus, Robert Wood Johnson Univ Hosp Hamilton; **Address:** 1255 Whitehorse-Mercerville Rd, B Bldg - Ste 510, Mercerville, NJ 08619-3800; **Phone:** 609-581-4480; **Board Cert:** Pediatrics 2009; Pediatric Endocrinology 2004; **Med School:** Emory Univ 1982; **Resid:** Pediatrics, Mt Sinai Hosp 1986; **Fellow:** Pediatric Endocrinology, Mt Sinai Hosp 2000

Pediatrics

Baiser, Dennis MD (Ped) *PCP* - **Spec Exp:** Developmental Disorders; Asthma; **Hospital:** Capital Hlth Sys - Mercer Campus, Robert Wood Johnson Univ Hosp Hamilton; **Address:** 1255 Whitehorse Mercerville Rd, B Bldg - Ste 510, Mercerville, NJ 08619-3800; **Phone:** 609-581-4480; **Board Cert:** Pediatrics 1983; **Med School:** NY Med Coll 1978; **Resid:** Pediatrics, Chldn's Hosp 1981; **Fac Appt:** Ped, Univ Pennsylvania

Palsky, Glenn S MD (Ped) *PCP* - **Hospital:** Capital Hlth Sys - Mercer Campus, Univ Med Ctr - Princeton; **Address:** 132 Franklin Corner Rd, Lawrenceville, NJ 08648-2526; **Phone:** 609-896-4141; **Board Cert:** Pediatrics 1978; **Med School:** Penn State Univ-Hershey Med Ctr 1973; **Resid:** Pediatrics, Albany Med Ctr 1977

Raymond, Gerald M MD (Ped) *PCP* - **Hospital:** Univ Med Ctr - Princeton; **Address:** 196 Princeton Heights Town Rd, West Windsor, NJ 08550; **Phone:** 609-799-5335; **Board Cert:** Pediatrics 1987; **Med School:** Penn State Univ-Hershey Med Ctr 1983; **Resid:** Pediatrics, Columbus Chldns Hosp 1986

Physical Medicine & Rehabilitation

Agri, Robyn F MD (PMR) - **Spec Exp:** Acupuncture; Pain Management; **Hospital:** St Lawrence Rehab Ctr, Capital Hlth Sys - Mercer Campus; **Address:** St Lawrence Rehabilitation Ctr, 2381 Lawrenceville Rd, Lawrenceville, NJ 08648-2024; **Phone:** 609-896-9500; **Board Cert:** Physical Medicine & Rehabilitation 1990; **Med School:** SUNY Upstate Med Univ 1985; **Resid:** Physical Medicine & Rehabilitation, Hosp Univ Penn 1989

Gribbin, Dorota M MD (PMR) - **Spec Exp:** Industrial Injuries; Sports Injuries; Pain Management; **Hospital:** Robert Wood Johnson Univ Hosp Hamilton, Univ Med Ctr - Princeton; **Address:** 2333 Whitehorse-Mercerville Rd, Ste 8, Mercerville, NJ 06819; **Phone:** 609-588-0540; **Board Cert:** Physical Medicine & Rehabilitation 2003; **Med School:** Poland 1984; **Resid:** Internal Medicine, Beth Israel Med Ctr 1989; Physical Medicine & Rehabilitation, New York Hosp-Cornell Med Ctr 1992; **Fellow:** Pain Medicine, Univ P&M Hosp 1985; **Fac Appt:** Asst Clin Prof PMR, Columbia P&S

Plastic Surgery

Drimmer, Marc A MD (PlS) - **Spec Exp:** Cosmetic Surgery; **Hospital:** Univ Med Ctr - Princeton; **Address:** 842 State Rd, Princeton, NJ 08540; **Phone:** 609-924-1026; **Board Cert:** Plastic Surgery 1981; **Med School:** Belgium 1974; **Resid:** Surgery, Beth Israel Med Ctr 1977; Plastic Surgery, Univ Hosp 1979

Leach, Thomas A MD (PlS) - **Spec Exp:** Cosmetic Surgery-Face; Cosmetic Surgery-Breast; Liposuction; **Hospital:** Univ Med Ctr - Princeton, Robert Wood Johnson Univ Hosp - New Brunswick; **Address:** 932 State Rd, Princeton, NJ 08540; **Phone:** 609-921-7161; **Board Cert:** Plastic Surgery 1994; **Med School:** UMDNJ-NJ Med Sch, Newark 1985; **Resid:** Surgery, UMDNJ Med Ctr 1990; **Fellow:** Plastic Surgery, UMDNJ Med Ctr 1992

Smotrich, Gary MD (PlS) - **Hospital:** Capital Hlth Sys - Mercer Campus, Robert Wood Johnson Univ Hosp Hamilton; **Address:** Lawrenceville Plastic Surgery, 3131 Princeton Pike Bldg 5 - Ste 205, Lawrenceville, NJ 08648-2300; **Phone:** 609-896-2525; **Board Cert:** Plastic Surgery 1991; **Med School:** Univ Conn 1982; **Resid:** Surgery, Boston Univ Med Ctr 1987; Plastic Surgery, U Louisville 1989

Psychiatry

Khouri, Philippe J MD (Psyc) - **Spec Exp:** Neuro-Psychiatry; Bipolar/Mood Disorders; Geriatric Psychiatry; **Hospital:** Univ Med Ctr - Princeton, Capital Health Sys - Fuld Campus; **Address:** 750 Brunswick Ave, Trenton, NJ 08638; **Phone:** 609-737-7797; **Board Cert:** Psychiatry 1977; Geriatric Psychiatry 2005; **Med School:** Lebanon 1972; **Resid:** Psychiatry, Strong Meml Hosp 1973; Psychiatry, Univ Tenn Med Ctr 1975; **Fellow:** Genetics and Metabolism, Nat Inst Mntl Hlth 1977; **Fac Appt:** Prof Psyc, Robert W Johnson Med Sch

Leifer, Marvin W MD (Psyc) - **Spec Exp:** Psychopharmacology; Anxiety & Mood Disorders; Depression; Bipolar/Mood Disorders; **Hospital:** Univ Med Ctr - Princeton; **Address:** 42 North Tulane St, Princeton, NJ 08542; **Phone:** 609-683-7929; **Board Cert:** Psychiatry 1977; **Med School:** SUNY Downstate 1970; **Resid:** Psychiatry, Albert Einstein 1974; **Fellow:** Psychopharmacology, Albert Einstein 1976

Schneider, Samuel MD (Psyc) - **Spec Exp:** Mood Disorders; Personality Disorders; Addiction/Substance Abuse; **Hospital:** Univ Med Ctr - Princeton; **Address:** 33 State Rd, Ste J, Princeton, NJ 08540-1304; **Phone:** 609-924-3980; **Board Cert:** Psychiatry 1984; Internal Medicine 1978; **Med School:** Penn State Univ-Hershey Med Ctr 1975; **Resid:** Internal Medicine, MS Hershey Med Ctr 1977; Psychiatry, Coll Med NJ 1983

Pulmonary Disease

Goldblatt, Kenneth H MD (Pul) - **Spec Exp:** Asthma; Emphysema; Sarcoidosis; **Hospital:** Univ Med Ctr - Princeton; **Address:** Princeton Healthcare Med Assoc, 253 Witherspoon St, Princeton, NJ 08540-3211; **Phone:** 609-497-4301; **Board Cert:** Internal Medicine 1975; Pulmonary Disease 1978; **Med School:** NY Med Coll 1972; **Resid:** Internal Medicine, CMDNJ-Rutgers 1975; **Fellow:** Pulmonary Disease, CMDNJ-Rutgers 1977; **Fac Appt:** Assoc Prof Med, UMDNJ-RW Johnson Med Sch

Harman, John MD (Pul) - **Hospital:** Capital Hlth Sys - Mercer Campus; **Address:** 2480 Pennington Rd, Ste 104, Pennington, NJ 08534; **Phone:** 609-737-7544; **Board Cert:** Internal Medicine 1972; **Med School:** Univ Pennsylvania 1969; **Resid:** Internal Medicine, Presby Hosp 1972; **Fellow:** Pulmonary Disease, Penn Hosp 1975

Seelagy, Marc M MD (Pul) - **Spec Exp:** Sleep Disorders; Lung Disease; Critical Care Medicine; **Hospital:** St Francis Med Ctr - Trenton, Robert Wood Johnson Univ Hosp Hamilton; **Address:** Allergy & Pulmonary Associates, 1542 Kuser Rd, Ste B7, Trenton, NJ 08619-3829; **Phone:** 609-581-1400; **Board Cert:** Internal Medicine 1989; Pulmonary Disease 2002; Critical Care Medicine 2003; Sleep Medicine 1995; **Med School:** Univ Chicago-Pritzker Sch Med 1986; **Resid:** Internal Medicine, Univ Colorado Hosp 1989; **Fellow:** Pulmonary Disease, Johns Hopkins Hosp 1993; Critical Care Medicine, Johns Hopkins Hosp 1993

Radiation Oncology

Baumann, John MD (RadRO) - **Spec Exp:** Breast Cancer; Cervical Cancer; Prostate Cancer; **Hospital:** Univ Med Ctr - Princeton, Hunterdon Med Ctr; **Address:** University Med Ctr - Radiation Oncology, 253 Witherspoon St, Princeton, NJ 08540; **Phone:** 609-497-4304; **Board Cert:** Radiation Oncology 1981; **Med School:** Harvard Med Sch 1977; **Resid:** Internal Medicine, Walter Reed AMC 1978; Radiation Oncology, Harvard Joint Program 1981; **Fellow:** Radiation Oncology, Harvard Joint Program

McKenna, Michael G MD (RadRO) - **Spec Exp:** Prostate Cancer; Breast Cancer; Head & Neck Cancer; **Hospital:** Robert Wood Johnson Univ Hosp Hamilton; **Address:** Cancer Inst NJ-Radiation Oncology, 2575 Klockner Rd, Hamilton, NJ 08690; **Phone:** 609-584-2800; **Board Cert:** Radiation Oncology 1993; **Med School:** Univ Mass Sch Med 1988; **Resid:** Radiation Oncology, Hosp Univ Penn 1992

Soffen, Edward MD (RadRO) - **Spec Exp:** Prostate Cancer; Breast Cancer; Brachytherapy; **Hospital:** Univ Med Ctr - Princeton, CentraState Med Ctr; **Address:** Med Ctr at Princeton, Dept Rad Onc, 253 Witherspoon St, Princeton, NJ 08540-3298; **Phone:** 609-497-4304; **Board Cert:** Radiation Oncology 1991; **Med School:** Temple Univ 1986; **Resid:** Radiation Oncology, Hosp Univ Penn 1990; **Fac Appt:** Asst Clin Prof RadRO, UMDNJ-RW Johnson Med Sch

Reproductive Endocrinology

O'Shaughnessy, Althea MD (RE) - **Spec Exp:** Infertility; **Hospital:** Capital Hlth Sys - Mercer Campus, Univ Med Ctr - Princeton; **Address:** Princeton Center for Infertility, 3131 Princeton Pike Bldg 6 - Ste 100, Lawrenceville, NJ 08648; **Phone:** 609-895-1114; **Board Cert:** Obstetrics & Gynecology 2009; Reproductive Endocrinology/Infertility 2009; **Med School:** Univ Rochester 1982; **Resid:** Obstetrics & Gynecology, Univ Conn Hlth Ctr 1986; **Fellow:** Reproductive Endocrinology, Downstate Med Ctr 1988

Rheumatology

Carney, Alexander MD (Rhu) - **Hospital:** Univ Med Ctr - Princeton; **Address:** 8 Quakerbridge Plaza, Ste H, Mercerville, NJ 08619; **Phone:** 609-588-9044; **Board Cert:** Internal Medicine 1972; **Med School:** Cornell Univ-Weill Med Coll 1966; **Resid:** Internal Medicine, Univ Iowa Hosp 1972; **Fellow:** Rheumatology, Univ Iowa Hosp 1974

Gordon, Richard D MD (Rhu) - **Spec Exp:** Rheumatoid Arthritis; Osteoporosis; Osteoarthritis; **Hospital:** Robert Wood Johnson Univ Hosp Hamilton; **Address:** Professional Ctr at Hamilton, 2121 Klockner Rd, Hamilton, NJ 08690; **Phone:** 609-587-9898; **Board Cert:** Internal Medicine 1978; Rheumatology 1980; **Med School:** Jefferson Med Coll 1975; **Resid:** Internal Medicine, Geo Wash Hosp/VA Hosp 1978; **Fellow:** Rheumatology, Georgetown Univ 1979; Rheumatology, St Vincents Hosp 1980

Surgery

Davidson, J Thomas MD (S) - **Spec Exp:** Vascular Surgery; **Hospital:** Univ Med Ctr - Princeton; **Address:** Princeton Surgical Assocs, 281 Witherspoon St, Ste 120, Princeton, NJ 08540-3210; **Phone:** 609-921-7223; **Board Cert:** Surgery 1974; **Med School:** Cornell Univ-Weill Med Coll 1966; **Resid:** Surgery, NYU Hosp-Bellevue Hosp 1973; **Fellow:** Vascular Surgery, NYU Hosp-Bellevue Hosp 1974; **Fac Appt:** Assoc Clin Prof S, UMDNJ-RW Johnson Med Sch

Dultz, Rachel P MD (S) - **Spec Exp:** Breast Surgery; Breast Cancer; **Hospital:** Univ Med Ctr - Princeton; **Address:** Princeton Breast Health Ctr, 300-B Princeton Heightstown Rd, East Windsor, NJ 08520; **Phone:** 609-688-2700; **Board Cert:** Surgery 2006; **Med School:** SUNY Downstate 1991; **Resid:** Surgery, RW Johnson Univ Hosp 1997; **Fellow:** Breast Surgery, Baylor Univ Med Ctr 1998

Jordan, Lawrence J MD (S) - **Spec Exp:** Laparoscopic Surgery; Biliary Surgery; Cancer Surgery; **Hospital:** Univ Med Ctr - Princeton; **Address:** Princeton Surgical Assocs, 281 Witherspoon St, Ste 120, Princeton, NJ 08540; **Phone:** 609-921-7223; **Board Cert:** Surgery 2010; **Med School:** Cornell Univ-Weill Med Coll 1983; **Resid:** Surgery, Columbia-Presby Med Ctr 1988

Schell, Harold S MD (S) - **Spec Exp:** Breast Cancer; Thyroid & Parathyroid Surgery; Gastrointestinal Surgery; **Hospital:** Capital Hlth Sys - Mercer Campus, Capital Health Sys - Fuld Campus; **Address:** 416 Bellevue Ave, Ste 406, Trenton, NJ 08618-4513; **Phone:** 609-392-8100; **Board Cert:** Surgery 2002; **Med School:** Boston Univ 1970; **Resid:** Surgery, St Vincent's Hosp 1975

Thoracic Surgery

Heim, John A MD (TS) - **Spec Exp:** Cardiothoracic Surgery; **Hospital:** Univ Med Ctr - Princeton; **Address:** Univ Med Ctr at Princeton, Dept Surgery, 243 Witherspoon St, Princeton, NJ 08540; **Phone:** 609-430-7200; **Board Cert:** Surgery 2002; Thoracic Surgery 2002; **Med School:** UMDNJ-RW Johnson Med Sch 1985; **Resid:** Surgery, Hartford Hosp 1991; **Fellow:** Thoracic Oncology, Meml Sloan Kettering Cancer Ctr 1992; Cardiothoracic Surgery, Rush Presby-St Lukes Med Ctr 1994; **Fac Appt:** Prof S, Robert W Johnson Med Sch

Laub, Glenn W MD (TS) - **Spec Exp:** Cardiac Surgery; Minimally Invasive Surgery; **Hospital:** St Francis Med Ctr - Trenton, Robert Wood Johnson Univ Hosp Hamilton; **Address:** 601 Hamilton Ave, rm 109, Trenton, NJ 08629-1915; **Phone:** 609-599-5307; **Board Cert:** Thoracic Surgery 1997; **Med School:** Dartmouth Med Sch 1981; **Resid:** Surgery, NYU-Bellevue Med Ctr 1986; Cardiothoracic Surgery, Allegheny Genl Hosp 1988; **Fac Appt:** Assoc Prof S, UMDNJ-RW Johnson Med Sch

Seinfeld, Fredric I MD (TS) - **Spec Exp:** Carotid Artery Surgery; Aneurysm; Esophageal Surgery; Cardiovascular Surgery; **Hospital:** St Francis Med Ctr - Trenton, Univ Med Ctr - Princeton; **Address:** 601 Hamilton Ave, Trenton, NJ 08629; **Phone:** 609-599-5308; **Board Cert:** Thoracic Surgery 2005; **Med School:** SUNY Buffalo 1976; **Resid:** Surgery, NYU Med Ctr 1981; Thoracic Surgery, Yale-New Haven Hosp 1984

Urology

Rossman, Barry R MD (U) - **Spec Exp:** Kidney Stones; Incontinence-Female; Prostate Cancer; Erectile Dysfunction; **Hospital:** Univ Med Ctr - Princeton, Robert Wood Johnson Univ Hosp - New Brunswick; **Address:** 281 Witherspoon St, Ste 100, Princeton, NJ 08542-3210; **Phone:** 609-924-6487; **Board Cert:** Urology 2009; **Med School:** Boston Univ 1983; **Resid:** Surgery, Montefiore Med Ctr 1985; Urology, Montefiore Med Ctr 1989; **Fac Appt:** Assoc Clin Prof U, UMDNJ-RW Johnson Med Sch

Vasselli, Anthony J MD (U) - **Hospital:** Univ Med Ctr - Princeton; **Address:** 299 Witherspoon St, Princeton, NJ 08540-3506; **Phone:** 609-252-0575; **Board Cert:** Urology 2006; **Med School:** NY Med Coll 1979; **Resid:** Urology, Albany Meml Hosp 1984

Vukasin, Alexander P MD (U) - **Spec Exp:** Laparoscopic Surgery; Urologic Cancer; Urology-Female; **Hospital:** Univ Med Ctr - Princeton, Robert Wood Johnson Univ Hosp - New Brunswick; **Address:** 281 Witherspoon St, Ste 100, Princeton, NJ 08540; **Phone:** 609-924-6487; **Board Cert:** Urology 2006; **Med School:** Yale Univ 1989; **Resid:** Urology, New York Hosp 1995; **Fac Appt:** Asst Clin Prof U, UMDNJ-RW Johnson Med Sch

Vascular & Interventional Radiology

Denny, Donald F MD (VIR) - **Spec Exp:** Dialysis Access; Uterine Fibroids; **Hospital:** Univ Med Ctr - Princeton; **Address:** Princeton Radiology Assocs, 3674 Route 27, Kendall Park, NJ 08824; **Phone:** 609-497-4310; **Board Cert:** Diagnostic Radiology 1982; Vascular & Interventional Radiology 2005; **Med School:** Hahnemann Univ 1978; **Resid:** Diagnostic Radiology, Yale-New Haven Hosp 1982; **Fellow:** Diagnostic Radiology, Brigham & Womens Hosp 1983; **Fac Appt:** Assoc Clin Prof Rad, Yale Univ

Vascular Surgery

Goldman, Kenneth A MD (VascS) - **Spec Exp:** Carotid Artery Surgery; Aneurysm-Aortic; Varicose Veins; Endovascular Surgery; **Hospital:** Univ Med Ctr - Princeton; **Address:** Princeton Surgical Assocs, 281 Witherspoon St, Ste 120, Princeton, NJ 08540-3210; **Phone:** 609-921-7223; **Board Cert:** Surgery 2003; Vascular Surgery 2004; **Med School:** NYU Sch Med 1988; **Resid:** Surgery, Bellevue Hosp 1993; **Fellow:** Vascular Surgery, NYU Med Ctr 1994

Middlesex

Adolescent Medicine

Snyder, Barbara K MD (AM) - **Spec Exp:** Eating Disorders; Pediatric Gynecology; **Hospital:** Robert Wood Johnson Univ Hosp - New Brunswick; **Address:** Childrens Health Inst New Jersey, 89 French St, Ste 2230, New Brunswick, NJ 08901; **Phone:** 732-235-6230; **Board Cert:** Pediatrics 1985; Adolescent Medicine 2002; **Med School:** Geo Wash Univ 1979; **Resid:** Pediatrics, Chldns National Med Ctr 1981; Pediatrics, Upstate Med Ctr 1982; **Fellow:** Adolescent Medicine, Univ Rochester 1988; **Fac Appt:** Assoc Prof Ped, Robert W Johnson Med Sch

Allergy & Immunology

Blum, Jay R MD (A&I) - **Spec Exp:** Rhinitis; Asthma; Hives; Urticaria; **Hospital:** St Peter's Univ Hosp, Robert Wood Johnson Univ Hosp - New Brunswick; **Address:** 85 Raritan Ave, Highland Park, NJ 08904-2439; **Phone:** 732-846-7861; **Board Cert:** Internal Medicine 1978; Allergy & Immunology 1979; **Med School:** Univ Pennsylvania 1974; **Resid:** Internal Medicine, Beth Israel Hosp 1977; **Fellow:** Allergy & Immunology, New York Hosp 1979

Kesarwala, Hemant MD (A&I) - **Spec Exp:** Food Allergy; Asthma; **Hospital:** St Peter's Univ Hosp, Robert Wood Johnson Univ Hosp - New Brunswick; **Address:** 3084 State Route 27, Ste 6, Kendall Park, NJ 08824-1657; **Phone:** 732-821-0595; **Board Cert:** Pediatrics 1979; Allergy & Immunology 1979; Pediatric Infectious Disease 2002; **Med School:** India 1971; **Resid:** Pediatrics, Lincoln Hosp 1976; **Fellow:** Infectious Disease, UMDNJ-Rutgers Med Sch 1978; Allergy & Immunology, Children's Hosp 1979; **Fac Appt:** Clin Prof Ped, Drexel Univ Coll Med

Leibner, Donald MD (A&I) - **Spec Exp:** Asthma & Allergy; Cough-Chronic; Insect Allergies; Nasal & Sinus Disorders; **Hospital:** Robert Wood Johnson Univ Hosp - New Brunswick, St Peter's Univ Hosp; **Address:** 579-A Cranbury Rd, Ste 103, East Brunswick, NJ 08816-5426; **Phone:** 732-390-4900; **Board Cert:** Pediatrics 2003; Allergy & Immunology 2005; **Med School:** SUNY Downstate 1981; **Resid:** Pediatrics, UMDNJ-Rutgers 1984; Pediatrics, Beth Israel Med Ctr 1982; **Fellow:** Allergy & Immunology, Long Island Coll Hosp 1986; **Fac Appt:** Asst Clin Prof Ped, Drexel Univ Coll Med

Cardiac Electrophysiology

Preminger, Mark W MD (CE) - **Spec Exp:** Arrhythmias; **Hospital:** St Luke's - Roosevelt Hosp Ctr - Roosevelt Div (page 94); **Address:** St Luke's Roosevelt Hosp Ctr, Ste 5200, 1111 Amsterdam Ave, New York, NY 10025; **Phone:** 212-523-4007; **Board Cert:** Internal Medicine 1989; Cardiovascular Disease 2001; Cardiac Electrophysiology 2002; **Med School:** Hahnemann Univ 1985; **Resid:** Internal Medicine, N Shore Univ Hosp/Cornell 1988; **Fellow:** Cardiovascular Disease, NY Hosp-Cornell Med Ctr 1991; Cardiac Electrophysiology, Philadelphia Heart Inst 1992; **Fac Appt:** Assoc Prof Med, Robert W Johnson Med Sch

Cardiovascular Disease

Kostis, John B MD (Cv) - **Spec Exp:** Hypertension; Coronary Artery Disease; Cholesterol/Lipid Disorders; **Hospital:** Robert Wood Johnson Univ Hosp - New Brunswick; **Address:** UMDNJ-Robert Wood Johnson Med School, 1 Robert Wood Johnson Pl, Box 19, New Brunswick, NJ 08903-0019; **Phone:** 732-235-7685; **Board Cert:** Internal Medicine 1973; Cardiovascular Disease 1973; **Med School:** Greece 1960; **Resid:** Internal Medicine, Evanglismos Hosp 1964; Internal Medicine, Cumberland Med Ctr 1967; **Fellow:** Cardiovascular Disease, Philadelphia Genl Hosp 1969; **Fac Appt:** Prof Med, UMDNJ-RW Johnson Med Sch

Lauer, Robert C MD (Cv) - **Spec Exp:** Nuclear Cardiology; Coronary Artery Disease; **Hospital:** JFK Med Ctr - Edison, Overlook Hosp (page 92); **Address:** Central Jersey Cardiology, 1511 Park Ave, Ste 2, South Plainfield, NJ 07080-5516; **Phone:** 908-756-4438; **Board Cert:** Internal Medicine 1981; Cardiovascular Disease 1985; **Med School:** Columbia P&S 1978; **Resid:** Internal Medicine, Columbia Presby Med Ctr 1981; **Fellow:** Cardiovascular Disease, Columbia Presby Med Ctr 1983; **Fac Appt:** Asst Clin Prof Med, UMDNJ-RW Johnson Med Sch

Mermelstein, Erwin MD (Cv) - **Spec Exp:** Cholesterol/Lipid Disorders; Cardiac Catheterization; Coronary Angioplasty/Stents; Congestive Heart Failure; **Hospital:** Robert Wood Johnson Univ Hosp - New Brunswick, St Peter's Univ Hosp; **Address:** 593 Cranbury Rd, East Brunswick, NJ 08816; **Phone:** 732-390-3333; **Board Cert:** Cardiovascular Disease 1983; Interventional Cardiology 1999; Internal Medicine 1981; **Med School:** Cornell Univ-Weill Med Coll 1978; **Resid:** Internal Medicine, NY Presby Hosp/Cornell 1981; **Fellow:** Cardiovascular Disease, Hosp Univ Penn 1983

Mondrow, Daniel N MD (Cv) - **Spec Exp:** Cardiac Catheterization; Nuclear Stress Testing; Critical Care Medicine; **Hospital:** JFK Med Ctr - Edison, Robert Wood Johnson Univ Hosp - New Brunswick; **Address:** 280 Main St, Metuchen, NJ 08840-2429; **Phone:** 732-494-3177; **Board Cert:** Internal Medicine 1979; Cardiovascular Disease 1985; **Med School:** SUNY Downstate 1976; **Resid:** Internal Medicine, Brookdale Hosp 1979; **Fellow:** Cardiovascular Disease, St Vincents Hosp 1981

Shell, Roger A MD (Cv) - **Spec Exp:** Coronary Artery Disease; Heart Valve Disease; Cholesterol/Lipid Disorders; **Hospital:** Robert Wood Johnson Univ Hosp - New Brunswick, St Peter's Univ Hosp; **Address:** 593 Cranberry Rd, East Brunswick, NJ 08816; **Phone:** 732-390-3333; **Board Cert:** Internal Medicine 1980; Cardiovascular Disease 1983; **Med School:** UMDNJ-Rutgers Med Sch 1977; **Resid:** Internal Medicine, Rutgers Med Sch 1980; **Fellow:** Cardiovascular Disease, Presby Hosp-Univ Penn 1982; **Fac Appt:** Asst Clin Prof Med, Robert W Johnson Med Sch

Shindler, Daniel M MD (Cv) - **Spec Exp:** Echocardiography; **Hospital:** Robert Wood Johnson Univ Hosp - New Brunswick; **Address:** Univ Med Group, 125 Paterson St, Ste 5200, New Brunswick, NJ 08901; **Phone:** 732-235-7854; **Board Cert:** Internal Medicine 1987; Cardiovascular Disease 2002; **Med School:** Spain 1979; **Resid:** Internal Medicine, US Public 1981; Internal Medicine, RW Johnson Hosp 1984; **Fellow:** Cardiovascular Disease, RW Johnson Hosp 1983; **Fac Appt:** Prof Med, UMDNJ-RW Johnson Med Sch

Child & Adolescent Psychiatry

Shampain, Lawrence R MD (ChAP) - **Spec Exp:** Trauma Psychiatry; Anxiety Disorders; **Hospital:** Somerset Med Ctr, UMDNJ-Univ Behavioral HealthCare; **Address:** 32B Wernik Place, Metuchen, NJ 08840; **Phone:** 732-548-1600; **Board Cert:** Psychiatry 1988; Child & Adolescent Psychiatry 1990; **Med School:** Hahnemann Univ 1982; **Resid:** Psychiatry, Mt Sinai Med Ctr 1985; **Fellow:** Child Psychiatry, UCLA Neuropsych Inst 1987

Child Neurology

Wollack, Jan B MD (ChiN) - **Spec Exp:** Epilepsy/Seizure Disorders; **Hospital:** Robert Wood Johnson Univ Hosp - New Brunswick; **Address:** 89 French St Fl 2nd, New Brunswick, NJ 08901; **Phone:** 732-235-6230; **Board Cert:** Pediatrics 1988; Child Neurology 1987; Neurodevelopmental Disabilities 2001; **Med School:** Columbia P&S 1981; **Resid:** Pediatrics, Columbia-Presby Med Ctr 1983; Neurology, Columbia-Presby Med Ctr 1986; **Fac Appt:** Assoc Prof Ped, UMDNJ-RW Johnson Med Sch

Clinical Genetics

Sklower Brooks, Susan MD (CG) - **Spec Exp:** Birth Defects; Inborn Errors of Metabolism; Developmental Disorders; Prenatal Diagnosis; **Hospital:** Robert Wood Johnson Univ Hosp - New Brunswick; **Address:** Child Hlth Inst of NJ, 89 French St, New Brunswick, NJ 08903-2160; **Phone:** 732-235-6230; **Board Cert:** Pediatrics 1979; Clinical Genetics 1982; Clinical Biochemical Genetics 1984; **Med School:** Mount Sinai Sch Med 1975; **Resid:** Pediatrics, Mount Sinai Hosp 1977; **Fellow:** Clinical Genetics, Mount Sinai Hosp 1979; **Fac Appt:** Prof Ped, UMDNJ-RW Johnson Med Sch

Colon & Rectal Surgery

Chinn, Bertram T MD (CRS) - **Spec Exp:** Laparoscopic Surgery; Colon & Rectal Cancer; Inflammatory Bowel Disease; Diverticulitis; **Hospital:** Overlook Hosp (page 92), Robert Wood Johnson Univ Hosp - New Brunswick; **Address:** 3900 Park Ave, Ste 101, Edison, NJ 08820; **Phone:** 732-494-6640; **Board Cert:** Surgery 2002; Colon & Rectal Surgery 2005; **Med School:** Jefferson Med Coll 1987; **Resid:** Surgery, Thomas Jefferson Univ Hosp 1992; **Fellow:** Colon & Rectal Surgery, UMDNJ-RW Johnson Med Ctr 1993; **Fac Appt:** Asst Clin Prof S, UMDNJ-RW Johnson Med Sch

Eisenstat, Theodore E MD (CRS) - **Spec Exp:** Colon Cancer; Inflammatory Bowel Disease; Anorectal Disorders; Hemorrhoids; **Hospital:** Robert Wood Johnson Univ Hosp - New Brunswick, JFK Med Ctr - Edison; **Address:** 3900 Park Ave, Ste 101, Edison, NJ 08820-3032; **Phone:** 732-494-6640; **Board Cert:** Surgery 1974; Colon & Rectal Surgery 1994; **Med School:** NY Med Coll 1968; **Resid:** Surgery, Thomas Jefferson Univ Hosp 1971; Surgery, Pennsylvania Hosp 1973; **Fellow:** Colon & Rectal Surgery, Muhlenberg Med Ctr 1978; **Fac Appt:** Clin Prof S, UMDNJ-RW Johnson Med Sch

Oliver, Gregory C MD (CRS) - **Spec Exp:** Colon & Rectal Cancer; Incontinence-Fecal; Ulcerative Colitis; Crohn's Disease; **Hospital:** JFK Med Ctr - Edison, Overlook Hosp (page 92); **Address:** 3900 Park Ave, Ste 101, Edison, NJ 08820; **Phone:** 732-494-6640; **Board Cert:** Colon & Rectal Surgery 1986; **Med School:** Geo Wash Univ 1976; **Resid:** Surgery, Geo Wash Univ Med Ctr 1983; Surgery, UMDNJ-Rutgers 1985; **Fac Appt:** Assoc Clin Prof S, UMDNJ-RW Johnson Med Sch

Rezac, Craig MD (CRS) - **Spec Exp:** Colon & Rectal Cancer; Inflammatory Bowel Disease; Diverticulitis; Pelvic & Perineal Surgery; **Hospital:** Robert Wood Johnson Univ Hosp - New Brunswick; **Address:** 125 Patterson St, New Brunswick, NJ 08901; **Phone:** 732-235-7920; **Board Cert:** Surgery 2002; Colon & Rectal Surgery 2003; **Med School:** Italy 1995; **Resid:** Surgery, RW Johnson Medical Ctr 2001; **Fellow:** Colon & Rectal Surgery, RW Johnson Med Ctr 2002; Laparoscopic Surgery, Hackensack Med Ctr 2003; **Fac Appt:** Asst Prof S, UMDNJ-RW Johnson Med Sch

Zinkin, Lewis D MD (CRS) - **Spec Exp:** Colon Cancer; Inflammatory Bowel Disease; **Hospital:** Robert Wood Johnson Univ Hosp - New Brunswick, St Peter's Univ Hosp; **Address:** 620 Cranbury Rd, Ste 111, East Brunswick, NJ 08816; **Phone:** 732-238-2662; **Board Cert:** Colon & Rectal Surgery 1978; **Med School:** UMDNJ-NJ Med Sch, Newark 1970; **Resid:** Surgery, St Vincents Hosp 1977; Colon & Rectal Surgery, Greater Baltimore Med Ctr 1978; **Fac Appt:** Assoc Clin Prof S, Robert W Johnson Med Sch

Dermatology

Milgraum, Sandy S MD (D) - **Spec Exp:** Skin Laser Surgery; Tattoo Removal; Cosmetic Dermatology; Pediatric Dermatology; **Hospital:** Robert Wood Johnson Univ Hosp - New Brunswick; **Address:** Academic Dermatology Ctr, 81 Brunswick Woods Drive, East Brunswick, NJ 08816-5601; **Phone:** 732-613-0300; **Board Cert:** Dermatology 1986; Pediatric Dermatology 2006; **Med School:** Australia 1983; **Resid:** Dermatology, Univ Mich Hosp 1986; **Fac Appt:** Assoc Prof D, Robert W Johnson Med Sch

Wrone, David A MD (D) - **Spec Exp:** Skin Laser Surgery; Cosmetic Surgery; Mohs' Surgery; Skin Cancer; **Hospital:** Univ Med Ctr - Princeton, Robert Wood Johnson Univ Hosp - New Brunswick; **Address:** 1956 Highway 27, Ste A, North Brunswick, NJ 08902; **Phone:** 609-683-4999; **Board Cert:** Dermatology 2001; **Med School:** Stanford Univ 1996; **Resid:** Dermatology, Univ Wisconsin Med Ctr 1998; Dermatology, Mass Genl Hosp 2001; **Fellow:** Mohs Surgery, UCLA Med Ctr 2002

Diagnostic Radiology

Compito, Gerard A MD (DR) - **Hospital:** Univ Med Ctr - Princeton; **Address:** 3674 Rt 27, Kendall Park, Kendall Park, NJ 08824; **Phone:** 609-921-3345; **Board Cert:** Diagnostic Radiology 1990; Neuroradiology 2005; **Med School:** SUNY Upstate Med Univ 1985; **Resid:** Diagnostic Radiology, NY Hosp-Cornell 1990; **Fellow:** Neuroradiology, NY Hosp-Cornell 1992

Epstein, Robert MD (DR) - **Spec Exp:** MRI; Musculoskeletal Imaging; **Hospital:** Robert Wood Johnson Univ Hosp - New Brunswick, St Peter's Univ Hosp; **Address:** Univ Radiology Grp, 579A Cranbury Rd Fl 3rd, East Brunswick, NJ 08816; **Phone:** 732-390-0040 x2021; **Board Cert:** Diagnostic Radiology 1995; **Med School:** Duke Univ 1990; **Resid:** Diagnostic Radiology, Thomas Jefferson Univ Hosp 1995; **Fellow:** Musculoskeletal Imaging, Hosp Univ Penn 1996; **Fac Appt:** Asst Clin Prof Rad, UMDNJ-RW Johnson Med Sch

Greer, Jeannete G MD (DR) - **Spec Exp:** Breast Imaging; **Hospital:** Somerset Med Ctr; **Address:** 239 Rte 22 E, Ste 302, Green Brook, NJ 08812; **Phone:** 732-968-5160; **Board Cert:** Diagnostic Radiology 1994; **Med School:** Harvard Med Sch 1989; **Resid:** Diagnostic Radiology, Thomas Jefferson Univ Hosp 1994; **Fellow:** Breast Imaging, Thomas Jefferson Univ Hosp 1995

Rosenfeld, David MD (DR) - **Spec Exp:** Pediatric Radiology; **Hospital:** Robert Wood Johnson Univ Hosp - New Brunswick, St Peter's Univ Hosp; **Address:** Univ Radiology Group, 579A Cranbury Rd Fl 3, East Brunswick, NJ 08816; **Phone:** 732-390-0040; **Board Cert:** Diagnostic Radiology 1972; **Med School:** Univ Pittsburgh 1967; **Resid:** Diagnostic Radiology, Montefiore Med Ctr 1971; **Fac Appt:** Clin Prof Rad, UMDNJ-RW Johnson Med Sch

Underberg-Davis, Sharon MD (DR) - **Spec Exp:** Pediatric Radiology; **Hospital:** St Peter's Univ Hosp, Robert Wood Johnson Univ Hosp - New Brunswick; **Address:** Univ Radiology Grp, 579A Cranbury Rd Fl 3, East Brunswick, NJ 08816; **Phone:** 732-390-0040; **Board Cert:** Diagnostic Radiology 1993; Pediatric Radiology 2004; **Med School:** Harvard Med Sch 1988; **Resid:** Diagnostic Radiology, Hosp Univ Penn 1993; **Fellow:** Pediatric Radiology, Chldns Hosp 1995

Endocrinology, Diabetes & Metabolism

Agrin, Richard MD (EDM) - **Spec Exp:** Thyroid Disorders; Parathyroid Disorders; Diabetes; **Hospital:** Robert Wood Johnson Univ Hosp - New Brunswick, Somerset Med Ctr; **Address:** 137 Louis St, New Brunswick, NJ 08901; **Phone:** 732-545-1065; **Board Cert:** Internal Medicine 1974; Endocrinology 1977; **Med School:** Univ Pennsylvania 1971; **Resid:** Internal Medicine, USPHS Hosp 1975; **Fellow:** Endocrinology, Boston Univ Hosp 1977; **Fac Appt:** Assoc Clin Prof Med, UMDNJ-RW Johnson Med Sch

Bucholtz, Harvey K MD (EDM) - **Spec Exp:** Diabetes; Thyroid Disorders; Osteoporosis; **Hospital:** JFK Med Ctr - Edison, Newark Beth Israel Med Ctr; **Address:** 2 Lincoln Hwy, Ste 501, Edison, NJ 08820; **Phone:** 732-549-7470; **Board Cert:** Internal Medicine 1973; Endocrinology 1975; **Med School:** SUNY Hlth Sci Ctr 1968; **Resid:** Internal Medicine, Univ Michigan Med Ctr 1971; **Fellow:** Endocrinology, Duke Univ Med Ctr 1975; **Fac Appt:** Asst Clin Prof Med, UMDNJ-NJ Med Sch, Newark

Maman, Arie MD (EDM) - **Spec Exp:** Thyroid Disorders; Diabetes; Pituitary Disorders; **Hospital:** Robert Wood Johnson Univ Hosp - New Brunswick, St Peter's Univ Hosp; **Address:** D3 Brier Hill Ct, East Brunswick, NJ 08816-3335; **Phone:** 732-613-0707; **Board Cert:** Internal Medicine 1977; Endocrinology, Diabetes & Metabolism 1979; **Med School:** France 1974; **Resid:** Internal Medicine, Jewish Hosp 1977; **Fellow:** Endocrinology, Univ Colorado Med Ctr 1979; **Fac Appt:** Assoc Clin Prof Med, UMDNJ-RW Johnson Med Sch

Schneider, Stephen H MD (EDM) - **Spec Exp:** Diabetes; Nutrition; Cholesterol/Lipid Disorders; **Hospital:** Robert Wood Johnson Univ Hosp - New Brunswick; **Address:** UMDNJ-RW Johnson Medical School, 51 French St, MEB 384, New Brunswick, NJ 08903; **Phone:** 732-235-7219; **Board Cert:** Internal Medicine 1975; Endocrinology, Diabetes & Metabolism 1979; **Med School:** Boston Univ 1972; **Resid:** Internal Medicine, Univ Hosp 1974; Internal Medicine, Boston City Hosp 1975; **Fellow:** Endocrinology, Diabetes & Metabolism, Boston City Hosp 1976; **Fac Appt:** Prof Med, UMDNJ-RW Johnson Med Sch

Spiler, Ira MD (EDM) - **Spec Exp:** Pituitary Disorders; Thyroid Disorders; Calcium Disorders; **Hospital:** Raritan Bay Med Ctr - Perth Amboy, Robert Wood Johnson Univ Hosp - New Brunswick; **Address:** 3 Hospital Plz, Ste 307, Old Bridge, NJ 08857-3095; **Phone:** 732-360-1122; **Board Cert:** Internal Medicine 1976; Endocrinology, Diabetes & Metabolism 1979; **Med School:** Albert Einstein Coll Med 1971; **Resid:** Internal Medicine, Bronx Municipal Hosp 1973; Internal Medicine, Boston City Hosp 1976; **Fellow:** Endocrinology, Tufts-New England Med Ctr 1978; **Fac Appt:** Assoc Clin Prof Med, UMDNJ-RW Johnson Med Sch

Family Medicine

Metz, John P MD (FMed) *PCP* - **Spec Exp:** Primary Care Sports Medicine; **Hospital:** JFK Med Ctr - Edison; **Address:** JFK Medical Ctr, Family Practice, 65 James St, Edison, NJ 08818; **Phone:** 732-321-7487; **Board Cert:** Family Medicine 2003; Sports Medicine 2001; **Med School:** Jefferson Med Coll 1994; **Resid:** Family Medicine, Malcolm Grow Med Ctr 1997; **Fellow:** Sports Medicine, Uniformed Srvs U Hlth Scis 2000

Picciano, Anne MD (FMed) *PCP* - **Hospital:** JFK Med Ctr - Edison; **Address:** 65 James St, Edison, NJ 08818; **Phone:** 732-321-7493; **Board Cert:** Family Medicine 2002; Adolescent Medicine 2003; **Med School:** Univ Pennsylvania 1987; **Resid:** Family Medicine, W Jersey Health Sys 1990; **Fac Appt:** Asst Clin Prof FMed, UMDNJ-RW Johnson Med Sch

Swee, David E MD (FMed) *PCP* - **Hospital:** Robert Wood Johnson Univ Hosp - New Brunswick; **Address:** 317 George St Fl 1st - Ste 100, New Brunswick, NJ 08901; **Phone:** 732-235-8993; **Board Cert:** Family Medicine 2007; **Med School:** Canada 1974; **Resid:** Family Medicine, Somerset Med Ctr 1977; **Fac Appt:** Prof FMed, UMDNJ-RW Johnson Med Sch

Tallia, Alfred F MD (FMed) *PCP* - **Hospital:** Robert Wood Johnson Univ Hosp - New Brunswick; **Address:** Family Medicine at Monument Square, 317 George St, Ste 100, New Brunswick, NJ 08901-2162; **Phone:** 732-235-8993; **Board Cert:** Family Medicine 2007; **Med School:** UMDNJ-RW Johnson Med Sch 1978; **Resid:** Family Medicine, Jefferson Univ Hosp 1981

Tierney, Peter C MD (FMed) *PCP* - **Hospital:** Univ Med Ctr - Princeton; **Address:** 666 Plainsboro Rd, Ste 1316, Plainsboro, NJ 08536; **Phone:** 609-275-8100; **Board Cert:** Family Medicine 2005; **Med School:** Univ VA Sch Med 1983; **Resid:** Family Medicine, Hunterdon Med Ctr 1986

Winter, Robin O MD (FMed) *PCP* - **Spec Exp:** Geriatric Medicine; **Hospital:** JFK Med Ctr - Edison; **Address:** JFK Med Ctr - Family Practice Ctr, 65 James St, Edison, NJ 08820-3947; **Phone:** 732-321-7487; **Board Cert:** Family Medicine 2005; Geriatric Medicine 2006; **Med School:** Albert Einstein Coll Med 1978; **Resid:** Family Medicine, Hunterdon Med Ctr 1981; **Fac Appt:** Clin Prof FMed, UMDNJ-RW Johnson Med Sch

Gastroenterology

Ben-Menachem, Tamir MD (Ge) - **Spec Exp:** Endoscopy; Pancreatic/Biliary Endoscopy (ERCP); Endoscopic Ultrasound; **Hospital:** Robert Wood Johnson Univ Hosp - New Brunswick, Overlook Hosp (page 92); **Address:** UMDNJ-RWJ Med Sch, 1 Robert Wood Johnson Place - MEB 478, New Brunswick, NJ 08901; **Phone:** 732-235-7784; **Board Cert:** Internal Medicine 2004; Gastroenterology 2007; **Med School:** Israel 1989; **Resid:** Internal Medicine, Henry Ford Hosp 1994; **Fellow:** Gastroenterology, Henry Ford Hosp 1997; **Fac Appt:** Assoc Prof Med, Robert W Johnson Med Sch

Hodes, Steven MD (Ge) - **Hospital:** Raritan Bay Med Ctr - Perth Amboy, JFK Med Ctr - Edison; **Address:** 205 May St, Ste 201, Edison, NJ 08837; **Phone:** 732-661-9225; **Board Cert:** Internal Medicine 1977; Gastroenterology 1979; **Med School:** Albert Einstein Coll Med 1974; **Resid:** Internal Medicine, Montefiore Med Ctr 1977; **Fellow:** Gastroenterology, Mt Sinai-Bronx VA Hosps 1979

Pitchumoni, Capecomorin S MD (Ge) - **Spec Exp:** Pancreatic Disease; Gastroesophageal Reflux Disease (GERD); Pancreatic Cancer; Hepatitis C; **Hospital:** St Peter's Univ Hosp; **Address:** St Peters Univ Hosp, 254 Easton Ave, CARES Bldg Fl 4 - Ste 4013, New Brunswick, NJ 08903-1766; **Phone:** 732-745-7939; **Board Cert:** Gastroenterology 1971; Internal Medicine 1977; **Med School:** India 1960; **Resid:** Internal Medicine, Norwalk Hosp 1968; **Fellow:** Gastroenterology, Yale New Haven Hosp 1969Metropolitan Hosp Ctr 1971; **Fac Appt:** Clin Prof Med, Robert W Johnson Med Sch

Plumser, Allan MD (Ge) - **Spec Exp:** Endoscopy; Pancreatic/Biliary Endoscopy (ERCP); Liver Disease; **Hospital:** Robert Wood Johnson Univ Hosp - New Brunswick, St Peter's Univ Hosp; **Address:** 465 Cranbury Rd, Ste 102, East Brunswick, NJ 08816; **Phone:** 732-390-1995; **Board Cert:** Internal Medicine 1981; Gastroenterology 1983; **Med School:** NY Med Coll 1978; **Resid:** Internal Medicine, SUNY Stonybrook Med Ctr 1981; **Fellow:** Gastroenterology, SUNY Stonybrook Med Ctr 1983

Geriatric Medicine

Bullock, Richard B MD (Ger) *PCP* - **Spec Exp:** Hypertension; Cholesterol/Lipid Disorders; Dementia; **Hospital:** JFK Med Ctr - Edison; **Address:** 225 May St, Ste E, Edison, NJ 08837-3266; **Phone:** 732-661-2020; **Board Cert:** Internal Medicine 1984; Geriatric Medicine 2000; **Med School:** Mount Sinai Sch Med 1981; **Resid:** Internal Medicine, Mt Sinai Hosp 1984; **Fac Appt:** Asst Clin Prof Med, Robert W Johnson Med Sch

Rao, Arun S MD (Ger) *PCP* - **Hospital:** St Peter's Univ Hosp; **Address:** St Peters Univ Hosp, Ctr Ambulatory Svcs, Div Geriatrics, 254 Easton Ave, New Brunswick, NJ 08901; **Phone:** 732-745-8600 x6656; **Board Cert:** Internal Medicine 2000; Geriatric Medicine 2002; **Med School:** UMDNJ-RW Johnson Med Sch 1997; **Resid:** Internal Medicine, RWJohnson Med Ctr 2000; **Fellow:** Geriatric Medicine, Univ Michigan Hosps 2002; **Fac Appt:** Asst Clin Prof Med, Cornell Univ-Weill Med Coll

Gynecologic Oncology

Carlson, John A MD (GO) - **Spec Exp:** Gynecologic Cancer; Ovarian Cancer; Gynecologic Surgery-Complex; **Hospital:** St Peter's Univ Hosp; **Address:** St Peter's Univ Hosp, 254 Easton Ave Cares Bldg, New Brunswick, NJ 08901; **Phone:** 732-937-6003; **Board Cert:** Obstetrics & Gynecology 1981; Gynecologic Oncology 1982; **Med School:** Georgetown Univ 1974; **Resid:** Obstetrics & Gynecology, Hosp Univ Penn 1978; **Fellow:** Gynecologic Oncology, MD Anderson Hosp 1980; **Fac Appt:** Prof ObG, Drexel Univ Coll Med

Goldberg, Michael I MD (GO) - **Spec Exp:** Ovarian Cancer; Uterine Cancer; **Hospital:** St Peter's Univ Hosp, Robert Wood Johnson Univ Hosp - New Brunswick; **Address:** 78 Easton Ave, New Brunswick, NJ 08901-1865; **Phone:** 732-828-3300; **Board Cert:** Obstetrics & Gynecology 1977; Gynecologic Oncology 1980; **Med School:** Italy 1970; **Resid:** Obstetrics & Gynecology, Maimonides Med Ctr 1975; **Fellow:** Gynecologic Oncology, Jackson Meml Hosp 1977; **Fac Appt:** Clin Prof ObG, UMDNJ-RW Johnson Med Sch

Rodriguez, Lorna MD/PhD (GO) - **Spec Exp:** Ovarian Cancer; Cervical Cancer; **Hospital:** Robert Wood Johnson Univ Hosp - New Brunswick; **Address:** Cancer Institute of New Jersey, 195 Little Albany St, rm 2009, New Brunswick, NJ 08903; **Phone:** 732-235-7615; **Board Cert:** Obstetrics & Gynecology 2009; Gynecologic Oncology 2010; **Med School:** Puerto Rico 1979; **Resid:** Obstetrics & Gynecology, Cooper Med Ctr 1983; **Fellow:** Gynecologic Oncology, Univ Michigan 1985; **Fac Appt:** Prof ObG, UMDNJ-RW Johnson Med Sch

Hand Surgery

Coyle, Michael P MD (HS) - **Spec Exp:** Arthritis Hand Surgery; Nerve Compression; Dupuytren's Contracture; **Hospital:** Robert Wood Johnson Univ Hosp - New Brunswick, St Peter's Univ Hosp; **Address:** 215 Easton Ave, New Brunswick, NJ 08901-1722; **Phone:** 732-545-0400; **Board Cert:** Orthopaedic Surgery 2005; Hand Surgery 2010; Orthopaedic Sports Medicine 2007; **Med School:** Columbia P&S 1968; **Resid:** Surgery, UCSF-Moffitt Hosp 1970; Orthopaedic Surgery, NY Orth Hosp 1976; **Fellow:** NY Orth Hosp 1973; Hand Surgery, NY Orth Hosp 1977; **Fac Appt:** Clin Prof OrS, UMDNJ-RW Johnson Med Sch

Hematology

Karp, George I MD (Hem) - **Spec Exp:** Coagulation/Bleeding Disorders; Anemia; Breast Cancer; **Hospital:** Robert Wood Johnson Univ Hosp - New Brunswick, St Peter's Univ Hosp; **Address:** Central NJ Onc Ctr, 205 Easton Ave, New Brunswick, NJ 08901; **Phone:** 732-828-9570; **Board Cert:** Internal Medicine 1979; Medical Oncology 1981; Hematology 1982; **Med School:** Columbia P&S 1976; **Resid:** Internal Medicine, Univ Chicago Hosps 1978; **Fellow:** Medical Oncology, Natl Cancer Inst 1979; Hematology, Dana Farber Cancer Inst 1982; **Fac Appt:** Clin Prof Med, Robert W Johnson Med Sch

Philipp, Claire S MD (Hem) - **Spec Exp:** Bleeding/Coagulation Disorders; **Hospital:** Robert Wood Johnson Univ Hosp - New Brunswick; **Address:** Robert Wood Johnson Med School, 125 Paterson St, CAB5231, New Brunswick, NJ 08901; **Phone:** 732-235-6531; **Board Cert:** Internal Medicine 1981; Hematology 1984; Medical Oncology 1985; **Med School:** Brown Univ 1978; **Resid:** Internal Medicine, Beth Israel Med Ctr 1981; **Fellow:** Hematology & Oncology, NYU Med Ctr 1984; **Fac Appt:** Prof Med, Robert W Johnson Med Sch

Strair, Roger MD/PhD (Hem) - **Spec Exp:** Leukemia; Lymphoma; Bone Marrow Transplant; Multiple Myeloma; **Hospital:** Robert Wood Johnson Univ Hosp - New Brunswick; **Address:** Cancer Inst of NJ, 195 Little Albany St, New Brunswick, NJ 08901; **Phone:** 732-235-6044; **Board Cert:** Internal Medicine 1984; Hematology 1986; Medical Oncology 1987; **Med School:** Albert Einstein Coll Med 1981; **Resid:** Internal Medicine, Brigham & Women's Hosp 1984; **Fellow:** Hematology & Oncology, Brigham & Women's Hosp 1988; **Fac Appt:** Assoc Prof Med, UMDNJ-RW Johnson Med Sch

Infectious Disease

Boruchoff, Susan E MD (Inf) - **Spec Exp:** Travel Medicine; AIDS/HIV; Viral Infections; **Hospital:** Robert Wood Johnson Univ Hosp - New Brunswick; **Address:** Clinical Academic Bldg, 125 Paterson St, Ste 5100B, New Brunswick, NJ 08901-1928; **Phone:** 732-235-7060; **Board Cert:** Internal Medicine 1985; Infectious Disease 1988; **Med School:** Columbia P&S 1982; **Resid:** Internal Medicine, Geo Wash Univ Hosp 1985; **Fellow:** Infectious Disease, Univ Mass Med Ctr 1988; **Fac Appt:** Prof Med, Robert W Johnson Med Sch

Middleton, John R MD (Inf) - **Spec Exp:** AIDS/HIV; Osteomyelitis; **Hospital:** Raritan Bay Med Ctr - Perth Amboy; **Address:** Raritan Bay Infectious Disease, 3 Hosp Plaza, Ste 208, Old Bridge, NJ 08857-3093; **Phone:** 732-360-2700; **Board Cert:** Internal Medicine 1973; Infectious Disease 1980; **Med School:** UMDNJ-NJ Med Sch, Newark 1970; **Resid:** Internal Medicine, NY Hosp-Cornell Med Ctr 1973; **Fellow:** Infectious Disease, RWJ Univ Hosp 1977; **Fac Appt:** Assoc Clin Prof Med, UMDNJ-Rutgers Med Sch

Sensakovic, John W MD/PhD (Inf) - **Spec Exp:** Lyme Disease; Fevers of Unknown Origin; Bone Infections; **Hospital:** Saint Michael's Med Ctr, JFK Med Ctr - Edison; **Address:** 113 James St, Edison, NJ 08820; **Phone:** 732-549-3449; **Board Cert:** Internal Medicine 1982; Infectious Disease 1984; **Med School:** UMDNJ-NJ Med Sch, Newark 1977; **Resid:** Internal Medicine, St Michael's Med Ctr 1980; **Fellow:** Infectious Disease, St Michael's Med Ctr 1982; **Fac Appt:** Prof Med, Seton Hall Univ Sch Hlth & Med Scis

Weinstein, Melvin P MD (Inf) - **Spec Exp:** Bone/Joint Infections; Infective Endocarditis; **Hospital:** Robert Wood Johnson Univ Hosp - New Brunswick; **Address:** 1 Robert Wood Johnson Pl, New Brunswick, NJ 08901-1928; **Phone:** 732-235-7713; **Board Cert:** Internal Medicine 1975; Infectious Disease 1978; Medical Microbiology 1983; **Med School:** Geo Wash Univ 1970; **Resid:** Internal Medicine, Hartford Hosp 1975; **Fellow:** Infectious Disease, Univ Colo Hosp 1977; **Fac Appt:** Prof Med, UMDNJ-RW Johnson Med Sch

Internal Medicine

Carson, Jeffrey MD (IM) *PCP* - **Hospital:** Robert Wood Johnson Univ Hosp - New Brunswick; **Address:** 125 Paterson St, Ste 5100, New Brunswick, NJ 08901; **Phone:** 732-235-6968; **Board Cert:** Internal Medicine 1980; **Med School:** Hahnemann Univ 1977; **Resid:** Internal Medicine, Hahnemann Univ Hosp 1980; **Fellow:** Internal Medicine, Hosp Univ Penn 1982; **Fac Appt:** Prof Med, UMDNJ-RW Johnson Med Sch

Cassidy, Brian MD (IM) *PCP* - **Hospital:** JFK Med Ctr - Edison; **Address:** 3910 Park Ave, Ste 8, Edison, NJ 08820; **Phone:** 732-767-3130; **Board Cert:** Internal Medicine 1988; **Med School:** Grenada 1985; **Resid:** Internal Medicine, Muhlenberg Med Ctr 1988

DeSilva Jr, Derrick M MD (IM) - **Spec Exp:** Complementary Medicine; Preventive Cardiology; **Hospital:** Raritan Bay Med Ctr - Perth Amboy; **Address:** 629 Amboy Ave Fl 2, Edison, NJ 08837; **Phone:** 732-738-8801; **Med School:** Dominican Republic 1982; **Resid:** Internal Medicine, Raritan Bay Med Ctr-Perth Amboy Div 1988

Gil, Constante MD (IM) *PCP* - **Spec Exp:** Hypertension; Stroke; Heart Failure; Diabetes; **Hospital:** Raritan Bay Med Ctr - Perth Amboy; **Address:** 220 Market St, Ste 2, Perth Amboy, NJ 08861; **Phone:** 732-826-1609; **Board Cert:** Internal Medicine 2000; **Med School:** Dominican Republic 1981; **Resid:** Internal Medicine, Raritan Bay Med Ctr-Perth Amboy Div 1989; **Fac Appt:** Assoc Clin Prof Med, UMDNJ-RW Johnson Med Sch

Guillen, Gregorio MD (IM) *PCP* - **Spec Exp:** Geriatric Medicine; **Hospital:** Raritan Bay Med Ctr - Perth Amboy, JFK Med Ctr - Edison; **Address:** 400 State St, Perth Amboy, NJ 08861; **Phone:** 732-442-6020; **Board Cert:** Internal Medicine 1998; **Med School:** Dominican Republic 1982; **Resid:** Internal Medicine, Raritan Bay Med Ctr 1990; **Fellow:** Geriatric Medicine, Univ Florida 1992

Schaer, Teresa M MD (IM) *PCP* - **Spec Exp:** Concierge Medicine; Geriatric Medicine; **Hospital:** St Peter's Univ Hosp, Robert Wood Johnson Univ Hosp - New Brunswick; **Address:** 12 Stults Rd, Ste 123, Dayton, NJ 08810; **Phone:** 732-230-3272; **Board Cert:** Internal Medicine 1984; Geriatric Medicine 2008; **Med School:** UCSD 1981; **Resid:** Internal Medicine, Bellevue Hosp Ctr 1984; **Fellow:** Geriatric Medicine, Geo Wash Univ Med Ctr 1986; **Fac Appt:** Assoc Clin Prof Med, Robert W Johnson Med Sch

Interventional Cardiology

Altmann, Dory B MD (IC) - **Spec Exp:** Coronary Artery Disease; Heart Valve Disease; **Hospital:** Robert Wood Johnson Univ Hosp - New Brunswick, St Peter's Univ Hosp; **Address:** Cardiology Assocs of New Brunswick, 593 Cranbury Rd, East Brunswick, NJ 08816; **Phone:** 732-390-3333; **Board Cert:** Internal Medicine 1989; Cardiovascular Disease 2000; Interventional Cardiology 2009; Nuclear Cardiology 1998; **Med School:** Yale Univ 1986; **Resid:** Internal Medicine, New England Med Ctr 1989; **Fellow:** Cardiovascular Disease, Mt Sinai Hosp 1992; Interventional Cardiology, Washington Hosp Ctr 1993; **Fac Appt:** Asst Clin Prof Med, UMDNJ-RW Johnson Med Sch

Maternal & Fetal Medicine

MacMillan, William E MD (MF) - **Spec Exp:** Fetal Diagnosis & Therapy; Diabetes in Pregnancy; Reproductive Genetics; Multiple Gestation; **Hospital:** Robert Wood Johnson Univ Hosp - New Brunswick; **Address:** Clin Academic Bldg, Ste 4200, 125 Paterson St, New Brunswick, NJ 08901; **Phone:** 732-235-6600; **Board Cert:** Obstetrics & Gynecology 2009; Maternal & Fetal Medicine 2009; **Med School:** Univ Wisc 1985; **Resid:** Obstetrics & Gynecology, Univ Wisc Affil Hosp 1989; **Fellow:** Maternal & Fetal Medicine, SUNY Stony Brook Affil Hosp 1991; **Fac Appt:** Asst Prof ObG, Robert W Johnson Med Sch

Medical Oncology

Aisner, Joseph MD (Onc) - **Spec Exp:** Lung Cancer; Solid Tumors; **Hospital:** Robert Wood Johnson Univ Hosp - New Brunswick; **Address:** Cancer Inst of New Jersey, 195 Little Albany St, rm 2006, New Brunswick, NJ 08903-2681; **Phone:** 732-235-6777; **Board Cert:** Internal Medicine 1973; Medical Oncology 1975; **Med School:** Wayne State Univ 1970; **Resid:** Internal Medicine, Georgetown Univ Hosp 1972; **Fellow:** Medical Oncology, Natl Cancer Inst 1975

DiPaola, Robert S MD (Onc) - **Spec Exp:** Genitourinary Cancer; Prostate Cancer; Urologic Cancer; **Hospital:** Robert Wood Johnson Univ Hosp - New Brunswick; **Address:** Cancer Inst of New Jersey, 195 Little Albany St, New Brunswick, NJ 08903; **Phone:** 732-235-6777; **Board Cert:** Internal Medicine 2001; Medical Oncology 2005; **Med School:** Univ Utah 1988; **Resid:** Internal Medicine, Duke Univ Med Ctr 1991; **Fellow:** Hematology & Oncology, Univ Penn Hosp 1994; **Fac Appt:** Assoc Prof Med, UMDNJ-RW Johnson Med Sch

Fang, Bruno S MD (Onc) - **Spec Exp:** Head & Neck Cancer; Lung Cancer; **Hospital:** Robert Wood Johnson Univ Hosp - New Brunswick, St Peter's Univ Hosp; **Address:** Central Jersey Oncology Ctr, 205 Easton Ave, New Brunswick, NJ 08901; **Phone:** 732-828-9570; **Board Cert:** Internal Medicine 2006; Hematology 2000; Medical Oncology 2000; **Med School:** Brazil 1991; **Resid:** Internal Medicine, Jackson Meml Hosp 1996; Internal Medicine, VA Med Ctr 1997; **Fellow:** Hematology & Oncology, Natl Cancer Inst/NIH 2000

Nissenblatt, Michael MD (Onc) - **Spec Exp:** Breast Cancer; Colon Cancer; Hereditary Cancer; Lymphoma; **Hospital:** Robert Wood Johnson Univ Hosp - New Brunswick, St Peter's Univ Hosp; **Address:** 205 Easton Ave, New Brunswick, NJ 08901-1722; **Phone:** 732-828-9570; **Board Cert:** Internal Medicine 1976; Medical Oncology 1979; **Med School:** Columbia P&S 1973; **Resid:** Internal Medicine, Johns Hopkins Hosp 1976; **Fellow:** Medical Oncology, Johns Hopkins Hosp 1978; **Fac Appt:** Clin Prof Med, Robert W Johnson Med Sch

Salwitz, James C MD (Onc) - **Hospital:** St Peter's Univ Hosp, Robert Wood Johnson Univ Hosp Hamilton; **Address:** Central Jersey Oncology Ctr, Brierhill Ct, J2 Bldg, East Brunswick, NJ 08816; **Phone:** 732-828-9570; **Board Cert:** Internal Medicine 1984; Medical Oncology 1987; **Med School:** UMDNJ-Rutgers Med Sch 1981; **Resid:** Internal Medicine, Northwestern Univ/McGaw Med Ctr 1984; **Fellow:** Medical Oncology, NIH-Natl Canc Inst 1987

Shypula, Gregory J MD (Onc) - **Spec Exp:** Hematology; **Hospital:** Raritan Bay Med Ctr - Perth Amboy, JFK Med Ctr - Edison; **Address:** 1030 St Georges Ave, Ste 307, Avenel, NJ 07001-1330; **Phone:** 732-750-1200; **Board Cert:** Internal Medicine 1989; Medical Oncology 2001; Hematology 2007; **Med School:** Poland 1981; **Resid:** Internal Medicine, T Marciniak Univ 1984; Internal Medicine, Raritan Bay Med Ctr-Perth Amboy Div 1988; **Fellow:** Hematology & Oncology, St Luke's-Roosevelt Hosp Ctr 1992; **Fac Appt:** Assoc Clin Prof Med, Columbia P&S

Toppmeyer, Deborah L MD (Onc) - **Spec Exp:** Breast Cancer; Hereditary Cancer; **Hospital:** Robert Wood Johnson Univ Hosp - New Brunswick; **Address:** Cancer Inst of New Jersey, 195 Little Albany St, New Brunswick, NJ 08903-2681; **Phone:** 732-235-9692; **Board Cert:** Internal Medicine 1988; Medical Oncology 2006; **Med School:** Albany Med Coll 1985; **Resid:** Internal Medicine, Univ Pittsburgh Hlth Ctr Hosp 1988; **Fellow:** Medical Oncology, Dana Farber Cancer Inst 1993; **Fac Appt:** Assoc Prof Med, Robert W Johnson Med Sch

Neonatal-Perinatal Medicine

Hiatt, I Mark MD (NP) - **Spec Exp:** Respiratory Failure; Prematurity/Low Birth Weight Infants; Ethics; **Hospital:** St Peter's Univ Hosp, Robert Wood Johnson Univ Hosp - New Brunswick; **Address:** St Peter's Univ Hosp, Div Neonatal Med, 254 Easton Ave, New Brunswick, NJ 08901; **Phone:** 732-745-8523; **Board Cert:** Pediatrics 1978; Neonatal-Perinatal Medicine 1979; **Med School:** Cornell Univ-Weill Med Coll 1972; **Resid:** Pediatrics, NY Hosp-Cornell Med Ctr 1975; **Fellow:** Neonatal-Perinatal Medicine, Babies Hosp-Columbia Univ 1977; **Fac Appt:** Prof Ped, Drexel Univ Coll Med

Mehta, Rajeev MD (NP) - **Spec Exp:** Neonatal Critical Care; **Hospital:** Robert Wood Johnson Univ Hosp - New Brunswick; **Address:** RW Johnson Med Sch-UMDNJ, 1 RW Johnson Pl, MEB 238, Dept Pediatrics, New Brunswick, NJ 08903-1766; **Phone:** 732-235-7036; **Board Cert:** Neonatal-Perinatal Medicine 2008; **Med School:** India 1979; **Resid:** Pediatrics, Queens Park/St Mary's/Dudley Rd Hosps 1985; Pediatrics, Univ Hosp 1990; **Fellow:** Neonatology, Bradford Royal Infirmary 1989; Neonatology, North Shore Univ Hosp 1993; **Fac Appt:** Assoc Prof Ped, UMDNJ-RW Johnson Med Sch

Nephrology

Covit, Andrew B MD (Nep) - **Spec Exp:** Hypertension; Kidney Failure; Renovascular Disease; **Hospital:** Robert Wood Johnson Univ Hosp - New Brunswick, St Peter's Univ Hosp; **Address:** 8 Old Bridge Tpke, South River, NJ 08882; **Phone:** 732-390-4888; **Board Cert:** Internal Medicine 1982; Nephrology 1986; **Med School:** SUNY Downstate 1979; **Resid:** Internal Medicine, NY Hosp 1982; **Fellow:** Nephrology, NY Hosp 1984; **Fac Appt:** Assoc Clin Prof Med, UMDNJ-RW Johnson Med Sch

Sherman, Richard A MD (Nep) - **Spec Exp:** Dialysis Care; Electrolyte Disorders; **Hospital:** Robert Wood Johnson Univ Hosp - New Brunswick; **Address:** 125 Patterson St, Ste 15-100, New Brunswick, NJ 08901; **Phone:** 732-235-6512; **Board Cert:** Internal Medicine 1978; Nephrology 1980; **Med School:** Albert Einstein Coll Med 1975; **Resid:** Internal Medicine, Metropolitan Hosp 1977; **Fellow:** Nephrology, Bronx Municipal Hosp Ctr 1979; **Fac Appt:** Prof Med, Robert W Johnson Med Sch

Neurological Surgery

Lee, Sun H MD/PhD (NS) - **Spec Exp:** Spinal Surgery-Complex; Brain Tumors; Minimally Invasive Surgery; Pituitary Tumors; **Hospital:** Robert Wood Johnson Univ Hosp - New Brunswick; **Address:** 125 Paterson St, CAB Bldg - Ste 2100, New Brunswick, NJ 08901; **Phone:** 732-235-7756; **Board Cert:** Neurological Surgery 2001; **Med School:** Korea 1979; **Resid:** Neurological Surgery, Seoul Nat'l Univ Hosp 1984; Neurological Surgery, Thomas Jefferson Univ Hosp 1998; **Fellow:** Neurological Surgery, Univ of Pittsburgh Med Ctr 1988; Neurological Surgery, Univ of Minnesota 1993; **Fac Appt:** Assoc Prof NS, Robert W Johnson Med Sch

Nosko, Michael MD/PhD (NS) - **Spec Exp:** Aneurysm-Cerebral; Brain Tumors; Pituitary Tumors; Cerebrovascular Neurosurgery; **Hospital:** Robert Wood Johnson Univ Hosp - New Brunswick, Univ Med Ctr - Princeton; **Address:** 125 Paterson St, CAB - Ste 2100, New Brunswick, NJ 08901-1962; **Phone:** 732-235-7757; **Board Cert:** Neurological Surgery 1993; **Med School:** Univ Toronto 1982; **Resid:** Neurological Surgery, Toronto Genl Hosp 1986; Neurological Surgery, Walter Mackenzie Ctr 1991; **Fellow:** Research, Alberta Heritage Fdn Med Rsch 1986; **Fac Appt:** Assoc Prof NS, UMDNJ-RW Johnson Med Sch

Przybylski, Gregory J MD (NS) - **Spec Exp:** Spinal Surgery; Multiple Sclerosis; Vascular Neurosurgery; Spinal Cord Tumors; **Hospital:** JFK Med Ctr - Edison, Jersey Shore Univ Med Ctr; **Address:** NJ Neuroscience Inst, 65 James St Fl 1st, Edison, NJ 08818; **Phone:** 732-321-7010; **Board Cert:** Neurological Surgery 2000; **Med School:** Jefferson Med Coll 1987; **Resid:** Neurological Surgery, Univ Pittsburgh 1994; **Fellow:** Spinal Surgery, Hosp St Vincent de Paul/Hosp St Roch 1995; Spinal Surgery, Med Coll Wisc 1996; **Fac Appt:** Prof NS, Seton Hall Univ Sch Hlth & Med Scis

Neurology

Belsh, Jerry M MD (N) - **Spec Exp:** Neuromuscular Disorders; Amyotrophic Lateral Sclerosis (ALS); **Hospital:** Robert Wood Johnson Univ Hosp - New Brunswick; **Address:** 97 Paterson St Fl 2 - rm 215, New Brunswick, NJ 08901-2160; **Phone:** 732-235-7340; **Board Cert:** Neurology 1981; **Med School:** Jefferson Med Coll 1975; **Resid:** Neurology, Hahnemann Med Coll Hosp 1977; Neurology, SUNY-Dwnst Med Ctr 1979; **Fellow:** Neuromuscular Medicine, Mt Sinai Hosp 1980; **Fac Appt:** Prof N, Robert W Johnson Med Sch

Gizzi, Martin S MD/PhD (N) - **Spec Exp:** Neuro-Ophthalmology; Stroke; Progressive Supranuclear Palsy (PSP); Stroke; **Hospital:** JFK Med Ctr - Edison; **Address:** NJ Neuroscience Insitute, 65 James St, Edison, NJ 08820-3947; **Phone:** 732-321-7010; **Board Cert:** Neurology 1990; Vascular Neurology 2008; **Med School:** Univ Miami Sch Med 1985; **Resid:** Neurology, Mount Sinai Hosp 1989; **Fellow:** Neuro-Ophthalmology, Mount Sinai Hosp 1991

Golbe, Lawrence I MD (N) - **Spec Exp:** Parkinson's Disease; Progressive Supranuclear Palsy (PSP); Movement Disorders; **Hospital:** Robert Wood Johnson Univ Hosp - New Brunswick; **Address:** 97 Paterson St Fl 2 - rm 204, New Brunswick, NJ 08901-2160; **Phone:** 732-235-7733; **Board Cert:** Neurology 1984; **Med School:** NYU Sch Med 1978; **Resid:** Internal Medicine, Hahnemann Univ Hosp 1980; Neurology, Bellevue Hosp 1983; **Fac Appt:** Prof N, UMDNJ-RW Johnson Med Sch

Lazar, Mark H MD (N) - **Spec Exp:** Headache; Pain Management; Acupuncture; Sarcoidosis; **Hospital:** Robert Wood Johnson Univ Hosp - New Brunswick; **Address:** 573 Cranbury Rd, Ste A5, East Brunswick, NJ 08816-4026; **Phone:** 732-254-5101; **Board Cert:** Neurology 1982; **Med School:** NYU Sch Med 1977; **Resid:** Neurology, NYU Med Ctr 1981; **Fellow:** Neurology, NY-Cornell Med Ctr 1982; Clinical Neurophysiology, Columbia-Presby Med Ctr 1983; **Fac Appt:** Assoc Clin Prof N, UMDNJ-RW Johnson Med Sch

Lepore, Frederick E MD (N) - **Spec Exp:** Neuro-Ophthalmology; Botox for Blepharospasm; Migraine; Pseudomotor Cerebri; **Hospital:** Robert Wood Johnson Univ Hosp - New Brunswick; **Address:** Dept Neurology, 97 Paterson St, rm 225, New Brunswick, NJ 08901-2160; **Phone:** 732-235-7733; **Board Cert:** Neurology 1981; **Med School:** Univ Rochester 1975; **Resid:** Internal Medicine, Univ Michigan Med Ctr 1976; Neurology, Univ Virginia Hlth Sci Ctr 1979; **Fellow:** Neuro-Ophthalmology, Bascom Palmer Eye Inst 1980; **Fac Appt:** Prof N, Robert W Johnson Med Sch

Oh, Youn K MD (N) - **Spec Exp:** Headache; Stroke; Seizure Disorders; Parkinson's Disease; **Hospital:** JFK Med Ctr - Edison, Robert Wood Johnson Univ Hosp at Rahway; **Address:** 34-36 Progress St, Ste B3, Edison, NJ 08820-1197; **Phone:** 908-757-6633; **Board Cert:** Neurology 1979; Psychiatry 1981; **Med School:** South Korea 1964; **Resid:** Psychiatry, Harvard Psy Svc/Boston City Hosp 1973; Neurology, UMDNJ-NJ Med Sch 1975; **Fac Appt:** Assoc Clin Prof N, UMDNJ-RW Johnson Med Sch

Rosenberg, Michael L MD (N) - **Spec Exp:** Neuro-Ophthalmology; Neuro-Otology; Balance Disorders; **Hospital:** JFK Med Ctr - Edison; **Address:** New Jersey Neuroscience Institute, 65 James St, Edison, NJ 08818; **Phone:** 732-321-7010; **Board Cert:** Neurology 1983; **Med School:** Baylor Coll Med 1976; **Resid:** Neurology, Letterman AMC 1981; **Fellow:** Neuro-Ophthalmology, Bascom-Palmer Eye Inst 1981; **Fac Appt:** Prof N, Seton Hall Univ Sch Hlth & Med Scis

Sage, Jacob MD (N) - **Spec Exp:** Parkinson's Disease; **Hospital:** Robert Wood Johnson Univ Hosp - New Brunswick; **Address:** UMDNJ, Dept Neurology, 97 Paterson St, New Brunswick, NJ 08901-2160; **Phone:** 732-235-7733; **Board Cert:** Neurology 1979; **Med School:** Univ Pittsburgh 1972; **Resid:** Neurology, Univ Pittsburgh Hosps 1978; **Fellow:** Neurological Chemistry, NY Hosp-Cornell 1980; **Fac Appt:** Prof N, UMDNJ-RW Johnson Med Sch

Neuroradiology

Keller, Irwin MD (NRad) - **Spec Exp:** Brain & Spinal Imaging; Interventional Neuroradiology; Aneurysm-Cerebral; **Hospital:** Robert Wood Johnson Univ Hosp - New Brunswick, St Peter's Univ Hosp; **Address:** 579A Cranbury Rd, East Brunswick, NJ 08816-5405; **Phone:** 732-390-0040; **Board Cert:** Diagnostic Radiology 1984; Neuroradiology 2005; **Med School:** NY Med Coll 1980; **Resid:** Diagnostic Radiology, Montefiore Hosp Med Ctr 1984; **Fellow:** Neuroradiology, NYU Med Ctr 1986; **Fac Appt:** Assoc Clin Prof Rad, UMDNJ-RW Johnson Med Sch

Roychowdhury, Sudipta MD (NRad) - **Spec Exp:** Interventional Neuroradiology; Pediatrics; **Hospital:** Robert Wood Johnson Univ Hosp - New Brunswick, St Peter's Univ Hosp; **Address:** University Radiology Group, 579A Cranbury Rd, East Brunswick, NJ 08816; **Phone:** 732-390-0040; **Board Cert:** Diagnostic Radiology 1997; Neuroradiology 1999; **Med School:** Northwestern Univ 1992; **Resid:** Diagnostic Radiology, Northwestern Univ 1997; **Fellow:** Neuroradiology, Hosp U Penn 1999; **Fac Appt:** Asst Clin Prof Rad, UMDNJ-RW Johnson Med Sch

Schonfeld, Steven MD (NRad) - **Spec Exp:** Spine Imaging & Intervention; Interventional Neuroradiology; **Hospital:** St Peter's Univ Hosp, Robert Wood Johnson Univ Hosp - New Brunswick; **Address:** University Radiology Group, 579A Cranbury Rd Fl 3, East Brunswick, NJ 08816; **Phone:** 732-390-0040; **Board Cert:** Diagnostic Radiology 1982; Neuroradiology 2005; **Med School:** Mount Sinai Sch Med 1978; **Resid:** Diagnostic Radiology, Montefiore Hosp Med Ctr 1982; **Fellow:** Neuroradiology, NYU Med Ctr 1984; **Fac Appt:** Assoc Clin Prof Rad, UMDNJ-RW Johnson Med Sch

Obstetrics & Gynecology

Bachmann, Gloria MD (ObG) - **Spec Exp:** Menopause Problems; Sexual Dysfunction; Pelvic Surgery; **Hospital:** Robert Wood Johnson Univ Hosp - New Brunswick; **Address:** Women's Hlth Inst, Clinical Academic Bldg, 125 Paterson St, Ste 2104, New Brunswick, NJ 08901-1962; **Phone:** 732-235-7633; **Board Cert:** Obstetrics & Gynecology 1981; **Med School:** Univ Pennsylvania 1974; **Resid:** Obstetrics & Gynecology, Hosp Univ Penn 1978; **Fac Appt:** Prof ObG, UMDNJ-RW Johnson Med Sch

Bochner, Ronnie MD (ObG) - **Spec Exp:** Gynecologic Surgery-Laparoscopic; Uterine Fibroids; Menopause Problems; **Hospital:** Robert Wood Johnson Univ Hosp - New Brunswick; **Address:** 3270 Rt 27, Ste 2200, Kendall Park, NJ 08824-1458; **Phone:** 732-422-8989; **Board Cert:** Obstetrics & Gynecology 2007; **Med School:** Mount Sinai Sch Med 1981; **Resid:** Obstetrics & Gynecology, LI Jewish Med Ctr 1985; **Fac Appt:** Asst Clin Prof ObG, Robert W Johnson Med Sch

Davis, Nicole D MD (ObG) - **Spec Exp:** Gynecology Only; **Hospital:** St Peter's Univ Hosp; **Address:** 620 Cranbury Rd, East Brunswick, NJ 08816; **Phone:** 732-257-0081; **Board Cert:** Obstetrics & Gynecology 2009; **Med School:** Yale Univ 1988; **Resid:** Obstetrics & Gynecology, New York Hosp 1992

Rathauser, Robert MD (ObG) - **Hospital:** Robert Wood Johnson Univ Hosp - New Brunswick; **Address:** 3270 Route 27, Ste 2200, Kendall Park, NJ 08824; **Phone:** 732-422-8989; **Board Cert:** Obstetrics & Gynecology 2009; **Med School:** NYU Sch Med 1979; **Resid:** Obstetrics & Gynecology, LI Jewish Med Ctr 1983; **Fac Appt:** Assoc Prof ObG, UMDNJ-RW Johnson Med Sch

Occupational Medicine

Gochfeld, Michael MD/PhD (OM) - **Spec Exp:** Environmental Medicine; Chemical Exposure; Mercury Toxic Exposure; **Hospital:** Robert Wood Johnson Univ Hosp - New Brunswick; **Address:** Enviro & Occupational Health - EOHSI, 170 Frelinghuysen Rd, Ste 200, Piscataway, NJ 08854; **Phone:** 732-445-0123 x627; **Board Cert:** Occupational Medicine 1983; **Med School:** Albert Einstein Coll Med 1965; **Resid:** Behavioral Medicine, Rockefeller Univ 1977; **Fac Appt:** Prof OM, UMDNJ-RW Johnson Med Sch

Kipen, Howard M MD (OM) - **Spec Exp:** Environmental Medicine; Occupational Medicine; Occupational Lung Disease; **Hospital:** Robert Wood Johnson Univ Hosp - New Brunswick; **Address:** UMDNJ-RWJ Med Sch, EOHSI, 170 Frelinghuysen Rd, Piscataway, NJ 08854; **Phone:** 732-445-0123 x600; **Board Cert:** Internal Medicine 1982; Occupational Medicine 1986; **Med School:** UCSF 1979; **Resid:** Internal Medicine, Columbia Presby Med Ctr 1982; Occupational Medicine, Mt Sinai Hosp 1984; **Fac Appt:** Prof Med, UMDNJ-RW Johnson Med Sch

Ophthalmology

Blondo, Dennis L MD (Oph) - **Hospital:** Raritan Bay Med Ctr - Old Bridge Div; **Address:** 28 Throckmorton Ln, Old Bridge, NJ 08857-2558; **Phone:** 732-679-6100; **Board Cert:** Ophthalmology 1979; **Med School:** Med Coll VA 1973; **Resid:** Ophthalmology, NYU Med Ctr 1977

Engel, J Mark MD (Oph) - **Spec Exp:** Pediatric Ophthalmology; **Hospital:** Robert Wood Johnson Univ Hosp - New Brunswick, St Peter's Univ Hosp; **Address:** Univ Chldns Eye Ctr, 4 Cornwall Ct, East Brunswick, NJ 08816; **Phone:** 732-613-9191; **Board Cert:** Ophthalmology 2003; **Med School:** Loyola Univ-Stritch Sch Med 1986; **Resid:** Internal Medicine, Evanston Hosp 1988; Ophthalmology, Interfaith Med Ctr 1991; **Fellow:** Pediatric Ophthalmology, Children's Meml Hosp 1992; **Fac Appt:** , UMDNJ-NJ Med Sch, Newark

Grabowski, Wayne M MD (Oph) - **Spec Exp:** Diabetic Eye Disease; Laser Vision Surgery; **Hospital:** Univ Med Ctr - Princeton; **Address:** 5 Centre Drive, Ste 1B, Monroetownship, NJ 08831; **Phone:** 609-409-2777; **Board Cert:** Ophthalmology 1982; **Med School:** Albany Med Coll 1977; **Resid:** Ophthalmology, Albany Med Ctr 1981; **Fellow:** Vitreoretinal Surgery, Wills Eye Hosp 1983

Napolitano, Joseph D MD (Oph) - **Spec Exp:** Pediatric Ophthalmology; Strabismus; Eye Muscle Disorders; **Hospital:** Robert Wood Johnson Univ Hosp - New Brunswick; **Address:** OMNI Eye Svcs, 485 Route 1 S A Bldg - Ste 140, Iselin, NJ 08830; **Phone:** 732-750-0400; **Board Cert:** Ophthalmology 2008; **Med School:** UMDNJ-RW Johnson Med Sch 1987; **Resid:** Ophthalmology, UMDNJ Affil Hosp 1992; **Fellow:** Pediatric Ophthalmology, Chldn's Hosp

Santamaria II, Jaime MD (Oph) - **Spec Exp:** Cataract Surgery; LASIK-Refractive Surgery; **Hospital:** Raritan Bay Med Ctr - Perth Amboy, NY-Presby Hosp/Columbia (page 104); **Address:** Santamaria Eye Center, 104 Market St, Perth Amboy, NJ 08861-4412; **Phone:** 732-826-5159; **Board Cert:** Ophthalmology 1979; **Med School:** Columbia P&S 1973; **Resid:** Ophthalmology, Columbia-Presby Med Ctr 1978; **Fac Appt:** Asst Clin Prof Oph, Columbia P&S

Orthopaedic Surgery

Butler, Mark S MD (OrS) - **Spec Exp:** Trauma; **Hospital:** Robert Wood Johnson Univ Hosp - New Brunswick, St Peter's Univ Hosp; **Address:** 215 Easton Ave, New Brunswick, NJ 08901; **Phone:** 732-545-0400; **Board Cert:** Orthopaedic Surgery 2004; **Med School:** UMDNJ-RW Johnson Med Sch 1984; **Resid:** Orthopaedic Surgery, RW Johnson Univ Hosp 1989

Garfinkel, Matthew J MD (OrS) - **Spec Exp:** Shoulder & Knee Surgery; Arthroscopic Surgery; Sports Medicine; **Hospital:** JFK Med Ctr - Edison; **Address:** 10 Parsonage Rd, Ste 500, Edison, NJ 08837-2429; **Phone:** 732-494-6226; **Board Cert:** Orthopaedic Surgery 2005; **Med School:** Cornell Univ-Weill Med Coll 1986; **Resid:** Orthopaedic Surgery, Montefiore/Weiler Einsten Med Ctr 1991; **Fellow:** Sports Medicine, Lankenau Hosp 1992

Lombardi, Joseph S MD (OrS) - **Spec Exp:** Spinal Surgery; Spinal Disc Replacement; **Hospital:** JFK Med Ctr - Edison; **Address:** 10 Parsonage Rd, Ste 500, Edison, NJ 08837-2475; **Phone:** 732-494-6226; **Board Cert:** Orthopaedic Surgery 2008; **Med School:** UMDNJ-RW Johnson Med Sch 1978; **Resid:** Orthopaedic Surgery, UMDNJ-Univ Hosp 1983; **Fellow:** Spinal Surgery, Long Beach Mem Med Ctr 1984

Piskun, Andrew MD (OrS) - **Spec Exp:** Trauma; Sports Injuries; Arthroscopic Surgery; **Hospital:** Robert Wood Johnson Univ Hosp - New Brunswick, St Peter's Univ Hosp; **Address:** 1132 S Washington Ave, Piscataway, NJ 08854-3335; **Phone:** 732-752-8484; **Board Cert:** Orthopaedic Surgery 1984; **Med School:** UMDNJ-RW Johnson Med Sch 1977; **Resid:** Orthopaedic Surgery, UMDNJ-RW Johnson Univ Hosp 1982; **Fac Appt:** Asst Clin Prof OrS, UMDNJ-RW Johnson Med Sch

Reich, Steven MD (OrS) - **Spec Exp:** Spinal Surgery; Spinal Injury; **Hospital:** Robert Wood Johnson Univ Hosp - New Brunswick, St Peter's Univ Hosp; **Address:** Orthopaedic Associates, 2186 Route 27, Ste 1A, New Brunswick, NJ 08902; **Phone:** 732-422-1222; **Board Cert:** Orthopaedic Surgery 2005; **Med School:** Albert Einstein Coll Med 1986; **Resid:** Orthopaedic Surgery, Hosp for Joint Dis 1991; **Fellow:** Spinal Surgery, Pennsylvania Hosp 1992; Spinal Surgery, Thomas Jefferson Univ Hosp 1992

Otolaryngology

Edelman, Bruce MD (Oto) - **Spec Exp:** Ear Disorders; Sinusitis; **Hospital:** St Peter's Univ Hosp; **Address:** B3 Cornwall Drive, East Brunswick, NJ 08816-3390; **Phone:** 732-238-0300; **Board Cert:** Otolaryngology 1990; **Med School:** NYU Sch Med 1984; **Resid:** Surgery, Albert Einstein 1986; Otolaryngology, NYU Med Ctr 1990; **Fellow:** Pediatric Otolaryngology, Children's Hosp 1991

Kay, Scott MD (Oto) - **Spec Exp:** Facial Nerve Disorders; Otology; Hearing Loss; Sinus Surgery; **Hospital:** Univ Med Ctr - Princeton; **Address:** 7 Schalks Crossing Rd, Ste 324, Plainsboro, NJ 08536; **Phone:** 609-897-0203; **Board Cert:** Otolaryngology 1993; **Med School:** Univ Pennsylvania 1986; **Resid:** Surgery, Mt Sinai Hosp 1988; Otolaryngology, Columbia-Presby Med Ctr 1992; **Fellow:** Facial Plastic Surgery, Shadyside Hosp 1993; **Fac Appt:** Prof S, Robert W Johnson Med Sch

Mazzara, Carl A MD (Oto) - **Spec Exp:** Rhinoplasty; Eyelid Surgery; Cancer Reconstruction; **Hospital:** JFK Med Ctr - Edison, Overlook Hosp (page 92); **Address:** 5 Lincoln Hwy, Edison, NJ 08820; **Phone:** 732-635-1800; **Board Cert:** Otolaryngology 1994; Facial Plastic & Reconstr Surgery 1995; **Med School:** Mount Sinai Sch Med 1988; **Resid:** Otolaryngology, UMDNJ- Univ Hosp 1992; **Fellow:** Facial Plastic & Reconstr Surgery, Inst Facial Plastic Surg 1993

Miller, Andrew J MD (Oto) - **Spec Exp:** Cosmetic Surgery-Face; **Hospital:** JFK Med Ctr - Edison; **Address:** Associates in Plastic Surgery, 1150 Amboy Ave, Edison, NJ 08837; **Phone:** 732-548-3200; **Board Cert:** Otolaryngology 2000; Facial Plastic & Reconstr Surgery 2002; **Med School:** Baylor Coll Med 1994; **Resid:** Otolaryngology, Tulane Univ Med Ctr 1999

Rosenbaum, Jeffrey M MD (Oto) - **Spec Exp:** Head & Neck Surgery; Cosmetic Surgery-Face; Salivary Gland Surgery; Thyroid & Parathyroid Surgery; **Hospital:** St Peter's Univ Hosp; **Address:** B3 Cornwall Drive, East Brunswick, NJ 08816-3352; **Phone:** 732-238-0300; **Board Cert:** Otolaryngology 1978; **Med School:** Albany Med Coll 1973; **Resid:** Surgery, Hartford Hosp 1975; Otolaryngology, NYU Med Ctr 1978; **Fellow:** Plastic Surgery, Wayne Co Genl Hosp 1979; **Fac Appt:** Assoc Prof Oto, NYU Sch Med

Pain Medicine

Grubb, William R MD (PM) - **Spec Exp:** Complex Regional Pain Syndrome; Pain-Cancer; **Hospital:** Robert Wood Johnson Univ Hosp - New Brunswick; **Address:** New Jersey Pain Institute, 125 Patterson St, Ste 3100, New Brunswick, NJ 08901; **Phone:** 732-937-8841; **Board Cert:** Anesthesiology 1990; Pain Medicine 2007; **Med School:** Geo Wash Univ 1985; **Resid:** Anesthesiology, George Washington Univ Med Ctr 1989; **Fellow:** Cardiac Anesthesiology, Univ S Florida 1994; **Fac Appt:** Asst Prof Anes, Robert W Johnson Med Sch

Levin, Alexander MD (PM) - **Spec Exp:** Pain-Chronic; **Hospital:** Robert Wood Johnson Univ Hosp - New Brunswick; **Address:** Pain Control Ctr of New Jersey, 561 Cranbury Rd, East Brunswick, NJ 08816-5400; **Phone:** 732-651-1300; **Board Cert:** Anesthesiology 1990; Pain Medicine 2007; **Med School:** Russia 1978; **Resid:** Anesthesiology, Westchester Med Ctr 1986; **Fellow:** Pain Medicine, Univ Cincinnati Med Ctr 1987

Pathology

Barnard, Nicola J MD (Path) - **Spec Exp:** Gynecologic Pathology; Breast Pathology; Surgical Pathology; **Hospital:** Robert Wood Johnson Univ Hosp - New Brunswick; **Address:** 1 Robert Wood Johnson Pl, Dept Surgical Pathology, New Brunswick, NJ 08903; **Phone:** 732-937-8592; **Board Cert:** Anatomic Pathology 1981; **Med School:** England, UK 1975; **Resid:** Anatomic Pathology, Yale-New Haven Hosp 1980; Anatomic Pathology, Beth Israel Deaconess Hosp 1982; **Fellow:** Clinical Pathology, Harvard Univ 1982; **Fac Appt:** Assoc Prof Path, Robert W Johnson Med Sch

Pediatric Cardiology

Agarwal, Kishan MD (PCd) - **Spec Exp:** Echocardiography; Heart Disease in Adolescents; Arrhythmias; **Hospital:** JFK Med Ctr - Edison, Children's Specialized Hosp; **Address:** 450 Plainfield Rd, Edison, NJ 08820-2628; **Phone:** 732-494-9500; **Board Cert:** Pediatrics 1990; Pediatric Cardiology 1990; **Med School:** India 1969; **Resid:** Pediatrics, St John's Episcopal Hosp 1977; Pediatrics, SUNY Downstate Med Ctr 1979; **Fellow:** Pediatric Cardiology, Mayo Clinic 1981; **Fac Appt:** Clin Prof Ped, UMDNJ-RW Johnson Med Sch

Gaffney, Joseph W MD (PCd) - **Spec Exp:** Echocardiography; Fetal Echocardiography; Critical Care; **Hospital:** Robert Wood Johnson Univ Hosp - New Brunswick, NYPresby-Morgan Stanley Children's Hosp (page 104); **Address:** Clin Academic Bldg, 125 Paterson St, Ste 6100, New Brunswick, NJ 08901; **Phone:** 732-235-7905; **Board Cert:** Pediatric Cardiology 2006; **Med School:** NY Med Coll 1981; **Resid:** Pediatrics, Brookdale Hosp Med Ctr 1984; **Fellow:** Pediatric Cardiology, Babies Hosp/Columbia-Presby 1987; **Fac Appt:** Assoc Prof Ped, UMDNJ-RW Johnson Med Sch

Kurer, Cheryl C MD (PCd) - **Spec Exp:** Arrhythmias; Congenital Heart Disease & Acquired; **Hospital:** St Peter's Univ Hosp, Chldns Hosp of Philadelphia; **Address:** CHOP Cardiac Ctr at St Peter's Univ Hosp, 254 Easton Ave, New Brunswick, NJ 08901-1766; **Phone:** 732-846-2855; **Board Cert:** Pediatrics 1987; Pediatric Cardiology 2006; **Med School:** Mount Sinai Sch Med 1983; **Resid:** Pediatrics, Mt Sinai Hosp 1986; **Fellow:** Pediatric Cardiology, Chldns Hosp 1989; **Fac Appt:** Assoc Clin Prof Ped, Univ Pennsylvania

Pediatric Critical Care Medicine

Anene, Okechukwu P MD (PCCM) - **Hospital:** JFK Med Ctr - Edison; **Address:** Children's Service Dept, JFK Medical Ctr, 65 James St, Edison, NJ 08818; **Phone:** 732-321-7000 x7010; **Board Cert:** Pediatric Critical Care Medicine 2004; Pediatrics 2009; **Med School:** Nigeria 1983; **Resid:** Pediatrics, UMDNJ-New Jersey Med Sch 1991; Pediatric Critical Care Medicine, Wayne St Univ-Detroit Med Ctr 1995; **Fellow:** Pediatric Critical Care Medicine, Chldn's Hosp of Michigan 1995; **Fac Appt:** Assoc Prof Ped, Seton Hall Univ Sch Hlth & Med Scis

Bojko, Thomas MD (PCCM) - **Spec Exp:** Asthma; Sepsis & Septic Shock; Pneumonia; Respiratory Failure; **Hospital:** Robert Wood Johnson Univ Hosp - New Brunswick; **Address:** 89 French St, rm 2232, New Brunswick, NJ 08901; **Phone:** 732-235-7400; **Board Cert:** Pediatrics 2007; Pediatric Critical Care Medicine 2002; **Med School:** Italy 1985; **Resid:** Pediatrics, Newark-Beth Israel Med Ctr 1991; **Fellow:** Pediatric Critical Care Medicine, NY Hosp-Cornell Med Ctr 1994; **Fac Appt:** Assoc Prof Ped, UMDNJ-RW Johnson Med Sch

Jonna, Siva P MD (PCCM) - **Spec Exp:** Pediatric Critical Care; **Hospital:** St Peter's Univ Hosp; **Address:** 254 Easton Ave, rm 5094, New Brunswick, NJ 08901; **Phone:** 732-745-8600 x8152; **Board Cert:** Pediatrics 2003; Pediatric Critical Care Medicine 2006; **Med School:** India 1981; **Resid:** Pediatrics, Howard Univ Hosp 1995; **Fellow:** Pediatric Critical Care Medicine, Georgetown Univ Hosp 1995

Pediatric Endocrinology

Marshall, Ian MD (PEn) - **Spec Exp:** Adrenal Disorders; Growth Disorders; Pubertal Disorders; **Hospital:** Robert Wood Johnson Univ Hosp - New Brunswick; **Address:** UMDNJ-RWJ Medical School, Div Pediatric Endocrinology, 89 French St Fl 2nd - Ste 2300, New Brunswick, NJ 08901; **Phone:** 732-235-6230; **Board Cert:** Pediatric Endocrinology 2003; **Med School:** South Africa 1991; **Resid:** Pediatrics, Schneider Chldns Hosp 1998; **Fellow:** Pediatric Endocrinology, NY Presby Hosp 2002; **Fac Appt:** Asst Prof Ped, Robert W Johnson Med Sch

Salas, Max MD (PEn) - **Spec Exp:** Growth Disorders; Pubertal Disorders; Diabetes; **Hospital:** St Peter's Univ Hosp; **Address:** 254 Easton Ave Fl 3rd, New Brunswick, NJ 08901-1766; **Phone:** 732-745-8574; **Board Cert:** Pediatrics 1968; Pediatric Endocrinology 1986; **Med School:** Mexico 1964; **Resid:** Pediatrics, Children's Hosp 1967; Pediatrics, Children's Hosp 1968; **Fellow:** Pediatric Endocrinology, Children's Hosp 1979; Pediatric Endocrinology, N Shore Univ Hosp 1980; **Fac Appt:** Assoc Prof Ped, Drexel Univ Coll Med

Skuza, Kathryn MD (PEn) - **Spec Exp:** Diabetes; Thyroid Disorders; **Hospital:** St Peter's Univ Hosp; **Address:** St Peter's Univ Hosp, 254 Easton Ave, Pediatric/Endocrine Dept, New Brunswick, NJ 08901; **Phone:** 732-745-8574; **Board Cert:** Pediatrics 1987; Pediatric Endocrinology 2004; **Med School:** Poland 1982; **Resid:** Pediatrics, UMDNJ-Chldns Hosp 1985; **Fellow:** Endocrinology, Diabetes & Metabolism, UMDNJ-Chldns Hosp 1988; **Fac Appt:** Asst Prof Ped, UMDNJ-NJ Med Sch, Newark

Pediatric Gastroenterology

Koniaris, Soula MD (PGe) - **Spec Exp:** Nutrition; **Hospital:** Robert Wood Johnson Univ Hosp - New Brunswick; **Address:** Chld Hlth Inst NJ-UMDNJ Brunswick, 89 French St Fl 2nd, Ped Gastroenterology Div, New Brunswick, NJ 08901; **Phone:** 732-235-7885; **Board Cert:** Pediatric Gastroenterology 2005; **Med School:** Univ Tenn Coll Med, Memphis 1988; **Resid:** Pediatrics, Montefiore Hosp Med Ctr 1991; **Fellow:** Pediatric Gastroenterology, North Shore Univ Hosp 1994; **Fac Appt:** Asst Prof Ped, UMDNJ-RW Johnson Med Sch

Pediatric Hematology-Oncology

Drachtman, Richard A MD (PHO) - **Spec Exp:** Pediatric Cancers; Sickle Cell Disease; **Hospital:** Robert Wood Johnson Univ Hosp - New Brunswick, Jersey Shore Univ Med Ctr; **Address:** Cancer Inst of New Jersey, 195 Little Albany St, New Brunswick, NJ 08903-2681; **Phone:** 732-235-5437; **Board Cert:** Pediatric Hematology-Oncology 2007; **Med School:** Ros Franklin Univ/Chicago Med Sch 1984; **Resid:** Pediatrics, N Shore Univ Hosp 1988; **Fellow:** Pediatric Hematology-Oncology, Mount Sinai Hosp 1991; **Fac Appt:** Prof Ped, UMDNJ-RW Johnson Med Sch

Kamen, Barton A MD/PhD (PHO) - **Spec Exp:** Drug Development; Leukemia; **Hospital:** Robert Wood Johnson Univ Hosp - New Brunswick; **Address:** Cancer Inst of New Jersey, 195 Little Albany St, rm 3507, New Brunswick, NJ 08903; **Phone:** 732-235-8864; **Board Cert:** Pediatrics 1981; Pediatric Hematology-Oncology 1987; **Med School:** Case West Res Univ 1976; **Resid:** Pediatrics, Yale-New Haven Hosp 1978; **Fellow:** Pediatric Hematology-Oncology, Yale-New Haven Hosp 1980; **Fac Appt:** Prof Ped, UMDNJ-RW Johnson Med Sch

Pediatric Infectious Disease

Tolan Jr, Robert W MD (PInf) - **Spec Exp:** Lyme Disease; Cytomegalovirus; Staphylococcal Infections; Toxic Shock Syndrome; **Hospital:** St Peter's Univ Hosp, Capital Health Sys - Fuld Campus; **Address:** Childrens Hosp at St Peters Univ Hosp, 254 Easton Ave, MOB 3110, New Brunswick, NJ 08901; **Phone:** 732-339-7841; **Board Cert:** Pediatrics 2005; Pediatric Infectious Disease 2009; **Med School:** Washington Univ, St Louis 1987; **Resid:** Pediatrics, Riley Childrens Hosp 1990; **Fellow:** Infectious Disease, Childrens Hosp/Barnes Jewish 1994; **Fac Appt:** Assoc Clin Prof Ped, Drexel Univ Coll Med

Whitley-Williams, Patricia MD (PInf) - **Spec Exp:** AIDS/HIV; **Hospital:** Robert Wood Johnson Univ Hosp - New Brunswick; **Address:** RWJ Med Sch, Dept Peds, One Robert Wood Johnson Pl, MEB, rm 322, New Brunswick, NJ 08901; **Phone:** 732-235-7894; **Board Cert:** Pediatrics 1980; Pediatric Infectious Disease 2005; **Med School:** Johns Hopkins Univ 1975; **Resid:** Pediatrics, Chldns Hosp Med Ctr 1978; **Fellow:** Pediatric Infectious Disease, Boston City Hosp 1980; **Fac Appt:** Prof Ped, UMDNJ-RW Johnson Med Sch

Pediatric Nephrology

Singh, Anup MD (PNep) - **Spec Exp:** Nephrotic Syndrome; Lupus/SLE; Hypertension in Children; Kidney Stones; **Hospital:** St Peter's Univ Hosp, Staten Island Univ Hosp - South; **Address:** St Peter's Univ Hospital, MOB-3, 254 Easton Ave, New Brunswick, NJ 08901; **Phone:** 732-565-5489; **Board Cert:** Pediatrics 2007; Pediatric Nephrology 2003; **Med School:** Philippines 1985; **Resid:** Pediatrics, SUNY-Downstate Med Ctr 1991; **Fellow:** Pediatric Nephrology, SUNY-Downstate Med Ctr 1994; **Fac Appt:** Assoc Prof Ped, Drexel Univ Coll Med

Weiss, Lynne MD (PNep) - **Spec Exp:** Hypertension; Kidney Disease; Kidney Failure-Chronic; **Hospital:** Robert Wood Johnson Univ Hosp - New Brunswick; **Address:** Robert Wood Johnson Univ Hosp, Pediatric Nephrology, 89 French St Fl 2nd, New Brunswick, NJ 08901; **Phone:** 732-235-7880; **Board Cert:** Pediatrics 1979; Pediatric Nephrology 1982; **Med School:** Hahnemann Univ 1974; **Resid:** Pediatrics, Michael Reese Hosp 1977; **Fellow:** Pediatric Nephrology, Michael Reese Hosp 1979; **Fac Appt:** Prof Ped, UMDNJ-RW Johnson Med Sch

Pediatric Otolaryngology

Traquina, Diana N MD (PO) - **Spec Exp:** Airway Disorders; Ear Disorders; Sinus Disorders; **Hospital:** Robert Wood Johnson Univ Hosp - New Brunswick; **Address:** 181 Somerset St Fl 2, New Brunswick, NJ 08901; **Phone:** 732-247-2401; **Board Cert:** Otolaryngology 1989; **Med School:** Yale Univ 1984; **Resid:** Surgery, Yale-New Haven Hosp 1986; Otolaryngology, Yale-New Haven Hosp 1989; **Fellow:** Pediatric Otolaryngology, Montefiore-Weiler Enstein Hosp 1990; **Fac Appt:** Assoc Prof Ped, UMDNJ-RW Johnson Med Sch

Pediatric Surgery

Gallucci, John MD (PS) - **Hospital:** St Peter's Univ Hosp; **Address:** St Peter's Univ Hosp, 254 Easton Ave, MOB4, New Brunswick, NJ 08901; **Phone:** 732-565-5482; **Board Cert:** Pediatric Surgery 2000; **Med School:** UMDNJ-RW Johnson Med Sch 1990; **Resid:** Surgery, Cooper Univ Hosp 1997; **Fellow:** Pediatric Surgery, McGill Univ Chldn's Hosp 2000

Pediatrics

Chefitz, Dalya L MD (Ped) - **Spec Exp:** Developmental Disorders; **Hospital:** Robert Wood Johnson Univ Hosp - New Brunswick; **Address:** 125 Paterson St, MEB 348, New Brunswick, NJ 08901; **Phone:** 732-235-7044; **Board Cert:** Pediatrics 2008; **Med School:** UMDNJ-RW Johnson Med Sch 1990; **Resid:** Pediatrics, UMDNJ-RW Johnson Univ Hosp. 1993; **Fac Appt:** Asst Clin Prof Ped, UMDNJ-RW Johnson Med Sch

Cohen, Richard I MD (Ped) *PCP* - **Hospital:** St Peter's Univ Hosp, Robert Wood Johnson Univ Hosp - New Brunswick; **Address:** 1598 US Highway 130, North Brunswick, NJ 08902-3040; **Phone:** 732-297-0603; **Board Cert:** Pediatrics 1974; **Med School:** Jefferson Med Coll 1968; **Resid:** Pediatrics, St Luke's Hosp 1970; **Fellow:** Pediatrics, Thomas Jeffferson Hosp 1972; **Fac Appt:** Asst Clin Prof Ped, UMDNJ-RW Johnson Med Sch

Yalamanchi, Krishan MD (Ped) - **Spec Exp:** Neurodevelopmental Disabilities; Brain Injury; Pediatric Rehabilitation; **Hospital:** Children's Specialized Hosp, Robert Wood Johnson Univ Hosp - New Brunswick; **Address:** 200 Somerset St, New Brunswick, NJ 08901; **Phone:** 732-258-7065; **Board Cert:** Pediatrics 2004; Neurodevelopmental Disabilities 2004; **Med School:** India 1981

Physical Medicine & Rehabilitation

Brown, David P DO (PMR) - **Spec Exp:** Sports Medicine; Electrodiagnosis; Electromyography; **Hospital:** JFK Med Ctr - Edison; **Address:** JFK Johnson Rehabilitation Inst, 65 James St, Edison, NJ 08820; **Phone:** 732-321-7070; **Board Cert:** Physical Medicine & Rehabilitation 1990; **Med School:** Philadelphia Coll Osteo Med 1985; **Resid:** Physical Medicine & Rehabilitation, Walter Reed AMC 1989; **Fac Appt:** Assoc Clin Prof PMR, Seton Hall Univ Sch Hlth & Med Scis

Fantasia, Michele E MD (PMR) - **Spec Exp:** Pediatric Rehabilitation; Spinal Cord Injury-Pediatric; Cerebral Palsy; Neuromuscular Disorders; **Hospital:** Children's Specialized Hosp, Robert Wood Johnson Univ Hosp - New Brunswick; **Address:** 200 Somerset St, New Brunswick, NJ 08901; **Phone:** 732-258-7065; **Board Cert:** Pediatrics 2007; Physical Medicine & Rehabilitation 2010; Spinal Cord Injury Medicine 2002; Pediatric Rehabilitation Medicine 2010; **Med School:** UMDNJ-NJ Med Sch, Newark 1993; **Resid:** Pediatrics, UMDNJ Med Ctr 1996; Physical Medicine & Rehabilitation, UMDNJ Med Ctr 1999; **Fac Appt:** Asst Prof PMR, UMDNJ-NJ Med Sch, Newark

Lopez, Eduardo MD (PMR) - **Spec Exp:** Neuro-Rehabilitation; **Hospital:** JFK Med Ctr - Edison; **Address:** JFK Johnson Rehab Inst, 65 James St, Edison, NJ 08818; **Phone:** 732-321-7070; **Board Cert:** Physical Medicine & Rehabilitation 2005; Spinal Cord Injury Medicine 2001; **Med School:** Puerto Rico 1987; **Resid:** Physical Medicine & Rehabilitation, SUNY Upstate Med Univ 1994; **Fellow:** Neurology, Med Coll VA Hosp 1995

Plastic Surgery

Borah, Gregory L MD (PlS) - **Spec Exp:** Cosmetic Surgery-Face; Cosmetic Surgery-Breast; Hand Surgery; **Hospital:** Robert Wood Johnson Univ Hosp - New Brunswick; **Address:** UMDNJ Medical Ctr-Div Plastic Surgery, 1 Robert Wood Johnson MEB 506, Box 19, New Brunswick, NJ 08901-1928; **Phone:** 732-235-7865; **Board Cert:** Plastic Surgery 1986; **Med School:** Harvard Med Sch 1978; **Resid:** Surgery, Mass Genl Hosp 1983; Plastic Surgery, Yale-New Haven Hosp 1985; **Fac Appt:** Prof PlS, UMDNJ-RW Johnson Med Sch

Cuber, Shain A MD (PlS) - **Spec Exp:** Cosmetic Surgery-Body; Breast Reconstruction; Cosmetic Surgery-Breast; Liposuction & Body Contouring; **Hospital:** JFK Med Ctr - Edison; **Address:** Assoc in Plastic Surgery, 1150 Amboy Ave, Edison, NJ 08837; **Phone:** 732-548-3200; **Board Cert:** Plastic Surgery 2002; **Med School:** NY Med Coll 1990; **Resid:** Surgery, Univ Texas Hlth Sci Ctr 1994; Plastic/Reconstructive Surgery, Univ Texas Hlth Sci Ctr 1997; **Fellow:** Hand & Microvascular Surgery, UMDNJ Med Ctr 1998

Herbstman, Robert A MD (PlS) - **Spec Exp:** Cosmetic Surgery-Face; Cosmetic Surgery-Body; Breast Reconstruction; **Hospital:** Robert Wood Johnson Univ Hosp - New Brunswick, Riverview Med Ctr; **Address:** 579A Cranbury Rt 535 South, Ste 202, East Brunswick, NJ 08816; **Phone:** 732-254-1919; **Board Cert:** Plastic Surgery 1992; **Med School:** Univ Rochester 1982; **Resid:** Surgery, RWJohnson Univ Med Ctr 1987; Plastic Surgery, UMDNJ-NJ Med Sch 1989; **Fac Appt:** Asst Clin Prof S, Robert W Johnson Med Sch

Kaufman, Matthew R MD (PlS) - **Spec Exp:** Facial Nerve Disorders; Head & Neck Cancer; Breast Reconstruction; Rhinoplasty; **Hospital:** St Peter's Univ Hosp, Somerset Med Ctr; **Address:** The Plastic Surgery Center, 561 Cranbury Rd, East Brunswick, NJ 08816; **Phone:** 732-613-2929; **Board Cert:** Otolaryngology 2004; Plastic Surgery 2007; **Med School:** SUNY Upstate Med Univ 1998; **Resid:** Otolaryngology, Mt Sinai Med Ctr 2003; Surgery, UCLA Med Ctr 2005; **Fac Appt:** Asst Clin Prof S, Drexel Univ Coll Med

Nini, Kevin T MD (PlS) - **Spec Exp:** Facial Plastic Surgery; Breast Surgery; Liposuction & Body Contouring; **Hospital:** St Peter's Univ Hosp, Robert Wood Johnson Univ Hosp - New Brunswick; **Address:** 78 Easton Ave Fl 2, New Brunswick, NJ 08901-5400; **Phone:** 732-418-0709; **Board Cert:** Plastic Surgery 1994; **Med School:** UMDNJ-RW Johnson Med Sch 1984; **Resid:** Surgery, Pennsylvania Hosp 1989; Plastic Surgery, Shands Hosp-Univ Fla 1991; **Fellow:** Plastic Surgery, Univ Miami Hosps 1992

Olson, Robert MD (PlS) - **Spec Exp:** Cleft Palate/Lip; Head & Neck Surgery; Wound Healing/Care; **Hospital:** St Peter's Univ Hosp, Robert Wood Johnson Univ Hosp - New Brunswick; **Address:** 78 Easton Ave, New Brunswick, NJ 08901-1838; **Phone:** 732-418-0709; **Board Cert:** Plastic Surgery 1982; **Med School:** Univ Pennsylvania 1974; **Resid:** Surgery, Peter Bent Brigham Hosp 1979; Plastic Surgery, Mayo Clinic 1981; **Fac Appt:** Assoc Prof S, UMDNJ-RW Johnson Med Sch

Wey, Philip D MD (PlS) - **Spec Exp:** Cosmetic Surgery-Face; Breast Cosmetic & Reconstructive Surgery; Liposuction & Body Contouring; **Hospital:** Robert Wood Johnson Univ Hosp - New Brunswick, St Peter's Univ Hosp; **Address:** 78 Easton Ave Fl 2, New Brunswick, NJ 08901-1838; **Phone:** 732-418-0709; **Board Cert:** Plastic Surgery 2007; **Med School:** Brown Univ 1986; **Resid:** Surgery, Northwestern Meml Hosp 1990; Plastic Surgery, New York Hosp 1992; **Fellow:** Breast Surgery, NYU/Meml Sloan-Kettering Cancer Ctr 1993; **Fac Appt:** Assoc Clin Prof S, UMDNJ-RW Johnson Med Sch

Psychiatry

Jones Jr, Frank A MD (Psyc) - **Spec Exp:** Depression; Anxiety Disorders; Mood Disorders; **Address:** 2186 Route 27, Ste 2A, North Brunswick, NJ 08902; **Phone:** 732-422-0800; **Board Cert:** Psychiatry 1977; **Med School:** Case West Res Univ 1972; **Resid:** Psychiatry, Boston State Hosp 1973; Psychiatry, Worcester State Hosp 1975; **Fac Appt:** Clin Prof Psyc, UMDNJ-RW Johnson Med Sch

Menza, Matthew A MD (Psyc) - **Spec Exp:** Psychopharmacology; Depression; Anxiety Disorders; **Hospital:** Robert Wood Johnson Univ Hosp - New Brunswick; **Address:** RW Johnson Med Sch, Dept Psychiatry, 671 Hoes Ln, Piscataway, NJ 08854; **Phone:** 732-235-7647; **Board Cert:** Psychiatry 1985; **Med School:** Temple Univ 1980; **Resid:** Psychiatry, NYU -Bellevue Hosp 1984; **Fellow:** Psychiatry, Harvard Med Sch 1985; **Fac Appt:** Prof Psyc, UMDNJ-RW Johnson Med Sch

Pulmonary Disease

Goldberg, Jory MD (Pul) - **Spec Exp:** Lung Disease; Asthma; **Hospital:** Univ Med Ctr - Princeton; **Address:** 18 Centre Drive, Ste 103, Monroetownship, NJ 08831-1564; **Phone:** 609-655-1700; **Board Cert:** Internal Medicine 1981; Pulmonary Disease 1984; Critical Care Medicine 2007; **Med School:** Mexico 1976; **Resid:** Internal Medicine, City Hosp Ctr Elmhurst 1979; Internal Medicine, Monmouth Hosp 1980; **Fellow:** Pulmonary Disease, Bergen County Hosp 1982

Harangozo, Andrea MD (Pul) - **Hospital:** Robert Wood Johnson Univ Hosp - New Brunswick, St Peter's Univ Hosp; **Address:** 593 Cranbury Rd, Ste 1-A, East Brunswick, NJ 08816-4029; **Phone:** 732-613-8880; **Board Cert:** Internal Medicine 1989; Pulmonary Disease 2005; Critical Care Medicine 2005; **Med School:** NYU Sch Med 1984; **Resid:** Internal Medicine, UMDNJ-RWJ Univ Hosp 1987; **Fellow:** Pulmonary Critical Care Medicine, UMDNJ-RWJ Univ Hosp 1990; **Fac Appt:** Asst Clin Prof Med, UMDNJ-RW Johnson Med Sch

Melillo, Nicholas MD (Pul) - **Spec Exp:** Chronic Obstructive Lung Disease (COPD); Lung Cancer; Asthma; Chronic Obstructive Lung Disease(COPD); **Hospital:** JFK Med Ctr - Edison; **Address:** Middlesex Pulmonary Assocs, 106 James St, Edison, NJ 08820-3945; **Phone:** 732-906-0091; **Board Cert:** Internal Medicine 1983; Pulmonary Disease 1986; Critical Care Medicine 2007; **Med School:** UMDNJ-NJ Med Sch, Newark 1979; **Resid:** Internal Medicine, St Michael's Med Ctr 1983; **Fellow:** Pulmonary Disease, St Michael's Med Ctr 1985; Critical Care Medicine, St Michael's Med Ctr 1986; **Fac Appt:** Assoc Clin Prof Med, Seton Hall Univ Sch Hlth & Med Scis

Riley, David MD (Pul) - **Spec Exp:** Pulmonary Fibrosis; Interstitial Lung Disease; **Hospital:** Robert Wood Johnson Univ Hosp - New Brunswick; **Address:** RWJ Univ Med Grp, 125 Patterson St, Ste 5100B, New Brunswick, NJ 08901; **Phone:** 732-235-7840; **Board Cert:** Internal Medicine 1980; Pulmonary Disease 1974; **Med School:** Univ MD Sch Med 1968; **Resid:** Internal Medicine, Baltimore City Hosps 1970; Internal Medicine, Johns Hopkins Hosp 1973; **Fellow:** Pulmonary Disease, Hosp Univ Penn 1972; **Fac Appt:** Prof Med, UMDNJ-RW Johnson Med Sch

Schiffman, Philip MD (Pul) - **Spec Exp:** Occupational Lung Disease; Sarcoidosis; Asthma; Amyotrophic Lateral Sclerosis (ALS); **Hospital:** Robert Wood Johnson Univ Hosp - New Brunswick, St Peter's Univ Hosp; **Address:** 593 Cranbury Road, Ste B, East Brunswick, NJ 08816; **Phone:** 732-613-8880; **Board Cert:** Internal Medicine 1975; Pulmonary Disease 1978; Critical Care Medicine 2007; **Med School:** SUNY Downstate 1972; **Resid:** Internal Medicine, LI Jewish Med Ctr 1975; Pulmonary Disease; **Fellow:** Pulmonary Disease, LAC/Harbor-UCLA Med Ctr 1977; **Fac Appt:** Clin Prof Med, UMDNJ-RW Johnson Med Sch

Radiation Oncology

Haffty, Bruce MD (RadRO) - **Spec Exp:** Breast Cancer; Head & Neck Cancer; Lung Cancer; **Hospital:** Robert Wood Johnson Univ Hosp - New Brunswick, Robert Wood Johnson Univ Hosp Hamilton; **Address:** The Cancer Institute of New Jersey, 195 Little Albany St, rm 2038, New Brunswick, NJ 08903; **Phone:** 732-253-3939; **Board Cert:** Radiation Oncology 1988; **Med School:** Yale Univ 1984; **Resid:** Radiation Oncology, Yale-New Haven Hosp 1988; **Fac Appt:** Prof RadRO, Robert W Johnson Med Sch

Macher, Mark MD (RadRO) - **Hospital:** JFK Med Ctr - Edison; **Address:** JFK Med Ctr, Mid-State Rad Oncology, 65 James St, Edison, NJ 08818; **Phone:** 732-321-7167; **Board Cert:** Radiation Oncology 1986; **Med School:** Howard Univ 1982; **Resid:** Diagnostic Radiology, New York Univ Med Ctr 1985; **Fellow:** Diagnostic Radiology, Univ Hosp 1986

Rheumatology

Lichtbroun, Alan S MD (Rhu) - **Spec Exp:** Rheumatoid Arthritis; Sjogren's Syndrome; Fibromyalgia; **Hospital:** Robert Wood Johnson Univ Hosp - New Brunswick, JFK Med Ctr - Edison; **Address:** 63 Brunswick Woods Dr, East Brunswick, NJ 08816-5601; **Phone:** 732-613-1900; **Board Cert:** Internal Medicine 1980; Rheumatology 1984; **Med School:** SUNY Downstate 1977; **Resid:** Internal Medicine, LI Jewish-Hillside Med Ctr 1980; **Fellow:** Rheumatology, Mt Sinai Hosp 1982; **Fac Appt:** Asst Clin Prof Med, UMDNJ-RW Johnson Med Sch

Surgery

August, David MD (S) - **Spec Exp:** Pancreatic Cancer; Esophageal Cancer; Stomach Cancer; Sarcoma-Soft Tissue; **Hospital:** Robert Wood Johnson Univ Hosp - New Brunswick; **Address:** Cancer Institute of NJ, 195 Little Albany St, New Brunswick, NJ 08903-1914; **Phone:** 732-235-7701; **Board Cert:** Surgery 2005; **Med School:** Yale Univ 1980; **Resid:** Surgery, Yale-New Haven Hosp 1986; **Fellow:** Surgical Oncology, Natl Cancer Inst 1984; **Fac Appt:** Prof S, UMDNJ-RW Johnson Med Sch

Brolin, Robert E MD (S) - **Spec Exp:** Obesity/Bariatric Surgery; Gastrointestinal Surgery; **Hospital:** Univ Med Ctr - Princeton; **Address:** 666 Plainsboro Rd, Ste 640, Plainsboro, NJ 08536; **Phone:** 609-785-5870; **Board Cert:** Surgery 2001; **Med School:** Univ Mich Med Sch 1974; **Resid:** Surgery, Univ Pittsburgh Med Ctr 1980; **Fac Appt:** Prof S, Univ Pittsburgh

Chung-Loy, Harold E MD (S) - **Spec Exp:** Laparoscopic Surgery; Breast Surgery; Vascular Surgery; **Hospital:** JFK Med Ctr - Edison, Robert Wood Johnson Univ Hosp at Rahway; **Address:** 98 James St, Ste 202, Edison, NJ 08820-3902; **Phone:** 732-548-1000; **Board Cert:** Surgery 2007; **Med School:** Howard Univ 1980; **Resid:** Surgery, Mount Sinai Hosp 1985; **Fellow:** Renal Transplant, Mount Sinai Hosp 1983

Dasmahapatra, Kumar MD (S) - **Spec Exp:** Cancer Surgery; Breast Surgery; Laparoscopic Surgery; Pancreatic Surgery; **Hospital:** Raritan Bay Med Ctr - Perth Amboy, JFK Med Ctr - Edison; **Address:** 225 May St, Ste A, Edison, NJ 08837; **Phone:** 732-346-5400; **Board Cert:** Surgery 2010; **Med School:** India 1973; **Resid:** Surgery, Grace Hosp 1979; **Fellow:** Surgical Oncology, Roswell Park Meml Inst 1982; **Fac Appt:** Assoc Clin Prof S, UMDNJ-NJ Med Sch, Newark

Gannon, Christopher J MD (S) - **Spec Exp:** Liver & Biliary Surgery; Liver Cancer; **Hospital:** Robert Wood Johnson Univ Hosp - New Brunswick; **Address:** Cancer Inst of NJ, 195 Little Albany St, New Brunswick, NJ 08903; **Phone:** 732-235-7563; **Board Cert:** Surgery 2005; **Med School:** Columbia P&S 1998; **Resid:** Surgery, Univ MAryland Hosps 2004

Goydos, James S MD (S) - **Spec Exp:** Cancer Surgery; Melanoma; Skin Cancer; **Hospital:** Robert Wood Johnson Univ Hosp - New Brunswick, St Peter's Univ Hosp; **Address:** Cancer Inst of NJ, 195 Little Albany St, rm 3000, New Brunswick, NJ 08903; **Phone:** 732-235-7563; **Board Cert:** Surgery 2004; **Med School:** UMDNJ-RW Johnson Med Sch 1988; **Resid:** Surgery, New Britain Gen Hosp 1993; **Fellow:** Surgical Oncology, Univ Pittsburgh 1995; **Fac Appt:** Assoc Prof S, Robert W Johnson Med Sch

Kearney, Thomas J MD (S) - **Spec Exp:** Breast Cancer; **Hospital:** Robert Wood Johnson Univ Hosp - New Brunswick, St Peter's Univ Hosp; **Address:** Cancer Institute New Jersey, 195 Little Albany St, New Brunswick, NJ 08901; **Phone:** 732-235-6777; **Board Cert:** Surgery 2000; **Med School:** Georgetown Univ 1984; **Resid:** Surgery, Cedars Sinai Med Ctr 1992; **Fellow:** Surgical Oncology, Univ Chicago-Pritzker Sch Med 1995; **Fac Appt:** Assoc Prof S, UMDNJ-RW Johnson Med Sch

Lowry, Stephen MD (S) - **Spec Exp:** Cancer Surgery; **Hospital:** Robert Wood Johnson Univ Hosp - New Brunswick; **Address:** 125 Patterson St, Ste 7300, New Brunswick, NJ 08901; **Phone:** 732-235-6096; **Board Cert:** Surgery 2001; **Med School:** Univ Mich Med Sch 1973; **Resid:** Surgery, Univ Utah Med Ctr 1975; Surgery, NCI-NIH 1978; **Fellow:** Surgical Oncology, Meml Sloan Kettering Cancer Ctr 1982

Thoracic Surgery

Anderson, Mark B MD (TS) - **Spec Exp:** Cardiac Surgery; **Hospital:** Robert Wood Johnson Univ Hosp - New Brunswick; **Address:** PO Box 19, New Brunswick, NJ 08903; **Phone:** 732-235-8725; **Board Cert:** Surgery 2003; Thoracic Surgery 2004; **Med School:** NY Med Coll 1988; **Resid:** Surgery, Lenox Hill Hosp 1993; **Fellow:** Thoracic Surgery, UCSD Med Ctr 1995

Urology

Fleisher, Michael H MD (U) - **Spec Exp:** Pediatric Urology; **Hospital:** St Peter's Univ Hosp, Jersey Shore Univ Med Ctr; **Address:** Pediatric Urology Assocs, 557 Cranbury Rd, East Brunswick, NJ 08816-5400; **Phone:** 732-613-9144; **Board Cert:** Urology 1984; **Med School:** SUNY Downstate 1977; **Resid:** Urology, SUNY Downstate Med Ctr 1982; **Fellow:** Transplant Medicine, Montefiore Hosp Med Ctr 1979; Pediatric Urology, Hosp Sick Chldn 1983; **Fac Appt:** Assoc Clin Prof U, Robert W Johnson Med Sch

Richards, Steven L MD (U) - **Spec Exp:** Kidney Stones; Erectile Dysfunction; Minimally Invasive Surgery; **Hospital:** Robert Wood Johnson Univ Hosp - New Brunswick, St Peter's Univ Hosp; **Address:** 333 Forestgate Drive, Ste 202, Jamesburg, NJ 08831; **Phone:** 732-561-2058; **Board Cert:** Urology 2001; **Med School:** Albert Einstein Coll Med 1993; **Resid:** Urology, Montefiore Med Ctr 1999

Solomon, Michael J MD (U) - **Hospital:** St Peter's Univ Hosp, Robert Wood Johnson Univ Hosp - New Brunswick; **Address:** 579A Cranbury Rd, Ste 105, East Brunswick, NJ 08816-4026; **Phone:** 732-390-8700; **Board Cert:** Urology 1981; **Med School:** Univ Pennsylvania 1973; **Resid:** Surgery, New England Med Ctr 1976; Urology, Lahey Clinic 1979; **Fellow:** Pediatric Urology, Mass Genl Hosp 1981; **Fac Appt:** Assoc Clin Prof U, UMDNJ-RW Johnson Med Sch

Vates III, Thomas S MD (U) - **Spec Exp:** Pediatric Urology; **Hospital:** Robert Wood Johnson Univ Hosp - New Brunswick, Monmouth Med Ctr; **Address:** Pediatric Urology Assocs, 557 Cranbury Rd, Ste 4, East Brunswick, NJ 08816; **Phone:** 732-613-9144; **Board Cert:** Urology 2007; **Med School:** Georgetown Univ 1989; **Resid:** Surgery, RW Johnson Univ Hosp 1991; Urology, RW Johnson Univ Hosp 1995; **Fellow:** Pediatric Urology, Chldns Hosp Michigan 1997

Weiss, Robert E MD (U) - **Spec Exp:** Bladder Cancer; Kidney Cancer; Testicular Cancer; Robotic Surgery; **Hospital:** Robert Wood Johnson Univ Hosp - New Brunswick, Univ Med Ctr - Princeton; **Address:** 1 Robert Wood Johnson Pl Ste MB588, New Brunswick, NJ 08901-1928; **Phone:** 732-235-9843; **Board Cert:** Urology 2004; **Med School:** NYU Sch Med 1985; **Resid:** Surgery, Mount Sinai Med Ctr 1987; Urology, Mount Sinai Med Ctr 1991; **Fellow:** Urologic Oncology, Meml Sloan Kettering Cancer Ctr 1994; **Fac Appt:** Assoc Prof U, UMDNJ-RW Johnson Med Sch

Vascular & Interventional Radiology

Nosher, John MD (VIR) - **Spec Exp:** Endovascular Surgery; Uterine Fibroid Embolization; Interventional Oncology; Liver Cancer; **Hospital:** Robert Wood Johnson Univ Hosp - New Brunswick; **Address:** UMDNJ-RW Johnson Med Sch-Dept Radiology, MEB 404, Box 19, New Brunswick, NJ 08903-0019; **Phone:** 732-390-0040; **Board Cert:** Diagnostic Radiology 1975; Vascular & Interventional Radiology 2005; **Med School:** Jefferson Med Coll 1970; **Resid:** Diagnostic Radiology, Columbia Presby Med Ctr 1975; **Fac Appt:** Clin Prof Rad, UMDNJ-RW Johnson Med Sch

Siegel, Randall L MD (VIR) - **Spec Exp:** Endovascular Surgery; Dialysis Access; Pediatric Interventional Radiology; **Hospital:** Robert Wood Johnson Univ Hosp - New Brunswick, St Peter's Univ Hosp; **Address:** University Radiology Group, 579A Cranbury Rd, East Brunswick, NJ 08816-5426; **Phone:** 732-390-0040; **Board Cert:** Diagnostic Radiology 1991; Vascular & Interventional Radiology 2005; **Med School:** Univ Pennsylvania 1986; **Resid:** Diagnostic Radiology, RWJ Univ Hosp 1991; **Fellow:** Vascular & Interventional Radiology, RWJ Univ Hosp 1992; **Fac Appt:** Asst Clin Prof Rad, UMDNJ-RW Johnson Med Sch

Vascular Surgery

Graham, Alan M MD (VascS) - **Spec Exp:** Endovascular Surgery; Aneurysm-Abdominal Aortic; Carotid Artery Surgery; **Hospital:** Robert Wood Johnson Univ Hosp - New Brunswick; **Address:** 1 Robert Wood Johnson Pl, MEB Bldg - rm 541, Box 19, New Brunswick, NJ 08901-1928; **Phone:** 732-235-8770; **Board Cert:** Vascular Surgery 2006; **Med School:** Canada 1979; **Resid:** Surgery, McGill Univ Med Ctr 1984; **Fellow:** Vascular Surgery, Univ Chicago Hosps 1985; **Fac Appt:** Prof S, UMDNJ-RW Johnson Med Sch

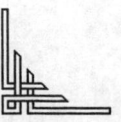
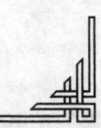

The Best in American Medicine
www.CastleConnolly.com

Monmouth

Monmouth

Allergy & Immunology

Gross, Gary L MD (A&I) - **Spec Exp:** Asthma; Cough-Chronic; Sinus Disorders; Atopic Dermatitis; **Hospital:** Jersey Shore Univ Med Ctr, Monmouth Med Ctr; **Address:** 802 W Park Ave, Ste 213, Ocean Township, NJ 07712-4556; **Phone:** 732-695-2555; **Board Cert:** Allergy & Immunology 1987; Pediatrics 1986; **Med School:** NYU Sch Med 1981; **Resid:** Pediatrics, Chldns Hosp 1984; **Fellow:** Allergy & Immunology, Chldns Hosp 1986; **Fac Appt:** Assoc Clin Prof Ped, Robert W Johnson Med Sch

Hirsch, Andrew C MD (A&I) - **Spec Exp:** Asthma; Sinusitis; Allergic Rhinitis; Eczema; **Hospital:** Riverview Med Ctr, Monmouth Med Ctr; **Address:** Allergy & Asthma Associates, 258 Broad St, Red Bank, NJ 07701-5623; **Phone:** 732-741-8900; **Board Cert:** Allergy & Immunology 2005; **Med School:** Temple Univ 1988; **Resid:** Pediatrics, New York Hosp 1991; **Fellow:** Allergy & Immunology, Thomas Jefferson Univ Hosp 1993

Picone, Frank J MD (A&I) - **Spec Exp:** Asthma; Sinus Disorders; Allergy; **Hospital:** Riverview Med Ctr, Monmouth Med Ctr; **Address:** 709 Sycamore Ave, Tinton Falls, NJ 07701; **Phone:** 732-747-8188; **Board Cert:** Pediatrics 1973; Allergy & Immunology 1975; **Med School:** UMDNJ-NJ Med Sch, Newark 1967; **Resid:** Pediatrics, Jackson Meml Hosp 1970; **Fellow:** Allergy & Immunology, Chldns Hosp Med Ctr 1974; **Fac Appt:** Asst Clin Prof Ped, Drexel Univ Coll Med

Sher, Ellen R MD (A&I) - **Spec Exp:** Asthma & Sinusitis; Nasal Allergies; Insect Allergies; Immune Deficiency; **Hospital:** Monmouth Med Ctr, Jersey Shore Univ Med Ctr; **Address:** 802 W Park Ave, Ste 213, Ocean Township, NJ 07712; **Phone:** 732-695-2555; **Board Cert:** Internal Medicine 1989; Allergy & Immunology 2003; **Med School:** Georgetown Univ 1986; **Resid:** Internal Medicine, Thomas Jefferson Univ Hosp 1989; **Fellow:** Pulmonary Disease, Thomas Jefferson Univ Hosp 1990; Allergy & Immunology, Natl Jewish Ctr Resp Dis 1992; **Fac Appt:** Asst Clin Prof Med, Drexel Univ Coll Med

Cardiovascular Disease

Beauregard, Lou-Anne M MD (Cv) - **Spec Exp:** Arrhythmias; Heart Disease in Women; **Hospital:** Robert Wood Johnson Univ Hosp - New Brunswick, CentraState Med Ctr; **Address:** Heart Specialists of Central Jersey, 100 Craig Rd Fl 2, Manalapan, NJ 07726; **Phone:** 732-866-0800; **Board Cert:** Internal Medicine 1983; Cardiovascular Disease 1985; Cardiac Electrophysiology 2002; Nuclear Cardiology 2005; **Med School:** Med Coll PA 1980; **Resid:** Internal Medicine, Temple Univ Hosp 1983; **Fellow:** Cardiovascular Disease, Med Coll Penn 1985; Cardiac Electrophysiology, Cooper Hosp 1986; **Fac Appt:** Assoc Clin Prof Med, Robert W Johnson Med Sch

Daniels, Jeffrey S MD (Cv) - **Hospital:** Monmouth Med Ctr, Jersey Shore Univ Med Ctr; **Address:** 215 Brighton Ave, Long Branch, NJ 07740; **Phone:** 732-222-5143; **Board Cert:** Internal Medicine 1983; Cardiovascular Disease 1985; **Med School:** Albany Med Coll 1980; **Resid:** Internal Medicine, Mt Sinai Hosp 1983; **Fellow:** Cardiovascular Disease, Mt Sinai Hosp 1985; **Fac Appt:** Asst Clin Prof Med, Drexel Univ Coll Med

Colon & Rectal Surgery

Arvanitis, Michael L MD (CRS) - **Spec Exp:** Laparoscopic Surgery; Colon & Rectal Cancer; Ulcerative Colitis; **Hospital:** Monmouth Med Ctr; **Address:** 1131 Broad St, Ste 105, Shrewsbury, NJ 07702-4329; **Phone:** 732-389-1331; **Board Cert:** Sports Medicine 2008; Colon & Rectal Surgery 2008; **Med School:** Hahnemann Univ 1982; **Resid:** Surgery, St Vincent's Hosp 1987; **Fellow:** Colon & Rectal Surgery, Cleveland Clinic 1988; **Fac Appt:** Assoc Prof S, Hahnemann Univ

Ross, Howard M MD (CRS) - **Spec Exp:** Laparoscopic Surgery; Colon & Rectal Cancer; Inflammatory Bowel Disease; **Hospital:** Riverview Med Ctr; **Address:** Riverview Surgical Assocs, 241 Monmouth Rd, West Longbranch, NJ 07764; **Phone:** 732-403-2075; **Board Cert:** Surgery 2000; Colon & Rectal Surgery 2001; **Med School:** Univ Rochester 1992; **Resid:** Surgery, Univ Conn Hlth Ctr 1994; **Fellow:** Colon & Rectal Surgery, Meml Sloan Kettering Cancer Ctr 1996; Colon & Rectal Surgery, Lahey Clinic 2000; **Fac Appt:** Asst Prof S, Univ Pennsylvania

Dermatology

Grossman, Kenneth A MD (D) - **Spec Exp:** Psoriasis; Skin Cancer; Cutaneous Lymphoma; Cosmetic Dermatology; **Hospital:** Riverview Med Ctr; **Address:** 180 White Rd, Ste 103, Little Silver, NJ 07739-1166; **Phone:** 732-842-5222; **Board Cert:** Internal Medicine 1980; Dermatology 1983; **Med School:** SUNY Hlth Sci Ctr 1977; **Resid:** Internal Medicine, Nassau County Med Ctr 1980; Dermatology, Montefiore Med Ctr 1983

Hametz, Irwin MD (D) - **Hospital:** CentraState Med Ctr; **Address:** 77-55 Schanck Rd, Ste B-3, Freehold, NJ 07728; **Phone:** 732-462-9800; **Board Cert:** Dermatology 1978; **Med School:** NY Med Coll 1973; **Resid:** Pediatrics, Long Island Jewish-Hillside Med Ctr 1975; Dermatology, Brown Univ Affil Hosps 1978; **Fac Appt:** Asst Clin Prof Med, UMDNJ-RW Johnson Med Sch

Orsini, William J MD (D) - **Hospital:** Monmouth Med Ctr; **Address:** 223 Monmouth Rd, W Long Branch, NJ 07764; **Phone:** 732-870-2992; **Board Cert:** Internal Medicine 1975; Dermatology 1977; **Med School:** UMDNJ-NJ Med Sch, Newark 1972; **Resid:** Internal Medicine, Monmouth Med Ctr 1975; Dermatology, Albany Med Ctr 1977

Diagnostic Radiology

Chalal, Jeffrey MD (DR) - **Hospital:** CentraState Med Ctr; **Address:** 901 W Main St, Ground Fl, Freehold, NJ 07728; **Phone:** 732-462-4844; **Board Cert:** Diagnostic Radiology 1982; **Med School:** Univ Pennsylvania 1977; **Resid:** Diagnostic Radiology, Columbia-Presby Med Ctr 1981; **Fellow:** Cross Sectional Imaging, Columbia-Presby Med Ctr 1982

Endocrinology, Diabetes & Metabolism

Nassberg, Barton MD (EDM) - **Spec Exp:** Thyroid Disorders; Diabetes; **Hospital:** Bayshore Community Hosp; **Address:** 723 N Beers St, Ste 2G, Holmdel, NJ 07733-1512; **Phone:** 732-739-0200; **Board Cert:** Internal Medicine 1982; Endocrinology, Diabetes & Metabolism 1985; **Med School:** Belgium 1979; **Resid:** Internal Medicine, Mountainside Hosp 1982; **Fellow:** Endocrinology, Diabetes & Metabolism, MS Hershey Med Ctr 1984

Family Medicine

Bernardo, Salvatore MD (FMed) *PCP* - **Hospital:** CentraState Med Ctr; **Address:** 4255 Route 9 N, Ste B, Freehold, NJ 07728; **Phone:** 732-683-9897; **Board Cert:** Family Medicine 2009; **Med School:** UMDNJ-NJ Med Sch, Newark 1993; **Resid:** Family Medicine, Somerset Med Ctr 1996

Catanese, Vincent J MD (FMed) *PCP* - **Spec Exp:** Hypertension; Diabetes; Functional Bowel Disorders; **Hospital:** Bayshore Community Hosp, Riverview Med Ctr; **Address:** 733 N Beers St, Ste U3, Holmdel, NJ 07733; **Phone:** 732-264-8484; **Board Cert:** Family Medicine 2005; **Med School:** Penn State Univ-Hershey Med Ctr 1978; **Resid:** Family Medicine, Conemaugh Valley Meml Hosp 1981

Liquori, Frances DO (FMed) *PCP* - **Hospital:** CentraState Med Ctr, Kimball Med Ctr; **Address:** Howell Family Med Ctr, 3701 Rte 9 N, Howell, NJ 07731-3396; **Phone:** 732-364-4555; **Board Cert:** Family Medicine 2001; **Med School:** Univ Osteo Med & Hlth Sci, Des Moines 1984; **Resid:** Family Medicine, Mountainside Hosp 1988

Gastroenterology

Binns, Joseph MD (Ge) - **Spec Exp:** Colonoscopy; **Hospital:** Riverview Med Ctr; **Address:** Red Bank Gastroenterology Assocs, 365 Broad St, Ste 1-E, Red Bank, NJ 07701; **Phone:** 732-842-4294; **Board Cert:** Internal Medicine 2000; Gastroenterology 2003; **Med School:** UMDNJ-RW Johnson Med Sch 1987; **Resid:** Internal Medicine, Pennsylvania Hosp 1990; **Fellow:** Gastroenterology, Graduate Hosp 1992

Fiest, Thomas DO (Ge) - **Spec Exp:** Colitis; Liver Disease; **Hospital:** Monmouth Med Ctr, Jersey Shore Univ Med Ctr; **Address:** 142 Highway 35, Eatontown, NJ 07724; **Phone:** 732-389-5004; **Board Cert:** Internal Medicine 1989; Gastroenterology 2005; **Med School:** Philadelphia Coll Osteo Med 1985; **Resid:** Internal Medicine, Monmouth Med Ctr 1990; **Fellow:** Gastroenterology, Jersey City Med Ctr 1993

Ludwig, Shelly L MD (Ge) - **Spec Exp:** Inflammatory Bowel Disease; Hepatitis C; Gastroesophageal Reflux Disease (GERD); Endoscopy; **Hospital:** CentraState Med Ctr, Robert Wood Johnson Univ Hosp - New Brunswick; **Address:** 535 Iron Bridge Rd, Ste 12, Freehold, NJ 07728-5301; **Phone:** 732-780-4224; **Board Cert:** Internal Medicine 1977; Gastroenterology 1979; **Med School:** Albert Einstein Coll Med 1974; **Resid:** Internal Medicine, LAC-Harbor UCLA Med Ctr 1977; **Fellow:** Gastroenterology, Wadsworth VA Hosp/UCLA 1979; **Fac Appt:** Assoc Clin Prof Med, Robert W Johnson Med Sch

Turtel, Penny S MD (Ge) - **Spec Exp:** Inflammatory Bowel Disease; Celiac Disease; Colon Polyps & Cancer; **Hospital:** Monmouth Med Ctr, Jersey Shore Univ Med Ctr; **Address:** 1907 Route 35, Ste 1, Oakhurst, NJ 07755-2760; **Phone:** 732-517-0060; **Board Cert:** Internal Medicine 1989; Gastroenterology 1999; **Med School:** Cornell Univ-Weill Med Coll 1986; **Resid:** Internal Medicine, Mount Sinai Hosp 1989; **Fellow:** Gastroenterology, Mount Sinai Hosp 1991

Geriatric Medicine

Israel, Jessica L MD (Ger) - **Spec Exp:** Palliative Care; **Hospital:** Monmouth Med Ctr; **Address:** Monmouth Medical Ctr, Dept Geriatrics, 300 Second Ave, Long Branch, NJ 07740; **Phone:** 732-923-7550; **Board Cert:** Geriatric Medicine 2006; **Med School:** Mount Sinai Sch Med 1995; **Resid:** Internal Medicine, Mt Sinai Med Ctr 1998; **Fellow:** Geriatric Medicine, Mt Sinai Med Ctr 2000

Hand Surgery

Lisser, Steven P MD (HS) - **Spec Exp:** Shoulder Surgery; Wrist/Hand Injuries; Ligament Reconstruction; Sports Medicine; **Hospital:** Riverview Med Ctr, Monmouth Med Ctr; **Address:** Orthopaedic, Sports Med & Rehab Ctr, 80 Oak Hill Rd, Red Bank, NJ 07701; **Phone:** 732-741-2313; **Board Cert:** Orthopaedic Surgery 2007; Hand Surgery 2007; Orthopaedic Sports Medicine 2007; **Med School:** Mount Sinai Sch Med 1987; **Resid:** Orthopaedic Surgery, Mt Sinai Med Ctr 1992; **Fellow:** Hand & Microvascular Surgery, Thom Jefferson Univ 1993; Sports Medicine & Shoulder Surgery, Univ Pennsylvania 1994

Hematology

Lerner, William A MD (Hem) - **Spec Exp:** Palliative Care; **Hospital:** Jersey Shore Univ Med Ctr, Ocean Med Ctr; **Address:** 1707 Atlantic Ave, Manasquan, NJ 08736-1147; **Phone:** 732-528-0760; **Board Cert:** Internal Medicine 1980; Hematology 1982; Medical Oncology 1983; Hospice & Palliative Medicine 2008; **Med School:** Belgium 1977; **Resid:** Internal Medicine, Albert Einstein Med Ctr 1980; **Fellow:** Hematology & Oncology, NYU Med Ctr 1983

Topilow, Arthur A MD (Hem) - **Spec Exp:** Lymphoma; Multiple Myeloma; **Hospital:** Jersey Shore Univ Med Ctr, Ocean Med Ctr; **Address:** 1707 Atlantic Ave, Manasquan, NJ 08736-1147; **Phone:** 732-528-0760; **Board Cert:** Internal Medicine 1971; Hematology 1972; Medical Oncology 1981; **Med School:** NY Med Coll 1967; **Resid:** Internal Medicine, Flower/NY Metro Hosp 1970; **Fellow:** Hematology, Flower/NY Metro Hosp 1972; **Fac Appt:** Assoc Clin Prof Med, UMDNJ-NJ Med Sch, Newark

Infectious Disease

Eng, Margaret H MD (Inf) - **Spec Exp:** AIDS/HIV; **Hospital:** Monmouth Med Ctr; **Address:** Monmouth Medical Ctr, Dept Medicine, 270 Broadway Ave, Long Branch, NJ 07740; **Phone:** 732-923-7139; **Board Cert:** Internal Medicine 1983; Infectious Disease 2000; **Med School:** Albert Einstein Coll Med 1980; **Resid:** Internal Medicine, Kings Co Hosp 1984; **Fellow:** Infectious Disease, Univ Maryland Med Ctr 1986

Internal Medicine

Courtney, Barbara E MD (IM) *PCP* - **Spec Exp:** Geriatric Medicine; **Hospital:** Monmouth Med Ctr; **Address:** Monmouth Med Grp, 370 Highway 35, Red Bank, NJ 07701; **Phone:** 732-842-0290; **Board Cert:** Internal Medicine 1980; Geriatric Medicine 2002; **Med School:** Hahnemann Univ 1977; **Resid:** Internal Medicine, Monmouth Med Ctr 1980; **Fac Appt:** Med

Glowacki, Jan S MD (IM) *PCP* - **Spec Exp:** Preventive Medicine; Diagnostic Problems; **Hospital:** Riverview Med Ctr, Monmouth Med Ctr; **Address:** 569 River Rd, Fair Haven, NJ 07704-3262; **Phone:** 732-530-0100; **Board Cert:** Internal Medicine 1980; **Med School:** Jefferson Med Coll 1977; **Resid:** Internal Medicine, Monmouth Med Ctr 1980

Granet, Kenneth M MD (IM) *PCP* - **Hospital:** Monmouth Med Ctr; **Address:** 1049 Broadway, Ste 4, West Long Branch, NJ 07764; **Phone:** 732-229-2020; **Board Cert:** Internal Medicine 1987; **Med School:** SUNY Downstate 1984; **Resid:** Internal Medicine, N Shore Univ Hosp 1987; **Fac Appt:** Asst Clin Prof Med, Drexel Univ Coll Med

Masterson, Raymond M MD (IM) *PCP* - **Spec Exp:** Hypertension; Diabetes; Cholesterol/Lipid Disorders; Peripheral Vascular Disease; **Hospital:** Jersey Shore Univ Med Ctr; **Address:** 700 Highway 11, Ste 9, Sea Girt, NJ 08750-2804; **Phone:** 732-974-0340; **Board Cert:** Internal Medicine 1986; **Med School:** Philippines 1978; **Resid:** Internal Medicine, St Michaels Med Ctr 1982

Interventional Cardiology

Watson, Rita MD (IC) - **Spec Exp:** Cardiac Catheterization; Peripheral Vascular Disease; Heart Valve Disease; Angioplasty; **Hospital:** Jersey Shore Univ Med Ctr, Monmouth Med Ctr; **Address:** 215 Brighton Ave, Long Branch, NJ 07740; **Phone:** 732-222-5143; **Board Cert:** Internal Medicine 1979; Cardiovascular Disease 1983; Interventional Cardiology 1999; **Med School:** Harvard Med Sch 1976; **Resid:** Internal Medicine, Hosp Univ Penn 1979; **Fellow:** Cardiovascular Disease, NHLBI-Natl Inst Hlth 1981

Maternal & Fetal Medicine

Gonzalez, David MD (MF) - **Spec Exp:** Pregnancy-High Risk; **Hospital:** Monmouth Med Ctr; **Address:** Monmouth Med Group, 73 S Bath Ave, Long Branch, NJ 07740; **Phone:** 732-870-3600; **Board Cert:** Obstetrics & Gynecology 2005; Maternal & Fetal Medicine 2005; **Med School:** Temple Univ 1990; **Resid:** Obstetrics & Gynecology, Univ Hosp-UMDNJ 1994; **Fellow:** Maternal & Fetal Medicine, Univ Hosp-UMDNJ 1996

Medical Oncology

Fitzgerald, Denis MD (Onc) - **Spec Exp:** Breast Cancer; Lung Cancer; Hemochromatosis; Lymphoma, Non-Hodgkin's; **Hospital:** Riverview Med Ctr; **Address:** 180 White Rd, Ste 101, Little Silver, NJ 07739; **Phone:** 732-530-8666; **Board Cert:** Internal Medicine 1981; Medical Oncology 1985; Hematology 1986; **Med School:** SUNY Hlth Sci Ctr 1978; **Resid:** Internal Medicine, St Vincents Hosp Med Ctr 1982; **Fellow:** Hematology & Oncology, Strong Meml Hosp 1985

Greenberg, Susan N MD (Onc) - **Spec Exp:** Breast Cancer; Lung Cancer; Palliative Care; **Hospital:** Jersey Shore Univ Med Ctr, Monmouth Med Ctr; **Address:** 39 Sycamore Ave, Little Silver, NJ 07739-1208; **Phone:** 732-576-8610; **Board Cert:** Internal Medicine 1981; Medical Oncology 1983; **Med School:** Med Coll PA Hahnemann 1978; **Resid:** Internal Medicine, Hosp Med Coll Penn 1981; **Fellow:** Hematology & Oncology, Columbia-Presby Med Ctr 1983

Kane, Michael J MD (Onc) - **Spec Exp:** Breast Cancer; Colon Cancer; Lung Cancer; **Hospital:** Bayshore Community Hosp; **Address:** Bayshore Hosp Cancer Program, 7200-B Cambridge St, Ste E5.101, Holmdel, NJ 07733; **Phone:** 732-888-1345; **Board Cert:** Internal Medicine 1986; Medical Oncology 1989; **Med School:** UMDNJ-NJ Med Sch, Newark 1983; **Resid:** Internal Medicine, Thomas Jefferson Univ Hosp 1986; **Fellow:** Medical Oncology, Mount Sinai Hosp 1988; **Fac Appt:** Assoc Clin Prof Med, UMDNJ-RW Johnson Med Sch

Sharon, David J MD (Onc) - **Spec Exp:** Breast Cancer; Lung Cancer; Gastrointestinal Cancer; Hematologic Malignancies; **Hospital:** Monmouth Med Ctr; **Address:** The Cancer Ctr - Monmouth Med Ctr, 100 State Highway 36, Ste 1B, West Long Branch, NJ 07764-6205; **Phone:** 732-222-1711; **Board Cert:** Internal Medicine 1980; Medical Oncology 1983; **Med School:** NY Med Coll 1977; **Resid:** Internal Medicine, Beth Israel Med Ctr 1980; **Fellow:** Medical Oncology, Mount Sinai Med Ctr 1982

Walsh, Christina MD (Onc) - **Spec Exp:** Cancer Genetics; Breast Cancer; **Hospital:** Riverview Med Ctr; **Address:** 180 White Rd, Ste 101, Little Silver, NJ 07739; **Phone:** 732-530-8666; **Board Cert:** Internal Medicine 1980; Hematology 1982; Medical Oncology 1985; **Med School:** Georgetown Univ 1977; **Resid:** Internal Medicine, Georgetown Univ Hosp 1980; **Fellow:** Hematology, Georgetown Univ Hosp 1981; Hematology & Oncology, NYU Medical Ctr 1984

Neonatal-Perinatal Medicine

Graff, Michael MD (NP) - **Spec Exp:** Neonatology; **Hospital:** Jersey Shore Univ Med Ctr, Ocean Med Ctr; **Address:** JSUMC-Dept Pediatrics, 1945 State Route 33, Neptune, NJ 07754; **Phone:** 732-776-4283; **Board Cert:** Pediatrics 1981; Neonatal-Perinatal Medicine 1983; **Med School:** Italy 1977; **Resid:** Pediatrics, NYU Medical Ctr 1980; **Fellow:** Neurology, Columbia Presby 1982; **Fac Appt:** Assoc Clin Prof Ped, UMDNJ-RW Johnson Med Sch

Nephrology

Flis, Raymond S DO (Nep) - **Spec Exp:** Hypertension; Kidney Disease; **Hospital:** Riverview Med Ctr, Monmouth Med Ctr; **Address:** 6 Industrial Way W, Ste B, Eatontown, NJ 07724-2268; **Phone:** 732-460-1200; **Board Cert:** Internal Medicine 1974; Nephrology 1976; **Med School:** Kirksville Coll Osteo Med 1971; **Resid:** Internal Medicine, Cooper Hosp 1974; **Fellow:** Nephrology, Thomas Jefferson Univ Hosp 1975; Nephrology, Temple Univ Hosp 1976; **Fac Appt:** Assoc Clin Prof Med, Drexel Univ Coll Med

Manning, Eric C MD/PhD (Nep) - **Spec Exp:** Hypertension; **Hospital:** Robert Wood Johnson Univ Hosp - New Brunswick, Somerset Med Ctr; **Address:** 719 Route 206, Ste 100, Hillsborough, NJ 08844; **Phone:** 908-904-9055; **Board Cert:** Internal Medicine 1989; Nephrology 2002; **Med School:** UC Davis 1985; **Resid:** Internal Medicine, Boston Univ Hosp 1988; **Fellow:** Nephrology, Boston Univ Hosp 1992

Neurological Surgery

Rosenblum, Bruce R MD (NS) - **Spec Exp:** Spinal Surgery; Brain Tumors; Pain-Back & Neck; Chiari's Deformity; **Hospital:** Riverview Med Ctr, Bayshore Community Hosp; **Address:** 160 Ave at the Commons, Shrewsbury, NJ 07702; **Phone:** 732-460-1522; **Board Cert:** Neurological Surgery 1991; **Med School:** Mount Sinai Sch Med 1982; **Resid:** Neurological Surgery, Mount Sinai Med Ctr 1988; **Fellow:** Stroke, Natl Inst Health 1986

Neurology

Gilson, Noah R MD (N) - **Spec Exp:** Multiple Sclerosis; Headache; Parkinson's Disease; **Hospital:** Monmouth Med Ctr, Riverview Med Ctr; **Address:** 107 Monmouth Rd, Ste 110, West Long Branch, NJ 07764; **Phone:** 732-935-1850; **Board Cert:** Neurology 1987; Vascular Neurology 2009; **Med School:** Loyola Univ-Stritch Sch Med 1982; **Resid:** Neurology, Mount Sinai Hosp 1986

Herman, Martin MD (N) - **Spec Exp:** Epilepsy; Stroke; **Hospital:** Monmouth Med Ctr, Riverview Med Ctr; **Address:** 107 Monmouth Rd, Ste 110, West Long Branch, NJ 07764-1000; **Phone:** 732-935-1850; **Board Cert:** Neurology 1973; **Med School:** Northwestern Univ 1964; **Resid:** Psychiatry, Strong Meml Hosp 1965; Neurology, Univ VA Hlth Sci Ctr 1970; **Fellow:** Clinical Neurophysiology, Columbia-Presby Hosp 1971; **Fac Appt:** Assoc Clin Prof N, Drexel Univ Coll Med

Holland, Neil R MD (N) - **Spec Exp:** Neuromuscular Disorders; Peripheral Neuropathy; Electro-diagnosis; Migraine; **Hospital:** Monmouth Med Ctr, Riverview Med Ctr; **Address:** 107 Monmouth Rd, Ste 110, West Long Branch, NJ 07764; **Phone:** 732-935-1850; **Board Cert:** Neurology 2000; Clinical Neurophysiology 2001; Electrodiagnostic Medicine 2007; Neuromuscular Medicine 2008; **Med School:** England, UK 1991; **Resid:** Neurology, Johns Hopkins Univ Hosp 1996; **Fellow:** Clinical Neurophysiology, Johns Hopkins Univ Hosp 1997; **Fac Appt:** Asst Prof N, Drexel Univ Coll Med

Silbert, Paul J MD (N) - **Spec Exp:** Parkinson's Disease; Migraine; Carpal Tunnel Syndrome; **Hospital:** Jersey Shore Univ Med Ctr; **Address:** 2100 Corlies Ave, Ste 10, Neptune, NJ 07753-6116; **Phone:** 732-776-8866; **Board Cert:** Neurology 1980; **Med School:** Jefferson Med Coll 1971; **Resid:** Neurology, Columbia-Presby Med Ctr 1975; **Fac Appt:** Asst Clin Prof N, Robert W Johnson Med Sch

Neuroradiology

Lu, Stanley MD (NRad) - **Hospital:** Monmouth Med Ctr; **Address:** Shrewsbury Diagnostic Imaging, 1131 Broad St, Shrewsbury, NJ 07702; **Phone:** 732-578-9640; **Board Cert:** Diagnostic Radiology 2004; Neuroradiology 2006; **Med School:** NYU Sch Med 1999; **Resid:** Dermatopathology, NYU Med Ctr 2004; **Fellow:** Neurological Radiology, Stanford Univ Med Ctr 2005

Obstetrics & Gynecology

Goldstein, Steven A MD (ObG) - **Spec Exp:** Ultrasound; Menopause Problems; Laparoscopic Hysterectomy; Minimally Invasive Surgery; **Hospital:** CentraState Med Ctr, Monmouth Med Ctr; **Address:** 501 Iron Bridge Rd, Ste 4, Freehold, NJ 07728; **Phone:** 732-431-1807; **Board Cert:** Obstetrics & Gynecology 2009; **Med School:** SUNY Downstate 1985; **Resid:** Obstetrics & Gynecology, RW Johnson Univ Hosp 1989

Seigel, Mark J MD (ObG) - **Spec Exp:** Adolescent Gynecology; Minimally Invasive Surgery; Menopause Problems; **Hospital:** CentraState Med Ctr, Monmouth Med Ctr; **Address:** 501 Iron Bridge Rd, Ste 4, Freehold, NJ 07728-5305; **Phone:** 732-431-1807; **Board Cert:** Obstetrics & Gynecology 2009; **Med School:** Geo Wash Univ 1980; **Resid:** Obstetrics & Gynecology, Columbia-Presby Med Ctr 1984

Ophthalmology

Engel, Mark L MD (Oph) - **Spec Exp:** Cataract Surgery; Glaucoma; **Hospital:** Bayshore Community Hosp, Riverview Med Ctr; **Address:** 733 N Beers St, Ste U4, Holmdel, NJ 07733-1528; **Phone:** 732-739-0707; **Board Cert:** Ophthalmology 1977; **Med School:** SUNY Downstate 1971; **Resid:** Ophthalmology, SUNY Downstate 1975

Goldberg, Daniel MD (Oph) - **Spec Exp:** LASIK-Refractive Surgery; Cornea Transplant; Cataract Surgery; Lens Implants; **Address:** Atlantic Laser Vision Center, 180 White Rd, Ste 202, Little Silver, NJ 07739-1166; **Phone:** 732-219-9220; **Board Cert:** Ophthalmology 1979; **Med School:** SUNY Downstate 1974; **Resid:** Ophthalmology, SUNY Downstate 1978; **Fellow:** Cornea, Eye & Ear Hosp 1979; **Fac Appt:** Assoc Clin Prof Oph, Drexel Univ Coll Med

Talansky, Marvin MD (Oph) - **Spec Exp:** Cataract Surgery; Diabetic Eye Disease; LASIK-Refractive Surgery; Eyelid Cosmetic Surgery; **Hospital:** Jersey Shore Univ Med Ctr, Monmouth Med Ctr; **Address:** 3333 Fairmont Ave, Asbury Park, NJ 07712; **Phone:** 732-988-4000; **Board Cert:** Ophthalmology 1978; **Med School:** Med Univ SC 1973; **Resid:** Ophthalmology, Storm Eye Inst 1978; **Fellow:** Retina, Storm Eye Inst 1986

Turtel, Lawrence S MD (Oph) - **Spec Exp:** Pediatric Ophthalmology; Strabismus; **Hospital:** Jersey Shore Univ Med Ctr, Monmouth Med Ctr; **Address:** 3333 Fairmount Ave, Asbury Park, NJ 07712; **Phone:** 732-988-4000; **Board Cert:** Ophthalmology 2003; **Med School:** Columbia P&S 1986; **Resid:** Ophthalmology, St Vincents Hosp 1990; **Fellow:** Pediatric Ophthalmology, Manhattan EE&T Hosp 1991

Orthopaedic Surgery

Bade III, Harry A MD (OrS) - **Spec Exp:** Joint Replacement; Shoulder Arthroscopic Surgery; Hand Surgery; Arthroscopic Surgery-Knee; **Hospital:** Monmouth Med Ctr, Riverview Med Ctr; **Address:** Professional Orthopedics Assoc, 776 Shrewsbury Ave, Ste 201, Tinton Falls, NJ 07724-3006; **Phone:** 732-530-4949 x218; **Board Cert:** Orthopaedic Surgery 1984; Orthopaedic Sports Medicine 2007; **Med School:** Jefferson Med Coll 1976; **Resid:** Surgery, Roosevelt Hosp 1978; Orthopaedic Surgery, Hosp for Special Surg 1981; **Fellow:** Shoulder Surgery, Hosp for Special Surg 1982; Hand Surgery, Roosevelt Hosp 1982

Grossman, Robert B MD (OrS) - **Spec Exp:** Knee Surgery; **Hospital:** Monmouth Med Ctr, Riverview Med Ctr; **Address:** 35 Gilbert St S, Tinton Falls, NJ 07701-4917; **Phone:** 732-530-1515; **Board Cert:** Orthopaedic Surgery 1978; **Med School:** Univ MD Sch Med 1972; **Resid:** Orthopaedic Surgery, Univ Vermont Med Ctr 1976; **Fellow:** Sports Medicine, Lenox Hill Hosp 1977; **Fac Appt:** Assoc Prof OrS, Hahnemann Univ

Otolaryngology

Rossos, Apostolos AP MD (Oto) - **Spec Exp:** Pediatric Otolaryngology; Sinus Disorders; Hearing Disorders; **Hospital:** CentraState Med Ctr, Robert Wood Johnson Univ Hosp Hamilton; **Address:** 501 Iron Bridge Rd, Ste 11, Freehold, NJ 07728-5305; **Phone:** 732-409-2500; **Board Cert:** Otolaryngology 1988; **Med School:** Grenada 1981; **Resid:** Surgery, UMDNJ Hosps 1983; Otolaryngology, UMDNJ Hosps 1986

Scaccia, Frank J MD (Oto) - **Spec Exp:** Cosmetic Surgery-Face; Rhinoplasty; Nasal & Sinus Surgery; **Hospital:** Riverview Med Ctr, Bayshore Community Hosp; **Address:** Riverside Plastic Surgery & Sinus Ctr, 70 E Front St Fl 3, Red Bank, NJ 07701; **Phone:** 732-747-5300; **Board Cert:** Otolaryngology 1993; Facial Plastic & Reconstr Surgery 1995; **Med School:** Wake Forest Univ 1985; **Resid:** Surgery, Monmouth Med Ctr 1988; Otolaryngology, Univ Hosp Cleveland 1992

Shah, Darsit K MD (Oto) - **Spec Exp:** Head & Neck Cancer & Surgery; Thyroid & Parathyroid Surgery; Parotid Surgery; Neuro-Otology; **Hospital:** Monmouth Med Ctr; **Address:** Central Jersey Otolaryngology, 1131 Broad St, Shrewsbury, NJ 07702; **Phone:** 732-389-3388; **Board Cert:** Otolaryngology 1997; **Med School:** Med Coll PA 1991; **Resid:** Surgery, Mt Sinai Hosp 1992; Otolaryngology, Mt Sinai Hosp 1996; **Fellow:** Neurotology, Michigan Ear Inst; **Fac Appt:** Asst Clin Prof Oto, Drexel Univ Coll Med

Pain Medicine

Bram, Harris MD (PM) - **Spec Exp:** Pain-Back & Neck; Complex Regional Pain Syndrome; **Hospital:** Monmouth Med Ctr, CentraState Med Ctr; **Address:** 200 White Rd, Ste 205, Little Silver, NJ 07739; **Phone:** 732-345-1180; **Board Cert:** Anesthesiology 1993; Pain Medicine 2004; **Med School:** Univ Ark 1988; **Resid:** Anesthesiology, Hahnemann Unin Hosp 1992; **Fellow:** Pain Medicine, TJefferson Univ Hosp 1993

Haber, Daran MD (PM) - **Spec Exp:** Pain-Back & Neck; Reflex Sympathetic Dystrophy (RSD); Pain-Musculoskeletal; Pain-Neuropathic; **Hospital:** Riverview Med Ctr; **Address:** One River View Plaza, Red Bank, NJ 07701-1864; **Phone:** 732-741-2700; **Board Cert:** Anesthesiology 1992; Pain Medicine 2007; **Med School:** Puerto Rico 1986; **Resid:** Anesthesiology, New Jersey Hosp 1989; Anesthesiology, Albert Einstein Coll Med 1989; **Fellow:** Anesthesiology, Albert Einstein Coll Med 1990; Pain Medicine, Yale-New Haven Hosp 1991

Staats, Peter MD (PM) - **Spec Exp:** Pain-Cancer; Pain-Back; **Hospital:** Riverview Med Ctr, CentraState Med Ctr; **Address:** Metzger Staats Pain Mgmt, 160 Avenue at the Commons, Ste 1, Shrewsbury, NJ 07702; **Phone:** 732-380-0200; **Board Cert:** Anesthesiology 1994; Pain Medicine 2005; **Med School:** Univ Mich Med Sch 1989; **Resid:** Anesthesiology, Johns Hopkins Hosp 1993; **Fellow:** Pain Medicine, Johns Hopkins Hosp 1994

Pediatric Endocrinology

Meyers-Seifer, Cynthia H MD (PEn) - **Spec Exp:** Diabetes; Thyroid Disorders; Growth Disorders; **Hospital:** Jersey Shore Univ Med Ctr, Riverview Med Ctr; **Address:** Jersey Shore Univ Med Ctr-Pediatrics, 1944 Route 33, Ste 204, Neptune, NJ 07753; **Phone:** 732-776-4860; **Board Cert:** Pediatrics 2005; Pediatric Endocrinology 2003; **Med School:** Stanford Univ 1984; **Resid:** Pediatrics, Stanford Univ Hosp 1986; Pediatrics, Univ Hosp 1987; **Fellow:** Anatomic Pathology, Univ Hosp-SUNY 1989; Pediatric Endocrinology, Yale Sch Med 1993

Pediatric Infectious Disease

Fisher, Margaret C MD (PInf) - **Spec Exp:** Pediatric Infections; **Hospital:** Monmouth Med Ctr; **Address:** The Children's Hosp at Monmouth Med Ctr, 300 Second Ave, Stanley 209, Long Branch, NJ 07740; **Phone:** 732-923-7251; **Board Cert:** Pediatrics 1980; Pediatric Infectious Disease 2008; **Med School:** UCLA 1975; **Resid:** Pediatrics, St Chris Hosp Chldn 1978; **Fellow:** Pediatric Infectious Disease, St Chris Hosp Chldn 1980; **Fac Appt:** Prof Ped, Drexel Univ Coll Med

Pediatric Otolaryngology

Tavill, Michael A MD (PO) - **Hospital:** Monmouth Med Ctr; **Address:** Central Jersey Otolaryngology, 1131 Broad St A Bldg, Shrewsbury, NJ 07702; **Phone:** 732-389-3388; **Board Cert:** Otolaryngology 1997; **Med School:** Case West Res Univ 1991; **Resid:** Otolaryngology, Hosp Univ Penn 1996; **Fellow:** Pediatric Otolaryngology, Childrens Hosp 1997

Pediatrics

Murphy, Robert D MD (Ped) *PCP* - **Spec Exp:** ADD/ADHD; Asthma; Vaccines; Infectious Disease; **Hospital:** Monmouth Med Ctr; **Address:** 223 Monmouth Rd, Ste 1, West Long Branch, NJ 07764-1029; **Phone:** 732-229-4540; **Board Cert:** Pediatrics 1982; **Med School:** Vanderbilt Univ 1977; **Resid:** Pediatrics, Yale-New Haven Hosp 1980

Physical Medicine & Rehabilitation

Braddom, Randall L MD (PMR) - **Spec Exp:** Electromyography; Pain-Neck; Pain-Low Back; Musculoskeletal Disorders; **Hospital:** Riverview Med Ctr; **Address:** Orthopaedic, Sports Medicine & Rehab Ctr, 80 Oak Hill Rd, rm 368, Red Bank, NJ 07701; **Phone:** 732-741-2313; **Board Cert:** Physical Medicine & Rehabilitation 1974; **Med School:** Ohio State Univ 1968; **Resid:** Physical Medicine & Rehabilitation, Ohio State Univ Hosp 1973; **Fac Appt:** Clin Prof PMR, UMDNJ-NJ Med Sch, Newark

Plastic Surgery

Chidyllo, Stephen A MD/DDS (PlS) - **Spec Exp:** Cosmetic Surgery-Face; Cosmetic Surgery-Breast; Body Contouring; Breast Reconstruction; **Hospital:** Monmouth Med Ctr, Riverview Med Ctr; **Address:** Central Jersey Plastic Surgery, 107 Monmouth Rd, Ste 106, West Long Branch, NJ 07764; **Phone:** 732-460-9566; **Board Cert:** Plastic Surgery 2003; **Med School:** Hahnemann Univ 1987; **Resid:** Surgery, NY Infirm-Beekman Downtown Hosp 1990; Plastic Surgery, Univ Illinois Med Ctr 1992; **Fellow:** Craniofacial Surgery, Eastern Va Med Sch 1993; **Fac Appt:** Assoc Clin Prof S, Drexel Univ Coll Med

Dudick, Stephen T MD (PlS) - **Spec Exp:** Breast Reconstruction & Augmentation; Cosmetic Surgery; Cleft Palate/Lip; Body Contouring after Weight Loss; **Hospital:** Jersey Shore Univ Med Ctr, Monmouth Med Ctr; **Address:** 252 Broad St, Red Bank, NJ 07701; **Phone:** 732-741-1303; **Board Cert:** Plastic Surgery 1993; **Med School:** Mexico 1975; **Resid:** Surgery, St Vincents Hosp 1981; Plastic Surgery, Indiana Univ Med Ctr 1983

Glicksman, Caroline A MD (PlS) - **Spec Exp:** Breast Reconstruction & Augmentation; Cosmetic Surgery-Breast; Liposuction & Body Contouring; Rhinoplasty; **Hospital:** Jersey Shore Univ Med Ctr; **Address:** 2164 Hwy 35, Bldg A, Sea Girt, NJ 08750; **Phone:** 732-974-2424; **Board Cert:** Plastic Surgery 1994; **Med School:** SUNY Downstate 1985; **Resid:** Surgery, Mt Sinai Hosp 1988; Plastic Surgery, NY Hosp-Cornell Med Ctr 1991; **Fellow:** Cosmetic Plastic Surgery, Mass Genl Hosp-Newton Wellesley Hosp 1992

Hetzler, Peter T MD (PlS) - **Spec Exp:** Breast Cosmetic & Reconstructive Surgery; Liposuction & Body Contouring; Melanoma; **Hospital:** Riverview Med Ctr, Monmouth Med Ctr; **Address:** 200 White Rd, Ste 211, Little Silver, NJ 07739-1162; **Phone:** 732-219-0447; **Board Cert:** Plastic Surgery 1991; **Med School:** Univ Mich Med Sch 1981; **Resid:** Surgery, MS Hershey Med Ctr 1986; Plastic/Reconstructive Surgery, MS Hershey Med Ctr 1988; **Fellow:** Microsurgery, York Hosp Trauma Ctr 1988; Cosmetic Plastic Surgery, Manhattan Eye & Ear Hosp 1989

Rose, Michael I MD (PlS) - **Spec Exp:** Body Contouring after Weight Loss; Cosmetic Surgery-Face; Eyelid Cosmetic & Reconstructive Surgery; Cosmetic Surgery-Breast; **Hospital:** Jersey Shore Univ Med Ctr, CentraState Med Ctr; **Address:** Plastic Surgery Center, 535 Sycamore Ave, Shrewsbury, NJ 07702; **Phone:** 732-741-0970; **Board Cert:** Surgery 2009; Plastic Surgery 2003; **Med School:** NYU Sch Med 1994; **Resid:** Surgery, NYU/Bellevue Med Ctr 2000; **Fellow:** Plastic Surgery, Emory Univ Med Ctr 2002

Samra, Said A MD (PlS) - **Spec Exp:** Reconstructive Surgery; Hand Surgery; Cosmetic Surgery; **Hospital:** Bayshore Community Hosp, Raritan Bay Med Ctr - Perth Amboy; **Address:** 733 N Beers St, Ste U-1, Holmdel, NJ 07733-1528; **Phone:** 732-739-2100; **Board Cert:** Plastic Surgery 1988; **Med School:** Syria 1973; **Resid:** Surgery, UMDNJ-NJ Med Sch 1980; Plastic Surgery, St Barnabas Hosp 1982; **Fellow:** Surgery, UMDNJ-NJ Med Sch 1978

Zaccaria, Alan MD (PlS) - **Spec Exp:** Breast Cosmetic & Reconstructive Surgery; Cosmetic Surgery-Face & Body; Botox Therapy; Wound Healing/Care; **Hospital:** Jersey Shore Univ Med Ctr, Monmouth Med Ctr; **Address:** 180 White Rd, Ste 102, Little Silver, NJ 07739; **Phone:** 732-530-8565; **Board Cert:** Surgery 2003; Plastic Surgery 2005; **Med School:** UMDNJ-RW Johnson Med Sch 1986; **Resid:** Surgery, Monmouth Med Ctr 1991; **Fellow:** Plastic Surgery, Univ Illinois 1993

Psychiatry

Rubin, Kenneth MD (Psyc) - **Spec Exp:** Mood Disorders; Anxiety Disorders; Dementia; **Hospital:** Monmouth Med Ctr; **Address:** 170 Morris Ave, Ste D, Long Branch, NJ 07740-6660; **Phone:** 732-870-3535; **Board Cert:** Psychiatry 1979; **Med School:** SUNY Downstate 1974; **Resid:** Psychiatry, Kings County Hosp 1977; **Fac Appt:** Assoc Clin Prof Psyc, Drexel Univ Coll Med

Pulmonary Disease

Davis, George MD (Pul) - **Spec Exp:** Critical Care; Chronic Obstructive Lung Disease (COPD); Sepsis; **Hospital:** Monmouth Med Ctr; **Address:** 279 3rd Ave, Ste 510, Long Branch, NJ 07740; **Phone:** 732-870-0650; **Board Cert:** Internal Medicine 1976; Pulmonary Disease 1980; Critical Care Medicine 2001; **Med School:** Hahnemann Univ 1972; **Resid:** Internal Medicine, Monmouth Med Ctr 1977; **Fellow:** Pulmonary Disease, Monmouth Med Ctr 1979

Markowitz, Daniel MD (Pul) - **Spec Exp:** Critical Care; **Hospital:** Jersey Shore Univ Med Ctr; **Address:** 2640 Hwy 70 6A Bldg, Manasquan, NJ 08736-2610; **Phone:** 732-528-5900; **Board Cert:** Internal Medicine 1974; Pulmonary Disease 1976; Critical Care Medicine 2001; **Med School:** Albert Einstein Coll Med 1971; **Resid:** Internal Medicine, Univ Mich Med Ctr 1974; **Fellow:** Pulmonary Critical Care Medicine, Univ Mich Med Ctr 1976

Reproductive Endocrinology

Damien, Miguel MD (RE) - **Hospital:** Riverview Med Ctr, Monmouth Med Ctr; **Address:** East Coast Infertility & IVF, 200 White Rd, Ste 214, Little Silver, NJ 07739; **Phone:** 732-758-6511 x111; **Board Cert:** Obstetrics & Gynecology 1998; Reproductive Endocrinology 1998; **Med School:** Dartmouth Med Sch 1982; **Resid:** Obstetrics & Gynecology, Beth Israel Deaconess Hosp 1986; **Fellow:** Reproductive Endocrinology, Harvard Med Sch 1988; Reproductive Endocrinology, Univ Conn 1989

Rheumatology

Schwartzberg, Mori MD (Rhu) - **Spec Exp:** Rheumatoid Arthritis; Spondylitis; Osteoarthritis; **Hospital:** Jersey Shore Univ Med Ctr; **Address:** 10 Neptune Blvd, Ste 106, Neptune, NJ 07753-4848; **Phone:** 732-988-5030; **Board Cert:** Internal Medicine 1976; Rheumatology 1978; **Med School:** SUNY Upstate Med Univ 1973; **Resid:** Internal Medicine, Nassau County Med Ctr 1976; **Fellow:** Rheumatology, Albert Einstein Med Ctr 1978; **Fac Appt:** Asst Clin Prof Med, UMDNJ-RW Johnson Med Sch

Wasser, Kenneth B MD (Rhu) - **Spec Exp:** Rheumatoid Arthritis; Lupus Nephritis; Psoriatic Arthritis; **Hospital:** Riverview Med Ctr, Monmouth Med Ctr; **Address:** 43 Gilbert St N, Ste 7, Tinton Falls, NJ 07701; **Phone:** 732-530-7999; **Board Cert:** Internal Medicine 1981; Rheumatology 1982; **Med School:** Case West Res Univ 1977; **Resid:** Internal Medicine, Univ Hosps 1980; Rheumatology, Univ Hosps 1982; **Fac Appt:** Asst Clin Prof Med, Drexel Univ Coll Med

Sports Medicine

Rice, Stephen G MD/PhD (SM) - **Spec Exp:** Primary Care Sports Medicine; Musculoskeletal Injuries; **Hospital:** Jersey Shore Univ Med Ctr; **Address:** Jersey Shore Sports Med Ctr, 51 Davis Ave, Ste S1-02, Neptune, NJ 07753; **Phone:** 732-776-2433; **Board Cert:** Pediatrics 1981; Sports Medicine 2004; **Med School:** NYU Sch Med 1974; **Resid:** Pediatrics, Chldn's Hosp Med Ctr 1977; **Fac Appt:** Assoc Clin Prof Ped, UMDNJ-RW Johnson Med Sch

Sclafani, Michael MD (SM) - **Spec Exp:** Knee Injuries/Ligament Surgery; Shoulder Instability; **Hospital:** Jersey Shore Univ Med Ctr; **Address:** Orthopedic Inst, 2315 Route 34 S, Manasquan, NJ 08736; **Phone:** 732-974-0404; **Board Cert:** Orthopaedic Surgery 2007; **Med School:** NYU Sch Med 1988; **Resid:** Orthopaedic Surgery, NYU Med Ctr 1993; **Fellow:** Sports Medicine, American Sports Med Inst 1994

Surgery

Arbour, Robert MD (S) - **Spec Exp:** Breast Surgery; Colon & Rectal Surgery; Biliary Surgery; Hernia; **Hospital:** Bayshore Community Hosp, Riverview Med Ctr; **Address:** 213 Main St, Matawan, NJ 07747-3285; **Phone:** 732-566-2363; **Board Cert:** Surgery 1972; **Med School:** UMDNJ-NJ Med Sch, Newark 1965; **Resid:** Surgery, Georgetown Univ Hosp 1971

Borao, Frank J MD (S) - **Spec Exp:** Laparoscopic Abdominal Surgery; Obesity/Bariatric Surgery; Gastroesophageal Reflux Disease (GERD); Critical Care; **Hospital:** Monmouth Med Ctr; **Address:** 1131 Broad St, Ste 105, Shrewsbury, NJ 07702; **Phone:** 732-389-1331; **Board Cert:** Surgery 2000; **Med School:** UMDNJ-NJ Med Sch, Newark 1994; **Resid:** Surgery, Monmouth Med Ctr 1999; **Fellow:** Laparoscopic Surgery, White Plains Hosp 2000; **Fac Appt:** Asst Clin Prof S, Hahnemann Univ

Goldfarb, Michael A MD (S) - **Spec Exp:** Breast Surgery; Telemedicine; **Hospital:** Monmouth Med Ctr; **Address:** 279 Third Ave, Ste 103, Long Branch, NJ 07740-6413; **Phone:** 732-870-6060; **Board Cert:** Surgery 1973; **Med School:** NYU Sch Med 1967; **Resid:** Surgery, Beth Israel Med Ctr 1972; **Fac Appt:** Prof S, Drexel Univ Coll Med

Schreiber, Martha L MD (S) - **Spec Exp:** Breast Disease; Breast Cancer; **Hospital:** Ocean Med Ctr, Jersey Shore Univ Med Ctr; **Address:** 1540 Hwy 138, Ste 201, Wall, NJ 07719; **Phone:** 732-280-0020; **Board Cert:** Surgery 2000; **Med School:** UMDNJ-RW Johnson Med Sch 1977; **Resid:** Surgery, Monmouth Med Ctr 1982

Thoracic Surgery

Neibart, Richard M MD (TS) - **Spec Exp:** Coronary Artery Surgery; Cardiac Surgery; **Hospital:** Jersey Shore Univ Med Ctr; **Address:** 1944 Route 33, Ste 201, Neptune, NJ 07753-4463; **Phone:** 732-776-4618; **Board Cert:** Surgery 1997; Thoracic Surgery 1999; **Med School:** Mount Sinai Sch Med 1982; **Resid:** Surgery, St Vincents Med Ctr 1987; **Fellow:** Thoracic Surgery, Jackson Meml Hosp 1989

Urology

Ebani, Jack MD (U) - **Spec Exp:** Prostate Cancer; Incontinence; **Hospital:** Jersey Shore Univ Med Ctr, Ocean Med Ctr; **Address:** 1820 Corlies Ave, Neptune, NJ 07753-4860; **Phone:** 732-774-4551; **Board Cert:** Urology 2006; **Med School:** SUNY Hlth Sci Ctr 1979; **Resid:** Surgery, North Shore Univ Hosp 1981; Urology, NYU Med Ctr 1985

Geltzeiler, Jules MD (U) - **Spec Exp:** Prostate Cancer; Incontinence; **Hospital:** Monmouth Med Ctr, Jersey Shore Univ Med Ctr; **Address:** NJ Urological Inst, 279 3rd Ave, Ste 101, Long Branch, NJ 07740-6205; **Phone:** 732-222-2111; **Board Cert:** Urology 2004; **Med School:** Hahnemann Univ 1979; **Resid:** Surgery, Monmouth Med Ctr 1981; Urology, Geo Wash Univ Med Ctr 1984; **Fac Appt:** Asst Clin Prof S, Drexel Univ Coll Med

Grebler, Arnold M MD (U) - **Spec Exp:** Urologic Cancer; Kidney Stones; Incontinence; Impotence; **Hospital:** Monmouth Med Ctr, Jersey Shore Univ Med Ctr; **Address:** NJ Urological Inst, 279 3rd Ave, Ste 101, Long Branch, NJ 07740; **Phone:** 732-222-2111; **Board Cert:** Urology 1982; **Med School:** Italy 1974; **Resid:** Surgery, Maimonides Med Ctr 1976; Urology, Maimonides Med Ctr 1979; **Fac Appt:** Assoc Clin Prof U, Hahnemann Univ

Litvin, Y Samuel MD (U) - **Spec Exp:** Infertility; Prostate Disease; **Hospital:** Monmouth Med Ctr, Riverview Med Ctr; **Address:** NJ Urological Inst, 279 3rd Ave, Ste 101, Long Branch, NJ 07740-6205; **Phone:** 732-222-2111; **Board Cert:** Urology 2003; **Med School:** UCLA 1986; **Resid:** Surgery, Beth Israel Med Ctr 1988; Urology, Beth Israel Med Ctr 1991

Rose, John G MD (U) - **Hospital:** Riverview Med Ctr, Bayshore Community Hosp; **Address:** 70 E Front St, Red Bank, NJ 07701-1851; **Phone:** 732-741-5923; **Board Cert:** Urology 1977; **Med School:** Cornell Univ-Weill Med Coll 1968; **Resid:** Surgery, Cornell Univ/NY Hosp 1970; Urology, Univ Virginia 1974

Rotolo, James MD (U) - **Spec Exp:** Prostate Disease; Urologic Cancer; Kidney Stones; **Hospital:** Ocean Med Ctr, Jersey Shore Univ Med Ctr; **Address:** 2401 Highway 35, Manasquan, NJ 08736; **Phone:** 732-223-7877; **Board Cert:** Urology 2010; **Med School:** Georgetown Univ 1984; **Resid:** Surgery, Georgetown Univ Hosp 1986; Urology, Georgetown Univ Hosp 1990

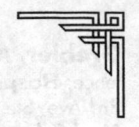

The Best in American Medicine
www.CastleConnolly.com

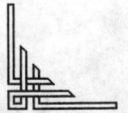
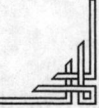

Morris

Morris

Adolescent Medicine

Rosenfeld, Walter D MD (AM) - **Spec Exp:** Eating Disorders; **Hospital:** Morristown Mem Hosp (page 92), Overlook Hosp (page 92); **Address:** Adolescent Medicine, 100 Madison Ave, Morristown, NJ 07962; **Phone:** 973-971-5199; **Board Cert:** Pediatrics 1980; Adolescent Medicine 2009; **Med School:** Temple Univ 1975; **Resid:** Pediatrics, Babies Hosp-Columbia Presby Med Ctr 1978; **Fellow:** Adolescent Medicine, Childrens Hosp 1979; **Fac Appt:** Prof Ped, UMDNJ-NJ Med Sch, Newark

Allergy & Immunology

Applebaum, Eric MD (A&I) - **Spec Exp:** Asthma; Food Allergy; Sinus Disorders; Rhinitis; **Hospital:** Morristown Mem Hosp (page 92), St Clare's Hosp - Denville; **Address:** 50 Cherry Hill Rd, Ste 301, Parsippany, NJ 07054-1101; **Phone:** 973-335-1700; **Board Cert:** Allergy & Immunology 2003; **Med School:** Albert Einstein Coll Med 1987; **Resid:** Internal Medicine, LI Jewish Med Ctr 1990; **Fellow:** Allergy & Immunology, LI Jewish Med Ctr 1992

Chernack, William J MD (A&I) - **Spec Exp:** Asthma; Sinus Disorders; Insect Allergies; **Hospital:** Morristown Mem Hosp (page 92), NYPresby-Morgan Stanley Children's Hosp (page 104); **Address:** 28 Franklin Pl, Morristown, NJ 07960-5305; **Phone:** 973-538-7271; **Board Cert:** Pediatrics 1975; Allergy & Immunology 1977; **Med School:** NY Med Coll 1970; **Resid:** Pediatrics, Columbia-Presby Med Ctr 1972; **Fellow:** Allergy & Immunology, Columbia-Presby Med Ctr 1974; **Fac Appt:** Asst Clin Prof Ped, Columbia P&S

Cardiac Electrophysiology

Winters, Stephen L MD (CE) - **Spec Exp:** Pacemakers/Defibrillators; Catheter Ablation; Atrial Fibrillation; Syncope; **Hospital:** Morristown Mem Hosp (page 92), Overlook Hosp (page 92); **Address:** Morristown Meml Hosp, 100 Madison Ave, Morristown, NJ 07962-6136; **Phone:** 973-971-4261; **Board Cert:** Internal Medicine 1982; Cardiovascular Disease 1985; Cardiac Electrophysiology 2002; **Med School:** Mount Sinai Sch Med 1979; **Resid:** Internal Medicine, Mt Sinai Med Ctr 1982; **Fellow:** Cardiovascular Disease, Mt Sinai Med Ctr 1985; Cardiac Electrophysiology, Mt Sinai Med Ctr 1986; **Fac Appt:** Assoc Prof Med, UMDNJ-NJ Med Sch, Newark

Cardiovascular Disease

Blick, Michael D MD (Cv) - **Spec Exp:** Cardiac Catheterization; **Hospital:** St Clare's Hosp - Dover, Morristown Mem Hosp (page 92); **Address:** Lakeland Cardiology, 765 Route 10 E, Randolph, NJ 07869; **Phone:** 973-989-2566; **Board Cert:** Internal Medicine 1985; Cardiovascular Disease 1987; **Med School:** Geo Wash Univ 1982; **Resid:** Internal Medicine, LI Jewish Med Ctr 1985; **Fellow:** Cardiovascular Disease, Philadelphia Heart Inst 1987

Blum, Mark A MD (Cv) - **Spec Exp:** Interventional Cardiology; Cholesterol/Lipid Disorders; Hypertrophic Cardiomyopathy; Preventive Cardiology; **Hospital:** Morristown Mem Hosp (page 92), Saint Barnabas Med Ctr; **Address:** 95 Madison Ave, Ste A-10, Morristown, NJ 07960; **Phone:** 973-889-9001; **Board Cert:** Internal Medicine 1986; Cardiovascular Disease 1989; Interventional Cardiology 1999; **Med School:** Mount Sinai Sch Med 1983; **Resid:** Internal Medicine, Montefiore Hosp Med Ctr 1985; Internal Medicine, Mt Sinai Hosp 1986; **Fellow:** Cardiovascular Disease, Mt Sinai Hosp 1988; Cardiovascular Disease, Newark Beth Israel Hosp 1989; **Fac Appt:** Asst Clin Prof Med, Mount Sinai Sch Med

Fisch, Arthur P MD (Cv) - **Spec Exp:** Echocardiography; Coronary Artery Disease; Heart Valve Disease; **Hospital:** Morristown Mem Hosp (page 92); **Address:** 182 South St, Ste 5, Morristown, NJ 07960-5350; **Phone:** 973-267-3944; **Board Cert:** Internal Medicine 1972; Cardiovascular Disease 1975; **Med School:** Boston Univ 1969; **Resid:** Internal Medicine, UCLA Med Ctr 1972; **Fellow:** Cardiovascular Disease, Hosp Univ Penn 1974

Lowell, Barry H MD (Cv) - **Spec Exp:** Interventional Cardiology; **Hospital:** St Clare's Hosp - Dover, Morristown Mem Hosp (page 92); **Address:** Morris Heart Assocs, 400 Valley Rd, Ste 102, Mount Arlington, NJ 07856; **Phone:** 973-770-7899; **Board Cert:** Internal Medicine 1986; Cardiovascular Disease 1989; Interventional Cardiology 1999; **Med School:** SUNY Stony Brook 1982; **Resid:** Internal Medicine, St Lukes Hosp 1985; **Fellow:** Cardiovascular Disease, St Lukes Hosp 1989

Raska, Karel MD (Cv) - **Spec Exp:** Preventive Cardiology; Hypertension; Echocardiography; **Hospital:** Morristown Mem Hosp (page 92); **Address:** 182 South St, Ste 5, Morristown, NJ 07960-5350; **Phone:** 973-267-3944; **Board Cert:** Cardiovascular Disease 2005; **Med School:** Harvard Med Sch 1989; **Resid:** Internal Medicine, Mass Genl Hosp 1992; **Fellow:** Cardiovascular Disease, Johns Hopkins Hosp 1995

Smart, Frank W MD (Cv) - **Spec Exp:** Congestive Heart Failure; Transplant Medicine-Heart; Ventricular Assist Device (LVAD); Pulmonary Hypertension; **Hospital:** Morristown Mem Hosp (page 92), Overlook Hosp (page 92); **Address:** Morristown Meml Hosp, Dept Cardiology, 100 Madison Ave, Box 5, Gagnon C Level, Morristown, NJ 07962; **Phone:** 973-971-4179; **Board Cert:** Internal Medicine 1988; Cardiovascular Disease 2001; **Med School:** Louisiana State U, New Orleans 1985; **Resid:** Internal Medicine, Ochsner Fdn Hosp 1988; **Fellow:** Cardiovascular Disease, Baylor Coll Med 1991; **Fac Appt:** Assoc Prof Med, Mount Sinai Sch Med

Child Neurology

Bennett, Harvey S MD (ChiN) - **Spec Exp:** Cerebral Palsy; Tourette's Syndrome; **Hospital:** Morristown Mem Hosp (page 92), Overlook Hosp (page 92); **Address:** Goryeb Children's Hosp, 100 Madison Ave, Box 24, Morristown, NJ 07962; **Phone:** 973-971-5700; **Board Cert:** Pediatrics 1979; Child Neurology 1991; **Med School:** Albert Einstein Coll Med 1975; **Resid:** Pediatrics, St Christopher's Hosp Chldn 1977; Child Neurology, Montefiore Med Ctr 1980; **Fac Appt:** Clin Prof N, Mount Sinai Sch Med

Grossman, Elliot A MD (ChiN) - **Spec Exp:** Migraine; ADD/ADHD; Tourette's Syndrome; Epilepsy; **Hospital:** Saint Barnabas Med Ctr, Morristown Mem Hosp (page 92); **Address:** 220 Ridgedale Ave, Ste A3, Florham Park, NJ 07932-1349; **Phone:** 973-966-6333; **Board Cert:** Pediatrics 1987; Child Neurology 1990; **Med School:** Meharry Med Coll 1980; **Resid:** Pediatrics, Bellevue Hosp 1982; Pediatrics, Boston Med Ctr 1983; **Fellow:** Pediatric Neurology, Boston Med Ctr 1986

Colon & Rectal Surgery

Moskowitz, Richard L MD (CRS) - **Spec Exp:** Colon & Rectal Cancer; Anorectal Disorders; Inflammatory Bowel Disease; **Hospital:** Morristown Mem Hosp (page 92), St Clare's Hosp - Dover; **Address:** 111 Madison Ave, Ste 312, Morristown, NJ 07960-6083; **Phone:** 973-267-1225; **Board Cert:** Surgery 2005; Colon & Rectal Surgery 1985; **Med School:** Penn State Univ-Hershey Med Ctr 1978; **Resid:** Surgery, LI Jewish-Hillside Med Ctr 1983; Colon & Rectal Surgery, Greater Baltimore Med Ctr 1984; **Fellow:** Colon & Rectal Surgery, St Marks Hosp 1985

Dermatology

Almeida, Laila N MD (D) - **Spec Exp:** Psoriasis; Acne; Skin Cancer; **Hospital:** St Clare's Hosp - Denville, NY-Presby Hosp/Columbia (page 104); **Address:** 199 Baldwin Rd, Ste 230, Parsippany, NJ 07054-2043; **Phone:** 973-335-2560; **Board Cert:** Internal Medicine 1986; Dermatology 1989; **Med School:** Univ Mich Med Sch 1983; **Resid:** Internal Medicine, Columbia-Presby 1986; Dermatology, Columbia-Presby 1989

Bisaccia, Emil MD (D) - **Spec Exp:** Skin Cancer; Cosmetic Dermatology; Botox Therapy; Mohs' Surgery; **Hospital:** Morristown Mem Hosp (page 92), NY-Presby Hosp/Columbia (page 104); **Address:** 182 South St, Ste 1, Morristown, NJ 07960; **Phone:** 973-267-0300; **Board Cert:** Dermatology 1984; Facial Plastic & Reconstr Surgery 1989; **Med School:** Med Coll OH 1979; **Resid:** Dermatology, Ohio State Univ Hosps 1982; Dermatology, Columbia Presby Hosp 1983; **Fac Appt:** Clin Prof D, Columbia P&S

Cooper, Lauren M MD (D) - **Spec Exp:** Sclerotherapy; Botox Therapy; Facial Rejuvenation; **Hospital:** Morristown Mem Hosp (page 92); **Address:** Affiliated Dermatologists, 182 South St, Morristown, NJ 07960; **Phone:** 973-267-0300; **Board Cert:** Dermatology 1988; **Med School:** NYU Sch Med 1984; **Resid:** Dermatology, Bellevue/NYU Med Ctr 1988

Marinaro, Robert E MD (D) - **Spec Exp:** Cosmetic Dermatology; Laser Surgery; **Hospital:** Morristown Mem Hosp (page 92); **Address:** 20 Community Pl, Morristown, NJ 07960-7501; **Phone:** 973-538-4544; **Board Cert:** Dermatology 1986; **Med School:** Univ Rochester 1981; **Resid:** Internal Medicine, Strong Meml Hosp 1983; Dermatology, Case Western Res Univ Hosps 1986

Diagnostic Radiology

Claps, Richard J MD (DR) - **Spec Exp:** Nuclear Medicine; Ultrasound; Mammography; **Hospital:** St Clare's Hosp - Denville; **Address:** 25 Pocono Rd, Denville, NJ 07834; **Phone:** 973-625-6000; **Board Cert:** Diagnostic Radiology 1973; Nuclear Medicine 1975; Nuclear Radiology 1978; **Med School:** NY Med Coll 1968; **Resid:** Diagnostic Radiology, Metropolitan Hosp 1972

Murphy, Robyn C MD (DR) - **Spec Exp:** Pediatric Radiology; **Hospital:** Morristown Mem Hosp (page 92); **Address:** Morristown Meml Hosp, Dept Radiology, 100 Madison Ave, Morristown, NJ 07960; **Phone:** 973-971-5370; **Board Cert:** Diagnostic Radiology 1997; Pediatric Radiology 1999; **Med School:** Med Coll VA 1992; **Resid:** Diagnostic Radiology, Columbia-Presby Med Ctr 1997; **Fellow:** Pediatric Radiology, NY-Presby Hosp 1998

Endocrinology, Diabetes & Metabolism

Nevin, Marie E MD (EDM) - **Hospital:** Morristown Mem Hosp (page 92); **Address:** 25 Lindsley Drive, Ste 203, Morristown, NJ 07960; **Phone:** 973-267-9099; **Board Cert:** Internal Medicine 1989; Endocrinology, Diabetes & Metabolism 2002; **Med School:** UMDNJ-NJ Med Sch, Newark 1986; **Resid:** Internal Medicine, Morristown Meml Hosp 1989; **Fellow:** Endocrinology, Mount Sinai Med Ctr 1991

Family Medicine

Holland Jr, Elbridge MD (FMed) *PCP* - **Hospital:** Overlook Hosp (page 92); **Address:** 492 Main St, Chatham, NJ 07928; **Phone:** 973-635-2432; **Board Cert:** Family Medicine 2002; Geriatric Medicine 2007; **Med School:** Univ Chicago-Pritzker Sch Med 1975; **Resid:** Family Medicine, Overlook Hosp 1978; **Fac Appt:** Asst Clin Prof FMed, UMDNJ-NJ Med Sch, Newark

Gastroenterology

Dalena, John M MD (Ge) - **Spec Exp:** Colon Cancer Screening; Endoscopy; Gastroesophageal Reflux Disease (GERD); Inflammatory Bowel Disease; **Hospital:** Morristown Mem Hosp (page 92); **Address:** 65 Ridgedale Ave, Cedar Knolls, NJ 07927; **Phone:** 973-401-0500; **Board Cert:** Internal Medicine 1988; Gastroenterology 2001; **Med School:** UMDNJ-NJ Med Sch, Newark 1985; **Resid:** Internal Medicine, Mount Sinai Hosp 1988; **Fellow:** Gastroenterology, UMDNJ-Univ Hosp 1990

Krupnick, Matthew MD (Ge) - **Spec Exp:** Colon Cancer; Crohn's Disease; Ulcerative Colitis; Gastroesophageal Reflux Disease (GERD); **Hospital:** St Clare's Hosp - Dover, St Clare's Hosp - Denville; **Address:** 369 W Blackwell St, Ste 120, Dover, NJ 07801; **Phone:** 973-361-7660; **Board Cert:** Gastroenterology 2005; **Med School:** Jefferson Med Coll 1990; **Resid:** Internal Medicine, NYU/Bellevue Med Ctr 1993; **Fellow:** Gastroenterology, NYU Med Ctr 1995

Samach, Michael MD (Ge) - **Spec Exp:** Colonoscopy; Gastroesophageal Reflux Disease (GERD); Hepatitis C; **Hospital:** Morristown Mem Hosp (page 92); **Address:** 101 Madison Ave, Ste 100, Morristown, NJ 07960; **Phone:** 973-455-0404; **Board Cert:** Internal Medicine 1974; Gastroenterology 1979; **Med School:** NYU Sch Med 1971; **Resid:** Internal Medicine, Montefiore Med Ctr 1974; **Fellow:** Gastroenterology, Montefiore Med Ctr 1978; **Fac Appt:** Asst Clin Prof Med, Mount Sinai Sch Med

Soriano, John G MD (Ge) - **Hospital:** St Clare's Hosp - Denville, Morristown Mem Hosp (page 92); **Address:** 16 Pocono Rd, Ste 201, Denville, NJ 07834; **Phone:** 973-627-4430; **Board Cert:** Internal Medicine 1986; Gastroenterology 2003; **Med School:** Mexico 1981; **Resid:** Internal Medicine, Morristown Meml Hosp 1987; **Fellow:** Gastroenterology, Long Island Coll Hosp 1989

Stein, Lawrence B MD (Ge) - **Spec Exp:** Hepatitis; Gastroesophageal Reflux Disease (GERD); Endoscopy; **Hospital:** Morristown Mem Hosp (page 92), Saint Barnabas Med Ctr; **Address:** 101 Madison Ave, Ste 102, Morristown, NJ 07960; **Phone:** 973-410-0960; **Board Cert:** Internal Medicine 1972; Gastroenterology 1973; **Med School:** Univ Minn 1965; **Resid:** Internal Medicine, Montefiore Med Ctr 1969; **Fellow:** Gastroenterology, Montefiore Med Ctr 1971

Geriatric Medicine

Ryan, Joseph MD (Ger) - **Spec Exp:** Dementia; **Hospital:** Morristown Mem Hosp (page 92); **Address:** 95 Madison Ave, Ste 411, Morristown, NJ 07962; **Phone:** 973-971-7022; **Board Cert:** Internal Medicine 1974; Gastroenterology 1981; **Med School:** SUNY Downstate 1970; **Resid:** Internal Medicine, Univ Hosp 1973; **Fellow:** Gastroenterology, St Vincent's Hosp & Med Ctr 1975; **Fac Appt:** Asst Prof Med, Columbia P&S

Gynecologic Oncology

Heller, Paul B MD (GO) - **Spec Exp:** Gynecologic Cancer; **Hospital:** Morristown Mem Hosp (page 92), Overlook Hosp (page 92); **Address:** Morristown Meml Hosp, Women's Cancer Ctr, 100 Madison Ave, Morristown, NJ 07960; **Phone:** 973-971-5900; **Board Cert:** Obstetrics & Gynecology 1975; Gynecologic Oncology 1982; **Med School:** NY Med Coll 1968; **Resid:** Obstetrics & Gynecology, Metroplitan Hosp 1971; Obstetrics & Gynecology, Beth Israel Med Ctr 1973; **Fellow:** Gynecologic Oncology, Metropolitan Hosp 1977; **Fac Appt:** Clin Prof ObG, Temple Univ

Tobias, Daniel H MD (GO) - **Spec Exp:** Gynecologic Cancer; Uterine Cancer; Laparoscopic Surgery; **Hospital:** Morristown Mem Hosp (page 92), Overlook Hosp (page 92); **Address:** Morristown Meml Hosp, Womens Cancer Ctr, 100 Madison Ave, Morristown, NJ 07962; **Phone:** 973-971-5900; **Board Cert:** Obstetrics & Gynecology 2000; Gynecologic Oncology 2002; **Med School:** Univ MO-Kansas City 1992; **Resid:** Obstetrics & Gynecology, Bronx Muni Hosp Ctr 1996; **Fellow:** Gynecologic Oncology, Mt Sinai Med Ctr 1999

Hand Surgery

Ende, Leigh MD (HS) - **Spec Exp:** Arthritis; Carpal Tunnel Syndrome; Hand & Upper Extremity Surgery; **Hospital:** St Clare's Hosp - Dover, Newton Meml Hosp; **Address:** 121 Center Grove Rd, Randolph, NJ 07869; **Phone:** 973-366-5565; **Board Cert:** Orthopaedic Surgery 2010; Hand Surgery 2010; **Med School:** Tulane Univ 1978; **Resid:** Orthopaedic Surgery, UMDNJ-Univ Hosp 1983; **Fellow:** Hand Surgery, Columbia Presby Med Ctr 1984

Miller, Jeffrey K MD (HS) - **Spec Exp:** Carpal Tunnel Syndrome; Dupuytren's Contracture; Wrist/Hand Injuries; Elbow Surgery; **Hospital:** Morristown Mem Hosp (page 92), Saint Barnabas Med Ctr; **Address:** 111 Madison Ave, Ste 302, Morristown, NJ 07960; **Phone:** 973-538-5200; **Board Cert:** Orthopaedic Surgery 2010; Hand Surgery 2010; **Med School:** Univ Pittsburgh 1981; **Resid:** Surgery, Geo Wash Univ Med Ctr; Orthopaedic Surgery, Boston Univ Med Ctr 1986; **Fellow:** Hand Surgery, Thomas Jefferson Med Ctr 1987

Hematology

Frank, Martin J MD (Hem) - **Hospital:** Chilton Meml Hosp; **Address:** Collins Pavilion, 97 West Pkwy, Pompton Plains, NJ 07444; **Phone:** 973-831-5451; **Board Cert:** Internal Medicine 1985; Medical Oncology 1989; **Med School:** Geo Wash Univ 1982; **Resid:** Hematology, Montefiore Med Ctr 1986

Infectious Disease

Allegra, Donald T MD (Inf) - **Spec Exp:** Tropical Diseases; AIDS/HIV; International Health; Travel Medicine; **Hospital:** St Clare's Hosp - Denville, Morristown Mem Hosp (page 92); **Address:** 765 Rte 10 E, Randolph, NJ 07869; **Phone:** 973-989-0068; **Board Cert:** Infectious Disease 1982; Internal Medicine 1978; **Med School:** Harvard Med Sch 1974; **Resid:** Internal Medicine, Univ Colorado Affil Hosps 1978; **Fellow:** Infectious Disease, Emory Univ Hosp 1981

McManus, Edward J MD (Inf) - **Hospital:** St Clare's Hosp - Denville, Morristown Mem Hosp (page 92); **Address:** 765 Route 10 E, Randolph, NJ 07869; **Phone:** 973-989-0068; **Board Cert:** Internal Medicine 1985; Infectious Disease 1988; **Med School:** UMDNJ-NJ Med Sch, Newark 1982; **Resid:** Internal Medicine, Univ Wisconsin Hosp 1986; **Fellow:** Infectious Disease, Nat Inst Health 1989

Internal Medicine

Collum, Robert G MD (IM) *PCP* - **Hospital:** St Clare's Hosp - Denville; **Address:** 16 Pocono Rd, Ste 317, Denville, NJ 07834; **Phone:** 973-627-2650; **Board Cert:** Internal Medicine 2005; **Med School:** Columbia P&S 1992; **Resid:** Internal Medicine, NY-Presby/Cornell Med Ctr 1995

Scaduto, Philip MD (IM) *PCP* - **Spec Exp:** Hypertension; Diabetes; Geriatric Medicine; Preventive Medicine; **Hospital:** St Clare's Hosp - Denville; **Address:** 223 W Main St, Boonton, NJ 07005-1166; **Phone:** 973-335-8656; **Board Cert:** Internal Medicine 1986; **Med School:** UMDNJ-NJ Med Sch, Newark 1983; **Resid:** Internal Medicine, UMDNJ-Univ Hosp 1986

Silva, Waldemar MD (IM) - **Hospital:** Chilton Meml Hosp; **Address:** 488 Newark Pompton Tpke, Pompton Plains, NJ 07444; **Phone:** 973-835-9100; **Board Cert:** Internal Medicine 1987; **Med School:** Harvard Med Sch 1982; **Resid:** Internal Medicine, Bronx Muni Hosp 1985

Storch, Kenneth J MD/PhD (IM) - **Spec Exp:** Nutrition; Diabetes; Cholesterol/Lipid Disorders; **Hospital:** Morristown Mem Hosp (page 92), Overlook Hosp (page 92); **Address:** Storch Med Nutrition Ctr, 7 Columbia Tpke, Florham Park, NJ 07932; **Phone:** 973-765-9355; **Board Cert:** Internal Medicine 1982; **Med School:** SUNY Downstate 1979; **Resid:** Internal Medicine, Staten Island Hosp 1982; **Fellow:** Nutrition & Metabolism, MIT 1986; Nutrition & Metabolism, New England Deaconess 1988; **Fac Appt:** Asst Clin Prof Med, UMDNJ-NJ Med Sch, Newark

Weine, Gary R MD (IM) *PCP* - **Spec Exp:** Hypertension; Cholesterol/Lipid Disorders; **Hospital:** Morristown Mem Hosp (page 92); **Address:** 95 Madison Ave, Ste 405, Morristown, NJ 07960-7336; **Phone:** 973-829-9998; **Board Cert:** Internal Medicine 1979; **Med School:** Cornell Univ-Weill Med Coll 1976; **Resid:** Internal Medicine, NY Hosp 1979; **Fac Appt:** Asst Clin Prof Med, UMDNJ-NJ Med Sch, Newark

Maternal & Fetal Medicine

Benito, Carlos W MD (MF) - **Spec Exp:** Pregnancy Loss; Prenatal Diagnosis; Premature Labor; **Hospital:** Morristown Mem Hosp (page 92), Overlook Hosp (page 92); **Address:** 95 Madison Ave, Ste 203, Dept Mat & Fetal Med, Morristown, NJ 07960; **Phone:** 973-971-7080; **Board Cert:** Obstetrics & Gynecology 2009; Maternal & Fetal Medicine 2009; **Med School:** UMDNJ-RW Johnson Med Sch 1993; **Resid:** Obstetrics & Gynecology, UMDNJ-RWJ Med Ctr 1997; **Fellow:** Maternal & Fetal Medicine, UMDNJ-RWJ Med Ctr 1999; **Fac Appt:** Assoc Prof ObG, Robert W Johnson Med Sch

Medical Oncology

Adler, Kenneth R MD (Onc) - **Spec Exp:** Breast Cancer; Myeloproliferative Disorders; Lymphoma; **Hospital:** Morristown Mem Hosp (page 92); **Address:** 100 Madison Ave Fl 2, Box 1089, Morristown, NJ 07962; **Phone:** 973-538-5210; **Board Cert:** Internal Medicine 1976; Hematology 1978; **Med School:** Albany Med Coll 1973; **Resid:** Internal Medicine, Albany Med Ctr 1976; **Fellow:** Hematology & Oncology, Albany Med Ctr 1978; **Fac Appt:** Asst Clin Prof Med, UMDNJ-NJ Med Sch, Newark

Farber, Charles M MD/PhD (Onc) - **Spec Exp:** Leukemia & Lymphoma; Breast Cancer; Ovarian Cancer; Multiple Myeloma; **Hospital:** Morristown Mem Hosp (page 92); **Address:** Carol G Simon Cancer Center, 100 Madison Ave, Box 1089, Morristown, NJ 07962-1089; **Phone:** 973-538-5210; **Board Cert:** Internal Medicine 2000; Medical Oncology 2000; **Med School:** NYU Sch Med 1986; **Resid:** Internal Medicine, NY Hosp 1988; **Fellow:** Hematology & Oncology, NY Hosp 1991; **Fac Appt:** Asst Clin Prof Med, UMDNJ-NJ Med Sch, Newark

Papish, Steven W MD (Onc) - **Spec Exp:** Breast Cancer; Lymphoma; Gynecologic Cancer; **Hospital:** Morristown Mem Hosp (page 92), St Clare's Hosp - Boonton Township; **Address:** Carol Simon Cancer Ctr, 100 Madison Ave, Box 1089, Morristown, NJ 07962-1089; **Phone:** 973-538-5210; **Board Cert:** Internal Medicine 1977; Hematology 1980; Medical Oncology 1981; **Med School:** Univ Pennsylvania 1974; **Resid:** Internal Medicine, Geo Wash Univ Med Ctr 1978; **Fellow:** Hematology, New England Med Ctr 1979; Medical Oncology, Dana Farber Canc Inst 1981

Neonatal-Perinatal Medicine

Skolnick, Lawrence MD (NP) - **Spec Exp:** Neonatal Care; **Hospital:** Morristown Mem Hosp (page 92), Overlook Hosp (page 92); **Address:** 100 Madison Ave, Morristown, NJ 07960-6136; **Phone:** 973-971-5488; **Board Cert:** Pediatrics 1977; Neonatal-Perinatal Medicine 1977; **Med School:** NYU Sch Med 1972; **Resid:** Pediatrics, Albert Einstein 1975; **Fellow:** Neonatal-Perinatal Medicine, Duke Univ Med Ctr 1977; **Fac Appt:** Assoc Clin Prof Ped, UMDNJ-NJ Med Sch, Newark

Nephrology

Fine, Paul L MD (Nep) - **Spec Exp:** Hypertension; Kidney Failure; Dialysis Care; **Hospital:** Morristown Mem Hosp (page 92), St Clare's Hosp - Denville; **Address:** 2 Franklin Pl, Morristown, NJ 07960-5305; **Phone:** 973-267-7673; **Board Cert:** Internal Medicine 1982; Nephrology 1984; **Med School:** Yale Univ 1979; **Resid:** Internal Medicine, New York Hosp 1982; **Fellow:** Nephrology, Kidney Ctr-Cornell Univ Med Ctr 1984

Najarian, James MD (Nep) - **Spec Exp:** Hypertension; Kidney Failure; Transplant Medicine-Kidney; Dialysis Care; **Hospital:** Morristown Mem Hosp (page 92), St Clare's Hosp - Denville; **Address:** 121 Center Grove Rd, Ste 13-14, Randolph, NJ 07869; **Phone:** 973-361-3737; **Board Cert:** Internal Medicine 1975; Nephrology 2006; **Med School:** Univ Wisc 1972; **Resid:** Internal Medicine, Beth Israel Hosp 1975; **Fellow:** Nephrology, Montefiore Med Ctr 1978

Neurological Surgery

Beyerl, Brian D MD (NS) - **Spec Exp:** Brain Tumors; Stereotactic Radiosurgery; Arteriovenous Malformations; **Hospital:** Morristown Mem Hosp (page 92), Overlook Hosp (page 92); **Address:** 310 Madison Ave, Ste 200, Morristown, NJ 07960; **Phone:** 973-285-7800; **Board Cert:** Neurological Surgery 1990; **Med School:** Johns Hopkins Univ 1980; **Resid:** Surgery, Johns Hopkins Univ Hosp 1981; Neurological Surgery, Mass Genl Hosp 1986; **Fac Appt:** Asst Clin Prof NS, UMDNJ-NJ Med Sch, Newark

Knightly, John J MD (NS) - **Spec Exp:** Spinal Surgery; Stereotactic Radiosurgery; Minimally Invasive Spinal Surgery; Trauma; **Hospital:** Overlook Hosp (page 92), Morristown Mem Hosp (page 92); **Address:** 310 Madison Ave, Ste 200, Morristown, NJ 07960; **Phone:** 973-285-7800; **Board Cert:** Neurological Surgery 1998; **Med School:** UMDNJ-NJ Med Sch, Newark 1985; **Resid:** Neurological Surgery, Bethesda Navval Hosp 1993; **Fellow:** Neurological Surgery, Barrow Neurol Inst 1993

Zampella, Edward J MD (NS) - **Spec Exp:** Stereotactic Radiosurgery; Pediatric Neurosurgery; Pain Management; Brain Tumors; **Hospital:** Overlook Hosp (page 92), Morristown Mem Hosp (page 92); **Address:** Atlantic Neurosurgical Specialists, 310 Madison Ave Fl 2, Morristown, NJ 07960; **Phone:** 973-285-7800; **Board Cert:** Neurological Surgery 1991; Pain Medicine 1997; **Med School:** Univ Alabama 1982; **Resid:** Neurological Surgery, Univ Alabama Hosp 1988; **Fellow:** Neurology, Natl Hosp Nervous Disorders-Queen Square 1985; **Fac Appt:** Assoc Prof NS, UMDNJ-NJ Med Sch, Newark

Neurology

Cerny, Kenneth R MD (N) - **Hospital:** Morristown Mem Hosp (page 92); **Address:** 310 Madison Ave, Ste 120, Morristown, NJ 07960; **Phone:** 973-285-1446; **Board Cert:** Neurology 1983; **Med School:** Columbia P&S 1976; **Resid:** Neurology, Barnes Hosp 1978; Neurology, Albert Einstein Med Ctr 1981

Fox, Stuart W MD (N) - **Spec Exp:** Neuromuscular Disorders; Headache; **Hospital:** Morristown Mem Hosp (page 92); **Address:** 310 Madison Ave, Ste 120, Morristown, NJ 07960-6092; **Phone:** 973-285-1446; **Board Cert:** Internal Medicine 1978; Neurology 1982; **Med School:** Cornell Univ-Weill Med Coll 1975; **Resid:** Internal Medicine, Univ Mich Med Ctr 1978; Neurology, Albert Einstein 1981; **Fellow:** Clinical Neurophysiology, LI Jewish-Hillside Hosp 1982; **Fac Appt:** Asst Clin Prof Med, Columbia P&S

Obstetrics & Gynecology

Banks, Judy L MD (ObG) - **Hospital:** Morristown Mem Hosp (page 92); **Address:** 256 Columbia Tpke, Ste 212, Florham Park, NJ 07932; **Phone:** 973-377-3374; **Board Cert:** Obstetrics & Gynecology 2003; **Med School:** Meharry Med Coll 1975; **Resid:** Obstetrics & Gynecology, Univ Hosp-UMDNJ 1980

Culligan, Patrick J MD (ObG) - **Spec Exp:** Uro-Gynecology; **Hospital:** Overlook Hosp (page 92), Morristown Mem Hosp (page 92); **Address:** 95 Madison Ave, Ste 204, Morristown, NJ 07962; **Phone:** 973-971-7267; **Board Cert:** Obstetrics & Gynecology 2001; **Med School:** Mercer Univ Sch Med 1993; **Resid:** Obstetrics & Gynecology, Greenville Hosp 1997; **Fellow:** Uro-Gynecology, Evanston Hosp 1999; **Fac Appt:** Assoc Clin Prof ObG, UMDNJ-NJ Med Sch, Newark

Dreyfuss, Patricia MD (ObG) - **Hospital:** St Clare's Hosp - Denville; **Address:** 115 Route 46 West, D Bldg - Ste 27, Mountain Lakes, NJ 07046; **Phone:** 973-334-3345; **Board Cert:** Obstetrics & Gynecology 1985; **Med School:** UMDNJ-Rutgers Med Sch 1979; **Resid:** Obstetrics & Gynecology, St Barnabas Hosp 1983

Gluck, Ian J MD (ObG) _PCP_ - **Hospital:** Morristown Mem Hosp (page 92); **Address:** 59 Franklin St, Morristown, NJ 07960; **Phone:** 973-538-1515; **Board Cert:** Obstetrics & Gynecology 1985; **Med School:** NY Med Coll 1979; **Resid:** Obstetrics & Gynecology, Grady Meml Hosp 1983; **Fac Appt:** Asst Clin Prof ObG, UMDNJ-NJ Med Sch, Newark

Iammatteo, Matthew D MD (ObG) - **Spec Exp:** Pregnancy-High Risk; Hysteroscopic Surgery; Laparoscopic Surgery; **Hospital:** Morristown Mem Hosp (page 92); **Address:** 111 Madison Ave, Ste 311, Morristown, NJ 07960; **Phone:** 973-971-9950; **Board Cert:** Obstetrics & Gynecology 2009; **Med School:** Dominica 1985; **Resid:** Obstetrics & Gynecology, St Michaels Med Ctr 1989

Mohr, Robert F MD (ObG) _PCP_ - **Spec Exp:** Gynecologic Surgery; Laparoscopic Surgery; Menopause Problems; **Hospital:** Morristown Mem Hosp (page 92), St Clare's Hosp - Denville; **Address:** 390 Route 10, Randolph, NJ 07869; **Phone:** 973-328-1262; **Board Cert:** Obstetrics & Gynecology 2003; **Med School:** Hahnemann Univ 1977; **Resid:** Obstetrics & Gynecology, Northwestern Meml Hosp 1981; **Fac Appt:** Asst Prof ObG, UMDNJ-Univ Med Dent NJ

Steer, Robert MD (ObG) - **Spec Exp:** Pregnancy-High Risk; Multiple Gestation; **Hospital:** Morristown Mem Hosp (page 92); **Address:** 60 Franklin St, Morristown, NJ 07960-5217; **Phone:** 973-993-1919; **Board Cert:** Obstetrics & Gynecology 2009; **Med School:** Cornell Univ-Weill Med Coll 1986; **Resid:** Obstetrics & Gynecology, New York Hosp 1990; **Fac Appt:** Assoc Clin Prof ObG, Mount Sinai Sch Med

Wallis, Joseph J DO (ObG) - **Spec Exp:** Laparoscopic Surgery; Endoscopy; Infertility; **Hospital:** St Clare's Hosp - Denville, St Clare's Hosp - Dover; **Address:** 600 Mt Pleasant Ave, Ste G, Dover, NJ 07801-1629; **Phone:** 973-989-9000; **Board Cert:** Obstetrics & Gynecology 1977; **Med School:** Philadelphia Coll Osteo Med 1970; **Resid:** Internal Medicine, St Michael's Med Ctr 1972; Obstetrics & Gynecology, St Michael's Med Ctr 1975

Ophthalmology

Chen, Lucy L MD (Oph) - **Spec Exp:** Pediatric Ophthalmology; Strabismus; **Hospital:** St Clare's Hosp - Sussex, Morristown Mem Hosp (page 92); **Address:** 95 Madison Ave, Ste 301, Morristown, NJ 07960-6092; **Phone:** 973-540-8814; **Board Cert:** Internal Medicine 1988; Ophthalmology 2004; **Med School:** Boston Univ 1985; **Resid:** Internal Medicine, NY Presby Hosp 1988; **Fellow:** Pediatric Ophthalmology, Wills Eye Hosp 1992

Kazam, Ezra S MD (Oph) - **Spec Exp:** Glaucoma; Cataract Surgery; Refractive Surgery; **Hospital:** Morristown Mem Hosp (page 92); **Address:** 2 Washington Pl, Morristown, NJ 07960-4220; **Phone:** 973-267-8755; **Board Cert:** Ophthalmology 1978; **Med School:** SUNY Downstate 1973; **Resid:** Ophthalmology, Montefiore Hosp 1977; **Fac Appt:** Asst Clin Prof Oph, Albert Einstein Coll Med

Pinke, Robert S MD (Oph) - **Spec Exp:** Cataract Surgery; Glaucoma; Laser Refractive Surgery; **Hospital:** St Clare's Hosp - Dover, St Clare's Hosp - Denville; **Address:** 66 Sunset Strip, Ste 107, Succasunna, NJ 07876; **Phone:** 973-584-4451; **Board Cert:** Ophthalmology 1989; **Med School:** Mount Sinai Sch Med 1984; **Resid:** Ophthalmology, Methodist Hosp-Baylor Coll Med 1988

Sachs, Ronald MD (Oph) - **Spec Exp:** Macular Degeneration; Diabetic Eye Disease/Retinopathy; Retinal Disorders; Retina/Vitreous Surgery; **Hospital:** Morristown Mem Hosp (page 92), St Clare's Hosp - Denville; **Address:** 8 Saddle Rd, Ste 201, Cedar Knolls, NJ 07927; **Phone:** 973-539-3600; **Board Cert:** Ophthalmology 2004; **Med School:** NYU Sch Med 1988; **Resid:** Ophthalmology, Montefiore Med Ctr 1992; **Fellow:** Retina, Albert Einstein Med Ctr 1993

Silverman, Cary M MD (Oph) - **Spec Exp:** LASIK-Refractive Surgery; Cataract Surgery; **Hospital:** Saint Barnabas Med Ctr; **Address:** EyeCare 20/20, 46 Eagle Rock Ave, East Hanover, NJ 07936; **Phone:** 973-560-1500; **Board Cert:** Ophthalmology 1987; **Med School:** UMDNJ-NJ Med Sch, Newark 1982; **Resid:** Ophthalmology, Hahnemann Univ Hosp 1986; **Fac Appt:** Clin Prof Oph, UMDNJ-RW Johnson Med Sch

Orthopaedic Surgery

Baydin, Jeffrey MD (OrS) - **Hospital:** Morristown Mem Hosp (page 92); **Address:** 50 Cherry Hill Rd, Ste 203, Parsippany, NJ 07054; **Phone:** 973-263-2828; **Board Cert:** Orthopaedic Surgery 1976; **Med School:** Tufts Univ 1969; **Resid:** Surgery, Boston City Hosp-Harvard 1971; Orthopaedic Surgery, Tufts-New England Med Ctr 1975

Dowling, William J MD (OrS) - **Spec Exp:** Joint Replacement; **Hospital:** Morristown Mem Hosp (page 92), Overlook Hosp (page 92); **Address:** 111 Madison Ave, Ste 400, Morristown, NJ 07960; **Phone:** 973-971-6470; **Board Cert:** Orthopaedic Surgery 1978; **Med School:** UMDNJ-NJ Med Sch, Newark 1971; **Resid:** Orthopaedic Surgery, UMDNJ-Newark 1976

Feldman, David J MD (OrS) - **Spec Exp:** Sports Medicine; **Hospital:** St Clare's Hosp - Denville; **Address:** 16 Pocono Rd, Ste 100, Denville, NJ 07834; **Phone:** 973-625-5700; **Board Cert:** Orthopaedic Surgery 1979; Orthopaedic Sports Medicine 2007; **Med School:** Boston Univ 1972; **Resid:** Surgery, Mt Sinai Med Ctr 1974; Orthopaedic Surgery, Mt Sinai Med Ctr 1977; **Fellow:** Pediatric Orthopaedic Surgery, Stanford Univ Med Ctr 1978

Montgomery, Kenneth MD (OrS) - **Spec Exp:** Hand Surgery; Shoulder Surgery; Knee Surgery; Rotator Cuff Surgery; **Address:** TriCounty Orthopaedics & Sports Medicine, PO Box 1446, Morristown, NJ 07962; **Phone:** 973-538-2334; **Board Cert:** Orthopaedic Surgery 2010; Orthopaedic Sports Medicine 2007; **Med School:** UCSF 1990; **Resid:** Orthopaedic Surgery, Hosp Special Surgery 1995; **Fellow:** Sports Medicine, Lenox Hill Hosp 1996; Obstetrics & Anesthesiology, Brigham & Women's Hosp 1997

Rieger, Mark MD (OrS) - **Spec Exp:** Pediatric Orthopaedic Surgery; Scoliosis; Hip Disorders-Pediatric; Adolescent Sports Medicine; **Hospital:** Morristown Mem Hosp (page 92), Saint Barnabas Med Ctr; **Address:** 218 Ridgedale Ave, Ste 104, Cedar Knolls, NJ 07927-2109; **Phone:** 973-538-7700; **Board Cert:** Orthopaedic Surgery 2002; **Med School:** Univ Conn 1983; **Resid:** Orthopaedic Surgery, LI Jewish Hosp 1988; **Fellow:** Pediatric Orthopaedic Surgery, DuPont Inst 1989; **Fac Appt:** Asst Clin Prof OrS, NYU Sch Med

Spielman, Joel H MD (OrS) - **Spec Exp:** Spinal Surgery; **Hospital:** St Clare's Hosp - Dover, St Clare's Hosp - Denville; **Address:** Ortho Assocs of West Jersey, 600 Mount Pleasant Ave, Dover, NJ 07801-1630; **Phone:** 973-989-0888; **Board Cert:** Orthopaedic Surgery 2005; **Med School:** Albert Einstein Coll Med 1986; **Resid:** Orthopaedic Surgery, Montefiore Med Ctr 1991; **Fellow:** Spinal Surgery, Hosp for Special Surg

Taffet, Berton MD (OrS) - **Hospital:** Morristown Mem Hosp (page 92); **Address:** 95 Madison Ave, Ste A07, Morristown, NJ 07960; **Phone:** 973-984-0404; **Board Cert:** Orthopaedic Surgery 2001; **Med School:** Albert Einstein Coll Med 1978; **Resid:** Orthopaedic Surgery, Mt Sinai Med Ctr 1983; **Fellow:** Joint Replacement Surgery, Univ Colorado Hosp 1984

Otolaryngology

Fleming, Gregory MD (Oto) - **Spec Exp:** Endoscopic Sinus Surgery; Sleep Disorders/Apnea; **Hospital:** Morristown Mem Hosp (page 92), Overlook Hosp (page 92); **Address:** 26 Madison Ave, Morristown, NJ 07960; **Phone:** 973-267-1850; **Board Cert:** Otolaryngology 1988; **Med School:** Univ Mass Sch Med 1982; **Resid:** Surgery, Univ Mass Med Ctr 1984; Otolaryngology, Mass EE Infirm 1988

Lachman, Reid MD (Oto) - **Hospital:** Morristown Mem Hosp (page 92); **Address:** 95 Madison Ave, Ste 105, Morristown, NJ 07960-7331; **Phone:** 973-644-0808; **Board Cert:** Otolaryngology 1986; **Med School:** NY Med Coll 1981; **Resid:** Otolaryngology, Albert Einstein Med Ctr 1986

Taylor, Howard MD (Oto) - **Spec Exp:** Hearing Loss; Sinus Surgery; Throat Disorders; Voice Disorders; **Hospital:** Chilton Meml Hosp; **Address:** 51 State Highway 23 S, Riverdale, NJ 07457-1625; **Phone:** 973-831-1220; **Board Cert:** Otolaryngology 1980; **Med School:** Columbia P&S 1976; **Resid:** Otolaryngology, Univ Chicago Hosps 1980; **Fellow:** Facial Plastic Surgery, Hosp Med Coll Penn 1981; **Fac Appt:** Asst Clin Prof Oto, UMDNJ-NJ Med Sch, Newark

Pain Medicine

Rudman, Michael E MD (PM) - **Spec Exp:** Pain-Back; Pain-Chronic; Complex Regional Pain Syndrome; **Hospital:** Morristown Mem Hosp (page 92); **Address:** Morristown Meml Hosp, Pain Mgmt Ctr, 95 Madison Ave, Ste 402, Morristown, NJ 07960; **Phone:** 973-971-6824; **Board Cert:** Pain Medicine 2007; Anesthesiology 1993; **Med School:** Penn State Univ-Hershey Med Ctr 1988; **Resid:** Anesthesiology, Hosp Univ Penn 1992

Pediatric Cardiology

Donnelly, Christine M MD (PCd) - **Spec Exp:** Fetal Echocardiography; Congenital Heart Disease; Cardiac Catheterization; **Hospital:** Morristown Mem Hosp (page 92), NYPresby-Morgan Stanley Children's Hosp (page 104); **Address:** 100 Madison Ave, Morristown, NJ 07960-6136; **Phone:** 973-971-5996; **Board Cert:** Pediatrics 1985; Pediatric Cardiology 1985; **Med School:** Columbia P&S 1978; **Resid:** Pediatrics, Columbia-Presby Med Ctr 1981; **Fellow:** Pediatric Cardiology, Columbia-Presby Med Ctr 1984; **Fac Appt:** Assoc Clin Prof Ped, Columbia P&S

Pediatric Endocrinology

Chin, Daisy MD (PEn) - **Spec Exp:** Thyroid Disorders; Growth Disorders; Pubertal Disorders; **Hospital:** Morristown Mem Hosp (page 92), Overlook Hosp (page 92); **Address:** Morristown Meml Hosp, 100 Madison Ave, Box 53, Morristown, NJ 07962; **Phone:** 973-971-4340; **Board Cert:** Pediatrics 2003; Pediatric Endocrinology 2007; **Med School:** SUNY Downstate 1992; **Resid:** Pediatrics, Columbia Presby Med Ctr 1995; **Fellow:** Pediatric Endocrinology, NYU Med Ctr 1998; **Fac Appt:** Asst Prof Ped, Columbia P&S

Starkman, Harold MD (PEn) - **Spec Exp:** Diabetes; Growth Disorders; **Hospital:** Morristown Mem Hosp (page 92); **Address:** 100 Madison Ave, Morristown Meml Hosp-Atlantic Hlth, Morristown, NJ 07962-6136; **Phone:** 973-971-4340; **Board Cert:** Pediatrics 1980; Pediatric Endocrinology 1983; **Med School:** Albert Einstein Coll Med 1976; **Resid:** Pediatrics, Mount Sinai Hosp 1978; Pediatrics, New York Hosp 1979; **Fellow:** Pediatric Endocrinology, New York Hosp 1980; Pediatric Endocrinology, Joslin Diabetes Center 1983; **Fac Appt:** Assoc Prof Ped, UMDNJ-NJ Med Sch, Newark

Pediatric Gastroenterology

Mones, Richard MD (PGe) - **Spec Exp:** Inflammatory Bowel Disease/Crohn's; Nutrition; **Hospital:** Morristown Mem Hosp (page 92), Overlook Hosp (page 92); **Address:** Morristown Meml Hosp-Atlantic Hlth, 100 Madison Ave, Box 82, Ped Gastro, Morristown, NJ 07962; **Phone:** 973-971-5676; **Board Cert:** Pediatrics 1976; Pediatric Gastroenterology 2005; **Med School:** NY Med Coll 1971; **Resid:** Pediatrics, Babies/Columbia-Presby Hosps 1973; **Fellow:** Pediatric Gastroenterology, Babies/Columbia-Presby Hosps 1977; **Fac Appt:** Assoc Clin Prof Ped, Columbia P&S

Rosh, Joel MD (PGe) - **Spec Exp:** Inflammatory Bowel Disease; Celiac Disease; Liver Disease; **Hospital:** Morristown Mem Hosp (page 92), Overlook Hosp (page 92); **Address:** Dept Peds Gastroenterology & Nutrition, 100 Madison Ave, Morristown, NJ 07960-6136; **Phone:** 973-971-5676; **Board Cert:** Pediatric Gastroenterology 2007; **Med School:** Albert Einstein Coll Med 1986; **Resid:** Pediatrics, Babies Hosp/Columbia-Presby Med Ctr 1989; **Fellow:** Pediatric Gastroenterology, Mount Sinai Med Ctr 1991; **Fac Appt:** Assoc Prof Ped, UMDNJ-NJ Med Sch, Newark

Pediatric Pulmonology

Atlas, Arthur B MD (PPul) - **Spec Exp:** Asthma; Cystic Fibrosis; Lung Disease; **Hospital:** Morristown Mem Hosp (page 92), Overlook Hosp (page 92); **Address:** Morristown Meml Hosp, Resp Ctr for Chldn, 100 Madison Ave, Box 107, Morristown, NJ 07962; **Phone:** 973-971-4142; **Board Cert:** Pediatric Pulmonology 2007; **Med School:** Mexico 1982; **Resid:** Pediatrics, St Louis Chldns Hosp 1986; **Fellow:** Allergy & Immunology, St Louis Chldns Hosp 1989; Pediatric Pulmonology, Chldns Hosp/Univ Pittsburgh 1991; **Fac Appt:** Asst Clin Prof Ped, UMDNJ-NJ Med Sch, Newark

Pediatrics

Caruso, Patrick A MD (Ped) - **Hospital:** Hackettstown Reg Med Ctr, Morristown Mem Hosp (page 92); **Address:** 657 Willow Grove St, Ste 401, Hackettstown, NJ 07834; **Phone:** 908-850-7800; **Board Cert:** Pediatrics 2004; **Med School:** Case West Res Univ 1983; **Resid:** Pediatrics, Univ Conn Hlth Ctr 1986; **Fac Appt:** Assoc Clin Prof Ped, Mount Sinai Sch Med

Gotfried, Fern MD (Ped) *PCP* - **Hospital:** Morristown Mem Hosp (page 92); **Address:** Franklin Pediatrics, 91 S Jefferson Rd Fl 2, Whippany, NJ 07981; **Phone:** 973-538-6116; **Board Cert:** Pediatrics 1986; Adolescent Medicine 2009; **Med School:** UMDNJ-Rutgers Med Sch 1980; **Resid:** Pediatrics, Strong Meml Hosp 1983; **Fellow:** Adolescent Medicine, Strong Meml Hosp 1985

Handler, Robert W MD (Ped) *PCP* - **Spec Exp:** Asthma; Allergy; Behavioral Disorders; **Hospital:** Morristown Mem Hosp (page 92), St Clare's Hosp - Denville; **Address:** 1140 Parsippany Blvd, Ste 102, Parsippany, NJ 07054; **Phone:** 973-263-0066; **Board Cert:** Pediatrics 1980; **Med School:** UMDNJ-NJ Med Sch, Newark 1975; **Resid:** Pediatrics, Chldns Hosp 1978; **Fac Appt:** Asst Clin Prof Ped, UMDNJ-NJ Med Sch, Newark

Suda, Anjuli MD (Ped) *PCP* - **Spec Exp:** Pulmonary Disease; **Hospital:** Chilton Meml Hosp; **Address:** 170 Kinnelon Rd, Ste 28, Kinnelon, NJ 07405; **Phone:** 973-838-0001; **Board Cert:** Pediatrics 1988; **Med School:** India 1976; **Resid:** Pediatrics, St Joseph's Hosp & Med Ctr 1985

Physical Medicine & Rehabilitation

Mulford, Gregory J MD (PMR) - **Spec Exp:** Sports Medicine; Electrodiagnosis; **Hospital:** Morristown Mem Hosp (page 92), Overlook Hosp (page 92); **Address:** Assoc in Rehab Medicine, 95 Mt Kemble Ave Thebaud Bldg Fl 4, Morristown, NJ 07960; **Phone:** 973-267-2293; **Board Cert:** Physical Medicine & Rehabilitation 1990; **Med School:** UMDNJ-RW Johnson Med Sch 1985; **Resid:** Physical Medicine & Rehabilitation, Columbia-Presby Hosp 1989; **Fac Appt:** Assoc Clin Prof PMR, UMDNJ-Univ Med Dent NJ

Skerker, Robert S MD (PMR) - **Spec Exp:** Sports Medicine; Orthopaedic Rehabilitation; Botox for Muscle Overactivity; **Hospital:** Morristown Mem Hosp (page 92); **Address:** Associates in Rehab Medicine, 95 Mt Kemble Ave, Bldg T-4, Morristown, NJ 07960; **Phone:** 973-267-2293; **Board Cert:** Physical Medicine & Rehabilitation 1991; **Med School:** Univ Mass Sch Med 1986; **Resid:** Physical Medicine & Rehabilitation, Univ Hosp 1990; **Fellow:** Sports Medicine, Hughston Sports Med Ctr 1991

Valenza, Joseph P MD (PMR) - **Spec Exp:** Pain Management; Complex Regional Pain Syndrome; Repetitive Strain Injuries; Spinal Cord Injury; **Hospital:** Kessler Inst for Rehab - Chester; **Address:** Kessler Inst for Rehab, Dept Pain Management, 201 Pleasant Hill Rd, Chester, NJ 07930; **Phone:** 973-252-6402; **Board Cert:** Physical Medicine & Rehabilitation 2007; Pain Medicine 2001; **Med School:** SUNY Downstate 1992; **Resid:** Physical Medicine & Rehabilitation, UMDNJ 1996; **Fac Appt:** Asst Clin Prof PMR, UMDNJ-NJ Med Sch, Newark

Plastic Surgery

Colon, Francisco G MD (PlS) - **Spec Exp:** Cosmetic Surgery-Face & Body; Reconstructive Plastic Surgery; **Hospital:** Saint Barnabas Med Ctr, Morristown Mem Hosp (page 92); **Address:** Peer-Group Plastic Surgery Ctr, 124 Columbia Tpke, Florham Park, NJ 07932; **Phone:** 973-822-3000; **Board Cert:** Plastic Surgery 2007; **Med School:** Columbia P&S 1987; **Resid:** Surgery, St Lukes Roosevelt Hosp 1992; Plastic Surgery, Beth Israel Deaconess Hosp 1992

Hawrylo, Richard R MD (PlS) - **Spec Exp:** Cosmetic Surgery-Breast; Cosmetic Surgery-Face & Eyelid; Abdominoplasty; Liposuction; **Hospital:** Saint Barnabas Med Ctr, Morristown Mem Hosp (page 92); **Address:** PeerGroup Plastic Surgery Ctr, 124 Columbia Tpke, Florham Park, NJ 07932; **Phone:** 973-822-3000; **Board Cert:** Plastic Surgery 1980; **Med School:** Wake Forest Univ 1972; **Resid:** Surgery, Bellevue/NYU Med Ctr 1977; Plastic Surgery, Bellevue/NYU Med Ctr 1979

Pyo, Daniel J MD (PlS) - **Spec Exp:** Cosmetic Surgery-Breast; Liposuction & Body Contouring; Facial Rejuvenation; **Hospital:** Morristown Mem Hosp (page 92), Saint Barnabas Med Ctr; **Address:** Plastic Surgery Ctr of NJ, 131 Madison Ave, Ste 120, Morristown, NJ 07960; **Phone:** 973-540-9055; **Board Cert:** Surgery 2009; Plastic Surgery 2009; **Med School:** Mount Sinai Sch Med 1990; **Resid:** Surgery, Strong Meml Hospital 1995; **Fellow:** Plastic Surgery, Yale-New Haven Hosp 1997

Rafizadeh, Farhad MD (PlS) - **Spec Exp:** Breast Reconstruction; Cosmetic Surgery-Face; Cosmetic Surgery-Breast; Facial Rejuvenation; **Hospital:** Morristown Mem Hosp (page 92), Saint Barnabas Med Ctr; **Address:** 101 Madison Ave, Ste 105, Morristown, NJ 07960; **Phone:** 973-267-0928; **Board Cert:** Plastic Surgery 1986; **Med School:** Switzerland 1975; **Resid:** Surgery, St Barnabas Med Ctr 1981; Surgery, Morristown Meml Hosp 1982; **Fellow:** Plastic Surgery, New York Hosp-Cornell Med Ctr 1984

Starker, Isaac MD (PlS) - **Spec Exp:** Cosmetic Surgery-Face & Body; Cosmetic Surgery-Breast; Breast Reconstruction; **Hospital:** Morristown Mem Hosp (page 92), Saint Barnabas Med Ctr; **Address:** 124 Columbia Tpke, Florham Park, NJ 07932; **Phone:** 973-822-3000; **Board Cert:** Plastic Surgery 1992; **Med School:** NYU Sch Med 1981; **Resid:** Surgery, St Lukes-Roosevelt Hosp Ctr 1986; Plastic Surgery, Montefiore Med Ctr 1988; **Fellow:** Hand Surgery, St Lukes-Roosevelt Hosp Ctr 1989

Weinstein, Larry MD (PlS) - **Spec Exp:** Breast Cosmetic & Reconstructive Surgery; Cosmetic Surgery-Face; Liposuction & Body Contouring; Facial Rejuvenation; **Hospital:** Morristown Mem Hosp (page 92), Overlook Hosp (page 92); **Address:** 385 State Rte 24, Ste 3K, Chester, NJ 07930-2910; **Phone:** 908-879-2222; **Board Cert:** Plastic Surgery 1993; **Med School:** Mexico 1979; **Resid:** Surgery, Univ Hosp/Morristown Meml Hosp 1984; Surgical Oncology, Meml Sloan-Kettering Cancer Ctr 1985; **Fellow:** Plastic Surgery, Univ Pittsburgh 1986; Plastic Surgery, SUNY-Brooklyn Med Ctr 1988

Psychiatry

Nadel, William MD (Psyc) - **Spec Exp:** Mood Disorders; **Address:** 203 River Edge Drive, Chattam, NJ 07928; **Phone:** 973-665-0066; **Board Cert:** Psychiatry 1975; **Med School:** Case West Res Univ 1968; **Resid:** Psychiatry, Montefiore Med Ctr 1972; **Fellow:** Social Psychiatry, Montefiore Med Ctr 1973

Sofair, Jane MD (Psyc) - **Spec Exp:** Anxiety & Depression; Women's Health; **Hospital:** Morristown Mem Hosp (page 92); **Address:** 35 Airport Rd, Ste 350, Morristown, NJ 07960; **Phone:** 973-292-0960; **Board Cert:** Psychiatry 1986; **Med School:** NYU Sch Med 1980; **Resid:** Psychiatry, NYU Med Ctr 1984

Pulmonary Disease

Benton, Marc L MD (Pul) - **Spec Exp:** Asthma & Emphysema; Sleep Disorders/Apnea; Cough; **Hospital:** Morristown Mem Hosp (page 92); **Address:** 300 Madison Ave, Ste 201, Madison, NJ 07940; **Phone:** 973-822-2772; **Board Cert:** Internal Medicine 1985; Pulmonary Disease 1988; Critical Care Medicine 2005; Sleep Medicine 1995; **Med School:** Mount Sinai Sch Med 1982; **Resid:** Internal Medicine, Mt Sinai Hosp 1985; **Fellow:** Pulmonary Disease, NYU Med Ctr 1988; **Fac Appt:** Asst Clin Prof Med, Mount Sinai Sch Med

Fiel, Stanley MD (Pul) - **Spec Exp:** Cystic Fibrosis; Chronic Obstructive Lung Disease (COPD); Asthma; Cystic Fibrosis; **Hospital:** Morristown Mem Hosp (page 92), Overlook Hosp (page 92); **Address:** 100 Madison Ave, Box 96, Morristown, NJ 07962; **Phone:** 973-971-5136; **Board Cert:** Internal Medicine 1976; Pulmonary Disease 1978; **Med School:** Med Coll PA 1973; **Resid:** Internal Medicine, Temple Univ Hosp 1976; Pulmonary Disease, Hosp Univ Penn 1978; **Fac Appt:** Prof Med, Mount Sinai Sch Med

O'Donnell, Timothy DO (Pul) - **Spec Exp:** Asthma; Lung Cancer; Interstitial Lung Disease; **Hospital:** Chilton Meml Hosp, Morristown Mem Hosp (page 92); **Address:** 63 Beaver Brook Rd, Ste 301, Lincoln Park, NJ 07035; **Phone:** 973-694-1300; **Board Cert:** Internal Medicine 1989; Pulmonary Disease 2002; Critical Care Medicine 2003; **Med School:** UMDNJ Sch Osteo Med 1985; **Resid:** Internal Medicine, NJ Med Sch/Univ Hosp 1989; **Fellow:** Pulmonary Critical Care Medicine, UMDNJ/Newark Beth Israel Med Ctr 1992

Radiation Oncology

Wong, James R MD (RadRO) - **Spec Exp:** Prostate Cancer; Breast Cancer; Head & Neck Cancer; Pancreatic Cancer; **Hospital:** Morristown Mem Hosp (page 92); **Address:** Morristown Meml Hosp, Dept Rad Oncology, 100 Madison Ave, Box 9, Morristown, NJ 07960; **Phone:** 973-971-5329; **Board Cert:** Radiation Oncology 1993; **Med School:** Harvard Med Sch 1986; **Resid:** Radiation Oncology, Harvard Jt Ctr for Rad Therapy 1992; **Fac Appt:** Assoc Clin Prof RadRO, Columbia P&S

Reproductive Endocrinology

Bergh, Paul A MD (RE) - **Spec Exp:** Infertility-IVF; **Hospital:** Morristown Mem Hosp (page 92), Saint Barnabas Med Ctr; **Address:** 111 Madison Ave, Ste 100, Morristown, NJ 07960; **Phone:** 973-971-4600; **Board Cert:** Obstetrics & Gynecology 2009; Reproductive Endocrinology 2009; **Med School:** UMDNJ-RW Johnson Med Sch 1983; **Resid:** Obstetrics & Gynecology, St Barnabas Hosp 1989; **Fellow:** Reproductive Endocrinology, Mount Sinai Med Ctr 1991; **Fac Appt:** Asst Clin Prof ObG, UMDNJ-RW Johnson Med Sch

Scott, Richard T MD (RE) - **Spec Exp:** Infertility; Infertility-IVF; Fertility Preservation in Cancer; **Hospital:** Morristown Mem Hosp (page 92), Saint Barnabas Med Ctr; **Address:** Reproductive Medicine Assocs, 111 Madison Ave, Ste 100, Morristown, NJ 07960-6083; **Phone:** 973-656-2831; **Board Cert:** Obstetrics & Gynecology 2009; Reproductive Endocrinology 2009; **Med School:** Univ VA Sch Med 1983; **Resid:** Obstetrics & Gynecology, Wilford Hall USAF Med Ctr 1987; **Fellow:** Reproductive Endocrinology, Jones Inst Reproductive Med 1989; **Fac Appt:** Clin Prof ObG, Robert W Johnson Med Sch

Rheumatology

Pasik, Deborah MD (Rhu) - **Spec Exp:** Rheumatoid Arthritis; Osteoporosis; Lupus/SLE; **Hospital:** Morristown Mem Hosp (page 92), Overlook Hosp (page 92); **Address:** Atlantic Rheumatology, 8 Saddle Rd, Ste 202, Cedar Knolls, NJ 07927; **Phone:** 973-984-9796; **Board Cert:** Internal Medicine 1985; Rheumatology 1988; **Med School:** Mount Sinai Sch Med 1982; **Resid:** Internal Medicine, Beth Israel Hosp 1985; **Fellow:** Rheumatology, NYU Med Ctr 1988

Surgery

Carter, Mitchel S MD (S) - **Spec Exp:** Laparoscopic Surgery; Laparoscopic Cholecystectomy; Gastroesophageal Reflux Disease (GERD); **Hospital:** Morristown Mem Hosp (page 92); **Address:** Allied Surgical Group, 261 James St, Ste 2G, Morristown, NJ 07960; **Phone:** 973-267-6400; **Board Cert:** Surgery 2003; **Med School:** Ros Franklin Univ/Chicago Med Sch 1979; **Resid:** Surgery, Albert Einstein Affil Hosp 1984

Diehl, William L MD (S) - **Spec Exp:** Breast Cancer; Pancreatic Cancer; Gastrointestinal Cancer; Colon Cancer; **Hospital:** Morristown Mem Hosp (page 92), St Clare's Hosp - Denville; **Address:** Allied Surgical Group, 261 James St, Ste 2G, Morristown, NJ 07960-6348; **Phone:** 973-267-6400; **Board Cert:** Surgery 2009; **Med School:** Mexico 1981; **Resid:** Surgery, Morristown Meml Hosp 1986; **Fellow:** Surgical Oncology, Meml Sloan Kettering Cancer Ctr 1988

Rolandelli, Rolando H MD (S) - **Spec Exp:** Crohn's Disease; Inflammatory Bowel Disease; Gastrointestinal Surgery; **Hospital:** Morristown Mem Hosp (page 92), Overlook Hosp (page 92); **Address:** 95 Madison Ave, Ste 304C, Morristown, NJ 07960; **Phone:** 973-971-7200; **Board Cert:** Surgery 2009; **Med School:** Argentina 1977; **Resid:** Surgery, Central Airforce Hosp 1982; Surgery, Grad Hosp 1990; **Fellow:** Metabolism, Univ Penn 1984

Sacco, Margaret M MD (S) - **Spec Exp:** Breast Surgery; Cancer Surgery; **Hospital:** Chilton Meml Hosp, St Clare's Hosp - Dover; **Address:** 22 Jackson Ave, Pompton Plains, NJ 07444; **Phone:** 973-835-0564; **Board Cert:** Surgery 2002; **Med School:** Hahnemann Univ 1986; **Resid:** Surgery, UMDNJ Univ Hosp 1991; **Fellow:** Surgical Oncology, UMDNJ-NJ Med Sch 1993

Strutin, Millard D MD (S) - **Hospital:** St Clare's Hosp - Denville, St Clare's Hosp - Dover; **Address:** NW Surgical Assocs, 121 Center Grove Rd, Randolph, NJ 07869; **Phone:** 973-328-1414; **Board Cert:** Surgery 2008; Surgical Critical Care 2002; **Med School:** Italy 1981; **Resid:** Surgery, UMDNJ Univ Hosp 1986

Whitman, Eric D MD (S) - **Spec Exp:** Melanoma; Endocrine Tumors; Cancer Surgery; Sarcoma; **Hospital:** Morristown Mem Hosp (page 92), Overlook Hosp (page 92); **Address:** 95 Madison Ave, Ste 307, Morristown, NJ 07962; **Phone:** 973-971-7111; **Board Cert:** Surgery 2002; **Med School:** Penn State Univ-Hershey Med Ctr 1985; **Resid:** Surgery, Hershey Med Ctr 1991; **Fellow:** Surgical Oncology, Natl Inst Hlth 1992

Thoracic Surgery

Brown III, John M MD (TS) - **Spec Exp:** Cardiac Surgery-Adult; Thoracic Cancers; Heart Valve Surgery; **Hospital:** Morristown Mem Hosp (page 92); **Address:** 100 Madison Ave, Morristown, NJ 07960-1956; **Phone:** 973-971-7300; **Board Cert:** Surgery 2001; Thoracic Surgery 2003; **Med School:** Cornell Univ-Weill Med Coll 1986; **Resid:** Surgery, NY Hosp-Cornell Univ Med Ctr 1991; **Fellow:** Thoracic Surgery, NY Hosp-Meml Sloan Kettering 1993

Parr, Grant V MD (TS) - **Spec Exp:** Cardiac Surgery; Heart Valve Surgery; Aneurysm-Thoracic Aortic; Atrial Fibrillation; **Hospital:** Morristown Mem Hosp (page 92), Overlook Hosp (page 92); **Address:** 100 Madison Ave, Morristown, NJ 07962-1956; **Phone:** 973-971-5597; **Board Cert:** Thoracic Surgery 2009; **Med School:** Cornell Univ-Weill Med Coll 1969; **Resid:** Surgery, Univ Hosps 1971; Surgery, Univ Alabama Hosp 1977; **Fellow:** Cardiothoracic Surgery, Univ Alabama Hosp 1977; **Fac Appt:** Asst Clin Prof S, Columbia P&S

Widmann, Mark D MD (TS) - **Spec Exp:** Minimally Invasive Thoracic Surgery; Video Assisted Thoracic Surgery (VATS); **Hospital:** Morristown Mem Hosp (page 92), Overlook Hosp (page 92); **Address:** PO Box 1348, Morristown, NJ 07962-1348; **Phone:** 973-644-4844; **Board Cert:** Thoracic Surgery 2007; **Med School:** Yale Univ 1987; **Resid:** Surgery, Yale-New Haven Hosp 1995; **Fellow:** Thoracic Surgery, Univ Iowa Hosps & Clinics 1998

Urology

Chaikin, David C MD (U) - **Spec Exp:** Voiding Dysfunction; Urology-Female; **Hospital:** Morristown Mem Hosp (page 92); **Address:** Morristown Urology, 261 James St, Ste 1A, Morristown, NJ 07960-6348; **Phone:** 973-539-1050; **Board Cert:** Urology 2007; **Med School:** Albert Einstein Coll Med 1992; **Resid:** Urology, Hosp Univ Penn 1997; **Fellow:** Female Urology, NY Hosp-Cornell Med Ctr 1999; **Fac Appt:** Asst Clin Prof U, Cornell Univ-Weill Med Coll

Colton, Marc D MD (U) - **Spec Exp:** Prostate Cancer; Urologic Cancer; Kidney Stones; Robotic Urologic Surgery; **Hospital:** St Clare's Hosp - Denville; **Address:** 16 Pocono Rd, Ste 205, Denville, NJ 07834-2907; **Phone:** 973-627-0060; **Board Cert:** Urology 2006; **Med School:** Med Coll PA 1989; **Resid:** Surgery, Temple Univ Hosp 1991; Urology, Temple Univ Hosp 1995

Connor, John Patrick MD (U) - **Spec Exp:** Pediatric Urology; **Hospital:** Morristown Mem Hosp (page 92), Overlook Hosp (page 92); **Address:** 261 James St, Ste 3A, Morristown, NJ 07960; **Phone:** 973-539-0333; **Board Cert:** Urology 2003; Pediatric Urology 2008; **Med School:** Ireland 1983; **Resid:** Surgery, UCLA Med Ctr 1986; Urology, Columbia-Presby Hosp 1990; **Fellow:** Urologic Oncology, Meml Sloan Kettering 1992; Pediatric Urology, Chldns Hosp Mich 1993; **Fac Appt:** Asst Prof U, Columbia P&S

Stone, Chester I MD (U) - **Spec Exp:** Prostate Cancer; **Hospital:** St Clare's Hosp - Dover, St Clare's Hosp - Denville; **Address:** 66 Sunset Strip, Ste 300, Succasunna, NJ 07876; **Phone:** 973-927-3388; **Board Cert:** Urology 1978; **Med School:** UMDNJ-NJ Med Sch, Newark 1971; **Resid:** Surgery, Maimonides Med Ctr 1973; Urology, Mount Sinai Med Ctr 1975

Vascular Surgery

Patel, Amit V MD (VascS) - **Hospital:** Morristown Mem Hosp (page 92); **Address:** Advanced Vascular Assocs, 131 Madison Ave Fl 2nd, Morristown, NJ 07960; **Phone:** 973-540-9700; **Board Cert:** Surgery 2004; Vascular Surgery 2006; **Med School:** Albert Einstein Coll Med 1988; **Resid:** Surgery, Montefiore Med Ctr 1993; **Fellow:** Vascular Surgery, Univ Penn 1994; **Fac Appt:** Asst Prof S, Albert Einstein Coll Med

Passaic

Passaic

Allergy & Immunology

Klein, Robert MD (A&I) - **Spec Exp:** Asthma; Sinusitis; Urticaria; Hereditary Angioedema; **Hospital:** NYPresby-Morgan Stanley Children's Hosp (page 104), St Mary's Hosp - Passaic; **Address:** 1005 Clifton Ave, Ste 4, Clifton, NJ 07013-3520; **Phone:** 973-773-7400; **Board Cert:** Pediatrics 1981; **Med School:** NY Med Coll 1976; **Resid:** Pediatrics, Beth Israel Hosp 1979; **Fellow:** Allergy & Immunology, Columbia-Presby Med Ctr 1984; **Fac Appt:** Asst Clin Prof Ped, Columbia P&S

Cardiovascular Disease

Julie, Edward MD (Cv) - **Spec Exp:** Interventional Cardiology; **Hospital:** St Mary's Hosp - Passaic, St Joseph's Regl Med Ctr - Paterson; **Address:** 1030 Clifton Ave, Clifton, NJ 07013-3500; **Phone:** 973-778-3777; **Board Cert:** Internal Medicine 1983; Cardiovascular Disease 1987; **Med School:** Albert Einstein Coll Med 1980; **Resid:** Internal Medicine, Mt Sinai Hosp 1983; **Fellow:** Cardiovascular Disease, NY Hosp 1986

Salimi, Mostafa MD (Cv) - **Hospital:** St. Joseph's Wayne Hosp, St Joseph's Regl Med Ctr - Paterson; **Address:** 246 Hamburg Tpke, Ste 201, Wayne, NJ 07470; **Phone:** 973-942-8176; **Board Cert:** Internal Medicine 1973; Cardiovascular Disease 1977; **Med School:** Iran 1964; **Resid:** Internal Medicine, VA Hospital 1970; **Fellow:** Cardiovascular Disease, George Washington Univ Hosp 1972

Siepser, Stuart L MD (Cv) - **Spec Exp:** Coronary Artery Disease; Hypertension; Nuclear Stress Testing; Cholesterol/Lipid Disorders; **Hospital:** Chilton Meml Hosp, Morristown Mem Hosp (page 92); **Address:** 1777 Hamburg Tpke, Ste 102, Wayne, NJ 07470-5243; **Phone:** 973-831-7455; **Board Cert:** Internal Medicine 1972; Cardiovascular Disease 1975; Nuclear Cardiology 2000; **Med School:** NYU Sch Med 1968; **Resid:** Internal Medicine, NYU Med Ctr 1970; Cardiovascular Disease, NYU Med Ctr 1972; **Fac Appt:** Asst Clin Prof Med, UMDNJ-NJ Med Sch, Newark

Strobeck, John E MD/PhD (Cv) - **Spec Exp:** Congestive Heart Failure; Nuclear Cardiology; Cardiac Imaging; **Hospital:** Valley Hosp (page 658); **Address:** Cardiac & Endovascular Assoc, 297 Lafayette Ave, Hawthorne, NJ 07506; **Phone:** 973-423-9388; **Board Cert:** Internal Medicine 1979; Cardiovascular Disease 1983; **Med School:** Univ Cincinnati 1974; **Resid:** Internal Medicine, Peter Bent Brigham Hosp 1976; **Fellow:** Cardiovascular Disease, Albert Einstein Coll Med 1978

Weiss, E Michael MD (Cv) - **Spec Exp:** Preventive Cardiology; Hypertension; Coronary Artery Disease; **Hospital:** St Mary's Hosp - Passaic, Univ Hosp-UMDNJ—Newark; **Address:** 842 Clifton Ave, Ste 5, Clifton, NJ 07013-1881; **Phone:** 973-777-2440; **Board Cert:** Internal Medicine 1984; Cardiovascular Disease 2007; **Med School:** Romania 1980; **Resid:** Internal Medicine, Hackensack Med Ctr 1983; **Fellow:** Cardiovascular Disease, Hackensack Med Ctr 1985; **Fac Appt:** Asst Clin Prof Med, UMDNJ-NJ Med Sch, Newark

Dermatology

Gold, Jonathan A MD (D) - **Spec Exp:** Acne & Rosacea; Eczema; **Hospital:** St Mary's Hosp - Passaic; **Address:** 1033 Clifton Ave, Clifton, NJ 07013; **Phone:** 973-777-6444; **Board Cert:** Dermatology 1987; **Med School:** Canada 1982; **Resid:** Dermatology, McGill Univ Med Ctr 1986; Dermatology, Montefiore Med Ctr 1987; **Fellow:** Dermatologic Pharmacology, NYU Med Ctr 1988

Maier, Herbert MD (D) - **Spec Exp:** Acne; Connective Tissue Disorders; Rosacea; **Hospital:** St. Joseph's Wayne Hosp; **Address:** 220 Hamburg Tpke Fl 2 - Ste 22, Wayne, NJ 07470-2132; **Phone:** 973-595-6338; **Board Cert:** Dermatology 1975; **Med School:** Geo Wash Univ 1967; **Resid:** Dermatology, Mount Sinai Med Ctr 1973

Pollack, Shoshannah S MD (D) - **Hospital:** Chilton Meml Hosp; **Address:** 1777 Hamburg Tpke, Ste 102, Wayne, NJ 07470; **Phone:** 973-835-1823; **Board Cert:** Dermatology 1990; **Med School:** Albert Einstein Coll Med 1986; **Resid:** Dermatology, Montefiore Med Ctr 1990

Tanzer, Floyd R MD (D) - **Spec Exp:** Acne; Eczema; **Hospital:** St Joseph's Regl Med Ctr - Paterson, Meadowlands Hosp Med Ctr; **Address:** 992 Clifton Ave, Clifton, NJ 07013-3502; **Phone:** 973-365-1800; **Board Cert:** Dermatology 1977; **Med School:** SUNY Downstate 1973; **Resid:** Dermatology, Kings Co Hosp 1977

Endocrinology, Diabetes & Metabolism

Berkowitz, Richard H MD (EDM) - **Spec Exp:** Diabetes; Cholesterol/Lipid Disorders; Thyroid Disorders; **Hospital:** Chilton Meml Hosp; **Address:** 2025 Hamburg Tpke, Ste D, Wayne, NJ 07470-6250; **Phone:** 973-839-5070; **Board Cert:** Internal Medicine 1975; Endocrinology 1977; **Med School:** SUNY Hlth Sci Ctr 1972; **Resid:** Internal Medicine, Montefiore Med Ctr 1974; Internal Medicine, UMDNJ-Univ Hosp 1975; **Fellow:** Endocrinology, Beth Israel Med Ctr 1977

Gastroenterology

Baum, Howard B MD (Ge) - **Spec Exp:** Endoscopy; Gastroesophageal Reflux Disease (GERD); Colonoscopy; **Hospital:** St Mary's Hosp - Passaic, St Joseph's Regl Med Ctr - Paterson; **Address:** 540 Broadway, Passaic, NJ 07055; **Phone:** 973-472-2100; **Board Cert:** Internal Medicine 1980; Gastroenterology 1983; **Med School:** Cornell Univ-Weill Med Coll 1977; **Resid:** Internal Medicine, Dartmouth-Hitchcock Med Ctr 1980; **Fellow:** Gastroenterology, NY Presby-Cornell Med Ctr

Bleicher, Robert MD (Ge) - **Spec Exp:** Inflammatory Bowel Disease; Irritable Bowel Syndrome; Liver Disease; **Hospital:** Chilton Meml Hosp; **Address:** 1825 Route 23 South, Wayne, NJ 07470; **Phone:** 973-633-1484; **Board Cert:** Internal Medicine 1981; Gastroenterology 1983; **Med School:** Columbia P&S 1978; **Resid:** Internal Medicine, Northwestern Meml Hosp 1981; **Fellow:** Gastroenterology, Northwestern Meml Hosp 1983

Farkas, John J MD (Ge) - **Hospital:** St Joseph's Regl Med Ctr - Paterson, St. Joseph's Wayne Hosp; **Address:** 716 Broad St Fl 1, Clifton, NJ 07013; **Phone:** 973-777-5717; **Board Cert:** Internal Medicine 1989; **Med School:** West Indies 1983; **Resid:** Internal Medicine, St Joseph's Hosp&Med Ctr 1986; **Fellow:** Gastroenterology, St Joseph's Hosp&Med Ctr 1988

Infectious Disease

Krieger, Richard MD (Inf) - **Spec Exp:** Lyme Disease; Endocarditis; **Hospital:** Chilton Meml Hosp, St. Joseph's Wayne Hosp; **Address:** 2035 Hamburg Tpke, Ste F, Wayne, NJ 07470-6251; **Phone:** 973-831-9228; **Board Cert:** Internal Medicine 1981; Infectious Disease 1984; **Med School:** UMDNJ-NJ Med Sch, Newark 1978; **Resid:** Internal Medicine, Med Coll Penn Hosp 1981; **Fellow:** Infectious Disease, Med Coll Penn Hosp 1983

Najjar, Sessine MD (Inf) - **Spec Exp:** Travel Medicine; **Hospital:** St Mary's Hosp - Passaic, Valley Hosp (page 658); **Address:** 975 Clifton Ave, Clifton, NJ 07013-2722; **Phone:** 973-778-8666; **Board Cert:** Internal Medicine 1979; Infectious Disease 1984; **Med School:** Lebanon 1974; **Resid:** Internal Medicine, Beekman Downtown Hosp 1977; **Fellow:** Infectious Disease, St Michaels Med Ctr 1979

Weiss, Gabriella A MD (Inf) - **Spec Exp:** Chronic Fatigue Syndrome; Lyme Disease; Bone Infections; **Hospital:** St Joseph's Regl Med Ctr - Paterson, St Mary's Hosp - Passaic; **Address:** 842 Clifto, Ste 4, Clifton, NJ 07013-1800; **Phone:** 973-777-2418; **Board Cert:** Internal Medicine 1985; **Med School:** Romania 1979; **Resid:** Internal Medicine, Hackensack Med Ctr 1984; **Fellow:** Infectious Disease, Hackensack Med Ctr 1985

Internal Medicine

De Giacomo, Frank C MD (IM) *PCP* - **Spec Exp:** Cholesterol/Lipid Disorders; **Hospital:** St Mary's Hosp - Passaic; **Address:** 540 Broadway, Passaic, NJ 07055-1956; **Phone:** 973-472-2100; **Board Cert:** Internal Medicine 1972; **Med School:** Harvard Med Sch 1965; **Resid:** Internal Medicine, Bellevue Hosp 1968; **Fellow:** Cardiovascular Disease, VA Hosp 1969

Gajdos, Robert MD (IM) *PCP* - **Hospital:** Mountainside Hosp, St Mary's Hosp - Passaic; **Address:** 1005 Clifton Ave, Clifton, NJ 07013-3520; **Phone:** 973-777-2005; **Board Cert:** Internal Medicine 1989; **Med School:** Grenada 1985; **Resid:** Internal Medicine, Mountainside Hosp 1989

Gold, Jeffrey L MD (IM) *PCP* - **Hospital:** St Joseph's Regl Med Ctr - Paterson, St Mary's Hosp - Passaic; **Address:** 1135 Broad St, Ste 205, Clifton, NJ 07013-3346; **Phone:** 973-471-8850; **Board Cert:** Internal Medicine 1983; **Med School:** Mexico 1977; **Resid:** Internal Medicine, St Josephs Hosp 1981; **Fac Appt:** Asst Clin Prof Med, UMDNJ-NJ Med Sch, Newark

Jawetz, Harold I MD (IM) - **Spec Exp:** Chronic Obstructive Lung Disease (COPD); Pulmonary Disease; Asthma; **Hospital:** St Mary's Hosp - Passaic, St Joseph's Regl Med Ctr - Paterson; **Address:** 540 Broadway, Passaic, NJ 07055-1956; **Phone:** 973-472-2100; **Board Cert:** Internal Medicine 1974; **Med School:** Albert Einstein Coll Med 1971; **Resid:** Internal Medicine, Montefiore Med Ctr 1974; **Fellow:** Pulmonary Disease, Montefiore Med Ctr 1978

Maternal & Fetal Medicine

Sullivan, Christopher A MD (MF) - **Spec Exp:** Pregnancy-High Risk; Perinatal Medicine; Diabetes in Pregnancy; Multiple Gestation; **Hospital:** St Joseph's Regl Med Ctr - Paterson, Holy Name Med Ctr (page 657); **Address:** 525 Union Blvd, Totowa, NJ 07512; **Phone:** 973-904-9778; **Board Cert:** Obstetrics & Gynecology 2009; Maternal & Fetal Medicine 2009; **Med School:** Albany Med Coll 1989; **Resid:** Obstetrics & Gynecology, St Barnabas Med Ctr 1993; **Fellow:** Maternal & Fetal Medicine, Univ of Miss Med Ctr 1995

Medical Oncology

Uhm, Kyudong MD (Onc) - **Hospital:** St Mary's Hosp - Passaic, St Joseph's Regl Med Ctr - Paterson; **Address:** 1117 Route 46 East, Ste 205, Clifton, NJ 07013; **Phone:** 973-471-0981; **Board Cert:** Internal Medicine 1978; Medical Oncology 1979; Hematology 1980; **Med School:** South Korea 1969; **Resid:** Internal Medicine, Englewood 1977; Hematology, Montefiore Hosp Med Ctr 1978; **Fellow:** Medical Oncology, Montefiore Hosp Med Ctr 1980

Nephrology

Vitting, Kevin E MD (Nep) - **Spec Exp:** Hypertension; Kidney Failure; **Hospital:** St Joseph's Regl Med Ctr - Paterson, St. Joseph's Wayne Hosp; **Address:** 342 Hamburg Tpke, Ste 201, Wayne, NJ 07470; **Phone:** 973-389-1119; **Board Cert:** Internal Medicine 1985; Nephrology 1988; **Med School:** UMDNJ-RW Johnson Med Sch 1982; **Resid:** Internal Medicine, Lenox Hill Hosp 1985; **Fellow:** Nephrology, Lenox Hill Hosp 1987; **Fac Appt:** Asst Clin Prof Med, Mount Sinai Sch Med

Neurology

Chodosh, Eliot H MD (N) - **Spec Exp:** Stroke; Multiple Sclerosis; **Hospital:** St. Joseph's Wayne Hosp, Chilton Meml Hosp; **Address:** 220 Hamburg Tpke, Ste 16, Wayne, NJ 07470-2193; **Phone:** 973-942-4778; **Board Cert:** Neurology 1987; **Med School:** Mexico 1981; **Resid:** Neurology, Boston Univ Med Ctr 1986; **Fellow:** Cerebrovascular Disease, Boston Univ Med Ctr 1987

Knep, Stanley MD (N) - **Spec Exp:** Electromyography; Parkinson's Disease; Headache; **Hospital:** St Joseph's Regl Med Ctr - Paterson, St Mary's Hosp - Passaic; **Address:** 905 Allwood Rd, Ste 105, Clifton, NJ 07013; **Phone:** 973-471-3680; **Board Cert:** Neurology 1977; **Med School:** South Africa 1965; **Resid:** Internal Medicine, Johannesburg Hosp 1970; Neurology, Albert Einstein 1975; **Fac Appt:** Asst Clin Prof N, Seton Hall Univ Sch Hlth & Med Scis

Obstetrics & Gynecology

Burns, Les A MD (ObG) *PCP* - **Spec Exp:** Menopause Problems; Pap Smear Abnormalities; Hysterectomy Alternatives; Pregnancy After Age 35; **Hospital:** Chilton Meml Hosp, St Joseph's Regl Med Ctr - Paterson; **Address:** 1784 Hamburg Tpke, Wayne, NJ 07470-4023; **Phone:** 973-831-9925; **Board Cert:** Obstetrics & Gynecology 2008; **Med School:** Hahnemann Univ 1981; **Resid:** Obstetrics & Gynecology, Danbury Hosp 1985

Kierce, Roger P MD (ObG) - **Hospital:** St Joseph's Regl Med Ctr - Paterson; **Address:** Willowbrook Obstetrics & Gynecology, 57 Willowbrook Blvd Fl 3 - Ste 301, Wayne, NJ 07470-7045; **Phone:** 973-754-4075; **Board Cert:** Obstetrics & Gynecology 2007; **Med School:** UMDNJ-NJ Med Sch, Newark 1986; **Resid:** Obstetrics & Gynecology, St Josephs Hosp 1990

Ophthalmology

Giliberti, Orazio L MD (Oph) - **Spec Exp:** Laser-Refractive Surgery; Cataract Surgery-Lens Implant; Corneal Disease & Surgery; Glaucoma; **Hospital:** Univ Hosp-UMDNJ—Newark, Clara Maass Med Ctr; **Address:** Giliberti Eye and Laser Center, 415 Totowa Rd, Totowa, NJ 07512-2081; **Phone:** 973-595-0011; **Board Cert:** Ophthalmology 1989; **Med School:** Grenada 1982; **Resid:** Ophthalmology, UMDNJ Affil Hosps 1987; **Fellow:** Ophthalmology, Pennsylvania Hosp 1984; Refractive Surgery, Vision Sculpting; **Fac Appt:** Asst Prof Oph, UMDNJ-NJ Med Sch, Newark

Vogel, Mitchell MD (Oph) - **Spec Exp:** Corneal Disease; Refractive Surgery; Uveitis; Cataract Surgery; **Hospital:** St Mary's Hosp - Passaic, Overlook Hosp (page 92); **Address:** 124 Gregory Ave, Ste 104, Passaic, NJ 07055-4856; **Phone:** 973-779-0808; **Board Cert:** Ophthalmology 2010; **Med School:** Temple Univ 1991; **Resid:** Ophthalmology, Nassau Co Med Ctr 1995; **Fellow:** Cornea, Univ Tex SW Med Ctr 1996

Orthopaedic Surgery

Drillings, Gary MD (OrS) - **Spec Exp:** Knee Injuries; Shoulder Injuries; Sports Medicine; **Hospital:** Chilton Meml Hosp; **Address:** 1777 Hamburg Tpke, Ste 305, Wayne, NJ 07470; **Phone:** 973-831-6666; **Board Cert:** Orthopaedic Surgery 2004; **Med School:** SUNY Upstate Med Univ 1985; **Resid:** Orthopaedic Surgery, Northwestern Med Ctr 1990; **Fellow:** Sports Medicine, Lenox Hill Hosp 1991

Emami, Arash MD (OrS) - **Spec Exp:** Spinal Surgery; Scoliosis; Minimally Invasive Spinal Surgery; Spinal Disc Replacement; **Hospital:** St Joseph's Regl Med Ctr - Paterson, NYU Hosp For Joint Diseases (page 106); **Address:** 504 Valley Rd, Fl 2 - Ste 203, Wayne, NJ 07470; **Phone:** 973-686-0700; **Board Cert:** Orthopaedic Surgery 2002; **Med School:** Univ Chicago-Pritzker Sch Med 1994; **Resid:** Orthopaedic Surgery, Univ Chicago Hosps 1999; **Fellow:** Spinal Surgery, UCSF Med Ctr 2000; **Fac Appt:** Asst Prof OrS, Seton Hall Univ Sch Hlth & Med Scis

Mc Inerney, Vincent MD (OrS) - **Spec Exp:** Hip Replacement; Minimally Invasive Surgery; Knee Replacement; Shoulder Replacement; **Hospital:** St Joseph's Regl Med Ctr - Paterson; **Address:** 504 Valley Rd, Wayne, NJ 07470; **Phone:** 973-694-2690; **Board Cert:** Orthopaedic Surgery 1984; **Med School:** UMDNJ-NJ Med Sch, Newark 1977; **Resid:** Orthopaedic Surgery, St Josephs Hosp Med Ctr 1981; **Fellow:** Sports Medicine, Mass Genl Hosp 1982

Reicher, Oscar MD (OrS) - **Spec Exp:** Reconstructive Surgery; Sports Medicine; **Hospital:** Chilton Meml Hosp, St. Joseph's Wayne Hosp; **Address:** 2035 Hamburg Tpke, Ste D, Wayne, NJ 07470; **Phone:** 973-616-0200; **Board Cert:** Orthopaedic Surgery 2007; **Med School:** Univ Pittsburgh 1979; **Resid:** Orthopaedic Surgery, Vanderbilt Univ Hosp 1984

Strongwater, Allan M MD (OrS) - **Spec Exp:** Pediatric Orthopaedic Surgery; Cerebral Palsy; Deformity Reconstruction; **Hospital:** St Joseph's Regl Med Ctr - Paterson, NYU Langone Med Ctr (page 106); **Address:** St Josephs Childrens Hospital, Dept Orthopaedic Surgery, 703 Main St - Xavier 702, Paterson, NJ 07503; **Phone:** 973-754-2414; **Board Cert:** Orthopaedic Surgery 2007; **Med School:** Rush Med Coll 1978; **Resid:** Orthopaedic Surgery, Yale-New Haven Hosp 1983; **Fellow:** Pediatric Orthopaedic Surgery, Hosp Joint Diseases 1984; **Fac Appt:** Clin Prof OrS, NYU Sch Med

Otolaryngology

Cece, John A MD (Oto) - **Spec Exp:** Sinus Surgery; Cosmetic Surgery-Face; Rhinoplasty; **Hospital:** Chilton Meml Hosp, St Mary's Hosp - Passaic; **Address:** 1211 Hamburg Tpke, Wayne, NJ 07470; **Phone:** 973-633-0808; **Board Cert:** Otolaryngology 1986; Facial Plastic & Reconstr Surgery 1992; **Med School:** UMDNJ-RW Johnson Med Sch 1981; **Resid:** Otolaryngology, Mt Sinai Med Ctr 1986

La Bagnara Jr, James MD (Oto) - **Spec Exp:** Thyroid & Parathyroid Surgery; Pediatric Otolaryngology; **Hospital:** St Joseph's Regl Med Ctr - Paterson, St. Joseph's Wayne Hosp; **Address:** 311 Lexington Ave, Paterson, NJ 07502-1010; **Phone:** 973-942-1300; **Board Cert:** Otolaryngology 1978; **Med School:** UMDNJ-NJ Med Sch, Newark 1974; **Resid:** Otolaryngology, UMDNJ Affil Hosp 1978; Otolaryngology, Newark EE Hosp 1981; **Fac Appt:** Assoc Clin Prof Oto, UMDNJ-NJ Med Sch, Newark

Mattel, Stephen F MD (Oto) - **Spec Exp:** Pediatric Otolaryngology; **Hospital:** Chilton Meml Hosp, Mountainside Hosp; **Address:** 1211 Hamburg Turnpike Ave, Ste 205, Wayne, NJ 07470; **Phone:** 973-633-0808; **Board Cert:** Otolaryngology 1981; **Med School:** NYU Sch Med 1977; **Resid:** Surgery, Mount Sinai Hosp 1978; Otolaryngology, Bellevue Hosp 1981

Pediatric Hematology-Oncology

Bonilla, Mary Ann MD (PHO) - **Hospital:** St Joseph's Regl Med Ctr - Paterson; **Address:** St Joseph's Chldns Hosp, 703 Main St, Xavier 7, Paterson, NJ 07503; **Phone:** 973-754-3230; **Board Cert:** Pediatrics 1986; Pediatric Hematology-Oncology 2005; **Med School:** Loyola Univ-Stritch Sch Med 1981; **Resid:** Pediatrics, Brookdale Hosp 1984; **Fellow:** Pediatric Hematology-Oncology, Meml Sloan Kettering Canc Ctr 1988; **Fac Appt:** Asst Prof Ped, Columbia P&S

Pediatric Nephrology

Salcedo-Contreras, Jose R MD (PNep) - **Spec Exp:** Hypertension; Dialysis Care; Kidney Failure; Lupus/SLE; **Hospital:** St Joseph's Regl Med Ctr - Paterson, Morristown Mem Hosp (page 92); **Address:** 703 Main St, Paterson, NJ 07503-2621; **Phone:** 973-754-2570; **Board Cert:** Pediatrics 1976; Pediatric Nephrology 1976; **Med School:** Mexico 1970; **Resid:** Pediatrics, UMDNJ-Martland Hosp 1974; **Fellow:** Pediatric Nephrology, Chldns Hosp Natl Med Ctr 1976; Nephrology, Armed Forces Inst Path 1977; **Fac Appt:** Assoc Clin Prof Ped, UMDNJ-NJ Med Sch, Newark

Pediatric Pulmonology

Nachajon, Roberto MD (PPul) - **Spec Exp:** Asthma; Cystic Fibrosis; Sleep Disorders; Bronchoscopy; **Hospital:** St Joseph's Regl Med Ctr - Paterson, Mount Sinai Med Ctr (page 102); **Address:** St Josephs Chldns Hosp, Div Pediatric Pulmonology, 703 Main St, Paterson, NJ 07503; **Phone:** 973-754-2550; **Board Cert:** Pediatric Pulmonology 2004; Sleep Medicine 2007; **Med School:** Uruguay 1985; **Resid:** Pediatrics, Chldns Hosp Uruguay 1990; Pediatrics, Beth Israel Med Ctr 1993; **Fellow:** Pediatric Pulmonology, Childrens Hosp 1996; **Fac Appt:** Asst Clin Prof Ped, Mount Sinai Sch Med

Pediatrics

Scofield, Lisa MD (Ped) *PCP* - **Hospital:** St Joseph's Regl Med Ctr - Paterson, Chilton Meml Hosp; **Address:** 57 Willowbrook Blvd, Ste 421, Wayne, NJ 07470; **Phone:** 973-754-4025; **Board Cert:** Pediatrics 2009; **Med School:** UMDNJ-NJ Med Sch, Newark 1990; **Resid:** Pediatrics, New York Hosp-Cornell 1994

Plastic Surgery

Ganchi, Parham A MD/PhD (PlS) - **Spec Exp:** Cosmetic Surgery-Face & Body; Cosmetic Surgery-Breast; Facial Rejuvenation; Body Contouring; **Hospital:** Chilton Meml Hosp, St. Joseph's Wayne Hosp; **Address:** 342 Hamburg Tpke, Ste 202, Wayne, NJ 07470; **Phone:** 973-942-6600; **Board Cert:** Surgery 2000; Plastic Surgery 2003; **Med School:** Duke Univ 1994; **Resid:** Surgery, Harvard Med Sch 1999; **Fellow:** Plastic Surgery, Harvard Plastic Surgery 2002

Psychiatry

Hindin, Lee MD (Psyc) - **Spec Exp:** Addiction Psychiatry; **Hospital:** Saint Barnabas Med Ctr; **Address:** Creative Intervention, 1149 Bloomfield Ave, Clifton, NJ 07012; **Phone:** 973-365-2300; **Board Cert:** Psychiatry 1984; **Med School:** UMDNJ-NJ Med Sch, Newark 1977; **Resid:** Psychiatry, UCLA-Neuropsyc Inst 1982

Pulmonary Disease

Amoruso, Robert C MD (Pul) - **Spec Exp:** Asthma; Critical Care; **Hospital:** St Joseph's Regl Med Ctr - Paterson, St. Joseph's Wayne Hosp; **Address:** 999 McBride Ave, Ste 201B, West Paterson, NJ 07424; **Phone:** 973-256-0287; **Board Cert:** Internal Medicine 1979; Pulmonary Disease 1982; **Med School:** Italy 1975; **Resid:** Internal Medicine, St Joseph's Hosp Med Ctr 1979; **Fellow:** Pulmonary Disease, College Hosp-UMDNJ 1981

Grizzanti, Joseph N DO (Pul) - **Spec Exp:** Lung Cancer; Asthma; Allergy; Immunologic Lung Disease; **Hospital:** Nyack Hosp, Englewood Hosp & Med Ctr (page 656); **Address:** 297 Lafayette Ave, Hawthorne, NJ 07506; **Phone:** 973-790-4111; **Board Cert:** Internal Medicine 1979; Pulmonary Disease 1982; Allergy & Immunology 1985; **Med School:** Philadelphia Coll Osteo Med 1976; **Resid:** Internal Medicine, Univ Hosp 1979; Allergy & Immunology, Montefiore-Albert Einstein 1984; **Fellow:** Pulmonary Disease, Montefiore-Albert Einstein 1981; **Fac Appt:** Assoc Clin Prof Med, Albert Einstein Coll Med

Radiation Oncology

Cole, Robert J MD (RadRO) - **Spec Exp:** Brachytherapy; Breast Cancer; Prostate Cancer; **Hospital:** St Mary's Hosp - Passaic, Robert Wood Johnson Univ Hosp - New Brunswick; **Address:** St Mary's Hosp, Dept Oncology, 350 Boulevard, Passaic, NJ 07055; **Phone:** 973-365-5088; **Board Cert:** Therapeutic Radiology 1983; **Med School:** Wake Forest Univ 1979; **Resid:** Therapeutic Radiology, Univ of VA Health Sci Ctr 1983

Reproductive Endocrinology

Ransom, Mark X MD (RE) - **Spec Exp:** Infertility-IVF; **Hospital:** St. Joseph's Wayne Hosp, Hackensack Univ Med Ctr (page 96); **Address:** 57 Willowbrook Blvd, Wayne, NJ 07470; **Phone:** 973-754-4055; **Board Cert:** Obstetrics & Gynecology 2009; Reproductive Endocrinology 2009; **Med School:** UMDNJ-RW Johnson Med Sch 1987; **Resid:** Obstetrics & Gynecology, RWJ Univ Hosp 1991; **Fellow:** Reproductive Endocrinology, RWJ Univ Hosp 1992

Rheumatology

Goldberg, Marc A MD (Rhu) - **Spec Exp:** Rheumatoid Arthritis; Osteoporosis; Osteoarthritis; **Hospital:** St Mary's Hosp - Passaic; **Address:** 200 Gregory Ave, Passaic, NJ 07055-3802; **Phone:** 973-473-2597; **Board Cert:** Internal Medicine 1972; Rheumatology 1976; **Med School:** Med Coll VA 1969; **Resid:** Internal Medicine, Univ Maryland Hosp 1972; Rheumatology, Johns Hopkins Hosp 1973; **Fellow:** Rheumatology, Hosp Univ Penn 1976

Lewko, Michael P MD (Rhu) - **Spec Exp:** Geriatric Rheumatology; Arthritis; Osteoporosis; Rheumatoid Arthritis; **Hospital:** St Joseph's Regl Med Ctr - Paterson; **Address:** 871 Allwood Rd, Clifton, NJ 07012; **Phone:** 973-405-5163; **Board Cert:** Internal Medicine 1988; Rheumatology 2002; Geriatric Medicine 2004; **Med School:** UMDNJ-Rutgers Med Sch 1985; **Resid:** Internal Medicine, RW Johnson Univ Hosp 1988; **Fellow:** Geriatric Medicine, Roger Williams Med Ctr 1989; Rheumatology, Hosp Univ Penn 1991; **Fac Appt:** Asst Clin Prof Med, Mount Sinai Sch Med

Surgery

Budd, Daniel C MD (S) - **Spec Exp:** Breast Cancer; Endocrine Surgery; Gastrointestinal Surgery; **Hospital:** Valley Hosp (page 658), Chilton Meml Hosp; **Address:** 707 Broadway, Paterson, NJ 07514; **Phone:** 973-742-3371; **Board Cert:** Surgery 1975; **Med School:** Duke Univ 1969; **Resid:** Surgery, Columbia-Presby Hosp 1974; **Fac Appt:** Assoc Clin Prof S, UMDNJ-NJ Med Sch, Newark

Feigenbaum, Howard MD (S) - **Spec Exp:** Gastrointestinal Surgery; Colon Surgery; Laparoscopic Surgery; Breast Surgery; **Hospital:** Chilton Meml Hosp, St. Joseph's Wayne Hosp; **Address:** 227 Hamburg Tpke, Pompton Lakes, NJ 07442-1838; **Phone:** 973-839-7999; **Board Cert:** Surgery 1998; **Med School:** NYU Sch Med 1971; **Resid:** Surgery, Bellevue Hosp 1977

Thoracic Surgery

Bronstein, Eric H MD (TS) - **Spec Exp:** Video Assisted Thoracic Surgery (VATS); Lung Cancer; Minimally Invasive Thoracic Surgery; **Hospital:** St Joseph's Regl Med Ctr - Paterson; **Address:** 703 Main St, Ste A2407, Paterson, NJ 07503; **Phone:** 973-754-2486; **Board Cert:** Surgery 2004; Thoracic Surgery 2006; **Med School:** SUNY Stony Brook 1987; **Resid:** Surgery, SUNY Downstate Med Ctr 1993; **Fellow:** Cardiothoracic Surgery, Geo Washington Univ Hosp 1997; **Fac Appt:** Asst Clin Prof S, Columbia P&S

Christakos, Manny E MD (TS) - **Spec Exp:** Cardiovascular Surgery; **Hospital:** St. Joseph's Wayne Hosp, St Mary's Hosp - Passaic; **Address:** 871 Allwood Rd Fl 2, Clifton, NJ 07012-1922; **Phone:** 973-779-2270; **Board Cert:** Thoracic Surgery 2002; **Med School:** SUNY Buffalo 1971; **Resid:** Surgery, EJ Meyer Meml Hosp 1976; Thoracic Surgery, UC Irvine Med Ctr 1980

Kaushik, Raj R MD (TS) - **Spec Exp:** Minimally Invasive Cardiac Surgery; Atrial Fibrillation; Laser Surgery; **Hospital:** St Mary's Hosp - Passaic, Mountainside Hosp; **Address:** St Mary's Hosp, Div Cardiac Surgery, 350 Boulevard, Ste 130, Passaic, NJ 07055; **Phone:** 973-365-4567; **Board Cert:** Thoracic Surgery 2009; **Med School:** India 1979; **Resid:** Surgery, Bridgeport Hosp 1985; Cardiothoracic Surgery, Newark Beth Israel Med Ctr 1988; **Fellow:** Cardiac Surgery, Baylor Univ 1989; Cardiac Surgery, Univ W Ontario Med Ctr 1990

Urology

Levine, Seth P MD (U) - **Spec Exp:** Prostate Cancer; **Hospital:** Chilton Meml Hosp, Valley Hosp (page 658); **Address:** 1777 Hamburg Tpke, Ste 304, Wayne, NJ 07470; **Phone:** 973-616-8400; **Board Cert:** Urology 1980; **Med School:** Tufts Univ 1971; **Resid:** Surgery, Mount Sinai Hosp 1973; Urology, Mount Sinai Hosp 1978

Somerset

Somerset

Allergy & Immunology

Caucino, Julie A DO (A&I) - **Spec Exp:** Asthma & Allergy; Food Allergy; Urticaria; **Hospital:** Univ Med Ctr - Princeton; **Address:** 24 Vreeland Drive, Skillnan, NJ 08558-2621; **Phone:** 609-921-2202; **Board Cert:** Internal Medicine 2000; Allergy & Immunology 2003; **Med School:** Kirksville Coll Osteo Med 1987; **Resid:** Internal Medicine, RWJ Univ Hosp 1991; **Fellow:** Allergy & Immunology, Albert Einstein Coll Med 1993

Fox, James A MD (A&I) - **Spec Exp:** Asthma; Urticaria; Food Allergy; Hereditary Angioedema; **Hospital:** Somerset Med Ctr, Hunterdon Med Ctr; **Address:** 3461 US Highway 22, Somerville, NJ 08876-6021; **Phone:** 908-725-4777; **Board Cert:** Pediatrics 1981; Allergy & Immunology 1983; **Med School:** Yale Univ 1977; **Resid:** Pediatrics, Bronx Municipal Hosp Ctr 1980; **Fellow:** Allergy & Immunology, Columbia-Presby Med Ctr 1982

Krol, Kristine MD (A&I) - **Spec Exp:** Insect Allergies; Drug Sensitivity; Food Allergy; Asthma; **Hospital:** Staten Island Univ Hosp - South, Somerset Med Ctr; **Address:** 177 W High St, Somerville, NJ 08876; **Phone:** 908-725-8666; **Board Cert:** Internal Medicine 1987; **Med School:** SUNY Downstate 1981; **Resid:** Internal Medicine, Staten Island Hosp 1985; **Fellow:** Allergy & Immunology, Mass Genl Hosp 1987; **Fac Appt:** Asst Clin Prof Med, SUNY Downstate

Pedinoff, Andrew J MD (A&I) - **Spec Exp:** Allergy; Asthma; Hay Fever; **Hospital:** Univ Med Ctr - Princeton, Robert Wood Johnson Univ Hosp - New Brunswick; **Address:** Princeton Allergy & Asthma Assoc, 24 Vreeland Drive, Skilman, NJ 08558; **Phone:** 609-921-2202; **Board Cert:** Allergy & Immunology 2003; **Med School:** Dominican Republic 1984; **Resid:** Pediatrics, Georgetown Univ Hosp 1987; **Fellow:** Allergy & Immunology, Georgetown Univ Hosp 1989; **Fac Appt:** Asst Clin Prof Ped, UMDNJ-RW Johnson Med Sch

Schulhafer, Edwin MD (A&I) - **Spec Exp:** Asthma; Sinus Disorders; Allergy; Migraine; **Hospital:** Somerset Med Ctr, Hunterdon Med Ctr; **Address:** 712 Courtyard Drive, Hillsborough, NJ 08844; **Phone:** 908-526-0200; **Board Cert:** Internal Medicine 1988; Allergy & Immunology 2006; **Med School:** UMDNJ-NJ Med Sch, Newark 1983; **Resid:** Internal Medicine, Overlook Hosp 1986; **Fellow:** Allergy & Immunology, Long Island Hosp 1988

Southern, D Loren MD (A&I) - **Spec Exp:** Asthma; Allergy; Hives; **Hospital:** Univ Med Ctr - Princeton; **Address:** 24 Vreeland Drive, Skillman, NJ 08558; **Phone:** 609-921-2202; **Board Cert:** Pediatrics 1976; **Med School:** Columbia P&S 1971; **Resid:** Pediatrics, Columbia-Presby Med Ctr 1974; **Fellow:** Allergy & Immunology, Columbia-Presby Med Ctr 1976

Cardiovascular Disease

Kulkarni, Rachana MD (Cv) - **Spec Exp:** Nuclear Cardiology; **Hospital:** Somerset Med Ctr; **Address:** 225 Jackson St, Bridgewater, NJ 08807; **Phone:** 908-526-8668; **Board Cert:** Cardiovascular Disease 2010; **Med School:** India 1988; **Resid:** Internal Medicine, UMDNJ-RWJ Univ Hosp 1995; **Fellow:** Cardiovascular Disease, UMDNJ-RWJ Univ Hosp 1998

Leeds, Richard S MD (Cv) - **Spec Exp:** Cardiac Catheterization; Invasive Cardiology; Non-Invasive Cardiology; **Hospital:** Somerset Med Ctr, Robert Wood Johnson Univ Hosp - New Brunswick; **Address:** 225 Jackson St, Bridgewater, NJ 08807; **Phone:** 908-526-8668; **Board Cert:** Cardiovascular Disease 1987; Internal Medicine 1984; **Med School:** NY Med Coll 1981; **Resid:** Internal Medicine, Beth Israel Med Ctr 1985; **Fellow:** Cardiovascular Disease, St Vincents Hosp 1987

Saulino, Patrick F MD (Cv) - **Spec Exp:** Cardiac Catheterization; Invasive Cardiology; Non-Invasive Cardiology; **Hospital:** Somerset Med Ctr, Robert Wood Johnson Univ Hosp - New Brunswick; **Address:** 225 Jackson Street, Bridgewater, NJ 08807; **Phone:** 908-526-8668; **Board Cert:** Internal Medicine 1984; Cardiovascular Disease 1987; **Med School:** Georgetown Univ 1981; **Resid:** Internal Medicine, Georgetown Univ Hosp 1984; Cardiovascular Disease, Georgetown Univ Hosp 1985; **Fellow:** Cardiovascular Disease, UMDNJ-RW Johnson Sch Med 1987; Cardiovascular Disease, Georgetown Univ Hosp 1988

Stroh, Jack MD (Cv) - **Spec Exp:** Angioplasty & Stent Placement; Hypertension; Cholesterol/Lipid Disorders; **Hospital:** Robert Wood Johnson Univ Hosp - New Brunswick, St Peter's Univ Hosp; **Address:** 75 Veronica Ave, Somerset, NJ 08873-5002; **Phone:** 732-247-7444; **Board Cert:** Internal Medicine 1987; Cardiovascular Disease 1989; Interventional Cardiology 2009; **Med School:** Albert Einstein Coll Med 1984; **Resid:** Internal Medicine, Boston Univ Med Ctr 1987; **Fellow:** Cardiovascular Disease, NYU Med Ctr 1990

Dermatology

Fox, Alissa MD (D) - **Spec Exp:** Acne; Psoriasis; **Hospital:** Somerset Med Ctr, Hunterdon Med Ctr; **Address:** 3461 US Highway 22, Branchburg, NJ 08876; **Phone:** 908-725-4777; **Board Cert:** Dermatology 1984; **Med School:** NYU Sch Med 1980; **Resid:** Dermatology, New York Hosp 1984

Pappert, Amy S MD (D) - **Hospital:** Robert Wood Johnson Univ Hosp - New Brunswick; **Address:** UMDNJ- RW Johnson Med School, Dept Dermatology, 1 World's Fair Drive, Ste 2400, Somerset, NJ 08873; **Phone:** 732-463-7546; **Board Cert:** Dermatology 2001; **Med School:** UMDNJ-RW Johnson Med Sch 1989; **Resid:** Dermatology, Columbia Presby Med Ctr 1994; **Fellow:** Research, Columbia Presby Med Ctr 1991; **Fac Appt:** Asst Prof D, UMDNJ-RW Johnson Med Sch

Diagnostic Radiology

Melville, Gordon MD (DR) - **Spec Exp:** Neuroradiology; MRI; **Hospital:** Somerset Med Ctr; **Address:** 16 Mountain Blvd, Warren, NJ 07059-6331; **Phone:** 908-769-7200; **Board Cert:** Diagnostic Radiology 1984; Neuroradiology 2006; **Med School:** Univ NC Sch Med 1979; **Resid:** Diagnostic Radiology, George Washington Univ Hosp 1984; **Fellow:** Neuroradiology, Mass Genl Hosp 1985; **Fac Appt:** Asst Clin Prof, Robert W Johnson Med Sch

Yang, Roger S MD (DR) - **Spec Exp:** Breast Imaging; Women's Imaging; **Hospital:** Somerset Med Ctr; **Address:** Somerset Med Ctr, Dept Radiology, 110 Rehill Ave, Somerville, NJ 08876; **Phone:** 908-685-2930; **Board Cert:** Diagnostic Radiology 1997; **Med School:** Northwestern Univ 1992; **Resid:** Diagnostic Radiology, Univ Hosp 1997; **Fellow:** Women's Imaging, Univ Hosp/Kings Co Hosp 1998; **Fac Appt:** Asst Clin Prof, SUNY Downstate

Family Medicine

Corson, Richard L MD (FMed) *PCP* - **Hospital:** Somerset Med Ctr; **Address:** 313 Courtyard Drive, Hillsborough, NJ 08844; **Phone:** 908-722-9962; **Board Cert:** Family Medicine 2004; **Med School:** UMDNJ-RW Johnson Med Sch 1983; **Resid:** Family Medicine, Somerset Med Ctr 1986

Frisoli, Anthony MD (FMed) *PCP* - **Spec Exp:** Sports Medicine; Geriatric Care; **Hospital:** Somerset Med Ctr; **Address:** 1973 Washington Valley Rd, Martinsville, NJ 08836; **Phone:** 732-560-9225; **Board Cert:** Family Medicine 2005; **Med School:** UMDNJ-Rutgers Med Sch 1983; **Resid:** Family Medicine, Somerset Med Ctr 1986

Ziering, Thomas S MD (FMed) *PCP* - **Spec Exp:** Anxiety & Depression; Gay/Lesbian/Transgender Health; Skin Diseases; Complementary Medicine; **Hospital:** Morristown Mem Hosp (page 92); **Address:** 39 Olcott Fl 2, Bernardsville, NJ 07924-2317; **Phone:** 908-221-1919; **Board Cert:** Family Medicine 2003; **Med School:** UMDNJ-NJ Med Sch, Newark 1987; **Resid:** Family Medicine, Somerset Med Ctr 1990; **Fac Appt:** Assoc Clin Prof FMed, Robert W Johnson Med Sch

Gastroenterology

Accurso, Charles A MD (Ge) - **Spec Exp:** Endoscopy; Irritable Bowel Syndrome; Gastroesophageal Reflux Disease (GERD); Peptic Acid Disorders; **Hospital:** Somerset Med Ctr; **Address:** 511 Courtyard Drive Bldg 500, Digestive Healthcare Ctr, Hillsborough, NJ 08844-2017; **Phone:** 908-218-9222; **Board Cert:** Internal Medicine 1987; Gastroenterology 1989; **Med School:** UMDNJ-NJ Med Sch, Newark 1984; **Resid:** Internal Medicine, Univ Hosp 1987; **Fellow:** Gastroenterology, Univ Hosp/NJ Med Sch 1989; **Fac Appt:** Asst Clin Prof Med, UMDNJ-NJ Med Sch, Newark

Ferges, Mitchell L MD (Ge) - **Spec Exp:** Liver Disease; **Hospital:** St Peter's Univ Hosp, Robert Wood Johnson Univ Hosp - New Brunswick; **Address:** 33 Clyde Rd, Ste 102, Somerset, NJ 08873; **Phone:** 732-873-9200; **Board Cert:** Internal Medicine 1978; Gastroenterology 1981; **Med School:** UMDNJ-RW Johnson Med Sch 1975; **Resid:** Internal Medicine, UMDNJ Rutgers Affil Hosps 1978; **Fellow:** Gastroenterology, UMDNJ Univ Hosp 1980

Hematology

Toomey, Kathleen C MD (Hem) - **Spec Exp:** Breast Cancer; **Hospital:** Somerset Med Ctr, St Peter's Univ Hosp; **Address:** Steepchase Cancer Ctr, 30 Rehill Ave, Ste 2500, Somerville, NJ 08876; **Phone:** 908-927-8700; **Board Cert:** Internal Medicine 1982; Medical Oncology 1987; Hematology 2003; **Med School:** Italy 1978; **Resid:** Internal Medicine, St Peters Med Ctr 1982; **Fellow:** Hematology & Oncology, UMDNJ-Rutgers Med Sch 1985

Infectious Disease

Herman, David J MD (Inf) - **Spec Exp:** Lyme Disease; AIDS/HIV; Travel Medicine; **Hospital:** Univ Med Ctr - Princeton, Somerset Med Ctr; **Address:** 105 Raider Blvd, Ste 101, Hillsborough, NJ 08844; **Phone:** 908-281-0221; **Board Cert:** Internal Medicine 1988; Infectious Disease 2000; **Med School:** Univ MO-Columbia Sch Med 1985; **Resid:** Internal Medicine, Northwestern Univ 1988; **Fellow:** Infectious Disease, Univ Minn 1991; **Fac Appt:** Asst Clin Prof Med, Robert W Johnson Med Sch

Nahass, Ronald MD (Inf) - **Spec Exp:** Hepatitis B & C; Lyme Disease; Wound Healing/Care; Bone Infections; **Hospital:** Robert Wood Johnson Univ Hosp - New Brunswick, Univ Med Ctr - Princeton; **Address:** 105 Raider Blvd, Ste 101, Hillsborough, NJ 08844-4254; **Phone:** 908-281-0221; **Board Cert:** Internal Medicine 1985; Infectious Disease 1988; **Med School:** UMDNJ-RW Johnson Med Sch 1982; **Resid:** Internal Medicine, RWJ Univ Hosp 1986; **Fellow:** Infectious Disease, RWJ Univ Hosp 1988; **Fac Appt:** Clin Prof Med, UMDNJ-RW Johnson Med Sch

Internal Medicine

Ashinsky, Douglas S MD (IM) *PCP* - **Spec Exp:** Diabetes; **Hospital:** Somerset Med Ctr, Overlook Hosp (page 92); **Address:** Warren Internal Medicine, 31-J Mountain Blvd, Warren, NJ 07059; **Phone:** 908-685-2505 x293; **Board Cert:** Internal Medicine 1989; **Med School:** NYU Sch Med 1984; **Resid:** Internal Medicine, Northport VA Med Ctr 1987

Bell, Kevin E MD (IM) *PCP* - **Spec Exp:** Lyme Disease; Hypertension; **Hospital:** Overlook Hosp (page 92); **Address:** 10 Mountain Blvd, Warren, NJ 07059-2639; **Phone:** 908-226-9000; **Board Cert:** Internal Medicine 1978; **Med School:** Columbia P&S 1975; **Resid:** Internal Medicine, Univ Wisconsin Med Ctr 1979; **Fac Appt:** Asst Clin Prof Med, Columbia P&S

Bonaventura, Lisa M MD (IM) *PCP* - **Hospital:** Morristown Mem Hosp (page 92); **Address:** 2345 Lamington Rd, Ste 104, Bedminster, NJ 07921-2612; **Phone:** 908-781-9661; **Board Cert:** Internal Medicine 1989; **Med School:** Univ Cincinnati 1986; **Resid:** Internal Medicine, Morristown Meml Hosp 1989

Ferrante, Maurice A MD (IM) *PCP* - **Hospital:** Overlook Hosp (page 92); **Address:** 8 Mountain Blvd, Warren, NJ 07059; **Phone:** 908-561-8600; **Board Cert:** Internal Medicine 2010; **Med School:** Jefferson Med Coll 1987; **Resid:** Internal Medicine, Univ Maryland Med Ctr 1990

Neiman, Deborah L MD (IM) *PCP* - **Spec Exp:** Obesity; Weight Management; **Hospital:** Somerset Med Ctr, Morristown Mem Hosp (page 92); **Address:** Internal Medicine Assocs of Somerset, 311 Omni Drive, Hillsborough, NJ 08844; **Phone:** 908-281-0632; **Board Cert:** Internal Medicine 1987; **Med School:** NY Med Coll 1984; **Resid:** Internal Medicine, Morristown Meml Hosp 1987

Sanchez-Catanese, Betty MD (IM) *PCP* - **Hospital:** Somerset Med Ctr; **Address:** 315 E Main St, Somerville, NJ 08876-3109; **Phone:** 908-722-3442; **Board Cert:** Internal Medicine 1987; **Med School:** NY Med Coll 1983; **Resid:** Internal Medicine, Northshore Univ Hosp 1986

Medical Oncology

Casper, Ephraim S MD (Onc) - **Spec Exp:** Gastrointestinal Cancer; Pancreatic Cancer; Sarcoma-Soft Tissue; Drug Development; **Hospital:** Overlook Hosp (page 92); **Address:** MSKCC at Basking Ridge, 136 Mountainview Blvd, Basking Ridge, NJ 07920; **Phone:** 908-542-3000; **Board Cert:** Internal Medicine 1977; Medical Oncology 1979; **Med School:** Rush Med Coll 1974; **Resid:** Internal Medicine, Rush Presby-St Lukes Hosp 1977; **Fellow:** Medical Oncology, Meml Sloan Kettering Cancer Ctr 1979; **Fac Appt:** Prof Med, Cornell Univ-Weill Med Coll

Hamilton, Audrey M MD (Onc) - **Spec Exp:** Hematologic Malignancies; **Hospital:** Meml Sloan-Kettering Cancer Ctr (page 112); **Address:** Meml Sloan Kettering Cancer Ctr, 136 Mountain View Blvd, Basking Ridge, NJ 07920; **Phone:** 908-542-3000; **Board Cert:** Internal Medicine 1986; Hematology 2004; Medical Oncology 2005; **Med School:** Harvard Med Sch 1983; **Resid:** Internal Medicine, Brigham & Womens Hosp 1986; **Fellow:** Hematology & Oncology, NY Hosp-Cornell Med Ctr 1989

Wu, Hen-Vai MD (Onc) - **Spec Exp:** Colon & Rectal Cancer; Lung Cancer; Lymphoma, Non-Hodgkin's; **Hospital:** Somerset Med Ctr, St Peter's Univ Hosp; **Address:** Steepchase Cancer Ctr, 30 Rehill Ave, Ste 2500, Somerville, NJ 08876; **Phone:** 908-927-8700; **Board Cert:** Internal Medicine 1977; Hematology 1978; Medical Oncology 1981; **Med School:** Taiwan 1972; **Resid:** Internal Medicine, Mount Vernon Hosp 1974; Internal Medicine, Helene Fuld Med Ctr 1975; **Fellow:** Hematology, Robert W Johnson Univ Hosp 1977; Medical Oncology, Robert W Johnson Univ Hosp 1980; **Fac Appt:** Asst Clin Prof Med, UMDNJ-Univ Med Dent NJ

Nephrology

Kabis, Suzanne M MD (Nep) - Spec Exp: Lupus Nephritis; Hypertension; Glomerulonephritis; **Hospital:** Robert Wood Johnson Univ Hosp - New Brunswick, St Peter's Univ Hosp; **Address:** 1350 Hamilton St, Somerset, NJ 08873; **Phone:** 732-246-2626; **Board Cert:** Internal Medicine 1982; Nephrology 1988; **Med School:** UMDNJ-Rutgers Med Sch 1979; **Resid:** Internal Medicine, NC Meml Hosp 1982; **Fellow:** Nephrology, NC Meml Hosp 1985; **Fac Appt:** Asst Clin Prof Med, Robert W Johnson Med Sch

Neurology

Friedlander, Devin S MD (N) - Spec Exp: Headache; Botox Therapy; **Hospital:** St Peter's Univ Hosp; **Address:** Princeton & Rutgers Neurology, 51 Veronica Ave, Somerset, NJ 08873; **Phone:** 732-246-1311; **Board Cert:** Neurology 2003; **Med School:** UMDNJ-RW Johnson Med Sch 1989; **Resid:** Neurology, Albert Einstein Med Ctr 1993; **Fellow:** Neurological Physiology, Lyons VA Med Ctr 1994

Gainey, Patrick J MD (N) - Hospital: St Peter's Univ Hosp; **Address:** 51 Veronica Ave, Somerset, NJ 08873; **Phone:** 732-246-1311; **Board Cert:** Neurology 1993; **Med School:** UMDNJ-RW Johnson Med Sch 1988; **Resid:** Neurology, UMDNJ Med Ctr 1990; **Fellow:** Neurology, UMDNJ Med Ctr 1993

Neuroradiology

Lee, S Howard MD (NRad) - Hospital: Somerset Med Ctr; **Address:** Radiology Dept, 110 Rehill Ave, Somerville, NJ 08876; **Phone:** 908-685-2930; **Board Cert:** Diagnostic Radiology 1971; Neuroradiology 2007; **Med School:** South Korea 1964; **Resid:** Radiology, Jefferson Hosp 1967; Radiology, Graduate Hosp 1970; **Fellow:** Neurological Radiology, Philadelphia Genl Hosp 1972; **Fac Appt:** Clin Prof Rad, Robert W Johnson Med Sch

Obstetrics & Gynecology

Sanderson, Rhonda A MD (ObG) - Spec Exp: Gynecology Only; **Hospital:** Overlook Hosp (page 92); **Address:** 8 Mountain Blvd, Warren, NJ 07059; **Phone:** 908-754-5775; **Board Cert:** Obstetrics & Gynecology 2006; **Med School:** Hahnemann Univ 1980; **Resid:** Obstetrics & Gynecology, Womens/Infants Hosp 1984

Ophthalmology

Angrist, Richard C MD (Oph) - Spec Exp: Cataract Surgery; Glaucoma; Eyelid/Tear Duct Disorders; Ophthalmic Plastic Surgery; **Hospital:** Robert Wood Johnson Univ Hosp - New Brunswick, Kimball Med Ctr; **Address:** 1527 State Highway 27, Ste 2600, Somerset, NJ 08873; **Phone:** 732-246-1050; **Board Cert:** Ophthalmology 1985; **Med School:** Albany Med Coll 1979; **Resid:** Ophthalmology, NY Eye& Ear Infirm 1983; **Fellow:** Ophthalmic Plastic & Reconstructive Surgery, Univ Wisconsin 1984

Salz, Alan G MD (Oph) - Spec Exp: LASIK-Refractive Surgery; Cataract Surgery-Lens Implant; **Hospital:** Somerset Med Ctr; **Address:** 201 Union Ave Bldg 2 - Ste F, Bridgewater, NJ 08807; **Phone:** 908-231-1110; **Board Cert:** Ophthalmology 1987; **Med School:** Boston Univ 1981; **Resid:** Ophthalmology, Wills Eye Hosp 1985

Orthopaedic Surgery

D'Agostini, Robert J MD (OrS) - **Spec Exp:** Joint Replacement; Sports Medicine; **Hospital:** Morristown Mem Hosp (page 92); **Address:** 1590 Route 206 N, Bedminster, NJ 07921; **Phone:** 908-234-2002; **Board Cert:** Orthopaedic Surgery 2008; Sports Medicine 2009; **Med School:** UMDNJ-RW Johnson Med Sch 1980; **Resid:** Orthopaedic Surgery, Georgetown Univ Hosp 1985

Dwyer, James W MD (OrS) - **Spec Exp:** Spinal Surgery; Minimally Invasive Spinal Surgery; Spinal Disc Replacement; Spinal Reconstructive Surgery; **Hospital:** Somerset Med Ctr, Univ Hosp-UMDNJ—Newark; **Address:** Somerset Orthopedic Assocs, 1081 Route 22 W, Bridgewater, NJ 08807; **Phone:** 908-722-0822; **Board Cert:** Orthopaedic Surgery 2003; **Med School:** UMDNJ-NJ Med Sch, Newark 1882; **Resid:** Orthopaedic Surgery, UMDNJ Affil Hosps 1989; **Fellow:** Spinal Surgery, Seton Med Ctr/St Marys Spine Ctr 1990; **Fac Appt:** Asst Clin Prof OrS, UMDNJ-NJ Med Sch, Newark

Johnson, Albert MD (OrS) - **Spec Exp:** Hand Surgery; Hip & Knee Replacement; **Hospital:** Somerset Med Ctr; **Address:** 1081 Route 22 W, Bridgewater, NJ 08807; **Phone:** 908-722-0822; **Board Cert:** Orthopaedic Surgery 1977; **Med School:** India 1967; **Resid:** Surgery, New England Med Ctr 1972; Orthopaedic Surgery, New England Med Ctr 1975; **Fellow:** Hand Surgery, St Luke's-Roosevelt Hosp Ctr 1975

Tria Jr, Alfred J MD (OrS) - **Spec Exp:** Knee Surgery; **Hospital:** St Peter's Univ Hosp, Robert Wood Johnson Univ Hosp Hamilton; **Address:** 1527 Route 27, Ste 1300, Somerset, NJ 08873; **Phone:** 732-249-4444; **Board Cert:** Orthopaedic Surgery 1980; **Med School:** Harvard Med Sch 1972; **Resid:** Surgery, Roosevelt Hosp 1975; Orthopaedic Surgery, New York Hosp 1978; **Fellow:** Knee Surgery, Hosp Special Surg 1979; **Fac Appt:** Clin Prof OrS, UMDNJ-RW Johnson Med Sch

Otolaryngology

Kunzman, Kenneth MD (Oto) - **Hospital:** Somerset Med Ctr; **Address:** 56 Union Ave, Ste 1, Somerville, NJ 08876; **Phone:** 908-722-1022; **Board Cert:** Otolaryngology 1973; **Med School:** UMDNJ-NJ Med Sch, Newark 1964; **Resid:** Surgery, Hartford Hosp 1966; Otolaryngology, Hosp Univ Penn 1969

Pediatric Pulmonology

Turcios, Nelson L MD (PPul) - **Spec Exp:** Breathing Disorders; Cough-Chronic; Cystic Fibrosis; Ciliary Dyskinesia; **Hospital:** Somerset Med Ctr, St Peter's Univ Hosp; **Address:** 282 E Main St, Pediatric Pulmonology & Cystic Fibrosis, Somerville, NJ 08876; **Phone:** 908-526-5212; **Board Cert:** Pediatrics 1982; Pediatric Pulmonology 2007; **Med School:** El Salvador 1973; **Resid:** Pediatrics, Univ Mississippi Med Ctr 1978; Pediatrics, Univ Maryland Hosp 1980; **Fellow:** Pediatric Pulmonology, Childrens Hosp 1982; **Fac Appt:** Assoc Prof Ped, UMDNJ-NJ Med Sch, Newark

Pediatrics

Katz, Andrea G MD (Ped) *PCP* - **Spec Exp:** Developmental & Behavioral Disorders; Chronic Illness; Obesity; **Hospital:** Overlook Hosp (page 92), Saint Barnabas Med Ctr; **Address:** 76 Stirling Rd, Ste 201, Overlook Hosp-Pediatrics Div, Warren, NJ 07059; **Phone:** 908-755-5437; **Board Cert:** Pediatrics 2006; **Med School:** NY Med Coll 1988; **Resid:** Pediatrics, NY Hosp-Cornell Med Ctr 1991

Yorke, Eric R MD (Ped) *PCP* - **Hospital:** Somerset Med Ctr, Morristown Mem Hosp (page 92); **Address:** Somerset Pediatric Group, 2345 Lamington Rd, Ste 101, Bedminster, NJ 07921; **Phone:** 908-470-1124; **Board Cert:** Pediatrics 2009; **Med School:** Columbia P&S 1982; **Resid:** Pediatrics, Babies Hosp-Columbia 1986

Plastic Surgery

Najmi, Jamsheed K MD (PlS) - **Spec Exp:** Cosmetic Surgery-Face; Breast Reconstruction; Liposuction & Body Contouring; **Hospital:** Somerset Med Ctr, Hunterdon Med Ctr; **Address:** 201 Union Ave Bldg 1 - Ste B, Bridgewater, NJ 08807-3001; **Phone:** 908-722-6450; **Board Cert:** Plastic Surgery 1984; **Med School:** India 1969; **Resid:** Surgery, St Barnabas Med Ctr 1980; Plastic Surgery, St Barnabas Med Ctr 1982

Perry, Arthur W MD (PlS) - **Spec Exp:** Rhinoplasty; Eyelid Surgery; Liposuction; Abdominoplasty; **Hospital:** Robert Wood Johnson Univ Hosp - New Brunswick, Somerset Med Ctr; **Address:** 3055 Route 27, Franklin Park, NJ 08823-1315; **Phone:** 732-422-9600; **Board Cert:** Plastic Surgery 1989; **Med School:** Albany Med Coll 1981; **Resid:** Surgery, Beth Israel Hosp 1984; Plastic Surgery, Univ Chicago Hosps 1987; **Fellow:** Burn Surgery, NY Hosp-Cornell 1985; Cosmetic Plastic Surgery, Univ Miami/Baker-Gordon Assocs 1987; **Fac Appt:** Assoc Clin Prof PlS, Robert W Johnson Med Sch

Psychiatry

Donnellan, Joseph A MD (Psyc) - **Spec Exp:** Eating Disorders; Obsessive-Compulsive Disorder; **Hospital:** Somerset Med Ctr; **Address:** 422 Courtyard Drive, Hillsborough, NJ 08844; **Phone:** 908-725-5595; **Board Cert:** Psychiatry 1991; **Med School:** UMDNJ-NJ Med Sch, Newark 1986; **Resid:** Psychiatry, UMDNJ Affil Hosp 1990; **Fac Appt:** Asst Clin Prof Psyc, UMDNJ-RW Johnson Med Sch

Rochford, Joseph MD (Psyc) - **Spec Exp:** Depression; Anxiety Disorders; Eating Disorders; **Hospital:** Somerset Med Ctr; **Address:** 407 Omni Drive, Hillsborough, NJ 08844; **Phone:** 908-359-2312; **Board Cert:** Psychiatry 1975; **Med School:** Yale Univ 1969; **Resid:** Psychiatry, Hosp Univ Penn 1973; **Fac Appt:** Assoc Clin Prof Psyc, UMDNJ-RW Johnson Med Sch

Pulmonary Disease

Arno, Louis MD (Pul) - **Hospital:** Somerset Med Ctr; **Address:** 489 Union Ave, Bridge Water, NJ 08807; **Phone:** 732-356-9950; **Board Cert:** Pulmonary Disease 2006; Internal Medicine 2002; **Med School:** Grenada 1986; **Resid:** Internal Medicine, Seton Hall Univ Hosp 1990; **Fellow:** Pulmonary Disease, Seton Hall Univ Hosp 1992; Critical Care Medicine, Seton Hall Univ Hosp 1993

Gerhard, Harvey MD (Pul) - **Hospital:** Morristown Mem Hosp (page 92); **Address:** The Pulmonary Group, 416 Mount Airy Rd, Basking Ridge, NJ 07920-2438; **Phone:** 908-766-6605; **Board Cert:** Internal Medicine 1977; **Med School:** Yale Univ 1974; **Resid:** Internal Medicine, Bellevue Hosp Ctr 1977; **Fellow:** Pulmonary Disease, Yale-New Haven Hosp 1979

Radiation Oncology

Braver, Joel K MD (RadRO) - **Spec Exp:** Prostate Cancer; Stereotactic Radiosurgery; Merkel Cell Carcinoma; **Hospital:** Somerset Med Ctr; **Address:** Steeplechase Cancer Ctr, Dept Radiation Oncology, 30 Rehill Ave, Ste 1100, Somerville, NJ 08876; **Phone:** 908-927-8777; **Board Cert:** Radiation Oncology 2006; **Med School:** UMDNJ-RW Johnson Med Sch 1991; **Resid:** Radiation Oncology, Montefiore Med Ctr 1996

Reproductive Endocrinology

Treiser, Susan L MD/PhD (RE) - **Spec Exp:** Infertility; Infertility-IVF; **Hospital:** St Peter's Univ Hosp; **Address:** IVF NJ Fertility & Gynecology Ctr, 81 Veronica Ave, Somerset, NJ 08873; **Phone:** 732-220-9060; **Board Cert:** Obstetrics & Gynecology 2008; Reproductive Endocrinology 2008; **Med School:** Georgetown Univ 1983; **Resid:** Obstetrics & Gynecology, UMDNJ Med Ctr 1988; **Fellow:** Reproductive Endocrinology, Columbia Presby Med Ctr 1990

Rheumatology

McWhorter, John E MD (Rhu) - **Spec Exp:** Arthritis; Osteoporosis; Lupus/SLE; Scleroderma; **Hospital:** Somerset Med Ctr, Hunterdon Med Ctr; **Address:** 201 Union Ave, Ste 2D, Bridgewater, NJ 08807-3002; **Phone:** 908-722-5380; **Board Cert:** Internal Medicine 1973; Rheumatology 1974; **Med School:** UMDNJ-NJ Med Sch, Newark 1968; **Resid:** Internal Medicine, Thomas Jefferson Univ Hosp 1971; Internal Medicine, Harlem Hosp 1972; **Fellow:** Rheumatology, Columbia-Presby Med Ctr 1975; **Fac Appt:** Asst Prof Med, UMDNJ-NJ Med Sch, Newark

Surgery

Drascher, Gary MD (S) - **Spec Exp:** Laparoscopic Surgery-Complex; Aneurysm; Carotid Artery Surgery; **Hospital:** Somerset Med Ctr, Robert Wood Johnson Univ Hosp - New Brunswick; **Address:** 515 Church St, Ste 1, Bound Brook, NJ 08805-1743; **Phone:** 732-356-0770; **Board Cert:** Surgery 2007; **Med School:** Mount Sinai Sch Med 1981; **Resid:** Internal Medicine, St Luke's-Roosevelt Hosp Ctr 1982; Surgery, St Luke's-Roosevelt Hosp Ctr 1987; **Fellow:** Vascular Surgery, Englewood Hosp 1989

Lanfranchi, Angela E MD (S) - **Spec Exp:** Breast Cancer; Breast Surgery; **Hospital:** Somerset Med Ctr; **Address:** Surgical Assocs Central NJ, 515 Church St, Ste 1, Bound Brook, NJ 08805; **Phone:** 732-356-0770; **Board Cert:** Surgery 2003; **Med School:** Georgetown Univ 1975; **Resid:** Family Medicine, Somerset Hosp 1978; Surgery, SUNY-Univ Affil Hosps 1982; **Fellow:** Vascular Surgery, Nassau Hosp 1983

McManus, Susan A MD (S) - **Spec Exp:** Breast Surgery; Cancer Surgery; **Hospital:** St Peter's Univ Hosp, Hunterdon Med Ctr; **Address:** 1553 Route 27, Ste 3100, Somerset, NJ 08873; **Phone:** 732-846-3300; **Board Cert:** Surgery 2006; **Med School:** Mexico 1979; **Resid:** Surgery, Beth Israel Med Ctr 1985; **Fac Appt:** Asst Clin Prof S, UMDNJ-RW Johnson Med Sch

Thoracic Surgery

Caccavale, Robert J MD (TS) - **Spec Exp:** Video Assisted Thoracic Surgery (VATS); **Hospital:** Somerset Med Ctr, St Peter's Univ Hosp; **Address:** 35 Clyde Rd, Ste 104, Somerset, NJ 08873; **Phone:** 732-247-3002; **Board Cert:** Thoracic Surgery 2008; **Med School:** SUNY Buffalo 1981; **Resid:** Surgery, NYU Med Ctr 1984; Surgery, Booth Meml Med Ctr 1986; **Fellow:** Thoracic Surgery, Downstate Med Ctr 1988; **Fac Appt:** Assoc Prof S, Robert W Johnson Med Sch

Urology

Barone, Joseph G MD (U) - **Spec Exp:** Robotic Surgery-Pediatric; Urinary Reconstruction; Incontinence; Hypospadias; **Hospital:** Robert Wood Johnson Univ Hosp - New Brunswick, Univ Med Ctr - Princeton; **Address:** One Worlds Fair Drive, Somerset, NJ 08873; **Phone:** 732-235-7960; **Board Cert:** Urology 2006; **Med School:** UMDNJ-Rutgers Med Sch 1989; **Resid:** Urology, R W Johnson Univ Hosp 1993; **Fellow:** Pediatric Urology, Emory Univ Med School 1994; **Fac Appt:** Assoc Prof S, UMDNJ-RW Johnson Med Sch

Catanese, Anthony J MD (U) - **Spec Exp:** Urologic Cancer; Kidney Surgery; **Hospital:** Somerset Med Ctr, St Peter's Univ Hosp; **Address:** 315 E Main St, Somerville, NJ 08876-3109; **Phone:** 908-722-6900; **Board Cert:** Urology 2009; **Med School:** NY Med Coll 1983; **Resid:** Surgery, NYU Med Ctr 1985; Urology, NYU Med Ctr 1989

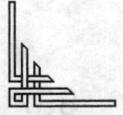
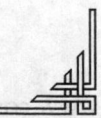

The Best in American Medicine
www.CastleConnolly.com

Union

Trinitas Regional Medical Center

225 WILLIAMSON STREET | ELIZABETH, NEW JERSEY 07207
PH 908.994.5000 | WWW.TRINITASRMC.ORG

Caring For You In Every Way

SPONSORSHIP: Trinitas Regional Medical Center is a voluntary not-for-profit Catholic teaching hospital sponsored by the Sisters of Charity of Saint Elizabeth in partnership with Elizabethtown Healthcare Foundation.

BEDS: 556   *Accredited by The Joint Commission*

MEDICAL STAFF

Trinitas Regional Medical Center has nearly 500 physicians and over 30 residents on its medical staff. Trinitas is a major clinical site for the Seton Hall School of Health and Medical Sciences' Internal Medicine Residency Program.

CENTERS OF EXCELLENCE:

Behavioral Health & Psychiatry: Behavioral Health services at Trinitas are among the most comprehensive in New Jersey and include a full range of inpatient and outpatient psychiatric care for seniors, adults, adolescents and children.

Cancer Care: The Trinitas Comprehensive Cancer Center offers the most advanced medical and radiation technology available, including Rapid Arc radiotherapy, to cancer patients. An interdisciplinary team works with each patient to develop a care plan encompassing the latest diagnostic treatment options, medical technology, clinical trials and integrative therapy.

Cardiology: Trinitas maintains a full-service cardiac facility for the intensive care of patients with heart disease, including elective angioplasty, a cardiac care unit, intermediate coronary care unit, cardiac catheterization lab, non-invasive cardiology services, full-service emergency department, and cardiac rehabilitation services.

Maternal & Child Health: Trinitas offers a Level II Intermediate Care Nursery, a 24-hour in-house pediatrician and obstetrician, and midwifery services. Inpatient care for child/adolescent psychiatric patients is also offered.

Renal Care: Trinitas is committed to patients experiencing kidney failure, and initiated the THRIVE early intervention program to reach high-risk patients.

Seniors Services: The Trinitas commitment to seniors takes many forms, most recently the establishment of the Acute Care for the Elderly (ACE) nursing unit. The Seniors First Membership Program offers special gifts and invitations to special events.

School of Nursing: The third largest school of nursing in the United States, the Trinitas School of Nursing, affiliated with Union County College, is known for an outstanding nursing education program that was recently designated a Center of Excellence in Nursing Education by the National League for Nursing.

Sleep Disorders: The Comprehensive Sleep Disorders Center provides monitored, fully-attended diagnostic sleep studies designed to rule out physical, non-stress related symptoms that may prevent restful sleep in adults and children. Two locations are offered, including the first hotel-based sleep center in New Jersey.

Women's Services: In addition to the latest modalities in digital mammography, breast biopsy, breast MRI, bone density screening and ultrasound, women can visit Trinitas for cosmetic and reconstructive surgery and innovative surgical care using the da Vinci® Robotic Surgical System for female incontinence and prolapse.

Wound Healing/Diabetes Management: The Trinitas Center for Wound Healing and Hyperbaric Medicine has one of the highest heal rates in the nation. Specially-trained certified nurses and physicians treat those with chronic, hard-to-heal wounds. Recognized by the American Diabetes Association, the Diabetes Management Center offers a high quality education program for diabetics.

Allergy & Immunology

Bielory, Leonard MD (A&I) - **Spec Exp:** Complementary Medicine; Asthma; Eye Allergy; Autoimmune Occular Disorders; **Hospital:** Univ Hosp-UMDNJ—Newark, Saint Barnabas Med Ctr; **Address:** 400 Mountain Ave, Springfield, NJ 07081; **Phone:** 973-912-9817; **Board Cert:** Internal Medicine 1984; Allergy & Immunology 1985; Clinical & Laboratory Immunology 1986; **Med School:** UMDNJ-NJ Med Sch, Newark 1980; **Resid:** Internal Medicine, Univ Md Hosp 1982; Hematology, Natl Inst Hlth 1983; **Fellow:** Allergy & Immunology, Natl Inst Hlth 1985; **Fac Appt:** Prof Med, UMDNJ-NJ Med Sch, Newark

Brown, David K MD (A&I) - **Spec Exp:** Asthma; Sinus Disorders; Headache; **Hospital:** Overlook Hosp (page 92); **Address:** 33 Overlook Rd Fl 3rd - Ste 307, Summit, NJ 07901-3563; **Phone:** 908-522-9696; **Board Cert:** Internal Medicine 1984; Allergy & Immunology 1987; **Med School:** Med Coll OH 1981; **Resid:** Internal Medicine, Overlook Hosp 1984; **Fellow:** Allergy & Immunology, St Luke's-Roosevelt Hosp Ctr 1986

Goodman, Alan J MD (A&I) - **Spec Exp:** Rhinitis; Sinus Disorders; Asthma; **Hospital:** Saint Barnabas Med Ctr; **Address:** 381 Chestnut St, Union, NJ 07083; **Phone:** 908-688-6200; **Board Cert:** Internal Medicine 1985; Allergy & Immunology 1999; **Med School:** SUNY Upstate Med Univ 1982; **Resid:** Internal Medicine, Washington Hosp Ctr 1985; **Fellow:** Allergy & Immunology, St Luke's-Roosevelt Hosp Ctr 1988

Le Benger, Kerry S MD (A&I) - **Spec Exp:** Asthma; Allergy; **Hospital:** Overlook Hosp (page 92), Saint Barnabas Med Ctr; **Address:** Summit Medical Group, 1 Diamond Hill Rd, Berkely Heights, NJ 07922; **Phone:** 908-277-8681; **Board Cert:** Internal Medicine 1983; Allergy & Immunology 1985; **Med School:** NY Med Coll 1980; **Resid:** Internal Medicine, Lenox Hill Hosp 1983; **Fellow:** Allergy & Immunology, New York Hosp 1985; **Fac Appt:** Asst Clin Prof Med, Mount Sinai Sch Med

Maccia, Clement MD (A&I) - **Spec Exp:** Rhinitis; Asthma; Urticaria; Eczema; **Hospital:** JFK Med Ctr - Edison, Robert Wood Johnson Univ Hosp - New Brunswick; **Address:** Asthma, Sinus & Allergy Centers, 19 Holly St, Cranford, NJ 07016-2158; **Phone:** 908-276-0666; **Board Cert:** Pediatrics 1980; Allergy & Immunology 1985; **Med School:** Italy 1971; **Resid:** Pediatrics, Muhlenberg Med Ctr 1974; **Fellow:** Allergy & Immunology, Univ Hosp 1976; **Fac Appt:** Clin Prof A&I, Robert W Johnson Med Sch

Mendelson, Joel S MD (A&I) - **Spec Exp:** Infectious Disease; Food Allergy; Urticaria; Eczema; **Hospital:** Saint Barnabas Med Ctr, Overlook Hosp (page 92); **Address:** 1124 Springfield Ave, Mountainside, NJ 07092; **Phone:** 908-233-4477; **Board Cert:** Pediatrics 1987; Allergy & Immunology 2009; Pediatric Infectious Disease 2005; **Med School:** Dominican Republic 1982; **Resid:** Pediatrics, St Luke's-Roosevelt Hosp 1985; **Fellow:** Allergy & Immunology, UMDNJ Med Ctr 1987; Infectious Disease, UMDNJ Med Ctr 1987; **Fac Appt:** Asst Prof Ped, Grenada

Cardiovascular Disease

Kalischer, Alan L MD (Cv) - **Spec Exp:** Echocardiography; Nuclear Cardiology; Coronary Artery Disease; Arrhythmias; **Hospital:** Overlook Hosp (page 92), JFK Med Ctr - Edison; **Address:** 313 South Ave, Ste 202, Fanwood, NJ 07023; **Phone:** 908-889-1900; **Board Cert:** Internal Medicine 1982; Cardiovascular Disease 1985; Echocardiography 2000; Nuclear Cardiology 2001; **Med School:** NY Med Coll 1977; **Resid:** Internal Medicine, Kings County Hosp 1980; **Fellow:** Cardiovascular Disease, Columbia-Presby Med Ctr 1984; **Fac Appt:** Asst Clin Prof Med, UMDNJ-RW Johnson Med Sch

Sachs, R Gregory MD (Cv) - **Spec Exp:** Heart Disease; Heart Valve Disease; Congenital Heart Disease-Adult; **Hospital:** Overlook Hosp (page 92), Morristown Mem Hosp (page 92); **Address:** 1 Diamond Hill Rd, Berkeley Heights, NJ 07922; **Phone:** 908-277-8713; **Board Cert:** Internal Medicine 1972; Cardiovascular Disease 1976; **Med School:** Georgetown Univ 1966; **Resid:** Internal Medicine, Georgetown Univ Hosp 1968; **Fellow:** Cardiovascular Disease, Emory Hosps 1970; Cardiovascular Disease, National Heart Hosp 1971; **Fac Appt:** Asst Clin Prof Med, Columbia P&S

Sheris, Steven J MD (Cv) - **Spec Exp:** Echocardiography; Cardiac Stress Testing; Nuclear Cardiology; **Hospital:** Overlook Hosp (page 92), Saint Barnabas Med Ctr; **Address:** Assocs in Cardiovascular Disease, 29 South St, New Providence, NJ 07974; **Phone:** 908-464-4200; **Board Cert:** Internal Medicine 2003; Cardiovascular Disease 2007; Nuclear Cardiology 2003; **Med School:** UMDNJ-Rutgers Med Sch 1988; **Resid:** Internal Medicine, Natl Naval Med Ctr 1994; **Fellow:** Cardiovascular Disease, Georgetown Univ Med Ctr 1997

Slama, Robert D MD (Cv) - **Spec Exp:** Echocardiography; Preventive Cardiology; Nuclear Cardiology; **Hospital:** Overlook Hosp (page 92), Morristown Mem Hosp (page 92); **Address:** Summit Med Grp, 1 Diamond Hill Rd, Berkeley Heights, NJ 07922; **Phone:** 908-277-8714; **Board Cert:** Internal Medicine 1974; Cardiovascular Disease 1977; **Med School:** Temple Univ 1971; **Resid:** Internal Medicine, Boston Med Ctr 1973; Internal Medicine, Georgetown Univ Hosp 1974; **Fellow:** Cardiovascular Disease, Boston Univ Med Ctr 1976

Stein, Elliott M MD (Cv) - **Hospital:** Overlook Hosp (page 92); **Address:** 211 Mountain Ave, Springfield, NJ 07081; **Phone:** 973-467-0005; **Board Cert:** Internal Medicine 1974; Cardiovascular Disease 1974; **Med School:** Jefferson Med Coll 1964; **Resid:** Internal Medicine, Mt Sinai Hosp 1969; Cardiovascular Disease, Mt Sinai Hosp 1971

Child & Adolescent Psychiatry

Greenberg, Rosalie MD (ChAP) - **Spec Exp:** Bipolar/Mood Disorders; ADD/ADHD; **Hospital:** Overlook Hosp (page 92); **Address:** 33 Overlook Rd, Ste 406, Summit, NJ 07901; **Phone:** 908-598-0200; **Board Cert:** Psychiatry 1982; Child & Adolescent Psychiatry 1983; **Med School:** Columbia P&S 1976; **Resid:** Psychiatry, Columbia-Presby Hosp 1979; **Fellow:** Child & Adolescent Psychiatry, Columbia-Presby Hosp 1981; **Fac Appt:** Asst Clin Prof Psyc, Columbia P&S

Child Neurology

Traeger, Eveline C MD (ChiN) - **Spec Exp:** Autism; ADD/ADHD; Learning Disorders; **Hospital:** Children's Specialized Hosp; **Address:** 150 New Providence Rd, Mountainside, NJ 07092; **Phone:** 908-233-3720 x5491; **Board Cert:** Child Neurology 2004; **Med School:** SUNY Buffalo 1984; **Resid:** Child Neurology, Yeshiva Univ 1986; Pediatrics, Jacobi Med Ctr 1988

Colon & Rectal Surgery

Groff, Walter MD (CRS) - **Spec Exp:** Colonoscopy; Rectal Cancer/Sphincter Preservation; **Hospital:** Overlook Hosp (page 92); **Address:** 33 Overlook Rd, Ste 412, Summit, NJ 07901-3564; **Phone:** 908-598-0220; **Board Cert:** Colon & Rectal Surgery 1980; **Med School:** Albany Med Coll 1970; **Resid:** Surgery, St Vincent's Hosp 1979; Colon & Rectal Surgery, Muhlenberg Med Ctr 1980; **Fac Appt:** Assoc Prof S, Columbia P&S

Dermatology

Eisenberg, Richard R MD (D) - **Spec Exp:** Skin Cancer; Melanoma; Acne; **Hospital:** Overlook Hosp (page 92); **Address:** 40 Stirling Rd, Ste 203, Watchung, NJ 07069; **Phone:** 908-753-4144; **Board Cert:** Internal Medicine 1985; Dermatology 1989; **Med School:** Cornell Univ-Weill Med Coll 1982; **Resid:** Internal Medicine, NY Hosp-Cornell Med Ctr 1985; Dermatology, NY Hosp-Cornell/Meml Sloan Kettering Cancer Ctr 1989

Weinberger, George I MD (D) - **Spec Exp:** Skin Cancer; **Hospital:** Saint Barnabas Med Ctr; **Address:** 190 Greenbrook Rd, N Plainfield, NJ 07060-3903; **Phone:** 908-561-8070; **Board Cert:** Dermatology 1977; **Med School:** UMDNJ-NJ Med Sch, Newark 1973; **Resid:** Dermatology, Henry Ford Hosp 1977

Diagnostic Radiology

Grosso, Sue Jane R MD (DR) - **Spec Exp:** Breast Imaging; **Hospital:** Overlook Hosp (page 92); **Address:** Summit Med Grp, 1 Diamond Hill Rd, Berkeley Heights, NJ 07922; **Phone:** 908-273-4300; **Board Cert:** Diagnostic Radiology 1991; **Med School:** Harvard Med Sch 1985; **Resid:** Diagnostic Radiology, NYU Med Ctr 1990; **Fellow:** Breast Imaging, NYU Med Ctr 1991

Endocrinology, Diabetes & Metabolism

Fuhrman, Robert MD (EDM) - **Spec Exp:** Diabetes; Thyroid Disorders; Osteoporosis; **Hospital:** Overlook Hosp (page 92); **Address:** 552 Westfield Ave, Westfield, NJ 07090-3312; **Phone:** 908-654-3377; **Board Cert:** Internal Medicine 1971; Endocrinology, Diabetes & Metabolism 1972; **Med School:** Ros Franklin Univ/Chicago Med Sch 1966; **Resid:** Internal Medicine, Mount Sinai Hosp 1970; Nuclear Medicine, VA Hospital 1970; **Fellow:** Endocrinology, Diabetes & Metabolism, Mount Sinai Hosp 1970; **Fac Appt:** Asst Clin Prof Med, UMDNJ-NJ Med Sch, Newark

Rosenbaum, Robert MD (EDM) - **Spec Exp:** Thyroid Disorders; Diabetes; Osteoporosis; **Hospital:** Overlook Hosp (page 92); **Address:** Summit Med Grp, One Diamond Hill Rd, Berkeley Heights, NJ 07922-2104; **Phone:** 908-273-4300; **Board Cert:** Internal Medicine 1978; Endocrinology, Diabetes & Metabolism 1981; **Med School:** Columbia P&S 1975; **Resid:** Internal Medicine, Montefiore Hosp Med Ctr 1978; **Fellow:** Endocrinology, Diabetes & Metabolism, Montefiore Hosp Med Ctr 1980; **Fac Appt:** Asst Clin Prof Med, Mount Sinai Sch Med

Selinger, Sharon E MD (EDM) - **Spec Exp:** Diabetes; Thyroid Disorders; Pituitary Disorders; Osteoporosis; **Hospital:** Overlook Hosp (page 92); **Address:** One Springfield Ave, Ste 1A, Summit, NJ 07901; **Phone:** 908-273-8300; **Board Cert:** Internal Medicine 1984; Endocrinology, Diabetes & Metabolism 1987; **Med School:** Cornell Univ-Weill Med Coll 1981; **Resid:** Internal Medicine, Montefiore Hosp Med Ctr 1984; **Fellow:** Endocrinology, Diabetes & Metabolism, Bellevue Hosp-NYU Med Ctr 1986

Silverman, Mitchell MD (EDM) - **Spec Exp:** Diabetes; Thyroid Disorders; Adrenal Disorders; **Hospital:** Saint Barnabas Med Ctr, Newark Beth Israel Med Ctr; **Address:** 2333 Morris Ave, Ste B-109, Union, NJ 07083; **Phone:** 908-964-5511; **Board Cert:** Internal Medicine 1983; Endocrinology 1987; **Med School:** Duke Univ 1980; **Resid:** Internal Medicine, Emory Univ Hosp 1983; **Fellow:** Endocrinology, Diabetes & Metabolism, NY Hosp-Meml Sloan-Kettering 1988

Family Medicine

Eisenstat, Steven DO (FMed) *PCP* - **Spec Exp:** Osteoporosis; Hypertension; Alzheimer's Disease; **Hospital:** Overlook Hosp (page 92); **Address:** 1050 Galloping Hill Rd, Ste 202, Union, NJ 07083-7980; **Phone:** 908-688-4845; **Board Cert:** Family Medicine 1993; Geriatric Medicine 1991; **Med School:** Ohio State Univ 1984; **Resid:** Family Medicine, Union Hosp 1987; **Fac Appt:** Asst Clin Prof FMed, NY Coll Osteo Med

Tabachnick, John F MD (FMed) *PCP* - **Hospital:** Overlook Hosp (page 92); **Address:** 563 Westfield Ave, Westfield, NJ 07090; **Phone:** 908-232-5858; **Board Cert:** Family Medicine 2007; **Med School:** Mount Sinai Sch Med 1979; **Resid:** Family Medicine, Overlook Hosp 1982; **Fac Appt:** Asst Clin Prof FMed, UMDNJ Sch Osteo Med

Gastroenterology

Goldenberg, David MD (Ge) - **Spec Exp:** Inflammatory Bowel Disease/Crohn's; Biliary Disease; Gastroesophageal Reflux Disease (GERD); **Hospital:** JFK Med Ctr - Edison, Somerset Med Ctr; **Address:** 1165 Park Ave, Plainfield, NJ 07060-3010; **Phone:** 908-754-2992; **Board Cert:** Internal Medicine 1977; Gastroenterology 1981; **Med School:** NY Med Coll 1974; **Resid:** Internal Medicine, Metropolitan Hosp 1977; **Fellow:** Gastroenterology, Emory Univ Hosp 1980

Kerner, Michael MD (Ge) - **Spec Exp:** Colonoscopy; Biliary Disease; Gastroesophageal Reflux Disease (GERD); Inflammatory Bowel Disease; **Hospital:** Overlook Hosp (page 92), Morristown Mem Hosp (page 92); **Address:** 25 Morris Ave, Springfield, NJ 07081-1406; **Phone:** 973-467-1313; **Board Cert:** Internal Medicine 1975; Gastroenterology 1977; **Med School:** Wake Forest Univ 1971; **Resid:** Internal Medicine, NYU Med Ctr 1974; **Fellow:** Gastroenterology, Manhattan VA-Bellevue Hosp 1976; **Fac Appt:** Asst Clin Prof Med, Mount Sinai Sch Med

Mahal, Pradeep MD (Ge) - **Spec Exp:** Gastrointestinal Cancer; **Hospital:** Overlook Hosp (page 92), Trinitas Reg Med Ctr (page 840); **Address:** 1308 Morris Ave, Ste 202, Union, NJ 07083; **Phone:** 908-851-6767; **Board Cert:** Gastroenterology 1981; Internal Medicine 1978; Geriatric Medicine 2002; Medical Oncology 1983; **Med School:** India 1975; **Resid:** Internal Medicine, UMDNJ Univ Hosp 1978; **Fellow:** Medical Oncology, MD Anderson Tumor Inst 1980; Gastroenterology, MD Anderson Tumor Inst 1980

Tempera, Patrick G MD (Ge) - **Spec Exp:** Biliary Disease; Pancreatic Disease; Gastroesophageal Reflux Disease (GERD); **Hospital:** Overlook Hosp (page 92), Somerset Med Ctr; **Address:** 1308 Morris Ave, Ste 103, Union, NJ 07083; **Phone:** 908-851-2771; **Board Cert:** Gastroenterology 2004; **Med School:** Grenada 1986; **Resid:** Surgery, Brooklyn Hosp 1987; Internal Medicine, Seton Hall Univ Hosp 1990; **Fellow:** Gastroenterology, Seton Hall Univ Hosp 1992; **Fac Appt:** Assoc Prof Med, Seton Hall Univ Sch Hlth & Med Scis

Geriatric Medicine

Khimani, Karim J MD (Ger) *PCP* - **Hospital:** Trinitas Reg Med Ctr (page 840); **Address:** 240 Williamson St, Ste 306, Elizabeth, NJ 07202; **Phone:** 908-352-5071; **Board Cert:** Internal Medicine 1986; Geriatric Medicine 2003; Hospice & Palliative Medicine 2008; **Med School:** Dominican Republic 1982; **Resid:** Internal Medicine, St Elizabeth Hosp 1985

Solomon, Robert B MD (Ger) *PCP* - **Spec Exp:** Alzheimer's Disease; Osteoporosis; **Hospital:** Trinitas Reg Med Ctr (page 840), Overlook Hosp (page 92); **Address:** 744 Galloping Hill Rd, Roselle Park, NJ 07204-1758; **Phone:** 908-241-0044; **Board Cert:** Internal Medicine 1980; Geriatric Medicine 2008; **Med School:** SUNY Hlth Sci Ctr 1977; **Resid:** Internal Medicine, Westchester Med Ctr 1980; **Fellow:** Geriatric Medicine, NY Hosp 1981

Hematology

Kessler, William MD (Hem) - **Hospital:** Trinitas Reg Med Ctr (page 840); **Address:** Med Offices, 225 Williamson St, Elizabeth, NJ 07207; **Phone:** 908-994-8773; **Board Cert:** Internal Medicine 1978; Hematology 1980; **Med School:** Albert Einstein Coll Med 1975; **Resid:** Internal Medicine, UMDNJ-Newark 1978; **Fellow:** Hematology, VA Hosp 1979

Infectious Disease

Farrer, William MD (Inf) - **Spec Exp:** AIDS/HIV; Diabetic Leg/Foot Infections; Travel Medicine; **Hospital:** Trinitas Reg Med Ctr (page 840); **Address:** 240 Williamson St, Ste 502, Elizabeth, NJ 07207-3625; **Phone:** 908-994-5300; **Board Cert:** Internal Medicine 1978; Infectious Disease 1980; **Med School:** Harvard Med Sch 1975; **Resid:** Internal Medicine, Montefiore Med Ctr 1978; **Fellow:** Infectious Disease, Montefiore Med Ctr 1980; **Fac Appt:** Assoc Prof Med, Seton Hall Univ Sch Hlth & Med Scis

Greenman, James L MD (Inf) - **Spec Exp:** AIDS/HIV; Lyme Disease; **Hospital:** Overlook Hosp (page 92); **Address:** Medical Diagnostic Associates, 525 Central Ave, Westfield, NJ 07090; **Phone:** 908-233-0895; **Board Cert:** Internal Medicine 1985; Infectious Disease 1988; **Med School:** Albert Einstein Coll Med 1982; **Resid:** Internal Medicine, Columbia-Presby Med Ctr 1985; **Fellow:** Infectious Disease, Montefiore Med Ctr 1988

Roland, Robert DO (Inf) - **Spec Exp:** AIDS/HIV; Travel Medicine; Hepatitis C; **Hospital:** Overlook Hosp (page 92), Robert Wood Johnson Univ Hosp at Rahway; **Address:** 1308 Morris Ave, Ste 204, Union, NJ 07083; **Phone:** 908-810-9200; **Board Cert:** Internal Medicine 1990; Infectious Disease 1992; **Med School:** Kirksville Coll Osteo Med 1985; **Resid:** Internal Medicine, Union Hosp 1989; **Fellow:** Infectious Disease, Kennedy Meml Hosp 1991; **Fac Appt:** Asst Clin Prof Med, NY Coll Osteo Med

Internal Medicine

Alterman, Lloyd H MD (IM) - **Spec Exp:** Hypertension; Kidney Disease-Chronic; **Hospital:** Overlook Hosp (page 92); **Address:** 33 Overlook Rd, Summit, NJ 07901; **Phone:** 908-219-3006; **Board Cert:** Internal Medicine 1980; Nephrology 1982; **Med School:** Wayne State Univ 1977; **Resid:** Internal Medicine, Overlook Hosp 1980; **Fellow:** Nephrology, Montefiore Med Ctr 1982

Feldman, Jeffrey N MD (IM) - **Spec Exp:** Hypertension; Cholesterol/Lipid Disorders; Diabetes; **Hospital:** Overlook Hosp (page 92); **Address:** 440 Chestnut St Fl 1, Union, NJ 07083-9306; **Phone:** 908-686-9330; **Board Cert:** Internal Medicine 1979; Nephrology 1982; **Med School:** Hahnemann Univ 1976; **Resid:** Internal Medicine, Bronx Municipal Hosp 1979; **Fellow:** Nephrology, SUNY Hlth Sci Ctr 1981

Goodgold, Abraham MD (IM) *PCP* - **Hospital:** Trinitas Reg Med Ctr (page 840), Robert Wood Johnson Univ Hosp at Rahway; **Address:** Elizabeth Medical Group, 310 W Jersey St, Elizabeth, NJ 07202-1832; **Phone:** 908-351-2222; **Board Cert:** Internal Medicine 1977; **Med School:** NYU Sch Med 1973; **Resid:** Infectious Disease, Montefiore Med Ctr 1976; **Fellow:** Endocrinology, Mt Sinai Med Ctr 1978

Maglaras, Nicholas C MD (IM) - **Hospital:** Trinitas Reg Med Ctr (page 840); **Address:** 236 E Westfield Ave, Ste 5, Roselle Park, NJ 07204; **Phone:** 908-245-8222; **Board Cert:** Internal Medicine 2003; Pulmonary Disease 2006; **Med School:** Grenada 1987; **Resid:** Internal Medicine, Elmhurst Hosp 1990; **Fellow:** Pulmonary Disease, Elmhurst Hosp 1992

Interventional Cardiology

Lux, Michael S MD (IC) - **Hospital:** Overlook Hosp (page 92), Morristown Mem Hosp (page 92); **Address:** Assocs in Cardiovascular Disease, 211 Mountain Ave, Springfield, NJ 07081-1581; **Phone:** 973-467-0005; **Board Cert:** Internal Medicine 1980; Cardiovascular Disease 1985; Interventional Cardiology 2002; **Med School:** NYU Sch Med 1977; **Resid:** Internal Medicine, Johns Hopkins Hosp 1980; **Fellow:** Cardiovascular Disease, Johns Hopkins Hosp 1983; **Fac Appt:** Asst Prof Med, Columbia P&S

Mich, Robert J MD (IC) - **Spec Exp:** Arrhythmias; **Hospital:** Morristown Mem Hosp (page 92), Overlook Hosp (page 92); **Address:** Assocs in Cardiovascular Disease, 29 South St Fl 1, New Providence, NJ 07974-1996; **Phone:** 908-464-4200; **Board Cert:** Internal Medicine 1984; Cardiovascular Disease 1985; Interventional Cardiology 2002; **Med School:** Johns Hopkins Univ 1979; **Resid:** Internal Medicine, John Hopkins Hosp 1982; **Fellow:** Cardiovascular Disease, Vanderbilt Univ Hosp 1984; Cardiovascular Disease, Mass Genl Hosp 1986

Medical Oncology

Gearhart, Bonni L MD (Onc) - **Spec Exp:** Breast Cancer; **Hospital:** Overlook Hosp (page 92); **Address:** Medical Diagnostic Assocs, Overlook Oncology Ctr, 99 Beauvoir Ave Fl 5th, Summit, NJ 07902; **Phone:** 908-608-0078; **Board Cert:** Internal Medicine 2005; Medical Oncology 2005; **Med School:** SUNY Stony Brook 1988; **Resid:** Internal Medicine, Vanderbilt Univ Med Ctr 1991; **Fellow:** Medical Oncology, UCSD Cancer Ctr 1993

Lowenthal, Dennis MD (Onc) - **Spec Exp:** Lung Cancer; Lymphoma; Prostate Cancer; Thoracic Cancers; **Hospital:** Overlook Hosp (page 92); **Address:** The Cancer Ctr at Overlook Hosp, 99 Beauvoir Ave, Summit, NJ 07902; **Phone:** 908-608-0078; **Board Cert:** Internal Medicine 1982; Medical Oncology 1985; Hematology 1986; **Med School:** Boston Univ 1979; **Resid:** Internal Medicine, Montefiore Med Ctr 1982; **Fellow:** Hematology, Montefiore Med Ctr 1983; Medical Oncology, Mem Sloan Kettering Cancer Ctr 1986; **Fac Appt:** Asst Clin Prof Med, Mount Sinai Sch Med

Moriarty, Daniel J MD (Onc) - **Spec Exp:** Gastrointestinal Cancer; **Hospital:** Overlook Hosp (page 92); **Address:** Med Diagnostic Assocs, 99 Beauvoir Ave, Summit, NJ 07902; **Phone:** 908-608-0078; **Board Cert:** Internal Medicine 1982; Medical Oncology 1987; **Med School:** Univ VT Coll Med 1976; **Resid:** Internal Medicine, Cambridge Hosp 1984; **Fellow:** Hematology & Oncology, St Elizabeth Hosp 1987

Wax, Michael MD (Onc) - **Hospital:** Overlook Hosp (page 92); **Address:** 1 Diamond Hill Rd, Berkeley Hieghts, NJ 07922; **Phone:** 908-277-8890; **Board Cert:** Internal Medicine 1980; Medical Oncology 1983; **Med School:** Med Coll PA Hahnemann 1977; **Resid:** Internal Medicine, Hosp Med Coll Penn 1980; **Fellow:** Hematology & Oncology, Univ Wash Med Ctr 1980; **Fac Appt:** Asst Clin Prof Med, Mount Sinai Sch Med

Neonatal-Perinatal Medicine

Giuliano, Michael A MD (NP) - **Hospital:** Hackensack Univ Med Ctr (page 96); **Address:** Hackensack Med Ctr, 30 Prospect Ave, Hackensack, NJ 07061; **Phone:** 201-996-5362; **Board Cert:** Pediatrics 2002; Neonatal-Perinatal Medicine 2002; **Med School:** SUNY Downstate 1981; **Resid:** Pediatrics, New York Hosp 1984; **Fellow:** Neonatal-Perinatal Medicine, New York Hosp/Cornell 1986

Nephrology

Goldstein, Carl MD (Nep) - **Spec Exp:** Hypertension; Glomerulonephritis; Kidney Failure; Metabolic Syndrome; **Hospital:** Overlook Hosp (page 92); **Address:** 215 North Ave W, Westfield, NJ 07090-1428; **Phone:** 908-232-4321; **Board Cert:** Internal Medicine 1981; Nephrology 1984; **Med School:** Washington Univ, St Louis 1978; **Resid:** Internal Medicine, Univ Minn Med Ctr 1981; **Fellow:** Nephrology, Hosp Univ Penn 1984; **Fac Appt:** Clin Prof Med, Mount Sinai Sch Med

McAnally, James F MD (Nep) - **Spec Exp:** Kidney Disease; Hypertension; Diabetes; **Hospital:** Trinitas Reg Med Ctr (page 840); **Address:** 240 Williamson St, Ste 307, Elizabeth, NJ 07202-3672; **Phone:** 908-994-9200; **Board Cert:** Internal Medicine 1978; Nephrology 1980; **Med School:** UMDNJ-NJ Med Sch, Newark 1975; **Resid:** Internal Medicine, CMDNJ-Newark Affil Hosp 1978; Internal Medicine, Georgetown Univ Hosp 1980; **Fellow:** Nephrology, Georgetown Univ Hosp 1980; **Fac Appt:** Assoc Clin Prof Med, Seton Hall Univ Sch Hlth & Med Scis

Neurological Surgery

Fineman, Sanford MD (NS) - **Spec Exp:** Brain Tumors; Pain Management; Spinal Surgery; **Hospital:** Robert Wood Johnson Univ Hosp at Rahway, Overlook Hosp (page 92); **Address:** 2333 Morris Ave, Ste B-8, Union, NJ 07083-5737; **Phone:** 908-688-8800; **Board Cert:** Neurological Surgery 1985; **Med School:** Temple Univ 1976; **Resid:** Neurological Surgery, Thomas Jefferson Univ Hosp 1981; **Fellow:** Neurological Surgery, Presby Hosp 1982

Friedlander, Marvin E MD (NS) - **Spec Exp:** Spinal Surgery; **Hospital:** Trinitas Reg Med Ctr (page 840), Overlook Hosp (page 92); **Address:** 700 Rahway Ave, Union, NJ 07083; **Phone:** 908-688-1999; **Board Cert:** Neurological Surgery 1994; **Med School:** SUNY Downstate 1982; **Resid:** Neurological Surgery, Kings Co Hosp 1989; **Fellow:** Metabolism, SUNY Downstate Med Ctr 1984

Hodosh, Richard M MD (NS) - **Spec Exp:** Acoustic Neuroma; Neurovascular Surgery; Spinal Surgery; **Hospital:** Overlook Hosp (page 92), Morristown Mem Hosp (page 92); **Address:** Atlantic Brain & Spine Institute, 99 Beauvoir Ave, Clinical Office MAC 1, ste 405, Summit, NJ 07901; **Phone:** 908-522-4979; **Board Cert:** Neurological Surgery 1980; **Med School:** Univ Cincinnati 1972; **Resid:** Neurological Surgery, Univ Tex Hlth Scis Ctr 1978; **Fellow:** Neuroradiology, Natl Hosp Neur Dis 1975; Neurological Surgery, Kanto Hosp 1976; **Fac Appt:** Clin Prof NS, UMDNJ-NJ Med Sch, Newark

Neurology

Bansil, Shalini M MD (N) - **Spec Exp:** Stroke; **Hospital:** Overlook Hosp (page 92); **Address:** Overlook Hospital, Director, Stroke Center, 99 Beauvoir Ave, Summit, NJ 07902; **Phone:** 908-522-5545; **Board Cert:** Neurology 1989; Vascular Neurology 2006; **Med School:** India 1981; **Resid:** Neurology, UMDNJ Med Ctr 1989; **Fellow:** Stroke, Beth Israel Med Ctr

Halperin, John MD (N) - **Spec Exp:** Neuromuscular Disorders; Lyme Disease; Multiple Sclerosis; **Hospital:** Overlook Hosp (page 92), Morristown Mem Hosp (page 92); **Address:** Dept Neurosciences, Overlook Hospital, Summit, NJ 07902; **Phone:** 908-522-2829; **Board Cert:** Internal Medicine 1978; Neurology 1982; Clinical Neurophysiology 2005; **Med School:** Harvard Med Sch 1975; **Resid:** Internal Medicine, Univ Chicago Hosps 1977; Neurology, Mass Genl Hosp 1980; **Fellow:** Neurology, Mass Genl Hosp 1983; **Fac Appt:** Prof N, Mount Sinai Sch Med

Politsky, Jeffrey M MD (N) - **Spec Exp:** Pediatric Neurology; Epilepsy/Seizure Disorders; Neurodegenerative Disorders; **Hospital:** Overlook Hosp (page 92), Hackensack Univ Med Ctr (page 96); **Address:** Atlantic Neuroscience Inst, 99 Beauvoir Ave, Summit, NJ 07901; **Phone:** 908-522-4990; **Board Cert:** Neurology 2005; **Med School:** Canada 1994; **Resid:** Neurology, Univ British Columbia 1999; **Fellow:** Epilepsy, Harvard Med Sch-Mass Genl Hosp 2001

Pollock, Jeffrey C MD (N) - **Hospital:** Overlook Hosp (page 92); **Address:** 47 Maple St, Ste 104, Summit, NJ 07901; **Phone:** 908-277-2722; **Board Cert:** Neurology 1987; **Med School:** Med Coll GA 1982; **Resid:** Neurology, UMDNJ Med Ctr 1986

Sachs, Stephen M MD (N) - **Spec Exp:** Headache; Stroke; Dementia; Parkinson's Disease; **Hospital:** Robert Wood Johnson Univ Hosp at Rahway, Trinitas Reg Med Ctr (page 840); **Address:** 700 N Broad St, Ste 201, Elizabeth, NJ 07208; **Phone:** 908-354-3994; **Board Cert:** Neurology 1977; **Med School:** Univ Pennsylvania 1971; **Resid:** Internal Medicine, Bellevue Hosp 1973; Neurology, Columbia-Presby Med Ctr 1976; **Fac Appt:** , UMDNJ-NJ Med Sch, Newark

Schanzer, Bernard MD (N) - **Spec Exp:** Stroke; Headache; Multiple Sclerosis; Amyotrophic Lateral Sclerosis (ALS); **Hospital:** Trinitas Reg Med Ctr (page 840), Robert Wood Johnson Univ Hosp at Rahway; **Address:** 700 N Broad St, Ste 201, Elizabeth, NJ 07208-2310; **Phone:** 908-354-3994; **Board Cert:** Neurology 1972; **Med School:** Belgium 1962; **Resid:** Internal Medicine, Maimonides Med Ctr 1965; Neurology, Bronx Muni Med Ctr 1970; **Fac Appt:** Assoc Clin Prof N, UMDNJ-NJ Med Sch, Newark

Neuroradiology

Horner, Neil B MD (NRad) - **Spec Exp:** MRI & CT of Brain & Spine; Spine Imaging & Intervention; Tumor Imaging; Brain Imaging; **Hospital:** Overlook Hosp (page 92), Mount Sinai Med Ctr (page 102); **Address:** Overlook Hosp, Dept Radiology, 99 Beauvoir Ave, Summit, NJ 07901; **Phone:** 908-522-2066; **Board Cert:** Diagnostic Radiology 1988; Nuclear Radiology 1989; Neuroradiology 2005; **Med School:** UMDNJ-Rutgers Med Sch 1983; **Resid:** Diagnostic Radiology, NYU Med Ctr 1988; **Fellow:** Neuroradiology, NYU Med Ctr 1989; Nuclear Radiology, NYU Med Ctr 1989; **Fac Appt:** Asst Clin Prof Rad, Mount Sinai Sch Med

Obstetrics & Gynecology

Beim, Robert B MD (ObG) - **Spec Exp:** Laparoscopic Surgery; Minimally Invasive Surgery; Colposcopy; **Hospital:** St Peter's Univ Hosp, JFK Med Ctr - Edison; **Address:** 190 Greenbrook Rd, N Plainfield, NJ 07060; **Phone:** 908-226-1555; **Board Cert:** Obstetrics & Gynecology 2007; **Med School:** SUNY Upstate Med Univ 1989; **Resid:** Obstetrics & Gynecology, Robert Wood Johnson Med Ctr 1993; **Fac Appt:** Asst Prof ObG, Drexel Univ Coll Med

Margulis, Elynne B MD (ObG) - **Spec Exp:** Infertility; **Hospital:** Overlook Hosp (page 92); **Address:** 522 E Broad St, Westfield, NJ 07090; **Phone:** 908-232-4449; **Board Cert:** Obstetrics & Gynecology 1985; **Med School:** Columbia P&S 1978; **Resid:** Obstetrics & Gynecology, Hosp Univ Penn 1982; **Fac Appt:** Asst Clin Prof ObG, Columbia P&S

Soffer, Jeffrey L MD (ObG) - **Hospital:** Overlook Hosp (page 92); **Address:** 522 E Broad St, Westfield, NJ 07090; **Phone:** 908-232-4449; **Board Cert:** Obstetrics & Gynecology 1983; **Med School:** Howard Univ 1975; **Resid:** Obstetrics & Gynecology, Hosp Univ Penn 1979

Ophthalmology

Confino, Joel MD (Oph) - **Spec Exp:** Laser Vision Surgery; Cataract Surgery; Corneal Disease & Transplant; **Hospital:** Overlook Hosp (page 92); **Address:** 592 Springfield Ave, Westfield, NJ 07090-1002; **Phone:** 908-789-8999; **Board Cert:** Ophthalmology 1985; **Med School:** Albert Einstein Coll Med 1980; **Resid:** Ophthalmology, Mt Sinai 1984; **Fellow:** Cornea & Ext Eye Disease, Univ California 1985

Natale, Benjamin DO (Oph) - **Spec Exp:** LASIK-Refractive Surgery; Cataract Surgery; **Hospital:** Saint Barnabas Med Ctr; **Address:** 1050 Galloping Hill Rd, Ste 104, Union, NJ 07083-7983; **Phone:** 908-964-7878; **Board Cert:** Ophthalmology 1991; **Med School:** Coll Osteo Med 1980; **Resid:** Family Medicine, Union Hosp 1982; Ophthalmology, Univ of Medicine & Dentistry 1985; **Fellow:** Refractive Surgery, Newark Eye & Ear Infirmary 1986

Orthopaedic Surgery

Barmakian, Joseph T MD (OrS) - **Spec Exp:** Carpal Tunnel Syndrome; Nerve & Tendon Reconstruction; Shoulder Reconstruction; **Hospital:** Overlook Hosp (page 92); **Address:** 523 Westfield Ave, Westfield, NJ 07090-3300; **Phone:** 908-654-1100; **Board Cert:** Orthopaedic Surgery 2003; Hand Surgery 2003; **Med School:** UMDNJ-RW Johnson Med Sch 1984; **Resid:** Surgery, Geo Wash Univ Med Ctr 1986; Orthopaedic Surgery, Columbia-Presby Med Ctr 1989; **Fellow:** Hand Surgery, Hosp for Joint Diseases 1990

Botwin, Clifford DO (OrS) - **Spec Exp:** Arthroscopic Surgery; Hip Surgery; Knee Surgery; **Hospital:** Overlook Hosp (page 92), Bayonne Med Ctr; **Address:** 900 Stuyvesant Ave, Union, NJ 07083-6936; **Phone:** 908-964-6600; **Resid:** Orthopaedic Surgery, Delaware Valley Hosp 1976

Drzala, Mark R MD (OrS) - **Spec Exp:** Spinal Surgery; **Hospital:** Mountainside Hosp, Overlook Hosp (page 92); **Address:** 33 Overlook Rd, Ste 305, Summit, NJ 07901; **Phone:** 908-608-9610; **Board Cert:** Orthopaedic Surgery 2001; **Med School:** UMDNJ-NJ Med Sch, Newark 1991; **Resid:** Orthopaedic Surgery, UMDNJ-NJ Med Sch 1997; **Fellow:** Spinal Surgery, San Francisco Orthopeds 1998

Gallick, Gregory MD (OrS) - **Spec Exp:** Sports Medicine; Knee Reconstruction; Shoulder Reconstruction; **Hospital:** Overlook Hosp (page 92); **Address:** 2780 Morris Ave, Ste 2-C, Union, NJ 07083; **Phone:** 908-686-6665; **Board Cert:** Orthopaedic Surgery 2009; **Med School:** UMDNJ-Rutgers Med Sch 1980; **Resid:** Surgery, Univ of Medicine & Dentistry 1981; Orthopaedic Surgery, Univ of Medicine & Dentistry 1985; **Fellow:** Interventional Cardiology, Southern California Sports Medicine 1986

Mackessy, Richard P MD (OrS) - **Spec Exp:** Hand Surgery; **Hospital:** Trinitas Reg Med Ctr (page 840), Robert Wood Johnson Univ Hosp at Rahway; **Address:** 210 W St Georges Ave, Linden, NJ 07036; **Phone:** 908-486-1111; **Board Cert:** Orthopaedic Surgery 2007; Hand Surgery 2007; **Med School:** UMDNJ-NJ Med Sch, Newark 1978; **Resid:** Surgery, St Vincents Hosp 1980; Orthopaedic Surgery, St Lukes Hosp 1983; **Fellow:** Hand Surgery, Thomas Jefferson Univ Hosp 1984

Sarokhan, Alan MD (OrS) - **Spec Exp:** Hip Replacement; Knee Replacement; Hand Surgery; **Hospital:** Overlook Hosp (page 92), Saint Barnabas Med Ctr; **Address:** Medical Arts Bldg, 33 Overlook Rd, Ste 201, Summit, NJ 07901-3562; **Phone:** 908-522-4555; **Board Cert:** Orthopaedic Surgery 2007; **Med School:** Harvard Med Sch 1977; **Resid:** Surgery, Peter Bent Brigham Hosp 1979; Orthopaedic Surgery, Harvard Affil Hosps 1982; **Fellow:** Hand Surgery, Roosevelt Hosp 1984

Otolaryngology

Carniol, Paul J MD (Oto) - **Spec Exp:** Facial Plastic Surgery; Facial Rejuvenation; Cosmetic Surgery; Skin Cancer; **Hospital:** Overlook Hosp (page 92); **Address:** Medical Arts Bldg, 33 Overlook Rd, Ste 401, Summit, NJ 07901; **Phone:** 908-598-1400; **Board Cert:** Otolaryngology 1981; Facial Plastic & Reconstr Surgery 1991; **Med School:** Univ Pennsylvania 1976; **Resid:** Surgery, North Shore Univ Hosp 1978; **Fellow:** Otolaryngology, Mass Eye & Ear Infirm 1981; Plastic Surgery, Hosp Univ Penn 1983; **Fac Appt:** Clin Prof S, UMDNJ-NJ Med Sch, Newark

Drake III, William MD (Oto) - **Spec Exp:** Endoscopic Sinus Surgery; Head & Neck Surgery; Thyroid & Parathyroid Surgery; Pediatric Otolaryngology; **Hospital:** Overlook Hosp (page 92); **Address:** Westfield Ear Nose & Throat Surg Assoc, 189 Elm St, Westfield, NJ 07090; **Phone:** 908-233-5500; **Board Cert:** Otolaryngology 1995; **Med School:** UMDNJ-NJ Med Sch, Newark 1989; **Resid:** Otolaryngology, Mt Sinai Med Ctr 1994

Eden, Avrim MD (Oto) - **Spec Exp:** Meniere's Disease; Hearing Loss; Balance Disorders; **Hospital:** Univ Hosp-UMDNJ—Newark, Overlook Hosp (page 92); **Address:** 1 Diamond Hill Rd, Berkeley Heights, NJ 07922-2104; **Phone:** 908-277-8681; **Board Cert:** Otolaryngology 1974; **Med School:** South Africa 1968; **Resid:** Otolaryngology, Univ Toronto Hosps 1974; **Fellow:** Otolaryngology, Univ Hosp Zurich 1975; **Fac Appt:** Clin Prof Oto, UMDNJ-NJ Med Sch, Newark

Kwartler, Jed A MD (Oto) - **Spec Exp:** Acoustic Neuroma; Balance Disorders; Cochlear Implants; Cholesteatoma; **Hospital:** Overlook Hosp (page 92), Hackensack Univ Med Ctr (page 96); **Address:** 1 Diamond Hill Rd, Berkeley Heights, NJ 07922; **Phone:** 908-277-8681; **Board Cert:** Otolaryngology 1988; **Med School:** UMDNJ-NJ Med Sch, Newark 1983; **Resid:** Surgery, UMDNJ/Univ Hosp 1985; Otolaryngology, UMDNJ/Univ Hosp 1988; **Fellow:** Otology & Neurotology, St Vincent's Hosp & Med Ctr 1990; **Fac Appt:** Assoc Clin Prof Oto, UMDNJ-NJ Med Sch, Newark

Scharf, Richard DO (Oto) - **Spec Exp:** Sinus Disorders/Surgery; Cosmetic Surgery-Face; Head & Neck Cancer; **Hospital:** Saint Barnabas Med Ctr, Bayonne Med Ctr; **Address:** 505 Chestnut St, Roselle Park, NJ 07204; **Phone:** 908-241-0200; **Board Cert:** Otolaryngology 1998; **Med School:** Univ Hlth Sci, Coll Osteo Med 1982; **Resid:** Otolaryngology, Flint Hosp 1990; **Fac Appt:** Assoc Clin Prof Oto, NY Coll Osteo Med

Pediatric Cardiology

Leichter, Donald MD (PCd) - **Spec Exp:** Congenital Heart Disease; Fetal Echocardiography; Echocardiography; **Hospital:** Overlook Hosp (page 92), NYPresby-Morgan Stanley Children's Hosp (page 104); **Address:** 47 Maple St, Ste 206, Summit, NJ 07901; **Phone:** 908-522-5566; **Board Cert:** Pediatrics 1988; Pediatric Cardiology 2003; **Med School:** Cornell Univ-Weill Med Coll 1980; **Resid:** Pediatrics, Chldns Hosp Natl Med Ctr 1983; **Fellow:** Pediatric Cardiology, Columbia Presby Med Ctr 1985; **Fac Appt:** Assoc Clin Prof Ped, Columbia P&S

Pediatric Endocrinology

Anhalt, Henry DO (PEn) - **Spec Exp:** Diabetes; Obesity; Growth Disorders; **Address:** 140 Prospect Ave, Ste 2, Hackensack, NJ 07061; **Phone:** 201-996-0777; **Board Cert:** Pediatric Endocrinology 2005; **Med School:** NY Coll Osteo Med 1988; **Resid:** Pediatrics, Winthrop Univ Hosp 1992; **Fellow:** Pediatric Endocrinology, Stanford Univ Med Ctr 1995; **Fac Appt:** Assoc Prof Ped, SUNY Hlth Sci Ctr

Pediatric Gastroenterology

Tyshkov, Michael MD (PGe) - **Spec Exp:** Nutrition; Crohn's Disease; Colitis; **Hospital:** Overlook Hosp (page 92), Staten Island Univ Hosp - North; **Address:** 33 Overlook Rd, Ste 207, Summit, NJ 07901; **Phone:** 908-273-2300; **Board Cert:** Pediatric Gastroenterology 2003; **Med School:** Russia 1977; **Resid:** Pediatrics, Flushing Hosp 1989; **Fellow:** Pediatric Gastroenterology, Westchester Co Med Ctr 1991; **Fac Appt:** Asst Clin Prof Ped, SUNY Downstate

Pediatrics

Ayyanathan, Karpukarasi MD (Ped) *PCP* - **Hospital:** Trinitas Reg Med Ctr (page 840), JFK Med Ctr - Edison; **Address:** Linden Pediatric Group, 517 Rahway Ave, Elizabeth, NJ 07202-2308; **Phone:** 908-527-1247; **Board Cert:** Pediatrics 1983; **Med School:** India 1975; **Resid:** Pediatrics, St Elizabeth Hosp 1977; Pediatrics, Rahway Hosp 1979

Corbo, Emanuel MD (Ped) *PCP* - **Spec Exp:** Vaccines; Asthma; Otitis Media; Pneumonia; **Hospital:** Overlook Hosp (page 92), Trinitas Reg Med Ctr (page 840); **Address:** 443 E Westfield Ave, Roselle Park, NJ 07204-2428; **Phone:** 908-245-2442; **Board Cert:** Pediatrics 2008; **Med School:** Grenada 1985; **Resid:** Pediatrics, Newark Beth Israel Med Ctr 1990; **Fellow:** Pediatrics, Newark Beth Israel Med Ctr 1991

Davis, Kenneth J MD (Ped) *PCP* - **Hospital:** Overlook Hosp (page 92), Trinitas Reg Med Ctr (page 840); **Address:** 701 Newark Ave, Ste 212, Elizabeth, NJ 07208-3550; **Phone:** 908-354-9500; **Board Cert:** Pediatrics 1985; **Med School:** Albert Einstein Coll Med 1980; **Resid:** Pediatrics, Bellevue Hosp 1983

Mehta, Uday C MD (Ped) - **Spec Exp:** Autism; ADD/ADHD; Neurodevelopmental Disabilities; **Hospital:** Children's Specialized Hosp, Robert Wood Johnson Univ Hosp - New Brunswick; **Address:** 150 New Providence Rd, Mountainside, NJ 07092; **Phone:** 908-301-5491; **Board Cert:** Pediatrics 1982; Developmental-Behavioral Pediatrics 2004; **Med School:** India 1971; **Resid:** Pediatrics, Overlook Hosp 1980; **Fellow:** Child Development, Chldns Hosp 1981; **Fac Appt:** Asst Clin Prof Ped, Robert W Johnson Med Sch

Panza, Robert MD (Ped) - **Hospital:** Overlook Hosp (page 92); **Address:** 566 Westfield Ave, Westfield, NJ 07090; **Phone:** 908-233-7171; **Board Cert:** Pediatrics 2004; **Med School:** Italy 1985; **Resid:** Pediatrics, Overlook Hosp 1989

Panzner, Elizabeth A MD (Ped) *PCP* - **Spec Exp:** Acne; Allergy; Asthma; **Hospital:** Saint Barnabas Med Ctr, Overlook Hosp (page 92); **Address:** 1050 Galloping Hill Rd, Ste 200, Union, NJ 07083-9417; **Phone:** 908-688-9900; **Board Cert:** Pediatrics 2004; **Med School:** Mexico 1984; **Resid:** Pediatrics, UMDNJ-Univ Hosp 1988

Saraiya, Narendra N MD (Ped) *PCP* - **Spec Exp:** Asthma; Anemia; Sickle Cell Disease; **Hospital:** Trinitas Reg Med Ctr (page 840); **Address:** 817 Rahway Ave, Elizabeth, NJ 07202; **Phone:** 908-353-5750; **Board Cert:** Pediatrics 1988; **Med School:** India 1971; **Resid:** Pediatrics, NY Methodist Hosp 1980; **Fellow:** Pediatric Hematology-Oncology, Maimonides Med Ctr 1982; Pediatric Hematology-Oncology, Chldns Hosp Buffalo 1984

Vigorita, John MD (Ped) *PCP* - **Hospital:** Overlook Hosp (page 92); **Address:** 33 Overlook Rd, Ste 101, Summit, NJ 07901; **Phone:** 908-273-1112; **Board Cert:** Pediatrics 2002; **Med School:** Mexico 1974; **Resid:** Pediatrics, Overlook Hosp 1978

Physical Medicine & Rehabilitation

Armento, Michael J MD (PMR) - **Spec Exp:** Pediatric Rehabilitation; Cerebral Palsy; Spina Bifida; Spinal Cord Injury-Pediatric; **Hospital:** Children's Specialized Hosp, Newark Beth Israel Med Ctr; **Address:** Children's Specialized Hospital, 150 New Providence Rd, Mountainside, NJ 07092; **Phone:** 908-301-5416; **Board Cert:** Physical Medicine & Rehabilitation 2003; Spinal Cord Injury Medicine 2002; Pediatric Rehabilitation Medicine 2004; **Med School:** UMDNJ-NJ Med Sch, Newark 1988; **Resid:** Physical Medicine & Rehabilitation, UMDNJ Affil Hosp 1992; **Fellow:** Pediatric Rehabilitation Medicine, Chldns Specializwd Hosp 1994; **Fac Appt:** Assoc Clin Prof Ped, UMDNJ-NJ Med Sch, Newark

Diamond, Martin MD (PMR) - **Spec Exp:** Cerebral Palsy; Neuromuscular Disorders; Electrodiagnosis; **Hospital:** Children's Specialized Hosp, Newark Beth Israel Med Ctr; **Address:** 150 New Providence Rd, Mountainside, NJ 07092-2590; **Phone:** 908-301-5416; **Board Cert:** Pediatrics 1983; Physical Medicine & Rehabilitation 1982; Pediatric Rehabilitation Medicine 2003; **Med School:** Univ Pittsburgh 1975; **Resid:** Pediatrics, Chldns Hosp Natl Med Ctr 1978; Physical Medicine & Rehabilitation, Sinai Hosp 1980; **Fac Appt:** Assoc Clin Prof PMR, UMDNJ-NJ Med Sch, Newark

Malanga, Gerard A MD (PMR) - **Spec Exp:** Pain-Back & Neck; Sports Injuries; Electrodiagnosis; Pain-Low Back; **Hospital:** Overlook Hosp (page 92), Morristown Mem Hosp (page 92); **Address:** 11 Overlook Rd, MAC #2, Ste B110, Summit, NJ 07901; **Phone:** 908-522-2808; **Board Cert:** Physical Medicine & Rehabilitation 2003; Pain Medicine 2002; Sports Medicine 2009; **Med School:** UMDNJ-NJ Med Sch, Newark 1987; **Resid:** Physical Medicine & Rehabilitation, UMDNJ Affil Hosp 1992; **Fellow:** Sports Medicine, Mayo Clinic 1993; **Fac Appt:** Assoc Clin Prof PMR, UMDNJ-NJ Med Sch, Newark

Novick, Ellen MD (PMR) - **Spec Exp:** Electrodiagnosis; Pain-Back & Neck; Sports Medicine; **Address:** 210 W St Georges Ave, Linden, NJ 07036; **Phone:** 908-486-1111; **Board Cert:** Physical Medicine & Rehabilitation 1986; **Med School:** Mount Sinai Sch Med 1982; **Resid:** Physical Medicine & Rehabilitation, Albert Einstein 1985; **Fac Appt:** Asst Clin Prof Med, UMDNJ-NJ Med Sch, Newark

Plastic Surgery

Gardner, James N MD (PlS) - **Spec Exp:** Breast Cosmetic & Reconstructive Surgery; Abdominoplasty; **Hospital:** Overlook Hosp (page 92), Univ Hosp-UMDNJ—Newark; **Address:** 33 Overlook Rd, Ste 310, Summit, NJ 07901; **Phone:** 908-918-1969; **Board Cert:** Plastic Surgery 2005; **Med School:** UMDNJ-RW Johnson Med Sch 1994; **Resid:** Surgery, UMDNJ Univ Hosp 1992; **Fellow:** Plastic Surgery, UMDNJ Univ Hosp 1994

Hyans, Peter MD (PIS) - **Spec Exp:** Cosmetic Surgery-Breast; Breast Reconstruction; Cosmetic Surgery-Face; Liposuction & Body Contouring; **Hospital:** Overlook Hosp (page 92), Saint Barnabas Med Ctr; **Address:** Summit Medical Grp, Plastic Surgery Ctr, Lawrence Pavilion, 1 Diamond Hill Rd, Berkeley Heights, NJ 07922; **Phone:** 908-277-8759; **Board Cert:** Plastic Surgery 2003; **Med School:** UMDNJ-RW Johnson Med Sch 1986; **Resid:** Surgery, Thomas Jefferson Univ Hosp 1991; **Fellow:** Plastic Surgery, Univ Cincinnati Hosp 1993

Tepper, Howard N MD (PIS) - **Spec Exp:** Cosmetic Surgery; Breast Surgery; Hand Surgery; **Hospital:** Overlook Hosp (page 92); **Address:** 522 E Broad St, Westfield, NJ 07090-2116; **Phone:** 908-654-6540; **Board Cert:** Plastic Surgery 1983; **Med School:** Albert Einstein Coll Med 1975; **Resid:** Surgery, Montefiore Hosp Med Ctr 1979; Plastic Surgery, Montefiore Hosp Med Ctr 1981; **Fellow:** Hand Surgery, St Luke's-Roosevelt Hosp Ctr 1979

Zeitels, Jerrold R MD (PIS) - **Spec Exp:** Liposuction & Body Contouring; Reconstructive Surgery; Hand Surgery; **Hospital:** Overlook Hosp (page 92), Robert Wood Johnson Univ Hosp at Rahway; **Address:** 522 E Broad St, Westfield, NJ 07090-2116; **Phone:** 908-654-6540; **Board Cert:** Plastic Surgery 1989; Hand Surgery 2009; **Med School:** Univ Chicago-Pritzker Sch Med 1980; **Resid:** Surgery, Univ Michigan Med Ctr 1985; Plastic Surgery, Hosp Univ Penn 1987

Psychiatry

Kaplan, Gabriel MD (Psyc) - **Spec Exp:** Psychopharmacology; ADD/ADHD; Depression; **Hospital:** Hoboken Univ Med Ctr - Hoboken; **Address:** 535 Morris Ave, Springfield, NJ 07081-1426; **Phone:** 201-659-6060; **Board Cert:** Psychiatry 1987; Child & Adolescent Psychiatry 1989; **Med School:** Argentina 1980; **Resid:** Psychiatry, NY Hosp-Cornell 1986; Child Psychiatry, NY Hosp-Cornell 1988; **Fac Appt:** Asst Clin Prof Psyc, UMDNJ-NJ Med Sch, Newark

Miller, David G MD (Psyc) - **Spec Exp:** Psychopharmacology; Depression; ADD/ADHD; Bipolar/Mood Disorders; **Address:** 28 Milburn Ave, Ste 5, Springfield, NJ 07081; **Phone:** 973-218-1770; **Board Cert:** Psychiatry 1985; **Med School:** Univ Rochester 1980; **Resid:** Psychiatry, Strong Meml Hosp 1984

Richardson, William T MD (Psyc) - **Spec Exp:** Adolescent Psychiatry; Family Therapy; Psychopharmacology; **Hospital:** Overlook Hosp (page 92), Morristown Mem Hosp (page 92); **Address:** 33 Overlook Rd, Ste 210, Summit, NJ 07901-3570; **Phone:** 908-598-0008; **Board Cert:** Psychiatry 1980; **Med School:** McGill Univ 1967; **Resid:** Psychiatry, Jewish Genl Hosp 1971; Psychiatry, Payne Whitney Clinic 1974

Silver, Bennett MD (Psyc) - **Spec Exp:** Child & Adolescent Psychiatry; ADD/ADHD; Anxiety Disorders; **Hospital:** Hoboken Univ Med Ctr - Hoboken; **Address:** 535 Morris Ave, Springfield, NJ 07081; **Phone:** 973-376-1020; **Board Cert:** Psychiatry 1979; **Med School:** SUNY Downstate 1974; **Resid:** Psychiatry, Mt Sinai Hosp 1978; **Fellow:** Child & Adolescent Psychiatry, Mt Sinai Hosp 1980

Villafranca, Manuel V MD (Psyc) - **Spec Exp:** Psychopharmacology; Depression; Anxiety Disorders; **Hospital:** Summit Oaks Hosp, Christ Hosp; **Address:** 220 Lenox Ave, Westfield, NJ 07090; **Phone:** 908-232-9369; **Board Cert:** Psychiatry 1982; **Med School:** Philippines 1971; **Resid:** Psychiatry, St Vincent's Hosp 1978; **Fellow:** Child & Adolescent Psychiatry, St Vincent's Hosp 1980

Pulmonary Disease

Cerrone, Federico MD (Pul) - **Spec Exp:** Asthma; Sleep Disorders; Chronic Obstructive Lung Disease (COPD); **Hospital:** Overlook Hosp (page 92), Morristown Mem Hosp (page 92); **Address:** 1 Springfield Ave, Summit, NJ 07901; **Phone:** 908-934-0555; **Board Cert:** Internal Medicine 1989; Pulmonary Disease 2002; Critical Care Medicine 2003; Sleep Medicine 2007; **Med School:** Georgetown Univ 1986; **Resid:** Internal Medicine, Bronx Municipal Hosp 1989; **Fellow:** Pulmonary Critical Care Medicine, Georgetown Univ Hosp 1992; **Fac Appt:** Asst Clin Prof Med, UMDNJ-NJ Med Sch, Newark

Hwang, Cheng-hong DO (Pul) *PCP* - **Spec Exp:** Critical Care Medicine; **Hospital:** Robert Wood Johnson Univ Hosp at Rahway; **Address:** 1457 Raritan Rd, Ste 201, Clark, NJ 07066; **Phone:** 908-272-2270; **Board Cert:** Internal Medicine 1983; Pulmonary Disease 1984; Critical Care Medicine 2005; **Med School:** Coll Osteo Med 1978; **Resid:** Internal Medicine, USPHS Hosp 1981; **Fellow:** Pulmonary Disease, UMDNJ-Univ Hosp 1983

Sussman, Robert MD (Pul) - **Spec Exp:** Asthma; Chronic Obstructive Lung Disease (COPD); Pulmonary Fibrosis; Lung Cancer; **Hospital:** Overlook Hosp (page 92), Morristown Mem Hosp (page 92); **Address:** 1 Springfield Ave, Summit, NJ 07901; **Phone:** 908-934-0555; **Board Cert:** Internal Medicine 1984; Pulmonary Disease 1988; Critical Care Medicine 1999; **Med School:** Albert Einstein Coll Med 1981; **Resid:** Internal Medicine, Montefiore Med Ctr 1984; **Fellow:** Pulmonary Disease, NYU/Bellevue Hosp 1987

Radiation Oncology

Schwartz, Louis E MD (RadRO) - **Spec Exp:** Stereotactic Radiosurgery; Prostate Cancer; Brain Tumors; **Hospital:** Overlook Hosp (page 92); **Address:** Overlook Hosp, Dept Rad Oncology, 33 Overlook Rd, Ste L05, Summit, NJ 07901-3561; **Phone:** 908-522-2871; **Board Cert:** Therapeutic Radiology 1979; Pediatrics 1981; **Med School:** SUNY Hlth Sci Ctr 1974; **Resid:** Pediatrics, NY Methodist Hosp 1976; Pediatrics, Chldns Hosp Med Ctr 1977; **Fellow:** Therapeutic Radiology, Columbia-Presby Hosp 1979

Rheumatology

Brodman, Richard R MD (Rhu) - **Spec Exp:** Lupus/SLE; Rheumatoid Arthritis; Osteoporosis; Osteoarthritis; **Hospital:** JFK Med Ctr - Edison; **Address:** 345 Somerset St, Ste 107, North Plainfield, NJ 07060-4774; **Phone:** 908-561-7440; **Board Cert:** Internal Medicine 1976; Rheumatology 1982; **Med School:** SUNY Downstate 1973; **Resid:** Internal Medicine, Rhode Island Hosp 1976; **Fellow:** Rheumatology, Brigham & Womens Hosp 1978; **Fac Appt:** Assoc Clin Prof Med, UMDNJ-RW Johnson Med Sch

Whitman III, Hendricks H MD (Rhu) - **Spec Exp:** Rheumatoid Arthritis; Scleroderma; **Hospital:** Overlook Hosp (page 92), Morristown Mem Hosp (page 92); **Address:** 1 Diamond Hill Rd, Bensley Pavillion, Berkeley Heights, NJ 07922; **Phone:** 908-277-8640; **Board Cert:** Internal Medicine 1978; Rheumatology 1980; **Med School:** Univ NC Sch Med 1975; **Resid:** Internal Medicine, NY Hosp-Cornell 1978; **Fellow:** Rheumatology, NY Hosp-Cornell 1980; **Fac Appt:** Asst Clin Prof Med, Cornell Univ-Weill Med Coll

Worth, David MD (Rhu) - **Spec Exp:** Rheumatoid Arthritis; Osteoporosis; **Hospital:** Overlook Hosp (page 92); **Address:** 2376 Morris Ave, Union, NJ 07083-5707; **Phone:** 908-686-6616; **Board Cert:** Internal Medicine 1974; Rheumatology 1978; **Med School:** Univ Rochester 1971; **Resid:** Internal Medicine, Montefiore Med Ctr 1974; **Fellow:** Rheumatology, Montefiore Med Ctr 1975; Rheumatology, Montefiore Med Ctr 1978; **Fac Appt:** Asst Clin Prof Med, UMDNJ-NJ Med Sch, Newark

Surgery

Colaco, Rodolfo MD (S) - **Spec Exp:** Hernia; Gallbladder Surgery; Laparoscopic Surgery; Breast Surgery; **Hospital:** Trinitas Reg Med Ctr (page 840); **Address:** 431 Elmora Ave, Elizabeth, NJ 07208; **Phone:** 908-353-4177; **Board Cert:** Surgery 2001; **Med School:** India 1974; **Resid:** Surgery, St Vincent Hosp 1980; Surgery, St Elizabeth Hosp 1983

Digioia, Julia M MD (S) - **Spec Exp:** Breast Disease; Breast Cancer; **Hospital:** Overlook Hosp (page 92), Jersey City Med Ctr; **Address:** Medical Arts Ctr, 33 Overlook Rd, Ste 205, Summit, NJ 07901; **Phone:** 908-522-3200; **Board Cert:** Surgery 2005; **Med School:** Italy 1979; **Resid:** Surgery, Jersey City Med Ctr 1984; **Fac Appt:** Asst Clin Prof S, UMDNJ-NJ Med Sch, Newark

Feteiha, Muhammad S MD (S) - **Spec Exp:** Minimally Invasive Surgery; Obesity/Bariatric Surgery; **Hospital:** Overlook Hosp (page 92), Trinitas Reg Med Ctr (page 840); **Address:** 155 Springfield Ave Fl 2, Springfield, NJ 07081-1225; **Phone:** 973-232-2300; **Board Cert:** Surgery 2001; **Med School:** Tufts Univ 1995; **Resid:** Surgery, Unv New Mexico Hlth Sci Ctr 2000; **Fellow:** Surgery, Columbia Presby Med Ctr 2001

Frost, James Henry MD (S) - **Spec Exp:** Breast Cancer; Colon Cancer; Laparoscopic Surgery; Vascular Surgery; **Hospital:** Overlook Hosp (page 92), Trinitas Reg Med Ctr (page 840); **Address:** 155 Morris Ave Fl 2, Springfield, NJ 07081; **Phone:** 973-232-2300; **Board Cert:** Surgery 2007; **Med School:** Mexico 1982; **Resid:** Surgery, Univ Illinois Med Ctr 1988

Lozner, Jerrold S MD (S) - **Spec Exp:** Breast Cancer & Surgery; Breast Surgery; **Hospital:** Overlook Hosp (page 92); **Address:** 1 Diamond Hill Rd, Berkeley Heights, NJ 07922; **Phone:** 908-277-8950; **Board Cert:** Surgery 2009; Thoracic Surgery 2001; **Med School:** Univ Louisville Sch Med 1971; **Resid:** Surgery, Univ Cincinnati Med Ctr 1976; **Fellow:** Cardiothoracic Surgery, Univ Cincinnati Med Ctr 1978; **Fac Appt:** Assoc Clin Prof S, Columbia P&S

Mandel, Marc S MD (S) - **Spec Exp:** Gastrointestinal Surgery; Breast Cancer & Surgery; Cancer Surgery; Abdominal Wall Reconstruction; **Hospital:** Overlook Hosp (page 92); **Address:** 11 Overlook Rd, Ste 160, Summit, NJ 07901; **Phone:** 908-598-0966; **Board Cert:** Surgery 2009; **Med School:** Albert Einstein Coll Med 1985; **Resid:** Surgery, Montefiore Med Ctr 1988; Surgery, Yale New Haven Hosp 1990; **Fac Appt:** Asst Clin Prof S, Columbia P&S

Nitzberg, Richard S MD (S) - **Spec Exp:** Laparoscopic Surgery; Vein Disorders; **Hospital:** Overlook Hosp (page 92); **Address:** 1 Diamond Hill Rd, Bensley Pavillion Fl 4th, Berkeley Heights, NJ 07922; **Phone:** 908-277-8950; **Board Cert:** Surgery 2009; Vascular Surgery 2001; **Med School:** Harvard Med Sch 1983; **Resid:** Surgery, Columbia-Presby Med Ctr 1988; **Fellow:** Vascular Surgery, New England Med Ctr 1990

Starker, Paul MD (S) - **Spec Exp:** Laparoscopic Surgery; Minimally Invasive Surgery; **Hospital:** Overlook Hosp (page 92); **Address:** 11 Overlook Rd, Ste 160, Summit, NJ 07901-3564; **Phone:** 908-608-9001; **Board Cert:** Surgery 2006; **Med School:** Columbia P&S 1980; **Resid:** Surgery, Columbia-Presby Med Ctr 1986; **Fellow:** Metabolism, Columbia-Presby Med Ctr 1982; **Fac Appt:** Asst Prof S, Columbia P&S

Urology

Lehrhoff, Bernard J MD (U) - **Spec Exp:** Prostate Cancer; Kidney Stones; Sexual Dysfunction; Bladder Cancer; **Hospital:** Overlook Hosp (page 92), Saint Michael's Med Ctr; **Address:** 275 Orchard St, Westfield, NJ 07090; **Phone:** 908-654-5100; **Board Cert:** Urology 1984; **Med School:** UMDNJ-NJ Med Sch, Newark 1976; **Resid:** Urology, Bellevue Hosp 1982; **Fac Appt:** Asst Clin Prof U, Columbia P&S

Ring, Kenneth S MD (U) - **Spec Exp:** Pediatric Urology; Urologic Cancer; Kidney Stones; **Hospital:** Overlook Hosp (page 92); **Address:** 275 Orchard St, Westfield, NJ 07090-3133; **Phone:** 908-654-5100; **Board Cert:** Urology 2001; **Med School:** Mount Sinai Sch Med 1985; **Resid:** Surgery, Mount Sinai Hosp 1987; Urology, Columbia-Presby Med Ctr 1991

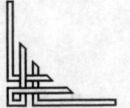
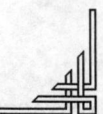

The Best in American Medicine
www.CastleConnolly.com

The State of Connecticut

The Best in American Medicine
www.CastleConnolly.com

Fairfield

Greenwich Hospital

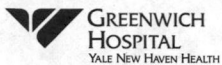

GENERAL OVERVIEW

Greenwich Hospital is a progressive, regional medical center and teaching institution with an internal medicine residency, serving lower Fairfield and Westchester counties. Care is provided on a beautiful, modern campus designed to create a healing environment for patients and visitors.

ACADEMIC AND CLINICAL AFFILIATIONS

As a member of the Yale New Haven Health System, Greenwich Hospital is a major affiliate of Yale School of Medicine and maintains affiliations with other leading medical providers. Patients have access to a comprehensive range of medical, surgical, diagnostic, *integrative medicine* and wellness programs. Greenwich Hospital also offers *robotic surgery* and *hyperbaric medicine and wound healing*. It has a State certified and Joint Commission accredited *Stroke Center*, and participates in international clinical trials.

OUTSTANDING CLINICAL SERVICES

Specialties include oncology care at the hospital's *Bendheim Cancer Center*; advanced breast care at the *Breast Center*; a comprehensive Maternity program including *Level III NICU* and *fertility services*; a *Pediatric Specialty Center*; *expert neuroscience and spine services* and a wide range of *surgical specialties* including *bariatric surgery*.

SERVICE EXCELLENCE

Greenwich Hospital is renowned for service excellence and has been awarded the *Press Ganey Summit Award* for highest ratings in Patient Satisfaction for the past five years.

5 Perryridge Road
Greenwich, CT 06830-4697
Tel: 203.863.3000
www.greenwichhospital.org

Physician Referral:
For a prompt, personal Physician Referral please call Greenwich Hospital at 203-863-3627 or *visit us online.*

Sponsorship:
Voluntary,
Not-for-profit

Beds:
174 bed-patients;
22 infants;
10 neonatal intensive care

Accreditation:
The Joint Commission

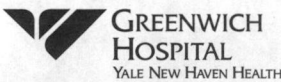

Real Life. Real Care.

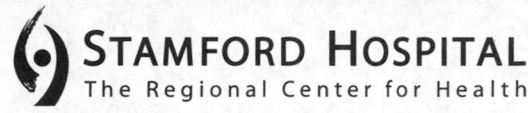
STAMFORD HOSPITAL
The Regional Center for Health

General Overview

Stamford Hospital provides area residents (Fairfield and Westchester Counties) access to the latest technology with a compassionate, patient-centered care approach in keeping with the Planetree philosophy. Stamford is a Level II trauma center with a nationally recognized adult intensive care unit. Our areas of expertise include:

Cancer Care	stamfordhospitalcancer.com
Heart Services	stamfordhospitalheart.com
Orthopedics	stamfordhospitalortho.com
Women's Health	stamfordhospitalwomenshealth.com

Our nurses have achieved the esteemed Magnet status—the highest honor in nursing.

Comprehensive Specialty Centers

Bennett Cancer Center provides compassionate, patient-centered care from diagnosis through post-treatment.

Center for Integrative Medicine and Wellness blends conventional and complementary care for patients.

Center for Robotic Surgery using the *da Vinci* Surgical System, enables surgeons to perform even the most complex and delicate procedures through very small incisions with unmatched precision.

Center for Sleep Medicine offers experts in diagnosing and treating pediatric and adult sleep disorders, including snoring, sleep apnea, insomnia, narcolepsy and restless leg syndrome.

Center for Surgical Weight Loss offers the region's only comprehensive weight management program.

CyberKnife Center, located at the only hospital in Fairfield and Westchester Counties, provides the technology to destroy tumors with pinpoint accuracy.

Diabetes & Endocrine Center brings together consultative services and complete clinical care, including comprehensive patient education, medical management and treatment.

Women's Breast Center, located at the only hospital in the state and first in the nation to receive accreditation from the American College of Surgeons for excellence in breast care.

Academic and Clinical Affiliations

Stamford Hospital is an affiliate of the New York–Presbyterian Healthcare System and a major teaching affiliate of the Columbia University College of Physicians & Surgeons.

Accreditation

Joint Commission on Accreditation of Healthcare Organization (JCAHO)

Beds

305

Sponsorship

Voluntary, Not-for-Profit

For a Physician Referral or more information, please call 1.877.233.9355 or visit stamfordhospital.org /doctor.

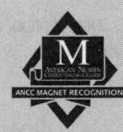

Stamford Hospital
30 Shelburne Road
Stamford, CT 06902
203.276.1000

stamfordhospital.org

Fairfield

Adolescent Medicine

Schneider, Marcie B MD (AM) - **Spec Exp:** Eating Disorders; Obesity; Menstrual Disorders; **Hospital:** Greenwich Hosp (page 862); **Address:** 239 Glenville Rd, Greenwich, CT 06831; **Phone:** 203-532-1919; **Board Cert:** Pediatrics 1987; Adolescent Medicine 2009; **Med School:** Albert Einstein Coll Med 1983; **Resid:** Pediatrics, Montefiore Med Ctr 1986; **Fellow:** Adolescent Medicine, N Shore Univ Hosp 1988; **Fac Appt:** Assoc Clin Prof Ped, Albert Einstein Coll Med

Allergy & Immunology

Bell, Jonathan MD (A&I) - **Spec Exp:** Asthma; Insect Allergies; Sinusitis; Hives; **Hospital:** Danbury Hosp; **Address:** 107 Newtown Rd, Ste 1B, Danbury, CT 06810-4156; **Phone:** 203-748-7433; **Board Cert:** Pediatrics 1986; Allergy & Immunology 1987; **Med School:** Georgetown Univ 1980; **Resid:** Pediatrics, St Christopher's Hosp Chldn 1983; **Fellow:** Pediatric Allergy & Immunology, Chldn's Hosp 1987; **Fac Appt:** Asst Clin Prof A&I, NY Med Coll

Lindner, Paul S MD (A&I) - **Spec Exp:** Asthma & Sinusitis; Hay Fever; Food Allergy; Drug Allergy; **Hospital:** Stamford Hosp (page 863); **Address:** 22 Fifth St, Stamford, CT 06905-5030; **Phone:** 203-978-0072; **Board Cert:** Internal Medicine 1989; Allergy & Immunology 2001; **Med School:** SUNY Buffalo 1985; **Resid:** Internal Medicine, Stamford Hosp 1989; **Fellow:** Allergy & Immunology, Nassau Co Med Ctr 1991

Litchman, Mark MD (A&I) - **Spec Exp:** Asthma; Immune Deficiency; Lupus/SLE; Vasculitis; **Hospital:** Greenwich Hosp (page 862), Stamford Hosp (page 863); **Address:** 2 1/2 Dearfield Drive, Greenwich, CT 06831-5335; **Phone:** 203-869-2080; **Board Cert:** Internal Medicine 1987; Allergy & Immunology 1999; Rheumatology 1988; **Med School:** Rush Med Coll 1984; **Resid:** Internal Medicine, Greenwich Hosp 1987; **Fellow:** Allergy & Immunology, Yale-New Haven Hosp 1989; Rheumatology, Yale-New Haven Hosp 1989; **Fac Appt:** Assoc Clin Prof Med, Yale Univ

Matczuk, Agnieszka MD (A&I) - **Spec Exp:** Pediatric Allergy & Immunology; **Hospital:** Greenwich Hosp (page 862); **Address:** 2 1/2 Deerfield Drive, Greenwich, CT 06831; **Phone:** 203-869-2080; **Board Cert:** Pediatrics 2008; Allergy & Immunology 2003; **Med School:** Poland 1993; **Resid:** Pediatrics, Beth Israel Med Ctr 2000; **Fellow:** Allergy & Immunology, Yale-New Haven Hosp 2002

Santilli, John MD (A&I) - **Spec Exp:** Allergy; Sinusitis; **Hospital:** St Vincent's Med Ctr - Bridgeport; **Address:** 4675 Main St, Bridgeport, CT 06606-1834; **Phone:** 203-374-6103; **Board Cert:** Pediatrics 1973; Allergy & Immunology 1983; **Med School:** Georgetown Univ 1968; **Resid:** Pediatrics, Georgetown Univ Hosp 1971; **Fellow:** Allergy & Immunology, Georgetown Univ Hosp 1973

Sproviero, Joseph MD (A&I) - **Hospital:** Norwalk Hosp, Greenwich Hosp (page 862); **Address:** 148 East Ave, Bldg 3G, Allergy & Asthma Assocs, Norwalk, CT 06851; **Phone:** 203-838-4034; **Board Cert:** Allergy & Immunology 1991; Internal Medicine 1989; **Med School:** Columbia P&S 1985; **Resid:** Internal Medicine, Yale New Haven Hosp 1988; **Fellow:** Allergy & Immunology, Yale-New Haven Hosp 1989; Rheumatology, Yale-New Haven Hosp 1990; **Fac Appt:** Asst Clin Prof Med, Yale Univ

Cardiac Electrophysiology

McPherson, Craig A MD (CE) - **Spec Exp:** Arrhythmias; Pacemakers/Defibrillators; Atrial Fibrillation; **Hospital:** Bridgeport Hosp, Yale-New Haven Hosp; **Address:** Bridgeport Hosp, Dept Electrophysiology, 267 Grant St, Bridgeport, CT 06610; **Phone:** 203-384-3442; **Board Cert:** Internal Medicine 1979; Cardiovascular Disease 1983; Cardiac Electrophysiology 2004; **Med School:** Tufts Univ 1976; **Resid:** Internal Medicine, Tufts-New England Med Ctr 1979; **Fellow:** Cardiovascular Disease, Yale-New Haven Hosp 1982; Cardiac Electrophysiology, Yale-New Haven Hosp 1983; **Fac Appt:** Clin Prof Med, Yale Univ

Cardiovascular Disease

Casale, Linda MD (Cv) - **Spec Exp:** Non-Invasive Cardiology; Women's Health; Echocardiography; **Hospital:** Bridgeport Hosp, Milford Hosp; **Address:** 1305 Post Rd, Fairfield, CT 06824; **Phone:** 203-292-2000; **Board Cert:** Cardiovascular Disease 2003; **Med School:** NY Med Coll 1986; **Resid:** Internal Medicine, Montefiore Med Ctr 1989; **Fellow:** Cardiovascular Disease, UC San Diego 1992

Copen, David L MD (Cv) - **Spec Exp:** Cardiac Catheterization; Coronary Artery Disease; Congestive Heart Failure; **Hospital:** Danbury Hosp; **Address:** 111 Osborne St Fl 3, Danbury, CT 06810-6099; **Phone:** 203-739-7155; **Board Cert:** Internal Medicine 1972; Cardiovascular Disease 1975; **Med School:** SUNY Downstate 1969; **Resid:** Internal Medicine, Yale-New Haven Hosp 1972; **Fellow:** Cardiovascular Disease, Mass Genl Hosp 1974; **Fac Appt:** Assoc Clin Prof Med, Yale Univ

Fisher, Lawrence I MD (Cv) - **Spec Exp:** Cardiac Catheterization; Pacemakers; Heart Valve Disease; **Hospital:** Danbury Hosp; **Address:** 25 Germantown Rd, Ste 2B, Danbury, CT 06810-6035; **Phone:** 203-794-0090; **Board Cert:** Internal Medicine 1988; Cardiovascular Disease 2001; **Med School:** SUNY Buffalo 1985; **Resid:** Internal Medicine, Bronx Muni Hosp 1988; **Fellow:** Cardiovascular Disease, Albert Einstein Coll Med 1990

Green, Jeffrey A MD (Cv) - **Hospital:** Stamford Hosp (page 863); **Address:** 80 Mill River St, Ste 1300, Stamford, CT 06902; **Phone:** 203-348-7410; **Board Cert:** Internal Medicine 2001; Cardiovascular Disease 2004; **Med School:** NY Med Coll 1998; **Resid:** Internal Medicine, Montefiore Med Ctr 2001; **Fellow:** Cardiovascular Disease, Montefiore Med Ctr 2004

Horowitz, Steven F MD (Cv) - **Spec Exp:** Nuclear Cardiology; Preventive Cardiology; Complementary Medicine; **Hospital:** Stamford Hosp (page 863); **Address:** Stamford Hospital, Dept Cardiology, 30 Shelburne Rd Fl 2, Stamford, CT 06904-9317; **Phone:** 203-276-7480; **Board Cert:** Internal Medicine 1975; Cardiovascular Disease 1979; **Med School:** NY Med Coll 1972; **Resid:** Internal Medicine, Beth Israel Hosp 1976; **Fellow:** Cardiovascular Disease, Mt Sinai Hosp 1978; Cardiology Research, Mt Sinai Hosp 1979

Keller, Andrew M MD (Cv) - **Spec Exp:** Echocardiography; Cardiac Imaging; **Hospital:** Danbury Hosp, NY-Presby Hosp/Weill Cornell (page 104); **Address:** Danbury Hospital, Div Cardiology, 111 Osborne St Fl 3, Danbury, CT 06810-6099; **Phone:** 203-739-7155; **Board Cert:** Internal Medicine 1982; Cardiovascular Disease 1985; **Med School:** Ohio State Univ 1979; **Resid:** Internal Medicine, Duke Univ Med Ctr Hosps 1982; **Fellow:** Cardiovascular Disease, Univ Texas-SW Med Ctr 1985; **Fac Appt:** Assoc Clin Prof Med, Columbia P&S

Kosinski, Edward J MD (Cv) - **Spec Exp:** Angioplasty & Stent Placement; **Hospital:** St Vincent's Med Ctr - Bridgeport, Bridgeport Hosp; **Address:** Cardiology Physicians, 4675 Main St, Bridgeport, CT 06606-4201; **Phone:** 203-683-5100; **Board Cert:** Internal Medicine 1976; Cardiovascular Disease 1979; **Med School:** Wake Forest Univ 1973; **Resid:** Internal Medicine, Columbia-Presby Med Ctr 1976; **Fellow:** Cardiovascular Disease, Peter Bent Brigham Hosp 1978; **Fac Appt:** Assoc Clin Prof Med, Columbia P&S

Marshalko, Stephen MD (Cv) - **Hospital:** Bridgeport Hosp, St Vincent's Med Ctr - Bridgeport; **Address:** 52 Beach Rd, Ste 105, Fairfield, CT 06824; **Phone:** 203-334-2100; **Board Cert:** Internal Medicine 2010; Cardiovascular Disease 2003; Interventional Cardiology 2004; **Med School:** Yale Univ 1996; **Resid:** Internal Medicine, Yale-New Haven Hosp 1999; **Fellow:** Cardiovascular Disease, Yale-New Haven Hosp 2000

Meizlish, Jay Lewis MD (Cv) - **Spec Exp:** Interventional Cardiology; Nuclear Cardiology; **Hospital:** Bridgeport Hosp; **Address:** 1305 Post Rd, Fairfield, CT 06824; **Phone:** 203-292-2000; **Board Cert:** Internal Medicine 1980; Cardiovascular Disease 1983; Nuclear Medicine 1984; Interventional Cardiology 2000; **Med School:** NYU Sch Med 1977; **Resid:** Internal Medicine, Harbor-UCLA Med Ctr 1980; **Fellow:** Cardiovascular Disease, Yale-New Haven Hosp 1983; Nuclear Medicine, Yale-New Haven Hosp

Neeson, Francis MD (Cv) - **Spec Exp:** Preventive Cardiology; Echocardiography; **Hospital:** Greenwich Hosp (page 862); **Address:** 75 Holly Hill Ln, Greenwich, CT 06830; **Phone:** 203-869-6960; **Board Cert:** Internal Medicine 1988; Cardiovascular Disease 2001; **Med School:** NYU Sch Med 1985; **Resid:** Internal Medicine, Bronx Muni Hosp 1988; **Fellow:** Cardiovascular Disease, Montefiore Med Ctr 1991

Taikowski, Richard L MD (Cv) - **Spec Exp:** Echocardiography; Congenital Heart Disease-Adult; Nuclear Cardiology; **Hospital:** Bridgeport Hosp, Milford Hosp; **Address:** 1305 Post Rd, Cardiac Specialists, Fairfield, CT 06824; **Phone:** 203-292-2000; **Board Cert:** Internal Medicine 1988; Cardiovascular Disease 2002; Echocardiography 2008; **Med School:** Boston Univ 1985; **Resid:** Internal Medicine, Boston Univ Med Ctr 1988; **Fellow:** Cardiovascular Disease, Mount Sinai Med Ctr 1991

Zarich, Stuart MD (Cv) - **Spec Exp:** Echocardiography; Diabetes & Heart Disease; Cholesterol/Lipid Disorders; **Hospital:** Bridgeport Hosp; **Address:** Bridgeport Hosp, Cardiology Div, 267 Grant St Fl 10, Bridgeport, CT 06605; **Phone:** 203-384-3844; **Board Cert:** Internal Medicine 1984; Cardiovascular Disease 1989; **Med School:** SUNY Upstate Med Univ 1981; **Resid:** Internal Medicine, Beth Israel Deaconess Hosp 1984; **Fellow:** Cardiovascular Disease, Beth Israel Deaconess Hosp/Harvard 1987; **Fac Appt:** Asst Clin Prof Med, Yale Univ

Child & Adolescent Psychiatry

Rosenfeld, Alvin A MD (ChAP) - **Spec Exp:** Psychotherapy; Sexual Development Problems; Overscheduled Children; Family Therapy; **Address:** 17 Sherwood Pl, Greenwich, CT 06830; **Phone:** 203-861-0700; **Board Cert:** Psychiatry 1976; Child & Adolescent Psychiatry 1978; **Med School:** Harvard Med Sch 1970; **Resid:** Psychiatry, Mass Mental Hlth Ctr 1973; **Fellow:** Child & Adolescent Psychiatry, Beth Israel Med Ctr 1975

Colon & Rectal Surgery

Littlejohn, Charles E MD (CRS) - **Spec Exp:** Colon & Rectal Cancer; **Hospital:** Stamford Hosp (page 863), Norwalk Hosp; **Address:** 70 Mill River St, Stamford, CT 06902; **Phone:** 203-323-8989; **Board Cert:** Colon & Rectal Surgery 1985; **Med School:** Dartmouth Med Sch 1978; **Resid:** Surgery, Univ Rochester Affil Hosps 1980; Surgery, UMDNJ Med Ctr 1983; **Fellow:** Colon & Rectal Surgery, UMDNJ Med Ctr 1984; **Fac Appt:** Asst Clin Prof S, Columbia P&S

McClane, Steven J MD (CRS) - **Spec Exp:** Colon & Rectal Cancer & Surgery; Inflammatory Bowel Disease; **Hospital:** Stamford Hosp (page 863), Norwalk Hosp; **Address:** 70 Mill River St, Stamford, CT 06902; **Phone:** 203-323-8989; **Board Cert:** Surgery 2000; Colon & Rectal Surgery 2009; **Med School:** Cornell Univ-Weill Med Coll 1992; **Resid:** Surgery, Hosp Univ Penn 1999; **Fellow:** Colon & Rectal Surgery, Cleveland Clinic 2000; **Fac Appt:** Asst Clin Prof S, Columbia P&S

Thornton, Scott MD (CRS) - **Spec Exp:** Laparoscopic Surgery; Colon & Rectal Cancer; **Hospital:** Bridgeport Hosp; **Address:** Park Avenue Surgical Assocs, 1305 Post Rd, Ste 215, Fairfield, CT 06824; **Phone:** 203-255-7088; **Board Cert:** Colon & Rectal Surgery 2005; Surgery 2003; **Med School:** Univ Pittsburgh 1986; **Resid:** Surgery, Univ Conn Sch Med 1991; Colon & Rectal Surgery, UMDNJ-NJ Med Sch 1992; **Fac Appt:** Clin Prof S, Yale Univ

Dermatology

Connors, Richard C MD (D) - **Spec Exp:** Skin Cancer; **Hospital:** Greenwich Hosp (page 862); **Address:** 1 Perryridge Rd, Greenwich, CT 06830-4607; **Phone:** 203-622-0808; **Board Cert:** Dermatology 1974; Dermatopathology 1976; **Med School:** Cornell Univ-Weill Med Coll 1967; **Resid:** Dermatology, New York Hosp 1974; **Fellow:** Dermatopathology, NYU Med Ctr 1975; **Fac Appt:** Assoc Clin Prof D, NYU Sch Med

Kolenik III, Steven A MD (D) - **Spec Exp:** Skin Cancer; Mohs' Surgery; **Hospital:** Norwalk Hosp, Yale-New Haven Hosp; **Address:** 761 Main Ave, Norwalk, CT 06851; **Phone:** 203-810-4151; **Board Cert:** Dermatology 2001; **Med School:** Yale Univ 1990; **Resid:** Dermatology, Yale-New Haven Hosp 1994; **Fellow:** Mohs Surgery, Yale-New Haven Hosp 1995; **Fac Appt:** Asst Clin Prof D, Yale Univ

Maiocco, Kenneth J MD (D) - **Spec Exp:** Skin Cancer; Cosmetic Dermatology; Dermatologic Surgery; **Hospital:** St Vincent's Med Ctr - Bridgeport, Bridgeport Hosp; **Address:** 4639 Main St, Bridgeport, CT 06606-1873; **Phone:** 203-374-5546; **Board Cert:** Dermatology 1976; **Med School:** Univ Rochester 1967; **Resid:** Surgery, St Vincents Med Ctr 1971; Dermatology, Geisinger Med Ctr 1975

Mayer, Fern E MD (D) - **Spec Exp:** Skin Cancer; Pediatric Dermatology; Immune Deficiency-Skin Disorders; **Hospital:** Stamford Hosp (page 863); **Address:** 132 Morgan St, Stamford, CT 06905; **Phone:** 203-969-0123; **Board Cert:** Dermatology 1990; **Med School:** NYU Sch Med 1986; **Resid:** Dermatology, Downstate Med Ctr 1990

Oshman, Robin G MD/PhD (D) - **Spec Exp:** Laser Hair Removal; Botox Therapy; Skin Cancer; Cosmetic Dermatology; **Hospital:** Yale-New Haven Hosp; **Address:** 101 Long Lots Rd, Westport, CT 06880-5426; **Phone:** 203-454-0743; **Board Cert:** Dermatology 1990; **Med School:** Brown Univ 1985; **Resid:** Dermatology, Mt Sinai Hosp 1989; **Fac Appt:** Asst Clin Prof D, Yale Univ

Pesce, Joseph R MD (D) - **Hospital:** St Vincent's Med Ctr - Bridgeport; **Address:** 4699 Main St, Ste 212, Bridgeport, CT 06606-1830; **Phone:** 203-372-8949; **Board Cert:** Dermatology 1972; **Med School:** Belgium 1967; **Resid:** Internal Medicine, Hosp of St Raphael 1968; Dermatology, Dartmouth/Hitchcock Med Ctr 1971

Pruzan-Clain, Debra L MD (D) - **Spec Exp:** Skin Cancer; Cosmetic Dermatology; Pediatric Dermatology; **Hospital:** Stamford Hosp (page 863); **Address:** 1290 Summer St, Ste 3600, Stamford, CT 06905; **Phone:** 203-325-3576; **Board Cert:** Dermatology 1990; **Med School:** Univ Pennsylvania 1986; **Resid:** Dermatology, SUNY Health Sci Ctr 1990; **Fac Appt:** Asst Prof D, Albert Einstein Coll Med

Sibrack, Laurence A MD (D) - **Spec Exp:** Skin Cancer; Cosmetic Dermatology; **Hospital:** Danbury Hosp, Yale-New Haven Hosp; **Address:** 73 Sand Pit Rd, Ste 207, Danbury, CT 06810; **Phone:** 203-792-4151; **Board Cert:** Dermatology 1978; **Med School:** Univ Mich Med Sch 1974; **Resid:** Dermatology, Yale-New Haven Hosp 1978; **Fac Appt:** Asst Prof D, Yale Univ

Diagnostic Radiology

Cohen, Steven M MD (DR) - **Spec Exp:** Ultrasound; Breast Imaging; CT Scan; MRI; **Hospital:** Bridgeport Hosp; **Address:** Bridgeport Hosp, Dept Radiology, 267 Grant St, Bridgeport, CT 06610; **Phone:** 203-337-9729; **Board Cert:** Diagnostic Radiology 1987; **Med School:** NY Med Coll 1983; **Resid:** Internal Medicine, Stamford Hosp 1984; Diagnostic Radiology, Montefiore Med Ctr 1987; **Fellow:** Ultrasound/CT/MRI, Thomas Jefferson Univ Hosp 1989; **Fac Appt:** Asst Prof Rad, Columbia P&S

Fey, Christopher P MD (DR) - **Hospital:** Greenwich Hosp (page 862); **Address:** Greenwich Radiology Group, 49 Lake Ave, Greenwich, CT 06830; **Phone:** 203-869-6220; **Board Cert:** Diagnostic Radiology 1998; Nuclear Medicine 2009; Nuclear Radiology 1999; **Med School:** Yale Univ 1993; **Resid:** Radiology, Beth Israel Deaconess Med Ctr 1998; **Fellow:** Nuclear Medicine, Harvard Univ Affil Hosp 1999

Greenstein, Caren E MD (DR) - **Spec Exp:** Breast Imaging; **Hospital:** Stamford Hosp (page 863); **Address:** Women's Breast Ctr, 32 Strawberry Hill Ct Fl 2, Stamford, CT 06902; **Phone:** 203-276-7112; **Board Cert:** Diagnostic Radiology 1989; **Med School:** Albert Einstein Coll Med 1984; **Resid:** Pathology, Montefiore Med Ctr 1985; Diagnostic Radiology, Montefiore Med Ctr 1989

Lee, Ronald P MD (DR) - **Spec Exp:** MRI; CT Scan; **Hospital:** Norwalk Hosp; **Address:** Norwalk Radiology, 148 East Ave, Ste 1R, Norwalk, CT 06851; **Phone:** 203-851-5645; **Board Cert:** Diagnostic Radiology 1991; **Med School:** NYU Sch Med 1986; **Resid:** Diagnostic Radiology, Bellevue Hosp/NYU Med Ctr 1991; **Fellow:** Magnetic Resonance Imaging, Johns Hopkins Hosp 1992

Strauss, Edward B MD (DR) - **Spec Exp:** Nuclear Medicine; Interventional Radiology; **Hospital:** Norwalk Hosp; **Address:** Norwalk Hosp, Radiology, 34 Maple St, Norwalk, CT 06856-3894; **Phone:** 203-852-2715; **Board Cert:** Diagnostic Radiology 1983; Nuclear Medicine 1984; Vascular & Interventional Radiology 2005; **Med School:** Yale Univ 1979; **Resid:** Diagnostic Radiology, Yale-New Haven Hosp 1983; **Fellow:** Nuclear Medicine, Yale-New Haven Hosp 1984

Sullivan, Scott J MD (DR) - **Spec Exp:** Neuroradiology; **Hospital:** Greenwich Hosp (page 862); **Address:** Greenwich Hosp-Dept Radiology, 5 Perryridge Rd, Greenwich, CT 06830; **Phone:** 203-863-3960; **Board Cert:** Diagnostic Radiology 1996; Neuroradiology 2004; **Med School:** Georgetown Univ 1991; **Resid:** Radiology, Yale-New Haven Hosp 1995; **Fellow:** Neuroradiology, Yale-New Haven Hosp 1996

Endocrinology, Diabetes & Metabolism

Goldberg-Berman, Judith C MD/PhD (EDM) - **Spec Exp:** Diabetes; Thyroid Disorders; Osteoporosis; **Hospital:** Greenwich Hosp (page 862); **Address:** 4 Dearfield Drive, Ste 102, Greenwich, CT 06831-5351; **Phone:** 203-622-9160; **Board Cert:** Internal Medicine 2000; Endocrinology, Diabetes & Metabolism 2000; **Med School:** Cornell Univ-Weill Med Coll 1987; **Resid:** Internal Medicine, NYU/Bellevue Hosp 1990; **Fellow:** Endocrinology, NY CornellHosp/Meml Sloan Kettering 1993

Guoth, Maria S MD (EDM) - **Hospital:** Bridgeport Hosp; **Address:** 5520 Park Ave, Ste 306, Trumball, CT 06611; **Phone:** 203-373-7388; **Board Cert:** Endocrinology, Diabetes & Metabolism 2007; **Med School:** Hungary 1980; **Resid:** Internal Medicine, LaGuardia Hosp 1994; **Fellow:** Endocrinology, Diabetes & Metabolism, Yale-New Haven Hosp 1997; **Fac Appt:** Asst Clin Prof Med, Yale Univ

Rosa, Joseph MD (EDM) - **Hospital:** St Vincent's Med Ctr - Bridgeport; **Address:** 4699 Main St, Ste 105, Bridgeport, CT 06606; **Phone:** 203-374-6162; **Board Cert:** Internal Medicine 1987; Endocrinology 1989; **Med School:** Mexico 1982; **Resid:** Internal Medicine, St Vincents Med Ctr 1986; **Fellow:** Endocrinology, Diabetes & Metabolism, Univ Conn Med Ctr 1988; **Fac Appt:** Assoc Prof Med, Columbia P&S

Savino, Robert R DO (EDM) - **Spec Exp:** Diabetes; **Hospital:** Danbury Hosp; **Address:** 25 German Town Rd, Danbury, CT 06810; **Phone:** 203-794-5620; **Board Cert:** Internal Medicine 2002; Endocrinology, Diabetes & Metabolism 2005; **Med School:** NY Coll Osteo Med 1988; **Resid:** Internal Medicine, LI Jewish Med Ctr 1992; **Fellow:** Endocrinology, Diabetes & Metabolism, Lahey-Hitchcock Med Ctr 1993; Endocrinology, Diabetes & Metabolism, Joslin Diabetes Ctr 1994; **Fac Appt:** Asst Clin Prof Med, Yale Univ

Family Medicine

Acosta, Rod MD (FMed) *PCP* - **Spec Exp:** Geriatric Care; Preventive Medicine; **Hospital:** Stamford Hosp (page 863); **Address:** Stamford Family Practice, 32 Strawberry Hill Ct, Stamford, CT 06902; **Phone:** 203-977-2566; **Board Cert:** Family Medicine 2001; Geriatric Medicine 2002; **Med School:** Univ Tex SW, Dallas 1984; **Resid:** Family Medicine, St Josephs Med Ctr 1987

Farrell, Matthew M MD (FMed) *PCP* - **Spec Exp:** Primary Care Sports Medicine; Sports Medicine-Aging Athlete; **Hospital:** Danbury Hosp; **Address:** 60 Old New Milford Rd, Ste 2A, Brookfield, CT 06804-2430; **Phone:** 203-775-6365; **Board Cert:** Adolescent Medicine 2001; Family Medicine 2007; Sports Medicine 2003; Geriatric Medicine 2006; **Med School:** Columbia P&S 1980; **Resid:** Family Medicine, Somerset Med Ctr 1983; **Fac Appt:** Asst Clin Prof FMed, Univ Conn

Filiberto, Cosmo MD (FMed) *PCP* - **Spec Exp:** Geriatric Care; Cholesterol/Lipid Disorders; Preventive Medicine; **Hospital:** St Vincent's Med Ctr - Bridgeport, Bridgeport Hosp; **Address:** 3715 Main St, Ste 200, Bridgeport, CT 06606-3611; **Phone:** 203-372-4065; **Board Cert:** Family Medicine 2006; Geriatric Medicine 2000; **Med School:** Italy 1976; **Resid:** Family Medicine, Lutheran Med Ctr 1980; **Fac Appt:** Asst Clin Prof FMed, Univ Conn

Mallozzi, Angelo MD (FMed) *PCP* - **Hospital:** Stamford Hosp (page 863); **Address:** 32 Strawberry Hill Court, Stamford, CT 06902; **Phone:** 203-977-2566; **Board Cert:** Family Medicine 2008; **Med School:** Italy 1978; **Resid:** Family Medicine, St Josephs Hosp 1982

Sekiguchi, Raymond T MD/PhD (FMed) *PCP* - **Spec Exp:** Pain Management; Pain-Back; Acupuncture; **Hospital:** Greenwich Hosp (page 862); **Address:** Greenwich Family Practice & Pain Center, 49 Lake Ave, Greenwich, CT 06830; **Phone:** 203-552-9037; **Board Cert:** Family Medicine 2003; **Med School:** Japan 1988; **Resid:** Family Medicine, N Shore Univ Hosp 1996; **Fellow:** Neuropathology, Univ Washington Med Ctr 1999

Gastroenterology

Bonheim, Nelson MD (Ge) - **Spec Exp:** Inflammatory Bowel Disease; Hepatitis C; Colon Cancer; **Hospital:** Greenwich Hosp (page 862); **Address:** 500 W Putnam Ave, Ste 100, Greenwich, CT 06830; **Phone:** 203-863-2900; **Board Cert:** Internal Medicine 1973; Gastroenterology 1975; **Med School:** Ros Franklin Univ/Chicago Med Sch 1970; **Resid:** Internal Medicine, Bronx Muni Hosp 1973; **Fellow:** Gastroenterology, NY Hosp-Cornell Med Ctr 1975; **Fac Appt:** Assoc Prof Med, Yale Univ

Dettmer, Robert M MD (Ge) - **Spec Exp:** Endoscopy; **Hospital:** Stamford Hosp (page 863); **Address:** Tulley Health Ctr, 32 Strawberry Hill Ct, Ste 41042, Stamford, CT 06902; **Phone:** 203-348-5355; **Board Cert:** Gastroenterology 2000; **Med School:** Albert Einstein Coll Med 1994; **Resid:** Internal Medicine, Columbia Presby Med Ctr 1998; **Fellow:** Gastroenterology, Columbia Presby Med Ctr 1999

Gardner, Peter W MD (Ge) - **Spec Exp:** Liver Disease; Inflammatory Bowel Disease; **Hospital:** Stamford Hosp (page 863), Greenwich Hosp (page 862); **Address:** 778 Long Ridge Rd, Ste 101, Stamford, CT 06902; **Phone:** 203-967-2100; **Board Cert:** Internal Medicine 1982; Gastroenterology 1987; **Med School:** Georgetown Univ 1979; **Resid:** Internal Medicine, St Vincents Med Ctr 1982; **Fellow:** Gastroenterology, Univ Conn Hlth Ctr 1984; **Fac Appt:** Asst Clin Prof Med, Columbia P&S

Grossman, Edward T MD (Ge) - **Spec Exp:** Inflammatory Bowel Disease; Malabsorption; **Hospital:** St Vincent's Med Ctr - Bridgeport, Bridgeport Hosp; **Address:** 425 Post Rd Fl 1, Fairfield, CT 06430-6059; **Phone:** 203-292-9000; **Board Cert:** Internal Medicine 1970; Gastroenterology 1973; **Med School:** Albert Einstein Coll Med 1963; **Resid:** Internal Medicine, Bronx Muni Hosp Ctr 1968; **Fellow:** Gastroenterology, NY Hosp-Cornell Med Ctr 1970; **Fac Appt:** Assoc Clin Prof Med, Yale Univ

Gruss, Claudia B MD (Ge) - **Spec Exp:** Colonoscopy; Gastroesophageal Reflux Disease (GERD); Inflammatory Bowel Disease; **Hospital:** Norwalk Hosp; **Address:** 73 Redding Rd, PO Box 270, Georgetown, CT 06829-0270; **Phone:** 203-544-9517; **Board Cert:** Internal Medicine 1980; Gastroenterology 1983; **Med School:** Brown Univ 1977; **Resid:** Internal Medicine, Rhode Island Hosp 1980; **Fellow:** Gastroenterology, Rhode Island Hosp 1982

Mauer, Kenneth MD (Ge) - **Spec Exp:** Endoscopy; Inflammatory Bowel Disease/Crohn's; Capsule Endoscopy; Colonoscopy; **Hospital:** St Vincent's Med Ctr - Bridgeport, Mount Sinai Med Ctr (page 102); **Address:** 425 Post Rd, Fairfield, CT 06824; **Phone:** 203-292-9000; **Board Cert:** Internal Medicine 1986; Gastroenterology 1989; **Med School:** NYU Sch Med 1983; **Resid:** Internal Medicine, Bronx Muni Hosp Ctr 1987; **Fellow:** Gastroenterology, Mount Sinai Hosp 1989

Meighan, Dennis DO (Ge) - **Hospital:** Norwalk Hosp; **Address:** 30 Stevens St, Norwalk, CT 06850-3859; **Phone:** 203-852-3455; **Board Cert:** Internal Medicine 1986; Gastroenterology 1989; **Med School:** Univ New Eng Coll Osteo Med 1982; **Resid:** Internal Medicine, Norwalk Hosp 1986; **Fellow:** Gastroenterology, Norwalk Hosp 1987

Sheinbaum, Richard C MD (Ge) - **Hospital:** Stamford Hosp (page 863); **Address:** 32 Strawberry Hill Ct, Ste 41042, Stamford, CT 06902; **Phone:** 203-348-5355; **Board Cert:** Internal Medicine 1983; Gastroenterology 1987; **Med School:** Temple Univ 1979; **Resid:** Surgery, Mt. Sinai Medical Hospital 1981; Internal Medicine, Stamford Hospital 1983; **Fellow:** Gastroenterology, Cedars-Sinai Medical Ctr 1985; **Fac Appt:** Asst Clin Prof Med, NY Med Coll

Taubin, Howard L MD (Ge) - **Spec Exp:** Colon Cancer Screening; Gastroesophageal Reflux Disease (GERD); Inflammatory Bowel Disease; Liver Disease; **Hospital:** Bridgeport Hosp, Yale-New Haven Hosp; **Address:** 2890 Main St, Stratford, CT 06614; **Phone:** 203-375-1200; **Board Cert:** Internal Medicine 1972; Gastroenterology 1973; **Med School:** Univ VA Sch Med 1965; **Resid:** Internal Medicine, Montefiore Hosp 1967; Internal Medicine, Yale-New Haven Hosp 1970; **Fellow:** Gastroenterology, Yale-New Haven Hosp 1973; **Fac Appt:** Assoc Clin Prof Med, Yale Univ

Zwas, Felice R MD (Ge) - **Hospital:** Greenwich Hosp (page 862); **Address:** 500 W Putnam Ave, Ste 100, Greenwich, CT 06831; **Phone:** 203-863-2900; **Board Cert:** Internal Medicine 1983; Gastroenterology 1985; **Med School:** Columbia P&S 1980; **Resid:** Internal Medicine, Columbia-Presby Med Ctr 1983; **Fellow:** Gastroenterology, Beth Israel Hosp 1985

Geriatric Medicine

Jones, Stephen G MD (Ger) *PCP* - **Spec Exp:** Alzheimer's Disease; **Hospital:** Greenwich Hosp (page 862); **Address:** 5 Perryridge Rd, Greenwich, CT 06830; **Phone:** 203-863-3415; **Board Cert:** Internal Medicine 2002; Geriatric Medicine 2004; **Med School:** SUNY Stony Brook 1985; **Resid:** Geriatric Medicine, SUNY-Stony Brook Hosp 1989; **Fac Appt:** Assoc Clin Prof Med, Yale Univ

Hand Surgery

Backe, Henry A MD (HS) - **Hospital:** St Vincent's Med Ctr - Bridgeport, Bridgeport Hosp; **Address:** 75 Kings Highway Cutoff, Fairfield, CT 06824; **Phone:** 203-337-2600; **Board Cert:** Orthopaedic Surgery 2006; Hand Surgery 2006; **Med School:** Temple Univ 1986; **Resid:** Orthopaedic Surgery, Temple Univ Hosp 1991; **Fellow:** Hand Surgery, Hosp for Joint Diseases 1992; Joint Reconstruction, Hosp Special Surgery 1993

Brown, Lionel G MD (HS) - **Spec Exp:** Hand Reconstruction; Carpal Tunnel Syndrome; **Hospital:** Danbury Hosp; **Address:** 35 Tamarack Ave, Danbury, CT 06811; **Phone:** 203-792-4263; **Board Cert:** Hand Surgery 2008; **Med School:** UCSF 1964; **Resid:** Surgery, UCSF Med Ctr 1976; **Fellow:** Hand Surgery, UCSF Med Ctr 1975

Rago, Thomas A MD (HS) - **Hospital:** Bridgeport Hosp, St Vincent's Med Ctr - Bridgeport; **Address:** 3101 Main St, Bridgeport, CT 06606; **Phone:** 203-374-5892; **Board Cert:** Orthopaedic Surgery 2007; Hand Surgery 2007; **Med School:** Columbia P&S 1977; **Resid:** Surgery, Roosevelt Hosp 1979; Orthopaedic Surgery, Presby Hosp 1982; **Fellow:** Hand Surgery, Columbia-Presby Med Ctr 1983

Hematology

Bar, Michael MD (Hem) - **Spec Exp:** Multiple Myeloma; Leukemia & Lymphoma; Bleeding/Coagulation Disorders; Gaucher Disease; **Hospital:** Stamford Hosp (page 863); **Address:** 34 Shelburne Rd, Bennett Cancer Ctr, Stamford, CT 06902; **Phone:** 203-325-2695; **Board Cert:** Internal Medicine 1986; Medical Oncology 1989; Hematology 2000; **Med School:** Columbia P&S 1983; **Resid:** Internal Medicine, Columbia-Presby Med Ctr 1986; **Fellow:** Hematology & Oncology, UCSF Med Ctr 1990; **Fac Appt:** Asst Clin Prof Med, Columbia P&S

Boyd, D Barry MD (Hem) - **Spec Exp:** Complementary Medicine; Acupuncture; Hematologic Malignancies; Breast Cancer; **Hospital:** Greenwich Hosp (page 862); **Address:** Boyd Ctr for Integrative Health, 15 Valley Drive Fl 2, Greenwich, CT 06831; **Phone:** 203-869-2111; **Board Cert:** Internal Medicine 1982; Medical Oncology 1987; **Med School:** Cornell Univ-Weill Med Coll 1979; **Resid:** Internal Medicine, NY Hosp-Cornell Med Ctr 1982; **Fellow:** Hematology & Oncology, NY Hosp-Cornell Med Ctr 1986; **Fac Appt:** Asst Clin Prof Med, Yale Univ

Cohen, Neil S MD (Hem) - **Spec Exp:** Leukemia; **Hospital:** Stamford Hosp (page 863); **Address:** 34 Shelburne Rd, Stamford, CT 06902-3658; **Phone:** 203-325-2695; **Board Cert:** Internal Medicine 1983; Medical Oncology 1987; Hematology 1988; **Med School:** NY Med Coll 1980; **Resid:** Internal Medicine, Stamford Hosp 1983; **Fellow:** Hematology & Oncology, U Mass Med Ctr 1987; Hematology & Oncology, N Shore Univ Hosp 1988; **Fac Appt:** Assoc Clin Prof Med, Columbia P&S

Duda, E Andrew MD (Hem) - **Hospital:** St Vincent's Med Ctr - Bridgeport, Bridgeport Hosp; **Address:** Medical Specialists of Fairfield, 425 Post Rd, Fairfield, CT 06824; **Phone:** 203-255-4545; **Board Cert:** Internal Medicine 1988; Medical Oncology 1989; Hematology 2002; **Med School:** Yale Univ 1984; **Resid:** Internal Medicine, Yale-New Haven Hosp 1987; **Fellow:** Hematology & Oncology, Dana Farber Cancer Ctr 1991; **Fac Appt:** Asst Clin Prof Med, Columbia P&S

Infectious Disease

Cipriani, Ralph MD (Inf) - **Spec Exp:** Lyme Disease; Fevers of Unknown Origin; **Hospital:** Greenwich Hosp (page 862); **Address:** 5 Perryridge Rd, Greenwich, CT 06830; **Phone:** 203-869-8838; **Board Cert:** Internal Medicine 1999; Infectious Disease 2001; **Med School:** Albert Einstein Coll Med 1996; **Resid:** Internal Medicine, Mt Sinai Hosp 1999; **Fellow:** Infectious Disease, Mt Sinai Hosp 2001; **Fac Appt:** Asst Clin Prof Med, NY Med Coll

Herbin, Joseph T MD (Inf) - **Spec Exp:** Lyme Disease; Infectious Disease in Elderly; **Hospital:** St Vincent's Med Ctr - Bridgeport; **Address:** 2150 Black Rock Tpke, Ste 201, Fairfield, CT 06825; **Phone:** 203-384-0451; **Board Cert:** Internal Medicine 1972; **Med School:** Switzerland 1965; **Resid:** Internal Medicine, St Vincent's Hosp & Med Ctr 1970; **Fellow:** Infectious Disease, Med Ctr Hosp 1971; **Fac Appt:** Asst Clin Prof Med, Columbia P&S

McLeod, Gavin MD (Inf) - **Spec Exp:** AIDS/HIV; Travel Medicine; Hospital Acquired Infections; Pneumonia; **Hospital:** Stamford Hosp (page 863); **Address:** 166 W Broad St, Ste 202, Stamford, CT 06902; **Phone:** 203-353-1427; **Board Cert:** Internal Medicine 1988; Infectious Disease 2002; **Med School:** Univ Conn 1985; **Resid:** Internal Medicine, North Shore Univ Hosp 1988; **Fellow:** Infectious Disease, New England Deaconess Med Ctr 1992; **Fac Appt:** Asst Clin Prof Med, Columbia P&S

Sabetta, James MD (Inf) - **Spec Exp:** Lyme Disease; Tropical Diseases; Bone & Joint Infections; Fevers of Unknown Origin; **Hospital:** Greenwich Hosp (page 862); **Address:** 5 Perryridge Rd, Ste 108, Greenwich, CT 06830; **Phone:** 203-869-8838; **Board Cert:** Internal Medicine 1981; Infectious Disease 1984; **Med School:** Brown Univ 1978; **Resid:** Internal Medicine, Rhode Island Hosp 1981; **Fellow:** Infectious Disease, Yale-New Haven Hosp 1984; **Fac Appt:** Assoc Clin Prof Med, Yale Univ

Saul, Zane MD (Inf) - **Spec Exp:** Lyme Disease; AIDS/HIV; **Hospital:** Bridgeport Hosp; **Address:** 2876-2890 Main St, Ste D, Stratford, CT 06614; **Phone:** 203-259-8087; **Board Cert:** Internal Medicine 2000; Infectious Disease 2000; **Med School:** Grenada 1985; **Resid:** Internal Medicine, Brooklyn Hosp 1988; **Fellow:** Infectious Disease, Hackensack Univ Med Ctr 1990

Yee, Arthur MD (Inf) - **Spec Exp:** Lyme Disease; Infections-Respiratory; Hospital Acquired Infections; **Hospital:** Norwalk Hosp; **Address:** 40 Cross St, Ste 400, Norwalk, CT 06851; **Phone:** 203-845-4838; **Board Cert:** Internal Medicine 1986; Infectious Disease 1988; **Med School:** Univ Conn 1982; **Resid:** Internal Medicine, Columbia-Presby Med Ctr 1985; **Fellow:** Infectious Disease, Hosp Univ Penn 1988; **Fac Appt:** Asst Clin Prof Med, Yale Univ

Internal Medicine

Altbaum, Robert A MD (IM) *PCP* - **Spec Exp:** Hypertension; Asthma; Osteoporosis; **Hospital:** Norwalk Hosp, Bridgeport Hosp; **Address:** 162 Kings Hwy N, Westport, CT 06880-2425; **Phone:** 203-226-0731; **Board Cert:** Internal Medicine 1978; **Med School:** Harvard Med Sch 1975; **Resid:** Internal Medicine, Mass Genl Hosp 1977; Internal Medicine, Yale-New Haven Hosp 1979

Bivona, James J MD (IM) *PCP* - **Hospital:** Stamford Hosp (page 863); **Address:** Stamford Primary Care, 1275 Summer St, Stamford, CT 06905; **Phone:** 203-325-2667; **Board Cert:** Internal Medicine 2000; **Med School:** Dominica 1997; **Resid:** Internal Medicine, Stamford Hosp 2000

Blumberg, Joel M MD (IM) *PCP* - **Spec Exp:** Preventive Cardiology; Hypertension; Cholesterol/Lipid Disorders; Echocardiography; **Hospital:** Greenwich Hosp (page 862); **Address:** 55 Holly Hill Ln, Greenwich, CT 06830; **Phone:** 203-661-4242; **Board Cert:** Internal Medicine 1972; Cardiovascular Disease 1974; **Med School:** NYU Sch Med 1966; **Resid:** Internal Medicine, Bellevue Hosp 1971; **Fellow:** Cardiovascular Disease, New York Hosp 1973; **Fac Appt:** Asst Clin Prof Med, Yale Univ

Costanzo, Joseph V MD (IM) *PCP* - **Hospital:** Stamford Hosp (page 863); **Address:** 80 Mill River St, Ste 2400, Stamford, CT 06902; **Phone:** 203-348-9455; **Board Cert:** Internal Medicine 2000; **Med School:** Harvard Med Sch 1987; **Resid:** Internal Medicine, Bronx Muni Hosp 1990

DoRosario, Arnold MD (IM) *PCP* - **Spec Exp:** Preventive Medicine; Geriatric Care; **Hospital:** St Vincent's Med Ctr - Bridgeport; **Address:** 4699 Main St, Ste 105, Bridgeport, CT 06606; **Phone:** 203-374-6162; **Board Cert:** Internal Medicine 1978; **Med School:** Spain 1975; **Resid:** Internal Medicine, St Vincent's Med Ctr 1978

Dreyer, Neil P MD (IM) *PCP* - **Spec Exp:** Hypertension; Preventive Medicine; **Hospital:** Stamford Hosp (page 863); **Address:** 51 Schuyler Ave, Stamford, CT 06902; **Phone:** 203-327-1187; **Board Cert:** Internal Medicine 1980; Nephrology 1974; **Med School:** NYU Sch Med 1967; **Resid:** Internal Medicine, Bronx Municipal Hosp Ctr 1972; **Fellow:** Nephrology, Montefiore Med Ctr 1973; **Fac Appt:** Asst Clin Prof Med, Columbia P&S

Fennell, Gail M MD (IM) *PCP* - **Spec Exp:** Women's Health; Hypertension; Cholesterol/Lipid Disorders; **Hospital:** Greenwich Hosp (page 862); **Address:** Greenwich Medical Group, 75 Holly Hill Ln, Greenwich, CT 06830; **Phone:** 203-413-1130; **Board Cert:** Internal Medicine 2006; **Med School:** Univ Conn 1992; **Resid:** Internal Medicine, Greenwich Hosp 1995

Hoffman, Pamela B MD (IM) *PCP* - **Spec Exp:** Geriatric Care; **Hospital:** St Vincent's Med Ctr - Bridgeport; **Address:** 2800 Main St, Bridgeport, CT 06606-4201; **Phone:** 203-576-5710; **Board Cert:** Internal Medicine 1983; **Med School:** Univ VA Sch Med 1978; **Resid:** Internal Medicine, St Vincent's Hosp & Med Ctr 1981; **Fellow:** Geriatric Medicine, Jewish Inst Geriatric Care 1983

Klein, Neil MD (IM) - **Spec Exp:** Inflammatory Bowel Disease/Crohn's; Ulcerative Colitis; **Hospital:** Stamford Hosp (page 863); **Address:** 1450 Washington Blvd, Stamford, CT 06902-2451; **Phone:** 203-327-9321; **Board Cert:** Internal Medicine 1974; Gastroenterology 1975; **Med School:** Cornell Univ-Weill Med Coll 1960; **Resid:** Internal Medicine, NY Hosp 1963; Internal Medicine, NY Hosp 1965; **Fellow:** Gastroenterology, NY Hosp 1967; **Fac Appt:** Clin Prof Med, Columbia P&S

Mickley, Diane W MD (IM) - **Spec Exp:** Eating Disorders; **Hospital:** Greenwich Hosp (page 862); **Address:** 7 Riversville Rd Fl 3, Greenwich, CT 06831; **Phone:** 203-531-1909; **Board Cert:** Internal Medicine 1974; **Med School:** Tufts Univ 1971; **Resid:** Internal Medicine, Barnes Jewish Hosp 1973; Internal Medicine, Montefiore Med Ctr 1974; **Fac Appt:** Assoc Clin Prof Med, Yale Univ

Mickley, Steven P MD (IM) *PCP* - **Hospital:** Greenwich Hosp (page 862); **Address:** Glenville Medical Associates, 7 Riversville Rd Fl 1, Greenwich, CT 06831-3697; **Phone:** 203-531-1808; **Board Cert:** Internal Medicine 1974; **Med School:** Harvard Med Sch 1971; **Resid:** Internal Medicine, Barnes Hospital 1973; Internal Medicine, USPHS 1974; **Fac Appt:** Asst Clin Prof Med, Yale Univ

Miner III, Charles MD (IM) - **Hospital:** Stamford Hosp (page 863), Norwalk Hosp; **Address:** 36 Old Kings Hwy S, Darien, CT 06820-4523; **Phone:** 203-655-8749; **Board Cert:** Internal Medicine 1982; **Med School:** Univ Cincinnati 1979; **Resid:** Internal Medicine, Lenox Hill Hosp 1982

Molloy, Edward M MD (IM) *PCP* - **Spec Exp:** Hypertension; Diabetes; Preventive Medicine; **Hospital:** St Vincent's Med Ctr - Bridgeport; **Address:** 134 Round Hill Rd, Fl 2, Fairfield, CT 06824; **Phone:** 203-255-0695; **Board Cert:** Internal Medicine 1974; **Med School:** UMDNJ-NJ Med Sch, Newark 1966; **Resid:** Internal Medicine, St Vincent's Hosp & Med Ctr 1972

Olin, Craig H MD (IM) *PCP* - **Spec Exp:** Preventive Medicine; Metabolic Disorders; **Hospital:** Stamford Hosp (page 863); **Address:** 5 High Ridge Park, Ste 104, Stamford, CT 06905; **Phone:** 203-968-9500; **Board Cert:** Internal Medicine 2006; **Med School:** NYU Sch Med 1993; **Resid:** Internal Medicine, New York Hosp-Cornell 1996

Osnoss, Kenneth MD (IM) *PCP* - **Spec Exp:** Asthma; Lung Disease; **Hospital:** Danbury Hosp; **Address:** 79 Sand Pit Rd, Danbury, CT 06810-6099; **Phone:** 203-749-5700; **Board Cert:** Internal Medicine 1978; Pulmonary Disease 1980; **Med School:** Tufts Univ 1975; **Resid:** Internal Medicine, Hosp Univ Penn 1978; **Fellow:** Pulmonary Disease, Hosp Univ Penn 1980

Skluth, Myra MD/PhD (IM) *PCP* - **Spec Exp:** Women's Health; Diabetes; Cardiovascular Disease; **Hospital:** Norwalk Hosp; **Address:** 10 Mott Ave, Ste 3A, Norwalk, CT 06850; **Phone:** 203-866-4455; **Board Cert:** Internal Medicine 1989; Geriatric Medicine 2006; Hospice & Palliative Medicine 2005; **Med School:** Albert Einstein Coll Med 1986; **Resid:** Internal Medicine, Montefiore Med Ctr 1989; **Fac Appt:** Asst Clin Prof Med, Yale Univ

Slogoff, Frederick B MD (IM) *PCP* - **Spec Exp:** Cardiovascular Disease; Preventive Medicine; Anxiety & Mood Disorders; **Hospital:** Stamford Hosp (page 863); **Address:** 5 High Ridge Park, Ste 104, Stamford, CT 06905; **Phone:** 203-968-9500; **Board Cert:** Internal Medicine 1999; **Med School:** Mount Sinai Sch Med 1996; **Resid:** Internal Medicine, New York Hosp 1999

Spano, Frank MD (IM) *PCP* - **Spec Exp:** Preventive Medicine; **Hospital:** Bridgeport Hosp, St Vincent's Med Ctr - Bridgeport; **Address:** Fairfield County Medical Group, 15 Corporate Drive, Ste 2-1, Trumbull, CT 06611; **Phone:** 203-459-5100; **Board Cert:** Internal Medicine 1987; **Med School:** Albert Einstein Coll Med 1984; **Resid:** Internal Medicine, Jacobi Hosp 1987

Thomas, Bryon S MD (IM) *PCP* - **Spec Exp:** Geriatric Care; **Hospital:** Danbury Hosp; **Address:** 79 Sand Pit Rd, Ste 102, Danbury, CT 06810; **Phone:** 203-749-5700; **Board Cert:** Internal Medicine 1978; Geriatric Medicine 2002; **Med School:** Univ Pittsburgh 1975; **Resid:** Internal Medicine, Mt Sinai Hosp 1978; **Fac Appt:** Asst Clin Prof Med, Yale Univ

Turetsky, Arthur S MD (IM) - **Hospital:** Bridgeport Hosp; **Address:** 15 Corporate Drive, Trumbull, CT 06611; **Phone:** 203-261-3980; **Board Cert:** Internal Medicine 1977; Pulmonary Disease 1980; Sleep Medicine 2009; **Med School:** Albert Einstein Coll Med 1974; **Resid:** Internal Medicine, Einstein Bronx Muncipal Hosp Ctr 1977; Pulmonary Disease, Bronx Municipal Hosp 1979; **Fac Appt:** Asst Clin Prof Med, Albert Einstein Coll Med

Walsh, Francis X MD (IM) *PCP* - **Spec Exp:** Kidney Disease; Hypertension; Dialysis Care; **Hospital:** Greenwich Hosp (page 862), Stamford Hosp (page 863); **Address:** 31 River Rd, Ste 200, Cos Cob, CT 06830-5694; **Phone:** 203-661-9433; **Board Cert:** Internal Medicine 1972; Nephrology 1974; **Med School:** NY Med Coll 1967; **Resid:** Internal Medicine, Greenwich Hosp 1970; **Fellow:** Nephrology, Duke Univ Med Ctr 1972; **Fac Appt:** Asst Clin Prof Med, Yale Univ

Zucker, Michael MD (IM) *PCP* - **Hospital:** Stamford Hosp (page 863); **Address:** 555 Newfield Ave, Stamford, CT 06905-3330; **Phone:** 203-359-4444; **Board Cert:** Internal Medicine 1988; **Med School:** NYU Sch Med 1985; **Resid:** Internal Medicine, Stamford Hospital 1988

Interventional Cardiology

Driesman, Mitchell MD (IC) - **Spec Exp:** Cardiac Catheterization; **Hospital:** Bridgeport Hosp; **Address:** 1305 Post Rd, Fairfield, CT 06430-6016; **Phone:** 203-292-2000; **Board Cert:** Internal Medicine 1980; Cardiovascular Disease 1983; Interventional Cardiology 2009; **Med School:** Brown Univ 1977; **Resid:** Internal Medicine, Tufts-New Eng Med Ctr 1980; **Fellow:** Cardiovascular Disease, Mt Sinai Hosp 1982; **Fac Appt:** Asst Clin Prof Med, Yale Univ

Howes, Christopher J MD (IC) - **Hospital:** Yale-New Haven Hosp, Yale Med Group; **Address:** 55 Holly Hill Ln, Ste 240, Cardiology Svcs of Greenwich, Greenwich, CT 06830; **Phone:** 203-863-4210; **Board Cert:** Internal Medicine 2002; Cardiovascular Disease 2007; Interventional Cardiology 2009; **Med School:** Albert Einstein Coll Med 1989; **Resid:** Internal Medicine, Yale-New Haven Hosp 1992; **Fellow:** Cardiovascular Disease, Yale-New Haven Hosp 1997; **Fac Appt:** Asst Prof Med, Yale Univ

Wasserman, Hal S MD (IC) - **Spec Exp:** Coronary Angioplasty/Stents; Mitral Valve Disease; Coronary Artery Disease; **Hospital:** Danbury Hosp, NY-Presby Hosp/Columbia (page 104); **Address:** 24 Hospital Ave, 7 Tower, Danbury, CT 06810; **Phone:** 203-739-7600; **Board Cert:** Internal Medicine 1985; Cardiovascular Disease 1987; Interventional Cardiology 2009; **Med School:** Columbia P&S 1982; **Resid:** Internal Medicine, Columbia-Presby Med Ctr 1985; **Fellow:** Cardiovascular Disease, Columbia-Presby Med Ctr 1988; **Fac Appt:** Assoc Clin Prof Med, Columbia P&S

Maternal & Fetal Medicine

Bobby, Paul D MD (MF) - **Spec Exp:** Pregnancy-High Risk; Prenatal Diagnosis; **Hospital:** Stamford Hosp (page 863); **Address:** Stamford Hosp, Dept Maternal/Fetal Med, 30 Shelburne Rd, Stamford, CT 06902; **Phone:** 203-276-7061; **Board Cert:** Obstetrics & Gynecology 2009; Maternal & Fetal Medicine 2009; **Med School:** Boston Univ 1990; **Resid:** Obstetrics & Gynecology, NYU Med Ctr 1994; **Fellow:** Maternal & Fetal Medicine, Montefiore Med Ctr 1996; **Fac Appt:** Assoc Clin Prof ObG, Albert Einstein Coll Med

Bond, Annette L MD (MF) - **Spec Exp:** Pregnancy-High Risk; Multiple Gestation; Prenatal Diagnosis; Hypertension in Pregnancy; **Hospital:** Greenwich Hosp (page 862); **Address:** Greenwich Hospital, 5 Perryridge Rd, rm 1-251, Greenwich, CT 06830; **Phone:** 203-863-3674; **Board Cert:** Obstetrics & Gynecology 2009; Maternal & Fetal Medicine 2009; **Med School:** Harvard Med Sch 1983; **Resid:** Obstetrics & Gynecology, NY Hosp-Cornell Med Ctr 1987; **Fellow:** Perinatal Medicine, NY Hosp-Cornell Med Ctr 1989

Laifer, Steven A MD (MF) - **Spec Exp:** Prenatal Diagnosis; Obesity in Pregnancy; **Hospital:** Bridgeport Hosp, Greenwich Hosp (page 862); **Address:** 267 Grant St Fl 5, Bridgeport, CT 06610-2805; **Phone:** 203-384-3544; **Board Cert:** Obstetrics & Gynecology 2009; Maternal & Fetal Medicine 2009; **Med School:** SUNY Downstate 1982; **Resid:** Obstetrics & Gynecology, Johns Hopkins Hosp 1987; **Fellow:** Maternal & Fetal Medicine, Magee Womens Hosp 1989; **Fac Appt:** Asst Clin Prof ObG, Yale Univ

Stiller, Robert J MD (MF) - **Spec Exp:** Prenatal Diagnosis; Ultrasound; Pregnancy-High Risk; Infectious Disease in Pregnancy; **Hospital:** Bridgeport Hosp, Greenwich Hosp (page 862); **Address:** Bridgeport Hospital, Ante Natal Testing, 267 Grant St, Bridgeport, CT 06610; **Phone:** 203-384-3544; **Board Cert:** Obstetrics & Gynecology 2010; Maternal & Fetal Medicine 2010; **Med School:** UMDNJ-Rutgers Med Sch 1979; **Resid:** Obstetrics & Gynecology, Univ Conn Med Ctr 1983; **Fellow:** Maternal & Fetal Medicine, Hosp U Penn 1985; **Fac Appt:** Assoc Clin Prof ObG, Yale Univ

Medical Oncology

Delprete, Salvatore A MD (Onc) - **Spec Exp:** Lung Cancer; Ovarian Cancer; Melanoma; Colon Cancer; **Hospital:** Stamford Hosp (page 863); **Address:** Bennett Cancer Ctr, 34 Shelburne Rd, Stamford, CT 06902-3658; **Phone:** 203-325-2695; **Board Cert:** Internal Medicine 1981; Medical Oncology 1985; Hematology 1986; **Med School:** Columbia P&S 1978; **Resid:** Internal Medicine, Dartmouth-Hitchcock Med Ctr 1981; **Fellow:** Pathology, Dartmouth-Hitchcock Med Ctr 1982; Hematology & Oncology, Dartmouth-Hitchcock Med Ctr 1984; **Fac Appt:** Assoc Clin Prof Med, NY Med Coll

Drucker, Beverly J MD/PhD (Onc) - **Spec Exp:** Breast Cancer; Head & Neck Cancer; Colon & Rectal Cancer; Clinical Trials; **Hospital:** Greenwich Hosp (page 862); **Address:** Hematology & Oncology Assocs Greenwich, 77 Lafayette Pl, Ste 260, Greenwich, CT 06830; **Phone:** 203-863-3737; **Board Cert:** Medical Oncology 2009; **Med School:** Columbia P&S 1994; **Resid:** Internal Medicine, Columbia Presby Med Ctr 1997; **Fellow:** Medical Oncology, John Hopkins 1999

Fischbach, Neal A MD (Onc) - **Spec Exp:** Breast Cancer; Lung Cancer; Colon Cancer; **Hospital:** Bridgeport Hosp, St Vincent's Med Ctr - Bridgeport; **Address:** Oncology Assocs of Bridgeport, 111 Beach Rd, Fairfield, CT 06824; **Phone:** 203-255-2766; **Board Cert:** Medical Oncology 2002; **Med School:** Harvard Med Sch 1995; **Resid:** Internal Medicine, UCSF Med Ctr 1999; **Fellow:** Hematology & Oncology, UCSF Med Ctr 2002

Folman, Robert S MD (Onc) - **Spec Exp:** Breast Cancer; Lung Cancer; Colon & Rectal Cancer; Genitourinary Cancer; **Hospital:** Bridgeport Hosp, St Vincent's Med Ctr - Bridgeport; **Address:** 5520 Park Ave, Trumbull, CT 06611-1351; **Phone:** 203-502-8400; **Board Cert:** Internal Medicine 1975; Medical Oncology 1977; **Med School:** SUNY Buffalo 1972; **Resid:** Internal Medicine, Buffalo Gen Hosp 1975; Internal Medicine, Meml Sloan Kettering Cancer Ctr 1976; **Fellow:** Medical Oncology, Meml Sloan Kettering Cancer Ctr 1977; **Fac Appt:** Asst Prof Med, Yale Univ

Frank, Richard C MD (Onc) - **Spec Exp:** Leukemia; Lymphoma; **Hospital:** Norwalk Hosp; **Address:** Whittingham Cancer Ctr, 24 Stevens St, Norwalk, CT 06856; **Phone:** 203-845-4899; **Board Cert:** Medical Oncology 2005; Hematology 2008; **Med School:** SUNY Stony Brook 1985; **Resid:** Internal Medicine, Columbia-Presby Med Ctr 1992; **Fellow:** Hematology & Oncology, Meml Sloan Kettering Cancer Ctr 1996

Hollister Jr, Dickerman MD (Onc) - **Spec Exp:** Breast Cancer; Lung Cancer; Colon Cancer; Leukemia & Lymphoma; **Hospital:** Greenwich Hosp (page 862); **Address:** 77 Lafayette Pl, Ste 260, Greenwich, CT 06830; **Phone:** 203-863-3737; **Board Cert:** Internal Medicine 1978; Hematology 1980; Medical Oncology 1981; **Med School:** Univ VA Sch Med 1975; **Resid:** Internal Medicine, NY Hosp-Cornell Med Ctr 1978; **Fellow:** Hematology & Oncology, NY Hosp-Cornell Med Ctr 1981; **Fac Appt:** Asst Clin Prof Med, Yale Univ

Kloss, Robert MD (Onc) - **Spec Exp:** Breast Cancer; Colon Cancer; Lung Cancer; **Hospital:** Danbury Hosp; **Address:** 95 Locust Ave Fl 1, Danbury, CT 06810-6010; **Phone:** 203-797-7029; **Board Cert:** Internal Medicine 1979; Medical Oncology 1981; Hospice & Palliative Medicine 2008; **Med School:** Jefferson Med Coll 1976; **Resid:** Internal Medicine, Univ Hosp 1979; **Fellow:** Hematology & Oncology, Columbia-Presby Med Ctr 1981

Lo, K M Steve MD (Onc) - **Spec Exp:** Breast Cancer; Lymphoma; **Hospital:** Stamford Hosp (page 863); **Address:** 34 Shelburne Rd, Stamford, CT 06902-3658; **Phone:** 203-325-2695; **Board Cert:** Internal Medicine 1989; Medical Oncology 2001; Hematology 2002; **Med School:** Harvard Med Sch 1985; **Resid:** Internal Medicine, Brigham & Women's Hosp 1988; **Fellow:** Hematology & Oncology, Dana Farber Cancer Inst 1991; Hematology, Dana Farber Cancer Inst 1992; **Fac Appt:** Asst Clin Prof Med, Columbia P&S

Weinstein, Paul MD (Onc) - **Spec Exp:** Breast Cancer; Lung Cancer; Colon Cancer; **Hospital:** Stamford Hosp (page 863); **Address:** 34 Shelburne Rd, Bennett Cancer Ctr, Hematology-Oncology, Stamford, CT 06902-3628; **Phone:** 203-325-2695; **Board Cert:** Internal Medicine 1973; Medical Oncology 1977; Hematology 1978; **Med School:** Ros Franklin Univ/Chicago Med Sch 1970; **Resid:** Internal Medicine, Montefiore Med Ctr 1973; **Fellow:** Hematology & Oncology, Montefiore Med Ctr 1975; **Fac Appt:** Assoc Clin Prof Med, Columbia P&S

Zelkowitz, Richard S MD (Onc) - **Spec Exp:** Breast Cancer; Hematology; **Hospital:** Norwalk Hosp; **Address:** 40 Cross St, Norwalk, CT 06851; **Phone:** 203-845-4890; **Board Cert:** Internal Medicine 1986; Hematology 1988; Medical Oncology 1989; **Med School:** NY Med Coll 1983; **Resid:** Internal Medicine, Westchester Co Med Ctr 1986; **Fellow:** Hematology & Oncology, Brown Univ Hosps 1989

Neonatal-Perinatal Medicine

Herzlinger, Robert A MD (NP) - **Spec Exp:** Neonatology; **Hospital:** Bridgeport Hosp, Yale-New Haven Hosp; **Address:** Bridgeport Hosp, 267 Grant St, Ste 6, Bridgeport, CT 06610-2870; **Phone:** 203-384-3486; **Board Cert:** Pediatrics 1974; Neonatal-Perinatal Medicine 1977; **Med School:** NY Med Coll 1969; **Resid:** Pediatrics, Westchester Co Med Ctr 1971; Pediatrics, Columbia-Presby Med Ctr 1972; **Fellow:** Neonatal-Perinatal Medicine, Columbia-Presby Med Ctr 1973; Neonatal-Perinatal Medicine, Montefiore Med Ctr 1976; **Fac Appt:** Assoc Clin Prof Ped, Yale Univ

Rakos, Gerald B MD (NP) - **Hospital:** Stamford Hosp (page 863); **Address:** Stamford Hospital, Dept Pediatrics, 30 Shelburne Rd, Box 9317, Stamford, CT 06904; **Phone:** 203-276-7085; **Board Cert:** Pediatrics 1985; Neonatal-Perinatal Medicine 1985; **Med School:** SUNY Upstate Med Univ 1980; **Resid:** Pediatrics, Univ Mass Medical Ctr 1983; **Fellow:** Neonatology, Montefiore Med Ctr 1985; **Fac Appt:** Asst Clin Prof Ped, Columbia P&S

Theofanidis, Stylianos MD (NP) - **Hospital:** Greenwich Hosp (page 862), Yale-New Haven Hosp; **Address:** 5 Perryridge Rd, Greenwich, CT 06830-4608; **Phone:** 203-863-3515; **Board Cert:** Neonatal-Perinatal Medicine 2004; **Med School:** Greece 1980; **Resid:** Pediatrics, St Lukes Hosp 1985; **Fellow:** Neonatal-Perinatal Medicine, NY Hosp-Cornell Med Ctr 1987; **Fac Appt:** Asst Clin Prof Ped, Yale Univ

Nephrology

Brown, Eric MD (Nep) - **Spec Exp:** Kidney Disease; Hypertension; Glomerulonephritis; **Hospital:** Stamford Hosp (page 863), Greenwich Hosp (page 862); **Address:** 30 Commerce Rd, Stamford, CT 06902-4550; **Phone:** 203-324-7666; **Board Cert:** Internal Medicine 1988; Nephrology 1999; **Med School:** Emory Univ 1985; **Resid:** Internal Medicine, Johns Hopkins Hosp 1988; **Fellow:** Nephrology, Yale-New Haven Hosp 1990; **Fac Appt:** Asst Clin Prof Med, Columbia P&S

Chan, Brenda MD (Nep) - **Spec Exp:** Dialysis Care; Kidney Failure-Chronic; Lupus Nephritis; Glomerulonephritis; **Hospital:** Stamford Hosp (page 863), Greenwich Hosp (page 862); **Address:** Stamford Nephrology, 30 Commerce Rd, Stamford, CT 06902; **Phone:** 203-324-7666; **Board Cert:** Nephrology 2007; **Med School:** Mount Sinai Sch Med 1990; **Resid:** Internal Medicine, Montefiore Med Ctr 1993; **Fellow:** Nephrology, Montefiore Med Ctr 1996

Feintzeig, Irwin D MD (Nep) - **Spec Exp:** Kidney Disease; Hypertension; Dialysis Care; **Hospital:** Bridgeport Hosp, St Vincent's Med Ctr - Bridgeport; **Address:** 900 Madison Ave, Ste 209, Bridgeport, CT 06606-5534; **Phone:** 203-335-0195; **Board Cert:** Internal Medicine 1982; Nephrology 1984; **Med School:** Univ Chicago-Pritzker Sch Med 1979; **Resid:** Internal Medicine, Temple Univ Hosp 1982; **Fellow:** Nephrology, Boston Univ Med Ctr 1985; **Fac Appt:** Asst Clin Prof Med, Yale Univ

Fogel, Mitchell A MD (Nep) - **Spec Exp:** Kidney Disease-Chronic; Glomerulonephritis; Dialysis Care; **Hospital:** St Vincent's Med Ctr - Bridgeport, Bridgeport Hosp; **Address:** 900 Madison Ave, Ste 209, Bridgeport, CT 06606-5534; **Phone:** 203-335-0195; **Board Cert:** Internal Medicine 1986; Nephrology 1988; **Med School:** Univ Pennsylvania 1982; **Resid:** Internal Medicine, Boston Univ Med Ctr 1985; **Fellow:** Nephrology, Boston Univ Med Ctr 1988; **Fac Appt:** Assoc Clin Prof Med, Columbia P&S

Garfinkel, Howard B MD (Nep) - **Spec Exp:** Hypertension; Kidney Disease; Kidney Stones; **Hospital:** Danbury Hosp; **Address:** 111 Osbourne St, Ste 210, Danbury, CT 06810; **Phone:** 203-739-7104; **Board Cert:** Internal Medicine 1972; Nephrology 1972; **Med School:** Tufts Univ 1965; **Resid:** Internal Medicine, Cleveland Metro Genl Hosp 1970; **Fellow:** Renal Disease, Tufts-New Eng Med Ctr 1972; **Fac Appt:** Assoc Clin Prof Med, Yale Univ

Hines, William H MD (Nep) - **Spec Exp:** Dialysis Care; Hypertension; Kidney Disease; **Hospital:** Stamford Hosp (page 863), Greenwich Hosp (page 862); **Address:** 30 Commerce Rd, Stamford, CT 06902-4550; **Phone:** 203-324-7666; **Board Cert:** Internal Medicine 1984; Nephrology 1986; **Med School:** Cornell Univ-Weill Med Coll 1981; **Resid:** Internal Medicine, Hosp Univ Penn 1984; **Fellow:** Nephrology, Hosp Univ Penn 1988; **Fac Appt:** Asst Clin Prof Med, Columbia P&S

Hunt, William A MD (Nep) - **Hospital:** Bridgeport Hosp; **Address:** 900 Madison Ave, Ste 209, Bridgeport, CT 06606-5534; **Phone:** 203-335-0195; **Board Cert:** Internal Medicine 1984; Nephrology 1986; **Med School:** Yale Univ 1981; **Resid:** Internal Medicine, Univ Hosps Cleveland 1984

Neurological Surgery

Apostolides, Paul J MD (NS) - **Spec Exp:** Minimally Invasive Spinal Surgery; Spinal Surgery; Spinal Disc Replacement; **Hospital:** Greenwich Hosp (page 862), Stamford Hosp (page 863); **Address:** Orthopaedic & Neurosurg Specialists PC, 6 Greenwich Office Park, Valley Drive, Greenwich, CT 06831; **Phone:** 203-869-1145; **Board Cert:** Neurological Surgery 2002; **Med School:** Univ Mass Sch Med 1991; **Resid:** Neurological Surgery, Barrow Neuro Inst/St Joseph's Hosp 1998; **Fellow:** Spinal Surgery, Barrow Neuro Inst/St Joseph's 1997

Fiore, Amory J MD (NS) - **Spec Exp:** Spinal Surgery; Minimally Invasive Surgery; **Hospital:** Greenwich Hosp (page 862); **Address:** 6 Greenwich Office Park, Valley Drive, Orthopaedic & Neurosurgery Specialists, Greenwich, CT 06831; **Phone:** 203-869-1145; **Board Cert:** Neurological Surgery 2006; **Med School:** Columbia P&S 1995; **Resid:** Neonatal-Perinatal Medicine, Presby Hosp 2001; **Fellow:** Spinal Surgery, The Emory Clinic 2002

Ghogawala, Zoher MD (NS) - **Spec Exp:** Minimally Invasive Spinal Surgery; Vascular Neurosurgery; Carotid Artery Surgery; Cerebrovascular Neurosurgery; **Hospital:** Greenwich Hosp (page 862), Yale Med Group; **Address:** 25 Valley Drive, Greenwich, CT 06831; **Phone:** 203-661-3333; **Board Cert:** Neurological Surgery 2004; **Med School:** Harvard Med Sch 1991; **Resid:** Neurological Surgery, Mass Genl Hosp 1999; **Fac Appt:** Asst Clin Prof NS, Yale Univ

Lipow, Kenneth MD (NS) - **Spec Exp:** Spinal Surgery; Brain Surgery; **Hospital:** Bridgeport Hosp, St Vincent's Med Ctr - Bridgeport; **Address:** CT Neurosurgical Specialists, 267 Grant St Fl 8, Bridgeport, CT 06610-2870; **Phone:** 203-384-4500; **Board Cert:** Neurological Surgery 1989; **Med School:** Albert Einstein Coll Med 1978; **Resid:** Neurological Surgery, Montefiore Med Ctr 1984

Mintz, Abraham MD (NS) - **Spec Exp:** Spinal Surgery; **Hospital:** St Vincent's Med Ctr - Bridgeport, Bridgeport Hosp; **Address:** 5520 Park Ave, Ste 210, Trumbull, CT 06611; **Phone:** 203-372-6460; **Board Cert:** Neurological Surgery 1992; **Med School:** Mexico 1982; **Resid:** Neurological Surgery, Jackson Meml Hosp 1989

Shahid, Syed J MD (NS) - **Spec Exp:** Brain Tumors; Spinal Surgery; Spinal Tumors; **Hospital:** Danbury Hosp, Norwalk Hosp; **Address:** 148 East Ave, Ste 3D, Norwalk, CT 06851; **Phone:** 203-853-0003; **Board Cert:** Neurological Surgery 1983; **Med School:** Pakistan 1972; **Resid:** Surgery, Kings County Hosp 1977; Neurological Surgery, Kings County Hosp 1980

Shear, Perry MD (NS) - **Hospital:** Bridgeport Hosp, St Vincent's Med Ctr - Bridgeport; **Address:** 75 Kings Highway Cutoff, Fairfield, CT 06824; **Phone:** 203-337-2629; **Board Cert:** Neurological Surgery 1996; **Med School:** Univ Toronto 1984; **Resid:** Neurological Surgery, Toronto Genl Hosp 1991

Neurology

Gross, Jeffrey L MD (N) - **Spec Exp:** Multiple Sclerosis; **Hospital:** St Vincent's Med Ctr - Bridgeport, Milford Hosp; **Address:** 75 Kings Highway Cutoff, Fairfield, CT 06824; **Phone:** 203-333-1133; **Board Cert:** Neurology 1985; **Med School:** Case West Res Univ 1978; **Resid:** Internal Medicine, Hosp Univ Penn 1980; Neurology, Hosp Univ Penn 1983; **Fellow:** Neuromuscular Disease, Hosp Univ Penn 1984

McAllister, Peter J MD (N) - **Spec Exp:** Headache; **Hospital:** St Vincent's Med Ctr - Bridgeport, Bridgeport Hosp; **Address:** Assoc Neurologists of S Connecticut, 75 Kings Highway Cutoff, Fairfield, CT 06430; **Phone:** 203-333-1133; **Board Cert:** Neurology 2007; **Med School:** Univ Conn 1991; **Resid:** Neurology, Med Coll Virginia 1995; **Fellow:** Neuromuscular Medicine, Med Coll Virginia 1996

Nahm, Frederick K MD/PhD (N) - **Spec Exp:** Cerebrovascular Disease; Stroke; **Hospital:** Greenwich Hosp (page 862); **Address:** Neurology of Greenwich, 49 Lake Ave, Ste LL3, Greenwich, CT 06830; **Phone:** 203-661-9383; **Board Cert:** Neurology 2003; **Med School:** Univ Mich Med Sch 1996; **Resid:** Neurology, Beth Israel Deaconess Med Ctr 2000; **Fellow:** Clinical Neurophysiology, Mass Genl Hosp 2001

Resor, Louise D MD (N) - **Hospital:** Stamford Hosp (page 863); **Address:** 166 W Broad St, Ste 203, Stamford, CT 06902; **Phone:** 203-978-0283; **Med School:** Washington Univ, St Louis 1974; **Resid:** Neurology, Columbia-Presby 1978; **Fellow:** Babies Hosp 1979

Rusk, Alice H MD (N) - **Spec Exp:** Movement Disorders; Parkinson's Disease; Dystonia; **Hospital:** Greenwich Hosp (page 862), Stamford Hosp (page 863); **Address:** Greenwich Neurology, 49 Lake Ave, Ste 206, Greenwich, CT 06830; **Phone:** 203-869-6446; **Board Cert:** Neurology 2006; **Med School:** Univ Conn 1991; **Resid:** Neurology, NY Hosp-Cornell Med Ctr 1995; **Fellow:** Clinical Neurophysiology, Columbia Presby Med Ctr 1996

Sena, Kanaga N MD (N) - **Spec Exp:** Stroke; Neuro-Rehabilitation; Headache; **Hospital:** Bridgeport Hosp, Griffin Hosp; **Address:** 2590 Main St, Stratford, CT 06615-5838; **Phone:** 203-377-5988; **Board Cert:** Neurology 1979; **Med School:** Sri Lanka 1969; **Resid:** Internal Medicine, Bridgeport Hosp 1973; Neurology, Yale-New Haven Hosp 1976; **Fac Appt:** Assoc Clin Prof N, Yale Univ

Siegel, Kenneth C MD (N) - **Spec Exp:** Parkinson's Disease; Headache; Stroke; Movement Disorders; **Hospital:** St Vincent's Med Ctr - Bridgeport, Milford Hosp; **Address:** Assoc Neurologists of S Connecticut, 75 Kings Highway Cutoff, Fairfield, CT 06824; **Phone:** 203-333-1133; **Board Cert:** Neurology 1975; **Med School:** Meharry Med Coll 1969; **Resid:** Neurology, Bellevue Med Ctr/NYU 1973; **Fac Appt:** Assoc Clin Prof N, Yale Univ

Nuclear Medicine

Gupta, Shiv M MD (NuM) - **Spec Exp:** Osteoporosis; **Hospital:** Danbury Hosp; **Address:** 24 Hospital Ave, Danbury, CT 06810; **Phone:** 203-739-7222; **Board Cert:** Nuclear Medicine 1981; **Med School:** India 1969; **Resid:** Nuclear Medicine, Univ Conn Hlth Ctr 1980; Internal Medicine, Danbury Hosp 1981; **Fellow:** Nuclear Medicine, Auckland Hosp 1978; **Fac Appt:** Clin Prof NuM, Univ Conn

Johns, William D MD (NuM) - **Hospital:** Danbury Hosp; **Address:** 24 Hospital Ave, Danbury, CT 06810; **Phone:** 203-739-7222; **Board Cert:** Internal Medicine 1986; Nuclear Medicine 1988; **Med School:** Univ Conn 1983; **Resid:** Internal Medicine, Danbury Hosp 1986; Nuclear Medicine, Brigham & Women's Hosp 1988

Obstetrics & Gynecology

Ayoub, Thomas V MD (ObG) - **Spec Exp:** Menopause Problems; **Hospital:** Norwalk Hosp; **Address:** Women's Healthcare of New England, 761 Main Ave, Ste 100, Norwalk, CT 06851; **Phone:** 203-644-1100; **Board Cert:** Obstetrics & Gynecology 2009; **Med School:** NYU Sch Med 1980; **Resid:** Obstetrics & Gynecology, Bellevue Hosp Ctr 1984

Besser, Gary S MD (ObG) - **Spec Exp:** Laparoscopic Surgery-Complex; Uro-Gynecology; Pelvic Surgery; Robotic Surgery; **Hospital:** Stamford Hosp (page 863), Norwalk Hosp; **Address:** Whittingham Pavilion, 190 W Broad St, Ste G-401, Stamford, CT 06902-3661; **Phone:** 203-325-4321; **Board Cert:** Obstetrics & Gynecology 2009; **Med School:** SUNY Downstate 1982; **Resid:** Obstetrics & Gynecology, Stamford Hosp 1986; **Fac Appt:** Assoc Prof ObG, Columbia P&S

Blair, Emily DO (ObG) - **Spec Exp:** Pregnancy-High Risk; **Hospital:** Bridgeport Hosp; **Address:** 1735 Post Rd, Fairfield, CT 06824; **Phone:** 203-256-3990; **Board Cert:** Obstetrics & Gynecology 2009; **Med School:** Univ Osteo Med & Hlth Sci, Des Moines 1986; **Resid:** Obstetrics & Gynecology, Bridgeport Hosp 1990; **Fac Appt:** Assoc Prof ObG, Univ Conn

Bruck, Lance MD (ObG) - **Spec Exp:** Minimally Invasive Surgery; Gynecologic Surgery; **Hospital:** Stamford Hosp (page 863); **Address:** Stamford Hosp-Dept Ob/Gyn, 30 Shelburne Rd, Stamford, CT 06902; **Phone:** 203-276-7853; **Board Cert:** Obstetrics & Gynecology 2009; **Med School:** NY Med Coll 1992; **Resid:** Obstetrics & Gynecology, Montefiore Med Ctr 1997; **Fac Appt:** Assoc Clin Prof ObG, Albert Einstein Coll Med

Donovan, Leslie MD (ObG) - **Spec Exp:** Adolescent Gynecology; Menopause Problems; Sexually Transmitted Diseases; Gynecology Only; **Hospital:** Greenwich Hosp (page 862); **Address:** Brookside Greenwich Gynecology Assocs, 159 W Putnam Ave, Greenwich, CT 06830; **Phone:** 203-869-7080; **Board Cert:** Obstetrics & Gynecology 2008; **Med School:** Univ Mass Sch Med 1993; **Resid:** Obstetrics & Gynecology, St Joseph's Med Ctr 1999

Schechter, Michael D MD (ObG) - **Hospital:** Greenwich Hosp (page 862); **Address:** Putnam Gynecology & Obstetrics, 500 W Putnam Ave, Greenwich, CT 06830; **Phone:** 203-622-0303; **Board Cert:** Obstetrics & Gynecology 2009; **Med School:** NYU Sch Med 1988; **Resid:** Obstetrics & Gynecology, St Lukes-Roosevelt Hosp 1992

Violi, Caterina MD (ObG) - **Spec Exp:** Endometriosis; Pelvic Organ Prolapse Repair; Pregnancy-High Risk; Laparoscopic Surgery-Complex; **Hospital:** Greenwich Hosp (page 862); **Address:** 2 1/2 Dearfield Drive, Ste 101, Greenwich, CT 06831; **Phone:** 203-861-9586; **Board Cert:** Obstetrics & Gynecology 2000; **Med School:** Univ Rochester 1994; **Resid:** Obstetrics & Gynecology, Winthrop Univ Hosp 1998

Weinstein Jr, David B MD (ObG) - **Spec Exp:** Pregnancy-High Risk; **Hospital:** Stamford Hosp (page 863); **Address:** Stamford Hospital, Whittingham Pavilion, 190 W Broad St, Ste G-401, Stamford, CT 06902; **Phone:** 203-325-4321; **Board Cert:** Obstetrics & Gynecology 2008; **Med School:** Univ Chicago-Pritzker Sch Med 1969; **Resid:** Obstetrics & Gynecology, NY Hosp-Cornell Med Ctr 1974; **Fac Appt:** Asst Clin Prof ObG, Cornell Univ-Weill Med Coll

Ophthalmology

DeBroff, Brian MD (Oph) - **Spec Exp:** Refractive Surgery; Cataract Surgery; Cataract-Pediatric; Anterior Segment Surgery; **Hospital:** Yale-New Haven Hosp, Bridgeport Hosp; **Address:** Eye Surgery Associates, 3060 Main St, Ste 101, Stratford, CT 06614; **Phone:** 203-375-5819; **Board Cert:** Ophthalmology 2005; **Med School:** Tufts Univ 1989; **Resid:** Ophthalmology, Univ Pittsburg/Eye & Ear Inst 1993; **Fellow:** Anterior Segment - External Disease, Gimbel Eye Ctr 1994; **Fac Appt:** Assoc Clin Prof Oph, Yale Univ

Finlay, Alexis E MD (Oph) - **Spec Exp:** Refractive Surgery; Cornea & Cataract Surgery; Lens Implants; **Hospital:** Greenwich Hosp (page 862), New York Eye & Ear Infirm (page 113); **Address:** 2 1/2 Dearfield Rd, Greenwich, CT 06831; **Phone:** 203-869-4446; **Board Cert:** Ophthalmology 1989; **Med School:** Hahnemann Univ 1981; **Resid:** Ophthalmology, NY E&E Informary 1985; **Fellow:** Ophthalmic Pathology, Johns Hopkins Hosp 1986

Gladstein, Gina F MD (Oph) - **Spec Exp:** Glaucoma; Cataract Surgery; **Hospital:** Greenwich Hosp (page 862); **Address:** Greenwich Ophthalmology Assocs, 4 Dearfield Drive, Greenwich, CT 06831; **Phone:** 203-869-3082; **Board Cert:** Ophthalmology 1989; **Med School:** Albert Einstein Coll Med 1983; **Resid:** Ophthalmology, Manhattan EE&T Hosp 1987; **Fellow:** Ophthalmology, Manhattan EE&T Hosp 1988

Kaplan, Jeffrey N MD (Oph) - **Spec Exp:** Corneal Disease; Cataract Surgery; **Hospital:** Bridgeport Hosp; **Address:** 4699 Main St, Ste 106, Bridgeport, CT 06606; **Phone:** 203-374-8182; **Board Cert:** Ophthalmology 1987; **Med School:** SUNY Stony Brook 1981; **Resid:** Ophthalmology, SUNY Downstate Med Ctr 1985; **Fellow:** Cornea, Dubroff Eye Ctr 1986

Mandava, Suresh MD (Oph) - **Spec Exp:** LASIK-Refractive Surgery; Cataract Surgery; Cornea Transplant; Cornea & External Eye Disease; **Hospital:** Greenwich Hosp (page 862); **Address:** 4 Dearfield Drive, Greenwich, CT 06831; **Phone:** 203-869-3082; **Board Cert:** Ophthalmology 2009; **Med School:** Yale Univ 1993; **Resid:** Ophthalmology, Manhattan EE&T 1997; **Fellow:** Cornea & Refractive Surgery, Univ Minnesota Med Ctr 1998

Manjoney, Delia MD (Oph) - **Spec Exp:** Cataract Surgery; Glaucoma; Eyelid Cosmetic Surgery; **Hospital:** St Vincent's Med Ctr - Bridgeport; **Address:** 2720 Main St, Bridgeport, CT 06606; **Phone:** 203-576-6500; **Board Cert:** Pediatrics 1982; Ophthalmology 1988; **Med School:** Univ VT Coll Med 1977; **Resid:** Pediatrics, Parkland Hosp/Chldns Med Ctr 1980; Ophthalmology, Colum Presby Med Ctr/Harkness 1986

Musto, Anthony MD (Oph) - **Spec Exp:** Cataract Surgery-Lens Implant; Eyelid Surgery; **Hospital:** Bridgeport Hosp; **Address:** 3060 Main St, Stratford, CT 06614-4945; **Phone:** 203-375-5819; **Board Cert:** Ophthalmology 1975; **Med School:** Georgetown Univ 1968; **Resid:** Ophthalmology, USPHS 1971; Ophthalmology, Manhattan Eye, Ear & Throat Infirm 1973; **Fac Appt:** Asst Clin Prof Oph, Yale Univ

Ostriker, Glenn E MD (Oph) - **Spec Exp:** Cataract Surgery; Glaucoma; **Hospital:** Stamford Hosp (page 863), NYU Langone Med Ctr (page 106); **Address:** 71 Strawberry Hill Ave, Ste 116, Stamford, CT 06902-2702; **Phone:** 203-348-6300; **Board Cert:** Ophthalmology 1987; **Med School:** NYU Sch Med 1982; **Resid:** Ophthalmology, NYU Med Ctr 1986; **Fellow:** Neurological Physiology, NYU Med Ctr 1983; **Fac Appt:** Assoc Clin Prof Oph, NYU Sch Med

Potter, William S MD (Oph) - **Spec Exp:** Pediatric Ophthalmology; Strabismus-Adult & Pediatric; Lens Implants; Amblyopia; **Hospital:** Greenwich Hosp (page 862), Stamford Hosp (page 863); **Address:** Greenwich Ophthalmology Assocs, 4 Dearfield Drive, Greenwich, CT 06831; **Phone:** 203-869-3082; **Board Cert:** Ophthalmology 1991; **Med School:** NY Med Coll 1985; **Resid:** Ophthalmology, NY E&E Infirmary 1989; **Fellow:** Strabismus, Wills Eye Hosp 1990

Reppucci, Vincent S MD (Oph) - **Spec Exp:** Retinal Disorders; Macular Degeneration; Diabetic Eye Disease; **Hospital:** Danbury Hosp, St Luke's - Roosevelt Hosp Ctr - Roosevelt Div (page 94); **Address:** 65 North St, Danbury, CT 06810; **Phone:** 203-792-6291; **Board Cert:** Ophthalmology 1989; **Med School:** Albert Einstein Coll Med 1983; **Resid:** Ophthalmology, Columbia-Presby Med Ctr 1987; **Fellow:** Vitreoretinal Surgery & Disease, New York Hosp-Cornell 1988; **Fac Appt:** Assoc Prof Oph, Cornell Univ-Weill Med Coll

Robbins, Kim P MD (Oph) - **Spec Exp:** Cataract Surgery; LASIK-Refractive Surgery; **Hospital:** Bridgeport Hosp; **Address:** 4695 Main St, Bridgeport, CT 06606; **Phone:** 203-371-5800; **Board Cert:** Ophthalmology 1985; **Med School:** NY Med Coll 1978; **Resid:** Internal Medicine, Stamford Hosp 1980; Ophthalmology, St Vincents Hosp 1983

Siderides, Elizabeth MD (Oph) - **Spec Exp:** Cataract Surgery; **Hospital:** Stamford Hosp (page 863); **Address:** Stamford Ophthalmology, 1351 Washington Blvd, Ste 101, Stamford, CT 06902-2453; **Phone:** 203-327-5808; **Board Cert:** Ophthalmology 1991; **Med School:** Columbia P&S 1985; **Resid:** Ophthalmology, NYU Med Ctr 1989; **Fellow:** Medical Retina, NYU Med Ctr 1990

Tom, David MD (Oph) - **Spec Exp:** Retinal Disorders; **Hospital:** Yale-New Haven Hosp, Greenwich Hosp (page 862); **Address:** New England Retina Assocs, 143 Sound Beach Ave, Old Greenwich, CT 06870; **Phone:** 203-288-2020; **Board Cert:** Ophthalmology 2008; **Med School:** Geo Wash Univ 1991; **Resid:** Ophthalmology, Yale-New Haven Hosp 1996; **Fellow:** Vitreoretinal Surgery, Manhattan EE & T 1997; **Fac Appt:** Asst Clin Prof Oph, Yale Univ

Wasserman, Eric L MD (Oph) - **Spec Exp:** Cataract Surgery; Glaucoma; **Hospital:** Stamford Hosp (page 863); **Address:** 1275 Summer St, Ste 200, Stamford, CT 06905-5315; **Phone:** 203-978-0800; **Board Cert:** Ophthalmology 1988; **Med School:** NY Med Coll 1979; **Resid:** Ophthalmology, NY Med Coll 1983; **Fellow:** Anterior Segment - External Disease, John H Sheets Eye Fdn 1984

Weber, Richard B MD (Oph) - **Spec Exp:** Retinal Disorders; **Hospital:** Stamford Hosp (page 863), Greenwich Hosp (page 862); **Address:** 1275 Summer St, Ste 103, Stamford, CT 06905; **Phone:** 203-353-1857; **Board Cert:** Internal Medicine 1979; Ophthalmology 1985; **Med School:** Albert Einstein Coll Med 1976; **Resid:** Internal Medicine, Bronx Muni Hosps 1979; Ophthalmology, Mass E&E Infirm 1984; **Fellow:** Retina, Mass E&E Infirm 1985

Orthopaedic Surgery

Bindelglass, David MD (OrS) - **Spec Exp:** Arthritis; Minimally Invasive Surgery; Hip Replacement; Knee Replacement; **Hospital:** Bridgeport Hosp, St Vincent's Med Ctr - Bridgeport; **Address:** 75 Kings Highway Cutoff, Fairfield, CT 06824; **Phone:** 203-337-2600; **Board Cert:** Orthopaedic Surgery 2005; **Med School:** Columbia P&S 1985; **Resid:** Surgery, Beth Israel Hosp 1987; Orthopaedic Surgery, Columbia-Presby Med Ctr 1990; **Fellow:** Orthopaedic Surgery, Kerlan-Jobe Ortho Clin 1991

Boone, Peter S MD (OrS) - **Spec Exp:** Sports Medicine; Knee Replacement; Hip Replacement; **Hospital:** St Vincent's Med Ctr - Bridgeport; **Address:** Orthopaedic & Sports Medicine Ctr, 888 White Plains Rd, Trumbull, CT 06611; **Phone:** 203-268-2882; **Board Cert:** Orthopaedic Surgery 2005; **Med School:** Univ Pennsylvania 1985; **Resid:** Surgery, Bellevue/NYU Med Ctr 1986; Orthopaedic Surgery, UMDNJ Med Ctr 1991; **Fellow:** Joint Replacement Surgery, Univ Indiana 1992

Clain, Michael R MD (OrS) - **Spec Exp:** Foot & Ankle Surgery; Sports Medicine; **Hospital:** Greenwich Hosp (page 862); **Address:** 6 Greenwich Office Park, 10 Valley Drive, Orthopaedic & Neurosurgery Specialists, Greenwich, CT 06831; **Phone:** 203-869-1145; **Board Cert:** Orthopaedic Surgery 2004; **Med School:** Columbia P&S 1984; **Resid:** Orthopaedic Surgery, Lenox Hill Hosp 1990; **Fellow:** Foot & Ankle Surgery, Baylor Coll Med 1991

Crowe, John F MD (OrS) - **Spec Exp:** Upper Extremity Surgery; Hip & Knee Replacement; Sports Medicine; **Hospital:** Greenwich Hosp (page 862); **Address:** 6 Greenwich Office Park, Greenwich, CT 06831-6086; **Phone:** 203-869-1145 x263; **Board Cert:** Orthopaedic Surgery 1977; **Med School:** Cornell Univ-Weill Med Coll 1971; **Resid:** Surgery, Roosevelt Hosp 1973; Orthopaedic Surgery, Hosp Special Surgery 1976; **Fellow:** Hand Surgery, Roosevelt Hosp 1979

Cunningham, James G MD (OrS) - **Spec Exp:** Arthroscopic Surgery; Shoulder Surgery; Knee Surgery; Sports Medicine; **Hospital:** Greenwich Hosp (page 862); **Address:** Orthopaedic & Neurosurg. Specialists PC, 6 Greenwich Offfice Park, Valley Drive, Greenwich, CT 06831; **Phone:** 203-869-1145; **Board Cert:** Orthopaedic Surgery 2009; Orthopaedic Sports Medicine 2007; **Med School:** NYU Sch Med 1983; **Resid:** Orthopaedic Surgery, Mt Sinai Med Ctr 1988; Surgery, Mt Sinai Med Ctr 1984; **Fellow:** Sports Medicine, New England Baptist Hosp 1989

D'Amico, Joseph MD (OrS) - **Spec Exp:** Knee Replacement; Hip Replacement; Sports Medicine; **Hospital:** Stamford Hosp (page 863); **Address:** 90 Morgan St, Ste 207, Stamford, CT 06905-5436; **Phone:** 203-325-4087; **Board Cert:** Orthopaedic Surgery 2003; **Med School:** Univ Tenn Coll Med, Memphis 1982; **Resid:** Orthopaedic Surgery, St Lukes-Roosevelt Med Ctr 1988

Henshaw, D Ross MD (OrS) - **Spec Exp:** Shoulder Surgery; Rotator Cuff Surgery; Cartilage Damage; Knee Surgery; **Hospital:** Danbury Hosp; **Address:** Danbury Orthopaedic Assocs, 226 White St, Danbury, CT 06810; **Phone:** 203-797-1500; **Board Cert:** Orthopaedic Surgery 2007; **Med School:** Columbia P&S 1998; **Resid:** Orthopaedic Surgery, Ny Presby-Columbia Med Ctr 2003; **Fellow:** Sports Medicine & Shoulder Surgery, Hosp for Special Surgery 2005

Hermele, Herbert I MD (OrS) - **Hospital:** Bridgeport Hosp, St Vincent's Med Ctr - Bridgeport; **Address:** 75 Kings Hwy Cutoff, Fairfield, CT 06824-5340; **Phone:** 203-337-2600; **Board Cert:** Orthopaedic Surgery 1975; **Med School:** Albert Einstein Coll Med 1969; **Resid:** Orthopaedic Surgery, Albert Einstein Affil Hosps 1974

Hindman, Steven MD (OrS) - **Hospital:** Greenwich Hosp (page 862); **Address:** 6 Greenwich Office Park, Greenwich, CT 06831-5151; **Phone:** 203-869-1145; **Board Cert:** Orthopaedic Surgery 1989; **Med School:** Albert Einstein Coll Med 1982

Hughes, Peter MD (OrS) - **Spec Exp:** Hip Replacement; Knee Replacement; Sports Medicine; **Hospital:** Stamford Hosp (page 863); **Address:** 90 Morgan St, Ste 207, Stamford, CT 06905; **Phone:** 203-325-4087; **Board Cert:** Orthopaedic Surgery 1978; **Med School:** NY Med Coll 1972; **Resid:** Orthopaedic Surgery, Metropolitan Hosp Ctr 1976; **Fellow:** Surgery, Hosp for Special Surg 1977; **Fac Appt:** Asst Clin Prof OrS, Columbia P&S

Kavanagh, Brian MD (OrS) - **Spec Exp:** Hip Replacement; Knee Replacement; Arthritis; **Hospital:** Greenwich Hosp (page 862); **Address:** 6 Greenwich Office Park, Greenwich Orthopedic Assoc, Greenwich, CT 06831-5151; **Phone:** 203-869-1145; **Board Cert:** Orthopaedic Surgery 2007; **Med School:** Univ Conn 1979; **Resid:** Orthopaedic Surgery, Mayo Clin 1984; **Fac Appt:** Asst Clin Prof OrS, Yale Univ

Miller, Seth R MD (OrS) - **Spec Exp:** Shoulder Surgery; Rotator Cuff Surgery; Sports Medicine; **Hospital:** Greenwich Hosp (page 862), NYU Hosp For Joint Diseases (page 106); **Address:** 6 Greenwich Office Park, 10 Valley Drive, Greenwich, CT 06831; **Phone:** 203-869-1145; **Board Cert:** Orthopaedic Surgery 2002; **Med School:** Mount Sinai Sch Med 1982; **Resid:** Surgery, Mt Sinai Hosp 1985; Orthopaedic Surgery, Columbia-Presby Med Ctr 1988; **Fellow:** Shoulder Surgery, Columbia-Presby Med Ctr 1989

Sethi, Paul MD (OrS) - **Spec Exp:** Sports Medicine; Knee Surgery; Shoulder Surgery; **Hospital:** Greenwich Hosp (page 862); **Address:** Ortho & Neurosurgery Specialists, 6 Greenwich Office Park, Greenwich, CT 06831; **Phone:** 203-869-1145; **Board Cert:** Orthopaedic Surgery 2005; Orthopaedic Sports Medicine 2007; **Med School:** Mount Sinai Sch Med 1997; **Resid:** Orthopaedic Surgery, Yale-New Haven Hosp 2002; **Fellow:** Sports Medicine, Kerlan Jobe Ortho Clin 2003; Arthroscopic Surgery, Kerlan Jobe Ortho Clin 2004

Spak, James I MD (OrS) - **Spec Exp:** Sports Medicine; **Hospital:** St Vincent's Med Ctr - Bridgeport; **Address:** Orthopaedic & Sports Med Ctr, 888 White Plains Rd, Trumbull, CT 06611; **Phone:** 203-268-2882; **Board Cert:** Orthopaedic Surgery 2000; **Med School:** Harvard Med Sch 1992; **Resid:** Orthopaedic Surgery, Brigham & Women's Hosp 1997; **Fellow:** Sports Medicine, Tahoe Fracture & Ortho Cl 1998; Trauma, Tahoe Fracture & Ortho Cl 1998

Stovell, Peter MD (OrS) - **Spec Exp:** Joint Replacement; Sports Medicine; **Hospital:** Norwalk Hosp; **Address:** 40 Cross St, Ste 300, Norwalk, CT 06851-5726; **Phone:** 203-845-2200; **Board Cert:** Orthopaedic Surgery 1976; **Med School:** Columbia P&S 1968; **Resid:** Surgery, St Luke's-Roosevelt Hosp Ctr 1970; Orthopaedic Surgery, Hosp for Special Surgery 1975

Troy, Allen MD (OrS) - **Spec Exp:** Foot & Ankle Surgery; Sports Medicine; **Hospital:** Stamford Hosp (page 863); **Address:** 61 4th St, Stamford, CT 06905-5010; **Phone:** 203-324-0307; **Board Cert:** Orthopaedic Surgery 2010; **Med School:** SUNY Downstate 1979; **Resid:** Orthopaedic Surgery, NYU Med Ctr 1984; **Fellow:** Foot & Ankle Surgery, Hosp Joint Disease 1985; **Fac Appt:** Asst Clin Prof OrS, Columbia P&S

Wilchinsky, Mark MD (OrS) - **Spec Exp:** Arthroscopic Surgery; Joint Replacement; **Hospital:** St Vincent's Med Ctr - Bridgeport, Griffin Hosp; **Address:** 888 White Plains Rd, Trumbull, CT 06611; **Phone:** 203-268-2882; **Board Cert:** Orthopaedic Surgery 2007; **Med School:** Tulane Univ 1979; **Resid:** Surgery, Univ Mass Med Ctr 1980; Orthopaedic Surgery, Univ Mass Med Ctr 1984; **Fac Appt:** Asst Prof OrS, Univ Mass Sch Med

Otolaryngology

Gordon, Neil A MD (Oto) - **Spec Exp:** Cosmetic Surgery-Face; **Hospital:** Bridgeport Hosp, Norwalk Hosp; **Address:** 539 Danbury Rd, Wilton, CT 06897; **Phone:** 203-661-1715; **Board Cert:** Otolaryngology 1996; Facial Plastic & Reconstr Surgery 1998; **Med School:** Albert Einstein Coll Med 1990; **Resid:** Otolaryngology, Yale-New Haven Hosp 1995; **Fellow:** Facial Plastic Surgery, Tulane Univ Med Ctr 1996

Klarsfeld, Jay MD (Oto) - **Spec Exp:** Sinus Disorders; Thyroid & Parathyroid Surgery; **Hospital:** Danbury Hosp; **Address:** 107 Newtown Rd, Ste 2A, Danbury, CT 06810-4151; **Phone:** 203-830-4700; **Board Cert:** Otolaryngology 1986; **Med School:** Mount Sinai Sch Med 1981; **Resid:** Surgery, Mt Sinai Hosp 1983; Otolaryngology, Mt Sinai Hosp 1986

Klenoff, Bruce MD (Oto) - **Spec Exp:** Ear Disorders/Surgery; Sinus Disorders/Surgery; Pediatric Otolaryngology; **Hospital:** Stamford Hosp (page 863); **Address:** Ear, Nose & Throat Ctr - Tully Hlth Ctr, 32 Strawberry Hill Ct, Fl 4 - Ste 4, Stamford, CT 06902; **Phone:** 203-353-0000; **Board Cert:** Otolaryngology 1976; **Med School:** Tufts Univ 1969; **Resid:** Surgery, St Elizabeth Hosp 1973; Otolaryngology, Mass Eye & Ear Infirm 1976; **Fac Appt:** Asst Clin Prof S, Columbia P&S

Levin, Richard MD (Oto) - **Spec Exp:** Sinus Disorders; Ear Infections; Facial Plastic & Reconstructive Surgery; **Hospital:** St Vincent's Med Ctr - Bridgeport, Bridgeport Hosp; **Address:** 1305 Post Rd, Fairfield, CT 06824; **Phone:** 203-259-4700; **Board Cert:** Otolaryngology 1993; **Med School:** Tufts Univ 1987; **Resid:** Otolaryngology, Mount Sinai Hosp 1993; **Fac Appt:** Asst Prof S, Yale Univ

Levine, Steven B MD (Oto) - **Spec Exp:** Sinus Disorders; Allergy & Immunotherapy; Snoring/Sleep Apnea; Facial Plastic Surgery; **Hospital:** Bridgeport Hosp; **Address:** 160 Hawley Ln, Ste 202, Trumbull, CT 06611; **Phone:** 203-380-3707; **Board Cert:** Otolaryngology 1986; **Med School:** Univ Rochester 1981; **Resid:** Surgery, Penn Hosp 1983; Otolaryngology, Hosp Univ Penn 1986; **Fellow:** Otolaryngology, NY Hosp 1986; **Fac Appt:** Asst Clin Prof S, Yale Univ

Lipton, Richard J MD (Oto) - **Spec Exp:** Head & Neck Surgery; **Hospital:** Danbury Hosp; **Address:** 107 Newtown Rd, Ste 2A, Danbury, CT 06810-4545; **Phone:** 203-830-4700; **Board Cert:** Otolaryngology 1990; **Med School:** Mayo Med Sch 1985; **Resid:** Surgery, Mayo Clinic 1986; Otolaryngology, Mayo Clinic 1990

Salzer, Stephen MD (Oto) - **Spec Exp:** Thyroid & Parathyroid Surgery; Pediatric Otolaryngology; Sinus Disorders/Surgery; Sleep Apnea; **Hospital:** Greenwich Hosp (page 862), Stamford Hosp (page 863); **Address:** 49 Lake Ave Fl 1, Greenwich, CT 06830-4519; **Phone:** 203-869-2030; **Board Cert:** Otolaryngology 1995; **Med School:** Johns Hopkins Univ 1989; **Resid:** Otolaryngology, Yale-New Haven Hosp 1994; **Fellow:** Otolaryngology, Laennec Hosp 1995

Pain Medicine

Kloth, David S MD (PM) - **Spec Exp:** Pain-Back; Pain-Cancer; **Hospital:** Danbury Hosp, St Mary's Hosp - Waterbury; **Address:** Connecticut Pain Care, 109 Newtown Rd, Danbury, CT 06810; **Phone:** 203-792-7246; **Board Cert:** Anesthesiology 1992; Pain Medicine 2007; **Med School:** NYU Sch Med 1987; **Resid:** Anesthesiology, Hosp U Penn 1991

Pediatric Cardiology

Berkwits, Kieve M MD (PCd) - **Spec Exp:** Congenital Heart Disease; **Hospital:** Bridgeport Hosp, St Vincent's Med Ctr - Bridgeport; **Address:** Bridgeport Hosp, Dept Peds, 267 Grant St, Box 5000, Bridgeport, CT 06610; **Phone:** 203-384-3783; **Board Cert:** Pediatrics 1986; Pediatric Cardiology 2003; **Med School:** Mexico 1979; **Resid:** Pediatrics, Beth Israel Med Ctr 1983; **Fellow:** Pediatric Cardiology, NY Hosp-Cornell Med Ctr 1985; **Fac Appt:** Asst Clin Prof Ped, Yale Univ

Snyder, Michael MD (PCd) - **Spec Exp:** Echocardiography; Fetal Echocardiography; **Hospital:** Stamford Hosp (page 863); **Address:** 1500 Boston Post Rd Fl 2, Darien, CT 06820-5936; **Phone:** 203-662-0313; **Board Cert:** Pediatrics 1984; Pediatric Cardiology 1985; **Med School:** Cornell Univ-Weill Med Coll 1979; **Resid:** Pediatrics, NY Hosp 1982; **Fellow:** Pediatric Cardiology, NY Hosp 1984; **Fac Appt:** Assoc Prof Ped, Columbia P&S

Pediatric Gastroenterology

Glassman, Mark MD (PGe) - **Spec Exp:** Inflammatory Bowel Disease/Crohn's; Gastroesophageal Reflux Disease (GERD); Diarrheal Diseases; Food Allergy; **Hospital:** Norwalk Hosp, Children's & Women's Phys.of Westchester; **Address:** 149 East Ave, Ste 39, Norwalk, CT 06851-5711; **Phone:** 203-853-7170; **Board Cert:** Pediatrics 1983; Pediatric Gastroenterology 2005; **Med School:** SUNY Buffalo 1978; **Resid:** Pediatrics, Yale-New Haven Hosp 1981; **Fellow:** Gastroenterology, Chldns Hosp 1983; **Fac Appt:** Prof Ped, NY Med Coll

Pediatric Hematology-Oncology

Ertl, John MD (PHO) - ; **Address:** 41 Germantown Rd, Ste 201, Danbury, CT 06810-4000; **Phone:** 203-744-1680; **Board Cert:** Pediatrics 1977; Pediatric Hematology-Oncology 1978; **Med School:** SUNY Downstate 1970; **Resid:** Pediatrics, Rhode Island Hosp 1973; **Fellow:** Pediatric Hematology-Oncology, UC Davis Medical Center 1977

Pediatric Pulmonology

Dworkin, Gregory MD (PPul) - **Spec Exp:** Asthma; Chronic Lung Disease; **Hospital:** Danbury Hosp; **Address:** 79 Sandpit Rd, Ste 201, Danbury, CT 06810; **Phone:** 203-790-5437; **Board Cert:** Pediatrics 1987; Pediatric Pulmonology 2004; **Med School:** Albany Med Coll 1982; **Resid:** Pediatrics, Mount Sinai 1985; Pediatrics, Mount Sinai 1986; **Fellow:** Pediatric Pulmonology, Mount Sinai 1989; **Fac Appt:** Asst Clin Prof Ped, NY Med Coll

Hen Jr, Jacob MD (PPul) - **Spec Exp:** Asthma; Critical Care; **Hospital:** Bridgeport Hosp, Yale-New Haven Hosp; **Address:** Bridgeport Hosp, Dept Peds, 267 Grant St, Box 5000, Bridgeport, CT 06610-2870; **Phone:** 203-384-3711; **Board Cert:** Pediatrics 1980; Pediatric Pulmonology 2006; Pediatric Critical Care Medicine 2003; **Med School:** UMDNJ-NJ Med Sch, Newark 1975; **Resid:** Pediatrics, UMDNJ-Univ Hosp 1977; **Fellow:** Pediatric Pulmonology, Yale-New Haven Hosp 1981; **Fac Appt:** Assoc Clin Prof Ped, Yale Univ

Sadeghi, Hossein MD (PPul) - **Spec Exp:** Asthma; Neonatal Chronic Lung Disease; Cystic Fibrosis; Bronchoscopy; **Hospital:** Stamford Hosp (page 863), Greenwich Hosp (page 862); **Address:** 32 Strawberry Hill Ct, Ste 11, Stamford, CT 06902-2777; **Phone:** 203-276-5949; **Board Cert:** Pediatrics 2003; Pediatric Pulmonology 2006; **Med School:** Australia 1990; **Resid:** Pediatrics, Royal Chldns Hosp 1992; Pediatrics, Med Coll Va Hosp 1995; **Fellow:** Pediatric Pulmonology, Westchester Co Med Ctr 1998; **Fac Appt:** Asst Clin Prof Ped, Columbia P&S

Pediatrics

Chessin, Robert D MD (Ped) *PCP* - **Spec Exp:** Child Development; Developmental Disorders; **Hospital:** Bridgeport Hosp, St Vincent's Med Ctr - Bridgeport; **Address:** 4699 Main St, Ste 215, Bridgeport, CT 06606-1830; **Phone:** 203-452-8322; **Board Cert:** Pediatrics 1978; Developmental-Behavioral Pediatrics 2004; **Med School:** Johns Hopkins Univ 1973; **Resid:** Pediatrics, Duke Univ Med Ctr 1976; **Fac Appt:** Assoc Clin Prof Ped, Yale Univ

Freedman, Richard M MD (Ped) *PCP* - **Spec Exp:** Neonatology; **Hospital:** Bridgeport Hosp, Yale-New Haven Hosp; **Address:** 4699 Main St, Ste 215, Bridgeport, CT 06606-1830; **Phone:** 203-452-8322; **Board Cert:** Pediatrics 1979; Neonatal-Perinatal Medicine 1981; **Med School:** Boston Univ 1975; **Resid:** Pediatrics, Yale-New Haven Hosp 1978; **Fellow:** Neonatology, Yale-New Haven Hosp 1980; **Fac Appt:** Assoc Clin Prof Ped, Yale Univ

Hedrick, David A MD (Ped) *PCP* - **Hospital:** Greenwich Hosp (page 862); **Address:** Children's Medical Group, 42 Sherwood Pl, Greenwich, CT 06830; **Phone:** 203-661-2440; **Board Cert:** Pediatrics 1981; **Med School:** Univ VA Sch Med 1976; **Resid:** Pediatrics, Children's Hosp of Pittsburgh 1079

Juan, Paul E MD (Ped) *PCP* - **Spec Exp:** Developmental Disorders; Asthma; **Hospital:** Greenwich Hosp (page 862); **Address:** Valley Pediatrics of Greenwich, 25 Valley Ave, Greenwich, CT 06830; **Phone:** 203-622-4301; **Board Cert:** Pediatrics 2009; **Med School:** NY Med Coll 1990; **Resid:** Pediatrics, Med Coll of Virginia 1993

Klenk, Rosemary MD (Ped) *PCP* - **Spec Exp:** ADD/ADHD; Eating Disorders; **Hospital:** Stamford Hosp (page 863), NY-Presby Hosp (page 104); **Address:** New England Pediatrics, 183 Cherry St, Ste 103, New Canaan, CT 06840; **Phone:** 203-972-5232; **Board Cert:** Pediatrics 1987; **Med School:** Cornell Univ-Weill Med Coll 1980; **Resid:** Pediatrics, Columbia-Presby Med Ctr 1983

Korval, Arnold MD (Ped) *PCP* - **Hospital:** Greenwich Hosp (page 862), Stamford Hosp (page 863); **Address:** 8 West End Ave, Old Greenwich, CT 06870-1642; **Phone:** 203-637-0186; **Board Cert:** Pediatrics 2009; **Med School:** St Louis Univ 1974; **Resid:** Pediatrics, Chldn's Hosp-Univ Penn 1977

Levine, Dorothy MD (Ped) *PCP* - **Spec Exp:** Complex Diagnosis; **Hospital:** Stamford Hosp (page 863), NY-Presby Hosp/Columbia (page 104); **Address:** New England Pediatrics, 183 Cherry St, Ste 103, New Canaan, CT 06840; **Phone:** 203-972-5232; **Board Cert:** Pediatrics 1985; **Med School:** Albert Einstein Coll Med 1980; **Resid:** Pediatrics, Columbia-Presby Med Ctr 1983; **Fac Appt:** Asst Clin Prof Ped, Columbia P&S

Mini, Katherine N MD (Ped) *PCP* - **Hospital:** Greenwich Hosp (page 862); **Address:** Chldn's Med Grp, 42 Sherwood Pl, Greenwich, CT 06830; **Phone:** 203-661-2440; **Board Cert:** Pediatrics 2005; **Med School:** Albert Einstein Coll Med 1994; **Resid:** Pediatrics, Yale-New Haven Hosp 1997

Mongillo, Nicholas MD (Ped) *PCP* - **Spec Exp:** AIDS/HIV; Sports Medicine; ADD/ADHD; **Hospital:** Bridgeport Hosp, Yale-New Haven Hosp; **Address:** 7365 Main St, Stratford, CT 06614; **Phone:** 203-381-9990; **Board Cert:** Pediatrics 2003; **Med School:** Grenada 1987; **Resid:** Pediatrics, Bridgeport Hosp 1990

Morelli, Alan MD (Ped) *PCP* - **Hospital:** Stamford Hosp (page 863); **Address:** New England Pediatrics, 166 W Broad St, Ste 103, Stamford, CT 06902; **Phone:** 203-323-1770; **Board Cert:** Pediatrics 1987; **Med School:** NY Med Coll 1982; **Resid:** Pediatrics, Yale-New Haven Hosp 1985

Schiz, Steven L MD (Ped) *PCP* - ; **Address:** Children's Medical Group, 42 Sherwood Pl, Greenwich, CT 06830-5633; **Phone:** 203-661-2440; **Board Cert:** Pediatrics 2009; **Med School:** Columbia P&S 1980; **Resid:** Pediatrics, Children's Hosp of Pittsburgh 1983

Schutzengel, Roy MD (Ped) *PCP* - **Spec Exp:** Growth Disorders; Developmental Disorders; **Hospital:** Bridgeport Hosp, St Vincent's Med Ctr - Bridgeport; **Address:** 3180 Main St, Ste G1, Bridgeport, CT 06606; **Phone:** 203-371-7111; **Board Cert:** Pediatrics 2004; **Med School:** Univ Pennsylvania 1984; **Resid:** Pediatrics, UC Davis Medical Center 1988; **Fellow:** Pediatric Endocrinology, Nat Inst Health 1986; Pediatric Hematology-Oncology, Yale-New Haven Hosp 1989

Physical Medicine & Rehabilitation

Grant, Linda MD (PMR) - **Hospital:** Greenwich Hosp (page 862); **Address:** Greenwich Hosp, Physical Med & Rehab, 5 Perryridge Rd, Greenwich, CT 06830; **Phone:** 203-863-3290; **Board Cert:** Physical Medicine & Rehabilitation 1990; **Med School:** UMDNJ-Rutgers Med Sch 1985; **Resid:** Physical Medicine & Rehabilitation, NYU Med Ctr 1989

Heftler, Jeffrey M MD (PMR) - **Spec Exp:** Pain Management; Spinal Rehabilitation; **Hospital:** Greenwich Hosp (page 862); **Address:** Orthopaedic & Neurosurgery Specialists, 6 Greenwich Office Park, Greenwich, CT 06831; **Phone:** 203-869-1145; **Board Cert:** Physical Medicine & Rehabilitation 2002; Pain Medicine 2003; **Med School:** UMDNJ-RW Johnson Med Sch 1997; **Resid:** Physical Medicine & Rehabilitation, Thos Jefferson Univ Med Ctr 2001; **Fellow:** Pain Management, Beth Israel Med Ctr 2002

Richter, Edwin MD (PMR) - **Spec Exp:** Neuro-Rehabilitation; Musculoskeletal Injuries; Amputee Rehabilitation; Lymphedema; **Hospital:** Stamford Hosp (page 863); **Address:** 32 Strawberry Hill Ct Fl 4 - Ste 9, Stamford, CT 06902; **Phone:** 203-316-0610; **Board Cert:** Physical Medicine & Rehabilitation 1992; **Med School:** NYU Sch Med 1987; **Resid:** Physical Medicine & Rehabilitation, NYU Med Ctr 1991; **Fac Appt:** Asst Clin Prof PMR, NYU Sch Med

Snowball, Halina MD (PMR) - **Spec Exp:** Pain Management; Acupuncture; **Hospital:** Greenwich Hosp (page 862); **Address:** Orthopaedic & Neurosurgery Specialists, 6 Greenwich Office Park, 10 Valley Drive, Greenwich, CT 06831; **Phone:** 203-869-1145; **Board Cert:** Physical Medicine & Rehabilitation 1990; **Med School:** Univ Fla Coll Med 1985; **Resid:** Physical Medicine & Rehabilitation, Stanford Univ Med Ctr 1989

Plastic Surgery

Attkiss, Keith J MD (PlS) - **Spec Exp:** Breast Cosmetic & Reconstructive Surgery; Liposuction & Body Contouring; **Hospital:** Greenwich Hosp (page 862); **Address:** 2 1/2 Dearfield Drive, Ste 203, Greenwich, CT 06831; **Phone:** 203-862-2700; **Board Cert:** Plastic Surgery 2001; **Med School:** Columbia P&S 1992; **Resid:** Surgery, UC Davies Med Ctr 1997; Plastic Surgery, Yale-New Haven Hosp 2000

Gewirtz, Harold S MD (PlS) - **Spec Exp:** Cosmetic Surgery-Face; Breast Cosmetic & Reconstructive Surgery; Liposuction & Body Contouring; Melanoma; **Hospital:** Stamford Hosp (page 863), Greenwich Hosp (page 862); **Address:** 70 Mill River St, Stamford, CT 06902-3725; **Phone:** 203-325-1381; **Board Cert:** Plastic Surgery 1984; Hand Surgery 1998; **Med School:** Johns Hopkins Univ 1975; **Resid:** Surgery, UCLA Med Ctr 1980; Plastic Surgery, NYU Med Ctr 1982; **Fac Appt:** Assoc Clin Prof PlS, Columbia P&S

Goldenberg, David M MD (PlS) - **Spec Exp:** Cosmetic Surgery; Breast Reconstruction; Wound Healing/Care; **Hospital:** Danbury Hosp; **Address:** 107 Newtown Rd, Ste 2C, Danbury, CT 06810-4151; **Phone:** 203-791-9661; **Board Cert:** Plastic Surgery 1990; **Med School:** NY Med Coll 1982; **Resid:** Surgery, Montefiore Med Ctr-Einstein Div 1986; **Fellow:** Plastic Surgery, Montefiore Med Ctr-Einstein Div 1988

Newman, Fredric A MD (PlS) - **Spec Exp:** Rhinoplasty; Breast Augmentation; Eyelid Surgery; Abdominoplasty; **Hospital:** Greenwich Hosp (page 862), Stamford Hosp (page 863); **Address:** 722 Post Rd, Ste 200, Darien, CT 06820; **Phone:** 203-656-9999; **Board Cert:** Plastic Surgery 1985; **Med School:** SUNY Downstate 1974; **Resid:** Surgery, Beth Israel Med Ctr 1977; Surgery, SUNY Downstate 1979; **Fellow:** Plastic/Reconstructive Surgery, NYU Med Ctr 1981; Plastic Surgery, Jackson Meml Hosp 1982; **Fac Appt:** Asst Prof PlS, NY Med Coll

O'Connell, Joseph B MD (PlS) - **Spec Exp:** Cosmetic Surgery-Liposuction; Cosmetic Surgery-Face; Cosmetic Surgery-Breast; Body Contouring; **Hospital:** Bridgeport Hosp; **Address:** 208 Post Rd W, Westport, CT 06880; **Phone:** 203-454-0044; **Board Cert:** Plastic Surgery 1992; **Med School:** Cornell Univ-Weill Med Coll 1981; **Resid:** Surgery, St Vincents Med Ctr 1986; **Fellow:** Plastic Surgery, New York Hosp 1988

Raskin, Elsa M MD (PlS) - **Spec Exp:** Eyelid Cosmetic & Reconstructive Surgery; Cosmetic Surgery-Face; Cosmetic Surgery-Breast; **Hospital:** Greenwich Hosp (page 862), Lenox Hill Hosp; **Address:** 2 1/2 Dearfield Drive, Ste 102, Greenwich, CT 06831-5335; **Phone:** 203-861-6620; **Board Cert:** Plastic Surgery 2002; **Med School:** Switzerland 1987; **Resid:** Ophthalmology, NY Eye & Ear Infirm 1995; Surgery, NYU Med Ctr 1999; **Fellow:** Plastic Surgery, Univ Pittsburgh Med Ctr 1996; Plastic/Reconstructive Surgery, NY Presby Hosp 2001

Rosenstock, Arthur MD (PIS) - **Spec Exp:** Cosmetic Surgery-Face; Eyelid Surgery; Cosmetic Surgery-Breast; **Hospital:** Stamford Hosp (page 863); **Address:** 1290 Summer St, Ste 3100, Stamford, CT 06905-5326; **Phone:** 203-359-1959; **Board Cert:** Plastic Surgery 1985; **Med School:** Belgium 1976; **Resid:** Surgery, Westchester Co Med Ctr 1981; **Fellow:** Plastic/Reconstructive Surgery, Med Coll Virginia 1983; **Fac Appt:** Asst Clin Prof S, Columbia P&S

Psychiatry

Boutaeva, Zinaida MD/PhD (Psyc) - **Spec Exp:** Substance Abuse; **Hospital:** Bridgeport Hosp, St Vincent's Med Ctr - Bridgeport; **Address:** 267 Grant St, Bridgeport, CT 06610; **Phone:** 203-384-3897; **Board Cert:** Psychiatry 2009; **Med School:** Russia 1995; **Resid:** Internal Medicine, Staten Island Univ Hosp 2004; Psychiatry, Maimonides Med Ctr 2007; **Fellow:** Addiction Psychiatry, Yale-New Haven Hosp 2008

Hart, Sidney MD (Psyc) - **Spec Exp:** Anxiety Disorders; Mood Disorders; Psychotherapy; **Hospital:** Greenwich Hosp (page 862); **Address:** 282 Railroad Ave Fl 2, Greenwich, CT 06830; **Phone:** 203-622-1722; **Board Cert:** Psychiatry 1973; **Med School:** Albert Einstein Coll Med 1964; **Resid:** Psychiatry, Bronx Municipal Hosp 1971; **Fellow:** Liaison Psychiatry, Montefiore Hosp Med Ctr 1973

Lorefice, Laurence S MD (Psyc) - **Spec Exp:** Depression; Bipolar/Mood Disorders; Obsessive-Compulsive Disorder; Anxiety Disorders; **Address:** 1037 E Putnam Ave, Riverside, CT 06878; **Phone:** 203-637-4006; **Board Cert:** Psychiatry 1979; **Med School:** Univ Pennsylvania 1975; **Resid:** Psychiatry, Mass General Hosp 1979

Morgan, Charles J MD (Psyc) - **Spec Exp:** Alcohol Abuse; Mood Disorders; Substance Abuse; **Hospital:** Bridgeport Hosp; **Address:** 267 Grant St, Bridgeport, CT 06610; **Phone:** 203-384-3897; **Board Cert:** Psychiatry 1990; **Med School:** Cornell Univ-Weill Med Coll 1983; **Resid:** Psychiatry, Yale-New Haven Hosp 1987

Mueller, F Carl MD (Psyc) - **Spec Exp:** Anxiety & Depression; Obsessive-Compulsive Disorder; Psychopharmacology; **Hospital:** Stamford Hosp (page 863); **Address:** 999 Summer St, Ste 200, Stamford, CT 06905-5513; **Phone:** 203-357-7773; **Board Cert:** Psychiatry 1987; Geriatric Psychiatry 2000; **Med School:** Univ Conn 1982; **Resid:** Psychiatry, Yale-New Haven Hosp 1985; **Fellow:** Psychiatry, Yale-New Haven Hosp 1986; **Fac Appt:** Asst Clin Prof Psyc, Yale Univ

Schechter, Justin MD (Psyc) - **Spec Exp:** Anxiety Disorders; Mood Disorders; Eating Disorders; Forensic Psychiatry; **Hospital:** Stamford Hosp (page 863); **Address:** 22 Fifth St, Stamford, CT 06905-5030; **Phone:** 203-323-7760; **Board Cert:** Psychiatry 1986; Forensic Psychiatry 2008; **Med School:** SUNY Stony Brook 1981; **Resid:** Psychiatry, Yale-New Haven Hosp 1985; **Fac Appt:** Asst Clin Prof Psyc, Yale Univ

Shapiro, Bruce MD (Psyc) - **Spec Exp:** Forensic Psychiatry; Psychopharmacology; Anxiety & Depression; Bipolar/Mood Disorders; **Address:** 666 W Glenbrook Rd, River Suite, Stamford, CT 06906; **Phone:** 203-327-4144; **Board Cert:** Psychiatry 1976; **Med School:** NY Med Coll 1972; **Resid:** Psychiatry, Metropolitan Hosp Ctr 1975; **Fac Appt:** Clin Prof Psyc, Columbia P&S

Sheftell, Fred D MD (Psyc) - **Spec Exp:** Headache; **Hospital:** Greenwich Hosp (page 862), Montefiore Med Ctr - Div. Moses (page 100); **Address:** 30 Buxton Farm Rd, Ste 230, Stamford, CT 06905; **Phone:** 203-968-1799; **Board Cert:** Psychiatry 1973; Headache Medicine 2006; **Med School:** NY Med Coll 1966; **Resid:** Psychiatry, Metropolitan Hosp Ctr 1970; **Fac Appt:** Asst Clin Prof Psyc, Albert Einstein Coll Med

Smith, Jo Ann MD (Psyc) - **Spec Exp:** Mood Disorders; Anxiety Disorders; Women's Health-Mental Health; **Hospital:** St Vincent's Med Ctr - Bridgeport; **Address:** 160 Hawley Ln, Ste 001, Trumbull, CT 06611-5300; **Phone:** 203-377-0111; **Board Cert:** Psychiatry 1980; **Med School:** SUNY Hlth Sci Ctr 1974; **Resid:** Psychiatry, Georgetown Univ Hosp 1979

Tamerin, John MD (Psyc) - **Spec Exp:** Psychotherapy; Bipolar/Mood Disorders; Substance Abuse; Alcohol Abuse; **Hospital:** NY-Presby Hosp/Weill Cornell (page 104), Greenwich Hosp (page 862); **Address:** 27 Stag Ln, Greenwich, CT 06831-3137; **Phone:** 203-661-8282; **Board Cert:** Psychiatry 1970; **Med School:** NYU Sch Med 1963; **Resid:** Psychiatry, Yale-New Haven Hosp 1965; Psychiatry, Mt Sinai Med Ctr 1967; **Fellow:** Child Psychiatry, Mt Sinai Med Ctr 1967; **Fac Appt:** Assoc Clin Prof Psyc, Cornell Univ-Weill Med Coll

Waynik, Mark MD (Psyc) - **Hospital:** St Vincent's Med Ctr - Bridgeport; **Address:** 52 Beach Rd, Ste 104, Fairfield, CT 06824; **Phone:** 203-254-2000; **Board Cert:** Psychiatry 1987; **Med School:** Mexico 1979; **Resid:** Psychiatry, Inst Living 1984

Pulmonary Disease

Brown, Robert B MD (Pul) - **Spec Exp:** Critical Care; **Hospital:** St Vincent's Med Ctr - Bridgeport; **Address:** 2800 Main St, Bridgeport, CT 06606; **Phone:** 203-576-5711; **Board Cert:** Internal Medicine 1981; Pulmonary Disease 1984; Critical Care Medicine 2007; **Med School:** SUNY Downstate 1978; **Resid:** Internal Medicine, Westchester Med Ctr 1981; **Fellow:** Pulmonary Disease, NY Med Coll 1984; **Fac Appt:** Asst Prof Med, NY Med Coll

Krasnogor, Lester J MD (Pul) - **Spec Exp:** Asthma; Emphysema; Cough-Chronic; Sleep Apnea; **Hospital:** Stamford Hosp (page 863); **Address:** 190 W Broad St, Stamford, CT 06902; **Phone:** 203-348-2437; **Board Cert:** Internal Medicine 1970; Pulmonary Disease 1972; **Med School:** NYU Sch Med 1963; **Resid:** Internal Medicine, Duke Univ Med Ctr 1965; Internal Medicine, Univ Pittsburgh Med Ctr 1969; **Fellow:** Pulmonary Disease, Yale-New Haven Hosp 1968; **Fac Appt:** Assoc Clin Prof Med, Columbia P&S

Krinsley, James MD (Pul) - **Spec Exp:** Asthma; Emphysema; Critical Care; **Hospital:** Stamford Hosp (page 863); **Address:** Pulmonary Associates, 190 W Broad St, Stamford, CT 06902; **Phone:** 203-348-2437; **Board Cert:** Internal Medicine 1983; Pulmonary Disease 1986; Critical Care Medicine 2009; **Med School:** Cornell Univ-Weill Med Coll 1980; **Resid:** Internal Medicine, NYU/VA Med Ctr 1983; **Fellow:** Pulmonary Disease, Yale-New Haven Hosp 1986; **Fac Appt:** Assoc Clin Prof Med, Columbia P&S

Kurtz, Caroline MD (Pul) - **Spec Exp:** Asthma; Emphysema; **Hospital:** Norwalk Hosp; **Address:** 30 Stevens St, Ste C, Norwalk, CT 06850; **Phone:** 203-855-3888; **Board Cert:** Internal Medicine 1988; Pulmonary Disease 2000; Critical Care Medicine 2000; **Med School:** NYU Sch Med 1984; **Resid:** Internal Medicine, Mt Sinai Hosp 1987; **Fellow:** Pulmonary Critical Care Medicine, Mt Sinai Hosp 1990

Marino, A Michael MD (Pul) - **Spec Exp:** Asthma; Bronchitis; Emphysema; Lung Cancer; **Hospital:** Greenwich Hosp (page 862); **Address:** 5 Perryridge Rd, Greenwich, CT 06830; **Phone:** 203-661-5379; **Board Cert:** Internal Medicine 1972; Pulmonary Disease 1972; **Med School:** Georgetown Univ 1964; **Resid:** Internal Medicine, VA Med Ctr 1967; **Fellow:** Pulmonary Disease, VA Med Ctr 1969; **Fac Appt:** Assoc Clin Prof Med, Yale Univ

McCalley, Stuart MD (Pul) - Spec Exp: Sleep Disorders; Chronic Obstructive Lung Disease (COPD); Asthma; Pulmonary Fibrosis; **Hospital:** Greenwich Hosp (page 862); **Address:** 75 Holly Hill Ln, Greenwich Medical Group, Greenwich, CT 06830; **Phone:** 203-869-6960; **Board Cert:** Internal Medicine 1972; Pulmonary Disease 1974; Sleep Medicine 2002; **Med School:** Case West Res Univ 1969; **Resid:** Internal Medicine, Univ Conn Hlth Ctr 1971; Internal Medicine, Univ Vermont Med Ctr 1972; **Fellow:** Pulmonary Disease, Bronx Muni Hosps 1974; **Fac Appt:** Asst Clin Prof Med, Yale Univ

Rudolph, Daniel J MD (Pul) - Hospital: Bridgeport Hosp; **Address:** Pulmonary & Internal Medicine, 15 Corporate Drive, Trumball, CT 06611; **Phone:** 203-261-3980; **Board Cert:** Internal Medicine 1985; Pulmonary Disease 1988; Critical Care Medicine 2000; **Med School:** NYU Sch Med 1982; **Resid:** Internal Medicine, SUNY Stony Brook Med Ctr 1985; **Fellow:** Pulmonary Disease, Montefiore Med Ctr 1986

Sachs, Paul MD (Pul) - Spec Exp: Pulmonary Rehabilitation; Asthma; **Hospital:** Stamford Hosp (page 863); **Address:** 190 W Broad St, Stamford, CT 06902-3633; **Phone:** 203-348-2437; **Board Cert:** Internal Medicine 1985; Pulmonary Disease 1988; Critical Care Medicine 2009; **Med School:** NYU Sch Med 1982; **Resid:** Internal Medicine, NY Hosp 1985; **Fellow:** Pulmonary Disease, Montefiore Med Ctr 1987

Winter, Stephen M MD (Pul) - Spec Exp: Respiratory Failure; Sepsis; Critical Care; Ethics; **Hospital:** Norwalk Hosp, VA Conn Hlthcre Sys; **Address:** Norwalk Hosp, Sect Pulm & Crit Care Med, 34 Maple St Fl 3, Norwalk, CT 06856; **Phone:** 203-852-2392; **Board Cert:** Internal Medicine 1984; Pulmonary Disease 1986; Critical Care Medicine 2007; **Med School:** Cornell Univ-Weill Med Coll 1981; **Resid:** Internal Medicine, NY Hosp 1984; **Fellow:** Pulmonary Disease, Yale-New Haven Hosp 1987; **Fac Appt:** Clin Prof Med, Yale Univ

Radiation Oncology

Dowling, Sean MD (RadRO) - Spec Exp: Breast Cancer; Gynecologic Cancer; **Hospital:** Stamford Hosp (page 863); **Address:** Dept Radiation Oncology, 34 Shelburne Rd, Stamford, CT 06902; **Phone:** 203-276-7886; **Board Cert:** Internal Medicine 1986; Radiation Oncology 1990; **Med School:** Yale Univ 1983; **Resid:** Internal Medicine, Yale-New Haven Hosp 1986; Radiation Oncology, Yale-New Haven Hosp 1989

Masino, Frank A MD (RadRO) - Spec Exp: Breast Cancer; Prostate Cancer; Brachytherapy; Stereotactic Radiosurgery; **Hospital:** Stamford Hosp (page 863); **Address:** 34 Shelburne Rd, Stamford, CT 06902-3628; **Phone:** 203-276-7886; **Board Cert:** Therapeutic Radiology 1982; **Med School:** Albert Einstein Coll Med 1978; **Resid:** Therapeutic Radiology, Yale-New Haven Hosp 1982

Pathare, Pradip Madhukar MD (RadRO) - Hospital: Norwalk Hosp; **Address:** Whittingham Cancer Center, 24 Stevans St, Norwalk, CT 06856; **Phone:** 203-852-2719; **Board Cert:** Radiology 1980; Therapeutic Radiology 1981; **Med School:** India 1975; **Resid:** Radiology, Misericordia/Lincoln Hosp 1979; Therapeutic Radiology, Yale-New Haven Hosp 1981; **Fac Appt:** Assoc Prof RadRO, Yale Univ

Spera, John A MD (RadRO) - Spec Exp: Breast Cancer; Prostate Cancer; Intensity Modulated Radiotherapy (IMRT); **Hospital:** Danbury Hosp; **Address:** Dept Rad Onc, 24 Hospital Ave, Danbury, CT 06810-6099; **Phone:** 203-739-7190; **Board Cert:** Radiation Oncology 1987; **Med School:** Georgetown Univ 1979; **Resid:** Surgery, Hosp Univ Penn 1981; Urology, Hosp Univ Penn 1983; **Fellow:** Radiation Oncology, Hosp Univ Penn 1987

Reproductive Endocrinology

Doyle, Michael B MD (RE) - **Spec Exp:** Infertility-IVF; Endometriosis; **Hospital:** Norwalk Hosp, St Vincent's Med Ctr - Bridgeport; **Address:** 4920 Main St, Ste 301, Bridgeport, CT 06606-1300; **Phone:** 203-373-1200; **Board Cert:** Obstetrics & Gynecology 2009; **Med School:** Georgetown Univ 1990; **Resid:** Obstetrics & Gynecology, Hosp Univ Penn 1993; **Fellow:** Reproductive Endocrinology, Yale New Haven Hosp 1995

Ginsburg, Frances W MD (RE) - **Spec Exp:** Infertility; Menopause Problems; Endometriosis; Menstrual Disorders; **Hospital:** Stamford Hosp (page 863); **Address:** Stamford Hosp, 30 Shelburne Ave, Box 9317, Stamford, CT 06904-9317; **Phone:** 203-276-7853; **Board Cert:** Obstetrics & Gynecology 2009; Reproductive Endocrinology 2009; **Med School:** NYU Sch Med 1980; **Resid:** Obstetrics & Gynecology, Bellevue Hosp Ctr-NYU 1984; **Fellow:** Reproductive Endocrinology, Bellevue Hosp Ctr-NYU 1986; **Fac Appt:** Asst Clin Prof ObG, Columbia P&S

Richlin, Spencer S MD (RE) - **Spec Exp:** Infertility-IVF; Reproductive Surgery; **Hospital:** Norwalk Hosp, Stamford Hosp (page 863); **Address:** Rma-Ct/Reproductive Med Assocs Of Ctr, 10 Glover Ave, Norwalk, CT 06850-1202; **Phone:** 203-750-7400; **Board Cert:** Obstetrics & Gynecology 2006; Reproductive Endocrinology/Infertility 2006; **Med School:** USC-Keck School of Medicine 1994; **Resid:** Obstetrics & Gynecology, Stamford Hosp 1999; **Fellow:** Reproductive Endocrinology, Emory Univ Hosp 2002

Witt, Barry R MD (RE) - **Spec Exp:** Infertility-IVF; **Hospital:** Greenwich Hosp (page 862), NYU Langone Med Ctr (page 106); **Address:** 55 Holly Hill Ln, Ste 270, Greenwich, CT 06830; **Phone:** 203-863-2990; **Board Cert:** Obstetrics & Gynecology 2009; Reproductive Endocrinology 2009; **Med School:** NY Med Coll 1984; **Resid:** Obstetrics & Gynecology, Montefiore-Weiler Einstein Med Ctr 1988; **Fellow:** Reproductive Endocrinology, Tulane Univ Med Ctr 1990; **Fac Appt:** Assoc Prof ObG, NYU Sch Med

Rheumatology

Danehower, Richard L MD (Rhu) - **Spec Exp:** Rheumatoid Arthritis; Temporal Arteritis; Psoriatic Arthritis; Osteoarthritis; **Hospital:** Greenwich Hosp (page 862); **Address:** 49 Lake Ave, Greenwich, CT 06830-4501; **Phone:** 203-869-5715; **Board Cert:** Internal Medicine 1971; Rheumatology 1974; **Med School:** Univ Pennsylvania 1965; **Resid:** Internal Medicine, Univ Michigan Med Ctr 1969; **Fellow:** Rheumatology, Univ Michigan Med Ctr 1970; **Fac Appt:** Asst Clin Prof Med, Yale Univ

Gladstein, Geoffrey S MD (Rhu) - **Hospital:** Bridgeport Hosp; **Address:** 5520 Park Ave, Ste 101, Trumbull, CT 06611; **Phone:** 203-371-5873; **Board Cert:** Internal Medicine 1976; Rheumatology 1978; **Med School:** Geo Wash Univ 1973; **Resid:** Internal Medicine, Albany Med Ctr 1976; **Fellow:** Rheumatology, Albany Med Ctr 1978

Miller, Kenneth A MD (Rhu) - **Spec Exp:** Rheumatoid Arthritis; Osteoporosis; Lyme Disease; Lupus/SLE; **Hospital:** Danbury Hosp, New Milford Hosp; **Address:** 27 Hospital Ave, Ste 205, Danbury, CT 06810-5954; **Phone:** 203-794-0599; **Board Cert:** Internal Medicine 1978; Rheumatology 1980; **Med School:** Rush Med Coll 1975; **Resid:** Internal Medicine, GW Univ Hosp 1978; **Fellow:** Rheumatology, Worcester City Hosp 1980

Nascimento, Joao M A MD (Rhu) - **Spec Exp:** Rheumatoid Arthritis; Lupus/SLE; Psoriatic Arthritis; **Hospital:** St Vincent's Med Ctr - Bridgeport, Bridgeport Hosp; **Address:** 3203 Main St, Bridgeport, CT 06606-4225; **Phone:** 203-371-0009; **Board Cert:** Internal Medicine 1989; Rheumatology 2002; **Med School:** Portugal 1984; **Resid:** Internal Medicine, Bridgeport Hosp 1989; **Fellow:** Rheumatology, Brown Univ Med Ctr 1991; **Fac Appt:** Asst Clin Prof Med, Columbia P&S

Novack, Stuart N MD (Rhu) - **Spec Exp:** Lupus/SLE; Osteoporosis; Rheumatoid Arthritis; **Hospital:** Norwalk Hosp; **Address:** Norwalk Medical Group, 40 Cross St Fl 4, Norwalk, CT 06851; **Phone:** 203-845-4830; **Board Cert:** Internal Medicine 1971; Rheumatology 1972; **Med School:** SUNY Hlth Sci Ctr 1966; **Resid:** Internal Medicine, Maimonides Med Ctr 1968; Internal Medicine, UCLA Med Ctr 1969; **Fellow:** Rheumatology, UCLA Med Ctr 1970; **Fac Appt:** Assoc Clin Prof Med, Yale Univ

Surgery

Bull, Sherman M MD (S) - **Spec Exp:** Breast Surgery; Cancer Surgery; Laparoscopic Cholecystectomy; Hernia; **Hospital:** Stamford Hosp (page 863); **Address:** 1351 Washington Blvd Fl 6, Stamford, CT 06902; **Phone:** 203-276-5959; **Board Cert:** Surgery 1969; **Med School:** Columbia P&S 1962; **Resid:** Surgery, Columbia-Presby Med Ctr 1967; **Fellow:** Pediatric Surgery, Children's Hosp 1969; **Fac Appt:** Asst Clin Prof S, Columbia P&S

Duerr, L Sean MD (S) - **Spec Exp:** Laparoscopic Abdominal Surgery; Hernia; **Hospital:** Bridgeport Hosp; **Address:** 2900 Main St, Ste 1F, Stratford, CT 06614; **Phone:** 203-378-4500; **Board Cert:** Surgery 2008; **Med School:** Univ VT Coll Med 1973; **Resid:** Surgery, Bridgeport Hosp 1977

Garvey, Richard J MD (S) - **Spec Exp:** Colon & Rectal Surgery; **Hospital:** Bridgeport Hosp; **Address:** 310 Mill Hill Ave, General Surgeons Of Bridgeport, Bridgeport, CT 06610-2863; **Phone:** 203-366-3211; **Board Cert:** Surgery 2009; **Med School:** Georgetown Univ 1974; **Resid:** Surgery, Boston Univ Med Ctr 1979

Kenler, Andrew S MD (S) - **Hospital:** Bridgeport Hosp; **Address:** Park Avenue Surgical Assocs, 5520 Park Ave, Ste 207, Trumbull, CT 06611; **Phone:** 203-373-9015; **Board Cert:** Surgery 2006; **Med School:** Cornell Univ-Weill Med Coll 1988; **Resid:** Orthopaedic Surgery, NE Deaconess Hosp 1991; Surgery, NE Deaconess Hosp 1995

Manasseh, Donna-Marie MD (S) - **Spec Exp:** Breast Surgery; **Hospital:** Stamford Hosp (page 863); **Address:** Tully Health Center, 32 Strawberry Hill Ct, Stamford, CT 06902; **Phone:** 203-276-4255; **Board Cert:** Surgery 2005; **Med School:** Harvard Med Sch 1996; **Resid:** Surgery, NY Presby Hosp 2002; **Fellow:** Surgical Breast Oncology, Meml Sloan Kettering Cancer Ctr 2005; **Fac Appt:** Asst Clin Prof S, Columbia P&S

Marcus, Stuart G MD (S) - **Spec Exp:** Gastrointestinal Cancer; Gastrointestinal Surgery; Hepatobiliary Surgery; Pancreatic Surgery; **Hospital:** St Vincent's Med Ctr - Bridgeport; **Address:** St Vincents Oncology Dept, 2800 Main St, Bridgeport, CT 06606; **Phone:** 203-576-6235; **Board Cert:** Surgery 2005; **Med School:** Duke Univ 1987; **Resid:** Surgery, NYU Med Ctr 1995; **Fellow:** Surgical Oncology, NCI-NIH 1992; **Fac Appt:** Assoc Clin Prof S, NYU Sch Med

McWhorter, Philip MD (S) - **Spec Exp:** Cancer Surgery; **Hospital:** Greenwich Hosp (page 862); **Address:** 77 Lafayette Pl, Ste 301, Greenwich, CT 06830; **Phone:** 203-863-4300; **Board Cert:** Surgery 1997; **Med School:** Cornell Univ-Weill Med Coll 1973; **Resid:** Surgery, NY Hosp 1977

Molinelli, Bruce M MD (S) - **Spec Exp:** Minimally Invasive Surgery; Laparoscopic Surgery; Hernia; Obesity/Bariatric Surgery; **Hospital:** Greenwich Hosp (page 862); **Address:** 77 Lafayette Pl, Ste 301, Greenwich, CT 06831; **Phone:** 203-863-4300; **Board Cert:** Surgery 2004; **Med School:** NYU Sch Med 1988; **Resid:** Surgery, St Lukes-Roosevelt Hosp 1993

Passeri, Daniel J MD (S) - **Spec Exp:** Cancer Surgery; Laparoscopic Surgery; **Hospital:** St Vincent's Med Ctr - Bridgeport, Bridgeport Hosp; **Address:** 888 White Plains Rd Fl 2 - Ste 206, Trumbull, CT 06611-4552; **Phone:** 203-459-2666; **Board Cert:** Surgery 2000; **Med School:** Yale Univ 1975; **Resid:** Surgery, Yale-New Haven Hosp 1980; **Fac Appt:** Assoc Clin Prof S, NY Med Coll

Ward, Barbara MD (S) - **Spec Exp:** Breast Cancer; Breast Surgery; Breast Disease; **Hospital:** Greenwich Hosp (page 862); **Address:** 77 Lafayette Pl, Ste 302, Greenwich, CT 06830-5426; **Phone:** 203-863-4250; **Board Cert:** Surgery 2002; **Med School:** Temple Univ 1983; **Resid:** Surgery, Yale-New Haven Hosp 1990; **Fellow:** Surgical Oncology, Natl Cancer Inst 1987; **Fac Appt:** Assoc Clin Prof S, Yale Univ

Thoracic Surgery

Ciaburri, Daniel G MD (TS) - **Spec Exp:** Coronary Artery Surgery; Heart Valve Surgery; **Hospital:** New York Methodist Hosp (page 404); **Address:** NY Methodist Hosp, Dept Cardiothoracic Surgery, 506 6th St, Brooklyn, NY 11215; **Phone:** 718-780-7700; **Board Cert:** Thoracic Surgery 2009; Surgery 2009; **Med School:** Univ Conn 1983; **Resid:** Surgery, NY Presby-Cornell Med Ctr 1988; **Fellow:** Cardiothoracic Surgery, NY Presby-Cornell Med Ctr 1990; **Fac Appt:** Asst Prof TS, Cornell Univ-Weill Med Coll

Hall, Timothy S MD (TS) - **Spec Exp:** Cardiothoracic Surgery; **Hospital:** Stamford Hosp (page 863); **Address:** Stamford Hosp, Dept Surgery, 30 Shelburn Rd, Stamford, CT 06902-3696; **Phone:** 203-276-7470; **Board Cert:** Surgery 2009; Thoracic Surgery 2001; Surgical Critical Care 2003; **Med School:** Temple Univ 1982; **Resid:** Surgery, Johns Hopkins Hosp 1988; Cardiothoracic Surgery, Johns Hopkins Hosp 1990; **Fellow:** Thoracic Surgery, Meml Sloan Kettering Cancer Ctr 1991

Lettera, James V MD (TS) - **Spec Exp:** Lung Cancer; Minimally Invasive Thoracic Surgery; Aneurysm-Aortic; Vascular Surgery; **Hospital:** Bridgeport Hosp, Norwalk Hosp; **Address:** 501 Kings Hwy E, Ste 112, Fairfield, CT 06825; **Phone:** 203-382-1900; **Board Cert:** Thoracic Surgery 2003; **Med School:** Georgetown Univ 1977; **Resid:** Surgery, St Vincent's Hosp Med Ctr 1982; Thoracic Surgery, Jackson Meml Hosp 1984; **Fac Appt:** Asst Clin Prof S, NY Med Coll

Rose, Daniel M MD (TS) - **Spec Exp:** Minimally Invasive Surgery; Cardiothoracic Surgery; **Hospital:** St Vincent's Med Ctr - Bridgeport, Bridgeport Hosp; **Address:** St Vincent's Med Ctr, 2800 Main St, Bridgeport, CT 06606; **Phone:** 203-576-5708; **Board Cert:** Thoracic Surgery 2001; **Med School:** Univ Colorado 1974; **Resid:** Surgery, Bellevue Hosp-NYU 1979; Cardiovascular Surgery, Natl Heart & Lung Inst 1980; **Fellow:** Cardiothoracic Surgery, Bellevue Hosp-NYU 1982; **Fac Appt:** Asst Prof S, SUNY Downstate

Squitieri, Rafael P MD (TS) - **Spec Exp:** Cardiothoracic Surgery; Aneurysm-Aortic; Maze Procedure for Atrial Fibrillation; Lung Cancer; **Hospital:** St Vincent's Med Ctr - Bridgeport; **Address:** St Vincent's Med Ctr, Dept Cardiology, 2800 Main St, Bridgeport, CT 06606; **Phone:** 203-576-5708; **Board Cert:** Surgery 1999; Thoracic Surgery 2002; **Med School:** Mount Sinai Sch Med 1993; **Resid:** Surgery, Morristown Meml Hosp 1998; **Fellow:** Thoracic Surgery, Mount Sinai Med Ctr 2001

Tittle, Shawn L MD (TS) - **Spec Exp:** Thoracic Cancers; Lung Cancer; Minimally Invasive Thoracic Surgery; **Hospital:** Danbury Hosp; **Address:** 111 Osbourne St, Ste 123, Danbury, CT 06810; **Phone:** 203-739-7131; **Board Cert:** Thoracic Surgery 2006; **Med School:** Wayne State Univ 1997; **Resid:** Surgery, St Mary's Hosp 2003; **Fellow:** Cardiothoracic Surgery, Yale/New Haven Hosp 2005; **Fac Appt:** Asst Prof S, NY Med Coll

Waters, Paul F MD (TS) - **Spec Exp:** Lung Cancer; Esophageal Surgery; Thoracic Cancers; Transplant-Lung; **Hospital:** Greenwich Hosp (page 862); **Address:** 77 Lafayette Pl, Ste 302, Greenwich, CT 06830; **Phone:** 203-863-4341; **Board Cert:** Surgery 2004; **Med School:** Univ Toronto 1974; **Resid:** Surgery, Univ Toronto Med Ctr 1979; Thoracic Surgery, Univ Toronto Med Ctr 1980; **Fellow:** Esophageal Surgery, Univ Chicago Hosps 1981

Urology

Andriani, Rudy MD (U) - **Spec Exp:** Urologic Cancer; Kidney Stones; Incontinence; **Hospital:** Stamford Hosp (page 863), Greenwich Hosp (page 862); **Address:** 166 W Broad St, Ste 404, Stamford, CT 06902-3661; **Phone:** 203-356-9692; **Board Cert:** Urology 2008; **Med School:** NY Med Coll 1981; **Resid:** Surgery, St Vincent's Hosp & Med Ctr 1983; Urology, Duke Univ Med Ctr 1987; **Fac Appt:** Asst Clin Prof U, Columbia P&S

Dodds, Peter MD (U) - **Hospital:** Norwalk Hosp; **Address:** 12 Elmcrest Ter, Urology Associates Of Norwalk, Norwalk, CT 06850-3964; **Phone:** 203-853-4200; **Board Cert:** Urology 2004; **Med School:** Columbia P&S 1977; **Resid:** Surgery, Yale-New Haven Hosp 1980; Urology, Yale-New Haven Hosp 1983

Muldoon, Lawrence D MD (U) - **Hospital:** St Vincent's Med Ctr - Bridgeport; **Address:** 425 Post Rd, Fairfield, CT 06824; **Phone:** 203-254-1576; **Board Cert:** Urology 2001; **Med School:** Northwestern Univ 1984; **Resid:** Surgery, Univ Hosps 1987; Urology, Univ Hosps 1990

Ranta, Jeffrey A MD (U) - **Spec Exp:** Prostate Cancer; Bladder Cancer; Kidney Stones; **Hospital:** Greenwich Hosp (page 862), Stamford Hosp (page 863); **Address:** 49 Lake Ave, Greenwich, CT 06830-4520; **Phone:** 203-869-1285; **Board Cert:** Urology 2004; **Med School:** Georgetown Univ 1979; **Resid:** Surgery, Georgetown Univ Hosp 1981; Urology, Lahey Clin 1984

Viner, Nicholas MD (U) - **Spec Exp:** Prostate Cancer; Kidney Stones; Bladder Cancer; **Hospital:** Bridgeport Hosp, St Vincent's Med Ctr - Bridgeport; **Address:** 160 Hawley Ln, Trumbull, CT 06611-6058; **Phone:** 203-375-3456; **Board Cert:** Urology 1977; **Med School:** Vanderbilt Univ 1968; **Resid:** Surgery, Greenwich Hosp 1970; Urology, Vanderbilt Univ Hosp 1974

Waxberg, Jonathan MD (U) - **Spec Exp:** Prostate Cancer; Minimally Invasive Surgery; Erectile Dysfunction; **Hospital:** Stamford Hosp (page 863); **Address:** 35 Hoyt St, Stamford, CT 06905-5602; **Phone:** 203-324-2268; **Board Cert:** Urology 2008; **Med School:** Univ Cincinnati 1980; **Resid:** Urology, Maimonides Med Ctr 1986; **Fac Appt:** Assoc Prof U, Yale Univ

Zuckerman, Howard L MD (U) - **Spec Exp:** Incontinence; Prostate Cancer; Pediatric Urology; **Hospital:** Bridgeport Hosp, St Vincent's Med Ctr - Bridgeport; **Address:** 160 Hawley Ln Ste 002 Bldg, Trumbull, CT 06611-5300; **Phone:** 203-375-3456; **Board Cert:** Urology 1977; **Med School:** St Louis Univ 1967; **Resid:** Surgery, Med Coll Virginia Hosp 1969; Urology, Albert Einstein Coll Med 1975

Vascular & Interventional Radiology

Hamet, Marc R MD (VIR) - **Spec Exp:** Osteoporosis Spine-Vertebroplasty; Uterine Fibroid Embolization; Endovascular Surgery; Carotid Artery Stent Placement; **Hospital:** Stamford Hosp (page 863); **Address:** Stamford Radiological Associates, PO Box 1092, Stamford, CT 06904-1092; **Phone:** 203-276-7860; **Board Cert:** Diagnostic Radiology 1995; Vascular & Interventional Radiology 2009; Neuroradiology 1999; **Med School:** Univ MD Sch Med 1991; **Resid:** Diagnostic Radiology, Univ Maryland Med Sys 1995; **Fellow:** Neuroradiology, Univ Maryland Med Sys 1996; Interventional Radiology, Johns Hopkins Hosp 1998

Hodges, Laura J MD (VIR) - **Spec Exp:** Uterine Fibroid Embolization; **Hospital:** Greenwich Hosp (page 862); **Address:** Greenwich Hospital, Dept Radiology, 5 Perryridge Rd, Greenwich, CT 06830; **Phone:** 203-863-3042; **Board Cert:** Diagnostic Radiology 1999; Vascular & Interventional Radiology 2002; **Med School:** Albert Einstein Coll Med 1994; **Resid:** Diagnostic Radiology, Yale-New Haven Hosp 1999; **Fellow:** Vascular & Interventional Radiology, NY Presby-Cornell Med Ctr 2000

Vascular Surgery

Dietzek, Alan M MD (VascS) - **Spec Exp:** Aneurysm-Aortic; Minimally Invasive Vascular Surgery; Arterial Bypass Surgery-Leg; Carotid Artery Surgery; **Hospital:** Danbury Hosp; **Address:** 111 Osborne St, Danbury, CT 06810; **Phone:** 203-739-7320; **Board Cert:** Surgery 1999; Vascular Surgery 2001; **Med School:** Loyola Univ-Stritch Sch Med 1983; **Resid:** Surgery, LI Jewish Med Ctr 1988; **Fellow:** Vascular Surgery, Montefiore Med Ctr 1990; **Fac Appt:** Asst Clin Prof S, NY Med Coll

Gagne, Paul J MD (VascS) - **Spec Exp:** Endovascular Surgery; Aneurysm-Abdominal Aortic; Carotid Artery Surgery; Vein Disorders; **Hospital:** Norwalk Hosp, Bridgeport Hosp; **Address:** Southern Connecticut Vascular Ctr, 999 Silver Lane, Ste 2B, Trumbull, CT 06611; **Phone:** 203-375-2861; **Board Cert:** Surgery 2001; Vascular Surgery 2005; **Med School:** NYU Sch Med 1986; **Resid:** Surgery, NYU Medical Center 1991; **Fellow:** Vascular Surgery, Univ Arkansas 1995

Huribal, Marsel MD (VascS) - **Hospital:** Bridgeport Hosp, St Vincent's Med Ctr - Bridgeport; **Address:** Southern CT Vascular Ctr, 999 Silver Ln, Ste 2B, Trumbull, CT 06611; **Phone:** 203-375-2861; **Board Cert:** Vascular Surgery 2008; **Med School:** Amer Univ Caribbean 1987; **Resid:** Surgery, Bridgeport Hosp 1994; **Fellow:** Vascular Surgery, SUNY Buffalo 1996; **Fac Appt:** Asst Clin Prof VascS, Yale Univ

Marsan, Ben U MD (VascS) - **Spec Exp:** Peripheral Vascular Disease; Vein Disorders; Aneurysm-Aortic; Endovascular Surgery; **Hospital:** Norwalk Hosp, Bridgeport Hosp; **Address:** Southern Connecticut Vascular Ctr, 999 Silver Lane, Ste 2B, Trumbull, CT 06611; **Phone:** 203-375-2861; **Board Cert:** Vascular Surgery 2009; **Med School:** Oregon Hlth & Sci Univ 1989; **Resid:** Surgery, Flushing Hosp Med Ctr 1995; **Fellow:** Vascular Surgery, SUNY Buffalo 1997

New Haven

New Haven

Addiction Psychiatry

Schottenfeld, Richard MD (AdP) - **Spec Exp:** Drug Abuse-Consultation; Alcohol Abuse-Consultation; **Hospital:** Yale-New Haven Hosp, Connecticut Mental Hlth Ctr; **Address:** Connecticut Mental Health Ctr, 34 Park St, rm S-204, New Haven, CT 06519; **Phone:** 203-974-7349; **Board Cert:** Psychiatry 1984; **Med School:** Yale Univ 1976; **Resid:** Psychiatry, Yale Psych Inst 1982; **Fellow:** Epidemiology, Yale Univ 1984; **Fac Appt:** Prof Psyc, Yale Univ

Allergy & Immunology

Adelsberg, Bernard Roy MD (A&I) - **Spec Exp:** Asthma & Allergy; Allergic Rhinitis; Food Allergy; **Hospital:** Hosp of St Raphael, Yale-New Haven Hosp; **Address:** CT Med Grp, 2416 Whitney Ave, Hamden, CT 06518-3248; **Phone:** 203-248-4331; **Board Cert:** Internal Medicine 1975; Allergy & Immunology 1979; Diagnostic Lab Immunology 1986; **Med School:** SUNY Downstate 1972; **Resid:** Internal Medicine, Mt Sinai Hosp 1975; **Fellow:** Immunology, Scripps Clinic And Research 1977

Askenase, Philip MD (A&I) - **Spec Exp:** Asthma; Urticaria; Sinusitis; **Hospital:** Yale-New Haven Hosp, Yale Med Group; **Address:** 40 Temple St, Ste 1A, New Haven, CT 06520-8013; **Phone:** 203-785-4143; **Board Cert:** Internal Medicine 1973; Allergy & Immunology 1974; **Med School:** Yale Univ 1965; **Resid:** Internal Medicine, Boston City Hosp 1967; **Fellow:** Allergy & Immunology, Yale/ New Haven Hosp 1971; **Fac Appt:** Prof Med, Yale Univ

Kaufman, Richard E MD (A&I) - **Spec Exp:** Asthma; Urticaria; Allergy; **Hospital:** Yale-New Haven Hosp, Hosp of St Raphael; **Address:** 960 Main St, Branford, CT 06405; **Phone:** 203-488-6358; **Board Cert:** Internal Medicine 1976; Allergy & Immunology 1979; **Med School:** Yale Univ 1971; **Resid:** Internal Medicine, Yale-New Haven Hosp 1976; **Fellow:** Immunology, Yale-New Haven Hosp 1978; **Fac Appt:** Assoc Clin Prof Med, Yale Univ

Cardiac Electrophysiology

Batsford, William P MD (CE) - **Spec Exp:** Arrhythmias; **Hospital:** Yale-New Haven Hosp, Yale Med Group; **Address:** Yale Univ School Medicine, Section Cardiovascular Medicine, 333 Cedar St, 3 FMP, Box 208017, New Haven, CT 06520-8017; **Phone:** 203-785-4126; **Board Cert:** Internal Medicine 1972; Cardiovascular Disease 1977; **Med School:** Albany Med Coll 1969; **Resid:** Internal Medicine, Hosp Univ Penn 1972; **Fac Appt:** Prof Med, Yale Univ

Schoenfeld, Mark MD (CE) - **Spec Exp:** Arrhythmias; **Hospital:** Hosp of St Raphael, Yale-New Haven Hosp; **Address:** 330 Orchard St, Ste 210, New Haven, CT 06511; **Phone:** 203-867-5400; **Board Cert:** Internal Medicine 1982; Cardiovascular Disease 1985; Cardiac Electrophysiology 2002; **Med School:** Harvard Med Sch 1979; **Resid:** Internal Medicine, Mass Genl Hosp 1982; **Fellow:** Cardiovascular Disease, Mass Genl Hosp 1985; Cardiac Electrophysiology, Mass Genl Hosp 1986; **Fac Appt:** Clin Prof Med, Yale Univ

Cardiovascular Disease

Cabin, Henry S MD (Cv) - **Spec Exp:** Interventional Cardiology; Cardiac Catheterization; **Hospital:** Yale-New Haven Hosp, Yale Med Group; **Address:** 333 Cedar St, PO Box 208017, New Haven, CT 06520-8017; **Phone:** 203-785-4129; **Board Cert:** Internal Medicine 1978; Cardiovascular Disease 1983; Interventional Cardiology 2000; **Med School:** Yale Univ 1975; **Resid:** Internal Medicine, Yale-New Haven Hosp 1978; **Fellow:** Internal Medicine, Natl Heart Lung and Blood Inst 1981; Cardiovascular Disease, Yale-New Haven Hosp 1982; **Fac Appt:** Prof Med, Yale Univ

Cleman, Michael W MD (Cv) - **Spec Exp:** Interventional Cardiology; Angioplasty; Cardiac Catheterization; **Hospital:** Yale-New Haven Hosp, Yale Med Group; **Address:** 333 Cedar St, Box 208017, New Haven, CT 06520-8017; **Phone:** 203-785-4129; **Board Cert:** Internal Medicine 1980; Cardiovascular Disease 1985; Interventional Cardiology 2000; **Med School:** Johns Hopkins Univ 1977; **Resid:** Internal Medicine, Univ Fla-Shands Hosp 1980; **Fellow:** Cardiovascular Disease, Yale-New Haven Hosp 1981; **Fac Appt:** Prof Med, Yale Univ

Freed, Lisa A MD (Cv) - **Spec Exp:** Heart Disease in Women; Mitral Valve Prolapse; **Hospital:** Yale-New Haven Hosp, Hosp of St Raphael; **Address:** Cardiology Assocs of New Haven, 40 Temple St, Ste 6A, New Haven, CT 06510; **Phone:** 203-789-2272; **Board Cert:** Cardiovascular Disease 2009; **Med School:** Johns Hopkins Univ 1992; **Resid:** Internal Medicine, NY Hosp-Cornell Med Ctr 1995; **Fellow:** Cardiovascular Disease, Mass Genl Hosp 1998; Cardiovascular Disease, Framingham Heart Study 1999

Child & Adolescent Psychiatry

Gammon, G Davis MD (ChAP) - **Hospital:** Yale-New Haven Hosp; **Address:** 67 Trumbull St, New Haven, CT 06510; **Phone:** 203-865-6540; **Board Cert:** Psychiatry 1981; Child & Adolescent Psychiatry 1992; **Med School:** Temple Univ 1976; **Resid:** Psychiatry, Yale-New Haven Hosp 1980; Child Psychiatry, Yale-New Haven Hosp 1984; **Fellow:** Epidemiology, Yale-New Haven Hosp 1983

King, Robert A MD (ChAP) - **Spec Exp:** Tourette's Syndrome; Obsessive-Compulsive Disorder; Psychoanalysis; **Hospital:** Yale-New Haven Hosp, Yale Med Group; **Address:** Yale Child Study Ctr, 230 S Frontage Rd, Box 207900, New Haven, CT 06510; **Phone:** 203-785-5880; **Board Cert:** Psychiatry 1974; Child & Adolescent Psychiatry 1981; **Med School:** Harvard Med Sch 1968; **Resid:** Pediatrics, Chldns Hosp 1969; Psychiatry, Mass Mental Hlth Ctr 1971; **Fellow:** Child Psychiatry, Chldns Hosp 1972; Child Psychiatry, Chldns Hosp Natl Med Ctr 1974; **Fac Appt:** Prof ChAP, Yale Univ

Leckman, James F MD (ChAP) - **Spec Exp:** Tourette's Syndrome; Obsessive-Compulsive Disorder; Autism; **Hospital:** Yale-New Haven Hosp, Yale Med Group; **Address:** Yale Child Study Ctr, 230 S Frontage Rd, Box 207900, New Haven, CT 06520-7900; **Phone:** 203-785-7971; **Board Cert:** Psychiatry 1980; Child & Adolescent Psychiatry 1982; **Med School:** Univ New Mexico 1973; **Resid:** Psychiatry, Yale Univ 1979; Child Psychiatry, Yale Chld Stdy Ctr 1980; **Fellow:** Psychiatry, Natl Inst Mental Hlth 1976; **Fac Appt:** Prof Psyc, Yale Univ

Madigan, Janet A MD (ChAP) - **Spec Exp:** Developmental Disorders; Psychotherapy; Psychoanalysis; Attachment Disorders; **Hospital:** Yale-New Haven Hosp; **Address:** 291 Whitney Ave, Ste 203, New Haven, CT 06511; **Phone:** 203-787-5420; **Board Cert:** Psychiatry 1982; Child & Adolescent Psychiatry 1986; **Med School:** NY Med Coll 1977; **Resid:** Psychiatry, Yale-New Haven Hosp 1981; **Fellow:** Child & Adolescent Psychiatry, Yale-New Haven Hosp 1983; **Fac Appt:** Asst Clin Prof Psyc, Yale Univ

Volkmar, Fred R MD (ChAP) - **Spec Exp:** Autism; Asperger's Syndrome; Developmental Disorders; Childhood Disintegrative Disorder; **Hospital:** Yale-New Haven Hosp, Greenwich Hosp (page 656); **Address:** Yale Child Study Ctr, 230 S Frontage Rd, Box 207900, Rm NIHB 200, New Haven, CT 06520-7900; **Phone:** 203-785-5759; **Board Cert:** Psychiatry 1981; Child & Adolescent Psychiatry 1988; **Med School:** Stanford Univ 1976; **Resid:** Psychiatry, Stanford Univ 1980; Child Psychiatry, Yale Child Study Ctr 1982; **Fac Appt:** Prof Psyc, Yale Univ

Child Neurology

Levy, Susan Ruth MD (ChiN) - **Spec Exp:** Epilepsy; Neurophysiology; Pediatric Neurology; Headache; **Hospital:** Yale-New Haven Hosp; **Address:** Child Neurology Assoc, 5 Durham Rd, Ste 1-7, Guilford, CT 06437-2076; **Phone:** 203-453-2181; **Board Cert:** Pediatrics 1984; Child Neurology 1986; **Med School:** Wake Forest Univ 1978; **Resid:** Pediatrics, N Carolina Baptist Hosp 1981; Pediatric Neurology, Univ Mass Med Ctr 1984; **Fellow:** Neurological Physiology, Mass Genl Hosp 1985; **Fac Appt:** Clin Prof N, Yale Univ

Ment, Laura R MD (ChiN) - **Spec Exp:** Developmental Disorders; Stroke; **Hospital:** Yale-New Haven Hosp, Yale Med Group; **Address:** Chldns Hosp Yale New Haven, Dept Pediatrics, Sch Med, 333 Cedar St, PO Box 208064, New Haven, CT 06520; **Phone:** 203-785-5708; **Board Cert:** Pediatrics 1979; Child Neurology 1980; **Med School:** Tufts Univ 1973; **Resid:** Pediatrics, Massachusetts Genl Hosp 1976; Pediatrics, Massachusetts Genl Hosp 1979; **Fellow:** Pediatrics, Hammersmith Hosp 1979

Shaywitz, Bennett A MD (ChiN) - **Spec Exp:** Learning Disorders; Dyslexia; Headache; **Hospital:** Yale-New Haven Hosp, Yale Med Group; **Address:** Yale Univ Sch Med, Dept Peds, 333 Cedar St, Box 208064, New Haven, CT 06520-8064; **Phone:** 203-785-4641; **Board Cert:** Pediatrics 1968; Child Neurology 1973; **Med School:** Washington Univ, St Louis 1963; **Resid:** Pediatrics, Bronx Muni Hosp Ctr 1967; **Fellow:** Child Neurology, Albert Einstein Coll Med 1970; **Fac Appt:** Prof Ped, Yale Univ

Testa, Francine M MD (ChiN) - **Spec Exp:** Epilepsy; **Hospital:** Yale-New Haven Hosp, Yale Med Group; **Address:** 5 Durham Rd, Ste 1-7, Guilford, CT 06437; **Phone:** 203-453-2181; **Board Cert:** Child Neurology 1994; **Med School:** SUNY Downstate 1986; **Resid:** Pediatrics, Yale-New Haven Hosp 1988; Child Neurology, NY Presby Hosp/Columbia 1991; **Fellow:** Neurological Physiology, Ny Presby Hosp/Columbia 1992; **Fac Appt:** Clin Prof N, Yale Univ

Clinical Genetics

Bale, Allen E MD (CG) - **Spec Exp:** Cancer Genetics; **Hospital:** Yale-New Haven Hosp, Yale Med Group; **Address:** 333 Cedar St, SHM Bldg - rm 1321, New Haven, CT 06519; **Phone:** 203-785-5745; **Board Cert:** Internal Medicine 1983; Clinical Genetics 1987; Clinical Molecular Genetics 2006; **Med School:** Univ Mass Sch Med 1979; **Resid:** Internal Medicine, Western Penn Hosp 1983; **Fellow:** Medical Genetics, Natl Inst of Health 1987; **Fac Appt:** Assoc Prof CG, Yale Univ

Mahoney, Maurice J MD (CG) - **Spec Exp:** Fetal Therapy; Prenatal Diagnosis; **Hospital:** Yale-New Haven Hosp, Yale Med Group; **Address:** Yale Genetics Consultation Serv, 333 Cedar St, rm WWW330, New Haven, CT 06520-8005; **Phone:** 203-785-2661; **Board Cert:** Pediatrics 1967; Clinical Genetics 1982; Clinical Biochemical Genetics 1982; **Med School:** Univ Pittsburgh 1962; **Resid:** Pediatrics, Johns Hopkins Hosp 1965; Pediatrics, Childrens Hosp 1966; **Fellow:** Clinical Genetics, Yale Univ Sch Med 1970; **Fac Appt:** Prof CG, Yale Univ

Seashore, Margretta MD (CG) - **Spec Exp:** Inherited Metabolic Disorders; **Hospital:** Yale-New Haven Hosp, Yale Med Group; **Address:** Yale Univ Sch Med, Dept Genetics, 333 Cedar St, rm 305, Box 208005, New Haven, CT 06520-8005; **Phone:** 203-785-2660; **Board Cert:** Pediatrics 1970; Clinical Biochemical Genetics 1982; Clinical Genetics 1982; **Med School:** Yale Univ 1965; **Resid:** Pediatrics, Yale-New Haven Hosp 1968; **Fellow:** Clinical Genetics, Yale-New Haven Hosp 1970; **Fac Appt:** Prof CG, Yale Univ

Colon & Rectal Surgery

Longo, Walter E MD (CRS) - **Spec Exp:** Colon & Rectal Cancer; Gastrointestinal Surgery; Inflammatory Bowel Disease; **Hospital:** Yale-New Haven Hosp, Yale Med Group; **Address:** Dept Surgery/Gastroenterology, 330 Cedar St, rm LH118, Box 208062, New Haven, CT 06520-8062; **Phone:** 203-785-2616; **Board Cert:** Surgery 2001; Colon & Rectal Surgery 2006; **Med School:** NY Med Coll 1984; **Resid:** Surgery, Yale-New Haven Hosp 1990; **Fellow:** Research, Yale-New Haven Hosp 1988; Colon & Rectal Surgery, Cleveland Clinic 1991; **Fac Appt:** Prof S, Yale Univ

Dermatology

Bolognia, Jean L MD (D) - **Spec Exp:** Melanoma; Skin Cancer; **Hospital:** Yale-New Haven Hosp, Yale Med Group; **Address:** 2 Church St S, Ste 305, New Haven, CT 06519; **Phone:** 203-789-1249; **Board Cert:** Dermatology 2005; **Med School:** Yale Univ 1980; **Resid:** Internal Medicine, Yale-New Haven Hosp 1982; Dermatology, Yale-New Haven Hosp 1985; **Fellow:** Dermatology, Yale-New Haven Hosp 1987; **Fac Appt:** Prof D, Yale Univ

Edelson, Richard L MD (D) - **Spec Exp:** Cutaneous Lymphoma; Immune Deficiency-Skin Disorders; **Hospital:** Yale-New Haven Hosp, Yale Med Group; **Address:** 2 Church St S, Ste 305, New Haven, CT 06519; **Phone:** 203-789-1249; **Board Cert:** Dermatology 1977; **Med School:** Yale Univ 1970; **Resid:** Dermatology, Mass Genl Hosp 1972; Dermatology, Natl Inst Hlth 1975; **Fac Appt:** Prof D, Yale Univ

Leffell, David J MD (D) - **Spec Exp:** Mohs' Surgery; Melanoma; Skin Cancer; Skin Laser Surgery; **Hospital:** Yale-New Haven Hosp, Yale Med Group; **Address:** Yale New Haven Hosp-Dept Dermatology, 40 Temple St, Ste 5A, PO Box 208059, New Haven, CT 06520; **Phone:** 203-785-3466; **Board Cert:** Internal Medicine 1984; Dermatology 2009; **Med School:** McGill Univ 1981; **Resid:** Internal Medicine, New York Hosp 1984; Dermatology, Yale-New Haven Hosp 1986; **Fellow:** Dermatology, Yale-New Haven Hosp 1987; Dermatologic Surgery, Univ Michigan Med Ctr 1988; **Fac Appt:** Prof D, Yale Univ

Savin, Ronald MD (D) - **Spec Exp:** Hair loss; Skin Tumors; Psoriasis; **Hospital:** Yale-New Haven Hosp, Hosp of St Raphael; **Address:** 134 Park St, New Haven, CT 06511-5416; **Phone:** 203-865-6143; **Board Cert:** Dermatology 1968; **Med School:** Univ Fla Coll Med 1961; **Resid:** Dermatology, Yale-New Haven Hosp 1965; **Fellow:** Dermatology, Yale-New Haven Hosp 1965; **Fac Appt:** Clin Prof D, Yale Univ

Diagnostic Radiology

McCarthy, Shirley M MD/PhD (DR) - **Spec Exp:** Gynecologic Cancer; Pelvic Imaging; **Hospital:** Yale-New Haven Hosp, Yale Med Group; **Address:** Yale-New Haven Hosp, 333 Cedar St, Ste TE2, New Haven, CT 06520-3206; **Phone:** 203-785-2384; **Board Cert:** Diagnostic Radiology 1983; **Med School:** Yale Univ 1979; **Resid:** Diagnostic Radiology, Yale-New Haven Hosp 1983; **Fellow:** Cross Sectional Imaging, UCSF Med Ctr 1984; **Fac Appt:** Prof Rad, Yale Univ

McClennan, Bruce MD (DR) - **Spec Exp:** Genitourinary Imaging; Abdominal Imaging; **Hospital:** Yale-New Haven Hosp, Yale Med Group; **Address:** Yale-New Haven Hosp, Dept Radiology, 333 Cedar St, Box 208042, New Haven, CT 06520-8042; **Phone:** 203-785-2384; **Board Cert:** Diagnostic Radiology 1972; **Med School:** SUNY Upstate Med Univ 1967; **Resid:** Diagnostic Radiology, Mary Imogene Bassett Hosp 1968; **Fellow:** Diagnostic Radiology, Columbia-Presby Med Ctr 1971; **Fac Appt:** Prof Rad, Yale Univ

Weinreb, Jeffrey C MD (DR) - **Spec Exp:** MRI; Breast Cancer; Abdominal Imaging; CT Body Scan; **Hospital:** Yale-New Haven Hosp, Yale Med Group; **Address:** Yale Univ Sch Medicine, Dept Radiology, 333 Cedar St, rm MRC147, Box 208042, New Haven, CT 06520-8042; **Phone:** 203-785-5913; **Board Cert:** Diagnostic Radiology 1983; **Med School:** Mount Sinai Sch Med 1978; **Resid:** Diagnostic Radiology, LI Jewish Med Ctr 1982; **Fellow:** Ultrasound/CT, Hosp Univ Penn 1983; **Fac Appt:** Prof Rad, Yale Univ

Endocrinology, Diabetes & Metabolism

Inzucchi, Silvio E MD (EDM) - **Spec Exp:** Diabetes; Pituitary Disorders; Growth Hormone Disorder-Adult; Cholesterol/Lipid Disorders; **Hospital:** Yale-New Haven Hosp, Yale Med Group; **Address:** Yale Univ Sch Med, Sect. Endocrinology, Box 208020, New Haven, CT 06520-8020; **Phone:** 203-737-1932; **Board Cert:** Internal Medicine 1988; Endocrinology, Diabetes & Metabolism 2006; **Med School:** Harvard Med Sch 1985; **Resid:** Internal Medicine, Yale-New Haven Hosp 1988; **Fellow:** Endocrinology, Diabetes & Metabolism, Yale-New Haven Hosp 1994; **Fac Appt:** Prof Med, Yale Univ

Wysolmerski, John J MD (EDM) - **Spec Exp:** Bone Disorders-Metabolic; Osteoporosis; Parathyroid Disorders; **Hospital:** Yale-New Haven Hosp, Yale Med Group; **Address:** Yale Sch Med-Div Endocrinology, Bone Ctr, 789 Howard Ave Fl 2, New Haven, CT 06520-8020; **Phone:** 203-737-1932; **Board Cert:** Internal Medicine 1989; **Med School:** Yale Univ 1986; **Resid:** Internal Medicine, New England Med Ctr 1989; **Fellow:** Endocrinology, Yale Univ Sch Med 1993; **Fac Appt:** Assoc Prof Med, Yale Univ

Gastroenterology

Dobbins, John Whitby MD (Ge) - **Spec Exp:** Pancreatic & Biliary Disease; Inflammatory Bowel Disease; **Hospital:** Yale-New Haven Hosp, Hosp of St Raphael; **Address:** Connecticut Gastroenterlogy Consultants PC, 40 Temple St, Ste A, New Haven, CT 06510; **Phone:** 203-777-0304; **Board Cert:** Internal Medicine 1973; Gastroenterology 2005; **Med School:** Univ Wash 1968; **Resid:** Internal Medicine, George Washington Univ Hosp 1973; **Fellow:** Gastroenterology, Yale/New Haven Hosp 1976; **Fac Appt:** Prof Med, Yale Univ

Fisher, Rosemarie Louise MD (Ge) - **Spec Exp:** Nutrition; Nutrition in Bowel Disorders; Inflammatory Bowel Disease/Crohn's; Endoscopy; **Hospital:** Yale-New Haven Hosp, St Mary's Hosp - Waterbury; **Address:** 40 Temple St, Ste 1A, New Haven, CT 06519-1369; **Phone:** 203-785-4183; **Board Cert:** Internal Medicine 1975; Gastroenterology 1977; **Med School:** Tufts Univ 1971; **Resid:** Internal Medicine, Montefiore Med Ctr 1973; **Fellow:** Gastroenterology, Yale-New Haven Hosp 1975; **Fac Appt:** Prof Med, Yale Univ

Jamidar, Priya A MD (Ge) - **Spec Exp:** Gallbladder Disease; Pancreatic Disease; Gastrointestinal Cancer; Pancreatic/Biliary Endoscopy (ERCP); **Hospital:** Yale-New Haven Hosp, Yale Med Group; **Address:** 40 Temple St Fl 1, New Haven, CT 06510; **Phone:** 203-785-6228; **Board Cert:** Internal Medicine 1988; Gastroenterology 2002; **Med School:** Ireland 1984; **Resid:** Internal Medicine, Univ Conn Hlth Ctr 1988; **Fellow:** Gastroenterology, USC/LAC Med Ctr 1990; Gastroenterology, Indiana Univ Med Ctr 1992; **Fac Appt:** Assoc Prof Med, Yale Univ

Proctor, Deborah D MD (Ge) - **Spec Exp:** Inflammatory Bowel Disease; Colon Cancer Screening; Endoscopy; **Hospital:** Yale-New Haven Hosp, Yale Med Group; **Address:** 40 Temple St, Ste 1A, Temple Medical Center, 1st Fl, New Haven, CT 06510; **Phone:** 203-785-4138; **Board Cert:** Gastroenterology 2003; **Med School:** Univ Cincinnati 1982; **Resid:** Internal Medicine, Beth Israel Hosp 1990; **Fellow:** Gastroenterology, Beth Israel Hosp 1992; **Fac Appt:** Prof Med, Yale Univ

Geriatric Medicine

Cooney Jr, Leo M MD (Ger) - **Spec Exp:** Geriatric Functional Assessment; Rheumatology; Mobility Evaluation & Treatment; **Hospital:** Yale-New Haven Hosp, Yale Med Group; **Address:** Yale-New Haven Hosp, Adler Geriatric Ctr, 20 York St, New Haven, CT 06510; **Phone:** 203-688-2204; **Board Cert:** Internal Medicine 1974; Rheumatology 1978; Geriatric Medicine 2000; **Med School:** Yale Univ 1969; **Resid:** Internal Medicine, Boston City Hosp 1971; Internal Medicine, Boston City Hosp 1974; **Fellow:** Rheumatology, Boston Med Ctr 1975; **Fac Appt:** Prof Med, Yale Univ

Gill, Thomas M MD (Ger) - **Spec Exp:** Geriatric Functional Assessment; **Hospital:** Yale-New Haven Hosp, Yale Med Group; **Address:** Yale New Haven Hosp, 20 York St, New Haven, CT 06504; **Phone:** 203-688-6361; **Board Cert:** Internal Medicine 2000; Geriatric Medicine 2000; **Med School:** Univ Chicago-Pritzker Sch Med 1987; **Resid:** Internal Medicine, Univ Wash 1990; **Fellow:** Internal Medicine, Yale-New Haven Hosp 1993; Geriatric Medicine, Yale-New Haven Hosp 1994; **Fac Appt:** Assoc Prof Med, Yale Univ

Street, Lynn MD (Ger) *PCP* - **Hospital:** Yale-New Haven Hosp; **Address:** University Towers, 100 York St, Ste 2E, New Haven, CT 06511; **Phone:** 203-787-3588; **Board Cert:** Internal Medicine 2001; Geriatric Medicine 2000; **Med School:** Yale Univ 1987; **Resid:** Internal Medicine, NYU-Bellvue Hosp 1990; **Fellow:** Epidemiology, RWJ Johnson Med Ctr 1992; Geriatric Medicine, Yale-New Haven Hosp 2000

Tinetti, Mary E MD (Ger) - **Spec Exp:** Falls in the Elderly; Geriatric Functional Assessment; **Hospital:** Yale-New Haven Hosp, Yale Med Group; **Address:** Yale-New Haven Hosp, Adler Geriatric Ctr, 20 York St, New Haven, CT 06510; **Phone:** 203-688-6361; **Board Cert:** Internal Medicine 1981; **Med School:** Univ Mich Med Sch 1978; **Resid:** Internal Medicine, Univ Minnesota 1981; **Fellow:** Geriatric Medicine, Univ Rochester 1984; **Fac Appt:** Prof Med, Yale Univ

Geriatric Psychiatry

van Dyck, Christopher H MD (GerPsy) - **Spec Exp:** Alzheimer's Disease; **Hospital:** Yale-New Haven Hosp, Yale Med Group; **Address:** One Church St, Ste 600, New Haven, CT 06510-3330; **Phone:** 203-688-6361; **Board Cert:** Psychiatry 1991; Geriatric Psychiatry 2005; **Med School:** Northwestern Univ 1984; **Resid:** Psychiatry, Yale-New Haven Hosp 1988; **Fellow:** Geriatric Psychiatry, Yale-New Haven Hosp 1990; **Fac Appt:** Assoc Prof Psyc, Yale Univ

Gynecologic Oncology

Azodi, Masoud MD (GO) - **Spec Exp:** Laparoscopic Surgery; Ovarian Cancer-Early Detection; Uterine Cancer; **Hospital:** Yale-New Haven Hosp, Yale Med Group; **Address:** Smilow Cancer Hosp, 35 Park St Fl 1, New Haven, CT 06519-1369; **Phone:** 203-200-4176; **Board Cert:** Gynecologic Oncology 2009; Obstetrics & Gynecology 2009; **Med School:** Wright State Univ 1992; **Resid:** Obstetrics & Gynecology, Aultman Hospital 1996; **Fellow:** Obstetrics & Gynecology, Yale-New Haven Hosp 1999; **Fac Appt:** Assoc Prof ObG, Yale Univ

Rutherford, Thomas J MD (GO) - **Spec Exp:** Ovarian Cancer; Uterine Cancer; Ovarian Cancer-Early Detection; Cervical Cancer; **Hospital:** Yale-New Haven Hosp, Yale Med Group; **Address:** Smilow Cancer Hosp, 35 Park St Fl 1, New Haven, CT 06519; **Phone:** 203-200-4176; **Board Cert:** Obstetrics & Gynecology 2009; Gynecologic Oncology 2009; **Med School:** Med Coll OH 1989; **Resid:** Obstetrics & Gynecology, Cooper Hosp 1993; **Fellow:** Gynecologic Oncology, Yale-New Haven Hosp 1995; **Fac Appt:** Assoc Prof ObG, Yale Univ

Santin, Alessandro MD (GO) - **Spec Exp:** Immunotherapy; Ovarian Cancer; Vulvar & Vaginal Cancer; **Hospital:** Yale-New Haven Hosp, Yale Med Group; **Address:** Yale Gynecologic Oncology, 800 Howard Ave, New Haven, CT 06519; **Phone:** 203-737-2280; **Med School:** Italy 1989; **Resid:** Obstetrics & Gynecology, Univ Brescia Sch Med 1993; **Fellow:** Gynecologic Oncology, UC Irvine 1995; Gynecologic Oncology, UAMS Med Ctr 2000; **Fac Appt:** Prof ObG, Yale Univ

Schwartz, Peter E MD (GO) - **Spec Exp:** Ovarian Cancer; Uterine Cancer; Gynecologic Surgery-Complex; Cervical Cancer; **Hospital:** Yale-New Haven Hosp, Yale Med Group; **Address:** Yale Univ Sch Med, Dept Ob/Gyn, 333 Cedar St, rm FMB-316, New Haven, CT 06510-3289; **Phone:** 203-785-4014; **Board Cert:** Obstetrics & Gynecology 1973; Gynecologic Oncology 1979; **Med School:** Albert Einstein Coll Med 1966; **Resid:** Obstetrics & Gynecology, Yale-New Haven Hosp 1970; **Fellow:** Gynecologic Oncology, MD Anderson Cancer Ctr 1975; **Fac Appt:** Prof ObG, Yale Univ

Hand Surgery

Thomson, J Grant MD (HS) - **Spec Exp:** Carpal Tunnel Syndrome; Hand Reconstruction; Microsurgery; **Hospital:** Yale-New Haven Hosp, Yale Med Group; **Address:** Yale Plastic Surgery, 333 Cedar St, Box 208041, New Haven, CT 06520-8041; **Phone:** 203-737-5130; **Board Cert:** Hand Surgery 2004; Plastic Surgery 2004; **Med School:** McGill Univ 1983; **Resid:** Surgery, Montreal Genl Hosp 1988; Plastic Surgery, Montreal Genl Hosp 1990; **Fellow:** Hand Surgery, Barnes Jewish Hosp 1991; **Fac Appt:** Assoc Prof PlS, Yale Univ

Hematology

Duffy, Thomas P MD (Hem) - **Spec Exp:** Mast Cell Diseases; Leukemia; Lymphoma; Mast Cell Diseases; **Hospital:** Yale-New Haven Hosp, Yale Med Group; **Address:** Yale Univ, Sect Hematology, 333 Cedar St, rm 403-WWW, Box 208021, New Haven, CT 06520-8021; **Phone:** 203-785-4744; **Board Cert:** Internal Medicine 1972; Hematology 1974; **Med School:** Johns Hopkins Univ 1962; **Resid:** Internal Medicine, Johns Hopkins Hosp 1965; **Fellow:** Hematology, Johns Hopkins Hosp 1970; **Fac Appt:** Prof Med, Yale Univ

Forget, Bernard MD (Hem) - **Spec Exp:** Thalassemia; Anemias & Red Cell Disorders; Leukemia; Sickle Cell Disease; **Hospital:** Yale-New Haven Hosp, Yale Med Group; **Address:** Yale Univ Sch Med, Div Hematology, PO Box 208021, New Haven, CT 06520-8021; **Phone:** 203-785-4144; **Board Cert:** Internal Medicine 1971; Hematology 1972; **Med School:** McGill Univ 1963; **Resid:** Internal Medicine, Mass Genl Hosp 1965; Clinical Pathology, Mass Genl Hosp 1968; **Fellow:** Hematology, Peter Bent Brigham Hosp 1971; **Fac Appt:** Prof Med, Yale Univ

Marks, Peter W MD/PhD (Hem) - **Spec Exp:** Hemophilia; Platelet Disorders; Bleeding/Coagulation Disorders; Leukemia; **Hospital:** Yale-New Haven Hosp, Yale Med Group; **Address:** Yale Hematology, 333 Cedar St, Box 208302, New Haven, CT 06520; **Phone:** 203-200-4363; **Board Cert:** Internal Medicine 2004; Hematology 2007; Medical Oncology 2007; **Med School:** NYU Sch Med 1991; **Resid:** Internal Medicine, Brigham & Women's Hosp 1994; **Fellow:** Hematology & Oncology, Brigham & Women's Hosp 1996; **Fac Appt:** Assoc Prof Med, Yale Univ

Sabbath, Kert David MD (Hem) - **Hospital:** St Mary's Hosp - Waterbury, Waterbury Hosp; **Address:** 1075 Chase Pkwy, Waterbury, CT 06708-2948; **Phone:** 203-755-6311; **Board Cert:** Internal Medicine 1982; Medical Oncology 1985; Hematology 1986; **Med School:** Boston Univ 1979; **Resid:** Internal Medicine, Boston Med Ctr 1982; **Fellow:** Hematology, Mass Genl Hosp 1985

Infectious Disease

Quagliarello, Vincent MD (Inf) - **Spec Exp:** Meningitis; Pneumonia; Endocarditis; **Hospital:** Yale-New Haven Hosp, Yale Med Group; **Address:** Yale Univ Sch Med, TAC S169A, 300 Cedar St, New Haven, CT 06520-8022; **Phone:** 203-785-3561; **Board Cert:** Internal Medicine 1984; Infectious Disease 1988; **Med School:** Washington Univ, St Louis 1980; **Resid:** Internal Medicine, Yale-New Haven Hosp 1984; **Fellow:** Infectious Disease, Univ VA Hlth Sci Ctr 1987; **Fac Appt:** Prof Med, Yale Univ

Internal Medicine

Eilbott, David J MD (IM) *PCP* - **Hospital:** Yale-New Haven Hosp, Hosp of St Raphael; **Address:** 500 E Main St, Ste 212, Branford, CT 06405-2937; **Phone:** 203-481-5665; **Board Cert:** Internal Medicine 1986; **Med School:** Univ Rochester 1981; **Resid:** Internal Medicine, Waterbury Hosp 1985; **Fellow:** Infectious Disease, SUNY Stony Brook 1988; **Fac Appt:** Asst Clin Prof Med, Yale Univ

Ellman, Matthew S MD (IM) *PCP* - **Spec Exp:** Preventive Medicine; **Hospital:** Yale-New Haven Hosp, Yale Med Group; **Address:** Yale Int Med Assocs, 789 Howard Ave, Dana Bldg - Fl 3, New Haven, CT 06510; **Phone:** 203-785-7411; **Board Cert:** Internal Medicine 2000; **Med School:** Harvard Med Sch 1987; **Resid:** Internal Medicine, Bellevue Hosp-NYU 1990; **Fellow:** Epidemiology, New Haven Hosp 1993; **Fac Appt:** Asst Prof Med, Yale Univ

Kernan, Walter MD (IM) *PCP* - **Spec Exp:** Stroke; Hypertension; **Hospital:** Yale-New Haven Hosp, Yale Med Group; **Address:** 20 York St, New Haven, CT 06520-1744; **Phone:** 203-688-2984; **Board Cert:** Internal Medicine 1987; **Med School:** Dartmouth Med Sch 1984; **Resid:** Internal Medicine, Johns Hopkins Hosp 1987; **Fellow:** Internal Medicine, Yale New Haven Hosp 1989; **Fac Appt:** Prof Med, Yale Univ

O'Connor, Patrick G MD (IM) *PCP* - **Spec Exp:** Substance Abuse; **Hospital:** Yale-New Haven Hosp, Yale Med Group; **Address:** Yale Univ School Medicine, PO Box 208093, New Haven, CT 06520-8093; **Phone:** 203-688-6532; **Board Cert:** Internal Medicine 1986; **Med School:** Albany Med Coll 1982; **Resid:** Internal Medicine, Univ Rochester Med Ctr 1985; **Fellow:** Internal Medicine, Yale-New Haven Hosp 1988; **Fac Appt:** Prof Med, Yale Univ

Maternal & Fetal Medicine

Copel, Joshua A MD (MF) - **Spec Exp:** Prenatal Diagnosis; Fetal Echocardiography; Pregnancy-High Risk; Fetal Diagnosis & Therapy; **Hospital:** Yale-New Haven Hosp, Yale Med Group; **Address:** Yale Univ Sch Med, Dept OB/GYN, 333 Cedar St, Box 208063, New Haven, CT 06520-3206; **Phone:** 203-785-5682; **Board Cert:** Obstetrics & Gynecology 2008; Maternal & Fetal Medicine 2008; **Med School:** Tufts Univ 1979; **Resid:** Obstetrics & Gynecology, Pennsylvania Hosp 1983; **Fellow:** Maternal & Fetal Medicine, Yale-New Haven Hosp 1985; **Fac Appt:** Prof ObG, Yale Univ

Funai, Edmund F MD (MF) - **Spec Exp:** Pregnancy-High Risk; Hypertension in Pregnancy; Premature Labor; **Hospital:** Yale-New Haven Hosp, Yale Med Group; **Address:** Yale-Dept Ob/Gyn & Reproductive Scis, Yale-New Haven Hosp, 333 Cedar St, FMB 308, New Haven, CT 06520-8063; **Phone:** 203-785-5682; **Board Cert:** Obstetrics & Gynecology 2008; Maternal & Fetal Medicine 2008; **Med School:** NY Med Coll 1992; **Resid:** Obstetrics & Gynecology, Lenox Hill Hosp 1996; **Fellow:** Maternal & Fetal Medicine, NYU Med Ctr 1998; **Fac Appt:** Assoc Prof ObG, Yale Univ

Lockwood, Charles MD (MF) - **Spec Exp:** Prematurity Prevention; Miscarriage-Recurrent; Multiple Gestation; Bleeding/Coagulation Disorders; **Hospital:** Yale-New Haven Hosp, Yale Med Group; **Address:** Yale Univ Sch Med, Dept Ob-Gyn, 333 Cedar St, rm FMB 302, New Haven, CT 06520-8063; **Phone:** 203-737-2970; **Board Cert:** Obstetrics & Gynecology 2007; Maternal & Fetal Medicine 2007; **Med School:** Univ Pennsylvania 1981; **Resid:** Obstetrics & Gynecology, Penn Hosp 1985; **Fellow:** Maternal & Fetal Medicine, Yale-New Haven Hosp 1987; Thrombosis, Mt Sinai Med Ctr 1991; **Fac Appt:** Prof ObG, Yale Univ

Magriples, Urania MD (MF) - **Spec Exp:** Pregnancy-High Risk; **Hospital:** Yale-New Haven Hosp, Yale Med Group; **Address:** Yale Univ Sch Med - Dept Ob/Gyn, 333 Cedar St, PO Box 208063, New Haven, CT 06520-8063; **Phone:** 203-785-5855; **Board Cert:** Obstetrics & Gynecology 2009; Maternal & Fetal Medicine 2009; **Med School:** Mount Sinai Sch Med 1987; **Resid:** Obstetrics & Gynecology, Yale-New Haven Hosp 1991; **Fellow:** Perinatal Medicine, Yale-New Haven Hosp 1994; **Fac Appt:** Assoc Prof ObG, Yale Univ

Paidas, Michael J MD (MF) - **Spec Exp:** Pregnancy-High Risk; Clotting Disorders in Pregnancy; Miscarriage-Recurrent; **Hospital:** Yale-New Haven Hosp, Yale Med Group; **Address:** Dept Ob/Gyn & Reproductive Scis, Yale-New Haven Hosp, 333 Cedar St, FMB 308, New Haven, CT 06520-8063; **Phone:** 203-785-5682; **Board Cert:** Obstetrics & Gynecology 2009; Maternal & Fetal Medicine 2009; **Med School:** Tufts Univ 1987; **Resid:** Obstetrics & Gynecology, Pennsylvania Hosp 1991; **Fellow:** Maternal & Fetal Medicine, Mount Sinai Med Ctr 1993; **Fac Appt:** Assoc Prof ObG, Yale Univ

Medical Oncology

Chu, Edward MD (Onc) - **Spec Exp:** Colon & Rectal Cancer; Gastrointestinal Cancer; Clinical Trials; **Hospital:** Yale-New Haven Hosp, Yale Med Group; **Address:** Yale Cancer Ctr, 333 Cedar St, Room WWW221, New Haven, CT 06520-8032; **Phone:** 203-785-6879; **Board Cert:** Internal Medicine 1986; Medical Oncology 1989; **Med School:** Brown Univ 1983; **Resid:** Internal Medicine, Roger Williams Hosp 1987; **Fellow:** Hematology & Oncology, Natl Cancer Inst 1990; Internal Medicine, Natl Cancer Inst 1992; **Fac Appt:** Prof Med, Yale Univ

Cooper, Dennis MD (Onc) - **Spec Exp:** Lymphoma; Stem Cell Transplant; Leukemia; **Hospital:** Yale-New Haven Hosp, Yale Med Group; **Address:** Yale Univ Sch Med, 333 Cedar St, FMP-121, Box 208032, New Haven, CT 06520-8032; **Phone:** 203-737-5751; **Board Cert:** Internal Medicine 1983; Medical Oncology 1985; **Med School:** Rush Med Coll 1979; **Resid:** Internal Medicine, Yale-New Haven Hosp 1982; Internal Medicine, Presby-Univ Hosp 1983; **Fellow:** Medical Oncology, Yale-New Haven Hosp 1985; **Fac Appt:** Assoc Prof Med, Yale Univ

DeVita Jr, Vincent T MD (Onc) - **Spec Exp:** Lymphoma Consultation; Hodgkin's Disease Consultation; **Hospital:** Yale-New Haven Hosp, Yale Med Group; **Address:** Yale Cancer Ctr, 333 Cedar St, rm WWW-211B, New Haven, CT 06520-8028; **Phone:** 203-737-1010; **Board Cert:** Internal Medicine 1974; Hematology 1972; Medical Oncology 1973; **Med School:** Geo Wash Univ 1961; **Resid:** Internal Medicine, Geo Wash Hosp 1963; Internal Medicine, Yale-New Haven Hosp 1966; **Fellow:** Medical Oncology, Natl Cancer Inst 1965; **Fac Appt:** Prof Med, Yale Univ

Foss, Francine M MD (Onc) - **Spec Exp:** Lymphoma, Cutaneous T Cell (CTCL); Stem Cell Transplant; Graft vs Host Disease; Multiple Myeloma; **Hospital:** Yale-New Haven Hosp, Yale Med Group; **Address:** Yale Cancer Ctr, 333 Cedar St, Box 208032, New Haven, CT 06520; **Phone:** 203-737-5312; **Board Cert:** Internal Medicine 1985; Medical Oncology 1987; **Med School:** Univ Mass Sch Med 1982; **Resid:** Internal Medicine, Brigham & Womens Hosp 1985; **Fellow:** Medical Oncology, Natl Cancer Inst 1988; **Fac Appt:** Prof Med, Yale Univ

Hochster, Howard S MD (Onc) - **Spec Exp:** Gastrointestinal Cancer; Gynecologic Cancer; Colon & Rectal Cancer; **Hospital:** Yale-New Haven Hosp; **Address:** Yale Cancer Ctr, 333 Cedar St, PO Box 208028, New Haven, CT 06520-8028; **Phone:** 203-785-4191; **Board Cert:** Internal Medicine 1983; Medical Oncology 1985; Hematology 1986; **Med School:** Yale Univ 1980; **Resid:** Internal Medicine, NYU Med Ctr 1983; **Fellow:** Hematology & Oncology, NYU Med Ctr 1985; Medical Oncology, Jules Bordet Inst 1986; **Fac Appt:** Prof Med, Yale Univ

Kelly, William K DO (Onc) - **Spec Exp:** Prostate Cancer; Genitourinary Cancer; Solid Tumors; **Hospital:** Yale-New Haven Hosp, Yale Med Group; **Address:** Yale Cancer Ctr, 333 Cedars St FMP130 Bldg, PO Box 208032, New Haven, CT 06520; **Phone:** 203-737-2572; **Board Cert:** Medical Oncology 2003; **Med School:** Philadelphia Coll Osteo Med 1986; **Resid:** Internal Medicine, Montefiore Med Ctr 1990; **Fellow:** Hematology & Oncology, Meml Sloan Kettering Cancer Ctr 1993; **Fac Appt:** Assoc Prof Med, Yale Univ

Lacy, Jill MD (Onc) - **Spec Exp:** Colon & Rectal Cancer; Brain Tumors; Gastrointestinal Cancer; Pancreatic Cancer; **Hospital:** Yale-New Haven Hosp, Yale Med Group; **Address:** Yale Univ Sch Med-Div Medical Oncology, 333 Cedar St, PO Box 208032, New Haven, CT 06520-8032; **Phone:** 203-785-4191; **Board Cert:** Internal Medicine 1982; Medical Oncology 2005; **Med School:** Yale Univ 1978; **Resid:** Internal Medicine, Yale-New Haven Hosp 1981; **Fellow:** Medical Oncology, Yale-New Haven Hosp 1985; **Fac Appt:** Assoc Prof Med, Yale Univ

Lundberg, Walter B MD (Onc) - **Spec Exp:** Lymphoma; Colon Cancer; Lung Cancer; **Hospital:** Hosp of St Raphael, Yale-New Haven Hosp; **Address:** 1450 Chapel St, Ste A, McGivney Center for Cancer Care, New Haven, CT 06511; **Phone:** 203-867-5420; **Board Cert:** Internal Medicine 1973; Hematology 1974; Blood Banking 1974; Medical Oncology 1975; **Med School:** Columbia P&S 1970; **Resid:** Internal Medicine, Columbia Presby Hosp 1972; Medical Oncology, Yale-New Haven Hosp 1976; **Fellow:** Internal Medicine, Harvard Med Sch 1971; Hematology, NIH 1974; **Fac Appt:** Assoc Clin Prof Med, Yale Univ

Lynch, Thomas J MD (Onc) - **Spec Exp:** Lung Cancer; Thoracic Cancers; **Hospital:** Yale-New Haven Hosp, Yale Med Group; **Address:** Smilow Cancer Hosp, 333 Cedar St, Office WWW 205, New Haven, CT 06510; **Phone:** 203-688-5864; **Board Cert:** Internal Medicine 1989; Medical Oncology 2003; **Med School:** Yale Univ 1986; **Resid:** Internal Medicine, Mass Genl Hosp 1989; **Fellow:** Medical Oncology, Dana-Farber Cancer Inst 1991; **Fac Appt:** Assoc Prof Med, Yale Univ

Neonatal-Perinatal Medicine

Ehrenkranz, Richard MD (NP) - **Spec Exp:** Nutrition; Lung Disease in Newborns; **Hospital:** Yale-New Haven Hosp, Yale Med Group; **Address:** Yale Univ-Dept Ped, PO Box 208064, New Haven, CT 06520-8064; **Phone:** 203-688-2320; **Board Cert:** Pediatrics 1977; Neonatal-Perinatal Medicine 1979; **Med School:** SUNY Downstate 1972; **Resid:** Pediatrics, Yale-New Haven Hosp 1974; **Fellow:** Neonatal-Perinatal Medicine, Yale-New Haven Hosp 1978; **Fac Appt:** Prof Ped, Yale Univ

Gross, Ian MD (NP) - **Spec Exp:** Breathing Disorders; Critical Care; **Hospital:** Yale-New Haven Hosp, Yale Med Group; **Address:** Yale Sch Med, Dept Pediatrics, 333 Cedar St, PO Box 208064, New Haven, CT 06520-8064; **Phone:** 203-688-2320; **Board Cert:** Pediatrics 1974; Neonatal-Perinatal Medicine 1977; **Med School:** South Africa 1967; **Resid:** Pediatrics, Univ Witwatersrand Affil Hosps 1971; Pediatrics, Chldns Hosp Med Ctr 1973; **Fellow:** Neonatal-Perinatal Medicine, Yale-New Haven Hosp 1974; **Fac Appt:** Prof Ped, Yale Univ

Nephrology

Aronson, Peter S MD (Nep) - **Spec Exp:** Electrolyte Disorders; Kidney Stones; Renal Tubular Acidosis; **Hospital:** Yale-New Haven Hosp, Yale Med Group; **Address:** Yale Sch Med, Dept Medicine, PO Box 208029, New Haven, CT 06520-8029; **Phone:** 203-785-4186; **Board Cert:** Internal Medicine 1973; Nephrology 1976; **Med School:** NYU Sch Med 1970; **Resid:** Internal Medicine, NC Meml Hosp 1972; Research, Natl Inst Hlth 1974; **Fellow:** Nephrology, Yale-New Haven Hosp 1977; **Fac Appt:** Prof Med, Yale Univ

Bia, Margaret MD (Nep) - **Spec Exp:** Transplant Medicine-Kidney; **Hospital:** Yale-New Haven Hosp, Yale Med Group; **Address:** Yale Univ, Sect of Nephrology, PO Box 208062, New Haven, CT 06520; **Phone:** 203-785-2565; **Board Cert:** Internal Medicine 1975; Nephrology 1978; **Med School:** Cornell Univ-Weill Med Coll 1972; **Resid:** Internal Medicine, Univ Hosp Penn 1975; **Fellow:** Renal Disease, Univ Hosp Penn 1976; **Fac Appt:** Prof Med, Yale Univ

Formica Jr, Richard N MD (Nep) - **Spec Exp:** Transplant Medicine-Kidney; Transplant-Pancreas; **Hospital:** Yale-New Haven Hosp; **Address:** PO Box 208029, 333 Cedar St, New Haven, CT 06520-8029; **Phone:** 203-785-4184; **Board Cert:** Internal Medicine 2007; Nephrology 2009; **Med School:** Boston Univ 1993; **Resid:** Internal Medicine, Boston Univ Hosp 1997; **Fellow:** Nephrology, Yale New-Haven Hosp 1997; **Fac Appt:** Assoc Prof S, Yale Univ

Kliger, Alan MD (Nep) - **Spec Exp:** Kidney Disease; Kidney Disease-Metabolic; **Hospital:** Hosp of St Raphael; **Address:** 136 Sherman Ave, New Haven, CT 06511-5238; **Phone:** 203-787-0117 x307; **Board Cert:** Internal Medicine 1973; Nephrology 1976; **Med School:** SUNY Upstate Med Univ 1970; **Resid:** Internal Medicine, SUNY Upstate Med Ctr 1973; **Fellow:** Nephrology, Georgetown Univ Hosp 1975; **Fac Appt:** Clin Prof Med, Yale Univ

Rastegar, Asghar MD (Nep) - **Spec Exp:** Glomerulonephritis; Amyloidosis; Electrolyte Disorders; **Hospital:** Yale-New Haven Hosp, Yale Med Group; **Address:** Yale Sch Med - Div Nephrology, 333 Cedar St, LMP1074, Box 208030, New Haven, CT 06520-8030; **Phone:** 203-737-2078; **Board Cert:** Internal Medicine 1972; Nephrology 1978; **Med School:** Univ Wisc 1968; **Resid:** Internal Medicine, Hosp Univ Penn 1973; **Fellow:** Nephrology, Hosp Univ Penn 1972; **Fac Appt:** Prof Med, Yale Univ

Neurological Surgery

Duncan, Charles C MD (NS) - **Spec Exp:** Pediatric Neurosurgery; **Hospital:** Yale-New Haven Hosp, Yale Med Group; **Address:** Yale Univ Sch Med, PO Box 208082, New Haven, CT 06520-8082; **Phone:** 203-785-2809; **Board Cert:** Neurological Surgery 1979; Pediatric Neurological Surgery 1996; **Med School:** Duke Univ 1971; **Resid:** Neurological Surgery, Duke Univ Med Ctr 1977; **Fac Appt:** Prof NS, Yale Univ

Piepmeier, Joseph MD (NS) - **Spec Exp:** Neuro-Oncology; Brain & Spinal Cord Tumors; **Hospital:** Yale-New Haven Hosp, Yale Med Group; **Address:** Yale Sch Med, Dept Neurosurgery, 333 Cedar St Fl TMP-410, New Haven, CT 06520; **Phone:** 203-785-2791; **Board Cert:** Neurological Surgery 1984; **Med School:** Univ Tenn Coll Med, Memphis 1975; **Resid:** Neurological Surgery, Yale-New Haven Hosp 1982; **Fac Appt:** Prof NS, Yale Univ

Spencer, Dennis D MD (NS) - **Spec Exp:** Epilepsy/Seizure Disorders; Brain Tumors; **Hospital:** Yale-New Haven Hosp, Yale Med Group; **Address:** Yale Univ Sch Med, Dept Neurosurgery, 333 Cedar St, TMP-4, New Haven, CT 06520; **Phone:** 203-785-4891; **Board Cert:** Neurological Surgery 1980; **Med School:** Washington Univ, St Louis 1971; **Resid:** Surgery, Barnes Hosp 1972; Neurological Surgery, Yale-New Haven Hosp 1976; **Fac Appt:** Prof NS, Yale Univ

Neurology

Blumenfeld, Hal MD/PhD (N) - **Spec Exp:** Epilepsy/Seizure Disorders; **Hospital:** Yale-New Haven Hosp, Yale Med Group; **Address:** Yale Dept of Neurology, 40 Temple St, Ste 6C, New Haven, CT 06520-8018; **Phone:** 203-785-4085; **Board Cert:** Neurology 2008; **Med School:** Columbia P&S 1992; **Resid:** Neurology, Mass Genl Hosp 1996; **Fellow:** Epilepsy, Yale-New Haven Hosp 1998; **Fac Appt:** Assoc Prof N, Yale Univ

Duckrow, Robert B MD (N) - **Spec Exp:** Epilepsy; **Hospital:** Yale-New Haven Hosp, Yale Med Group; **Address:** 800 Howard Ave, New Haven, CT 06520; **Phone:** 203-785-4085; **Board Cert:** Neurology 1984; Clinical Neurophysiology 2004; **Med School:** Yale Univ 1975; **Resid:** Neurology, Yale-New Haven Hosp 1979; **Fellow:** Metabolic Neurology, Univ Miami Hosp 1981; **Fac Appt:** Assoc Prof N, Yale Univ

Goldstein, Jonathan M MD (N) - **Spec Exp:** Myasthenia Gravis; Peripheral Neuropathy; **Hospital:** Yale-New Haven Hosp, Yale Med Group; **Address:** 800 Howard Ave, New Haven, CT 06520; **Phone:** 203-785-4085; **Board Cert:** Neurology 1991; **Med School:** Brown Univ 1986; **Resid:** Neurology, Yale-New Haven Hosp 1990; **Fellow:** Clinical Neurophysiology, Yale-New Haven Hosp 1991; Neurological Immunology, Yale-New Haven Hosp 1992; **Fac Appt:** Assoc Prof N, Yale Univ

Greer, David M MD (N) - **Spec Exp:** Stroke; Cerebrovascular Disease; **Hospital:** Yale-New Haven Hosp; **Address:** Yale Univ Sch Medicine, Dept Neurology, 333 Cedar St, PO Box 208018, New Haven, CT 06520-8018; **Phone:** 203-737-1057; **Board Cert:** Neurology 2000; Vascular Neurology 2008; **Med School:** Univ Fla Coll Med 1995; **Resid:** Neurology, Mass General Hosp 1999; **Fellow:** Vascular Neurology, Mass General Hosp 2001

Katz, Amiram MD (N) - **Spec Exp:** Seizure Disorders; Lyme Disease; Diving Medicine; Sleep Medicine; **Hospital:** Norwalk Hosp, Yale-New Haven Hosp; **Address:** 325 Boston Post Rd, Ste 1B, Orange, CT 06477; **Phone:** 203-795-5425; **Board Cert:** Neurology 1993; **Med School:** Israel 1976; **Resid:** Neurology, Sheba Hospital 1980; Neurology, Tel Aviv Med Ctr 1984; **Fellow:** Clinical Neurophysiology, Cleveland Clinic 1988; Epilepsy, Yale Univ 1991; **Fac Appt:** Asst Clin Prof N, Yale Univ

Obstetrics & Gynecology

Fine, Emily A MD (ObG) - **Spec Exp:** Menopause Problems; Vulvar Disease; **Hospital:** Yale-New Haven Hosp; **Address:** 60 Washington Ave, Ste 201, Hamden, CT 06518; **Phone:** 203-230-2939; **Board Cert:** Obstetrics & Gynecology 1984; **Med School:** Yale Univ 1978; **Resid:** Obstetrics & Gynecology, Yale-New Haven Hosp 1982; **Fac Appt:** Asst Clin Prof ObG, Yale Univ

Lynch, Vincent A MD (ObG) - **Spec Exp:** Laparoscopic Surgery; Menopause Problems; Heart Disease in Pregnancy; **Hospital:** Yale-New Haven Hosp, Yale Med Group; **Address:** 46 Prince St, Ste 207, New Haven, CT 06519; **Phone:** 203-787-2264; **Board Cert:** Obstetrics & Gynecology 1986; **Med School:** NY Med Coll 1967; **Resid:** Obstetrics & Gynecology, Yale-New Haven Hosp 1972; **Fac Appt:** Clin Prof ObG, Yale Univ

Ophthalmology

Bernardino, C Roberto MD (Oph) - **Spec Exp:** Oculoplastic Surgery; Orbital Surgery; Thyroid Eye Disease; Anophthalmia; **Hospital:** Yale-New Haven Hosp, Yale Med Group; **Address:** Yale Eye Center, 40 Temple St, Ste 3B, New Haven, CT 06510; **Phone:** 203-785-2020; **Board Cert:** Ophthalmology 2003; **Med School:** Jefferson Med Coll 1997; **Resid:** Ophthalmology, Wills Eye Hosp 2001; **Fellow:** Oculoplastic Surgery, Mass Eye & Ear Infirm 2003; **Fac Appt:** Assoc Prof Oph, Yale Univ

Lesser, Robert L MD (Oph) - **Spec Exp:** Neuro-Ophthalmology; Myasthenia Gravis; Pseudotumor Cerebri; Temporal Arteritis; **Hospital:** Yale-New Haven Hosp, St Mary's Hosp - Waterbury; **Address:** The Eye Care Group, 40 Temple St, Ste 5B, New Haven, CT 06510; **Phone:** 203-789-2020; **Board Cert:** Ophthalmology 1975; **Med School:** Cornell Univ-Weill Med Coll 1967; **Resid:** Ophthalmology, Yale-New Haven Hosp 1974; **Fellow:** Neuro-Ophthalmology, Bascom Palmer Eye Inst 1972; **Fac Appt:** Clin Prof Oph, Yale Univ

Tsai, James C MD (Oph) - **Spec Exp:** Glaucoma; **Hospital:** Yale-New Haven Hosp, Yale Med Group; **Address:** Yale Eye Center, 40 Temple St, New Haven, CT 06520-8061; **Phone:** 203-785-2020; **Board Cert:** Ophthalmology 2006; **Med School:** Stanford Univ 1989; **Resid:** Ophthalmology, Doheny Eye Inst/USC 1993; **Fellow:** Glaucoma, Bascom Palmer Eye Inst 1994; Glaucoma, Moorfields Eye Hosp 1995; **Fac Appt:** Prof Oph, Yale Univ

Orthopaedic Surgery

Baumgaertner, Michael R MD (OrS) - **Spec Exp:** Trauma; Hip & Knee Reconstruction; Fractures-Complex & Non Union; **Hospital:** Yale-New Haven Hosp, Yale Med Group; **Address:** 800 Howard Ave, Yale Physicians Bldg, Fl 1, New Haven, CT 06520; **Phone:** 203-737-5667; **Board Cert:** Orthopaedic Surgery 2010; **Med School:** UCSD 1982; **Resid:** Orthopaedic Surgery, UCSF Med Ctr 1987; **Fellow:** Plastic Surgery, Univ Mass Med Ctr 1988; Trauma, AO Foundation 1989; **Fac Appt:** Prof OrS, Yale Univ

Friedlaender, Gary E MD (OrS) - **Spec Exp:** Bone & Soft Tissue Tumors; Limb Surgery/Reconstruction; Fractures-Complex & Non Union; Tissue Banking; **Hospital:** Yale-New Haven Hosp, Yale Med Group; **Address:** 800 Howard Ave, Yale Physicians Fl 1, New Haven, CT 06519; **Phone:** 203-737-5667; **Board Cert:** Orthopaedic Surgery 1975; **Med School:** Univ Mich Med Sch 1969; **Resid:** Surgery, Michigan Med Ctr 1971; Orthopaedic Surgery, Yale-New Haven Hosp 1974; **Fellow:** Musculoskeletal Oncology, Mass Genl Hosp 1983; **Fac Appt:** Prof OrS, Yale Univ

Jokl, Peter MD (OrS) - **Spec Exp:** Knee Surgery; Sports Medicine; Shoulder Surgery; **Hospital:** Yale-New Haven Hosp, Yale Med Group; **Address:** Yale Sports Med, Dept Orthopaedics, 800 Howard Ave, New Haven, CT 06519-1369; **Phone:** 203-785-2579; **Board Cert:** Orthopaedic Surgery 1974; **Med School:** Yale Univ 1968; **Resid:** Orthopaedic Surgery, Yale-New Haven Hosp 1972; **Fac Appt:** Prof OrS, Yale Univ

Marsh, James S MD (OrS) - **Spec Exp:** Pediatric Orthopaedic Surgery; **Hospital:** Yale-New Haven Hosp, Hosp of St Raphael; **Address:** 34 York St, Ste 8, Guilford, CT 06437; **Phone:** 203-453-1088; **Med School:** Harvard Med Sch 1981; **Resid:** Orthopaedic Surgery, Stanford Univ 1986; **Fellow:** Pediatric Orthopaedic Surgery, Mass Genl Hosp 1987; **Fac Appt:** Assoc Prof OrS, Yale Univ

Smith, Brian Gerard MD (OrS) - **Spec Exp:** Pediatric Orthopaedic Surgery; Spinal Deformity; Scoliosis; Foot Deformities; **Hospital:** Yale-New Haven Hosp, Yale Med Group; **Address:** 800 Howard Ave, Yale Physicians Bldg Fl 1, New Haven, CT 06519; **Phone:** 203-737-5667; **Board Cert:** Orthopaedic Surgery 2010; **Med School:** Georgetown Univ 1982; **Resid:** Orthopaedic Surgery, Georgetown Univ Hosp 1987; **Fellow:** Pediatric Orthopaedic Surgery, Children's Hosp 1992; **Fac Appt:** Assoc Prof OrS, Yale Univ

Otolaryngology

Kveton, John MD (Oto) - **Spec Exp:** Ear Disorders/Surgery; Cochlear Implants; Acoustic Neuroma; Hearing Loss; **Hospital:** Yale-New Haven Hosp, Hosp of St Raphael; **Address:** 46 Prince St, Ste 601, New Haven, CT 06519-1634; **Phone:** 203-752-1726; **Board Cert:** Otolaryngology 1982; Neurotology 2004; **Med School:** St Louis Univ 1978; **Resid:** Otolaryngology, Yale-New Haven Hosp 1982; **Fellow:** Neurotology, The Otology Group 1983; **Fac Appt:** Clin Prof Oto, Yale Univ

Michaelides, Elias M MD (Oto) - **Spec Exp:** Neuro-Otology; Hearing Loss; Pediatric Otolaryngology; Otology; **Hospital:** Yale-New Haven Hosp, Yale Med Group; **Address:** 800 Howard Ave, Yale Physicians Bldg, Fl 4, New Haven, CT 06519; **Phone:** 203-785-7656; **Board Cert:** Otolaryngology 1999; Neurotology 2008; **Med School:** SUNY Stony Brook 1993; **Resid:** Otolaryngology, Med Coll Va 1998; **Fellow:** Otology, Michigan Ear Inst 2000; **Fac Appt:** Asst Prof S, Yale Univ

Sasaki, Clarence T MD (Oto) - **Spec Exp:** Head & Neck Cancer; Skull Base Surgery; Voice Disorders; Zenker Diverticulum; **Hospital:** Yale-New Haven Hosp, Yale Med Group; **Address:** Yale Sch Med, Dept Otolaryngology, 333 Cedar St, Box 208041, New Haven, CT 06520-8041; **Phone:** 203-785-2592; **Board Cert:** Otolaryngology 1973; **Med School:** Yale Univ 1966; **Resid:** Surgery, Mary Hitchcock Hosp 1968; Otolaryngology, Yale-New Haven Hosp 1973; **Fellow:** Head and Neck Surgery, Univ of Milan 1978; Skull Base Surgery, Univ Zurich 1982; **Fac Appt:** Prof Oto, Yale Univ

Vining, Eugenia M MD (Oto) - **Spec Exp:** Sinus Disorders/Surgery; Skull Base Tumors; Sinus Tumors; **Hospital:** Yale-New Haven Hosp, Hosp of St Raphael; **Address:** 46 Prince St, Ste 601, New Haven, CT 06519; **Phone:** 203-752-1726; **Board Cert:** Otolaryngology 1993; **Med School:** Yale Univ 1987; **Resid:** Otolaryngology, Yale-New Haven Hosp 1991; Otolaryngology, Yale-New Haven Hosp 1992; **Fellow:** Sinus Surgery, Univ Penn 1993

Pain Medicine

Saberski, Lloyd MD (PM) - **Hospital:** Hosp of St Raphael, Yale-New Haven Hosp; **Address:** Adavanced Diagnostic Pain Management, 150 Sargent Drive, New Haven, CT 06511; **Phone:** 203-624-4208; **Board Cert:** Internal Medicine 1985; Anesthesiology 1988; Pain Medicine 2004; **Med School:** NY Med Coll 1982; **Resid:** Internal Medicine, Albany Meml Hosp 1985; Anesthesiology, Albany Meml Hosp 1987; **Fellow:** Pain Medicine, Albany Meml Hosp 1988; **Fac Appt:** Asst Prof Anes, Yale Univ

Pediatric Cardiology

Friedman, Alan H MD (PCd) - **Spec Exp:** Echocardiography; Fetal Echocardiography; Cardiac Imaging; Sports Medicine; **Hospital:** Yale-New Haven Hosp, Yale Med Group; **Address:** Yale Univ, Dept Pediatrics, 333 Cedar St, 302 LCI, New Haven, CT 06520-8064; **Phone:** 203-785-2022; **Board Cert:** Pediatric Cardiology 2004; **Med School:** Wayne State Univ 1987; **Resid:** Pediatrics, Chldns Meml Hosp 1991; **Fellow:** Pediatric Cardiology, New Haven Hosp 1994; **Fac Appt:** Prof Ped, Yale Univ

Pediatric Endocrinology

Carpenter, Thomas O MD (PEn) - **Spec Exp:** Calcium Disorders; Bone Disorders-Metabolic; Thyroid Disorders; Parathyroid Disorders; **Hospital:** Yale-New Haven Hosp, Yale Med Group; **Address:** Yale Sch Med, Dept Pediatrics, 333 Cedar St, Box 208064, New Haven, CT 06520-8064; **Phone:** 203-764-9199; **Board Cert:** Pediatrics 1982; Pediatric Endocrinology 1999; **Med School:** Univ Alabama 1977; **Resid:** Pediatrics, Univ Alabama Hosp 1980; **Fellow:** Pediatric Endocrinology, Children's Hosp 1983; **Fac Appt:** Prof Ped, Yale Univ

Rivkees, Scott A MD (PEn) - **Spec Exp:** Thyroid Disorders; Adrenal Disorders; Neuroendocrinology; Growth Disorders; **Hospital:** Yale-New Haven Hosp, Yale Med Group; **Address:** Yale Dept Pediatrics, 464 Congress Ave, PO Box 208081, New Haven, CT 06520-8081; **Phone:** 203-737-5971; **Board Cert:** Pediatrics 1987; Pediatric Endocrinology 2005; **Med School:** UMDNJ-NJ Med Sch, Newark 1982; **Resid:** Pediatrics, Mass Genl Hosp 1985; **Fellow:** Pediatric Endocrinology, Mass Genl Hosp 1986; **Fac Appt:** Prof Ped, Yale Univ

Tamborlane, William V MD (PEn) - **Spec Exp:** Diabetes; **Hospital:** Yale-New Haven Hosp; **Address:** Yale Pediatric Endocrinology, 333 Cedar St, rm 3091-LMP, New Haven, CT 06510-3289; **Phone:** 203-764-6747; **Board Cert:** Pediatrics 1978; Pediatric Endocrinology 1986; **Med School:** Georgetown Univ 1972; **Resid:** Pediatrics, Georgetown Univ Hosp 1975; **Fellow:** Pediatric Endocrinology, Yale-New Haven Hosp 1977; **Fac Appt:** Prof Ped, Yale Univ

Pediatric Hematology-Oncology

Kadan-Lottick, Nina S MD (PHO) - **Spec Exp:** Cancer Survivors-Late Effects of Therapy; **Hospital:** Yale-New Haven Hosp, Yale Med Group; **Address:** Yale Pediatric Hematology/Oncology, PO Box 208064, 333 Cedar St, LMP 2073, New Haven, CT 06520; **Phone:** 203-785-4640; **Board Cert:** Pediatrics 2004; Pediatric Hematology-Oncology 2009; **Med School:** Johns Hopkins Univ 1993; **Resid:** Pediatrics, Johns Hopkins Hosp 1996; **Fellow:** Pediatric Hematology-Oncology, Chldns Hosp 1999; Cancer Epidemiology, Univ Minnesota 2000; **Fac Appt:** Asst Prof Ped, Yale Univ

McNamara, Joseph M MD (PHO) - **Hospital:** Yale-New Haven Hosp, Yale Med Group; **Address:** Pediatric Hematology/Oncology Assocs, 405 Church St, Guilford, CT 06437; **Phone:** 203-453-2013; **Board Cert:** Pediatrics 1987; Pediatric Hematology-Oncology 2005; **Med School:** Italy 1982; **Resid:** Pediatrics, Misericordia Hosp 1985; **Fellow:** Pediatric Hematology-Oncology, Schneider Chldns Hosp 1987

Pediatric Infectious Disease

Andiman, Warren A MD (PInf) - **Spec Exp:** AIDS/HIV; Viral Infections; Lyme Disease; Infectious Mononucleosis; **Hospital:** Yale-New Haven Hosp, Yale Med Group; **Address:** 333 Cedar St, rm 418 LSOG, Box 208064, Yale Univ Sch Med, New Haven, CT 06520-8064; **Phone:** 203-785-4730; **Board Cert:** Pediatrics 1975; **Med School:** Albert Einstein Coll Med 1969; **Resid:** Pediatrics, Babies Hosp-Columbia Presby 1971; **Fellow:** Pediatric Infectious Disease, Yale Univ Sch Med 1973; **Fac Appt:** Prof Ped, Yale Univ

Baltimore, Robert MD (PInf) - **Spec Exp:** Neonatal Infections; Hospital Acquired Infections; Tuberculosis; **Hospital:** Yale-New Haven Hosp, Yale Med Group; **Address:** Yale Univ Sch Med, Dept Pediatrics, 333 Cedar St, Box 208064, New Haven, CT 06520-8064; **Phone:** 203-785-4750; **Board Cert:** Pediatrics 1975; Pediatric Infectious Disease 2008; **Med School:** SUNY Buffalo 1968; **Resid:** Pediatrics, Univ Chicago Hosps 1971; **Fellow:** Infectious Disease, Boston City Hosp-Harvard 1976; **Fac Appt:** Prof Ped, Yale Univ

Shapiro, Eugene D MD (PInf) - **Spec Exp:** Lyme Disease; Vaccines; **Hospital:** Yale-New Haven Hosp, Yale Med Group; **Address:** Yale Univ, Dept Pediatrics, 333 Cedar St, Box 208064, New Haven, CT 06520-8064; **Phone:** 203-688-4518; **Board Cert:** Pediatrics 1980; Pediatric Infectious Disease 2009; **Med School:** UCSF 1976; **Resid:** Pediatrics, Chldns Hosp 1979; **Fellow:** Pediatric Infectious Disease, Chldns Hosp 1981; Research, Yale Univ 1983; **Fac Appt:** Prof Ped, Yale Univ

Pediatric Pulmonology

Bazzy-Asaad, Alia MD (PPul) - **Hospital:** Yale-New Haven Hosp, Yale Med Group; **Address:** 333 Cedar St, PO Box 208064, New Haven, CT 06520-8064; **Phone:** 203-785-2480; **Board Cert:** Pediatrics 1987; Pediatric Pulmonology 2009; **Med School:** Amer Univ Beirut 1978; **Resid:** Pediatrics, Amer Univ Beirut 1980; **Fellow:** Pediatric Pulmonology, NY Presby Hosp 1983; **Fac Appt:** Assoc Prof Ped, Yale Univ

Pediatric Rheumatology

McCarthy, Paul L MD (PRhu) - **Spec Exp:** Lupus/SLE; Juvenile Arthritis; Dermatomyositis; Vasculitis; **Hospital:** Yale-New Haven Hosp, Yale Med Group; **Address:** Yale Schl Med, 333 Cedar St, Box 208064, New Haven, CT 06520-3206; **Phone:** 203-688-2475; **Board Cert:** Pediatrics 1974; Pediatric Rheumatology 2007; **Med School:** Georgetown Univ 1969; **Resid:** Pediatrics, Chldns Hosp 1972; **Fellow:** Pediatrics, Chldns Hosp 1974; **Fac Appt:** Prof Ped, Yale Univ

Pediatric Surgery

Moss, R Lawrence MD (PS) - **Spec Exp:** Congenital Anomalies; Cancer Surgery; Minimally Invasive Surgery; **Hospital:** Yale-New Haven Hosp, Yale Med Group; **Address:** Dept Surgery-Ped Surgery, PO Box 208062, rm FMB132, New Haven, CT 06520-8062; **Phone:** 203-785-2701; **Board Cert:** Surgery 1999; Pediatric Surgery 2003; Surgical Critical Care 2000; **Med School:** UCSD 1986; **Resid:** Surgery, Virginia Mason Med Ctr 1991; Surgical Critical Care, Chldns Meml Hosp 1992; **Fellow:** Pediatric Surgery, Chldns Meml Hosp 1994; **Fac Appt:** Prof S, Yale Univ

Pediatrics

Angoff, Ronald MD (Ped) *PCP* - **Hospital:** Hosp of St Raphael, Yale-New Haven Hosp; **Address:** 200 Orchard St, Ste 108, New Haven, CT 06511; **Phone:** 203-865-3737; **Board Cert:** Pediatrics 1978; **Med School:** Univ Cincinnati 1973; **Resid:** Pediatrics, Yale-New Haven Hosp 1975; **Fellow:** Child Development, Yale-New Haven Hosp 1977; **Fac Appt:** Assoc Prof Ped, Yale Univ

Canny, Christopher R MD (Ped) *PCP* - **Spec Exp:** Behavioral Disorders; Developmental Disorders; **Hospital:** Yale-New Haven Hosp, Hosp of St Raphael; **Address:** 9 Washington Ave, Hamden, CT 06518; **Phone:** 203-287-0552; **Board Cert:** Pediatrics 2002; **Med School:** Washington Univ, St Louis 1976; **Resid:** Pediatrics, Yale-New Haven Hosp 1978; **Fellow:** Child Development, Yale Child Study Ctr 1980; **Fac Appt:** Assoc Clin Prof Ped, Yale Univ

Gruskay, Jeffrey MD (Ped) *PCP* - **Hospital:** Milford Hosp, Yale-New Haven Hosp; **Address:** 20 Commerce Park, Milford, CT 06460; **Phone:** 203-882-2066; **Board Cert:** Pediatrics 1985; Neonatal-Perinatal Medicine 1987; **Med School:** Yale Univ 1981; **Resid:** Pediatrics, Childrens Hosp 1984; **Fellow:** Neonatal-Perinatal Medicine, Childrens Hosp 1986; **Fac Appt:** Assoc Clin Prof Ped, Yale Univ

Morgan Jr, James L MD (Ped) *PCP* - **Spec Exp:** Sports Medicine; **Hospital:** Yale-New Haven Hosp, Hosp of St Raphael; **Address:** 240 Indian River Rd, Ste B1, Orange, CT 06477; **Phone:** 203-795-6025; **Board Cert:** Pediatrics 1983; **Med School:** Med Coll VA 1978; **Resid:** Pediatrics, Chldn's Hosp 1982

Robert, Marie F MD (Ped) *PCP* - **Hospital:** Yale-New Haven Hosp, Yale Med Group; **Address:** 240 Indian River Rd, Ste B1, Orange, CT 06477; **Phone:** 203-795-6025; **Board Cert:** Pediatrics 1984; **Med School:** McGill Univ 1976; **Resid:** Pediatrics, Chldn's Hosp 1978; Allergy & Immunology, Yale-New Haven Hosp 1979; **Fellow:** Infectious Disease, Yale Univ 1984

Shaywitz, Sally E MD (Ped) - **Spec Exp:** Learning Disorders-Studies Only; Dyslexia-Studies Only; **Hospital:** Yale-New Haven Hosp, Yale Med Group; **Address:** Yale Univ Dept Pediatrics, 333 Cedar St, PO Box 208064, New Haven, CT 06520-8064; **Phone:** 203-785-4641; **Board Cert:** Pediatrics 1971; **Med School:** Albert Einstein Coll Med 1966; **Resid:** Pediatrics, Albert Einstein Coll Med 1970; **Fellow:** Pediatrics, Bronx Muni Hosp Ctr 1968; Behavioral Pediatrics, Albert Einstein Coll Med 1970; **Fac Appt:** Prof Ped, Yale Univ

Plastic Surgery

Ariyan, Stephan MD (PlS) - **Spec Exp:** Melanoma; Head & Neck Cancer; **Hospital:** Yale-New Haven Hosp; **Address:** New Haven Hosp, 60 Temple St, Ste 4B, New Haven, CT 06510-2716; **Phone:** 203-786-3000; **Board Cert:** Plastic Surgery 1978; **Med School:** NY Med Coll 1966; **Resid:** Surgery, Yale-New Haven Hosp 1975; Plastic Surgery, Yale-New Haven Hosp 1976; **Fellow:** Surgical Oncology, Yale-New Haven Hosp 1971; **Fac Appt:** Clin Prof S, Yale Univ

Persing, John A MD (PlS) - **Spec Exp:** Craniofacial Surgery; Vascular Malformations; Cosmetic Surgery; **Hospital:** Yale-New Haven Hosp, Yale Med Group; **Address:** Yale Plastic Surgery, 330 Cedar St Boardroom Bldg Fl 3, New Haven, CT 06519-3218; **Phone:** 203-785-2570; **Board Cert:** Plastic Surgery 1985; Neurological Surgery 1986; **Med School:** Univ VT Coll Med 1974; **Resid:** Surgery, Univ Arizona Med Ctr 1976; Neurological Surgery, Univ Virginia Med Ctr 1982; **Fellow:** Plastic Surgery, Univ Virginia Med Ctr 1984; **Fac Appt:** Prof PlS, Yale Univ

Restifo, Richard MD (PlS) - **Spec Exp:** Breast Surgery; Abdominoplasty; Liposuction & Body Contouring; **Hospital:** St Vincent's Med Ctr - Bridgeport, Yale-New Haven Hosp; **Address:** 59 Elm St, Ste 560, New Haven, CT 06510; **Phone:** 203-772-1444; **Board Cert:** Plastic Surgery 2005; **Med School:** Harvard Med Sch 1986; **Resid:** Surgery, Georgetown Univ Hosp 1991; Plastic Surgery, Univ Pittsburgh Med Ctr 1993

Stahl, Richard S MD (PlS) - **Spec Exp:** Abdominal Wall Reconstruction; Chest Wall Reconstruction; Breast Reconstruction; Chest Wall Deformities; **Hospital:** Yale-New Haven Hosp, Hosp of St Raphael; **Address:** 5 Durham Rd, Guilford, CT 06437; **Phone:** 203-458-4440; **Board Cert:** Surgery 2001; Plastic Surgery 1984; **Med School:** Vanderbilt Univ 1976; **Resid:** Surgery, Yale New Haven Hosp 1981; **Fellow:** Plastic Surgery, Emory Univ Med Ctr 1983; **Fac Appt:** Clin Prof S, Yale Univ

Psychiatry

Lewis, Dorothy Otnow MD (Psyc) - **Spec Exp:** Dissociative Disorders; Aggression Disorders; **Hospital:** Yale-New Haven Hosp, Bellevue Hosp Ctr; **Address:** 100 York St, 8H, New Haven, CT 06511; **Phone:** 203-624-3933; **Board Cert:** Psychiatry 1972; **Med School:** Yale Univ 1963; **Resid:** Psychiatry, Yale-New Haven Hosp 1967; **Fellow:** Child & Adolescent Psychiatry, Yale-New Haven Hosp 1969; Psychiatric Research, Natl Inst Mental Hlth 1967; **Fac Appt:** Clin Prof Psyc, Yale Univ

McGlashan, Thomas H MD (Psyc) - **Spec Exp:** Schizophrenia-Early Detection/Treatment; Personality Disorders; Schizophrenia-Clinical Trials; Personality Disorders-Clinical Trials; **Hospital:** Connecticut Mental Hlth Ctr, Yale-New Haven Hosp; **Address:** Yale Univ Sch Med, Dept Psychiatry, 301 Cedar St, New Haven, CT 06519; **Phone:** 203-737-2077; **Board Cert:** Psychiatry 1973; **Med School:** Univ Pennsylvania 1967; **Resid:** Psychiatry, Mass Mental Hlth Ctr 1971; **Fac Appt:** Prof Psyc, Yale Univ

Riordan, Charles E MD (Psyc) - **Spec Exp:** Addiction/Substance Abuse; **Hospital:** Hosp of St Raphael; **Address:** Stony Creek Medical Center, 6 Business Park Drive, Ste 203A, Branford, CT 06405; **Phone:** 203-483-5300; **Board Cert:** Psychiatry 1970; **Med School:** Harvard Med Sch 1963; **Resid:** Psychiatry, St Vincent's Hosp & Med Ctr 1967; **Fac Appt:** Clin Prof Psyc, Yale Univ

Pulmonary Disease

Friedman, Lloyd Neal MD (Pul) - **Spec Exp:** Tuberculosis; **Hospital:** Milford Hosp, Yale-New Haven Hosp; **Address:** Milford Hospital, 300 Seaside Ave, Milford, CT 06460; **Phone:** 203-876-4288; **Board Cert:** Internal Medicine 1983; Pulmonary Disease 1988; Critical Care Medicine 1999; **Med School:** Yale Univ 1979; **Resid:** Internal Medicine, Beth Israel Med Ctr 1980; Internal Medicine, Oregon Hlth Scis Univ 1983; **Fellow:** Pulmonary Intensive Care, Yale-New Haven Hosp 1988; **Fac Appt:** Clin Prof Med, Yale Univ

Redlich, Carrie MD (Pul) - **Spec Exp:** Occupational Lung Disease; **Hospital:** Yale-New Haven Hosp, Yale Med Group; **Address:** Yale Occupational & Environmental Med, 135 College St Fl 3 - Ste 392, New Haven, CT 06510; **Phone:** 203-785-4197; **Board Cert:** Internal Medicine 1986; Occupational Medicine 1990; Pulmonary Disease 2002; **Med School:** Yale Univ 1982; **Resid:** Internal Medicine, Yale-New Haven Hosp 1986; Occupational Medicine, Yale-New Haven Hosp 1987; **Fellow:** Pulmonary Disease, Univ Washington 1989; **Fac Appt:** Assoc Prof Med, Yale Univ

Rochester, Carolyn L MD (Pul) - **Spec Exp:** Chronic Obstructive Lung Disease (COPD); **Hospital:** VA Conn Hlthcre Sys, Yale-New Haven Hosp; **Address:** Yale Univ Sch Med, Pulm & Crit Care Sect, 300 Cedar St, Box 208057, New Haven, CT 06520-8057; **Phone:** 203-785-3207; **Board Cert:** Internal Medicine 1986; Pulmonary Disease 2002; Critical Care Medicine 2006; **Med School:** Columbia P&S 1983; **Resid:** Internal Medicine, Columbia Presby Med Ctr 1986; **Fellow:** Pulmonary Disease, Columbia Presby Med Ctr 1988; **Fac Appt:** Asst Prof Med, Yale Univ

Tanoue, Lynn MD (Pul) - **Spec Exp:** Lung Cancer; **Hospital:** Yale-New Haven Hosp, Yale Med Group; **Address:** Yale Univ Sch Med, Div Pulm & Critical Care, 333 Cedar St, Box 208057, New Haven, CT 06520-8057; **Phone:** 203-785-6359; **Board Cert:** Internal Medicine 1985; Pulmonary Disease 1988; Critical Care Medicine 2002; **Med School:** Yale Univ 1982; **Resid:** Internal Medicine, Yale-New Haven Hosp 1985; **Fellow:** Pulmonary Disease, Yale-New Haven Hosp 1988; Critical Care Medicine, Yale-New Haven Hosp 1988; **Fac Appt:** Assoc Prof Med, Yale Univ

Radiation Oncology

Higgins, Susan A MD (RadRO) - **Spec Exp:** Gynecologic Cancer; Vulvar/Vaginal Cancer; Breast Cancer; Gastrointestinal Cancer; **Hospital:** Yale-New Haven Hosp, Yale Med Group; **Address:** Yale Therapeutic Radiology, 15 York St Hunter Bldg Fl 1, New Haven, CT 06520; **Phone:** 203-785-7033; **Board Cert:** Radiation Oncology 2004; **Med School:** Univ Rochester 1990; **Resid:** Radiology, Yale-New Haven Hosp 1993; **Fac Appt:** Assoc Prof RadRO, Yale Univ

Knisely, Jonathan MD (RadRO) - **Spec Exp:** Brain Tumors; Stereotactic Radiosurgery; Gastrointestinal Cancer; **Hospital:** Yale-New Haven Hosp, Yale Med Group; **Address:** Dept Therapeutic Radiology, 15 York St, Hunter Bldg-HRT 133, New Haven, CT 06520-8040; **Phone:** 203-785-2957; **Board Cert:** Internal Medicine 1989; Radiation Oncology 1993; **Med School:** Univ Pennsylvania 1986; **Resid:** Internal Medicine, Michael Reese Hosp 1989; Radiation Oncology, Univ Toronto Med Ctr 1992; **Fac Appt:** Assoc Prof RadRO, Yale Univ

Peschel, Richard E MD (RadRO) - **Spec Exp:** Prostate Cancer; **Hospital:** Yale-New Haven Hosp, Yale Med Group; **Address:** Yale-New Haven Hosp, Dept Therapeutic Radiology, 15 York St, rm HRT 142, New Haven, CT 06510; **Phone:** 203-785-2957; **Board Cert:** Therapeutic Radiology 1982; **Med School:** Yale Univ 1977; **Resid:** Radiation Oncology, Yale-New Haven Hosp 1981; **Fac Appt:** Prof RadRO, Yale Univ

Roberts, Kenneth MD (RadRO) - **Spec Exp:** Pediatric Cancers; Lymphoma; Hodgkin's Disease; **Hospital:** Yale-New Haven Hosp, Yale Med Group; **Address:** Yale Univ Sch Med, Dept Radiation Therapy, 15 York St, New Haven, CT 06520-8040; **Phone:** 203-785-2957; **Board Cert:** Internal Medicine 1987; Medical Oncology 1989; Radiation Oncology 1995; **Med School:** Duke Univ 1984; **Resid:** Internal Medicine, Ohio State Univ Hosps 1987; Radiation Oncology, Duke Univ Med Ctr 1992; **Fellow:** Hematology & Oncology, Duke Univ Med Ctr 1989; **Fac Appt:** Assoc Prof Rad, Yale Univ

Weidhaas, Joanne B MD (RadRO) - **Spec Exp:** Breast Cancer; Gynecologic Cancer; **Hospital:** Yale-New Haven Hosp; **Address:** Smilow Cancer Hospital, Dept Radiation Oncology, 35 Park St, New Haven, CT 06520; **Phone:** 203-737-2165; **Board Cert:** Radiation Oncology 2005; **Med School:** Tufts Univ 1999; **Resid:** Radiation Oncology, Meml Sloan Kettering Cancer Ctr 2005; **Fac Appt:** Asst Prof RadRO, Yale Univ

Wilson, Lynn D MD (RadRO) - **Spec Exp:** Lymphoma, Cutaneous T Cell (CTCL); Lymphoma, Cutaneous B Cell (CBCL); Lung Cancer; Head & Neck Cancer; **Hospital:** Yale-New Haven Hosp, Yale Med Group; **Address:** Yale Univ Sch Med, Dept Therapeutic Rad, PO Box 208040, New Haven, CT 06520-8040; **Phone:** 203-688-4344; **Board Cert:** Radiation Oncology 2004; **Med School:** Geo Wash Univ 1990; **Resid:** Therapeutic Radiology, Yale-New Haven Hosp 1994; **Fac Appt:** Prof RadRO, Yale Univ

Reproductive Endocrinology

Patrizio, Pasquale MD (RE) - **Spec Exp:** Infertility-IVF; Fertility Preservation in Cancer; **Hospital:** Yale-New Haven Hosp, Yale Med Group; **Address:** Yale Fertility Ctr, Dept OB/GYN, 150 Sargent Drive, New Haven, CT 06511; **Phone:** 203-785-4708; **Board Cert:** Obstetrics & Gynecology 2007; Reproductive Endocrinology 2010; **Med School:** Italy 1983; **Resid:** Obstetrics & Gynecology, Univ Naples 1987; Reproductive Endocrinology, Univ Pisa 1990; **Fellow:** Infertility, UC Irvine 1995; **Fac Appt:** Prof ObG, Yale Univ

Taylor, Hugh S MD (RE) - **Spec Exp:** Infertility-IVF; Endometriosis; Menopause Problems; Vaginal/Uterine Abnormalities; **Hospital:** Yale-New Haven Hosp, Yale Med Group; **Address:** Yale Univ School Med, Dept OB/GYN, 333 Cedar St, New Haven, CT 06520; **Phone:** 203-785-4708; **Board Cert:** Obstetrics & Gynecology 1999; Reproductive Endocrinology 2002; **Med School:** Univ Conn 1988; **Resid:** Obstetrics & Gynecology, Yale-New Haven Hosp 1997; **Fellow:** Reproductive Endocrinology, Yale-New Haven Hosp 1998; **Fac Appt:** Prof ObG, Yale Univ

Rheumatology

Craft, Joseph MD (Rhu) - **Spec Exp:** Lupus Nephritis; Lupus/SLE; Lyme Disease; **Hospital:** Yale-New Haven Hosp, Yale Med Group; **Address:** Yale Univ, Dept Med-Rheum Section, 300 Cedar St, rm S-541D - PO Box 208031, New Haven, CT 06520-8031; **Phone:** 203-785-2454; **Board Cert:** Internal Medicine 1980; Rheumatology 2008; **Med School:** Univ NC Sch Med 1977; **Resid:** Internal Medicine, Yale-New Haven Hosp 1980; **Fellow:** Rheumatology, Yale-New Haven Hosp 1985; **Fac Appt:** Prof Med, Yale Univ

Hutchinson, Gordon J MD (Rhu) - **Spec Exp:** Rheumatoid Arthritis; Lyme Disease; Polymyositis; **Hospital:** Hosp of St Raphael, Yale-New Haven Hosp; **Address:** 136 Sherman Ave, Ste 104, New Haven, CT 06511; **Phone:** 203-785-0885; **Board Cert:** Internal Medicine 1980; Rheumatology 1982; **Med School:** Switzerland 1976; **Resid:** Internal Medicine, Hosp St Raphael 1980; **Fellow:** Rheumatology, Yale Univ Med Ctr 1982; **Fac Appt:** Assoc Clin Prof Med, Yale Univ

Liebling, Anne MD (Rhu) - **Spec Exp:** Arthritis; Juvenile Arthritis; Fibromyalgia; **Hospital:** Yale-New Haven Hosp, Yale Med Group; **Address:** 60 Temple St, Ste 6A, New Haven, CT 06510; **Phone:** 203-789-2255; **Board Cert:** Internal Medicine 2000; Pediatric Rheumatology 2009; Rheumatology 2000; **Med School:** SUNY Downstate 1986; **Resid:** Internal Medicine & Pediatrics, Univ Chicago Hosps 1990; **Fellow:** Rheumatology, Univ Chicago Hosps 1993; Pediatric Rheumatology, Univ Chicago Hosps 1993

Schoen, Robert T MD (Rhu) - **Spec Exp:** Rheumatoid Arthritis; Lyme Disease; Osteoporosis; **Hospital:** Yale-New Haven Hosp; **Address:** 60 Temple St, Ste 6A, New Haven, CT 06510-2716; **Phone:** 203-789-2255; **Board Cert:** Internal Medicine 1979; Rheumatology 1982; **Med School:** Columbia P&S 1976; **Resid:** Internal Medicine, Yale New Haven Hosp 1979; **Fellow:** Rheumatology, Brigham & Womens Hosp 1981; **Fac Appt:** Clin Prof Med, Yale Univ

Surgery

Barcewicz, Paul MD (S) - **Spec Exp:** Cancer Surgery; Laparoscopic Surgery; Soft Tissue Tumors; Endoscopy; **Hospital:** Hosp of St Raphael, Yale-New Haven Hosp; **Address:** 6 Woodland Ave, Madison, CT 06443; **Phone:** 203-245-2977; **Board Cert:** Surgery 2002; **Med School:** Univ Rochester 1977; **Resid:** Surgery, Hartford Hosp 1982; **Fellow:** Surgical Oncology, Roswell Park Cancer Ctr 1984; **Fac Appt:** Asst Clin Prof S, Yale Univ

Emre, Sukru MD (S) - **Spec Exp:** Transplant-Liver-Adult & Pediatric; Hepatobiliary Surgery; Liver Cancer; Portal Hypertension; **Hospital:** Yale-New Haven Hosp, Yale Med Group; **Address:** 333 Cedar St, FMB 121, New Haven, CT 06520; **Phone:** 203-785-2565; **Med School:** Turkey 1977; **Resid:** Surgery, Univ Istanbul 1982; **Fellow:** Hepatobiliary Surgery, Univ Istanbul 1988; Transplant Surgery, Mount Sinai Med Ctr 1994; **Fac Appt:** Prof S, Yale Univ

Kurtzman, Scott H MD (S) - **Spec Exp:** Breast Cancer & Surgery; Sarcoma; **Hospital:** Waterbury Hosp, Univ of Conn Hlth Ctr, John Dempsey Hosp; **Address:** 1625 Straits Tpke, Ste 200, Middlebury, CT 06762; **Phone:** 203-568-2929; **Board Cert:** Surgery 2009; **Med School:** Albany Med Coll 1981; **Resid:** Surgery, Univ Maryland Hosp 1983; Surgery, UMDNJ Affil Hosp 1989; **Fellow:** Surgical Oncology, Natl Cancer Inst 1985; Surgical Oncology, Meml Sloan Kettering Cancer Ctr 1990; **Fac Appt:** Assoc Prof S, Univ Conn

Lannin, Donald R MD (S) - **Spec Exp:** Breast Cancer; Breast Surgery; **Hospital:** Yale-New Haven Hosp, Yale Med Group; **Address:** Yale-New Haven Breast Ctr, 800 Howard Ave, Yale Physicians Bldg, Lower Level 38, New Haven, CT 06520-8062; **Phone:** 203-785-2328; **Board Cert:** Surgery 2002; **Med School:** Univ Minn 1974; **Resid:** Surgery, Univ Minnesota Med Ctr 1982; **Fac Appt:** Prof S, Yale Univ

Salem, Ronald R MD (S) - **Spec Exp:** Cancer Surgery; Liver & Biliary Surgery; Gastrointestinal Cancer; Liver Cancer; **Hospital:** Yale-New Haven Hosp, Yale Med Group; **Address:** Dept Surgery, 333 Cedar St, TMP 202, New Haven, CT 06520-8062; **Phone:** 203-785-3577; **Board Cert:** Surgery 2000; **Med School:** Zimbabwe 1978; **Resid:** Surgery, Hammersmith Hosp 1985; Surgery, New England Deaconess Hosp 1989; **Fac Appt:** Assoc Prof S, Yale Univ

Udelsman, Robert MD (S) - **Spec Exp:** Parathyroid Cancer; Adrenal Tumors; Thyroid Cancer; Parathyroid Disorders; **Hospital:** Yale-New Haven Hosp, Yale Med Group; **Address:** Yale School Medicine, Dept Surgery, 330 Cedar St, FMB 102, New Haven, CT 06511; **Phone:** 203-785-2697; **Board Cert:** Surgery 1999; **Med School:** Geo Wash Univ 1981; **Resid:** Surgery, Natl Inst Hlth 1986; Surgery, Johns Hopkins Hosp 1989; **Fellow:** Gastrointestinal Surgery, Johns Hopkins Hosp 1990; Surgical Oncology, Natl Cancer Inst 1985; **Fac Appt:** Prof S, Yale Univ

Thoracic Surgery

Elefteriades, John MD (TS) - **Spec Exp:** Aneurysm-Thoracic Aortic; Transplant-Heart; Ventricular Assist Device (LVAD); **Hospital:** Yale-New Haven Hosp, Yale Med Group; **Address:** Yale Sch of Medicine, Dept Cardiothoracic Surgery, PO Box 208039, New Haven, CT 06520; **Phone:** 203-785-2705; **Board Cert:** Thoracic Surgery 2004; **Med School:** Yale Univ 1976; **Resid:** Surgery, Yale-New Haven Hosp 1981; Cardiothoracic Surgery, Yale-New Haven Hosp 1983; **Fellow:** Cardiothoracic Surgery, Yale-New Haven Hosp 1983; **Fac Appt:** Prof S, Yale Univ

Hashim, Sabet W MD (TS) - **Spec Exp:** Mitral Valve Surgery; Heart Valve Surgery; Maze Procedure for Atrial Fibrillation; **Hospital:** Yale-New Haven Hosp, Yale Med Group; **Address:** Yale Univ Cardiothoracic Surgery, 333 Cedar St, Boardman 204, PB Box 208039, New Haven, CT 06520-8039; **Phone:** 203-785-6214; **Board Cert:** Thoracic Surgery 2001; **Med School:** Lebanon 1975; **Resid:** Surgery, St Lukes Roosevely Hosp 1979; Cardiothoracic Surgery, Yale-New Haven Hosp 1981

Kopf, Gary S MD (TS) - **Spec Exp:** Cardiac Surgery; Pediatric Cardiothoracic Surgery; Congenital Heart Disease; **Hospital:** Yale-New Haven Hosp, Yale Med Group; **Address:** Yale Univ Sch Med, Dept of Surgery, Box 208039, New Haven, CT 06520-8039; **Phone:** 203-785-2702; **Board Cert:** Thoracic Surgery 2000; **Med School:** Harvard Med Sch 1970; **Resid:** Surgery, Peter Bent Brigham Hosp 1977; Cardiothoracic Surgery, Chldns Hosp Med Ctr 1980; **Fellow:** Cardiothoracic Surgery, Peter Bent Brigham Hosp 1980; **Fac Appt:** Prof S, Yale Univ

Sanchez, Juan A MD (TS) - **Spec Exp:** Lung Surgery; Esophageal Surgery; Cardiac Surgery; Thymoma; **Hospital:** St Mary's Hosp - Waterbury, Bridgeport Hosp; **Address:** 56 Franklin St, Waterbury, CT 06706; **Phone:** 203-709-6315; **Board Cert:** Thoracic Surgery 2004; Surgery 2008; **Med School:** Univ Fla Coll Med 1984; **Resid:** Surgery, Georgetown Univ 1989; Thoracic Surgery, Yale-New Haven Hosp 1993; **Fellow:** Research, Columbia-Presby Med Ctr 1990; Transplant Surgery, Yale-New Haven Hosp 1991

Urology

Colberg, John W MD (U) - **Spec Exp:** Prostate Cancer; Bladder Cancer; Kidney Cancer; Testicular Cancer; **Hospital:** Yale-New Haven Hosp, Yale Med Group; **Address:** Yale Urology Group, 800 Howard Ave Fl 3, New Haven, CT 06520-8062; **Phone:** 203-785-2815; **Board Cert:** Urology 2001; **Med School:** Washington Univ, St Louis 1985; **Resid:** Surgery, Yale-New Haven Hosp 1987; Urology, Yale-New Haven Hosp 1990; **Fac Appt:** Assoc Prof U, Yale Univ

Flanagan, Michael J MD (U) - **Spec Exp:** Prostate Disease; Incontinence; Incontinence-Fecal; **Hospital:** Waterbury Hosp, St Mary's Hosp - Waterbury; **Address:** Urology Specialists, 1579 Straits Tpke, Ste 2A, Middlebury, CT 06762; **Phone:** 203-757-8361; **Board Cert:** Urology 2003; **Med School:** UMDNJ-Univ Med Dent NJ 1985; **Resid:** Surgery, Waterbury Hosp 1988; Urology, Temple Univ Hosp 1992

Foster Jr, Harris E MD (U) - **Spec Exp:** Urology-Female; Urodynamics; Neurogenic Bladder; Voiding Dysfunction; **Hospital:** Yale-New Haven Hosp, Yale Med Group; **Address:** Yale Urology Grp, 800 Howard Ave Fl 3, New Haven, CT 06520-8062; **Phone:** 203-785-2815; **Board Cert:** Urology 2003; **Med School:** Univ Miami Sch Med 1987; **Resid:** Surgery, Univ Michigan Med Ctr 1989; Urology, Univ Michigan Med Ctr 1992; **Fac Appt:** Prof U, Yale Univ

Weiss, Robert M MD (U) - **Spec Exp:** Pediatric Urology; Testicular Cancer; Penile Cancer; Bladder Cancer; **Hospital:** Yale-New Haven Hosp, Yale Med Group; **Address:** Yale Univ Sch Med, Dept Urology, 800 Howard Ave, Box 208041, New Haven, CT 06520-8041; **Phone:** 203-785-2815; **Board Cert:** Urology 1970; **Med School:** SUNY Downstate 1960; **Resid:** Surgery, Beth Israel Hosp 1962; Urology, Columbia Presby Hosp 1967; **Fellow:** Pharmacology, Columbia Presby Hosp 1965; **Fac Appt:** Prof U, Yale Univ

Vascular & Interventional Radiology

Aruny, John E MD (VIR) - **Spec Exp:** Thrombolytic Therapy; Dialysis Access; Vascular Disease; Vein Disorders; **Hospital:** Yale-New Haven Hosp, Yale Med Group; **Address:** Yale Univ School of Medicine, 333 Cedar St, New Haven, CT 06520; **Phone:** 203-785-7026; **Board Cert:** Diag Rad with Spec Comp in Nuc Rad 1989; Vascular & Interventional Radiology 2009; **Med School:** Mexico 1983; **Resid:** Diagnostic Radiology, Westch Co Med Ctr 1989; **Fellow:** Interventional Radiology, Brigham & Women's Hosp 1992; **Fac Appt:** Assoc Prof Rad, Yale Univ

White, Robert I MD (VIR) - **Spec Exp:** Uterine Fibroid Embolization; Pelvic Congestion Syndrome; Varicocele Embolization; Hereditary Hemorrhagic Telangiectasia; **Hospital:** Yale-New Haven Hosp, Yale Med Group; **Address:** Yale Univ Sch Med, Vasc & Interventional Rad, PO Box 208042, New Haven, CT 06520-8042; **Phone:** 203-737-5395; **Board Cert:** Diagnostic Radiology 1970; **Med School:** Baylor Coll Med 1963; **Resid:** Internal Medicine, Johns Hopkins Hosp 1967; Diagnostic Radiology, Johns Hopkins Hosp 1969; **Fellow:** Cardiovascular Disease, Johns Hopkins Hosp 1958; Cardiovascular Radiology, Univ Minn Med Ctr 1971; **Fac Appt:** Prof Rad, Yale Univ

Vascular Surgery

DeNatale, Ralph MD (VascS) - **Hospital:** Hosp of St Raphael, Yale-New Haven Hosp; **Address:** Conneticut Vascular Ctr, 280 State St, North Haven, CT 06473; **Phone:** 203-288-2886; **Board Cert:** Vascular Surgery 2009; **Med School:** Italy 1979; **Resid:** Surgery, Hosp St Raphael 1984; Vascular Surgery, Baylor Coll Med 1985; **Fellow:** Cardiovascular Surgery, Baylor Coll Med 1986

Gusberg, Richard J MD (VascS) - **Spec Exp:** Endovascular Surgery; Aneurysm-Aortic; Renovascular Disease; **Hospital:** Yale-New Haven Hosp, Yale Med Group; **Address:** Yale Univ School of Med-Dept Surgery, 333 Cedar St, Box 208062, New Haven, CT 06520-8062; **Phone:** 203-785-6217; **Board Cert:** Vascular Surgery 2008; **Med School:** Columbia P&S 1970; **Resid:** Surgery, Columbia-Presby Med Ctr 1975; **Fellow:** Vascular Surgery, Columbia-Presby Med Ctr 1976; **Fac Appt:** Prof S, Yale Univ

Sumpio, Bauer E MD/PhD (VascS) - **Spec Exp:** Diabetic Leg/Foot; Endovascular Surgery; **Hospital:** Yale-New Haven Hosp, Yale Med Group; **Address:** Yale Univ School Medicine, Dept Surgery, 333 Cedar St, rm FMB137, Box 208062, New Haven, CT 06520; **Phone:** 203-785-6217; **Board Cert:** Vascular Surgery 2009; Surgery 2009; **Med School:** Cornell Univ-Weill Med Coll 1980; **Resid:** Surgery, Yale-New Haven Hosp 1986; **Fellow:** Vascular Surgery, Univ N Carolina Hosp 1987; **Fac Appt:** Prof S, Yale Univ

Sweeney, Thomas F MD (VascS) - **Spec Exp:** Minimally Invasive Vascular Surgery; Varicose Veins; Vein Disorders; **Hospital:** Yale-New Haven Hosp, Hosp of St Raphael; **Address:** 280 State St, North Haven, CT 06473; **Phone:** 203-288-2886; **Board Cert:** Vascular Surgery 2008; **Med School:** Yale Univ 1973; **Resid:** Surgery, Yale-New Haven Hosp 1977; **Fellow:** Vascular Surgery, Yale-New Haven Hosp 1978; **Fac Appt:** Assoc Clin Prof S, Yale Univ

The Best in American Medicine
www.CastleConnolly.com

Centers of Excellence

Addiction Psychiatry

BEHAVIORAL HEALTH

About the Behavioral Health Program:

The Behavioral Health Program at NYU Langone Medical Center offers the most up-to-date treatments available for a wide range of disorders including: Stress/anxiety, schizophrenia, depression (including medicine resistant depression), shyness, insomnia, low self esteem, women's issues, sexual difficulties, panic attacks and phobias, manic-depression, obsession and compulsions and attention-deficit/hyperactivity disorder. The program serves its patients through a variety of approaches including career counseling, assertiveness training, marital/couples counseling, and individual, group or family therapy. *We specialize in the following areas:*

Inpatient services

An inpatient unit serves an adult population and includes a special Young Adult Program. The service combines comprehensive diagnostic assessment and treatment including psychopharmacology, neuropsychology, psychotherapies and electroconvulsive therapy – a treatment in which seizures are electronically induced in anesthetized patients for therapeutic effect. A multidisciplinary team approach provides a continuum of behavioral and therapeutic modalities.

Outpatient Psychiatry

The Outpatient Psychiatry Program at our Tisch Hospital provides expert treatment to individuals suffering from a broad range of mental disorders and emotional problems including anxiety, depression (including medicine resistant depression) , insomnia, manic-depression, reproductive psychiatry, attention-deficit hyperactivity disorder and schizophrenia. Our multidisciplinary team of licensed psychiatrists, psychologists and social workers offer the most up-to-date and scientifically validated treatments such as psychotherapy, medication, or a combination of the two. For those who prefer it, direct treatment with a member of faculty is also available as an option.

Scientific Innovation

At NYU Langone Medical Center, scientific innovation goes hand in hand with patient care. Our physician-scientists continue to lead the way in psychopharmacology and continue to test new treatments for depression and bipolar disorder, with potentially life-altering results for the millions who suffer from these debilitating illnesses.

Sleep Disorders

The Sleep Disorders Consultation and Treatment Service provides thorough evaluation for a full range of sleep problems including insomnia, nightmares, narcolepsy, sleepwalking and restless leg syndrome. Both behavioral and medication treatments are available to treat sleep disorders.

PSYCHIATRY

About the Department of Psychiatry:
The Department of Psychiatry is dedicated to improving the health and well-being of its patient population by delivering peerless psychiatric services and care. The Department is home to some of the nation's most respected clinical psychiatrists and psychologists, with specialties in psychoanalysis, psychopharmacology, behavioral therapy, child psychiatry, geriatric psychiatry, neuropsychiatry, PTSD, and positron emission topography, a nuclear medicine imaging technique that produces a three-dimensional image of brain functions. *We specialize in the following areas:*

Inpatient services
The Inpatient Service Unit combines comprehensive diagnostic assessment and treatment including psychopharmacology, neuropsychology, psychotherapies and electroconvulsive therapy – a treatment in which seizures are electronically induced in anesthetized patients for therapeutic effect.

Outpatient Psychiatry
The Outpatient Psychiatry Program at NYU Langone Medical Center's Tisch Hospital provides expert treatment to individuals suffering from a broad range of mental disorders and emotional problems including anxiety, depression (including medicine resistant depression) , insomnia, manic-depression, reproductive psychiatry, attention-deficit hyperactivity disorder and schizophrenia. Our multidisciplinary team of licensed psychiatrists, psychologists and social workers offer the most up-to-date and scientifically validated treatments such as psychotherapy, medication, or a combination.

Post Traumatic Stress Disorder
Here at the Department of Psychiatry we offer assessment and treatment of PTSD in victims of sexual and physical assault, natural disasters, terrorism and combat trauma. Treatment includes end-based cognitive behavioral therapy and evaluation of strategies for the prevention of insomnia, stress, anxiety and depression.

Memory Impairment
The Pearl Barlow Center for Memory Evaluation and Treatment specializes in treating patients with memory impairments caused by neurological, psychological and physical ailments, as well as memory issues resulting from medication side effects, anxiety, depression and the effects of normal aging, including illnesses such as Alzheimer's disease. The multidisciplinary medical approach integrated with the most advanced research capabilities is the most comprehensive and first of its kind in the treatment of memory disorders in New York City.

Human Sexuality
The Human Sexuality Treatment Program provides a comprehensive evaluation of a full range of sexual disorders including erectile disorder, premature ejaculation, male orgasmic disorder, female orgasmic and arousal disorders, vaginismus, dyspareunia, lack of desire, the unconsummated marriage and sexual incompatibility between partners. Experienced, skilled clinicians carry out treatment in complete confidence and in the best tradition of the doctor-patient relationship.

Adolescent Medicine

AIDS/HIV

INFECTIOUS DISEASES

About the Division of Infectious Diseases and Immunology:
Developing effective treatment for infectious diseases is among the miracles of the last century's science, but today we are faced with deadly new infections and old ones that were never tamed. These and the rapidly emerging problem of resistance to antibiotics place the study and treatment of infectious diseases at the forefront of modern medicine. NYU Langone Medical Center faculty and fellows within the Division of Infectious Diseases and Immunology have expertise in the diagnosis, treatment and prevention of rare and common acute and chronic infectious diseases. Physicians within the Division are actively involved in the management of complicated bone and joint infections, prevention of infection in cancer and transplant patients and developing strategies for managing hepatitis B and C. The Division also offers the opportunity for patients with HIV to enroll in clinical trials of new drugs that are not yet widely available. ***We specialize in the following areas:***

HIV Prevention
The NYU Division of Infectious Diseases and Immunology has developed a uniquely effective program in HIV prevention that has gained wide recognition and has extended the hospital's expertise from New York City to West and East Africa.

AIDS Clinical Trials
The NYU AIDS Clinical Trials Unit is one of 35 such units designated and supported by the National Institute of Allergy and Infectious Diseases and is a dedicated resource for healthcare providers, researchers and scientists working in the field of HIV/AIDS research. It is one of the most productive units in the nation and enrolls adult and pediatric patients in clinical trials supported by the NIH. The data produced by the unit has supported the licensing of several drugs and plays an essential role in defining optimal therapies and preventing complications.

Population Biology of Infectious Diseases
This novel program combines laboratory and clinical studies with epidemiology (examines factors affecting the health and illness of populations) and genetics to reach maximum results. Research doctors in the Division of Infectious Diseases and Immunology are extensively involved in local and international research into the early diagnosis, treatment and prevention of chronic infections such as tuberculosis and Helicobacter (bacteria associated with stomach ulcers).

Medical and Molecular Parasitology
The NYU Division of Infectious Diseases and Immunology works alongside NYU Langone Medical Center's Department of Medical Parasitology to bring malaria and other parasitic diseases under control.

PEDIATRIC INFECTIOUS DISEASES

About the Division of Pediatric Infectious Diseases, Department of Pediatrics:
The Division of Pediatric Infectious Diseases (PID) of NYU Langone Medical Center, offers one of the largest programs in New York City for mothers and children with HIV infection at Bellevue Hospital Center an affiliate of NYU Langone. Initiated in 1982, this program furthers the understanding of the transmission of HIV from mothers to children and contributes to their improved care and longevity. The Division was one of the first NIH-funded Pediatric AIDS Clinical Trials Group sites and has cared for almost 500 HIV-infected children. It currently is funded as an HIV Clinical Trials site called IMPAACT (International Maternal Pediatric Adolescent AIDS Clinical Trials) devoted to the treatment of HIV infection, as well as its complications. Additionally, PID treats patients with other infectious diseases such as herpes viruses, respiratory viruses, hepatitis, bacterial, fungal and parasitic infections (tropical and local). We are also experienced in travel medicine and congenital infectious diseases.
We specialize in the following areas:

Adolescent HIV Clinic
The Bellevue Adolescent Clinic provides free, confidential HIV testing, pre- and post-test counseling, complete medical evaluations, comprehensive medical care and, if requested, referrals to clinical trials for HIV-positive teenagers. NYU Langone Medical Center was designated a Reaching for Excellence in Adolescent Care and Health (REACH) site, an NIH/HRSA-funded project. The clinic's primary objective is to increase the understanding of the natural history of HIV in teens and disease management.

Infectious Diseases Clinic
The Pediatric Infectious Diseases Clinic is one of the major providers of care for women and children at risk for HIV infection and other infectious diseases. Medical services are provided for children by the PID Clinic attending physicians, postdoctoral fellows and a pediatrician, with a dermatologist and pedodontist available. The clinic screens mothers for risk factors and provides counseling, testing and follow-up care for those receiving prenatal care.

Pediatric Infectious Disease
Children requiring intravenous infusions during the course of their illness are cared for at the Pediatric Infectious Disease Day Hospital. The hospital also provides the medical, nursing, psychological and social support services these children require. Pediatrics patients can also use the hospital for non-acute care outside of regular clinic hours.

TB Clinic
The TB Clinic evaluates approximately 200 new cases of latent and active tuberculosis a year and is a referral center for TB in the city. The Clinic is staffed by residents, a pediatric nurse practitioner, two PID attending physicians with particular expertise and experience with tuberculosis.

Viral Hepatitis Clinic
The Viral Hepatitis Clinic meets twice a week in Bellevue Hospital and follows approximately 250 children with chronic hepatitis C infection. The Clinic is a referral center for viral hepatitis infections in children and is the principal referral center for the NYC Pediatric Viral Hepatitis Network, a consortium of health facilities that is funded by the NY City Council.

The Best in American Medicine
www.CastleConnolly.com

Arthritis and Orthopaedics

NYU **Hospital for Joint Diseases**
NYU LANGONE MEDICAL CENTER

301 East 17th Street *(at Second Avenue)*
New York, NY 100036
www.NYUHJD.org
212-598-6000 fax: 212-260-1203

The Hospital for Joint Diseases (HJD) at NYU Langone Medical Center is one of the nation's leading orthopaedic and rheumatologic, specialty hospitals dedicated to the prevention and treatment of musculoskeletal diseases. The hospital provides some of the most advanced orthopaedic programs in the region for musculoskeletal disorders and the largest pediatric orthopaedic program in New York City. HJD is consistently ranked among the leading orthopaedic centers nationwide by U.S. News and World Report. *We specialize in the following areas:*

Orthopaedic Surgery

HJD faculty includes world-renowned surgeons working to treat a wide variety of orthopaedic and rheumatologic conditions. Areas of specialty include trauma and fractures, adult reconstructive surgery, hip and knee replacement, spine surgery, sports medicine, hand and wrist disorders, musculoskeletal oncology, foot and ankle care, shoulder and elbow problems, minimally invasive surgery of hip, knee, shoulder and spine, robotic-assisted joint replacement and pediatric orthopaedics.

Rheumatology

HJD is devoted to the care of patients with clinical problems involving joints, soft tissues and the combined conditions of connective tissues. Conditions treated include rheumatoid arthritis, osteoarthritis, lupus, pediatric rheumatology and Lyme disease.

Neurology

HJD provides a broad range of diagnostic and therapeutic services to patients with neurological disorders. Our outstanding clinical staff includes specialists in multiple sclerosis, pain management, spine and nerve pain, attention deficit disorder and cerebral palsy. Our Neurorehabilitation and Traumatic Brain Injury programs are centers of innovation and excellence for the treatment of neurobehavioral disorders. Additionally, the Initiative for Women with Disabilities is a center committed to providing high quality medical, gynecological and wellness programs promoting services for women with disabilities and chronic conditions in a fully accessible environment. We also provide multidisciplinary treatment to both children and adults with ADD at our Attention Deficit Disorder Center.

Radiology

HDJ provides complete inpatient and outpatient diagnostic orthopaedic radiology services, including MRI, computed tomography, ultrasonography and conventional radiography, as well as a multitude of musculoskeletal interventional procedures. Our neurointerventional specialist also performs the highly effective new vertebroplasty (a medical spinal repair procedure) for treatment of osteoporotic compression fractures. The faculty includes several internationally known musculoskeletal radiologists with expertise in all aspects of osteo-radiology.

Behavioral Health

Birthing Services

PROGRAM FOR IVF REPRODUCTIVE SURGERY AND INFERTILITY

**About the Division of Reproductive Endocrinology and Infertility,
Department of Obstetrics and Gynecology:**

The Division of Reproductive Endocrinology and Infertility at NYU Langone Medical Center can help patients realize their dreams of parenthood with its unique experience in all aspects of reproductive endocrinology, including the diagnosis and treatment of endometriosis, fibroids, problems with ovulation or sperm function and recurring pregnancy loss. The Medical Center offers the most advanced technology to assist infertile women and men who wish to conceive children. The combination of academic, scientific and technical expertise found at the Medical Center has created one of the most respected fertility programs and clinical divisions in the country. Our clinical work includes some of the world's finest technicians and physicians who have pioneered new innovations and been honored for their outstanding contributions to the field of reproductive medicine. *We specialize in the following areas:*

Patient-Centered Care

From the initial diagnosis through all stages of treatment, couples at NYU Langone Medical Center receive state-of-the-art compassionate care based on their specific needs. After a comprehensive evaluation to determine the cause of infertility, couples are counseled on whether assisted reproduction is necessary. Often surgery or stimulation of a woman's ovaries with medication can correct disorders that lead to infertility.

In Vitro Fertilization (IVF)

When medical conditions prevent the sperm from reaching the egg, skilled physicians and laboratory staff at the Fertility Center at NYU Langone Medical Center assist patients with retrieving their eggs, insemination in the lab and then insertion back into the patient's uterus as embryos. Preimplantation Genetic Screening (PGS)- The NYU Fertility Center offers tests for aneuploidy (an abnormal number of chromosomes). Embryos can also be tested for single-gene defects or can be tested for gender. This advanced technology allows prospective parents who are carriers of genetic conditions to avoid selective pregnancy termination. Some of the genetic disorders identified with PGS include: cystic fibrosis, Down syndrome, hemophilia, Huntington's disease, Marfan's disease, muscular dystrophy and sickle cell anemia. The state-of-the-art technology is also used to increase chances of delivery in certain women with a history of recurrent miscarriage or previous IVF failures.

Complex Cases

The NYU Fertility Center specializes in complex cases of infertility. Many patients have undergone IVF unsuccessfully elsewhere and some were even told that they should stop trying IVF. The Center offers the most advanced care available for patients still wanting to conceive.

IVF for Male Factor Infertility

The Fertility Center at NYU Langone Medical Center provides male patients with experienced urologists who can provide expert fertility treatment. As part of the diagnosis process, men receive a complete evaluation, including a fertility history, physical exam, blood testing and semen analysis. Surgical treatment of male infertility is performed onsite at the Center's surgical suites on an outpatient basis and may include the following procedures: testicular biopsy, vasectomy reversal, epididymal tissue repair, varicose vein repair and Microsurgical Sperm Aspiration used to obtain sperm when infertility is caused by blockage.

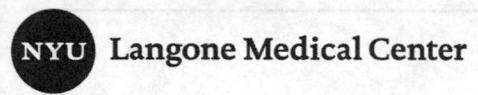

Breast Disease

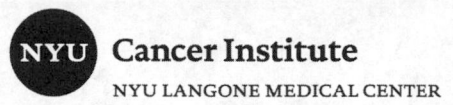

NYU Langone Medical Center
550 First Avenue , New York, NY 10016
www.NYULMC.org

NYU Clinical Cancer Center
160 East 34th Street, New York, NY 10016
www.NYUCI.org

**The Stephen D. Hassenfeld Children's Center
for Cancer and Blood Disorders**
160 East 32nd Street, New York, NY 10016
www.NYUMC.org/Hassenfeld

The NYU Cancer Institute is an NCI-designated cancer center and provides personalized patient care that is both compassionate and state of the art. The doctors and researchers work together to develop innovative therapies for patients. The Cancer Institute is world-renowned for excellence in cancer-focused research, personalized care, education and community outreach. Its mission is to discover the origins of human cancer and to use that knowledge to eradicate the personal and societal burden of cancer in our community, the nation and the world. For more information about our expert physicians, call 212-731-5000. *We specialize in the following areas:*

Patient-Focused Setting
The NYU Clinical Cancer Center is the principal outpatient facility of The Cancer Institute and serves as home to our patients and their caregivers. The center and its multidisciplinary team of experts provide access to the latest treatment options and clinical trials along with a variety of programs in cancer risk reduction/prevention, screening, diagnostics, genetic counseling and supportive services. In addition the NYUCI emphasizes the importance of a holistic approach to management services in complementary medicine, psychosocial support, survivorship and palliative care.

Renowned Expertise
The NYU Cancer Institute brings together experts from a variety of disciplines to create collaborative research endeavors and clinical care teams. The Cancer Institute offers a full continuum of personalized care, from prevention through diagnosis, treatment and post-treatment support. The compassion and expertise of our team members helps patients better manage the symptoms of their diseases as well as meet their special needs. Additionally, we have created special emphasis programs in diseases such as breast cancer, melanoma, GI cancer, prostate cancer, hematologic malignancies and lung cancer among others, as well as, translational programs in cancer healthcare disparities, molecularly targeted therapy, and the cell signaling pathways involved in cancer.

A Translational Approach
NYU Langone Medical Center scientists and other researchers excel in uncovering how cancer develops at the molecular level, and how we can harness that knowledge to reduce the risk of cancer and treat the disease. The Medical Center constantly seeks to create new opportunities for collaboration between investigators within our own institution, those located elsewhere in the NYU network of campuses, and researchers at other institutions.

The Stephen D. Hassenfeld Children's Center for Cancer and Blood Disorders
The center is a leading pediatric outpatient facility for the treatment of childhood cancers and blood diseases. Its unique interdisciplinary and family-centered approach combines the most advanced medical treatments with psychosocial and emotional support services for young patients and their families.

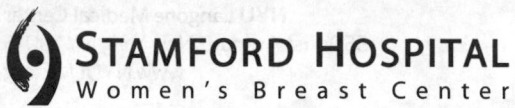

STAMFORD HOSPITAL
Women's Breast Center

Women's Breast Center

Stamford Hospital's Women's Breast Center is the first center in the nation to be recognized as a national Accreditation Program for Breast Centers. Our Center offers women a multi-disciplinary approach to care by focusing on imaging, pathology, medical and radiation oncology, genetic testing, nursing, and surgical care to treat diseases of the breast. Our facility is one of five out of the state's 133 breast imaging centers to have been designated a Breast Imaging Center of Excellence by the American College of Radiology.

Advanced Technology

All digital diagnostic care includes breast MRI with the highest resolution images available in Fairfield County, digital mammography that can image large breasted women, advanced computer assisted detection software, and equipment and procedures for minimally invasive biopsies.

Multi-disciplinary Team Approach

Our expert team is comprised of fellowship-trained female breast surgeons, reconstructive plastic surgeons, breast imaging fellowship-trained radiologists, breast pathologists, medical and radiation oncologists, nurse navigator and genetic counselor. The team meets on a weekly basis to discuss the best possible individualized treatment for each patient.

Personalized Care

In the event a problem is identified, our patients will have immediate follow up testing, see a surgeon within 24–26 hours and have the support of a dedicated nurse navigator to guide them through the process, from diagnosis through treatment and beyond. We work closely with the Integrative Medicine and Wellness team and the Bennett Cancer Center, in providing support services. We offer a warm setting for breast care designed with soft touches to make each and every patient feel as relaxed and comfortable as possible.

Academic and Clinical Affiliations

Stamford Hospital is an affiliate of the New York–Presbyterian Healthcare System and a major teaching affiliate of the Columbia University College of Physicians & Surgeons.

Accreditation

Joint Commission on Accreditation of Healthcare Organization (JCAHO)

Beds

305

Sponsorship

Voluntary, Not-for-Profit

For a Physician Referral or more information, please call 1.877.233.9355 or visit stamfordhospital.org /doctor.

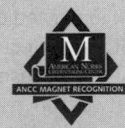

Stamford Hospital
30 Shelburne Road
Stamford, CT 06902
203.276.1000

stamfordhospital.org

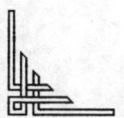
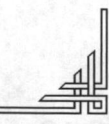

The Best in American Medicine
www.CastleConnolly.com

Cancer Care

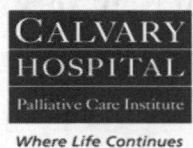

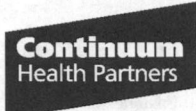

Continuum Cancer Centers of New York

(212) 844-6027

The hospitals of Continuum – Beth Israel Medical Center, St. Luke's and Roosevelt Hospitals and the New York Eye and Ear Infirmary – are leading providers of cancer care through Continuum Cancer Centers of New York. This year as part of a major expansion of our cancer care services, Beth Israel Medical Center opened The Beth Israel Comprehensive Cancer Center-West Side Campus, a state-of-the-art facility comprising 88,000 square feet located in Manhattan. Our integrated system allows us to build on the clinical strengths found at each of our partner hospitals.

The goal – and result – is delivery of care in ways that are more efficient, more attractive and more convenient for patients. Specifically, it means that cancer patients at any Continuum hospital can benefit from system-wide cancer expertise, facilities and resources. Continuum Cancer Centers feature world-renowned cancer specialists, including top-rated surgeons, medical oncologists, radiation oncologists, radiologists, pathologists, and oncology nurses.

Comprehensive diagnostic and treatment services are available for breast cancer, prostate cancer, head and neck and thyroid cancers, skin cancer, lung cancer, colorectal and other gastrointestinal cancers, lymphoma/Hodgkin's Disease, gynecological cancers, and cancers of the brain and central nervous system. Delivered efficiently in a friendly and supportive environment, our services include prevention programs – such as community education, screenings and early detection – expert diagnosis, outpatient treatment, inpatient services and home care. In addition, our Research Program offers patients access to investigational protocols through a wide number of clinical trials. Our physicians are leaders in both non-invasive and minimally invasive cancer treatments that focus on maximizing both the cure rate and the quality of life.

Support Services also play an important role at Continuum Cancer Centers. Our nurses, social workers, psychiatrists, chaplains, pharmacists, rehabilitation therapists and nutritionists all have specialized knowledge and expertise in the field of oncology. For help finding the services and care you need, please call us at (212) 844–6027.

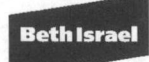 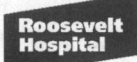 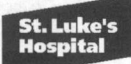 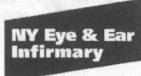

www.chpnyc.org

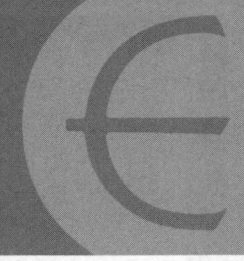

ENGLEWOOD
HOSPITAL AND MEDICAL CENTER℠
AN AFFILIATE OF MOUNT SINAI SCHOOL OF MEDICINE

350 Engle Street, Englewood, New Jersey 07631
Physician Referral: 1.866.980.EHMC
www.englewoodhospital.com and www.bestoncologydocs.com

CANCER CARE AT ENGLEWOOD HOSPITAL AND MEDICAL CENTER

The highly skilled cancer care experts at Englewood Hospital provide personalized, compassionate treatment to every patient. We are home to the latest research and technology, offering outpatients and inpatients the most advanced diagnostic capabilities and powerful, precise treatment options for all stages of various cancers.

Multidisciplinary Care: Once a diagnosis is made, a team of experts, including oncologists, hematologists, radiologists, surgeons, nurses, physical therapists, nutritionists and other healthcare professionals take part in designing and implementing a patient's treatment plan. Treatment plans for new patients who have been diagnosed or who have initiated a course of treatment at another hospital are also reviewed and/or reconfirmed by the team, including on-site pathologists. This innovative, multidisciplinary approach to treating each patient extends for the entire length of their treatment.

Nationally Recognized Breast Care: The Leslie Simon Breast Care and Cytodiagnosis Center is a leader in comprehensive, reliable and compassionate means for the early diagnosis and treatment of breast cancer. For women diagnosed with breast cancer, we offer the expertise, advanced methods and personal support to help them along their journey.

We were the first breast care facility in New Jersey to be recognized by the National Accreditation Program for Breast Centers. The American College of Radiology designated us a Center of Excellence, and the Intersocietal Commission for the Accreditation of Magnetic Resonance Laboratories has accredited our program for breast magnetic resonance imaging (MRI).

Higlights include:

- A dedicated breast MRI unit used to obtain conventional images and perform MRI biopsy
- Digital mammography, which offers a greater level of detail than traditional film mammography
- Vast experience in performing Fine Needle Aspiration (FNA); a cytopathologist is always on-site to perform the test and immediately interpret the results

- A High Risk Breast Cancer Program that provides risk assessment, genetic counseling and testing, and a personalized screening and prevention plan for women at increased risk of developing breast cancer
- A Mammography Screening Center that allows diagnostic and screening mammography patients to wait in separate areas
- A Telephone system that allows screening mammography patients to access their results within 24 hours
- A Patient Navigator program that helps breast cancer patients access services and programs offering both tangible support, such as free wigs, and emotional support, such as support groups that connect patients with survivors
- The services of Englewood Hospital's Center for Integrative Healing, which include oncology massage, acupuncture, holistic nutrition, stress management, and guided imagery for surgery and pain management

Advanced Imaging: We provide the highest level of accuracy in imaging to help diagnose all types of cancer and to measure the effects of cancer treatment. Our superior equipment includes an Aurora Dedicated Breast MRI System and combination PET/CT technology.

Surgical Expertise and Technology: Englewood Hospital is home to many of the area's top surgeons, including experts in breast, prostate, gynecologic and GI oncology procedures. A leader in minimally invasive and bloodless surgery, our experts use the latest technology, including DaVinci® Robotic-assisted procedures when appropriate, to ensure the best patient outcomes possible.

Infusion Center: For patients undergoing chemotherapy, our 8,000-square-foot infusion facility offers personal care in a modern environment. Highlights include 28 individual treatment areas, each with its own TV and a chair for a family member or friend; Wi-Fi access; and a nutrition center.

Research: The cancer care experts are also involved in ongoing oncology research studies regarding the proper treatment for breast, colon and rectal cancers; determining genetic abnormalities that may contribute to the development of certain types of cancer; possible environmental causes of breast cancer; and more.

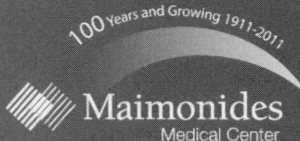

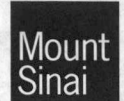
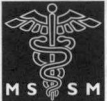

Mount Sinai

MSSM

MOUNT SINAI
SCHOOL OF
MEDICINE

THE TISCH CANCER INSTITUTE
AT THE MOUNT SINAI MEDICAL CENTER

One Gustave L. Levy Place
Fifth Avenue and 100th Street
New York, NY 10029-6574
Physician Referral: 1-800-MD-SINAI (637-4624)
www.tischcancerinstitute.org

THE TISCH CANCER INSTITUTE, part of The Mount Sinai Medical Center, is located on the Upper East Side of Manhattan, bordering East and Central Harlem. The Mount Sinai Medical Center was founded in 1852 and encompasses one of the oldest teaching hospitals in the country. In an atmosphere of learning, cutting-edge basic and clinical research, and superb patient care, The Tisch Cancer Institute coordinates a full-service diagnostic and treatment program for cancer patients. Because new treatments are developed at the Institute, patients often have access to these therapies before they are available anywhere else in the world.

A Heritage of Breakthroughs – Teams of physicians and scientists at The Tisch Cancer Institute at Mount Sinai work together to rapidly translate laboratory research into new patient treatments. Among the advances pioneered at Mount Sinai are the first successful treatment of tumors of the bladder by transurethral electrocoagulation, the first demonstration of how asbestos can cause cancerous changes in the DNA of cells, and the first development of an ultrasound-guided technique to insert radioactive seeds into the prostate to treat prostate cancer.

Services and Programs – The Tisch Cancer Institute employs a multidisciplinary treatment approach, providing access to clinical breakthroughs, innovative techniques, leading-edge technologies, and a wide range of diagnostic, therapeutic, and support services for all types of cancer. The Institute treats: breast cancer; head and neck cancer; thoracic cancer (including lung and esophagus); gynecologic cancer; hematological malignancies (including multiple myeloma, myelodysplastic syndrome and myeloproliferative disorders); brain tumors; and prostate, bladder, kidney, and liver cancer. In addition to surgical treatment, the Institute provides radiation and medical oncology therapies as well as bone marrow transplantation.

> **THE RUTTENBERG TREATMENT CENTER**
>
> The Derald H. Ruttenberg Treatment Center houses the ambulatory cancer program of The Tisch Cancer Institute and is operated by the Mount Sinai Hospital. The Ruttenberg Center provides physician evaluation and management services as well as chemotherapy and laboratory diagnostics. The members of The Tisch Cancer Institute—laboratory scientists and clinical investigators—are developing cancer therapies and prevention strategies to improve cancer care, and patients at the Center are the first to benefit from these treatments.

The Institute's multidisciplinary treatment approach involves collaboration with colleagues across the Medical Center, drawing upon the knowledge of a vast network of specialists who are outstanding in their fields. These experts consist of award-winning physicians and surgeons specializing in cardiac care, neurology, urology, pediatrics, digestive diseases, obstetrics and gynecology, and other therapeutic areas. Oncologists, surgeons, radiation oncologists, and specialists from across the medical spectrum work together to provide the highest quality care to all cancer patients. Furthermore, Mount Sinai's nursing staff is an important part of the Medical Center's focus on delivering exceptional patient care, and it has received the prestigious Magnet Award for nursing excellence.

Mount Sinai is renowned for its palliative care program, which provides the highest level of care, focusing on the relief of pain, symptoms, and stress in cancer patients in both an inpatient and outpatient setting.

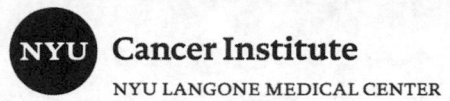

NYU Cancer Institute
NYU LANGONE MEDICAL CENTER

NYU Langone Medical Center
550 First Avenue , New York, NY 10016
www.NYULMC.org

NYU Clinical Cancer Center
160 East 34th Street, New York, NY 10016
www.NYUCI.org

**The Stephen D. Hassenfeld Children's Center
for Cancer and Blood Disorders**
160 East 32nd Street, New York, NY 10016
www.NYUMC.org/Hassenfeld

The NYU Cancer Institute is an NCI-designated cancer center and provides personalized patient care that is both compassionate and state of the art. The doctors and researchers work together to develop innovative therapies for patients. The Cancer Institute is world-renowned for excellence in cancer-focused research, personalized care, education and community outreach. Its mission is to discover the origins of human cancer and to use that knowledge to eradicate the personal and societal burden of cancer in our community, the nation and the world. For more information about our expert physicians, call 212-731-5000. *We specialize in the following areas:*

Patient-Focused Setting
The NYU Clinical Cancer Center is the principal outpatient facility of The Cancer Institute and serves as home to our patients and their caregivers. The center and its multidisciplinary team of experts provide access to the latest treatment options and clinical trials along with a variety of programs in cancer risk reduction/prevention, screening, diagnostics, genetic counseling and supportive services. In addition the NYUCI emphasizes the importance of a holistic approach to management services in complementary medicine, psychosocial support, survivorship and palliative care.

Renowned Expertise
The NYU Cancer Institute brings together experts from a variety of disciplines to create collaborative research endeavors and clinical care teams. The Cancer Institute offers a full continuum of personalized care, from prevention through diagnosis, treatment and post-treatment support. The compassion and expertise of our team members helps patients better manage the symptoms of their diseases as well as meet their special needs. Additionally, we have created special emphasis programs in diseases such as breast cancer, melanoma, GI cancer, prostate cancer, hematologic malignancies and lung cancer among others, as well as, translational programs in cancer healthcare disparities, molecularly targeted therapy, and the cell signaling pathways involved in cancer.

A Translational Approach
NYU Langone Medical Center scientists and other researchers excel in uncovering how cancer develops at the molecular level, and how we can harness that knowledge to reduce the risk of cancer and treat the disease. The Medical Center constantly seeks to create new opportunities for collaboration between investigators within our own institution, those located elsewhere in the NYU network of campuses, and researchers at other institutions.

The Stephen D. Hassenfeld Children's Center for Cancer and Blood Disorders
The center is a leading pediatric outpatient facility for the treatment of childhood cancers and blood diseases. Its unique interdisciplinary and family-centered approach combines the most advanced medical treatments with psychosocial and emotional support services for young patients and their families.

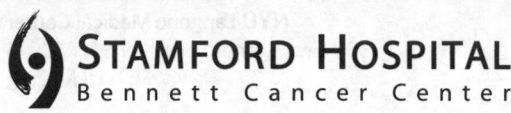

STAMFORD HOSPITAL
Bennett Cancer Center

Bennett Cancer Center

Stamford Hospital's Carl & Dorothy Bennett Cancer Center provides compassionate, patient-centered care from diagnosis through post treatment. We are accredited as a Teaching Hospital Cancer Program, the highest designation available to a community hospital. A multidisciplinary team of physicians, oncology nurses, nurse navigators and radiation therapists, offers advanced surgical, medical and technological services in a warm, caring environment.

Expertise Combined With Comfort
Our physicians' skill, knowledge and expertise are equaled only by their compassion in dealing with our patients. They are represented on the consulting staff of Memorial Sloan-Kettering Cancer Center and teaching faculty of Columbia University College of Physicians and Surgeons. They are also active participants in national research groups. The Center is involved with more clinical trials than any other area hospital.

Genetic Counseling
We offer the only full-time cancer genetic counselor in Fairfield County, ensuring timely delivery of genetic counseling services and superior interaction with other specialists, as well as the most current information in both genetics and oncology.

Treatment Beyond the Disease
We provide chemotherapy and immunotherapy in an outpatient setting, where patients can be treated in private suites with a home-like ambiance or a group room in the company of others. Cancer cases are reviewed by a multidisciplinary team of physicians and staff. This offers patients the benefit of different specialists combining their expertise.

Our Integrative Medicine Program and other support services including the *Transitions: Choices in Recovery* post-treatment survivorship program, offer a wide range of complementary therapies along with stress management, individual, family and group therapy.

Technology That Doesn't Forget Humanity
We are the only hospital in Fairfield and Westchester Counties to offer CyberKnife™ stereoatactic radiosurgery to treat tumors with pinpoint accuracy. Additional technology includes simulator and linear accelerator machines with both Intensity Modulated Radiation Therapy and Image-Guided Radiation Therapy. Our diagnostic imaging services include a 64-slice CT scan, ultrasound, nuclear medicine, PET CT and MRI.

Academic and Clinical Affiliations
Stamford Hospital is an affiliate of the New York–Presbyterian Healthcare System and a major teaching affiliate of the Columbia University College of Physicians & Surgeons.

Accreditation
Joint Commission on Accreditation of Healthcare Organization (JCAHO)

Beds
305

Sponsorship
Voluntary, Not-for-Profit

For a Physician Referral or more information, please call 1.877.233.9355 or visit stamfordhospital.org /doctor.

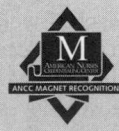

Stamford Hospital
30 Shelburne Road
Stamford, CT 06902
203.276.1000

stamfordhospital.org

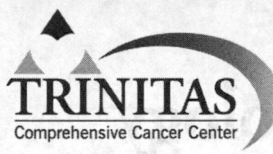

Cardiac Electrophysiology

Cardiovascular Disease

GAGNON CARDIOVASCULAR INSTITUTE

Morristown Memorial Hospital • Overlook Hospital

THE PASSION TO LEAD

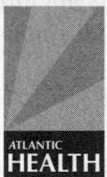

**Goryeb Children's Hospital • Atlantic Neuroscience Institute
Carol G. Simon Cancer Center • Gagnon Cardiovascular Institute
Atlantic Rehabilitation Institute**

P.O. Box 1905, Morristown, NJ 07962 • www.atlantichealth.org

To find a doctor, call 800-247-9580 or visit us online

Superior Cardiovascular Care

◢ **National Leadership in Cardiac Care, Close To Home** – Expert care and comprehensive cardiovascular services are available at Gagnon Cardiovascular Institute, which encompasses all cardiovascular services at Overlook Hospital and at Morristown Memorial Hospital. Morristown Memorial has the state's largest cardiac surgery program, with more heart surgeries performed there than at any other New Jersey hospital. Overlook Hospital has been approved to perform elective angioplasty and its newly established Women's Heart Awareness Program is designed to educate women about heart disease through screenings and analysis, information and education. We also offer the innovative "Live from the Cardiac Classroom" in cooperation with Liberty Science Center, where students can view heart surgery live via satellite.

◢ **Gagnon Cardiovascular Institute** – Housed in a new 250,000 square-foot building at Morristown Memorial and in a state-of-the-art facility at Overlook Hospital, Gagnon Cardiovascular Institute is staffed by more than 700 top-ranked, board-certified cardiac and vascular care specialists, nurses and technologists. The Institute's flagship facility at Morristown Memorial, which opened January 2009, features 106 private patient rooms, new operating and procedure rooms, the most advanced diagnostic tools and convenient access to all facets of cardiac care.

◢ **Newest Diagnostic and Treatment Options** – Gagnon Cardiovascular Institute offers the latest in non-invasive and cardiac imaging technologies, including 320 slice CT Image Cardiac CT Angiography and Volume Computed Tomography (VCT); cardiac MRI; advanced electrophysiology capabilities such as catheter ablation and mapping; leading technology for interventional procedures and advanced diagnostics; robotic surgery, a groundbreaking technology now in use at Morristown Memorial; and 24/7 critical transport services care.

◢ **Interventional Cardiology** – Every year, Morristown Memorial and Overlook doctors perform more than 7,500 successful cardiac catheterizations and angioplasties, saving thousands of lives.

◢ **Balloon Angioplasty**	◢ **Valvuloplasty**	◢ **Atherectomy**
◢ **Rotoblator**	◢ **Coronary Stenting**	◢ **Atrial Septal Defect Repair**

◢ **Cardiac Rhythm Management Program** – The cardiac rhythm management team performs comprehensive electrophysiology studies, radiofrequency ablations for supraventricular and ventricular tachycardias, pacemaker and defibrillator implantations and tilt table testing, and offers a comprehensive atrial fibrillation treatment program. The team also participates in important clinical trials to advance the standard of patient care.

◢ **Heart Success Program** – The Heart Success Program is a comprehensive inpatient and outpatient management program designed to provide specialized care for patients with advanced heart failure, cardiomyopathies and pulmonary hypertension. Our expert team evaluates patients and develops comprehensive plans of care. Our services include:

◢ **Bio impedance cardiography**	◢ **Cardiac rehab specifically designed for**
◢ **Acoustic cardiography (EP)**	**heart failure patients**
◢ **Metabolic stress testing**	◢ **Integrative medicine for heart failure**
◢ **Device optimization (EP)**	◢ **Pulmonary arterial hypertension evaluation**
◢ **Remote fluid status monitoring**	◢ **Integrative medicine**
◢ **Transplant and VAD evaluation**	◢ **Vascular**

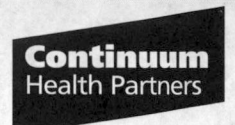

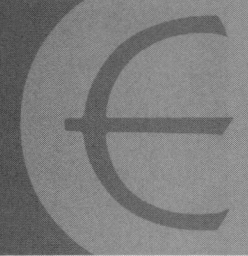

ENGLEWOOD
HOSPITAL AND MEDICAL CENTER℠
AN AFFILIATE OF MOUNT SINAI SCHOOL OF MEDICINE

350 Engle Street, Englewood, New Jersey 07631
Physician Referral: 1.866.980.EHMC
www.englewoodhospital.com and www.bestheartdocs.com

CARDIAC CARE AT ENGLEWOOD HOSPITAL

Celebrating a Decade of Cardiac Excellence, our Heart and Vascular Institute offers patients access to world-renowned experts in all areas of heart and cardiovascular care, including cardiac surgery, interventional cardiology, cardiac electrophysiology and vascular surgery. Our experts provide the latest medical, interventional and surgical treatments for coronary artery disease, valve disease, cardiac arrhythmias and other disorders of the cardiovascular system.

AN INDIVIDUAL APPROACH TO DIAGNOSIS AND TREATMENT

By taking a team approach and individualizing patient care, we are able to focus on the diagnosis and treatment of all manifestations of cardiovascular disease. At Englewood Hospital, top cardiologists, vascular surgeons, electrophysiologists, emergency medicine personnel, cardiac rehabilitation specialists and Magnet Award-winning nurses work together to offer a wide range of services, from treating sleep disorders to coronary bypass surgery.

A LEADER IN BYPASS SURGERY AND HEART ATTACK CARE

Englewood Hospital has continuously achieved among the lowest mortality rates in New Jersey for isolated coronary artery bypass graft surgery.[1] We have received this distinction from New Jersey's Department of Health and Senior Services despite accepting a high proportion of highly complex cardiac cases, including those who have been turned away by other institutions. These results were accomplished with one of the lowest average lengths of stay in the state, another measure of the quality care achieved.

According to statistics from the Center for Medicare Services (CMS), heart attack patients who received treatment at Englewood Hospital and Medical Center had a better chance of surviving over a 30-day period than those treated at any other New Jersey hospital. The same data places the Medical Center among the top three in the U.S. for one-month heart attack survival rate.[2] Furthermore, the hospital has been a leader in heart attack care with a "door to balloon" time better than 20 minutes below the national average over the past seen years.

GROUND BREAKING TREATMENTS AND TECHNOLOGY

Englewood Hospital acquired the Sensei® robot in 2008, and became the first facility in New Jersey to offer this technology. This specialized tool is used for catheter-based mapping within the chambers of a patient's heart, for more precise and stable catheter manipulation during complex cardiac procedures to diagnose abnormal heart rhythms. Benefits include increased accuracy, less tissue damage, reduced exposure to radiation, and shorter procedure times.

The Institute's CT Angiography Center utilizes a state-of-the-art 64-slice detection scanner – the first scanner fast enough to accurately reveal blockages in the coronary arteries. Our center is one of the few that have computerized reporting and routine correlation with invasive angiographic data, enabling doctors to begin treatment before problems occur.

[1]. As defined by the Dept. of Health and Senior Services, Cardiac Surgery in NJ, 2006
[2]. CMS data for Medicare patients discharged between July 2006 and June 2007.

Our Cardiac Program is proud to hold the following distinctions:

- Ranked #1 with a 100% survival rate in isolated coronary artery bypass graft surgery – a perfect record – in the past four Cardiac Surgery Report Cards by the State of New Jersey Department of Health and Senior Services

- Ranked #1 in New Jersey and #3 in the U.S. for 30-day Heart Attack Survival Rate by the Centers for Medicare & Medicaid Services

- HealthGrades® five-star rated for Coronary Bypass Surgery for two consecutive years (2010-2011) This designation ranks us among the top 10 in NJ for Cardiac Surgery.

- HealthGrades® five-star rated for Treatment of Heart Attack for three consecutive years (2009-2011) This designation ranks us in the top 10 in NJ for Cardiology Services.

- Award for "An Outstanding Cardiovascular Experience" from J.D. Power and Associates®

- CareChex® Medical Excellence Award (2009-2011) This designation places us in the top 10% in New Jersey.

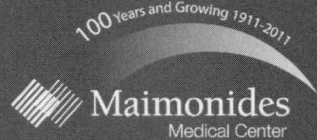
Having pioneered numerous heart care innovations through the years, the Cardiac Institute offers diagnostic studies and therapeutic treatments, procedures and surgeries. It has been ranked by the Centers for Medicare and Medicaid Services among those hospitals achieving excellent ratings in both heart attack and heart failure patient outcomes.

Cardiology
Among the most published and respected in the field, the Maimonides cardiology team continuously sets higher standards for patient care. Edgar Lichstein, MD, Chair of Medicine, has been chief investigator of NIH-sponsored cardiac drug trials, and our Congestive Heart Failure (CHF) Program is among the most effective in the nation.

Interventional Cardiology
Led by Cardiac Institute Chair Jacob Shani, MD, numerous therapeutic devices were developed and implemented here. Our Electrophysiology Lab has a superb record of achievement in diagnosing and treating arrhythmias. A close collaboration with the Department of Emergency Medicine ensures that chest pain patients are evaluated immediately and that interventional procedures are used to stop heart attacks in progress whenever necessary.

Cardiothoracic Surgery
The Maimonides Cardiothoracic Surgery program has an illustrious history, setting the national standard for advances in service. Under the direction of Greg Ribakove, MD, minimally invasive and robotic heart surgeries are offered in state-of-the-art facilities. In collaboration with Electrophysiology, Cardiothoracic Surgery has established an Atrial Fibrillation Center of Excellence. Maimonides provides one of the most prestigious cardiothoracic residency programs in the US.

Historic Moments
- In 1967, the first successful human heart transplant in the nation was performed at Maimonides.
- The intra-aortic balloon pump was developed here in 1970.
- Surgical techniques that protect the spine during cardiothoracic surgery were perfected here in 1982.
- Revolutionary cardiac catheterization devices were invented here in 1992 and 1997.
- Maimonides was the first hospital in US to implement fully automatic external cardiac defibrillators in 2001.

Physicians at Maimonides are among the small percentage in the US who use computers to enter patient orders, thereby reducing the risk of errors, increasing efficiency, and speeding the healing process. Maimonides has appeared on the American Hospital Association's "Most Wired" and "Most Wireless" lists more often than any other health care institution in the metropolitan area. Advanced technology allows our doctors to focus more attention on caring for their patients.

Maimonides Medical Center
Passionate about medicine.
Compassionate about people.

www.maimonidesmed.org/cardiac

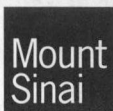
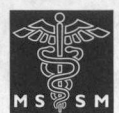

MOUNT SINAI SCHOOL OF MEDICINE

THE MOUNT SINAI MEDICAL CENTER
MOUNT SINAI HEART—CARDIOVASCULAR HEALTH
One Gustave L. Levy Place
Fifth Avenue and 100th Street
New York, NY 10029-6574
Physician Referral: 1-800-MD-SINAI (637-4624)
www.mountsinai.org/heart

At **MOUNT SINAI HEART**, we take both a personal and a global view of cardiovascular health. Our integrated system of care brings together the world's most accomplished physicians, research scientists, and educators who deliver creative programs and an unwavering commitment to the prevention and treatment of cardiovascular disease. With access to the latest discoveries and a diversity of the most experienced minds, our doctors ensure that patients receive the best individualized care. The rapid translation of innovative research into prevention, diagnosis, and therapy means that patients receive multidisciplinary treatment of unprecedented quality. Our programs treat patients from the earliest stages of life (our pediatric cardiologists can detect cardiac disease in the unborn fetus) well into the advanced elderly years (through specialized geriatric cardiology).

We specialize in consultative cardiology, cardiac catheterization, heart and lung transplantation, cardiovascular surgery, heart failure, pulmonary hypertension, lipid management, and hypertension, as well as:

Noninvasive diagnostic imaging – State-of-the-art echocardiography, nuclear cardiology, PET, CT, and MRI technology;

Coronary artery disease – We are ranked as New York State's highest volume and safest center for coronary angioplasty and other catheter-based procedures;

Cardiac rhythm disturbances – Expert management of all aspects of heart rhythm disorders is provided under the auspices of pioneers in the field, including for atrial fibrillation (AFib), the most common abnormal heart rhythm, and ventricular tachycardias, the most common cause of sudden cardiac death, as well as implantable devices, such as pacemakers and defibrillators;

Valvular heart disease – Medical and surgical options, including a leading valve-repair program and long-term follow-up care;

Aortic diseases – Pioneering techniques for stent-graft repair of thoracic and abdominal aortic aneurysms and for surgical correction of the most complex aortic pathology;

Congenital heart disease – Expertise in pediatric cardiology and in minimally invasive approaches to the correction of congenital heart defects in children and adults;

Cardiac failure and transplantation – A multidisciplinary team approach to comprehensive, compassionate care for patients with the most advanced forms of heart failure and cardiomyopathy;

Comprehensive cardiac disease prevention and rehabilitation – A unique synergism provides unparalleled patient care and breakthroughs in cardiovascular disease prevention and treatment, while promoting cardiovascular health globally through six projects around the world;

LEADING SURGEONS, INNOVATIVE TREATMENTS
Under the direction of internationally renowned cardiologist Valentin Fuster, MD, PhD, Mount Sinai Heart is recognized worldwide for expert evaluation, management, and prevention of cardiovascular disease through integrated patient care, education, and research. Mount Sinai Heart encompasses the Zena and Michael A. Wiener Cardiovascular Institute and the Marie-Josée and Henry R. Kravis Center for Cardiovascular Health at Mount Sinai, both preeminent resources for the study and treatment of heart and blood vessel diseases.

Vascular medicine and surgery – Noninvasive diagnostic procedures and an interdisciplinary approach to disease management, including medical, surgical, catheter-based, and gene therapy techniques for arterial obstruction, limb salvage, venous, and lymphatic diseases. A pioneer in large-artery stenting, Mount Sinai fostered the development of stenting of abdominal aortic aneurysms.

Mount Sinai's Cardiac Catheterization Laboratory – Studies the heart with the most precise technologies available, including diagnostic angiography, angioplasty, and biopsy. In a statewide study, our Cath Lab was found to be the busiest and safest, with the lowest 30-day risk-adjusted mortality rate for percutaneous coronary intervention (angioplasty).

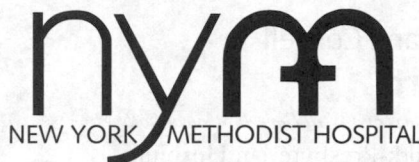
NEW YORK METHODIST HOSPITAL

THE INSTITUTE FOR CARDIOLOGY AND CARDIAC SURGERY

New York Methodist Hospital
506 Sixth Street, Brooklyn, N.Y. 11215
Phone 866 84-HEART (866-844-3278)
http://www.nym.org

SPECIALISTS AND MEDICAL SERVICES

The Institute is the Hospital's program for the prevention, diagnosis and treatment of all types of heart disease. The Institute brings together a panel of specialists and a range of services in all areas related to cardiac disease. These services, which range from screening and diagnostic procedures to emergency and ongoing treatment for heart attacks and chronic heart disease, are provided at the Hospital's specialized laboratories and clinical units, on both an inpatient and outpatient basis. New York Methodist houses state-of-the-art diagnostic and surgical facilities, including three cardiac catheterization laboratories and the most modern cardiac surgery suite in the area. The Institute's staff of physicians includes specialists in all areas of cardiology, electrophysiology, interventional cardiology and cardiac surgery.

PROGRAMS OFFERED

The programs and services offered by the Institute include consultative services, a chest pain emergency center (located in the Emergency Department), diagnostic evaluation (including cardiac MRI) and medical treatment for heart disease, interventional cardiology procedures (angioplasty and stents), electrophysiology (pacemakers, implantable defibrillators, ablation, etc.), and cardiac surgery.

* * *

Referrals to the specialists or to cardiac programs and services can be made through an individual's primary care physician or requested directly through the Institute's referral service. More information (and on-line physician referral) is available at the Hospital's website, http://www.nym.org.

THE NEW YORK METHODIST-CORNELL HEART CENTER

The New York Methodist-Cornell Heart Center is one of only three programs approved to perform cardiac surgery in Brooklyn. It is staffed by physicians from the prestigious Weill Cornell Medical Center of NewYork-Presbyterian Hospital. The Center is located in a new state-of-the-art cardiac surgery suite.

Procedures performed at the Center include coronary bypass surgery, off-pump bypass surgery, valve replacement and repair, thoracic aneurysm repair, minimally invasive cardiac surgery and bloodless heart surgery.

St. Francis Hospital The Heart Center®
100 Port Washington Blvd.
Roslyn, New York 11576
www.stfrancisheartcenter.com
(516) 562-6000 1-888-HEARTNY

A Leader in Cardiac Care

St. Francis Hospital, The Heart Center® is New York State's only specialty designated cardiac center and is one of the busiest heart centers in the nation. Located in Roslyn, New York, on Long Island's North Shore, St. Francis Hospital has been ranked among the best hospitals in the United States for the fourth consecutive year by *U.S. News & World Report* in heart and heart surgery and geriatrics, and for the first time, neurology and neurosurgery.

St. Francis Hospital:

• Has a highly experienced team of physicians and surgeons with one of the highest volumes in the nation for cardiac surgery, interventional and arrythmia procedures.

• Offers innovative approaches to cardiac surgery, including minimally invasive procedures and off-pump coronary artery bypass surgery, designed to minimize trauma and reduce surgical complications

• Performs one of the region's highest volumes of catheter-based techniques to close atrial septal defects (ASDs) and patent foramen ovale (PFO)

• Operates a nationally recognized Arrhythmia and Pacemaker Center staffed with electrophysiologists with over a decade of experience in radiofrequency ablation, a permanent cure for certain arrhythmias, including atrial fibrillation

• Maintains a high volume center for the implantation of cardiac pacemakers and defibrillators

• Offers the only world-class program in cardiac imaging that fully integrates all technologies including advanced methods in cardiac MRI, coronary CT angiography, PET/CT and three-dimensional echocardiography

• Has received the Magnet Award for excellence in nursing services

• Is a premier center for clinical trials and studies of the application of image-guided methods of diagnosis and treatment of heart disease

St. Francis Hospital has near-perfect patient satisfaction ratings, with over 99 percent of patients saying they would recommend the Hospital to family and friends.

"Our large cardiac caseload and our growing research program put us in an excellent position to introduce new techniques that can benefit thousands of people in need each year."

–Alan D. Guerci, M.D.
President and Chief Executive Officer
St. Francis Hospital, The Heart Center®

St. Francis Hospital The Heart Center®
100 Port Washington Blvd.
Roslyn, New York 11576
www.stfrancisheartcenter.com
(516) 562-6000   1-888-HEARTNY

Non-Invasive Cardiac Imaging
Using the latest in non-invasive cardiac imaging technology, St. Francis Hospital's physicians can evaluate blood flow, heart muscle strength, anatomy, and coronary artery blockages, allowing them to more effectively guide a patient's course of treatment.

Among the most recent advances in St. Francis Hospital's range of services are:

Coronary CT Angiography
St. Francis Hospital was the first hospital on Long Island to offer Multidetector Computed Tomography (MDCT) for non-invasive coronary artery imaging. This technology provides previously unobtainable non-invasive visualization of the coronary arteries and plaque build-up in the walls of the arteries.

Cardiac MRI
The only center on Long Island with a dedicated program and world-class expertise in cardiac MRI, St. Francis Hospital has the ability to non-invasively evaluate heart anatomy, function, blood flow, scarring and inflammation using advanced techniques on two state-of-the-art scanners. Cardiac MRI allows physicians to evaluate effects of heart attack and coronary artery blockages and noncoronary causes of heart failure to determine whether or not patients will benefit from heart surgery or other therapies. World-renowned cardiac MRI authority Nathaniel Reichek, M.D., leads St. Francis Hospital's clinical and research applications with cardiac MRI.

Three-Dimensional Echocardiography
St. Francis Hospital is an internationally recognized leader in three-dimensional echocardiography for quantifying the effects of heart disease and is the leading center in the New York metropolitan area in this field. By creating three-dimensional reconstructions of the heart and blood flow within it, this technology provides diagnostic information that far surpasses that available with conventional echocardiography in many patients.

Nuclear Imaging
Conventional nuclear imaging involves the injection of nuclear isotopes and imaging by a gamma camera that circles the patient's body, improving the accuracy of stress testing. St. Francis Hospital offers the latest advances in nuclear cardiology, such as single-photon emission computed tomography with CT attenuation correction (SPECT/CT). The nuclear cardiology laboratory at St. Francis Hospital is also a leader in developing new types of computer analysis to improve the value of SPECT imaging, and was among the first facilities in the U.S. to receive accreditation from The Intersocietal Commission for the Accreditation of Nuclear Medicine Laboratories. In 2009, St. Francis became the only Long Island hospital offering cardiac positron emission tomography with CT, or PET/CT, a new advanced approach which further enhances diagnostic assessment and clinical decision making.

Non-Invasive Imaging at St. Francis Hospital
Non-invasive imaging services at St. Francis Hospital include:

- multidetector computed tomographic coronary angiography
- cardiac MRI
- SPECT/CT nuclear Imaging
- Cardiac PET imaging
- transesophageal echocardiography
- three-dimensional echocardiography
- Stress testing with nuclear, echocardiographic or MRI imaging.

St. Francis Hospital's cutting-edge non-invasive imaging technology is also being applied in its research programs on cardiovascular disease. Drawing on its depth of experience with various imaging modalities, the Hospital has launched a multi-disciplinary effort at its St. Francis Cardiac Research Institute to improve methods for the diagnosis and treatment of cardiac disease. Past research efforts at the Hospital include The St. Francis Heart Study—a pioneering effort and the largest study of CT calcium scoring to be conducted at any single center—which supported the use of CT calcium scoring for atherosclerotic plaque detection as a tool in cardiac risk evaluation.

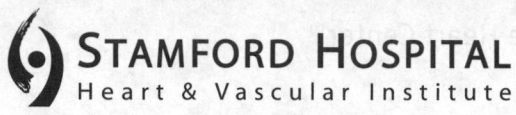

STAMFORD HOSPITAL
Heart & Vascular Institute

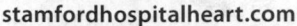
stamfordhospitalheart.com

Heart and Vascular Institute

Stamford Hospital's Heart and Vascular Institute is the only comprehensive cardiovascular program to include open heart surgery and elective and primary angioplasty in lower Fairfield County. We offer the finest cardiac services, including cardiovascular screening, diagnostic services, advanced cardiac non-surgical and surgical treatment, cardiac rehabilitation and integrative services and wellness programs.

Nationally Recognized Critical Care Unit

Stamford Hospital's Critical Care Unit has been recognized as one of the best in the country and earned the prestigious, national Codman Award, from the Joint Commission, for development of a life-saving protocol.

Cardiac Catheterization

Our two brand-new, state-of-the-art Cardiac Catheterization Labs, enable diagnosis and treatment of heart conditions, emergency angioplasty to open blocked coronary arteries during heart attacks, electrophysiology procedures that diagnose and treat heart arrhythmias, and the insertion of pacemakers and internal defibrillators. Emergency and elective angioplasty are performed for the treatment of acute myocardial infarction (heart attack) and coronary blockages.

Open Heart Surgery

Our expert team is equipped to handle any emergent and non-emergent surgical issue including CABG, valve repairs and replacements and aneurysm's using state-of-the-art surgical techniques. We have a dedicated team of surgeons, cardiac anesthesiologist, physician assistants, registered nurses and a clinical coordinator who provide patient-centered care.

Cardiac Rehabilitation

Located at the Tully Health Center, we help patients with heart disease recover faster and return to full, productive lives. Together with medical and surgical treatment, cardiac rehab includes exercise, education, counseling and behavioral change strategies that lead to a healthier life.

Integrative Cardiology and Wellness Programs

Offered through our Center for Integrative Medicine and Wellness, this program will offer multiple lifestyle techniques to complement and support the treatment of heart disease. The program is built on the belief that health and wellness involve healing of the spirit, mind and body not solely the treatment of heart disease.

Academic and Clinical Affiliations
Stamford Hospital is an affiliate of the New York–Presbyterian Healthcare System and a major teaching affiliate of the Columbia University College of Physicians & Surgeons.

Accreditation
Joint Commission on Accreditation of Healthcare Organization (JCAHO)

Beds
305

Sponsorship
Voluntary, Not-for-Profit

For a Physician Referral or more information, please call 1.877.233.9355 or visit stamfordhospital.org/doctor.

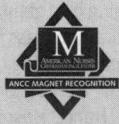

Stamford Hospital
30 Shelburne Road
Stamford, CT 06902
203.276.1000

stamfordhospital.org

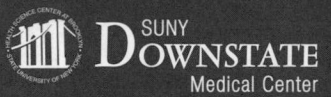

Child & Adolescent Psychiatry

Clinical Genetics

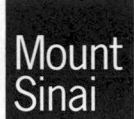
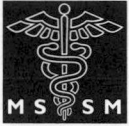

**MOUNT SINAI
SCHOOL OF
MEDICINE**

THE MOUNT SINAI MEDICAL CENTER
GENETICS AND GENOMIC SCIENCES
One Gustave L. Levy Place
Fifth Avenue and 100th Street
New York, NY 10029-6574
Physician Referral: 1-800-MD-SINAI (637-4624)
www.mountsinai.org

THE DEPARTMENT OF GENETICS AND GENOMIC SCIENCES at The Mount Sinai Medical Center is one of the largest medical genetics centers in the nation, providing expert diagnostic, therapeutic, and counseling services for patients and families with genetic disorders, birth defects, and pregnancy loss. The Department performs sophisticated diagnostic tests in its state-of-the-art DNA, biochemical, and cytogenetics laboratories, certified by NY State, CLIA, and CAP.

The Department has more than 50 internationally recognized physician and scientist faculty members, including American Board of Medical Genetics Certified Clinical and Diagnostic Laboratory geneticists, 10 experienced genetic counselors, and a full support and research staff of more than 150 people who provide expert clinical services.

Programs and services offered by the Department include:

- Comprehensive Genetic Diagnostic and Counseling Services
- Clinical and Laboratory Evaluation of Patients with Genetic Disorders, Birth Defects, and Reproductive Loss
- Prenatal diagnostic services
- Ethnicity-based carrier screening programs
- The Center for Jewish Genetic Disease
- Program for Inherited Metabolic Diseases
- Cancer genetic counseling program
- Cardiovascular Genetics Program
- Cleft and Craniofacial Program
- The Comprehensive Gaucher Disease Treatment Program
- The International Center for Fabry Disease
- The International Center for Types A and B Niemann-Pick Disease

Advances In Diagnosis And Disease Treatment – In the past several years, Mount Sinai researchers have identified the genes responsible for various genetic diseases and developed new treatments for inherited disorders. The following are some examples and results of this important work:

- We have identified the genes responsible for over a dozen diseases, most recently a debilitating juvenile arthritis, several dystonias, and an inherited form of obesity. The identification of these genes leads to precise diagnosis, understanding disease pathogenesis, and new treatments for these diseases. We have also recently identified a gene linked to prostate cancer.

GROUNDBREAKING RESEARCH AND NEW FORMS OF TREATMENT
Diseases and conditions run in families. In fact, there are more than 10,000 known genetic disorders, and current research is identifying the genetic susceptibilities or predispositions for many common diseases and cancers. The Faculty in the Department of Genetics and Genomic Sciences at Mount Sinai is performing research to develop new and improved methods for the diagnosis, prevention, and treatment of rare and common diseases. The Human Genome Project, and advances in gene analysis technology and stem cell biology, have accelerated this research.

- Our researchers have identified three genes causing Noonan syndrome, a common genetic disorder that causes congenital heart defects. Affected families can now receive early diagnosis and prevention.

- Research pioneered by the Department of Genetics and Genomic Sciences resulted in the development of a safe, effective, FDA-approved treatment for Fabry disease, an inherited metabolic disorder that can cause kidney failure, heart disease, stroke, and premature death.

- Departmental faculty have developed a treatment for Niemann-Pick Type B disease, a hereditary disorder that results in death in childhood or early adulthood.

Colon & Rectal Surgery

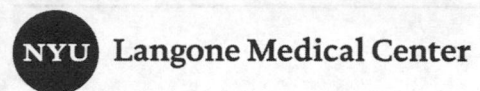

Langone Medical Center

550 First Avenue (*at 31st Street*)
New York, NY 10016
www.NYULMC.org
Physician Referral: **(888)7-NYU-MED** (*888-769-8633*)

COLON AND RECTAL SURGERY

About the Division of Colon and Rectal Surgery:

The colorectal surgeons at NYU Langone Medical Center, perform more than 5,000 outpatient and inpatient procedures each year using laser, laparoscopic, endoscopic and other minimally invasive techniques. Candidates for surgery receive same-day care that includes imaging, radiation and nutritional support. The program provides an integrated team approach, resulting in an environment that offers complete, patient-centered care. *We specialize in the following areas:*

Adrenalectomies

Surgeons at NYU Langone Medical Center are skilled at performing adrenalectomies, the surgical removal of one or both of the adrenal glands. This procedure is usually advised for patients with tumors of the adrenal glands. Adrenal gland tumors may be malignant or benign. Only functioning tumors excrete excessive amounts of one or more hormones. Adrenalectomy, once exclusively performed by conventional (open) surgery, is now routinely being performed with laparoscopy. In this manner, adrenalectomy can be accomplished through four very small incisions with patients usually being discharged within 36 hours.

Colorectal Cancer

NYU Langone Medical Center offers the most advanced screening options available for the diagnosis of colon cancer, the second leading cause of cancer death in the U.S. Additionally, the Medical Center continues to investigate colorectal cancer screenings in special populations such as women, veterans, immigrants, minorities and patients with HIV, and offer the use of virtual colonoscopy for the detection of colorectal polyps and cancer.

Laparoscopic Techniques

Surgeons at NYU Langone Medical Center use tiny incisions to remove a segment of the colon, which dramatically speeds recovery and reduces the need for pain medication. In addition treating colon cancer laparoscopically, this technique is used to treat pancreatic tumors, splenic related conditions, hiatus hernias, small bowel tumors and adrenalectomies.

Liver Lesions

Our surgeons effectively treat liver lesions with painless radiofrequency ablation. When the need arises, minimally invasive resections when feasible or open liver surgery is routinely performed at NYU Langone.

Robotic Surgery

NYU Langone Medical Center was the first hospital in New York City to use the minimally invasive da Vinci Si HD robotic surgical system and it is now used in operations of the colon. The robotic technology allows for a 40 percent higher definition view of the surgical field as well as an additional surgical arm to hold surgical instruments. The device also allows physicians to import and display medical test results from any computer or diagnostic medical device.

Virtual Colonoscopy

NYU Langone Medical Center offers the latest developments in colon cancer detection, including virtual colonoscopy. The noninvasive procedure makes use of sophisticated imaging techniques to generate a 3-D reconstruction of the inner surface of the colon, which can then be evaluated for abnormalities by specially trained radiologists.

Dermatology

DERMATOLOGY

About the Ronald O. Perelman Department of Dermatology:
With a history dating back to 1882, The Ronald O. Perelman Department of Dermatology at NYU Langone Medical Center is a national and international leader in dermatology, utilizing the most up-to-date advances in medicine and science to diagnose and treat skin disorders. The Department provides dermatologic care for more than 100,000 patients each year. In addition, faculty members conduct research focused on the most significant dermatologic problems including the prevention, detection and treatment of melanoma and other skin cancers. Our services include adult and pediatric medical dermatology, dermatologic/skin cancer surgery and cosmetic dermatology.
We specialize in the following areas:

Dermatologic / Skin Cancer Surgery and Cosmetic Dermatology
NYU Langone Medical Center's dermatologists provide specialized care for the treatment of malignant and benign skin lesions and offers cutting-edge therapies for aesthetic and cosmetic concerns. Mohs surgery represents an advanced technique for the removal of the most common forms of skin cancer to minimize the chance of recurrence. This microscopically controlled tissue-sparing procedure is performed by a specially-trained dermatologic surgeon.

General Dermatology
Dermatologic Associates at NYU Langone Medical Center offers multi-subspecialty dermatology care by physicians providing consultations and continuing care in a private office setting. Dermatologic Associates provides care for all patients with disorders of the skin, hair, and nails as well as for patients with complex illnesses, difficult to diagnose conditions or those experiencing treatment dilemmas. Examples include inflammatory skin diseases such as psoriasis and lupus, cancers and other skin tumors, hair loss, infections and allergic skin diseases such as eczema, contact dermatitis and hives.

Pediatric and Adolescent Dermatology
NYU Langone Medical Center also boasts a specialized professional practice dedicated to the treatment of diseases affecting the skin, hair, and nails of infants, children and adolescents such as acne, atopic dermatitis/eczema, hair loss, hemangiomas, moles, birthmarks, vitiligo and genetic disorders affecting the skin.

Charles C. Harris Skin and Cancer Unit / Dermatology Clinical Trials Unit
The Charles C. Harris Skin and Cancer Unit at our Tisch Hospital is an outpatient dermatology teaching center, combining unique patient care with superior medical education. The resident and attending physicians provide diagnostic and treatment services for skin diseases for patients of all ages, including common conditions such as acne, eczema and warts as well as complex medical conditions such as connective tissue disorders, pigmented lesions, skin allergies and skin cancers. The affiliated Dermatopharmacology Unit is one of the nation's most distinguished clinical research centers in dermatology. It is primarily responsible for carrying out clinical trials relating to inflammatory and autoimmune conditions such as psoriasis and lupus, skin cancer, acne, and infections.

Dermatopathology
Highly trained dermatopathologists at the Medical Center examine skin tissues submitted by physicians from biopsies and surgeries to diagnose skin diseases and malignancies. One of the busiest academic skin pathology units in the country, the Dermatopathology Section also provides consultative services for the review of skin pathology specimens performed elsewhere.

Diabetes Management/
Wound Care

Diagnostic Radiology

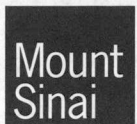
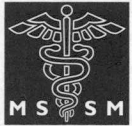

NYU **Langone Medical Center**

RADIOLOGY

The Radiology Department at NYU Langone Medical Center is committed to providing the most advanced imaging services by capturing the best images with the lowest dose possible. As an academic medical center, our radiologists are in a unique position to take the lead in helping to define and advance radiology in today's rapidly advancing technological environment.

Expertise
NYU Langone Medical Center's board certified radiologists and licensed technologists specialize in imaging and are involved in a variety of innovative collaborations and research initiatives. Our experienced eagle-eyed radiologists, with the assistance of the newest technology, are renowned for their interpretation and insight. Our staff consists of over100 sub-specialized academic radiologists, many of whom are acknowledged leaders and innovators in their field.

Advanced Technology
NYU Langone Medical Center uses some of the most advanced imaging equipment in the world. We offer high and ultra high-field MRI imaging systems (known as 1.5T and 3T magnets). Our MRI scanners are shorter and wider than ever—making for a more patient friendly experience. Our Center for Biomedical Imaging, a research facility features a 7T magnet.

Recognition for Safety and Quality
We continually follow a set of rigorous quality standards and maintain accreditation by the American College of Radiology (ACR). We are designated by the ACR as a "Breast Imaging Center of Excellence;" we have achieved high practice standards in image quality, personal qualifications, facility equipment, and quality control procedures and quality assurance programs.

Patient Focused Approach:
We are conveniently located and participate in an extensive number of insurance plans. We create timely delivery of reports and images and physicians can view patient exam status, reports and images online from their office. In addition to our convenient day time hours, weekend, evenings and often same day appointments are available. We provide language interpretation services, as needed.

We specialize in the following areas:
We offer an extensive range of diagnostic services in MRI, CT, ultrasound, PET/CT, X-ray, and interventional radiology and nuclear medicine. Subspecialized radiologists provide diagnostic interpretation in abdominal, biomedical, breast, cardiac, chest, emergency, general, musculoskeletal, neuroradiology, neuro interventional, nuclear medicine, pediatric, vascular interventional and women's imaging. Our Specialty Procedures Include: Coronary artery disease and virtual colonoscopy screening programs, Stereotactic biopsy capability, minimally invasive techniques including radiofrequency ablation and chemoembolization, Radioimmunotherapy, and Bone densitometry.

The Best in American Medicine
www.CastleConnolly.com

Gastroenterology

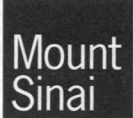
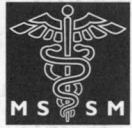

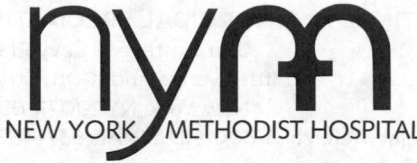

NEW YORK METHODIST HOSPITAL

THE INSTITUTE FOR DIGESTIVE AND LIVER DISORDERS

New York Methodist Hospital
506 Sixth Street, Brooklyn, N.Y. 11215
Phone 866 DIGEST-1 (866 344-3781)
http://www.nym.org

SPECIALISTS AND MEDICAL SERVICES

The Institute's panel of physician specialists includes gastroenterologists, hepatologists, surgeons, laparoscopic surgeons, radiologists, medical and radiation oncologists and pathologists. Nutritionists and psychologists are also members of the team. The latest advances in the diagnosis and treatment of the gastrointestinal tract and the liver are available. These include endoscopic ultrasound, pediatric and adult capsule endoscopy and advanced laparoscopic surgery. In addition, the Endoscopy Suite at New York Methodist Hospital enables physicians to perform highly advanced diagnostic and treatment procedures that can detect and describe disorders of the gastrointestinal tract and bile ducts as well as perform the non-surgical removal of bile duct gallstones.

PROGRAMS OFFERED

Among the programs and services offered by the Institute are a Colorectal Cancer Program, Heartburn (GERD) Program, Chronic Hepatitis B & C Program, Liver Transplantation Evaluation Program, Ulcer Program, Bowel Disorders Program and Pediatric Gastroenterology Program. Gallbladder and pancreatic conditions are also treated.

***

Referrals to the Institute's specialists, programs andservices can be made through an individual's primary care physician or requested directly through the Institute's telephone referral service. More information (and on-line physician referral) is available at the Hospital's website, http://www.nym.org.

THE PEDIATRIC GASTROENTEROLOGY PROGRAM

Problems commonly seen by physicians affiliated with the program include regurgitation, colic, constipation, diarrhea, recurrent abdominal pain, jaundice, blood in the stools, failure to thrive and formula intolerances. Children with these disorders present a special challenge because, along with the medical treatment that they receive, they need special care to ensure that their normal growth and development is not disrupted.

Special procedures that can be used to evaluate and diagnose pediatric gastrointestinal disorders include upper and lower endoscopies, liver biopsies and suction rectal biopsies. These procedures are performed by board certified specials in pediatric gastroenterology.

992

NewYork-Presbyterian

The University Hospital of Columbia and Cornell

NewYork-Presbyterian Digestive Disease Services

Affiliated with Columbia University College of Physicians and Surgeons and Weill Cornell Medical College

NewYork-Presbyterian Hospital
Weill Cornell Medical Center
525 East 68th Street
New York, NY 10065

NewYork-Presbyterian Hospital
Columbia University Medical Center
622 West 168th Street
New York, NY 10032

OVERVIEW:

The Digestive Disease Services of NewYork-Presbyterian Hospital provide expert capabilities in research, education and clinical care of patients with gastrointestinal, liver and bile duct, pancreatic and nutritional disorders.

The Hospital offers a wide range of diagnostic tests including,

- Routine procedures, such as endoscopy, capsule endoscopy, colonoscopy and flexible sigmoidoscopy.

- Endoscopic retrograde cholangiopancreatography (ERCP) to evaluate the ducts of the gallbladder, pancreas and liver

- Endoscopic ultrasonography (EUS) to provide detailed images of the upper and lower gastrointestinal tract and for the staging of patients with esophageal, gastric and rectal cancers. The Hospital is one of the few centers using EUS for needle aspiration of pancreatic cysts and tumors.

- Laparoscopy for direct examination of the liver, gallbladder and spleen and in the diagnosis, staging and treatment of pancreatic, gastric, esophageal and colorectal cancer.

The Hospital is a leader in treating gastrointestinal (GI) conditions. For example,

- The Minimal Access Surgery Center (MASC) is at the forefront of developing and applying new technologies, such as robotics, computerized image processing and enhanced optics. It is improving the outcomes of GI surgical patients and speeding their recovery from conditions such as GERD, gallbladder disease, and benign and malignant colon and rectal disease.

- Our surgeons also perform endoscopic sewing (endocinch) and radiofrequency treatment (Stretta procedure) for GERD.

- Our surgeons are internationally renowned in the use of laparoscopic methods for cancer and other colorectal conditions. They are highly experienced with the Whipple procedure to remove a pancreas tumor, which improves the survival rates and life expectancies of patients with pancreatic cancer and other less common pancreas problems.

Additionally, our physicians are involved in numerous clinical trials, (including studies on Cox-2 inhibitors) for preventing colorectal cancer and familial polyposis (a precursor to colorectal cancer), and antiviral therapy for chronic hepatitis C.

Physician Referral: For a physician referral or to learn more about the NewYork-Presbyterian Digestive Disease Services call toll free **1-877-NYP-WELL** (1-877-697-9355) or visit our website at **www.nyp.org/digestive**

COMPREHENSIVE CARE

Patients benefit from the collaboration of gastroenterologists, hepatologists, surgeons and diagnostic and pathology experts who develop optimal treatment plans. Areas of expertise include:

- GI Cancer, including esophageal, colorectal, liver, pancreatic and gastric tumors

- Inflammatory Bowel Diseases (Ulcerative Colitis and Crohn's Disease)

- Liver Diseases. The Hospital has a comprehensive Hepatitis C Center and the Center for Liver Disease and Transplantation

- Esophageal Disorders, including gastroesophageal reflux disease (GERD) and Barrett's esophagus

- Pancreatic and Biliary Disorders

- Celiac Disease

- Polyps of the Colon

- Peptic Ulcer Disease/Helicobacter Pylori Infections

- Gallbladder and Bile Duct Disorders

- Restorative surgery to avoid colostomies in diseases like rectal cancer, Crohn's disease, ulcerative colitis, and incontinence

- Anal diseases, such as hemorrhoids, fistulas, vascular tumors, abscesses and others

GASTROENTEROLOGY

About the Division of Gastroenterology, Department of Medicine:
The Division of Gastroenterology at NYU Langone Medical Center is dedicated to the diagnosis and treatment of patients with diseases of the gastrointestinal tract. Its physicians offer a rich body of knowledge in the diagnosis and management of inflammatory bowel disease, peptic ulcer disease, esophageal disorders, gastrointestinal cancer, and liver, biliary and pancreatic diseases.
We specialize in the following areas:

Colorectal Cancer
NYU Langone Medical Center offers the most advanced screening options available for the diagnosis of colon cancer, the second leading cause of cancer death in the U.S. Additionally, members of the Division continue to investigate colorectal cancer screenings in special populations such as women, veterans, immigrants, minorities and patients with HIV, and offer the use of virtual colonoscopy for the detection of colorectal polyps and cancer.

Esophageal Diseases
The Esophageal Disease Center at NYU Langone Medical Center offers patients state-of-the-art diagnosis and treatment of esophageal disorders and an ongoing program of translational and clinical research. The Center focuses on gastroesophageal reflux disease, esophageal motility disorders, Barrett's esophagus, adenocarcinoma of the esophagus and swallowing disorders. The Center offers diagnostic studies, such as esophageal manometry, impedance testing for swallowing, pH catheter and impedance testing for reflux and BRAVO capsule pH testing, as well as therapies, such Barrett's ablation and esophageal dilations, including those for achalasia.

Gastrointestinal Cancers
Gastrointestinal cancers are the most common group of cancers in the United States, accounting for approximately 20 percent of all non-skin cancers. They include cancers of the esophagus, stomach, colon/rectum, small intestine, liver, pancreas, gallbladder, and biliary tract. NYU Cancer Institute physicians treat patients with all types of gastrointestinal cancers, including those with complex cases such as those with recurrent disease or those whose disease persists despite treatments received elsewhere. Patients have the opportunity to participate in numerous clinical trials.

Complex Treatments and Diagnosis
Members of the Division have specific interest and expertise in the diagnosis of gastrointestinal bleeding of obscure origin, including the use of enteroscopy and capsule endoscopy. They have specific interest in diagnosis and treatment of patients with complex pancreatic-biliary diseases, including the use of ERCP and endoscopic ultrasound.

Virtual Colonoscopy
NYU Langone Medical Center offers the latest developments in colon cancer detection, including virtual colonoscopy. The noninvasive procedure makes use of sophisticated imaging techniques to generate a 3-D reconstruction of the colon, which can then be evaluated for abnormalities by specially trained radiologists. The study gives a complete evaluation of the entire surface of the colon and can be performed more quickly, with little discomfort and extremely accurate readings.

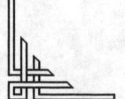

The Best in American Medicine
www.CastleConnolly.com

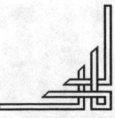

Geriatric Medicine

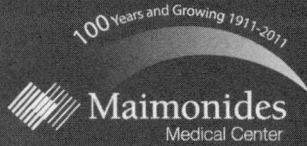

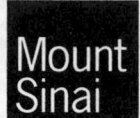
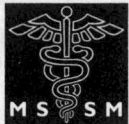

THE MOUNT SINAI MEDICAL CENTER
THE BROOKDALE DEPARTMENT OF
GERIATRICS AND PALLIATIVE MEDICINE

One Gustave L. Levy Place
Fifth Avenue and 100th Street
New York, NY 10029-6574
Physician Referral: 1-800-MD-SINAI (637-4624)
www.mountsinai.org

The Best in Clinical Care

In recognition of the care offered to older patients, The Mount Sinai Medical Center's **BROOKDALE DEPARTMENT OF GERIATRICS AND PALLIATIVE MEDICINE** is cited time and time again as the finest in the nation. In 2010, *U.S. News & World Report* ranked our geriatrics specialty #1 and our medical school program #2 in the United States.

We offer a full spectrum of patient care, including a specialized inpatient care team for the elderly to minimize complications sometimes associated with an older person's hospital stay, a primary care geriatrics practice for older adults living in the community, a hospital-based consultation service for patients throughout Mount Sinai, a number of community-linked programs and partnerships, and a palliative care team dedicated to ensuring the highest quality care and support for patients and families facing serious illnesses.

The Martha Stewart Center for Living, a modern facility designed by renowned architect C.C. Pei, provides clinical care and education for patients and serves as a training ground for physicians.

Groundbreaking Research – Mount Sinai's researchers continue to advance the understanding, prevention, and treatment of age-related disorders. The extensive research on aging conducted by the Brookdale Department of Geriatrics and Palliative Medicine includes studies on health services, medical decision making and ethical dilemmas, palliative care, the neurobiology of aging, and clinical interventions to promote independence in old age. The Department's expertise serves as a renowned educational resource for all Mount Sinai affiliates and other institutions in teaching geriatrics and palliative medicine to medical students, medical residents, geriatrics and palliative care fellows, established physicians, and health profession trainees in other disciplines.

History Of Excellence – The Mount Sinai Medical Center is a pioneer in geriatric medicine. In 1909, a Mount Sinai physician coined the term "geriatrics," and in 1914, he wrote the first textbook on medical care for older adults. Today, the Brookdale Department of Geriatrics and Palliative Medicine continues to break new ground, offering comprehensive care, disease prevention, and the promotion of healthy and productive aging. The Department's enhanced expertise in assessing and managing patients with dementia greatly complements its established, interdisciplinary approach to patient care, in which medical staff and social workers address each patient's needs as a team.

THE FIRST FREESTANDING DEPARTMENT OF GERIATRICS AT A U.S. MEDICAL SCHOOL

Mount Sinai's Brookdale Department of Geriatrics and Palliative Medicine was the first freestanding department of geriatrics established by a U.S. medical school, and it continues to be one of the very best. It offers unparalleled inpatient and outpatient care, as well as numerous treatment programs designed to meet the unique needs of older adults. Mount Sinai is also home to world-class researchers dedicated to advancing our understanding of Alzheimer's disease and other common geriatric conditions. At the Department's heart are its patients. The geriatricians of The Mount Sinai Medical Center work hard to improve life and longevity for New York's elderly.

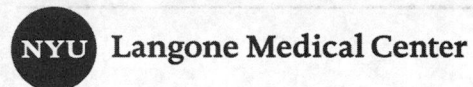
GERIATRIC MEDICINE

About the Section of Geriatrics, Division of General Internal Medicine, Department of Medicine:
The goal of geriatric medicine at NYU Langone Medical Center is to keep us all — for as long as possible — healthy, functional and vital members of our families and communities. NYU Langone Medical Center has a distinguished history in this vital specialty as a federally designated research center and leader in the care of geriatrics. Finding new answers and applying them to patient care are equally important. *We specialize in the following areas:*

Inpatient Geriatrics Services
Using a team approach, a senior geriatrician leads nurses, pharmacists, geropsychiatrists, rehabilitation experts, and fellowship trainees in caring for geriatric patients with complex conditions. NYU Langone Medical Center has also just started a new service to improve the care delivered to all older patients. If screening reveals a hospitalized patient is suffering from a geriatric problem (such as cognitive impairment), special consultation is offered to the patient's health care team.

The NYU Healthy Aging Initiative
Geriatric Medicine has a strong interest in healthy aging – assessing older individuals and advising them on what they can do to avoid developing problems such as cognitive or functional impairment. This is a fundamental part of the care provided by geriatricians within NYU Langone Medical Center's faculty group practice. In addition, we are currently piloting a Healthy Aging Clinic, with plans to expand it to NYU in the near future.

The William and Sylvia Silberstein Aging and Dementia Research Center
The Silberstein Aging and Dementia Research Center is a National Institute on Aging- designated Center of Excellence in Alzheimer's treatment. The facility provides comprehensive diagnostic evaluations to determine if memory loss is "normal" or more serious; a memory enhancement program for age-related memory decline; clinical trials for mild memory loss and for Alzheimer's treatment; state-of-the-art brain imaging techniques; methods to minimize disability in Alzheimer's patients; and comprehensive counseling and support groups for patients, caregivers and family members.

The Pearl Barlow Center for Memory Evaluation and Treatment
The Pearl Barlow Center for Memory Evaluation and Treatment is the clinical care and diagnostic unit of the Silberstein Alzheimer's Institute at NYU Medical Center. The Pearl Barlow Center for Memory Evaluation and Treatment specializes in treating patients with memory impairments caused by neurological, psychological and physical ailments, as well as memory issues resulting from medication side effects, anxiety, depression and the effects of normal aging, including illnesses such as Alzheimer's disease. The multidisciplinary medical approach integrated with the most advanced research capabilities is the most comprehensive and first of its kind in the treatment of memory disorders in New York City.

Geriatric Psychiatry

PSYCHIATRY

About the Department of Psychiatry:
The Department of Psychiatry is dedicated to improving the health and well-being of its patient population by delivering peerless psychiatric services and care. The Department is home to some of the nation's most respected clinical psychiatrists and psychologists, with specialties in psychoanalysis, psychopharmacology, behavioral therapy, child psychiatry, geriatric psychiatry, neuropsychiatry, PTSD, and positron emission topography, a nuclear medicine imaging technique that produces a three-dimensional image of brain functions. *We specialize in the following areas:*

Inpatient services
The Inpatient Service Unit combines comprehensive diagnostic assessment and treatment including psychopharmacology, neuropsychology, psychotherapies and electroconvulsive therapy – a treatment in which seizures are electronically induced in anesthetized patients for therapeutic effect.

Outpatient Psychiatry
The Outpatient Psychiatry Program at NYU Langone Medical Center's Tisch Hospital provides expert treatment to individuals suffering from a broad range of mental disorders and emotional problems including anxiety, depression (including medicine resistant depression) , insomnia, manic-depression, reproductive psychiatry, attention-deficit hyperactivity disorder and schizophrenia. Our multidisciplinary team of licensed psychiatrists, psychologists and social workers offer the most up-to-date and scientifically validated treatments such as psychotherapy, medication, or a combination.

Post Traumatic Stress Disorder
Here at the Department of Psychiatry we offer assessment and treatment of PTSD in victims of sexual and physical assault, natural disasters, terrorism and combat trauma. Treatment includes end-based cognitive behavioral therapy and evaluation of strategies for the prevention of insomnia, stress, anxiety and depression.

Memory Impairment
The Pearl Barlow Center for Memory Evaluation and Treatment specializes in treating patients with memory impairments caused by neurological, psychological and physical ailments, as well as memory issues resulting from medication side effects, anxiety, depression and the effects of normal aging, including illnesses such as Alzheimer's disease. The multidisciplinary medical approach integrated with the most advanced research capabilities is the most comprehensive and first of its kind in the treatment of memory disorders in New York City.

Human Sexuality
The Human Sexuality Treatment Program provides a comprehensive evaluation of a full range of sexual disorders including erectile disorder, premature ejaculation, male orgasmic disorder, female orgasmic and arousal disorders, vaginismus, dyspareunia, lack of desire, the unconsummated marriage and sexual incompatibility between partners. Experienced, skilled clinicians carry out treatment in complete confidence and in the best tradition of the doctor-patient relationship.

Gynecologic Oncology

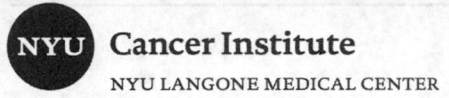

Hand Surgery

NYU **Hospital for Joint Diseases**

NYU LANGONE MEDICAL CENTER

301 East 17th Street *(at Second Avenue)*
New York, NY 100036

www.NYUHJD.org

212-598-6000 fax: 212-260-1203

HAND SURGERY

The Hospital for Joint Diseases (HJD) at NYU Langone Medical Center provides comprehensive care for patients with hand and wrist disorders including: fractures, congenital anomalies, soft tissue and skeletal trauma, degenerative and rheumatoid arthritis, sports-related injuries, vascular disorders, tumors and occupational disorders. Care is provided by specialists encompassing all aspects of diagnosis and treatment affecting the hand and wrist. *We specialize in the following areas:*

Orthopaedic Hand Program
Through its Division of Hand Surgery, the Hospital for Joint Diseases at NYU Langone Medical Center provides specific emphasis on fractures of the wrist and distal radius and reconstructive hand surgery. Hand surgery experts specialize in post traumatic injuries, arthritis and congenital, neuromuscular and neoplastic conditions. Offering one of the largest Hand Programs in the United States, NYU Langone Medical Center provides comprehensive care for the many problems that affect the upper extremity including: acute traumatic injuries (fractures, dislocations and tendon, nerve and vascular lacerations), post-traumatic and arthritic deformities, acquired problems (nerve compressions and tumors), congenital deformities and neuromuscular disorders such as cerebral palsy. The board-certified and fellowship-trained orthopaedists perform more than 5,000 operative procedures on adults and children each year.

Rehabilitation
After surgery, the outpatient Hand Therapy Unit at the Rusk Institute of Rehabilitation Medicine at NYU Langone Medical Center helps surgical patients recover full or partial use of their hands, providing comprehensive rehabilitation for a variety of ailments associated with the hand and upper body. The Unit specializes in fractures, traumatic injuries, tendonitis, sports injuries, work-related injuries, repetitive stress injuries, carpal tunnel syndrome, tendon and nerve repairs and arthritis. The Unit is staffed by expert occupational therapists that specialize in treatments of the hand and upper extremities.

Research
The research focus of the Hospital for Joint Diseases' Hand Service program at NYU Langone Medical Center is on a variety of clinical problems, including wrist fractures, non-unions of the scaphoid (bone between the hand and the forearm), Kienbock's disease (death and fracture of bone tissue due to interruption of blood supply), intercarpal subluxations (incomplete or partial dislocation) and neuropathies (disorders of the nerves) of the upper extremities.

Hematology

⌐ NewYork-Presbyterian
⌐ The University Hospital of Columbia and Cornell

NewYork-Presbyterian Cancer Centers

Affiliated with Columbia University College of Physicians and Surgeons and Weill Cornell Medical College

Herbert Irving Comprehensive Cancer Center	Weill Cornell Cancer Center
NewYork-Presbyterian Hospital	NewYork-Presbyterian Hospital
Columbia University Medical Center	Weill Cornell Medical Center
161 Fort Washington Avenue	525 East 68th Street
New York, NY 10032	New York, NY 10065

OVERVIEW:

The Cancer Centers of NewYork-Presbyterian Hospital draw on the traditions of innovation and excellence established by the scientific and clinical endeavors of the Herbert Irving Comprehensive Cancer Center at NewYork-Presbyterian Hospital/Columbia University Medical Center and the Weill Cornell Cancer Center of NewYork-Presbyterian Hospital/Weill Cornell Medical Center. The outstanding accomplishments of these centers in all areas of cancer research, diagnosis, treatment, and prevention, are world-renowned.

The Herbert Irving Comprehensive Cancer Center is one of only two National Cancer Institute-designated comprehensive cancer centers in Manhattan. It is committed to eradicating cancer through research, education, and patient care. The Center also promotes interdisciplinary laboratory, clinical, and population-based research, and facilitates the application of this research to cancer prevention, diagnosis, and treatment.

Weill Cornell Cancer Center brings together specialists in the diagnosis, treatment, and prevention of cancer, and conducts a wide range of basic science and clinical research to help make the newest and most promising cancer treatments possible.

The Cancer Centers, which treat over 7,000 newly diagnosed patients annually, include the following specialty programs:

- AIDS-related Malignancies
- Bone Marrow Transplant
- Brain Cancer
- Breast Cancer
- Dermatologic/Skin Cancer
- Esophageal Cancer
- Gastrointestinal Cancers
- Genitourinary Cancers including bladder, kidney and prostate
- Gynecologic Cancers
- Head and Neck Cancers
- Hodgkin's Lymphoma and Non Hodgkin's Lymphoma
- Lung Cancer
- Myelodysplastic Syndrome
- Myeloma
- Myeloproliferative Disease
- Neurological Cancer
- Ophthalmic Cancer
- Pancreatic Cancer
- Pediatric Hematology/Oncology
- Radiation Oncology
- Sarcomas and Mesotheliomas

Research programs are supported by grants from the National Cancer Institute, the National Institutes of Health, other federal agencies, the Leukemia and Lymphoma Society, the Lymphoma Research Foundation, the Avon Breast Cancer Research Foundation, the Komen Breast Cancer Foundation, and other private foundations and philanthropic organizations. Patients have access to over 500 clinical trials.

Physician Referral: For a physician referral call toll free **1-877-NYP-WELL** (1-877-697-9355) or to learn more about our Cancer Centers visit our website at **www.nyp.org/cancer**

ADVANCED SURGICAL AND THERAPEUTIC SERVICES INCLUDE:

- Double cord transplants and use of mesenchymal stem cells to treat graft vs. host disease
- Sentinel node biopsy to assess spread of breast cancer
- Skin sparing mastectomy and nipple sparing techniques for breast cancer and oncoplastic procedures
- Interventional endoscopy and laparoscopic surgery for colon and other gastrointestinal cancers
- Stereotactic biopsies for breast and brain cancer:
  - Gamma radiation and novel medical therapies for recurrent brain cancer
  - Robotic Prostatectomy for prostate, kidney, bladder, and gynecologic cancers
  - Partial breast radiation using MammoSite balloon brachytherapy
  - State of the art interventional endoscopy
  - Interleukin-2 Vaccine Program
  - Minimally invasive lung sparing surgery and lobectomies for lung cancer
  - Novel therapeutics for lymphomas, leukemias, and myelomas

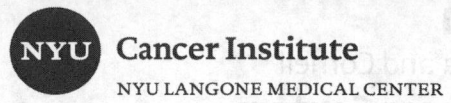

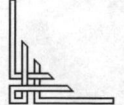
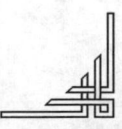

The Best in American Medicine
www.CastleConnolly.com

Home Healthcare

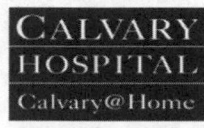

CALVARY HOSPITAL
1740 Eastchester Road
Bronx, NY 10461
Tel: (718) 518-2000
www.calvaryhospital.org

CALVARY@HOME
HOME CARE, HOSPICE, AND NURSING HOME HOSPICE

Calvary@Home, the umbrella for our Home Care, Hospice, and Nursing Home Hospice program, brings compassionate care to patients who can be cared for at home. Our interdisciplinary team includes physicians, nurses, aides, social workers, spiritual care providers, volunteers, bereavement support workers, and other providers as needed. In 2009, The Joint Commission gave Calvary@Home a Gold Seal of Approval™. Calvary@Home cares for nearly 2,000 patients and families each year.

The National Hospice and Palliative Care Organization and the National Island Peer Review Organization place Calvary@Home above state and national averages for relief of pain, patient/family education, and other parameters.

Certified Home Health Agency
Established in 1985, serves patients with all acute, chronic or life-limiting illnesses. We provide a full range of specialized home healthcare experts to support patients and families. Home care patients approaching the end of life have access to palliative care services such as pain and symptom management, assistance with advance care planning, and psychosocial support. We strive to ensure continuity of care by assigning a core group of caregivers to each patient. Our community health nurses work with the patient's person physicians to deliver appropriate care.

Areas We Serve

Manhattan	Bronx
Queens	Westchester

Hospice
Established in 1998, brings comprehensive care to people at home with all end-stage illnesses. Calvary assembles a core group of permanent staff to care for each patient, creating continuity of service for patients and families. Patients who require short-stay inpatient care can be admitted to Calvary in a seamless process. In addition to nurses, physicians and aides, social workers, spiritual counselors, and volunteers make home visits to ensure that physical, psychosocial, emotional and spiritual needs are met. We provide bereavement services for 13 months for families. Staffing exceeds national recommendations.

Areas We Serve

Manhattan	Bronx	Queens
Brooklyn	Nassau	Rockland
Westchester		

Nursing Home Hospice
Brings comprehensive palliative care to nursing home residents suffering from all end-stage illnesses. Provides appropriate care to all dually eligible (Medicare/Medicaid) residents, and bereavement services for loved ones. Calvary Nursing Home Hospice has contracts with 25 facilities in:

Manhattan	Bronx	Queens
Brooklyn	Nassau	Rockland
Westchester		

For information about Calvary@Home, please call 718-518-2465.

Palliative Home Care

In 2010, Calvary launched an innovative program to provide Palliative Care services to its Home Care patients. These services are generally not available to home care patients approaching the end of life.

Calvary's Palliative Program provides pain and symptom management, assistance with advance care planning, and psychosocial support to its existing Home Care patients.

In the Hospital's three-year pilot, Calvary will provide palliative home care training to clinicians and aides, educate providers on how to identify appropriate patients for referral, pilot-test the palliative home care model with 75 patients, and develop disease- and discipline-specific guidelines.

To assess the impact of palliative home care on quality of life and on medical costs, Calvary will compare rates of re-hospitalizations, medical crises, and completion of advance directives for patients enrolled in palliative home care to rates for a comparable group of previous Calvary home care patients.

This innovative program has received major funding from The Altman Foundation, Fan Fox & Leslie R. Samuels Foundation, and the United Hospital Fund.

Infectious Disease

INFECTIOUS DISEASES

About the Division of Infectious Diseases and Immunology:
Developing effective treatment for infectious diseases is among the miracles of the last century's science, but today we are faced with deadly new infections and old ones that were never tamed. These and the rapidly emerging problem of resistance to antibiotics place the study and treatment of infectious diseases at the forefront of modern medicine. NYU Langone Medical Center faculty and fellows within the Division of Infectious Diseases and Immunology have expertise in the diagnosis, treatment and prevention of rare and common acute and chronic infectious diseases. Physicians within the Division are actively involved in the management of complicated bone and joint infections, prevention of infection in cancer and transplant patients and developing strategies for managing hepatitis B and C. The Division also offers the opportunity for patients with HIV to enroll in clinical trials of new drugs that are not yet widely available. *We specialize in the following areas:*

HIV Prevention
The NYU Division of Infectious Diseases and Immunology has developed a uniquely effective program in HIV prevention that has gained wide recognition and has extended the hospital's expertise from New York City to West and East Africa.

AIDS Clinical Trials
The NYU AIDS Clinical Trials Unit is one of 35 such units designated and supported by the National Institute of Allergy and Infectious Diseases and is a dedicated resource for healthcare providers, researchers and scientists working in the field of HIV/AIDS research. It is one of the most productive units in the nation and enrolls adult and pediatric patients in clinical trials supported by the NIH. The data produced by the unit has supported the licensing of several drugs and plays an essential role in defining optimal therapies and preventing complications.

Population Biology of Infectious Diseases
This novel program combines laboratory and clinical studies with epidemiology (examines factors affecting the health and illness of populations) and genetics to reach maximum results. Research doctors in the Division of Infectious Diseases and Immunology are extensively involved in local and international research into the early diagnosis, treatment and prevention of chronic infections such as tuberculosis and Helicobacter (bacteria associated with stomach ulcers).

Medical and Molecular Parasitology
The NYU Division of Infectious Diseases and Immunology works alongside NYU Langone Medical Center's Department of Medical Parasitology to bring malaria and other parasitic diseases under control.

Internal Medicine

INTERNAL MEDICINE

About the Division of General Internal Medicine, Department of Medicine:

Famous equally for cutting-edge research and for nurturing lifelong physician-patient relationships, the internal medicine physicians of NYU Langone Medical Center are dedicated to treating the whole patient and not just their disease. Internists at the Medical Center meet the highest standards of the medical profession, addressing physical and psychological aspects of health and disease through clear communication and integration of diverse elements of care. NYU Langone Medical Center attracts internists whose passion is the care of patients with multiple problems and who specialize in keeping people healthy. *We specialize in the following areas:*

Primary and Specialized Healthcare

The Division of General Internal Medicine offers physical examinations, as well as specialized care in illnesses involving the heart, lungs, gastrointestinal tract, joints, bones, muscles, endocrine organs and kidneys. Our faculty believe in integrating the care of multiple conditions, and place a premium on coordinating care that is often spread across a wide variety of doctor's offices. A wide range of laboratory, imaging and advanced diagnostic testing, ranging from throat cultures to the complex mapping of the electrical surface of the heart, are available on-site or by referral. We also provides comprehensive women's healthcare, including cancer screening and osteoporosis prevention and treatment.

Geriatrics

Our geriatric specialists provide comprehensive and multidisciplinary care, consultation and follow-up for elderly patients ranging across the full spectrum from prevention and healthy aging to the treatment and care of chronic conditions including dementia, functional impairment and degenerative disorders.

Center for Healthful Behavior Change (CHBC)

The Center for Healthful Behavior Change (CHBC) focuses on developing evidence-based behavioral interventions aimed at improving patient health by altering unhealthy behaviors. The CHBC originates, tests and spreads innovative evidence-based behavioral interventions into everyday clinical practice and community settings for patients with high blood pressure and other conditions associated with cardiovascular risk including obesity and high cholesterol.

Interventional Cardiology

Maternal & Fetal Medicine

MATERNAL-FETAL MEDICINE

About the Division of Maternal-Fetal Medicine

The Division of Maternal-Fetal Medicine at NYU Langone Medical Center is committed to ensuring that both mother and fetus receive the specialized care that they need. The Division focuses on multifetal pregnancies, genetic counseling, women who have miscarried, preterm deliveries and other medical complications that can occur during pregnancy. We also specialize in helping women who have other medical conditions that may complicate a pregnancy such as diabetes, heart problems, high blood pressure, and lupus, among others. ***We specialize in the following areas:***

Education

NYU Langone Medical Center's Maternal-Fetal specialists offer patient-centered care for high-risk women. We offer the latest state-of-the-art techniques for in-utero diagnosis and treatment and overall care of complex obstetrical patients.

Patient Care

The Department of Fetal-Medicine focuses on making sure that each patient delivers a healthy baby. Using minimally invasive techniques, doctors at NYU Langone Medical Center are able to repair a number of life-threatening conditions in a child before it is even born, reducing the risks of preterm labor and the need for cesarean births. Our physicians have developed numerous new treatment protocols for high-risk obstetrics around the nation and the world.

Research

The Division of Maternal-Fetal Medicine has generated new treatment modalities for high-risk obstetrics patients and introduced new methods of diagnosis and treatment for the care of the fetus.

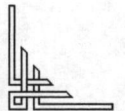
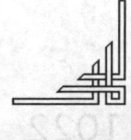

The Best in American Medicine
www.CastleConnolly.com

Medical Oncology

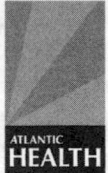

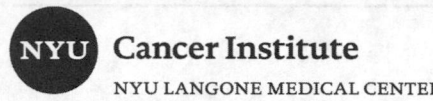

NYU **Cancer Institute**

NYU LANGONE MEDICAL CENTER

NYU Langone Medical Center
550 First Avenue , New York, NY 10016
www.NYULMC.org

NYU Clinical Cancer Center
160 East 34th Street, New York, NY 10016
www.NYUCI.org

**The Stephen D. Hassenfeld Children's Center
for Cancer and Blood Disorders**
160 East 32nd Street, New York, NY 10016
www.NYUMC.org/Hassenfeld

The NYU Cancer Institute is an NCI-designated cancer center and provides personalized patient care that is both compassionate and state of the art. The doctors and researchers work together to develop innovative therapies for patients. The Cancer Institute is world-renowned for excellence in cancer-focused research, personalized care, education and community outreach. Its mission is to discover the origins of human cancer and to use that knowledge to eradicate the personal and societal burden of cancer in our community, the nation and the world. For more information about our expert physicians, call 212-731-5000. *We specialize in the following areas:*

Patient-Focused Setting
The NYU Clinical Cancer Center is the principal outpatient facility of The Cancer Institute and serves as home to our patients and their caregivers. The center and its multidisciplinary team of experts provide access to the latest treatment options and clinical trials along with a variety of programs in cancer risk reduction/prevention, screening, diagnostics, genetic counseling and supportive services. In addition the NYUCI emphasizes the importance of a holistic approach to management services in complementary medicine, psychosocial support, survivorship and palliative care.

Renowned Expertise
The NYU Cancer Institute brings together experts from a variety of disciplines to create collaborative research endeavors and clinical care teams. The Cancer Institute offers a full continuum of personalized care, from prevention through diagnosis, treatment and post-treatment support. The compassion and expertise of our team members helps patients better manage the symptoms of their diseases as well as meet their special needs. Additionally, we have created special emphasis programs in diseases such as breast cancer, melanoma, GI cancer, prostate cancer, hematologic malignancies and lung cancer among others, as well as, translational programs in cancer healthcare disparities, molecularly targeted therapy, and the cell signaling pathways involved in cancer.

A Translational Approach
NYU Langone Medical Center scientists and other researchers excel in uncovering how cancer develops at the molecular level, and how we can harness that knowledge to reduce the risk of cancer and treat the disease. The Medical Center constantly seeks to create new opportunities for collaboration between investigators within our own institution, those located elsewhere in the NYU network of campuses, and researchers at other institutions.

The Stephen D. Hassenfeld Children's Center for Cancer and Blood Disorders
The center is a leading pediatric outpatient facility for the treatment of childhood cancers and blood diseases. Its unique interdisciplinary and family-centered approach combines the most advanced medical treatments with psychosocial and emotional support services for young patients and their families.

Minimally Invasive Surgery

Neonatal-Perinatal Medicine

NYU **Langone Medical Center**

NEONATAL PERINATAL MEDICINE

About the Neonatology Program, Department of Pediatrics:
The Neonatology Program at NYU Langone Medical Center understands that infants have different and unique emotional and developmental needs from those of adults. The Program combines family-centered care and state-of-the art technology to offer positive early experiences and simultaneously, enhance the quality of medical care for newborns and infants. *We specialize in the following areas:*

Neonatal Intensive Care
The Neonatal Intensive Care Unit (NICU) at NYU Langone Medical Center provides the most advanced care in New York City, including general and cardiac surgery, neurosurgery and craniofacial surgery. In addition to providing maternal-fetal medicine services and a NICU, the Program offers early intervention evaluation services and comprehensive family support and education. The developmentally appropriate environment includes covered incubators, drawn shades and parents holding pre-term infants skin-to-skin. Studies from NYU Langone Medical Center show that this approach has decreased the need for ventilator support and the risk of chronic lung disease. It has also enhanced weight gain and improved overall neurological development.

Continuing Care
Because many premature babies may be at an increased risk for problems in growth and development, the Neonatal Comprehensive Continuing Care Program (NCCCP) follows these infants from birth through pre-school, providing evaluation and assessment of problems as soon as they arise.

Hypothermia Program
The Hypothermia Program at NYU Langone Medical Center is a full multidisciplinary service with neonatal transport and inpatient and outpatient follow-up services. The Program provides rapid assessment and treatment implementation for those infants affected.

Infant Apnea and SIDS
The Infant Apnea and SIDS Program at the Bellevue Hospital Center, an affiliate of NYU Langone Medical Center, provides treatment to critically ill infants from the Neonatal Intensive Care Unit and other children at risk for apnea, sudden infant death syndrome (SIDS) and other acute life-threatening events. The Program offers parent CPR education and support for as long as the infant requires monitored care.

Neonatal Transport
As a designated New York State Regional Perinatal Center, The Division of Neonatology cares for over 1/5 of New York City's mothers and infants. To do so and provide effective care for infants in need, the program offers an active transport program to bring mothers and/or their newborn infants into NYU Langone Medical Center's Tisch Hospital NICU for specialized intensive care.

Neurological Surgery

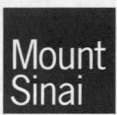 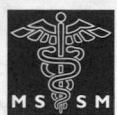
THE MOUNT SINAI MEDICAL CENTER
NEUROSURGERY

One Gustave L. Levy Place
Fifth Avenue and 100th Street
New York, NY 10029-6574
Physician Referral: 1-800-MD-SINAI (637-4624)
www.mountsinai.org

THE DEPARTMENT OF NEUROSURGERY at Mount Sinai, established in 1920, has earned a distinguished international reputation. Areas of clinical expertise include the treatment of skull base tumors, primary and metastatic brain tumors, pituitary adenomas and acoustic neuromas, and deep brain stimulation for movement disorders. The Department also provides advanced endovascular and microsurgical treatment of aneurysms, treatments for arteriovenous malformations and stroke, microvascular decompression for trigeminal neuralgia and hemifacial spasm, and advanced minimally invasive resection of spine and spinal cord tumors and degenerative spine disease.

The Comprehensive Brain Tumor Program collaborates with The Tisch Cancer Institute and the Departments of Neurology, Radiation Oncology, Radiology, and Pathology to provide comprehensive therapies for primary and metastatic brain tumors. We have pioneered minimally invasive approaches using imaging technology, frameless stereotaxy, and skull base endoscopy, awake and asleep brain mapping, and advanced microneurosurgery. Stereotactic radiosurgery, a minimally invasive treatment that does not require open surgery, gene therapy, and clinical trials are also possible options.

The Neuroendocrine Program sees more than 200 new pituitary tumor patients each year and more then 300 follow-up patients annually, and has performed more than 2,500 transphenoidal pituitary operations.

The Minimally Invasive and Endoscopic Skull Base Surgery Program provides comprehensive, highly advanced treatment for lesions located near the complex structures at the base of the skull. This multidisciplinary program unites surgical specialists in neurosurgery, otolaryngology, head and neck cancer, craniofacial surgery, oral and maxillofacial surgery, and microvascular and reconstructive procedures. We have pioneered the development of minimally invasive techniques including, transnasal endoscopic tumor resection and stereotactic radiosurgery for complex skull base lesions. This program offers renowned treatment of pituitary adenomas, acoustic neuromas, meningiomas, chordomas, craniopharyngiomas, cholesterol granulomas, chondrosarcomas, and all the pathologies of the skull base.

The Cerebrovascular Program has a highly experienced team that provides a complete range of services for the diagnosis and treatment of patients with neurovascular disorders of the brain and spinal cord, including aneurysms, arteriovenous malformations (AVMs), carotid and intracranial stenoses, and other conditions. Our team includes physicians specializing in microsurgical techniques, endovascular techniques, stereotactic radiosurgery, and neurocritical care, all working together to prevent or minimize the neurological impact of neurovascular disorders and to maximize recovery. Some current treatments include microsurgical treatment of aneurysms and AVMs with clipping and resection, endovascular treatment of aneurysms with coils and/or stents, endovascular treatment of AVMs with liquid acrylics, stereotactic radiosurgical treatment of AVMs, endovascular treatment of stenoses with stents and angioplasty and microsurgical treatment of stenoses and occlusions with bypass. We treat a high volume of patients using endovascular methods, and have the largest experience in the stent-assisted embolization of cerebral aneurysms and stent treatment of carotid artery disease amongst neurovascular centers in New York.

The Functional and Restorative Neurosurgery Program uses the latest technology to precisely target areas of abnormal activity in the brain and spinal cord. Our physicians are focused on developing minimally invasive neurosurgical techniques that either modulate neural function, replace lost neuronal populations, or halt the neurodegenerative process altogether. Currently, deep brain stimulation dominates this field, but many technologies with great potential are on the horizon. Our physicians have been honored by the Dystonia Medical Research Foundation for their pioneering work treating dystonia with deep brain stimulation. We also use gene therapy for the treatment of patients with Parkinson's disease, epilepsy, essential tremor, facial nerve disorders, and chronic pain syndromes.

The Neurosurgery Spinal Disorders Program offers treatment for all disorders of the spinal column and spinal cord, including degenerative disorders (disc herniations, spinal stenosis, spinal instability), trauma, infections, congenital disorders (including scoliosis), and tumors. Our neurosurgeons have pioneered endoscopic, minimally invasive approaches for tumors resection and treatment of degenerative diseases. These approaches reduce pain, and hospital stays, and facilitate an early return to normal activity.

NEUROSURGERY

About the Department of Neurosurgery:

Offering some of the most technologically and minimally invasive advanced surgical procedures available, we also feature cutting-edge research and medical education through our renowned inter-disciplinary team. *We specialize in the following areas*:

Brain Tumor

We specialize in both malignant and benign brain tumors, including skull base tumors. Expertise includes glioblastoma, ependymoma, hemangioblastoma, other gliomas, meningiomas and vestibular schwannomas (acoustic neuromas).

Cerebrovascular Surgery

The Division of Cerebrovascular Surgery is a premier center for brain aneurysms, giant intracranial aneurysms, brain vascular malformations and cavernomas (blood-filled clusters of vessels).

Epilepsy

The Comprehensive Epilepsy Center is the largest epilepsy center in the U.S. and offers advanced surgical and medical options. Complementary management including diet, yoga, biofeedback, meditation, lifestyle changes is also offered.

Spinal Neurosurgery

The Division of Spine Surgery provides treatment for spinal diseases such as degenerative diseases, spinal tumors, spinal trauma and spinal infections. Our surgeons have expertise in the newest minimally invasive approaches.

Neurosurgical Technology

Our neurosurgeons remove deep-seated tumors, vascular malformations and other sites of dysfunction with outstanding results using the Leksell Gamma Knife,. Aided by 3-D MRI technology, the Perfexion®, the most advanced model, is used to bombard targeted areas with precise doses of radiation, while still preserving healthy tissue.

The Department of Neurosurgery also provides state-of-the-art care and research through the following divisions:

- Facial Pain: provides patients a thorough examination and if required, nerve injections and minimally invasive surgery.
- Functional Neurosurgery: offers diagnosis and treatment of Parkinson's disease and conditions that involve involuntary muscle contractions.
- Pediatric Neurosurgery: provides treatment to children with brain and spinal cord tumors, congenital and development disorders.
- Peripheral Nerve Surgery: focuses on the diagnosis and treatment of nerve compressions, nerve tremors, Brachial Plexus (never fiber) and nerve injuries.

Neuro-Critical Care

We provide intensive care and treatment of critical neurosurgical illnesses such as respiratory failure, hypotension, hypertension, coagulopathy (blood clotting disorder) as well as infections including pneumonia, sepsis, wound infections and meningitis. High-caliber care for patients with seizures and raised intracranial pressure is also offered. Our physicians are available 24 hours a day for immediate consultation.

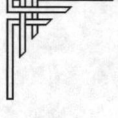

The Best in American Medicine
www.CastleConnolly.com

Neurology

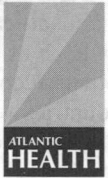

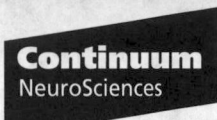
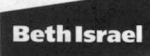

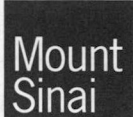
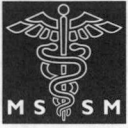

MOUNT SINAI SCHOOL OF MEDICINE

THE MOUNT SINAI MEDICAL CENTER
NEUROLOGY
One Gustave L. Levy Place
Fifth Avenue and 100th Street
New York, NY 10029-6574
Physician Referral: 1-800-MD-SINAI (637-4624)
www.mountsinai.org

THE ESTELLE AND DANIEL MAGGIN DEPARTMENT OF NEUROLOGY at Mount Sinai provides compassionate, state-of-the-art, interdisciplinary care for disorders of the brain and nervous system.

The Robert and John M. Bendheim Parkinson and Movement Disorders Center is one of the world's leading multidisciplinary centers for the study of Parkinson's disease and related disorders, and serves as a forum for collaboration among internationally acclaimed neuroscientists. The Center offers advanced clinical care, translational research, and basic science programs aimed at discovering the cause of and cure for Parkinson's, dystonia, and other movement disorders. The Center incorporates a renowned deep-brain stimulation program and has played a major role in evaluating cell-based and gene therapies for the treatment of movement disorders.

The Corinne Goldsmith Dickinson Center for Multiple Sclerosis is an internationally recognized comprehensive center, uniting the efforts of leading physicians and scientists from many disciplines to understand the causes and consequences of multiple sclerosis (MS). The Center provides services in all aspects of diagnosis, disease management, rehabilitation, and patient support, and the opportunity for patients to participate in potentially groundbreaking clinical trials.

The Clinical Program for Cerebrovascular Disorders comprises an outstanding team of medical experts who specialize in the most advanced approaches in the evaluation, treatment, and rehabilitation of patients with cerebrovascular diseases. Services include the early diagnosis of stroke, a specialized Neurointensive Care Unit, and an advanced inpatient stroke unit. Physicians are available at all times for emergency consultation with referring physicians.

The NeuroAIDS Program provides diagnosis and treatment for neurological disorders associated with HIV disease. This program is one of the few in the world to treat the various complications of the disease that affect the central and peripheral nervous systems in as many as 70 percent of patients.

The Epilepsy Center provides specific expertise in the diagnosis and treatment of epilepsy and related disorders. The Center encompasses outstanding epileptologists, a new modern inpatient epilepsy monitoring unit, and full outpatient EEG and diagnostic capabilities.

The ALS/Muscular Dystrophy Program provides diagnosis and treatment of muscular dystrophy and amyotrophic lateral sclerosis (ALS). Our clinical care team specializes in improving the quality of life for patients, and scientists engage in both clinical and laboratory research aimed at finding better treatment and cures.

THE ESTELLE AND DANIEL MAGGIN DEPARTMENT OF NEUROLOGY The Mount Sinai Medical Center is renowned for its unique integration of outstanding patient care and cutting-edge research laboratories, which together work to find better treatment for Parkinson's disease, MS, stroke, and other neurological disorders. One of the nation's top programs for research and patient care, the department is led by some of the most prominent figures in American neurology and receives annual research grants of more than $20 million.

The Division of Neuromuscular Diseases provides diagnosis, treatment, and compassionate care for patients with disorders in neuromuscular transmission, muscle diseases, peripheral nerve problems, and spasticity resulting from stroke or damage to the central nervous system.

Mount Sinai's Neurological Tumor Program is world-acclaimed for the treatment of pituitary adenomas, acoustic neuromas, meningiomas, and cancerous brain tumors. The program's multispecialty group of physicians works together to provide outstanding care through state-of-the-art surgical procedures, radiation therapy, chemotherapy, and supportive therapy. Our physicians have pioneered the treatment of tumors with stereotactic radiosurgery, as well as developed a number of experimental treatment protocols to improve patients' lives.

The Eye Movement and Vestibular Disorder Program at Mount Sinai provides outstanding diagnosis and treatment for visual problems, balance problems, and motion sickness. Our physicians participate in NASA programs, employing equipment used to assess these disorders in space.

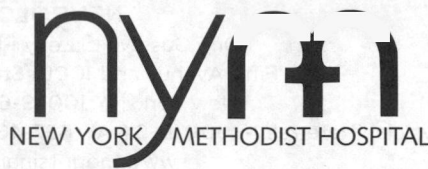

NEW YORK / METHODIST HOSPITAL

THE INSTITUTE FOR NEUROSCIENCES

New York Methodist Hospital
506 Sixth Street, Brooklyn, N.Y. 11215
Phone: 866-DO-NEURO (866-366-3876)
http://www.nym.org

SPECIALISTS AND MEDICAL SERVICES

The Institute for Neurosciences at New York Methodist Hospital brings together a unique group of specialists and medical services, offering diagnosis and treatment of a broad range of neurological conditions, ranging from frequent headaches to Parkinson's disease to multiple sclerosis.

The Institute's panel of physician specialists includes neurologists, neurosurgeons, psychiatrists, endocrinologists, neuroradiologists, radiation oncologists, physiatrists, geriatricians, psychologists and rehabilitation therapists.

All diagnostic and therapeutic procedures are performed at New York Methodist Hospital or at individual physicians' offices. State-of-the-art equipment to perform computed tomography (CT), magnetic resonance imaging (MRI), and magnetic resonance angiography (MRA) is located in the Hospital's Radiology Department. In addition, equipment and specialists trained to perform neurological diagnostic tests, such as electroencephalography (EEG), electromyography (EMG), and evoked potential examinations are available on the main campus.

The Institute also has a satellite office in Staten Island, located at 1 Harvey Avenue. It can be reached by calling 718-494-4360.

PROGRAMS OFFERED:

Special programs and services offered by the Institute include an Alzheimer's disease/memory center, a neuropathy program, pediatric and adult epilepsy programs that offer diagnosis via video EEG, a Parkinson's disease and other movement disorders program, a pituitary program, a multiple sclerosis center, a neuro-oncology service, inpatient and outpatient psychiatry programs, rehabilitation services and a State-designated Stroke Center. Neurosurgeons on the Institute's panel perform highly sophisticated procedures, including deep brain stimulation surgery, vascular neurosurgery, skull base surgery and spinal surgery. A stereotactic radiosurgery service is also available at the Hospital's regional radiation oncology center.

***

Referrals to the Institute, its programs and physicians can be made through an individual's primary care physician or requested directly through the Institute's telephone referral service. More information (and on-line physician referral) is available at the Hospital's website, http://www.nym.org.

THE MULTIPLE SCLEROSIS CENTER

The Multiple Sclerosis Center is headed by a neurologist trained in the most advanced MS treatments and clinical research. The center offers compassionate multidisciplinary care with a team of specialists.

After a comprehensive evaluation, treatment is tailored for each individual patient, based on the type of MS, the symptoms, and the patient's lifestyle.

NEUROLOGY

About the Department of Neurology:
NYU Langone Medical Center evaluates and treats children and adults with a broad spectrum of neurological diseases. Specialty groups deliver integrated care to patients with stroke, epilepsy, cerebrovacular diseases, behavioral disorders and dementia, brain tumors, genetic and degenerative diseases, nerve and muscle problems, headache and pain syndromes and movement disorders. We are home to the largest multiple sclerosis (MS) program in New York and the first primary Stroke Center in New York City. *We specialize in the following areas:*

Autonomic Diseases
Our specialized center evaluates and treats children and adults with familial dysautonomia and other inherited or acquired autonomic nervous system diseases including orthostatic hypotension and rare forms of hereditary sensory neuropathy.

Epilepsy
The Comprehensive Epilepsy Center offers the most advanced surgical and medical options in the treatment of epilepsy. Complementary management approaches such as diet alteration, lifestyle changes and other remedies are part of a comprehensive management plan. Our primary goal is to help patients with unmanageable epilepsy achieve complete control, or at least a reduction in the frequency of seizures and/or the medical side effects to achieve the highest possible quality of life.

Multiple Sclerosis
The Comprehensive MS Care Center provides state-of-the-art diagnostic evaluations and follow-up care. We feature an onsite team of highly trained professionals, as well as consulting services, to provide comprehensive care.

Neurogenetics
The Division of Neurogenetics focuses on inherited diseases of the nervous system. Services include diagnosis and management of inherited diseases, biochemical and molecular testing and genetic counseling.

Neuro-oncology
The NYU Cancer Institute, an NCI-designated cancer center, is home to one of the nation's leading brain and spinal cord tumor treatment programs, with medical experts experienced in neuro-oncology, neurosurgery, neuroradiology.

Neuromuscular Diseases
The Neuromuscular Division offers multidisciplinary inpatient and outpatient programs for neuromuscular diseases with emphasis on: acquired peripheral neuropathy, Charcot Marie Tooth neuropathy, myasthenia gravis, Amyotrophic lateral sclerosis, spinal muscular atrophy and post-polio syndrome, muscular dystrophy and Lyme neuroborreliosis.

Parkinson's Disease and Movement Disorders
The Parkinson and Movement Disorders Center helps individuals and families achieve the highest possible quality of life. We have an active research program that explores best treatments options for Parkinson's disease.

Stroke Care
The first primary stroke center in New York City, the multidisciplinary Comprehensive Stroke Care Center at NYU Langone Medical Center provides rapid diagnosis, immediate and effective intervention and early rehabilitation.

St. Francis Hospital The Heart Center®

100 Port Washington Blvd.
Roslyn, New York 11576
www.stfrancisheartcenter.com
(516) 562-6000   Physician referral: 1-888-HEARTNY
A member of Catholic Health Services of Long Island

Top-Ranked Neurological Services

St. Francis Hospital, The Heart Center® was recognized by *U.S. News & World Report* as one of the nation's best hospitals for neurology and neurosurgery in 2010-11. The Department of Neurology at St. Francis provides high quality neurological care to hospital and emergency room patients with acute and chronic neurological issues. Under the leadership of department chair, Anthony Cohen, M.D., our team of highly skilled board certified neurologists diagnose, treat and manage patients with various ailments including stroke, neuromuscular disorders, seizure disorders, movement disorders, multiple sclerosis, Alzheimer's disease, and headache. Many of the neurologists have subspecialty training in these areas. Combining their knowledge and expertise in the field with advanced technology and diagnostic testing, the staff provides the most comprehensive care available.

An Award-Winning Stroke Center

Under its Director, Paul Wright, M.D., and team of experienced physicians, the Stroke Center at St. Francis Hospital has become a leader in the diagnosis, treatment, and support of stroke patients. The hospital provides advanced treatment in emergency settings, facilitating the diagnosis and expeditious management of stroke victims. The Stroke Center is staffed with critically trained nurses, with specific expertise in the management of acute stroke patients. By creating an environment with superior neurological care and compassionate and Magnet Award-winning nursing staff, St. Francis strives to be at the forefront of leading hospitals regionally and nationally.

An Innovative Neurosurgery Program

Richard Johnson, M.D., Director of Neurosurgery, leads a team of more than 15 neurosurgeons who specialize in treating debilitating conditions that affect the brain and spine. The hospital offers advanced minimally invasive procedures such as the X-STOP for patients suffering from lumbar spinal stenosis. Other minimally invasive therapies that can decompress and fuse the spine for patients suffering from chronic back pain and herniated disks are also offered at the hospital. For patients with cervical myelopathy or a compression of the cervical spine, St. Francis surgeons can now operate through the front of the neck to remove bone, ligaments or discs that press against the spine. Using pieces of bone or a carbon fiber composite, they can reconstruct and stabilize the spine. St. Francis also offers an outstanding intracranial neurosurgical service, having acquired the latest technology and equipment for removal of brain tumors and other intracranial lesions.

Conditions Treated

- Stroke
- Headache and facial pain
- Multiple Sclerosis
- Parkinson's disease
- Lou Gehrig's disease
- Epilepsy
- Neck pain
- Back pain
- Coma
- Infections of the nervous system
- Alzheimer's
- Dementia
- Dizziness
- Vertigo
- Brain tumors
- Spinal cord injuries and tumors

Key treatments:

Electro-myograph (EMG) and Nerve Conduction Studies - This test records electrical activity in the muscles and is a diagnostic tool used to evaluate the peripheral nervous system. It is usually performed along with an assessment of conductivity of peripheral nerves (NCS). The test can confirm or reject the suspicion of disorder of muscles or nerves, such as neuropathy, myopathy, myasthenia gravis, Lou Gehrig's Disease, radiculopathy, and carpal tunnel syndrome.

Electro-encephalography (EEG) - The primary test used to diagnose seizures and epilepsy. Electrodes are placed over the surface of the head and recording brain activity for 20 to 30 minutes.

Somato-Sensory Evoked Potential - Used as an assessment of the functional state of the conductivity in the central nervous system (unlike the imaging studies that assess the anatomical appearance). The test involves electrical stimulation of extremities with recording signals arriving at the brain. It is used to assess patients in a coma and those with conditions that can not be confirmed on CT or MRI.

Neuroradiology

Nuclear Medicine

Obstetrics & Gynecology

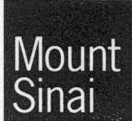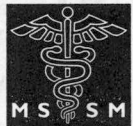

THE MOUNT SINAI MEDICAL CENTER
OBSTETRICS, GYNECOLOGY, AND REPRODUCTIVE SCIENCE

One Gustave L. Levy Place
Fifth Avenue and 100th Street
New York, NY 10029-6574
Physician Referral: 1-800-MD-SINAI (637-4624)
www.mountsinai.org

Building on more than a century of leadership in providing health care to women, the **DEPARTMENT OF OBSTETRICS, GYNECOLOGY, AND REPRODUCTIVE SCIENCE** at The Mount Sinai Medical Center offers special expertise in:

General obstetrics – Genetic counseling, prenatal care, labor and delivery management, and postpartum care. In addition to our talented physicians, other health care professionals are integrated into our practice, including genetic counselors, nutritionists, social workers, nurse midwives, childbirth educators, and lactation/breastfeeding specialists.

High-risk obstetrics – Advanced techniques in prenatal diagnosis and consultations in the management of complicated pregnancies. Our ultrasound unit is recognized for its expertise in fetal anatomy ultrasound assessments. The latest technology, including 4D imaging, is employed. Antepartum testing, including amniocentesis, chorionic villus sampling, and fetal blood sampling, are all routinely performed at Mount Sinai.

Reproductive endocrinology and infertility – Diagnosis and treatment of both female and male factor infertility. Treatment options for women include fertility medications, intrauterine insemination, in vitro fertilization, intracytoplasmic sperm injection, and ovum donation.

General gynecology – Cancer screening, management of abnormal Pap smears, family planning, and surgical management of fibroids, endometriosis, and other benign gynecologic conditions.

Gynecologic infectious diseases – Treatment and prevention of sexually transmitted infections and consultations on obstetrical and gynecological infections.

Gynecologic oncology – Care for women with cancers of the ovary, uterus, cervix, vulva, and vagina.

Minimally invasive surgery – For many conditions.

Urogynecology and reconstructive pelvic surgery – Lower urinary tract disorders.

INNOVATIVE APPROACHES TO PRENATAL CARE AND THE TREATMENT OF GYNECOLOGIC CANCERS
Known worldwide for excellence and innovative approaches to prenatal diagnosis and fetal therapy, Mount Sinai's Department of Obstetrics, Gynecology, and Reproductive Science has a long tradition of advancing clinical practice through patient-oriented research. Faculty members are pioneering work in diverse areas, including first- and second-trimester screening for fetal chromosomal abnormalities, vaccines for the prevention of sexually transmitted infections, minimally invasive surgical techniques, and new approaches to the diagnosis and treatment of gender-specific cancers.

WOMEN'S HEALTH - OBSTETRICS AND GYNECOLOGY

About the Department of Obstetrics and Gynecology:
NYU Langone Medical Center provides comprehensive programs and services designed specifically for women. Services range from primary care to the most specialized programs. Supported by sophisticated research and advanced training, we offer a full range of women's health care.
We specialize in the following areas:

Fertility-Related Services
We offer state-of-the-art programs in egg donation, egg freezing and wellness (acupuncture, mind/body, psychology and yoga). Diagnosis and treatment includes ovulation induction, assisted reproductive technologies and surgical options that incorporate the latest endoscopic techniques. The Center also tests for genetic abnormalities, as well as immunity and infectious diseases.

Gynecologic Oncology
The NCI-designated NYU Cancer Institute's Women's Cancer Program specializes in the treatment of cervical cancer, endometrial cancer, ovarian cancer, uterine cancer, vaginal cancer and vulvar cancer. The Program also provides treatment for uterine sarcoma, molar pregnancy and gestational trophoblastic disease.

Maternal Fetal Medicine
We offer prenatal care for high-risk pregnancies and detailed consultations before, during and after pregnancy. Special attention is given to multifetal pregnancies and to women who have other medical conditions that may complicate a pregnancy such as diabetes, heart problems, high blood pressure and lupus.

Obstetrics
We offer a broad range of services including: prenatal care that gives equal emphasis to the well-being of the mother and of the fetus; fetal monitoring through ultrasound and other techniques; childbirth preparedness and breastfeeding classes; and consultation for high-risk pregnancies, including treatment for women who experience recurrent pregnancy loss.

Specialty Services
In addition to routine gynecological care, we offer many other services including: pelvic ultrasound; aspiration of breast cysts; evaluation of infertility (including the special needs of same-sex couples); colposcopy (a diagnostic evaluation of abnormal pap smears); LEEP (a loop electrosurgical procedure used to diagnose and treat cervical cancer); cryotherapy for vaginal warts; and bone density testing.

Urogynecology and Reconstructive Pelvic Surgery
We focus on using state-of-the-art diagnostic methods for all forms of incontinence and pelvic disorders, as well as correcting malformations of the reproductive tract found at birth, during childhood or in young adults. Our urogynecologists are experts in providing comprehensive care for women with conditions such as overactive bladder, urinary and/or fecal incontinence and pelvic organ prolapse.

The Best in American Medicine
www.CastleConnolly.com

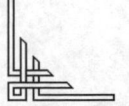
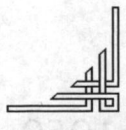

Occupational Medicine

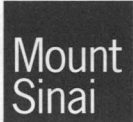
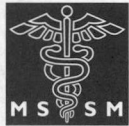

Mount Sinai

M S ⚕ S M

MOUNT SINAI
SCHOOL OF
MEDICINE

THE MOUNT SINAI MEDICAL CENTER
OCCUPATIONAL AND ENVIRONMENTAL MEDICINE

One Gustave L. Levy Place
Fifth Avenue and 100th Street
New York, NY 10029-6574
Physician Referral: 1-800-MD-SINAI (637-4624)
www.mountsinai.org

The mission of the **MOUNT SINAI - IRVING J. SELIKOFF CENTER FOR OCCUPATIONAL AND ENVIRONMENTAL MEDICINE** is the diagnosis, treatment and prevention of occupational disease in the workplace. To achieve this goal, we utilize a preventive medicine model that includes three integrated components:

Clinical Care – Our services include the diagnosis, treatment, and management of occupational diseases for current and retired workers, including, for example, work-related musculoskeletal disease, asbestos-related disease, lead toxicity and others. We offer comprehensive occupational medicine evaluations to facilitate a safe return to work with proper accommodations when appropriate. Our services include medical evaluation and support for Workers' Compensation claims when necessary. Our social workers provide counseling regarding the financial, social, and psychological aspects of occupational disease.

Disease Prevention Services – Our team educates patients, health care professionals, workers, unions, employers, and communities on the signs and symptoms of occupational disease. We provide comprehensive industrial hygiene and ergonomic services to evaluate exposures and recommend effective preventive measures. We also provide technical assistance and consultation services for employers, unions, and public health agencies.

Surveillance and Data Management – We study the pattern and prevalence of occupational disease and identify new links between workplace exposure and disease.

IMPROVING PUBLIC HEALTH

To promote disease prevention, the Center treats each newly identified case of occupational disease as a potential sentinel health event—that is, as a signal that there may be similar cases of disease in the patient's coworkers. This approach, coupled with our efforts to reduce workplace hazards, places the Center's impact well beyond individual patient evaluations. To help achieve our goal of improving public health by preventing occupational and environmental disease, we work closely with labor unions, employers, government and service organizations, health care providers and community organizations.

The Mount Sinai - Irving J. Selikoff Center for Occupational and Environmental Medicine has two clinical centers in New York. One is located in Manhattan, one is in Lower Westchester County, and there is a satellite clinic in Queens.

Ophthalmology

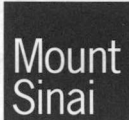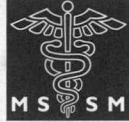

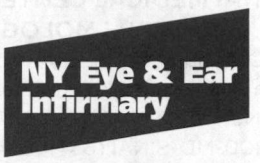

NY Eye & Ear Infirmary

Continuum Health Partners, Inc.

THE NEW YORK EYE AND EAR INFIRMARY

310 East 14th Street
New York, New York 10003
Tel. 212.979.4000   Fax. 212.228.0664
http://www.nyee.edu

PROVIDING EXCEPTIONAL EYE CARE

The Department of Ophthalmology is the region's most comprehensive center for the delivery of primary through tertiary eye care. It is also by far the largest provider of eye care in the metropolitan area—with some 155,000 outpatient visits and 19,200 surgical cases performed each year. 375 board-certified ophthalmologists located throughout New York City and its tri-state area comprise the attending Medical Staff.

IN A HIGHLY SPECIALIZED SETTING

As a specialty hospital, the Infirmary is uniquely qualified to handle the most complicated cases. It serves as a nationwide referral center with a commitment to teaching, research, and high-technology based patient care. Computerized ocular imaging equipment includes the new combination of scanning laser ophthalmoscopy with optical coherence tomography, to provide highest resolution in-depth images which detect the smallest defects and assist in the earliest and most accurate diagnosis of diseases such as glaucoma and macular degeneration. Highly experienced staff using state-of-the-art instrumentation have made the Infirmary's 17 operating rooms a national benchmark in efficiency in eye surgery cases.

FOR PATIENTS OF ALL AGES

Staff at the Infirmary are sensitive to the specific needs of patients of all ages. Senior citizens are the vast majority of the Infirmary's 8,000 yearly cataract patients, as well as individuals receiving treatment for age-related macular degeneration. Young children are now 25 percent of the patient population, with conditions such as strabismus, acquired and congenital cataracts, corneal diseases and ocular trauma. For those rare cases of children who have a disease ordinarily associated with age, the Infirmary runs New York's only Pediatric Glaucoma Service. Active adults of all ages utilize the New York Metropolitan Eye Trauma Center and Oculoplastic and Orbital Surgery Services.

Ophthalmology Clinical Services

Ambulatory Care Services
Comprehensive Eye Care
Cornea & Refractive Surgery
Eye Trauma
Glaucoma
Low Vision
Neuro-Ophthalmology
Oculoplastic &
Orbital Surgery
Ocular Tumor
Pediatric Ophthalmology
& Strabismus
Retinal-Vitreal
Uveitis/Ocular Immunology

Facilities

Ambulatory Surgery Center
Metropolitan Eye Trauma Center
Retina Center

About The New York Eye and Ear Infirmary

Founded in 1820, it is the nation's first and foremost, continuously operating specialty hospital. More than 10 million people have sought treatment here since its inception.

Physician Referral
1.800.449.HOPE (4673)

The Best in American Medicine
www.CastleConnolly.com

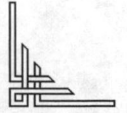

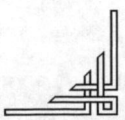

Orthopaedic Surgery

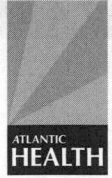

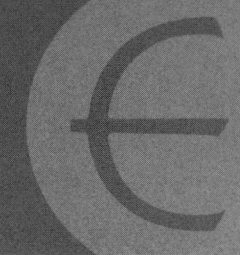

1060   Sponsored Page

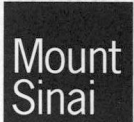
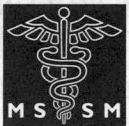

MOUNT SINAI
SCHOOL OF
MEDICINE

THE MOUNT SINAI MEDICAL CENTER
ORTHOPAEDICS

One Gustave L. Levy Place
Fifth Avenue and 100th Street
New York, NY 10029-6574
Physician Referral: 1-800-MD-SINAI (637-4624)
www.mountsinai.org

Beyond its reputation for depth and breadth of expertise, **THE LENI AND PETER W. MAY DEPARTMENT OF ORTHOPAEDICS** at The Mount Sinai Medical Center is known for personalized care. The faculty and staff invest the time to get to know their patients as individuals, ensuring that they receive direct care from subspecialty-trained orthopedists. The faculty share expertise in surgery of the foot and ankle, knee, hip, hand, elbow, shoulder, and spine; total joint replacement; microvascular surgery; cancer surgery; and minimally invasive surgery. Taking a whole-patient approach to care, they work in close collaboration with specialists in geriatrics, neurology, oncology, pathology, and rehabilitation medicine.

Investigation and Innovation – Recent years have seen successive refinements in the techniques of orthopedic surgery at Mount Sinai, including joint replacement, minimally invasive fracture repair, and microvascular surgery. Faculty members have been instrumental in the design and perfection of hip and shoulder prostheses. Additionally, Mount Sinai has broadened the applications of arthroscopic surgery—the fiber optic technology that first heralded the arrival of minimally invasive surgery.

Mount Sinai orthopedic bone, spine and tendon scientists are known for their studies of diseases of the skeletal system. Researchers are currently investigating disc degeneration in the spine; rotator cuff degeneration; methods of determining bone strength; how genetic alterations change the skeleton's function; and the fundamental molecular mechanisms of arthritis.

Use of Cutting-Edge Techniques – Mount Sinai uses innovative, minimally invasive approaches for joint replacement and fracture repair. The Department's oncology service is renowned for saving limbs with both bone and joint malignancies.

The Sports Service is one of few departments in New York that provides patients with the option of arthroscopic surgery of the hip. Patients have the ability to return to activities faster and with less pain with this minimally invasive procedure. Our arthroscopists also specialize in cartilage preservation techniques, including cartilage transplantation, allowing patients to preserve their own joints and delaying the need for joint replacement surgery.

GROUNDBREAKING PROCEDURES ENHANCE QUALITY OF LIFE

Today at Mount Sinai, arthroscopy is used to repair not only the knee but virtually every joint. Converting what used to be major open surgery to outpatient procedures has dramatically shortened rehabilitation and return to work times. More significantly, it has allowed many more patients to get help for painful, function-limiting conditions. That is the case for many elderly or frail patients who are physically unable to undergo major surgery. The fact that such procedures are now more widely accessible is enhancing the quality of life for many patients and allowing them to lead more active lives.

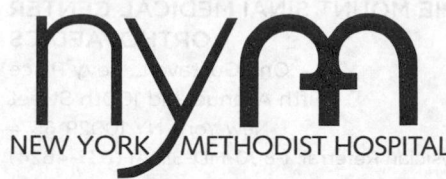

THE INSTITUTE FOR ORTHOPEDIC MEDICINE AND SURGERY

New York Methodist Hospital
506 Sixth Street, Brooklyn, N.Y. 11215
Phone: 866-ORTHO-11 (866-678-4611)
http://www.nym.org.

SPECIALISTS AND MEDICAL SERVICES

The Institute for Orthopedic Medicine and Surgery at New York Methodist Hospital brings together a unique team of specialists, facilities, and medical services to provide comprehensive treatment of a broad range of orthopedic disorders.

The Institute's panel of physicians includes specialists in adult and pediatric orthopedic surgery, emergency medicine, rheumatology, podiatric medicine and surgery, endocrinology, sports medicine, pain management, orthopedic oncology, and neurosurgery. Other important health care team members include podiatrists and physical and occupational therapists. All diagnostic and therapeutic procedures are performed at New York Methodist Hospital or in the offices of the referred physicians.

PROGRAMS OFFERED

In addition to emergency orthopedic services, programs offered through the Institute include joint replacement, arthroscopic knee surgery and cartilage restoration and medical treatments for arthritis, medical and surgical treatment for hand and shoulder injuries and degenerative conditions, spine surgery, physical therapy and pain management. Podiatric physicians specialize in all foot disorders, including reconstructive foot surgery. In addition, the Institute offers complementary medicine services including chiropractic care, acupuncture, and medical massage.

* * *

Referrals to the Institute, its programs and physicians can be made through an individual's primary care physician or requested directly through the Institute's telephone referral service. More information (and on-line physician referral) is available at the Hospital's website, http: //www.nym.org.

THE COMPREHENSIVE BACK AND NECK PAIN CENTER

NYM's Comprehensive Back and Neck Pain Center is dedicated to providing patients with the best clinical treatment for disorders of the back and neck. Diagnosis and treatment are centrally coordinated, so that patients avoid duplication of screening and testing procedures, if they need to see more than one specialist.

The Center focuses on conservative treatment, most commonly medication and/or rehabilitation (physical or occupational) therapy. Many other modalities are also available. If surgery is recommended, minimally invasive procedures may be applicable. Treatment decisions are made with consideration for the nature and severity of the condition, as well as the patient's lifestyle and preferences.

ORTHOPAEDIC SERVICES

Our Department of Orthopaedic Surgery, based at our Hospital for Joint Diseases, one of the nation's leading orthopaedic hospitals, has been consistently recognized as one of the top orthopaedic departments in the country by U.S. News and World Report. Our expert physicians combine extensive experience and research with the latest technology for bone and joint problems that affect patients' ability to function. *We specialize in the following areas:*

Joint Replacement
Patients have access to physicians and surgeons specialized in treating degenerative joint conditions through our Joint Replacement Center, one of the busiest in the world, performing over 2,500 joint replacements annually. We are experts in knee, hip & shoulder replacements, complex joint revisions, and minimally invasive surgeries.

Spine
We provide comprehensive treatment of adult and pediatric spine disorders including lower back and neck pain, scoliosis, osteoporosis and complex spine problems. The Spine Center performs minimally invasive spinal fusions and is one of the first in the country to successfully perform artificial disc implantation.

Pediatric Orthopaedics
We provide specialized orthopaedic care for children with neuromuscular diseases such as cerebral palsy, spina bifida and muscular dystrophies, and congenital conditions including clubfoot, hip dysplasia and limb deformities.

Hip Care
We are dedicated to treating a wide range of conditions that affect the hip, whether developmental, traumatic or degenerative, allowing doctors to see the issues from a broad perspective.

Bone Healing
We evaluate and treat complex problem fractures and are leaders in technologies and procedures to help patients facing a long, difficult recovery from complex fracture reconstruction or fracture healing problems.

Foot & Ankle
The Diabetes Foot & Ankle Center focuses on the prevention and recurrence of foot and ankle problems. Dedicated medical professionals provide the most advanced treatment for those complications.

Immediate Care
The Samuels Orthopaedic Immediate Care Center is New York City's only walk-in orthopaedic clinic. Staffed by members of the Department of Orthopaedic Surgery, the "I-Care" Center uses state-of-the-art diagnostic equipment to evaluate and treat urgent problems, including hand & foot injuries, hip, arm or leg fractures, dislocation or joint injury, sprains, and bone or joint infection.

Dance Injuries
The Harkness Center for Dance Injuries offers many subsidized and free services for dancers, including clinics staffed by orthopaedists and dance physical therapists. The Center also offers state-of-the-art rehabilitation technology and free injury prevention screenings and lectures.

Occupational & Industrial Orthopaedics
We provide clinical, educational, research and consulting services in the prevention and treatment of musculoskeletal injuries and disorders that arise from work or the work environment.

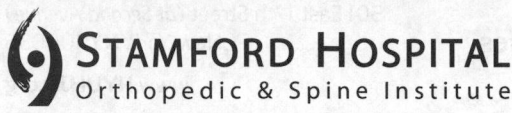
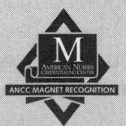

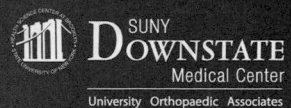

Otolaryngology

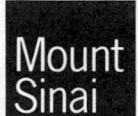 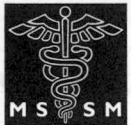

MOUNT SINAI SCHOOL OF MEDICINE

THE MOUNT SINAI MEDICAL CENTER
OTOLARYNGOLOGY – EAR, NOSE, AND THROAT
One Gustave L. Levy Place
Fifth Avenue and 100th Street
New York, NY 10029-6574
Physician Referral: 1-800-MD-SINAI (637-4624)
www.mountsinai.org

Mount Sinai's **DEPARTMENT OF OTOLARYNGOLOGY HEAD AND NECK SURGERY** – is recognized as one of the finest head and neck surgery programs in the nation. Consistently ranked among the top twenty programs in the country, Mount Sinai's department of Otolaryngology-Head and Neck Surgery is one of the oldest in the country. Since the early nineteenth century, Mount Sinai faculty have pioneered surgical advances in endoscopy, otology, skull-base surgery, laryngology, rhinology, facial plastic surgery, and head and neck oncology and reconstruction. Over the past decade, the department has expanded to include cutting-dge technology in robotic and endoscopic surgery, basic science research, and translational science programs.

Robotic Head and Neck Surgery – The Department of Otolaryngology-Head and Neck Surgery is a world leader in robotic head and neck surgery using the da Vinci® Surgical Robotic System. Mount Sinai surgeons and researchers have published new techniques in robotic surgery that have changed the paradigm for management of head and neck cancer. These techniques allow for endoscopic surgery without external incisions shortening hospital stay and improving quality-of-life outcomes.

Endoscopic Laser Surgery of the Larynx and Trachea – Surgeons and researchers at the Mount Sinai School of Medicine have introduced new techniques in laryngeal and tracheal surgery including endoscopic laser surgery, tracheal transplantation, and reconstructive surgery that allows for removal of malignant disease with voice and swallowing preservation.

The Grabsheid Voice Center – For more than a century, Mount Sinai has provided professional singers and patients in need with cutting-edge technology using endoscopic laser surgery and minimally invasive surgical techniques. Surgeons at the Grabsheid Voice Center have pioneered office-based surgical techniques that offer patients the opportunity to undergo therapy without the need for general anesthesia.

Cranial Base Surgery – Techniques in endoscopic trans-nasal surgery have revolutionized the management of skull base tumors and cerebrospinal leaks. Surgeons at Mount Sinai have developed procedures for accessing the cranial base and frontal lobes of the brain through the nose. Outcomes using these methods have demonstrated that patients have excellent outcomes with lower complications rates.

Thyroid and Parathyroid Surgery – The Mount Sinai Thyroid and Parathyroid Center is nationally recognized for excellence in clinical care and clinical outcomes research. Minimally invasive and robotic surgical techniques have provided patients the opportunity for surgery to be performed through an minimally invasive incision. Cure rates for thyroid cancer using these techniques are higher than 95 percent. Parathyroid surgery is performed using similar techniques and intraoperative parathyroid hormone monitoring.

Otology and Neurotology – The multidisciplinary team has long been recognized as one of the best in the nation. Outcomes for acoustic tumors and hearing restoration procedures are among the best in the country. Otologic surgeons at Mount Sinai have pioneered surgical techniques for the management of chronic ear disease and cochlear implantation that have resulted is excellent outcomes.

THE MULTIDISCIPLINARY HEAD AND NECK ONCOLOGY TEAM
Recognized as one of the finest programs in the country, members of the multidisciplinary team include 35 physicians, surgeons, and ancillary staff from 12 different departments focused on the care of patients. The head and neck oncology program offers world-renown courses, training fellowships, and research fellowships that are respected as the finest in the country. Mount Sinai's multi-disciplinary head and neck cancer team has gained national recognition for its expertise and innovation in the management of head, neck, and skull-base cancer. The Mount Sinai team of experts in minimally invasive and endoscopic head and neck surgery comprises a group of surgeons and oncologists focused on curative treatment for head and neck malignancies. The expert team works to treat tumors of the oral cavity, jaw, and larynx, and preserve each patient's quality of life. Speech and swallowing rehabilitation therapists work with patients to help them recover. Mount Sinai is on the cutting edge of head and neck cancer therapy, reconstruction, and rehabilitation.

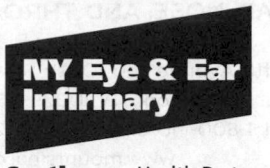
THE NEW YORK EYE AND EAR INFIRMARY

310 East 14th Street
New York, New York 10003
Tel. 212.979.4000   Fax. 212.228.0664
http://www.nyee.edu

PROVIDING EXCEPTIONAL CARE OF THE EAR, NOSE, THROAT, AND HEAD & NECK

Established in 1820 the Department of Otolaryngology/Head & Neck Surgery is the first training program in this specialty in the Western Hemisphere. Over nearly two centuries the department has evolved to be an international referral center for the medical and surgical treatment of diseases of the ear, nose, and throat.

OUTSTANDING SERVICES:

Ear Institute (Otology – Neuro-otology): Specializing in the care of chronic ear disease including hearing loss, cochlear implantation, dizziness, tinnitus, intra cranial tumors and facial nerve disorders. Our advanced otologic and vestibular diagnostic labs assist physicians in treatment.

Facial Plastic Surgery: In-office or ambulatory procedures utilizing computer imaging, new techniques and materials produce outstanding results with minimal incisions, rapid recovery and a natural, youthful appearance.

Facial Paralysis: Comprehensive center treating all causes and offering reconstruction of the paralyzed face.

Head & Neck Oncology: A multi-disciplinary team including board-certified surgeons, medical & radiation oncologists, nutritionists and rehabilitation specialists insure rapid recovery from complex, life-saving surgical procedures and return to daily activities.

Pediatric Otolaryngology: Treating children has long been a priority at the Infirmary. Pediatric care ranges from middle ear infection, tonsil and adenoid disease, and neck masses to complex sinus and airway diseases.

Rhinology and Sinus Surgery: Internationally known specialists utilize minimally invasive techniques to treat disorders from sinusitis to intra cranial tumors.

Thyroid Center: A comprehensive program to streamline the diagnosis and treatment of thyroid diseases and cancers. A highly skilled team of surgeons, endocrinologists and radiologists manage the patient's care.

Voice & Swallowing Institute: Combining the expertise of physicians, speech pathologists and a voice physiologist to diagnose and treat voice problems – not only for performing artists but also for teachers, stockbrokers, receptionists, salespeople – anyone for whom voice is an important part of life.

Otolaryngology Clinical Services

General Otolaryngology *plus*
Facial Plastic & Reconstructive Surgery
Cochlear Implantation
Voice & Vocal Dynamics
Head & Neck Oncology
Laryngology
Otology & Neuro-otology
Pediatric Otolaryngology
Rhinology & Sinus Surgery
Swallowing Disorders
Thyroid Center

Facilities

Ambulatory Care Services
Faculty Practice
Teaching Practice
Hearing Aid Dispensary
Vestibular Rehabilitation

About The New York Eye and Ear Infirmary

The Infirmary is the nation's oldest, continuously operating specialty hospital and one of the most experienced in terms of the number of patients it treats and complexity of its cases. Each year the otolaryngology department performs more than 6,000 surgeries and sees more than 70,000 visits from outpatients

Physician Referral
1.800.449.HOPE (4673)

OTOLARYNGOLOGY

About the Department of Otolaryngology:
The Department of Otolaryngology at NYU Langone Medical Center provides the highest quality treatment for ear, nose, throat, head and neck disorders. Focusing on patient care and innovative research, we have one of the premier Head and Neck Surgery programs in the country.
We specialize in the following areas:

Cochlear Implants
We provide patients extensive assessments, device programming and speech rehabilitation offering both pre- and post-operative speech and language evaluation and therapy. The Center was the first in the U.S. to use a multichannel cochlear implant in a profoundly deaf adult and the first in the Northeast to perform an auditory brainstem implant.

Facial Plastic and Reconstructive Surgery
We provide care for patients requiring facial reconstructive surgery for a wide variety of facial deformities or those patients seeking facial cosmetic surgery. Specialties include functional and aesthetic rhinoplasty, facial rejuvenation surgery, injectable fillers, Botulinum Toxin (Botox) for facial spasm or wrinkles and chemical peels and microdermabrasion.

General Otolaryngology and Sleep Surgery
We provide care for adult patients suffering from voice, sleep, allergy and nasal breathing disorders, as well as general otolaryngology. Children's services are provided through the Division of Pediatric Otolaryngology.

Head and Neck Surgery and Oncology
We provide care for patients with cancer of the head and neck including cancer of the: larynx, oral cavity, throat, nasal cavity and sinuses, salivary glands and lymph nodes in the neck. We also provide microvascular reconstruction, thyroid neoplasms treatment and anterior cranial base surgery.

Neutology/Skull Base Program
Using a multispecialty approach, we provide care of patients with hearing loss, facial nerve palsy, vertigo and tinnitus and treat lesions such as acoustic neuromas and skull base meningiomas. As one of the highest volume centers in the country, featured services include Facial Palsy Rehabilitation, Auditory Brainstem Implants, Cochlear implants, laser surgery and endoscopic anterior and lateral skull base surgery.

Voice and Swallowing Disorders
We provide diagnosis, treatment and therapy for voice and swallowing disorders including sore throat, chronic cough, hoarseness, voice loss, swallowing dysfunction, benign growths and cancerous tumors, vocal cord paralysis, the aging voice, recurrent or chronic laryngitis, gastroesophageal reflux and injuries from overuse and misuse of the voice.

Audiology: offers treatment for patients suffering with hearing or balance disorders; **Head and Neck Speech Pathology:** provides treatment for voice, speech or swallowing problems; **Rhinology:** provides treatment for all diseases of the paranasal sinuses, nose and related structures; **Skull Base Surgery:** offers a minimally invasive and advanced surgical approach to tumors of the anterior and posterior skull base.

Pediatric Cardiology

PEDIATRIC CARDIOLOGY

About the Division of Pediatric Cardiology, Department of Pediatrics:
The Division of Pediatric Cardiology, at the Cardiac and Vascular Institute at NYU Langone Medical Center, is at the forefront of innovation in clinical care, research and teaching. A special emphasize on early and accurate diagnosis during fetal life allows for better preparation and quicker response for the treatment of neonates with congenital heart disease. Excellent surgical and ICU capabilities result in better outcomes for a wide range of patients with congenital heart disease from the fetus to the adult. The Division's staff is vigilant in helping children stay in contact with their parents during their stay at the Medical Center, as well welcoming parents to stay overnight in their child's room on the pediatric floor whenever possible. Social workers and child life experts are always on hand to give families the information and support they need to cope with their child's disease during and after their stay at the Medical Center. *We specialize in the following areas:*

Cardiothoracic Surgery
The Division offers corrective and palliative procedures for all types of congenital and acquired heart disease for a wide range of ages from fetal life to the adult population.

Pediatric Cardiac Critical Care
NYU Langone Medical Center provides cardiac intensive care for children with heart disease. Our staff of pediatric cardiologists, pediatric cardiac intensivists, neonatologists, cardiac anesthesiologists, respiratory therapists and pediatric intensive care nurses are experienced, highly skilled and compassionate.

Pediatric Cardiac Electrophysiology
Specialists within the Division provide a wide array of diagnostic and therapeutic services including arrhythmia detection, cardiac ablation and pacemaker placement.

Pediatric Cardiopulmonary Exercise Laboratory
The lab assesses the cardio-respiratory response of exercise in children as young as three and four years old. It features some of the most sophisticated equipment in the region for measuring oxygen consumption, cardiac output and lung capacity.

Pediatric Interventional Cardiac Catheterization
The Division offers diagnosis and treatment of complex heart conditions in a nonsurgical setting, sometimes used in combination (hybrid) with open-heart surgery. Full range of interventional procedures including stent implantation and transcatheter device closure are available.

Pediatric Non-Invasive Cardiac Imaging
The Division of Pediatric Cardiology at the Cardiac and Vascular Institute at NYU Langone Medical Center offers Cardiac Echocardiography, Magnetic Resonance Imaging (MRI) and Computer Tomography (CT) to diagnose and monitor a wide range of cardiac abnormalities.

Fetal Cardiac Program
An active program of fetal cardiac imaging program is collaborating closely with NYU Langone Neonatologists, Geneticists and the OB/GYN department.

Pediatric Emergency Medicine

PEDIATRIC EMERGENCY MEDICINE

About the Division of Pediatric Emergency Medicine, Department of Pediatrics:
The Division of Pediatric Emergency Medicine at NYU Langone Medical Center offers patients compassionate and state-of-the-art emergency medical care. Or physicians are specially trained in pediatric emergency medicine and are expert in managing emergencies specific to infants, children, adolescents and young adults. They are recognized as national leaders for the training of Pediatric Emergency Medicine physicians, as well as for research and advocacy. ***We specialize in the following areas:***

Pediatric Emergency Medicine
The Tisch Hospital Pediatric Emergency Medicine Program at NYU Langone Medical Center provides the highest level of state-of-the-art care to all pediatric patients. Ill and injured children seeking care receive treatment in an area that is child friendly and family focused. The pediatric sub-specialty physicians and pediatric surgical physicians are available for consultation in the Emergency Department 24 hours a day, 365 days a year.

Pediatric Emergency Services
Pediatric Emergency Services (PES) at Bellevue Hospital Center, an affiliate of NYU Langone Medical Center, is dedicated to the care of acutely ill and injured children. Each year approximately 25,000 children and young adults are evaluated in the PES which is staffed around the clock by board-certified pediatric emergency medicine physicians and nurses who specialize in the emergency care of children. The PES manages patients with a wide range of medical, surgical and psychiatric problems, including asthma, appendicitis, child abuse, orthopaedic injuries, major trauma, poisoning and suicide.

Pediatric Transport
The Pediatric Transport Program at NYU Langone Medical Center transfers critically ill pediatric patients from outlying facilities to the Medical Center. In-house teams are available 24 hours a day, 7 days a week to allow a rapid response for medical transports. Patients are transported from more than 50 hospitals. The transport team assembled includes personnel with expertise in respiratory therapy and pediatric critical care nursing, in addition to the highest level of physician staff as appropriate. Patients are provided with the most advanced care from the beginning of the transport at the referring facility to their final destination, where they are cared for by physicians in a comprehensive network of sub-specialties.

Pediatric Gastroenterology

550 First Avenue *(at 31st Street)*
New York, NY 10016
www.NYULMC.org

Physician Referral: **(888)7-NYU-MED** *(888-769-8633)*

PEDIATRIC GASTROENTEROLOGY

About the Division of Pediatric Gastroenterology, Department of Pediatrics:
The pediatric gastroenterologists at NYU Langone Medical Center are dedicated to providing the highest quality medical care and state-of-the-art techniques in the evaluation and management of gastrointestinal, liver and nutritional disorders from infancy to young adulthood. With access to the latest in endoscopic procedures performed at one of the country's leading academic medical centers, patients receive comprehensive and multidisciplinary treatments for a wide range of conditions. Our pediatric gastroenterologists are particularly adept at providing family-centered, integrated care with a focus on the physical and psychological well-being of the child. *We specialize in the following areas:*

Clinical Care
Most children will occasionally experience one or more gastrointestinal symptoms during their childhood years. Some children, however, develop recurrent symptoms, which interrupt their normal lives and are the presenting features of important, treatable diseases. The gastrointestinal and nutritional concerns impacting on the health and quality of life of children on the autism spectrum is an area of particular interest and at NYU Langone. We are at the forefront in the evaluation and management of celiac disease and food allergies, including allergic involvement of the esophagus (eosinophilic esophagitis) and our experts use the latest techniques to pinpoint problems and to determine the most effective therapy.We offer a vast range of therapeutic services, as well as access to clinical nutrition services, pediatric rehabilitation and some of the country's best surgeons.

Specialty Care
Pediatric gastroenterologists at NYU Langone Medical Center evaluate and treat a variety of disorders including: abdominal pain, celiac spruce, congenital bowel dysfunction, congenital liver disorders and chronic liver disease, chronic constipation, feeding problems in infants, failure to thrive, food allergies, lactose intolerance, gastrointestinal bleeding, gastroesophageal reflux, hepatitis, malabsorption syndromes, pancreatitis, peptic ulcer disease, ulcerative colitis and Crohn's disease.

Pediatric Hematology-Oncology

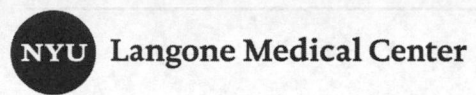
PEDIATRIC HEMATOLOGY/ONCOLOGY

About the Division of Pediatric Hematology/Oncology, Department of Pediatrics and the NCI-designated NYU Cancer Institute

Our Division of Pediatric Hematology and Oncology is an academically oriented program that is committed to providing modern, family-centered and highly personalized care to children with cancer and blood disorders. Teams of specialists deliver personalized care in a healing environment that promotes the physical, emotional and spiritual well-being of children and their families, using the tools of modern biology to identify the causes of childhood cancer and blood disorders and rapidly translate scientific discovery into better treatments. *We specialize in the following areas:*

Hematologic Malignancies

Our Pediatric Hematologic Malignancies Program offers new treatments for childhood acute lymphoblastic leukemia (ALL). We currently lead nationwide clinical trials for those with newly diagnosed leukemia and recurrent diseases, and participate in a number of clinical trials that offer new treatment agents.

Hematology

We offer state-of-the-art treatment for children and adolescents with all blood disorders including Sickle Cell Disease, other hemoglobinopathies, bleeding disorders and aplastic anemia.

Pediatric Neuro-Oncology

We provide comprehensive care for infants, children, adolescents and young adults with primary central nervous system, slow-growing and malignant tumors. We offer a multidisciplinary approach to provide the safest and most effective curative treatment for patients with newly diagnosed and recurrent tumors.

Pediatric Special Hematology Laboratory

We offer comprehensive homeostasis and red cell testing. Test procedures incorporate the latest developments in the field. We provide fast, precise test information that leads to effective treatments while maintaining rigorous quality control standards.

Psychosocial Services

To help children and families cope with their disease and to prevent later psychological trauma, our holistic approach to care includes: art therapy, relaxation training, play therapy, psychiatric evaluation, neuropsychological assessment, individual and group counseling and patient education.

Sarcoma and Solid Tumor Program

Our Pediatric Hematologic Malignancies Program offers cutting-edge medical, surgical and radiotherapy treatments for bone and soft tissue sarcomas, and all pediatric solid tumors including Wilms' Tumor and neuroblastoma. We are developing national trials for the treatment of sarcomas and offer a number of clinical trials that offer new treatment agents.

The Stephen D. Hassenfeld Children's Center for Cancer and Blood Center's

We are constantly developing new ways to treat childhood cancer. Our mission is to provide children, with cancer and blood disorders, the best research-driven care in a comprehensive and compassionate manner. Our unique interdisciplinary and family-centered approach combines the most advanced medical treatments.

Pediatric Infectious Disease

PEDIATRIC INFECTIOUS DISEASES

About the Division of Pediatric Infectious Diseases, Department of Pediatrics:
The Division of Pediatric Infectious Diseases (PID) of NYU Langone Medical Center, offers one of the largest programs in New York City for mothers and children with HIV infection at Bellevue Hospital Center an affiliate of NYU Langone. Initiated in 1982, this program furthers the understanding of the transmission of HIV from mothers to children and contributes to their improved care and longevity. The Division was one of the first NIH-funded Pediatric AIDS Clinical Trials Group sites and has cared for almost 500 HIV-infected children. It currently is funded as an HIV Clinical Trials site called IMPAACT (International Maternal Pediatric Adolescent AIDS Clinical Trials) devoted to the treatment of HIV infection, as well as its complications. Additionally, PID treats patients with other infectious diseases such as herpes viruses, respiratory viruses, hepatitis, bacterial, fungal and parasitic infections (tropical and local). We are also experienced in travel medicine and congenital infectious diseases.
We specialize in the following areas:

Adolescent HIV Clinic
The Bellevue Adolescent Clinic provides free, confidential HIV testing, pre- and post-test counseling, complete medical evaluations, comprehensive medical care and, if requested, referrals to clinical trials for HIV-positive teenagers. NYU Langone Medical Center was designated a Reaching for Excellence in Adolescent Care and Health (REACH) site, an NIH/HRSA-funded project. The clinic's primary objective is to increase the understanding of the natural history of HIV in teens and disease management.

Infectious Diseases Clinic
The Pediatric Infectious Diseases Clinic is one of the major providers of care for women and children at risk for HIV infection and other infectious diseases. Medical services are provided for children by the PID Clinic attending physicians, postdoctoral fellows and a pediatrician, with a dermatologist and pedodontist available. The clinic screens mothers for risk factors and provides counseling, testing and follow-up care for those receiving prenatal care.

Pediatric Infectious Disease
Children requiring intravenous infusions during the course of their illness are cared for at the Pediatric Infectious Disease Day Hospital. The hospital also provides the medical, nursing, psychological and social support services these children require. Pediatrics patients can also use the hospital for non-acute care outside of regular clinic hours.

TB Clinic
The TB Clinic evaluates approximately 200 new cases of latent and active tuberculosis a year and is a referral center for TB in the city. The Clinic is staffed by residents, a pediatric nurse practitioner, two PID attending physicians with particular expertise and experience with tuberculosis.

Viral Hepatitis Clinic
The Viral Hepatitis Clinic meets twice a week in Bellevue Hospital and follows approximately 250 children with chronic hepatitis C infection. The Clinic is a referral center for viral hepatitis infections in children and is the principal referral center for the NYC Pediatric Viral Hepatitis Network, a consortium of health facilities that is funded by the NY City Council.

Pediatric Pulmonology

NYU Langone Medical Center

PEDIATRIC PULMONOLOGY

About Pediatric Pulmonology, Department of Pediatrics:
The Division of Pediatric Pulmonology at NYU Langone Medical Center provides comprehensive care to children with a variety of conditions affecting the respiratory system, from infancy to adolescence and young adulthood. Physicians in the Division are committed to providing both family-centered and multidisciplinary care, collaborating with specialists in other divisions throughout the medical center. For example, physicians in the Division work closely with the NYU Infant Apnea/SIDS Program to follow children discharged from the Neonatal Intensive Care Unit; with the division of Pediatric Gastroenterology and the Swallowing Center to follow children with feeding difficulties and swallowing dysfunction; the division of Pediatric Surgery, to follow children with congenital lung lesions through minimally invasive surgery; and with the Division of Orthopedics to optimize the care of children with neuromuscular disease undergoing spine surgery. *We specialize in the following areas:*

Pulmonologists in the Division care for children with a wide range of problems, including asthma, bronchopulmonary dysplasia (chronic lung disease of prematurity), cystic fibrosis, chronic respiratory failure and pulmonary complications of neuromuscular disease, congenital lung malformations, chest wall deformities, interstitial lung disease, and obstructive sleep apnea. We also provide consultation for chronic cough, noisy breathing, and exercise intolerance.

Flexible bronchoscopy
Using specialized pediatric equipment, the airways of even the tiniest infants can be examined in the state-of –the art endoscopy suite at NYU Langone Medical Center. Procedures are often performed in a multidisciplinary fashion, if multiple specialists are involved in the care of the child. Equipment is mobile, and, if required, procedures can also be performed at the bedside in the Intensive Care Unit.

Pediatric Rheumatology

PEDIATRIC RHEUMATOLOGY

About the Division of Pediatric Rheumatology, Department of Pediatrics:

The pediatric rheumatology specialists at the NYU Langone Medical Center are devoted to the complete care of children with rheumatic disease. In conjunction with our multi-disciplinary therapeutic team of specialists we treat children with a variety of rheumatologic conditions including Juvenile Idiopathic Arthritis (JIA), systemic lupus erythematosus, juvenile dermatomyositis, Kawasaki's disease and others. Through early diagnosis and appropriately intensive treatment we aim to achieve disease quiescence as quickly and safely as possible with the ultimate goal of returning children to full physical functioning. Patients are seen at our private practice offices, as well as in weekly clinics at the Hospital for Joint Diseases, Bellevue Medical Center and Woodhull Medical Center.

In addition to our clinical services, we are also committed to the continued formal education of residents, rheumatology fellows and medical students, as well as the general public with our community outreach programs though various organizations. In collaboration with the adult rheumatology division, we have initiated an annual pediatric rheumatology CME course which is well-attended by general physicians as well as rheumatologists. Our emphasis on providing high-level clinical services and teaching is also complemented by the division's collaboration with national pediatric rheumatology research organizations in several clinical research projects pertaining to drug exposure is children with rheumatic disease. *We specialize in the following areas:*

Juvenile Idiopathic Arthritis
An umbrella term for several different patterns of arthritis in children, juvenile idiopathic arthritis (JIA) refers to arthritic disorders caused by an autoimmune reaction. Our Pediatric rheumatologists diagnose and treat the different types of JIA. The use of methotrexate in combination with new discovered biologic agents, such as Etanercept and Infliximab, gives even greater reason for optimism. Juvenile arthritis, once a cripple of children, is fast becoming a highly manageable disease.

Pediatric Arthritis
Arthritis is the term used to describe inflammation and swelling of the tissues in a joint. Perhaps surprisingly, viruses are the most common cause of arthritis in children. This type of arthritis is usually temporary and passes quickly without permanent damage. However, a bacterial joint infection is a more urgent matter. Called septic arthritis, this painful condition requires urgent care to prevent the spread of infection and the possibility of permanent damage to the joint. At its first sign, the NYU Langone's expert staff is quick to take steps to fight the infection at its source.

Pediatric Surgery

PEDIATRIC SURGERY

About the Division of Pediatric Surgery:
The Division of Pediatric Surgery at NYU Langone Medical Center provides comprehensive pediatric surgical care from the smallest preterm infant to the adolescent. Our board-certified pediatric surgeons are experts at utilizing minimally invasive, resulting in shorter hospitals stays and faster recoveries, as well as conventional techniques, to treat a broad range of surgical problems. Care begins even before the child is admitted and may continue long after the child is discharged. In addition to the highly-skilled surgeons and surgical nurses, the Medical Center offers a wide array of Child Life Services to help children and their families become familiar with the hospital environment and lessen fears that often accompany a hospital stay. *We specialize in the following areas:*

Surgical Expertise
NYU Langone Medical Center is renowned for its achievements in the full spectrum of pediatric surgical specialties, including abdominal and thoracic surgery, neonatal surgery, surgery for all congenital anomalies, cancer surgery, urology, neurosurgery, orthopedics, plastic and reconstructive surgery, repair of cleft lips and palates, ophthalmology, and ENT among others. All surgical specialists are trained in the latest technological advances within their respective disciplines.

Pediatric Anesthesia
The thought of anesthesia invariably provokes parental anxiety. We are proud to have an expert group of fellowship trained pediatric anesthesiologists to serve our pediatric population. The anesthesiologists are involved in preoperative and postoperative care as well as administering anesthesia and have developed close working relationships with the pediatric surgeons.

Child Life Services
The pediatric unit at our Tisch Hospital is home to The Child Life Program that focuses on creating a supportive environment for children undergoing surgery. The program offers a total care approach for the child and support services for the families. Child Life personnel meet the parents and their child immediately prior to surgery and provide a continuum of care to the entire family throughout the hospital experience.

Pre-Admission Orientation and Information
Informational packets about what to expect are given to families during the pre-admission testing process. Parents and their children are also encouraged to attend an orientation session with a member of the Child Life Program staff.

Facilities
Day Surgery facilities include an expansive playroom with computers, games and Child Life personnel to care for the family. A separate recovery room area has been established to provide a calming environment during emergence from anesthesia. Inpatients are exposed to a multitude of Child Life Programs.

Pediatrics

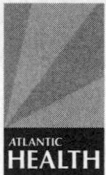

**Goryeb Children's Hospital • Atlantic Neuroscience Institute
Carol G. Simon Cancer Center • Gagnon Cardiovascular Institute
Atlantic Rehabilitation Institute**

P.O. Box 1905, Morristown, NJ 07962 • www.atlantichealth.org

To find a doctor, call 800-247-9580 or visit us online

Nationally Recognized Pediatric Care

At Goryeb Children's Hospital, we know there is nothing more important than a child's health. That's why we are committed to delivering the finest personalized pediatric specialty care in a patient- and family-centered environment to more than 50,000 children, from infants to young adults, each year. Your child will benefit from the expertise of nationally recognized, board-certified pediatric specialists who are actively involved in clinical research, enabling them to offer your child the newest medications, treatments and technologies. We have over 100 specialty physicians in 20 concentrated areas of pediatric medical and surgical care.

Services available through Goryeb Children's Hospital include:

◢ **Pediatric Cardiology – The Children's Heart Center** provides comprehensive, evaluation of children with suspected congenital and acquired heart disease. Services include diagnosis, treatment and diagnostic testing using the latest technology.

◢ **Pediatric Critical Care – The Pediatric Intensive Care Unit (PICU)** provides care to children with life-threatening illness and injury. The PICU features advanced technologies for continuous monitoring of respiratory, cardiac and neurological functions. The PICU also includes a specialized pediatric transport team to rapidly and safely bring children to our facility by ambulance or helicopter.

◢ **Pediatric Endocrinology – The Pediatric and Adolescent Endocrine and BD Diabetes Centers** provide care to children and teens with a variety of metabolic and hormonal disorders. The BD Diabetes Center – the largest pediatric diabetes center in the region – helps children and their families learn how to manage type 1 and type 2 diabetes and offers the most effective tools for living with diabetes.

◢ **Pediatric Gastroenterology - The Division of Pediatric Gastroenterology, Hepatology and Nutrition** uses a multidisciplinary team approach in the diagnosis and management of children with digestive disorders, including feeding problems, recurrent abdominal pain, gastroesophageal reflux and liver disorders. The Center for Pediatric Inflammatory Bowel Disease is the largest in the state of New Jersey.

◢ **Pediatric Hematology and Oncology – The Valerie Fund Children's Center at Morristown Memorial and Overlook hospitals** provides personalized, comprehensive medical care to patients with cancer and blood disorders. Our multidisciplinary team of professionals have access to the most advanced therapeutic options for patients and their families.

◢ **Pediatric Neurology – The Division of Pediatric Neurology** provides comprehensive care for children with neurologic disorders including, but not limited to, epilepsy and seizure disorders, attention deficit hyperactivity disorder, autistic disorders, cerebral palsy, and developmental and learning disabilities.

◢ **Pediatric Pulmonology - The Respiratory Center for Children** offers comprehensive care for children with all forms of lung disease. We have the largest pediatric pulmonary center in New Jersey with certified nurse asthma educators and a free-standing pediatric sleep lab and exercise lab.

◢ **Pediatric Surgery- The Division of Pediatric Surgery** provides comprehensive surgical care for children using state-of-the-art techniques and innovative approaches. We have general pediatric surgeons with expertise in all areas of general and thoracic surgery, as well as specialty surgeons with expertise in pediatric neurosurgery and orthopedic surgery. Our surgeons work closely with pediatric radiologists and pediatric anesthesiologists and use minimally invasive surgical techniques whenever possible.

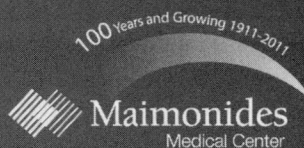
Sponsored Page

NewYork-Presbyterian

The University Hospital of Columbia and Cornell

NewYork-Presbyterian
Morgan Stanley Children's Hospital
Columbia University Medical Center
3959 Broadway
New York, NY 10032

 NewYork-Presbyterian
Phyllis and David Komansky
Center for Children's Health
Weill Cornell Medical Center
525 East 68th Street
New York, NY 10065

Accreditation: The Joint Commission

OVERVIEW:

The pediatric services of NewYork-Presbyterian Hospital are comprised of NewYork-Presbyterian Morgan Stanley Children's Hospital, which is affiliated with Columbia University College of Physicians and Surgeons, and the NewYork-Presbyterian Phyllis and David Komansky Center for Children's Health, which is affiliated with Weill Cornell Medical College. Together, they serve as one of the nation's premier centers for comprehensive pediatric care. Skilled and experienced physicians, surgeons, nurses and other pediatric healthcare professionals manage some of the most complex medical conditions of children at every stage of development. Their expertise includes general pediatric care and the full range of medical and surgical subspecialties:

- Adolescent Medicine
- Allergy and Immunology
- Anesthesiology
- Blood Disorders
- Blood and Marrow Transplantation
- Cancer
- Cardiology and Cardiac Surgery
- Craniofacial and Plastic Surgery
- Critical Care
- Dermatology
- Digestive Disease
- Ear, Nose and Throat
- Emergency Department, including specialized units for burns and trauma injuries
- Endocrinology, Diabetes and Metabolism
- Epilepsy
- Genetics
- Infectious Diseases

- Kidney Disease
- Liver Disease
- Lung Disease
- Neonatal Medicine
- Neurology and Neurological Surgery
- Nutrition
- Obesity and Bariatric Surgery
- Ophthalmology
- Oral and Maxillofacial Surgery and Pediatric Dentistry
- Organ Transplantation
- Orthopaedic Surgery
- Pain Medicine
- Pediatric Surgery
- Pregnancy and Newborn Services
- Primary Care/General Pediatrics
- Psychiatry
- Radiology
- Rheumatology
- Urology

FOR MORE INFORMATION:
To find a physician or for more information, call
1-800-245-KIDS (1-800-245-5437) or visit our website at
www.childrensnyp.org

HIGHLIGHTS AT A GLANCE:

- A national leader in pediatric open-heart surgery with one the largest pediatric heart transplant programs in the nation.

- A pediatric kidney transplant program, which includes a Living Donor Program and leading edge therapies to help reduce the side effects of anti-rejection drugs.

- Pediatric cardiac surgeons at the forefront of ventricular assist devices for infants and small children as a bridge to recovery or transplantation.

- One of three Level 1-designated Regional Pediatric Trauma Centers in New York State and the only one in New York City.

- A New York State Department of Health-designated Regional Perinatal Center of expertise for the care of women with high-risk pregnancies.

- One of the largest Type 1 diabetes programs in New York State.

- Outstanding neonatal intensive care programs setting standards of care nationwide for extremely ill newborns.

- The only program in the New York tri-state area that has active programs in both liver and small bowel transplantation.

Physical Medicine &

Rehabilitation

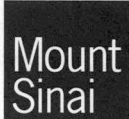 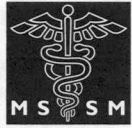

MOUNT SINAI SCHOOL OF MEDICINE

THE MOUNT SINAI MEDICAL CENTER
REHABILITATION MEDICINE
One Gustave L. Levy Place
Fifth Avenue and 100th Street
New York, NY 10029-6574
Physician Referral: 1-800-MD-SINAI (637-4624)
www.mountsinai.org

THE DEPARTMENT OF REHABILITATION MEDICINE at Mount Sinai is a Center of Excellence in the delivery of complete care for people with disabilities. A wide range of comprehensive patient care services is available for individuals with spinal cord injuries, brain injuries, and a variety of neuromuscular, musculoskeletal, and chronic conditions. We are accredited by the Commission on Accreditation of Rehabilitation Facilities (CARF) for our inpatient spinal cord and brain injury programs—the only such accredited programs at non-VA hospitals in New York City—as well as for our comprehensive rehabilitation medicine program.

Pivotal to successful rehabilitation, the multidisciplinary team approach at Mount Sinai takes advantage of all areas of expertise to provide the highest quality of coordinated care. Our experienced professionals evaluate each patient and meet regularly to develop and implement individualized treatment plans in partnership with patients and their families. Our goal is to make each individual with a disability maximally self-sufficient and mobile, and able to return to community life.

The Mount Sinai Rehabilitation Center team is led by Kristjan T. Ragnarsson, MD, whose leadership and innovative approach to patient care has had a major impact in the field of rehabilitation medicine. The Center includes physicians, primary rehabilitation nurses, nurse practitioners, and professional staff in physical therapy, occupational therapy, speech therapy, nutrition, social work, psychology, therapeutic recreation, and vocational counseling. Special rehabilitation medicine programs include the following:

- **The Spinal Cord Injury Rehabilitation Program** provides comprehensive care to individuals with spinal cord injuries. This includes a full range of innovative medical and rehabilitation services. For example, our "Do It" program is a unique outpatient program that facilitates community integration.

- **The Brain Injury Rehabilitation Program** provides comprehensive care to individuals with brain injuries. It is well recognized that the treatment of individuals with cognitive and behavioral challenges is critical to community integration. Our program contains specialists uniquely qualified to meet these challenges.

- **The Sports Therapy Center** is a comprehensive outpatient physical and occupational therapy facility offering individualized treatments for people with a variety of musculoskeletal conditions. It is conveniently located in midtown Manhattan.

MODEL SYSTEMS OF CARE

The Department of Rehabilitation Medicine provides comprehensive services that serve as national models of care. • Consistently ranked among the top rehabilitation centers by *U.S. News & World Report.*

- One of 14 programs designated by the National Institute of Disability and Rehabilitation Research (NIDRR) as a Model System of Care for Spinal Cord Injury, the only such designated program in New York State.

- One of 16 programs designated by NIDRR as a Model System of Care for Traumatic Brain Injury, the only such designated program in New York State.

- The only NIDRR-designated Research and Training Center for Traumatic Brain Injury Intervention.

- The first CDC Injury Control Research Center focusing on traumatic brain injury research.

Plastic Surgery

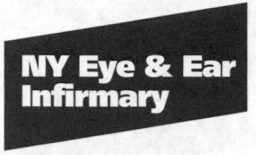

Psychiatry

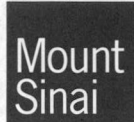
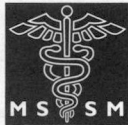

**THE MOUNT SINAI MEDICAL CENTER
PSYCHIATRY**
One Gustave L. Levy Place
Fifth Avenue and 100th Street
New York, NY 10029-6574
Physician Referral: 1-800-MD-SINAI (637-4624)
www.mountsinai.org

THE DEPARTMENT OF PSYCHIATRY at Mount Sinai strives to bring tomorrow's breakthrough treatments from clinical neuroscience research to clinical care today. We provide services for infants, children, adolescents, adults, and seniors, offering mental health evaluation and treatment for autism, attention-deficit hyperactivity disorder (ADHD), behavioral disorders, schizophrenia, Alzheimer's disease, mood and anxiety disorders, obsessive-compulsive disorder (OCD), substance abuse, post-traumatic stress disorder (PTSD), eating disorders, and personality disorders.

Clinical Services – The Department of Psychiatry is organized around key Centers of Excellence that link academic thought leaders to clinicians throughout the department. We offer a full range of diagnostic and treatment services, including psychotherapy, psychopharmacology, emergency services, electroconvulsive therapy, neuropsychological testing, and management of difficult clinical cases. We also provide mental health services in the Mount Sinai's World Trade Center Medical Monitoring and Treatment Program.

Specialty Programs – The Seaver Autism Center of Excellence offers a comprehensive assessment and treatment program that provides the finest patient care informed by the latest research. Our expert clinical staff is experienced in autism spectrum disorders, specializing in personalized and evidence-based treatment for very young children and high-functioning adults, as well as those individuals considered most difficult to assess and treat. The Attention-Deficit Hyperactivity Disorder (ADHD) Center serves children and adults providing state-of-the-art psychiatric evaluation, psychological testing, behavioral and cognitive-behavioral treatments, and medication management. Our Center for Eating and Weight Disorders serves adults and children, offering innovative, and evidence based treatment for anorexia nervosa, bulimia nervosa, binge eating disorder, and obesity.

The Mood and Anxiety Disorders Program (MAP) is devoted to understanding the causes of mood and anxiety disorders and aims to advance the latest integrative treatment strategies for patients who suffer from major depression, bipolar disorder, PTSD, panic attacks, generalized anxiety disorder, and social phobia. MAP at Mount Sinai uses state-of-the-art brain imaging, and genetic, and clinical trials methods to enhance our understanding of brain processes associated with these disorders.

TRANSLATING KNOWLEDGE INTO NEW SOLUTIONS
Mount Sinai is at the forefront of unlocking the interactions between biological processes and the myriad states of the human mind. Among our major research programs in psychiatry are the Alzheimer's Disease Research Center, which conducts both basic science and clinical research, and The Seaver Autism Center for Research and Treatment, which is dedicated to unraveling the biological causes of this disorder and to developing innovative treatment strategies. In shedding important new light on mental illness, psychiatrists at Mount Sinai are frequently able to offer the treatments of tomorrow—therapies that will not be widely available for years.

The Obsessive Compulsive Disorders (OCD) Center of Excellence provides state-of-the-art diagnostic evaluation and specializes in treating severe or treatment-resistant OCD. The Center offers comprehensive evaluations, expert consultations, novel and evidence-based treatments, and research studies. We offer outpatient services for children, adolescents, and adults. We specialize in biological interventions for patients who have not responded to conventional therapies.

Pulmonary Disease

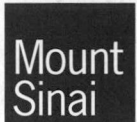
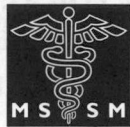

**MOUNT SINAI
SCHOOL OF
MEDICINE**

THE MOUNT SINAI MEDICAL CENTER
PULMONARY MEDICINE
One Gustave L. Levy Place
Fifth Avenue and 100th Street
New York, NY 10029-6574
Physician Referral: 1-800-MD-SINAI (637-4624)
www.mountsinai.org

The mission of Mount Sinai's **DIVISION OF PULMONARY, CRITICAL CARE, AND SLEEP MEDICINE** is to offer state-of-the-art clinical care to patients with all forms of lung disease and critical illness, cutting-edge research that will translate into improved patient care and outcomes, and hands-on training of future leaders in the field.

To achieve this goal, every faculty member is charged with the success of a specific program. Mount Sinai's Sarcoidosis Service, the largest of its kind in the world, is a Center of Excellence for sarcoidosis research. It is the only site in the United States that performs the diagnostic Kveim-Siltzbach skin test for sarcoidosis, which eliminates the need for more invasive, uncomfortable, and expensive procedures.

Through its Pulmonary Physiology Laboratory, Mount Sinai has been instrumental in establishing normal values for various pulmonary function tests and is currently conducting clinical studies of new tests for obesity, sarcoidosis, asthma, and lung cancer. Pulmonary specialists at Mount Sinai are investigating asthma and emphysema, lung cancer, collagen vascular diseases, pulmonary infections, and occupational lung diseases. Mount Sinai has the largest screening program for workers and anyone in the general population exposed to polluted air at the World Trade Center catastrophe site. Our critical care physicians are experts in treating liver disease and acute and chronic respiratory failure, using the most modern forms of delivery of intensive care and providing compassionate end-of-life care.

Our programs and services include:

- **The Asthma Program** uses a multidisciplinary team approach, focusing on patient education and skill-building to foster self-management;

- **The Chronic Obstructive Pulmonary Disease Program** offers a coordinated approach of exercise, treatment, and education that improves quality of life and clinical outlook, for one of the nation's most underdiagnosed conditions;

- **The Critical Care Medicine Program** features state-of-the-art medical intensive care and respiratory care units;

- **The Interventional Pulmonary Service** performs cutting-edge diagnostic and therapeutic procedures for patients with advanced pulmonary diseases;

- **The Occupational Lung Disorders Program** specializes in the diagnosis and management of occupational lung disorders, such as occupational asthma and bronchitis, asbestosis, silicosis, and heavy metal lung injury;

- **The Pulmonary Fibrosis/Interstitial Lung Disease Program** treats patients with chronic inflammatory and scarring disorders of the lungs, including collagen vascular-associated pulmonary diseases;

- **The Pulmonary Physiology Laboratory**, which has recently doubled in capacity, performs the full range of physiological testing for lung disease;

- **The Pulmonary Rehabilitation Program** provides occupational, physical, and cardiopulmonary rehabilitation programs for patients with disabling lung disorders, as well as pre- and post-operative consultation and therapy;

- **The Thoracic Oncology Service** provides multidisciplinary medical care for lung cancer, as a joint effort with the Department of Cardiothoracic Surgery; and,

- **The Sarcoidosis Service,** which has passed its 20,000 enrollee count, offers standard care as well as the opportunity to participate in new clinical trials to 60 new enrollees per week.

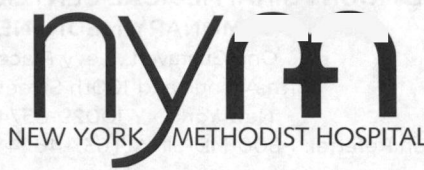

NEW YORK METHODIST HOSPITAL

THE INSTITUTE FOR ASTHMA AND OTHER LUNG DISEASES

New York Methodist Hospital
506 Sixth Street, Brooklyn, N.Y. 11215
Phone: 866-ASK-LUNG (866-275-5864)
http://www.nym.org

SPECIALISTS AND MEDICAL SERVICES

The Institute for Asthma and Other Lung Diseases brings together a unique group of specialists and medical services to offer comprehensive diagnosis and treatment of a broad range of lung conditions. The Institute's panel of physician specialists includes both pediatric and adult pulmonologists and allergists. A larger constellation of physicians—medical oncologists, radiologists, radiation oncologists, and surgeons—is available as needed. For diagnostic purposes, state-of-the-art specialty facilities—including the interventional bronchoscopy suite, the pulmonary function laboratory and the Sleep Disorders Center—are conveniently located on the Hospital campus. These facilities are used to diagnose and treat a variety of lung disorders and are staffed by registered respiratory therapists, board-certified pulmonary function technologists, and exercise physiologists.

PROGRAMS OFFERED

In addition to the treatment of pediatric and adult asthma, physicians affiliated with the Institute diagnose and care for patients with chronic obstructive lung disease (COPD), interstitial lung disease, infectious lung disease, pulmonary hypertension and lung cancer. Highly sophisticated interventional pulmonary services and advanced thoracic surgery procedures are performed at the Hospital.

* * *

Referrals to the Institute, its programs and physicians can be made through an individual's primary care physician or requested directly through the Institute's telephone referral service. More information (and on-line physician referral) is available at the Hospital's website, http://www.nym.org.

THE INTERVENTIONAL PULMONOLOGY CENTER

New York Methodist Hospital's new Interventional Pulmonology Program is the only one of its kind in Brooklyn. This service offers state-of-the-art diagnostic and therapeutic pulmonary procedures, many of which are minimally invasive.

Minimally invasive procedures are efficient and desirable because they typically cause less pain and are less time consuming than conventional investigative surgery. Furthermore, these procedures enable earlier diagnosis of certain forms of lung cancer, thereby enhancing the chances for successful treatment.

For more information, call the Center at 718-788-5835.

PULMONOLOGY

About the Division of Pulmonary, Critical Care and Sleep Medicine:

The NYU Langone Medical Center Pulmonary, Critical Care and Sleep Medicine Division offers a full continuum of services available for diagnosis, treatment and research of both the inpatient and ambulatory patient. Available services include Pulmonary Function Laboratories, a specialized inpatient pulmonary unit at Bellevue Hospital, specialized medical critical care units at Bellevue, our Tisch Hospital and our Hospital for Joint Diseases which are staffed by dedicated pulmonary/critical care physicians, and a multidisciplinary interventional bronchoscopy program integrated with thoracic radiology at Bellevue and Tisch Hospitals. Research grant support includes National Institute of Health and Centers for Disease Control and Prevention grant programs. *We specialize in the following areas:*

Asthma

NYU Langone Medical Center treats all aspects of asthma and airway disorders. The Bellevue Asthma Clinic at Bellevue Hospital Center, an affiliate of NYU Langone Medical Center, offers an active research program dealing exclusively with particulate matter pollution and asthma. In addition, there is an ongoing gene banking program to study disease modifying genes in asthma and community-based studies of the health effects of the World Trade Center destruction.

Pulmonary Services

The Division of Pulmonary Medicine at NYU Langone Medical Center provides clinical chest services at Tisch Hospital and its affiliate hospital, Bellevue Hospital Center, which cares for patients with tuberculosis, lung cancer, asthma, and interstitial fibrosis. The NYU Langone Medical Center Pulmonary Services consults on interstitial lung diseases, sarcoidosis, pulmonary hypertension, COPD, lung cancer, occupational lung diseases, bronchiectasis, and myobacterial other than TB. Current research is on bacterial pneumonia in HIV-1+ individuals and high-risk smokers with lung cancer.

Interventional Bronchoscopy

The Interventional Bronchoscopy Program offered at Tisch Hospital at NYU Langone Medical Center employs leading-edge techniques to diagnose and treat tumors and inflammatory conditions of the lung.

NYU Lung Cancer Biomarker Center

High-risk smokers can participate in a CT-scan lung cancer screening research program identifying molecular and protein biomarkers in blood and sputum.

Sleep Disorders

The Sleep Disorders Center at NYU Langone Medical Center offers clinical and research services for physicians and patients in the diagnosis and treatment of severe or prolonged difficulties regarding sleep. The Center is also equipped for limited home or in-hospital monitoring for patient screening and follow-up.

Radiation Oncology

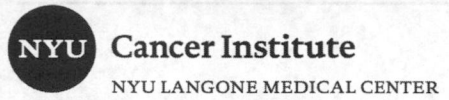

NYU **Cancer Institute**
NYU LANGONE MEDICAL CENTER

NYU Langone Medical Center
550 First Avenue , New York, NY 10016
www.NYULMC.org

NYU Clinical Cancer Center
160 East 34th Street, New York, NY 10016
www.NYUCI.org

**The Stephen D. Hassenfeld Children's Center
for Cancer and Blood Disorders**
160 East 32nd Street, New York, NY 10016
www.NYUMC.org/Hassenfeld

The NYU Cancer Institute is an NCI-designated cancer center and provides personalized patient care that is both compassionate and state of the art. The doctors and researchers work together to develop innovative therapies for patients. The Cancer Institute is world-renowned for excellence in cancer-focused research, personalized care, education and community outreach. Its mission is to discover the origins of human cancer and to use that knowledge to eradicate the personal and societal burden of cancer in our community, the nation and the world. For more information about our expert physicians, call 212-731-5000. *We specialize in the following areas:*

Patient-Focused Setting
The NYU Clinical Cancer Center is the principal outpatient facility of The Cancer Institute and serves as home to our patients and their caregivers. The center and its multidisciplinary team of experts provide access to the latest treatment options and clinical trials along with a variety of programs in cancer risk reduction/prevention, screening, diagnostics, genetic counseling and supportive services. In addition the NYUCI emphasizes the importance of a holistic approach to management services in complementary medicine, psychosocial support, survivorship and palliative care.

Renowned Expertise
The NYU Cancer Institute brings together experts from a variety of disciplines to create collaborative research endeavors and clinical care teams. The Cancer Institute offers a full continuum of personalized care, from prevention through diagnosis, treatment and post-treatment support. The compassion and expertise of our team members helps patients better manage the symptoms of their diseases as well as meet their special needs. Additionally, we have created special emphasis programs in diseases such as breast cancer, melanoma, GI cancer, prostate cancer, hematologic malignancies and lung cancer among others, as well as, translational programs in cancer healthcare disparities, molecularly targeted therapy, and the cell signaling pathways involved in cancer.

A Translational Approach
NYU Langone Medical Center scientists and other researchers excel in uncovering how cancer develops at the molecular level, and how we can harness that knowledge to reduce the risk of cancer and treat the disease. The Medical Center constantly seeks to create new opportunities for collaboration between investigators within our own institution, those located elsewhere in the NYU network of campuses, and researchers at other institutions.

The Stephen D. Hassenfeld Children's Center for Cancer and Blood Disorders
The center is a leading pediatric outpatient facility for the treatment of childhood cancers and blood diseases. Its unique interdisciplinary and family-centered approach combines the most advanced medical treatments with psychosocial and emotional support services for young patients and their families.

Rehabilitation Medicine

Reproductive Endocrinology

PROGRAM FOR IVF REPRODUCTIVE SURGERY AND INFERTILITY

About the Division of Reproductive Endocrinology and Infertility, Department of Obstetrics and Gynecology:

The Division of Reproductive Endocrinology and Infertility at NYU Langone Medical Center can help patients realize their dreams of parenthood with its unique experience in all aspects of reproductive endocrinology, including the diagnosis and treatment of endometriosis, fibroids, problems with ovulation or sperm function and recurring pregnancy loss. The Medical Center offers the most advanced technology to assist infertile women and men who wish to conceive children. The combination of academic, scientific and technical expertise found at the Medical Center has created one of the most respected fertility programs and clinical divisions in the country. Our clinical work includes some of the world's finest technicians and physicians who have pioneered new innovations and been honored for their outstanding contributions to the field of reproductive medicine. *We specialize in the following areas:*

Patient-Centered Care

From the initial diagnosis through all stages of treatment, couples at NYU Langone Medical Center receive state-of-the-art compassionate care based on their specific needs. After a comprehensive evaluation to determine the cause of infertility, couples are counseled on whether assisted reproduction is necessary. Often surgery or stimulation of a woman's ovaries with medication can correct disorders that lead to infertility.

In Vitro Fertilization (IVF)

When medical conditions prevent the sperm from reaching the egg, skilled physicians and laboratory staff at the Fertility Center at NYU Langone Medical Center assist patients with retrieving their eggs, insemination in the lab and then insertion back into the patient's uterus as embryos. Preimplantation Genetic Screening (PGS)- The NYU Fertility Center offers tests for aneuploidy (an abnormal number of chromosomes). Embryos can also be tested for single-gene defects or can be tested for gender. This advanced technology allows prospective parents who are carriers of genetic conditions to avoid selective pregnancy termination. Some of the genetic disorders identified with PGS include: cystic fibrosis, Down syndrome, hemophilia, Huntington's disease, Marfan's disease, muscular dystrophy and sickle cell anemia. The state-of-the-art technology is also used to increase chances of delivery in certain women with a history of recurrent miscarriage or previous IVF failures.

Complex Cases

The NYU Fertility Center specializes in complex cases of infertility. Many patients have undergone IVF unsuccessfully elsewhere and some were even told that they should stop trying IVF. The Center offers the most advanced care available for patients still wanting to conceive.

IVF for Male Factor Infertility

The Fertility Center at NYU Langone Medical Center provides male patients with experienced urologists who can provide expert fertility treatment. As part of the diagnosis process, men receive a complete evaluation, including a fertility history, physical exam, blood testing and semen analysis. Surgical treatment of male infertility is performed onsite at the Center's surgical suites on an outpatient basis and may include the following procedures: testicular biopsy, vasectomy reversal, epididymal tissue repair, varicose vein repair and Microsurgical Sperm Aspiration used to obtain sperm when infertility is caused by blockage.

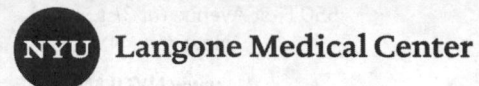
PROGRAM FOR IVF REPRODUCTIVE SURGERY AND INFERTILITY

About the Division of Reproductive Endocrinology and Infertility, Department of Obstetrics and Gynecology:
The Division of Reproductive Endocrinology and Infertility at NYU Langone Medical Center can help patients realize their dreams of parenthood with its unique experience in all aspects of reproductive endocrinology, including the diagnosis and treatment of endometriosis, fibroids, problems with ovulation or sperm function and recurring pregnancy loss. The Medical Center offers the most advanced technology to assist infertile women and men who wish to conceive children. The combination of academic, scientific and technical expertise found at the Medical Center has created one of the most respected fertility programs and clinical divisions in the country. Our clinical work includes some of the world's finest technicians and physicians who have pioneered new innovations and been honored for their outstanding contributions to the field of reproductive medicine. **We specialize in the following areas:**

Patient-Centered Care
From the initial diagnosis through all stages of treatment, couples at NYU Langone Medical Center receive state-of-the-art compassionate care based on their specific needs. After a comprehensive evaluation to determine the cause of infertility, couples are counseled on whether assisted reproduction is necessary. Often surgery or stimulation of a woman's ovaries with medication can correct disorders that lead to infertility.

In Vitro Fertilization (IVF)
When medical conditions prevent the sperm from reaching the egg, skilled physicians and laboratory staff at the Fertility Center at NYU Langone Medical Center assist patients with retrieving their eggs, insemination in the lab and then insertion back into the patient's uterus as embryos. Preimplantation Genetic Screening (PGS)- The NYU Fertility Center offers tests for aneuploidy (an abnormal number of chromosomes). Embryos can also be tested for single-gene defects or can be tested for gender. This advanced technology allows prospective parents who are carriers of genetic conditions to avoid selective pregnancy termination. Some of the genetic disorders identified with PGS include: cystic fibrosis, Down syndrome, hemophilia, Huntington's disease, Marfan's disease, muscular dystrophy and sickle cell anemia. The state-of-the-art technology is also used to increase chances of delivery in certain women with a history of recurrent miscarriage or previous IVF failures.

Complex Cases
The NYU Fertility Center specializes in complex cases of infertility. Many patients have undergone IVF unsuccessfully elsewhere and some were even told that they should stop trying IVF. The Center offers the most advanced care available for patients still wanting to conceive.

IVF for Male Factor Infertility
The Fertility Center at NYU Langone Medical Center provides male patients with experienced urologists who can provide expert fertility treatment. As part of the diagnosis process, men receive a complete evaluation, including a fertility history, physical exam, blood testing and semen analysis. Surgical treatment of male infertility is performed onsite at the Center's surgical suites on an outpatient basis and may include the following procedures: testicular biopsy, vasectomy reversal, epididymal tissue repair, varicose vein repair and Microsurgical Sperm Aspiration used to obtain sperm when infertility is caused by blockage.

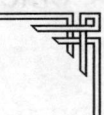

The Best in American Medicine
www.CastleConnolly.com

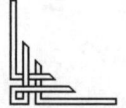
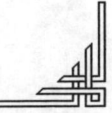

Rheumatology

NYU **Hospital for Joint Diseases**
NYU LANGONE MEDICAL CENTER

301 East 17th Street *(at Second Avenue)*
New York, NY 100036
www.NYUHJD.org
212-598-6000 fax: 212-260-1203

RHEUMATOLOGY

The rheumatologists at NYU Langone Medical Center are dedicated to the diagnosis and treatment of patients with rheumatic illnesses with a focus on autoimmune diseases. *U.S. News and World Report* has repeated recognized us as among the most prestigious rheumatology programs in the country and we were ranked #8 nationwide in the 2010/2011 "Best Hospitals" issue of *U.S. News and World Report Best Hospitals.* **We specialize in the following areas:**

Arthritis And Autoimmunity
We offer a comprehensive program for the prevention, diagnosis and treatment of all rheumatologic conditions. Patients also have access to orthopaedic and other subspecialty services, sophisticated diagnostic testing, physical and occupational therapy and complementary medicine.

Behçet's Syndrome
We have the only North American Behçet's Center for research and the evaluation and treatment of patients with Behçet's Syndrome, a disease that involves inflammation of the blood vessels.

Biological Treatment
Biological treatments for inflammatory arthritis, rheumatoid arthritis, lupus, psoriatic arthritis, vasculitis, and osteoporosis are administered within the Medical Center's infusion centers.

Lupus
The Lupus Center and Translational Laboratory is devoted to the treatment and research of patients with this disease. Patients have access to world renowned specialists in lupus, lupus and pregnancy, and related sub-specialties.

Osteoporosis
We offer comprehensive care for the prevention, evaluation and treatment of osteoporosis, including state-of-the art bone densitometers, and programs in balance training and physical therapy and exercise instruction.

Psoriatic Arthritis
The Psoriatic Arthritis Center is a collaborative effort with the Department of Dermatology. Patients are seen by both a rheumatologist and dermatologist who specialize in psoriasis and psoriatic arthritis.

Research
Our research focuses on osteoarthritis, rheumatoid arthritis, lupus, osteoporosis, psoriatic arthritis, Behçets and other autoimmune diseases positioning us at the forefront of basic science and translational research, personalized medicine and genetics of rheumatic diseases. The Peter D. Seligman Center for Advanced Therapeutics conducts clinical studies using a wide variety of newly developed therapies.

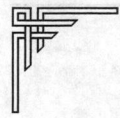
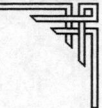

Sleep Disorders

The Best in American Medicine
www.CastleConnolly.com

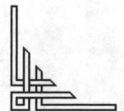
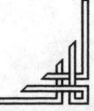

Sleep Disorders

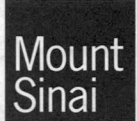
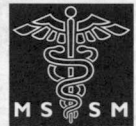

THE MOUNT SINAI MEDICAL CENTER
SLEEP MEDICINE

One Gustave L. Levy Place
Fifth Avenue and 100th Street
New York, NY 10029-6574
Physician Referral: 1-800-MD-SINAI (637-4624)
www.mountsinai.org

MOUNT SINAI
SCHOOL OF
MEDICINE

Mount Sinai's **CENTER FOR SLEEP MEDICINE** is a comprehensive, full-service program that specializes in the compassionate and personalized care of individuals with sleep disorders. The Center for Sleep Medicine is accredited by the American Academy of Sleep Medicine.

We use state-of-the-art equipment to diagnose and treat all aspects of sleep pathology, including breathing-related disorders, insomnia, restless leg syndrome, periodic limb movements, and narcolepsy. An initial consultation includes a clinical history and physical examination. In some cases, the diagnosis and treatment plan can be completed in a single visit. In other cases, the evaluation requires a sleep study—typically over one or two nights—or other tests. Overnight tests are completed by 7 am, so it is usually not necessary to miss a day of work. In rare instances, daytime studies are also recommended.

Services available at the Comprehensive Center for Sleep Medicine include:

- Consultations with board-certified sleep specialists.

- Overnight sleep testing and daytime testing provided by experienced physicians and technicians. During a sleep study, the patient is monitored by painless, noninvasive technology called polysomnography that records breathing, heart rate, brain waves, oxygen levels, and eye and leg movement.

- Treatment for a sleep disorder that may include a device to aid the patient's breathing while sleeping called Continuous Positive Airway Pressure or Bilevel Positive Airway Pressure, medication, or light therapy, as well as neuropsychiatric interventions. If indicated, consultations with other specialists are available to aid in diagnosis and therapy.

- Mechanical, behavioral, surgical, dental, and pharmacological therapies. Consultations can also be arranged with pulmonologists; ear, nose, and throat surgeons; bariatric surgeons; dentists; and psychiatrists.

MOUNT SINAI SPECIALIZES IN TREATING OBSTRUCTIVE SLEEP APNEA

Approximately 20 million Americans suffer from obstructive sleep apnea, which occurs when muscles of the back of the mouth and the throat relax during sleep, causing a complete (apnea) or partial (hypopnea) blockage of the airway. Apneic episodes lead to frequent awakenings and lowering of the oxygen level, causing the heart to work harder. When untreated, this disorder can lead to hypertension, heart failure, and stroke, as well as bouts of daytime sleepiness that increase the risk of motor vehicle and industrial accidents. Sleepiness is often misperceived as a natural consequence of aging. If you are overweight and snore, you may have sleep apnea or another sleep disorder.

Trinitas Regional Medical Center

COMPREHENSIVE SLEEP DISORDERS CENTER

210 WILLIAMSON STREET | ELIZABETH, NEW JERSEY 07207
PH 908.994.8694 | WWW.NJSLEEPDISORDERSCENTER.COM

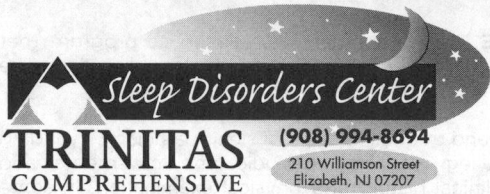

Sleep Disorders Center
TRINITAS
COMPREHENSIVE

(908) 994-8694
210 Williamson Street
Elizabeth, NJ 07207

Accredited by The American Academy of Sleep Medicine

Getting a good night's sleep is an essential part of healthy living, but for the millions of Americans who suffer from sleep disorders, getting enough rest can be difficult, if not impossible. Left untreated, sleep disorders can have harmful, even life-threatening effects on health, well-being and safety.

The Comprehensive Sleep Disorders Center at Trinitas Regional Medical Center provides a monitored, fully attended diagnostic sleep study designed to rule out physical, non-stress related symptoms that may prevent restful sleep. The medical director is board certified in Internal Medicine, Critical Care, Sleep Medicine and Pulmonary Medicine. A team of trained sleep specialists supervises each study and coordinates follow-up care with the patient's physician. These professionals can quickly diagnose any sleep problem and, working closely with each patient's primary physician, provide expert treatment and follow-up.

Located within the main campus of Trinitas Regional Medical Center, the state-of-the-art Comprehensive Sleep Disorders Center is designed to diagnose sleep disorders, including insomnia, sleep apnea, restless leg syndrome, snoring and narcolepsy, among others. The private, comfortable testing is performed in home-like suites with soft designer sheets, pillows and a private shower. Studies are provided for adults and children as young as 18 months. Daytime studies are available to meet patient needs.

In 2010, a second sleep center was unveiled in Homewood Suites by Hilton, Cranford. The site is the first hotel-based sleep center in New Jersey.

Both locations offer state-of-the-art diagnostic sleep studies performed by specially trained sleep pulmonologists, registered polysomnographers and licensed, credentialed respiratory therapists.

The Trinitas Comprehensive Sleep Disorders Center is a fully staffed center accredited by The American Academy of Sleep Medicine - the "gold standard" accrediting body for sleep centers - offering the benefits of two distinct locations. With one location on the campus of Trinitas Regional Medical Center, a comprehensive, state-of-the-art medical facility and the other at a nearby nationally known hotel chain, patients who have sleep studies performed at Trinitas receive the high level of attention or treatment that is simply not possible to receive at a neighborhood sleep center.

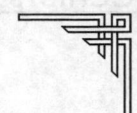

The Best in American Medicine
www.CastleConnolly.com

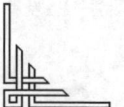
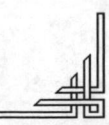

Sports Medicine

Stroke Care

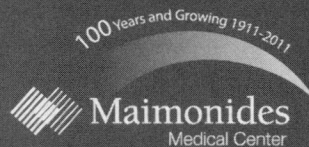

NEUROLOGY

About the Department of Neurology:

NYU Langone Medical Center evaluates and treats children and adults with a broad spectrum of neurological diseases. Specialty groups deliver integrated care to patients with stroke, epilepsy, cerebrovacular diseases, behavioral disorders and dementia, brain tumors, genetic and degenerative diseases, nerve and muscle problems, headache and pain syndromes and movement disorders. We are home to the largest multiple sclerosis (MS) program in New York and the first primary Stroke Center in New York City. *We specialize in the following areas:*

Autonomic Diseases

Our specialized center evaluates and treats children and adults with familial dysautonomia and other inherited or acquired autonomic nervous system diseases including orthostatic hypotension and rare forms of hereditary sensory neuropathy.

Epilepsy

The Comprehensive Epilepsy Center offers the most advanced surgical and medical options in the treatment of epilepsy. Complementary management approaches such as diet alteration, lifestyle changes and other remedies are part of a comprehensive management plan. Our primary goal is to help patients with unmanageable epilepsy achieve complete control, or at least a reduction in the frequency of seizures and/or the medical side effects to achieve the highest possible quality of life.

Multiple Sclerosis

The Comprehensive MS Care Center provides state-of-the-art diagnostic evaluations and follow-up care. We feature an onsite team of highly trained professionals, as well as consulting services, to provide comprehensive care.

Neurogenetics

The Division of Neurogenetics focuses on inherited diseases of the nervous system. Services include diagnosis and management of inherited diseases, biochemical and molecular testing and genetic counseling.

Neuro-oncology

The NYU Cancer Institute, an NCI-designated cancer center, is home to one of the nation's leading brain and spinal cord tumor treatment programs, with medical experts experienced in neuro-oncology, neurosurgery, neuroradiology.

Neuromuscular Diseases

The Neuromuscular Division offers multidisciplinary inpatient and outpatient programs for neuromuscular diseases with emphasis on: acquired peripheral neuropathy, Charcot Marie Tooth neuropathy, myasthenia gravis, Amyotrophic lateral sclerosis, spinal muscular atrophy and post-polio syndrome, muscular dystrophy and Lyme neuroborreliosis.

Parkinson's Disease and Movement Disorders

The Parkinson and Movement Disorders Center helps individuals and families achieve the highest possible quality of life. We have an active research program that explores best treatments options for Parkinson's disease.

Stroke Care

The first primary stroke center in New York City, the multidisciplinary Comprehensive Stroke Care Center at NYU Langone Medical Center provides rapid diagnosis, immediate and effective intervention and early rehabilitation.

Surgery

The Best in American Medicine
www.CastleConnolly.com

Surgery

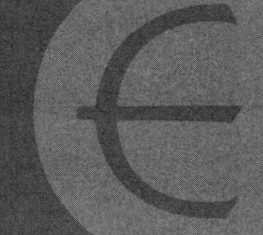

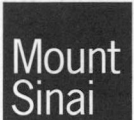
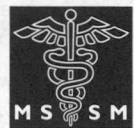

THE MOUNT SINAI MEDICAL CENTER
DEPARTMENT OF SURGERY

One Gustave L. Levy Place
Fifth Avenue and 100th Street
New York, NY 10029-6574
Physician Referral: 1-800-MD-SINAI (637-4624)
www.mountsinai.org/surgery

THE DEPARTMENT OF SURGERY at Mount Sinai continues to be at the forefront of minimally invasive surgery. Mount Sinai surgeons build upon the legacy of those who have gone before, caring for the very sickest of patients while developing new therapies and training tomorrow's physicians to save and enhance lives. Patients today are experiencing less pain, shorter hospital stays, and faster recovery times than was ever imaginable just 20 years ago.

Bariatric Surgery – The latest minimally invasive techniques are used to perform laparoscopic gastric bypass, lap band placement, duodenal switch, and sleeve gastrectomy. In addition, a full inter-disciplinary team follows all aspects of pre- and post-operative care.

Colon and Rectal Surgery – Leaders in the treatment of gastrointestinal disorders, our surgeons care for a wide range of diseases, including: inflammatory bowel disease (Crohn's disease and ulcerative colitis), diverticulitis, and colon and rectal cancers. We offer many important procedures not commonly available.

General Surgery – Treatment is individualized based on the patient's condition, with options from advanced laparoscopic procedures to complex operations.

Laparoscopic and Minimally Invasive Surgery – Mount Sinai surgeons include the world's most respected and innovative surgeons, who perform more laparoscopic procedures than surgeons at any other hospital in New York.

Pediatric Surgery – Surgeries involving children can be met with even more apprehension than those for adults. Fortunately, Mount Sinai surgeons offer a full range of pediatric surgical procedures in a family-focused, child-sensitive environment.

Plastic and Reconstructive Surgery – Surgical care from aesthetic to complex reconstruction is offered for benign and malignant disease, as well as for deformities that are either congenital or acquired. The aim is to restore function and correct deformities caused by birth defects, aging, accident, or illness.

Surgical Oncology – Patients are seen promptly and are cared for by a team of medical and surgical experts, enabling them to benefit from the opinions of dozens of nationally renowned doctors.

Vascular Surgery – A recognized world leader in the development of new techniques for the treatment of aortic aneurysms, Mount Sinai continues to perform extensive research to advance the field of vascular surgery. A wide array of advanced patient services are available, ensuring that conditions are managed successfully.

TOP-RANKING MINIMALLY INVASIVE SURGEONS

In surveys of leading minimally invasive surgeons in a variety of specialties, Mount Sinai's physicians are consistently at the top of the list in surgery of the colon and rectum, liver and bile ducts, thyroid, hernia, chest, and blood vessels. Compared with traditional open surgery, minimally invasive procedures result in less tissue trauma, less scarring, and shorter postoperative recovery time. Although the techniques vary from procedure to procedure and among different surgical subspecialties, minimally invasive surgical procedures typically employ video cameras and lens systems to provide anatomic visualization within a region of the body.

NYU **Cardiac and Vascular Institute**

NYU LANGONE MEDICAL CENTER

550 First Avenue *(at 31st Street)*
New York, NY 10016

www.NYULMC.org

Physician Referral: **(888)7-NYU-MED** *(888-769-8633)*

CARDIAC SURGERY

NYU Langone Medical Center is one of the tri-state area's largest cardiac surgery centers and a nationally recognized leader in advanced treatments and technologies for adult, pediatric and congenital heart disease. Our world renowned surgeons pioneered minimally invasive heart surgery and valve repair or replacement, and have performed over 5,000 minimally invasive heart surgery procedures. We also perform other state-of-the-art surgical procedures for structural and valvular heart disease, coronary artery disease, congenital heart disease, and aortic aneurysm disease, as well as specialize in cardiac surgery for high-risk and elderly patients. Our team's multidisciplinary approach to high quality patient-centered care and their commitment to research are just a few of the many factors that set us apart.

Center for Structural and Valvular Heart Disease
Mitral Valve Repair. We are a leader in the field of mitral valve repair and it was our heart surgeons who first introduced mitral valve repair to the U.S. more than 30 years ago. We have since refined the technique and performed over 3,800 mitral valve repair procedures –the most mitral valve repair procedures in the country.

High Risk Cardiac Surgery. Our cardiac surgery team are specialists in the surgical care of high-risk patients, including re-operative surgery in the elderly. Surgical procedures for high-risk patients include coronary bypass surgery, heart valve repair or replacement, surgical repair of the failing heart and ventricular assist device implantation.

Minimally Invasive Cardiac Surgery. Over 5,000 minimally invasive heart surgery procedures have been performed here since 1996. The preferred approach for the majority of our valve surgery patients, the benefits include dramatic reduced pain, lower risk of bleeding and infection, and a quicker recovery.

Center for Aortic Diseases
We are dedicated to providing a collaborative multidisciplinary approach to the medical and surgical treatments of complex aortic disease and long-term management of patients with residual aortic dissection and connective tissue disorders. We offer a range of treatment and therapeutic options including open surgery and stent graft therapy for patients with aortic aneurysms, aortic dissections and inherited diseases of the aorta, such as Marfan's syndrome.

Center for Pediatric and Adult Congenital Heart Disease
The Division of Pediatric & Adult Congenital Cardiac Surgery treats patients of all ages with inherited and acquired cardiac defects. Our surgeons are experts in reconstructive procedures for those with complex cardiovascular disorders. We offer a team approach of specialists in pediatric and adult cardiology, neonatal and pediatric cardiac intensive care, pediatric cardiac anesthesiology, nursing, and extracorporeal perfusion.

THORACIC SURGERY

About the Division of Thoracic Surgery:
The Thoracic Surgeons at NYU Langone Medical Center offer the most advanced diagnosis and treatment options for patients with both benign and malignant lesions of the lung, esophagus, mediastinum and chest wall. All of the thoracic attending surgeons at the Medical Center are experts in minimally invasive, video-assisted thoracic surgery which minimizes patient discomfort and shortens recuperation time. *We specialize in the following areas:*

Airway Stenting
Patients experiencing trouble breathing may require airway stenting in order to maintain an open airway (windpipe). Treatment of primary and metastatic lung cancer often includes the use of hollow tubes (stents) to maintain an unobstructed airway. At NYU Langone Medical Center, stent placement is performed in the operating room by an experienced team that includes a surgeon, anesthesiologist and nursing staff. The procedure can be performed through either rigid or flexible bronchoscopy, using either temporary (plastic) or more permanent (metal) stents. Post-operative patients are carefully monitored by a multidisciplinary team to ensure their comfort and care.

Minimally Invasive Thoracic Surgery
The Division of Thoracic Surgery at NYU Langone Medical Center offers a minimally invasive surgery program, incorporating both video-assisted and "open chest" techniques along with the newest methods for post-operative pain relief. The use of video-assisted equipment allows for a smaller incision without spreading the rib spaces leading to greater patient comfort, a shorter recovery time and decreased length of stay for patients. Procedures offered include video-assisted thoracoscopy for biopsy with or without removal of a portion of the lungs as well as repair of hiatal hernias and minimally invasive esophagectomy.

Pioneering Treatments
NYU Langone Medical Center leads the way in pioneering new treatments for the early detection of airway malignancies, diagnosis and treatment strategies for endobronchial abnormalities, investigation of non-surgical techniques selectively used for destruction of lung cancer nodules and the use of stents (and replaceable stents) to relieve blockages of the windpipe and esophagus.

Research
NYU Langone is committed to state-of-the-art surgical management and developing novel treatment strategies using clinical trials. We also leverage the resources at the New York Thoracic Surgery Laboratory house at Bellevue Hospital to search for genes and proteins in malignancies of the chest in order to detect them earlier or develop novel targeted therapies.

VASCULAR SURGERY

Staffed by one of the largest vascular surgery teams in the country, we offer expert patient care with an emphasis on minimally invasive therapies. Our physicians have extensive experience in performing the most up-to-date procedures including stents, angioplasty for carotid artery disease, aortic aneurysms and blockages in arteries throughout the body. In addition to its expertise in arterial disease, NYU is proud to offer one of the few Academic Vein Centers in the United States.
We specialize in the following areas:

Aortic Pathology
We offer minimally invasive surgical solutions as well as treatments for complex aortic problems. Patients usually require no blood transfusions and are able to leave the hospital just one or two days after surgery. We are also a training center for endovascular management of abdominal and thoracic aneurysms.

Carotid Artery Disease
We remain a leader in both the screening for carotid disease and the prevention of stroke for those being treated for carotid artery occlusive disease, known to predispose patients to stroke. Our physicians were central to pioneering carotid endarterectomy as an open surgical procedure, as well as playing a pivotal role in the development of the carotid stenting procedure.

Peripheral Arterial Disease
Our doctors have a wealth of experience in treating peripheral arterial disease (PAD) and specialize in new and innovative technologies such as laser and "Silverhawk" atherectomy procedures as well as cryoplasty. Additionally, we are one of the only centers in the tristate area with access to drug-eluting stents which are coated with special medicines that may prevent scar formation and re-occlusion of the stent.

Vascular Screenings
Our doctors are committed to improving the public awareness and understanding of vascular disease through preventative screenings. The disease is among the leading causes of death in the U.S., yet is generally asymptomatic until a stroke or aneurysm rupture. Effective screenings performed include ultrasound scans of the aorta, ultrasound scans of the carotid arteries and blood pressure measurements.

Venous Disease
The Vein Center at NYU Langone Medical Center is considered an authority in the minimally invasive treatment of venous disease, treating patients with all forms of venous pathology ranging from venous insufficiency and varicose veins to occlusive disease and deep vein thrombosis.

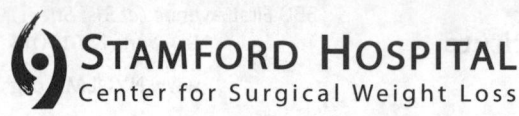

STAMFORD HOSPITAL
Center for Surgical Weight Loss

Center for Surgical Weight Loss

At Stamford Hospital's Center for Surgical Weight Loss, patients benefit from a comprehensive program led by an expert team of weight management specialists. Surgeons, physicians, dedicated nurse practitioner, registered dietitian, behaviorist and exercise physiologist provide patients with the knowledge and skills needed to achieve the best possible results. In addition to surgical procedures, the Center offers medically supervised weight management for patients who do not qualify for surgery or simply prefer to take a different approach.

Surgical Procedures

The Center offers four types of weight loss surgery: gastric bypass, gastric banding, sleeve gastrectomy and duodenal switch, all of which are performed laparoscopically (tiny incisions) and result in less pain and scarring with a faster recovery.

Stamford Hospital also offers laparoscopic revisional surgery to help manage weight regain following bariatric procedures and is involved in ongoing research into new techniques, including "incisionless" surgery and endolumenal therapies for obesity.

Integrated Care

We offer an extraordinary breadth of expertise across many medical and support disciplines to guide a patient to success. *Our comprehensive plan includes:*

Surgical Preparatory Program

We offer educational seminars, consultations, complimentary 90-day membership at our Health & Fitness Institute and support groups.

Center for Integrative Medicine and Wellness

Patients learn mind-body, guided imagery techniques to prepare emotionally and physically for surgery as well as to help heal and recover faster and more comfortably. In addition, acupuncture, stress management and nutritional counseling support are offered.

Health & Fitness Institute

An innovative wellness facility, offering medically supervised fitness and lifestyle change, includes a dedicated exercise physiologist on staff who specializes in working with bariatric patients. The use of state-of-the-art exercise equipment, 25-yard lap pool, warm water therapeutic pool and Jacuzzi helps patients achieve weight loss and fitness goals.

Academic and Clinical Affiliations

Stamford Hospital is an affiliate of the New York–Presbyterian Healthcare System and a major teaching affiliate of the Columbia University College of Physicians & Surgeons.

Accreditation

Joint Commission on Accreditation of Healthcare Organization (JCAHO)

Beds

305

Sponsorship

Voluntary, Not-for-Profit

For a Physician Referral or more information, please call 1.877.233.9355 or visit stamfordhospital.org /doctor.

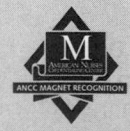

Stamford Hospital
30 Shelburne Road
Stamford, CT 06902
203.276.1000

stamfordhospital.org

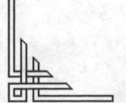
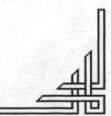

The Best in American Medicine
www.CastleConnolly.com

Therapeutic Radiology

RADIOLOGY

The Radiology Department at NYU Langone Medical Center is committed to providing the most advanced imaging services by capturing the best images with the lowest dose possible. As an academic medical center, our radiologists are in a unique position to take the lead in helping to define and advance radiology in today's rapidly advancing technological environment.

Expertise

NYU Langone Medical Center's board certified radiologists and licensed technologists specialize in imaging and are involved in a variety of innovative collaborations and research initiatives. Our experienced eagle-eyed radiologists, with the assistance of the newest technology, are renowned for their interpretation and insight. Our staff consists of over100 sub-specialized academic radiologists, many of whom are acknowledged leaders and innovators in their field.

Advanced Technology

NYU Langone Medical Center uses some of the most advanced imaging equipment in the world. We offer high and ultra high-field MRI imaging systems (known as 1.5T and 3T magnets). Our MRI scanners are shorter and wider than ever—making for a more patient friendly experience. Our Center for Biomedical Imaging, a research facility features a 7T magnet.

Recognition for Safety and Quality

We continually follow a set of rigorous quality standards and maintain accreditation by the American College of Radiology (ACR). We are designated by the ACR as a "Breast Imaging Center of Excellence;" we have achieved high practice standards in image quality, personal qualifications, facility equipment, and quality control procedures and quality assurance programs.

Patient Focused Approach:

We are conveniently located and participate in an extensive number of insurance plans. We create timely delivery of reports and images and physicians can view patient exam status, reports and images online from their office. In addition to our convenient day time hours, weekend, evenings and often same day appointments are available. We provide language interpretation services, as needed.

We specialize in the following areas:

We offer an extensive range of diagnostic services in MRI, CT, ultrasound, PET/CT, X-ray, and interventional radiology and nuclear medicine. Subspecialized radiologists provide diagnostic interpretation in abdominal, biomedical, breast, cardiac, chest, emergency, general, musculoskeletal, neuroradiology, neuro interventional, nuclear medicine, pediatric, vascular interventional and women's imaging. Our Specialty Procedures Include: Coronary artery disease and virtual colonoscopy screening programs, Stereotactic biopsy capability, minimally invasive techniques including radiofrequency ablation and chemoembolization, Radioimmunotherapy, and Bone densitometry.

Thoracic Surgery

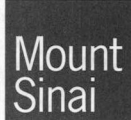 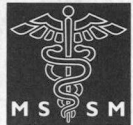

THE MOUNT SINAI MEDICAL CENTER
CARDIOTHORACIC SURGERY
One Gustave L. Levy Place
Fifth Avenue and 100th Street
New York, NY 10029-6574
Physician Referral: 1-800-MD-SINAI (637-4624)
www.mountsinai.org/heart

THE DEPARTMENT OF CARDIOTHORACIC SURGERY at Mount Sinai is one of the nation's most prestigious programs. Cardiothoracic surgical patients benefit from an integrated and personalized care plan designed in coordination with expert cardiologists, anesthesiologists, perfusionists, and intensive care physicians. Mount Sinai is a quaternary referral center, meaning its surgeons often operate on the sickest and most complicated patients.

The Mitral Valve Repair Reference Center at Mount Sinai is one of the largest and most advanced in the nation. The superiority of mitral valve repair over replacement with a mechanical or bioprosthetic valve is now well established. Directed by David H. Adams, MD, Mount Sinai's Mitral Valve Repair Reference Center offers patients one of the highest percentages of successful valve repair in the world. In patients with mitral valve prolapse, Mount Sinai's success rate in avoiding valve replacement approaches 100 percent. Our physicians are experts in mitral valve repair for patients with advanced cardiomyopathy. For patients who have associated atrial fibrillation, Mount Sinai offers the latest in concomitant arrhythmia surgery, including the MAZE procedure. Mitral valve repair with minimally invasive approaches is also performed when appropriate. Learn more about our Reference Center at www.mitralvalverepair.org.

The Aortic Valve Repair Program offers patients with aortic valve disease an alternative to replacement of their aortic valve and the freedom from taking blood-thinning medications. Our surgeons are thoroughly versed in nonthrombogenic alternatives to mechanical valve replacement, including such valve-sparing procedures as the David and Yacoub procedures. Mount Sinai's Paul Stelzer, MD, is one of the most experienced surgeons in the nation in using the Ross procedure, in which the diseased aortic valve is replaced with the patient's own pulmonary valve. This technique has improved durability over other replacement options, particularly in younger patients.

LEADING SURGEONS, UNPARALLELED POSSIBILITIES

The Department of Cardiothoracic Surgery at Mount Sinai is chaired by David H. Adams, MD, the Marie-Josée and Henry R. Kravis Professor. Dr. Adams is a world-renowned mitral repair surgeon. Randall B. Griepp, MD, Professor of Cardiothoracic Surgery, is an internationally recognized leader in thoracic aortic surgery. Paul Stelzer, MD, is a specialist in aortic root surgery whose experience with the Ross procedure is unmatched, exceeding 20 years and 475 cases. These leaders work in concert with other members of Mount Sinai Heart, which is under the direction of world-renowned cardiologist Valentin Fuster, MD, PhD, to deliver unparalleled possibilities for patients with cardiovascular disease.

The Thoracic Aortic Surgery Program is known around the world for its leadership role in surgical therapy of complex aortic disease. This program specializes in the operative management of all diseases of the ascending aorta, arch, and descending thoracic aorta. Ascending aortic replacement, trifurcation-graft arch replacement, acute aortic dissection repair, and thoracoabdominal aortic surgery are all commonly performed at Mount Sinai. Special emphasis is placed on cerebral and spinal protection, where we have a significant clinical and scientific research interest led by our pioneering director, Randall B. Griepp, MD. Our surgeons have also been involved in the early development of minimally invasive aortic stent grafting.

The Cardiac Transplant and Assist Program, one of the largest in the nation, is now under the direction of Anelechi Anyanwu, MD. We have been involved in the field of mechanical cardiac assistance from its inception, and have experience with most of the available FDA-approved devices. We have also played an active role in multi-institutional studies exploring permanent mechanical heart support.

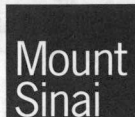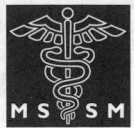

THORACIC SURGERY at The Mount Sinai Medical Center is world renowned for its state-of-the-art surgery, multidisciplinary team approach to treatment, and commitment to compassionate patient care. Protocol-driven therapy ensures that Mount Sinai patients are given access to many clinical trials.

Our team of dedicated thoracic surgeons are experts in the treatment of all primary cancers of the chest, lung, esophagus, mediastinum, and airway, and all metastatic tumors of the chest. We also diagnose and treat patients who are affected by benign esophageal disorders such as gastroesophageal reflux disease, achalasia, and motility disorders.

Mount Sinai is a leader in the development and implementation of the latest technologies and treatment options for disorders of the lung and esophagus, including:

- Video-assisted thoracic surgery (VATS)
- VATS lobectomy
- VATS thymectomy
- VATS sympathectomy for excessive sweating of the hands
- Minimally invasive esophagectomy
- Robotic surgery
- Minimally invasive anti-reflux surgery
- Endobronchial ultrasound—a new noninvasive method for staging lung cancers
- Complex airway resection and reconstruction
- Stent and laser treatment of the airway and esophagus
- Sterotactic and radiofrequency ablation of lung tumors
- Navigational bronchoscopy—an innovative, noninvasive technique for lung biopsies
- Lung volume reduction surgery

TAKING CARE OF ONE PATIENT AT A TIME
At Mount Sinai we believe in personalized care. Each patient benefits from a team approach that includes thoracic surgeons, anesthesiologists, medical oncologists, radiation oncologists, and oncology-dedicated nurses. Coordinating information among team members to ensure seamless delivery of care is a top priority.

Screening and Diagnosis – Mount Sinai is New York City's leading center for comprehensive screening for lung and esophageal cancer, including CT scans for early detection, advanced endoscopic techniques to detect early lesions and recurrence, PET scans, and innovative MRI technology with ultrasensitive resolution. Our developing program for the screening and detection of esophageal cancer is the first of its kind in New York City.

Translational Research – Mount Sinai's thoracic surgeons and physician-scientists are conducting state-of-the-art translational thoracic research, including genomic analysis of tumors to better understand and predict behavior, in order to develop more directed, personalized therapeutic approaches to treatment with novel targeted therapies.

Outreach Programs – Mount Sinai is a leader in bringing cutting-edge treatments to the community. Our community-based programs include: the Asian-American Thoracic Program, Women and Lung Cancer Program, and the Mount Sinai Airway Program.

Transplant Program – Our transplant program is one of two accredited programs in the New York metropolitan area dedicated to lung transplantation for a wide variety of conditions. Patients enrolled in this program receive a multidisciplinary team approach to their condition.

THORACIC SURGERY

About the Division of Thoracic Surgery:
The Thoracic Surgeons at NYU Langone Medical Center offer the most advanced diagnosis and treatment options for patients with both benign and malignant lesions of the lung, esophagus, mediastinum and chest wall. All of the thoracic attending surgeons at the Medical Center are experts in minimally invasive, video-assisted thoracic surgery which minimizes patient discomfort and shortens recuperation time. *We specialize in the following areas:*

Airway Stenting
Patients experiencing trouble breathing may require airway stenting in order to maintain an open airway (windpipe). Treatment of primary and metastatic lung cancer often includes the use of hollow tubes (stents) to maintain an unobstructed airway. At NYU Langone Medical Center, stent placement is performed in the operating room by an experienced team that includes a surgeon, anesthesiologist and nursing staff. The procedure can be performed through either rigid or flexible bronchoscopy, using either temporary (plastic) or more permanent (metal) stents. Post-operative patients are carefully monitored by a multidisciplinary team to ensure their comfort and care.

Minimally Invasive Thoracic Surgery
The Division of Thoracic Surgery at NYU Langone Medical Center offers a minimally invasive surgery program, incorporating both video-assisted and "open chest" techniques along with the newest methods for post-operative pain relief. The use of video-assisted equipment allows for a smaller incision without spreading the rib spaces leading to greater patient comfort, a shorter recovery time and decreased length of stay for patients. Procedures offered include video-assisted thoracoscopy for biopsy with or without removal of a portion of the lungs as well as repair of hiatal hernias and minimally invasive esophagectomy.

Pioneering Treatments
NYU Langone Medical Center leads the way in pioneering new treatments for the early detection of airway malignancies, diagnosis and treatment strategies for endobronchial abnormalities, investigation of non-surgical techniques selectively used for destruction of lung cancer nodules and the use of stents (and replaceable stents) to relieve blockages of the windpipe and esophagus.

Research
NYU Langone is committed to state-of-the-art surgical management and developing novel treatment strategies using clinical trials. We also leverage the resources at the New York Thoracic Surgery Laboratory house at Bellevue Hospital to search for genes and proteins in malignancies of the chest in order to detect them earlier or develop novel targeted therapies.

Transplantation

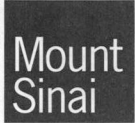 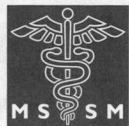

**THE MOUNT SINAI MEDICAL CENTER
TRANSPLANTATION**
One Gustave L. Levy Place
Fifth Avenue and 100th Street
New York, NY 10029-6574
Physician Referral: 1-800-MD-SINAI (637-4624)
www.mountsinai.org

Scientific breakthroughs, technological advances, and improved clinical therapies make it possible to save more lives through organ transplantation than ever before. The Mount Sinai Medical Center's **RECANATI MILLER/TRANSPLANTATION INSTITUTE (RMTI)** has been a world leader in these advances. The RMTI brings together clinical programs in adult and pediatric liver, kidney, pancreas, and intestinal transplantation. It is one of the largest transplant centers in the United States and performs more than 350 transplant procedures annually. In addition, RMTI surgeons also perform complex hepatobiliary surgical procedures.

History of Achievement – The kidney transplant program was instituted at Mount Sinai in 1967 and is now one of the largest adult and pediatric programs in the nation, having performed more than 2,000 transplants. The first liver transplant to be performed in New York State was in 1988 at Mount Sinai. There have been many other "firsts" in the program's 22-year history, including the first pediatric liver transplant and the first adult-to-adult living-donor liver transplant in New York State. Our surgeons have successfully performed more than 3,000 liver transplants.

Tradition of Excellence – Mount Sinai is one of the few hospitals in the country that offers comprehensive, multi-organ transplant services for both children and adults. Our physicians are able to accept and care for the sickest and most complex patients.

Innovative Programs

- HIV/Protocol Study – Since 2001, the RMTI has been one of the only National Institutes of Health-sponsored transplant centers to participate in a national study on transplantation for carefully selected patients with HIV.

- Living Donor Program – Mount Sinai has an active living-donor program and recently established the first Center for Living Donation where dedicated resources ensure the well-being of these heroes that give one, or a part, of their own organs to save another person's life. We also participate in local and national paired-exchange and donor-chain initiatives.

- Multi-organ Transplantation and Intestinal Rehabilitation Program – We have performed many combined transplant procedures. Our rehabilitation program offers patients with intestinal failure the opportunity, when possible, to avoid transplantation through medical and/or surgical interventions.

- Translational Research – Our scientists are actively investigating new and innovative ways to detect, prevent and treat rejection. We have nationally recognized and well-funded transplant, genomic, and proteomic projects.

Urology

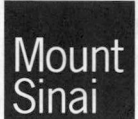 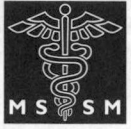

THE MOUNT SINAI MEDICAL CENTER
UROLOGY
One Gustave L. Levy Place
Fifth Avenue and 100th Street
New York, NY 10029-6574
Physician Referral: 1-800-MD-SINAI (637-4624)
www.mountsinai.org

MOUNT SINAI
SCHOOL OF
MEDICINE

THE MILTON AND CARROLL PETRIE DEPARTMENT OF UROLOGY at The Mount Sinai Medical Center offers the latest technologic advances for the diagnosis and treatment of urologic diseases and conditions, while supporting a strong translational and clinical research program.

Prostate Cancer – The Department of Urology's Barbara and Maurice Deane Prostate Health and Research Center offers a full range of surgical and radiation treatments for the management of localized prostate cancer, including one of the busiest robotic prostatectomy programs. For more advanced disease, options include hormonal therapy, Sipuleucel – T vaccine and new chemotherapy regimens. Current gene therapy research also offers hope for the future.

Bladder Cancer – As recognized leaders in the assessment and treatment of all forms of bladder cancer, Mount Sinai uro-oncologists employ knowledge of tumor markers and new diagnostic techniques and work with Department of Urology surgeons to determine the most effective treatment approaches. Robotics surgeons can perform cystectomies with a variety of diversions, resulting in minimal impact on quality of life.

Kidney Cancer – A majority of kidney tumors can be removed by Department of Urology surgeons via minimally invasive robotic surgical techniques, reducing pain and recovery time. Laparoscopic surgery may be utilized to remove all or a portion of a kidney. Other less-invasive modalities—such as freezing, may be recommended to treat small kidney cancers while reserving maximum function.

Prostatic Enlargement (benign prostatic hyperplasia) – The Deane Center offers the latest technologies and treatments, including Holmium Laser Ablation, the Button TURP and transurethral microwave dilation therapy, highly effective approaches to relieving urinary problems associated with an enlarged prostate, including urinary frequency, pain, burning, and retention. Many of these procedures are offered in an outpatient setting.

Urinary Dysfunction – Mount Sinai provides comprehensive resources for the evaluation and treatment, both medical and surgical, of urinary incontinence, neuro-urologic problems, and pelvic pain syndrome for both men and women. Many procedures can now be performed on an outpatient basis in a new, state-of-the-art facility within the Deane Center. Urologic Stone Disease–Mount Sinai's expertise in kidney stone disease ranges from stone prevention to minimally invasive therapies with lasers, sonic energies, and extracorporeal shock wave lithotripsy. Pediatric Conditions – Mount Sinai has a strong reputation in the area of pediatric urology, offering expertise in minimally invasive reconstructive procedures for both infants and children.

Male Infertility – Mount Sinai offers state-of-the-art approaches using medications and in vitro fertilization techniques that result in high success rates.

Sexuality-Related Health Concerns – For both men and women, sexuality-related issues are addressed with both medical and surgical approaches.

THE BARBARA AND MAURICE DEANE PROSTATE HEALTH AND RESEARCH CENTER offers a multidisciplinary approach for the assessment and treatment of all aspects of prostate disease, including cancer, benign enlargement, and inflammation. The Center strives to empower the patient and his family, as well as help them to better understand various prostate conditions so they can choose the most appropriate treatment and derive lasting benefits.

Mount Sinai offers a comprehensive **Minimally Invasive Urologic Surgery Program** and is a recognized leader in the greater New York area for performing complex robotic and laparoscopic procedures to treat urologic cancers. Areas of focus also include the treatment and management of stone disease and reconstructive procedures for various urologic cancers and anatomic abnormalities.

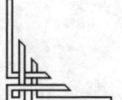
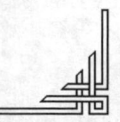

The Best in American Medicine
www.CastleConnolly.com

Vascular & Interventional Radiology

NYU **Cardiac and Vascular Institute**
NYU LANGONE MEDICAL CENTER

550 First Avenue *(at 31st Street)*
New York, NY 10016
www.NYULMC.org

Physician Referral: **(888)7-NYU-MED** *(888-769-8633)*

VASCULAR SURGERY

Staffed by one of the largest vascular surgery teams in the country, we offer expert patient care with an emphasis on minimally invasive therapies. Our physicians have extensive experience in performing the most up-to-date procedures including stents, angioplasty for carotid artery disease, aortic aneurysms and blockages in arteries throughout the body. In addition to its expertise in arterial disease, NYU is proud to offer one of the few Academic Vein Centers in the United States.
We specialize in the following areas:

Aortic Pathology
We offer minimally invasive surgical solutions as well as treatments for complex aortic problems. Patients usually require no blood transfusions and are able to leave the hospital just one or two days after surgery. We are also a training center for endovascular management of abdominal and thoracic aneurysms.

Carotid Artery Disease
We remain a leader in both the screening for carotid disease and the prevention of stroke for those being treated for carotid artery occlusive disease, known to predispose patients to stroke. Our physicians were central to pioneering carotid endarterectomy as an open surgical procedure, as well as playing a pivotal role in the development of the carotid stenting procedure.

Peripheral Arterial Disease
Our doctors have a wealth of experience in treating peripheral arterial disease (PAD) and specialize in new and innovative technologies such as laser and "Silverhawk" atherectomy procedures as well as cryoplasty. Additionally, we are one of the only centers in the tristate area with access to drug-eluting stents which are coated with special medicines that may prevent scar formation and re-occlusion of the stent.

Vascular Screenings
Our doctors are committed to improving the public awareness and understanding of vascular disease through preventative screenings. The disease is among the leading causes of death in the U.S., yet is generally asymptomatic until a stroke or aneurysm rupture. Effective screenings performed include ultrasound scans of the aorta, ultrasound scans of the carotid arteries and blood pressure measurements.

Venous Disease
The Vein Center at NYU Langone Medical Center is considered an authority in the minimally invasive treatment of venous disease, treating patients with all forms of venous pathology ranging from venous insufficiency and varicose veins to occlusive disease and deep vein thrombosis.

Vascular Surgery

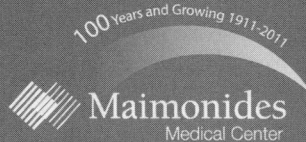

Women's Health

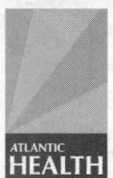

Trinitas Regional Medical Center

WOMEN'S SERVICES

225 WILLIAMSON STREET | ELIZABETH, NEW JERSEY 07207
PH 908.994.5138 | WWW.TRINITASRMC.ORG

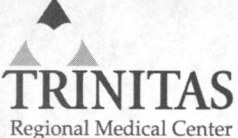

TRINITAS
Regional Medical Center

Trinitas Regional Medical Center offers a number of advanced services just for women that range from the latest in imaging and diagnostic technology, to state-of-the-art, minimally invasive procedures used for hysterectomies and in the treatment of incontinence and prolapse.

WOMEN'S IMAGING CENTER

Our new, technologically advanced, FDA-approved and MQSA (Mammography Quality Standards Act) certified facility provides the services - digital mammography, stereotactic needle biopsy, ultrasound and bone densitometry - that are essential in addressing women's concerns.

The staff in the Women's Imaging Center has had specialized training, and they will work with you and your physician to provide services in a comfortable and professional environment. State-of-the-art digital mammography equipment further enhances the diagnostic quality of the images of the breast tissue and the accuracy of the interpretation of the mammogram. All studies are interpreted by Board Certified Radiologists.

Procedures may be scheduled by calling 908-994-5984.

TREATMENT FOR INCONTINENCE AND PROLAPSE

Trinitas is a pioneer in the latest, minimally invasive procedures for the treatment of female incontinence and vaginal prolapse. A new approach to prolapse includes a single-incision approach that shortens surgical time, minimizes tissue trauma and reduces recovery time. The treatment of incontinence is also accomplished with highly effective, minimally invasive techniques, many

performed for the first time in New Jersey at Trinitas Regional Medical Center. Single-incision techniques involve the placement of an internal supporting sling that is highly effective in eliminating stress incontinence. Procedures are commonly performed on an outpatient basis.

MINIMALLY INVASIVE HYSTERECTOMY

Trinitas Regional Medical Center offers a non-surgical option for women who undergo hysterectomy to treat excessive menstrual or uterine bleeding. Endometrial Ablation involves removing only the lining of a woman's uterus using warmed water.

In the event that surgery is necessary, Trinitas now offers a precise, minimally invasive option for hysterectomy through the use of the da Vinci® Surgical System. The da Vinci system provides surgeons with an alternative to both traditional open surgery and conventional laparoscopy, putting a surgeon's hands at the controls of a state-of-the-art robotic platform. The da Vinci® Surgical System enables surgeons to perform even the most complex and delicate procedures through very small incisions with unmatched precision. Benefits for patients include significantly less pain, less blood loss, less scarring, shorter recovery time, a faster return to normal daily activities and, in many cases, better clinical outcomes.

Wound Care

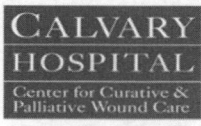

CALVARY HOSPITAL
1740 Eastchester Road
Bronx, NY 10461
Tel: (718) 518-2000
www.calvaryhospital.org

CENTER FOR CURATIVE AND PALLIATIVE WOUND CARE

Founded in 1899, Calvary Hospital is the nation's only acute care specialty hospital dedicated to caring for inpatients with advanced cancer. We serve people of all faith traditions in a restraint-free environment that offers 24/7 visiting hours and extensive bereavement support for families and friends. In addition to inpatient care, we offer outpatient care, home care, hospice, nursing home hospice, and wound care. All Calvary care is guided by our core values of compassion, respect for the dignity of every patient, and non-abandonment of patients and families.

Calvary Wound Care: A Proud Tradition
In the course of caring for people with advanced cancer, Calvary has developed outstanding expertise in the care of complex, intractable wounds. We extend this care to people in the community through our outpatient clinic. In 2004, we established the Center for Curative and Palliative Wound Care, where we treat patients with chronic wounds secondary to diabetes, neuropathy, chronic venous insufficiency, immobility, lymphedema, peripheral vascular disease, cancer, and other inflammatory or hematological disorders that can cause wounds. Through December 2010, Calvary recorded more than 26,700 patient visits to this pioneering center.

A Personalized Approach
Our personalized approach to wound management goes beyond established curative protocols to address the larger goals of patient care, by seeking to enhance quality of life for patients and families. We strive to relieve the suffering of patients when wounds do not respond to standard interventions, or when demands of treatment are beyond their tolerance or stamina.

The Center for Curative and Palliative Wound Care offers treatment options for wounds associated with such underlying medical conditions as:

Venous or Arterial Disease	Diabetes	Neuropathy
Immobility	Autoimmune Disease	Arthritis
Chronic Inflammatory Conditions	Blood Disorders	Lymphedema

We also treat post-operative wounds and wounds caused by cancer, chemotherapy, and/or radiation therapy. Wound care personnel are available to consult with nursing homes and long-term care facilities on request. Specially trained visiting nurses and therapists provide expert wound care services for patients at home.

We are a community resource for Bronx Hispanic residents, who record the highest prevalence for diabetes in New York and among one of the highest in the country. To help people identify and prevent serious foot-related problems before they occur, the Wound Care Center hosted free foot screenings by expert medical professionals for adult diabetics in 2008 and 2009. These screenings helped hundreds of adult diabetics from all over the metropolitan area.

Support for Families
Family members often serve as caregivers. Our physicians and nurses strive to build a foundation of trust and open communication with patients and families. We teach family members to clean wounds and change dressings, and we are always available to answer questions or offer guidance about wound care.

Pastoral care, family care, nutrition counseling, and other Calvary services are available to patients and families of the Center for Curative and Palliative Wound Care.

Research is integral to the mission of the Center, which is now pursuing a number of protocols focusing on novel treatments for wounds related to diabetes and other disorders.

For information or to refer a patient to the Wound Care Center, please call (718) 518-2577.

WOUND CARE

About the Division of Wound Healing and Regenerative Medicine:
The Division of Wound Healing and Regenerative Medicine at NYU Langone Medical Center treats chronic, non-healing wounds in a personal and caring environment that involves patients and their families at every level of care. We are dedicated to all aspects of healing, particularly on establishing the highest standards for persons with wounds including those with diabetes, disabilities and the elderly. The Helen L. and Martin S. Kimmel Wound Healing Center specializes in treating chronic wounds such as diabetic foot ulcers, pressure ulcers (bed sores), venous ulcers and sickle cell ulcers and is one of the only dedicated inpatient units in the world specifically for chronic wounds.
We specialize in the following areas:

Clinical Care
The clinical team at the Division of Wound Healing and Regenerative Medicine at NYU Langone Medical Center—consisting of doctors, nurses, physician assistants and social workers—brings patients the most comprehensive, innovative and compassionate care possible. Utilizing the most advanced, evidence-based techniques, patients have access to more than 20 specialists, including but not limited to, cardiologists, vascular surgeons, plastic surgeons, orthopaedists, podiatrists and physical therapists.

Research
Researchers at the Division of Wound Healing and Regenerative Medicine at NYU Langone Medical Center started a human wound cell bank, which resulted in the discovery of one of the first genes that inhibits wound healing in humans. Researchers also made the discovery that human skin equivalent therapy, previously thought to act as a skin graft, accelerates healing through its effects of the controlled release of a series of growth factors from cells, e.g, human keratinocytes and fibroblasts. This discovery led clinical research on cellular therapies for chronic wounds, which has resulted in decreased amputations in persons with diabetic foot ulcers and is the only treatment approved in randomized control trials for venous ulcers.

Wound Electronic Medical Records
NYU Langone Medical Center has designed a Wound Electronic Medical Record (WEMR) to acquire and display the data and provide the decision support necessary to improve the care of patients with chronic wounds. As part of this medical record, photographs of the wounds are taken during each clinical visit to record the progress of healing. Using these photographs and a computer program, the team calculates wound area as a method of tracking the healing rate. As part of each visit, patients can view these photographs and a graph of the wound area to see improvement over time.

Trinitas Regional Medical Center

CENTER FOR WOUND HEALING & HYPERBARIC MEDICINE

240 WILLIAMSON STREET, SUITE 104 | ELIZABETH, NEW JERSEY 07207
PH 908.994.5480 | WWW.WOUNDHEALINGCENTER.ORG

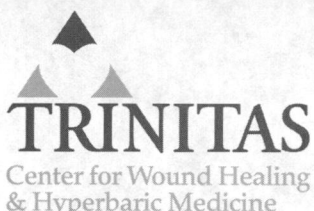

AWARD-WINNING CARE FOR HARD-TO-HEAL WOUNDS

At the Center for Wound Healing & Hyperbaric Medicine, our unique team of highly trained physicians, nurses and foot specialists can help sufferers get their lives back. We specialize in non-healing wounds - those that have resisted healing after months and even years of traditional treatment. This is accomplished with a success rate that is consistently 90% and above, and the vast majority of our patients leave the Center completely healed in an average of just 28 days.

The treatment options offered at the Center include the Vacuum-Assisted Closure (VAC) Therapy System, Hyperbaric Oxygen Therapy, and Apligraf cultured living skin.

Wounds don't heal for a variety of reasons. Diabetes, smoking, poor circulation, heart problems, poor nutrition and many medications may prevent healing. As one of the nation's leading centers for wound healing, we see a complex array of hard-to-heal wounds in patients from all races, nationalities and economic backgrounds. Hard-to-heal wounds come in all shapes and sizes, and can affect many parts of the body.

The five main types of wounds treated at Trinitas are pressure ulcers, venous ulcers, diabetic ulcers, arterial ulcers and trauma wounds. Our approach to wound healing is holistic in that we look at the entire person, not just the wound. How is the wound affecting the patient's life? What other lifestyle factors might hinder successful wound healing? What genetic factors contribute to the patient's overall well-being?

By using well-researched, proven techniques, our multi-disciplinary team provides healing and relief for patients who previously thought their wounds were irreparable or would ultimately result in amputation.

The Center for Wound Healing & Hyperbaric Medicine, named by Praxis Clinical Services as "Center of the Year," was the first in the state to use such innovative technologies as the Apligraf living skin device. The expertise of the Center's physicians in pioneering wound closure technologies such as the Vacuum Assisted Closure (VAC) was shared recently at a number of national wound healing conferences. The Center ranks as one of the top Centers for Wound Healing in the nation.

The Best in American Medicine
www.CastleConnolly.com

SECTION FIVE

Appendices

Appendix A:
Medical Boards

Intro to ABMS and Osteopathic Specialties

The following pages contain descriptions of the "official" medical specialties, approved by the American Board of Medical Specialists (for M.D.s) or by the American Osteopathic Association (for D.O.s). These are important because they are the only specialties recognized by the official governing boards. There may be physicians who call themselves one kind of specialist or another, but they may not be certified by the "official" boards. There are, in fact, over 100 such "self-designated" boards, some simply groups of physicians interested in a given area of medicine with no qualifications for membership to other groups with very specific qualifications for membership.

It is important for the medical consumer to seek out physicians certified by the ABMS or AOA to assure their doctor has had the appropriate training and passed the board certification exam.

ABMS

The ABMS is an organization of ABMS approved medical specialty boards. The mission of the ABMS is to maintain and improve the quality of medical care by assisting the Member Boards in their efforts to develop and utilize professional and educational standards for the evaluation and certification of physician specialists. The intent of certification of physicians is to provide assurance to the public that a physician specialist certified by a Member Board of the ABMS has successfully completed an approved educational program and evaluation process which includes an examination designed to assess the knowledge, skills, and experience required to provide quality patient care in that specialty. The ABMS serves to coordinate the activities of its Member Boards and to provide information to the public, the government, the profession and its Members concerning issues involving specialization and certification in medicine.

Following is a list of the addresses of the various medical specialty boards approved by the ABMS. Note that there are 24 board organizations for 25 medical specialties. Psychiatry and Neurology share the same board.

Appendix A: Medical Boards

To find out if a physician is certified, consumers can call the individual boards which may charge a fee for the information, or they can contact the ABMS at 866-275-2267 (no fee) or www.abms.org.

American Board of Allergy and Immunology
111 South Independence Mall East
Suite 701
Philadelphia, PA 19106
(215) 592-9466, (866) 264-5568

General Certification in Allergy and Immunology. Certifications awarded since 1989 are valid for 10 years. For those certified prior to 1989 there is no recertification requirement.

American Board of Anesthesiology
4208 Six Forks Rd, Ste 900
Raleigh, NC 27607-5735
(919) 745-2200

General Certification in Anesthesiology; with Special and Added Qualifications in Critical Care Medicine, Hospice & Palliative Medicine and Pain Management. Certifications awarded since 2000 are valid for 10 years.

American Board of Colon and Rectal Surgery
20600 Eureka Road, Suite 600
Taylor, MI 48180
(734) 282-9400

General Certification in Colon and Rectal Surgery. Certifications awarded since 1990 are valid for 10 years.

American Board of Dermatology
Henry Ford Health System
1 Ford Place
Detroit, MI 48202-3450
(313) 874-1088

General Certification in Dermatology; with Special Qualifications in Clinical and Laboratory Dermatological Immunology, Dermatopathology, and Pediatric Dermatology. Certifications awarded since 1991 are valid for 10 years.

American Board of Emergency Medicine

3000 Coolidge Road
East Lansing, MI 48823-6319
(517) 332-4800

General Certification in Emergency Medicine; with Special and Added Qualifications in Hospice & Palliative Medicine, Medical Toxicology, Pediatric Emergency Medicine, Sports Medicine and Undersea and Hyperbaric Medicine. Certifications awarded since 1980 are valid for 10 years.

American Board of Family Practice

1648 McGrathiania Parkway, 5th Floor
Lexington, KY 40511
(859) 269-5626, (888) 995-5700

General Certification in Family Practice; with Added Qualifications in Adolescent Medicine, Geriatric Medicine, Hospice & Palliative Medicine, Sleep Medicine and Sports Medicine. Certifications awarded since 1970 are valid for 7 years.

American Board of Internal Medicine

510 Walnut Street, Suite 1700
Philadelphia, PA 19106-3699
(215) 446-3500, (800) 441-ABIM

General Certification in Internal Medicine; with Special Qualifications in Cardiovascular Disease, Endocrinology, Diabetes and Metabolism, Gastroenterology, Hematology, Infectious Disease, Medical Oncology, Nephrology, Pulmonary Disease, and Rheumatology; and Added Qualifications in Adolescent Medicine, Advanced Heart Failure & Transplane Cardiology, Clinical Cardiac Electrophysiology, Critical Care Medicine, Geriatric Medicine, Interventional Cardiology, Sleep Medicine, Sports Medicine and Transplant Hepatology. Certifications awarded since 1990 are valid for 10 years.

American Board of Medical Genetics

9650 Rockville Pike
Bethesda, MD 20814-3998
(301) 634-7315

General Certification in Clinical Genetics (MD), PhD Medical Genetics, Clinical Biochemical Genetics, Clinical Cytogenetics and Clinical Molecular Genetics; with Added Qualifications in Medical Biochemical Genetics, Molecular Genetic Pathology. Certifications awarded since 2002 are valid for 2 years.

Appendix A: Medical Boards

American Board of Neurological Surgery
6550 Fannin Street, Suite 2139
Houston, TX 77030-2701
(713) 441-6015

General Certification in Neurological Surgery. Certifications awarded since 1999 are valid for 10 years.

American Board of Nuclear Medicine
4555 Forest Park Boulevard, Suite 119
St. Louis, MO 63108
(314) 367-2225

General Certification in Nuclear Medicine. Certifications awarded since 1992 are valid for 10 years.

American Board of Obstetrics and Gynecology
2915 Vine Street, Suite 300
Dallas, TX 75204
(214) 871-1619

General Certification in Obstetrics and Gynecology; with Special Qualifications in Gynecologic Oncology, Maternal and Fetal Medicine, Reproductive Endocrinology/Infertility; and Added Qualifications in Hospice & Palliative Medicine and Critical Care Medicine. Certifications awarded since 1986 are valid for 6 years.

American Board of Ophthalmology
111 Presidential Boulevard, Suite 241
Bala Cynwyd, PA 19004-1075
(610) 664-1175

General certification in Ophthalmology. Certifications awarded since 1992 are valid for 10 years. For those certified prior to 1992 there is no recertification requirement.

American Board of Orthopaedic Surgery
400 Silver Cedar Court
Chapel Hill, NC 27514
(919) 929-7103

General Certification in Orthopaedic Surgery; with Added Qualification in Hand Surgery and Orthopaedic Sports Medicine. Certifications awarded since 1986 are valid for 10 years.

American Board of Otolaryngology
5615 Kirby Drive, Suite 600
Houston, TX 77005
(713) 850-0399

General Certification in Otolaryngology; with Added Qualifications in Neurotology, Pediatric Otolaryngology, Plastic Surgery within the Head and Neck and Sleep Medicine. Certifications awarded since 2002 are valid for 10 years.

American Board of Pathology
4830 Kennedy Boulevard
Suite 690
Tampa, FL 33622
(813) 286-2444

General Certification in Anatomic and Clinical Pathology, Anatomic Pathology and Clinical Pathology; with Special Qualifications in Blood Banking/Transfusion Medicine, Chemical Pathology, Dermatopathology, Forensic Pathology, Hematology, Medical Microbiology, Molecular Genetic Pathology, Neuropathology and Pediatric Pathology; and Added Qualifications in Cytopathology. Certifications awarded since 1997 are valid for 10 years.

American Board of Pediatrics
111 Silver Cedar Court
Chapel Hill, NC 27514-1651
(919) 929-0461

General Certification in Pediatrics; with Special Qualifications in Adolescent Medicine, Developmental-Behavioral Pediatrics, Neonatal-Perinatal Medicine, Pediatric Cardiology, Pediatric Critical Care Medicine, Pediatric Emergency Medicine, Pediatric Endocrinology, Pediatric Gastroenterology, Pediatric Hematology-Oncology, Pediatric Infectious Diseases, Pediatric Nephrology, Pediatric Pulmonology, and Pediatric Rheumatology; and Added Qualifications in Medical Toxicology, Neurodevelopmental Disabilities, Pediatric Transplant Hepatology, Sleep Medicine and Sports Medicine. Certifications awarded since 1988 valid for 7 years.

American Board of Physical Medicine and Rehabilitation

3015 Allegro Park Lane, S.W.

Rochester, MN 55902-4139

(507) 282-1776

General Certification in Physical Medicine and Rehabilitation; with Special Qualifications in Pain Medicine, Pediatric Rehabilitation Medicine, and Spinal Cord Injury Medicine; and Added Qualifications in Hospice & Palliative Medicine, Neuromuscular Medicine and Sports Medicine. Certifications awarded since 1993 are valid for 10 years.

American Board of Plastic Surgery

Seven Penn Center, Suite 400

1635 Market Street

Philadelphia, PA 19103-2204

(215) 587-9322

General Certification in Plastic Surgery; with Added Qualifications in Hand Surgery and Head & Neck Surgery. Certifications awarded since 1995 are valid for 10-years.

American Board of Preventive Medicine

111 W. Jackson, Suite 1110

Chicago, IL 60604

(312) 939-ABPM [2276]

General Certification in Aerospace Medicine, Occupational Medicine and Public Health and General Preventive Medicine; with Added Qualifications in Undersea and Hyperbaric Medicine and Medical Toxicology. Certifications awarded since 1997 are valid for 10 years.

American Board of Psychiatry and Neurology

2150 E. Lake Cook Road, Suite 900

Buffalo Grove, IL 60089

(847) 229-6500

General Certification in Psychiatry, Neurology and Neurology with Special Qualification in Child Neurology; with Special Qualifications in Child and Adolescent Psychiatry, Epilepsy, Hospice & Palliative Medicine, Pain Medicine and Sleep Medicine; and Added Qualifications in Addiction Psychiatry, Clinical Neurophysiology, Forensic Psychiatry, Geriatric Psychiatry, Hospice & Palliative Medicine, Neurodevelopmental Disabilities, Psychosomatic Medicine and Vascular Neurology. Certifications awarded since 1994 are valid for 10 years.

American Board of Radiology
5441 E. Williams Boulevard, Suite 200
Tucson, AZ 85711
(520) 790-2900

General Certification in Diagnostic Radiology or Radiation Oncology; with Special Competency in Nuclear Radiology; and Added Qualifications in Hospice & Palliative Medicine, Neuroradiology, Pediatric Radiology and Vascular and Interventional Radiology. Radiological Physics is a non-clinical certification. Certificates are valid for 10 years.

American Board of Surgery
1617 John F. Kennedy Boulevard, Suite 860
Philadelphia, PA 19103-1847
(215) 568-4000

General Certification in Surgery and Vascular Surgery; with Special Qualifications in Pediatric Surgery and Surgery of the Hand; and Added Qualifications in Hospice & Palliative Medicine and Surgical Critical Care. Certifications awarded since 1976 are valid for 10 years.

American Board of Thoracic Surgery
633 North St. Clair Street, Suite 2320
Chicago, IL 60611
(312) 202-5900

General Certification in Thoracic Surgery; and Added Qualifications in Congenital Cardiac Surgery. Certifications awarded since 1976 are valid for 10 years.

American Board of Urology
2216 Ivy Road, Suite 210
Charlottesville, VA 22903
(434) 979-0059

General Certification in Urology; and Added Qualifications in Pediatric Urology. Certifications awarded as of 1985 are valid for 10 years.

Osteopathic

The American Osteopathic Association (AOA) is a member association representing more than 67,000 osteopathic physicians (D.O.s). The AOA serves as the primary certifying body for D.O.s, and is the accrediting agency for all osetopathic medical colleges and healthcare facilities. The AOA's mission is to advance the philosophy and practice of osteopathic medicine by promoting excellence in education, research, and the delivery of quality, cost-effective healthcare within a distinct, unified profession.

American Osteopathic Association
142 E Ontario Street
Chicago, IL 60611

Consumers may call the American Osteopathic Association at (800) 621-1773 or visit the website, www.osteopathic.org, for general certification information.

American Osteopathic Board of Anesthesiology

General certification in Anesthesiology; with Added Qualifications in Addiction Medicine, Critical Care Medicine, and Pain Management. Certifications awarded since 2004 are valid for 10 years. For those certified prior to 2004 there is no recertification requirement.

American Osteopathic Board of Dermatology

General certification in Dermatology; with Added Qualifications in Dermatopathology and Mohs'-Micrographic Surgery. Certifications awarded since 2004 are valid for 10 years.

American Osteopathic Board of Emergency Medicine

General certification in Emergency Medicine; with Added Qualifications in Emergency Medical Services, Medical Toxicology, and Sports Medicine. Certifications awarded since 1994 are valid for 10 years.

American Osteopathic Board of Family Physicians

General certification in Family Practice and Osteopathic Manipulative Treatment (OMT); with Added Qualifications in Geriatric Medicine, Hospice & Palliative Medicine, Sleep Medicine, Sports Medicine and Undersea & Hyperbaric Medicine. Certifications awarded since March 1,1997 are valid for 8 years.

American Osteopathic Board of Internal Medicine

General certification in Internal Medicine; with Special Qualifications in Allergy/Immunology, Cardiology, Endocrinology, Gastroenterology, Hematology, Infectious Disease, Nephrology, Oncology, Pulmonary Disease, Rheumatology; with Added Qualifications in Addiction Medicine, Critical Care Medicine, Clinical Cardiac Electrophysiology, Hospice & Palliative Medicine, Geriatric Medicine, Interventional Cardiology, Sleep Medicine, Sports Medicine and Undersea & Hyperbaric Medicine. Certifications awarded since 1993 are valid for 10 years.

American Osteopathic Board of Neurology and Psychiatry

General certification in Neurology and Psychiatry; with Special Qualifications in Child/Adolescent Psychiatry and Child/Adolescent Neurology; with Added Qualifications in Addiction Medicine, Geriatric Psychiatry, Hospice & Palliative Medicine, Neurophysiology, and Sleep Medicine. Certifications awarded since 1995 are valid for 10 years.

American Osteopathic Board of Neuromusculoskeletal Medicine

General certification in Neuromusculoskelatal Medicine & Osteopathic Manipulative Medicine; with Added qualifications in Sports Medicine.

American Osteopathic Board of Nuclear Medicine

General certification in Nuclear Medicine. Certifications awarded since 1995 are valid for 10 years. This certification is no longer issued.

American Osteopathic Board of Obstetrics and Gynecology

General certification in Obstetrics and Gynecology; with Special Qualifications in Gynecologic Oncology; Maternal and Fetal Medicine and Reproductive Endocrinology. Certifications awarded since June 2002 are valid for 6 years.

American Osteopathic Board of Ophthalmology and Otolaryngology - Head & Neck Surgery

General certification in Ophthalmology, Otolaryngology, Facial Plastic Surgery and Otolaryngology/Facial Plastic Surgery; with Added Qualifications in Otolaryngic Allergy and Sleep Medicine. Certifications awarded in Ophthalmology since 2000 are valid for 10 years. For those certified prior to 2000 there is no recertification requirement. Certifications awarded in Otolaryngology and/or Otolaryngology/Facial Plastic Surgery since 2002 are valid for 10 years.

American Osteopathic Board of Orthopaedic Surgery

General certification in Orthopaedic Surgery; with Added Qualifications in Hand Surgery. Certifications awarded since 1994 are valid for 10 years.

American Osteopathic Board of Pathology

General certification in Laboratory Medicine, Anatomic Pathology and Anatomic Pathology and Laboratory Medicine; with Special Qualifications in Forensic Pathology; and with Added Qualifications in Dermatopathology. Certifications awarded since 1995 are valid for 10 years.

American Osteopathic Board of Pediatrics

General certification in Pediatrics with Special Qualifications in Adolescent and Young Adult Medicine, Neonatology, Pediatric Allergy/Immunology and Pediatric Endocrinology; with Added Qualifications in Sports Medicine. Certifications awarded since 1995 are valid for 7 years.

American Osteopathic Board of Physical Medicine and Rehabilitation Medicine

General certification in Physical Medicine and Rehabilitation; with Added Qualifications in Hospice & Palliative Medicine and Sports Medicine. Certifications awarded since 2004 are valid
for 10 years.

American Osteopathic Board of Preventive Medicine

General certification in Preventive Medicine/Aerospace Medicine, Preventive Medicine/Occupational-Environmental Medicine and Preventive Medicine/Public Health; with Added Qualifications in Occupational Medicine and Undersea & Hyperbaric Medicine. Certifications awarded since 1994 are valid for 10 years.

American Osteopathic Board of Proctology

General certification in Proctology. Certifications awarded since 2004 are valid for 10 years.

American Osteopathic Board of Radiology

General certification in Diagnostic Radiology and Radiation Oncology; with Added Qualifications in Angiography & Interventional Radiology, Body Imaging, Diagnostic Ultrasound, Neuroradiology, Nuclear Radiology, Pediatric Radiology. Certifications awarded since 2002 are valid for 10 years.

American Osteopathic Board of Surgery

General certification in General Vascular Surgery, Surgery, Neurological Surgery, Plastic and Reconstructive Surgery, Thoracic Cardiovascular Surgery, Urological Surgery; with Added Qualifications in Surgical Critical Care. Certifications awarded since 1997 are valid for 10 years.

Appendix B:
Self-Designated Medical Specialties

This list of self-designated medical specialty groups was obtained from the American Board of Medical Specialties. However, it is important to point out that these groups are not recognized by the ABMS, the governing board for the recognized twenty-four medical specialty boards (listed in Appendix A).

The organizations listed below range from highly organized groups that are attempting to formalize training and certification in their field to informal groups interested in a particular aspect of medicine.

If you wish to obtain information from any of these groups you will have to do some detective work. Because so many are informal, the location, phone and mailing addresses change frequently, depending upon the person who is functioning as secretary or administrator.

The best way to track down one of these groups is to consult the doctor listings to find a doctor who has expressed a special interest in that field, and call his or her office. You might also call a nearby academic health center in the area to see if they have a faculty or staff member known to be involved in that particular medical interest. If that fails, take the same approach with your community hospital.

A

Abdominal Surgeons

Acupuncture Medicine

Addiction Medicine

Addictionology

Adolescent Psychiatry

Aesthetic Plastic Surgery

Alcoholism and Other Drug
        Dependencies (AMSAODD)

Algology (Chronic Pain)

Alternative Medicine

Ambulatory Anesthesia

Ambulatory Foot Surgery

Anesthesia

Arthroscopic Surgery

Arthroscopy (Board of North America)

B

Bariatric Medicine

Bionic Psychology

Bloodless Medicine & Surgery

C

Chelation Therapy

Chemical Dependence

Clinical Chemistry

Clinical Ecology

Clinical Medicine and Surgery

Clinical Neurology

Clinical Neurophysiology

Clinical Neurosurgery

Clinical Nutrition

Clinical Orthopaedic Surgery

Clinical Pharmacology

Clinical Polysomnography

Clinical Psychiatry

Clinical Psychology

Clinical Toxicology

Cosmetic Plastic Surgery

Cosmetic Surgery

Council of Non-Board Certified Physicians

Critical Care in Medicine & Surgery

D

Disability Analysis

Disability Evaluating Physicians

E

Electrodiagnostic Medicine

Electroencephalography

Electromyography & Electrodiagnosis

Environmental Medicine

Epidemiology (College)

Eye Surgery

F

Facial Cosmetic Surgery

Facial Plastic & Reconstructive Surgery

Family Practice, Certification

Forensic Examiners

Forensic Psychiatry

Forensic Toxicology

H

Hand Surgery

Head, Facial & Neck Pain & TMJ Orthopaedics

Health Physics

Homeopathic Physicians

Homeotherapeutics

Hypnotic Anesthesiology, National Board for

I

Independent Medical Examiners

Industrial Medicine & Surgery

Insurance Medicine

International Cosmetic & Plastic
        Facial Reconstructive Standards

Interventional Radiology

L

Laser Surgery
Law in Medicine
Longevity Medicine/Surgery

M

Malpractice Physicians
Maxillofacial Surgeons
Medical Accreditation (American Federation for)
Medical Hypnosis
Medical Laboratory Immunology
Medical-Legal Analysis of Medicine & Surgery
Medical Legal & Workers
     Comp. Medicine & Surgery
Medical-Legal Consultants
Medical Management
Medical Microbiology
Medical Preventics (Academy)
Medical Psychotherapists
Medical Toxicology
Microbiology (Medical Microbiology)
Military Medicine
Mohs' Micrographic Surgery &
     Cutaneous Oncology

N

Neuroimaging
Neurologic & Orthopaedic Dental
     Medicine and Surgery
Neurological & Orthopaedic Medicine
Neurological & Orthopaedic Surgery
Neurological Microsurgery
Neurology
Neuromuscular Thermography
Neuro-Orthopaedic Dental Medicine
Neuro-Orthopaedic Electrodiagnosis
Neuro-Orthopaedic Laser Surgery
Neuro-Orthopaedic Psychiatry
Neuro-Orthopaedic Thoracic Medicine
Neurorehabilitation
Nutrition

O

Orthopaedic Medicine
Orthopaedic Microneurosurgery
Otorhinolaryngology

P

Pain Management (American Academy of)
Pain Management Specialties
Pain Medicine
Palliative Medicine
Percutaneous Diskectomy
Plastic Esthetic Surgeons
Prison Medicine
Professional Disability Consultants
Psychiatric Medicine
Psychiatry (American National Board of)
Psychoanalysis (American Examining
     Board in)
Psychological Medicine (International)

Q

Quality Assurance & Utilization Review

R

Radiology & Medical Imaging
Rheumatologic Surgery
Rheumatological & Reconstructive Medicine
Ringside Medicine & Surgery

S

Skin Specialists
Sleep Medicine (Polysomnography)
Spinal Cord Injury
Spinal Surgery
Sports Medicine
Sports Medicine/Surgery

T

Toxicology
Trauma Surgery
Traumatologic Medicine & Surgery
Tropical Medicine

U

Ultrasound Technology
Urologic Allied Health Professionals
Urological Surgery

W

Weight Reduction Medicine

APPENDIX C:
Hospital Listings

The following is an alphabetical listing of all hospitals that have at least one Castle Connolly Top Doctor in this guide. Institutions listed in **Bold** are profiled in this Guide in association with Castle Connolly's Partnership for Excellence program. The abbreviations as they appear in the listings are in italics below. Due to the many changes taking place in the hospital industry, the names on this list may have changed subsequent to publication of this guide.

Bayonne Medical Center   (201) 858-5000
Bayonne Med Ctr
29 E 29th St   Bayonne, NJ 07002   HUDSON

Bayshore Community Hospital   (732) 739-5900
Bayshore Community Hosp
7727 North Beers Street   Holmdel, NJ 07733   MONMOUTH

Bellevue Hospital Center   (212) 562-1000
Bellevue Hosp Ctr
462 First Avenue   New York, NY 10016   NEW YORK (MANHATTAN)

Beth Israel Medical Center - Kings Highway Division   (718) 252-3000
Beth Israel Med Ctr- Kings Hwy Div
3201 Kings Highway   Brooklyn, NY 11234   KINGS (BROOKLYN)

Beth Israel Medical Center - Milton & Caroll Petrie Division   (212) 420-2000
Beth Israel Med Ctr - Petrie Division
First Avenue @ 16th Street   New York, NY 10003   NEW YORK (MANHATTAN)

Blythedale Children's Hospital   (914) 592-7555
Blythedale Children's Hosp
95 Bradhurst Avenue   Valhalla, NY 10595   WESTCHESTER

Bridgeport Hospital   (203) 384-3000
Bridgeport Hosp
267 Grant St   Bridgeport, CT 06610   FAIRFIELD

Bronx Children's Psychiatric Center   (718) 239-3621
Bronx Children's Psych Ctr
1000 Waters Place   Bronx, NY 10461   BRONX

Bronx Lebanon Hospital Center   (718) 590-1800
Bronx Lebanon Hosp Ctr
1276 Fulton Ave   Bronx, NY 10457   BRONX

Bronx Psychiatric Center   (718) 931-0600
Bronx Psych Ctr
1500 Waters Place   Bronx, NY 10461   BRONX

Brookdale University Hospital Medical Center   (718) 240-5000
Brookdale Univ Hosp Med Ctr
One Brookdale Plaza   Brooklyn, NY 11212   KINGS (BROOKLYN)

Brookhaven Memorial Hospital & Medical Center   (631) 654-7100
Brookhaven Meml Hosp & Med Ctr
101 Hospital Road   Patchogue, NY 11772   SUFFOLK

Brooklyn Hospital Center-Downtown   (718) 250-8000
Brooklyn Hosp Ctr-Downtown
121 DeKalb Avenue   Brooklyn, NY 11201   KINGS (BROOKLYN)

Burke Rehabilitation Hospital   (914) 597-2500
Burke Rehab Hosp
785 Mamaroneck Avenue   White Plains, NY 10605   WESTCHESTER

Calvary Hospital   (718) 518-2000
Calvary Hosp
1740 Eastchester Road   Bronx, NY 10461   BRONX

Capital Health System - Fuld Campus   (609) 394-6000
Capital Health Sys - Fuld Campus
750 Brunswick Avenue   Trenton, NJ 08638-4174   MERCER

Capital Health System - Mercer Campus   (609) 394-4000
Capital Hlth Sys - Mercer Campus
446 Bellevue Avenue   Trenton, NJ 08618   MERCER

CentraState Medical Center   (732) 431-2000
CentraState Med Ctr
901 West Main Street   Freehold, NJ 07728   MONMOUTH

Children's Specialized Hospital   (908) 233-3720
Children's Specialized Hosp
150 New Providence Rd   Mountainside, NJ 07092   UNION

Chilton Memorial Hospital   (973) 831-5000
Chilton Meml Hosp
97 West Parkway   Pompton Plains, NJ 07444   MORRIS

Christ Hospital   (201) 795-8200
Christ Hosp
176 Palisade Avenue   Jersey City, NJ 07306   HUDSON

Clara Maass Medical Center   (973) 450-2000
Clara Maass Med Ctr
One Clara Maass Drive   Belleville, NJ 07109   ESSEX

Community Hospital - Dobbs Ferry   (914) 693-0700
Comm Hosp - Dobbs Ferry
128 Ashford Ave   Dobbs Ferry, NY 10522-1924   WESTCHESTER

Coney Island Hospital   (718) 616-3000
Coney Island Hosp
2601 Ocean Parkway   Brooklyn, NY 11235   KINGS (BROOKLYN)

Connecticut Mental Health Center   (203) 789-7092
Connecticut Mental Hlth Ctr
34 Park St   New Haven, CT 06508-1842   NEW HAVEN

Danbury Hospital   (203) 739-7000
Danbury Hosp
24 Hospital Avenue   Danbury, CT 06810   FAIRFIELD

Eastern Long Island Hospital   (631) 477-1000
Eastern Long Island Hosp
201 Manor Place   Greenport, NY 11944   SUFFOLK

Elmhurst Hospital Center   (718) 334-4000
Elmhurst Hosp Ctr
79-01 Broadway   Elmhurst, NY 11373   QUEENS

Englewood Hospital & Medical Center   (201) 894-3000
Englewood Hosp & Med Ctr
350 Engle Street   Englewood, NJ 07631   BERGEN

Flushing Hospital Medical Center   (718) 670-5000
Flushing Hosp Med Ctr
45th Ave @ Parsons Blvd   Flushing, NY 11355   QUEENS

Forest Hills Hospital   (718) 830-4000
Forest Hills Hosp
102-01 66th Rd   Forest Hills, NY 11375   QUEENS

Four Winds Hospital   (914) 763-8151
Four Winds Hosp
800 Cross River Road   Katonah, NY 10536   WESTCHESTER

Franklin Hospital   (516) 256-6000
Franklin Hosp
900 Franklin Avenue   Valley Stream, NY 11580   NASSAU

Glen Cove Hospital   (516) 674-7300
Glen Cove Hosp
101 St Andrew's Ln   Glen Cove, NY 11542   NASSAU

Good Samaritan Hospital - Suffern   (845) 368-5000
Good Samaritan Hosp - Suffern
255 Lafayette Ave   Suffern, NY 10901   ROCKLAND

Good Samaritan Hospital Medical Center - West Islip   (631) 376-3000
Good Samaritan Hosp Med Ctr - West Islip
1000 Montauk Highway   West Islip, NY 11795   SUFFOLK

Gracie Square Hospital   (212) 988-4400
Gracie Square Hosp
420 E 76th St   New York, NY 10021   NEW YORK (MANHATTAN)

Greenwich Hospital   (203) 863-3000
Greenwich Hosp
Five Perryridge Road   Greenwich, CT 06830   FAIRFIELD

Hackensack University Medical Center   (201) 996-2000
Hackensack Univ Med Ctr
30 Prospect Avenue   Hackensack, NJ 07601   BERGEN

Hackettstown Regional Medical Center   (908) 852-5100
Hackettstown Reg Med Ctr
651 Willow Grove St   Hackettstwon, NJ 07840   WARREN

Harlem Hospital Center   (212) 939-1000
Harlem Hosp Ctr
506 Lenox Avenue   New York, NY 10037   NEW YORK (MANHATTAN)

Helen Hayes Hospital   (845) 786-4000
Helen Hayes Hosp
Route 9 W   West Haverstraw, NY 10993   ROCKLAND

Hoboken University Medical Center   (201) 418-1000
Hoboken Univ Med Ctr - Hoboken
308 Willow Ave   Hoboken, NJ 07030   HUDSON

Holy Name Medical Center   (201) 833-3000
Holy Name Med Ctr
718 Teaneck Road   Teaneck, NJ 07666-4281   BERGEN

Hospital for Special Surgery   (212) 606-1000
Hosp For Special Surgery
535 East 70th Street   New York, NY 10021   NEW YORK (MANHATTAN)

Hospital of St Raphael   (203) 789-3000
Hosp of St Raphael
1450 Chapel Street   New Haven, CT 06511   NEW HAVEN

Hudson Valley Hospital Center   (914) 737-9000
Hudson Valley Hosp Ctr
1980 Crompond Road   Cortland Manor, NY 10567   WESTCHESTER

Huntington Hospital   (631) 351-2000
Huntington Hosp
270 Park Avenue   Huntington, NY 11743   SUFFOLK

Interfaith Medical Center - St John's Episcopal Hospital   (718) 613-4000
Interfaith Med Ctr - St John's Episcopal Hosp
1545 Atlantic Avenue   Brooklyn, NY 11213   KINGS (BROOKLYN)

Jacobi Medical Center   (718) 918-5000
Jacobi Med Ctr
1400 Pelham Parkway South   Bronx, NY 10461   BRONX

Jamaica Hospital Medical Center   (718) 206-6000
Jamaica Hosp Med Ctr
8900 Van Wyck Expressway   Jamaica, NY 11418   QUEENS

Jersey City Medical Center   (201) 915-2000
Jersey City Med Ctr
355 Grand Street   Jersey City, NJ 07302   HUDSON

Jersey Shore University Medical Center   (732) 775-5500
Jersey Shore Univ Med Ctr
1945 Route 33   Neptune, NJ 07753   MONMOUTH

JFK Medical Center - Edison   (732) 321-7000
JFK Med Ctr - Edison
65 James St   Edison, NJ 08818   MIDDLESEX

John T Mather Memorial Hospital   (631) 473-1320
John T Mather Meml Hosp
75 N Country Rd   Port Jefferson, NY 11777   SUFFOLK

Kessler Institute for Rehabilitation - Chester   (973) 252-6400
Kessler Inst for Rehab - Chester
201 Pleasant Hill Rd   Chester, NJ 07930   MORRIS

Kessler Institute for Rehabilitation - West Orange   (973) 243-6800
Kessler Inst for Rehab - W Orange
1199 Pleasant Valley Way   West Orange, NJ 07052-1499   ESSEX

Kings County Hospital Center   (718) 245-3131
Kings County Hosp Ctr
451 Clarkson Avenue   Brooklyn, NY 11203   KINGS (BROOKLYN)

Kingsbrook Jewish Medical Center   (718) 604-5000
Kingsbrook Jewish Med Ctr
585 Schenectady Avenue   Brooklyn, NY 11203   KINGS (BROOKLYN)

Lawrence Hospital Center   (914) 787-1000
Lawrence Hosp Ctr
55 Palmer Avenue   Bronxville, NY 10708   WESTCHESTER

Lenox Hill Hospital   (212) 434-2000
Lenox Hill Hosp
100 East 77th Street   New York, NY 10021   NEW YORK (MANHATTAN)

Lenox Hill Hospital (Manhattan Eye, Ear & Throat Hosp)   (212) 838-9200
Lenox Hill Hosp (Manh Eye, Ear & Throat Hosp)
210 East 64th Street   New York, NY 10021   NEW YORK (MANHATTAN)

Lincoln Medical & Mental Health Center   (718) 579-5000
Lincoln Med & Mental Hlth Ctr
234 East 149th St.   Bronx, NY 10451   BRONX

Long Beach Medical Center   (516) 897-1000
Long Beach Med Ctr
455 East Bay Drive   Long Beach, NY 11561   NASSAU

Long Island College Hospital   (718) 780-1000
Long Island Coll Hosp
339 Hicks Street   Brooklyn, NY 11201   KINGS (BROOKLYN)

Long Island Jewish Medical Center   (718) 470-7000
Long Island Jewish Med Ctr
270-05 76th Avenue   New Hyde Park, NY 11040   NASSAU

Lutheran Medical Center - Brooklyn   (718) 630-7000
Lutheran Med Ctr - Brooklyn
150 55th Street   Brooklyn, NY 11220   KINGS (BROOKLYN)

Maimonides Medical Center   (718) 283-6000
Maimonides Med Ctr
4802 Tenth Avenue   Brooklyn, NY 11219   KINGS (BROOKLYN)

Meadowlands Hospital Medical Center   (201) 392-3100
Meadowlands Hosp Med Ctr
55 Meadowland Parkway   Secaucus, NJ 07096   HUDSON

Memorial Sloan-Kettering Cancer Center   (212) 639-2000
Meml Sloan-Kettering Cancer Ctr
1275 York Avenue   New York, NY 10021   NEW YORK (MANHATTAN)

Mercy Medical Center - Rockville Centre   (516) 705-2525
Mercy Med Ctr - Rockville Centre
1000 North Village Avenue   Rockville Centre, NY 11570   NASSAU

Metropolitan Hospital Center - NY   (212) 423-6262
Metropolitan Hosp Ctr - NY
1901 First Avenue   New York, NY 10029   NEW YORK (MANHATTAN)

Milford Hospital   (203) 876-4000
Milford Hosp
300 Seaside Ave   Milford, CT 06460   NEW HAVEN

Monmouth Medical Center   (732) 222-5200
Monmouth Med Ctr
300 2nd Ave   Long Branch, NJ 07740-6300   MONMOUTH

Montefiore Medical Center - Henry and Lucy Moses Division   (718) 920-4321
Montefiore Med Ctr - Div. Moses
111 East 210 Street   Bronx, NY 10467   BRONX

Montefiore Medical Center - Jack D. Weiler Division   (718) 904-2000
Montefiore Med Ctr - Div. Weiler
1825 Eastchester Road   Bronx, NY 10461   BRONX

Montefiore Medical Center - North Division   (718) 920-9000
Montefiore Med Ctr - Div. North
600 E 233rd St   Bronx, NY 10466   BRONX

Morristown Memorial Hospital   (973) 971-5000
Morristown Mem Hosp
100 Madison Avenue   Morristown, NJ 07960-6095   MORRIS

Mount Sinai Hospital of Queens   (718) 932-1000
Mount Sinai Hosp of Queens
25-10 30th Avenue   Long Island City, NY 11102   QUEENS

Mount Sinai Medical Center   (212) 241-6500
Mount Sinai Med Ctr
One Gustave L. Levy Pl   New York, NY 10029   NEW YORK (MANHATTAN)

Mount Vernon Hospital   (914) 664-8000
Mount Vernon Hosp
12 N Seventh Ave   Mount Vernon, NY 10550   WESTCHESTER

Mountainside Hospital   (973) 429-6000
Mountainside Hosp
1 Bay Ave   Montclair, NJ 07042   ESSEX

Nassau University Medical Center   (516) 572-0123
Nassau Univ Med Ctr
2201 Hempstead Tpke   East Meadow, NY 11554   NASSAU

New York Community Hospital   (718) 692-5300
New York Comm Hosp
2525 Kings Highway   Brooklyn, NY 11229   KINGS (BROOKLYN)

New York Downtown Hospital   (212) 312-5000
NY Downtown Hosp
170 William Street   New York, NY 10038   NEW YORK (MANHATTAN)

New York Eye & Ear Infirmary   (212) 979-4000
New York Eye & Ear Infirm
310 East 14th Street   New York, NY 10003   NEW YORK (MANHATTAN)

New York Hospital Queens   (718) 670-1231
NY Hosp Queens
56-45 Main Street   Flushing, NY 11355   QUEENS

New York Methodist Hospital   (718) 780-3000
New York Methodist Hosp
506 Sixth Street   Brooklyn, NY 11215   KINGS (BROOKLYN)

New York Presbyterian Hosp/Westchester Div   (914) 682-9100
NY-Presby Hosp/Westchester Div
21 Bloomingdale Rd   White Plains, NY 10605   WESTCHESTER

New York State Psychiatric Institute   (212) 543-5000
NY State Psychiatric Inst
1051 Riverside Dr   New York, NY 10032   NEW YORK (MANHATTAN)

New York Westchester Square Medical Center   (718) 430-7300
NY Westchester Sq Med Ctr
2475 St Raymond Ave   Bronx, NY 10461   BRONX

Newark Beth Israel Medical Center   (973) 926-7000
Newark Beth Israel Med Ctr
201 Lyons Ave   Newark, NJ 07112   ESSEX

NewYork-Presbyterian Hospital   (212) 305-2500
NY-Presby Hosp
161 Fort Washington Ave   New York, NY 10032   NEW YORK (MANHATTAN)

NewYork-Presbyterian Hospital/Columbia   (212) 305-2500
NY-Presby Hosp/Columbia
622 W 168th St   New York, NY 10032   NEW YORK (MANHATTAN)

NewYork-Presbyterian Hospital/The Allen Hospital   (212) 932-4000
NY-Presby Hosp/The Allen Hosp
5141 Broadway   New York, NY 10034   NEW YORK (MANHATTAN)

NewYork-Presbyterian Hospital/Weill Cornell   (212) 746-5454
NY-Presby Hosp/Weill Cornell
525 E 68th St   New York, NY 10021   NEW YORK (MANHATTAN)

NewYork-Presbyterian/Morgan Stanley Children's Hospital   (212) 305-2500
NYPresby-Morgan Stanley Children's Hosp
622 W 168th St   New York, NY 10032   NEW YORK (MANHATTAN)

North Shore University Hospital   (516) 562-0100
N Shore Univ Hosp
300 Community D r   Manhasset, NY 11030   NASSAU

North Shore-LIJ Health System   (516) 465-2600
NS-LIJ Hlth Sys
125 Community Drive   Great Neck, NY 11021   NASSAU

Northern Westchester Hospital   (914) 666-1200
Northern Westchester Hosp
400 East Main Street   Mount Kisco, NY 10549   WESTCHESTER

Norwalk Hospital   (203) 852-2000
Norwalk Hosp
34 Maple Street   Norwalk, CT 06856   FAIRFIELD

Nyack Hospital   (845) 348-2000
Nyack Hosp
160 North Midland Avenue   Nyack, NY 10960   ROCKLAND

NYU Hospital for Joint Diseases   (212) 598-6000
NYU Hosp For Joint Diseases
301 East 17th Street   New York, NY 10003   NEW YORK (MANHATTAN)

NYU Langone Medical Center   (212) 263-7300
NYU Langone Med Ctr
550 First Avenue   New York, NY 10016   NEW YORK (MANHATTAN)

NYU Rusk Institute   (212) 263-2606
NYU Rusk Inst
400 East 34th Street   New York, NY 10016   NEW YORK (MANHATTAN)

Ocean Medical Center   (732) 840-2200
Ocean Med Ctr
425 Jack Martin Blvd   Brick, NJ 08724   OCEAN

Overlook Hospital   (908) 522-2000
Overlook Hosp
99 Beauvoir Ave   Summit, NJ 07901   UNION

Palisades Medical Center   (201) 854-5000
Palisades Med Ctr
7600 River Road   North Bergen, NJ 07047   HUDSON

Peconic Bay Medical Center   (631) 548-6000
Peconic Bay Med Ctr
1300 Roanoke Avenue   Riverhead, NY 11901   SUFFOLK

Peninsula Hospital Center   (718) 734-2000
Peninsula Hosp Ctr
51-15 Beach Channel Drive   Far Rockaway, NY 11691   QUEENS

Phelps Memorial Hospital Center   (914) 366-3000
Phelps Meml Hosp Ctr
701 N Broadway   Sleepy Hollow, NY 10591   WESTCHESTER

Plainview Hospital   (516) 719-3000
Plainview Hosp
888 Old Country Rd   Plainview, NY 11803   NASSAU

Queens Hospital Center - Jamaica   (718) 883-3000
Queens Hosp Ctr - Jamaica
82-68 164th Street   Jamaica, NY 11432   QUEENS

Raritan Bay Medical Center - Old Bridge Division   (732) 360-1000
Raritan Bay Med Ctr - Old Bridge Div
One Hospital Plaza   Old Bridge, NJ 08857   MIDDLESEX

Raritan Bay Medical Center - Perth Amboy Division   (732) 442-3700
Raritan Bay Med Ctr - Perth Amboy
530 New Brunswick Avenue   Perth Amboy, NJ 08861-3654   MIDDLESEX

Richmond University Medical Center   (718) 818-1234
Richmond Univ Med Ctr
355 Bard Ave   Staten Island, NY 10310-1699   RICHMOND (STATEN ISLAND)

Riverview Medical Center
Riverview Med Ctr
1 Riverview Plaza   Red Bank, NJ 07701

(732) 741-2700

MONMOUTH

Robert Wood Johnson University Hospital - Hamilton
Robert Wood Johnson Univ Hosp Hamilton
1 Hamilton Health Pl   Hamilton, NJ 08690

(609) 586-7900

MERCER

Robert Wood Johnson University Hospital - New Brunswick
Robert Wood Johnson Univ Hosp - New Brunswick
1 Robert Wood Johnson Pl   New Brunswick, NJ 08903

(732) 828-3000

MIDDLESEX

Robert Wood Johnson University Hospital at Rahway
Robert Wood Johnson Univ Hosp at Rahway
865 Stone St   Rahway, NJ 07065

(732) 381-4200

UNION

Rockefeller University
Rockefeller Univ
1230 York Avenue   New York, NY 10021

(212) 327-8000

NEW YORK (MANHATTAN)

Rockland Psychiatric Center
Rockland Psych Ctr
140 Old Orangeburg Rd   Orangeburg, NY 10962-1196

(845) 359-1000

ROCKLAND

Saint Barnabas Medical Center
Saint Barnabas Med Ctr
94 Old Short Hills Rd   Livingston, NJ 07039-5672

(973) 322-5000

ESSEX

Saint Joseph's Medical Center - Yonkers
Saint Joseph's Med Ctr - Yonkers
127 South Broadway   Yonkers, NY 10701

(914) 378-7000

WESTCHESTER

Saint Michael's Medical Center
Saint Michael's Med Ctr
111 Central Avenue Blvd   Newark, NJ 07102

(973) 877-5000

ESSEX

Saint Vincent Catholic Medical Centers - St. Vincent's Westchester
St Vincent Cath Med Ctrs - Westchester
275 North Street   Harrison, NY 10528

(914) 967-6500

WESTCHESTER

Silver Hill Hospital
Silver Hill Hosp
208 Valley Rd   New Canaan, CT 06840-3899

(203) 966-3561

FAIRFIELD

Somerset Medical Center
Somerset Med Ctr
110 Rehill Ave   Somerville, NJ 08876

(908) 685-2200

SOMERSET

Sound Shore Medical Center - Westchester   (914) 632-5000
Sound Shore Med Ctr - Westchester
16 Guion Pl   New Rochelle, NY 10801   WESTCHESTER

South Nassau Communities Hospital   (516) 632-3000
South Nassau Comm Hosp
1 Healthy Way   Oceanside, NY 11572   NASSAU

South Oaks Hospital   (631) 264-4000
S Oaks Hosp
400 Sunrise Hwy   Amityville, NY 11701   SUFFOLK

Southampton Hospital   (631) 726-8200
Southampton Hosp
240 Meeting House Ln   Southampton, NY 11968   SUFFOLK

Southside Hospital   (631) 968-3000
Southside Hosp
301 E Main St   Bay Shore, NY 11706   SUFFOLK

St Barnabas Hospital - Bronx   (718) 960-9000
St Barnabas Hosp - Bronx
4422 Third Avenue   Bronx, NY 10457   BRONX

St Catherine's of Siena Medical Center   (631) 862-3000
St Catherine's of Siena Med Ctr
50 Rt 25A   Smithtown, NY 11787   SUFFOLK

St Charles Hospital   (631) 474-6000
St Charles Hosp
200 Belle Terre Rd   Port Jefferson, NY 11777   SUFFOLK

St Clare's Hospital - Denville   (973) 625-6000
St Clare's Hosp - Denville
25 Pocono Road   Denville, NJ 07834   MORRIS

St Clare's Hospital - Dover   (973) 625-6000
St Clare's Hosp - Dover
400 W Blackwell St   Dover, NJ 07801   MORRIS

St Clare's Hospital - Sussex   (973) 702-2600
St Clare's Hosp - Sussex
20 Walnut St   Sussex, NJ 07461   SUSSEX

St Francis Hospital - Jersey City   (201) 418-1000
St Francis Hosp - Jersey City
25 McWilliams Place   Jersey City, NJ 07302   HUDSON

St Francis Hospital - The Heart Center   (516) 562-6000
St Francis Hosp - The Heart Ctr
100 Port Washington Boulevard   Roslyn, NY 11576   NASSAU

St Francis Medical Center - Trenton   (609) 599-5000
St Francis Med Ctr - Trenton
601 Hamilton Avenue   Trenton, NJ 08629   MERCER

St John's Episcopal Hospital - South Shore   (718) 869-7000
St John's Epis Hosp - S Shore
327 Beach 19th Street   Far Rockaway, NY 11691   QUEENS

St John's Riverside Hospital   (914) 964-4444
St John's Riverside Hosp
967 N Broadway   Yonkers, NY 10701   WESTCHESTER

St Joseph's Hospital-Nassau   (516) 579-6000
St Joseph's Hosp-Nassau
4295 Hempstead Turnpike   Bethpage, NY 11714   NASSAU

St Joseph's Regional Medical Center - Paterson   (973) 754-2000
St Joseph's Regl Med Ctr - Paterson
703 Main St   Paterson, NJ 07503   PASSAIC

St Lawrence Rehabilitation Center   (609) 896-9500
St Lawrence Rehab Ctr
2381 Lawrencville Rd   Lawrencville, NJ 08648   MERCER

St Luke's - Roosevelt Hospital Center - Roosevelt Division   (212) 523-4000
St Luke's - Roosevelt Hosp Ctr - Roosevelt Div
1000 Tenth Avenue   New York, NY 10019   NEW YORK (MANHATTAN)

St Luke's - Roosevelt Hospital Center - St Luke's Hospital   (212) 523-4000
St Luke's - Roosevelt Hosp Ctr - St Luke's Hosp
1111 Amsterdam Ave   New York, NY 10025   NEW YORK (MANHATTAN)

St Mary's Hospital - Passaic   (973) 365-4300
St Mary's Hosp - Passaic
350 Boulevard   Passaic, NJ 07055   PASSAIC

St Mary's Hospital - Waterbury   (203) 709-6000
St Mary's Hosp - Waterbury
56 Franklin St   Waterbury, CT 06706-1200   FAIRFIELD

St Peter's University Hospital   (732) 745-8600
St Peter's Univ Hosp
254 Easton Ave   New Brunswick, NJ 08901-1780   MIDDLESEX

St Vincent's Medical Center - Bridgeport   (203) 576-6000
St Vincent's Med Ctr - Bridgeport
2800 Main St   Bridgeport, CT 06606   FAIRFIELD

St. Joseph's Wayne Hospital   (973) 942-6900
St. Joseph's Wayne Hosp
224 Hamburg Turnpike   Wayne, NJ 07470   PASSAIC

St. Mary's Hospital For Children   (718) 281-8800
St Mary's Hosp for Chldn
29-01 216th St   Bayside, NY 11360-2899   QUEENS

Stamford Hospital   (203) 276-1000
Stamford Hosp
30 Shelburne Rd @ W Broad St, Box 9317   Stamford, CT 06904   FAIRFIELD

Staten Island University Hospital - North   (718) 226-9000
Staten Island Univ Hosp - North
475 Seaview Avenue   Staten Island, NY 10305   RICHMOND (STATEN ISLAND)

Staten Island University Hospital - South   (718) 226-2000
Staten Island Univ Hosp - South
375 Seguine Avenue   Staten Island, NY 10309   RICHMOND (STATEN ISLAND)

Steven and Alexandra Cohen Children's Medical Center of New York   (718) 470-3000
Steven & Alexandra Cohen Chldn's Med Ctr of NY
269-01 76th Ave   New Hyde Park, NY 11040   NASSAU

Stony Brook University Medical Center   (631) 444-4000
Stony Brook Univ Med Ctr
101 Nicolls Rd   Stony Brook, NY 11794-8410   SUFFOLK

Stony Lodge Hospital   (914) 941-7400
Stony Lodge Hosp
40 Croton Dam Road   Ossining, NY 10562   WESTCHESTER

Summit Oaks Hospital   (908) 522-7000
Summit Oaks Hosp
19 Prospect St   Summit, NJ 07902   UNION

SUNY Downstate Medical Center (University Hospital of Brooklyn)   (718) 703-5900
SUNY Downstate Med Ctr
445 Lenox Rd   Brooklyn, NY 11203   KINGS (BROOKLYN)

Syosset Hospital   (516) 496-6400
Syosset Hosp
221 Jericho Tpke   Syosset, NY 11791-4536   NASSAU

Trinitas Regional Medical Center   (908) 994-5000
Trinitas Reg Med Ctr
225 Williamson St   Elizabeth, NJ 07207   UNION

University Hospital-UMDNJ-Newark   (973) 972-4300
Univ Hosp-UMDNJ—Newark
150 Bergen St   Newark, NJ 07103-2406   ESSEX

University Medical Center at Princeton   (609) 497-4000
Univ Med Ctr - Princeton
253 Witherspoon St   Princeton, NJ 08540   MERCER

VA Connecticut Healthcare System   (203) 932-5711
VA Conn Hlthcre Sys
950 Campbell Ave   West Haven, CT 06516   NEW HAVEN

VA Hudson Valley Health Care System-FDR/Montrose   (914) 737-4400
VA Hudson Valley-FDR/Montrose
622 Albany Post Rd   Montrose, NY 10548   WESTCHESTER

VA Medical Center - Bronx   (718) 584-9000
VA Med Ctr - Bronx
130 W Kingsbridge Rd   Bronx, NY 10468   BRONX

VA Medical Center - Brooklyn   (718) 836-6600
VA Med Ctr - Bklyn
800 Poly Pl   Bay Ridge, NY 11209   KINGS (BROOKLYN)

VA Medical Center - Manhattan   (212) 686-7500
VA Med Ctr - Manhattan
423 E 23rd St   New York, NY 10010   NEW YORK (MANHATTAN)

Valley Hospital   (201) 447-8000
Valley Hosp
223 N Van Dien Ave   Ridgewood, NJ 07450-2736   BERGEN

Waterbury Hospital   (203) 574-6000
Waterbury Hosp
56 Franklin St0   Waterbury, CT 06706-1200   NEW HAVEN

Westchester Medical Center   (914) 493-7000
Westchester Med Ctr
95 Grasslands Road   Valhalla, NY 10595   WESTCHESTER

White Plains Hospital Center   (914) 681-0600
White Plains Hosp Ctr
Davis Ave at E Post Rd   White Plains, NY 10601   WESTCHESTER

Wills Eye Hospital   (215) 928-3000
Wills Eye Hosp
840 Walnut St   Philadelphia, PA 19107-5598   PHILADELPHIA

Winthrop - University Hospital   (516) 663-0333
Winthrop - Univ Hosp
259 1st StMineola,   NY 11501   NASSAU

Woodhull Medical & Mental Health Center   (718) 963-8000
Woodhull Med & Mental Hlth Ctr
760 Broadway   Brooklyn, NY 11206   KINGS (BROOKLYN)

Wyckoff Heights Medical Center   (718) 963-7272
Wyckoff Heights Med Ctr
374 Stockholm Street   Brooklyn, NY 11237   KINGS (BROOKLYN)

Yale-New Haven Hospital   (203) 688-4242
Yale-New Haven Hosp
20 York St   New Haven, CT 06510   NEW HAVEN

Zucker Hillside Hospital   (718) 470-8000
Zucker Hillside Hosp
75-59 263rd St   Glen Oaks, NY 11004   QUEENS

Appendix D:
Selected Resources

AMERICAN AMBULANCE ASSOCIATION (AAA)
The American Ambulance Association represents emergency and non-emergency medical transportation providers, advocating high quality pre-hospital care and keeping these providers aware of legislation and news that may affect them.

8400 Westpark Drive
Second Floor
McLean, VA 22102

800-523-4447
703-610-9018
fax 703-610-0210
www.the-aaa.org/

AMERICA'S HEALTH INSURANCE PLANS (AHIP)
America's Health Insurance Plans is a national trade association representing nearly 1,300 member companies providing health benefits to more than 200 million Americans.

601 Pennsylvania Ave, NW
South Building Suite 500
Washington, DC 20004

202-778-3200
fax: 202-331-7487
www.ahip.org/

AMERICAN BOARD OF MEDICAL SPECIALTIES (ABMS)
The ABMS is the authoritative body for the recognition of medical specialties, coordinating 24 medical specialty boards (including 25 medical specialties) and providing information on the board certification of doctors.

222 N LaSalle St, Ste 1500
Chicago, IL 60601

847-491-9091 or 866-ASK-ABMS
fax 312-436-2700
www.abms.org

AMERICAN HOSPITAL ASSOCIATION (AHA)
A national health advocacy organization, the AHA represents hospitals and healthcare networks in legislative and regulatory matters. In 1973 the AHA adopted the Patient Bill of Rights to help patients understand their rights and responsibilities.

155 N Wacker Drive
Chicago, IL 60606

800-424-4301 or 312-422-3000
fax 312-422-4796
www.aha.org/

325 7th St. NW
Washington, DC 20004

800-424-4301 or 202-638-1100
fax 202-626-3245

AMERICAN MEDICAL ASSOCIATION (AMA)
The AMA is an association that maintains information on physicians practicing throughout the nation. Healthcare consumers can use their database to check the location, licensing, education and specialty of many doctors in the United States.

515 North State Street
Chicago, IL 60654

800-621-8335
www.ama-assn.org/

CENTER FOR MEDICAL CONSUMERS
Provides volume and outcome data on certain medical procedures performed in New York state.

239 Thompson St.　　　　　　　　　　212-674-7105
New York, NY 10012　　　　　　　　　　fax 212-674-7100

CenterForMedicalConsumers@gmail.com　　www.medicalconsumers.org

CENTERS FOR DISEASE CONTROL AND PREVENTION (CDC)
Part of the Department of Health and Human Services, the CDC's mission is to prevent and manage diseases and illnesses. Its website contains information on a range of illnesses and the research being pursued to manage them. It also provides free faxed reports on disease risk and prevention in various parts of the world.

Public Inquiries/MASO　　　　　　　　　1-800-CDC-INFO
Mailstop E11
1600 Clifton Road
Atlanta, GA 30333

toll free number for international travelers 877 FYI-TRIP or 404-639-3534
fax information service for international travelers 888-232-3299
www.cdc.gov/netinfo.htm

THE CENTERWATCH CLINICAL TRIALS LISTING SERVICE
Profiles centers conducting clinical research by therapeutic area and geographic region, including more than 41,000 international industry and government-sponsored clinical trials and new FDA approved drug therapies, as well as 5,200 clinical trials that are actively recruiting patients.

100 N. Washington Street, Ste 301　　　　617-948-5100
Boston, MA 02114　　　　　　　　　　fax 617-948-5101
　　　　　　　　　　　　　　　　　www.centerwatch.com

HEALTH CARE CHOICES
Provides information on volume and outcomes of certain medical procedures performed in hospitals in various states throughout the country.

P.O. Box 21039　　　　　　　　　　　212-724-9395
Columbus Circle Station　　　　　　　　www.healthcarechoices.org
New York, NY 10023

INTERNATIONAL ASSOCIATION FOR MEDICAL ASSISTANCE TO TRAVELLERS (IAMAT)
IAMAT is a non-profit organization that disseminates information on health and sanitary conditions worldwide. Membership is free but donations are appreciated. Members will receive a membership card making them eligible to access English speaking physicians all over the world. The organization also provides information on immunization requirements, malaria, and other tropical diseases, and sanitary and climactic conditions around the world. For information, send request in writing.

1623 Military Road #279　　　　　　　716-754-4883
Niagra Falls, NY 14304-1745　　　　　　www.iamat.org

JOINT COMMISSION ON ACCREDITATION OF HEALTHCARE ORGANIZATIONS
The Joint Commission (JCAHO) is an independent, not-for-profit organization, which evaluates the quality and safety of care for nearly 17,000 health care organizations. To maintain and earn accreditation, organizations must have an extensive on-site review by a team of JCAHO health care professionals, at least once every three years. JCAHO is governed by a board that includes physicians, nurses, and consumers. JCAHO sets the standards by which health care quality is measured in America and around the world.

One Renaissance Boulevard　　　　　　630-792-5000
Oakbrook Terrace, IL 60181　　　　　　fax 630-792-5005
　　　　　　　　　　　　　　　　　www.jcaho.org

MEDIC ALERT FOUNDATION

The Medic Alert Foundation (a non-profit organization) provides an "ID tag" engraved with personal medical facts, as well as a 24-hour emergency response center which can release additional personal medical details. Membership is $30/year (plus $9.95 initial setup fee) and members need to purchase the "ID tag" which sells for as low as $35.

2323 Colorado Avenue	888-633-4298
Turlock, CA 95382	Fax 209-669-2450
	www.medicalert.org

MEDLINE

One Medline Place	1-800-MEDLINE (800-633-5463)
Mundelein, IL 60060	fax 1-800-351-1512
	www.medline.com

A medical database including millions of medical references and abstracts from thousands of scientific and medical journals.

THE NATIONAL CANCER INSTITUTE (NCI)

Part of the NIH, the NCI sponsors cancer clinical trials at more than 100 sites in the United States. Trials are carried out in major medical research centers, such as teaching hospitals, as well as in community hospitals, specialized medical clinics and even in doctors' offices.

Clinical Studies Support Center (CSSC)	800-4-CANCER (800-422-6237)
6116 Executive Boulevard	www.nci.nih.gov
Bethesda, MD 20892-8322	www.cancer.gov
	cancergovstaff@mail.nih.gov

NATIONAL CENTER FOR COMPLEMENTARY AND ALTERNATIVE MEDICINE CLEARINGHOUSE (NCCAMC)

The NCCAMC facilitates the evaluation of alternative medical treatment modalities to help determine their effectiveness and bring alternative medicine into mainstream medicine. This agency does not provide referrals.

9000 Rockville Pike	888-644-6226
Bethesda, MD 20892	fax 866-464-3616
	www.nccam.nih.gov
	info@nccam.nih.gov

NATIONAL CONSUMERS LEAGUE (NCL)

NCL is a private, nonprofit consumer advocacy organization. NCL strives to investigate, educate, and advocate on a variety of issues including healthcare. Membership is $35 annually, but individuals can also write to the organization for a list of publications that non-members can purchase.

1701 K Street, NW, Suite 1200	202-835-3323
Washington, DC 20006	fax 202-835-0747
	www.nclnet.org
	info@nclnet.org

THE NATIONAL INSTITUTES OF HEALTH (NIH)

An organization operated by the U.S. government, the NIH operates its own hospital at which the care provided is usually related to clinical studies its researchers are undertaking. Information about the Warren G. Magnuson Clinical Center is also available.

Patient Recruitment Referral Center	800-411-1222 or 301-496-4000
9000 Rockville Pike	www.nih.gov
Bethesda, MD 20892	www.clinicaltrials.gov
	nihinfo@od.nih.gov

NATIONAL INSURANCE INFORMATION INSTITUTE

The National Insurance Information Institute Helpline advises consumers on how to choose an insurance company or broker. It also offers an analysis of life insurance and assists in insurance complaints.

110 William Street
New York, NY 10038

800-942-4242 or 212-346-5500
www.iii.org

THE PATIENT ADVOCATE FOUNDATION

A national non-profit organization that provides consultation, referrals and case management to patients to ensure that they are not denied access to healthcare, insurance coverage, employment and public assistance programs during an illness. In particular, the organization maintains comprehensive information on cancer treatment options that are available to consumers through a separate website: www.oncology.com.

421 Butler Farm Rd
Hampton, VA 23666

800-532-5274
fax 757-873-8999
www.patientadvocate.org/
help@patientadvocate.org

PEOPLE'S MEDICAL SOCIETY

The People's Medical Society, a nonprofit organization, is focused on educating the healthcare consumer about healthcare issues and medical rights. Their website provides information on useful books and publications as well as the latest healthcare developments.

P.O. Box 868
Allentown, PA 18105

610-770-1670
www.peoplesmed.org
cbi@peoplesmed.org

PERSONS UNITED LIMITING SUBSTANDARDS AND ERRORS IN HEALTHCARE (P.U.L.S.E.)

A support group for the survivors of medical malpractice and substandard healthcare, this nonprofit group also advocates patient education and patient-doctor communication.

PO Box 353
3300 Park Avenue
Wantagh, NY 11793-0353

800-96-pulse (800-967-8573) or
516-579-4711
fax: 516-520-8105
www.PULSEamerica.org
www.PULSEofNY.com
pulse516@aol.com

Colorado Office

719-250-1286
PULSECOLO@YAHOO.COM

PUBLIC CITIZEN'S HEALTH AND RESEARCH GROUP

A non-profit organization, the Public Citizen's Group acts as a watchdog agency by advocating accountability and the open use of doctors' disciplinary backgrounds.

1600 20th Street NW
Washington, DC 20009

202-588-1000
www.citizen.org/hrg/

VERITAS MEDICINE

An organization that allows individuals to perform confidential, personalized searches of their clinical trials database and to access information on new treatment and drug options. The text is submitted by Harvard-affiliated doctors.

11 Cambridge Center
Cambridge, MA 02142

617-234-1500 or
877-5-TRIALS (877-587-4257)
fax 617-234-1555
www.veritasmedicine.com
info@veritasmedicine.com

Appendix E:
State Agencies

While there is a wealth of information available through these state agencies, much of it is not user-friendly. Complicated contractual agreements and other legal documents contain information that might prove to be valuable, providing a consumer can locate it and then review it with some understanding. Often a department will suggest that a consumer visit the office for guidance in reviewing the documents. However, some of these agencies provide useful information on doctors, hospitals, and HMOs. They may also offer statistical reports and consumer-oriented studies.

CONNECTICUT

DOCTORS

Department of Public Health State of Connecticut
Practitioner Licensing and Investigations Section
410 Capitol Avenue, MS#12MQA
P.O. Box 340308
Hartford, CT 06134-0308
(860) 509-7603
www.dph.state.ct.us
Attn: Physician renewal of verification

Department of Public Health State of Connecticut
Legal Office
410 Capitol Avenue, MS#12LEG
P.O. Box 340308
Hartford, CT 06134-0308
(860) 509-7600

HOSPITALS

Department of Public Health State of Connecticut
Facilities Licensing and Investigations Section
410 Capitol Avenue, MS#12HSR
P.O. Box 340308
Hartford, CT 06134-0308
(860) 509-7400

HMOs

Department of Insurance (Location address)
153 Market Street, 7th Floor
Hartford, CT 06103-0816
(860) 297-3800

Department of Insurance (Mailing address)
P.O. Box 816
Hartford, CT 06142-0816
(860) 297-3800

www.ct.gov/cid/site/default.asp

Office of Health Care Access
410 Capitol Avenue, MS#13HCA
P.O. Box 340308
Hartford, CT 06134-0308
800-797-9688

TDD 860-418-7058

www.ct.gov/ohca/site/default.asp

NEW JERSEY

DOCTORS

New Jersey State Board of Medical Examiners (Location address)
140 East Front Street, 2nd Floor
Trenton, NJ 08608
(609) 826-7100

New Jersey State Board of Medical Examiners (Mailing address)
P.O. Box 183
Trenton, NJ 08625-0183

http://www.state.nj.us/lps/ca/bme/index.html
bme@dca.lps.state.nj.us

HOSPITALS

Department of Health
Division of Health Facilities Evaluation and Licensing
P.O. Box 367
120 S Stockton Street
Trenton, NJ 08625-0367
(609) 292-7837

http://www.nj.gov/health/

HMOs

Department of Health
Division of Health Facilities Evaluation and Licensing
P.O. Box 367
120 S Stockton Street
Trenton, NJ 08625-0367
(609) 292-7837

Department of Health
Office of Managed Care
20 West State St, 11th Fl
P.O. Box 325
Trenton, NJ 08625
(609) 292-7272

http://www.state.nj.us/dobi/managed.htm

Department of Banking & Insurance (Location address)
Division of Insurance, Life and Health Division
Managed Healthcare Bureau
20 West State St
P.O. Box 325
Trenton, NJ 08625
(609) 292-7272

http://www.state.nj.us/dobi/

Department of Banking & Insurance (Mailing address)
Division of Insurance, Life and Health Division
Managed Healthcare Bureau
20 West State St
P.O. Box 325
Trenton, NJ 08625
(609) 292-7272

Office of Managed Care Hotline: 1-888-393-1062
Office of managed Care Fax: (609) 633-0807
Consumer Protection Services Main Line: (609) 292-7272

NEW YORK

DOCTORS
New York State Department of Health
Office of Professional Medical Conduct
433 River Street, Suite 303
Troy, NY 12180
(518) 402-0836
www.health.state.ny.us
opmc@health.state.ny.us

New York State Education Department
Division of Professional Licensing Services
State Education Building - 2nd floor
89 Washington Avenue
Albany, NY 12234
(518) 474-3817
http://www.op.nysed.gov/home.html

op4info@mail.nysed.gov

Hospitals

Office of Health Systems Management
Corning Tower, Fl 14
Empire State Plaza
Albany, NY 12237
(518) 474-7028

New York State Department of Health
Bureau of Biometrics
Corning Tower, Room 2348
Empire State Plaza
Albany, NY 12237
(518) 474-3189

HMOs

New York State Insurance Department
Health Bureau
1 Commerce Plaza, Suite 1909
Albany, NY 12257
(518) 474-6272

New York State Insurance Department
Life Policy Bureau
1 Commerce Plaza, Suite 1910
Albany, NY 12257
(518) 474-4552

New York State Department of Health
Office of Managed Care
Corning Tower, Room 1911
Albany, NY 12237
(518) 473-4178

New York State Department of Health
Records Access Office
Corning Tower, Room 2364
Empire State Plaza
Albany, NY 12237
(518) 486-9144

SECTION SIX

Indices

The Best in American Medicine
www.CastleConnolly.com

Subject Index

A

Academic Medical Center 14

Advertising 8

Alternative medicine 43-45, 51

Alternative therapy 40, 45

American Board of Medical Specialties (ABMS) 4, 14, 16, 18, 19, 41, 53

American Board of Radiology 17, 19

American Medical Association (AMA) 32, 33, 51, 53

American Medical News 25

B

Bachelor of Medicine 8

Baseline tests 32, 34

Board certification 12, 17-19, 23

Board eligibility 19

C

Capitation 60, 63, 64

Chiropractors 8

Chronic condition 51

Clinical trials 39, 40, 45-46

Community hospitals 12, 21-22

Compendium of Certified Medical Specialists 16

Continuing Medical Education (CME) 18

Credentialing 14, 20

H

Harvard/Beth Israel Center 43

Health Maintenance Organization (HMO) 58-67

Hippocratic Oath xiii

Hospital appointment 15, 20-21

Hospital referral services 7

I

Indemnity insurance 14, 32

IPA 60, 62-63

J

J.D. Power and Associates 66

L

LEXIS/NEXIS 54, 58

Licensed nurse practitioners 24

Licensure 14, 17, 24

Louis Harris Associates 66

Lupus 4, 6

Lyme disease 4, 6, 23

M

Malpractice insurance 21

Managed care 4, 6, 20, 32, 33, 42, 51, 60-66

Medical history 34-35

Medical records 30, 35, 48, 52-53

Medical school faculty appointment 22

Medical schools 16-17, 21-22, 26

Medical societies 2, 7

MedStat Group 66

Midlevel providers 24

Multi-specialty group 24

N

National Practitioner Data Bank 50, 54

New England Journal of Medicine 44

O

Office and practice arrangements 15, 24

P

Physician's assistants 24

Placebo 40, 45

Podiatrists 8

PPO 60-63, 66

Preventive medicine 4, 6, 9

Primary care physicians 3-5

PSO 60

Psychologists 8

Public Citizen Health Research Group 50, 54

Q

Questionable doctors 53

R

S

T

U

W

The Best in American Medicine
www.CastleConnolly.com

Special Expertise Index

This index lists the areas that the physicians listed in the Guide have identified as their "special expertise." These are not medical specialties. They are specific elements of disease, procedures, techniques and treatments for which these physicians are best known and are referred patients.

Spec	Name	St	Pg

A

Abdominal Imaging

Spec	Name	St	Pg
DR	Baer, J	NY	153
DR	Brancaccio, W	NY	568
DR	Lubat, E	NJ	666
DR	McClennan, B	CT	904
DR	Megibow, A	NY	156
DR	Newhouse, J	NY	156
DR	Swirsky, M	NY	373
DR	Weinreb, J	CT	905
DR	Wolf, E	NY	373

Abdominal Wall Reconstruction

Spec	Name	St	Pg
PlS	Stahl, R	CT	917
PS	Weinberg, G	NY	392
S	Mandel, M	NJ	856

Abdominoplasty

Spec	Name	St	Pg
PlS	Almeyda, E	NY	301
PlS	Feinberg, J	NY	536
PlS	Friedman, D	NY	303
PlS	Gallagher, P	NY	536
PlS	Gardner, J	NJ	853
PlS	Goldstein, R	NY	395
PlS	Hawrylo, R	NJ	813
PlS	Lesesne, C	NY	305
PlS	Matarasso, A	NY	305
PlS	Newman, F	CT	890
PlS	Perrotti, J	NY	305
PlS	Perry, A	NJ	835
PlS	Pitman, G	NY	306
PlS	Restifo, R	CT	917
PlS	Wells, S	NY	308

Abuse/Neglect

Spec	Name	St	Pg
AM	Diaz, A	NY	124
AM	Johnson, R	NJ	703
Ger	Lachs, M	NY	175

Acanthamoeba Keratitis

Spec	Name	St	Pg
Oph	Auran, J	NY	239

Achalasia

Spec	Name	St	Pg
Ge	Lambroza, A	NY	169

Acne

Spec	Name	St	Pg
D	Almeida, L	NJ	803
D	Aprile, G	NY	497
D	Aranoff, S	NY	144
D	Berson, D	NY	145
D	Blank, E	NJ	733
D	Bruckstein, R	NY	497
D	Davis, J	NY	146
D	Deitz, M	NY	412
D	Demar, L	NY	146
D	Dolitsky, C	NY	497
D	Eisenberg, R	NJ	844
D	Falcon, R	NY	498
D	Feldman, P	NY	412
D	Fox, A	NJ	830
D	Fried, S	NJ	664
D	Giardina-Beckett, M	NJ	664
D	Goldberg, N	NY	601
D	Hefter, H	NY	498
D	Hisler, B	NY	498
D	Huh, J	NY	567
D	Lerman, J	NY	602
D	Lukash, B	NY	602
D	Maier, H	NJ	819
D	Notaro, A	NY	568
D	Rosen, D	NY	371
D	Rosenthal, E	NY	603
D	Rozanski, R	NJ	706
D	Scherl, S	NJ	665
D	Seidenberg, R	NY	151
D	Stillman, M	NY	603
D	Sweeney, E	NJ	665
D	Tanzer, F	NJ	820
D	Tom, J	NY	568
D	Treiber, R	NY	603
D	Waldorf, D	NY	553
D	Walther, R	NY	152
D	Wattenberg, D	NY	153
D	Wexler, P	NY	153
Ped	Panzner, E	NJ	852

Acne & Rosacea

Spec	Name	St	Pg
D	Baldwin, H	NY	412
D	Danziger, S	NY	412
D	Felderman, L	NY	146
D	Gold, J	NJ	819
D	Liftin, A	NJ	706

Acoustic Neuroma

Spec	Name	St	Pg
NS	Davis, R	NY	575
NS	Golfinos, J	NY	217
NS	Gutin, P	NY	218
NS	Hodosh, R	NJ	848
NS	Jafar, J	NY	218
NS	Sisti, M	NY	220
NS	Stieg, P	NY	220
Oto	Chandrasekhar, S	NY	268
Oto	Feghali, J	NY	388
Oto	Kohan, D	NY	270
Oto	Kveton, J	CT	914
Oto	Kwartler, J	NJ	851
Oto	Linstrom, C	NY	272
Oto	Roland, J	NY	273
Oto	Selesnick, S	NY	274
Oto	Storper, I	NY	275

Acupuncture

Spec	Name	St	Pg
AdP	Smith, M	NY	367
FMed	Kligler, B	NY	162
FMed	Sekiguchi, R	CT	871
Hem	Boyd, D	CT	873
IM	Ehrlich, M	NY	191
IM	Gazzara, P	NY	478
IM	Lu, B	NY	422
IM	Strauss, M	NY	197
N	Lazar, M	NJ	768
PM	Agin, C	NY	580
PM	Moqtaderi, F	NY	277
PM	Ngeow, J	NY	277
PMR	Agri, R	NJ	750
PMR	Atakent, P	NY	442
PMR	Dillard, J	NY	298
PMR	Gasalberti, R	NY	468
PMR	Snowball, H	CT	890
Rhu	Meed, S	NY	336
SM	Hamner, D	NY	339

Acute Coronary Syndromes

Spec	Name	St	Pg
Cv	Infantino, M	NY	132
Cv	Menegus, M	NY	369

ADD/ADHD

Spec	Name	St	Pg
ChAP	Abright, A	NY	138
ChAP	Bartlett, J	NJ	705

Special Expertise Index

Special Expertise Index

Special Expertise Index

Special Expertise Index

Spec	Name	St	Pg	Spec	Name	St	Pg	Spec	Name	St	Pg
A&I	Satnick, S	NY	563	Ped	Murphy, R	NJ	793	Pul	Castellano, M	NY	484
A&I	Schneider, A	NY	407	Ped	Panzner, E	NJ	852	Pul	Cerrone, F	NJ	855
A&I	Schulhafer, E	NJ	829	Ped	Poon, E	NY	296	Pul	Chadha, J	NY	469
A&I	Sicklick, M	NY	490	Ped	Puder, D	NY	558	Pul	Cohen, M	NY	540
A&I	Slankard, M	NY	126	Ped	Rosenfeld, S	NY	297	Pul	Cooke, J	NY	325
A&I	Southern, D	NJ	829	Ped	Saraiya, N	NJ	853	Pul	De Matteo, R	NY	642
A&I	Tolston, E	NY	126	Ped	Schechter, M	NY	394	Pul	Delorenzo, L	NY	642
A&I	Tuerk-Mendelsohn, L	NY	594	Ped	Zoltan, I	NY	394	Pul	DiPasquale, L	NJ	691
A&I	Weinstock, G	NY	490	PPul	Aguila, H	NJ	721	Pul	Donath, J	NY	470
A&I	Weiss, S	NJ	703	PPul	Amin, N	NY	634	Pul	Eden, E	NY	325
A&I	Winant, J	NJ	741	PPul	Atlas, A	NJ	811	Pul	Elamir, M	NJ	737
A&I	Young, S	NY	126	PPul	Bisberg, D	NJ	721	Pul	Fein, A	NY	540
FMed	Ibelli, V	NY	554	PPul	Boyer, J	NY	635	Pul	Fiel, S	NJ	814
FMed	Karatoprak, O	NJ	667	PPul	Bye, M	NY	291	Pul	Fishman, D	NY	325
FMed	Klein, S	NY	502	PPul	Dimaio, M	NY	291	Pul	Gagliardi, A	NY	325
FMed	Levites, K	NY	570	PPul	Dozor, A	NY	635	Pul	Garay, S	NY	325
IM	Altbaum, R	CT	874	PPul	Dworkin, G	CT	888	Pul	Goldberg, J	NJ	778
IM	Carosella, C	NY	613	PPul	Giusti, R	NY	440	Pul	Goldblatt, K	NJ	751
IM	Cusumano, S	NY	509	PPul	Hen, J	CT	888	Pul	Gordon, R	NY	540
IM	Fortunato, F	NJ	711	PPul	Kanengiser, S	NJ	686	Pul	Greenberg, M	NJ	724
IM	Horovitz, L	NY	193	PPul	Kattan, M	NY	291	Pul	Grizzanti, J	NJ	825
IM	Horovitz, L	NY	193	PPul	Kottler, W	NJ	721	Pul	Groopman, J	NY	445
IM	Jawetz, H	NJ	821	PPul	Lamm, C	NY	291	Pul	Gulrajani, R	NY	445
IM	Kapoor, S	NY	614	PPul	Lee, H	NY	441	Pul	Hammer, A	NY	446
IM	Melman, M	NY	615	PPul	Lowenthal, D	NY	635	Pul	Jacobowitz, M	NY	643
IM	Minkowitz, S	NY	195	PPul	Marcus, M	NY	441	Pul	Karetzky, M	NY	397
IM	Osnoss, K	CT	875	PPul	Nachajon, R	NJ	824	Pul	Klapholz, A	NY	325
IM	Simon, T	NY	423	PPul	Narula, P	NY	441	Pul	Klapper, P	NY	397
IM	Spero, M	NY	197	PPul	Quittell, L	NY	291	Pul	Klares, S	NY	643
PA&I	Ehrlich, P	NY	280	PPul	Sadeghi, H	CT	888	Pul	Kolodny, E	NY	326
PA&I	Fagin, J	NY	528	PPul	Schaeffer, J	NY	532	Pul	Kozel, J	NY	737
PA&I	Fost, A	NJ	719	PPul	Ting, A	NY	291	Pul	Krasnogor, L	CT	892
PA&I	Rappaport, I	NY	281	Pul	Abott, M	NY	444	Pul	Krinsley, J	CT	892
PA&I	Torre, A	NJ	719	Pul	Acquista, A	NY	323	Pul	Kurtz, C	CT	892
PCCM	Bojko, T	NJ	773	Pul	Adams, F	NY	323	Pul	Labissiere, J	NJ	724
PCCM	Greenwald, B	NY	283	Pul	Adler, J	NY	324	Pul	Lee, M	NY	326
Ped	Andrade, J	NY	392	Pul	Aldrich, T	NY	396	Pul	Leeman, B	NY	540
Ped	Bailey, M	NY	636	Pul	Amoruso, R	NJ	824	Pul	Lehrman, S	NY	643
Ped	Baiser, D	NJ	750	Pul	Appel, D	NY	397	Pul	Levine, S	NJ	691
Ped	Buchalter, M	NJ	687	Pul	Baskin, M	NY	324	Pul	Libby, D	NY	326
Ped	Burstin, H	NY	294	Pul	Bergman, M	NY	445	Pul	Lowy, J	NY	326
Ped	Chernobilsky, L	NY	582	Pul	Bernardini, D	NY	585	Pul	Mandel, M	NY	643
Ped	Chianese, M	NY	533	Pul	Bernstein, C	NY	445	Pul	Maniatis, T	NY	484
Ped	Corbo, E	NJ	852	Pul	Bevelaqua, F	NY	324	Pul	Marino, A	CT	892
Ped	Glatt, H	NY	534	Pul	Binder, R	NY	642	Pul	Marino, W	NY	397
Ped	Goldstein, S	NY	468	Pul	Birns, R	NJ	691	Pul	Martins, P	NY	484
Ped	Green, A	NY	534	Pul	Blair, L	NY	324	Pul	McCalley, S	CT	893
Ped	Gruenwald, L	NJ	722	Pul	Blum, A	NY	540	Pul	Meixler, S	NY	643
Ped	Handler, R	NJ	812	Pul	Bondi, E	NY	445	Pul	Melillo, N	NJ	778
Ped	Hirschman, A	NY	393	Pul	Brauntuch, G	NJ	691	Pul	Menon, L	NY	397
Ped	Juan, P	CT	888	Pul	Breidbart, D	NY	540	Pul	Mensch, A	NY	540
Ped	Kaplan, M	NY	583	Pul	Brill, J	NY	642	Pul	Mermelstein, S	NY	541
Ped	Kotin, N	NY	295	Pul	Bromberg, A	NJ	691	Pul	Miarrostami, R	NY	446
Ped	Kushner, S	NJ	688	Pul	Burschtin, O	NY	324	Pul	Nash, T	NY	326
Ped	Levitzky, S	NY	295	Pul	Casino, J	NY	642	Pul	Nath, S	NY	470

Special Expertise Index

Spec	Name	St	Pg
Pul	Newmark, I	NY	541
Pul	O'Donnell, T	NJ	814
Pul	Osei, C	NY	559
Pul	Pinsker, K	NY	397
Pul	Polkow, M	NJ	692
Pul	Posner, D	NY	327
Pul	Prager, K	NY	327
Pul	Prezant, D	NY	397
Pul	Raskin, J	NY	327
Pul	Rose, H	NJ	692
Pul	Rosen, M	NY	541
Pul	Sachs, P	CT	893
Pul	Safirstein, B	NJ	725
Pul	Saleh, A	NY	446
Pul	Sasso, L	NY	485
Pul	Schiffman, P	NJ	778
Pul	Schreiber, M	NY	643
Pul	Schulster, R	NY	541
Pul	Sender, J	NY	398
Pul	Shah, S	NJ	725
Pul	Silverman, J	NY	470
Pul	Simon, C	NJ	692
Pul	Sklarek, H	NY	585
Pul	Stein, S	NY	327
Pul	Steinberg, H	NY	541
Pul	Sukumaran, M	NY	328
Pul	Sussman, R	NJ	855
Pul	Tessler, S	NY	446
Pul	Thomashow, B	NY	328
Pul	Volcovici, G	NY	328
Pul	Weinberg, H	NY	644
Pul	Wyner, P	NY	541
Pul	Yip, C	NY	328
Pul	Zupnick, H	NY	542
Rhu	Lans, D	NY	645

Asthma & Allergy

Spec	Name	St	Pg
A&I	Adelsberg, B	CT	901
A&I	Buchbinder, E	NY	124
A&I	Caucino, J	NJ	829
A&I	Corriel, R	NY	489
A&I	Fonacier, L	NY	490
A&I	Grubman, S	NY	125
A&I	Leibner, D	NJ	757
A&I	Silverman, B	NY	407
FMed	Leeds, G	NY	162
Pul	Amin, H	NY	445

Asthma & Chronic Lung Disease

Spec	Name	St	Pg
PPul	Loughlin, G	NY	291

Asthma & Emphysema

Spec	Name	St	Pg
Pul	Benton, M	NJ	813

Spec	Name	St	Pg
Pul	Demetis, S	NY	445

Asthma & Sinusitis

Spec	Name	St	Pg
A&I	Bassett, C	NY	124
A&I	Harish, Z	NJ	660
A&I	Lindner, P	CT	865
A&I	Sher, E	NJ	785
PA&I	Hicks, P	NJ	685

Asthma in Pregnancy

Spec	Name	St	Pg
A&I	Ricketti, A	NJ	741
MF	Chazotte, C	NY	381
PA&I	Hicks, P	NJ	685

Asthma-Adult & Pediatric

Spec	Name	St	Pg
A&I	Novick, B	NY	490
PA&I	Colenda, M	NJ	685

Atopic Dermatitis

Spec	Name	St	Pg
A&I	Gross, G	NJ	785
A&I	Rosenstreich, D	NY	367
A&I	Silverman, B	NY	407
D	Aprile, G	NY	497
D	Bagel, J	NJ	741
D	Rosenthal, E	NY	603
D	Schwartz, R	NJ	706
PA&I	Sampson, H	NY	281
Ped	Kushner, S	NJ	688

Atrial Fibrillation

Spec	Name	St	Pg
CE	Chinitz, L	NY	126
CE	Gomes, J	NY	127
CE	Jadonath, R	NY	491
CE	Krumerman, A	NY	368
CE	Levine, J	NY	491
CE	McPherson, C	CT	866
CE	Mehta, D	NY	127
CE	Rashba, E	NY	563
CE	Steinberg, J	NY	127
CE	Suri, R	NY	128
CE	Winters, S	NJ	801
Cv	Friedman, H	NY	130
Cv	Goldschmidt, H	NJ	661
Cv	Gupta, P	NY	409
Cv	Halperin, J	NY	131
Cv	Kerstein, J	NY	409
Cv	Koss, J	NY	493
Cv	Matilsky, M	NY	565
Cv	Sahar, D	NY	369
Cv	Tenenbaum, J	NY	137
TS	Elmann, E	NJ	696
TS	Fernandez, H	NY	546
TS	Graver, L	NY	471

Spec	Name	St	Pg
TS	Kaushik, R	NJ	826
TS	Michler, R	NY	400
TS	Parr, G	NJ	815

Atrial Septal Defect

Spec	Name	St	Pg
PCd	Levchuck, S	NY	528
PCd	Love, B	NY	282
PCd	Sommer, R	NY	282

Attachment Disorders

Spec	Name	St	Pg
ChAP	Madigan, J	CT	902

Autism

Spec	Name	St	Pg
ChAP	Cohen, L	NY	599
ChAP	Leckman, J	CT	902
ChAP	Leventhal, B	NY	139
ChAP	Pomeroy, J	NY	566
ChAP	Shatkin, J	NY	140
ChAP	Volkmar, F	CT	902
ChiN	De Carlo, R	NY	476
ChiN	Jacobson, R	NY	600
ChiN	Kaufman, D	NY	141
ChiN	Kosofsky, B	NY	141
ChiN	Kutscher, M	NY	600
ChiN	Nass, R	NY	141
ChiN	Traeger, E	NJ	843
FMed	Morrow, R	NY	375
Ped	Adesman, A	NY	533
Ped	Kanter, A	NJ	688
Ped	McCarton, C	NY	295
Ped	Mehta, U	NJ	852
Psyc	Cohen, A	NY	311
Psyc	Di Buono, M	NY	484
Psyc	Hollander, E	NY	314
Psyc	Moraille, P	NJ	737

Autoimmune Disease

Spec	Name	St	Pg
D	Granstein, R	NY	147
N	Miller, A	NY	226
PHO	Bussel, J	NY	286
Rhu	Gorevic, P	NY	335
Rhu	Guma, M	NJ	693
Rhu	Solomon, G	NY	338
Rhu	Sonpal, G	NY	471

Autoimmune Disease in Pregnancy

Spec	Name	St	Pg
ObG	Mack, L	NY	519

Autoimmune Occular Disorders

Spec	Name	St	Pg
A&I	Bielory, L	NJ	842

Special Expertise Index

Special Expertise Index

Special Expertise Index

Spec	Name	St	Pg
S	Blackwood, M	NJ	726
S	Estabrook, A	NY	342
S	Osborne, M	NY	345
S	Schnabel, F	NY	346

Breast Cosmetic & Reconstructive Surgery

Spec	Name	St	Pg
PlS	Alizadeh, K	NY	535
PlS	Ascherman, J	NY	301
PlS	Attkiss, K	CT	890
PlS	Chun, J	NY	302
PlS	Gardner, J	NJ	853
PlS	Gewirtz, H	CT	890
PlS	Hetzler, P	NJ	794
PlS	Karp, N	NY	305
PlS	Lukash, F	NY	538
PlS	Schulman, N	NY	306
PlS	Silberman, M	NY	538
PlS	Vickery, C	NY	308
PlS	Weinstein, L	NJ	813
PlS	Weiss, P	NY	308
PlS	Wey, P	NJ	777
PlS	Zaccaria, A	NJ	794

Breast Disease

Spec	Name	St	Pg
ObG	Segarra, P	NY	237
S	Auguste, L	NY	545
S	Axelrod, D	NY	340
S	Bernik, S	NY	340
S	Bernstein, M	NY	449
S	Cioroiu, M	NY	341
S	Cohen, B	NY	588
S	Digioia, J	NJ	856
S	Estabrook, A	NY	342
S	Fleischer, L	NY	560
S	Fou, A	NY	646
S	Huston, J	NJ	727
S	Osborne, M	NY	345
S	Pass, H	NY	647
S	Schreiber, M	NJ	796
S	Simmons, R	NY	347
S	Swistel, A	NY	347
S	Ward, B	CT	896
S	Wright, A	NY	451
S	Zingale, R	NY	588

Breast Feeding Problems

Spec	Name	St	Pg
NP	Hand, I	NY	465
NP	Roth, P	NY	480
NP	Schanler, R	NY	514
Ped	Musiker, S	NY	583
PGe	Jelin, A	NY	438

Breast Imaging

Spec	Name	St	Pg
DR	Berson, B	NY	153
DR	Calem-Grunat, J	NJ	665
DR	Cohen, S	CT	869
DR	Dershaw, D	NY	154
DR	Goldfischer, M	NJ	666
DR	Greenstein, C	CT	869
DR	Greer, J	NJ	760
DR	Gross, J	NJ	666
DR	Grosso, S	NJ	844
DR	Herman, Z	NY	155
DR	Hricak, H	NY	155
DR	Levy, L	NJ	666
DR	Levy, M	NY	155
DR	Liberman, L	NY	156
DR	LoRusso, D	NY	604
DR	Morris, E	NY	156
DR	Novick, M	NY	459
DR	Sanders, L	NJ	707
DR	Sorabella, P	NJ	666
DR	Yang, R	NJ	830

Breast MRI

Spec	Name	St	Pg
DR	Levy, L	NJ	666
DR	Morris, E	NY	156
DR	Rosenfeld, S	NY	157
DR	Sonnenblick, E	NY	158

Breast Pathology

Spec	Name	St	Pg
Path	Barnard, N	NJ	772
Path	Bleiweiss, I	NY	278

Breast Reconstruction

Spec	Name	St	Pg
PlS	Ablaza, V	NJ	723
PlS	Ahn, C	NY	301
PlS	Bernard, R	NY	638
PlS	Bikoff, D	NJ	689
PlS	Birnbaum, J	NY	301
PlS	Breitbart, A	NY	535
PlS	Chidyllo, S	NJ	794
PlS	Choi, M	NY	302
PlS	Cordeiro, P	NY	302
PlS	Cuber, S	NJ	777
PlS	Disa, J	NY	303
PlS	Friedman, D	NY	303
PlS	Goldenberg, D	CT	890
PlS	Grant, R	NY	304
PlS	Herbstman, R	NJ	777
PlS	Hoffman, L	NY	304
PlS	Hyans, P	NJ	854
PlS	Israeli, R	NY	537
PlS	Kaufman, M	NJ	777
PlS	Keller, A	NY	537

Spec	Name	St	Pg
PlS	Kessler, M	NY	537
PlS	Kolker, A	NY	305
PlS	Leipziger, L	NY	537
PlS	Mehrara, B	NY	305
PlS	Najmi, J	NJ	835
PlS	Palaia, D	NY	639
PlS	Rafizadeh, F	NJ	813
PlS	Razaboni, R	NY	306
PlS	Rosen, A	NJ	723
PlS	Roth, M	NY	443
PlS	Sabry, M	NY	306
PlS	Salzberg, C	NY	639
PlS	Sklansky, B	NY	538
PlS	Stahl, R	CT	917
PlS	Starker, I	NJ	813
PlS	Sultan, M	NY	307
PlS	Ting, J	NY	308

Breast Reconstruction & Augmentation

Spec	Name	St	Pg
PlS	DiGregorio, V	NY	536
PlS	Dudick, S	NJ	794
PlS	Gayle, L	NY	303
PlS	Glicksman, C	NJ	794
PlS	LoVerme, P	NJ	723

Breast Surgery

Spec	Name	St	Pg
PlS	Broumand, S	NY	302
PlS	Cherofsky, A	NY	484
PlS	Choi, M	NY	302
PlS	Disa, J	NY	303
PlS	Duboys, E	NY	584
PlS	Goldstein, R	NY	395
PlS	Nini, K	NJ	777
PlS	Ofodile, F	NJ	689
PlS	Restifo, R	CT	917
PlS	Rosenberg, M	NY	639
PlS	Salzberg, C	NY	639
PlS	Tepper, H	NJ	854
PlS	Zevon, S	NY	309
S	Agarwal, N	NY	398
S	Ahlborn, T	NJ	694
S	Arbour, R	NJ	796
S	Blackwood, M	NJ	726
S	Borriello, R	NY	449
S	Bull, S	CT	895
S	Busch-Devereaux, E	NY	587
S	Cahan, A	NY	646
S	Cassell, L	NY	341
S	Chung-Loy, H	NJ	779
S	Cleary, J	NY	646
S	Colaco, R	NJ	856
S	Dasmahapatra, K	NJ	779
S	Dresner, L	NY	449

Special Expertise Index

Spec	Name	St	Pg
TS	Saunders, C	NJ	728
TS	Schubach, S	NY	547

Cardiac Surgery-Adult

Spec	Name	St	Pg
TS	Bilfinger, T	NY	588
TS	Brown, J	NJ	815
TS	Connolly, M	NJ	728
TS	Krieger, K	NY	351
TS	McMurtry, K	NJ	738

Cardiac Surgery-High Risk

Spec	Name	St	Pg
TS	Fernandez, H	NY	546

Cardiac Toxicity in Cancer Therapy

Spec	Name	St	Pg
Onc	Speyer, J	NY	212

Cardiac Tumors, Myxomas

Spec	Name	St	Pg
TS	Grossi, E	NY	350

Cardiothoracic Surgery

Spec	Name	St	Pg
TS	Bains, M	NY	348
TS	Burack, J	NY	451
TS	DeAnda, A	NY	349
TS	Girardi, L	NY	350
TS	Hall, T	CT	896
TS	Hartman, A	NY	547
TS	Heim, J	NJ	753
TS	Lang, S	NY	472
TS	Lundy, E	NY	560
TS	McGinn, J	NY	486
TS	Mosca, R	NY	351
TS	Port, J	NY	352
TS	Rose, D	CT	896
TS	Squitieri, R	CT	896

Cardiovascular Disease

Spec	Name	St	Pg
FMed	Klein, S	NY	502
IM	Gambarin, B	NY	421
IM	Legato, M	NY	194
IM	Mutterperl, M	NJ	735
IM	Sherman, F	NY	423
IM	Skluth, M	CT	875
IM	Slogoff, F	CT	875

Cardiovascular Imaging

Spec	Name	St	Pg
DR	Wolff, S	NY	158

Cardiovascular Surgery

Spec	Name	St	Pg
TS	Christakos, M	NJ	826
TS	Seinfeld, F	NJ	753

Career Related Problems

Spec	Name	St	Pg
Psyc	Borbely, A	NY	310

Caribbean Health Care

Spec	Name	St	Pg
FMed	Krotowski, M	NY	415

Carotid Artery Stent Placement

Spec	Name	St	Pg
Cv	Cohen, H	NY	129
IC	Petrossian, G	NY	511
IC	Roubin, G	NY	199
NRad	Tenner, M	NY	623
VIR	Hamet, M	CT	897

Carotid Artery Surgery

Spec	Name	St	Pg
NS	Ghogawala, Z	CT	880
NS	Langer, D	NY	516
NS	Quest, D	NY	219
S	Drascher, G	NJ	836
S	Fried, K	NJ	695
S	McGovern, P	NJ	737
S	Vitale, G	NY	546
TS	Seinfeld, F	NJ	753
TS	Syracuse, D	NJ	728
VascS	Adelman, M	NY	362
VascS	Arnold, T	NY	589
VascS	Ascher, E	NY	453
VascS	Babu, S	NY	650
VascS	Bernik, T	NY	362
VascS	Brener, B	NJ	729
VascS	Chaudhry, S	NY	549
VascS	Deitch, J	NY	486
VascS	Dietzek, A	CT	898
VascS	Faries, P	NY	362
VascS	Faust, G	NY	549
VascS	Gagne, P	CT	898
VascS	Geuder, J	NJ	698
VascS	Goldman, K	NJ	754
VascS	Graham, A	NJ	781
VascS	Green, R	NY	362
VascS	Grossi, R	NY	363
VascS	Harrington, E	NY	363
VascS	Harrington, M	NY	363
VascS	Jacobowitz, G	NY	363
VascS	Karanfilian, R	NY	651
VascS	Lipsitz, E	NY	401
VascS	Marin, M	NY	363
VascS	Nowygrod, R	NY	364
VascS	Pollina, R	NY	589
VascS	Purtill, W	NY	550
VascS	Riles, T	NY	364
VascS	Suggs, W	NY	401
VascS	Todd, G	NY	364
VascS	Weiser, R	NY	453

Spec	Name	St	Pg
VascS	Wolodiger, F	NJ	699

Carpal Tunnel Syndrome

Spec	Name	St	Pg
HS	Ark, J	NJ	743
HS	Botwinick, N	NY	179
HS	Brown, L	CT	872
HS	Ende, L	NJ	805
HS	Gurland, M	NJ	670
HS	Kamler, K	NY	506
HS	King, W	NY	179
HS	Kulick, R	NY	378
HS	Lane, L	NY	506
HS	Lee, S	NY	179
HS	Lenzo, S	NY	179
HS	Miller, J	NJ	805
HS	Palmieri, T	NY	506
HS	Pruzansky, M	NY	180
HS	Raskin, K	NY	180
HS	Rosenstein, R	NJ	670
HS	Rosenwasser, M	NY	180
HS	Teplitz, G	NY	507
HS	Thomson, J	CT	907
N	Alweiss, G	NJ	678
N	Belok, L	NY	221
N	Silbert, P	NJ	791
N	Weintraub, M	NY	623
NS	Zonenshayn, M	NY	428
OrS	Altman, W	NJ	682
OrS	Barmakian, J	NJ	850
OrS	Green, S	NY	258
OrS	Grenis, M	NJ	748

Cartilage Damage

Spec	Name	St	Pg
DR	Potter, H	NY	157
OrS	Cushner, F	NY	256
OrS	Gladstone, J	NY	257
OrS	Henshaw, D	CT	885
SM	Rodeo, S	NY	339

Cartilage Damage & Transplant

Spec	Name	St	Pg
OrS	Levitz, C	NY	524
OrS	Williams, R	NY	267
SM	Gehrmann, R	NJ	726
SM	Levy, A	NJ	726
SM	Plancher, K	NY	339

Cataract Surgery

Spec	Name	St	Pg
Oph	Accardi, F	NY	238
Oph	Angrist, R	NJ	833
Oph	Asbell, P	NY	238
Oph	Auran, J	NY	239
Oph	Benedetto, D	NJ	736
Oph	Biser, S	NY	625

Special Expertise Index

Spec	Name	St	Pg
Oph	Braunstein, R	NY	239
Oph	Broderick, R	NY	520
Oph	Burke, P	NJ	680
Oph	Chaiken, B	NY	240
Oph	Chern, R	NY	240
Oph	Chin, P	NJ	681
Oph	Chu, W	NY	240
Oph	Cohen, L	NY	240
Oph	Confino, J	NJ	850
Oph	Constad, W	NJ	736
Oph	Cykiert, R	NY	241
Oph	D'Aversa, G	NY	521
Oph	Davidson, L	NJ	716
Oph	DeBroff, B	CT	882
Oph	DeLuca, J	NJ	681
Oph	Deutsch, J	NY	432
Oph	Dieck, W	NY	625
Oph	Dinnerstein, S	NY	241
Oph	Engel, M	NJ	791
Oph	Feinstein, N	NY	432
Oph	Fong, R	NY	242
Oph	Friedman, R	NY	243
Oph	Fromer, M	NY	243
Oph	Gibralter, R	NY	243
Oph	Girardi, A	NY	521
Oph	Gladstein, G	CT	883
Oph	Glassman, M	NY	625
Oph	Goldberg, D	NJ	791
Oph	Goldberg, L	NY	521
Oph	Grasso, C	NY	466
Oph	Grayson, D	NY	243
Oph	Greenbaum, A	NY	626
Oph	Haight, D	NY	244
Oph	Harmon, G	NY	244
Oph	Hatsis, A	NY	521
Oph	Hayworth, R	NY	386
Oph	Jaffe, H	NY	433
Oph	Kaplan, J	CT	883
Oph	Kasper, W	NY	521
Oph	Kazam, E	NJ	809
Oph	Kelly, S	NY	244
Oph	Klapper, D	NY	244
Oph	Klein, N	NY	245
Oph	Koplin, R	NY	245
Oph	Kramer, P	NY	481
Oph	Lebowitz, M	NY	433
Oph	Leib, M	NY	245
Oph	Liebmann, J	NY	245
Oph	Lippman, J	NY	626
Oph	Liva, D	NJ	681
Oph	Mackool, R	NY	467
Oph	Magramm, I	NY	246
Oph	Malik, S	NY	521
Oph	Mandava, S	CT	883
Oph	Mandelbaum, S	NY	246

Spec	Name	St	Pg
Oph	Manjoney, D	CT	883
Oph	Marks, A	NY	522
Oph	Martin, J	NY	578
Oph	Matossian, C	NJ	747
Oph	Mayers, M	NY	386
Oph	McKee, H	NY	626
Oph	Merriam, J	NY	247
Oph	Michalos, P	NY	578
Oph	Mignone, B	NY	626
Oph	Miller, B	NY	626
Oph	Miller, P	NJ	717
Oph	Mitchell, J	NY	247
Oph	Moazed, K	NY	247
Oph	Natale, B	NJ	850
Oph	Nattis, R	NY	578
Oph	Nelson, D	NY	522
Oph	Nightingale, J	NY	248
Oph	O'Malley, G	NY	578
Oph	Obstbaum, S	NY	248
Oph	Ostriker, G	CT	883
Oph	Pearlstein, E	NY	433
Oph	Perry, H	NY	522
Oph	Pinke, R	NJ	809
Oph	Prince, A	NY	248
Oph	Prywes, A	NY	522
Oph	Ray, A	NY	627
Oph	Reich, R	NY	433
Oph	Relland, M	NY	249
Oph	Robbins, K	CT	883
Oph	Romanelli, J	NY	578
Oph	Rosenbaum, P	NY	386
Oph	Rosenthal, K	NY	522
Oph	Rothberg, C	NY	579
Oph	Rubin, L	NY	522
Oph	Rudick, A	NY	249
Oph	Saffra, N	NY	433
Oph	Safran, S	NJ	747
Oph	Salzman, J	NY	627
Oph	Santamaria, J	NJ	771
Oph	Sciortino, P	NY	433
Oph	Seidenfeld, A	NY	467
Oph	Seidman, M	NY	434
Oph	Sherman, S	NY	250
Oph	Sherman, S	NY	434
Oph	Shulman, J	NY	250
Oph	Siderides, E	CT	884
Oph	Silberman, D	NY	434
Oph	Silbert, G	NJ	681
Oph	Silverman, C	NJ	809
Oph	Smith, E	NY	434
Oph	Solomon, E	NJ	681
Oph	Stabile, J	NJ	681
Oph	Stein, A	NY	434
Oph	Stein, M	NY	627
Oph	Sturm, R	NY	522

Spec	Name	St	Pg
Oph	Talansky, M	NJ	791
Oph	Tiwari, R	NY	387
Oph	Vogel, M	NJ	822
Oph	Wasserman, E	CT	884
Oph	Weinstein, J	NY	523
Oph	Weiss, M	NY	252
Oph	Whitmore, W	NY	252
Oph	Wolf, K	NY	387
Oph	Young, J	NY	253
Oph	Zaidman, G	NY	628
Oph	Zellner, J	NY	434
Oph	Zerykier, A	NY	481
Oph	Zweibel, L	NY	579
Oph	Zweifach, P	NY	253

Cataract Surgery-Lens Implant

Spec	Name	St	Pg
Oph	Ackerman, J	NY	431
Oph	Berke, S	NY	520
Oph	Buxton, D	NY	239
Oph	Dodick, J	NY	241
Oph	Fishman, A	NY	466
Oph	Giliberti, O	NJ	822
Oph	Glatt, H	NJ	717
Oph	Musto, A	CT	883
Oph	Salz, A	NJ	833
Oph	Wong, M	NJ	748
Oph	Wong, R	NJ	748

Cataract-Pediatric

Spec	Name	St	Pg
Oph	DeBroff, B	CT	882
Oph	Hall, L	NY	244
Oph	Medow, N	NY	246

Catheter Ablation

Spec	Name	St	Pg
CE	Lerman, B	NY	127
CE	Steinberg, J	NY	127
CE	Winters, S	NJ	801

Celiac Disease

Spec	Name	St	Pg
Ge	Cooper, R	NY	165
Ge	Gettenberg, G	NY	416
Ge	Green, P	NY	167
Ge	Rubin, M	NY	172
Ge	Schrader, Z	NJ	709
Ge	Turtel, P	NJ	787
PGe	Benkov, K	NY	285
PGe	Kazlow, P	NY	285
PGe	Levy, J	NY	285
PGe	Newman, L	NY	633
PGe	Pettei, M	NY	530
PGe	Rosh, J	NJ	811

Special Expertise Index

Special Expertise Index

Special Expertise Index

Special Expertise Index

Spec	Name	St	Pg
Cv	Shell, R	NJ	758
Cv	Shimony, R	NY	136
Cv	Siegal, M	NY	136
Cv	Siepser, S	NJ	819
Cv	Silver, M	NY	598
Cv	Stein, R	NY	137
Cv	Tenenbaum, J	NY	137
Cv	Tenet, W	NY	495
Cv	Tyberg, T	NY	137
Cv	Unger, A	NY	137
Cv	Varriale, P	NY	137
Cv	Weg, I	NY	495
Cv	Wein, P	NY	410
Cv	Weisenseel, A	NY	138
Cv	Weiss, E	NJ	819
Cv	Weiss, M	NY	598
Cv	Weissman, R	NY	598
Cv	Wolk, M	NY	138
IC	Altmann, D	NJ	765
IC	Angeli, S	NJ	673
IC	Innerfield, M	NY	555
IC	Lichtstein, E	NJ	673
IC	Lituchy, A	NY	511
IC	Stone, G	NY	199
IC	Wasserman, H	CT	876
IC	Weinberger, J	NY	199
IM	Ascheim, R	NY	189
IM	Kennish, A	NY	194
IM	Lauricella, J	NJ	672
IM	Lipton, M	NY	195

Coronary Artery Surgery

Spec	Name	St	Pg
TS	Adams, D	NY	348
TS	Argenziano, M	NY	348
TS	Ciaburri, D	NY	896
TS	Connolly, M	NJ	728
TS	Culliford, A	NY	349
TS	Esposito, R	NY	546
TS	Galloway, A	NY	350
TS	Goldenberg, B	NJ	728
TS	Graver, L	NY	471
TS	Hartman, A	NY	547
TS	Isom, O	NY	350
TS	Krieger, K	NY	351
TS	Lansman, S	NY	648
TS	Lee, L	NJ	696
TS	Michler, R	NY	400
TS	Neibart, R	NJ	796
TS	Schubach, S	NY	547
TS	Spielvogel, D	NY	648
TS	Swistel, D	NY	352
TS	Tortolani, A	NY	451
TS	Tranbaugh, R	NY	353
TS	Zapolanski, A	NJ	696

Cosmetic & Reconstructive Surgery

Spec	Name	St	Pg
PlS	Duboys, E	NY	584
PlS	Ponamgi, S	NJ	689
PlS	Reiffel, R	NY	639

Cosmetic Dermatology

Spec	Name	St	Pg
D	Albom, M	NY	144
D	Aranoff, S	NY	144
D	Ashinoff, R	NJ	664
D	Avram, M	NY	144
D	Baldwin, H	NY	412
D	Basuk, P	NY	567
D	Biro, D	NY	412
D	Bisaccia, E	NJ	803
D	Brademas, M	NY	145
D	Brancaccio, R	NY	412
D	Brandt, F	NY	145
D	Brauner, G	NJ	664
D	Bruckstein, R	NY	497
D	Buchness, M	NY	145
D	Burke, K	NY	145
D	Clark, S	NY	146
D	Davis, I	NY	601
D	Davis, J	NY	146
D	Demar, L	NY	146
D	Downie, J	NJ	706
D	Felderman, L	NY	146
D	Gendler, E	NY	147
D	Geronemus, R	NY	147
D	Goldberg, D	NY	147
D	Gordon, M	NY	147
D	Greenberg, R	NY	147
D	Grodberg, M	NJ	665
D	Grossman, K	NJ	786
D	Hatcher, V	NY	148
D	Hefter, H	NY	498
D	Hochman, H	NY	148
D	Jacobs, M	NY	148
D	Katz, B	NY	148
D	Katz, S	NY	371
D	Kauvar, A	NY	148
D	Kenet, B	NY	148
D	Kline, M	NY	148
D	Kopec, A	NJ	733
D	Kriegel, D	NY	149
D	Lederman, J	NY	476
D	Levine, L	NY	498
D	Liftin, A	NJ	706
D	Lombardo, P	NY	149
D	Maiocco, K	CT	868
D	Marinaro, R	NJ	803
D	Marmur, E	NY	149
D	Mermelstein, H	NY	602

Spec	Name	St	Pg
D	Milgraum, S	NJ	760
D	Narins, R	NY	602
D	Newburger, A	NY	603
D	Oshman, R	CT	868
D	Ostad, A	NY	150
D	Polis, L	NY	150
D	Pruzan-Clain, D	CT	869
D	Prystowsky, J	NY	150
D	Rapaport, J	NJ	665
D	Rigel, D	NY	150
D	Romano, J	NY	151
D	Rozanski, R	NJ	706
D	Sarnoff, D	NY	498
D	Scherl, S	NJ	665
D	Schultz, N	NY	151
D	Seidenberg, R	NY	151
D	Shelton, R	NY	151
D	Sibrack, L	CT	869
D	Sklar, J	NY	499
D	Sobel, H	NY	152
D	Sturza, J	NY	603
D	Tesser, M	NY	152
D	Vine, J	NJ	742
D	Vogel, L	NY	152
D	Waldorf, D	NY	553
D	Waldorf, H	NY	554
D	Warner, R	NY	152
D	Wattenberg, D	NY	153
D	Weiss, D	NJ	665
D	Zweibel, S	NY	603

Cosmetic Surgery

Spec	Name	St	Pg
D	Safai, B	NY	151
D	Wrone, D	NJ	760
Oto	Carniol, P	NJ	851
PlS	Ascherman, J	NY	301
PlS	Bromley, G	NY	301
PlS	Choi, M	NY	302
PlS	Drimmer, M	NJ	750
PlS	Dudick, S	NJ	794
PlS	Elkowitz, M	NY	536
PlS	Feldman, D	NY	443
PlS	Forley, B	NY	303
PlS	Ginsberg, G	NY	303
PlS	Goldenberg, D	CT	890
PlS	Granick, M	NJ	723
PlS	Grant, R	NY	304
PlS	Karp, N	NY	305
PlS	Kleinman, A	NY	638
PlS	Persing, J	CT	917
PlS	Razaboni, R	NY	306
PlS	Sabry, M	NY	306
PlS	Samra, S	NJ	794
PlS	Sklansky, B	NY	538
PlS	Spector, J	NY	307

Spec	Name	St	Pg
PlS	Taub, P	NY	308
PlS	Tepper, H	NJ	854

Cosmetic Surgery-Body

Spec	Name	St	Pg
PlS	Ahn, C	NY	301
PlS	Bernard, R	NY	638
PlS	Cherofsky, A	NY	484
PlS	Cuber, S	NJ	777
PlS	Gayle, L	NY	303
PlS	Gold, A	NY	537
PlS	Herbstman, R	NJ	777
PlS	Hunter, J	NY	304
PlS	Vickery, C	NY	308
PlS	Weiss, P	NY	308

Cosmetic Surgery-Breast

Spec	Name	St	Pg
PlS	Almeyda, E	NY	301
PlS	Aston, S	NY	301
PlS	Bikoff, D	NJ	689
PlS	Borah, G	NJ	776
PlS	Breitbart, A	NY	535
PlS	Chidyllo, S	NJ	794
PlS	Cuber, S	NJ	777
PlS	DeVita, G	NY	536
PlS	Foster, C	NY	303
PlS	Freund, R	NY	303
PlS	Ganchi, P	NJ	824
PlS	Glicksman, C	NJ	794
PlS	Godfrey, P	NY	304
PlS	Gold, A	NY	537
PlS	Hawrylo, R	NJ	813
PlS	Hidalgo, D	NY	304
PlS	Hunter, J	NY	304
PlS	Hyans, P	NJ	854
PlS	Khoury, F	NY	638
PlS	Kolker, A	NY	305
PlS	Leach, T	NJ	750
PlS	Leipziger, L	NY	537
PlS	O'Connell, J	CT	890
PlS	Pyo, D	NJ	813
PlS	Rafizadeh, F	NJ	813
PlS	Raskin, E	CT	890
PlS	Rose, M	NJ	794
PlS	Rosenblatt, W	NY	306
PlS	Rosenstock, A	CT	891
PlS	Roth, D	NY	639
PlS	Roth, M	NY	443
PlS	Skolnik, R	NY	307
PlS	Starker, I	NJ	813
PlS	Sultan, M	NY	307
PlS	Suzman, M	NY	639

Cosmetic Surgery-Face

Spec	Name	St	Pg
Oto	Brunner, E	NJ	749

Spec	Name	St	Pg
Oto	Cece, J	NJ	823
Oto	Chaudhry, M	NY	436
Oto	Gordon, N	CT	886
Oto	Guida, R	NY	269
Oto	Li, R	NJ	749
Oto	Miller, A	NJ	772
Oto	Miller, P	NY	272
Oto	Morrow, T	NJ	718
Oto	Romo, T	NY	273
Oto	Rosenbaum, J	NJ	772
Oto	Rosenberg, D	NY	273
Oto	Scaccia, F	NJ	792
Oto	Scharf, R	NJ	851
Oto	Sclafani, A	NY	274
Oto	Snyder, G	NY	467
Oto	Soletic, R	NY	526
PlS	Ahn, C	NY	301
PlS	Anton, J	NY	584
PlS	Baker, D	NY	301
PlS	Bernard, R	NY	638
PlS	Borah, G	NJ	776
PlS	Chidyllo, S	NJ	794
PlS	Chiu, D	NY	302
PlS	Chun, J	NY	302
PlS	D'Amico, R	NJ	689
PlS	DeVita, G	NY	536
PlS	DiGregorio, V	NY	536
PlS	Friedman, D	NY	303
PlS	Gewirtz, H	CT	890
PlS	Herbstman, R	NJ	777
PlS	Hidalgo, D	NY	304
PlS	Hoffman, L	NY	304
PlS	Hyans, P	NJ	854
PlS	Imber, G	NY	304
PlS	Karpinski, R	NY	305
PlS	Khoury, F	NY	638
PlS	Leach, T	NJ	750
PlS	Lesesne, C	NY	305
PlS	LoVerme, P	NJ	723
PlS	Lukash, F	NY	538
PlS	McCarthy, J	NY	305
PlS	Najmi, J	NJ	835
PlS	O'Connell, J	CT	890
PlS	Palaia, D	NY	639
PlS	Pitman, G	NY	306
PlS	Rafizadeh, F	NJ	813
PlS	Raskin, E	CT	890
PlS	Romita, M	NY	306
PlS	Rose, M	NJ	794
PlS	Rosenstock, A	CT	891
PlS	Roth, D	NY	639
PlS	Salzberg, C	NY	639
PlS	Scott, S	NY	306
PlS	Sherman, J	NY	307
PlS	Siebert, J	NY	307

Spec	Name	St	Pg
PlS	Silberman, M	NY	538
PlS	Skolnik, R	NY	307
PlS	Spinelli, H	NY	307
PlS	Staffenberg, D	NY	395
PlS	Sultan, M	NY	307
PlS	Suzman, M	NY	639
PlS	Tabbal, N	NY	308
PlS	Verga, M	NY	308
PlS	Vickery, C	NY	308
PlS	Weinstein, L	NJ	813
PlS	Weiss, P	NY	308
PlS	Wells, S	NY	308
PlS	Wey, P	NJ	777
PlS	Zubowski, R	NJ	690

Cosmetic Surgery-Face & Body

Spec	Name	St	Pg
PlS	Aston, S	NY	301
PlS	Breitbart, A	NY	535
PlS	Colon, F	NJ	812
PlS	DiBernardo, B	NJ	723
PlS	Friedlander, B	NJ	723
PlS	Funt, D	NY	536
PlS	Ganchi, P	NJ	824
PlS	Kessler, M	NY	537
PlS	Rosenblatt, W	NY	306
PlS	Schulman, N	NY	306
PlS	Starker, I	NJ	813
PlS	Zaccaria, A	NJ	794

Cosmetic Surgery-Face & Breast

Spec	Name	St	Pg
PlS	Birnbaum, J	NY	301
PlS	Colen, H	NY	302
PlS	Gotkin, R	NY	537
PlS	Jacobs, E	NY	304
PlS	Perrotti, J	NY	305
PlS	Rosen, A	NJ	723
PlS	Simpson, R	NY	538
PlS	Sternschein, M	NJ	690
PlS	Thorne, C	NY	308

Cosmetic Surgery-Face & Eyelid

Spec	Name	St	Pg
PlS	Hawrylo, R	NJ	813
PlS	Roth, M	NY	443

Cosmetic Surgery-Face & Eyes

Spec	Name	St	Pg
PlS	Feinberg, J	NY	536
PlS	Gold, A	NY	537
PlS	Leipziger, L	NY	537
PlS	Matarasso, A	NY	305
PlS	Silich, R	NY	307

Cosmetic Surgery-Face & Neck

Spec	Name	St	Pg
PlS	Cutolo, L	NY	484

Special Expertise Index

Special Expertise Index

Spec	Name	St	Pg
Psyc	Appelbaum, P	NY	310
Psyc	Aronson, T	NY	584
Psyc	Asnis, G	NY	396
Psyc	Bailine, S	NY	538
Psyc	Behr, R	NY	538
Psyc	Benjamin, J	NY	538
Psyc	Berkowitz, H	NY	443
Psyc	Bhatt, A	NY	539
Psyc	Brenner, R	NY	468
Psyc	Carone, P	NY	539
Psyc	Chung, H	NY	311
Psyc	Crasta, J	NY	539
Psyc	Di Buono, M	NY	484
Psyc	Douglas, C	NY	312
Psyc	Dulit, R	NY	640
Psyc	Eitan, N	NY	444
Psyc	Faber, M	NJ	724
Psyc	Friedman, R	NY	313
Psyc	Gelfand, J	NY	396
Psyc	Glassman, A	NY	313
Psyc	Harlam, D	NY	640
Psyc	Heller, S	NY	314
Psyc	Hoffman, J	NY	314
Psyc	Idupuganti, S	NY	444
Psyc	Jones, F	NJ	777
Psyc	Kaplan, G	NJ	854
Psyc	Karasu, T	NY	315
Psyc	Kowallis, G	NY	315
Psyc	Kurani, D	NJ	724
Psyc	Lebinger, M	NY	396
Psyc	Leifer, M	NJ	751
Psyc	Liang, V	NY	584
Psyc	Lorefice, L	CT	891
Psyc	Marin, D	NY	316
Psyc	Markowitz, J	NY	316
Psyc	McGrath, P	NY	316
Psyc	Menza, M	NJ	778
Psyc	Meyers, B	NY	641
Psyc	Miller, D	NJ	854
Psyc	Milone, R	NY	641
Psyc	Moore, J	NY	317
Psyc	Nass, J	NY	584
Psyc	Nucci, A	NJ	724
Psyc	Nunes, E	NY	317
Psyc	Papp, L	NY	318
Psyc	Rochford, J	NJ	835
Psyc	Rosen, A	NY	319
Psyc	Rosen, B	NY	585
Psyc	Rosenthal, J	NY	319
Psyc	Sami, S	NY	539
Psyc	Samuels, S	NJ	690
Psyc	Schein, J	NY	320
Psyc	Schleifer, S	NJ	724
Psyc	Schore, A	NY	320
Psyc	Schwartz, B	NY	396

Spec	Name	St	Pg
Psyc	Seaman, C	NY	320
Psyc	Selzer, J	NY	469
Psyc	Shapiro, P	NY	320
Psyc	Shinbach, K	NY	321
Psyc	Siever, L	NY	321
Psyc	Teusink, J	NY	322
Psyc	Upadhyay, Y	NY	585
Psyc	Villafranca, M	NJ	854
Psyc	Viswanathan, R	NY	444
Psyc	Vivek, S	NY	469
Psyc	Wager, S	NY	322
Psyc	Zolkind, N	NY	642
Psyc	Zornitzer, M	NJ	724

Depression in Adolescents

ChAP	Perlmutter, I	NY	495

Depression in Schizophrenia

Psyc	Siris, S	NY	469

Depression in the Elderly

GerPsy	Cohen, C	NY	418
Psyc	Farkas, E	NJ	690
Psyc	Marin, D	NY	316
Psyc	Roose, S	NY	319

Depression-TMS Therapy

Psyc	Manevitz, A	NY	316

Dermatologic Surgery

D	Aranoff, S	NY	144
D	De Pietro, W	NY	497
D	Demento, F	NY	497
D	Greenspan, A	NY	147
D	Hefter, H	NY	498
D	Heldman, J	NJ	665
D	Kenet, B	NY	148
D	Levy, R	NY	602
D	Maiocco, K	CT	868
D	Orentreich, D	NY	149
D	Paltzik, R	NY	498
D	Ratner, D	NY	150
D	Safai, B	NY	151
D	Siegel, D	NY	568

Dermatomyositis

D	Franks, A	NY	146
PRhu	Ilowite, N	NY	391
PRhu	Kimura, Y	NJ	687
PRhu	McCarthy, P	CT	916
Rhu	Mitnick, H	NY	336

Spec	Name	St	Pg
Dermatopathology			
D	Shim-Chang, H	NY	151
D	Silvers, D	NY	152
Path	Gottlieb, G	NY	278
Path	McNutt, N	NY	279

Developmental & Behavioral Disorders

Ped	Ferrier, G	NY	294
Ped	Kaminer, R	NY	393
Ped	Katz, A	NJ	834
Ped	Marino, R	NY	534
Ped	Stein, B	NY	297
Ped	Stein, R	NY	394

Developmental Disorders

CG	Shapiro, L	NY	600
CG	Sklower Brooks, S	NJ	759
ChAP	Burkes, L	NY	138
ChAP	Hertzig, M	NY	139
ChAP	Madigan, J	CT	902
ChAP	Newcorn, J	NY	140
ChAP	Pomeroy, J	NY	566
ChAP	Rubinstein, B	NY	599
ChAP	Schreiber, K	NY	599
ChAP	Volkmar, F	CT	902
ChiN	Andriola, M	NY	566
ChiN	Kosofsky, B	NY	141
ChiN	Ment, L	CT	903
ChiN	Schubert, R	NY	411
N	Kuzniecky, R	NY	224
NP	Manginello, F	NJ	676
Ped	Adesman, A	NY	533
Ped	Arnstein, E	NY	392
Ped	Baiser, D	NJ	750
Ped	Berman, M	NY	636
Ped	Canny, C	CT	916
Ped	Chefitz, D	NJ	776
Ped	Chessin, R	CT	888
Ped	Gould, E	NY	534
Ped	Hankin, D	NY	534
Ped	Igel, G	NY	393
Ped	Juan, P	CT	888
Ped	Kaplan, M	NY	583
Ped	McCarton, C	NY	295
Ped	Poon, E	NY	296
Ped	Puder, D	NY	558
Ped	Rosenfeld, S	NY	297
Ped	Schutzengel, R	CT	889
Ped	Strassberg, B	NY	394
Psyc	Moraille, P	NJ	737

Special Expertise Index

Spec	Name	St	Pg
Diabetes Ketoacidosis			
PCCM	Greenwald, B	NY	283
Diabetes Surgery-Rubino's Procedure			
S	Rubino, F	NY	346
Diabetic Eye Disease			
Oph	Casper, D	NY	240
Oph	Cohen, S	NJ	716
Oph	Fisher, Y	NY	242
Oph	Grabowski, W	NJ	770
Oph	Reppucci, V	CT	883
Oph	Salzman, J	NY	627
Oph	Talansky, M	NJ	791
Diabetic Eye Disease/Retinopathy			
Oph	Angioletti, L	NY	238
Oph	Barile, G	NY	239
Oph	Berman, D	NY	432
Oph	Bhagat, N	NJ	716
Oph	Brecher, R	NY	432
Oph	Cangemi, F	NJ	716
Oph	Chang, S	NY	240
Oph	Cohen, B	NY	240
Oph	D'Amico, D	NY	241
Oph	Del Priore, L	NY	241
Oph	Douros, S	NY	432
Oph	Eichler, J	NJ	716
Oph	Elbaba, F	NY	578
Oph	Fastenberg, D	NY	521
Oph	Feinstein, N	NY	432
Oph	Fleischman, J	NY	625
Oph	Fromer, M	NY	243
Oph	Fuchs, W	NY	243
Oph	Gentile, R	NY	243
Oph	Kramer, P	NY	481
Oph	Lee, C	NY	245
Oph	Lewis, H	NY	245
Oph	Lombardo, J	NY	433
Oph	MacKay, C	NY	246
Oph	Muldoon, T	NY	248
Oph	Pizzarello, L	NY	578
Oph	Rosenthal, J	NY	249
Oph	Sachs, R	NJ	809
Oph	Schiff, W	NY	250
Oph	Schubert, H	NY	250
Oph	Shabto, U	NY	250
Oph	Slamovits, T	NY	387
Oph	Solomon, S	NY	627
Oph	Spaide, R	NY	251
Oph	Svitra, P	NY	523

Spec	Name	St	Pg
Oph	Tiwari, R	NY	387
Oph	Walsh, J	NY	252
Oph	Weber, P	NY	579
Oph	Wolf, K	NY	387
Oph	Wong, R	NY	253
Oph	Yagoda, A	NY	253
Oph	Yannuzzi, L	NY	253
Oph	Zarbin, M	NJ	717
Oph	Zerykier, A	NY	481
Diabetic Kidney Disease			
EDM	Bloomgarden, Z	NY	158
Nep	Charytan, C	NY	383
Nep	Gorkin, J	NY	383
Nep	Kozin, A	NY	556
Nep	Kozlowski, J	NJ	676
Nep	Laitman, R	NY	383
Nep	Mattana, J	NY	515
Nep	Parnes, E	NY	427
Nep	Ruddy, M	NJ	746
Nep	Shein, L	NY	427
Nep	Singhal, P	NY	515
Nep	Spitalewitz, S	NY	427
Diabetic Leg/Foot			
OrS	Weinfeld, S	NY	266
VascS	Faust, G	NY	549
VascS	Sumpio, B	CT	923
VascS	Teodorescu, V	NY	364
Diabetic Leg/Foot Infections			
Inf	Farrer, W	NJ	846
NuM	Palestro, C	NY	519
Diabetic Neuropathy			
N	Brannagan, T	NY	221
N	Weintraub, M	NY	623
Diagnostic Problems			
ChAP	Burkes, L	NY	138
Cv	Goldman, M	NY	131
Cv	Sklaroff, H	NY	137
IM	Fulop, R	NY	478
IM	Glowacki, J	NJ	788
IM	Walfish, J	NY	197
Inf	Smith, S	NJ	710
Inf	Wormser, G	NY	612
Oph	Boniuk, V	NY	520
Oph	Lederman, M	NY	626
Ped	Asnes, R	NJ	687
Ped	Brown, J	NY	636
Ped	Zoltan, I	NY	394

Spec	Name	St	Pg
Dialysis Access			
VIR	Aruny, J	CT	922
VIR	Cynamon, J	NY	401
VIR	Denny, D	NJ	753
VIR	Siegel, R	NJ	781
Dialysis Access Surgery			
S	Greenstein, S	NY	399
S	Lois, W	NY	450
S	Rajdeo, H	NY	647
S	Shapiro, M	NJ	695
VascS	Arnold, T	NY	589
VascS	Chaudhry, S	NY	549
VascS	Pollina, R	NY	589
VascS	Schwartz, K	NY	651
Dialysis Care			
IM	Constantiner, A	NY	191
IM	Lebofsky, M	NY	614
IM	Rubenstein, J	NY	510
IM	Walsh, F	CT	876
Nep	Adler, S	NY	620
Nep	Ames, R	NJ	214
Nep	Byrd, L	NJ	713
Nep	Chan, B	CT	879
Nep	Chou, S	NY	426
Nep	Croll, J	NY	383
Nep	Delano, B	NY	426
Nep	Devita, M	NY	215
Nep	Feintzeig, I	CT	879
Nep	Fine, P	NJ	807
Nep	Fishbane, S	NY	515
Nep	Fogel, M	CT	879
Nep	Garrick, R	NY	620
Nep	Garvey, M	NY	215
Nep	Grasso, M	NJ	713
Nep	Grodstein, G	NJ	676
Nep	Hines, W	CT	879
Nep	Kostadaras, A	NY	465
Nep	Kozlowski, J	NJ	676
Nep	Levin, D	NJ	677
Nep	Lipner, H	NY	426
Nep	Lyman, N	NJ	713
Nep	Lynn, R	NY	383
Nep	Mailloux, L	NY	515
Nep	Matalon, R	NY	215
Nep	Mattoo, N	NY	465
Nep	Michelis, M	NY	215
Nep	Mittman, N	NY	426
Nep	Najarian, J	NJ	807
Nep	Pannone, J	NY	426
Nep	Parnes, E	NY	427
Nep	Pattner, A	NJ	677
Nep	Rigolosi, R	NJ	677

E

Spec columns on right:

Spec	Name	St	Pg
HS	Hurst, L	NY	571
HS	Miller, J	NJ	805
OrS	Hotchkiss, R	NY	259

Special Expertise Index

Special Expertise Index

Special Expertise Index

Special Expertise Index

Special Expertise Index

Special Expertise Index

Spec	Name	St	Pg
Oph	Bogaty, S	NY	577
Oph	Broderick, R	NY	520
Oph	Charles, N	NY	240
Oph	Cook, J	NY	520
Oph	Davidson, L	NJ	716
Oph	Dieck, W	NY	625
Oph	Dinnerstein, S	NY	241
Oph	Engel, M	NJ	791
Oph	Esposito, D	NY	242
Oph	Feinstein, N	NY	432
Oph	Fong, R	NY	242
Oph	Freedman, J	NY	432
Oph	Friedman, A	NY	243
Oph	Giliberti, O	NJ	822
Oph	Girardi, A	NY	521
Oph	Gladstein, G	CT	883
Oph	Glassman, M	NY	625
Oph	Grasso, C	NY	466
Oph	Grayson, D	NY	243
Oph	Harmon, G	NY	244
Oph	Hayworth, R	NY	386
Oph	Jaffe, H	NY	433
Oph	Kasper, W	NY	521
Oph	Kazam, E	NJ	809
Oph	Klapper, D	NY	244
Oph	Klein, N	NY	245
Oph	Kramer, P	NY	481
Oph	Liebmann, J	NY	245
Oph	Liva, D	NJ	681
Oph	Lombardo, J	NY	433
Oph	Manjoney, D	CT	883
Oph	Matossian, C	NJ	747
Oph	McDermott, J	NY	246
Oph	McKee, H	NY	626
Oph	Mignone, B	NY	626
Oph	Miller, B	NY	626
Oph	Miller, P	NJ	717
Oph	Mitchell, J	NY	247
Oph	Mogil, L	NY	433
Oph	Nelson, D	NY	522
Oph	Obstbaum, S	NY	248
Oph	Ostriker, G	CT	883
Oph	Pinke, R	NJ	809
Oph	Prince, A	NY	248
Oph	Prywes, A	NY	522
Oph	Ray, A	NY	627
Oph	Ritch, R	NY	249
Oph	Romanelli, J	NY	578
Oph	Rosenbaum, P	NY	386
Oph	Rothberg, C	NY	579
Oph	Rubin, L	NY	522
Oph	Rudick, A	NY	249
Oph	Safran, S	NJ	747
Oph	Salzman, J	NY	627
Oph	Serle, J	NY	250

Spec	Name	St	Pg
Oph	Sherman, S	NY	250
Oph	Sherman, S	NY	434
Oph	Shulman, J	NY	250
Oph	Sidoti, P	NY	250
Oph	Smith, S	NY	251
Oph	Solomon, I	NY	627
Oph	Soloway, B	NY	251
Oph	Stein, A	NY	434
Oph	Sturm, R	NY	522
Oph	Tello, C	NY	252
Oph	Tiwari, R	NY	387
Oph	Tsai, J	CT	913
Oph	Wasserman, E	CT	884
Oph	Weinberg, M	NJ	681
Oph	Whitmore, W	NY	252
Oph	Zerykier, A	NY	481
Oph	Zweibel, L	NY	579
Oph	Zweifach, P	NY	253

Glaucoma-Pediatric

Spec	Name	St	Pg
Oph	Buxton, D	NY	239
Oph	Medow, N	NY	246
Oph	Raab, E	NY	248

Gliomas

Spec	Name	St	Pg
N	Rosenfeld, S	NY	228
NS	Boockvar, J	NY	216
Onc	Ratner, L	NY	210

Glomerulonephritis

Spec	Name	St	Pg
Nep	Adler, S	NY	620
Nep	Appel, G	NY	214
Nep	Brown, E	CT	879
Nep	Chan, B	CT	879
Nep	Cohen, D	NY	214
Nep	Devita, M	NY	215
Nep	Fogel, M	CT	879
Nep	Goldstein, C	NJ	848
Nep	Kabis, S	NJ	833
Nep	Liu, D	NY	215
Nep	Mattana, J	NY	515
Nep	Rastegar, A	CT	911
Nep	Sherman, R	NY	215
Nep	Winston, J	NY	216
PNep	Johnson, V	NY	289
PNep	Kaplan, M	NY	440
PNep	Lieberman, K	NJ	686
PNep	Perelstein, E	NY	289
PNep	Seigle, R	NY	290

Glycogen Storage Diseases

Spec	Name	St	Pg
PEn	Slonim, A	NY	284

Gout

Spec	Name	St	Pg
Rhu	Agus, B	NY	334
Rhu	Berger, J	NY	645
Rhu	Crane, R	NY	334
Rhu	Faller, J	NY	334
Rhu	Fields, T	NY	334
Rhu	Fomberstein, B	NY	398
Rhu	Leibowitz, E	NJ	693
Rhu	Meredith, G	NY	544
Rhu	Reinitz, E	NY	645
Rhu	Sharon, E	NY	470
Rhu	Smiles, S	NY	337
Rhu	Weinstein, J	NY	398
Rhu	Yee, A	NY	338

Graft vs Host Disease

Spec	Name	St	Pg
Hem	Rowley, S	NJ	671
Onc	Foss, F	CT	909

Graves' Disease

Spec	Name	St	Pg
EDM	Davies, T	NY	159

Growth Disorders

Spec	Name	St	Pg
Ped	Rosenbaum, M	NY	297
Ped	Schutzengel, R	CT	889
Ped	Siegal, E	NY	558
PEn	Anhalt, H	NJ	852
PEn	Avruskin, T	NY	438
PEn	Carey, D	NY	529
PEn	Chin, D	NJ	811
PEn	Franklin, B	NY	283
PEn	Kohn, B	NY	283
PEn	Marshall, I	NJ	774
PEn	Meyers-Seifer, C	NJ	793
PEn	Oberfield, S	NY	284
PEn	Rapaport, R	NY	284
PEn	Rivkees, S	CT	915
PEn	Salas, M	NJ	774
PEn	Starkman, H	NJ	811
PEn	Torrado-Jule, C	NY	483
PEn	Vogiatzi, M	NY	284
PEn	Wilson, T	NY	581

Growth Disorders in Childhood Cancer

Spec	Name	St	Pg
PEn	Sklar, C	NY	284

Growth Hormone Disorder-Adult

Spec	Name	St	Pg
EDM	Inzucchi, S	CT	905

H

Special Expertise Index

Spec	Name	St	Pg
Hairy Cell Leukemia			
Hem	Tallman, M	NY	184
Hand & Elbow Nerve Disorders			
HS	Strauch, R	NY	180
Hand & Microvascular Surgery			
PlS	Chiu, D	NY	302
Hand & Upper Extremity Surgery			
HS	Athanasian, E	NY	178
HS	Carlson, M	NY	179
HS	Ende, L	NJ	805
HS	Kulick, R	NY	378
HS	Magill, R	NY	611
HS	Schefer, A	NY	611
Hand & Upper Extremity Tumors			
HS	Athanasian, E	NY	178
Hand & Wrist Injuries			
HS	Lenzo, S	NY	179
OrS	Altman, W	NJ	682
OrS	Grenis, M	NJ	748
Hand & Wrist Surgery			
HS	Caligiuri, D	NY	419
HS	Fragner, P	NY	611
HS	Glickel, S	NY	179
HS	Strauch, R	NY	180
OrS	Green, S	NY	258
Hand Reconstruction			
HS	Brown, L	CT	872
HS	King, W	NY	179
HS	Lane, L	NY	506
HS	Strauch, R	NY	180
HS	Thomson, J	CT	907
HS	Weiland, A	NY	180
OrS	Hausman, M	NY	259
PlS	Kasabian, A	NY	537
PlS	Scott, S	NY	306
Hand Rehabilitation			
HS	Palmieri, T	NY	506
Hand Surgery			
HS	Ark, J	NJ	743
HS	Yang, S	NY	181

Spec	Name	St	Pg
OrS	Bade, H	NJ	792
OrS	Green, S	NY	258
OrS	Hotchkiss, R	NY	259
OrS	Jayaram, N	NY	482
OrS	Johnson, A	NJ	834
OrS	Kleinman, P	NY	387
OrS	Mackessy, R	NJ	850
OrS	Montero, C	NY	524
OrS	Montgomery, K	NJ	810
OrS	Pianka, G	NY	263
OrS	Sarokhan, A	NJ	851
OrS	Stuchin, S	NY	265
PlS	Bikoff, D	NJ	689
PlS	Borah, G	NJ	776
PlS	Choi, M	NY	302
PlS	Dagum, A	NY	584
PlS	Gayle, L	NY	303
PlS	Kessler, M	NY	537
PlS	Liebling, R	NY	395
PlS	Reiffel, R	NY	639
PlS	Samra, S	NJ	794
PlS	Tepper, H	NJ	854
PlS	Ting, J	NY	308
PlS	Zeitels, J	NJ	854
Hashimoto's Disease			
EDM	Davies, T	NY	159
Hay Fever			
A&I	Harish, Z	NJ	660
A&I	Klein, N	NY	407
A&I	Lindner, P	CT	865
A&I	Minikes, N	NJ	660
A&I	Pedinoff, A	NJ	829
A&I	Tuerk-Mendelsohn, L	NY	594
Head & Neck Autoimmune Disease			
Oto	Lebovics, R	NY	272
Head & Neck Cancer			
Hem	Meyer, R	NY	183
Onc	Drucker, B	CT	877
Onc	Fang, B	NJ	766
Onc	Mehrotra, B	NY	513
Onc	Oster, M	NY	209
Onc	Pfister, D	NY	209
Onc	Posner, M	NY	210
Oto	Carew, J	NY	268
Oto	Caruana, S	NY	268
Oto	Close, L	NY	268
Oto	Costantino, P	NY	269
Oto	DeLacure, M	NY	269

Spec	Name	St	Pg
Oto	Fox, M	NY	630
Oto	Har-El, G	NY	270
Oto	Kraus, D	NY	271
Oto	Lawson, W	NY	271
Oto	Persky, M	NY	272
Oto	Rosner, L	NY	526
Oto	Sasaki, C	CT	914
Oto	Schantz, S	NY	274
Oto	Scharf, R	NJ	851
Oto	Shemen, L	NY	274
Oto	Smith, R	NY	388
Oto	Strome, M	NY	275
PlS	Ariyan, S	CT	917
PlS	Kaufman, M	NJ	777
RadRO	Cooper, J	NY	447
RadRO	Dalton, J	NY	470
RadRO	Fass, D	NY	644
RadRO	Haffty, B	NJ	778
RadRO	Harrison, L	NY	329
RadRO	Ingenito, A	NJ	692
RadRO	Lee, N	NY	329
RadRO	McKenna, M	NJ	752
RadRO	Meek, A	NY	586
RadRO	Ng, J	NY	329
RadRO	Pollack, J	NY	542
RadRO	Wilson, L	CT	919
RadRO	Wong, J	NJ	814
RadRO	Zelefsky, M	NY	330
S	Datta, R	NY	545
Head & Neck Cancer & Surgery			
Oto	Frank, D	NY	525
Oto	Genden, E	NY	269
Oto	Krespi, Y	NY	271
Oto	Lagmay, V	NY	436
Oto	Portnoy, W	NY	273
Oto	Shah, D	NJ	792
Oto	Singh, B	NY	275
Oto	Urken, M	NY	275
S	Shah, J	NY	346
Head & Neck Cancer Reconstruction			
Oto	DeLacure, M	NY	269
Oto	Genden, E	NY	269
Oto	Portnoy, W	NY	273
Oto	Urken, M	NY	275
Head & Neck Imaging			
DR	Holliday, R	NY	155
DR	Jacobs, M	NY	155
DR	Lee, H	NJ	707
DR	Reede, D	NY	413

Special Expertise Index

Special Expertise Index

Special Expertise Index

Spec	Name	St	Pg
FMed	Catanese, V	NJ	786
FMed	Eisenstat, S	NJ	845
FMed	Fisher, G	NY	460
FMed	Ibelli, V	NY	554
FMed	Krotowski, M	NY	415
FMed	Leeds, G	NY	162
FMed	Levites, K	NY	570
FMed	Levy, A	NY	162
FMed	Molnar, T	NY	461
FMed	Moynihan, B	NY	502
FMed	Roth, A	NY	461
Ger	Bullock, R	NJ	763
Ger	Kellogg, F	NY	175
IM	Altbaum, R	CT	874
IM	Alterman, L	NJ	846
IM	Ammazzalorso, M	NY	508
IM	Bell, K	NJ	832
IM	Blum, D	NY	463
IM	Blumberg, J	CT	874
IM	Brewer, M	NY	463
IM	Butt, A	NY	421
IM	Cardiello, G	NJ	734
IM	Carosella, C	NY	613
IM	Case, D	NY	190
IM	Cohn, S	NY	421
IM	Constantiner, A	NY	191
IM	Cusumano, S	NY	509
IM	Dhalla, S	NY	191
IM	Ditchek, A	NY	421
IM	Dreyer, N	CT	874
IM	Fazio, N	NY	613
IM	Federbush, R	NY	509
IM	Feldman, J	NJ	846
IM	Fennell, G	CT	874
IM	Gil, C	NJ	765
IM	Gribbon, J	NJ	711
IM	Haggerty, M	NJ	711
IM	Hendricks, J	NY	478
IM	Isaacs, E	NY	614
IM	Kaiser, S	NY	422
IM	Kernan, W	CT	908
IM	Lebofsky, M	NY	614
IM	Logan, B	NY	195
IM	Mann, S	NY	195
IM	Masterson, R	NJ	788
IM	Melman, M	NY	615
IM	Minkowitz, S	NY	195
IM	Mojtabai, S	NY	380
IM	Molloy, E	CT	875
IM	Mutterperl, M	NJ	735
IM	Pecker, M	NY	196
IM	Pollak, H	NY	510
IM	Rosch, E	NY	615
IM	Rucker, S	NY	510
IM	Scaduto, P	NJ	806
IM	Solomon, G	NY	197
IM	Soltren, R	NY	615
IM	Tal, A	NY	423
IM	Teffera, F	NY	381
IM	Underberg, J	NY	197
IM	Volpe, A	NJ	673
IM	Walsh, F	CT	876
IM	Weine, G	NJ	806
IM	Weinstein, M	NY	510
IM	Witt, M	NY	198
IM	Zeale, P	NY	198
Nep	Adler, S	NY	620
Nep	Ames, R	NY	214
Nep	August, P	NY	214
Nep	Bellucci, A	NY	515
Nep	Blumenfeld, J	NY	214
Nep	Brown, E	CT	879
Nep	Buzzeo, L	NY	620
Nep	Byrd, L	NJ	713
Nep	Charytan, C	NY	383
Nep	Chou, S	NY	426
Nep	Coco, M	NY	383
Nep	Covit, A	NJ	767
Nep	Croll, J	NY	383
Nep	De Fabritus, A	NY	214
Nep	Devita, M	NY	215
Nep	Fein, D	NJ	676
Nep	Feintzeig, I	CT	879
Nep	Fine, P	NJ	807
Nep	Flis, R	NJ	790
Nep	Galler, M	NY	465
Nep	Gardenswartz, M	NY	215
Nep	Garfinkel, H	CT	879
Nep	Garrick, R	NY	620
Nep	Goldstein, C	NJ	848
Nep	Gorkin, J	NY	383
Nep	Grasso, M	NJ	713
Nep	Grodstein, G	NJ	676
Nep	Hines, W	CT	879
Nep	Kabis, S	NJ	833
Nep	Kleiner, M	NY	480
Nep	Kostadaras, A	NY	465
Nep	Kozin, A	NY	556
Nep	Kozlowski, J	NJ	676
Nep	Levin, D	NJ	677
Nep	Lipner, H	NY	426
Nep	Liu, D	NY	215
Nep	Lynn, R	NY	383
Nep	Mailloux, L	NY	515
Nep	Manning, E	NJ	790
Nep	Mattana, J	NY	515
Nep	Mattoo, N	NY	465
Nep	McAnally, J	NJ	848
Nep	Michelis, M	NY	215
Nep	Mittman, N	NY	426
Nep	Najarian, J	NJ	807
Nep	Neelakantappa, K	NY	426
Nep	Pannone, J	NY	426
Nep	Parnes, E	NY	427
Nep	Pattner, A	NJ	677
Nep	Reda, D	NY	620
Nep	Rie, J	NY	620
Nep	Rigolosi, R	NJ	677
Nep	Ruddy, M	NJ	746
Nep	Saltzman, M	NY	620
Nep	Schwarz, R	NY	575
Nep	Scott, D	NY	465
Nep	Shapiro, K	NY	556
Nep	Shapiro, W	NY	427
Nep	Shein, L	NY	427
Nep	Sherman, R	NY	215
Nep	Singhal, P	NY	515
Nep	Sipzner, R	NJ	714
Nep	Spinowitz, B	NY	466
Nep	Spitalewitz, S	NY	427
Nep	Tartini, A	NJ	677
Nep	Thomsen, S	NJ	735
Nep	Uday, K	NY	383
Nep	Vitting, K	NJ	821
Nep	Wagner, J	NY	515
Nep	Wang, J	NY	216
Nep	Wei, F	NJ	746
Nep	Weizman, H	NJ	677
Nep	Yablon, S	NY	556
Nep	Yoo, J	NY	383
PNep	Johnson, V	NY	289
PNep	Kaplan, M	NY	440
PNep	Perelstein, E	NY	289
PNep	Roberti, I	NJ	721
PNep	Salcedo-Contreras, J	NJ	824
PNep	Satlin, L	NY	289
PNep	Schoeneman, M	NY	440
PNep	Trachtman, H	NY	532
PNep	Weiss, L	NJ	775

Hypertension in Children

PNep	Saland, J	NY	289
PNep	Singh, A	NJ	775

Hypertension in Pregnancy

MF	Bond, A	CT	877
MF	Funai, E	CT	908
Nep	August, P	NY	214
Nep	Gardenswartz, M	NY	215

Hypertrophic Cardiomyopathy

Cv	Blum, M	NJ	801
Cv	Weissman, R	NY	598
PCd	Addonizio, L	NY	281

Special Expertise Index

Spec	Name	St	Pg
RE	Navot, D	NJ	693
RE	Noyes, N	NY	332
RE	Patrizio, P	CT	919
RE	Ransom, M	NJ	825
RE	Richlin, S	CT	894
RE	Rosenfeld, D	NY	543
RE	Rosenwaks, Z	NY	332
RE	Sandler, B	NY	332
RE	Sauer, M	NY	332
RE	Schmidt-Sarosi, C	NY	333
RE	Scott, R	NJ	814
RE	Seifer, D	NY	447
RE	Spandorfer, S	NY	333
RE	Stangel, J	NY	644
RE	Sultan, K	NY	333
RE	Taylor, H	CT	919
RE	Treiser, S	NJ	836
RE	Witt, B	CT	894

Infertility-IVF Failure

ObG	Scher, J	NY	237

Infertility-Male

ObG	Melnick, H	NY	236
U	Bar-Chama, N	NY	353
U	Basralian, K	NJ	696
U	Fisch, H	NY	355
U	Girardi, S	NY	548
U	Goldstein, M	NY	355
U	Lessing, J	NY	486
U	Lizza, E	NY	357
U	Matthews, G	NY	649
U	McCullough, A	NY	357
U	Mellinger, B	NY	549
U	Mulhall, J	NY	357
U	Nagler, H	NY	357
U	Roberts, L	NY	650
U	Sadeghi-Nejad, H	NJ	697
U	Schiff, H	NY	359
U	Schlegel, P	NY	359

Infertility-Male in Spinal Cord Injury

U	Linsenmeyer, T	NJ	729

Inflammatory Arthritis

Rhu	Gibofsky, A	NY	335

Inflammatory Bowel Disease

CRS	Arnell, T	NY	142
CRS	Chinn, B	NJ	759
CRS	Eisenstat, T	NJ	759
CRS	Longo, W	CT	904

Spec	Name	St	Pg
CRS	McClane, S	CT	868
CRS	Milsom, J	NY	143
CRS	Moskowitz, R	NJ	802
CRS	Nizin, J	NJ	663
CRS	Ozuner, G	NY	553
CRS	Penzer, J	NY	143
CRS	Rezac, C	NJ	759
CRS	Ross, H	NJ	786
CRS	Rothberg, R	NJ	706
CRS	Sonoda, T	NY	143
CRS	Zinkin, L	NJ	759
Ge	Abemayor, E	NY	607
Ge	Aisenberg, J	NY	163
Ge	Baiocco, P	NY	163
Ge	Bartolomeo, R	NY	503
Ge	Bleicher, R	NJ	820
Ge	Blumstein, M	NY	503
Ge	Bonheim, N	CT	871
Ge	Brandt, L	NY	375
Ge	Chinitz, M	NY	607
Ge	Dalena, J	NJ	804
Ge	Dobbins, J	CT	905
Ge	Dworkin, B	NY	607
Ge	Finkelstein, W	NJ	708
Ge	Gardner, P	CT	871
Ge	Goldblatt, R	NY	608
Ge	Greenberg, R	NY	504
Ge	Grossman, E	CT	871
Ge	Gruss, C	CT	871
Ge	Itzkowitz, S	NY	168
Ge	Jaffin, B	NY	168
Ge	Kahn, O	NY	608
Ge	Katz, S	NY	504
Ge	Kerner, M	NJ	845
Ge	Kressner, M	NY	609
Ge	Landau, S	NY	609
Ge	Liss, M	NY	609
Ge	Ludwig, S	NJ	787
Ge	Maizel, B	NY	417
Ge	Margulis, S	NJ	668
Ge	Marin, G	NJ	743
Ge	Meirowitz, R	NJ	743
Ge	Milman, P	NY	505
Ge	Mogan, G	NJ	708
Ge	Nagler, J	NY	171
Ge	Nussbaum, M	NY	461
Ge	Panella, V	NJ	669
Ge	Proctor, D	CT	905
Ge	Ramgopal, M	NY	461
Ge	Roston, A	NY	609
Ge	Roth, J	NJ	669
Ge	Rubin, K	NJ	669
Ge	Rubin, M	NY	172
Ge	Sable, R	NY	376
Ge	Sachs, J	NJ	743

Spec	Name	St	Pg
Ge	Salik, J	NY	172
Ge	Scherl, E	NY	172
Ge	Shapiro, N	NY	609
Ge	Sloan, W	NJ	709
Ge	Spielberg, A	NY	571
Ge	Spira, R	NJ	709
Ge	Taffet, S	NY	610
Ge	Taubin, H	CT	872
Ge	Turtel, P	NJ	787
Ge	Weissman, G	NY	505
Ge	Zimbalist, E	NY	417
IM	Bains, Y	NJ	711
PGe	Chawla, A	NY	581
PGe	Daum, F	NY	530
PGe	Halata, M	NY	633
PGe	Kazlow, P	NY	285
PGe	Levine, J	NY	530
PGe	McFarlane-Ferreira, Y	NY	438
PGe	Newman, L	NY	633
PGe	Rabinowitz, S	NY	483
PGe	Rosh, J	NJ	811
PGe	Schwarz, S	NY	438
PGe	Sunaryo, F	NJ	720
PS	Alexander, F	NJ	687
S	Eng, K	NY	342
S	Rolandelli, R	NJ	815

Inflammatory Bowel Disease-Consult

Ge	Sachar, D	NY	172

Inflammatory Bowel Disease/Crohn's

CRS	Procaccino, J	NY	497
CRS	Steinhagen, R	NY	143
Ge	Ben-Zvi, J	NY	164
Ge	Chapman, M	NY	165
Ge	Erber, W	NY	415
Ge	Fisher, R	CT	905
Ge	Fiske, S	NJ	708
Ge	Frank, M	NY	166
Ge	Goldenberg, D	NJ	845
Ge	Goldin, H	NY	167
Ge	Gutwein, I	NY	376
Ge	Kenny, R	NJ	708
Ge	Kimball, A	NY	168
Ge	Lebwohl, O	NY	169
Ge	Mauer, K	CT	871
Ge	Mayer, I	NY	417
Ge	Mayer, L	NY	170
Ge	Milano, A	NY	171
Ge	Ullman, T	NY	173
Ge	Weg, A	NY	462
Ge	Wickremesinghe, P	NY	478

Special Expertise Index

Spec	Name	St	Pg
IM	Klein, N	CT	875
PEn	Slonim, A	NY	284
PGe	Benkov, K	NY	285
PGe	Birnbaum, A	NY	633
PGe	Glassman, M	CT	887
PGe	Kessler, B	NY	581
PGe	Markowitz, J	NY	530
PGe	Mones, R	NJ	811
PGe	Sockolow, R	NY	285
PGe	Spivak, W	NY	285
PGe	Weinstein, T	NY	530
PS	Dolgin, S	NY	532

Inflammatory Muscle Disease

Rhu	Abramson, S	NY	333
Rhu	Guma, M	NJ	693

Inherited Disorders of Nervous System

N	Kolodny, E	NY	224

Inherited Metabolic Disorders

CG	Desnick, R	NY	142
CG	Seashore, M	CT	903

Insect Allergies

A&I	Bell, J	CT	865
A&I	Chernack, W	NJ	801
A&I	Geraci-Ciardullo, K	NY	594
A&I	Krol, K	NJ	829
A&I	Lang, P	NY	490
A&I	Leibner, D	NJ	757
A&I	Shepherd, G	NY	126
A&I	Sher, E	NJ	785

Intensity Modulated Radiotherapy (IMRT)

RadRO	Gejerman, G	NJ	692
RadRO	Katz, A	NY	586
RadRO	Lee, N	NY	329
RadRO	Potters, L	NY	543
RadRO	Rosenbaum, A	NY	330
RadRO	Spera, J	CT	893

International Health

Inf	Allegra, D	NJ	805
PrM	Cahill, J	NY	309
PrM	Cahill, K	NY	309

Interstitial Cystitis

U	Lieberman, E	NY	548
U	Marks, J	NY	357
U	Moldwin, R	NY	549

Interstitial Lung Disease

Path	Travis, W	NY	280
Pul	Addrizzo-Harris, D	NY	324
Pul	Arcasoy, S	NY	324
Pul	Binder, R	NY	642
Pul	Fishman, D	NY	325
Pul	Libby, D	NY	326
Pul	Maniatis, T	NY	484
Pul	O'Donnell, T	NJ	814
Pul	Riley, D	NJ	778
Pul	Saleh, A	NY	446
Pul	Sasso, L	NY	485
Pul	Sklarek, H	NY	585
Pul	Stover-Pepe, D	NY	328
Pul	Teirstein, A	NY	328

Interventional Cardiology

CE	Cohen, M	NY	594
Cv	Blum, M	NJ	801
Cv	Cabin, H	CT	901
Cv	Charney, R	NY	595
Cv	Chengot, M	NY	564
Cv	Ciccone, J	NJ	704
Cv	Cleman, M	CT	902
Cv	Cohen, H	NY	129
Cv	Dervan, J	NY	564
Cv	Ezratty, A	NY	492
Cv	Feit, A	NY	408
Cv	Goldstein, J	NJ	704
Cv	Goldweit, R	NJ	661
Cv	Green, S	NY	493
Cv	Greenberg, M	NY	368
Cv	Jeremias, A	NY	564
Cv	Julie, E	NJ	819
Cv	Kantrowitz, N	NY	409
Cv	Klapholz, M	NJ	704
Cv	Koss, J	NY	493
Cv	Landers, D	NJ	661
Cv	Lowell, B	NJ	802
Cv	Meizlish, J	CT	867
Cv	Menegus, M	NY	369
Cv	Pappas, T	NY	494
Cv	Pucillo, A	NY	597
Cv	Radwaner, B	NY	135
Cv	Reison, D	NJ	662
Cv	Rossakis, C	NJ	662
Cv	Shamoon, F	NJ	704
Cv	Sherman, W	NY	136
Cv	Shlofmitz, R	NY	494
Cv	Swamy, S	NY	476
Cv	Vazzana, T	NY	476
Cv	Wangenheim, P	NJ	705

Spec	Name	St	Pg
IC	Lituchy, A	NY	511
IC	Miller, K	NJ	712
PCd	Biancaniello, T	NY	581
PCd	Hellenbrand, W	NY	282
PCd	Hsu, D	NY	389
PCd	Levchuck, S	NY	528
PCd	Love, B	NY	282
PCd	Messina, J	NJ	685
PCd	Reitman, M	NY	528
TS	Williams, M	NY	353

Interventional Neuroradiology

NRad	Berenstein, A	NY	230
NRad	Fiorella, D	NY	576
NRad	Keller, I	NJ	769
NRad	Meyers, P	NY	231
NRad	Ortiz, O	NY	518
NRad	Pile-Spellman, J	NY	518
NRad	Roychowdhury, S	NJ	769
NRad	Schonfeld, S	NJ	769
NS	Patel, A	NY	219

Interventional Oncology

VIR	Nosher, J	NJ	781

Interventional Pulmonology

Pul	Malovany, R	NJ	691

Interventional Radiology

DR	Poplausky, M	NY	604
DR	Strauss, E	CT	869
DR	Weck, S	NY	500
VIR	Brown, K	NY	361
VIR	Crystal, K	NY	549

Intraocular Lenses

Oph	Rubin, L	NY	522

Invasive Cardiology

Cv	Hershman, R	NY	493
Cv	Leeds, R	NJ	829
Cv	Saulino, P	NJ	830
Cv	Swamy, S	NY	476
Cv	Vazzana, T	NY	476

Irritable Bowel Syndrome

Ge	Abemayor, E	NY	607
Ge	Accurso, C	NJ	831
Ge	Bleicher, R	NJ	820
Ge	Duva, J	NY	571
Ge	Field, S	NY	166
Ge	Friedlander, C	NY	166

Special Expertise Index

Spec	Name	St	Pg
Nep	Kleiner, M	NY	480
Nep	Kliger, A	CT	911
Nep	Lipner, H	NY	426
Nep	McAnally, J	NJ	848
Nep	Michelis, M	NY	215
Nep	Neelakantappa, K	NY	426
Nep	Pattner, A	NJ	677
Nep	Reda, D	NY	620
Nep	Rigolosi, R	NJ	677
Nep	Salifu, M	NY	427
Nep	Saltzman, M	NY	620
Nep	Schwarz, R	NY	575
Nep	Scott, D	NY	465
Nep	Sudhakar, T	NJ	746
Nep	Tartini, A	NJ	677
Nep	Thomsen, S	NJ	735
Nep	Yoo, J	NY	383
PNep	Nash, M	NY	289
PNep	Saland, J	NY	289
PNep	Seigle, R	NY	290
PNep	Weiss, L	NJ	775
PNep	Whyte, D	NY	582

Kidney Disease-Chronic

Spec	Name	St	Pg
IM	Alterman, L	NJ	846
Nep	De Fabritus, A	NY	214
Nep	Devita, M	NY	215
Nep	Fishbane, S	NY	515
Nep	Fogel, M	CT	879
Nep	Pannone, J	NY	426
Nep	Winston, J	NY	216
PNep	Kaskel, F	NY	391

Kidney Disease-Diabetic

Spec	Name	St	Pg
Nep	Shapiro, K	NY	556
Nep	Spinowitz, B	NY	466

Kidney Disease-Hereditary

Spec	Name	St	Pg
PNep	Satlin, L	NY	289

Kidney Disease-Metabolic

Spec	Name	St	Pg
Nep	Kliger, A	CT	911

Kidney Disease-Pediatric & Adult

Spec	Name	St	Pg
Nep	Rosen, M	NY	620

Kidney Failure

Spec	Name	St	Pg
Ger	Russell, R	NY	377
Nep	Adler, S	NY	620
Nep	Bellucci, A	NY	515
Nep	Covit, A	NJ	767

Spec	Name	St	Pg
Nep	Fine, P	NJ	807
Nep	Goldstein, C	NJ	848
Nep	Gorkin, J	NY	383
Nep	Liu, D	NY	215
Nep	Lyman, N	NJ	713
Nep	Matalon, R	NY	215
Nep	Mattoo, N	NY	465
Nep	Najarian, J	NJ	807
Nep	Shapiro, W	NY	427
Nep	Sipzner, R	NJ	714
Nep	Vitting, K	NJ	821
Nep	Winston, J	NY	216
Nep	Yablon, S	NY	556
PNep	Nash, M	NY	289
PNep	Perelstein, E	NY	289
PNep	Roberti, I	NJ	721
PNep	Salcedo-Contreras, J	NJ	824
PNep	Seigle, R	NY	290
PNep	Weiss, R	NY	634

Kidney Failure-Chronic

Spec	Name	St	Pg
IM	Rubenstein, J	NY	510
Nep	Chan, B	CT	879
Nep	Croll, J	NY	383
Nep	Delano, B	NY	426
Nep	Kozin, A	NY	556
Nep	Shapiro, W	NY	427
Nep	Sherman, R	NY	215
Nep	Stern, L	NY	216
Nep	Wagner, J	NY	515
PNep	Lieberman, K	NJ	686
PNep	Schoeneman, M	NY	440
PNep	Weiss, L	NJ	775

Kidney Imaging

Spec	Name	St	Pg
NuM	Scharf, S	NY	232

Kidney Stones

Spec	Name	St	Pg
IM	Constantiner, A	NY	191
IM	Rucker, S	NY	510
IM	Zackson, D	NY	198
Nep	Aronson, P	CT	911
Nep	Bellucci, A	NY	515
Nep	Charytan, C	NY	383
Nep	Garfinkel, H	CT	879
Nep	Kostadaras, A	NY	465
Nep	Rie, J	NY	620
Nep	Spinowitz, B	NY	466
Nep	Wei, F	NJ	746
PNep	Roberti, I	NJ	721
PNep	Singh, A	NJ	775
U	Andriani, R	CT	897
U	Berdini, J	NJ	697
U	Berman, S	NY	353

Spec	Name	St	Pg
U	Birkhoff, J	NY	353
U	Boorjian, P	NJ	728
U	Brodherson, M	NY	354
U	Bruno, A	NY	548
U	Colton, M	NJ	816
U	DelPizzo, J	NY	354
U	Dillon, R	NY	354
U	Eshghi, A	NY	649
U	Fine, E	NY	354
U	Giella, J	NY	560
U	Grasso, M	NY	355
U	Grebler, A	NJ	797
U	Gribetz, M	NY	355
U	Grunberger, I	NY	452
U	Harris, S	NY	548
U	Housman, A	NY	649
U	Irwin, M	NY	452
U	Kaminetsky, J	NY	356
U	Katz, H	NJ	738
U	Katz, J	NJ	728
U	Klein, G	NY	356
U	Landman, J	NY	356
U	Layne, J	NY	548
U	Lehrhoff, B	NJ	857
U	Lessing, J	NY	486
U	Leventhal, A	NY	548
U	Loo, M	NY	357
U	Marks, J	NY	357
U	Meisenberg, G	NY	452
U	Munver, R	NJ	697
U	Palese, M	NY	358
U	Peng, B	NY	358
U	Provet, J	NY	358
U	Putignano, J	NY	650
U	Raboy, A	NY	486
U	Ranta, J	CT	897
U	Richards, S	NJ	780
U	Ring, K	NJ	857
U	Rosenthal, S	NY	452
U	Rossman, B	NJ	753
U	Rotolo, J	NJ	797
U	Rudin, L	NY	560
U	Saada, S	NY	452
U	Savino, M	NY	486
U	Shepard, B	NY	549
U	Shulman, Y	NJ	738
U	Sosa, R	NY	360
U	Steigman, E	NJ	738
U	Stone, P	NY	401
U	Strauss, B	NJ	729
U	Tarasuk, A	NY	472
U	Viner, N	CT	897
U	Wasserman, G	NJ	698
U	Williams, J	NY	361
U	Ziegelbaum, M	NY	549

Special Expertise Index

Spec	Name	St	Pg
S	Carter, M	NJ	815
S	Christoudias, G	NJ	695
S	Grieco, M	NY	545

Laparoscopic Hernia Repair

Spec	Name	St	Pg
S	Christoudias, G	NJ	695

Laparoscopic Hysterectomy

Spec	Name	St	Pg
ObG	Goldstein, S	NJ	791
ObG	Mendelowitz, L	NY	624

Laparoscopic Kidney Surgery

Spec	Name	St	Pg
U	DelPizzo, J	NY	354
U	Esposito, M	NJ	697

Laparoscopic Surgery

Spec	Name	St	Pg
CRS	Arnell, T	NY	142
CRS	Arvanitis, M	NJ	785
CRS	Chinn, B	NJ	759
CRS	Greenwald, M	NY	496
CRS	Krakovitz, E	NY	600
CRS	Milsom, J	NY	143
CRS	Ozuner, G	NY	553
CRS	Ross, H	NJ	786
CRS	Sonoda, T	NY	143
CRS	Temple, L	NY	143
CRS	Thornton, S	CT	868
CRS	Waxenbaum, S	NJ	663
CRS	Whelan, R	NY	144
CRS	Wishner, J	NY	601
GO	Azodi, M	CT	906
GO	Barakat, R	NY	177
GO	Brown, C	NY	177
GO	Chuang, L	NY	611
GO	Curtin, J	NY	177
GO	Denehy, T	NJ	709
GO	Dottino, P	NY	177
GO	Herzog, T	NY	177
GO	Holcomb, K	NY	177
GO	Poynor, E	NY	178
GO	Rahaman, J	NY	178
GO	Serur, E	NY	418
GO	Tobias, D	NJ	805
ObG	Banzon, M	NJ	735
ObG	Beim, R	NJ	849
ObG	Brodman, M	NY	233
ObG	Cooperman, A	NJ	715
ObG	Englert, C	NJ	680
ObG	Florio, P	NY	623
ObG	Goldstein, M	NY	234
ObG	Grano, V	NY	623
ObG	Haselkorn, J	NY	519
ObG	Hurst, W	NJ	680

Spec	Name	St	Pg
ObG	Iammatteo, M	NJ	808
ObG	Krim, E	NY	519
ObG	Luciani, R	NJ	715
ObG	Lynch, V	CT	912
ObG	Meacham, K	NY	624
ObG	Mohr, R	NJ	808
ObG	Nimaroff, M	NY	519
ObG	Olanescu, A	NY	466
ObG	Sailon, P	NY	237
ObG	Sassoon, R	NY	237
ObG	Wallis, J	NJ	808
PS	Friedman, D	NJ	687
PS	Gandhi, R	NJ	687
RE	Copperman, A	NY	331
RE	Fateh, M	NY	331
RE	Grifo, J	NY	331
RE	Grunfeld, L	NY	331
RE	Kofinas, G	NY	447
RE	Matera, C	NY	332
RE	Sultan, K	NY	333
S	Adler, H	NY	448
S	Amory, S	NY	340
S	Andrei, V	NJ	726
S	Ballantyne, G	NJ	694
S	Barcewicz, P	CT	920
S	Bellemare, S	NY	398
S	Bessler, M	NY	341
S	Bufalini, B	NJ	695
S	Carter, M	NJ	815
S	Chamberlain, R	NJ	726
S	Chung-Loy, H	NJ	779
S	Cohen, B	NY	588
S	Colaco, R	NJ	856
S	Cosgrove, J	NY	399
S	Dasmahapatra, K	NJ	779
S	Denoto, G	NY	545
S	Fahoum, B	NY	449
S	Feigenbaum, H	NJ	825
S	Fielding, G	NY	342
S	Fleischer, L	NY	560
S	Fried, K	NJ	695
S	Frost, J	NJ	856
S	Gecelter, G	NY	545
S	Genato, R	NY	449
S	Gorecki, P	NY	450
S	Greenstein, S	NY	399
S	Herron, D	NY	343
S	Hornyak, S	NY	485
S	Jordan, L	NJ	752
S	Kassel, B	NY	647
S	Kennedy, T	NY	399
S	Khalife, M	NY	545
S	Kimmelstiel, F	NY	344
S	Lau, H	NY	647
S	Licata, J	NJ	695

Spec	Name	St	Pg
S	Molinelli, B	CT	895
S	Nitzberg, R	NJ	856
S	Pahuja, M	NY	485
S	Passeri, D	CT	896
S	Rajdeo, H	NY	647
S	Rajpal, S	NY	450
S	Rangraj, M	NY	647
S	Reiner, D	NY	546
S	Reiner, M	NY	346
S	Ren-Fielding, C	NY	346
S	Romero, C	NY	546
S	Sas, N	NY	399
S	Schechner, R	NY	399
S	Schwartzman, A	NY	450
S	Shah, P	NY	347
S	Shapiro, M	NY	588
S	Silvestri, F	NJ	695
S	Slater, G	NY	347
S	Starker, P	NJ	856
S	Sung, K	NY	471
S	Sussman, B	NJ	695
S	Zenilman, M	NY	451
S	Zingale, R	NY	588
U	Eshghi, A	NY	649
U	Grasso, M	NY	355
U	Hajjar, J	NJ	697
U	Katz, S	NJ	697
U	Kavoussi, L	NY	548
U	Palese, M	NY	358
U	Savino, M	NY	486
U	Silver, D	NY	453
U	Sosa, R	NY	360
U	Vukasin, A	NJ	753
U	Ziegelbaum, M	NY	549
VascS	Wolodiger, F	NJ	699

Laparoscopic Surgery-Complex

Spec	Name	St	Pg
ObG	Besser, G	CT	882
ObG	Goldman, G	NY	234
ObG	Quartell, A	NJ	715
ObG	Ullman, J	NY	625
ObG	Violi, C	CT	882
S	Drascher, G	NJ	836

Laparoscopy/Hysteroscopy

Spec	Name	St	Pg
ObG	Armbruster, R	NY	623
ObG	Duvivier, R	NY	385

Laryngeal & Vocal Cord Surgery

Spec	Name	St	Pg
Oto	Sulica, R	NY	275

Special Expertise Index

Spec	Name	St	Pg
Lens Implants			
Oph	Finlay, A	CT	882
Oph	Goldberg, D	NJ	791
Oph	Potter, W	CT	883
Oph	Silbert, G	NJ	681
Lens Implants-Multifocal			
Oph	Dieck, W	NY	625
Oph	Mackool, R	NY	467
Oph	Malik, S	NY	521
Oph	Wong, M	NJ	748
Leukemia			
Hem	Cohen, N	CT	873
Hem	Cook, P	NY	181
Hem	Duffy, T	CT	907
Hem	Forget, B	CT	907
Hem	Halperin, I	NY	182
Hem	Kempin, S	NY	183
Hem	Leonard, J	NY	183
Hem	Marks, P	CT	907
Hem	Mears, J	NY	183
Hem	Meyer, R	NY	183
Hem	Nimer, S	NY	183
Hem	Ossias, A	NY	184
Hem	Rai, K	NY	507
Hem	Raphael, B	NY	184
Hem	Schulman, P	NY	572
Hem	Strair, R	NJ	764
Hem	Tallman, M	NY	184
Hem	Troy, K	NY	184
Hem	Wisch, N	NY	184
Onc	Berman, E	NY	202
Onc	Cooper, D	CT	909
Onc	Feldman, E	NY	203
Onc	Frank, R	CT	878
Onc	Gabrilove, J	NY	204
Onc	Goldberg, S	NJ	674
Onc	Jakubowski, A	NY	206
Onc	Jurcic, J	NY	206
Onc	Liu, D	NY	618
Onc	Maslak, P	NY	207
Onc	Ostrow, S	NY	575
Onc	Raza, A	NY	210
Onc	Scheinberg, D	NY	211
Onc	Seiter, K	NY	619
Path	Knowles, D	NY	279
PHO	Aledo, A	NY	286
PHO	Cairo, M	NY	286
PHO	Carroll, W	NY	286
PHO	Guarini, L	NY	439
PHO	Kamalakar, P	NJ	720
PHO	Kamen, B	NJ	774
PHO	Kernan, N	NY	287

Spec	Name	St	Pg
PHO	Kulpa, J	NY	439
PHO	Marcus, J	NY	287
PHO	Redner, A	NY	531
PHO	Sundaram, R	NY	439
PHO	Weiner, M	NY	288
Leukemia & Lymphoma			
Hem	Allen, S	NY	507
Hem	Bar, M	CT	872
Hem	Dosik, H	NY	419
Hem	Hymes, K	NY	182
Hem	Kolitz, J	NY	507
Hem	Vogel, J	NY	184
Onc	Coleman, M	NY	203
Onc	Decter, J	NY	203
Onc	Farber, C	NJ	806
Onc	Hollister, D	CT	878
Onc	Silverman, L	NY	211
PHO	Halpern, S	NJ	685
PHO	Harris, M	NJ	686
PHO	Rausen, A	NY	288
PHO	Steinherz, P	NY	288
PHO	Tugal, O	NY	634
PHO	Weinblatt, M	NY	531
Leukemia-Chronic Lymphocytic			
Onc	Bernhardt, B	NY	617
Liaison Psychiatry			
Psyc	Heisman, A	NY	444
Psyc	Kalash, G	NY	469
Psyc	Shapiro, P	NY	320
Psyc	Vivek, S	NY	469
Ligament Reconstruction			
HS	Lisser, S	NJ	787
OrS	Hannafin, J	NY	258
SM	Levy, A	NJ	726
Limb Deformities			
OrS	Feldman, D	NY	257
OrS	Rozbruch, S	NY	264
OrS	Sabharwal, S	NJ	718
OrS	Widmann, R	NY	267
Limb Lengthening			
OrS	Rozbruch, S	NY	264
OrS	Widmann, R	NY	267
Limb Lengthening (Ilizarov Procedure)			
OrS	Egol, K	NY	256

Spec	Name	St	Pg
OrS	Sabharwal, S	NJ	718
OrS	Vitale, M	NY	266
Limb Sparing Surgery			
OrS	Benevenia, J	NJ	717
VascS	Ascher, E	NY	453
VascS	Chaudhry, S	NY	549
VascS	Manno, J	NJ	698
VascS	Marin, M	NY	363
VascS	Mendes, D	NY	363
Limb Surgery/Reconstruction			
OrS	Friedlaender, G	CT	913
OrS	Rozbruch, S	NY	264
Liposuction			
D	Bank, D	NY	601
D	Kenet, B	NY	148
D	Narins, R	NY	602
D	Orentreich, D	NY	149
D	Sklar, J	NY	499
D	Sobel, H	NY	152
D	Urbanek, R	NY	476
D	Wexler, P	NY	153
PlS	Almeyda, E	NY	301
PlS	Anton, J	NY	584
PlS	Birnbaum, J	NY	301
PlS	Breitbart, A	NY	535
PlS	Cutolo, L	NY	484
PlS	Funt, D	NY	536
PlS	Gotkin, R	NY	537
PlS	Hawrylo, R	NJ	813
PlS	Hoffman, L	NY	304
PlS	Leach, T	NJ	750
PlS	Matarasso, A	NY	305
PlS	Ofodile, F	NJ	689
PlS	Perry, A	NJ	835
PlS	Pitman, G	NY	306
PlS	Schulman, M	NY	306
PlS	Verga, M	NY	308
PlS	Zevon, S	NY	309
Liposuction & Body Contouring			
PlS	Alizadeh, K	NY	535
PlS	Aston, S	NY	301
PlS	Attkiss, K	CT	890
PlS	Broumand, S	NY	302
PlS	Colen, H	NY	302
PlS	Cuber, S	NJ	777
PlS	Diktaban, T	NY	303
PlS	Friedlander, B	NJ	723
PlS	Friedman, D	NY	303
PlS	Gewirtz, H	CT	890

Special Expertise Index

Lung Cancer-Early Detection

Lung Disease

Special Expertise Index

Spec	Name	St	Pg
N	Petito, F	NY	227
Plnf	Andiman, W	CT	915
Plnf	Boscamp, J	NJ	686
Plnf	Krilov, L	NY	531
Plnf	Munoz, J	NY	634
Plnf	Nachman, S	NY	582
Plnf	Shapiro, E	CT	916
Plnf	Sood, S	NY	532
Plnf	Tolan, R	NJ	775
PRhu	Eichenfield, A	NY	292
PRhu	Ilowite, N	NY	391
PRhu	Lazarus, H	NY	292
Rhu	Craft, J	CT	920
Rhu	Faller, J	NY	334
Rhu	Hutchinson, G	CT	920
Rhu	Magid, S	NY	336
Rhu	Meed, S	NY	336
Rhu	Miller, K	CT	894
Rhu	Schoen, R	CT	920

Lyme Disease-Neuro Complications

Psyc	Fallon, B	NY	312

Lymph Node Pathology

Path	Knowles, D	NY	279
Path	Orazi, A	NY	279

Lymphedema

PHO	Blei, F	NY	286
PMR	Francis, K	NJ	722
PMR	Richter, E	CT	890

Lymphoma

Hem	Avvento, L	NY	572
Hem	Cook, P	NY	181
Hem	Diaz, M	NY	182
Hem	Duffy, T	CT	907
Hem	Goldenberg, A	NY	182
Hem	Kempin, S	NY	183
Hem	Leonard, J	NY	183
Hem	Lester, T	NY	611
Hem	Mears, J	NY	183
Hem	Meyer, R	NY	183
Hem	Moskovits, T	NY	183
Hem	Ossias, A	NY	184
Hem	Rai, K	NY	507
Hem	Raphael, B	NY	184
Hem	Sabnani, I	NJ	709
Hem	Savage, D	NY	184
Hem	Schulman, P	NY	572
Hem	Strair, R	NJ	764
Hem	Topilow, A	NJ	788

Spec	Name	St	Pg
Hem	Troy, K	NY	184
Hem	Wisch, N	NY	184
Onc	Adler, K	NJ	806
Onc	Ahmed, T	NY	617
Onc	Akhund, B	NY	574
Onc	Astrow, A	NY	424
Onc	Attas, L	NJ	674
Onc	Berman, E	NY	202
Onc	Bernhardt, B	NY	617
Onc	Budman, D	NY	512
Onc	Camacho, F	NY	381
Onc	Caron, P	NY	617
Onc	Caruso, R	NY	574
Onc	Cohen, S	NY	203
Onc	Cooper, D	CT	909
Onc	Cortes, E	NY	464
Onc	Dutcher, J	NY	381
Onc	Feldman, S	NY	617
Onc	Frank, R	CT	878
Onc	Goldberg, J	NY	617
Onc	Goy, A	NJ	674
Onc	Greenberg, H	NY	465
Onc	Grossbard, L	NY	204
Onc	Grossbard, M	NY	204
Onc	Gulati, S	NY	204
Onc	Hassoun, H	NY	205
Onc	Liu, D	NY	618
Onc	Lo, K	CT	878
Onc	Lonberg, M	NY	555
Onc	Lowenthal, D	NJ	847
Onc	Lundberg, W	CT	910
Onc	Nissenblatt, M	NJ	766
Onc	Offit, K	NY	208
Onc	Ostrow, S	NY	575
Onc	Papish, S	NJ	806
Onc	Pasmantier, M	NY	209
Onc	Phillips, E	NY	618
Onc	Portlock, C	NY	209
Onc	Saponara, E	NY	619
Onc	Sara, G	NY	211
Onc	Sierocki, J	NJ	745
Onc	Sparano, J	NY	382
Onc	Straus, D	NY	212
Onc	Yi, P	NJ	746
Onc	Zelenetz, A	NY	213
Path	Knowles, D	NY	279
PHO	Aledo, A	NY	286
PHO	Cairo, M	NY	286
PHO	Marcus, J	NY	287
PHO	Parker, R	NY	581
PHO	Weiner, M	NY	288
RadRO	Bosworth, J	NY	542
RadRO	Goodman, R	NJ	725
RadRO	Ingenito, A	NJ	692
RadRO	Marin, L	NY	542

Spec	Name	St	Pg
RadRO	Roberts, K	CT	919
RadRO	Yahalom, J	NY	330

Lymphoma Consultation

Onc	DeVita, V	CT	909

Lymphoma, Cutaneous B Cell (CBCL)

RadRO	Wilson, L	CT	919

Lymphoma, Cutaneous T Cell (CTCL)

Onc	Foss, F	CT	909
Onc	Horwitz, S	NY	205
RadRO	Wilson, L	CT	919

Lymphoma, Non-Hodgkin's

NuM	Goldsmith, S	NY	231
Onc	Fitzgerald, D	NJ	789
Onc	Ramirez, M	NY	382
Onc	Wu, H	NJ	832

M

Macular Degeneration

Oph	Angioletti, L	NY	238
Oph	Berman, D	NY	432
Oph	Bhagat, N	NJ	716
Oph	Brecher, R	NY	432
Oph	Cangemi, F	NJ	716
Oph	Cohen, B	NY	240
Oph	Cohen, S	NJ	716
Oph	Del Priore, L	NY	241
Oph	Douros, S	NY	432
Oph	Eichler, J	NJ	716
Oph	Elbaba, F	NY	578
Oph	Fastenberg, D	NY	521
Oph	Feinstein, N	NY	432
Oph	Fleischman, J	NY	625
Oph	Gentile, R	NY	243
Oph	MacKay, C	NY	246
Oph	Paccione, J	NY	248
Oph	Reppucci, V	CT	883
Oph	Rosenthal, J	NY	249
Oph	Sachs, R	NJ	809
Oph	Schubert, H	NY	250
Oph	Slakter, J	NY	251
Oph	Smith, R	NY	251
Oph	Solomon, S	NY	627
Oph	Spaide, R	NY	251

Special Expertise Index

Special Expertise Index

Spec	Name	St	Pg
TS	Tittle, S	CT	896
TS	Widmann, M	NJ	816
TS	Zairis, I	NJ	696

Minimally Invasive Urologic Surgery

Spec	Name	St	Pg
U	Esposito, M	NJ	697
U	Hall, S	NY	355
U	Landman, J	NY	356
U	Lanteri, V	NJ	697
U	Munver, R	NJ	697

Minimally Invasive Vascular Surgery

Spec	Name	St	Pg
VascS	Benvenisty, A	NY	362
VascS	Brener, B	NJ	729
VascS	Dietzek, A	CT	898
VascS	Jacobowitz, G	NY	363
VascS	Schneider, D	NY	364
VascS	Sweeney, T	CT	923
VascS	Todd, G	NY	364

Miscarriage-Recurrent

Spec	Name	St	Pg
MF	Lockwood, C	CT	909
MF	Paidas, M	CT	909
ObG	Friedman, L	NY	234
ObG	Ordorica, S	NY	236
ObG	Scher, J	NY	237
ObG	Young, B	NY	238
RE	David, S	NY	331
RE	Stangel, J	NY	644

Mitral Valve Disease

Spec	Name	St	Pg
Cv	D'Agostino, R	NY	492
Cv	Teichholz, L	NJ	663
IC	Wasserman, H	CT	876
IM	Kennish, A	NY	194

Mitral Valve Minimally Invasive Surgery

Spec	Name	St	Pg
TS	Culliford, A	NY	349
TS	Esposito, R	NY	546

Mitral Valve Prolapse

Spec	Name	St	Pg
Cv	Andersen, H	NY	128
Cv	Freed, L	CT	902
Cv	Kobren, S	NY	493

Mitral Valve Surgery

Spec	Name	St	Pg
TS	Adams, D	NY	348
TS	DeRose, J	NY	400
TS	Filsoufi, F	NY	349

Spec	Name	St	Pg
TS	Grossi, E	NY	350
TS	Hashim, S	CT	921
TS	Naka, Y	NY	351
TS	Smith, C	NY	352

Mobility Evaluation & Treatment

Spec	Name	St	Pg
Ger	Cooney, L	CT	906

Mohs' Surgery

Spec	Name	St	Pg
D	Albom, M	NY	144
D	Ashinoff, R	NJ	664
D	Biro, D	NY	412
D	Bisaccia, E	NJ	803
D	Carucci, J	NY	145
D	Connolly, A	NJ	706
D	Davis, I	NY	601
D	Franck, J	NY	498
D	Geronemus, R	NY	147
D	Goldberg, D	NY	147
D	Kauvar, A	NY	148
D	Kline, M	NY	148
D	Kolenik, S	CT	868
D	Kriegel, D	NY	149
D	Leffell, D	CT	904
D	Marmur, E	NY	149
D	Morman, M	NJ	665
D	Ostad, A	NY	150
D	Prioleau, P	NY	150
D	Prystowsky, J	NY	150
D	Ratner, D	NY	150
D	Robins, P	NY	150
D	Sarnoff, D	NY	498
D	Shelton, R	NY	151
D	Siegel, D	NY	568
D	Spinowitz, A	NY	499
D	Vine, J	NJ	742
D	Waldorf, H	NY	554
D	Wrone, D	NJ	760
D	Zweibel, S	NY	603

Mood Disorders

Spec	Name	St	Pg
ChAP	Bartlett, J	NJ	705
ChAP	Foley, C	NY	495
ChAP	Rubinstein, B	NY	599
Psyc	Asnis, G	NY	396
Psyc	Attia, E	NY	310
Psyc	Badikian, A	NY	639
Psyc	Bauman, J	NY	640
Psyc	Ferran, E	NY	312
Psyc	Finkel, J	NY	312
Psyc	Fyer, M	NY	313
Psyc	Goldberg, J	NY	444
Psyc	Goldman, N	NY	313
Psyc	Hart, S	CT	891

Spec	Name	St	Pg
Psyc	Jacoby, J	NJ	737
Psyc	Jones, F	NJ	777
Psyc	Katz, J	NY	539
Psyc	Kocsis, J	NY	315
Psyc	Kremberg, M	NY	315
Psyc	Licht, A	NY	444
Psyc	Mann, J	NY	316
Psyc	Morgan, C	CT	891
Psyc	Nadel, W	NJ	813
Psyc	Narula, A	NJ	690
Psyc	Rosenfeld, D	NJ	690
Psyc	Rubin, K	NJ	795
Psyc	Russakoff, L	NY	641
Psyc	Schechter, J	CT	891
Psyc	Schneider, S	NJ	751
Psyc	Schwartz, M	NY	585
Psyc	Selzer, J	NY	469
Psyc	Smith, J	CT	892
Psyc	Taylor, N	NY	322
Psyc	Wachtel, A	NY	322

Movement Disorders

Spec	Name	St	Pg
N	Bressman, S	NY	221
N	Fahn, S	NY	222
N	Golbe, L	NJ	768
N	Goodgold, A	NY	223
N	Kaufman, D	NY	384
N	Maniscalco, A	NY	429
N	Olanow, C	NY	227
N	Oribe, E	NY	227
N	Rusk, A	CT	881
N	Salgado, M	NY	430
N	Siegel, K	CT	881
N	Waters, C	NY	229
NS	de Lotbiniere, A	NY	621
NS	Schulder, M	NY	516

Moya Moya

Spec	Name	St	Pg
N	Mohr, J	NY	226

MRI

Spec	Name	St	Pg
DR	Cohen, B	NY	154
DR	Cohen, S	CT	869
DR	Epstein, R	NJ	760
DR	Ford, R	NJ	742
DR	Geller, M	NY	554
DR	Hammel, J	NY	499
DR	Hertz, M	NY	603
DR	Jewel, K	NJ	707
DR	Kazam, E	NY	155
DR	Kirshy, D	NY	568
DR	Knopp, E	NY	155
DR	Krinsky, G	NJ	666
DR	Laks, M	NY	372

Special Expertise Index

Special Expertise Index

Spec	Name	St	Pg
Neurofibromatosis			
CG	Bialer, M	NY	496
CG	Davis, J	NY	142
Neurogenetics			
ChiN	Pavlakis, S	NY	411
Neurogenic Bladder			
U	Blaivas, J	NY	354
U	Foster, H	CT	922
U	Vapnek, J	NY	360
Neurologic Complications-HIV/Infections			
N	Britton, C	NY	221
Neurologic Critical Care			
N	Mayer, S	NY	226
PCCM	Conway, E	NY	283
Neurologic Imaging			
NuM	Strashun, A	NY	430
NuM	Vanheertum, R	NY	232
Neurologic Rehabilitation			
PMR	Ahn, J	NY	298
PMR	Gifford, I	NY	443
Neuromuscular Disorders			
ChiN	De Vivo, D	NY	140
N	Belsh, J	NJ	768
N	Buckner, C	NY	428
N	Cohen, D	NY	576
N	Daras, M	NY	222
N	Dickoff, D	NY	621
N	Fox, S	NJ	808
N	Gerber, O	NY	576
N	Halperin, J	NJ	849
N	Herbert, J	NY	224
N	Herskovitz, S	NY	384
N	Heublum, M	NY	224
N	Holland, N	NJ	790
N	Kelemen, J	NY	517
N	Kula, R	NY	517
N	Lange, D	NY	225
N	Maccabee, P	NY	429
N	Maniscalco, A	NY	429
N	Mitsumoto, H	NY	226
N	Ober, D	NY	556
N	Olarte, M	NY	227
N	Roohi, F	NY	429
N	Ruderman, M	NJ	715

Spec	Name	St	Pg
N	Sander, H	NY	228
N	Simpson, D	NY	229
N	Sivak, M	NY	229
N	Stubgen, J	NY	229
N	Weinberg, H	NY	230
N	Witte, A	NJ	747
PMR	Bach, J	NJ	722
PMR	Cole, J	NJ	722
PMR	Diamond, M	NJ	853
PMR	Fantasia, M	NJ	776
PMR	Strauss, N	NY	300
Neuropathology			
Path	Mirra, S	NY	437
Path	Rosenblum, M	NY	280
Path	Zagzag, D	NY	280
Neurophysiology			
ChiN	Cracco, J	NY	411
ChiN	Levy, S	CT	903
Neuroradiology			
DR	Budin, J	NJ	665
DR	Jacobs, M	NY	155
DR	Knopp, E	NY	155
DR	Leslie, D	NY	604
DR	Melville, G	NJ	830
DR	Sullivan, S	CT	869
DR	Yoon, S	NY	500
DR	Yoon, S	NY	500
NS	Riina, H	NY	219
Neurovascular Surgery			
NS	Hodosh, R	NJ	848
NS	Langer, D	NY	516
NS	Quest, D	NY	219
Newborn Care			
Ped	Goldstein, J	NY	294
Ped	Oghia, H	NY	442
Ped	Versfelt, M	NY	637
Nipple Sparing Mastectomy			
S	Swistel, A	NY	347
Non-Invasive Cardiology			
Cv	Altschul, L	NY	564
Cv	Anto, M	NY	491
Cv	Casale, L	CT	866
Cv	Conroy, D	NJ	660
Cv	Elkind, B	NJ	733
Cv	Epstein, S	NY	130

Spec	Name	St	Pg
Cv	Fishbach, M	NY	595
Cv	Gabelman, G	NY	596
Cv	Greengart, A	NY	409
Cv	Kay, R	NY	596
Cv	Leeds, R	NJ	829
Cv	Medina, E	NY	597
Cv	Robbins, M	NY	457
Cv	Roth, R	NY	553
Cv	Saulino, P	NJ	830
Cv	Schreiber, C	NY	494
Cv	Shimony, R	NY	136
Cv	Southren, D	NY	553
Cv	Vazzana, T	NY	476
Cv	Winter, S	NY	476
IM	Lipton, M	NY	195
Noonan Syndrome			
PCd	Gelb, B	NY	282
Nuclear Cardiology			
Cv	Altschul, L	NY	564
Cv	Bergmann, S	NY	128
Cv	Blake, J	NY	128
Cv	Blood, D	NJ	660
Cv	Borek, M	NY	564
Cv	Borer, J	NY	408
Cv	Chengot, M	NY	564
Cv	Eisenberg, S	NJ	661
Cv	Gabelman, G	NY	596
Cv	Heitner, J	NY	409
Cv	Horowitz, S	CT	866
Cv	Kalischer, A	NJ	842
Cv	Kaufman, D	NY	368
Cv	Keltz, T	NY	596
Cv	Kirtane, S	NY	457
Cv	Koss, J	NY	493
Cv	Kulkarni, R	NJ	829
Cv	Lauer, R	NJ	758
Cv	Meizlish, J	CT	867
Cv	Prabhu, H	NY	410
Cv	Romanello, P	NY	135
Cv	Rossakis, C	NJ	662
Cv	Schreiber, C	NY	494
Cv	Shamoon, F	NJ	704
Cv	Sheris, S	NJ	843
Cv	Slama, R	NJ	843
Cv	Steingart, R	NY	137
Cv	Strobeck, J	NJ	819
Cv	Swamy, S	NY	476
Cv	Taikowski, R	CT	867
NuM	Sanger, J	NY	231
NuM	Strashun, A	NY	430

Special Expertise Index

Spec	Name	St	Pg
EDM	Bloomgarden, D	NY	604
EDM	Blum, D	NY	604
EDM	Bockman, R	NY	159
EDM	Bucholtz, H	NJ	761
EDM	Cam, J	NJ	733
EDM	Cohen, N	NY	477
EDM	Cosman, F	NY	554
EDM	Felig, P	NY	159
EDM	Friedman, S	NY	500
EDM	Fuhrman, R	NJ	844
EDM	Gewirtz, G	NJ	707
EDM	Goldberg-Berman, J	CT	870
EDM	Grajower, M	NY	373
EDM	Greene, L	NY	159
EDM	Greenfield, M	NY	501
EDM	Hochstein, M	NJ	667
EDM	Hupart, K	NY	501
EDM	Kantor, A	NY	605
EDM	Kukar, N	NY	460
EDM	Leibowitz, J	NY	605
EDM	Park, C	NY	160
EDM	Peck, V	NY	161
EDM	Resta, C	NY	460
EDM	Rosenbaum, R	NJ	844
EDM	Rosman, L	NY	460
EDM	Rothman, J	NY	477
EDM	Schmidt, P	NY	414
EDM	Selinger, S	NJ	844
EDM	Shane, E	NY	161
EDM	Sherry, S	NJ	707
EDM	Silverberg, A	NY	414
EDM	Silverberg, S	NY	161
EDM	Siris, E	NY	161
EDM	Tohme, J	NJ	667
EDM	Vaswani, A	NY	501
EDM	Weinerman, S	NY	502
EDM	Wiesen, M	NJ	667
EDM	Wysolmerski, J	CT	905
EDM	Young, I	NY	162
FMed	Blyskal, S	NY	570
FMed	Eisenstat, S	NJ	845
FMed	Ibelli, V	NY	554
FMed	Vincent, M	NY	415
Ger	Malik, R	NY	377
Ger	Solomon, R	NJ	846
IM	Alpert, B	NY	612
IM	Altbaum, R	CT	874
IM	Joseph, J	NY	463
IM	Zackson, D	NY	198
NuM	Gupta, S	CT	881
ObG	Berman, A	NY	232
ObG	Krim, E	NY	519
ObG	Leiter, G	NY	235
ObG	Rothbaum, D	NY	520
PEn	Vogiatzi, M	NY	284

Spec	Name	St	Pg
Rhu	Bauer, B	NY	334
Rhu	Blau, S	NY	543
Rhu	Brodman, R	NJ	855
Rhu	Cannarozzi, N	NJ	725
Rhu	Cohen, D	NY	543
Rhu	Garner, B	NY	448
Rhu	Goldberg, M	NJ	825
Rhu	Goldstein, M	NY	485
Rhu	Gordon, R	NJ	752
Rhu	Green, S	NY	448
Rhu	Guma, M	NJ	693
Rhu	Hoffman, M	NY	544
Rhu	Honig, S	NY	335
Rhu	Jarrett, M	NY	485
Rhu	Kaell, A	NY	587
Rhu	Lans, D	NY	645
Rhu	Lewko, M	NJ	825
Rhu	Lipstein-Kresch, E	NY	544
Rhu	Marcus, R	NJ	694
Rhu	Mascarenhas, B	NY	645
Rhu	McWhorter, J	NJ	836
Rhu	Miller, K	CT	894
Rhu	Mitnick, H	NY	336
Rhu	Novack, S	CT	895
Rhu	Pasik, D	NJ	814
Rhu	Porges, A	NY	544
Rhu	Rackoff, P	NY	337
Rhu	Scarpa, N	NJ	737
Rhu	Schiff, C	NY	448
Rhu	Schoen, R	CT	920
Rhu	Smiles, S	NY	337
Rhu	Sonpal, G	NY	471
Rhu	Stern, R	NY	338
Rhu	Worth, D	NJ	856

Osteoporosis Spine-Kyphoplasty

Spec	Name	St	Pg
OrS	Lane, J	NY	260

Osteoporosis Spine-Vertebroplasty

Spec	Name	St	Pg
VIR	Hamet, M	CT	897

Otitis Media

Spec	Name	St	Pg
Ped	Corbo, E	NJ	852
Ped	Kushner, S	NJ	688
PO	Keller, J	NY	634

Otology

Spec	Name	St	Pg
Oto	Grosso, J	NY	525
Oto	Hanson, M	NY	436
Oto	Kay, S	NJ	772
Oto	Litman, R	NY	580
Oto	Mattucci, K	NY	525

Spec	Name	St	Pg
Oto	Michaelides, E	CT	914

Otology & Neuro-Otology

Spec	Name	St	Pg
Oto	Jahn, A	NY	270
Oto	Meiteles, L	NY	630

Otosclerosis

Spec	Name	St	Pg
Oto	Gordon, M	NY	525
Oto	Selesnick, S	NY	274
Oto	Sperling, N	NY	437

Ovarian Cancer

Spec	Name	St	Pg
GO	Abu-Rustum, N	NY	176
GO	Barakat, R	NY	177
GO	Brown, C	NY	177
GO	Caputo, T	NY	177
GO	Carlson, J	NJ	763
GO	Chuang, L	NY	611
GO	Curtin, J	NY	177
GO	Denehy, T	NJ	709
GO	Economos, K	NY	418
GO	Fishman, D	NY	177
GO	Goldberg, M	NJ	763
GO	Herzog, T	NY	177
GO	Koulos, J	NY	178
GO	Lovecchio, J	NY	506
GO	Maiman, M	NY	478
GO	Menzin, A	NY	506
GO	Rodriguez, L	NJ	763
GO	Rutherford, T	CT	906
GO	Santin, A	CT	907
GO	Schwartz, P	CT	907
GO	Smith, H	NY	378
GO	Wallach, R	NY	178
Onc	Aghajanian, C	NY	201
Onc	Astrow, A	NY	424
Onc	Delprete, S	CT	877
Onc	Farber, C	NJ	806
Onc	Oratz, R	NY	209
Onc	Pasmantier, M	NY	209
Onc	Sabbatini, P	NY	210
Onc	Speyer, J	NY	212
Onc	Spriggs, D	NY	212
Path	Tornos, C	NY	580

Ovarian Cancer Genetics

Spec	Name	St	Pg
ObG	Krause, C	NY	235

Ovarian Cancer Ultrasound Diagnosis

Spec	Name	St	Pg
DR	Hann, L	NY	154

Special Expertise Index

Special Expertise Index

Spec	Name	St	Pg
S	Newman, E	NY	345
S	Pachter, H	NY	345

Pancreatic Cancer(Familial)

Spec	Name	St	Pg
Ge	Kurtz, R	NY	169

Pancreatic Disease

Spec	Name	St	Pg
Ge	Basuk, P	NY	163
Ge	Cohen, J	NY	165
Ge	Grendell, J	NY	504
Ge	Gress, F	NY	416
Ge	Jacobson, I	NY	168
Ge	Jamidar, P	CT	905
Ge	Pitchumoni, C	NJ	762
Ge	Stein, J	NY	173
Ge	Stevens, P	NY	173
Ge	Tempera, P	NJ	845

Pancreatic Islet Cell Transplant

Spec	Name	St	Pg
S	Kapur, S	NY	343

Pancreatic Surgery

Spec	Name	St	Pg
S	Attiyeh, F	NY	340
S	Chabot, J	NY	341
S	Coppa, G	NY	545
S	Dasmahapatra, K	NJ	779
S	Inabnet, W	NY	343
S	Kennedy, T	NY	399
S	Marcus, S	CT	895
S	Rao, A	NY	450
S	Ratner, L	NY	345
S	Reiner, M	NY	346
S	Savino, J	NY	648
S	Zenilman, M	NY	451

Pancreatic/Biliary Endoscopy (ERCP)

Spec	Name	St	Pg
Ge	Ben-Menachem, T	NJ	762
Ge	Ben-Zvi, J	NY	164
Ge	Carr-Locke, D	NY	164
Ge	Chessler, R	NJ	668
Ge	Clain, D	NY	165
Ge	Cohen, J	NY	165
Ge	Cohen, S	NY	165
Ge	Freiman, H	NY	166
Ge	Friedrich, I	NJ	668
Ge	Gutwein, I	NY	376
Ge	Haber, G	NY	167
Ge	Heier, S	NY	608
Ge	Iswara, K	NY	416
Ge	Jamidar, P	CT	905
Ge	Lebovics, E	NY	609
Ge	May, L	NY	554

Spec	Name	St	Pg
Ge	Plumser, A	NJ	762
Ge	Prakash, A	NJ	734
Ge	Roston, A	NY	609
Ge	Sohn, W	NY	417
Ge	Stevens, P	NY	173
Ge	Wayne, P	NY	610

Panic Disorder

Spec	Name	St	Pg
Psyc	Brenner, R	NY	468
Psyc	Farkas, E	NJ	690
Psyc	Fyer, A	NY	313
Psyc	Heller, S	NY	314
Psyc	Idupuganti, S	NY	444
Psyc	Kurani, D	NJ	724
Psyc	Lebinger, M	NY	396
Psyc	Papp, L	NY	318
Psyc	Vivek, S	NY	469
Psyc	Zornitzer, M	NJ	724

Panic Disorder in Schizophrenia

Spec	Name	St	Pg
Psyc	Siris, S	NY	469

Pap Smear Abnormalities

Spec	Name	St	Pg
ObG	Burns, L	NJ	822
ObG	Diamond, S	NY	233
ObG	Friedman, L	NY	234
ObG	Friedman, R	NY	234
ObG	Grano, V	NY	623
ObG	Gruss, L	NY	234
ObG	Krause, C	NY	235
ObG	Mack, L	NY	519

Paragangliomas

Spec	Name	St	Pg
Oto	Myssiorek, D	NY	272

Parasitic Infections

Spec	Name	St	Pg
Ge	Connor, B	NY	165
Inf	Hartman, B	NY	186
Inf	Murray, H	NY	187
Inf	Tanowitz, H	NY	379
Inf	Weiss, L	NY	380
PrM	Cahill, J	NY	309
PrM	Cahill, K	NY	309

Parathyroid Cancer

Spec	Name	St	Pg
Oto	Shemen, L	NY	274
S	Udelsman, R	CT	921

Parathyroid Disorders

Spec	Name	St	Pg
EDM	Agrin, R	NJ	761
EDM	Bilezikian, J	NY	158

Spec	Name	St	Pg
EDM	Bockman, R	NY	159
EDM	Hoffman, R	NY	477
EDM	Schmidt, P	NY	414
EDM	Shane, E	NY	161
EDM	Silverberg, S	NY	161
EDM	Wysolmerski, J	CT	905
IM	Zackson, D	NY	198
PEn	Carpenter, T	CT	915
S	Udelsman, R	CT	921

Parathyroid Surgery

Spec	Name	St	Pg
Oto	Kuhel, W	NY	271
Oto	Kuriloff, D	NY	271
S	Mendoza, E	NY	471
S	Shapiro, M	NJ	695

Parenting Issues

Spec	Name	St	Pg
AM	Alderman, E	NY	367
AM	Lopez, R	NY	124
AM	Marks, A	NY	124
ChAP	Turecki, S	NY	140
Ped	Oppedisano, C	NY	394

Parkinson's Disease

Spec	Name	St	Pg
GerPsy	Serby, M	NY	176
N	Blady, D	NJ	714
N	Bodis-Wollner, I	NY	428
N	Bressman, S	NY	221
N	Cohen, J	NY	384
N	Dickoff, D	NY	621
N	Fahn, S	NY	222
N	Foo, S	NY	223
N	Forster, G	NY	223
N	Gendelman, S	NY	223
N	Gerber, O	NY	576
N	Gilson, N	NJ	790
N	Golbe, L	NJ	768
N	Goodgold, A	NY	223
N	Gross, E	NY	622
N	Herbstein, D	NY	224
N	Kay, A	NY	429
N	Kessler, J	NY	517
N	Knep, S	NJ	822
N	Levin, K	NJ	678
N	Levy, L	NY	518
N	Morris, J	NY	622
N	Oh, Y	NJ	769
N	Olanow, C	NY	227
N	Rabin, A	NY	678
N	Rusk, A	CT	881
N	Sachs, S	NJ	849
N	Sadeghi, H	NJ	735
N	Sage, J	NJ	769
N	Salgado, M	NY	430

Special Expertise Index

Special Expertise Index

Spec	Name	St	Pg
Disorders			
ChAP	Perry, R	NY	140

Spec	Name	St	Pg
Pet Allergy			
A&I	Bassett, C	NY	124

Spec	Name	St	Pg
PET Imaging			
DR	Bobroff, L	NY	554
DR	Cohen, B	NY	154
DR	Kirshy, D	NY	568
DR	Neistadt, L	NY	156
DR	Sherman, S	NY	500
NuM	Agress, H	NJ	679
NuM	Brunetti, J	NJ	679
NuM	Carrasquillo, J	NY	231
NuM	Fawwaz, R	NY	231
NuM	Freeman, L	NY	385
NuM	Gerard, P	NY	430
NuM	Goldsmith, S	NY	231
NuM	Larson, S	NY	231
NuM	Vanheertum, R	NY	232
NuM	Yung, E	NY	519

Spec	Name	St	Pg
PET Imaging-Brain			
NuM	Strashun, A	NY	430
NuM	Vanheertum, R	NY	232

Spec	Name	St	Pg
Peyronie's Disease			
U	Mellinger, B	NY	549
U	Mulhall, J	NY	357
U	Sadeghi-Nejad, H	NJ	697

Spec	Name	St	Pg
Pheochromocytoma			
EDM	Seltzer, T	NY	161
Nep	Ruddy, M	NJ	746
S	Fahey, T	NY	342

Spec	Name	St	Pg
Photodynamic Therapy			
D	Bickers, D	NY	145
D	Scherl, S	NJ	665

Spec	Name	St	Pg
Photosensitive Skin Diseases			
D	DeLeo, V	NY	146

Spec	Name	St	Pg
Phototherapy			
D	Bickers, D	NY	145
D	Greenspan, A	NY	147

Spec	Name	St	Pg
Phyllodes Tumors			
S	Bernik, S	NY	340

Spec	Name	St	Pg
Physicians' Health-Psychiatric			
AdP	Rosenberg, K	NY	123

Spec	Name	St	Pg
Pituitary Disorders			
EDM	Baranetsky, N	NJ	707
EDM	Bitton, R	NY	500
EDM	Brand, H	NY	569
EDM	Carlson, H	NY	569
EDM	Cobin, R	NJ	666
EDM	Friedman, S	NY	500
EDM	Gelato, M	NY	569
EDM	Goldman, M	NJ	667
EDM	Gordon, J	NY	500
EDM	Greene, L	NY	159
EDM	Inzucchi, S	CT	905
EDM	Jacobs, T	NY	160
EDM	Kleinberg, D	NY	160
EDM	Maman, A	NJ	761
EDM	Margulies, P	NY	501
EDM	Marshall, M	NY	605
EDM	Rosenthal, D	NY	501
EDM	Rosman, L	NY	460
EDM	Selinger, S	NJ	844
EDM	Spiler, I	NJ	761
EDM	Wardlaw, S	NY	162
EDM	Warman, J	NY	414
EDM	Wehmann, R	NJ	667
EDM	Young, I	NY	162
NRad	Khandji, A	NY	230
PEn	Kohn, B	NY	283
PEn	Sklar, C	NY	284

Spec	Name	St	Pg
Pituitary Tumors			
NS	Bederson, J	NY	216
NS	Boockvar, J	NY	216
NS	Bruce, J	NY	217
NS	Cardoso, E	NY	428
NS	de Lotbiniere, A	NY	621
NS	Eisenberg, M	NY	516
NS	Huang, P	NY	218
NS	Lee, S	NJ	767
NS	Murali, R	NY	621
NS	Nosko, M	NJ	768
NS	Schwartz, T	NY	219

Spec	Name	St	Pg
Plasmapheresis			
Nep	Stam, L	NY	427

Spec	Name	St	Pg
Plastic & Reconstructive Surgery			
PlS	Israeli, R	NY	537
PlS	Kasabian, A	NY	537

Spec	Name	St	Pg
Platelet Disorders			
Hem	Aledort, L	NY	181
Hem	Billett, H	NY	378
Hem	Marks, P	CT	907
Hem	Vogel, J	NY	184
PHO	Parker, R	NY	581

Spec	Name	St	Pg
Pneumonia			
CCM	Siegel, R	NY	371
Inf	Cunha, B	NY	507
Inf	McLeod, G	CT	873
Inf	Quagliarello, V	CT	908
Inf	Simberkoff, M	NY	189
PCCM	Bojko, T	NJ	773
Ped	Corbo, E	NJ	852
PPul	Bye, M	NY	291
Pul	Baskin, M	NY	324
Pul	Bergman, M	NY	445
Pul	Bondi, E	NY	445
Pul	Fein, A	NY	540
Pul	Leeman, B	NY	540
Pul	Levine, S	NJ	691
Pul	Nash, T	NY	326
Pul	Niederman, M	NY	541

Spec	Name	St	Pg
Poison Control			
PrM	Hoffman, R	NY	309

Spec	Name	St	Pg
Poland Syndrome			
PlS	Colen, H	NY	302
PlS	Keller, A	NY	537

Spec	Name	St	Pg
Polycystic Kidney Disease			
Nep	Blumenfeld, J	NY	214
Nep	Gardenswartz, M	NY	215
PNep	Satlin, L	NY	289

Spec	Name	St	Pg
Polycystic Ovarian Syndrome			
EDM	Albin, J	NY	604
EDM	Gelato, M	NY	569
RE	Brenner, S	NY	543
RE	Chang, P	NY	330
RE	Klein, J	NY	644
RE	Lesorgen, P	NJ	693
RE	Lydic, M	NY	586
RE	Schmidt-Sarosi, C	NY	333

Spec	Name	St	Pg
Polycythemia Rubra Vera			
Hem	Fruchtman, S	NY	182

Spec	Name	St	Pg
Polymyalgia Rheumatica			
Rhu	Belilos, E	NY	543

Spec	Name	St	Pg
Rhu	Lesser, R	NY	448
Rhu	Magid, S	NY	336
Rhu	Stern, R	NY	338

Polymyositis

Spec	Name	St	Pg
Rhu	Bernstein, L	NY	448
Rhu	Hutchinson, G	CT	920
Rhu	Zalkowitz, A	NJ	694

Polypharmacology (Excess Medications)

Spec	Name	St	Pg
Ger	Sherman, F	NY	176

Porphyria

Spec	Name	St	Pg
CG	Desnick, R	NY	142

Portal Hypertension

Spec	Name	St	Pg
S	Emre, S	CT	920

Post Polio Syndrome/Rehabilitation

Spec	Name	St	Pg
PMR	Bach, J	NJ	722
PMR	Moldover, J	NY	299
PMR	Zimmerman, J	NJ	689

Post Traumatic Stress Disorder

Spec	Name	St	Pg
ChAP	Fornari, V	NY	458
ChAP	Perlmutter, I	NY	495
Psyc	Caracci, G	NJ	723
Psyc	Eth, S	NY	312
Psyc	Levin, A	NY	640
Psyc	Markowitz, J	NY	316
Psyc	Schroeder, K	NY	559

Power Doppler Imaging

Spec	Name	St	Pg
DR	Adler, R	NY	153

Preconception Planning

Spec	Name	St	Pg
MF	Monheit, A	NY	574
ObG	Brightman, R	NY	232
ObG	Brustman, L	NY	233

Pregnancy & Hematologic Abnormalities

Spec	Name	St	Pg
Hem	Rand, J	NY	379
MF	Berkowitz, R	NY	200

Pregnancy & Rheumatic Disease

Spec	Name	St	Pg
Rhu	Lockshin, M	NY	336

Pregnancy After Age 35

Spec	Name	St	Pg
MF	Hutson, J	NY	200
ObG	Burns, L	NJ	822
ObG	Friedman, L	NY	234

Pregnancy Loss

Spec	Name	St	Pg
MF	Benito, C	NJ	806
MF	Meirowitz, N	NY	511
MF	Roshan, D	NY	201

Pregnancy Loss-Recurrent

Spec	Name	St	Pg
RE	Bronson, R	NY	586
RE	Lydic, M	NY	586

Pregnancy-High Risk

Spec	Name	St	Pg
MF	Alvarez, M	NJ	673
MF	Berck, D	NY	616
MF	Bobby, P	CT	876
MF	Bond, A	CT	877
MF	Bush, J	NY	424
MF	Chandra, P	NY	424
MF	Chazotte, C	NY	381
MF	Chervenak, F	NY	200
MF	Copel, J	CT	908
MF	D'Alton, M	NY	200
MF	Devine, P	NY	616
MF	Eddleman, K	NY	200
MF	Fleischer, A	NY	511
MF	Funai, E	CT	908
MF	Gimovsky, M	NJ	712
MF	Gonzalez, D	NJ	789
MF	Grunebaum, A	NY	200
MF	Henderson, C	NY	381
MF	Inglis, S	NY	464
MF	Kirshenbaum, N	NY	616
MF	Klein, V	NY	511
MF	Lescale, K	NY	616
MF	Lysikiewicz, A	NY	200
MF	Magriples, U	CT	909
MF	Meirowitz, N	NY	511
MF	Monheit, A	NY	574
MF	Mootabar, H	NY	617
MF	Paidas, M	CT	909
MF	Patrick, S	NY	201
MF	Principe, D	NJ	674
MF	Rebarber, A	NY	201
MF	Rochelson, B	NY	512
MF	Roshan, D	NY	201
MF	Saltzman, D	NY	201
MF	Stiller, R	CT	877
MF	Sullivan, C	NJ	821
MF	Warren, W	NJ	712
ObG	Apuzzio, J	NJ	715

Spec	Name	St	Pg
ObG	Armbruster, R	NY	623
ObG	Benedict, L	NY	519
ObG	Blair, E	CT	882
ObG	Brightman, R	NY	232
ObG	Burns, E	NY	623
ObG	Buterman, I	NY	233
ObG	Coven, R	NJ	680
ObG	Dor, N	NY	431
ObG	Faust, M	NJ	680
ObG	Florio, P	NY	623
ObG	Friedman, A	NJ	747
ObG	Gubernick, M	NY	234
ObG	Haratz-Rubinstein, N	NY	431
ObG	Iammatteo, M	NJ	808
ObG	Kessler, A	NY	235
ObG	Kim, J	NY	235
ObG	Lederman, S	NY	431
ObG	Luciani, R	NJ	715
ObG	Mack, L	NY	519
ObG	Maidman, J	NY	236
ObG	Meacham, K	NY	624
ObG	Mendelowitz, L	NY	624
ObG	Ordorica, S	NY	236
ObG	Rezvani, F	NJ	680
ObG	Sassoon, R	NY	237
ObG	Scher, J	NY	237
ObG	Steer, R	NJ	808
ObG	Toles, A	NY	520
ObG	Vasudeva, K	NY	520
ObG	Violi, C	CT	882
ObG	Weinstein, D	CT	882

Pregnancy-High Risk, Consultation

Spec	Name	St	Pg
ObG	Minkoff, H	NY	431

Pregnancy-Teenage

Spec	Name	St	Pg
MF	Chandra, P	NY	424

Preimplantation Genetic Diagnosis

Spec	Name	St	Pg
RE	Grazi, R	NY	447

Premature Labor

Spec	Name	St	Pg
MF	Benito, C	NJ	806
MF	Chandra, P	NY	424
MF	Devine, P	NY	616
MF	Funai, E	CT	908
MF	Patrick, S	NY	201
ObG	Baker, D	NY	576

Prematurity Prevention

Spec	Name	St	Pg
MF	Lockwood, C	CT	909

Special Expertise Index

Spec	Name	St	Pg
Prematurity/Low Birth Weight Infants			
NP	Boxer, H	NY	514
NP	Campbell, D	NY	382
NP	Golombek, S	NY	619
NP	Gudavalli, M	NY	425
NP	Hand, I	NY	465
NP	Hiatt, I	NJ	767
NP	La Gamma, E	NY	619
NP	Manginello, F	NJ	676
NP	Perlman, J	NY	213
NP	Shahrivar, F	NY	214
NP	Sun, S	NJ	713
ObG	Brustman, L	NY	233
Ped	Preis, O	NY	442
Ped	Weinberger, S	NY	297

Spec	Name	St	Pg
Prenatal Diagnosis			
CG	Anyane-Yeboa, K	NY	141
CG	Gilbert, F	NY	142
CG	Gross, S	NY	370
CG	Hyman, D	NY	566
CG	Mahoney, M	CT	903
CG	Shapiro, L	NY	600
CG	Sklower Brooks, S	NJ	759
MF	Benito, C	NJ	806
MF	Bobby, P	CT	876
MF	Bond, A	CT	877
MF	Copel, J	CT	908
MF	D'Alton, M	NY	200
MF	Devine, P	NY	616
MF	Frieden, F	NJ	674
MF	Inglis, S	NY	464
MF	Laifer, S	CT	877
MF	Lescale, K	NY	616
MF	Lysikiewicz, A	NY	200
MF	Meirowitz, N	NY	511
MF	Rochelson, B	NY	512
MF	Saltzman, D	NY	201
MF	Smith, L	NJ	712
MF	Stiller, R	CT	877
ObG	Apuzzio, J	NJ	715
ObG	Lederman, S	NY	431

Spec	Name	St	Pg
Prenatal Genetic Diagnosis			
RE	Grifo, J	NY	331

Spec	Name	St	Pg
Prenatal Ultrasound			
CG	Gross, S	NY	370
MF	Frieden, F	NJ	674
MF	Lysikiewicz, A	NY	200
MF	Stone, J	NY	201

Spec	Name	St	Pg
Preventive Cardiology			
AM	Jacobson, M	NY	489
Cv	Andersen, H	NY	128
Cv	Berdoff, R	NY	128
Cv	Blum, M	NJ	801
Cv	Blumenthal, D	NY	129
Cv	Brown, D	NY	564
Cv	Chesner, M	NY	491
Cv	Eisenberg, S	NJ	661
Cv	Elkind, B	NJ	733
Cv	ElMasri, B	NY	130
Cv	Epstein, S	NY	130
Cv	Fass, A	NY	595
Cv	Friedman, S	NY	130
Cv	Frishman, W	NY	595
Cv	Fuchs, R	NY	130
Cv	Fuster, V	NY	130
Cv	Gabelman, G	NY	596
Cv	Gardin, J	NJ	661
Cv	Gelbfish, J	NY	408
Cv	Gelles, J	NY	408
Cv	Giardina, E	NY	131
Cv	Gleckel, L	NY	492
Cv	Goldberg, N	NY	131
Cv	Goldberg, S	NY	492
Cv	Horowitz, S	CT	866
Cv	Kay, R	NY	596
Cv	Keltz, T	NY	596
Cv	Landzberg, J	NJ	662
Cv	Lewis, B	NY	133
Cv	Mahalingam, B	NJ	741
Cv	Matos, M	NY	597
Cv	Mercando, A	NY	597
Cv	Mintz, G	NY	494
Cv	Nash, I	NY	134
Cv	Neeson, F	CT	867
Cv	O'Brien, F	NY	134
Cv	Paiusco, A	NY	410
Cv	Phillips, M	NY	369
Cv	Porder, J	NY	134
Cv	Radwaner, B	NY	135
Cv	Raska, K	NJ	802
Cv	Reichstein, R	NY	135
Cv	Saroff, A	NJ	704
Cv	Schiffer, M	NY	135
Cv	Seinfeld, D	NY	136
Cv	Siegel, S	NY	136
Cv	Slama, R	NJ	843
Cv	Southren, D	NY	553
Cv	Spadaro, L	NY	495
Cv	Stein, R	NY	137
Cv	Swamy, S	NY	476
Cv	Unger, A	NY	137
Cv	Wein, P	NY	410
Cv	Weintraub, H	NY	138

Spec	Name	St	Pg
Cv	Weisenseel, A	NY	138
Cv	Weiss, E	NJ	819
Cv	Winter, S	NY	476
Cv	Zimmerman, F	NY	598
FMed	Blyskal, S	NY	570
FMed	Rednor, J	NJ	742
IC	Abittan, M	NY	510
IC	Innerfield, M	NY	555
IM	Blumberg, J	CT	874
IM	Case, D	NY	190
IM	DeSilva, D	NJ	765
IM	Lipton, M	NY	195
IM	Underberg, J	NY	197
PCd	Langsner, A	NJ	720

Spec	Name	St	Pg
Preventive Medicine			
Cv	Porder, J	NY	134
FMed	Acosta, R	CT	870
FMed	Aponte, A	NY	570
FMed	Coloka-Kump, R	NY	374
FMed	Edelstein, M	NY	502
FMed	Filiberto, C	CT	870
FMed	Fisher, G	NY	460
FMed	Gottesfeld, P	NY	606
FMed	Greenblatt, L	NY	570
FMed	Istrico, R	NY	460
FMed	Lyon, V	NY	163
FMed	Morrow, R	NY	375
FMed	Moskowitz, G	NY	415
FMed	Sadovsky, R	NY	415
FMed	Sutton, I	NY	606
FMed	Vincent, M	NY	415
Ger	Callahan, E	NY	174
Ger	Fogel, J	NY	175
Ger	Korc, B	NY	175
Ger	Paris, B	NY	417
IM	Baskin, D	NY	190
IM	Beyda, A	NY	463
IM	Bush, M	NY	190
IM	Cacciola, T	NJ	672
IM	Carmichael, L	NY	190
IM	Charap, P	NY	190
IM	Cohen, R	NY	191
IM	De Cosimo, D	NJ	711
IM	DoRosario, A	CT	874
IM	Dreyer, N	CT	874
IM	Ehrlich, M	NY	191
IM	Ellman, M	CT	908
IM	Etingin, O	NY	191
IM	Feltheimer, S	NY	192
IM	Fisher, L	NY	192
IM	Friedling, S	NY	573
IM	Friedman, J	NY	192
IM	Fukilman, O	NY	463
IM	Gelberg, B	NY	509

Special Expertise Index

Spec	Name	St	Pg
Psychiatry in Physical Illness			
Psyc	Basch, S	NY	310
Psyc	Bronheim, H	NY	311
Psyc	Fallon, B	NY	312
Psyc	Goodman, B	NY	314
Psyc	Gurevich, M	NY	539
Psyc	Kalash, G	NY	469
Psyc	Muskin, P	NY	317
Psyc	Schroeder, K	NY	559
Psyc	Shapiro, P	NY	320
Psyc	Strain, J	NY	321
Psyc	Wallack, J	NY	322
Psyc	Weill, T	NY	323
Psychiatry in Terminal Illness			
Psyc	Klagsbrun, S	NY	640
Psychiatry of Prostate Cancer			
Psyc	Roth, A	NY	319
Psychoanalysis			
ChAP	Hyler, I	NY	599
ChAP	King, R	CT	902
ChAP	Madigan, J	CT	902
Psyc	Basch, S	NY	310
Psyc	Bone, S	NY	310
Psyc	Buckley, P	NY	311
Psyc	Bukberg, J	NY	311
Psyc	Chertoff, H	NJ	690
Psyc	Goldenberg, D	NY	313
Psyc	Kalinich, L	NY	314
Psyc	Levitan, S	NY	315
Psyc	Lew, A	NY	641
Psyc	Mahon, E	NY	316
Psyc	Michels, R	NY	317
Psyc	Olds, D	NY	318
Psyc	Rees, E	NY	318
Psyc	Samberg, E	NY	320
Psyc	Sawyer, D	NY	320
Psyc	Scharf, R	NY	320
Psyc	Shaw, R	NY	320
Psyc	Stone, M	NY	321
Psyc	Strain, J	NY	321
Psyc	Welsh, H	NY	323
Psychodynamic Psychotherapy			
Psyc	Berman, S	NY	538
Psyc	Winters, R	NY	323
Psychoneuroimmunology			
Psyc	Schleifer, S	NJ	724

Spec	Name	St	Pg
Psychopharmacology			
ChAP	Coffey, B	NY	139
ChAP	Cohen, L	NY	599
ChAP	Kron, L	NY	139
ChAP	Leventhal, B	NY	139
ChAP	Lewis, O	NY	139
ChAP	Newcorn, J	NY	140
ChAP	Perry, R	NY	140
ChAP	Rubinstein, B	NY	599
ChAP	Seaver, R	NY	599
ChAP	Slater, J	NY	599
ChAP	Williams, D	NY	495
Onc	Budman, D	NY	512
Psyc	Addonizio, G	NY	639
Psyc	Adler, L	NY	309
Psyc	Alper, K	NY	309
Psyc	Arkow, S	NY	310
Psyc	Asnis, G	NY	396
Psyc	Bailine, S	NY	538
Psyc	Basch, S	NY	310
Psyc	Berman, S	NY	538
Psyc	Bhatt, A	NY	539
Psyc	Brodie, J	NY	311
Psyc	Brown, R	NY	311
Psyc	Caracci, G	NJ	723
Psyc	First, M	NY	312
Psyc	Fox, H	NY	313
Psyc	Friedman, R	NY	313
Psyc	Frogel, M	NY	539
Psyc	Gabel, R	NY	640
Psyc	Gershell, W	NY	313
Psyc	Glassman, A	NY	313
Psyc	Goldstein, S	NY	313
Psyc	Gorman, L	NY	314
Psyc	Harlam, D	NY	640
Psyc	Hoffman, J	NY	314
Psyc	Jacoby, J	NJ	737
Psyc	Kahn, D	NY	314
Psyc	Kaplan, G	NJ	854
Psyc	Katus, E	NY	539
Psyc	Kocsis, J	NY	315
Psyc	Leifer, M	NJ	751
Psyc	Levin, A	NY	640
Psyc	Levitan, S	NY	315
Psyc	Levy, M	NY	559
Psyc	Lindenmayer, J	NY	315
Psyc	Lipton, B	NY	316
Psyc	Markowitz, J	NY	316
Psyc	McGrath, P	NY	316
Psyc	McMullen, R	NY	316
Psyc	Mendelowitz, A	NY	469
Psyc	Menza, M	NJ	778
Psyc	Meyers, B	NY	641
Psyc	Miller, D	NJ	854
Psyc	Milone, R	NY	641

Spec	Name	St	Pg
Psyc	Mueller, F	CT	891
Psyc	Muskin, P	NY	317
Psyc	Nininger, J	NY	317
Psyc	Nucci, A	NJ	724
Psyc	Opler, L	NY	641
Psyc	Papp, L	NY	318
Psyc	Perry, B	NY	641
Psyc	Preven, D	NY	318
Psyc	Richardson, W	NJ	854
Psyc	Rosen, A	NY	319
Psyc	Rosen, B	NY	585
Psyc	Rubinstein, M	NY	319
Psyc	Scharf, R	NY	320
Psyc	Seaman, C	NY	320
Psyc	Shapiro, B	CT	891
Psyc	Shinbach, K	NY	321
Psyc	Siever, L	NY	321
Psyc	Silver, J	NY	321
Psyc	Stabinsky, S	NY	641
Psyc	Sullivan, A	NY	469
Psyc	Sussman, N	NY	321
Psyc	Tardiff, K	NY	322
Psyc	Villafranca, M	NJ	854
Psyc	Wager, S	NY	322
Psyc	Wallack, J	NY	322
Psyc	Winters, R	NY	323
Psyc	Zornitzer, M	NJ	724
Psychosomatic Disorders			
AM	Marks, A	NY	124
ChAP	Williams, D	NY	495
FMed	Lansing, M	NJ	742
Psyc	Coplan, J	NY	444
Psyc	Fallon, B	NY	312
Psyc	Gelfand, J	NY	396
Psyc	Goodman, B	NY	314
Psyc	Kalash, G	NY	469
Psyc	Lipton, B	NY	316
Psyc	Muhlbauer, H	NY	317
Psychotherapy			
ChAP	Hyler, I	NY	599
ChAP	Kron, L	NY	139
ChAP	Lewis, O	NY	139
ChAP	Madigan, J	CT	902
ChAP	Rosenfeld, A	CT	867
Psyc	Addonizio, G	NY	639
Psyc	Arkow, S	NY	310
Psyc	Bemporad, J	NY	640
Psyc	Bone, S	NY	310
Psyc	Bukberg, J	NY	311
Psyc	Caracci, G	NJ	723
Psyc	Cohen, A	NY	311
Psyc	Cournos, F	NY	312

Special Expertise Index

Spec	Name	St	Pg
Psyc	First, M	NY	312
Psyc	Fox, H	NY	313
Psyc	Frogel, M	NY	539
Psyc	Gabel, R	NY	640
Psyc	Hart, S	CT	891
Psyc	Kahn, D	NY	314
Psyc	Kalinich, L	NY	314
Psyc	Karasu, T	NY	315
Psyc	Katus, E	NY	539
Psyc	Levitan, S	NY	315
Psyc	Lew, A	NY	641
Psyc	Lipton, B	NY	316
Psyc	Meyers, B	NY	641
Psyc	Nininger, J	NY	317
Psyc	Olds, D	NY	318
Psyc	Opler, L	NY	641
Psyc	Preven, D	NY	318
Psyc	Rees, E	NY	318
Psyc	Rosenbloom, C	NY	319
Psyc	Sadock, V	NY	320
Psyc	Scharf, R	NY	320
Psyc	Seaman, C	NY	320
Psyc	Shaw, R	NY	320
Psyc	Stabinsky, S	NY	641
Psyc	Sullivan, A	NY	469
Psyc	Swiller, H	NY	321
Psyc	Tamerin, J	CT	892
Psyc	Tardiff, K	NY	322
Psyc	Tolchin, J	NY	322
Psyc	Welsh, H	NY	323
Psyc	Zornitzer, M	NJ	724

Psychotherapy & Psychopharmacology

ChAP	Moreau, D	NY	140
Psyc	Goodman, B	NY	314
Psyc	Gurevich, M	NY	539
Psyc	Schwartz, M	NY	585
Psyc	Stein, S	NY	321
Psyc	Sullivan, T	NY	641

Psychotherapy-Men's Issues

Psyc	Farkas, E	NJ	690

Pubertal Disorders

PEn	Chin, D	NJ	811
PEn	Frank, G	NY	530
PEn	Marshall, I	NJ	774
PEn	Salas, M	NJ	774
PEn	Speiser, P	NY	468
PEn	Vogiatzi, M	NY	284

Pulmonary Disease

A&I	Goldstein, S	NY	490
IM	Bregman, Z	NY	190
IM	Jawetz, H	NJ	821
IM	Spero, M	NY	197
IM	Warren, R	NJ	744
NP	Golombek, S	NY	619
NP	Perl, H	NJ	676
Ped	Kotin, N	NY	295
Ped	Suda, A	NJ	812
Pul	Ankobiah, W	NY	469
Pul	Engler, M	NJ	691

Pulmonary Disease/Immunocompromised

Pul	Stover-Pepe, D	NY	328

Pulmonary Embolism

DR	Ginsberg, M	NY	154
DR	Naidich, D	NY	156
Pul	Arcasoy, S	NY	324

Pulmonary Fibrosis

Pul	Adams, F	NY	323
Pul	DiCosmo, B	NY	642
Pul	Hammer, A	NY	446
Pul	McCalley, S	CT	893
Pul	Padilla, M	NY	326
Pul	Polkow, M	NJ	692
Pul	Posner, D	NY	327
Pul	Riley, D	NJ	778
Pul	Sussman, R	NJ	855

Pulmonary Hypertension

Cv	Dresdale, R	NY	492
Cv	Horn, E	NY	132
Cv	Klapholz, M	NJ	704
Cv	Lachmann, J	NY	493
Cv	Pinney, S	NY	134
Cv	Poon, M	NY	565
Cv	Smart, F	NJ	802
Cv	Zucker, M	NJ	705
Pul	Demetis, S	NY	445
Pul	Padilla, M	NY	326
Pul	Shah, S	NJ	725
Pul	Steiger, D	NY	327

Pulmonary Infections

Pul	Stover-Pepe, D	NY	328

Pulmonary Infectious Disease

Pul	Leeman, B	NY	540

Pulmonary Pathology

Path	Travis, W	NY	280

Pulmonary Rehabilitation

Pul	Novitch, R	NY	643
Pul	Raskin, J	NY	327
Pul	Sachs, P	CT	893
Pul	Silverman, J	NY	470

R

Radiation Therapy-Intraoperative

RadRO	Harrison, L	NY	329

Radiofrequency Ablation

CE	Costeas, C	NJ	703
CE	Rubin, D	NY	594

Radiofrequency Tumor Ablation

VIR	Brown, K	NY	361

Radioimmunotherapy of Cancer

NuM	Carrasquillo, J	NY	231
NuM	Fawwaz, R	NY	231

Rare Skin Disorders

D	Grossman, M	NY	601
D	Shupack, J	NY	151

Raynaud's Disease

D	Franks, A	NY	146
Rhu	Schwartzman, S	NY	337

Reconstructive Microsurgery

Oto	DeLacure, M	NY	269

Reconstructive Microvascular Surgery

OrS	Hausman, M	NY	259
PlS	Ting, J	NY	308

Reconstructive Plastic Surgery

PlS	Colon, F	NJ	812
PlS	Cutting, C	NY	302
PlS	Dagum, A	NY	584
PlS	Dubner, S	NY	536
PlS	Ginsberg, G	NY	303

Special Expertise Index

Spec	Name	St	Pg
Pul	Winter, S	CT	893

Retina-Artificial

Spec	Name	St	Pg
Oph	Del Priore, L	NY	241

Retina/Vitreous Consultation

Oph	Barile, G	NY	239
Oph	Fisher, Y	NY	242

Retina/Vitreous Surgery

Oph	Bhagat, N	NJ	716
Oph	Chang, S	NY	240
Oph	Chess, J	NY	386
Oph	Cohen, B	NY	240
Oph	Cohen, S	NJ	716
Oph	Coleman, D	NY	240
Oph	Douros, S	NY	432
Oph	Elbaba, F	NY	578
Oph	Fastenberg, D	NY	521
Oph	Friedman, R	NY	243
Oph	Gentile, R	NY	243
Oph	Lee, C	NY	245
Oph	Muldoon, T	NY	248
Oph	Rosenthal, J	NY	249
Oph	Sachs, R	NJ	809
Oph	Weseley, P	NY	252
Oph	Yannuzzi, L	NY	253

Retinal Detachment

Oph	Berman, D	NY	432
Oph	Cangemi, F	NJ	716
Oph	D'Amico, D	NY	241
Oph	Del Priore, L	NY	241
Oph	Lewis, H	NY	245
Oph	Schiff, W	NY	250
Oph	Schubert, H	NY	250
Oph	Wong, R	NY	253
Oph	Zarbin, M	NJ	717

Retinal Disorders

Oph	Angioletti, L	NY	238
Oph	Barile, G	NY	239
Oph	Carr, R	NY	239
Oph	Chang, S	NY	240
Oph	D'Amico, D	NY	241
Oph	Eichler, J	NJ	716
Oph	Engel, H	NY	242
Oph	Ferrone, P	NY	521
Oph	Friedman, A	NY	242
Oph	Fromer, M	NY	243
Oph	Fuchs, W	NY	243
Oph	Gentile, R	NY	243
Oph	Odel, J	NY	248

Spec	Name	St	Pg
Oph	Paccione, J	NY	248
Oph	Reppucci, V	CT	883
Oph	Sachs, R	NJ	809
Oph	Saffra, N	NY	433
Oph	Schubert, H	NY	250
Oph	Slakter, J	NY	251
Oph	Smith, R	NY	251
Oph	Spaide, R	NY	251
Oph	Stein, A	NY	434
Oph	Stoller, G	NY	579
Oph	Tom, D	CT	884
Oph	Topilow, H	NJ	681
Oph	Unterricht, S	NY	434
Oph	Walsh, J	NY	252
Oph	Weber, P	NY	579
Oph	Weber, R	CT	884
Oph	Weiss, M	NY	252

Retinitis Pigmentosa

Oph	MacKay, C	NY	246
Oph	Solomon, S	NY	627

Retinoblastoma

Oph	Abramson, D	NY	238
Oph	Finger, P	NY	242
PHO	Dunkel, I	NY	286
PHO	Rausen, A	NY	288

Retinopathy of Prematurity

NP	Hendricks-Munoz, K	NY	213
Oph	Cangemi, F	NJ	716
Oph	Horowitz, M	NY	626
Oph	Most, R	NY	627
Oph	Shabto, U	NY	250
Oph	Topilow, H	NJ	681

Retroperitoneal Fibrosis

Rhu	Solitar, B	NY	337
U	Stifelman, M	NY	360

Rhabdomyosarcoma

PHO	Wexler, L	NY	288

Rheumatic Fever

Rhu	Gibofsky, A	NY	335

Rheumatic Heart Disease

PCd	Cooper, R	NY	528

Rheumatoid Arthritis

HS	Miller-Breslow, A	NJ	670
IM	Kazdin, H	NY	422

Spec	Name	St	Pg
IM	Miguel, E	NJ	672
PRhu	Lehman, T	NY	292
Rhu	Adlersberg, J	NY	333
Rhu	Agus, B	NY	334
Rhu	Barone, R	NY	644
Rhu	Belilos, E	NY	543
Rhu	Belmont, H	NY	334
Rhu	Berger, J	NY	645
Rhu	Bernstein, L	NY	448
Rhu	Bienenstock, H	NY	448
Rhu	Blau, S	NY	543
Rhu	Blume, R	NY	334
Rhu	Brodman, R	NJ	855
Rhu	Burns, M	NY	645
Rhu	Cannarozzi, N	NJ	725
Rhu	Carsons, S	NY	543
Rhu	Crane, R	NY	334
Rhu	Danehower, R	CT	894
Rhu	Faller, J	NY	334
Rhu	Fields, T	NY	334
Rhu	Fischer, H	NY	335
Rhu	Fomberstein, B	NY	398
Rhu	Furie, R	NY	544
Rhu	Garner, B	NY	448
Rhu	Gibofsky, A	NY	335
Rhu	Goldberg, M	NJ	825
Rhu	Goldstein, M	NY	485
Rhu	Goodman, S	NY	335
Rhu	Gordon, R	NJ	752
Rhu	Green, S	NY	448
Rhu	Greenwald, R	NY	544
Rhu	Greisman, S	NY	335
Rhu	Hamburger, M	NY	587
Rhu	Hoffman, M	NY	544
Rhu	Honig, S	NY	335
Rhu	Horowitz, M	NY	335
Rhu	Hutchinson, G	CT	920
Rhu	Jarrett, M	NY	485
Rhu	Keiser, H	NY	398
Rhu	Kerr, L	NY	336
Rhu	Kopelman, R	NJ	693
Rhu	Kramer, N	NJ	725
Rhu	Lans, D	NY	645
Rhu	Lee, S	NY	336
Rhu	Leibowitz, E	NJ	693
Rhu	Lesser, R	NY	448
Rhu	Lewko, M	NJ	825
Rhu	Lichtbroun, A	NJ	779
Rhu	Lipstein-Kresch, E	NY	544
Rhu	Magid, S	NY	336
Rhu	Marcus, R	NJ	694
Rhu	Markenson, J	NY	336
Rhu	Meredith, G	NY	544
Rhu	Miller, K	CT	894
Rhu	Mitnick, H	NY	336

Special Expertise Index

Spec	Name	St	Pg
Rotator Cuff Surgery			
HS	Monsanto, E	NY	419
OrS	Abrams, J	NJ	748
OrS	Berman, M	NJ	682
OrS	Bigliani, L	NY	254
OrS	Cordasco, F	NY	255
OrS	Flatow, E	NY	257
OrS	Harwin, S	NY	258
OrS	Henshaw, D	CT	885
OrS	Kraushaar, B	NY	557
OrS	Lubliner, J	NY	261
OrS	Maddalo, A	NY	629
OrS	Miller, S	CT	885
OrS	Montgomery, K	NJ	810
OrS	Pidoriano, A	NY	629
OrS	Pollock, R	NJ	683
OrS	Soifer, T	NY	435
OrS	Ticker, J	NY	524
OrS	Warren, R	NY	266
OrS	Weinstein, R	NY	629
OrS	Wickiewicz, T	NY	266
OrS	Zuckerman, J	NY	267
SM	Cavaliere, G	NY	646
Running Injuries			
PMR	Gotlin, R	NY	298
SM	Hamner, D	NY	339
SM	Maharam, L	NY	339
SM	Metzl, J	NY	339

S

Spec	Name	St	Pg
Salivary Gland Surgery			
Oto	Fox, M	NY	630
Oto	Myssiorek, D	NY	272
Oto	Rosenbaum, J	NJ	772
Salivary Gland Tumors			
Oto	Komisar, A	NY	270
Oto	Smith, R	NY	388
Oto	Urken, M	NY	275
Salivary Gland Tumors & Surgery			
Oto	Frank, D	NY	525
Oto	Sacks, S	NY	274
S	Shah, J	NY	346
Sarcoidosis			
CCM	Efferen, L	NY	458

Spec	Name	St	Pg
N	Lazar, M	NJ	768
Oph	Frohman, L	NJ	716
Pul	Adams, F	NY	323
Pul	Bevelaqua, F	NY	324
Pul	Blair, L	NY	324
Pul	Breidbart, D	NY	540
Pul	Brill, J	NY	642
Pul	Demetis, S	NY	445
Pul	Eden, E	NY	325
Pul	Goldblatt, K	NJ	751
Pul	Gulrajani, R	NY	445
Pul	Lee, M	NY	326
Pul	Miller, R	NJ	724
Pul	Padilla, M	NY	326
Pul	Pinsker, K	NY	397
Pul	Polkow, M	NJ	692
Pul	Posner, D	NY	327
Pul	Safirstein, B	NJ	725
Pul	Schiffman, P	NJ	778
Pul	Sender, J	NY	398
Pul	Silverman, J	NY	470
Pul	Smith, P	NY	446
Pul	Teirstein, A	NY	328
Rhu	Agus, B	NY	334
Rhu	Yee, A	NY	338
Sarcoma			
Onc	Blum, R	NY	202
Onc	Fanucchi, M	NY	203
Onc	Scoppetuolo, M	NJ	713
OrS	Healey, J	NY	259
PHO	Gorlick, R	NY	390
PHO	Meyers, P	NY	287
S	Bloom, N	NY	341
S	Brennan, M	NY	341
S	Kurtzman, S	CT	920
S	Whitman, E	NJ	815
Sarcoma-Soft Tissue			
Onc	Casper, E	NJ	832
OrS	Benevenia, J	NJ	717
OrS	Healey, J	NY	259
OrS	Wittig, J	NY	267
PHO	Wexler, L	NY	288
S	Ashikari, A	NY	646
S	August, D	NJ	779
S	Rosenberg, V	NY	346
S	Singer, S	NY	347
Scar Revision			
D	Rapaport, J	NJ	665

Spec	Name	St	Pg
Schizophrenia			
GerPsy	Cohen, C	NY	418
Psyc	Benjamin, J	NY	538
Psyc	Harlam, D	NY	640
Psyc	Kahn, D	NY	314
Psyc	Kaufmann, C	NY	315
Psyc	Lindenmayer, J	NY	315
Psyc	Mendelowitz, A	NY	469
Psyc	Schwartz, B	NY	396
Psyc	Siris, S	NY	469
Psyc	Sullivan, T	NY	641
Schizophrenia-Clinical Trials			
Psyc	McGlashan, T	CT	918
Schizophrenia-Early Detection/Treatment			
Psyc	McGlashan, T	CT	918
Sciatica			
PM	Lefkowitz, M	NY	437
PM	Waldman, S	NY	278
Scleroderma			
D	Franks, A	NY	146
PRhu	Haines, K	NJ	686
PRhu	Lehman, T	NY	292
Rhu	Bernstein, L	NY	448
Rhu	Blau, S	NY	543
Rhu	Kerr, L	NY	336
Rhu	McWhorter, J	NJ	836
Rhu	Radin, A	NY	337
Rhu	Spiera, H	NY	338
Rhu	Spiera, R	NY	338
Rhu	Whitman, H	NJ	855
Rhu	Yegudin-Ash, J	NY	645
Sclerotherapy			
D	Cooper, L	NJ	803
D	Mermelstein, H	NY	602
Scoliosis			
OrS	Bendo, J	NY	254
OrS	Boachie-Adjei, O	NY	254
OrS	Cammisa, F	NY	255
OrS	Casden, A	NY	255
OrS	Emami, A	NJ	823
OrS	Errico, T	NY	256
OrS	Feldman, D	NY	257
OrS	Goldstein, J	NY	257
OrS	Hyman, J	NY	259
OrS	Lonner, B	NY	260

Spec	Name	St	Pg
OrS	Merola, A	NY	435
OrS	Moskovich, R	NY	262
OrS	Neuwirth, M	NY	262
OrS	Olsewski, J	NY	388
OrS	Rawlins, B	NY	263
OrS	Rieger, M	NJ	810
OrS	Roye, D	NY	263
OrS	Schwab, F	NY	264
OrS	Smith, B	CT	914
OrS	Spivak, J	NY	265
OrS	Tindel, N	NY	265
OrS	Vitale, M	NY	266
OrS	Widmann, R	NY	267

Seizure Disorders

Spec	Name	St	Pg
ChiN	Molofsky, W	NY	141
N	Bronster, D	NY	221
N	Ettinger, A	NY	517
N	Jutkowitz, R	NY	480
N	Katz, A	CT	912
N	Najjar, S	NY	481
N	Oh, Y	NJ	769

Sentinel Node Surgery

Spec	Name	St	Pg
S	Blackwood, M	NJ	726
S	Cohen, B	NY	588
S	Geller, P	NY	343
S	Nowak, E	NY	345
S	O'Hea, B	NY	588
S	Osborne, M	NY	345
S	Swistel, A	NY	347
S	Tartter, P	NY	347

Sepsis

Spec	Name	St	Pg
CCM	Benjamin, E	NY	144
CCM	Nierman, D	NY	458
Pul	Davis, G	NJ	795
Pul	Multz, A	NY	541
Pul	Rosen, M	NY	541
Pul	Winter, S	CT	893
S	Barie, P	NY	340

Sepsis & Septic Shock

Spec	Name	St	Pg
PCCM	Bojko, T	NJ	773
PCCM	Davis, A	NJ	720
PCCM	Goltzman, C	NY	632
PCCM	Greenwald, B	NY	283
PCCM	Ushay, H	NY	390

Sexual Addiction

Spec	Name	St	Pg
Psyc	First, M	NY	312

Sexual Behavior-Compulsive

Spec	Name	St	Pg
Psyc	Krueger, R	NY	315

Sexual Development Problems

Spec	Name	St	Pg
ChAP	Rosenfeld, A	CT	867
PEn	Castro-Magana, M	NY	529

Sexual Differentiation Disorders

Spec	Name	St	Pg
PEn	Saenger, P	NY	633
PEn	Wilson, T	NY	581

Sexual Dysfunction

Spec	Name	St	Pg
AdP	Rosenberg, K	NY	123
FMed	Levy, A	NY	162
IM	Lamm, S	NY	194
ObG	Bachmann, G	NJ	769
ObG	Berman, A	NY	232
Psyc	Sadock, V	NY	320
Psyc	Schore, A	NY	320
U	Glassman, C	NY	649
U	Gribetz, M	NY	355
U	Kaminetsky, J	NY	356
U	Klein, G	NY	356
U	Lehrhoff, B	NJ	857
U	Seidman, B	NJ	729
U	Shulman, Y	NJ	738
U	Strauss, B	NJ	729

Sexually Transmitted Diseases

Spec	Name	St	Pg
Inf	Johnson, D	NY	508
Inf	Lerner, C	NY	187
Inf	McCormack, W	NY	420
Inf	Robbins, N	NY	379
Inf	Scheer, M	NY	508
ObG	Donovan, L	CT	882
PInf	Neu, N	NY	289

Short Stature in Children

Spec	Name	St	Pg
PEn	Agdere, L	NY	438
PEn	Saenger, P	NY	633

Shoulder & Elbow Surgery

Spec	Name	St	Pg
OrS	Alpert, S	NY	579
OrS	Mendoza, F	NY	261
SM	Levine, W	NY	339

Shoulder & Knee Injuries

Spec	Name	St	Pg
OrS	Maddalo, A	NY	629
SM	Gross, M	NJ	694
SM	Savatsky, G	NJ	694

Shoulder & Knee Reconstruction

Spec	Name	St	Pg
OrS	Splain, S	NY	435

Shoulder & Knee Surgery

Spec	Name	St	Pg
OrS	Garfinkel, M	NJ	771
OrS	Gladstone, J	NY	257
OrS	Nicholas, S	NY	262
OrS	Schob, C	NJ	718
OrS	Shebairo, R	NY	524
SM	Nisonson, B	NY	339

Shoulder Arthroscopic Surgery

Spec	Name	St	Pg
HS	Barron, O	NY	178
OrS	Bade, H	NJ	792
OrS	Craig, E	NY	256
OrS	Fealy, S	NY	257
OrS	Flatow, E	NY	257
OrS	Hannafin, J	NY	258
OrS	Kraushaar, B	NY	557
OrS	Pollock, R	NJ	683
OrS	Rubin, C	NY	557
OrS	Ticker, J	NY	524
OrS	Williams, R	NY	267

Shoulder Injuries

Spec	Name	St	Pg
OrS	Altman, W	NJ	682
OrS	Austin, K	NY	557
OrS	Drillings, G	NJ	822
OrS	Flatow, E	NY	257
OrS	Pollock, R	NJ	683
SM	Gehrmann, R	NJ	726
SM	Halpern, B	NY	339

Shoulder Instability

Spec	Name	St	Pg
SM	Cavaliere, G	NY	646
SM	Sclafani, M	NJ	796

Shoulder Reconstruction

Spec	Name	St	Pg
HS	Barron, O	NY	178
OrS	Barmakian, J	NJ	850
OrS	Decter, E	NJ	718
OrS	Gallick, G	NJ	850

Shoulder Replacement

Spec	Name	St	Pg
OrS	Craig, E	NY	256
OrS	Dines, D	NY	523
OrS	Fealy, S	NY	257
OrS	Flatow, E	NY	257
OrS	Mc Inerney, V	NJ	823
OrS	Warren, R	NY	266
SM	Plancher, K	NY	339

Special Expertise Index

Spec	Name	St	Pg
A&I	Schneider, A	NY	407
A&I	Tolston, E	NY	126
IM	Lu, B	NY	422
Oto	Edelman, B	NJ	771
Oto	Moisa, I	NY	525
PA&I	Fost, A	NJ	719
PA&I	Torre, A	NJ	719
PO	Keller, J	NY	634
PO	Rothschild, M	NY	290

Sjogren's Syndrome

Rhu	Carsons, S	NY	543
Rhu	Kramer, N	NJ	725
Rhu	Lichtbroun, A	NJ	779
Rhu	Rackoff, P	NY	337
Rhu	Rosenstein, E	NJ	726

Skin Allergies

A&I	Fonacier, L	NY	490
A&I	Richheimer, M	NY	563

Skin Cancer

D	Almeida, L	NJ	803
D	Aranoff, S	NY	144
D	Basuk, P	NY	567
D	Berkowitz, R	NY	601
D	Berry, R	NY	412
D	Berson, D	NY	145
D	Bickers, D	NY	145
D	Bisaccia, E	NJ	803
D	Bolognia, J	CT	904
D	Bronin, A	NY	601
D	Bruckstein, R	NY	497
D	Buchness, M	NY	145
D	Burke, K	NY	145
D	Bystryn, J	NY	145
D	Clark, R	NY	567
D	Clark, S	NY	146
D	Connolly, A	NJ	706
D	Connors, R	CT	868
D	Corey, T	NJ	664
D	Davis, I	NY	601
D	Demar, L	NY	146
D	Demento, F	NY	497
D	Dolitsky, C	NY	497
D	Eisenberg, R	NJ	844
D	Falcon, R	NY	498
D	Felderman, L	NY	146
D	Fishman, M	NJ	664
D	Fried, S	NJ	664
D	Geronemus, R	NY	147
D	Goldberg, D	NY	147
D	Granstein, R	NY	147
D	Greenspan, A	NY	147

Spec	Name	St	Pg
D	Grossman, K	NJ	786
D	Halpern, A	NY	148
D	Hisler, B	NY	498
D	Hochman, H	NY	148
D	Huh, J	NY	567
D	Jacobs, M	NY	148
D	Klar, T	NY	602
D	Kline, M	NY	148
D	Kolenik, S	CT	868
D	Krivo, J	NY	498
D	Lebwohl, M	NY	149
D	Lederman, J	NY	476
D	Leffell, D	CT	904
D	Levy, R	NY	602
D	Lombardo, P	NY	149
D	Lukash, B	NY	602
D	Machler, B	NJ	706
D	Mackler, K	NY	602
D	Maiocco, K	CT	868
D	Marghoob, A	NY	567
D	Mayer, F	CT	868
D	McCormack, P	NY	476
D	Morman, M	NJ	665
D	Moynihan, G	NY	567
D	Myskowski, P	NY	149
D	Notaro, A	NY	568
D	Orbuch, P	NY	149
D	Oshman, R	CT	868
D	Ostad, A	NY	150
D	Pereira, F	NY	459
D	Podwal, M	NY	150
D	Possick, P	NJ	665
D	Prioleau, P	NY	150
D	Pruzan-Clain, D	CT	869
D	Prystowsky, J	NY	150
D	Ramsay, D	NY	150
D	Ratner, D	NY	150
D	Rigel, D	NY	150
D	Robins, P	NY	150
D	Rosen, D	NY	371
D	Safai, B	NY	151
D	Sarnoff, D	NY	498
D	Schliftman, A	NY	603
D	Schwartz, R	NJ	706
D	Sibrack, L	CT	869
D	Siegel, D	NY	568
D	Simon, S	NY	413
D	Skrokov, R	NY	568
D	Spinowitz, A	NY	499
D	Stillman, M	NY	603
D	Sweeney, E	NJ	665
D	Tanenbaum, D	NY	152
D	Tesser, M	NY	152
D	Treiber, R	NY	603
D	Waldorf, D	NY	553

Spec	Name	St	Pg
D	Waldorf, H	NY	554
D	Walther, R	NY	152
D	Weinberger, G	NJ	844
D	Wrone, D	NJ	760
D	Zweibel, S	NY	603
Onc	Pavlick, A	NY	209
Onc	Pfister, D	NY	209
Oto	Carniol, P	NJ	851
PlS	Granick, M	NJ	723
PlS	Groeger, W	NY	537
PlS	Roth, D	NY	639
PlS	Sklansky, B	NY	538
RadRO	Cooper, J	NY	447
RadRO	Lee, N	NY	329
S	Goydos, J	NJ	779

Skin Cancer & Moles

D	Danziger, S	NY	412
D	Katz, S	NY	371

Skin Cancer Reconstruction

PlS	Lesesne, C	NY	305

Skin Cancer-Head & Neck

Onc	Posner, M	NY	210

Skin Diseases

D	Bagel, J	NJ	741
D	Brademas, M	NY	145
FMed	Moynihan, B	NY	502
FMed	Sutton, I	NY	606
FMed	Ziering, T	NJ	831
IM	Bernard, R	NY	573
IM	Fazio, N	NY	613

Skin Diseases in Transplants/Cancer

D	Grossman, M	NY	601

Skin Diseases-Immunologic

D	Liteplo, R	NY	371

Skin Infections

D	Buchness, M	NY	145
D	Rudikoff, D	NY	371

Skin Laser Surgery

D	Avram, M	NY	144
D	Bank, D	NY	601
D	Basuk, P	NY	567
D	Biro, D	NY	412
D	Brancaccio, R	NY	412

Special Expertise Index

Spec	Name	St	Pg
D	Brauner, G	NJ	664
D	Bruckstein, R	NY	497
D	Clark, S	NY	146
D	De Pietro, W	NY	497
D	Downie, J	NJ	706
D	Geronemus, R	NY	147
D	Greenberg, R	NY	147
D	Grossman, M	NY	148
D	Grossman, M	NY	148
D	Hochman, H	NY	148
D	Katz, B	NY	148
D	Kriegel, D	NY	149
D	Leffell, D	CT	904
D	Levine, L	NY	498
D	Levy, R	NY	602
D	Lombardo, P	NY	149
D	McCormack, P	NY	476
D	Milgraum, S	NJ	760
D	Ostad, A	NY	150
D	Polis, L	NY	150
D	Rapaport, J	NJ	665
D	Safai, B	NY	151
D	Sarnoff, D	NY	498
D	Schultz, N	NY	151
D	Shelton, R	NY	151
D	Waldorf, H	NY	554
D	Wattenberg, D	NY	153
D	Weiss, D	NJ	665
D	Wrone, D	NJ	760
D	Zweibel, S	NY	603
Oto	Brunner, E	NJ	749
Oto	Guida, R	NY	269
PlS	Gotkin, R	NY	537

Skin Tumors

Spec	Name	St	Pg
D	Feldman, P	NY	412
D	Savin, R	CT	904

Skin/Soft Tissue Infection

Spec	Name	St	Pg
Inf	Aufiero, P	NJ	744
Inf	Scheer, M	NY	508
Inf	Soroko, T	NJ	710

Skin/Soft Tissue Infections

Spec	Name	St	Pg
Inf	Brause, B	NY	185
Inf	Helfgott, D	NY	186
Inf	Smith, P	NY	189

Skull Base Surgery

Spec	Name	St	Pg
NS	Bruce, J	NY	217
NS	Chen, C	NY	217
NS	Davis, R	NY	575
NS	Eisenberg, M	NY	516
NS	Golfinos, J	NY	217
NS	Murali, R	NY	621
NS	Schulder, M	NY	516
NS	Sen, C	NY	220
NS	Stieg, P	NY	220
Oto	Close, L	NY	268
Oto	Frank, D	NY	525
Oto	Lalwani, A	NY	271
Oto	Lawson, W	NY	271
Oto	Meiteles, L	NY	630
Oto	Sasaki, C	CT	914
Oto	Storper, I	NY	275

Skull Base Tumors

Spec	Name	St	Pg
NS	Bilsky, M	NY	216
NS	Chen, C	NY	217
NS	Jafar, J	NY	218
NS	Sen, C	NY	220
Oto	Costantino, P	NY	269
Oto	Har-El, G	NY	270
Oto	Kraus, D	NY	271
Oto	Persky, M	NY	272
Oto	Vining, E	CT	914
S	Shah, J	NY	346

Sleep & Snoring Disorders

Spec	Name	St	Pg
Oto	Youngerman, J	NY	526
Pul	Kupfer, Y	NY	446
Pul	Lombardo, G	NY	446

Sleep Apnea

Spec	Name	St	Pg
Oto	Josephson, J	NY	270
Oto	Salzer, S	CT	887
PO	April, M	NY	290
PO	Goldsmith, A	NY	440
PPul	Lee, H	NY	441
PPul	Marcus, M	NY	441
Pul	Garay, S	NY	325
Pul	Krasnogor, L	CT	892
Pul	Lombardo, G	NY	446

Sleep Disorders

Spec	Name	St	Pg
Oto	Schley, W	NY	274
Oto	Volpi, D	NY	276
Ped	Cohen, M	NY	294
Ped	Kotin, N	NY	295
PO	Dolitsky, J	NY	290
PPul	Kanengiser, S	NJ	686
PPul	Lamm, C	NY	291
PPul	Nachajon, R	NJ	824
Psyc	Aronoff, M	NY	310
Pul	Blum, A	NY	540
Pul	Casino, J	NY	642
Pul	Cerrone, F	NJ	855
Pul	Chadha, J	NY	469
Pul	DiPasquale, L	NJ	691
Pul	Elamir, M	NJ	737
Pul	Engler, M	NJ	691
Pul	George, L	NY	445
Pul	Gordon, R	NY	540
Pul	Hammer, A	NY	446
Pul	Karetzky, M	NJ	397
Pul	Lehrman, G	NY	643
Pul	McCalley, S	CT	893
Pul	Rose, H	NJ	692
Pul	Seelagy, M	NJ	751

Sleep Disorders/Apnea

Spec	Name	St	Pg
Oto	Edelstein, D	NY	269
Oto	Fleming, G	NJ	810
Oto	Habib, M	NY	436
Oto	Kates, M	NY	630
Oto	Krespi, Y	NY	271
Oto	Schneider, K	NY	274
Oto	Setzen, M	NY	526
Oto	Shapiro, B	NY	631
Oto	Sinnreich, A	NY	482
Oto	Stewart, M	NY	275
Oto	Strome, M	NY	275
Oto	Tawfik, B	NY	526
PO	Keller, J	NY	634
PO	Respler, D	NJ	686
PPul	Arens, R	NY	391
PPul	Loughlin, G	NY	291
Psyc	Kavey, N	NY	315
Pul	Appel, D	NY	397
Pul	Benton, M	NJ	813
Pul	Burschtin, O	NY	324
Pul	Greenberg, H	NY	540
Pul	Klapholz, A	NY	325
Pul	Mandel, M	NY	643
Pul	Rapoport, D	NY	327
Pul	Wohlberg, G	NY	586

Sleep Disorders/Cardiac Risk

Spec	Name	St	Pg
Cv	Goldweit, R	NJ	661

Sleep Medicine

Spec	Name	St	Pg
N	Katz, A	CT	912
Oto	Krevitt, L	NY	271
Psyc	Kavey, N	NY	315
Pul	Rapoport, D	NY	327

Small Cell Lung Cancer

Spec	Name	St	Pg
Onc	Krug, L	NY	207

Spec	Name	St	Pg
Smallpox			
D	Rudikoff, D	NY	371
Smoking Cessation			
AdP	Paul, E	NY	123
FMed	Kelly, S	NY	606
Psyc	Glassman, A	NY	313
Psyc	Wineburg, E	NY	323
Pul	Appel, D	NY	397
Pul	George, L	NY	445
Pul	Smith, P	NY	446
Snoring/Sleep Apnea			
Oto	Krespi, Y	NY	271
Oto	Levine, S	CT	886
Oto	Moisa, I	NY	525
Oto	Perlman, P	NY	526
Oto	Ryback, H	NY	630
Oto	Schneider, K	NY	274
Oto	Setzen, M	NY	526
Oto	Shemen, L	NY	274
Oto	Tawfik, B	NY	526
Oto	Volpi, D	NY	276
Soft Tissue Pathology			
Path	Schiller, A	NY	280
Soft Tissue Tumors			
DR	Panicek, D	NY	156
Path	Kahn, L	NY	527
S	Barcewicz, P	CT	920
Solid Tumors			
Hem	Kopel, S	NY	419
Hem	Wolf, D	NY	185
Onc	Aisner, J	NJ	766
Onc	Bashevkin, M	NY	424
Onc	Forte, F	NJ	674
Onc	Kelly, W	CT	910
Onc	Puccio, C	NY	618
PHO	Gorlick, R	NY	390
PHO	Guarini, L	NY	439
PHO	Kamalakar, P	NJ	720
PHO	Redner, A	NY	531
PS	Alexander, F	NJ	687
RadRO	Donahue, B	NY	447
Solid Tumors-Pediatric			
PHO	Marcus, J	NY	287
Spasticity Management			
N	Azhar, S	NY	428

Spec	Name	St	Pg
PMR	Kirshblum, S	NJ	722
PMR	Rosenberg, C	NY	583
Special Health Care Needs			
Ped	Mezey, A	NY	442
Ped	Oppenheim, J	NY	442
Spina Bifida			
CG	Marion, R	NY	370
ChiN	Cracco, J	NY	411
PMR	Armento, M	NJ	853
PMR	Gold, J	NY	298
Spinal Access Surgery			
VascS	Fantini, G	NY	362
VascS	Nalbandian, M	NY	363
Spinal Cord Disorders			
N	Goodgold, A	NY	223
N	Levine, D	NY	225
NS	Cardoso, E	NY	428
Spinal Cord Injury			
Ger	Schor, J	NY	610
NS	Heary, R	NJ	714
PMR	Ahn, J	NY	298
PMR	Bryce, T	NY	298
PMR	Kirshblum, S	NJ	722
PMR	Nelson, M	NY	637
PMR	Ragnarsson, K	NY	299
PMR	Root, B	NY	535
PMR	Stein, A	NY	535
PMR	Valenza, J	NJ	812
Spinal Cord Injury & Colonic Motility			
Ge	Korsten, M	NY	376
Spinal Cord Injury-Complex			
NS	Frempong-Boadu, A	NY	217
Spinal Cord Injury-Pediatric			
PMR	Armento, M	NJ	853
PMR	Fantasia, M	NJ	776
Spinal Cord Surgery-Pediatric			
NS	Feldstein, N	NY	217
Spinal Cord Tumors			
NS	Frempong-Boadu, A	NY	217
NS	Kornel, E	NY	621

Spec	Name	St	Pg
NS	Moore, F	NY	219
NS	Przybylski, G	NJ	768
NS	Snow, R	NY	220
NS	Steinberger, A	NY	220
Spinal Deformity			
NS	Heary, R	NJ	714
OrS	Bitan, F	NY	254
OrS	Dowling, T	NY	579
OrS	Lonner, B	NY	260
OrS	Schwab, F	NY	264
OrS	Smith, B	CT	914
Spinal Disc Replacement			
NS	Apostolides, P	CT	880
NS	Chiurco, A	NJ	746
NS	Davis, R	NY	575
NS	Goulart, H	NJ	677
NS	Hartl, R	NY	218
NS	Kaiser, M	NY	218
OrS	Bendo, J	NY	254
OrS	Bitan, F	NY	254
OrS	Cammisa, F	NY	255
OrS	Casden, A	NY	255
OrS	Dwyer, J	NJ	834
OrS	Emami, A	NJ	823
OrS	Errico, T	NY	256
OrS	Goldstein, J	NY	257
OrS	Hecht, A	NY	259
OrS	Lombardi, J	NJ	771
OrS	Sandhu, H	NY	264
Spinal Disorders			
N	Haimovic, I	NY	517
N	Hainline, B	NY	517
N	Neophytides, A	NY	227
N	Schaefer, J	NY	228
N	Smallberg, G	NY	229
N	Swerdlow, M	NY	385
N	Weinberg, H	NY	230
NS	Lavyne, M	NY	219
OrS	Mendes, J	NJ	718
OrS	Moskovich, R	NY	262
Spinal Disorders-Degenerative			
NS	Anant, A	NY	427
NS	Huang, P	NY	218
NS	Onesti, S	NY	428
NS	Oppenheim, J	NY	556
OrS	Bitan, F	NY	254
Spinal Injury			
OrS	Reich, S	NJ	771

Special Expertise Index

Special Expertise Index

Spec	Name	St	Pg
NS	Lansen, T	NY	621
NS	LaSala, P	NY	384
NS	Lee, T	NY	621
NS	Rajaraman, V	NJ	678
NS	Sisti, M	NY	220
NS	Spitzer, D	NY	556
NS	Zampella, E	NJ	807
NS	Zonenshayn, M	NY	428
RadRO	Braver, J	NJ	836
RadRO	Isaacson, S	NY	329
RadRO	Knisely, J	CT	919
RadRO	Masino, F	CT	893
RadRO	Meek, A	NY	586
RadRO	Mullen, E	NY	542
RadRO	Schwartz, L	NJ	855

Stomach Cancer

Spec	Name	St	Pg
S	August, D	NJ	779
S	Brennan, M	NY	341
S	Coit, D	NY	341
S	Fong, Y	NY	342
S	Reed, W	NY	546

Strabismus

Spec	Name	St	Pg
Oph	Campolattaro, B	NY	239
Oph	Caputo, A	NJ	716
Oph	Chen, L	NJ	809
Oph	Cossari, A	NY	577
Oph	Deutsch, J	NY	432
Oph	Gallin, P	NY	243
Oph	Horowitz, M	NY	626
Oph	Magramm, I	NY	246
Oph	Muchnick, R	NY	247
Oph	Napolitano, J	NJ	771
Oph	Rubin, S	NY	522
Oph	Steele, M	NY	251
Oph	Turtel, L	NJ	791
Oph	Wagner, R	NJ	717
Oph	Wagner, R	NJ	717
Oph	Wang, F	NY	252
Oph	Weingarten, P	NY	557
Oph	Wisnicki, H	NY	253

Strabismus-Adult & Pediatric

Spec	Name	St	Pg
Oph	Eggers, H	NY	241
Oph	Hall, L	NY	244
Oph	Most, R	NY	627
Oph	Potter, W	CT	883
Oph	Raab, E	NY	248

Stress Echocardiography

Spec	Name	St	Pg
Cv	Cramer, M	NY	491
Cv	Golier, F	NY	596
Cv	Mueller, R	NY	134

Stress Management

Spec	Name	St	Pg
ChAP	Bartlett, J	NJ	705
Cv	Hodges, D	NJ	661
Psyc	Aronoff, M	NY	310

Stroke

Spec	Name	St	Pg
ChiN	Kosofsky, B	NY	141
ChiN	Ment, L	CT	903
ChiN	Molofsky, W	NY	141
ChiN	Pavlakis, S	NY	411
Ger	Jacobs, L	NY	377
Ger	Schor, J	NY	610
IM	Butt, A	NY	421
IM	Gil, C	NJ	765
IM	Kernan, W	CT	908
N	Anselmi, G	NJ	735
N	Azhar, S	NY	428
N	Bansil, S	NJ	848
N	Blady, D	NJ	714
N	Brust, J	NY	222
N	Charney, J	NY	222
N	Chodosh, E	NJ	822
N	Cohen, D	NY	576
N	Cohen, J	NY	384
N	Coll, R	NY	222
N	Fellus, J	NJ	714
N	Fink, M	NY	223
N	Foo, S	NY	223
N	Gerber, O	NY	576
N	Gizzi, M	NJ	768
N	Gizzi, M	NJ	768
N	Greer, D	CT	912
N	Gropen, T	NY	429
N	Herman, M	NJ	790
N	Horvath, S	NY	224
N	Kay, A	NY	429
N	Klein, P	NJ	678
N	Koppel, B	NY	224
N	Levin, K	NJ	678
N	Levine, D	NY	225
Cv	Levine, S	NY	225
N	Libman, R	NY	518
N	Marks, S	NY	622
N	Mayer, S	NY	226
N	Mohr, J	NY	226
N	Morris, J	NY	622
N	Nahm, F	CT	881
N	Neophytides, A	NY	227
N	Oh, Y	NJ	769
N	Oribe, E	NY	227
N	Rosenbaum, D	NY	430
N	Rudolph, S	NY	430
N	Sachs, S	NJ	849
N	Sadeghi, H	NJ	735
N	Schaefer, J	NY	228
N	Schanzer, B	NJ	849
N	Sena, K	CT	881
N	Sheinart, K	NY	228
N	Siegel, K	CT	881
N	Singh, A	NY	622
N	Sobol, N	NY	430
N	Sparr, S	NY	385
N	Tuhrim, S	NY	229
N	Vas, G	NY	430
N	Vester, J	NJ	747
N	Weinberg, H	NY	230
N	Weinberger, J	NY	230
NRad	Drayer, B	NY	230
NRad	Fiorella, D	NY	576
NRad	Tenner, M	NY	623
NS	Riina, H	NY	219
NS	Woo, H	NY	575

Stroke Rehabilitation

Spec	Name	St	Pg
PMR	Ahn, J	NY	298
PMR	Atakent, P	NY	442
PMR	Flanagan, S	NY	298
PMR	Greenwald, B	NY	299
PMR	Stein, A	NY	535
PMR	Stein, J	NY	300

Substance Abuse

Spec	Name	St	Pg
ChAP	Pincus, E	NJ	663
IM	O'Connor, P	CT	908
N	Brust, J	NY	222
Psyc	Boutaeva, Z	CT	891
Psyc	Morgan, C	CT	891
Psyc	Nunes, E	NY	317
Psyc	Pines, J	NY	318
Psyc	Tamerin, J	CT	892

Substance Abuse Effects in Newborn

Spec	Name	St	Pg
NP	Rosen, T	NY	213

Substance Abuse in ADHD Patients

Spec	Name	St	Pg
AdP	Levin, F	NY	123

Sudden Death Prevention

Spec	Name	St	Pg
CE	Levine, J	NY	491

Sudden Infant Death Syndrome

Special Expertise Index

Special Expertise Index

Special Expertise Index

Special Expertise Index

The Best in American Medicine
www.CastleConnolly.com

Alphabetical Listing of Doctors

Name	Specialty	Pg
A		
Abelow, Arthur (NY)	Ge	375
Abemayor, Elie (NY)	Ge	607
Abenavoli, Tancredi (NY)	IM	612
Aberg, Judith (NY)	Inf	185
Abittan, Meyer (NY)	IC	510
Ablaza, Valerie (NJ)	PlS	723
Abott, Michael (NY)	Pul	444
Abramowitz, Avram (NY)	Onc	464
Abrams, Jeffrey (NJ)	OrS	748
Abramson, David (NY)	Oph	238
Abramson, Sara (NY)	DR	153
Abramson, Steven (NY)	Rhu	333
Abright, Arthur (NY)	ChAP	138
Abrol, Sunil (NY)	TS	451
Abu-Rustum, Nadeem (NY)	GO	176
Abularrage, Joseph (NY)	Ped	468
Accardi, Frank (NY)	Oph	238
Accettola, Albert (NY)	OrS	481
Accurso, Charles (NJ)	Ge	831
Acker, Peter (NY)	Ped	635
Ackerman, Jacob (NY)	Oph	431
Ackert, John (NY)	Ge	163
Acosta, Rod (CT)	FMed	870
Acquista, Angelo (NY)	Pul	323
Adam, Henry (NY)	Ped	392
Adams, David (NY)	TS	348
Adams, Francis (NY)	Pul	323
Adams, Marc (NY)	RadRO	485
Addonizio, Gerard (NY)	Psyc	639
Addonizio, Linda (NY)	PCd	281
Addrizzo-Harris, Doreen (NY)	Pul	324
Adelman, Mark (NY)	VascS	362
Adelman, Ronald (NY)	Ger	174
Adelsberg, Bernard (CT)	A&I	901
Ades, Joseph (NY)	IM	612
Adesman, Andrew (NY)	Ped	533

Name	Specialty	Pg
Adler, Edward (NY)	OrS	253
Adler, Harry (NY)	S	448
Adler, Howard (NY)	Ge	163
Adler, Jack (NY)	Pul	324
Adler, Kenneth (NJ)	Onc	806
Adler, Lenard (NY)	Psyc	309
Adler, Mitchell (NY)	IM	189
Adler, Ronald (NY)	DR	153
Adler, Stephen (NY)	Nep	620
Adlersberg, Jay (NY)	Rhu	333
Afridi, Shariq (NJ)	Ge	743
Agarwal, Kishan (NJ)	PCd	773
Agarwal, Nanakram (NY)	S	398
Agdere, Levon (NY)	PEn	438
Aghajanian, Carol (NY)	Onc	201
Agin, Carole (NY)	PM	580
Agress, Harry (NJ)	NuM	679
Agri, Robyn (NJ)	PMR	750
Agrin, Richard (NJ)	EDM	761
Aguila, Helen (NJ)	PPul	721
Agus, Bertrand (NY)	Rhu	334
Aharon, Raphael (NY)	Oph	466
Ahlborn, Thomas (NJ)	S	694
Ahluwalia, Brij M Singh (NY)	N	621
Ahmed, Fakhiuddin (NY)	Onc	424
Ahmed, Tauseef (NY)	Onc	617
Ahn, Christina (NY)	PlS	301
Ahn, Jung (NY)	PMR	298
Aisenberg, James (NY)	Ge	163
Aisner, Joseph (NJ)	Onc	766
Ajl, Stephen (NY)	Ped	441
Akhund, Birjis (NY)	Onc	574
Akinboboye, Olakunle (NY)	Cv	457
Albin, Joan (NY)	EDM	604
Albom, Michael (NY)	D	144
Alderman, Elizabeth (NY)	AM	367
Aldrich, Thomas (NY)	Pul	396

Alphabetical Listing of Doctors

Name	Specialty	Pg	Name	Specialty	Pg
Aledo, Alexander (NY)	PHO	286	Amorosi, Edward (NY)	Hem	181
Aledort, Louis (NY)	Hem	181	Amoruso, Robert (NJ)	Pul	824
Alexander, Frederick (NJ)	PS	687	Amory, Spencer (NY)	S	340
Alexiades, Michael (NY)	OrS	254	Anant, Ashok (NY)	NS	427
Alfonso, Antonio (NY)	S	449	Andaz, Shahriyour (NY)	TS	546
Alizadeh, Kaveh (NY)	PlS	535	Andersen, Holly (NY)	Cv	128
Allegra, Donald (NJ)	Inf	805	Anderson, Mark (NJ)	TS	780
Allen, Carol (NY)	EDM	373	Andiman, Warren (CT)	PInf	915
Allen, Jeffrey (NY)	ChiN	140	Andrade, Joseph (NY)	Ped	392
Allen, Steven (NY)	Hem	507	Andrei, Valeriu (NJ)	S	726
Allendorf, Dennis (NY)	Ped	293	Andriani, Rudy (CT)	U	897
Almeida, Laila (NJ)	D	803	Andriola, Mary (NY)	ChiN	566
Almeleh, Jack (NY)	Psyc	309	Anene, Okechukwu (NJ)	PCCM	773
Almeyda, Elizabeth (NY)	PlS	301	Angeli, Stephen (NJ)	IC	673
Aloia, John (NY)	EDM	500	Angioletti, Louis (NY)	Oph	238
Alper, Kenneth (NY)	Psyc	309	Angoff, Ronald (CT)	Ped	916
Alpert, Barbara (NY)	IM	612	Angrist, Richard (NJ)	Oph	833
Alpert, Scott (NY)	OrS	579	Anhalt, Henry (NJ)	PEn	852
Altbaum, Robert (CT)	IM	874	Ankobiah, William (NY)	Pul	469
Altchek, David (NY)	SM	338	Annabi, Iyad (NY)	FMed	606
Alterman, Lloyd (NJ)	IM	846	Ansell, Jack (NY)	Hem	181
Altholz, Jeffrey (NY)	IM	613	Anselmi, Gregory (NJ)	N	735
Altman, Robin (NY)	Ped	636	Anto, Maliakal (NY)	Cv	491
Altman, Wayne (NJ)	OrS	682	Anton, John (NY)	PlS	584
Altmann, Dory (NJ)	IC	765	Antonelle, Robert (NY)	Ge	607
Altorki, Nasser (NY)	TS	348	Antony, Michael (NY)	Ge	375
Altschul, Larry (NY)	Cv	564	Anyane-Yeboa, Kwame (NY)	CG	141
Alvarez, Manuel (NJ)	MF	673	Apatoff, Brian (NY)	N	221
Alweiss, Gary (NJ)	N	678	Aponte, Alex (NY)	FMed	570
Ames, Richard (NY)	Nep	214	Apostolides, Paul (CT)	NS	880
Amin, Hossam (NY)	Pul	445	Appel, David (NY)	Pul	397
Amin, Mahendra (NY)	IM	463	Appel, Gerald (NY)	Nep	214
Amin, Milan (NY)	Oto	267	Appelbaum, Jeffrey (NY)	N	466
Amin, Nikhil (NY)	PPul	634	Appelbaum, Paul (NY)	Psyc	310
Amin, Ravindra (NY)	GerPsy	418	Applebaum, Eric (NJ)	A&I	801
Amis, E Stephen (NY)	DR	371	April, Max (NY)	PO	290
Amler, David (NY)	Ped	636	Aprile, Georgette (NY)	D	497
Ammazzalorso, Michael (NY)	IM	508	Apuzzio, Joseph (NJ)	ObG	715
Amodio, John (NY)	DR	413	Apuzzo, Thomas (NY)	FMed	606

Alphabetical Listing of Doctors

Name	Specialty	Pg	Name	Specialty	Pg
Aranoff, Shera (NY)	D	144	Askanas, Alexander (NY)	Cv	128
Arbour, Robert (NJ)	S	796	Askenase, Philip (CT)	A&I	901
Arcasoy, Selim (NY)	Pul	324	Asnes, Russell (NJ)	Ped	687
Arcati, Anthony (NY)	FMed	502	Asnis, Deborah (NY)	Inf	419
Arcati, Robert (NY)	FMed	502	Asnis, Gregory (NY)	Psyc	396
Arden, Martha (NY)	AM	489	Asnis, Stanley (NY)	OrS	523
Arena, Francis (NY)	Onc	512	Asprinio, David (NY)	OrS	628
Arens, Raanan (NY)	PPul	391	Aston, Sherrell (NY)	PlS	301
Argenziano, Michael (NY)	TS	348	Astrow, Alan (NY)	Onc	424
Aries, Philip (NY)	Oph	577	Atakent, Pinar (NY)	PMR	442
Ariyan, Stephan (CT)	PlS	917	Athanail, Steven (NY)	FMed	414
Ark, Jon (NJ)	HS	743	Athanasian, Edward (NY)	HS	178
Arkow, Stan (NY)	Psyc	310	Atkin, Suzanne (NJ)	IM	710
Armbruster, Robert (NY)	ObG	623	Atlas, Arthur (NJ)	PPul	811
Armenakas, Noel (NY)	U	353	Attas, Lewis (NJ)	Onc	674
Armento, Michael (NJ)	PMR	853	Attia, Evelyn (NY)	Psyc	310
Arnell, Tracey (NY)	CRS	142	Attiyeh, Fadi (NY)	S	340
Arno, Louis (NJ)	Pul	835	Attkiss, Keith (CT)	PlS	890
Arnold, Thomas (NY)	VascS	589	Auerbach, Mitchell (NY)	Ge	607
Arnon, Rica (NY)	PCd	281	Aufiero, Patrick (NJ)	Inf	744
Arnstein, Ellis (NY)	Ped	392	August, David (NJ)	S	779
Aronne, Louis (NY)	IM	189	August, Phyllis (NY)	Nep	214
Aronoff, Michael (NY)	Psyc	310	Auguste, Louis (NY)	S	545
Aronson, Peter (CT)	Nep	911	Auran, James (NY)	Oph	239
Aronson, Thomas (NY)	Psyc	584	Austin, John (NY)	DR	153
Arpadi, Stephen (NY)	Ped	293	Austin, Kenneth (NY)	OrS	557
Aruny, John (CT)	VIR	922	Aviv, Jonathan (NY)	Oto	268
Arvanitis, Michael (NJ)	CRS	785	Avram, Marc (NY)	D	144
Asarian, Armand (NY)	CRS	411	Avruskin, Theodore (NY)	PEn	438
Asbell, Penny (NY)	Oph	238	Avvento, Louis (NY)	Hem	572
Ascheim, Robert (NY)	IM	189	Axelrod, Deborah (NY)	S	340
Ascher, Enrico (NY)	VascS	453	Axelrod, Felicia B (NY)	Ped	293
Ascher-Walsh, Charles (NY)	ObG	232	Axelrod, Sheldon (NY)	U	649
Ascherman, Jeffrey (NY)	PlS	301	Ayoub, Thomas (CT)	ObG	881
Ashamalla, Hani (NY)	RadRO	447	Ayyanathan, Karpukarasi (NJ)	Ped	852
Ashikari, Andrew (NY)	S	646	Azhar, Salman (NY)	N	428
Ashinoff, Robin (NJ)	D	664	Azodi, Masoud (CT)	GO	906
Ashinsky, Douglas (NJ)	IM	831			
Ashley, Richard (NY)	U	548			

Alphabetical Listing of Doctors

Name	Specialty	Pg
B		
Babitz, Lisa (NY)	IM	190
Babu, Sateesh (NY)	VascS	650
Bacall, Charles (NY)	ObG	232
Baccash, Emil (NY)	Ger	417
Bach, John (NJ)	PMR	722
Bacha, Emile (NY)	TS	348
Bachmann, Gloria (NJ)	ObG	769
Backe, Henry (CT)	HS	872
Bade, Harry (NJ)	OrS	792
Badikian, Arthur (NY)	Psyc	639
Badshah, Cyrus (NY)	Inf	185
Baer, Jeanne (NY)	DR	153
Bagel, Jerry (NJ)	D	741
Bahr, Gerald (NY)	CCM	144
Bailey, Michele (NY)	Ped	636
Bailine, Samuel (NY)	Psyc	538
Bains, Manjit (NY)	TS	348
Bains, Yatinder (NJ)	IM	711
Baiocco, Peter (NY)	Ge	163
Baiser, Dennis (NJ)	Ped	750
Bajorin, Dean (NY)	Onc	202
Baker, Azzam (NJ)	Ped	736
Baker, Daniel (NY)	PlS	301
Baker, David (NY)	ObG	576
Baldwin, Hilary (NY)	D	412
Bale, Allen (CT)	CG	903
Balk, Sophie (NY)	Ped	392
Balkin, Michael (NY)	EDM	569
Ballantyne, Garth (NJ)	S	694
Balot, Barry (NY)	IM	573
Baltimore, Robert (CT)	PInf	915
Bangaru, Babu (NY)	PGe	285
Bank, David (NY)	D	601
Banks, Judy (NJ)	ObG	808
Bansal, Rajendra (NY)	Oph	625
Bansil, Shalini (NJ)	N	848
Banzon, Manuel (NJ)	ObG	735

Name	Specialty	Pg
Bar, Michael (CT)	Hem	872
Bar-Chama, Natan (NY)	U	353
Barakat, Richard (NY)	GO	177
Baram, Daniel (NY)	Pul	585
Baranetsky, Nicholas (NJ)	EDM	707
Barbaccia, Ann (NY)	ObG	519
Barbasch, Avi (NY)	Onc	202
Barbuto, Joseph (NY)	Psyc	310
Barcewicz, Paul (CT)	S	920
Barie, Philip (NY)	S	340
Barile, Gaetano (NY)	Oph	239
Barker, Barbara (NY)	Oph	239
Barley, Christopher (NY)	IM	190
Barmakian, Joseph (NJ)	OrS	850
Barnard, Nicola (NJ)	Path	772
Barone, Clement (NY)	DR	153
Barone, Joseph (NJ)	U	837
Barone, Richard (NY)	Rhu	644
Barron, O Alton (NY)	HS	178
Bartlett, Jacqueline (NJ)	ChAP	705
Bartolomeo, Robert (NY)	Ge	503
Barzegar, Hooshang (NY)	ObG	431
Basch, Samuel (NY)	Psyc	310
Bashevkin, Michael (NY)	Onc	424
Baskin, David (NY)	IM	190
Baskin, Martin (NY)	Pul	324
Baskind, Lawrence (NY)	Ped	636
Basralian, Kevin (NJ)	U	696
Bassett, Clifford (NY)	A&I	124
Bastawros, Mary (NY)	Ped	483
Basuk, Pamela (NY)	D	567
Basuk, Paul (NY)	Ge	163
Bateman, David (NY)	NP	213
Batsford, William (CT)	CE	901
Bauer, Bertha (NY)	Rhu	334
Baum, Howard (NJ)	Ge	820
Bauman, Jonathan (NY)	Psyc	640
Bauman, Phillip (NY)	OrS	254
Baumann, John (NJ)	RadRO	751

Name	Specialty	Pg	Name	Specialty	Pg
Baumgaertner, Michael (CT)	OrS	913	Bennett, Harvey (NJ)	ChiN	802
Baydin, Jeffrey (NJ)	OrS	809	Benson, Mitchell (NY)	U	353
Bazzy-Asaad, Alia (CT)	PPul	916	Bent, John (NY)	PO	391
Beauregard, Lou-Anne (NJ)	Cv	785	Benton, Marc (NJ)	Pul	813
Beccia, David (NY)	U	589	Benvenisty, Alan (NY)	VascS	362
Becker, Alfred (NY)	Rhu	559	Berbari, Nicholas (NY)	IM	509
Bederson, Joshua (NY)	NS	216	Berck, David (NY)	MF	616
Bednarek, Karl (NY)	Ge	163	Berdini, Jeffrey (NJ)	U	697
Behm, Dutsi (NY)	IM	421	Berdoff, Russell (NY)	Cv	128
Behr, Raymond (NY)	Psyc	538	Berenstein, Alejandro (NY)	NRad	230
Behrens, Myles (NY)	Oph	239	Berezin, Marc (NY)	SM	560
Beim, Robert (NJ)	ObG	849	Berezin, Stuart (NY)	PGe	633
Belamarich, Peter (NY)	Ped	392	Berger, Bernard (NY)	D	567
Beldner, Steven (NY)	HS	178	Berger, Jack (NY)	Rhu	645
Belilos, Elise (NY)	Rhu	543	Berger, Jeffrey (NY)	IM	509
Bell, Jonathan (CT)	A&I	865	Berger, Judith (NY)	Inf	379
Bell, Kevin (NJ)	IM	832	Berger, Marvin (NY)	Cv	128
Bellemare, Sarah (NY)	S	398	Bergh, Paul (NJ)	RE	814
Bello, Jacqueline (NY)	NRad	385	Bergman, Donald (NY)	EDM	158
Bello, Mary (NJ)	FMed	667	Bergman, Michael (NY)	Pul	445
Bellucci, Alessandro (NY)	Nep	515	Bergmann, Steven (NY)	Cv	128
Belmont, H Michael (NY)	Rhu	334	Bergtraum, Marcia (NY)	ChiN	496
Belok, Lennart (NY)	N	221	Berke, Andrew (NY)	IC	511
Belsh, Jerry (NJ)	N	768	Berke, Stanley (NY)	Oph	520
Bemporad, Jules (NY)	Psyc	640	Berkey, Peter (NY)	Inf	611
Ben-Menachem, Tamir (NJ)	Ge	762	Berkowitz, Howard (NY)	Psyc	443
Ben-Zvi, Jeffrey (NY)	Ge	164	Berkowitz, Leonard (NY)	Inf	419
Benardete, Ethan (NY)	NS	427	Berkowitz, Norman (NY)	Ped	636
Bendo, John (NY)	OrS	254	Berkowitz, Rhonda (NY)	D	601
Benedetto, Dominick (NJ)	Oph	736	Berkowitz, Richard (NY)	MF	200
Benedict, Leonard (NY)	ObG	519	Berkowitz, Richard (NJ)	EDM	820
Benedicto, Milagros (NY)	ObG	466	Berkwits, Kieve (CT)	PCd	887
Benevenia, Joseph (NJ)	OrS	717	Berman, Alvin (NY)	ObG	232
Beniaminovitz, Ainat (NY)	Cv	553	Berman, Daniel (NY)	IM	613
Benisovich, Vladimir (NY)	Onc	464	Berman, David (NY)	Oph	432
Benito, Carlos (NJ)	MF	806	Berman, Ellin (NY)	Onc	202
Benjamin, Ernest (NY)	CCM	144	Berman, Mark (NJ)	OrS	682
Benjamin, John (NY)	Psyc	538	Berman, Morton (NY)	Ped	636
Benkov, Keith (NY)	PGe	285	Berman, Russell (NY)	S	340

Alphabetical Listing of Doctors

Name	Specialty	Pg	Name	Specialty	Pg
Berman, Sandra (NY)	IM	421	Bia, Margaret (CT)	Nep	911
Berman, Sheldon (NY)	Psyc	538	Biagiotti, Wendy (NY)	FMed	374
Berman, Steven (NY)	U	353	Bialer, Martin (NY)	CG	496
Bernard, Robert (NY)	IM	573	Biancaniello, Thomas (NY)	PCd	581
Bernard, Robert (NY)	PlS	638	Bickers, David (NY)	D	145
Bernardini, Dennis (NY)	Pul	585	Bielory, Leonard (NJ)	A&I	842
Bernardino, C Roberto (CT)	Oph	913	Bienenstock, Harry (NY)	Rhu	448
Bernardo, Salvatore (NJ)	FMed	786	Bierman, Fredrick (NY)	PCd	528
Bernhardt, Bernard (NY)	Onc	617	Bigliani, Louis (NY)	OrS	254
Bernik, Stephanie (NY)	S	340	Bikoff, David (NJ)	PlS	689
Bernik, Thomas (NY)	VascS	362	Bilezikian, John (NY)	EDM	158
Bernstein, Brett (NY)	Ge	164	Bilfinger, Thomas (NY)	TS	588
Bernstein, Chaim (NY)	Pul	445	Billett, Henny (NY)	Hem	378
Bernstein, Charles (NY)	D	476	Bilsky, Mark (NY)	NS	216
Bernstein, David (NY)	Ge	503	Bindelglass, David (CT)	OrS	884
Bernstein, Harvey (NY)	Ped	582	Binder, Ralph (NY)	Pul	642
Bernstein, Larry (NY)	A&I	457	Binns, Joseph (NJ)	Ge	787
Bernstein, Lawrence (NY)	Rhu	448	Birch, Thomas (NJ)	Inf	671
Bernstein, Michael (NY)	S	449	Bird, Hector (NY)	ChAP	138
Bernstein, Robert (NY)	D	145	Birkhoff, John (NY)	U	353
Bernstein, William (NY)	Ped	558	Birnbaum, Audrey (NY)	PGe	633
Berry, Richard (NY)	D	412	Birnbaum, Jay (NY)	PlS	301
Berson, Barry (NY)	DR	153	Birns, Douglas (NY)	U	353
Berson, Diane (NY)	D	145	Birns, Robert (NJ)	Pul	691
Besser, Gary (CT)	ObG	882	Biro, David (NY)	D	412
Besser, Louis (NY)	Cv	475	Bisaccia, Emil (NJ)	D	803
Besser, Walter (NY)	OrS	467	Bisberg, Dorothy (NJ)	PPul	721
Bessey, Palmer (NY)	S	340	Biser, Seth (NY)	Oph	625
Bessler, Marc (NY)	S	341	Bitan, Fabien (NY)	OrS	254
Bethel, Colin (NJ)	PS	721	Bitton, Rachelle (NY)	EDM	500
Better, Donna (NY)	PCd	528	Biviano, Bernard (NY)	S	471
Bevelaqua, Frederick (NY)	Pul	324	Bivona, James (CT)	IM	874
Beyda, Allan (NY)	IM	463	Blackwood, M Michele (NJ)	S	726
Beyda, Bernadette (NY)	D	459	Blady, David (NJ)	N	714
Beyerl, Brian (NJ)	NS	807	Blair, Bryan (NY)	U	649
Bhagat, Neelakshi (NJ)	Oph	716	Blair, Emily (CT)	ObG	882
Bharathan, Thayyullathil (NY)	IM	421	Blair, Lester (NY)	Pul	324
Bhatt, Anjani (NY)	EDM	500	Blaivas, Jerry (NY)	U	354
Bhatt, Ashok (NY)	Psyc	539	Blake, James (NY)	Cv	128

Name	Specialty	Pg	Name	Specialty	Pg
Blanck, Richard (NY)	N	516	Bodenheimer, Henry (NY)	Ge	164
Blanco, Jody (NY)	ObG	232	Bodenstein, Lawrence (NY)	PS	292
Blank, Ellen (NJ)	D	733	Bodis-Wollner, Ivan (NY)	N	428
Blau, Sheldon (NY)	Rhu	543	Bodner, William (NY)	RadRO	398
Blei, Francine (NY)	PHO	286	Bogaty, Stanley (NY)	Oph	577
Bleiberg, Melvyn (NY)	Cv	594	Bogen, Steven (NY)	Psyc	640
Bleicher, Robert (NJ)	Ge	820	Bogin, Marc (NY)	Cv	475
Bleiweiss, Ira (NY)	Path	278	Boim, Marilynn (NJ)	PEn	749
Blick, Michael (NJ)	Cv	801	Bojko, Thomas (NJ)	PCCM	773
Blitzer, Andrew (NY)	Oto	268	Bolognia, Jean (CT)	D	904
Blondo, Dennis (NJ)	Oph	770	Bomback, Fredric (NY)	Ped	636
Blood, David (NJ)	Cv	660	Bonagura, Vincent (NY)	PA&I	527
Bloom, Norman (NY)	S	341	Bonaventura, Lisa (NJ)	IM	832
Bloom, Patricia (NY)	Ger	174	Bond, Annette (CT)	MF	877
Bloomfield, Diane (NY)	Ped	392	Bondi, Elliott (NY)	Pul	445
Bloomgarden, David (NY)	EDM	604	Bone, Stanley (NY)	Psyc	310
Bloomgarden, Zachary (NY)	EDM	158	Bonheim, Nelson (CT)	Ge	871
Blum, Alan (NY)	Pul	540	Bonilla, Mary Ann (NJ)	PHO	823
Blum, Conrad (NY)	EDM	158	Boniuk, Vivien (NY)	Oph	520
Blum, Daniel (NY)	IM	463	Boockvar, John (NY)	NS	216
Blum, David (NY)	EDM	604	Boodish, Wesley (NJ)	Ped	722
Blum, Jay (NJ)	A&I	757	Bookner, Scott (NY)	Ped	636
Blum, Mark (NJ)	Cv	801	Boone, Peter (CT)	OrS	884
Blum, Ronald (NY)	Onc	202	Boorjian, Peter (NJ)	U	728
Blumberg, Joel (CT)	IM	874	Borah, Gregory (NJ)	PlS	776
Blume, Ralph (NY)	Rhu	334	Borao, Frank (NJ)	S	796
Blumenfeld, Hal (CT)	N	912	Borbely, Antal (NY)	Psyc	310
Blumenfeld, Jon (NY)	Nep	214	Borcich, Anthony (NY)	Ge	164
Blumenthal, David (NY)	Cv	129	Borek, Mark (NY)	Cv	564
Blumstein, Meyer (NY)	Ge	503	Borer, Jeffrey (NY)	Cv	408
Blyskal, Stanley (NY)	FMed	570	Borg, Morton (NY)	PCd	281
Boachie-Adjei, Oheneba (NY)	OrS	254	Borgen, Patrick (NY)	S	449
Bobby, Paul (CT)	MF	876	Borkowsky, William (NY)	PInf	288
Bobroff, Lewis (NY)	DR	554	Borriello, Raffaele (NY)	S	449
Bochner, Bernard (NY)	U	354	Boruchoff, Susan (NJ)	Inf	764
Bochner, Ronnie (NJ)	ObG	770	Boscamp, Jeffrey (NJ)	PInf	686
Bockman, Richard (NY)	EDM	159	Bosco, Joseph (NY)	OrS	254
Boczko, Judd (NY)	U	649	Bosl, George (NY)	Onc	202
Boczko, Stanley (NY)	U	354	Bosso, John (NY)	A&I	553

Alphabetical Listing of Doctors

Name	Specialty	Pg	Name	Specialty	Pg
Bostrom, Mathias (NY)	OrS	254	Brenner, Steven (NY)	RE	543
Bosworth, Jay (NY)	RadRO	542	Bressman, Susan (NY)	N	221
Botwin, Clifford (NJ)	OrS	850	Brewer, Marlon (NY)	IM	463
Botwinick, Nelson (NY)	HS	179	Brick, David (NY)	PCd	281
Bourla, Steven (NY)	Nep	515	Brickman, Alan (NY)	EDM	413
Boutaeva, Zinaida (CT)	Psyc	891	Brickner, Gary (NJ)	ObG	747
Boxer, Harriet (NY)	NP	514	Brief, Rochelle (NY)	PMR	558
Boxer, Mitchell (NY)	A&I	489	Brightman, Rebecca (NY)	ObG	232
Boyd, D Barry (CT)	Hem	873	Brill, Joseph (NY)	Pul	642
Boyer, Joseph (NY)	PPul	635	Brill, Paula (NY)	DR	154
Braddom, Randall (NJ)	PMR	793	Brillon, David (NY)	EDM	159
Brademas, Mary Ellen (NY)	D	145	Brisson, Paul (NY)	OrS	255
Bradley, Thomas (NY)	Onc	512	Britton, Carolyn (NY)	N	221
Braff, Robert (NY)	Cv	129	Broderick, Robert (NY)	Oph	520
Bram, Harris (NJ)	PM	792	Brodherson, Michael (NY)	U	354
Brancaccio, Ronald (NY)	D	412	Brodie, Jonathan (NY)	Psyc	311
Brancaccio, William (NY)	DR	568	Brodman, Michael (NY)	ObG	233
Brand, Howard (NY)	EDM	569	Brodman, Richard (NJ)	Rhu	855
Brandeis, Steven (NY)	CRS	142	Brody, Samuel (NY)	Ger	462
Brandt, Fredric (NY)	D	145	Brolin, Robert (NJ)	S	779
Brandt, Lawrence (NY)	Ge	375	Bromberg, Assia (NJ)	Pul	691
Brannagan, Thomas (NY)	N	221	Bromley, Gary (NY)	PlS	301
Branovan, Daniel (NY)	Oto	268	Bronheim, Harold (NY)	Psyc	311
Brauner, Gary (NJ)	D	664	Bronin, Andrew (NY)	D	601
Braunstein, Richard (NY)	Oph	239	Bronson, Michael (NY)	OrS	255
Brauntuch, Glenn (NJ)	Pul	691	Bronson, Richard (NY)	RE	586
Brause, Barry (NY)	Inf	185	Bronstein, Eric (NJ)	TS	826
Braver, Joel (NJ)	RadRO	836	Bronster, David (NY)	N	221
Brecher, Rubin (NY)	Oph	432	Broumand, Stafford (NY)	PlS	302
Breen, William (NY)	Cv	491	Brovender, Bruce (NY)	Ped	293
Bregman, Zachary (NY)	IM	190	Brower, Mark (NY)	Hem	181
Breidbart, David (NY)	Pul	540	Brown, Andrew (NY)	PMR	298
Breitbart, Arnold (NY)	PlS	535	Brown, Arthur (NY)	Inf	185
Breitbart, William (NY)	Psyc	311	Brown, Carol (NY)	GO	177
Brem, Harold (NY)	S	341	Brown, David (NJ)	PMR	776
Brener, Bruce (NJ)	VascS	729	Brown, David (NJ)	A&I	842
Brener, Sorin (NY)	IC	423	Brown, David (NY)	Cv	564
Brennan, Murray (NY)	S	341	Brown, Eric (CT)	Nep	879
Brenner, Ronald (NY)	Psyc	468	Brown, Jeffrey (NY)	Ped	636

Name	Specialty	Pg	Name	Specialty	Pg
Brown, Jeffrey (NY)	NS	516	Bullock, Richard (NJ)	Ger	763
Brown, John (NJ)	TS	815	Buly, Robert (NY)	OrS	255
Brown, Karen (NY)	VIR	361	Burack, Joshua (NY)	TS	451
Brown, Lionel (CT)	HS	872	Burak, George (NY)	OrS	628
Brown, Mitchell (NJ)	Ger	734	Burke, Karen (NY)	D	145
Brown, Richard (NY)	Psyc	311	Burke, Patricia (NJ)	Oph	680
Brown, Robert (CT)	Pul	892	Burkes, Lynn (NY)	ChAP	138
Brown, Robert (NY)	Ge	164	Burns, Elisa (NY)	ObG	623
Browner-Elhanan, Karen (NY)	AM	407	Burns, Les (NJ)	ObG	822
Bruce, Jeffrey (NY)	NS	217	Burns, Mark (NY)	Rhu	645
Bruck, Lance (CT)	ObG	882	Burns, Paul (NY)	PM	558
Bruckner, Howard (NY)	Onc	202	Burns, Paul (NJ)	TS	727
Bruckstein, Alex (NY)	Ge	477	Burschtin, Omar (NY)	Pul	324
Bruckstein, Robert (NY)	D	497	Burstin, Harris (NY)	Ped	294
Brunckhorst, Keith (NY)	Onc	202	Burton, Daniel (NY)	A&I	124
Brunetti, Jacqueline (NJ)	NuM	679	Busch-Devereaux, Erna (NY)	S	587
Brunner, Eugenie (NJ)	Oto	749	Bush, Jacqueline (NY)	MF	424
Brunnquell, Stephen (NJ)	IM	672	Bush, Michael (NY)	IM	190
Bruno, Anthony (NY)	U	548	Busillo, Christopher (NY)	Inf	185
Brust, John (NY)	N	222	Bussel, James (NY)	PHO	286
Brustein, Harris (NY)	Oph	625	Buterman, Irving (NY)	ObG	233
Brustman, Lois (NY)	ObG	233	Butler, David (NJ)	ObG	679
Bryce, Thomas (NY)	PMR	298	Butler, Mark (NJ)	OrS	771
Buatti, Elizabeth (NY)	IM	380	Butt, Ahmar (NY)	IM	421
Buchalter, Maury (NJ)	Ped	687	Buxton, Douglas (NY)	Oph	239
Buchbinder, Ellen (NY)	A&I	124	Buyon, Jill (NY)	Rhu	334
Buchholtz, Michael (NY)	Hem	572	Buzzeo, Louis (NY)	Nep	620
Buchness, Mary Ruth (NY)	D	145	Bye, Michael (NY)	PPul	291
Bucholtz, Harvey (NJ)	EDM	761	Byk, Cheryl (NJ)	DR	707
Buckley, Peter (NY)	Psyc	311	Byrd, Lawrence (NJ)	Nep	713
Buckner, Cary (NY)	N	428	Bystryn, Jean-Claude (NY)	D	145
Budd, Daniel (NJ)	S	825			
Budin, Joel (NJ)	DR	665			
Budman, Cathy (NY)	Psyc	539			
Budman, Daniel (NY)	Onc	512			
Bufalini, Bruno (NJ)	S	695	Cabin, Henry (CT)	Cv	901
Bukberg, Judith (NY)	Psyc	311	Caccavale, Robert (NJ)	TS	837
Bukberg, Phillip (NY)	EDM	159	Caccese, William (NY)	Ge	503
Bull, Sherman (CT)	S	895	Cacciola, Thomas (NJ)	IM	672

C

Alphabetical Listing of Doctors

Name	Specialty	Pg	Name	Specialty	Pg
Cafferty, Maureen (NY)	N	222	Carniol, Paul (NJ)	Oto	851
Cahan, Anthony (NY)	S	646	Caron, Philip (NY)	Onc	617
Cahill, John (NY)	PrM	309	Carone, Patrick (NY)	Psyc	539
Cahill, Kevin (NY)	PrM	309	Carosella, Christine (NY)	IM	613
Cahill, Linda (NY)	Ped	392	Carpenter, Duncan (NJ)	NS	677
Cairo, Mitchell (NY)	PHO	286	Carpenter, Thomas (CT)	PEn	915
Calem-Grunat, Jaclyn (NJ)	DR	665	Carr, Ronald (NY)	Oph	239
Caligiuri, Daniel (NY)	HS	419	Carr-Locke, David (NY)	Ge	164
Callahan, Eileen (NY)	Ger	174	Carrasquillo, Jorge (NY)	NuM	231
Callahan, Lisa (NY)	SM	338	Carroll, William (NY)	PHO	286
Calman, Neil (NY)	FMed	162	Carson, Jeffrey (NJ)	IM	765
Cam, Jenny (NJ)	EDM	733	Carsons, Steven (NY)	Rhu	543
Camacho, Fernando (NY)	Onc	381	Carter, Mitchel (NJ)	S	815
Camacho, Margarita (NJ)	TS	727	Caruana, Salvatore (NY)	Oto	268
Cammisa, Frank (NY)	OrS	255	Carucci, John (NY)	D	145
Campbell, Deborah (NY)	NP	382	Caruso, Patrick (NJ)	Ped	812
Campolattaro, Brian (NY)	Oph	239	Caruso, Rocco (NY)	Onc	574
Camunas, Jorge (NY)	TS	349	Casale, Linda (CT)	Cv	866
Cancellieri, Russell (NY)	A&I	563	Casden, Andrew (NY)	OrS	255
Cangemi, Francis (NJ)	Oph	716	Case, David (NY)	IM	190
Cannarozzi, Nicholas (NJ)	Rhu	725	Casino, Joseph (NY)	Pul	642
Canny, Christopher (CT)	Ped	916	Casper, Daniel (NY)	Oph	240
Cantor, Michael (NY)	Ge	164	Casper, Ephraim (NJ)	Onc	832
Capobianco, Luigi (NY)	FMed	502	Casper, Theodore (NY)	Pul	397
Capozzi, James (NY)	OrS	523	Cassell, Lauren (NY)	S	341
Caputo, Anthony (NJ)	Oph	716	Cassidy, Brian (NJ)	IM	765
Caputo, Thomas (NY)	GO	177	Casson, Ira (NY)	N	466
Caracci, Giovanni (NJ)	Psyc	723	Castellano, Bartolomeo (NY)	Oto	482
Cardiello, Gary (NJ)	IM	734	Castellano, Michael (NY)	Pul	484
Cardoso, Erico (NY)	NS	428	Castro-Magana, Mariano (NY)	PEn	529
Carew, John (NY)	Oto	268	Castro-Malaspina, Hugo (NY)	Hem	181
Carey, Dennis (NY)	PEn	529	Catanese, Anthony (NJ)	U	837
Carlin, Elizabeth (NJ)	NP	676	Catanese, James (NY)	Cv	595
Carlson, Gabrielle (NY)	ChAP	565	Catanese, Vincent (NJ)	FMed	786
Carlson, Harold (NY)	EDM	569	Caucino, Julie (NJ)	A&I	829
Carlson, John (NJ)	GO	763	Cavaliere, Gregg (NY)	SM	646
Carlson, Michelle (NY)	HS	179	Cavallaro, Barbara (NJ)	ObG	680
Carmichael, L David (NY)	IM	190	Cece, John (NJ)	Oto	823
Carney, Alexander (NJ)	Rhu	752	Cemaletin, Nevber (NY)	Cv	129

Name	Specialty	Pg	Name	Specialty	Pg
Cerny, Kenneth (NJ)	N	807	Chen, Chun (NY)	NS	217
Cerrone, Federico (NJ)	Pul	855	Chen, Jonathan (NY)	TS	349
Cerulli, Maurice (NY)	Ge	503	Chen, Lucy (NJ)	Oph	809
Cervia, Joseph (NY)	Inf	507	Chengot, Mathew (NY)	Cv	564
Chabot, John (NY)	S	341	Chern, Relly (NY)	Oph	240
Chachoua, Abraham (NY)	Onc	202	Chernack, William (NJ)	A&I	801
Chadda, Kul (NY)	Cv	491	Chernobilsky, Lev (NY)	Ped	582
Chadha, Jang B S (NY)	Pul	469	Cherofsky, Alan (NY)	PlS	484
Chai, Emily (NY)	Ger	174	Cherry, Sheldon (NY)	ObG	233
Chaiken, Barry (NY)	Oph	240	Chertoff, Harvey (NJ)	Psyc	690
Chaikin, David (NJ)	U	816	Chervenak, Francis (NY)	MF	200
Chalal, Jeffrey (NJ)	DR	786	Chesner, Michael (NY)	Cv	491
Chamberlain, Ronald (NJ)	S	726	Chess, Jeremy (NY)	Oph	386
Chambers, Joseph (NY)	GO	418	Chessin, Robert (CT)	Ped	888
Chan, Brenda (CT)	Nep	879	Chessler, Richard (NJ)	Ge	668
Chandler, Michael (NY)	A&I	125	Chianese, Maurice (NY)	Ped	533
Chandra, Pradeep (NY)	Onc	424	Chiariello, Mario (NY)	S	449
Chandra, Prasanta (NY)	MF	424	Chideckel, Norman (NY)	VascS	362
Chandrasekhar, Sujana (NY)	Oto	268	Chidyllo, Stephen (NJ)	PlS	794
Chang, Christine (NY)	Ger	174	Chin, Daisy (NJ)	PEn	811
Chang, Peter (NY)	RE	330	Chin, Jean (NY)	ObG	233
Chang, Stanley (NY)	Oph	240	Chin, Patrick (NJ)	Oph	681
Chapman, Mark (NY)	Ge	165	Chinitz, Larry (NY)	CE	126
Chapman, Paul (NY)	Onc	203	Chinitz, Marvin (NY)	Ge	607
Chapnick, Edward (NY)	Inf	420	Chinn, Bertram (NJ)	CRS	759
Charap, Mitchell (NY)	IM	190	Chitkara, Dev (NY)	Oto	580
Charap, Peter (NY)	IM	190	Chiu, David (NY)	PlS	302
Charles, James (NJ)	N	735	Chiurco, Anthony (NJ)	NS	746
Charles, Norman (NY)	Oph	240	Chodosh, Eliot (NJ)	N	822
Charney, Jonathan (NY)	N	222	Choi, Mihye (NY)	PlS	302
Charney, Richard (NY)	Cv	595	Cholst, Ina (NY)	RE	331
Charnoff, Judah (NY)	Cv	408	Chou, Shyan-Yih (NY)	Nep	426
Charytan, Chaim (NY)	Nep	383	Choudhury, Muhammad (NY)	U	649
Chase, Mark (NJ)	OrS	717	Chrisanderson, Donna (NJ)	IM	711
Chaudhry, M Rashid (NY)	Oto	436	Christakos, Manny (NJ)	TS	826
Chaudhry, Saqib (NY)	VascS	549	Christoudias, George (NJ)	S	695
Chawla, Anupama (NY)	PGe	581	Chu, Edward (CT)	Onc	909
Chazotte, Cynthia (NY)	MF	381	Chu, Wing (NY)	Oph	240
Chefitz, Dalya (NJ)	Ped	776	Chuang, Linus (NY)	GO	611

Alphabetical Listing of Doctors

Name	Specialty	Pg	Name	Specialty	Pg
Chun, Audrey (NY)	Ger	175	Cohen, David (NY)	D	146
Chun, Jin (NY)	PlS	302	Cohen, Howard (NY)	Cv	129
Chung, Henry (NY)	Psyc	311	Cohen, Jacob (NY)	Ge	503
Chung-Loy, Harold (NJ)	S	779	Cohen, Joel (NY)	N	384
Ciaburri, Daniel (NY)	TS	896	Cohen, Jonathan (NY)	Ge	165
Ciccone, John (NJ)	Cv	704	Cohen, Lawrence (NY)	Ge	165
Ciccone, Patrick (NJ)	U	728	Cohen, Lee (NY)	ChAP	599
Cicogna, Cristina (NJ)	Inf	671	Cohen, Leeber (NY)	Oph	240
Cioroiu, Michael (NY)	S	341	Cohen, Marc (NJ)	IC	712
Cipriani, Ralph (CT)	Inf	873	Cohen, Martin (NY)	CE	594
Cirello, Richard (NJ)	FMed	708	Cohen, Michael (NY)	Pul	540
Citron, Marc (NY)	Onc	512	Cohen, Michael (NY)	Cv	129
Clain, David (NY)	Ge	165	Cohen, Michel (NY)	Ped	294
Clain, Michael (CT)	OrS	884	Cohen, Neil (CT)	Hem	873
Claps, Richard (NJ)	DR	803	Cohen, Neil (NY)	EDM	477
Clark, Richard (NY)	D	567	Cohen, Richard (NY)	IM	191
Clark, Sheryl (NY)	D	146	Cohen, Richard (NJ)	Ped	776
Cleary, Joseph (NY)	S	646	Cohen, Robert (NY)	IM	191
Cleman, Michael (CT)	Cv	902	Cohen, Seth (NY)	Ge	165
Cleri, Dennis (NJ)	Inf	744	Cohen, Seymour (NY)	Onc	203
Close, Lanny (NY)	Oto	268	Cohen, Steven (CT)	DR	869
Coady, Deborah (NY)	ObG	233	Cohen, Steven (NY)	D	371
Cobelli, Neil (NY)	OrS	387	Cohen, Steven (NJ)	Oph	716
Cobin, Rhoda (NJ)	EDM	666	Cohn, Steven (NY)	IM	421
Coco, Maria (NY)	Nep	383	Cohn, Symra (NY)	IM	191
Coffey, Barbara (NY)	ChAP	139	Cohn, William (NY)	Ge	570
Cofsky, Richard (NY)	Inf	420	Coit, Daniel (NY)	S	341
Cohen, Alice (NJ)	Hem	709	Colaco, Rodolfo (NJ)	S	856
Cohen, Arnold (NY)	Psyc	311	Colangelo, Daniel (NY)	IM	613
Cohen, Barry (NY)	IM	421	Colberg, John (CT)	U	921
Cohen, Barry (NJ)	Nep	746	Cole, Jeffrey (NJ)	PMR	722
Cohen, Ben (NY)	Oph	240	Cole, Robert (NJ)	RadRO	825
Cohen, Bradley (NY)	S	588	Cole, William (NY)	Cv	129
Cohen, Burton (NY)	DR	154	Coleman, D Jackson (NY)	Oph	240
Cohen, Carl (NY)	GerPsy	418	Coleman, Morton (NY)	Onc	203
Cohen, Charmian (NY)	EDM	373	Colen, Helen (NY)	PlS	302
Cohen, Daniel (NY)	Rhu	543	Colenda, Maryann (NJ)	PA&I	685
Cohen, Daniel (NY)	N	576	Coll, Raymond (NY)	N	222
Cohen, David (NY)	Nep	214	Coller, Barry (NY)	Hem	181

Name	Specialty	Pg	Name	Specialty	Pg
Collum, Robert (NJ)	IM	805	Coppa, Gene (NY)	S	545
Coloka-Kump, Rodika (NY)	FMed	374	Copperman, Alan (NY)	RE	331
Colon, Francisco (NJ)	PlS	812	Coppola, John (NY)	Cv	129
Colton, Marc (NJ)	U	816	Corapi, Mark (NY)	IM	509
Compito, Catherine (NY)	OrS	255	Corazza, Douglas (NJ)	IM	744
Compito, Gerard (NJ)	DR	760	Corbo, Emanuel (NJ)	Ped	852
Comrie, Millicent (NY)	ObG	431	Cordasco, Frank (NY)	OrS	255
Condo, Dominick (NJ)	IM	734	Cordeiro, Peter (NY)	PlS	302
Confino, Joel (NJ)	Oph	850	Cordero, Evelyn (NY)	FMed	374
Connery, Cliff (NY)	TS	349	Coren, Charles (NY)	PS	532
Connolly, Adrian (NJ)	D	706	Corey, Timothy (NJ)	D	664
Connolly, Mark (NJ)	TS	728	Corn, Beth (NY)	A&I	125
Connor, Bradley (NY)	Ge	165	Cornell, Charles (NY)	OrS	256
Connor, John (NJ)	U	816	Cornell, James (NJ)	CCM	664
Connor, Thomas (NJ)	PCd	719	Corpuz, Marilou (NY)	Inf	379
Connors, Richard (CT)	D	868	Correia, Joaquim (NJ)	CE	703
Conroy, Daniel (NJ)	Cv	660	Corriel, Robert (NY)	A&I	489
Constad, William (NJ)	Oph	736	Corson, Richard (NJ)	FMed	830
Constantiner, Arturo (NY)	IM	191	Cortes, Engracio (NY)	Onc	464
Constantinides, Minas (NY)	Oto	268	Cosgrove, John (NY)	S	399
Conte, Charles (NY)	S	545	Cosman, Felicia (NY)	EDM	554
Conway, Edward (NY)	PCCM	283	Cossari, Alfred (NY)	Oph	577
Cook, Jack (NY)	Oph	520	Costa, Leon (NJ)	OrS	748
Cook, Perry (NY)	Hem	181	Costantino, Peter (NY)	Oto	269
Cook, Stuart (NJ)	N	714	Costanzo, Joseph (CT)	IM	874
Cooke, Joseph (NY)	Pul	325	Costeas, Constantinos (NJ)	CE	703
Cooney, Leo (CT)	Ger	906	Costin, Andrew (NJ)	Cv	741
Cooper, Arthur (NY)	PS	292	Coupey, Susan (NY)	AM	367
Cooper, Dennis (CT)	Onc	909	Cournos, Francine (NY)	Psyc	312
Cooper, Jay (NY)	RadRO	447	Courtney, Barbara (NJ)	IM	788
Cooper, Jerome (NY)	Cv	595	Coven, Barbara (NY)	Ped	636
Cooper, Lauren (NJ)	D	803	Coven, Roger (NJ)	ObG	680
Cooper, Robert (NY)	Ge	165	Covey, Alexander (NY)	IM	573
Cooper, Rubin (NY)	PCd	528	Covit, Andrew (NJ)	Nep	767
Cooper, Seymour (NY)	Ped	533	Cox, Kathryn (NY)	ObG	233
Cooperman, Alan (NJ)	ObG	715	Coyle, Michael (NJ)	HS	763
Copel, Joshua (CT)	MF	908	Coyle, Patricia (NY)	N	576
Copen, David (CT)	Cv	866	Cracchiolo, Bernadette (NJ)	GO	709
Coplan, Jeremy (NY)	Psyc	444	Cracco, Joan (NY)	ChiN	411

Alphabetical Listing of Doctors

Name	Specialty	Pg	Name	Specialty	Pg
Craft, Joseph (CT)	Rhu	920	D'Agostino, Richard (NY)	OrS	523
Craig, Edward (NY)	OrS	256	D'Agostino, Ronald (NY)	Cv	492
Cramer, Marvin (NY)	Cv	491	D'Alton, Mary (NY)	MF	200
Crane, Richard (NY)	Rhu	334	D'Amico, Donald (NY)	Oph	241
Crane, Stephen (NJ)	ObG	715	D'Amico, Joseph (CT)	OrS	885
Crasta, Jovita (NY)	Psyc	539	D'Amico, Richard (NJ)	PlS	689
Crawford, Bernard (NY)	TS	349	D'Anna, John (NY)	S	485
Crawford, James (NY)	Path	527	D'Aversa, Gerard (NY)	Oph	521
Cristofaro, Robert (NY)	OrS	628	D'Ayala, Marcus (NY)	VascS	453
Croen, Kenneth (NY)	IM	613	Dagum, Alexander (NY)	PlS	584
Croll, James (NY)	Nep	383	Dalena, John (NJ)	Ge	804
Cross, Jennifer (NY)	Ped	294	Dalton, Jack (NY)	RadRO	470
Crowe, John (CT)	OrS	884	Daly, Jane (NY)	Onc	464
Cruz, Merle (NJ)	Cv	733	Damien, Miguel (NJ)	RE	795
Crystal, Howard (NY)	N	428	Danehower, Richard (CT)	Rhu	894
Crystal, Kenneth (NY)	VIR	549	Daniels, Jeffrey (NJ)	Cv	785
Cuber, Shain (NJ)	PlS	777	Danziger, Stephen (NY)	D	412
Culliford, Alfred (NY)	TS	349	Daras, Michael (NY)	N	222
Culligan, Patrick (NJ)	ObG	808	Das, Seshadri (NY)	EDM	477
Cunha, Burke (NY)	Inf	507	Dasgupta, Indira (NY)	PHO	390
Cunningham, James (CT)	OrS	885	Dasmahapatra, Kumar (NJ)	S	779
Cunningham-Rundles, Charlotte (NY)	A&I	125	Datta, Rajiv (NY)	S	545
			Daum, Fredric (NY)	PGe	530
Cunningham-Rundles, Ward (NY)	IM	191	Davenport, Deborah (NY)	ObG	576
Cuomo, Frances (NY)	OrS	256	David, Sami (NY)	RE	331
Curtin, John (NY)	GO	177	Davidson, Dennis (NY)	NP	514
Cushner, Fred (NY)	OrS	256	Davidson, J Thomas (NJ)	S	752
Cusumano, Barbara (NY)	Ped	582	Davidson, Lawrence (NJ)	Oph	716
Cusumano, Stephen (NY)	IM	509	Davies, Terry (NY)	EDM	159
Cutolo, Louis (NY)	PlS	484	Davis, Alan (NJ)	PCCM	720
Cutting, Court (NY)	PlS	302	Davis, George (NJ)	Pul	795
Cykiert, Robert (NY)	Oph	241	Davis, Ira (NY)	D	601
Cynamon, Jacob (NY)	VIR	401	Davis, Jessica (NY)	CG	142
Cziner, David (NY)	Cv	595	Davis, Joyce (NY)	D	146
			Davis, Kenneth (NJ)	Ped	852
			Davis, Nicole (NJ)	ObG	770
D			Davis, Owen (NY)	RE	331
			Davis, Raphael (NY)	NS	575
D'Agostini, Robert (NJ)	OrS	834	Davison, Edward (NY)	Cv	492

Name	Specialty	Pg	Name	Specialty	Pg
De Angelis, Lisa (NY)	N	222	Dennett, Ronald (NY)	IM	613
De Antonio, Joseph (NJ)	Ge	743	Denny, Donald (NJ)	VIR	753
De Carlo, Regina (NY)	ChiN	476	Denoto, George (NY)	S	545
De Cosimo, Diana (NJ)	IM	711	Derespinis, Patrick (NY)	Oph	481
De Fabritus, Albert (NY)	Nep	214	DeRose, Joseph (NY)	TS	400
De Giacomo, Frank (NJ)	IM	821	Dershaw, D David (NY)	DR	154
de Lotbiniere, Alain (NY)	NS	621	Dervan, John (NY)	Cv	564
De Matteo, Robert (NY)	Pul	642	DeSilva, Derrick (NJ)	IM	765
De Pietro, William (NY)	D	497	Desnick, Robert (NY)	CG	142
De Vivo, Darryl (NY)	ChiN	140	Desposito, Franklin (NJ)	CG	705
DeAnda, Abelardo (NY)	TS	349	Dettmer, Robert (CT)	Ge	871
DeAraujo, Maria (NY)	PMR	395	Deutsch, Adam (NY)	Cv	129
DeBroff, Brian (CT)	Oph	882	Deutsch, James (NY)	Oph	432
Decter, Edward (NJ)	OrS	718	Devereux, Richard (NY)	Cv	130
Decter, Julian (NY)	Onc	203	Devine, Patricia (NY)	MF	616
Dedousis, John (NJ)	IM	734	Devinsky, Orrin (NY)	N	222
Degenhardt, Alexandra (NY)	N	429	DeVita, Gregory (NY)	PlS	536
Deitch, Edwin (NJ)	S	727	Devita, Maria (NY)	Nep	215
Deitch, Jonathan (NY)	VascS	486	DeVita, Vincent (CT)	Onc	909
Deitz, Marcia (NY)	D	412	DeVito, Bethany (NY)	Ge	503
Del Priore, Lucian (NY)	Oph	241	Devlin, Michael (NY)	Psyc	312
DeLacure, Mark (NY)	Oto	269	Dhalla, Satish (NY)	IM	191
Deland, Jonathan (NY)	OrS	256	Dharmarajan, Thiruvinvamvalai (NY)		Ger
Delaney, Brian (NY)	FMed	374	377		
Delaney, Veronica (NY)	Nep	620	Di Buono, Mark (NY)	Psyc	484
Delano, Barbara (NY)	Nep	426	Di Giacinto, George (NY)	NS	217
DeLeo, Vincent (NY)	D	146	Di Giacomo, William (NJ)	IM	711
Delerme, Milton (NY)	Oph	241	Di Leo, Frank (NY)	Oph	578
Della Rocca, Robert (NY)	Oph	241	Diamant, Esther (NY)	Ped	558
Delman, Michael (NY)	IM	573	Diamond, Ezriel (NY)	RadRO	542
Delorenzo, Lawrence (NY)	Pul	642	Diamond, Martin (NJ)	PMR	853
DelPizzo, Joseph (NY)	U	354	Diamond, Sharon (NY)	ObG	233
Delprete, Salvatore (CT)	Onc	877	Diamond, Steven (NJ)	PHO	685
DeLuca, Joseph (NJ)	Oph	681	Diaz, Angela (NY)	AM	124
Demar, Leon (NY)	D	146	Diaz, Michael (NY)	Hem	182
Demento, Frank (NY)	D	497	DiBernardo, Barry (NJ)	PlS	723
Demetis, Spiro (NY)	Pul	445	Dickler, Maura (NY)	Onc	203
DeNatale, Ralph (CT)	VascS	922	Dickoff, David (NY)	N	621
Denehy, Thad (NJ)	GO	709	DiCosmo, Bruno (NY)	Pul	642

Alphabetical Listing of Doctors

Alphabetical Listing of Doctors

Name	Specialty	Pg	Name	Specialty	Pg
Engel, Murray (NY)	N	222	Falco, Thomas (NY)	Cv	564
Engler, Mitchell (NJ)	Pul	691	Falcon, Ronald (NY)	D	498
Englert, Christopher (NJ)	ObG	680	Falk, Theodore (NJ)	A&I	660
Ennis, Ronald (NY)	RadRO	329	Faller, Jason (NY)	Rhu	334
Epstein, Lawrence (NY)	PM	631	Fallon, Brian (NY)	Psyc	312
Epstein, Nancy (NY)	NS	516	Fang, Bruno (NJ)	Onc	766
Epstein, Robert (NJ)	DR	760	Fantasia, Michele (NJ)	PMR	776
Epstein, Stanley (NY)	Cv	130	Fantini, Gary (NY)	VascS	362
Erber, William (NY)	Ge	415	Fanucchi, Michael (NY)	Onc	203
Ergin, M Arisan (NJ)	TS	696	Farber, Bruce (NY)	Inf	508
Ernst, Jerome (NY)	IM	380	Farber, Charles (NY)	Ge	504
Errico, Thomas (NY)	OrS	256	Farber, Charles (NJ)	Onc	806
Ertl, John (CT)	PHO	887	Faries, Peter (NY)	VascS	362
Escher, Jeffrey (NY)	Ger	610	Farkas, Edward (NJ)	Psyc	690
Esformes, Ira (NJ)	OrS	682	Farkas, John (NJ)	Ge	820
Eshghi, A Majid (NY)	U	649	Farrell, Matthew (CT)	FMed	870
Eskreis, David (NY)	Ge	503	Farrell, Robert (NY)	U	472
Esposito, Donna (NY)	Oph	242	Farrer, William (NJ)	Inf	846
Esposito, Michael (NJ)	U	697	Fass, Arthur (NY)	Cv	595
Esposito, Rick (NY)	TS	546	Fass, Daniel (NY)	RadRO	644
Esposito, Stephen (NY)	Ge	461	Fast, Avital (NY)	PMR	395
Estabrook, Alison (NY)	S	342	Fastenberg, David (NY)	Oph	521
Esteban-Cruciani, Nora (NY)	Ped	393	Fateh, Majid (NY)	RE	331
Eth, Spencer (NY)	Psyc	312	Faust, Glenn (NY)	VascS	549
Etingin, Orli (NY)	IM	191	Faust, Michael (NY)	Ge	166
Ettinger, Alan (NY)	N	517	Faust, Michael (NJ)	ObG	680
Evans, Mark (NY)	ObG	233	Fawwaz, Rashid (NY)	NuM	231
Eviatar, Lydia (NY)	ChiN	496	Fazio, Nelson (NY)	IM	613
Ezratty, Ari (NY)	Cv	492	Fazio, Richard (NY)	Ge	477
			Fealy, Stephen (NY)	OrS	257
			Federbush, Richard (NY)	IM	509
F			Fefferman, Nancy (NY)	DR	154
			Feghali, Joseph (NY)	Oto	388
Faber, Mark (NJ)	Psyc	724	Feigenbaum, Howard (NJ)	S	825
Fagin, James (NY)	PA&I	528	Fein, Alan (NY)	Pul	540
Fahey, Thomas (NY)	S	342	Fein, Deborah (NJ)	Nep	676
Fahn, Stanley (NY)	N	222	Fein, Frederick (NY)	Cv	492
Fahoum, Bashar (NY)	S	449	Feinberg, Joseph (NY)	PMR	298
Fakharzadeh, Frederick (NJ)	HS	670	Feinberg, Joseph (NY)	PlS	536

Name	Specialty	Pg	Name	Specialty	Pg
Feinberg, Todd (NY)	N	223	Fialk, Mark (NY)	Onc	617
Feinstein, Neil (NY)	Oph	432	Fiedler, Robert (NY)	IM	192
Feintzeig, Irwin (CT)	Nep	879	Fiel, Stanley (NJ)	Pul	814
Feit, Alan (NY)	Cv	408	Field, Barry (NY)	Ge	607
Feit, David (NJ)	Ge	668	Field, Steven (NY)	Ge	166
Feld, Michael (NY)	Cv	595	Fielding, George (NY)	S	342
Felderman, Lenora (NY)	D	146	Fields, Theodore (NY)	Rhu	334
Feldman, Alan (NJ)	EDM	742	Fiest, Thomas (NJ)	Ge	787
Feldman, B Robert (NY)	A&I	125	Figgie, Mark (NY)	OrS	257
Feldman, David (NY)	PlS	443	Filiberto, Cosmo (CT)	FMed	870
Feldman, David (NJ)	OrS	809	Filippone, Mark (NJ)	PMR	736
Feldman, David (NY)	OrS	257	Filsoufi, Farzan (NY)	TS	349
Feldman, Eric (NY)	Onc	203	Fine, Emily (CT)	ObG	912
Feldman, Jeffrey (NJ)	IM	846	Fine, Eugene (NY)	U	354
Feldman, Philip (NY)	D	412	Fine, Paul (NJ)	Nep	807
Feldman, Sheldon (NY)	S	342	Fine, Robert (NY)	Onc	203
Feldman, Stuart (NY)	Onc	617	Fine, Stanley (NY)	A&I	457
Feldstein, Neil (NY)	NS	217	Fineman, Sanford (NJ)	NS	848
Felig, Philip (NY)	EDM	159	Finger, Paul (NY)	Oph	242
Fellus, Jonathan (NJ)	N	714	Fink, Matthew (NY)	N	223
Felsenstein, Jerome M (NY)	D	601	Finkel, Jay (NY)	Psyc	312
Feltheimer, Seth (NY)	IM	192	Finkelstein, Martin (NY)	Ger	175
Fennell, Gail (CT)	IM	874	Finkelstein, Warren (NJ)	Ge	708
Fennoy, Ilene (NY)	PEn	283	Finlay, Alexis (CT)	Oph	882
Ferges, Mitchell (NJ)	Ge	831	Fiore, Amory (CT)	NS	880
Fernandes, David (NY)	Ped	441	Fiore, John (NY)	Onc	574
Fernandes, John (NJ)	PCd	719	Fiorella, David (NY)	NRad	576
Fernandez, Harold (NY)	TS	546	Fiorentino, Thomas (NY)	IM	613
Fernbach, Barry (NJ)	Hem	671	First, Michael (NY)	Psyc	312
Ferran, Elena Nascimbeni (NY)	Ge	166	Fisch, Arthur (NJ)	Cv	802
Ferran, Ernesto (NY)	Psyc	312	Fisch, Harry (NY)	U	355
Ferrante, Maurice (NJ)	IM	832	Fischbach, Neal (CT)	Onc	877
Ferrick, Kevin (NY)	CE	368	Fischer, Harry (NY)	Rhu	335
Ferrier, Genevieve (NY)	Ped	294	Fish, Bernard (NY)	PCd	631
Ferriter, Pierce (NY)	OrS	257	Fishbach, Mitchell (NY)	Cv	595
Ferrone, Philip (NY)	Oph	521	Fishbane, Steven (NY)	Nep	515
Festa, Robert (NY)	Ped	582	Fisher, George (NY)	FMed	460
Feteiha, Muhammad (NJ)	S	856	Fisher, Laura (NY)	IM	192
Fey, Christopher (CT)	DR	869	Fisher, Lawrence (CT)	Cv	866

Alphabetical Listing of Doctors

Name	Specialty	Pg	Name	Specialty	Pg
Fisher, Margaret (NJ)	PInf	793	Fonacier, Luz (NY)	A&I	490
Fisher, Martin (NY)	AM	489	Fong, Raymond (NY)	Oph	242
Fisher, Rosemarie (CT)	Ge	905	Fong, Yuman (NY)	S	342
Fisher, Yale (NY)	Oph	242	Foo, Sun-Hoo (NY)	N	223
Fishkin, Michael (NY)	FMed	570	Foong, Anthony (NY)	Ge	166
Fishman, Allen (NY)	Oph	466	Ford, Robert (NJ)	DR	742
Fishman, David (NY)	GO	177	Forget, Bernard (CT)	Hem	907
Fishman, Donald (NY)	Pul	325	Forlenza, Thomas (NY)	Onc	479
Fishman, Miriam (NJ)	D	664	Forley, Bryan (NY)	PlS	303
Fiske, Steven (NJ)	Ge	708	Forman, Mark (NJ)	TS	728
Fitzgerald, Denis (NJ)	Onc	789	Forman, Scott (NY)	Oph	625
Flamm, Eugene (NY)	NS	384	Formenti, Silvia (NY)	RadRO	329
Flanagan, Michael (CT)	U	922	Formica, Richard (CT)	Nep	911
Flanagan, Steven (NY)	PMR	298	Fornari, Victor (NY)	ChAP	458
Flatow, Evan (NY)	OrS	257	Forster, George (NY)	N	223
Fleischer, Adiel (NY)	MF	511	Fort, Pavel (NY)	PEn	529
Fleischer, Lee (NY)	S	560	Forte, Francis (NJ)	Onc	674
Fleischer, Marian (NY)	CRS	412	Fortunato, Franklin (NJ)	IM	711
Fleischman, Jay (NY)	Oph	625	Foss, Francine (CT)	Onc	909
Fleischman, Jean (NY)	Pul	470	Fost, Arthur (NJ)	PA&I	719
Fleisher, Michael (NJ)	U	780	Foster, Craig (NY)	PlS	303
Fleming, Gregory (NJ)	Oto	810	Foster, Harris (CT)	U	922
Flis, Raymond (NJ)	Nep	790	Fou, Adora (NY)	S	646
Flood, Mary (NY)	Inf	186	Fox, Alissa (NJ)	D	830
Florakis, George (NY)	Oph	242	Fox, Herbert (NY)	Psyc	313
Flores, Lucio (NY)	VascS	453	Fox, James (NJ)	A&I	829
Flores, Raja (NY)	TS	350	Fox, John (NY)	IC	198
Florio, Philip (NY)	ObG	623	Fox, Joyce (NY)	CG	496
Flug, Frances (NJ)	PHO	685	Fox, Mark (NY)	Oto	630
Flynn, Maryirene (NY)	OrS	482	Fox, Martin (NY)	Oph	242
Flynn, Patrick (NY)	PCd	281	Fox, Stewart (NY)	TS	546
Fochios, Steven (NY)	Ge	166	Fox, Stuart (NJ)	N	808
Fogel, Joyce (NY)	Ger	175	Fracchia, John (NY)	U	355
Fogel, Mitchell (CT)	Nep	879	Frager, Joseph (NY)	Ge	375
Fogler, Richard (NY)	S	449	Fragner, Paul (NY)	HS	611
Fojas, Antonio (NY)	IM	380	Frances, Richard (NY)	AdP	123
Foley, Carmel (NY)	ChAP	495	Francfort, John (NY)	S	588
Folman, Robert (CT)	Onc	877	Francis, Kathleen (NJ)	PMR	722
Fomberstein, Barry (NY)	Rhu	398	Franck, Jeanne (NY)	D	498

Alphabetical Listing of Doctors

Name	Specialty	Pg	Name	Specialty	Pg
Fyer, Minna (NY)	Psyc	313	Gardner, Peter (CT)	Ge	871
			Garfinkel, Howard (CT)	Nep	879
			Garfinkel, Matthew (NJ)	OrS	771
			Gargano, Robert (NY)	Oto	580
G			Gargiulo, Juan (NY)	PM	580
Gabbay, Vilma (NY)	ChAP	139	Garner, Bruce (NY)	Rhu	448
Gabel, Richard (NY)	Psyc	640	Garner, Steven (NY)	DR	413
Gabelman, Gary (NY)	Cv	596	Garrick, Renee (NY)	Nep	620
Gabrilove, Janice (NY)	Onc	204	Garvey, Michael (NY)	Nep	215
Gaffney, Joseph (NJ)	PCd	773	Garvey, Richard (CT)	S	895
Gagliardi, Anthony (NY)	Pul	325	Garvin, James (NY)	PHO	287
Gagne, Paul (CT)	VascS	898	Garzon, Maria (NY)	D	147
Gainey, Patrick (NJ)	N	833	Gasalberti, Richard (NY)	PMR	468
Gajdos, Robert (NJ)	IM	821	Gately, Adrian (NY)	Ped	441
Galanter, Marc (NY)	AdP	123	Gayle, Lloyd (NY)	PlS	303
Galinkin, Lawrence (NY)	Ped	533	Gaynor, Mitchell (NY)	Onc	204
Gallagher, Mary (NY)	PEn	283	Gazzara, Paul (NY)	IM	478
Gallagher, Pamela (NY)	PlS	536	Gearhart, Bonni (NJ)	Onc	847
Galland, Leo (NY)	IM	192	Gecelter, Gary (NY)	S	545
Galler, Marilyn (NY)	Nep	465	Geders, Jane (NY)	Ge	608
Gallick, Gregory (NJ)	OrS	850	Gehrmann, Robin (NJ)	SM	726
Gallin, Pamela (NY)	Oph	243	Geisler, Edward (NY)	U	400
Galloway, Aubrey (NY)	TS	350	Gejerman, Glen (NJ)	RadRO	692
Gallucci, John (NJ)	PS	775	Gekowski, Kathleen (NJ)	Inf	744
Gamache, Francis (NY)	NS	217	Gelato, Marie (NY)	EDM	569
Gambarin, Boris (NY)	IM	421	Gelb, Bruce (NY)	PCd	282
Gammon, G Davis (CT)	ChAP	902	Gelberg, Burt (NY)	IM	509
Gamss, Jeffrey (NY)	Ge	416	Gelbfish, Joseph (NY)	Cv	408
Ganchi, Parham (NJ)	PlS	824	Gelfand, Janice (NY)	Psyc	396
Gandhi, Lajpat (NY)	ChAP	566	Geller, Eric (NJ)	N	714
Gandhi, Rajinder (NJ)	PS	687	Geller, Mark (NY)	DR	554
Gannon, Christopher (NJ)	S	779	Geller, Peter (NY)	S	343
Garan, Hasan (NY)	CE	127	Gelles, Jeremiah (NY)	Cv	408
Garay, Kenneth (NJ)	Oto	683	Gelmann, Edward (NY)	Onc	204
Garay, Stuart (NY)	Pul	325	Geltzeiler, Jules (NJ)	U	796
Garber, Perry (NY)	Oph	521	Genato, Romulo (NY)	S	449
Gardenswartz, Mark (NY)	Nep	215	Gendelman, Seymour (NY)	N	223
Gardin, Julius (NJ)	Cv	661	Genden, Eric (NY)	Oto	269
Gardner, James (NJ)	PlS	853	Gendler, Ellen (NY)	D	147

Name	Specialty	Pg	Name	Specialty	Pg
Genieser, Nancy (NY)	DR	154	Gilbert, Fred (NY)	CG	142
Genn, David (NY)	Ge	608	Gildengers, Jaime (NJ)	S	737
Gennace, Ronald (NJ)	OrS	682	Gilder, Mark (NJ)	CRS	706
Gentile, Ronald (NY)	Oph	243	Giliberti, Orazio (NJ)	Oph	822
Gentilesco, Michael (NY)	ObG	576	Gill, Thomas (CT)	Ger	906
George, Liziamma (NY)	Pul	445	Gilson, Noah (NJ)	N	790
Geraci-Ciardullo, Kira (NY)	A&I	594	Gimovsky, Martin (NJ)	MF	712
Geraghty, Michael (NY)	Onc	425	Gindea, Aaron (NY)	Cv	492
Gerard, Perry (NY)	NuM	430	Ginsberg, Gerald (NY)	PlS	303
Gerber, Oded (NY)	N	576	Ginsberg, Michelle (NY)	DR	154
Gerberg, Lynda (NY)	Ped	534	Ginsburg, Frances (CT)	RE	894
Gerbino-Rosen, Ginny (NY)	ChAP	370	Ginsburg, Howard (NY)	PS	292
Gerdes, Hans (NY)	Ge	167	Ginsburg, Mark (NY)	TS	350
Gerhard, Harvey (NJ)	Pul	835	Gioia, Leonard (NY)	EDM	569
German, Harold (NY)	IM	573	Girardi, Anthony (NY)	Oph	521
Geronemus, Roy (NY)	D	147	Girardi, Leonard (NY)	TS	350
Gershell, William (NY)	Psyc	313	Girardi, Sarah (NY)	U	548
Gerson, Charles (NY)	Ge	167	Gitler, Bernard (NY)	Cv	596
Gesner, Matthew (NY)	PInf	440	Gitler, Ellen (NY)	EDM	605
Gettenberg, Gary (NY)	Ge	416	Giuffrida, Regina (NY)	ObG	623
Geuder, James (NJ)	VascS	698	Giugliano, James (NY)	FMed	570
Gevirtz, Clifford (NY)	PM	631	Giuliano, Michael (NJ)	NP	848
Gewanter, Richard (NY)	RadRO	542	Giusti, Robert (NY)	PPul	440
Gewirtz, George (NJ)	EDM	707	Gizzi, Martin (NJ)	N	768
Gewirtz, Harold (CT)	PlS	890	Gladstein, Geoffrey (CT)	Rhu	894
Gewitz, Michael (NY)	PCd	632	Gladstein, Gina (CT)	Oph	883
Gewolb, Eric (NJ)	Psyc	736	Gladstein, Michael (NY)	D	459
Gharibo, Christopher (NY)	PM	276	Gladstone, James (NY)	OrS	257
Ghavamian, Reza (NY)	U	400	Glanzman, Barry (NY)	Ge	571
Ghogawala, Zoher (CT)	NS	880	Glaser, Amy (NY)	Ped	441
Giardina, Elsa-Grace (NY)	Cv	131	Glaser, Jordan (NY)	Inf	478
Giardina, Patricia (NY)	PHO	287	Glaser, Morton (NY)	Pul	585
Giardina-Beckett, MarieAnne (NJ)	D	664	Glashow, Jonathan (NY)	OrS	257
Gibofsky, Allan (NY)	Rhu	335	Glassberg, Kenneth (NY)	U	355
Gibralter, Richard (NY)	Oph	243	Glassman, Alexander (NY)	Psyc	313
Giegerich, Edmund (NY)	EDM	413	Glassman, Charles (NY)	U	649
Giella, John (NY)	U	560	Glassman, Charles (NY)	IM	555
Gifford, Irina (NY)	PMR	443	Glassman, Lawrence (NY)	TS	547
Gil, Constante (NJ)	IM	765	Glassman, Mark (CT)	PGe	887

Alphabetical Listing of Doctors

Name	Specialty	Pg	Name	Specialty	Pg
Glassman, Morris (NY)	Oph	625	Goldberg-Berman, Judith (CT)	EDM	870
Glatt, Herbert (NJ)	Oph	717	Goldblatt, Kenneth (NJ)	Pul	751
Glatt, Hershel (NY)	Ped	534	Goldblatt, Robert (NY)	Ge	608
Gleckel, Louis (NY)	Cv	492	Goldblum, Lester (NY)	Ge	504
Glick, Ronald (NJ)	OrS	748	Golden, Flavia (NY)	IM	192
Glickel, Steven (NY)	HS	179	Goldenberg, Alan (NY)	EDM	569
Glicksman, Caroline (NJ)	PlS	794	Goldenberg, Alec (NY)	Hem	182
Gliedman, Paul (NY)	RadRO	447	Goldenberg, Bruce (NJ)	TS	728
Gliklich, Jerry (NY)	Cv	131	Goldenberg, David (NJ)	Ge	845
Glowacki, Jan (NJ)	IM	788	Goldenberg, David (CT)	PlS	890
Gluck, Ian (NJ)	ObG	808	Goldenberg, David (NY)	Psyc	313
Gochfeld, Michael (NJ)	OM	770	Goldfarb, C Richard (NY)	NuM	231
Godfrey, Norman (NY)	PlS	304	Goldfarb, Joel (NJ)	Ge	668
Godfrey, Philip (NY)	PlS	304	Goldfarb, Michael (NJ)	S	796
Goland, Robin (NY)	EDM	159	Goldfarb, Steven (NY)	IM	573
Golbe, Lawrence (NJ)	N	768	Goldfischer, Mindy (NJ)	DR	666
Gold, Alan (NY)	PlS	537	Goldin, Howard (NY)	Ge	167
Gold, David (NY)	PGe	581	Goldman, Gary (NY)	ObG	234
Gold, Jeffrey (NJ)	IM	821	Goldman, Ira (NY)	Ge	504
Gold, Joan (NY)	PMR	298	Goldman, Jack (NY)	IM	613
Gold, Jonathan (NJ)	D	819	Goldman, Joel (NY)	EDM	414
Gold, Scott (NY)	Oto	269	Goldman, Kenneth (NJ)	VascS	754
Goldberg, Arthur (NY)	Onc	204	Goldman, Martin (NY)	Cv	131
Goldberg, Daniel (NJ)	Oph	791	Goldman, Michael (NJ)	EDM	667
Goldberg, David (NY)	D	147	Goldman, Neil (NY)	Psyc	313
Goldberg, Harvey (NY)	Cv	131	Goldman, Neil (NY)	A&I	594
Goldberg, Jeffrey (NY)	Psyc	444	Goldschmidt, Howard (NJ)	Cv	661
Goldberg, Jonathan (NY)	Onc	617	Goldsmith, Ari (NY)	PO	440
Goldberg, Jory (NJ)	Pul	778	Goldsmith, Stanley (NY)	NuM	231
Goldberg, Leslie (NY)	Oph	521	Goldstein, Carl (NJ)	Nep	848
Goldberg, Marc (NJ)	Rhu	825	Goldstein, Jeffrey (NY)	OrS	257
Goldberg, Michael (NJ)	GO	763	Goldstein, Jonathan (NJ)	Cv	704
Goldberg, Myron (NY)	Ge	167	Goldstein, Jonathan (CT)	N	912
Goldberg, Neil (NY)	D	601	Goldstein, Judith (NY)	Ped	294
Goldberg, Nieca (NY)	Cv	131	Goldstein, Marc (NY)	U	355
Goldberg, Robert (NY)	Onc	555	Goldstein, Mark (NY)	Rhu	485
Goldberg, Roy (NY)	Ger	377	Goldstein, Martin (NY)	ObG	234
Goldberg, Steven (NY)	Cv	492	Goldstein, Paul (NY)	IM	192
Goldberg, Stuart (NJ)	Onc	674	Goldstein, Robert (NY)	PlS	395

Name	Specialty	Pg	Name	Specialty	Pg
Goldstein, Stanley (NY)	A&I	490	Gorfine, Stephen (NY)	CRS	142
Goldstein, Steven (NY)	Oto	388	Gorkin, Janet (NY)	Nep	383
Goldstein, Steven (NJ)	ObG	791	Gorlick, Richard (NY)	PHO	390
Goldstein, Steven (NY)	Ped	468	Gorman, Lauren (NY)	Psyc	314
Goldstein, Steven (NY)	ObG	234	Gorman, Robert (NJ)	FMed	708
Goldstein, Susanna (NY)	Psyc	313	Gorski, Lydia (NY)	IM	509
Goldweit, Richard (NJ)	Cv	661	Gotfried, Fern (NJ)	Ped	812
Golfinos, John (NY)	NS	217	Gotkin, Robert (NY)	PlS	537
Golier, Francis (NY)	Cv	596	Gotlin, Robert (NY)	PMR	298
Golombek, Sergio (NY)	NP	619	Gottesfeld, Peter (NY)	FMed	606
Goltzman, Carey (NY)	PCCM	632	Gottesman, Lester (NY)	CRS	143
Goluboff, Erik (NY)	U	355	Gottlieb, Beth (NY)	PRhu	532
Gomes, J Anthony (NY)	CE	127	Gottlieb, Geoffrey (NY)	Path	278
Gomez, William (NJ)	OrS	748	Gotto, Antonio (NY)	Cv	131
Gomolin, Irving (NY)	Ger	505	Gottridge, Joanne (NY)	IM	509
Gonzalez, David (NJ)	MF	789	Gouge, Thomas (NY)	S	343
Goodgold, Abraham (NJ)	IM	846	Goulart, Hamilton (NJ)	NS	677
Goodgold, Albert (NY)	N	223	Gould, Eric (NY)	Ped	534
Goodman, Alan (NJ)	A&I	842	Gould, Perry (NY)	Ge	504
Goodman, Berney (NY)	Psyc	314	Gould, Richard (NY)	Ge	608
Goodman, Kenneth (NY)	DR	499	Goy, Andre (NJ)	Onc	674
Goodman, Mark (NY)	Cv	493	Goydos, James (NJ)	S	779
Goodman, Michael (NY)	IM	509	Grabowski, Wayne (NJ)	Oph	770
Goodman, Robert (NY)	NS	217	Grace, William (NY)	Onc	204
Goodman, Robert (NJ)	RadRO	725	Graff, Michael (NJ)	NP	790
Goodman, Susan (NY)	Rhu	335	Graham, Alan (NJ)	VascS	781
Goodstein, Carolyn (NJ)	A&I	660	Grajower, Martin (NY)	EDM	373
Goodwin, Charles (NY)	OrS	258	Gralla, Richard (NY)	Onc	512
Gordon, Jeffrey (NY)	EDM	500	Granatir, Charles (NJ)	OrS	736
Gordon, Marc (NY)	N	517	Granet, Kenneth (NJ)	IM	788
Gordon, Mark (NY)	S	646	Granick, Mark (NJ)	PlS	723
Gordon, Marsha (NY)	D	147	Grano, Vanessa (NY)	ObG	623
Gordon, Michael (NY)	Oto	525	Granstein, Richard (NY)	D	147
Gordon, Neil (CT)	Oto	886	Grant, Linda (CT)	PMR	889
Gordon, Richard (NJ)	Rhu	752	Grant, Robert (NY)	PlS	304
Gordon, Richard (NY)	Pul	540	Grasso, Cono (NY)	Oph	466
Gorecki, Piotr (NY)	S	450	Grasso, Michael (NY)	U	355
Gorenstein, Lyall (NY)	TS	560	Grasso, Michael (NJ)	Nep	713
Gorevic, Peter (NY)	Rhu	335	Graver, L Michael (NY)	TS	471

Alphabetical Listing of Doctors

Name	Specialty	Pg	Name	Specialty	Pg
Gray, William (NY)	IC	198	Greenwald, Blaine (NY)	GerPsy	462
Grayson, Douglas (NY)	Oph	243	Greenwald, Brian (NY)	PMR	299
Grazi, Richard (NY)	RE	447	Greenwald, Bruce (NY)	PCCM	283
Greaney, Edward (NY)	IM	192	Greenwald, David (NY)	Ge	375
Grebler, Arnold (NJ)	U	797	Greenwald, Marc (NY)	CRS	496
Greeley, Norman (NY)	A&I	407	Greenwald, Robert (NY)	Rhu	544
Green, Abraham (NY)	Ped	534	Greer, David (CT)	N	912
Green, Jeffrey (CT)	Cv	866	Greer, Jeannete (NJ)	DR	760
Green, Mark (NY)	N	223	Greif, Richard (NY)	Cv	596
Green, Peter (NY)	Ge	167	Greisman, Stewart (NY)	Rhu	335
Green, Richard (NY)	VascS	362	Grelsamer, Ronald (NY)	OrS	258
Green, Robert (NY)	Oto	269	Grendell, James (NY)	Ge	504
Green, Stephen (NY)	Cv	493	Grenell, Steven (NY)	N	384
Green, Steven (NY)	OrS	258	Grenis, Michael (NJ)	OrS	748
Green, Stuart (NY)	Rhu	448	Gress, Frank (NY)	Ge	416
Greenbaum, Allen (NY)	Oph	626	Gribbin, Dorota (NJ)	PMR	750
Greenberg, Harly (NY)	Pul	540	Gribbon, John (NJ)	IM	711
Greenberg, Howard (NY)	Onc	465	Gribetz, Michael (NY)	U	355
Greenberg, Judith (NY)	ChAP	566	Grieco, Michael (NY)	S	545
Greenberg, Mark (NY)	Cv	368	Griepp, Randall (NY)	TS	350
Greenberg, Martin (NJ)	Pul	724	Grifo, James (NY)	RE	331
Greenberg, Robert (NY)	D	147	Grijnsztein, Jacob (NY)	Ped	534
Greenberg, Robert (NJ)	GerPsy	734	Grizzanti, Joseph (NJ)	Pul	825
Greenberg, Ronald (NY)	Ge	504	Grodberg, Michele (NJ)	D	665
Greenberg, Rosalie (NJ)	ChAP	843	Grodman, Richard (NY)	Cv	475
Greenberg, Steven (NY)	Oph	626	Grodstein, Gerald (NJ)	Nep	676
Greenberg, Steven (NY)	Cv	493	Groeger, William (NY)	PlS	537
Greenberg, Susan (NJ)	Onc	789	Groff, Walter (NJ)	CRS	843
Greenblatt, Louis (NY)	FMed	570	Groopman, Jacob (NY)	Pul	445
Greene, Jeffrey (NY)	Inf	186	Gropen, Toby (NY)	N	429
Greene, Loren Wissner (NY)	EDM	159	Grosman, Irwin (NY)	Ge	416
Greenfield, Martin (NY)	EDM	501	Gross, Dennis (NY)	D	147
Greengart, Alvin (NY)	Cv	409	Gross, Elliott (NY)	N	622
Greenman, James (NJ)	Inf	846	Gross, Gary (NJ)	A&I	785
Greenspan, Alan (NY)	D	147	Gross, Harvey (NJ)	FMed	667
Greenspan, Joel (NY)	Inf	508	Gross, Ian (CT)	NP	910
Greenstein, Bruce (NY)	PlS	395	Gross, Jay (NY)	CE	368
Greenstein, Caren (CT)	DR	869	Gross, Jeffrey (CT)	N	880
Greenstein, Stuart (NY)	S	399	Gross, Joshua (NJ)	DR	666

Name	Specialty	Pg	Name	Specialty	Pg
Gross, Michael (NJ)	SM	694	Guma, Michael (NJ)	Rhu	693
Gross, Susan (NY)	CG	370	Gumprecht, Jeffrey (NY)	Inf	186
Grossbard, Lionel (NY)	Onc	204	Gundy, Edward (NY)	OrS	628
Grossbard, Michael (NY)	Onc	204	Guoth, Maria (CT)	EDM	870
Grossi, Eugene (NY)	TS	350	Gupta, Jagdish (NY)	Ge	416
Grossi, Robert (NY)	VascS	363	Gupta, Prem (NY)	Cv	409
Grossman, Bernard (NJ)	Onc	745	Gupta, Sanjeev (NY)	Ge	376
Grossman, Edward (CT)	Ge	871	Gupta, Shiv (CT)	NuM	881
Grossman, Elliot (NJ)	ChiN	802	Gurevich, Michael (NY)	Psyc	539
Grossman, Kenneth (NJ)	D	786	Gurland, Frances (NJ)	Psyc	690
Grossman, Marc (NY)	D	601	Gurland, Judith (NY)	Oph	386
Grossman, Melanie (NY)	D	148	Gurland, Mark (NJ)	HS	670
Grossman, Robert (NJ)	OrS	792	Gusberg, Richard (CT)	VascS	922
Grossman, Susan (NY)	Nep	480	Gusmorino, Paul (NY)	PM	276
Grosso, John (NY)	Oto	525	Gusset, George (NY)	Ge	416
Grosso, Sue Jane (NJ)	DR	844	Gutin, Philip (NY)	NS	218
Grubb, William (NJ)	PM	772	Gutowski, W Thomas (NJ)	OrS	749
Gruber, Michael (NY)	N	223	Gutwein, Isadore (NY)	Ge	376
Grubman, Samuel (NY)	A&I	125	Guyer, David (NY)	Cv	131
Gruenstein, Steven (NY)	Hem	182	Guzman, Rodolfo (NY)	EDM	373
Gruenwald, Laurence (NJ)	Ped	722			
Grunberger, Ivan (NY)	U	452			
Grunebaum, Amos (NY)	MF	200			
Grunfeld, Lawrence (NY)	RE	331	# H		
Grunzweig, Milton (NY)	IM	422	Haas, Jonathan (NY)	RadRO	542
Gruskay, Jeffrey (CT)	Ped	916	Haas, Steven (NY)	OrS	258
Gruss, Claudia (CT)	Ge	871	Haber, Daran (NJ)	PM	792
Gruss, Leslie (NY)	ObG	234	Haber, Gregory (NY)	Ge	167
Guarini, Ludovico (NY)	PHO	439	Haber, Patricia (NY)	Ped	393
Guarracini, Mary (NY)	PMR	558	Haber, Stuart (NY)	IM	193
Gubernick, Martin (NY)	ObG	234	Habib, Mohsen (NY)	Oto	436
Gudavalli, Madhu (NY)	NP	425	Haddad, Joseph (NY)	PO	290
Guida, Louis (NY)	A&I	563	Haffty, Bruce (NJ)	RadRO	778
Guida, Robert (NY)	Oto	269	Haft, Jacob (NJ)	Cv	661
Guillem, Jose (NY)	CRS	143	Hagaman, John (NJ)	Cv	741
Guillen, Gregorio (NJ)	IM	765	Hages, Harry (NJ)	Ped	687
Guillory, Samuel (NY)	Oph	244	Haggerty, Mary (NJ)	IM	711
Gulati, Subhash (NY)	Onc	204	Hahn, John (NJ)	Ge	734
Gulrajani, Ramesh (NY)	Pul	445	Haig, Scott (NY)	OrS	628

Alphabetical Listing of Doctors

Name	Specialty	Pg	Name	Specialty	Pg
Haight, David (NY)	Oph	244	Hannafin, Jo (NY)	OrS	258
Haimovic, Itzhak (NY)	N	517	Hanson, Matthew (NY)	Oto	436
Haines, Kathleen (NJ)	PRhu	686	Har-El, Gady (NY)	Oto	270
Hainline, Brian (NY)	N	517	Haramati, Linda (NY)	DR	372
Hajjar, John (NJ)	U	697	Haramati, Nogah (NY)	DR	372
Halaas, Jeffrey (NY)	Onc	618	Harangozo, Andrea (NJ)	Pul	778
Halata, Michael (NY)	PGe	633	Harary, Albert (NY)	Ge	168
Hall, Lisabeth (NY)	Oph	244	Haratz-Rubinstein, Natan (NY)	ObG	431
Hall, Simon (NY)	U	355	Harin, Anantham (NY)	NP	480
Hall, Timothy (CT)	TS	896	Harish, Ziv (NJ)	A&I	660
Hallal, Edward (NY)	IM	573	Harlam, Dean (NY)	Psyc	640
Halmi, Katherine (NY)	Psyc	640	Harlow, Paul (NJ)	Ped	688
Halperin, Ira (NY)	Hem	182	Harman, John (NJ)	Pul	751
Halperin, John (NJ)	N	849	Harmon, Gregory (NY)	Oph	244
Halperin, Jonathan (NY)	Cv	131	Haroldson, Olaf (NJ)	Oto	749
Halpern, Allan (NY)	D	148	Harooni, Robert (NY)	Ge	461
Halpern, Brian (NY)	SM	339	Harpaz, Noam (NY)	Path	278
Halpern, Neil (NY)	CCM	144	Harper, Harry (NJ)	Onc	674
Halpern, Steven (NJ)	PHO	685	Harrington, Elizabeth (NY)	VascS	363
Hamburger, Max (NY)	Rhu	587	Harrington, Martin (NY)	VascS	363
Hamet, Marc (CT)	VIR	897	Harris, Dena (NY)	ObG	234
Hametz, Irwin (NJ)	D	786	Harris, Leon (NY)	Pul	559
Hamilton, Audrey (NJ)	Onc	832	Harris, Loren (NY)	TS	486
Hamilton, William (NY)	OrS	258	Harris, Michael (NJ)	PHO	686
Hammel, Jay (NY)	DR	499	Harris, Steven (NY)	U	548
Hammer, Arthur (NY)	Pul	446	Harrison, Aaron (NY)	Ge	571
Hammer, Glenn (NY)	Inf	186	Harrison, Louis (NY)	RadRO	329
Hammer, Scott (NY)	Inf	186	Hart, Catherine (NY)	IM	193
Hammerman, Hillel (NY)	Ge	167	Hart, Sidney (CT)	Psyc	891
Hammerschlag, Paul (NY)	Oto	270	Hartl, Roger (NY)	NS	218
Hamner, Daniel (NY)	SM	339	Hartman, Alan (NY)	TS	547
Hand, Ivan (NY)	NP	465	Hartman, Barry (NY)	Inf	186
Handelsman, Dan (NY)	PEn	632	Hartz, Cindi (NY)	Ped	637
Handelsman, Richard (NY)	IM	555	Hartzband, Mark (NJ)	OrS	682
Handler, Robert (NJ)	Ped	812	Harwin, Steven (NY)	OrS	258
Hankin, Dorie (NY)	Ped	534	Haselkorn, Joan (NY)	ObG	519
Hanley, Gerard (NY)	Cv	409	Hashim, Sabet (CT)	TS	921
Hann, Lucy (NY)	DR	154	Hassoun, Hani (NY)	Onc	205
Hanna, Moneer (NY)	U	548	Hatcher, Virgil (NY)	D	148

Name	Specialty	Pg	Name	Specialty	Pg
Hatsis, Alexander (NY)	Oph	521	Henschke, Claudia (NY)	DR	155
Hauptman, Allen (NY)	IM	193	Henshaw, D Ross (CT)	OrS	885
Hausman, Michael (NY)	OrS	259	Hensle, Terry (NY)	U	356
Havens, Jennifer (NY)	ChAP	139	Herbert, Joseph (NY)	N	224
Hawrylo, Richard (NJ)	PlS	813	Herbin, Joseph (CT)	Inf	873
Hayes, Leslie (NY)	AM	407	Herbstein, Diego (NY)	N	224
Hayes, Mary Katherine (NY)	RadRO	329	Herbstman, Robert (NJ)	PlS	777
Hayworth, Robin (NY)	Oph	386	Herman, David (NJ)	Inf	831
Hayworth, Scott (NY)	ObG	624	Herman, Martin (NJ)	N	790
Healey, John (NY)	OrS	259	Herman, Zeva (NY)	DR	155
Heary, Robert (NJ)	NS	714	Hermele, Herbert (CT)	OrS	885
Hecht, Alan (NY)	Cv	132	Herold, Betsy (NY)	PInf	390
Hecht, Andrew (NY)	OrS	259	Herr, Harry (NY)	U	356
Hedrick, David (CT)	Ped	888	Herron, Daniel (NY)	S	343
Heerdt, Alexandra (NY)	S	343	Hersh, Peter (NJ)	Oph	681
Hefter, Harold (NY)	D	498	Hershman, Dawn (NY)	Onc	205
Heftler, Jeffrey (CT)	PMR	889	Hershman, Ronnie (NY)	Cv	493
Heier, Stephen (NY)	Ge	608	Herskovitz, Steven (NY)	N	384
Heim, John (NJ)	TS	753	Hertan, Hilary (NY)	Ge	376
Heiman, Peter (NY)	Psyc	396	Hertz, Marc (NY)	DR	603
Heinemann, Murk (NY)	Oph	244	Hertzig, Margaret (NY)	ChAP	139
Heisman, Alexander (NY)	Psyc	444	Herzlinger, Robert (CT)	NP	878
Heitner, John (NY)	Cv	409	Herzog, David (NY)	IM	614
Helbraun, Mark (NJ)	CRS	663	Herzog, Thomas (NY)	GO	177
Heldman, Jay (NJ)	D	665	Hes, Dyan (NY)	Ped	441
Helfet, David (NY)	OrS	259	Hetzler, Peter (NJ)	PlS	794
Helfgott, David (NY)	Inf	186	Heublum, Michael (NY)	N	224
Hellenbrand, William (NY)	PCd	282	Hiatt, I Mark (NJ)	NP	767
Heller, Debra (NJ)	Path	719	Hicks, Patricia (NJ)	PA&I	685
Heller, Keith (NY)	S	343	Hidalgo, David (NY)	PlS	304
Heller, Paul (NJ)	GO	804	Hiesiger, Emile (NY)	N	224
Heller, Stanley (NY)	Psyc	314	Higgins, Susan (CT)	RadRO	918
Hellerman, James (NY)	EDM	605	Higgins, William (NY)	IM	614
Hembree, Wylie (NY)	EDM	159	Hindenburg, Alexander (NY)	Onc	513
Hen, Jacob (CT)	PPul	888	Hindin, Lee (NJ)	Psyc	824
Henderson, Cassandra (NY)	MF	381	Hindman, Steven (CT)	OrS	885
Hendricks, Judith (NY)	IM	478	Hines, William (CT)	Nep	879
Hendricks-Munoz, Karen (NY)	NP	213	Hirsch, Andrew (NJ)	A&I	785
Henick, David (NJ)	Oto	683	Hirsch, Glenn (NY)	ChAP	139

Alphabetical Listing of Doctors

Name	Specialty	Pg	Name	Specialty	Pg
Hirsch, Lissa (NY)	ObG	234	Holtzman, Robert (NY)	NS	218
Hirschfeld, Alan (NY)	NS	218	Hong, Andrew (NY)	PS	533
Hirschman, Alan (NY)	Ped	393	Hong, Joon Ho (NY)	S	450
Hirschman, Richard (NY)	Onc	205	Honig, Stephen (NY)	Rhu	335
Hirshaut, Yashar (NY)	Onc	205	Hopkins, Arthur (NY)	IM	614
Hirt, Paula (NY)	ObG	577	Horbar, Gary (NY)	IM	193
Hisler, Barbara (NY)	D	498	Hordof, Allan (NY)	PCd	282
Ho, Bryan (NJ)	Oto	683	Horn, Evelyn (NY)	Cv	132
Hochman, Herbert (NY)	D	148	Horner, Neil (NJ)	NRad	849
Hochstein, Martin (NJ)	EDM	667	Hornyak, Stephen (NY)	S	485
Hochster, Howard (CT)	Onc	910	Horovitz, Len (NY)	IM	193
Hockstein, Steven (NY)	ObG	235	Horowitz, Harold (NY)	Inf	186
Hoda, Syed (NY)	Path	279	Horowitz, Marc (NY)	Oph	626
Hodes, David (NY)	Pul	559	Horowitz, Mark (NY)	U	452
Hodes, Steven (NJ)	Ge	762	Horowitz, Mark (NY)	Rhu	335
Hodges, David (NJ)	Cv	661	Horowitz, Steven (CT)	Cv	866
Hodges, Laura (CT)	VIR	898	Horvath, Susanna (NY)	N	224
Hodgson, W John (NY)	S	399	Horwitz, Steven (NY)	Onc	205
Hodosh, Richard (NJ)	NS	848	Hotchkiss, Edward (NY)	IM	509
Hoffman, Darryl (NY)	TS	350	Hotchkiss, Robert (NY)	OrS	259
Hoffman, Eileen (NY)	IM	193	Housman, Arno (NY)	U	649
Hoffman, Janet (NY)	DR	499	Howes, Christopher (CT)	IC	876
Hoffman, Joel (NY)	Psyc	314	Hricak, Hedvig (NY)	DR	155
Hoffman, Lloyd (NY)	PlS	304	Hsu, Daphne (NY)	PCd	389
Hoffman, Michael (NY)	Rhu	544	Hsuih, Terence CH (NY)	IM	422
Hoffman, Pamela (CT)	IM	874	Huang, Paul (NY)	NS	218
Hoffman, Richard (NY)	EDM	477	Hubbard, Christopher (NY)	OrS	259
Hoffman, Robert (NY)	PrM	309	Hubschmann, Otakar (NJ)	NS	714
Hoffman, Ronald (NY)	Oto	270	Hudis, Clifford (NY)	Onc	205
Holcomb, Kevin (NY)	GO	177	Hughes, Peter (CT)	OrS	885
Holder, Jonathan (NY)	OrS	628	Huh, Julie (NY)	D	567
Holland, Claudia (NY)	ObG	235	Hunt, William (CT)	Nep	879
Holland, Elbridge (NJ)	FMed	803	Hunter, John (NY)	PlS	304
Holland, James (NY)	Onc	205	Huo, Jerry (NY)	Oto	467
Holland, Neil (NJ)	N	790	Hupart, Kenneth (NY)	EDM	501
Hollander, Eric (NY)	Psyc	314	Huprikar, Shirish (NY)	Inf	187
Hollander, Gerald (NY)	Cv	409	Huribal, Marsel (CT)	VascS	898
Holliday, Roy (NY)	DR	155	Hurst, Lawrence (NY)	HS	571
Hollister, Dickerman (CT)	Onc	878	Hurst, Wendy (NJ)	ObG	680

Name	Specialty	Pg	Name	Specialty	Pg
Hurwitz, Diana (NY)	D	601	Isola, Luis (NY)	Hem	182
Huston, Jan (NJ)	S	727	Isom, O Wayne (NY)	TS	350
Hutchinson, Gordon (CT)	Rhu	920	Israel, Alan (NJ)	Hem	671
Hutson, J Milton (NY)	MF	200	Israel, Jessica (NJ)	Ger	787
Hwang, Cheng-hong (NJ)	Pul	855	Israeli, Ron (NY)	PlS	537
Hyans, Peter (NJ)	PlS	854	Issenberg, Henry (NY)	PCd	632
Hyatt, Alexander (NJ)	Ped	688	Istrico, Richard (NY)	FMed	460
Hyde, Phyllis (NY)	Hem	419	Iswara, Kadirawel (NY)	Ge	416
Hyler, Irene (NY)	ChAP	599	Itzkowitz, Steven (NY)	Ge	168
Hyman, David (NY)	CG	566			
Hyman, George (NY)	Oph	432			
Hyman, Jeffrey (NY)	IM	422			
Hyman, Joshua (NY)	OrS	259	**J**		
Hymes, Kenneth (NY)	Hem	182	Jabs, Douglas (NY)	Oph	244
			Jackson, Rosemary (NY)	Ped	441
			Jacob, Jessica (NY)	ObG	519
			Jacobowitz, Glenn (NY)	VascS	363
I			Jacobowitz, Marilyn (NY)	Pul	643
Iammatteo, Matthew (NJ)	ObG	808	Jacobs, Elliot (NY)	PlS	304
Ibelli, Vincent (NY)	FMed	554	Jacobs, Jonathan (NY)	Inf	187
Idupuganti, Sudharam (NY)	Psyc	444	Jacobs, Joseph (NY)	Oto	270
Igel, Gerard (NY)	Ped	393	Jacobs, Laurie (NY)	Ger	377
Ilowite, Norman (NY)	PRhu	391	Jacobs, Michael (NY)	D	148
Ilson, David (NY)	Onc	205	Jacobs, Morton (NY)	DR	155
Imber, Gerald (NY)	PlS	304	Jacobs, Thomas (NY)	EDM	160
Inabnet, William (NY)	S	343	Jacobson, Ira (NY)	Ge	168
Inamdar, Sarla (NY)	Ped	294	Jacobson, Marc (NY)	AM	489
Infantino, Michael (NY)	Cv	132	Jacobson, Ronald (NY)	ChiN	600
Ingenito, Anthony (NJ)	RadRO	692	Jacoby, Jacob (NJ)	Psyc	737
Inglis, Steven (NY)	MF	464	Jadonath, Ram (NY)	CE	491
Ingrassia, Joseph (NY)	FMed	554	Jafar, Jafar (NY)	NS	218
Innerfield, Michael (NY)	IC	555	Jaffe, Alan (NY)	Ge	608
Inra, Lawrence (NY)	Cv	132	Jaffe, Fredrick (NY)	OrS	260
Inwald, Gary (NY)	PMR	299	Jaffe, Herbert (NY)	Oph	433
Inzucchi, Silvio (CT)	EDM	905	Jaffin, Barry (NY)	Ge	168
Irwin, Mark (NY)	U	452	Jagannath, Sundar (NY)	Onc	206
Isaacs, Ellen (NY)	IM	614	Jahn, Anthony (NY)	Oto	270
Isaacson, Steven (NY)	RadRO	329	Jahre, Caren (NY)	NRad	230
Isay, Richard (NY)	Psyc	314	Jaile-Marti, Jesus (NY)	NP	619

Alphabetical Listing of Doctors

Name	Specialty	Pg	Name	Specialty	Pg
Jain, Subhash (NY)	PM	277	Kabis, Suzanne (NJ)	Nep	833
Jakubowski, Ann (NY)	Onc	206	Kacker, Ashutosh (NY)	Oto	270
Jamidar, Priya (CT)	Ge	905	Kadan-Lottick, Nina (CT)	PHO	915
Jarnagin, William (NY)	S	343	Kaell, Alan (NY)	Rhu	587
Jarowski, Charles (NY)	Onc	206	Kafantaris, Vivian (NY)	ChAP	458
Jarrett, Mark (NY)	Rhu	485	Kahn, David (NY)	Psyc	314
Jawetz, Harold (NJ)	IM	821	Kahn, Leonard (NY)	Path	527
Jay, Judith (NY)	Oto	630	Kahn, Max (NY)	Ped	294
Jayaram, Nadubeethi (NY)	OrS	482	Kahn, Oren (NY)	Ge	608
Jelin, Abraham (NY)	PGe	438	Kairam, Indira (NY)	Ge	168
Jelveh, Mansoor (NY)	Cv	493	Kaiser, Michael (NY)	NS	218
Jennis, Andrew (NJ)	Onc	675	Kaiser, Paul (NJ)	N	747
Jeremias, Allen (NY)	Cv	564	Kaiser, Stephen (NY)	IM	422
Jewel, Kenneth (NJ)	DR	707	Kalafatic, Alfredo (NY)	CRS	496
Johns, William (CT)	NuM	881	Kalash, Glenn (NY)	Psyc	469
Johnson, Albert (NJ)	OrS	834	Kalchthaler, Thomas (NY)	Ger	610
Johnson, Diane (NY)	Inf	508	Kaleya, Ronald (NY)	S	647
Johnson, Robert (NJ)	AM	703	Kalikow, Kevin (NY)	ChAP	599
Johnson, Valerie (NY)	PNep	289	Kalinich, Lila (NY)	Psyc	314
Jokl, Peter (CT)	OrS	913	Kalischer, Alan (NJ)	Cv	842
Jones, Frank (NJ)	Psyc	777	Kalman, Jill (NY)	Cv	132
Jones, Jacqueline (NY)	PO	290	Kamalakar, Peri (NJ)	PHO	720
Jones, Stephen (CT)	Ger	872	Kamelhar, David (NY)	Pul	325
Jonna, Siva (NJ)	PCCM	773	Kamen, Barton (NJ)	PHO	774
Jordan, Barry (NY)	N	622	Kamen, Mazen (NY)	Cv	132
Jordan, Lawrence (NJ)	S	752	Kaminer, Ruth (NY)	Ped	393
Joseph, John (NY)	IM	463	Kaminetsky, Jed (NY)	U	356
Joseph, Patricia (NY)	S	560	Kaminsky, Donald (NY)	IM	193
Josephson, Jordan (NY)	Oto	270	Kamler, Kenneth (NY)	HS	506
Josephson, Lynn (NY)	S	647	Kane, Michael (NJ)	Onc	789
Joy, Mark (NY)	IM	422	Kanengiser, Steven (NJ)	PPul	686
Juan, Paul (CT)	Ped	888	Kang, Harriet (NY)	ChiN	600
Julie, Edward (NJ)	Cv	819	Kang, Pritpal (NY)	Cv	409
Jurcic, Joseph (NY)	Onc	206	Kanner, Ronald (NY)	N	517
Jutkowitz, Robert (NY)	N	480	Kanter, Alan (NJ)	Ped	688
			Kantor, Alan (NY)	EDM	605
			Kantrowitz, Niki (NY)	Cv	409
			Kaplan, Gabriel (NJ)	Psyc	854
			Kaplan, Jeffrey (CT)	Oph	883

K

Name	Specialty	Pg	Name	Specialty	Pg
Kaplan, Kenneth (NY)	Cv	596	Katz, Harry (NJ)	Oto	683
Kaplan, Martin (NY)	Ped	583	Katz, Henry (NY)	Ge	608
Kaplan, Matthew (NY)	PNep	440	Katz, Herbert (NJ)	U	738
Kaplan, Ronald (NY)	PM	277	Katz, Jack (NY)	Psyc	539
Kaplan, Sherri (NY)	D	602	Katz, Jeffrey (NJ)	U	728
Kaplan, Steven (NY)	U	356	Katz, Seymour (NY)	Ge	504
Kaplitt, Michael (NY)	NS	218	Katz, Steven (NJ)	U	697
Kaplovitz, Harry (NY)	PCd	437	Katz, Stuart (NY)	Cv	132
Kapoor, Satish (NY)	IM	614	Katz, Susan (NY)	D	371
Kappel, Bruce (NY)	Onc	513	Katzenelenbogen, Moshe (NY)	IM	422
Kapur, Sandip (NY)	S	343	Katzenstein, Martin (NY)	NP	382
Karamitsos, Harry (NY)	ObG	235	Kaufman, Alan (NY)	A&I	367
Karanfilian, Richard (NY)	VascS	651	Kaufman, David (NY)	IM	193
Karas, Evan (NY)	OrS	629	Kaufman, David (NY)	ChiN	141
Karasu, Sylvia (NY)	Psyc	314	Kaufman, David (NY)	Cv	368
Karasu, T Byram (NY)	Psyc	315	Kaufman, David (NY)	N	384
Karatoprak, Ohan (NJ)	FMed	667	Kaufman, Matthew (NJ)	PlS	777
Karetzky, Monroe (NY)	Pul	397	Kaufman, Richard (CT)	A&I	901
Karmen, Carol (NY)	IM	614	Kaufmann, Charles (NY)	Psyc	315
Karp, Adam (NY)	Ger	175	Kaushik, Raj (NJ)	TS	826
Karp, George (NJ)	Hem	764	Kauvar, Arielle (NY)	D	148
Karp, Nolan (NY)	PlS	305	Kavanagh, Brian (CT)	OrS	885
Karpeh, Martin (NY)	S	343	Kavey, Neil (NY)	Psyc	315
Karpinski, Richard (NY)	PlS	305	Kavoussi, Louis (NY)	U	548
Kasabian, Armen (NY)	PlS	537	Kay, Arthur (NY)	N	429
Kase, Steven (NY)	Oto	630	Kay, Richard (NY)	Cv	596
Kaskel, Frederick (NY)	PNep	391	Kay, Scott (NJ)	Oto	772
Kasper, William (NY)	Oph	521	Kazam, Elias (NY)	DR	155
Kassel, Barry (NY)	S	647	Kazam, Ezra (NJ)	Oph	809
Kates, Matthew (NY)	Oto	630	Kazdin, Hal (NY)	IM	422
Kato, Tomoaki (NY)	S	344	Kazim, Michael (NY)	Oph	244
Kattan, Meyer (NY)	PPul	291	Kazlow, Philip (NY)	PGe	285
Katus, Eli (NY)	Psyc	539	Kearney, Thomas (NJ)	S	780
Katz, Aaron (NY)	U	356	Keefe, David (NY)	RE	331
Katz, Alan (NY)	RadRO	586	Keilson, Marshall (NY)	N	429
Katz, Amiram (CT)	N	912	Keiser, Harold (NY)	Rhu	398
Katz, Andrea (NJ)	Ped	834	Keith, Marie (NY)	Ped	294
Katz, Bruce (NY)	D	148	Kelemen, John (NY)	N	517
Katz, Edward (NY)	Cv	132	Keller, Adina (NY)	ObG	624

Alphabetical Listing of Doctors

Name	Specialty	Pg	Name	Specialty	Pg
Keller, Alex (NY)	PlS	537	Kessler, William (NJ)	Hem	846
Keller, Andrew (CT)	Cv	866	Khalife, Michael (NY)	S	545
Keller, Irwin (NJ)	NRad	769	Khan, Arfa (NY)	DR	499
Keller, Jeffrey (NY)	PO	634	Khandji, Alexander (NY)	NRad	230
Keller, Peter (NY)	Cv	368	Khilnani, Neil (NY)	VIR	361
Keller, Steven (NY)	TS	400	Khimani, Karim (NJ)	Ger	845
Kellogg, F Russell (NY)	Ger	175	Khouri, Philippe (NJ)	Psyc	751
Kelly, Anna (NY)	NRad	230	Khoury, F Frederic (NY)	PlS	638
Kelly, Michael (NJ)	SM	694	Khoury, Paul (NY)	DR	603
Kelly, Stephen (NY)	Oph	244	Khulpateea, Neekianund (NY)	GO	418
Kelly, Stephen (NY)	FMed	606	Kierce, Roger (NJ)	ObG	822
Kelly, William (CT)	Onc	910	Kiernan, Howard (NY)	OrS	260
Kelsen, David (NY)	Onc	206	Kim, Hong (NY)	U	452
Keltz, Theodore (NY)	Cv	596	Kim, Joyce (NY)	ObG	235
Kemeny, M Margaret (NY)	S	471	Kim, Tae (NY)	PlS	638
Kemeny, Nancy (NY)	Onc	206	Kimball, Annetta (NY)	Ge	168
Kempin, Sanford (NY)	Hem	183	Kimmelstiel, Fred (NY)	S	344
Kenan, Samuel (NY)	OrS	523	Kimura, Yukiko (NJ)	PRhu	687
Kenet, Barney (NY)	D	148	King, Robert (CT)	ChAP	902
Kenigsberg, Daniel (NY)	RE	586	King, William (NY)	HS	179
Kenler, Andrew (CT)	S	895	Kinkhabwala, Milan (NY)	S	399
Kennedy, Gary (NY)	GerPsy	378	Kipen, Howard (NJ)	OM	770
Kennedy, James (NY)	IM	193	Kirschenbaum, Alexander (NY)	U	356
Kennedy, Timothy (NY)	S	399	Kirschenbaum, Ira (NY)	OrS	387
Kennish, Arthur (NY)	IM	194	Kirshblum, Steven (NJ)	PMR	722
Kenny, Raymond (NJ)	Ge	708	Kirshenbaum, Nancy (NY)	MF	616
Kent, Joan (NY)	ObG	235	Kirshy, David (NY)	DR	568
Kernan, Nancy (NY)	PHO	287	Kirtane, Sanjay (NY)	Cv	457
Kernan, Walter (CT)	IM	908	Kizelshteyn, Grigory (NY)	PM	631
Kerner, Michael (NJ)	Ge	845	Klagsbrun, Samuel (NY)	Psyc	640
Kerr, Leslie (NY)	Rhu	336	Klapholz, Ari (NY)	Pul	325
Kerstein, Joshua (NY)	Cv	409	Klapholz, Marc (NJ)	Cv	704
Kesarwala, Hemant (NJ)	A&I	757	Klapper, Daniel (NY)	Oph	244
Kessler, Alan (NY)	ObG	235	Klapper, Philip (NY)	Pul	397
Kessler, Bradley (NY)	PGe	581	Klar, Tobi (NY)	D	602
Kessler, Edmund (NY)	PS	533	Klares, Scott (NY)	Pul	643
Kessler, Jeffrey (NY)	N	517	Klarsfeld, Jay (CT)	Oto	886
Kessler, Leonard (NY)	Onc	513	Klausner, Stanley (NY)	S	588
Kessler, Martin (NY)	PlS	537	Kleber, Herbert (NY)	AdP	123

Name	Specialty	Pg	Name	Specialty	Pg
Kleeman, Harris (NY)	Cv	410	Kofinas, George (NY)	RE	447
Klein, George (NY)	U	356	Kohan, Darius (NY)	Oto	270
Klein, Irwin (NY)	EDM	501	Kohn, Brenda (NY)	PEn	283
Klein, Jeffrey (NY)	RE	644	Kolenik, Steven (CT)	D	868
Klein, Natalie (NY)	Inf	508	Kolitz, Jonathan (NY)	Hem	507
Klein, Neil (CT)	IM	875	Kolker, Adam (NY)	PlS	305
Klein, Noah (NY)	Oph	245	Kolker, Harvey (NY)	Ped	583
Klein, Norman (NY)	A&I	407	Kolodny, Edwin (NY)	N	224
Klein, Patricia (NJ)	N	678	Kolodny, Erwin (NY)	Pul	326
Klein, Robert (NJ)	A&I	819	Kolsky, Neil (NJ)	Ped	688
Klein, Steven (NY)	FMed	502	Komisar, Arnold (NY)	Oto	270
Klein, Victor (NY)	MF	511	Koniaris, Soula (NJ)	PGe	774
Klein, Walter (NJ)	Ge	668	Konka, Sudarsanam (NY)	IM	422
Kleinberg, David (NY)	EDM	160	Kopec, Anna (NJ)	D	733
Kleiner, Morton (NY)	Nep	480	Kopel, Samuel (NY)	Hem	419
Kleinman, Andrew (NY)	PlS	638	Kopelman, Rima (NJ)	Rhu	693
Kleinman, Paul (NY)	OrS	387	Kopf, Gary (CT)	TS	921
Klenk, Rosemary (CT)	Ped	888	Koplin, Richard (NY)	Oph	245
Klenoff, Bruce (CT)	Oto	886	Koppel, Barbara (NY)	N	224
Kliger, Alan (CT)	Nep	911	Korc, Beatriz (NY)	Ger	175
Kligfield, Paul (NY)	Cv	133	Koreen, Amy (NY)	Psyc	584
Kligler, Benjamin (NY)	FMed	162	Korenstein, Deborah (NY)	IM	194
Kline, Gary (NY)	TS	547	Kornel, Ezriel (NY)	NS	621
Kline, Mitchell (NY)	D	148	Korsten, Mark (NY)	Ge	376
Kloss, Robert (CT)	Onc	878	Korval, Arnold (CT)	Ped	889
Kloth, David (CT)	PM	887	Kosinski, Edward (CT)	Cv	867
Klyde, Barry (NY)	EDM	160	Kosofsky, Barry (NY)	ChiN	141
Knackmuhs, Gary (NJ)	Inf	671	Kososky, Charles (NJ)	N	747
Knapp, Albert (NY)	Ge	168	Koss, Jerome (NY)	Cv	493
Knep, Stanley (NJ)	N	822	Kostadaras, Ari (NY)	Nep	465
Knightly, John (NJ)	NS	807	Kostis, John (NJ)	Cv	757
Knisely, Jonathan (CT)	RadRO	919	Kotin, Neal (NY)	Ped	295
Knopp, Edmond (NY)	DR	155	Kotler, Donald (NY)	Ge	168
Knowles, Daniel (NY)	Path	279	Kotler, Lisa (NJ)	ChAP	663
Kobren, Steven (NY)	Cv	493	Kottler, William (NJ)	PPul	721
Kocher, Jeffrey (NJ)	Inf	672	Kottmeier, Stephen (NY)	SM	587
Kocsis, James (NY)	Psyc	315	Koufman, Jamie (NY)	Oto	271
Koenig, Eli (NY)	NP	425	Koulos, John (NY)	GO	178
Koenigsberg, Mordecai (NY)	DR	372	Kowallis, George (NY)	Psyc	315

Alphabetical Listing of Doctors

Name	Specialty	Pg	Name	Specialty	Pg
Kozel, Joseph (NJ)	Pul	737	Krown, Susan (NY)	Onc	207
Kozicky, Orest (NY)	Ge	609	Krueger, Richard (NY)	Psyc	315
Kozin, Arthur (NY)	Nep	556	Krug, Lee (NY)	Onc	207
Kozlowski, Jeffrey (NJ)	Nep	676	Kruger, Bernard (NY)	Onc	207
Kozuch, Peter (NY)	Onc	206	Krumerman, Andrew (NY)	CE	368
Krakovitz, Evan (NY)	CRS	600	Krumholz, Michael (NY)	Ge	169
Kramer, Mitchell (NY)	ObG	577	Krupnick, Matthew (NJ)	Ge	804
Kramer, Neil (NJ)	Rhu	725	Krutchik, Allan (NJ)	Onc	675
Kramer, Philip (NY)	Oph	481	Kuhel, William (NY)	Oto	271
Kranzler, L Stephan (NY)	N	622	Kukar, Narinder (NY)	EDM	460
Krasinski, Keith (NY)	PInf	288	Kula, Roger (NY)	N	517
Krasnogor, Lester (CT)	Pul	892	Kulick, Roy (NY)	HS	378
Kraus, Dennis (NY)	Oto	271	Kulkarni, Rachana (NJ)	Cv	829
Krause, Cynthia (NY)	ObG	235	Kulpa, Jolanta (NY)	PHO	439
Kraushaar, Barry (NY)	OrS	557	Kulsakdinun, Chaiyaporn (NY)	OrS	387
Kreitzer, Joel (NY)	PM	277	Kummer, Bart (NY)	Ge	169
Kreitzer, Paula (NY)	PEn	530	Kunzman, Kenneth (NJ)	Oto	834
Krellenstein, Daniel (NY)	TS	351	Kupersmith, Mark (NY)	Oph	245
Kremberg, M Roy (NY)	Psyc	315	Kupfer, Yizhak (NY)	Pul	446
Krespi, Yosef (NY)	Oto	271	Kurani, Devendra (NJ)	Psyc	724
Kressner, Michael (NY)	Ge	609	Kurer, Cheryl (NJ)	PCd	773
Krevitt, Lane (NY)	Oto	271	Kurfist, Lee (NY)	Ped	583
Kriegel, David (NY)	D	149	Kuriloff, Daniel (NY)	Oto	271
Krieger, Ben (NY)	Ped	442	Kurtz, Caroline (CT)	Pul	892
Krieger, Karl (NY)	TS	351	Kurtz, Lewis (NY)	S	545
Krieger, Richard (NJ)	Inf	820	Kurtz, Robert (NY)	Ge	169
Krieger, Sharon (NY)	IM	614	Kurtzman, Scott (CT)	S	920
Krilov, Leonard (NY)	PInf	531	Kushner, Brian (NY)	PHO	287
Krim, Eileen (NY)	ObG	519	Kushner, Evan (NJ)	IM	672
Krinsky, Glenn (NJ)	DR	666	Kushner, Susan (NJ)	Ped	688
Krinsley, James (CT)	Pul	892	Kutcher, Rosalyn (NY)	DR	604
Kris, Mark (NY)	Onc	206	Kutin, Neil (NY)	PS	582
Kristal, Leonard (NY)	D	498	Kutnick, Richard (NY)	Cv	133
Krivo, James (NY)	D	498	Kutscher, Martin (NY)	ChiN	600
Krol, Kristine (NJ)	A&I	829	Kuzniecky, Ruben (NY)	N	224
Kron, Leo (NY)	ChAP	139	Kveton, John (CT)	Oto	914
Kronn, David (NY)	CG	600	Kwartler, Jed (NJ)	Oto	851
Kronzon, Itzhak (NY)	Cv	133			
Krotowski, Mark (NY)	FMed	415			

Name	Specialty	Pg

L

Name	Specialty	Pg
La Bagnara, James (NJ)	Oto	823
La Gamma, Edmund (NY)	NP	619
La Marca, Charles (NY)	Oto	467
La Quaglia, Michael (NY)	PS	292
Labar, Douglas (NY)	N	225
Labissiere, Jean-Claude (NJ)	Pul	724
Labow, Daniel (NY)	S	344
Lachman, Reid (NJ)	Oto	810
Lachmann, Elisabeth (NY)	PMR	299
Lachmann, Justine (NY)	Cv	493
Lachs, Mark (NY)	Ger	175
Lacqua, Frank (NY)	CRS	412
Lacy, Jill (CT)	Onc	910
Lafaro, Rocco (NY)	TS	648
Lafferty, James (NY)	Cv	475
Lagmay, Victor (NY)	Oto	436
Lahita, Robert (NJ)	Rhu	725
Laifer, Steven (CT)	MF	877
Laitman, Robert (NY)	Nep	383
Laks, Mitchell (NY)	DR	372
Lalli, Corradino (NY)	IM	573
Lalwani, Anil (NY)	Oto	271
Lambroza, Arnon (NY)	Ge	169
Lamm, Carin (NY)	PPul	291
Lamm, Steven (NY)	IM	194
Lan, Vivian (NJ)	IM	672
Landau, Leon (NY)	Hem	379
Landau, Steven (NY)	Ge	609
Landers, David (NJ)	Cv	661
Landesman, Sheldon (NY)	Inf	420
Landman, Jaime (NY)	U	356
Landrigan, Philip (NY)	OM	238
Landzberg, Joel (NJ)	Cv	662
Lane, Joseph (NY)	OrS	260
Lane, Lewis (NY)	HS	506
Lanfranchi, Angela (NJ)	S	836
Lang, Paul (NY)	A&I	490
Lang, Samuel (NY)	TS	472
Lange, Dale (NY)	N	225
Langer, David (NY)	NS	516
Langer, Paul (NJ)	Oph	717
Langsner, Alan (NJ)	PCd	720
Lanman, Geraldine (NY)	Ger	505
Lannin, Donald (CT)	S	920
Lans, David (NY)	Rhu	645
Lansen, Thomas (NY)	NS	621
Lansing, Martha (NJ)	FMed	742
Lansman, Steven (NY)	TS	648
Lanteri, Vincent (NJ)	U	697
Lara, Jonathan (NJ)	Path	719
Laraque, Danielle (NY)	Ped	295
Larsen, John (NY)	PInf	288
Larson, Signe (NY)	Ped	295
Larson, Steven (NY)	NuM	231
LaSala, Patrick (NY)	NS	384
Latov, Norman (NY)	N	225
Lau, Har Chi (NY)	S	647
Lau, Henry (NJ)	Cv	662
Laub, Glenn (NJ)	TS	753
Laucella, Michael (NY)	DR	568
Lauer, Robert (NJ)	Cv	758
Lauer, Simeon (NY)	Oph	245
Lauricella, Joseph (NJ)	IM	672
Lavyne, Michael (NY)	NS	219
Lawson, William (NY)	Oto	271
Lax, James (NY)	Ge	169
Layne, Jeffrey (NY)	U	548
Lazar, Eliot (NY)	Cv	133
Lazar, Mark (NJ)	N	768
Lazar, Robert (NY)	Ge	571
Lazarus, George (NY)	Ped	295
Lazarus, Herbert (NY)	PRhu	292
Lazzaro, Richard (NY)	TS	451
Le Benger, Kerry (NJ)	A&I	842
Leach, Thomas (NJ)	PlS	750
Leahy, Mary (NY)	IM	555

Alphabetical Listing of Doctors

Name	Specialty	Pg	Name	Specialty	Pg
Leavens-Maurer, Jill (NY)	Ped	534	Leeman, Benjamin (NY)	Pul	540
Leb, Alvin (NY)	Ge	416	Leff, Sanford (NY)	Cv	410
Lebinger, Martin (NY)	Psyc	396	Leffell, David (CT)	D	904
Lebofsky, Martin (NY)	IM	614	Lefkovitz, Zvi (NY)	DR	604
Lebovics, Edward (NY)	Ge	609	Lefkowitz, Mathew (NY)	PM	437
Lebovics, Robert (NY)	Oto	272	Legato, Marianne (NY)	IM	194
Lebowicz, Joseph (NY)	Onc	425	Lehach, Joan (NY)	A&I	367
Lebowitz, Mark (NY)	Oph	433	Lehman, Thomas (NY)	PRhu	292
Lebwohl, Mark (NY)	D	149	Lehrhoff, Bernard (NJ)	U	857
Lebwohl, Oscar (NY)	Ge	169	Lehrman, Gary (NY)	Pul	643
Lechner, Michael (NY)	IM	614	Lehrman, Stuart (NY)	Pul	643
Leckman, James (CT)	ChAP	902	Leib, Martin (NY)	Oph	245
Lederman, Jeffrey (NY)	Inf	612	Leibner, Donald (NJ)	A&I	757
Lederman, Josiane (NY)	D	476	Leiboff, Arnold (NY)	CRS	567
Lederman, Martin (NY)	Oph	626	Leibowitz, Evan (NJ)	Rhu	693
Lederman, Sanford (NY)	ObG	431	Leibowitz, Jonas (NY)	EDM	605
Lee, Alexander (NY)	PMR	299	Leichter, Donald (NJ)	PCd	851
Lee, April (NY)	AM	475	Leifer, Bennett (NJ)	Ger	670
Lee, Carol (NY)	Oph	245	Leifer, Marvin (NJ)	Psyc	751
Lee, Douglas (NY)	ObG	577	Leipsner, George (NJ)	FMed	668
Lee, Francis (NY)	OrS	260	Leipzig, Rosanne (NY)	Ger	175
Lee, Haesoon (NY)	PPul	441	Leipziger, Lyle (NY)	PlS	537
Lee, Huey-Jen (NJ)	DR	707	Leiter, Gila (NY)	ObG	235
Lee, James (NY)	S	344	Leitner, Stuart (NJ)	Onc	712
Lee, Kwang (NY)	Psyc	584	Lemercier, Maud (NY)	S	647
Lee, Leonard (NJ)	TS	696	Lenci, Margaret (NY)	Rhu	645
Lee, Marjorie (NY)	Pul	326	Lense, Lloyd (NY)	Cv	565
Lee, Nancy (NY)	RadRO	329	Lenzo, Salvatore (NY)	HS	179
Lee, Paul (NY)	TS	472	Leon, Martin (NY)	IC	198
Lee, Roberta (NY)	IM	194	Leonard, John (NY)	Hem	183
Lee, Ronald (CT)	DR	869	Leong, Pauline (NY)	IM	510
Lee, S Howard (NJ)	NRad	833	Lepor, Herbert (NY)	U	356
Lee, Sicy (NY)	Rhu	336	Lepore, Frederick (NJ)	N	768
Lee, Steve (NY)	HS	179	Lerma, Pauline (NJ)	Onc	745
Lee, Sun (NJ)	NS	767	Lerman, Bruce (NY)	CE	127
Lee, Thomas (NY)	PS	582	Lerman, Jay (NY)	D	602
Lee, Thomas (NY)	NS	621	Lerman, Jay (NY)	DR	413
Leeds, Gary (NY)	FMed	162	Lerner, Chester (NY)	Inf	187
Leeds, Richard (NJ)	Cv	829	Lerner, Elliot (NJ)	NRad	679

Name	Specialty	Pg	Name	Specialty	Pg
Lerner, Seth (NY)	U	649	Levine, William (NY)	SM	339
Lerner, William (NJ)	Hem	788	Levitan, Stephan (NY)	Psyc	315
Lescale, Keith (NY)	MF	616	Levites, Kenneth (NY)	FMed	570
Lesesne, Carroll (NY)	PIS	305	Levitt, Miriam (NY)	Ped	637
Leslie, Denise (NY)	DR	604	Levitz, Craig (NY)	OrS	524
Lesorgen, Philip (NJ)	RE	693	Levitzky, Susan (NY)	Ped	295
Lesser, Robert (NY)	Rhu	448	Levy, Adam (NY)	PHO	390
Lesser, Robert (CT)	Oph	913	Levy, Albert (NY)	FMed	162
Lessing, Jeffrey (NY)	U	486	Levy, Andrew (NJ)	SM	726
Lester, Thomas (NY)	Hem	611	Levy, Howard (NY)	OrS	260
Lettera, James (CT)	TS	896	Levy, I Martin (NY)	OrS	387
Levchuck, Sean (NY)	PCd	528	Levy, Joseph (NY)	PGe	285
Leventhal, Arnold (NY)	U	548	Levy, Lauren (NJ)	DR	666
Leventhal, Bennett (NY)	ChAP	139	Levy, Lewis (NY)	N	518
Levey, Robert (NY)	IM	422	Levy, Michael (NY)	Psyc	559
Levin, Alexander (NJ)	PM	772	Levy, Miriam (NY)	DR	155
Levin, Andrew (NY)	Psyc	640	Levy, Morton (NY)	Ped	534
Levin, David (NJ)	Nep	677	Levy, Ross (NY)	D	602
Levin, Frances (NY)	AdP	123	Levy, Susan (CT)	ChiN	903
Levin, Kenneth (NJ)	N	678	Lew, Arthur (NY)	Psyc	641
Levin, Richard (CT)	Oto	886	Lewin, Margaret (NY)	IM	194
Levin, Sheryl (NY)	PMR	395	Lewin, Neal (NY)	IM	194
Levin Carmine, Linda (NY)	AM	489	Lewin, Sharon (NY)	IM	194
Levine, David (NY)	N	225	Lewis, Benjamin (NY)	Cv	133
Levine, David (NY)	OrS	260	Lewis, Blair (NY)	Ge	169
Levine, Dorothy (CT)	Ped	889	Lewis, Dorothy (CT)	Psyc	917
Levine, Evan (NY)	Cv	596	Lewis, Hilel (NY)	Oph	245
Levine, Jeremiah (NY)	PGe	530	Lewis, Owen (NY)	ChAP	139
Levine, Jerome (NJ)	Inf	672	Lewis, Ronald (NY)	OrS	524
Levine, Joseph (NY)	CE	491	Lewis, Theophilus (NY)	S	450
Levine, Laurie (NY)	D	498	Lewko, Michael (NJ)	Rhu	825
Levine, Martin (NJ)	FMed	733	Li, Ronald (NJ)	Oto	749
Levine, Mitchell (NY)	NS	516	Liang, Vera (NY)	Psyc	584
Levine, Randy (NY)	Hem	183	Libby, Daniel (NY)	Pul	326
Levine, Richard (NY)	ObG	235	Liberman, Laura (NY)	DR	156
Levine, Selwyn (NJ)	Pul	691	Libman, Richard (NY)	N	518
Levine, Seth (NJ)	U	826	Libutti, Steven (NY)	S	399
Levine, Steven (CT)	Oto	886	Licata, Joseph (NJ)	S	695
Levine, Steven (NY)	N	225	Licciardi, Frederick (NY)	RE	332

Alphabetical Listing of Doctors

Name	Specialty	Pg	Name	Specialty	Pg
Licht, Arnold (NY)	Psyc	444	Liquori, Frances (NJ)	FMed	787
Lichtbroun, Alan (NJ)	Rhu	779	Lisman, Richard (NY)	Oph	246
Lichter, Stephen (NY)	Onc	425	Liss, Donald (NJ)	PMR	689
Lichtstein, Elliott (NJ)	IC	673	Liss, Mark (NY)	Ge	609
Lieb, Mark (NY)	Cv	597	Lisser, Steven (NJ)	HS	787
Lieberman, David (NY)	Oph	433	Litchman, Mark (CT)	A&I	865
Lieberman, Elliott (NY)	U	548	Liteplo, Ronald (NY)	D	371
Lieberman, Kenneth (NJ)	PNep	686	Litman, Nathan (NY)	PInf	391
Lieberman, Michael (NY)	S	344	Litman, Richard (NY)	Oto	580
Liebert, Peter (NY)	PS	635	Litman, Steven (NY)	PM	580
Liebling, Anne (CT)	Rhu	920	Littlejohn, Charles (CT)	CRS	868
Liebling, Melissa (NJ)	DR	666	Lituchy, Andrew (NY)	IC	511
Liebling, Ralph (NY)	PlS	395	Litvin, Y Samuel (NJ)	U	797
Liebmann, Jeffrey (NY)	Oph	245	Liu, David (NY)	Nep	215
Liftin, Alan (NJ)	D	706	Liu, DeLong (NY)	Onc	618
Lightdale, Charles (NY)	Ge	169	Liu, George (NY)	IM	195
Ligresti, Louise G (NJ)	Onc	675	Liva, Douglas (NJ)	Oph	681
Liguori, Michael (NY)	IM	195	Livingston, Philip (NY)	Onc	207
Lin, Michael (NY)	N	225	Lizza, Eli (NY)	U	357
Lind, Lawrence (NY)	ObG	236	Lloyd, J Mervyn (NJ)	OrS	682
Lindenmayer, Jean-Pierre (NY)	Psyc	315	Lo, K M Steve (CT)	Onc	878
Lindner, Paul (CT)	A&I	865	Lo Galbo, Peter (NY)	A&I	553
Lindsay, Gaius (NY)	U	452	Lockshin, Michael (NY)	Rhu	336
Linsenmeyer, Todd (NJ)	U	729	Lockwood, Charles (CT)	MF	909
Linstrom, Christopher (NY)	Oto	272	Lodge, Henry (NY)	IM	195
Lipetz, Jason (NY)	PMR	535	Logan, Bruce (NY)	IM	195
Lipner, Henry (NY)	Nep	426	Lois, William (NY)	S	450
Lipow, Kenneth (CT)	NS	880	Lomasky, Steven (NY)	EDM	501
Lippman, Alan (NJ)	Onc	712	Lombardi, Joseph (NJ)	OrS	771
Lippman, Jay (NY)	Oph	626	Lombardo, Gerard (NY)	Pul	446
Lipsitz, Evan (NY)	VascS	401	Lombardo, James (NY)	Oph	433
Lipson, David (NJ)	PlS	689	Lombardo, Peter (NY)	D	149
Lipstein-Kresch, Esther (NY)	Rhu	544	Lomonaco, Salvatore (NY)	ChAP	370
Lipsztein, Roberto (NY)	RadRO	470	Lonberg, Mathew (NY)	Onc	555
Lipton, Brian (NY)	Psyc	316	London, Ronald (NY)	Ped	393
Lipton, Jeffrey (NY)	PHO	531	Longo, Walter (CT)	CRS	904
Lipton, Mark (NY)	IM	195	Lonner, Baron (NY)	OrS	260
Lipton, Richard (NY)	N	385	Loo, Marcus (NY)	U	357
Lipton, Richard (CT)	Oto	887	Lopez, Clark (NY)	FMed	415

Name	Specialty	Pg	Name	Specialty	Pg
Lopez, Eduardo (NJ)	PMR	776	Lustbader, Ian (NY)	Ge	170
Lopez, Ralph (NY)	AM	124	Lustig, Ilana (NY)	ObG	236
Lorber, Daniel (NY)	EDM	460	Lutchman, Gordon (NY)	S	450
Lorefice, Laurence (CT)	Psyc	891	Lutwick, Larry (NY)	Inf	420
Loren, Gary (NJ)	PM	749	Lutz, Gregory (NY)	PMR	299
Lorich, Dean (NY)	OrS	260	Lutzker, Letty (NJ)	NuM	715
LoRusso, Diane (NY)	DR	604	Lux, Michael (NJ)	IC	847
Loughlin, Gerald (NY)	PPul	291	Lyden, John (NY)	OrS	261
Louie, Eddie (NY)	Inf	187	Lydic, Michael (NY)	RE	586
Loulmet, Didier (NY)	TS	351	Lyman, Neil (NJ)	Nep	713
Love, Barry (NY)	PCd	282	Lynch, Thomas (CT)	Onc	910
Lovecchio, John (NY)	GO	506	Lynch, Vincent (CT)	ObG	912
LoVerme, Paul (NJ)	PlS	723	Lynn, Robert (NY)	Nep	383
Low, Ronald (NJ)	Oto	684	Lyon, Valerie (NY)	FMed	163
Lowe, Franklin (NY)	U	357	Lysikiewicz, Andrzej (NY)	MF	200
Lowell, Barry (NJ)	Cv	802			
Lowenthal, Dennis (NJ)	Onc	847			
Lowenthal, Diana (NY)	PPul	635			
Lowry, Stephen (NJ)	S	780	**M**		
Lowy, Joseph (NY)	Pul	326	Ma, Dong (NY)	PMR	299
Lozner, Jerrold (NJ)	S	856	Macaulay, William (NY)	OrS	261
Lu, Bing (NY)	IM	422	Maccabee, Paul (NY)	N	429
Lu, Stanley (NJ)	NRad	791	Maccia, Clement (NJ)	A&I	842
Lubat, Edward (NJ)	DR	666	Macher, Mark (NJ)	RadRO	779
Lubell, Harry (NY)	Ped	637	Machler, Brian (NJ)	D	706
Lubitz, Arthur (NY)	A&I	125	Macina, Lucy (NY)	Ger	506
Lublin, Fred (NY)	N	225	Mack, Laurence (NY)	ObG	519
Lubliner, Jerry (NY)	OrS	261	MacKay, Cynthia (NY)	Oph	246
Lucak, Susan (NY)	Ge	170	Mackenzie, C Ronald (NY)	IM	195
Lucariello, Richard (NY)	Cv	368	Mackessy, Richard (NJ)	OrS	850
Luciani, Richard (NJ)	ObG	715	Mackler, Karen (NY)	D	602
Luciano, Daniel (NY)	N	225	Mackool, Richard (NY)	Oph	467
Ludwig, Shelly (NJ)	Ge	787	Maclaren, Noel (NY)	PEn	284
Lukash, Barbara (NY)	D	602	MacMillan, William (NJ)	MF	766
Lukash, Frederick (NY)	PlS	538	Madajewicz, Stefan (NY)	Onc	381
Luks, Howard (NY)	SM	646	Maddalo, Anthony (NY)	OrS	629
Lundberg, Walter (CT)	Onc	910	Madigan, Janet (CT)	ChAP	902
Lundy, Edward (NY)	TS	560	Magid, Steven (NY)	Rhu	336
Lusman, Paul (NY)	A&I	563	Magill, Richard (NY)	HS	611

Alphabetical Listing of Doctors

Name	Specialty	Pg	Name	Specialty	Pg
Maglaras, Nicholas (NJ)	IM	847	Manevitz, Alan (NY)	Psyc	316
Magramm, Irene (NY)	Oph	246	Manginello, Frank (NJ)	NP	676
Magriples, Urania (CT)	MF	909	Mani, John (NY)	OrS	435
Magro, Cynthia (NY)	Path	279	Maniatis, Theodore (NY)	Pul	484
Magun, Arthur (NY)	Ge	170	Maniscalco, Anthony (NY)	N	429
Mahal, Pradeep (NJ)	Ge	845	Manjoney, Delia (CT)	Oph	883
Mahalingam, Banu (NJ)	Cv	741	Mankes, Seth (NY)	DR	568
Maharam, Lewis (NY)	SM	339	Mann, Charles (NY)	ObG	577
Maher, Elizabeth (NY)	Oph	386	Mann, David (NY)	EDM	414
Maheshwari, Vivek (NJ)	S	727	Mann, J John (NY)	Psyc	316
Mahler, Richard (NY)	EDM	160	Mann, Ronald (NY)	OrS	629
Mahon, Eugene (NY)	Psyc	316	Mann, Samuel (NY)	IM	195
Mahoney, Maurice (CT)	CG	903	Manners, Richard (NY)	Ped	583
Maidman, Jack (NY)	ObG	236	Manning, Eric (NJ)	Nep	790
Maier, Herbert (NJ)	D	819	Manno, Joseph (NJ)	VascS	698
Mailloux, Lionel (NY)	Nep	515	Mansour, E Hani (NJ)	S	727
Maiman, Mitchell (NY)	GO	478	Mansouri, Hormoz (NY)	S	546
Maiocco, Kenneth (CT)	D	868	Marcus, Judith (NY)	PHO	287
Maizel, Barry (NY)	Ge	417	Marcus, Michael (NY)	PPul	441
Malach, Barbara (NY)	IM	479	Marcus, Norman (NY)	PM	277
Malamud, Stephen (NY)	Onc	207	Marcus, Ralph (NJ)	Rhu	694
Malanga, Gerard (NJ)	PMR	853	Marcus, Richard (NJ)	Ped	722
Maldonado, Thomas (NY)	VascS	363	Marcus, Stuart (CT)	S	895
Malik, Asim (NY)	IM	423	Marder, Karen (NY)	N	226
Malik, Rubina (NY)	Ger	377	Marghoob, Ashfaq (NY)	D	567
Malik, Sajid (NY)	Oph	521	Margulies, Paul (NY)	EDM	501
Malits, Bella (NY)	PM	631	Margulis, Elynne (NJ)	ObG	849
Mallozzi, Angelo (CT)	FMed	870	Margulis, Stephen (NJ)	Ge	668
Maloney, Romelle (NY)	ObG	624	Margulis, Steven (NY)	IM	615
Malovany, Robert (NJ)	Pul	691	Marin, Deborah (NY)	Psyc	316
Malpeso, James (NY)	IC	479	Marin, Geobel (NJ)	Ge	743
Maman, Arie (NJ)	EDM	761	Marin, Lorraine (NY)	RadRO	542
Manasseh, Donna-Marie (CT)	S	895	Marin, Michael (NY)	VascS	363
Mancini, Donna (NY)	Cv	133	Marinaro, Robert (NJ)	D	803
Mandava, Suresh (CT)	Oph	883	Marino, A Michael (CT)	Pul	892
Mandel, Eric (NY)	Oph	246	Marino, John (NY)	Onc	513
Mandel, Marc (NJ)	S	856	Marino, Ronald (NY)	Ped	534
Mandel, Michael (NY)	Pul	643	Marino, William (NY)	Pul	397
Mandelbaum, Sidney (NY)	Oph	246	Marion, James (NY)	Ge	170

Name	Specialty	Pg	Name	Specialty	Pg
Marion, Robert (NY)	CG	370	Matalon, Martin (NY)	ObG	577
Markell, Mariana (NY)	Nep	426	Matalon, Robert (NY)	Nep	215
Markenson, Joseph (NY)	Rhu	336	Matarasso, Alan (NY)	PlS	305
Markovics, Sharon (NY)	A&I	490	Matczuk, Agnieszka (CT)	A&I	865
Markowitz, Arlene (NY)	Oto	272	Matera, Cristina (NY)	RE	332
Markowitz, Arnold (NY)	Ge	170	Matilsky, Michael (NY)	Cv	565
Markowitz, Daniel (NJ)	Pul	795	Matos, Jeffrey (NY)	CE	127
Markowitz, David (NY)	Ge	170	Matos, Marshall (NY)	Cv	597
Markowitz, James (NY)	PGe	530	Matossian, Cynthia (NJ)	Oph	747
Markowitz, John (NY)	Psyc	316	Matta, Raymond (NY)	Cv	133
Markowitz, Steven (NY)	CE	127	Mattana, Joseph (NY)	Nep	515
Marks, Alan (NY)	Oph	522	Mattel, Stephen (NJ)	Oto	823
Marks, Andrea (NY)	AM	124	Mattes, Leonard (NY)	Cv	133
Marks, David (NJ)	N	715	Matthews, Gerald (NY)	U	649
Marks, Jon (NY)	U	357	Mattison, Timothy (NY)	D	602
Marks, Peter (CT)	Hem	907	Mattoo, Nirmal (NY)	Nep	465
Marks, Stephen (NY)	N	622	Mattucci, Kenneth (NY)	Oto	525
Marmur, Ellen (NY)	D	149	Mauer, Kenneth (CT)	Ge	871
Marron-Corwin, Mary (NY)	NP	213	Mauri, Thomas (NY)	OrS	524
Marsan, Ben (CT)	VascS	898	Mauskop, Alexander (NY)	N	226
Marsh, Franklin (NY)	Ge	170	Maxfield, Roger (NY)	Pul	326
Marsh, James (CT)	OrS	913	May, Louis (NY)	Ge	554
Marshalko, Stephen (CT)	Cv	867	Mayer, Daniel (NY)	A&I	563
Marshall, Ian (NJ)	PEn	774	Mayer, Fern (CT)	D	868
Marshall, Merville (NY)	EDM	605	Mayer, Ira (NY)	Ge	417
Martimucci, William (NY)	Ger	610	Mayer, Lloyd (NY)	Ge	170
Martin, Jeffrey (NY)	Oph	578	Mayer, Stephan (NY)	N	226
Martinez, Homar (NJ)	Inf	710	Mayers, Marguerite (NY)	Ped	393
Martins, Publius (NY)	Pul	484	Mayers, Martin (NY)	Oph	386
Marush, Arthur (NY)	IM	423	Maytal, Joseph (NY)	ChiN	496
Marx, Robert (NY)	OrS	261	Mazlin, Jeffrey (NY)	ObG	236
Mascarenhas, Bento (NY)	Rhu	645	Mazza, David (NY)	A&I	125
Masci, Joseph (NY)	Inf	462	Mazzara, Carl (NJ)	Oto	772
Masciello, Michael (NY)	Cv	565	Mc Inerney, Vincent (NJ)	OrS	823
Maselli, Frank (NY)	FMed	374	McAllister, Peter (CT)	N	881
Masino, Frank (CT)	RadRO	893	McAnally, James (NJ)	Nep	848
Maslak, Peter (NY)	Onc	207	McCain, Donald (NJ)	S	695
Masson, Lalitha (NJ)	ObG	735	McCalley, Stuart (CT)	Pul	893
Masterson, Raymond (NJ)	IM	788	McCann, Peter (NY)	OrS	261

Alphabetical Listing of Doctors

Name	Specialty	Pg	Name	Specialty	Pg
McCarthy, Joseph (NY)	PlS	305	McNamara, Joseph (CT)	PHO	915
McCarthy, Paul (CT)	PRhu	916	McNutt, N Scott (NY)	Path	279
McCarthy, Shirley (CT)	DR	904	McPherson, Craig (CT)	CE	866
McCarton, Cecelia (NY)	Ped	295	McVeigh, Anne Marie (NY)	Oph	246
McClane, Steven (CT)	CRS	868	McWhorter, John (NJ)	Rhu	836
McClelland, Shearwood (NY)	OrS	261	McWhorter, Philip (CT)	S	895
McClennan, Bruce (CT)	DR	904	Meacham, Kevin (NY)	ObG	624
McClung, John (NY)	Cv	597	Mears, John Gregory (NY)	Hem	183
McConnell, Robert (NY)	EDM	160	Mechanick, Jeffrey (NY)	EDM	160
McCormack, Patricia (NY)	D	476	Medici, Mark (NY)	OrS	557
McCormack, William (NY)	Inf	420	Medina, Emma (NY)	Cv	597
McCormick, Beryl (NY)	RadRO	329	Medow, Norman (NY)	Oph	246
McCormick, Paul (NY)	NS	219	Meed, Steven (NY)	Rhu	336
McCullough, Andrew (NY)	U	357	Meek, Allen (NY)	RadRO	586
McDermott, John (NY)	Oph	246	Meere, Patrick (NY)	OrS	261
McFarlane-Ferreira, Yvonne (NY)	PGe	438	Megibow, Alec (NY)	DR	156
McGinn, Joseph (NY)	TS	486	Mehrara, Babak (NY)	PlS	305
McGlashan, Thomas (CT)	Psyc	918	Mehrotra, Bhoomi (NY)	Onc	513
McGovern, Catherine (NY)	ObG	624	Mehta, Davendra (NY)	CE	127
McGovern, Margaret (NY)	CG	566	Mehta, Rajeev (NJ)	NP	767
McGovern, Patrick (NJ)	S	737	Mehta, Rekha (NY)	Ge	376
McGovern, Peter (NJ)	RE	693	Mehta, Uday (NJ)	Ped	852
McGovern, Thomas (NY)	U	357	Meier, Diane (NY)	Ger	175
McGowan, James (NY)	Psyc	316	Meighan, Dennis (CT)	Ge	871
McGowan, Joseph (NY)	Inf	508	Meirowitz, Natalie (NY)	MF	511
McGrath, Patrick (NY)	Psyc	316	Meirowitz, Robert (NJ)	Ge	743
McHugh, Margaret (NY)	Ped	295	Meisenberg, Gene (NY)	U	452
McIlveen, Stephen (NJ)	OrS	682	Meisler, Susan (NY)	Ped	637
McKee, Heather (NY)	Oph	626	Meiteles, Lawrence (NY)	Oto	630
McKenna, Michael (NJ)	RadRO	752	Meixler, Steven (NY)	Pul	643
McKiernan, James (NY)	U	357	Meizlish, Jay (CT)	Cv	867
McKinley, Matthew (NY)	Ge	504	Melamed, Jonathan (NY)	Path	279
McLaughlin, Mark (NJ)	NS	746	Melillo, Nicholas (NJ)	Pul	778
McLeod, Gavin (CT)	Inf	873	Meller, Jose (NY)	Cv	134
McManus, Edward (NJ)	Inf	805	Mellinger, Brett (NY)	U	549
McManus, Susan (NJ)	S	836	Mellman, Lisa (NY)	Psyc	317
McMeeking, Alexander (NY)	Inf	187	Melman, Martin (NY)	IM	615
McMullen, Robert (NY)	Psyc	316	Melnick, Hugh (NY)	ObG	236
McMurtry, Kirk (NJ)	TS	738	Melone, Charles (NY)	HS	179

Name	Specialty	Pg	Name	Specialty	Pg
Melton, R Christine (NY)	Oph	246	Meyers, Paul (NY)	PHO	287
Melville, Gordon (NJ)	DR	830	Meyers, Philip (NY)	NRad	231
Menchell, David (NY)	A&I	457	Meyers-Seifer, Cynthia (NJ)	PEn	793
Mendelowitz, Alan (NY)	Psyc	469	Mezey, Andrew (NY)	Ped	442
Mendelowitz, Lawrence (NY)	ObG	624	Miarrostami, Rameen (NY)	Pul	446
Mendelsohn, Michael (NY)	Oto	525	Mich, Robert (NJ)	IC	847
Mendelsohn, Sara (NY)	OM	520	Michaelides, Elias (CT)	Oto	914
Mendelson, Joel (NJ)	A&I	842	Michaelson, Richard (NJ)	Onc	713
Mendes, Donna (NY)	VascS	363	Michalos, Peter (NY)	Oph	578
Mendes, John (NJ)	OrS	718	Michel, Ketly (NY)	ObG	236
Mendoza, Ernesto (NY)	S	471	Michelassi, Fabrizio (NY)	S	344
Mendoza, Francis (NY)	OrS	261	Michelis, Mary Ann (NJ)	A&I	660
Mendoza, Glenn (NY)	NP	556	Michelis, Michael (NY)	Nep	215
Menegus, Mark (NY)	Cv	369	Michels, Robert (NY)	Psyc	317
Menezes, Placido (NY)	OrS	435	Michler, Robert (NY)	TS	400
Menitove, Stephen (NY)	Pul	559	Mickley, Diane (CT)	IM	875
Menon, Latha (NY)	Pul	397	Mickley, Steven (CT)	IM	875
Mensch, Alan (NY)	Pul	540	Middlesworth, William (NY)	PS	293
Ment, Laura (CT)	ChiN	903	Middleton, John (NJ)	Inf	764
Menza, Matthew (NJ)	Psyc	778	Mieszerski, Laura (NY)	ObG	624
Menzin, Andrew (NY)	GO	506	Mignone, Biagio (NY)	Oph	626
Merav, Avraham (NY)	TS	648	Miguel, Eduardo (NJ)	IM	672
Mercando, Anthony (NY)	Cv	597	Milano, Andrew (NY)	Ge	171
Meredith, Gary (NY)	Rhu	544	Mildvan, Donna (NY)	Inf	187
Merer, David (NY)	PO	634	Miles, Daniel (NY)	ChiN	141
Merhige, Kenneth (NY)	Oph	247	Milgraum, Sandy (NJ)	D	760
Merker, Edward (NY)	FMed	606	Milgrim, Laurence (NJ)	Oto	684
Mermelstein, Erwin (NJ)	Cv	758	Milite, James (NY)	Oph	247
Mermelstein, Harold (NY)	D	602	Miller, Aaron (NY)	N	226
Mermelstein, Steve (NY)	Pul	541	Miller, Andrew (NJ)	Oto	772
Merola, Andrew (NY)	OrS	435	Miller, Brian (NY)	Oph	626
Merriam, John (NY)	Oph	247	Miller, Daniel (NY)	FMed	606
Messana, Ida (NY)	IM	463	Miller, David (NJ)	Psyc	854
Messina, John (NJ)	PCd	685	Miller, David (NY)	Cv	134
Metz, John (NJ)	FMed	761	Miller, Dennis (NY)	Inf	187
Metzl, Jordan (NY)	SM	339	Miller, Jeffrey (NJ)	HS	805
Meyer, Monica (NJ)	ObG	680	Miller, Kenneth (CT)	Rhu	894
Meyer, Richard (NY)	Hem	183	Miller, Kenneth (NJ)	IC	712
Meyers, Barnett (NY)	Psyc	641	Miller, Philip (NJ)	Oph	717

Alphabetical Listing of Doctors

Name	Specialty	Pg	Name	Specialty	Pg
Miller, Philip (NY)	Oto	272	Mojtabai, Shaparak (NY)	IM	380
Miller, Richard (NJ)	Pul	724	Moldover, Jonathan (NY)	PMR	299
Miller, Scott (NY)	PHO	439	Moldwin, Robert (NY)	U	549
Miller, Seth (CT)	OrS	885	Molinelli, Bruce (CT)	S	895
Miller, Seth (NY)	Ge	505	Mollin, Joel (NY)	DR	459
Miller, Theodore (NY)	DR	156	Molloy, Edward (CT)	IM	875
Miller, Vincent (NY)	Onc	207	Molnar, Thomas (NY)	FMed	461
Miller-Breslow, Anne (NJ)	HS	670	Molofsky, Walter (NY)	ChiN	141
Mills, Carl (NY)	U	589	Moncrief, Robyn (NY)	S	344
Mills, Christopher (NY)	S	344	Mondrow, Daniel (NJ)	Cv	758
Mills, Nancy (NY)	Onc	618	Mones, Richard (NJ)	PGe	811
Milman, Perry (NY)	Ge	505	Mongillo, Nicholas (CT)	Ped	889
Milone, Richard (NY)	Psyc	641	Monheit, Alan (NY)	MF	574
Milowsky, Matthew (NY)	Onc	207	Monrad, E Scott (NY)	Cv	369
Milsom, Jeffrey (NY)	CRS	143	Monsanto, Enrique (NY)	HS	419
Milstein, David (NY)	NuM	385	Montero, Carlos (NY)	OrS	524
Min, Albert (NY)	Ge	171	Montgomery, Kenneth (NJ)	OrS	810
Mindel, Joel (NY)	Oph	247	Monti, Louis (NY)	Ped	295
Miner, Charles (CT)	IM	875	Moore, Anne (NY)	Onc	208
Mini, Katherine (CT)	Ped	889	Moore, Frank (NY)	NS	219
Minikes, Neil (NJ)	A&I	660	Moore, Joanne (NY)	Psyc	317
Minkoff, Howard (NY)	ObG	431	Moorthy, Chitti (NY)	RadRO	644
Minkowitz, Susan (NY)	IM	195	Mootabar, Hamid (NY)	MF	617
Mintz, Abraham (CT)	NS	880	Moqtaderi, Farideh (NY)	PM	277
Mintz, Guy (NY)	Cv	494	Moraille, Pascale (NJ)	Psyc	737
Mirra, Suzanne (NY)	Path	437	Moreau, Donna (NY)	ChAP	140
Miskovitz, Paul (NY)	Ge	171	Morehouse, Helen (NY)	DR	372
Mitchell, John (NY)	Oph	247	Morelli, Alan (CT)	Ped	889
Mitnick, Hal (NY)	Rhu	336	Morello, Robert (NY)	Oph	626
Mitnick, Julie (NY)	DR	156	Moreta, Henry (NY)	N	576
Mitsumoto, Hiroshi (NY)	N	226	Moretti, Michael (NY)	MF	479
Mittler, Mark (NY)	NS	516	Morgan, Charles (CT)	Psyc	891
Mittman, Neal (NY)	Nep	426	Morgan, Daniel (NY)	OrS	435
Moazed, Kambiz (NY)	Oph	247	Morgan, James (CT)	Ped	917
Mogan, Glen (NJ)	Ge	708	Moriarty, Daniel (NJ)	Onc	847
Mogil, Laurey (NY)	Oph	433	Morman, Manuel (NJ)	D	665
Mohr, JP (NY)	N	226	Morris, Elizabeth (NY)	DR	156
Mohr, Robert (NJ)	ObG	808	Morris, James (NY)	N	622
Moisa, Idel (NY)	Oto	525	Morris, Robert (NY)	Oph	578

Name	Specialty	Pg	Name	Specialty	Pg
Morrison, R Sean (NY)	Ger	176	Mullen, Michael (NY)	Inf	187
Morrison, Susan (NJ)	PA&I	719	Multz, Alan (NY)	Pul	541
Morrissey, Kevin (NY)	S	344	Munoz, Jose (NY)	PInf	634
Morrow, Monica (NY)	S	345	Munver, Ravi (NJ)	U	697
Morrow, Robert (NY)	FMed	375	Muraca, Glenn (NY)	FMed	461
Morrow, Todd (NJ)	Oto	718	Murali, Raj (NY)	NS	621
Mosca, Ralph (NY)	TS	351	Murphy, Barbara (NY)	Nep	215
Moscatello, Augustine (NY)	Oto	630	Murphy, Ramon (NY)	Ped	296
Moses, Brett (NJ)	Oto	749	Murphy, Robert (NJ)	Ped	793
Moses, Jeffrey (NY)	IC	199	Murphy, Robyn (NJ)	DR	803
Moseson, Michael (NY)	CRS	497	Murray, Henry (NY)	Inf	187
Moshe, Solomon (NY)	ChiN	370	Murray, Simon (NJ)	IM	744
Moskovich, Ronald (NY)	OrS	262	Musiker, Seymour (NY)	Ped	583
Moskovits, Norbert (NY)	Cv	410	Muskin, Philip (NY)	Psyc	317
Moskovits, Tibor (NY)	Hem	183	Musto, Anthony (CT)	Oph	883
Moskowitz, Bruce (NY)	Oph	247	Mutterperl, Mitchell (NJ)	IM	735
Moskowitz, George (NY)	FMed	415	Myskowski, Patricia (NY)	D	149
Moskowitz, Richard (NJ)	CRS	802	Myssiorek, David (NY)	Oto	272
Moss, Charles (NJ)	VascS	698			
Moss, R Lawrence (CT)	PS	916			
Most, Richard (NY)	Oph	627			
Motiwala, Rajeev (NY)	N	226	**N**		
Motzer, Robert (NY)	Onc	208			
Moulton, Thomas (NY)	PHO	390	Nachajon, Roberto (NJ)	PPul	824
Moussa, Ghias (NJ)	Cv	733	Nachman, Sharon (NY)	PInf	582
Moynihan, Brian (NY)	FMed	502	Nadel, William (NJ)	Psyc	813
Moynihan, Gavan (NY)	D	567	Nadelman, Robert (NY)	Inf	612
Muchnick, Richard (NY)	Oph	247	Nagler, Harris (NY)	U	357
Mueller, F Carl (CT)	Psyc	891	Nagler, Jerry (NY)	Ge	171
Mueller, Richard (NY)	Cv	134	Nahass, Ronald (NJ)	Inf	831
Muggia, Franco (NY)	Onc	208	Nahm, Frederick (CT)	N	881
Muhlbauer, Helen (NY)	Psyc	317	Naidich, David (NY)	DR	156
Mukherjee, Tanmoy (NY)	RE	332	Najarian, James (NJ)	Nep	807
Muldoon, Lawrence (CT)	U	897	Najjar, Sessine (NJ)	Inf	820
Muldoon, Thomas (NY)	Oph	248	Najjar, Souhel (NY)	N	481
Mulford, Gregory (NJ)	PMR	812	Najmi, Jamsheed (NJ)	PlS	835
Mulgaonkar, Shamkant (NJ)	Nep	714	Naka, Yoshifumi (NY)	TS	351
Mulhall, John (NY)	U	357	Nalbandian, Matthew (NY)	VascS	363
Mullen, Edward (NY)	RadRO	542	Namerow, David (NJ)	Ped	688
			Nanus, David (NY)	Onc	208

Alphabetical Listing of Doctors

Name	Specialty	Pg	Name	Specialty	Pg
Napolitano, Joseph (NJ)	Oph	771	Nevin, Marie (NJ)	EDM	803
Narins, Rhoda (NY)	D	602	New, Maria (NY)	PEn	284
Narula, Amarjot (NJ)	Psyc	690	Newburger, Amy (NY)	D	603
Narula, Pramod (NY)	PPul	441	Newcorn, Jeffrey (NY)	ChAP	140
Narwal, Shivinder (NY)	PGe	438	Newhouse, Jeffrey (NY)	DR	156
Nascimento, Joao (CT)	Rhu	894	Newman, Elliot (NY)	S	345
Nash, Bernard (NY)	Inf	572	Newman, Fredric (CT)	PlS	890
Nash, Ira (NY)	Cv	134	Newman, Lawrence (NY)	N	227
Nash, Martin (NY)	PNep	289	Newman, Leonard (NY)	PGe	633
Nash, Thomas (NY)	Pul	326	Newman, Scott (NY)	PlS	638
Nass, Jack (NY)	Psyc	584	Newman, Stephen (NY)	N	518
Nass, Richard (NY)	Oto	272	Newman-Cedar, Meryl (NY)	Ped	296
Nass, Ruth (NY)	ChiN	141	Newmark, Ian (NY)	Pul	541
Nassberg, Barton (NJ)	EDM	786	Newton, Michael (NY)	Oph	248
Natale, Benjamin (NJ)	Oph	850	Ng, John (NY)	RadRO	329
Nath, Sunil (NY)	Pul	470	Ngeow, Jeffrey (NY)	PM	277
Nattis, Richard (NY)	Oph	578	Nguyen, Khanh (NY)	TS	351
Navot, Daniel (NJ)	RE	693	Nicholas, Stephen (NY)	OrS	262
Nealon, Nancy (NY)	N	226	Nichols, Jeffrey (NY)	Ger	176
Neelakantappa, Kotresha (NY)	Nep	426	Nickerson, Katherine (NY)	Rhu	336
Neeson, Francis (CT)	Cv	867	Nicosia, Thomas (NY)	Cv	494
Neibart, Eric (NY)	Inf	188	Niederman, Michael (NY)	Pul	541
Neibart, Richard (NJ)	TS	796	Nierman, David (NY)	CCM	458
Neiman, Deborah (NJ)	IM	832	Nightingale, Jeffrey (NY)	Oph	248
Neistadt, L Daniel (NY)	DR	156	Nikias, George (NJ)	Ge	669
Nelson, David (NY)	Oph	522	Nimaroff, Michael (NY)	ObG	519
Nelson, Deena (NY)	IM	196	Nimer, Stephen (NY)	Hem	183
Nelson, John (NY)	Hem	611	Nini, Kevin (NJ)	PlS	777
Nelson, John (NY)	OrS	629	Nininger, James (NY)	Psyc	317
Nelson, Judith (NY)	Pul	326	Nisonson, Barton (NY)	SM	339
Nelson, Mario (NY)	PMR	637	Nissenblatt, Michael (NJ)	Onc	766
Nelson, William (NY)	ObG	624	Nitti, Victor (NY)	U	358
Neophytides, Andreas (NY)	N	227	Nitzberg, Richard (NJ)	S	856
Nepola, Neil (NY)	FMed	477	Nizin, Joel (NJ)	CRS	663
Nerwen, Clifford (NY)	Ped	535	Nori, Dattatreyudu (NY)	RadRO	330
Neschis, Ronald (NY)	Psyc	641	Norton, Larry (NY)	Onc	208
Neu, Natalie (NY)	PInf	289	Nosher, John (NJ)	VIR	781
Neuberg, Gerald (NY)	Cv	369	Nosko, Michael (NJ)	NS	768
Neuwirth, Michael (NY)	OrS	262	Notar-Francesco, Vincent (NY)	Ge	417

Alphabetical Listing of Doctors

Name	Specialty	Pg	Name	Specialty	Pg
Ossias, A Lawrence (NY)	Hem	184	Pannone, John (NY)	Nep	426
Ostad, Ariel (NY)	D	150	Panza, Robert (NJ)	Ped	852
Oster, Martin (NY)	Onc	209	Panzner, Elizabeth (NJ)	Ped	852
Ostrer, Harry (NY)	CG	142	Papadakos, Stylianos (NY)	IC	464
Ostriker, Glenn (CT)	Oph	883	Papish, Steven (NJ)	Onc	806
Ostrow, Stanley (NY)	Onc	575	Papp, Laszlo (NY)	Psyc	318
Ott, Allen (NY)	ObG	577	Pappas, Steven (NY)	IM	615
Ott, Patrick (NY)	Onc	209	Pappas, Thomas (NY)	Cv	494
Ottaviano, Lawrence (NY)	Ge	171	Pappert, Amy (NJ)	D	830
Owens, George (NY)	U	650	Pardi, Desiree (NY)	IM	196
Oz, Mehmet (NY)	TS	351	Parekh, Aruna (NY)	NP	575
Ozkaynak, M Fevzi (NY)	PHO	633	Parikh, Manish (NY)	IC	199
Ozuner, Gokhan (NY)	CRS	553	Parikh, Sanjay (NY)	PO	391
			Paris, Barbara (NY)	Ger	417
			Parisier, Simon (NY)	Oto	272
P			Park, Bernard (NJ)	TS	696
			Park, Constance (NY)	EDM	160
Paccione, Jeffrey (NY)	Oph	248	Park, Tae (NY)	RadRO	586
Pace, Benjamin (NY)	S	471	Parker, Robert (NY)	PHO	581
Pachter, H Leon (NY)	S	345	Parks, Michael (NY)	OrS	262
Pacia, Steven (NY)	N	227	Parles, James (NY)	Ped	583
Packer, Samuel (NY)	Oph	522	Parnell, Vincent (NY)	PS	533
Padgett, Douglas (NY)	OrS	262	Parnes, Eliezer (NY)	Nep	427
Padilla, Maria (NY)	Pul	326	Parness, Ira (NY)	PCd	282
Paget, Stephen (NY)	Rhu	337	Parr, Grant (NJ)	TS	815
Pahuja, Murlidhar (NY)	S	485	Parrish, Edward (NY)	Rhu	337
Paidas, Michael (CT)	MF	909	Pascal, Mark (NJ)	Onc	675
Paiusco, A Dino (NY)	Cv	410	Pasik, Deborah (NJ)	Rhu	814
Pak, Jayoung (NJ)	ChiN	705	Pasmantier, Mark (NY)	Onc	209
Palaia, David (NY)	PlS	639	Pasquale, Jack (NY)	IM	463
Palatt, Terry (NY)	TS	589	Pass, Harvey (NY)	TS	351
Palese, Michael (NY)	U	358	Pass, Helen (NY)	S	647
Palestro, Christopher (NY)	NuM	519	Passeri, Daniel (CT)	S	896
Palmer, Melissa (NY)	Ge	505	Patel, Aman (NY)	NS	219
Palmieri, Thomas (NY)	HS	506	Patel, Amit (NJ)	VascS	816
Palsky, Glenn (NJ)	Ped	750	Patel, Jitendra (NY)	Rhu	448
Paltzik, Robert (NY)	D	498	Pathare, Pradip (CT)	RadRO	893
Panella, Vincent (NJ)	Ge	669	Patrick, Sharon (NY)	MF	201
Panicek, David (NY)	DR	156	Patrizio, Pasquale (CT)	RE	919

Name	Specialty	Pg	Name	Specialty	Pg
Pattner, Austin (NJ)	Nep	677	Perry, Richard (NY)	ChAP	140
Paty, Philip (NY)	S	345	Perry-Bottinger, Lynne (NY)	Cv	597
Paul, Edward (NY)	AdP	123	Persing, John (CT)	PlS	917
Pavlakis, Steven (NY)	ChiN	411	Persky, Mark (NY)	Oto	272
Pavlick, Anna (NY)	Onc	209	Pesce, Joseph (CT)	D	869
Pavlov, Helene (NY)	DR	157	Peschel, Richard (CT)	RadRO	919
Pawel, Michael (NY)	Psyc	318	Peterson, Stephen (NY)	IM	615
Pearl, Michael (NY)	GO	571	Petito, Frank (NY)	N	227
Pearlstein, Eric (NY)	Oph	433	Petra, Eugene (NY)	Nep	480
Pechman, Karen (NY)	PMR	638	Petrone, Sylvia (NJ)	S	727
Peck, Valerie (NY)	EDM	161	Petrossian, George (NY)	IC	511
Pecker, Mark (NY)	IM	196	Petrylak, Daniel (NY)	Onc	209
Pecora, Andrew (NJ)	Onc	675	Pettei, Michael (NY)	PGe	530
Pedinoff, Andrew (NJ)	A&I	829	Pfeffer, Cynthia (NY)	Psyc	318
Pedley, Timothy (NY)	N	227	Pfister, David (NY)	Onc	209
Pegler, Cynthia (NY)	AM	124	Philipp, Claire (NJ)	Hem	764
Pelavin, Martin (NJ)	IM	673	Phillips, Elizabeth (NY)	Onc	618
Pellicci, Paul (NY)	OrS	262	Phillips, Howard (NY)	Oph	627
Pellicone, John (NY)	Pul	559	Phillips, Malcolm (NY)	Cv	369
Peng, Benjamin (NY)	U	358	Phillips, Robin (NY)	ObG	236
Penzer, Jason (NY)	CRS	143	Pianka, George (NY)	OrS	263
Pepe, John (NY)	Nep	480	Picciano, Anne (NJ)	FMed	761
Pereira, Frederick (NY)	D	459	Piccione, Paul (NY)	Ge	417
Pereira, Stephen (NJ)	S	695	Piccirilli, Dora (NY)	FMed	606
Perelstein, Eduardo (NY)	PNep	289	Pici, Ralph (NY)	PMR	638
Perez-Soler, Roman (NY)	Onc	382	Picone, Frank (NJ)	A&I	785
Perin, Noel (NY)	NS	219	Pidoriano, Arthur (NY)	OrS	629
Perl, Harold (NJ)	NP	676	Piepmeier, Joseph (CT)	NS	911
Perlman, Barry (NY)	Psyc	641	Pile-Spellman, John (NY)	NRad	518
Perlman, David (NY)	Inf	188	Pincus, Emile (NJ)	ChAP	663
Perlman, Donald (NJ)	A&I	703	Pincus, Robert (NY)	Oto	273
Perlman, Jeffrey (NY)	NP	213	Pines, Jeffrey (NY)	Psyc	318
Perlman, Philip (NY)	Oto	526	Pinke, Robert (NJ)	Oph	809
Perlmutter, Ilisse (NY)	ChAP	495	Pinney, Sean (NY)	Cv	134
Perron, Reed (NJ)	N	678	Pinsker, Kenneth (NY)	Pul	397
Perrotti, John (NY)	PlS	305	Pinsky, Steven (NY)	PM	527
Perry, Arthur (NJ)	PlS	835	Piskun, Andrew (NJ)	OrS	771
Perry, Bradford (NY)	Psyc	641	Pitchumoni, Capecomorin (NJ)	Ge	762
Perry, Henry (NY)	Oph	522	Pitman, Gerald (NY)	PlS	306

Alphabetical Listing of Doctors

Name	Specialty	Pg	Name	Specialty	Pg
Pizzarello, Louis (NY)	Oph	578	Portlock, Carol (NY)	Onc	209
Pizzurro, Joseph (NJ)	OrS	683	Portnoy, William (NY)	Oto	273
Plancher, Kevin (NY)	SM	339	Porwancher, Richard (NJ)	Inf	744
Plesset, Maxwell (NY)	IM	615	Posner, David (NY)	Pul	327
Plestis, Konstadinos (NY)	TS	352	Posner, Jerome (NY)	N	227
Plumser, Allan (NJ)	Ge	762	Posner, Marshall (NY)	Onc	210
Pochapin, Mark (NY)	Ge	171	Possick, Paul (NJ)	D	665
Podwal, Mark (NY)	D	150	Post, Martin (NY)	Cv	134
Policastro, Anthony (NY)	S	647	Postley, John (NY)	IM	196
Polin, Richard (NY)	NP	213	Potaznik, Daniel (NY)	PHO	483
Polis, Laurie (NY)	D	150	Potter, Hollis (NY)	DR	157
Politsky, Jeffrey (NJ)	N	849	Potter, William (CT)	Oph	883
Polkow, Melvin (NJ)	Pul	692	Potters, Louis (NY)	RadRO	543
Pollack, Geoffrey (NY)	Oto	273	Powell, Jeffrey (NY)	EDM	605
Pollack, Jed (NY)	RadRO	542	Poynor, Elizabeth (NY)	GO	178
Pollack, Shoshannah (NJ)	D	820	Prabhu, H Sudhakar (NY)	Cv	410
Pollak, Harvey (NY)	IM	510	Prager, Kenneth (NY)	Pul	327
Pollina, Robert (NY)	VascS	589	Prakash, Anaka (NJ)	Ge	734
Pollock, Alan (NY)	Inf	188	Preis, Oded (NY)	Ped	442
Pollock, Jeffrey (NJ)	N	849	Preminger, Mark (NY)	CE	757
Pollock, Roger (NJ)	OrS	683	Press, Robert (NY)	Inf	188
Pollowitz, James (NY)	A&I	594	Presti, Salvatore (NY)	PCd	437
Polsky, Bruce (NY)	Inf	188	Pretto, Zorayda (NY)	EDM	605
Pomeroy, John (NY)	ChAP	566	Preven, David (NY)	Psyc	318
Pomp, Alfons (NY)	S	345	Prezant, David (NY)	Pul	397
Ponamgi, Suri (NJ)	PlS	689	Prezioso, Paula (NY)	Ped	296
Ponterio, Jane (NY)	ObG	481	Price, Andrew (NY)	OrS	263
Poon, Eric (NY)	Ped	296	Price, Thomas (NY)	Cv	597
Poon, Michael (NY)	Cv	565	Prince, Alice (NY)	Ped	296
Poplausky, Maurice (NY)	DR	604	Prince, Andrew (NY)	Oph	248
Popovich, Joseph (NJ)	S	737	Prince, Martin (NY)	DR	157
Poppas, Dix (NY)	U	358	Principe, David (NJ)	MF	674
Popper, Laura (NY)	Ped	296	Prioleau, Philip (NY)	D	150
Porder, Joseph (NY)	Cv	134	Procaccino, John (NY)	CRS	497
Poretsky, Leonid (NY)	EDM	161	Proctor, Deborah (CT)	Ge	905
Porges, Andrew (NY)	Rhu	544	Provenzano, Anthony (NY)	Onc	618
Port, Abraham (NY)	DR	499	Provet, John (NY)	U	358
Port, Jeffrey (NY)	TS	352	Pruzan-Clain, Debra (CT)	D	869
Portenoy, Russell (NY)	PM	277	Pruzansky, Mark (NY)	HS	180

Name	Specialty	Pg
Prystowsky, Janet (NY)	D	150
Prywes, Arnold (NY)	Oph	522
Przybylski, Gregory (NJ)	NS	768
Puccio, Carmelo (NY)	Onc	618
Pucillo, Anthony (NY)	Cv	597
Puder, Douglas (NY)	Ped	558
Pujol-Morato, Fernando (NY)	Inf	420
Pumill, Rick (NJ)	Cv	662
Purtill, William (NY)	VascS	550
Putignano, Joseph (NY)	U	650
Putman, Donald (NJ)	PCd	720
Putterman, Eric (NY)	SM	587
Pyo, Daniel (NJ)	PlS	813

Q

Name	Specialty	Pg
Qadir, Shuja (NY)	Cv	457
Quaegebeur, Jan (NY)	PS	293
Quagliarello, John (NY)	RE	332
Quagliarello, Vincent (CT)	Inf	908
Quartell, Anthony (NJ)	ObG	715
Quest, Donald (NY)	NS	219
Quinn, Joseph (NY)	Ped	583
Quittell, Lynne (NY)	PPul	291

R

Name	Specialty	Pg
Raab, Edward (NY)	Oph	248
Rabin, Aaron (NJ)	N	678
Rabinowicz, Morris (NY)	Ped	535
Rabinowitz, Simon (NY)	PGe	483
Raboy, Adley (NY)	U	486
Rackoff, Paula (NY)	Rhu	337
Radin, Allen (NY)	Rhu	337
Radwaner, Bradley (NY)	Cv	135
Raffalli, John (NY)	Inf	612
Rafizadeh, Farhad (NJ)	PlS	813
Ragnarsson, Kristjan (NY)	PMR	299

Name	Specialty	Pg
Ragno, Philip (NY)	Cv	494
Rago, Thomas (CT)	HS	872
Ragone, Philip (NY)	N	518
Ragukonis, Thomas (NJ)	PM	684
Rahaman, Jamal (NY)	GO	178
Rahmin, Michael (NJ)	Ge	669
Rai, Kanti (NY)	Hem	507
Raina, Suresh (NJ)	S	727
Rajaraman, Viswanathan (NJ)	NS	678
Rajdeo, Heena (NY)	S	647
Rajpal, Sanjeev (NY)	S	450
Rakos, Gerald (CT)	NP	878
Rakowitz, Frederic (NY)	IM	510
Rakowski, Thomas (NJ)	Onc	675
Raman, Bharathi (NY)	Ger	176
Ramanathan, Kumudha (NY)	DR	413
Ramaswamy, Prema (NY)	PCd	438
Rambler, Louis (NJ)	DR	666
Ramgopal, Mekala (NY)	Ge	461
Ramirez, Mark (NY)	Onc	382
Ramsay, David (NY)	D	150
Ranawat, Chitranjan (NY)	OrS	263
Rand, Jacob (NY)	Hem	379
Rand, James (NY)	Ge	461
Randolph, Audrey (NY)	PMR	638
Rangraj, Madhu (NY)	S	647
Raniolo, Robert (NY)	S	647
Ransom, Mark (NJ)	RE	825
Ranta, Jeffrey (CT)	U	897
Rao, Addagada (NY)	S	450
Rao, Arun (NJ)	Ger	763
Rao, Yalamanchi (NY)	A&I	407
Rao, Yalamanchili (NY)	A&I	475
Raoof, Suhail (NY)	Pul	446
Rapaport, Jeffrey (NJ)	D	665
Rapaport, Robert (NY)	PEn	284
Raphael, Bruce (NY)	Hem	184
Rapoport, David (NY)	Pul	327
Rapoport, Samuel (NY)	N	228

Alphabetical Listing of Doctors

Name	Specialty	Pg	Name	Specialty	Pg
Rappaport, Irwin (NY)	PA&I	281	Reichman, Lee (NJ)	Pul	724
Raptis, George (NY)	Onc	210	Reichstein, Robert (NY)	Cv	135
Rashba, Eric (NY)	CE	563	Reiffel, James (NY)	Cv	135
Raska, Karel (NJ)	Cv	802	Reiffel, Robert (NY)	PlS	639
Raskin, Elsa (CT)	PlS	890	Reilly, James (NY)	ObG	481
Raskin, Jonathan (NY)	Pul	327	Reilly, John (NY)	OrS	482
Raskin, Keith (NY)	HS	180	Reilly, Kevin (NY)	ObG	386
Rastegar, Asghar (CT)	Nep	911	Reilly, Thomas (NY)	IM	463
Rathauser, Robert (NJ)	ObG	770	Reiner, Dan (NY)	S	546
Ratner, Desiree (NY)	D	150	Reiner, Mark (NY)	S	346
Ratner, LLoyd (NY)	S	345	Reinitz, Elizabeth (NY)	Rhu	645
Ratner, Lynn (NY)	Onc	210	Reisberg, Barry (NY)	GerPsy	176
Raucher, Harold (NY)	Ped	296	Reisner, Michelle (NJ)	Ger	734
Rausen, Aaron (NY)	PHO	288	Reison, Dennis (NJ)	Cv	662
Rawlins, Bernard (NY)	OrS	263	Reitman, Milton (NY)	PCd	528
Ray, Audell (NY)	Oph	627	Reizis, Igal (NY)	ObG	431
Raymond, Gerald (NJ)	Ped	750	Relkin, Norman (NY)	N	228
Raza, Azra (NY)	Onc	210	Relland, Maureen (NY)	Oph	249
Razaboni, Rosa (NY)	PlS	306	Remy, Prospere (NY)	Ge	376
Reader, Robert (NY)	S	345	Ren-Fielding, Christine (NY)	S	346
Rebarber, Andrei (NY)	MF	201	Rentrop, K Peter (NY)	Cv	135
Recht, Michael (NY)	DR	157	Repice, Michael (NY)	Rhu	587
Rechter, Lesley (NY)	FMed	502	Reppucci, Vincent (CT)	Oph	883
Reckler, Jon (NY)	U	358	Resmovits, Marvin (NY)	Ped	535
Reda, Dominick (NY)	Nep	620	Resnick, David (NY)	A&I	126
Reda, Edward (NY)	U	650	Resnick, Richard (NY)	Psyc	318
Reddy, Mallikarjuna (NY)	FMed	461	Resor, Louise (CT)	N	881
Reding, Michael (NY)	N	622	Respler, Don (NJ)	PO	686
Redlich, Carrie (CT)	Pul	918	Resta, Christine (NY)	EDM	460
Redner, Arlene (NY)	PHO	531	Restifo, Richard (CT)	PlS	917
Rednor, Jeffrey (NJ)	FMed	742	Rettig, Michael (NY)	HS	180
Reed, Mary (NY)	Onc	382	Reuter, Victor (NY)	Path	279
Reed, William (NY)	S	546	Rezac, Craig (NJ)	CRS	759
Reede, Deborah (NY)	DR	413	Rezvani, Fred (NJ)	ObG	680
Rees, Ellen (NY)	Psyc	318	Rho, Dae (NY)	PMR	300
Regard, Monique (NY)	ObG	624	Rice, Stephen (NJ)	SM	795
Reich, Raymond (NY)	Oph	433	Rich, Daniel (NY)	OrS	524
Reich, Steven (NJ)	OrS	771	Richards, Steven (NJ)	U	780
Reicher, Oscar (NJ)	OrS	823	Richardson, William (NJ)	Psyc	854

Name	Specialty	Pg	Name	Specialty	Pg
Richel, Peter (NY)	Ped	637	Rochelson, Burton (NY)	MF	512
Richheimer, Michael (NY)	A&I	563	Rochester, Carolyn (CT)	Pul	918
Richlin, Spencer (CT)	RE	894	Rochford, Joseph (NJ)	Psyc	835
Richman, Daniel (NY)	PM	277	Rodeo, Scott (NY)	SM	339
Richter, Edwin (CT)	PMR	890	Rodgers, I Rand (NY)	Oph	249
Ricketti, Anthony (NJ)	A&I	741	Rodino, William (NY)	VascS	486
Ridge, Gerald (NY)	IM	615	Rodke, Gae (NY)	ObG	236
Rie, Jonathan (NY)	Nep	620	Rodriguez, Lorna (NJ)	GO	763
Riechers, Roger (NY)	U	650	Rodriguez-Sains, Rene (NY)	Oph	249
Rieger, Mark (NJ)	OrS	810	Roelke, Marc (NJ)	CE	704
Rifkin, Matthew (NY)	DR	568	Rogal, Gary (NJ)	Cv	704
Rigel, Darrell (NY)	D	150	Rogers, David (NY)	VIR	472
Rigolosi, Robert (NJ)	Nep	677	Roland, J Thomas (NY)	Oto	273
Rigtrup, Edward (NJ)	Ped	722	Roland, Robert (NJ)	Inf	846
Riina, Howard (NY)	NS	219	Rolandelli, Rolando (NJ)	S	815
Riles, Thomas (NY)	VascS	364	Romagnoli, Mario (NY)	Inf	188
Riley, David (NJ)	Pul	778	Romanelli, John (NY)	Oph	578
Ring, Kenneth (NJ)	U	857	Romanello, Paul (NY)	Cv	135
Riordan, Charles (CT)	Psyc	918	Romano, Alicia (NY)	PEn	632
Ritch, Robert (NY)	Oph	249	Romano, Angela (NY)	PCd	528
Ritterband, David (NY)	Oph	249	Romano, John (NY)	D	151
Rivkees, Scott (CT)	PEn	915	Romano, Rosario (NY)	IM	574
Rivlin, Richard (NY)	IM	196	Romas, Nicholas (NY)	U	358
Rizk, Samieh (NY)	Oto	273	Romero, Carlos (NY)	S	546
Rizvi, Hasan (NY)	Onc	575	Romeu, Jose (NY)	Ge	171
Rizvi, Naiyer (NY)	Onc	210	Romita, Mauro (NY)	PlS	306
Robbins, Kim (CT)	Oph	883	Rommer, James (NJ)	IM	711
Robbins, Michael (NY)	Cv	457	Romo, Thomas (NY)	Oto	273
Robbins, Noah (NY)	Inf	379	Roohi, Fereydoon (NY)	N	429
Robert, Marie (CT)	Ped	917	Roose, Steven (NY)	Psyc	319
Roberti, Isabel (NJ)	PNep	721	Root, Barry (NY)	PMR	535
Roberts, Kenneth (CT)	RadRO	919	Rosa, Joseph (CT)	EDM	870
Roberts, Larry (NY)	U	650	Rosch, Elliott (NY)	IM	615
Roberts, Matthew (NY)	OrS	263	Rose, Daniel (CT)	TS	896
Robilotti, James (NY)	Ge	171	Rose, Donald (NY)	OrS	263
Robins, Perry (NY)	D	150	Rose, Henry (NJ)	Pul	692
Robinson, Michael (NY)	PMR	558	Rose, Howard (NY)	OrS	263
Robinson, Newell (NY)	TS	547	Rose, John (NJ)	U	797
Robson, Mark (NY)	Onc	210	Rose, Michael (NJ)	PlS	794

Alphabetical Listing of Doctors

Name	Specialty	Pg	Name	Specialty	Pg
Rosell, Frank (NY)	TS	486	Rosenfeld, Richard (NY)	PO	440
Rosello, Lori (NY)	Ped	296	Rosenfeld, Stanley (NY)	DR	157
Rosemarin, Jack (NY)	Ge	609	Rosenfeld, Steven (NY)	N	228
Rosen, Allen (NJ)	PlS	723	Rosenfeld, Suzanne (NY)	Ped	297
Rosen, Arie (NJ)	Oto	684	Rosenfeld, Walter (NJ)	AM	801
Rosen, Arnold (NY)	Psyc	319	Rosengart, Todd (NY)	TS	589
Rosen, Bruce (NY)	Psyc	585	Rosenstein, Elliot (NJ)	Rhu	726
Rosen, Douglas (NY)	D	371	Rosenstein, Roger (NJ)	HS	670
Rosen, Evelyn (NY)	GerPsy	418	Rosenstock, Arthur (CT)	PlS	891
Rosen, Mark (NY)	Pul	541	Rosenstreich, David (NY)	A&I	367
Rosen, Michael (NY)	Nep	620	Rosenthal, David (NY)	EDM	501
Rosen, Nedra (NY)	IM	196	Rosenthal, Elizabeth (NY)	D	603
Rosen, Norman (NY)	Onc	618	Rosenthal, Jeanne (NY)	Oph	249
Rosen, Robert (NY)	VIR	361	Rosenthal, Jesse (NY)	Psyc	319
Rosen, Tove (NY)	NP	213	Rosenthal, Kenneth (NY)	Oph	522
Rosenbaum, Alfred (NY)	RadRO	330	Rosenthal, Richard (NY)	Psyc	319
Rosenbaum, Daniel (NY)	N	430	Rosenthal, Sheldon (NY)	U	452
Rosenbaum, Jeffrey (NJ)	Oto	772	Rosenwaks, Zev (NY)	RE	332
Rosenbaum, Marlon (NY)	Cv	135	Rosenwasser, Melvin (NY)	HS	180
Rosenbaum, Michael (NY)	Ped	297	Roses, Daniel (NY)	S	346
Rosenbaum, Pearl (NY)	Oph	386	Rosh, Joel (NJ)	PGe	811
Rosenbaum, Robert (NJ)	EDM	844	Roshan, Daniel (NY)	MF	201
Rosenberg, Craig (NY)	PMR	583	Rosman, Lawrence (NY)	EDM	460
Rosenberg, David (NY)	Oto	273	Rosner, Bruce (NJ)	Ge	743
Rosenberg, Gene (NJ)	U	697	Rosner, Louis (NY)	Oto	526
Rosenberg, Kenneth (NY)	AdP	123	Rosner, Richard (NY)	Psyc	319
Rosenberg, Michael (NJ)	N	769	Rosner, Saran (NY)	NS	621
Rosenberg, Michael (NY)	PlS	639	Ross, Howard (NJ)	CRS	786
Rosenberg, Vladimiro (NY)	S	346	Ross, Marc (NY)	PMR	443
Rosenberg, Zehava (NY)	DR	157	Rossakis, Constantine (NJ)	Cv	662
Rosenblatt, Ruth (NY)	DR	157	Rossi, Dennis (NY)	DR	499
Rosenblatt, William (NY)	PlS	306	Rossman, Barry (NJ)	U	753
Rosenbloom, Charles (NY)	Psyc	319	Rossos, Apostolos (NJ)	Oto	792
Rosenblum, Bruce (NJ)	NS	790	Roston, Alfred (NY)	Ge	609
Rosenblum, Marc (NY)	Path	280	Roth, Alan (NY)	FMed	461
Rosenfeld, Alvin (CT)	ChAP	867	Roth, Andrew (NY)	Psyc	319
Rosenfeld, David (NJ)	Psyc	690	Roth, Douglas (NY)	PlS	639
Rosenfeld, David (NY)	RE	543	Roth, Joseph (NJ)	Ge	669
Rosenfeld, David (NJ)	DR	760	Roth, Malcolm (NY)	PlS	443

Name	Specialty	Pg	Name	Specialty	Pg
Roth, Neil (NY)	SM	340	Ruddy, Michael (NJ)	Nep	746
Roth, Patrick (NJ)	NS	678	Ruderman, Marvin (NJ)	N	715
Roth, Philip (NY)	NP	480	Rudick, A Joseph (NY)	Oph	249
Roth, Richard (NY)	Cv	553	Rudikoff, Donald (NY)	D	371
Rothbaum, David (NY)	ObG	520	Rudin, Eric (NY)	EDM	605
Rothberg, Charles (NY)	Oph	579	Rudin, Leonard (NY)	U	560
Rothberg, Robert (NJ)	CRS	706	Rudman, Michael (NJ)	PM	810
Rothman, Howard (NJ)	Cv	662	Rudolph, Daniel (CT)	Pul	893
Rothman, Ivan (NY)	Onc	513	Rudolph, Steven (NY)	N	430
Rothman, Jeffrey (NY)	EDM	477	Ruggiero, Joseph (NY)	Onc	210
Rothschild, Michael (NY)	PO	290	Ruoff, Michael (NY)	Ge	172
Rothstein, Stephen (NY)	Oto	273	Rush, Thomas (NY)	Inf	612
Rotolo, James (NJ)	U	797	Rusk, Alice (CT)	N	881
Roubin, Gary (NY)	IC	199	Russakoff, L Mark (NY)	Psyc	641
Rowley, Scott (NJ)	Hem	671	Russell, Robin (NY)	Ger	377
Roychowdhury, Sudipta (NJ)	NRad	769	Russo, John (NJ)	IM	711
Roye, David (NY)	OrS	263	Russo, Paul (NY)	U	358
Rozanski, Reuben (NJ)	D	706	Rutherford, Thomas (CT)	GO	906
Rozbruch, Jacob (NY)	OrS	264	Rutkovsky, Edward (NY)	Cv	494
Rozbruch, S Robert (NY)	OrS	264	Rutkovsky, Lisa (NY)	PCd	468
Rozenblit, Alla (NY)	DR	372	Ruzal-Shapiro, Carrie (NY)	DR	157
Rubenstein, Andrew (NJ)	ObG	680	Ryan, Joseph (NJ)	Ger	804
Rubenstein, Jack (NY)	IM	510	Ryback, Hyman (NY)	Oto	630
Rubin, Cheryl (NY)	OrS	557	Rydzinski, Mayer (NY)	Cv	458
Rubin, David (NY)	CE	594			
Rubin, James (NY)	A&I	126			
Rubin, Kenneth (NJ)	Psyc	795			
Rubin, Kenneth (NJ)	Ge	669	## S		
Rubin, Laurence (NY)	Oph	522	Saada, Simon (NY)	U	452
Rubin, Lorry (NY)	PInf	531	Saal, Stuart (NY)	Nep	215
Rubin, Marc (NJ)	Ge	743	Sabatino, Dominick (NY)	PHO	531
Rubin, Moshe (NY)	Ge	172	Sabbath, Kert (CT)	Hem	907
Rubin, Steven (NY)	Oph	522	Sabbatini, Paul (NY)	Onc	210
Rubino, Francesco (NY)	S	346	Saberski, Lloyd (CT)	PM	914
Rubinoff, Mitchell (NJ)	Ge	669	Sabetta, James (CT)	Inf	873
Rubinstein, Arye (NY)	A&I	367	Sabharwal, Sanjeev (NJ)	OrS	718
Rubinstein, Boris (NY)	ChAP	599	Sable, Robert (NY)	Ge	376
Rubinstein, Mort (NY)	Psyc	319	Sabnani, Indu (NJ)	Hem	709
Rucker, Steve (NY)	IM	510	Saboeiro, Gregory (NY)	VIR	361

Alphabetical Listing of Doctors

Name	Specialty	Pg	Name	Specialty	Pg
Sabry, M Zakir (NY)	PlS	306	Salem, Ronald (CT)	S	921
Sacchi, Terrence (NY)	IC	423	Salerno, William (NJ)	Cv	662
Sacco, Margaret (NJ)	S	815	Salgado, Miran (NY)	N	430
Sachar, David (NY)	Ge	172	Salifu, Moro (NY)	Nep	427
Sachs, Jonathan (NJ)	Ge	743	Salik, James (NY)	Ge	172
Sachs, Paul (CT)	Pul	893	Salimi, Mostafa (NJ)	Cv	819
Sachs, R Gregory (NJ)	Cv	843	Salky, Barry (NY)	S	346
Sachs, Ronald (NJ)	Oph	809	Salmon, Jane (NY)	Rhu	337
Sachs, Stephen (NJ)	N	849	Salsitz, Edwin (NY)	IM	196
Sacker, Ira (NY)	Ped	297	Saltz, Leonard (NY)	Onc	211
Sacks, Michael (NY)	Psyc	319	Saltzman, Daniel (NY)	MF	201
Sacks, Steven (NY)	Oto	274	Saltzman, Martin (NY)	Nep	620
Sacks-Berg, Anne (NY)	Inf	572	Saltzman, Simone (NY)	Inf	379
Sadan, Sara (NY)	Onc	618	Saltzman-Gabelman, Lori (NY)	IM	615
Sadanandan, Swayam (NY)	PHO	439	Salvati, Eduardo (NY)	OrS	264
Sadarangani, Balvinder (NY)	ObG	237	Salwitz, James (NJ)	Onc	766
Sadeghi, Hooshang (NJ)	N	735	Salz, Alan (NJ)	Oph	833
Sadeghi, Hossein (CT)	PPul	888	Salzberg, C Andrew (NY)	PlS	639
Sadeghi-Nejad, Hossein (NJ)	U	697	Salzer, Richard (NJ)	OrS	683
Sadiq, Saud (NY)	N	228	Salzer, Stephen (CT)	Oto	887
Sadock, Virginia (NY)	Psyc	320	Salzman, Jacquelin (NY)	Oph	627
Sadovsky, Richard (NY)	FMed	415	Samach, Michael (NJ)	Ge	804
Saenger, Paul (NY)	PEn	633	Samadi, David (NY)	U	359
Safai, Bijan (NY)	D	151	Samberg, Eslee (NY)	Psyc	320
Saffra, Norman (NY)	Oph	433	Sami, Sherif (NY)	Psyc	539
Safirstein, Benjamin (NJ)	Pul	725	Sampson, Hugh (NY)	PA&I	281
Safran, Steven (NJ)	Oph	747	Samra, Said (NJ)	PlS	794
Sage, Jacob (NJ)	N	769	Samson, C Michael (NY)	Oph	249
Sagorin, Charles (NJ)	Onc	713	Samuel, Steven (NJ)	Cv	741
Sagy, Mayer (NY)	PCCM	529	Samuels, Steven (NJ)	Psyc	690
Saha, Chanchal (NY)	TS	547	Samuels, Steven (NY)	Inf	572
Sahar, David (NY)	Cv	369	San Filippo, J Anthony (NY)	S	648
Sailon, Peter (NY)	ObG	237	San Roman, Gerardo (NY)	ObG	577
Saiman, Lisa (NY)	PInf	289	Sanchez, Juan (CT)	TS	921
Saland, Jeffrey (NY)	PNep	289	Sanchez, Miguel (NJ)	Path	684
Salas, Max (NJ)	PEn	774	Sanchez-Catanese, Betty (NJ)	IM	832
Salcedo-Contreras, Jose (NJ)	PNep	824	Sander, Howard (NY)	N	228
Saleh, Anthony (NY)	Pul	446	Sander, Norbert (NY)	IM	380
Salem, Noel (NJ)	Rhu	694	Sanders, Abraham (NY)	Pul	327

Name	Specialty	Pg	Name	Specialty	Pg
Sanders, Linda (NJ)	DR	707	Scaduto, Philip (NJ)	IM	806
Sanderson, Rhonda (NJ)	ObG	833	Scardino, Peter (NY)	U	359
Sandhaus, Jeffrey (NY)	U	472	Scarpa, Nicholas (NJ)	Rhu	737
Sandhu, Harvinder (NY)	OrS	264	Schaebler, David (NJ)	Onc	745
Sandler, Benjamin (NY)	RE	332	Schaefer, John (NY)	N	228
Sandoval, Claudio (NY)	PHO	633	Schaefer, Steven (NY)	Oto	274
Sands, Andrew (NY)	OrS	264	Schaeffer, Henry (NY)	Ped	442
Sanford, Marie (NY)	Ped	297	Schaeffer, Janis (NY)	PPul	532
Sanger, Joseph (NY)	NuM	231	Schaeffer, Mark (NJ)	IM	744
Santamaria, Jaime (NJ)	Oph	771	Schaer, Teresa (NJ)	IM	765
Santilli, John (CT)	A&I	865	Schanler, Richard (NY)	NP	514
Santin, Alessandro (CT)	GO	907	Schantz, Stimson (NY)	Oto	274
Saponara, Eduardo (NY)	Onc	619	Schanzer, Bernard (NJ)	N	849
Sara, Gabriel (NY)	Onc	211	Scharf, Richard (NJ)	Oto	851
Saraiya, Narendra (NJ)	Ped	853	Scharf, Robert (NY)	Psyc	320
Sarno, John (NY)	PM	278	Scharf, Stephen (NY)	NuM	232
Sarnoff, Deborah (NY)	D	498	Schattman, Glenn (NY)	RE	333
Saroff, Alan (NJ)	Cv	704	Schaul, Neil (NY)	N	518
Sarokhan, Alan (NJ)	OrS	851	Schechner, Richard (NY)	S	399
Sas, Norman (NY)	S	399	Schechter, Justin (CT)	Psyc	891
Sasaki, Clarence (CT)	Oto	914	Schechter, Michael (CT)	ObG	882
Sasso, Louis (NY)	Pul	485	Schechter, Miriam (NY)	Ped	394
Sassoon, Robert (NY)	ObG	237	Scheer, Max (NY)	Inf	508
Satlin, Lisa (NY)	PNep	289	Schefer, Alan (NY)	HS	611
Satnick, Steven (NY)	A&I	563	Schein, Jonah (NY)	Psyc	320
Sauer, Mark (NY)	RE	332	Scheinberg, David (NY)	Onc	211
Saul, Zane (CT)	Inf	873	Schell, Harold (NJ)	S	753
Saulino, Patrick (NJ)	Cv	830	Scher, David (NY)	OrS	264
Saunders, Craig (NJ)	TS	728	Scher, Howard (NY)	Onc	211
Savage, David (NY)	Hem	184	Scher, Jonathan (NY)	ObG	237
Savatsky, Gary (NJ)	SM	694	Scherl, Ellen (NY)	Ge	172
Savatta, Domenico (NJ)	U	729	Scherl, Michael (NJ)	Oto	684
Savin, Ronald (CT)	D	904	Scherl, Sharon (NJ)	D	665
Savino, John (NY)	S	648	Scherr, Douglas (NY)	U	359
Savino, Michael (NY)	U	486	Schiano, Thomas (NY)	Ge	172
Savino, Robert (CT)	EDM	870	Schick, David (NY)	Cv	369
Sawczuk, Ihor (NJ)	U	698	Schiff, Carl (NY)	Rhu	448
Sawyer, David (NY)	Psyc	320	Schiff, Howard (NY)	U	359
Scaccia, Frank (NJ)	Oto	792	Schiff, Peter (NY)	RadRO	330

Alphabetical Listing of Doctors

Name	Specialty	Pg	Name	Specialty	Pg
Schiff, Russell (NY)	PCd	529	Schor, Joshua (NY)	Ger	610
Schiff, William (NY)	Oph	250	Schore, Arthur (NY)	Psyc	320
Schiffer, Mark (NY)	Cv	135	Schottenfeld, Richard (CT)	AdP	901
Schiffman, Philip (NJ)	Pul	778	Schrader, Zalman (NJ)	Ge	709
Schiller, Alan (NY)	Path	280	Schrager, Alan (NY)	U	650
Schiller, Myles (NY)	PCd	389	Schreiber, Carl (NY)	Cv	494
Schiller, Robert (NY)	FMed	163	Schreiber, Klaus (NY)	ChAP	599
Schiowitz, Emanuel (NY)	FMed	415	Schreiber, Martha (NJ)	S	796
Schiz, Steven (CT)	Ped	889	Schreiber, Michael (NY)	Pul	643
Schlam, Everett (NJ)	FMed	708	Schroeder, Karl (NY)	Psyc	559
Schlegel, Peter (NY)	U	359	Schubach, Scott (NY)	TS	547
Schleider, Michael (NJ)	Onc	675	Schubert, Hermann (NY)	Oph	250
Schleifer, Steven (NJ)	Psyc	724	Schubert, Romaine (NY)	ChiN	411
Schlesinger, Iris (NY)	OrS	629	Schulder, Michael (NY)	NS	516
Schley, W Shain (NY)	Oto	274	Schulhafer, Edwin (NJ)	A&I	829
Schliftman, Alan (NY)	D	603	Schulman, Ira (NY)	Cv	135
Schluger, Neil (NY)	Pul	327	Schulman, Matthew (NY)	PlS	306
Schlussel, Richard (NY)	U	359	Schulman, Norman (NY)	PlS	306
Schmerin, Michael (NY)	Ge	172	Schulman, Philip (NY)	Hem	572
Schmidt, Hans (NJ)	S	695	Schulster, Rita (NY)	Pul	541
Schmidt, Philip (NY)	EDM	414	Schultz, Neal (NY)	D	151
Schmidt-Sarosi, Cecilia (NY)	RE	333	Schulze, Paul (NY)	Cv	136
Schnabel, Freya (NY)	S	346	Schuss, Steven (NJ)	Ped	688
Schneck, Gideon (NY)	Oph	579	Schuster, Michael (NY)	Hem	572
Schneebaum, Cary (NY)	Ge	172	Schutzengel, Roy (CT)	Ped	889
Schneider, Arlene (NY)	A&I	407	Schwab, Frank (NY)	OrS	264
Schneider, Darren (NY)	VascS	364	Schwartz, Allan (NY)	Cv	136
Schneider, Kenneth (NY)	Oto	274	Schwartz, Amit (NY)	NS	428
Schneider, Lewis (NY)	Ge	173	Schwartz, Bruce (NY)	Psyc	396
Schneider, Marcie (CT)	AM	865	Schwartz, Charles (NY)	Cv	475
Schneider, Robert (NY)	Onc	619	Schwartz, Evan (NY)	OrS	467
Schneider, Samuel (NJ)	Psyc	751	Schwartz, Gary (NY)	Ge	505
Schneider, Stephen (NJ)	EDM	761	Schwartz, Joel (NY)	NRad	557
Schneider, Steven (NY)	IM	197	Schwartz, Judith (NY)	ObG	237
Schob, Clifford (NJ)	OrS	718	Schwartz, Kenneth (NY)	VascS	651
Schoen, Robert (CT)	Rhu	920	Schwartz, Lawrence (NY)	DR	157
Schoeneman, Morris (NY)	PNep	440	Schwartz, Louis (NJ)	RadRO	855
Schoenfeld, Mark (CT)	CE	901	Schwartz, Michael (NY)	Psyc	585
Schonfeld, Steven (NJ)	NRad	769	Schwartz, Myron (NY)	S	346

Name	Specialty	Pg	Name	Specialty	Pg
Schwartz, Paula (NY)	Onc	513	Seidenfeld, Andrew (NY)	Oph	467
Schwartz, Peter (CT)	GO	907	Seidenstein, Michael (NJ)	OrS	718
Schwartz, Robert (NJ)	D	706	Seidman, Barry (NJ)	U	729
Schwartz, Simeon (NY)	Onc	619	Seidman, Mitchell (NY)	Oph	434
Schwartz, Theodore (NY)	NS	219	Seifer, David (NY)	RE	447
Schwartz, William (NY)	Cv	136	Seigel, Mark (NJ)	ObG	791
Schwartzberg, Mori (NJ)	Rhu	795	Seigle, Robert (NY)	PNep	290
Schwartzman, Alexander (NY)	S	450	Seinfeld, David (NY)	Cv	136
Schwartzman, Sergio (NY)	Rhu	337	Seinfeld, Fredric (NJ)	TS	753
Schwarz, Richard (NY)	Nep	575	Seiter, Karen (NY)	Onc	619
Schwarz, Steven (NY)	PGe	438	Sekiguchi, Raymond (CT)	FMed	871
Schweitzer, Philip (NY)	Ge	376	Selesnick, Samuel (NY)	Oto	274
Schwinn, Hans (NY)	FMed	570	Seliger, Glenn (NY)	N	557
Scibetta, Maria (NJ)	IM	673	Selinger, Sharon (NJ)	EDM	844
Scigliano, Eileen (NY)	Hem	184	Selman, Jay (NY)	N	622
Sciortino, Patrick (NY)	Oph	433	Seltzer, Terry (NY)	EDM	161
Sclafani, Anthony (NY)	Oto	274	Selwyn, Peter (NY)	IM	380
Sclafani, Lisa (NY)	S	588	Selzer, Jeffrey (NY)	Psyc	469
Sclafani, Michael (NJ)	SM	796	Seminara, Donna (NY)	Ger	478
Sclafani, Salvatore (NY)	VIR	453	Sen, Chandranath (NY)	NS	220
Scofield, Lisa (NJ)	Ped	824	Sena, Kanaga (CT)	N	881
Scoppetuolo, Michael (NJ)	Onc	713	Sender, Joel (NY)	Pul	398
Scott, Claude (NY)	OrS	435	Sensakovic, John (NJ)	Inf	764
Scott, David (NY)	Nep	465	Sepkowitz, Douglas (NY)	Inf	420
Scott, Richard (NJ)	RE	814	Sepkowitz, Kent (NY)	Inf	188
Scott, Susan (NY)	PlS	306	Seplowitz, Alan (NY)	EDM	161
Scott, W Norman (NY)	OrS	264	Serby, Michael (NY)	GerPsy	176
Scuderi, Giles (NY)	OrS	265	Sergiou, Harry (NY)	Ped	442
Sculco, Thomas (NY)	OrS	265	Serle, Janet (NY)	Oph	250
Scully, Brian (NY)	Inf	188	Serur, Eli (NY)	GO	418
Seaman, Cheryl (NY)	Psyc	320	Sethi, Paul (CT)	OrS	885
Seashore, Margretta (CT)	CG	903	Sett, Suvro (NY)	TS	648
Seaver, Robert (NY)	ChAP	599	Setton, Avi (NY)	NRad	518
Seebacher, J Robert (NY)	OrS	629	Setzen, Michael (NY)	Oto	526
Seedor, John (NY)	Oph	250	Sgaglione, Nicholas (NY)	OrS	524
Seelagy, Marc (NJ)	Pul	751	Shabry, Fryderyka (NY)	ChAP	411
Segal-Maurer, Sorana (NY)	Inf	462	Shabsigh, Ridwan (NY)	U	453
Segarra, Pedro (NY)	ObG	237	Shabto, Uri (NY)	Oph	250
Seidenberg, Roy (NY)	D	151	Shah, Darsit (NJ)	Oto	792

Alphabetical Listing of Doctors

Name	Specialty	Pg	Name	Specialty	Pg
Shah, Jatin (NY)	S	346	Sheinfeld, Joel (NY)	U	359
Shah, Paresh (NY)	S	347	Shell, Roger (NJ)	Cv	758
Shah, Smita (NJ)	Pul	725	Shelmet, John (NJ)	EDM	742
Shahid, Syed (CT)	NS	880	Shelton, Ronald (NY)	D	151
Shahrivar, Farrokh (NY)	NP	214	Shemen, Larry (NY)	Oto	274
Shamoon, Fayez (NJ)	Cv	704	Shenoy, Rajesh (NY)	PCd	389
Shamoon, Harry (NY)	EDM	373	Shepard, Barry (NY)	U	549
Shampain, Lawrence (NJ)	ChAP	758	Shepherd, Gillian (NY)	A&I	126
Shanahan, Andrew (NJ)	IC	745	Sher, Ellen (NJ)	A&I	785
Shane, Elizabeth (NY)	EDM	161	Sheridan, Bernadette (NY)	FMed	415
Shani, Jacob (NY)	IC	424	Sheris, Steven (NJ)	Cv	843
Shapir, Yehuda (NY)	PCd	529	Sherling, Bruce (NY)	Pul	643
Shapiro, Barry (NY)	Oto	631	Sherman, Frederic (NY)	IM	423
Shapiro, Bruce (CT)	Psyc	891	Sherman, Fredrick (NY)	Ger	176
Shapiro, Ellen (NY)	U	359	Sherman, Howard (NY)	Ge	377
Shapiro, Eugene (CT)	PInf	916	Sherman, John (NY)	PlS	307
Shapiro, Kenneth (NY)	Nep	556	Sherman, Mark (NY)	OrS	482
Shapiro, Lawrence (NY)	EDM	501	Sherman, Raymond (NY)	Nep	215
Shapiro, Lawrence (NY)	CG	600	Sherman, Richard (NJ)	Nep	767
Shapiro, Marc (NY)	S	588	Sherman, Scott (NY)	DR	500
Shapiro, Michael (NJ)	S	695	Sherman, Spencer (NY)	Oph	250
Shapiro, Neil (NY)	Ge	609	Sherman, Steven (NY)	Oph	434
Shapiro, Peter (NY)	Psyc	320	Sherman, Warren (NY)	Cv	136
Shapiro, Richard (NY)	S	347	Sherman, William (NY)	Onc	211
Shapiro, Warren (NY)	Nep	427	Sherry, Stephen (NJ)	EDM	707
Sharma, Samin (NY)	IC	199	Sheth, Parag (NY)	PMR	300
Sharon, David (NJ)	Onc	789	Shike, Moshe (NY)	Ge	173
Sharon, Ezra (NY)	Rhu	470	Shikowitz, Mark (NY)	Oto	526
Shatkin, Jess (NY)	ChAP	140	Shim-Chang, Helen (NY)	D	151
Shaw, Ronda (NY)	Psyc	320	Shimony, Rony (NY)	Cv	136
Shaywitz, Bennett (CT)	ChiN	903	Shinbach, Kent (NY)	Psyc	321
Shaywitz, Sally (CT)	Ped	917	Shindler, Daniel (NJ)	Cv	758
Shear, Perry (CT)	NS	880	Shinnar, Shlomo (NY)	ChiN	370
Shebairo, Raymond (NY)	OrS	524	Shlofmitz, Richard (NY)	Cv	494
Sheftell, Fred (CT)	Psyc	891	Short, Joan (NY)	Ped	483
Sheikh, Shahid (NY)	Cv	598	Shugar, Joel (NY)	Oto	275
Shein, Leon (NY)	Nep	427	Shulman, Julius (NY)	Oph	250
Sheinart, Kara (NY)	N	228	Shulman, Melanie (NY)	N	228
Sheinbaum, Richard (CT)	Ge	872	Shulman, Yale (NJ)	U	738

Name	Specialty	Pg	Name	Specialty	Pg
Shum, Kee (NY)	Onc	465	Silverman, Bernard (NY)	A&I	407
Shupack, Jerome (NY)	D	151	Silverman, Cary (NJ)	Oph	809
Shypula, Gregory (NJ)	Onc	766	Silverman, David (NY)	IM	197
Sibony, Patrick (NY)	Oph	579	Silverman, Joel (NY)	Pul	470
Sibrack, Laurence (CT)	D	869	Silverman, Lewis (NY)	Onc	211
Sibulkin, David (NY)	D	151	Silverman, Mitchell (NJ)	EDM	844
Sicherer, Scott (NY)	PA&I	281	Silverman, Rubin (NY)	Cv	369
Sicklick, Marc (NY)	A&I	490	Silvers, David (NY)	D	152
Siderides, Elizabeth (CT)	Oph	884	Silvestri, Fred (NJ)	S	695
Sidoti, Paul (NY)	Oph	250	Simberkoff, Michael (NY)	Inf	189
Siebert, John (NY)	PlS	307	Simmons, Rache (NY)	S	347
Siegal, Elliot (NY)	Ped	558	Simon, Clifford (NJ)	Pul	692
Siegal, Frederick (NY)	A&I	126	Simon, Jonathan (NJ)	Rhu	726
Siegal, Michael (NY)	Cv	136	Simon, Lawrence (NY)	S	560
Siegel, Daniel (NY)	D	568	Simon, Lloyd (NY)	IM	574
Siegel, Judy (NY)	U	650	Simon, Sheldon (NY)	OrS	265
Siegel, Kenneth (CT)	N	881	Simon, Steven (NY)	D	413
Siegel, Randall (NJ)	VIR	781	Simon, Todd (NY)	IM	423
Siegel, Robert (NY)	CCM	371	Simonson, Barry (NY)	OrS	524
Siegel, Stephen (NY)	Cv	136	Simpson, David (NY)	N	229
Siegler, Eugenia (NY)	Ger	176	Simpson, Roger (NY)	PlS	538
Siepser, Stuart (NJ)	Cv	819	Singer, Carol (NY)	Inf	508
Sierocki, John (NJ)	Onc	745	Singer, Lewis (NY)	PCCM	389
Siever, Larry (NY)	Psyc	321	Singer, Samuel (NY)	S	347
Silberman, Deborah (NY)	Oph	434	Singh, Anup (NJ)	PNep	775
Silberman, Mark (NY)	PlS	538	Singh, Avtar (NY)	N	622
Silbert, Glenn (NJ)	Oph	681	Singh, Bhuvanesh (NY)	Oto	275
Silbert, Paul (NJ)	N	791	Singhal, Pravin (NY)	Nep	515
Silich, Robert (NY)	PlS	307	Sinnreich, Abraham (NY)	Oto	482
Silva, Jose (NY)	U	360	Sipzner, Robert (NJ)	Nep	714
Silva, Waldemar (NJ)	IM	806	Siracuse, Jeffrey (NY)	NP	425
Silver, Bennett (NJ)	Psyc	854	Siris, Ethel (NY)	EDM	161
Silver, David (NY)	U	453	Siris, Samuel (NY)	Psyc	469
Silver, Jonathan (NY)	Psyc	321	Siskind, Steven (NY)	Cv	458
Silver, Lester (NY)	PlS	307	Sison, Joseph (NJ)	NP	676
Silver, Michael (NY)	Cv	598	Sisti, Michael (NY)	NS	220
Silverberg, Arnold (NY)	EDM	414	Sivak, Mark (NY)	N	229
Silverberg, Nanette (NY)	D	151	Skerker, Robert (NJ)	PMR	812
Silverberg, Shonni (NY)	EDM	161	Sklansky, B Donald (NY)	PlS	538

Alphabetical Listing of Doctors

Name	Specialty	Pg	Name	Specialty	Pg
Sklar, Charles (NY)	PEn	284	Smith, Harriet (NY)	GO	378
Sklar, Jeffrey (NY)	D	499	Smith, Jo Ann (CT)	Psyc	892
Sklarek, Howard (NY)	Pul	585	Smith, Julia (NY)	Onc	212
Sklarin, Nancy (NY)	Onc	211	Smith, Leon (NJ)	MF	712
Sklaroff, Herschel (NY)	Cv	137	Smith, Michael (NY)	AdP	367
Sklower, Jay (NJ)	FMed	733	Smith, Paul (NY)	Inf	189
Sklower Brooks, Susan (NJ)	CG	759	Smith, Peter (NY)	Pul	446
Skluth, Myra (CT)	IM	875	Smith, R Theodore (NY)	Oph	251
Skolnick, Lawrence (NJ)	NP	807	Smith, Richard (NY)	Oto	388
Skolnik, Richard (NY)	PlS	307	Smith, Scott (NY)	Oph	251
Skopicki, Hal (NY)	Cv	565	Smith, Sharon (NY)	IM	197
Skripkus, Aldona (NJ)	Ped	736	Smith, Stephen (NJ)	Inf	710
Skrokov, Robert (NY)	D	568	Smithy, William (NY)	CRS	567
Skupski, Daniel (NY)	MF	464	Smotkin, David (NY)	GO	378
Skuza, Kathryn (NJ)	PEn	774	Smotrich, Gary (NJ)	PlS	750
Sladowski, Catherine (NJ)	ObG	716	Snow, Robert (NY)	NS	220
Slakter, Jason (NY)	Oph	251	Snowball, Halina (CT)	PMR	890
Slama, Robert (NJ)	Cv	843	Snyder, Barbara (NJ)	AM	757
Slamovits, Thomas (NY)	Oph	387	Snyder, David (NY)	N	229
Slankard, Marjorie (NY)	A&I	126	Snyder, Gary (NY)	Oto	467
Slater, Gary (NY)	S	347	Snyder, Jon (NY)	ObG	237
Slater, James (NY)	IC	199	Snyder, Michael (CT)	PCd	887
Slater, Jonathan (NY)	ChAP	599	Sobel, Howard (NY)	D	152
Slater, William (NY)	Cv	137	Sobol, Norman (NY)	N	430
Slavit, David (NY)	Oto	275	Sockolow, Robbyn (NY)	PGe	285
Slim, Jihad (NJ)	Inf	710	Sofair, Jane (NJ)	Psyc	813
Sloan, William (NJ)	Ge	709	Soffen, Edward (NJ)	RadRO	752
Sloane, Lori (NY)	Rhu	645	Soffer, Jeffrey (NJ)	ObG	850
Slogoff, Frederick (CT)	IM	875	Softness, Barney (NY)	Ped	297
Slonim, Alfred (NY)	PEn	284	Sogani, Pramod (NY)	U	360
Slovin, Susan (NY)	Onc	212	Sohn, Won (NY)	Ge	417
Small, Eric (NY)	SM	646	Soifer, Todd (NY)	OrS	435
Smallberg, Gerald (NY)	N	229	Sokal, Myron (NY)	NP	426
Smart, Frank (NJ)	Cv	802	Sokol, Sergio (NY)	Cv	494
Smilen, Scott (NY)	ObG	237	Soletic, Raymond (NY)	Oto	526
Smiles, Stephen (NY)	Rhu	337	Solitar, Bruce (NY)	Rhu	337
Smith, Brian (CT)	OrS	914	Solomon, Edward (NJ)	Oph	681
Smith, Craig (NY)	TS	352	Solomon, Gary (NY)	Rhu	338
Smith, Edward (NY)	Oph	434	Solomon, Gregory (NY)	IM	197

Name	Specialty	Pg	Name	Specialty	Pg
Solomon, Ira (NY)	Oph	627	Sparano, Joseph (NY)	Onc	382
Solomon, Joel (NY)	Oph	251	Sparr, Steven (NY)	N	385
Solomon, Michael (NJ)	U	780	Spector, Jason (NY)	PlS	307
Solomon, Robert (NY)	NS	220	Speiser, Phyllis (NY)	PEn	468
Solomon, Robert (NJ)	Ger	846	Spencer, Dennis (CT)	NS	911
Solomon, Ronald (NY)	HS	419	Spencer, Elizabeth Kay (NY)	ChAP	140
Solomon, Sherry (NY)	Oph	627	Spera, John (CT)	RadRO	893
Solomon, William (NY)	Onc	425	Spergel, Gabriel (NY)	EDM	414
Soloway, Barrie (NY)	Oph	251	Sperling, Neil (NY)	Oto	437
Soloway, Bruce (NY)	FMed	375	Spero, Charles (NY)	OrS	435
Soltren, Rafael (NY)	IM	615	Spero, Marc (NY)	IM	197
Som, Peter (NY)	DR	158	Speyer, James (NY)	Onc	212
Sommer, Robert (NY)	PCd	282	Spielberg, Alan (NY)	Ge	571
Sommers, Gara (NJ)	GO	670	Spielman, Joel (NJ)	OrS	810
Somogyi, Anthony (NY)	IM	463	Spielvogel, David (NY)	TS	648
Sonett, Joshua (NY)	TS	352	Spiera, Harry (NY)	Rhu	338
Sonnenblick, Emily (NY)	DR	158	Spiera, Robert (NY)	Rhu	338
Sonoda, Toyooki (NY)	CRS	143	Spiler, Ira (NJ)	EDM	761
Sonpal, Girish (NY)	Rhu	471	Spindola-Franco, Hugo (NY)	DR	372
Sood, Sunil (NY)	PInf	532	Spinelli, Henry (NY)	PlS	307
Sorabella, Philip (NJ)	DR	666	Spinowitz, Alan (NY)	D	499
Sorbera, Carmine (NY)	Cv	598	Spinowitz, Bruce (NY)	Nep	466
Soriano, John (NJ)	Ge	804	Spira, Robert (NJ)	Ge	709
Soroko, Theresa (NJ)	Inf	710	Spitalewitz, Samuel (NY)	Nep	427
Sorra, Toomas (NY)	Ge	417	Spitz, Henry (NY)	Psyc	321
Sosa, R Ernest (NY)	U	360	Spitzer, Daniel (NY)	NS	556
Soskel, Neil (NY)	FMed	502	Spivak, Jeffrey (NY)	OrS	265
Soslow, Robert (NY)	Path	280	Spivak, William (NY)	PGe	285
Sosulski, Richard (NY)	Ped	583	Splain, Shepard (NY)	OrS	435
Soter, Nicholas (NY)	D	152	Spotnitz, Henry (NY)	TS	352
Sotsky, Gerald (NJ)	Cv	662	Sprecher, Stanley (NY)	DR	459
Southern, D Loren (NJ)	A&I	829	Spriggs, David (NY)	Onc	212
Southren, David (NY)	Cv	553	Sproviero, Joseph (CT)	A&I	865
Souweidane, Mark (NY)	NS	220	Squitieri, Rafael (CT)	TS	896
Spadaro, Louise (NY)	Cv	495	Staats, Peter (NJ)	PM	793
Spaide, Richard (NY)	Oph	251	Stabile, John (NJ)	Oph	681
Spak, James (CT)	OrS	886	Stabinsky, Susan (NY)	Psyc	641
Spandorfer, Steven (NY)	RE	333	Staffenberg, David (NY)	PlS	395
Spano, Frank (CT)	IM	875	Stahl, Richard (CT)	PlS	917

Alphabetical Listing of Doctors

Name	Specialty	Pg	Name	Specialty	Pg
Stam, Lawrence (NY)	Nep	427	Steingart, Richard (NY)	Cv	137
Stanford, Paulette (NJ)	AM	703	Steinhagen, Randolph (NY)	CRS	143
Stangel, John (NY)	RE	644	Steinherz, Laurel (NY)	PCd	283
Starc, Thomas (NY)	PCd	282	Steinherz, Peter (NY)	PHO	288
Starke, Charles (NY)	IM	615	Stelzer, Paul (NY)	TS	352
Starker, Isaac (NJ)	PlS	813	Stern, Harvey (NY)	DR	373
Starker, Paul (NJ)	S	856	Stern, Leonard (NY)	Nep	216
Starkman, Harold (NJ)	PEn	811	Stern, Richard (NY)	Rhu	338
Starpoli, Anthony (NY)	Ge	173	Sternschein, Michael (NJ)	PlS	690
Starr, Michael (NY)	Oph	251	Stevens, Peter (NY)	Ge	173
Staszewski, Harry (NY)	Hem	507	Stewart, Allan (NY)	TS	352
Steele, Andrew (NY)	NP	515	Stewart, Michael (NY)	Oto	275
Steele, Mark (NY)	Oph	251	Stidham, Katrina (NY)	Oto	631
Steer, Robert (NJ)	ObG	808	Stieg, Philip (NY)	NS	220
Steiger, David (NY)	Pul	327	Stifelman, Michael (NY)	U	360
Steigman, Elliot (NJ)	U	738	Stiller, Robert (CT)	MF	877
Stein, Adam (NY)	PMR	535	Stillman, Michael (NY)	D	603
Stein, Alan (NY)	Inf	420	Stilwell, Anne (NY)	PM	482
Stein, Arnold (NY)	Oph	434	Stock, Jeffrey (NJ)	U	729
Stein, Barry (NY)	Ped	297	Stock, Richard (NY)	RadRO	330
Stein, Cy (NY)	Onc	382	Stolar, Charles (NY)	PS	293
Stein, David (NY)	Ge	377	Stoller, Gerald (NY)	Oph	579
Stein, Elliott (NJ)	Cv	843	Stone, Chester (NJ)	U	816
Stein, Jeffrey (NY)	Ge	173	Stone, Gregg (NY)	IC	199
Stein, Jeffrey (NY)	VascS	364	Stone, Joanne (NY)	MF	201
Stein, Joel (NY)	PMR	300	Stone, Michael (NY)	Psyc	321
Stein, Lawrence (NJ)	Ge	804	Stone, Peter (NY)	U	401
Stein, Mark (NY)	U	400	Stoopler, Mark (NY)	Onc	212
Stein, Mitchell (NY)	Oph	627	Storch, Kenneth (NJ)	IM	806
Stein, Perry (NY)	PMR	443	Storper, Ian (NY)	Oto	275
Stein, Richard (NY)	Cv	137	Stovell, Peter (CT)	OrS	886
Stein, Ruth (NY)	Ped	394	Stover-Pepe, Diane (NY)	Pul	328
Stein, Sidney (NY)	Pul	327	Strain, James (NY)	Psyc	321
Stein, Stefan (NY)	Psyc	321	Strair, Roger (NJ)	Hem	764
Steinberg, Harry (NY)	Pul	541	Strange, Theodore (NY)	IM	479
Steinberg, Jonathan (NY)	CE	127	Strashun, Arnold (NY)	NuM	430
Steinberg, L Gary (NY)	PCd	282	Strassberg, Barbara (NY)	Ped	394
Steinberger, Alfred (NY)	NS	220	Strauch, Robert (NY)	HS	180
Steiner, Henry (NY)	S	450	Straus, David (NY)	Onc	212

Name	Specialty	Pg	Name	Specialty	Pg
Strauss, Barry (NY)	Onc	575	Sunaryo, Francis (NJ)	PGe	720
Strauss, Bernard (NJ)	U	729	Sundaram, Revathy (NY)	PHO	439
Strauss, Edward (CT)	DR	869	Sung, Kap-Jae (NY)	S	471
Strauss, Elton (NY)	OrS	265	Sunshine, Robert (NY)	U	549
Strauss, H William (NY)	NuM	232	Suri, Ranjit (NY)	CE	128
Strauss, Michael (NY)	IM	197	Surks, Martin (NY)	EDM	374
Strauss, Nancy (NY)	PMR	300	Surow, Jason (NJ)	Oto	684
Street, Lynn (CT)	Ger	906	Sussman, Barry (NJ)	S	695
Stringel, Gustavo (NY)	PS	635	Sussman, Norman (NY)	Psyc	321
Strobeck, John (NJ)	Cv	819	Sussman, Robert (NJ)	Pul	855
Stroh, Jack (NJ)	Cv	830	Sutton, Ira (NY)	FMed	606
Strome, Marshall (NY)	Oto	275	Suzman, Michael (NY)	PlS	639
Strongwater, Allan (NJ)	OrS	823	Svitra, Paul (NY)	Oph	523
Strongwater, Richard (NY)	FMed	606	Swamy, Samala (NY)	Cv	476
Strutin, Millard (NJ)	S	815	Swee, David (NJ)	FMed	762
Stubblefield, Michael (NY)	PMR	300	Sweeney, Eugene (NJ)	D	665
Stubgen, Joerg-Patrick (NY)	N	229	Sweeney, Thomas (CT)	VascS	923
Stuchin, Steven (NY)	OrS	265	Swerdlow, Michael (NY)	N	385
Sturm, Richard (NY)	Oph	522	Swiderski, Deborah (NY)	IM	380
Sturza, Jeffrey (NY)	D	603	Swiller, Hillel (NY)	Psyc	321
Suchy, Frederick (NY)	PGe	285	Swirsky, Michael (NY)	DR	373
Suda, Anjuli (NJ)	Ped	812	Swistel, Alexander (NY)	S	347
Sudhakar, Telechery (NJ)	Nep	746	Swistel, Daniel (NY)	TS	352
Sugarman, Lynn (NJ)	Ped	688	Syracuse, Donald (NJ)	TS	728
Suggs, William (NY)	VascS	401	Szabo, Albert (NY)	N	622
Sukumaran, Muthiah (NY)	Pul	328	Szabo, Andrew (NY)	EDM	162
Sulica, Radu Lucian (NY)	Oto	275			
Sullivan, Ann (NY)	Psyc	469			
Sullivan, Christopher (NJ)	MF	821	**T**		
Sullivan, James (NY)	CRS	497			
Sullivan, James (NY)	Rhu	544	Tabachnick, John (NJ)	FMed	845
Sullivan, Scott (CT)	DR	869	Tabar, Viviane (NY)	NS	220
Sullivan, Timothy (NY)	Psyc	641	Tabbal, Nicolas (NY)	PlS	308
Sullum, Stanford (NY)	ObG	237	Tabershaw, Richard (NY)	OrS	579
Sultan, Khalid (NY)	RE	333	Taffet, Berton (NJ)	OrS	810
Sultan, Mark (NY)	PlS	307	Taffet, Sanford (NY)	Ge	610
Sultan, Ronald (NJ)	S	738	Tagawa, Scott (NY)	Onc	212
Sumpio, Bauer (CT)	VascS	923	Taikowski, Richard (CT)	Cv	867
Sun, Shyan-chu (NJ)	NP	713	Taitsman, James (NJ)	OrS	749

Alphabetical Listing of Doctors

Name	Specialty	Pg	Name	Specialty	Pg
Tal, Avraham (NY)	IM	423	Temple, Larissa (NY)	CRS	143
Talansky, Arthur (NY)	Ge	505	Tenenbaum, Joseph (NY)	Cv	137
Talansky, Marvin (NJ)	Oph	791	Tenet, William (NY)	Cv	495
Tallia, Alfred (NJ)	FMed	762	Tennenbaum, Steven (NJ)	U	698
Tallman, Martin (NY)	Hem	184	Tenner, Michael (NY)	NRad	623
Tamborlane, William (CT)	PEn	915	Teodorescu, Victoria (NY)	VascS	364
Tamerin, John (CT)	Psyc	892	Teperman, Lewis (NY)	S	347
Tan, Mark (NY)	Rhu	587	Tepler, Melvin (NY)	OrS	436
Tanchajja, Supoj (NY)	S	450	Teplitz, Glenn (NY)	HS	507
Tancredi, Laurence (NY)	Psyc	322	Tepper, Howard (NJ)	PlS	854
Taneja, Samir (NY)	U	360	Terjanian, Terenig (NY)	Onc	480
Tanenbaum, Diane (NY)	D	152	Tesser, Mark (NY)	D	152
Tanoue, Lynn (CT)	Pul	918	Tessler, Sidney (NY)	Pul	446
Tanowitz, Herbert (NY)	Inf	379	Testa, Francine (CT)	ChiN	903
Tanzer, Floyd (NJ)	D	820	Teusink, J Paul (NY)	Psyc	322
Tarasuk, Albert (NY)	U	472	Tewari, Ashutosh (NY)	U	360
Tardiff, Kenneth (NY)	Psyc	322	Theofanidis, Stylianos (CT)	NP	879
Tartaglia, Joseph (NY)	Cv	598	Thomas, Bryon (CT)	IM	876
Tartell, Jay (NY)	DR	459	Thomas, David (NY)	PMR	300
Tartini, Albert (NJ)	Nep	677	Thomas, Gary (NY)	PM	278
Tartter, Paul (NY)	S	347	Thomas, Mark (NY)	PMR	395
Tassiopoulos, Apostolos (NY)	VascS	589	Thomashow, Byron (NY)	Pul	328
Taub, Peter (NY)	PlS	308	Thomsen, Stephen (NJ)	Nep	735
Taubin, Howard (CT)	Ge	872	Thomson, J Grant (CT)	HS	907
Taubman, Lowell (NY)	IM	510	Thorne, Charles (NY)	PlS	308
Tavill, Michael (NJ)	PO	793	Thornton, Scott (CT)	CRS	868
Tawfik, Bernard (NY)	Oto	526	Tibaldi, Joseph (NY)	EDM	460
Tay, Steven (NY)	IM	197	Ticker, Jonathan (NY)	OrS	524
Taylor, Howard (NJ)	Oto	810	Tierney, Peter (NJ)	FMed	762
Taylor, Hugh (CT)	RE	919	Tiger, Louis (NY)	Rhu	544
Taylor, James (NY)	TS	547	Tillem, Steven (NY)	U	472
Taylor, Noel (NY)	Psyc	322	Timpone, Leonard (NY)	IM	510
Te, Alexis (NY)	U	360	Tindel, Nathaniel (NY)	OrS	265
Teffera, Fassil (NY)	IM	381	Tinetti, Mary (CT)	Ger	906
Teichholz, Louis (NJ)	Cv	663	Ting, Andrew (NY)	PPul	291
Teirstein, Alvin (NY)	Pul	328	Ting, Jess (NY)	PlS	308
Tello, Celso (NY)	Oph	252	Tinger, Alfred (NY)	RadRO	644
Telzak, Edward (NY)	Inf	380	Tischler, Henry (NY)	OrS	436
Tempera, Patrick (NJ)	Ge	845	Tiszenkel, Howard (NY)	CRS	458

Name	Specialty	Pg	Name	Specialty	Pg
Tittle, Shawn (CT)	TS	896	Troy, Kevin (NY)	Hem	184
Tiwari, Ram (NY)	Oph	387	Tsai, James (CT)	Oph	913
Tobias, Daniel (NJ)	GO	805	Tuchman, Alan (NY)	N	229
Tobias, Geoffrey (NJ)	Oto	684	Tuerk-Mendelsohn, Lois (NY)	A&I	594
Tobias, Hillel (NY)	Ge	173	Tugal, Oya (NY)	PHO	634
Todd, George (NY)	VascS	364	Tuhrim, Stanley (NY)	N	229
Tohme, Jack (NJ)	EDM	667	Turbin, Roger (NJ)	Oph	717
Tolan, Robert (NJ)	PInf	775	Turcios, Nelson (NJ)	PPul	834
Tolchin, Joan (NY)	Psyc	322	Turecki, Stanley (NY)	ChAP	140
Tolchin, Sara (NY)	Ped	394	Turetsky, Arthur (CT)	IM	876
Toles, Allen (NY)	ObG	520	Turitto, Gioia (NY)	CE	408
Tolston, Evelyn (NY)	A&I	126	Turk, Jon (NY)	Oto	526
Tom, David (CT)	Oph	884	Turner, Ira (NY)	N	518
Tom, Jack (NY)	D	568	Turro, James (NY)	IM	616
Tomao, Frank (NY)	Onc	513	Turtel, Andrew (NY)	OrS	265
Toomey, Kathleen (NJ)	Hem	831	Turtel, Lawrence (NJ)	Oph	791
Topilow, Arthur (NJ)	Hem	788	Turtel, Penny (NJ)	Ge	787
Topilow, Harvey (NJ)	Oph	681	Tuttle, R Michael (NY)	EDM	162
Toppmeyer, Deborah (NJ)	Onc	767	Tyberg, Theodore (NY)	Cv	137
Torman, Julie (NY)	Ge	610	Tyshkov, Michael (NJ)	PGe	852
Tornos, Carmen (NY)	Path	580			
Torrado-Jule, Carmen (NY)	PEn	483			
Torre, Arthur (NJ)	PA&I	719			
Tortolani, Anthony (NY)	TS	451	**U**		
Tostanoski, Jean (NY)	Oph	627			
Touliopoulos, Steven (NY)	OrS	467	Uday, Kalpana (NY)	Nep	383
Tozzi, Robert (NJ)	PCd	685	Udell, Ira (NY)	Oph	523
Trachtman, Howard (NY)	PNep	532	Udelsman, Robert (CT)	S	921
Traeger, Eveline (NJ)	ChiN	843	Uhm, Kyudong (NJ)	Onc	821
Traister, Michael (NY)	Ped	297	Ullman, Joel (NY)	ObG	625
Tranbaugh, Robert (NY)	TS	353	Ullman, Thomas (NY)	Ge	173
Traquina, Diana (NJ)	PO	775	Underberg, James (NY)	IM	197
Traube, Charles (NY)	Cv	410	Underberg-Davis, Sharon (NJ)	DR	760
Traube, Morris (NY)	Ge	173	Unger, Allen (NY)	Cv	137
Travis, William (NY)	Path	280	Unger, Walter (NY)	D	152
Treiber, Ruth (NY)	D	603	Unis, George (NY)	OrS	266
Treiser, Susan (NJ)	RE	836	Unterricht, Sam (NY)	Oph	434
Tria, Alfred (NJ)	OrS	834	Upadhyay, Yogendra (NY)	Psyc	585
Troy, Allen (CT)	OrS	886	Urban, William (NY)	OrS	436
			Urbanek, Richard (NY)	D	476

Alphabetical Listing of Doctors

Name	Specialty	Pg	Name	Specialty	Pg
Urken, Mark (NY)	Oto	275	Vester, John (NJ)	N	747
Ushay, H Michael (NY)	PCCM	390	Vialotti, Charles (NJ)	RadRO	692
Uy, Vena (NJ)	ObG	735	Vickery, Carlin (NY)	PlS	308
			Vieira, Jeffrey (NY)	IM	423
			Vigorita, John (NJ)	Ped	853
			Vigorita, Vincent (NY)	Path	437
V			Villafranca, Manuel (NJ)	Psyc	854
Vad, Vijay (NY)	PMR	300	Villamena, Patricia (NY)	Pul	328
Vahdat, Linda (NY)	Onc	212	Vincent, Miriam (NY)	FMed	415
Vaidya, Sudhir (NY)	FMed	606	Vinciguerra, Vincent (NY)	Onc	514
Vaillancourt, Philippe (NY)	PM	580	Vine, Anthony (NY)	S	348
Valda, Victor (NJ)	PS	687	Vine, John (NJ)	D	742
Valenza, Joseph (NJ)	PMR	812	Viner, Nicholas (CT)	U	897
Valinoti, Anne Marie (NJ)	IM	673	Vingan, Roy (NJ)	NS	678
Vallarino, Ramon (NY)	PMR	443	Vining, Eugenia (CT)	Oto	914
Vallone, Ambrose (NY)	PCd	529	Vintzileos, Anthony (NY)	MF	512
Vambutas, Andrea (NY)	Oto	526	Violi, Caterina (CT)	ObG	882
van Dyck, Christopher (CT)	GerPsy	906	Visconti, Ernest (NY)	Ped	483
Van Engel, Daniel (NJ)	N	679	Viswanathan, Kusum (NY)	PHO	439
Van Slooten, David (NJ)	N	679	Viswanathan, Ramaswamy (NY)	Psyc	444
Van Zee, Kimberly (NY)	S	347	Vitale, Gerard (NY)	S	546
Vanheertum, Ronald (NY)	NuM	232	Vitale, Michael (NY)	OrS	266
Vapnek, Jonathan (NY)	U	360	Vitenson, Jack (NJ)	U	698
Vargas, Ileana (NY)	PEn	284	Vitting, Kevin (NJ)	Nep	821
Varriale, Philip (NY)	Cv	137	Vivek, Seeth (NY)	Psyc	469
Varsos, George (NY)	RadRO	470	Vogel, James (NY)	Hem	184
Vas, George (NY)	N	430	Vogel, Louis (NY)	D	152
Vasselli, Anthony (NJ)	U	753	Vogel, Mitchell (NJ)	Oph	822
Vastola, A Paul (NY)	Oto	437	Vogelman, Arthur (NY)	Ge	462
Vasudeva, Kusum (NY)	ObG	520	Vogiatzi, Maria (NY)	PEn	284
Vaswani, Ashok (NY)	EDM	501	Vogl, Steven (NY)	Onc	382
Vates, Thomas (NJ)	U	780	Volcovici, Guido (NY)	Pul	328
Vazzana, Thomas (NY)	Cv	476	Volkmar, Fred (CT)	ChAP	902
Velcek, Francisca (NY)	PS	293	Volpe, Anthony (NJ)	IM	673
Veloso, Manuel (NY)	ObG	520	Volpi, David (NY)	Oto	276
Vera, Reinaldo (NY)	ChAP	411	Vukasin, Alexander (NJ)	U	753
Verga, Michele (NY)	PlS	308			
Versfelt, Mary (NY)	Ped	637			
Vesole, David (NJ)	Hem	671			

Name	Specialty	Pg
W		
Wachtel, Alan (NY)	Psyc	322
Wager, Marc (NY)	Ped	637
Wager, Steven (NY)	Psyc	322
Wagle, Sharad (NJ)	Psyc	691
Wagman, Raquel (NJ)	RadRO	725
Wagner, John (NY)	Nep	515
Wagner, Rudolph (NJ)	Oph	717
Wainstein, Sasha (NY)	U	453
Waintraub, Stanley (NJ)	Onc	675
Walczyk, John (NY)	D	499
Waldman, Seth (NY)	PM	278
Waldorf, Donald (NY)	D	553
Waldorf, Heidi (NY)	D	554
Walfish, Jacob (NY)	IM	197
Wallach, Frances (NY)	Inf	189
Wallach, Robert (NY)	GO	178
Wallack, Joel (NY)	Psyc	322
Wallack, Marc (NY)	S	348
Wallerstein, Robert (NJ)	CG	663
Wallis, Joseph (NJ)	ObG	808
Walser, Lawrence (NY)	Pul	585
Walsh, B Timothy (NY)	Psyc	322
Walsh, Christina (NJ)	Onc	789
Walsh, Christine (NY)	PCd	389
Walsh, Francis (CT)	IM	876
Walsh, Joseph (NY)	Oph	252
Walsh, Raymond (NY)	OrS	436
Walther, Robert (NY)	D	152
Waner, Milton (NY)	Oto	276
Wang, Frederick (NY)	Oph	252
Wang, Jen Chin (NY)	Onc	514
Wang, John (NY)	Nep	216
Wang, Timothy (NY)	Ge	174
Wangenheim, Paul (NJ)	Cv	705
Wapner, Ronald (NY)	MF	201
Ward, Barbara (CT)	S	896
Ward, Robert (NY)	PO	290

Name	Specialty	Pg
Wardlaw, Sharon (NY)	EDM	162
Warman, Jacob (NY)	EDM	414
Warner, Robert (NY)	D	152
Warren, Floyd (NY)	Oph	252
Warren, Michelle (NY)	RE	333
Warren, Ronald (NJ)	IM	744
Warren, Russell (NY)	OrS	266
Warren, Wendy (NJ)	MF	712
Wasnick, Robert (NY)	U	589
Wasser, Kenneth (NJ)	Rhu	795
Wasserman, Barry (NJ)	Oph	748
Wasserman, Eric (CT)	Oph	884
Wasserman, Gary (NJ)	U	698
Wasserman, Hal (CT)	IC	876
Wasserman, Kenneth (NJ)	IM	673
Wasserman, Patricia (NY)	Path	527
Waters, Cheryl (NY)	N	229
Waters, Paul (CT)	TS	897
Watson, Rita (NJ)	IC	789
Wattenberg, Debra (NY)	D	153
Wax, Michael (NJ)	Onc	847
Waxberg, Jonathan (CT)	U	897
Waxenbaum, Steven (NJ)	CRS	663
Waye, Jerome (NY)	Ge	174
Wayne, Peter (NY)	Ge	610
Waynik, Mark (CT)	Psyc	892
Weber, Pamela (NY)	Oph	579
Weber, Richard (CT)	Oph	884
Weck, Steven (NY)	DR	500
Wedderburn, Raymond (NY)	S	348
Weg, Arnold (NY)	Ge	462
Weg, Ira (NY)	Cv	495
Wehmann, Robert (NJ)	EDM	667
Wei, Fong (NJ)	Nep	746
Weidhaas, Joanne (CT)	RadRO	919
Weiland, Andrew (NY)	HS	180
Weill, Terry (NY)	Psyc	323
Wein, Paul (NY)	Cv	410
Weinberg, Gerard (NY)	PS	392

Alphabetical Listing of Doctors

Name	Specialty	Pg	Name	Specialty	Pg
Weinberg, Harlan (NY)	Pul	644	Weisenseel, Arthur (NY)	Cv	138
Weinberg, Harold (NY)	N	230	Weiser, Martin (NY)	CRS	144
Weinberg, Jeffrey (NY)	PMR	484	Weiser, Robert (NY)	VascS	453
Weinberg, Marc (NY)	Cv	565	Weisholtz, Steven (NJ)	Inf	672
Weinberg, Martin (NJ)	Oph	681	Weiss, Carol (NY)	AdP	123
Weinberger, George (NJ)	D	844	Weiss, Darryl (NJ)	D	665
Weinberger, Jesse (NY)	N	230	Weiss, E Michael (NJ)	Cv	819
Weinberger, Judah (NY)	IC	199	Weiss, Gabriella (NJ)	Inf	821
Weinberger, Michael (NY)	PM	278	Weiss, Gerson (NJ)	RE	693
Weinberger, Sylvain (NY)	Ped	297	Weiss, Louis (NY)	Inf	380
Weinblatt, Mark (NY)	PHO	531	Weiss, Lynne (NJ)	PNep	775
Weine, Gary (NJ)	IM	806	Weiss, Melvin (NY)	Cv	598
Weiner, Howard (NY)	NS	221	Weiss, Michael (NY)	Oph	252
Weiner, Kevin (NY)	PMR	300	Weiss, Paul (NY)	PlS	308
Weiner, Lon (NY)	OrS	266	Weiss, Rita (NY)	Onc	514
Weiner, Michael (NY)	PHO	288	Weiss, Robert (NY)	Ge	174
Weiner, Richard (NY)	Ped	394	Weiss, Robert (NJ)	U	780
Weinerman, Stuart (NY)	EDM	502	Weiss, Robert (NY)	PNep	634
Weinfeld, Steven (NY)	OrS	266	Weiss, Robert (CT)	U	922
Weingarten, Jacqueline (NY)	PCCM	390	Weiss, Steven (NJ)	A&I	703
Weingarten, Phyllis (NY)	Oph	557	Weissman, Gary (NY)	Ge	505
Weinreb, Jeffrey (CT)	DR	905	Weissman, Ronald (NY)	Cv	598
Weinstein, David (CT)	ObG	882	Weisstuch, Joseph (NY)	Nep	216
Weinstein, Jay (NY)	IM	198	Weizman, Howard (NJ)	Nep	677
Weinstein, Joseph (NY)	Oph	523	Welch, Peter (NY)	Inf	612
Weinstein, Joshua (NY)	Rhu	398	Wells, Scott (NY)	PlS	308
Weinstein, Larry (NJ)	PlS	813	Welsh, Howard (NY)	Psyc	323
Weinstein, Mark (NY)	IM	510	Welshinger, Marie (NY)	GO	462
Weinstein, Melvin (NJ)	Inf	764	Wenig, Bruce (NY)	Path	280
Weinstein, Paul (CT)	Onc	878	Wert, Sanford (NY)	OrS	436
Weinstein, Richard (NY)	OrS	629	Wertkin, Martin (NY)	S	648
Weinstein, Samuel (NY)	TS	400	Weseley, Peter (NY)	Oph	252
Weinstein, Toba (NY)	PGe	530	Wesson, Michael (NJ)	RadRO	692
Weinstock, Gary (NY)	A&I	490	Westrich, Geoffrey (NY)	OrS	266
Weintraub, Howard (NY)	Cv	138	Wetherbee, Roger (NY)	Inf	189
Weintraub, Joshua (NY)	VIR	361	Wetzler, Graciela (NY)	PGe	439
Weintraub, Michael (NY)	N	623	Wexler, Craig (NY)	EDM	569
Weisbrot, Deborah (NY)	ChAP	566	Wexler, Leonard (NY)	PHO	288
Weiselberg, Lora (NY)	Onc	514	Wexler, Patricia (NY)	D	153

Name	Specialty	Pg	Name	Specialty	Pg
Wey, Philip (NJ)	PlS	777	Wisnicki, H Jay (NY)	Oph	253
Whelan, Richard (NY)	CRS	144	Wisoff, Jeffrey (NY)	NS	221
White, Robert (CT)	VIR	922	Wisotsky, David (NJ)	Ped	689
White, Ronald (NJ)	CRS	664	Witt, Barry (CT)	RE	894
Whitley-Williams, Patricia (NJ)	PInf	775	Witt, Marvin (NY)	IM	198
Whitman, Eric (NJ)	S	815	Witte, Arnold (NJ)	N	747
Whitman, Hendricks (NJ)	Rhu	855	Wittig, James (NY)	OrS	267
Whitmore, Wayne (NY)	Oph	252	Wiznia, Andrew (NY)	PA&I	389
Whyte, Dilys (NY)	PNep	582	Wohlberg, Gary (NY)	Pul	586
Wickiewicz, Thomas (NY)	OrS	266	Wolf, David (NY)	Hem	185
Wickremesinghe, Prasanna (NY)	Ge	478	Wolf, David (NY)	Ge	610
Widmann, Mark (NJ)	TS	816	Wolf, Ellen (NY)	DR	373
Widmann, Roger (NY)	OrS	267	Wolf, Kenneth (NY)	Oph	387
Wiesen, Mark (NJ)	EDM	667	Wolf, Steven (NY)	ChiN	141
Wilbur, Sabrina (NY)	CE	408	Wolf-Klein, Gisele (NY)	Ger	506
Wilchinsky, Mark (CT)	OrS	886	Wolfe, Lawrence (NY)	PHO	531
Williams, Daniel (NY)	ChAP	495	Wolfe, Mary (NY)	IM	616
Williams, John (NY)	U	361	Wolfe, Scott (NY)	HS	180
Williams, Mathew (NY)	TS	353	Wolff, Steven (NY)	DR	158
Williams, Riley (NY)	OrS	267	Wolfson, Robert (NY)	IM	616
Willner, Joseph (NJ)	N	679	Wolintz, Arthur (NY)	Oph	434
Wilner, Philip (NY)	Psyc	323	Wolk, Michael (NY)	Cv	138
Wilson, Arnold (NY)	OrS	388	Wollack, Jan (NJ)	ChiN	758
Wilson, Lynn (CT)	RadRO	919	Wolodiger, Fred (NJ)	VascS	699
Wilson, Thomas (NY)	PEn	581	Wong, James (NJ)	RadRO	814
Winant, John (NJ)	A&I	741	Wong, Martha (NY)	Ped	394
Winchester, James (NY)	Nep	216	Wong, Michael (NJ)	Oph	748
Windsor, Russell (NY)	OrS	267	Wong, Raymond (NY)	Oph	253
Wineburg, Elliot (NY)	Psyc	323	Wong, Richard (NJ)	Oph	748
Winston, Jonathan (NY)	Nep	216	Woo, Henry (NY)	NS	575
Winter, Robin (NJ)	FMed	762	Woo, Peak (NY)	Oto	276
Winter, Stephen (CT)	Pul	893	Wormser, Gary (NY)	Inf	612
Winter, Steven (NY)	Cv	476	Worth, David (NJ)	Rhu	856
Winterkorn, Jacqueline (NY)	Oph	252	Wright, Albert (NY)	S	451
Winters, Richard (NY)	Psyc	323	Wrone, David (NJ)	D	760
Winters, Stephen (NJ)	CE	801	Wu, Chia (NJ)	Cv	705
Wisch, Nathaniel (NY)	Hem	184	Wu, Hen-Vai (NJ)	Onc	832
Wiseman, Paul (NY)	IM	198	Wu, Jason (NY)	Ped	442
Wishner, Jerald (NY)	CRS	601	Wyner, Perry (NY)	Pul	541

Alphabetical Listing of Doctors

Name	Specialty	Pg	Name	Specialty	Pg
Wysoki, Randee (NY)	ObG	625	Young, Joshua (NY)	Oph	253
Wysolmerski, John (CT)	EDM	905	Young, Stuart (NY)	A&I	126
Wyszynski, Bernard (NY)	Psyc	396	Youngerman, Jay (NY)	Oto	526
			Yudin, Howard (NY)	FMed	607
			Yung, Elizabeth (NY)	NuM	519

Y

Name	Specialty	Pg
Yablon, Steven (NY)	Nep	556
Yadoo, Moshe (NY)	Ped	468
Yaffe, Bruce (NY)	IM	198
Yagoda, Arnold (NY)	Oph	253
Yahalom, Joachim (NY)	RadRO	330
Yalamanchi, Krishan (NJ)	Ped	776
Yale, Suzanne (NY)	ObG	237
Yamane, Michael (NJ)	IM	745
Yancovitz, Stanley (NY)	Inf	189
Yang, Roger (NJ)	DR	830
Yang, S Steven (NY)	HS	181
Yankelevitz, David (NY)	DR	158
Yankelowitz, Stanley (NY)	Oto	388
Yannuzzi, Lawrence (NY)	Oph	253
Yarberry Allen, Patricia (NY)	ObG	238
Yasgur, David (NY)	OrS	629
Yee, Arthur (CT)	Inf	874
Yee, Arthur (NY)	Rhu	338
Yegudin-Ash, Julia (NY)	Rhu	645
Yeh, Timothy (NJ)	PCCM	720
Yellin, Joseph (NY)	N	430
Yi, Peter (NJ)	Onc	746
Yiengpruksawan, Anusak (NJ)	S	696
Yip, Chun (NY)	Pul	328
Yoo, Jinil (NY)	Nep	383
Yoon, Sydney (NY)	DR	500
Yorke, Eric (NJ)	Ped	835
Youner, Craig (NY)	DR	459
Young, Bruce (NY)	ObG	238
Young, Constance (NY)	ObG	386
Young, George (NY)	U	361
Young, Iven (NY)	EDM	162

Z

Name	Specialty	Pg
Zaccaria, Alan (NJ)	PlS	794
Zackson, David (NY)	IM	198
Zager, Robert (NJ)	Hem	710
Zagzag, David (NY)	Path	280
Zahtz, Gerald (NY)	Oto	527
Zaidman, Gerald (NY)	Oph	628
Zairis, Ignatios (NJ)	TS	696
Zalkowitz, Alan (NJ)	Rhu	694
Zaloom, Robert (NY)	Cv	410
Zalvan, Craig (NY)	Oto	631
Zambetti, George (NY)	OrS	267
Zampella, Edward (NJ)	NS	807
Zapolanski, Alex (NJ)	TS	696
Zarbin, Marco (NJ)	Oph	717
Zaremski, Benjamin (NY)	Cv	138
Zarich, Stuart (CT)	Cv	867
Zarowitz, William (NY)	IM	616
Zauber, N Peter (NJ)	Hem	710
Zbar, Lloyd (NJ)	Oto	718
Zeale, Peter (NY)	IM	198
Zeitels, Jerrold (NJ)	PlS	854
Zeitlin, Alan (NY)	S	471
Zeldis, Steven (NY)	Cv	495
Zelefsky, Michael (NY)	RadRO	330
Zelenetz, Andrew (NY)	Onc	213
Zelicof, Steven (NY)	OrS	630
Zelkowitz, Richard (CT)	Onc	878
Zellner, James (NY)	Oph	434
Zelman, Warren (NY)	Oto	527
Zeltsman, Vadim (NY)	TS	547

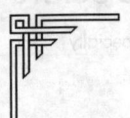

The Best in American Medicine
www.CastleConnolly.com

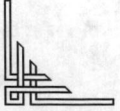

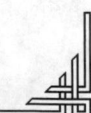

Acknowledgments

The publishers would like to thank the entire staff for their many hours and days of intense and precise work on this guide in order to further its goal of assisting consumers in making the best healthcare choices.

Castle Connolly Executive Management:

Chairman	John K. Castle
President & CEO	John J. Connolly, Ed.D.
Vice President, Chief Medical & Research Officer	Jean Morgan, M.D.
Vice President, Chief Strategy & Operations Officer	William Liss-Levinson, Ph.D.
Research Coordinators	Maryann Hynd, RN
	Sara Sezer
	Terysia Herbert
	Mandy Guerrero
	Jerville Weekes
Book Layout, Database Management	Russell Hodgson
Office Manager, Book Coordination	Marcie Samartino
Corporate Services Manager	Jennifer Mojave
Social Media/Public Relations Coordinator	Nicki Hughes

We also would like to extend our gratitude to the American Board of Medical Specialties (ABMS) for allowing us to use excerpts, especially the descriptions of medical specialties and subspecialties, from the text of their publication "Which Medical Specialist for You?"

Other Publications from Castle Connolly Medical Ltd.:
America's Top Doctors®; *America's Top Doctors® for Cancer*; and *Top Doctors®: New York Metro Area* and others...
Order online at http://www.castleconnolly.com/books

The Best in American Medicine
www.CastleConnolly.com

Special Products and Services
provided by Castle Connolly Medical Ltd

Corporate Membership

This service enables an employer to assist employees in identifying Top Doctors to care for themselves and their families. It is a low-cost, non-intrusive service that will result in better care and, ultimately, lower costs.

For $2-$5 per employee/family per year, employees have complete access to the Castle Connolly website and database of Top Doctors nominated by their peers and screened by the Castle Connolly physician-led research team.

Instead of simply picking a doctor's name from the phone book or a plan directory, the employee can compare physician names to the Castle Connolly database of 26,000 plus Top Doctors and select from among the best. This will result in overall better care, lower costs and improved morale.

For further information, contact:

Jennifer Mojave

Corporate Services Manager

212.367.8400, ext. 35

or

jmojave@castleconnolly.com

The Doctor-Patient Advisor (Corporate)

The Doctor-Patient Advisor program is a higher level service at still a low cost- $.50-$10 (depending on employee numbers) per employee - per month. Employees can call Castle Connolly and speak with a Registered Nurse who, utilizing the Castle Connolly data base, will identify top doctors and hospitals to meet the client's needs.

For further information, contact:

Jennifer Mojave

Corporate Services Manager

212.367.8400, ext. 35

or

jmojave@castleconnolly.com

The New Movers Program

Perhaps nothing is more challenging to a family that is transferred or takes a position in a new community, than finding appropriate healthcare resources, especially physicians. While they can turn to recommendations from new neighbors and friends, or pick names from the phone book or a plan directory, that is hardly adequate, especially when there are special healthcare needs in the family.

The Castle Connolly New Movers Program is designed to alleviate that concern, or even fear, as well as the time-consuming struggle to identify the right – and best – doctors and hospitals in the new community or region.

The cost is $2,500.00 per family and includes identifying primary care physicians (Pediatricians, OB/GYN, Internists) as well as other specialists that may be needed (e.g., Ophthalmologists, Allergists, Endocrinologists, etc.).

For further information, contact:

Jennifer Mojave

Corporate Services Manager

212.367.8400, ext. 35

or

jmojave@castleconnolly.com

Doctor-Patient Advisor (Consumers)

Doctor-Patient Advisor is a Castle Connolly Medical Ltd. service providing one-on-one consultations with a physician or nurse practitioner to individuals who have serious or complex medical problems or to anyone who feels he/she needs assistance finding the right physician for any purpose. Each client will receive personalized assistance in identifying the appropriate specialists for his/her condition, utilizing the Castle Connolly Medical Ltd. database of physicians and hospitals, as well as individual searches, to locate the best resources to meet the client's needs.

Fee: $375. For further information call (212) 367-8400 x 16.

Strategic Partnerships

Castle Connolly Medical Ltd. has a number of strategic partnerships that may be of interest to consumers and physicians

Empowered Doctor

Empowered Doctor develops practice websites for physicians, all of whom must first be screened and vetted by the physician-led research department of Castle Connolly Medical Ltd. Websites are designed for new patients to easily find the physician and request an appointment, as well as to serve as a resource for existing patients. Website features include: Practice brochures; appointment and prescription refill request forms; patient intake forms; a patient education library; and a library of the latest news stories related to the physician's medical specialty.

For further information call toll free (866) 375-4007, or visit www.empowereddoctor.net.

The Best in American Medicine
www.CastleConnolly.com

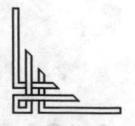
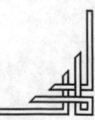

DrScore.com

Founded by Steven Feldman, M.D., DrScore.com is an interactive online survey site where patients can rate their physicians, as well as find a physician based on their service level preference. The mission of DrScore.com is to improve medical care by giving patients a forum for rating their physician and by giving doctors an affordable, objective, non-intrusive means of documenting the quality of care that they provide. Visitors on Castle Connolly's website who are searching for "topdoctors" have the option to also rate these and other physicians they have been to as patients, as well as to see if these physicians have been rated previously by other consumers on DrScore.com. Visitors to DrScore.com will be able to see if their doctors and/or other doctors are Castle Connolly "top doctors."

For more information, visit www.drscore.com.

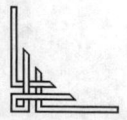
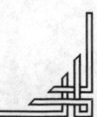

The Best in American Medicine
www.CastleConnolly.com

Consumer's Medical Resource (CMR)

Consumer's Medical Resource was started in 1996 to offer high-quality, high-impact employee benefit programs to help employees and their dependents, and has been a pioneer in Medical Decision Support® services. CMR addresses all medical conditions at any point within the continuum of care, by providing personalized, evidence-based medical research, information, and support services to employees who face serious, complicated, and chronic illness, or would like to become well-informed healthcare consumers. Leveraging a state-of-the-art integrated model of Web, phone, and print-based services, CMR enables employees to fully understand and evaluate their options so they can make the most informed medical decisions possible with their doctors. The company is privately held and currently provides services to more than 600,000 Americans, achieving extremely high levels of user and customer satisfaction, improved clinical quality outcomes, and generated excellent ROI.

Castle Connolly and CMR are working together to provide Castle Connolly's various corporate services to CMR client companies and their employees.

Castle Connolly LifeStream MD

Castle Connolly Medical Ltd. has a strategic relationship with Castle Connolly LifeStream MD to provide a unique health advisory service designed for families and executives, especially those who travel regularly or may have more than one residence.

Each client is assigned a Castle Connolly LifeStream MD physician who is available to them by phone 24/7/365. A client call from anywhere in the world is answered in ten seconds or less and within ten minutes or less, the client is connected with their Castle Connolly LifeStream MD physician advisor. Castle Connolly LifeStream MDs work in teams of three per client. Each team has available a secure, password protected web-based emergency personal medical record for their clients to be referenced while providing advice and may assist other physicians in accessing this information with the members permission. Castle Connolly LifeStream MD constructs and periodically updates this personal medical record in conjunction with the client's primary care physician. The Castle Connolly LifeStream MD physician acts as a health manager assisting in navigation of an increasingly complex health care environment. The Castle Connolly LifeStream MD physician does not replace the member's primary physician or specialists, but provides additional independent counsel and services that provide security to our members either at home or while traveling.

In the United States, the Castle Connolly LifeStream MD physician will use the Castle Connolly database of Top Doctors to refer the client to an excellent physician and hospital for non-urgent care or will direct them to an excellent hospital for urgent care. Assistance in securing timely appointments with specialists and records transfer is facilitated as needed.

Outside of the United States, Castle Connolly LifeStream MD has an affiliation with International SOS, the world's largest and leading provider of medical travel assistance. While traveling abroad, International SOS will guide the client to the very best local care center and doctors, provide assistance, and, if necessary, provide medical transport to the best regional facility or, as necessary, orchestrate air evacuation to the U.S. The Castle Connolly LifeStream MD physician assists with access to our members' medical records and provides communication between physicians at the point of care, our client's primary and specialist physicians, and family members.

The annual cost of this service is: $7,500 per individual; $10,000 per couple; $12,500 per family of four; and $15,000 for a family of eight. The price is negotiable for families larger than eight.

For information, contact 877-760-3418;
or visit http://www.lifestreammd.com.

National Physician of the Year Awards

National Physician of the Year Awards Castle Connolly Medical Ltd. proudly hosted its fifth annual *National Physician of the Year Awards* on March 22, 2010 at The Hudson theatre New York City. It was a spectacular evening which allowed us to recognize both the outstanding honorees and the excellence of the many thousands of physicians throughout the nation.

The Genesis of the National Physician of the Year Award.

Each year we receive thousands of nominations from physicians and the medical leadership of major medical centers, specialty hospitals, teaching hospitals and regional and community medical centers across the United States as an integral part of our research, screening and selection process to identify *America's Top Doctors*®. The selected physicians, while spread across all fifty states and involved in more than 70 medical specialties and subspecialties, all share one distinguishing professional attribute: an unwavering dedication to their patients and to medicine as a whole. Each and every one of these outstanding medical professionals is a symbol of the clinical excellence that characterizes American medicine. In honor of these exemplary physicians, Castle Connolly Medical Ltd. has created the *National Physician of the Year Awards* to recognize the thousands of excellent, dedicated physicians across the United States. Our Medical Advisory Board selected the honorees from the hundreds nominated in a special nomination process conducted months before the event.

The honorees, Drs. John B. Buse, Larry Norton and Ching-Hon Pui are superb examples of excellence in clinical medical practice. In addition to these awards for Clinical Excellence, Castle Connolly Medical Ltd. honored Drs. Basil I. Hirschowitz and Leonard Apt for their lifetime achievement in medicine. Matthew Reeve and Alexandra Reeve Givens, board members of the Christopher & Dana Reeve Foundation, are tireless fundraisers for this organization and exemplary recipients for our fifth National Health Leadership Award.

Each honoree received Imaginatio, a beautiful and distinctive porcelain figurine from the world renowned Lladro. Portraying an angel with soaring wings, this statue represents the hope and comfort all the honorees have brought to the world through their devotion to their patients and communities.

**National Physician of the Year Awards Honorees
For Clinical Excellence**

<u>John B. Buse, M.D., Ph.D., Endocrinology</u>
University of North Carolina Hospitals, Chapel Hill, NC

<u>Larry Norton, M.D., Medical Oncology</u>
Memorial Sloan-Kettering Cancer Center, New York, NY

<u>Ching-Hon Pui, M.D., Pediatric Hematology/Oncology</u>
St. Jude Children's Research Hospital, Memphis, TN

<u>Lifetime Achievement</u>
<u>Basil Hirshowitz, M.D., Gastroenterology</u>
University of Alabama, Birmingham, AL

<u>Leonard Apt, M.D., Pediatric Ophthalmology</u>
UCLA School of Medicine, Jules Stein Eye Institute, Los Angeles, CA

<u>National Health Leadership</u>
Matthew Reeve and Alexandra Reeve Givens, Board Members
Christopher & Dana Reeve Foundation

Previous National Physician of the Year Award Honorees

2009

Clinical Excellence

Carol R. Bradford, M.D., Professor and Chair
Department of Otolaryngology
University of Michigan Medical System

Diane E. Meier, M.D., Director, Center to Advance Palliative Care
Mount Sinai School of Medicine

Judd W. Moul, M.D., Chief of Urology
Duke University Medical Center

Lifetime Achievement

Emil J. Freireich, M.D., D. Sc. (Hon.),
Ruth Harriet Ainsworth Chair, Distinguished Teaching Professor
Director, Special Medical Education Programs
Director, Adult Leukemia Research Program
The University of Texas M.D. Anderson Cancer Center

Thomas E. Starzl, M.D., Ph.D.
Professor of Surgery, Emeritus
Distinguished Service Professor
University of Pittsburgh Medical Center

National Health Leadership

Page Morton Black
Chairman of the Board, Parkinson's Disease Foundation

****

2008

Clinical Excellence
Robert W. Carlson, M.D.
Medical Oncology
Stanford University Medical Center

Stanley Chang, M.D.
Ophthalmology
New York-Presbyterian Hospital

L. Dade Lunsford, M.D.
Neurological Surgery
University of Pittsburgh Medical Center

Lifetime Achievement
Jacqueline A. Noonan, M.D.
Pediatric Cardiology
University of Kentucky Medical Center

Robert W. Schrier, M.D.
Nephrology
University of Colorado Health Sciences Center

National Health Leadership
Suzanne and Robert Wright
Vice-Chair of the Board, General Electric Company
Co-founders of Autism Speaks™

****

2007

Clinical Excellence
Delos M. Cosgrove, M.D.
Chairman, Board of Governors
CEO and President
The Cleveland Clinic

Joseph G. McCarthy, M.D.
Lawrence D. Bell Professor of Plastic Surgery
Director, The Institute of Reconstructive Plastic Surgery
NYU Medical Center

Patrick C. Walsh, M.D.
University Distinguished Service Professor and Director of Urology
The James Buchanan Brady Urological Institute
The Johns Hopkins Hospital

Lifetime Achievement
Maria Delivoria-Papadopoulos, M.D.
Director, The Neonatal Intensive Care Unit
St. Christopher's Hospital for Children;
Professor of Pediatrics, Physiology and Obstetrics/Gynecology
Drexel University College of Medicine

National Health Leadership
The Honorable Nancy G. Brinker
Founder of Susan G. Komen for the Cure
Former U.S. Ambassador to Hungary

****

2006

Clinical Excellence
Bart Barlogie, M.D., Ph.D.
Director, Myeloma Institute for Research Therapy
University of Arkansas for Medical Services

Marilyn J. Bull, M.D.
Morris Green Professor of Pediatrics
Riley Hospital for Children

Michael J. Zinner, M.D.
Moseley Professor of Surgery
Harvard Medical School
Surgeon-in-Chief, Brigham & Women's Hospital

Lifetime Achievement
Michael E. DeBakey, M.D.
Chancellor Emeritus, Baylor College of Medicine

National Health Leadership
Princess Yasmin Aga Khan
Honorary Vice Chair
Alzheimer's Association

The Best in American Medicine
www.CastleConnolly.com

Castle Connolly and Social Media

Castle Connolly maintains Facebook and Twitter accounts in an effort to keep consumers informed of the latest news at Castle Connolly Medical Ltd. Consumers who use our print guides, online database or refer to our regional magazine features can find up-to-date information about Castle Connolly by logging onto these social networking sites:

Become a Fan on Facebook: www.facebook.com/TopDoctors
or
Follow us on Twitter: www.twitter.com/castleconnolly

To find out more about our *National Physician of the Year Award* honorees, distribution dates for our newest publications and news of Castle Connolly Top Doctors featuring in local, regional and national media, visit Facebook and Twitter.

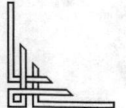

The Best in American Medicine
www.CastleConnolly.com

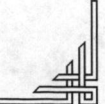

Castle Connolly's Top Cosmetic Doctors Online

Castle Connolly has developed a website and database – www.topcosmeticdoctors.com – to enable consumers to search and identify top cosmetic specialists who have been nominated by their peers through an extensive, annual survey process involving tens of thousands of American physicians. Nominated physicians' medical education, training, hospital appointments, disciplinary histories - and much more - are screened and reviewed by our physician-led research team. Those selected as top doctors may appear in a number of Castle Connolly guides/online databases, including www.topcosmeticdoctors.com. They are specially trained in cosmetic procedures and spend the majority of their time in their medical practice doing cosmetic work.The top cosmetic doctors whose profiles are included on this site are in one of only six medical specialties: Dermatology, Facial Plastic Surgery, Ophthalmology, Otolaryngology, Plastic Surgery, or Surgery. The website also includes valuable information on how to select the right cosmetic doctor for you, as well as detailed information about some of the most common procedures.

For more information visit: www.topcosmeticdoctors.com

Premium Membership at www.CastleConnolly.com

Reap the benefits of membership with Castle Connolly. Gain access to ALL online top doctor listings and get discounts on book purchases from our extensive catalog.

- Search among more than 26,000 Castle Connolly Top Doctor listings
- Search among select hospitals and centers of excellence
- Receive a 30% discount on all book purchases

Membership Levels:

- One year - $24.95
- Two years - $34.95

For more information visit: www.CastleConnolly.com/membership

Other Products From Castle Connolly

Castle Connolly Guides

Titles Include:
- *America's Top Doctors®*
- *America's Top Doctors® for Cancer*
- *Cancer Made Easier*

And Many More

To order other Castle Connolly guides at a 15% discount please visit

http://www.CastleConnolly.com/books

When ordering use discount code: **NY14DOM**

Castle Connolly Top Doctors Available Online

- Free Access to 20 -25% of Castle Connolly Top Doctors
- Purchase Access to the entire database of more than 23,000 doctor profiles

http://www.castleconnolly.com/membership

Customer Feedback Offer

We would appreciate your help to improve our guide. Send your feedback, comments or questions to webmaster@castleconnolly.com.

Diane Berson MD
Manhattan Dermatologist
(212) 327-0346